Pediatric Hepatology and Liver Transplantation

Lorenzo D'Antiga
Editor

Pediatric Hepatology and Liver Transplantation

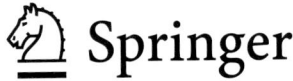 Springer

Editor
Lorenzo D'Antiga
Paediatric Hepatology, Gastroenterology and Transplantation
Hospital Papa Giovanni XXIII
Bergamo
Italy

ISBN 978-3-319-96399-0   ISBN 978-3-319-96400-3   (eBook)
https://doi.org/10.1007/978-3-319-96400-3

Library of Congress Control Number: 2019930554

© Springer Nature Switzerland AG 2019

This work is subject to copyright. All rights are reserved by the Publisher, whether the whole or part of the material is concerned, specifically the rights of translation, reprinting, reuse of illustrations, recitation, broadcasting, reproduction on microfilms or in any other physical way, and transmission or information storage and retrieval, electronic adaptation, computer software, or by similar or dissimilar methodology now known or hereafter developed.

The use of general descriptive names, registered names, trademarks, service marks, etc. in this publication does not imply, even in the absence of a specific statement, that such names are exempt from the relevant protective laws and regulations and therefore free for general use.

The publisher, the authors, and the editors are safe to assume that the advice and information in this book are believed to be true and accurate at the date of publication. Neither the publisher nor the authors or the editors give a warranty, express or implied, with respect to the material contained herein or for any errors or omissions that may have been made. The publisher remains neutral with regard to jurisdictional claims in published maps and institutional affiliations.

This Springer imprint is published by the registered company Springer Nature Switzerland AG
The registered company address is: Gewerbestrasse 11, 6330 Cham, Switzerland

To Martina, the sun of my life,
and to our children Francesco, Mattia, Anna and Maddalena
who make our days full of joy, projects and hope for the future

To Mum and Dad†
so trustful and proud, since the very beginning

To my brothers
Luca, who, as a young employee, made my studies at the Medical School affordable,
Alvise† and Angelo, always supportive during my career,
and Maria Giovanna†, who passed away at 4 months of age from an unknown liver disease

To my mentors
Lucia, Giorgina, Anil
and many others I am still learning from

To all doctors who take tender care of the sick ones
and consider it a privilege

Foreword

Paediatric hepatology has gone from obscurity to a status of specialty in its own merit over the span of seven decades. Though jaundice in babies and children had been occasionally reported in the past, liver disorders in childhood were considered extremely rare and almost always lethal. The real burden of paediatric liver disease was first recognised in the late 1950s and became a focus of attention only in the 1960s and 1970s.

Visionary men, like Morio Kasai, Daniel Alagille and Alex Mowat, put paediatric hepatology firmly on the map of paediatrics by the 1970s, recognising the importance of concentrating expertise in specialised centres, in order to elucidate physiopathological mechanisms, with consequent improved management and outcome for children with liver disease. This has resulted over a relatively short period of time in a vortex of new information, including the discovery of several causes of juvenile liver disease, leading not only to successful specific managements, but also to a better understanding of the liver physiology, based on the discovery of the deleterious effect of genetic defects affecting synthesis, transport and function of proteins manufactured by the liver.

In parallel, grew the awareness that liver disorders of adulthood can affect children as well, but that in children they present important differences, which need to be taken into account for successful treatment, examples of these conditions being autoimmune liver disease, viral hepatitides and acute liver failure.

Despite improved knowledge, the prognosis of paediatric liver disease remained severe for decades, with mortality rates between 50 and 60% within a few years from diagnosis for many conditions, until the advent of liver transplantation as a standard mode of treatment for children with end-stage liver disease in the early 1990s, which rapidly led to long-term survival rates of over 95%.

Current tasks are to clarify the physiopathological mechanisms of those juvenile liver diseases that remain without a recognised cause, to perfect medical management to avoid transplantation—including isolated hepatocyte or gene therapy—and to overcome the problems of rejection and long-term complications for those patients who need a liver transplant.

D'Antiga's *Pediatric Hepatology and Liver Transplantation* stems from the Editor's ambitious aim to provide a comprehensive, practical and up-to-date description of paediatric liver disorders and their management, spanning from historical notes, liver anatomy and physiology, to the discovery of new conditions and their management, to liver transplantation, to the peculiarities in children and adolescents of liver disorders that affect also adults.

This textbook will be highly valuable not only to gastroenterologists, paediatric hepatologists and transplant surgeons, but also to medical students, residents and adult physicians looking after patients with liver disease, as improved knowledge and management of hitherto lethal paediatric liver conditions has led to survival into adulthood and transition to adult services.

Lorenzo D'Antiga's aim was ambitious: the result excellent.

Giorgina Mieli-Vergani
London, UK

Preface

The liver may be considered "a timid, clever and resilient organ", because of its circulation enclosed between two capillary beds and the hidden excretion in the middle of the digestive tract, its pivotal role in human metabolism and its resistance to suffering if not to the exhaustion of the reserves. These intrinsic features and the relative rarity of hepatic disorders in infancy make liver disease in children a narrow and rather unknown field.

The liver goes through a perinatal immaturity phase during which it is prone to insults of various kinds but then matures and acquires the silent and stable control of most of the functions of body homeostasis and intermediate metabolism. The reasons why the functions and the diseases of the liver are still little known, and the expertise is prerogative of few specialized centres, probably reside in the lack of non-invasive tests allowing to understand the punctual state of health of this organ.

The purpose of this book is to try shedding some light on this field, spreading the experience made in the major international centres of paediatric hepatology and transplantation. Indeed the strength of this work stands on the contribution of the greatest experts working in the field all over the world, who kindly agreed to grant their expertise preparing a chapter of this book. It has been a great pleasure and honour having a prompt acceptance from persons I consider the top experts in various hepatology subspecialties and from whom I keep learning. Once again I experienced that friendship and mutual respect is a key component of any team project.

I am also particularly grateful for having the chance to deepen my experience in the field of education I have always been very fond of. In that respect the attempt of this work is to give a comprehensive (although certainly incomplete) scenario of what a physician involved in the care of paediatric liver disease might face, opening the lens of the camera to a wide angle, and helping the reader place information within the broader topic of child health and global health. For this reason the first chapter, taking advantage of the World Health Organisation data, focuses on the relevance of liver disease worldwide, both in adults and in children. Part III is entirely devoted to paediatric liver disease in continents having different epidemiology and standards of care, appearing less frequently in the current literature but certainly taking care of the largest proportion of children with liver disease in the world. Another novelty of this book is the balanced examination of both paediatric liver disease and liver transplantation, discussed in the first two parts, since these topics are inherently related, given that most chronic liver disorders eventually require organ replacement. Several chapters are dedicated to emerging issues in the field, such as long-term graft dysfunction, quality of life and transition to adult care, but also to newly developed strategies to manage our patients, such as next-generation sequencing testing, cell and gene therapy.

My wish is to provide a helpful tool for a range of practitioners looking after children with liver disease, from residents making their first approach to paediatric liver disease through to specialists working in transplantation centres. I really hope this book can contribute to the care of children with liver disease.

Bergamo, Italy   Lorenzo D'Antiga

The Editor would be pleased to receive from the readers any suggestion aimed to improve the next edition of this book. Please send your precious comments to the following mailing address: dantiga.book@gmail.com.

Contents

Part I Paediatric Hepatology

1. Liver Disease in Paediatric Medicine: An Overview 3
    Valeria Casotti and Lorenzo D'Antiga

2. Basic Principles of Liver Physiology 21
    Valeria Casotti and Lorenzo D'Antiga

3. The Anatomy and Histology of the Liver and Biliary Tract 41
    Maria Guido, Samantha Sarcognato, Diana Sacchi, and Kathrin Ludwig

4. Laboratory Evaluation of Hepatobiliary Disease 57
    Henrik Arnell and Björn Fischler

5. Diagnostic and Interventional Radiology 67
    R. Agazzi, P. Tessitore, and S. Sironi

6. Practical Approach to the Jaundiced Infant........................ 99
    Ekkehard Sturm and Steffen Hartleif

7. Biliary Atresia and Other Congenital Disorders of the Extrahepatic
    Biliary Tree 129
    Pietro Betalli and Mark Davenport

8. Acute Liver Failure in Children 145
    Naresh Shanmugam and Anil Dhawan

9. Chronic Viral Hepatitis 155
    Giuseppe Indolfi and Lorenzo D'Antiga

10. Autoimmune Liver Disease 175
    Giorgina Mieli-Vergani and Diego Vergani

11. Fibrocystic Liver Disease 201
    Laura Cristoferi, Giovanni Morana, Mario Strazzabosco, and Luca Fabris

12. Gallstone Disease....................................... 219
    Fabiola Di Dato, Giusy Ranucci, and Raffaele Iorio

13. Genetic Cholestatic Disorders 227
    Emanuele Nicastro and Lorenzo D'Antiga

14. Wilson's Disease 247
    Piotr Socha and Wojciech Janczyk

15. Liver Disease in Cystic Fibrosis.............................. 255
    Dominique Debray

16. Inherited Metabolic Disorders............................... 271
    Nedim Hadzic and Roshni Vara

17	**Nonalcoholic Fatty Liver Disease and Steatohepatitis in Children** 279
	Antonella Mosca, Silvio Veraldi, Andrea Dellostrologo, Mariateresa Sanseviero, and Valerio Nobili
18	**Complications of Liver Cirrhosis** 293
	A. Holvast and H. J. Verkade
19	**Portal Hypertension** 299
	Angelo Di Giorgio and Lorenzo D'Antiga
20	**Vascular Liver Disease** 329
	Simon C. Ling and Ines Loverdos
21	**Liver Tumours and Nodular Lesions** 345
	Chayarani Kelgeri, Khalid Sharif, and Ulrich Baumann
22	**The Liver in Systemic Illness** 361
	Melanie Schranz, Maria Grazia Lucà, Lorenzo D'Antiga, and Stefano Fagiuoli
23	**Nutrition and Liver Disease** 397
	Florence Lacaille
24	**Intensive Care Management of Children with Liver Disease** 409
	Isabella Pellicioli, Angelo Di Giorgio, and Lorenzo D'Antiga

Part II Paediatric Liver Transplantation

25	**Precision Medicine in Liver Transplantation** 435
	Alastair Baker
26	**Liver Allograft Donor Selection and Allocation** 455
	James E. Squires and George V. Mazariegos
27	**Surgical Techniques** 465
	Michele Colledan and Stefania Camagni
28	**Pediatric Living Donor Liver Transplantation** 487
	Mureo Kasahara, Seisuke Sakamoto, and Akinari Fukuda
29	**Listing for Transplantation; Postoperative Management and Long-Term Follow-Up** 515
	Nathalie Marie Rock and Valérie Anne McLin
30	**Surgical Complications Following Transplantation** 535
	Michele Colledan, Domenico Pinelli, and Laura Fontanella
31	**Immunosuppression in Pediatric Liver Transplant** 555
	Patrick McKiernan and Ellen Mitchell
32	**Pathology of Allograft Liver Dysfunction** 565
	Aurelio Sonzogni, Lisa Licini, and Lorenzo D'Antiga
33	**Chronic Rejection and Late Allograft Hepatitis** 585
	Deirdre Kelly
34	**Cytomegalovirus and Epstein-Barr Virus Infection and Disease** 593
	Emanuele Nicastro and Lorenzo D'Antiga
35	**Liver Transplantation for Inherited Metabolic Disorders** 603
	Alberto Burlina and Lorenzo D'Antiga

36	**Immune Tolerance After Liver Transplantation**	625
	Sandy Feng and Alberto Sanchez-Fueyo	
37	**Long-Term Outcome and Transition**.................................	653
	Marianne Samyn	
38	**Neurodevelopment and Health Related Quality of Life of the Transplanted Child**	665
	Vicky Lee Ng and Jessica Woolfson	

Part III Paediatric Hepatology Across the World

39	**Pediatric Liver Disease in Latin America**.............................	687
	Daniel D'Agostino, Maria Camila Sanchez, and Gustavo Boldrini	
40	**Pediatric Liver Disease in the African Continent**	699
	Mortada H. F. El-Shabrawi and Naglaa M. Kamal	
41	**Pediatric Liver Disease in the Asian Continent**	743
	Anshu Srivastava and Rishi Bolia	

Part IV Future Perspectives

42	**Next-Generation Sequencing in Paediatric Hepatology**	767
	Lorenzo D'Antiga	
43	**Cell Therapy in Acute and Chronic Liver Disease**.......................	781
	Massimiliano Paganelli	
44	**Gene Therapy in Pediatric Liver Disease**.............................	799
	Andrès F. Muro, Lorenzo D'Antiga, and Federico Mingozzi	

Editor and Contributors

About the Editor

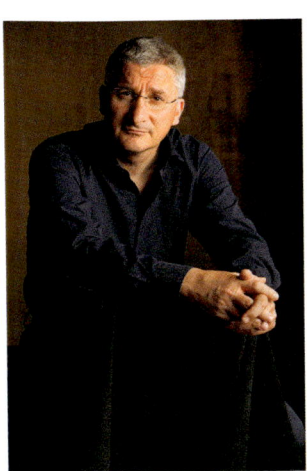

Lorenzo D'Antiga is a Paediatric Hepatologist and Gastroenterologist working in Italy. His current position is Director of Child Health and of the Paediatric Liver, GI and Transplantation Unit of the Papa Giovanni XXIII Hospital of Bergamo. He trained as a Paediatrician at the University of Padua and as a Paediatric Hepatologist in the United Kingdom at King's College Hospital London. He has worked as Consultant Gastroenterologist and Hepatologist as well as Paediatric Intensivist, specializing in organ failure and transplantation. ESPGHAN member for 15 years, he contributed to the field of paediatric hepatology with publications, scientific presentations and invited lectures. He has been member of the Council of the ESPGHAN as Education Secretary (till 2014) and Member of the Education Committee of the UEG (till 2014). He serves as Senior Associate Editor for *Journal of Pediatric Gastroenterology and Nutrition* and as Associate Editor of *Liver Transplantation*.

Contributors

R. Agazzi Interventional Radiology, Department of Diagnostic Radiology, Hospital Papa Giovanni XIII, Bergamo, Italy

Henrik Arnell Department of Paediatrics, Karolinska University Hospital and CLINTEC, Karolinska Institutet, Stockholm, Sweden

Alastair Baker Paediatric Liver Centre, King's College Hospital, London, UK

Ulrich Baumann Liver Unit and Small Bowel Transplant, Birmingham Women's and Children's Hospital, Birmingham, UK

Hannover Medical School, Hannover, Germany

Pietro Betalli Department of Paediatric Surgery, Papa Giovanni XXIII Hospital, Bergamo, Italy

Rishi Bolia Department of Pediatric Gastroenterology, Sanjay Gandhi Postgraduate Institute of Medical Sciences, Lucknow, India

Alberto Burlina Division of Inherited Metabolic Diseases, Reference Centre Expanded Newborn Screening, Department of Woman's and Child's Health, University of Padova, Padova, Italy

Stefania Camagni Department of Organ Failure and Transplantation, Hospital Papa Giovanni XXIII, Bergamo, Italy

Valeria Casotti Paediatric Hepatology, Gastroenterology and Transplantation, Hospital Papa Giovanni XXIII, Bergamo, Italy

Michele Colledan Department of Organ Failure and Transplantation, Hospital Papa Giovanni XXIII, Bergamo, Italy

Laura Cristoferi Division of Gastroenterology, Department of Medicine and Surgery, University of Milan-Bicocca, Milan, Italy

International Center for Digestive Health, University of Milan-Bicocca, Milan, Italy

Daniel D'Agostino School of Medicine, USAL University, Buenos Aires, Argentina

Division of Pediatric GI and Hepatology, Pediatric Liver and Intestinal Transplantation Program, Hospital Italiano, Buenos Aires, Argentina

Department of Pediatric, Hospital Italiano, Buenos Aires, Argentina

Lorenzo D'Antiga Paediatric Hepatology, Gastroenterology and Transplantation, Hospital Papa Giovanni XXIII, Bergamo, Italy

Mark Davenport Department of Paediatric Surgery, King's College Hospital, London, UK

Dominique Debray Pediatric Liver Unit, Reference Center for Biliary Atresia and Cholestatic Genetic Diseases, Hôpital Necker-Enfants Malades, Paris, France

Andrea Dellostrologo Hepatology, Gastroenterology and Nutrition Unit, "Bambino Gesù" Children's Hospital, Rome, Italy

Anil Dhawan Paediatric Liver GI and Nutrition Center and Mowat Labs, King's College Hospital, London, UK

Fabiola Di Dato Department of Translational Medical Science, Section of Paediatrics, University of Naples Federico II, Naples, Italy

Angelo Di Giorgio Paediatric Hepatology, Gastroenterology and Transplantation, Hospital Papa Giovanni XXIII, Bergamo, Italy

Mortada H. F. El-Shabrawi Faculty of Medicine, Cairo University, Cairo, Egypt

Luca Fabris International Center for Digestive Health, University of Milan-Bicocca, Milan, Italy

Digestive Disease Section, Yale University, New Haven, CT, USA

Department of Molecular Medicine, University of Padua, Padua, Italy

Stefano Fagiuoli Gastroenterology, Hepatology and Transplantation, ASST Papa Giovanni XXIII, Bergamo, Italy

Sandy Feng Division of Transplantation, Department of Surgery, University of California San Francisco, San Francisco, CA, USA

Björn Fischler Department of Paediatrics, Karolinska University Hospital and CLINTEC, Karolinska Institutet, Stockholm, Sweden

Laura Fontanella Department of Organ Failure and Transplantation, Hospital Papa Giovanni XXIII, Bergamo, Italy

Akinari Fukuda Organ Transplantation Center, National Center for Child Health and Development, Tokyo, Japan

Maria Guido Department of Medicine—DIMED, Anatomic Pathology Unit, University of Padova, Padova, Italy

Gustavo Boldrini Division of Pediatric GI and Hepatology, Pediatric Liver and Intestinal Transplantation Program, Hospital Italiano, Buenos Aires, Argentina

Department of Pediatrics, Hospital Italiano, Buenos Aires, Argentina

Nedim Hadzic Kings College Hospital, London, UK

Steffen Hartleif University Children's Hospital Tübingen, Tübingen, Germany

A. Holvast Pediatric Hepatology, Beatrix Children's Hospital-UMCG, University of Groningen, Groningen, The Netherlands

Giuseppe Indolfi Meyer Children's University Hospital, Firenze, Italy

Raffaele Iorio Department of Translational Medical Science, Section of Paediatrics, University of Naples Federico II, Naples, Italy

Wojciech Janczyk The Children's Memorial Health Institute, Warsaw, Poland

Naglaa M. Kamal Faculty of Medicine, Cairo University, Cairo, Egypt

Mureo Kasahara Organ Transplantation Center, National Center for Child Health and Development, Tokyo, Japan

Chayarani Kelgeri Liver Unit and Small Bowel Transplant, Birmingham Women's and Children's Hospital, Birmingham, UK

Deirdre Kelly The Liver Unit, Birmingham Womens and Childrens Hospital and University of Birmingham, Birmingham, UK

Florence Lacaille Pediatric Gastroenterology-Hepatology-Nutrition Unit, Hôpital Universitaire Necker-Enfants Malades, University Paris Cité Sorbonne Paris Descartes Medical School, Paris, France

Lisa Licini Department of Pathology, Papa Giovanni XXIII Hospital, Bergamo, Italy

Simon C. Ling Division of Gastroenterology, Hepatology and Nutrition, The Hospital for Sick Children, Toronto, ON, Canada

Department of Paediatrics, University of Toronto, Toronto, ON, Canada

Ines Loverdos Unidad de Gastroenterología, Hepatología y Nutrición pediátrica, Corporació Sanitària Universitària Parc Taulí. Sabadell, Barcelona, Spain

Maria Grazia Lucà Gastroenterology, Hepatology and Transplantation, ASST Papa Giovanni XXIII, Bergamo, Italy

Kathrin Ludwig Department of Medicine—DIMED, Unit of Pathology and Cytopathology, University Hospital of Padova, Padova, Italy

George V. Mazariegos UPMC Children's Hospital of Pittsburgh, Pittsburgh, PA, USA

Patrick McKiernan Division of Pediatric Gastroenterology Hepatology and Nutrition, Children's Hospital of Pittsburgh of UPMC and University of Pittsburgh, Pittsburgh, PA, USA

V. A. McLin Pediatric Gastroenterology, Hepatology and Nutrition Unit, Swiss Pediatric Liver Center, University Hospitals of Geneva, Geneva, Switzerland

Giorgina Mieli-Vergani MowatLabs, Paediatric Liver, GI and Nutrition Centre, King's College Hospital, London, UK

Federico Mingozzi Spark Therapeutic Inc, Philadelphia, PA, USA

Inserm, Évry, France

Genethon, Évry, France

Ellen Mitchell Division of Pediatric Gastroenterology Hepatology and Nutrition, Children's Hospital of Pittsburgh of UPMC and University of Pittsburgh, Pittsburgh, PA, USA

Giovanni Morana Division of Radiology, Treviso Regional Hospital, Treviso, Italy

Antonella Mosca Hepatology, Gastroenterology and Nutrition Unit, "Bambino Gesù" Children's Hospital, Rome, Italy

Andrès F. Muro Mouse Molecular Genetics Laboratory, International Center for Genetic Engineering and Biotechnology (ICGEB), Trieste, Italy

Vicky Lee Ng The Hospital for Sick Children, University of Toronto, Toronto, ON, Canada

Emanuele Nicastro Paediatric Hepatology, Gastroenterology and Transplantation, Hospital Papa Giovanni XXIII, Bergamo, Italy

Valerio Nobili Hepatology, Gastroenterology and Nutrition Unit, "Bambino Gesù" Children's Hospital, Rome, Italy

Department of Pediatrics, Facoltà di Medicina e Psicologia, Sapienza University of Rome, Rome, Italy

Massimiliano Paganelli Pediatric Gastroenterology, Hepatology and Nutrition, Sainte-Justine University Hospital Center, Montreal, QC, Canada

Hepatology & Cell Therapy Laboratory, Sainte-Justine Research Center, Montreal, QC, Canada

Department of Pediatrics, Université de Montréal, Montreal, QC, Canada

Isabella Pellicioli Pediatric Intensive Care Unit, Hospital Papa Giovanni XXIII, Bergamo, Italy

Domenico Pinelli Department of Organ Failure and Transplantation, Hospital Papa Giovanni XXIII, Bergamo, Italy

Giusy Ranucci Department of Translational Medical Science, Section of Paediatrics, University of Naples Federico II, Naples, Italy

Nathalie Marie Rock Pediatric Gastroenterology, Hepatology and Nutrition Unit, Swiss Pediatric Liver Center, University Hospitals of Geneva, Geneva, Switzerland

Diana Sacchi Department of Medicine—DIMED, Anatomic Pathology Unit, University of Padova, Padova, Italy

Seisuke Sakamoto Organ Transplantation Center, National Center for Child Health and Development, Tokyo, Japan

Marianne Samyn Paediatric Liver, GI and Nutrition Centre, King's College Hospital NHS Foundation Trust, London, UK

Maria Camila Sanchez Division of Pediatric GI and Hepatology, Pediatric Liver and Intestinal Transplantation Program, Hospital Italiano, Buenos Aires, Argentina

Department of Pediatrics, Hospital Italiano, Buenos Aires, Argentina

Alberto Sanchez-Fueyo Institute of Liver Studies, King's College, London, London, UK

Mariateresa Sanseviero Hepatology, Gastroenterology and Nutrition Unit, "Bambino Gesù" Children's Hospital, Rome, Italy

Samantha Sarcognato Department of Medicine—DIMED, Anatomic Pathology Unit, University of Padova, Padova, Italy

Melanie Schranz Gastroenterology, Hepatology and Transplantation, ASST Papa Giovanni XXIII, Bergamo, Italy

Naresh Shanmugam Institute of Advanced Paediatrics, Dr. Rela Institute and Medical Centre, Chennai, India

Khalid Sharif Liver Unit and Small Bowel Transplant, Birmingham Women's and Children's Hospital, Birmingham, UK

S. Sironi Department of Diagnostic Radiology, Hospital Papa Giovanni XIII, Bergamo, Italy

Piotr Socha The Children's Memorial Health Institute, Warsaw, Poland

Aurelio Sonzogni Department of Pathology, Papa Giovanni XXIII Hospital, Bergamo, Italy

James E. Squires UPMC Children's Hospital of Pittsburgh, Pittsburgh, PA, USA

Anshu Srivastava Department of Pediatric Gastroenterology, Sanjay Gandhi Postgraduate Institute of Medical Sciences, Lucknow, India

Mario Strazzabosco Division of Gastroenterology, Department of Medicine and Surgery, University of Milan-Bicocca, Milan, Italy

International Center for Digestive Health, University of Milan-Bicocca, Milan, Italy

Digestive Disease Section, Yale University, New Haven, CT, USA

Ekkehard Sturm University Children's Hospital Tübingen, Tübingen, Germany

P. Tessitore Department of Diagnostic Radiology, Hospital Papa Giovanni XIII, Bergamo, Italy

Roshni Vara Paediatric Inherited Metabolic Disease, Evelina Children's Hospital, London, UK

Silvio Veraldi Hepatology, Gastroenterology and Nutrition Unit, "Bambino Gesù" Children's Hospital, Rome, Italy

Diego Vergani MowatLabs, Institute of Liver Studies, King's College Hospital, London, UK

H. J. Verkade Pediatric Hepatology, Beatrix Children's Hospital-UMCG, University of Groningen, Groningen, The Netherlands

Jessica Woolfson The Hospital for Sick Children, University of Toronto, Toronto, ON, Canada

Part I

Paediatric Hepatology

*"Cure the sick, raise the dead, cleanse the lepers, cast out devils.
You received without charge; give without charge"*

(Matthew 10:8)

Liver Disease in Paediatric Medicine: An Overview

Valeria Casotti and Lorenzo D'Antiga

Key Points
- Aepidemiological studies of global mortality reveal that liver disease is the 11th cause of death in the world population, but only a minority relates to the paediatric age.
- Probably in children liver disease is the cause of global mortality in less than 1% of cases, and it is mainly due to viral hepatitis.
- In Western countries, liver disease is the 20th cause of death during childhood.
- Liver disease in children presents most often in the first 2 years of age and is mainly caused by biliary atresia and genetic cholestatic disorders.
- Chronic liver disease in children eventually requires liver transplantation in a large proportion of cases.

Research Needed in the Field
- To improve our knowledge on the aepidemiology of liver disease in different continents and at different latitudes, to better focus on specific needs of different populations
- To improve the prevention of HAV infection in developing countries
- To develop strategies able to achieve the global eradication of HCV infection
- To develop effective treatments to control HBV infection worldwide, including children vertically infected by the virus
- To improve our knowledge on pathophysiology of biliary atresia, the most common indication to liver transplantation, still orphan of an effective cure

V. Casotti (✉) · L. D'Antiga
Paediatric Hepatology, Gastroenterology and Transplantation, Hospital Papa Giovanni XXIII, Bergamo, Italy
e-mail: vcasotti@asst-pg23.it; ldantiga@asst-pg23.it

1.1 How It All Began: The Study of the Liver in the Third Millennium BC

1.1.1 The Liver of Mari in Mesopotamia

As far as we can go back to the history of human culture and tradition, the first information we gathered on examinations of the liver dates back to the third millennium BC. In the ancient Near East (the current Middle East), around the year 3000 BC, the practice of divination was widely diffused. In particular the Babylonians believed that the gods would manifest their answer in the healthy liver of a sacrificial animal. Such belief was connected with the production of liver clay models carrying inscriptions describing the meaning of the features the liver had, as shown in those excavated in 1935 in the Royal Palace of Mari, a city of Mesopotamia (Fig. 1.1).

This practice of slaughtering animals to observe the liver and predict the future is mentioned also in the *Book of Ezekiel* 21:21: 'For the king of Babylon stands at the split in the road, at the fork of the two roads, to practice divination: he shakes the arrows, consults the idols, and observes the liver'.

The liver was the organ used to hand down the practice of predicting the future not only among the Babylonians but also by the Etruscans, Greeks and Romans. The liver was considered the site of the soul, the vital organ and the central place of all forms of mental and emotional activity. Only much later the heart began to serve this function in these civilisations.

The association between divination and anatomy came from the interest of the priests in locating the souls of men and animals. Therefore, the former theologians became the first students of human and comparative anatomy. Priests realised that, although the basic configuration remained, two livers never looked the same. Prediction of the future was therefore based on specific findings of the liver surface. These priests developed sheep liver clay models that were used to instruct those aspiring to the priesthood. Wooden

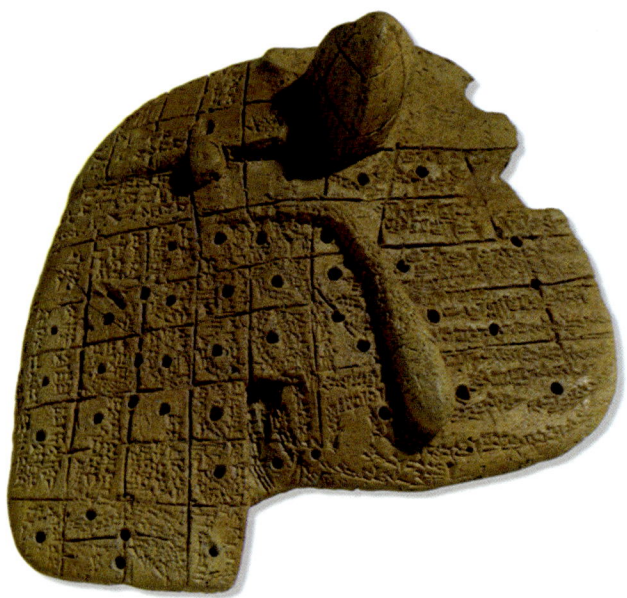

Fig. 1.1 The liver tablet—clay model of a sheep liver, Old Babylonian 1900–1600 BC. British Museum, London—BM92668. Reproduced with permission

pegs were placed in the holes of the clay tablet to record features found in a sacrificed animal's liver, to predict the outcome of a person's concern.

From the translation of the inscriptions, we know that the right and left lobes were designated as 'right and left wings'. The gallbladder fossa was called 'the river edge of the liver' and the umbilical fissure, 'River of the liver'. The caudate lobe was identified as the 'middle of the liver', and the gallbladder was given the name 'bitter part'. The hepatic duct was known as 'output' and the common bile duct as 'the junction'. The *porta hepatis* was called 'the gate'; the secondary hepatic ducts were named 'branches', and the portal triads were represented as 'holes' or 'passages'. The most important feature of the liver, namely, the groove found on the left lobe of the liver of the sheep, was called 'the left split' but also 'the presence', indicating that this is a mark left by the presence of the deity during the ritual. Modern liver anatomical terminology finds its roots in the nomenclature used by Babylonians.

Omens and liver models depict popular beliefs, state religion and how ancient inhabitants of Mesopotamia saw their relationship with the gods. The conception of the future, and the fact that men could act to prevent negative outcomes, is the reason for the long life of this practice and its presence in almost every aspect of life. In the light of what has been considered so far, the Mari liver models, dated around 1900–1600 BC, offer a fascinating insight into ancient Mesopotamian life and testify that the interest for the liver anatomy characterised their culture and religious tradition.

1.1.2 The Liver of Piacenza in Etruria

The practice of hepatoscopy survived for millennia and spread to other Mediterranean cultures, as attested by various liver omens and models from different periods, found in Mari (Mesopotamia, the current Middle East), Hattusa (Hittite city, the current Turkey) and Etruria (the current Italy).

In Hattusa, some 40 liver models have been excavated. In Etruria, a sculpture of a liver, known as the 'Liver of Piacenza', was discovered in 1877 near the town of Piacenza in Northern Italy. The Liver of Piacenza is a real-size bronze model of a sheep liver covered by Etruscan inscriptions, dated to the late second century BC. It is divided into 16 sections inscribed with names of Etruscan deities, among which the most famous are Neptune, Bacchus, Mars and Hercules (Fig. 1.2).

1.1.3 The Myth of Prometheus

Religions and myths always overlapped or even merged over the centuries. Indeed Hercules is also the protagonist of a Greek myth well known also by the Roman tradition: the myth of Prometheus. This mythological figure is often mentioned when it comes to discuss the regenerative capacity of the liver. What is less known of this myth is that Prometheus is presented as a sort of a saviour of the humankind, who created the men, took tender care of the human beings and defended them against all odds and against the gods of the Olympus.

According to Aeschylus, the ancient Greek playwright, Prometheus was a titan very faithful to Zeus, who, as a reward, gave him the opportunity to freely access the Olympus. Zeus, for the estimation he put in Prometheus, gave him the task of forging man. Prometheus moulded it

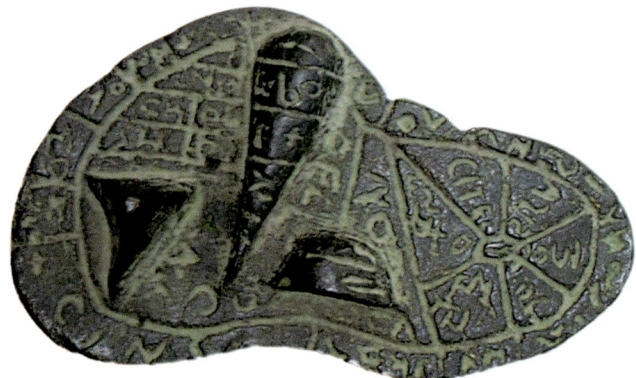

Fig. 1.2 The Liver of Piacenza: bronze model of a sheep liver indicating the seats of the deities. From Decima di Gossolengo, Piacenza, Italy. Etruscan, late second to early first century BC

from the mud and animated it with the divine fire. The 'man of forethought' (this is the meaning of Προμηθεύς in ancient Greek) felt a deep friendship for men and distributed to them several good qualities he received from Athena, including intelligence and memory. Besides, the titan closed in a vase all the evils that could torment men, such as fatigue, sickness, old age, madness, passion and death. Zeus did not approve Prometheus' kindness for his creatures, considering the titan's gifts too powerful for the mankind. Moreover Prometheus demonstrated to prefer men to Zeus, who therefore decided to destroy the humanity taking away the fire from men and hiding it. The men, without fire, were dying of cold. Prometheus went secretly to the Olympus, lit a torch and brought the fire back to the men. Zeus decided to punish the titan fiercely. He got Prometheus chained up in the highest and most exposed rock and sent an eagle that would pierce his abdomen and tear out pieces of his liver, which grew back during the night (Fig. 1.3).

Meanwhile, as reported in Hesiod's *Theogony* and *Works of the Days*, Pandora found the vase that was jealously guarded by Prometheus' brother and opened it, so that all the evils were spread to the mankind; only the hope remained in the vase and served as consolation for the humanity. Eventually, after several years, Hercules passed near the rock where Prometheus was chained, pierced with an arrow the eagle that tormented Prometheus and freed him, breaking the

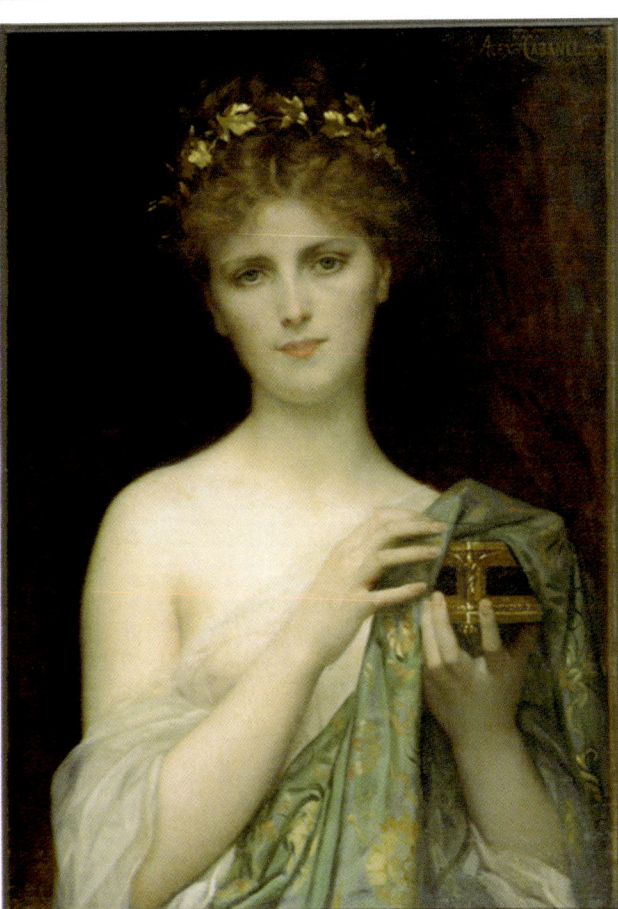

Fig. 1.4 *Pandora*. Oil on canvas, completed by Alexandre Cabanel in 1873. The Walters Art Museum, Online collection

chains. Nevertheless the men remained affected by fatigue, sickness, old age, madness, passion and death, and the commitment to take care of the suffering mankind was so passed on to the human beings (Fig. 1.4).

1.2 Liver Disease Aepidemiology in the Twenty-First Century

Liver disease occurs throughout the world irrespective of age, sex, region or race. Many conditions are acute, but cirrhosis is a common end result of a variety of liver diseases and can have different clinical manifestations and complications. According to the World Health Organization (WHO), about 46% of global diseases and 59% of the mortality are because of chronic illnesses, and almost 35 million people in the world die of chronic diseases. In the following section, we present the burden of liver disease worldwide, to include the following discussion on paediatric hepatology and liver transplantation in the context of the global health situation.

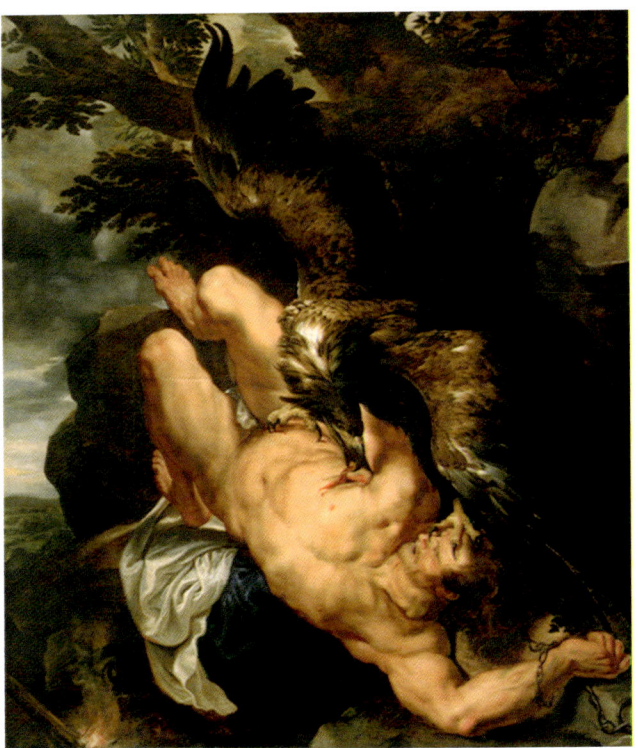

Fig. 1.3 *Prometheus Bound*. Oil painting, completed by Peter Paul Rubens in 1618. Philadelphia Museum of Art, Pennsylvania

1.2.1 The Global Causes of Death and a Focus on Liver Disease

In adulthood, it is reported that 29 million people are affected by liver diseases; moreover, cirrhosis and end-stage liver diseases are responsible for around 170,000 deaths every year.

Looking at the WHO Global Health Estimates data updated in 2015, liver cirrhosis and liver cancer are included in the 20 leading causes of deaths in adulthood, as shown in Table 1.1 [1].

In a study performed in the USA, looking at the burden of digestive diseases in the general population, the authors found that liver disease was the ninth leading digestive disease diagnosis at ambulatory care visits; however, if visits with liver disease are combined with the 3.5 million visits for viral hepatitis, then liver disease would have been the third leading diagnosis. Among all digestive diseases, liver disease was the second leading cause of death in adulthood, after colorectal cancer. In this study, also data from patients <15 years are reported, showing a prevalence of 14:100,000 of liver disease diagnosis at hospital discharge, a mortality rate of 0.2:100,000 and a number of years of potential life loss of 10,700 years for all patients (Figs. 1.5 and 1.6) [2].

Paediatric liver disease aepidemiology is poorly studied, and the exact prevalence of these diseases is unknown. The available data reported that each year approximately 15,000 paediatric patients are hospitalised for liver diseases in the USA, but liver disease is not cited in the first 15 causes of death in children. It is possible that the relative lack of aepidemiological research studies leads to underestimate the true prevalence of chronic liver disease in children; it is known that incidence and prevalence is lower compared to adults, but the impact of these conditions is high. In fact, chronic hepatobiliary diseases have significant effects on health and quality of life, on the family unit or disruption, on the number of years of life gained or lost, on mortality and need for liver transplantation and finally on health-care expenditure. Overall lack of awareness of the varied manifestations of hepatobiliary diseases in children often delays their diagnosis, thus contributing to increased morbidity and mortality, as a result of progression to end-stage liver disease. Paediatric liver disorders are particularly important because several paediatric conditions are precursors for adult chronic liver diseases, cirrhosis and hepatocellular carcinoma [3, 4].

1.2.2 Global Causes of Death in Children

From the more recent data by the United Nations International Children's Emergency Fund (UNICEF) ('2017 Revision on Levels and Trends in Child mortality'), children under 15 years of age represent around 26% of the world's inhabitants, with 9% under age 5. In the last years, there was a substantial improvement in life expectancy, and a significant progress in reducing child mortality, in particular the under-five mortality rate, an important indicator of development and children's well-being. The total number of under-five deaths dropped from 12.6 million in 1990 to 5.6 million in 2016—15,000 every day compared to 35,000; the global under-five mortality rate declined by 56%, from 93 deaths per 1,000 live births in 1990 to 41 in 2016. Children face the highest risk of dying in their first month of life, at a rate of 19 deaths per 1,000 live births. By comparison, the probability of dying after the first month but before reaching age 1 is 12, and after age 1 but before turning 5 is 11 deaths per 1,000 live births.

Disparities in child survival exist across regions and countries, with about 80% of under-five deaths occurring in two regions, sub-Saharan Africa and Southern Asia.

Most under-five deaths are caused by diseases that are readily preventable or treatable with proven, cost-effective interventions.

Table 1.1 Leading causes of death in 2015

	2015: Global health estimates: 20 leading causes of death per year			
Rank	Cause	Deaths (000s)	% of total deaths	CDR (per 100,000 population)
0	All causes	56,441	100,0	768,5
1	Ischaemic heart disease	8,756	15,5	119,2
2	Stroke	6,241	11,1	85,0
3	Lower respiratory infections	3,190	5,7	43,4
4	Chronic obstructive pulmonary disease	3,170	5,6	43,2
5	Trachea, bronchus, lung cancers	1,695	3,0	23,1
6	Diabetes mellitus	1,586	2,8	21,6
7	Alzheimer's disease and other dementias	1,542	2,7	21,0
8	Diarrhoeal diseases	1,389	2,5	18,9
9	Tuberculosis	1,373	2,4	18,7
10	Road injury	1,342	2,4	18,3
11	Cirrhosis of the liver	1,162	2,1	15,8
12	Kidney diseases	1,129	2,0	15,4
13	HIV/AIDS	1,060	1,9	14,4
14	Preterm birth complications	1,058	1,9	14,4
15	Hypertensive heart disease	942	1,7	12,8
16	Liver cancer	788	1,4	10,7
17	Self-harm	788	1,4	10,7
18	Colon and rectum cancers	774	1,4	10,5
19	Stomach cancer	754	1,3	10,3
20	Birth asphyxia and birth trauma	691	1,2	9,4

Modified from WHO: Global Health Estimates 2015 summary tables
CDR crude death rate

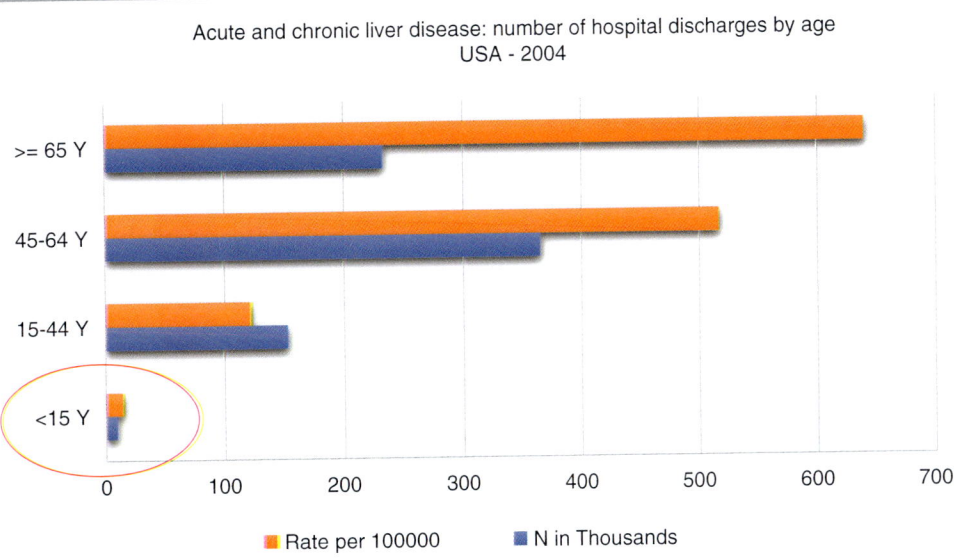

Fig. 1.5 Liver disease impact in hospitalised patients by age. Data referring to the paediatric age are circled. Data extracted from Everhart et al. Gastroenterology 2009 (see [2])

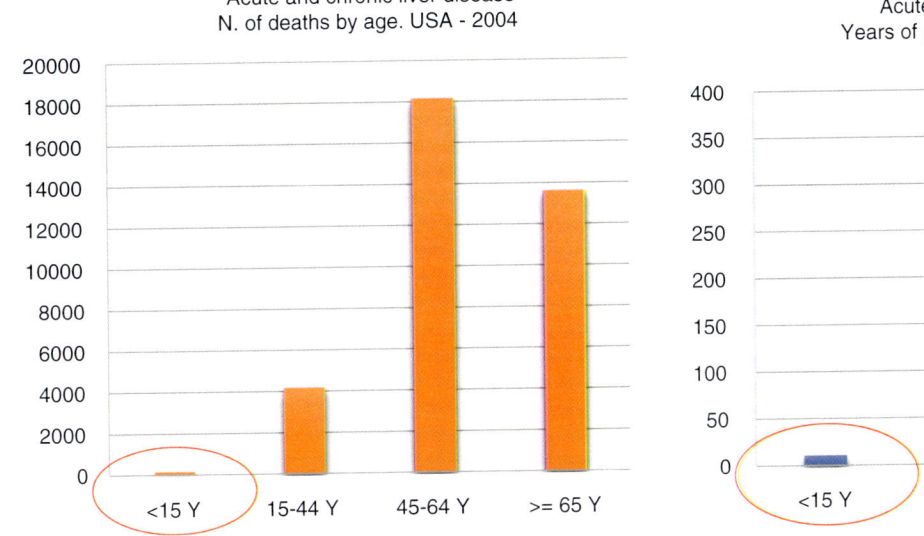
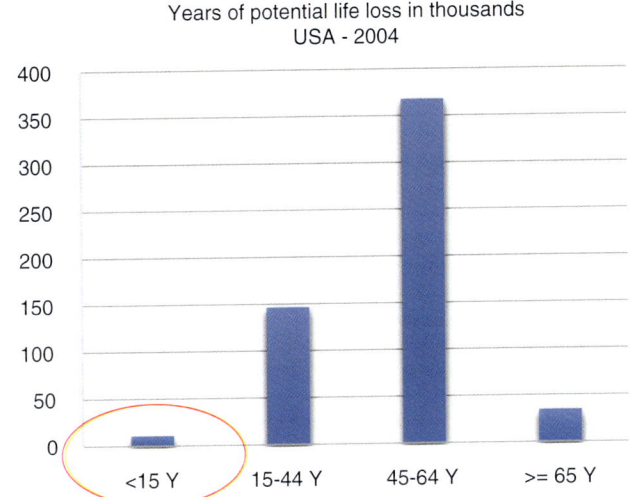

Fig. 1.6 Liver disease impact in mortality and life loss by age. Data referring to the paediatric age are circled. Data extracted from Everhart et al. Gastroenterology 2009 (see [2])

In particular, the WHO disease classification distinguishes three main categories:

- Group 1: Communicable, maternal, perinatal and nutritional conditions, including:
  – Infectious and parasitic diseases
  – Respiratory infections
  – Neonatal conditions
  – Nutritional deficiencies
- Group 2: Non-communicable diseases, including:
  – Malignant neoplasms
  – Other neoplasms
  – Diabetes mellitus
  – Endocrine, blood, immune disorders
  – Mental and substance use disorders
  – Neurological conditions (epilepsy)
  – Sense organ diseases
  – Cardiovascular diseases
  – Respiratory diseases
  – Digestive diseases
  – Genitourinary diseases
  – Skin diseases
  – Musculoskeletal diseases
  – Congenital anomalies
  – Sudden infant death syndrome
- Group 3: Injuries

In the next figures (from Figs. 1.7, 1.8, and 1.9), the WHO data, referred to the childhood mortality at the last Global Health Estimates (updated in 2015), are represented for the

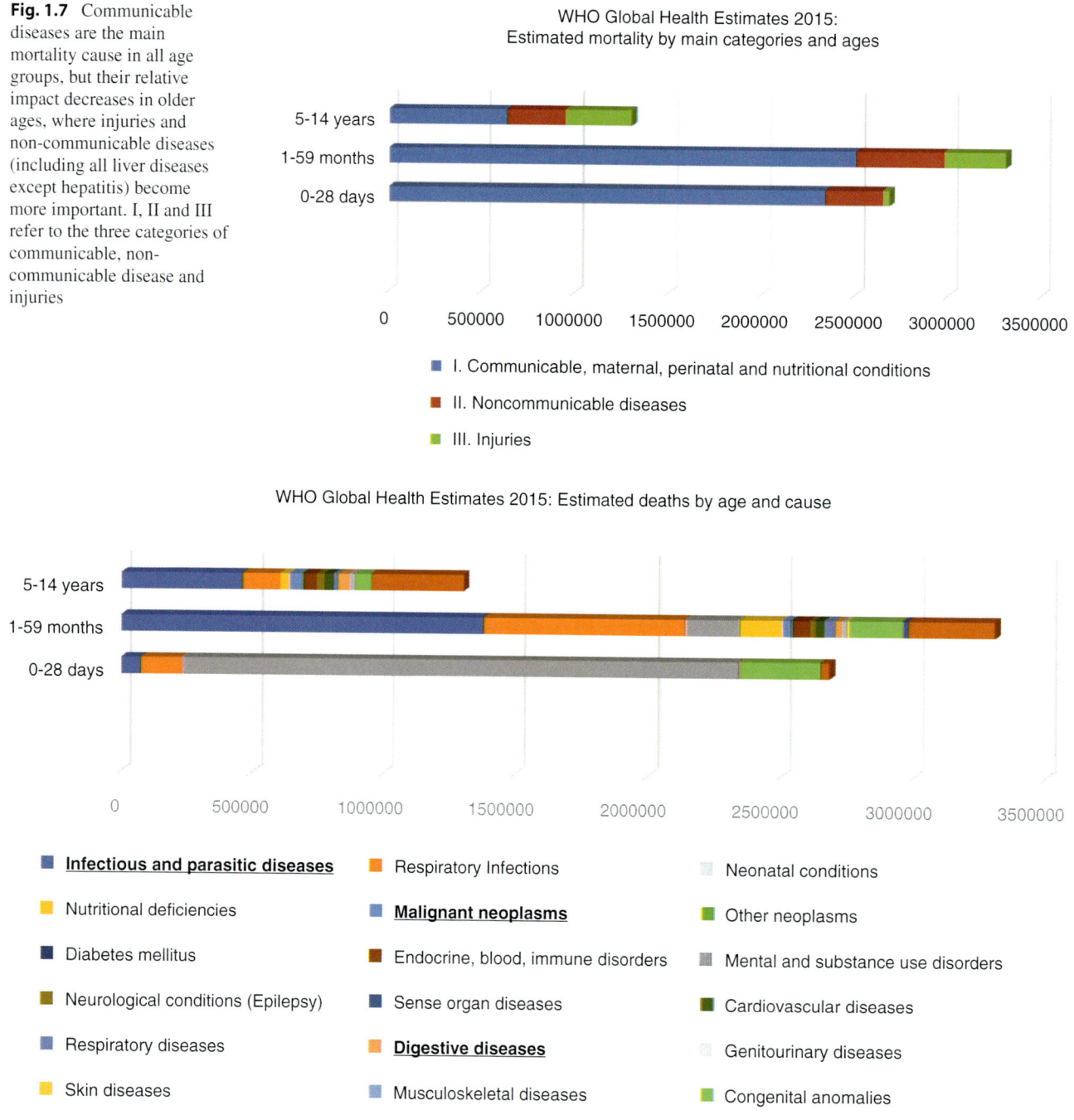

Fig. 1.7 Communicable diseases are the main mortality cause in all age groups, but their relative impact decreases in older ages, where injuries and non-communicable diseases (including all liver diseases except hepatitis) become more important. I, II and III refer to the three categories of communicable, non-communicable disease and injuries

Fig. 1.8 The mortality by main causes and age is shown in this figure; the underlined categories are those including the different liver diseases

main categories. From these data, it is possible to derive information about the impact of liver disease in this global scenario [5–8].

Based on this classification, the WHO in 2016 reported the cause-specific estimates of deaths for children under age 5. These are expressed by distinguishing the causes of death during the neonatal (0–27 days) and postneonatal (1–59 months) periods (Table 1.2).

As shown in this table, the leading causes of death among children under age 5 (accounting for almost a third of global under-five deaths and about 40% of under-five deaths in sub-Saharan Africa) included preterm birth complications (18%), pneumonia (16%), intrapartum-related events (12%), diarrhoea (8%), neonatal sepsis (7%) and malaria (5%). Liver diseases are included in the group of 'other diseases' in neonatal period and in the

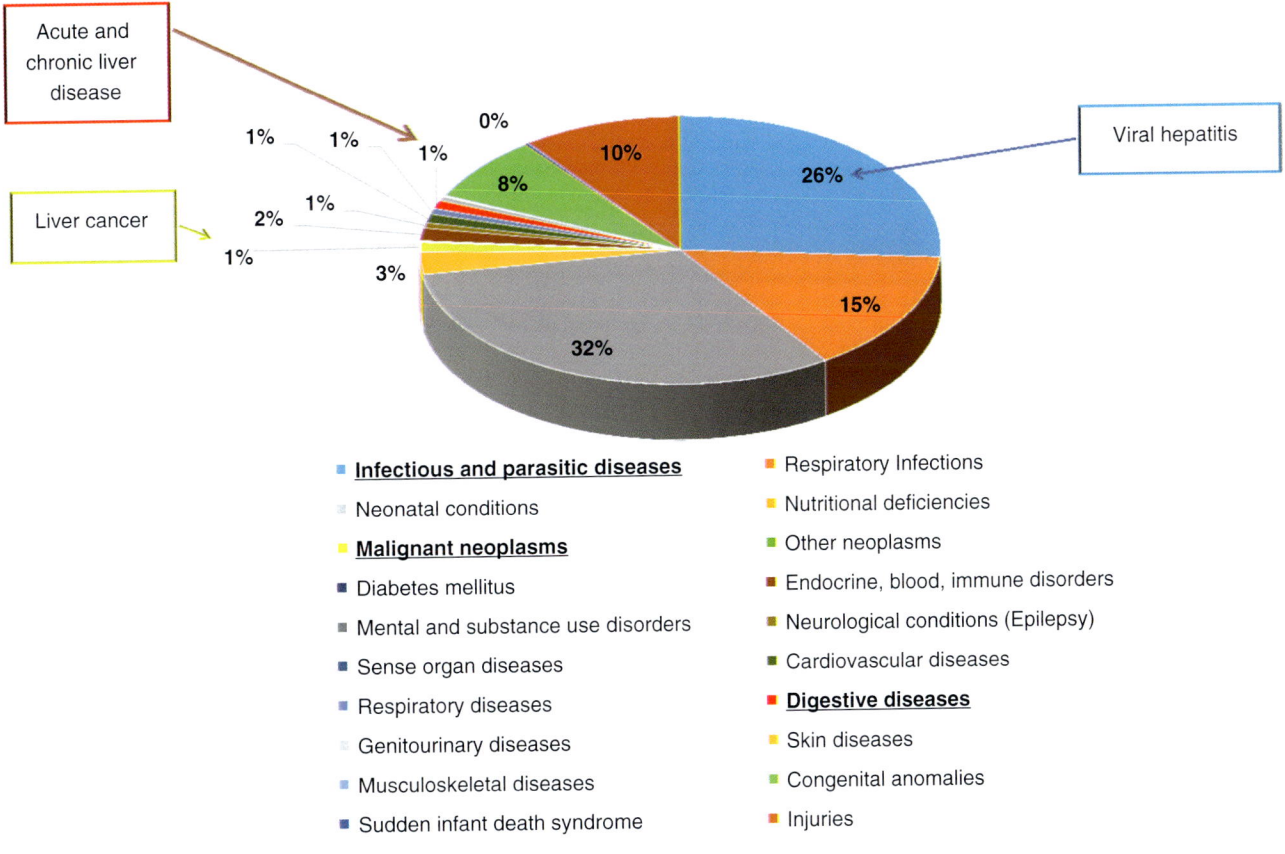

Fig. 1.9 WHO Global Health Estimates 2015: 0–14 year mortality by cause

Table 1.2 Causes of death among children under 5 years of age

Neonatal deaths 0–27 days (46%)		Postneonatal deaths 1–59 months (54%)	
Prematurity	16%	Pneumonia	13%
Intrapartum complications	11%	Other group 1 conditions	10%
Neonatal sepsis	7%	Diarrhoea	9%
Congenital anomalies	5%	*Congenital anomalies*[a]	8%
Pneumonia	3%	Injuries	6%
Other	3%	Malaria	5%
Neonatal tetanus	1%	Prematurity	2%
		Measles	1%
		HIV/AIDS	1%

Data are extracted from the Global Health Estimates technical paper, WHO-MCEE methods and data sources for child causes of death 2000–2015
[a]Includes other non-communicable diseases. Categories reported in italic include liver diseases

group of 'congenital anomalies' among children 12–59 months.

Looking at the older ages, the WHO data show that the probability of dying among children aged 5–14 was 7.5 deaths per 1,000 children; mortality in this age group is low, but 1 million children still died in 2016. The communicable diseases are a less prominent cause of death than among younger children, and other causes including injuries and non-communicable diseases become important.

In particular, injuries account for more than a quarter of the deaths, non-communicable diseases for about another quarter and infectious diseases and other communicable diseases, perinatal and nutritional causes, for about half of the deaths.

In this context, the liver disease aepidemiology includes:

- In the group of communicable diseases: viral hepatitis (HAV, HBV, HCV, HEV)
- In the group of non-communicable diseases: haemochromatosis, Reye's syndrome, Wilson's disease, alcoholic liver disease, toxic liver disease, hepatic failure, chronic hepatitis (not elsewhere classified), fibrosis and cirrhosis of liver, other inflammatory liver diseases, other diseases of liver, liver disorders in diseases classified elsewhere and metabolic disorders

These conditions are subcategorised within the groups of infectious, malignant and digestive diseases, as shown in Fig. 1.8.

In particular, the group of infectious diseases include the different forms of hepatitis; the group of malignant neoplasms include the liver and biliary tract cancers, the group of digestive diseases include all forms of other liver disease and cirrhosis (Fig. 1.9).

1.2.3 The Global Burden of Liver Disease in Children

Among the category 'infectious and parasitic diseases', liver diseases correspond to viral hepatitis. Of a total of 1,915,434 deaths due to infections in paediatric age, 21,328 (=1%) are due to the different forms of viral hepatitis, as shown in Fig. 1.10.

Among the category 'non-communicable diseases', the liver is involved in the group of malignant diseases and in that of digestive diseases.

On a total of 86,769 death in paediatric age because of malignancy, 1,983 (2.2%) are due to different forms of liver cancer, as shown in Fig. 1.11.

Finally, looking at the digestive diseases, on a total of 74,391 deaths in paediatric age, 27,882 (37%) were due to the different forms of cirrhosis, and 3,064 (4%) to gallbladder and biliary diseases, as shown in Fig. 1.12 [5–8].

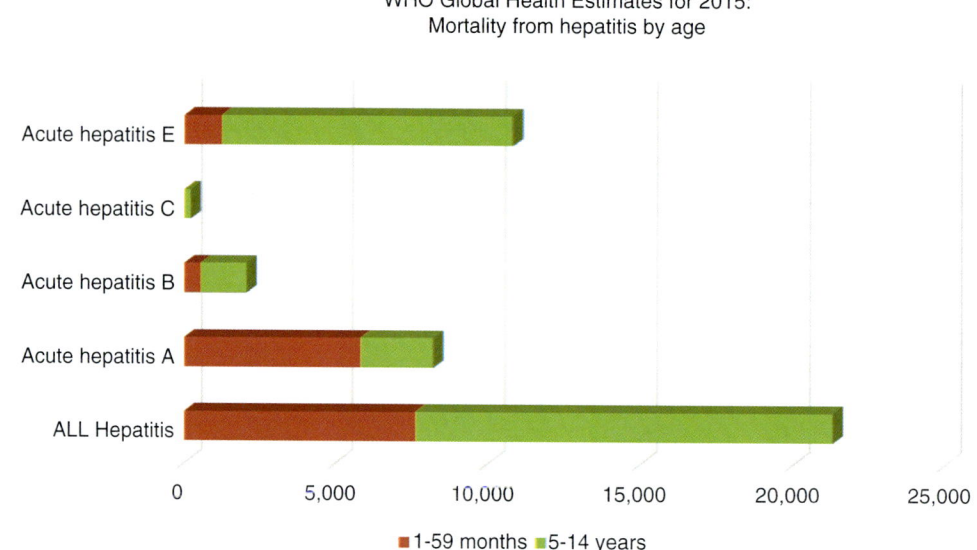

Fig. 1.10 The mortality for hepatitis is distinguished by different age groups (1–59 months, 5–14 years). No deaths were observed for this cause in the age group 0–28 days

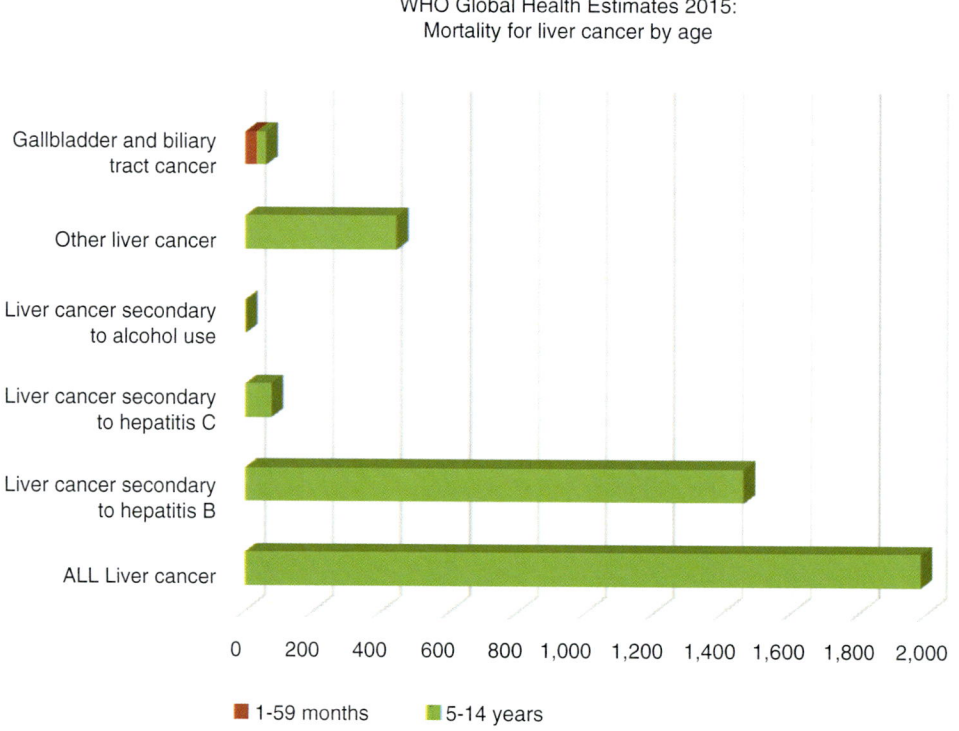

Fig. 1.11 The mortality for liver cancer is distinguished by different age groups (1–59 months, 5–14 years). No deaths were observed for these causes in the age group 0–28 days

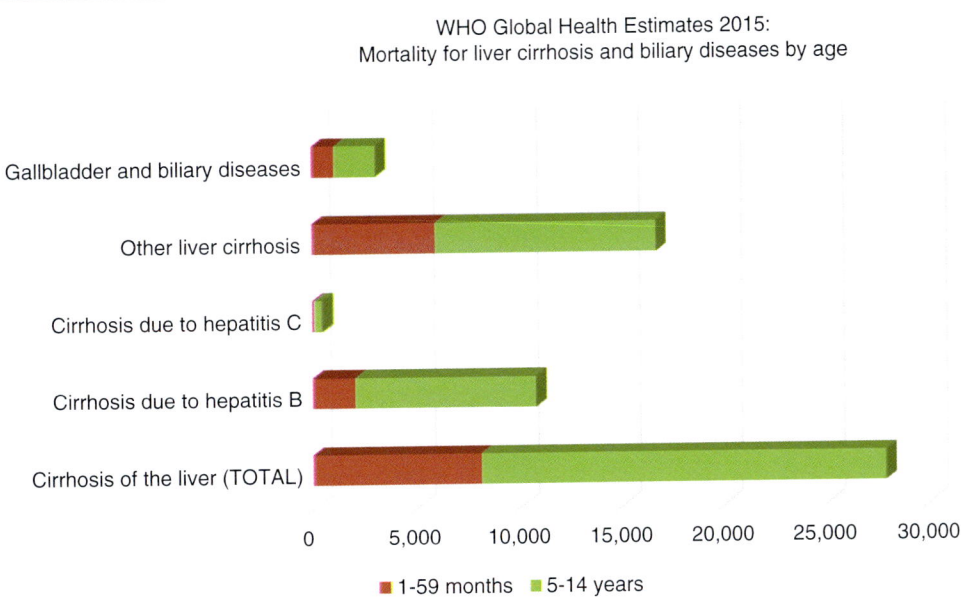

Fig. 1.12 The mortality for liver cirrhosis and biliary diseases is distinguished by different age groups (1–59 months, 5–14 years). No deaths were observed for this cause in the age group 0–28 days

1.2.4 Causes of Death in Western Countries (USA and Europe)

Besides the WHO reports, several recent studies in the USA and Europe focused the attention on mortality and morbidity by selected causes in paediatric population.

A recent paper by National Vital Statistics Reports represents final 2015 data on US number of deaths, death rates, life expectancy, infant mortality and trends, by selected characteristics such as age, sex, state of residence and cause of death. A total of 2,712,630 deaths were reported in the USA; the age-adjusted death rate was 733.1 deaths per 100,000 US standard population. Life expectancy at birth was 78.8 years. Looking at these data, it is possible to focus the attention on childhood mortality and on the low impact of liver diseases in this scenario, as shown in Table 1.3 [9].

More recently, an aepidemiological study was conducted in European regions, including data from 51 countries, assessing the distribution and trends of the main causes of death among children aged 5–9 years and 10–14 years from 1990 to 2016.

For children aged 5–9 years, all-cause mortality rates (per 100,000 population) were estimated to be 46.3 in 1990 and 19.5 in 2016, reflecting a 58% decline. For children aged 10–14 years, all-cause mortality rates (per 100,000 population) were 37.9 in 1990 and 20.1 in 2016, reflecting a 47.1% decline.

In 2016, 10,740 deaths in children aged 5–9 years and 10,279 deaths in those aged 10–14 years were estimated. The leading causes of death were similar between the two age groups. Liver cirrhosis is the 20th cause of death among children aged 5–9 years and the 16th cause in the group 10–14 years.

These data are shown in Figs. 1.13 and 1.14 [10].

1.3 Aepidemiology of Paediatric Liver Disease in Western Countries

In the last few decades, paediatric hepatology has developed from a newborn discipline to a highly specialised field in which unexpected progresses in genetics, molecular biology and pathophysiology of liver disease have been achieved. Liver disease in children is considered rare, and the care and follow-up of paediatric patients with hepatopathies are demanded to specialised centres. The opening of the frontiers has favoured immigration of people to the Western countries, changing the ethnical and cultural composition of our societies and consequently also the incidence of diseases once unfamiliar. For instance, inborn errors of metabolism are more frequent in communities having the tradition of consanguineous marriage, whereas viral hepatitis is common in children of Asian or African origin, where such infections are highly prevalent.

The discipline of paediatric hepatology has recently seen many advances in the understanding, diagnosing and treating paediatric liver diseases. At the same time other areas of paediatrics have improved leading to the emergence of new disorders caused by the complications of children who once would not have survived. This is, for instance, the case of the increasing number of newborn and infants treated for severe prematurity and presenting with liver disease. The field of liver diseases in ex preterm babies, still rather unknown, is expanding and will probably represent a new important area of interest for the paediatric hepatologist. The same can be stated for diseases following the use of chemotherapy and radiotherapy for the treatment of malignancies.

Table 1.3 Childhood mortality in the USA in 2015 by age and cause

Cause	<1 year	1–4 years	5–14 years	Total 0–14 years
Septicaemia	180	54	64	298
Viral hepatitis	1	0	1	2
HIV disease	2	2	1	5
Enterocolitis due to Clostridium difficile	2	2	3	7
Malignant neoplasms total	53	354	865	1272
Malignant neoplasms of liver and biliary tract	2	14	19	35
Anaemia	17	25	33	75
Diabetes mellitus	3	5	23	31
Nutritional deficiencies	9	4	1	14
Obesity	0	1	4	5
Cardiovascular diseases	400	196	300	896
Influenza and pneumonia	174	88	83	345
Chronic lower respiratory diseases	26	40	173	239
Aspiration pneumonia	8	10	16	34
Chronic liver disease and cirrhosis	3	2	1	6
Nephritis, nephrotic syndrome and nephrosis	85	16	17	118
Perinatal conditions	11,613	50	21	11,684
Congenital malformations and genetic disease	4825	435	337	5597
Accidents (unintentional)	1291	1235	1518	4044
Intentional self-provoked injuries (suicide)	0	0	413	413
Assault (homicide)	263	369	298	930
Complications of medical and surgical care	12	18	17	47
All causes	23,455	3965	5411	32,831

Modified by Murphy 2015, National Vital Statistics Reports

The spectrum of diseases diagnosed at a centre depends on many factors. One is the diagnostic capacity of the centre itself, in terms of professional skills and resources; another is the composition of the population living in the area, and a third is the type and amount of referrals from other centres. For these reasons it is not possible to consider a single centre as representative of the changing spectrum of liver diseases in a country, and even less in the global community.

Nonetheless all children with rare conditions need high-quality service programmes that have sufficient patient volume to guarantee the clinical expertise, and ancillary services necessary to address their specialised needs. Although their impact in global children survival is low (mainly because the global prevalence is low), these diseases are heterogeneous and may have a significant impact on morbidity and quality of life of affected patients [11].

The overall incidence of liver diseases in neonates (neonatal cholestasis) in the USA is approximately 1 in every 2500 live births, with extrahepatic biliary atresia, metabolic disorders and neonatal hepatitis being the most common causes; in older children, common causes of chronic liver disease (CLD) include metabolic disorders, chronic intrahepatic cholestasis, obesity-related steatohepatitis, drug- and toxin-induced disorders and autoimmune liver disease (Table 1.4).

In Australia, the most common cause of CLD starting in the neonatal age in children is biliary atresia, occurring in approximately 1 in 8,000 live births, with other common causes being alpha-1-antitrypsin deficiency and Alagille syndrome. Similarly, in Brazil, biliary atresia is the most common cause of CLD in children. In contrast, a study in Pakistan found viral hepatitis to be the most common cause of neonatal onset CLD, followed by metabolic disorders and biliary atresia, while a study in India found metabolic disorders to be the most common cause of CLD in children [12].

In a study performed at King's College Hospital of London, patients referred to a tertiary centre for suspected hepatopathies in the period 1985–2000 were collected and classified according to the diagnoses:

1. Hepatitis of infancy ('idiopathic neonatal hepatitis' 'neonatal giant cell hepatitis')
2. Alpha-1-antitrypsin deficiency
3. Extrahepatic biliary atresia
4. Alagille syndrome
5. Autoimmune hepatitis and sclerosing cholangitis
6. Wilson disease
7. Cystic fibrosis
8. Progressive familial intrahepatic cholestasis

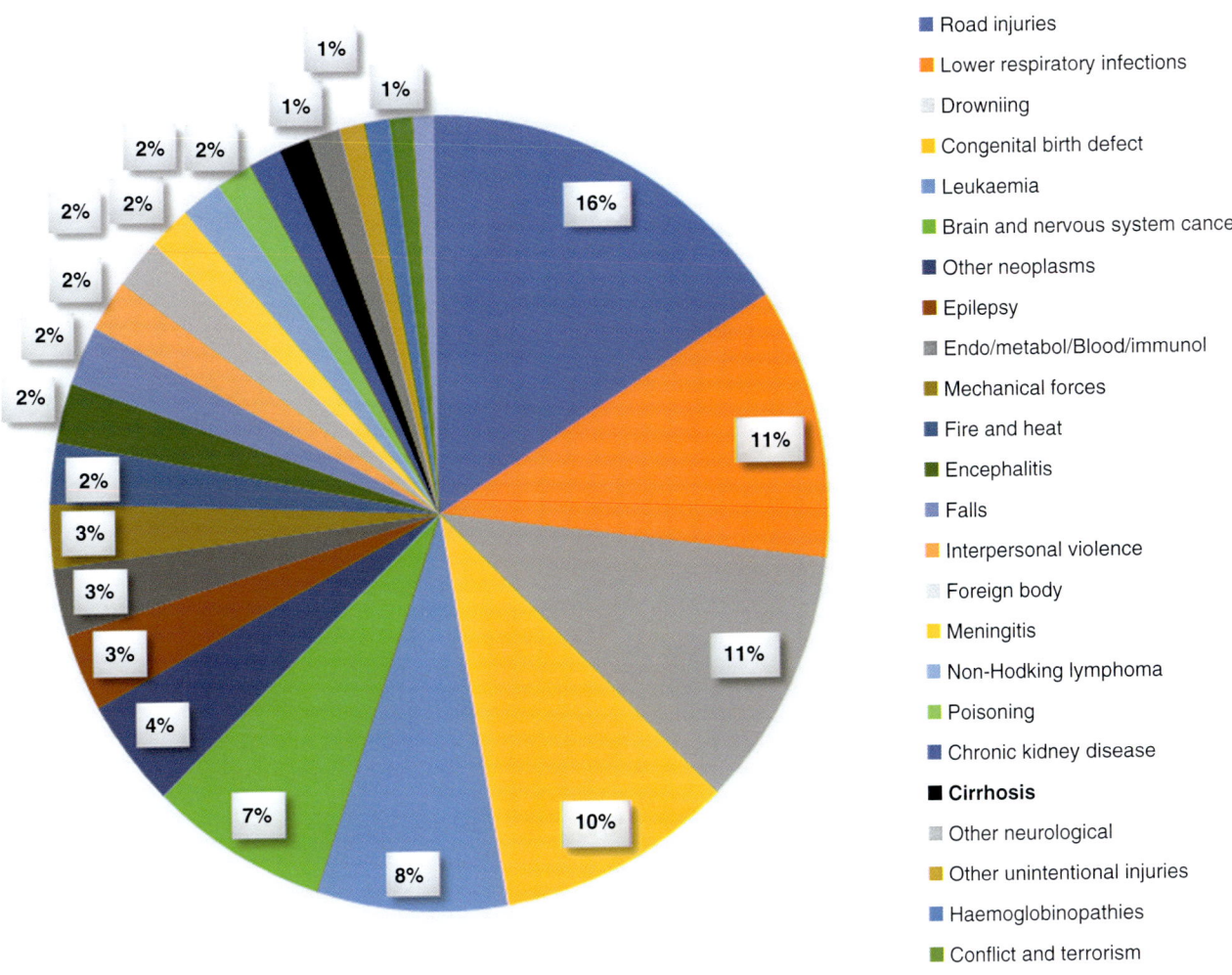

Fig. 1.13 Mortality by cause in the WHO European region, in the age group 5–9 years (data extracted by Kyu et al. systematic analysis for the Global Burden of Disease Study 2016)

9. Metabolic disorders (including all the inborn errors of metabolism involving the liver and not described singularly in other categories)
10. Cryptogenic cirrhosis
11. Prematurity-related liver disease
12. Ductal plate malformation
13. Viral hepatitis
14. Biliary anomalies (including choledochal cyst, inspissated bile syndrome, unspecified dilatation of the bile ducts, cholelithiasis, spontaneous perforation of the bile ducts)
15. Tumours (including primary and metastatic malignancies presenting with liver disease)
16. Septo-optic dysplasia (including any midline abnormalities causing hypopituitarism and liver disease)
17. NonA-NonB acute liver failure
18. Portal vein thrombosis and Budd-Chiari syndrome
19. Others (including other cases with less common diagnosis).

The database counted 3276 children who were described in this study (D'Antiga, unpublished data).

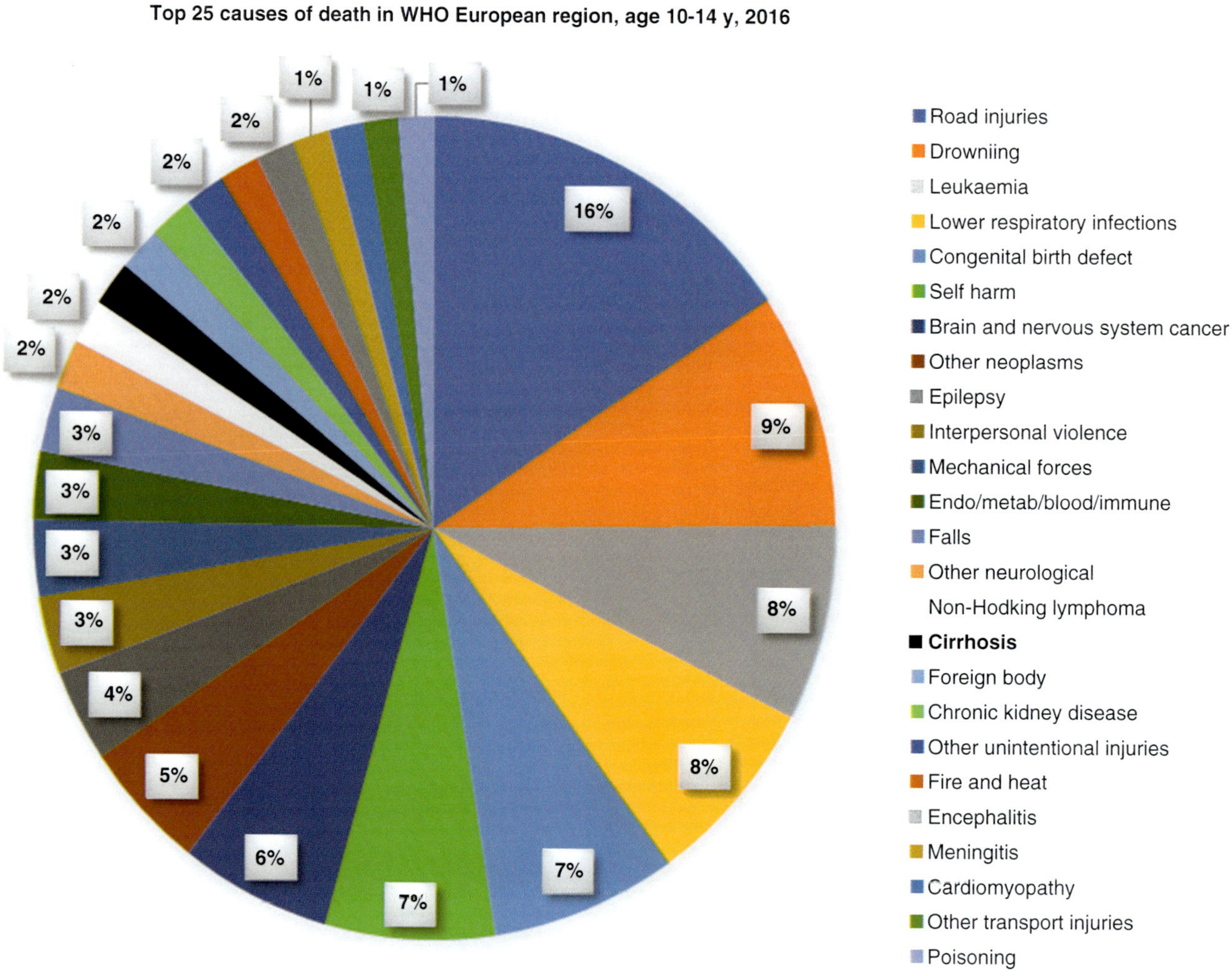

Top 25 causes of death in WHO European region, age 10-14 y, 2016

- Road injuries
- Drowniing
- Leukaemia
- Lower respiratory infections
- Congenital birth defect
- Self harm
- Brain and nervous system cancer
- Other neoplasms
- Epilepsy
- Interpersonal violence
- Mechanical forces
- Endo/metab/blood/immune
- Falls
- Other neurological
- Non-Hodking lymphoma
- **Cirrhosis**
- Foreign body
- Chronic kidney disease
- Other unintentional injuries
- Fire and heat
- Encephalitis
- Meningitis
- Cardiomyopathy
- Other transport injuries
- Poisoning

Fig. 1.14 Mortality by cause in the WHO European region, in the age group 10–14 years (data extracted by Kyu et al. systematic analysis for the Global Burden of Disease Study 2016)

The results show that liver disease in childhood presents mostly between 1 and 2 years of age (Fig. 1.15).

At the time of data collection (year 2000), in newborns and infants, the most common cause of liver disease was hepatitis of infancy, whereas between 1 and 10 years of age, it was viral hepatitis. After the tenth year, autoimmune hepatitis and sclerosing cholangitis were the most common diagnoses. In this study the data analysis did not include children affected by NAFLD, which is currently one of the most frequent causes of liver diseases in adolescents. This was due to the lack of referrals of these patients to the tertiary centre in which the study was conducted.

The impact of different liver diseases and the age at presentation are synthesised in Figs. 1.16 and 1.17. The hypothetical number of NAFLD/NASH cases, according to the known prevalence in Western countries, is reported aside. Figure 1.18 shows the different diagnoses divided by age group [19].

However, with the introduction of high-throughput genetic testing, the aepidemiology of liver disease in children is rapidly changing, especially for the definitions of many cases formerly classified as 'neonatal hepatitis' or 'cryptogenic liver disease' (see also chapters on cholestatic disorders and next-generation sequencing, Chaps. 13 and 42 respectively) (Fig. 1.19).

1 Liver Disease in Paediatric Medicine: An Overview

Table 1.4 Incidence/prevalence of different causes of liver disease in the paediatric population

Disease	Incidence/prevalence
Cholestatic diseases	1:2,500 live birth (l.b.)
Biliary atresia	1:8,000–1:21,000 l.b.
Alagille syndrome	1:70,000 l.b.
PFIC/BRIC	1:7,000 l.b.
Caroli disease/congenital hepatic fibrosis	1:6,000–1:40,000
Neonatal haemochromatosis	<1:1,000,000 l.b.
Idiopathic neonatal hepatitis	1:4,800–1:9000 l.b.
Wilson disease	1:30,000–1:50.000 l.b.
Cystic fibrosis	1:2,000 l.b.
Alpha-1-antitrypsin deficiency	1:1,800 l.b.
Metabolic diseases	1:1,800 l.b.
Disorders of carbohydrate metabolism	– Fructosaemia 1:20,000 l.b. – Galactosaemia 1:63,000 l.b. – GSD I–III and IV: 1:100,000–1:1,000,000
Tyrosinemia	1:100,000–1:120,000 l.b.
Peroxisomal disorders	1:25,000 l.b.
Urea cycle disorders	1:30,000 l.b.
Organic acidosis	1:1,000 l.b.
Lysosomal storage disorders	– Gaucher disease: 1:5,700 l.b. – Niemann-Pick A/B: 1:1,000,000 l.b – Niemann-Pick C: 1:130,000–1:150,000 l.b. – CESD: 1:300,000 l.b. – Wolman disease: 1:500,000 l.b.
Congenital disorders of glycosylation	1:10,000–1:100,000 l.b.
Mitochondrial hepatopathies	1:20,000 children under 16 years of age
Tumours	1,8:1,000,000
NAFLD/NASH	Prevalence 5–17% in general paediatric population, up to 70–90% in young obese
Autoimmune liver disease (including AIH/ASC and PSC)	Prevalence 1:200,000
Infections	
Hepatitis A (HAV)	1.4 million cases occur annually
Hepatitis B (HBV)	Global prevalence 2–20%. Horizontal transmission responsible for 37–52%; perinatal transmission 13–26%
Hepatitis C (HCV)	Prevalence from 1:500 (age 6–11 years) to 1:250 (age 12–19 years)

PFIC progressive familial intrahepatic cholestasis, *BRIC* benign recurrent intrahepatic cholestasis, *GSD* glycogen storage disease, *CESD* cholesteryl ester storage disease, *NAFLD* non-alcoholic fatty liver disease, *NASH* non-alcoholic steatohepatitis, *AIH* autoimmune hepatitis, *ASC* autoimmune sclerosing cholangitis, *PSC* primary sclerosing cholangitis. Extracted from [13–18]

1.3.1 Prevalence of Liver Disease Among Children Presenting to an Emergency Department

Many acute systemic conditions may present with transient, benign raise of transaminases. Previous studies looking at children coming to the emergency department with an acute illness, who had liver function tests (LFTs) tested, showed that some 30% had raised transaminases. LFTs remained abnormal in 8%. At the end, excluding those lost to follow-up, 5% had a chronic liver disease, including NAFLD/NASH. The others normalised liver enzymes, and it can be hypothesised that, in many children, common viral infections play a role in the transient increase in transaminases during acute illnesses (Fig. 1.20).

Despite extensive investigation, the cause of elevated transaminases may remain unknown in 10–15% of cases [20–22].

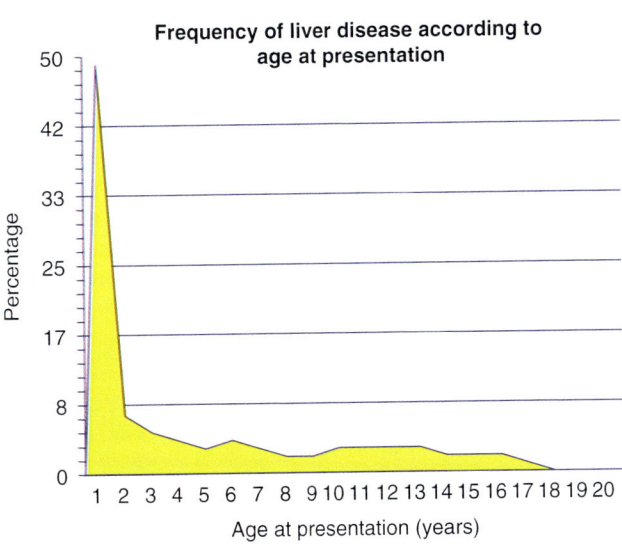

Fig. 1.15 Distribution of liver diseases in childhood at different presentation ages. The higher percentage of hepatopathies occurs in the first 2 years of age

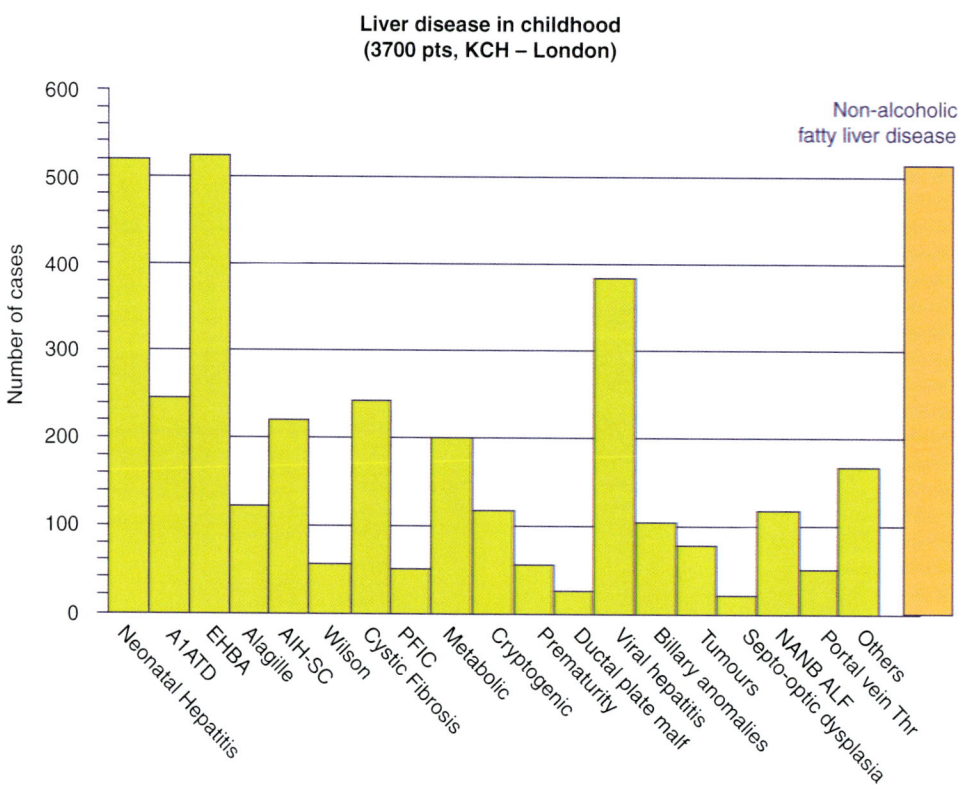

Fig. 1.16 Liver disease distribution in a paediatric population. A1ATD, alpha-1-antitrypsin deficiency; EHBA, biliary atresia; AIH-SC, autoimmune hepatitis and sclerosing cholangitis; PFIC, progressive familial intrahepatic cholestasis; Ductal plate malf, ductal plate malformation; biliary anomalies, choledochal cyst and inspissated bile syndrome; NANB ALF, nonA-nonB acute liver failure (D'Antiga L, unpublished data)

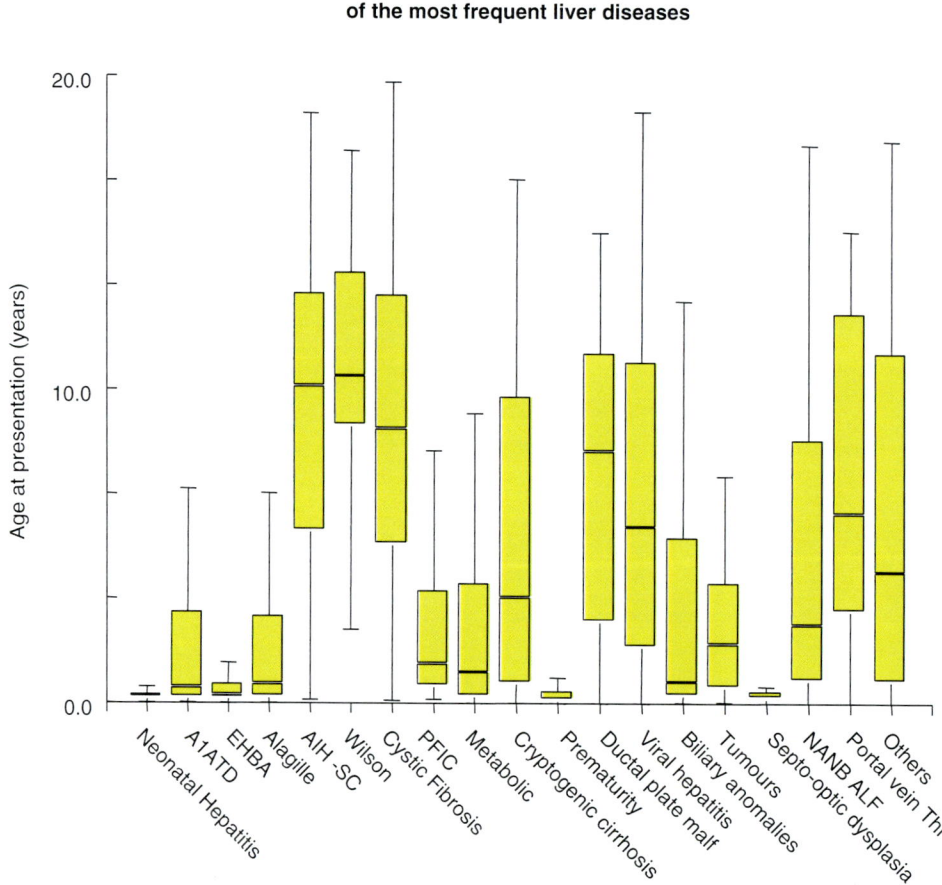

Fig. 1.17 Age at presentation of the most frequent liver diseases. The upper value is the largest observation that is less or equal to the 75th percentile plus 1.5 times the interquartile range (IQR). The lower value is the smallest observation that is greater than or equal to the 25th percentile minus 1.5 times IQR. The top and bottom of the box are the 25th and the 75th percentiles. The line drawn through the middle of the box is the median. A1ATD, alpha-1-antitrypsin deficiency; EHBA, biliary atresia; AIH-SC, autoimmune hepatitis and sclerosing cholangitis; PFIC, progressive familial intrahepatic cholestasis; Ductal plate malf, ductal plate malformation; Biliary anomalies, choledochal cyst and inspissated bile syndrome; NANB ALF, nonA-nonB liver failure (D'Antiga L, unpublished data)

1 Liver Disease in Paediatric Medicine: An Overview

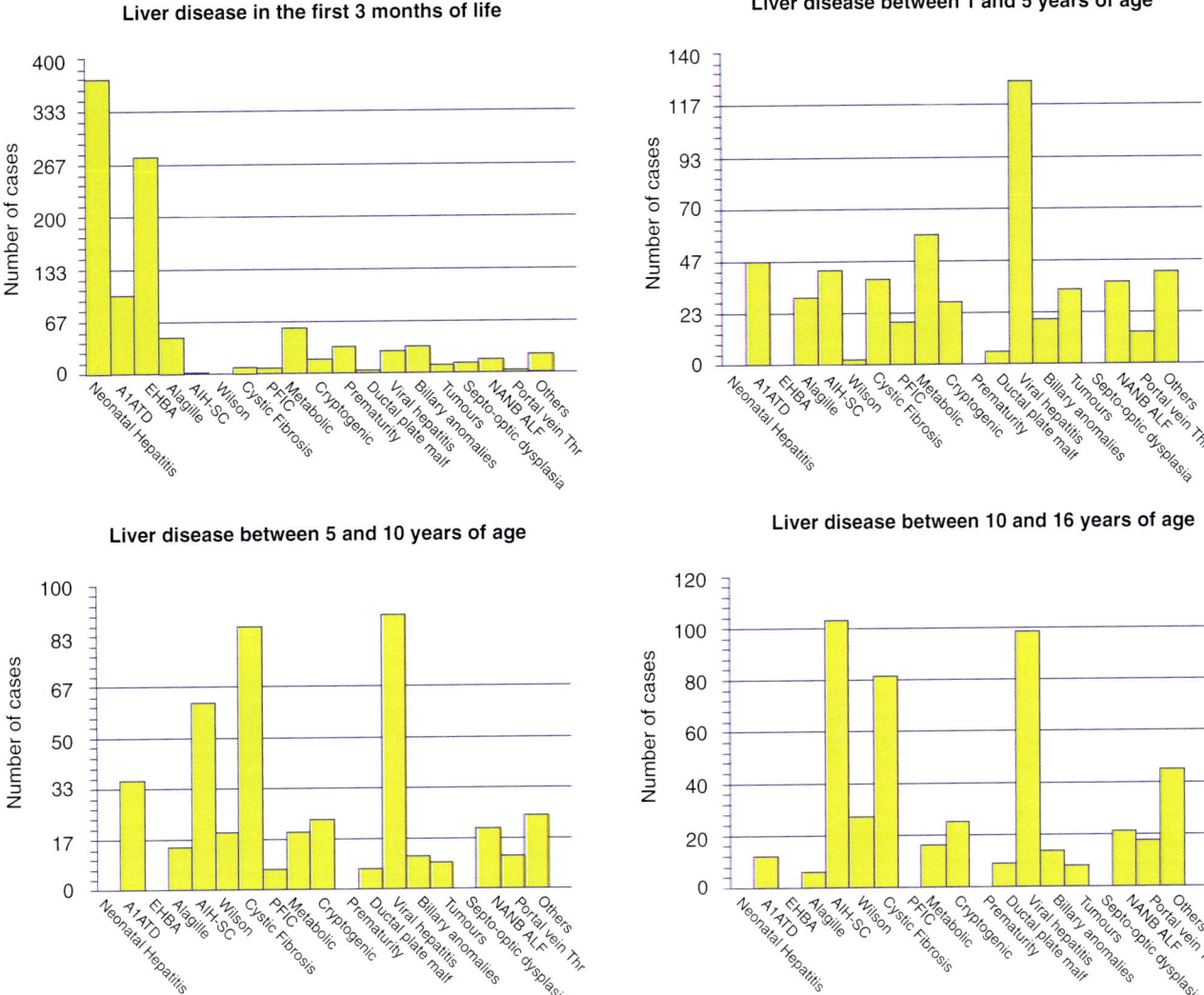

Fig. 1.18 Frequency of liver disease at different presenting ages. A1ATD, alpha-1-antitrypsin deficiency; EHBA, biliary atresia; AIH-SC, autoimmune hepatitis and sclerosing cholangitis; PFIC, progressive familial intrahepatic cholestasis; Ductal plate malf, ductal plate malformation; Biliary anomalies, choledochal cyst and inspissated bile syndrome; NANB ALF, nonA-nonB acute liver failure (D'Antiga L, unpublished data)

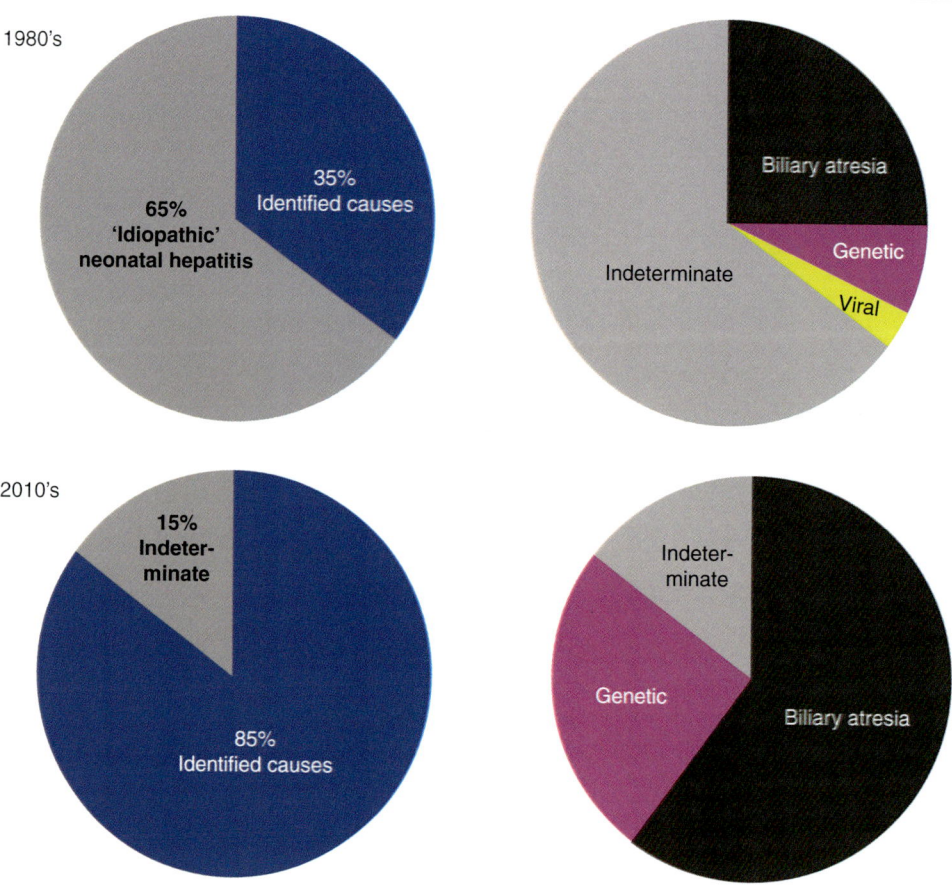

Fig. 1.19 Diagnostic yield in patients with neonatal cholestasis in two different eras, before and after the introduction in Bergamo of next-generation sequencing. Note the increased diagnosis of genetic disorders and of referral of biliary atresia patients

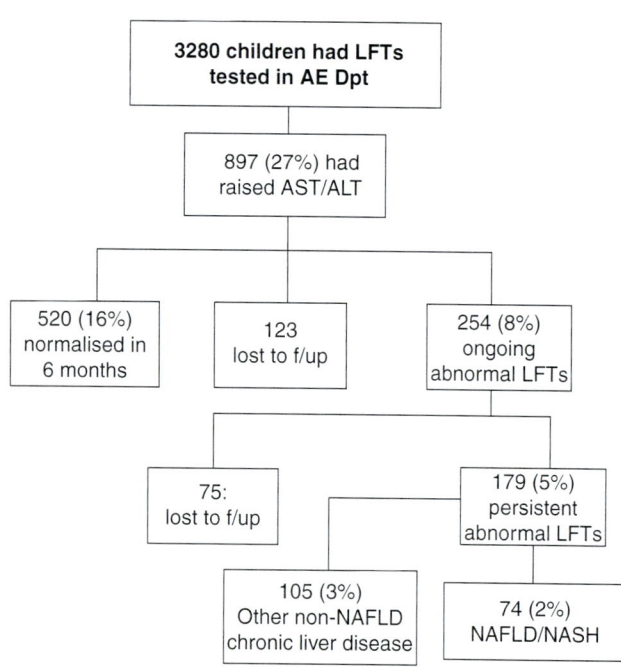

Fig. 1.20 Rate of chronic liver disease among children coming to the accident and emergency department for an acute illness. AE, accident and emergency department. LFTs, liver function tests. NAFLD, non-alcoholic fatty liver disease. NASH, non-alcoholic steatohepatitis. Modified from Nobili et al. [22]

References

1. United Nations Department of Economic and Social Affairs/Population Division World population prospects: the 2017 revision, key findings and advance tables.
2. Everhart JE, Ruhl CE. Burden of digestive diseases in the United States part III: liver, biliary tract, and pancreas. Gastroenterology. 2009;136:1134–44.
3. Arya G, Balistreri W. Pediatric liver disease in the United States: epidemiology and impact. J Gastroenterol Hepatol. 2002;17:521–5.
4. Della Corte C, Mosca A, Vania A, Alterio A, Alisi A, Nobili V. Pediatric liver diseases: current challenges and future perspectives. Expert Rev Gastroenterol Hepatol. 2016;10(2):255–65.
5. Levels & trends in child mortality: REPORT 2017 estimates developed by the UN Inter-agency Group for Child Mortality Estimation. United Nations.
6. World population monitoring 2001; Population, environment and development. New York: United Nations; 2001.
7. MCEE-WHO methods and data sources for child causes of death 2000-2015. Global Health Estimates Technical Paper WHO/HIS/IER/GHE/2016.
8. MCEE-WHO methods and data sources for child causes of death 2000-2015. Department of Evidence, Information and Research (WHO, Geneva) and Maternal Child Epidemiology Estimation (MCEE). Global Health Estimates Technical Paper, February 2016.
9. Murphy SL, Xu J, Kochanek KD, Curtin SC, Arias E. Deaths: final data for 2015, vol. 66, no. 6. National Vital Statistics Reports, 2017.
10. Kyu HH, Stein CE, Boschi Pinto C, et al. Causes of death among children aged 5–14 years in the WHO European Region: a system-

atic analysis for the Global Burden of Disease Study 2016. Lancet Child Adolesc Health. 2018;2:321–37.
11. Perrin JM, Anderson E, Van Cleave J. The rise in chronic conditions among infants, children, and youth can be met with continued health system innovations. Health Aff. 2014;33:2099–105.
12. Yang C, Perumpail BJ, Yoo ER, Ahmed A, Kerner JA. Nutritional needs and support for children with chronic liver disease. Nutrients. 2017;9:1127.
13. Vajro P, Maddaluno S, Veropalumbo C. Persistent hypertransaminasemia in asymptomatic children: a stepwise approach. World J Gastroenterol. 2013;19(18):2740–51.
14. Abdel Hady M, Kelly D. Chronic hepatitis B in children and adolescents: epidemiology and management. Pediatr Drugs. 2013;15:311–7.
15. Berardis S, Sokal E. Pediatric non-alcoholic fatty liver disease: an increasing public health issue. Eur J Pediatr. 2014;173:131–9.
16. Gower E, Estes C, Blach S, Razavi-Shearer K, Razavi H. Global epidemiology and genotype distribution of the hepatitis C virus infection. J Hepatol. 2014;61:S45–57.
17. Kanyenda TJ, Abdullahi LH, Hussey GD, Kagina BM. Epidemiology of hepatitis A virus in Africa among persons aged 1–10 years: a systematic review protocol. Syst Rev. 2015;4:129. SC04-SC07
18. Suchy FJ, Sokol RJ, Balistreri WF. Liver diseases in children. 4th ed. Cambridge University Press; 2014.
19. D'Antiga L, Dhawan A, Baker A, Hadzic N, Thompson R, Cheesman P, Mieli Vergani G. Liver disorders in childhood: a 15-year audit at a supraregional centre in the United Kingdom (data not published).
20. Matsui A. Hypertransaminasemia: the end of a thread. J Gastroenterol. 2005;40:859–60.
21. Iorio R, Sepe A, Giannattasio A, Cirillo F, Vegnente A. Hypertransaminasemia in childhood as a marker of genetic liver disorders. J Gastroenterol. 2005;40:820–6.
22. Nobili V, Reale A, Alisi A, Morino G, Trenta I, Pisani M, Marcellini M, Raucci U. Elevated serum ALT in children presenting to the emergency unit: relationship with NAFLD. Dig Liver Dis. 2009;41(19):749–52.

Basic Principles of Liver Physiology

Valeria Casotti and Lorenzo D'Antiga

Key Points
- The liver is the most important organ for the regulation of body homeostasis, in which the majority of metabolic processes occur, including glucose, amino acids and lipid metabolisms.
- The liver plays a central role in detoxifications of substances coming from the gut and the bloodstream (nutrient products, bacterial products, drugs, xenobiotics and other toxic products).
- Since the metabolically active liver requires continuous synthesis of ATP, hepatocytes contain a relatively high density of mitochondria compared with other cells. This is why mitochondrial disorders are generally highly expressed in the liver.
- A unique function of the liver is that of producing and recirculating bile, required for lipid digestion and excretion of toxic byproducts such as bilirubin and xenobiotics.
- Many liver functions, including hepatic lipid and glucose metabolism, bile acid homeostasis, embryonic development, reproduction, inflammation, cell differentiation, tissue regeneration and repair, are regulated by nuclear receptors (i.e. FXR, LXR, PPAR, CAR, PXR, TGR5).
- At birth, the liver is immature and more exposed to generic noxae. Full expression of the drug-metabolizing enzymes CYP450 and UGT is reached around 1 year of age.

Research Needed in the Field
- To increase our knowledge on cellular signalling and nuclear receptors and their relation with liver disease
- To develop strategies aimed at counteracting the process of fibrosis formation in the liver
- To increase our knowledge on liver maturation during pre- and postnatal life and its relation to paediatric liver disease developing at early ages

2.1 Introduction

The liver is the most important organ for the regulation of body homeostasis, in which the majority of metabolic processes occur. At birth, the liver constitutes about 4% of body weight; at the end of the growth, it accounts for 2.5–3% of body weight. The blood flow is ensured for 75% from the portal vein and for 25% from the hepatic artery. For all its metabolic performances, the liver has a high energy requirement, around 20% of the total oxygen need of the body.

The functional development of the liver requires a complicated orchestration of changes in hepatic enzymes and metabolic pathways that result in the mature capacity to undertake metabolism, biotransformation and transport.

The main liver functions can be summarised as follows:

- Selection, processing and detoxification of substances coming from the bowel and other organs (nutrient products, bacterial products, xenobiotics and toxic products)
- Glucose, amino acids and lipid homeostasis
- Synthesis, processing, recycling and degradation of lipoproteins
- Synthesis of the majority of plasmatic proteins (albumin, acute-phase proteins, coagulation proteins)
- Urea synthesis and ammonium detoxification
- Exocrine function: synthesis of biliary salts
- Haemoglobin degradation and bilirubin excretion [1, 2]

V. Casotti (✉) · L. D'Antiga
Paediatric Hepatology, Gastroenterology and Transplantation, Hospital Papa Giovanni XXIII, Bergamo, Italy
e-mail: vcasotti@asst-pg23.it; ldantiga@asst-pg23.it

© Springer Nature Switzerland AG 2019
L. D'Antiga (ed.), *Pediatric Hepatology and Liver Transplantation*, https://doi.org/10.1007/978-3-319-96400-3_2

2.2 Anatomo-functional Characteristics of the Liver

The liver can be viewed as two interdependent organs with a dual afferent blood supply:

- The *biliary tree* tissue, supplied by arterial blood, draining into a typical capillary network. The flow is regulated by systemic pressure and intrahepatic resistance; hepatic artery branches divide into axial (accompanying) vessels that branch into peri-biliary (connecting) arterioles. These taper to form the peri-biliary capillary plexus (PCP), which supplies bile ducts. The biliary tree is lined by a single layer of biliary epithelial cells (BEC: cholangiocytes) under hormonal and neural control, is an excretory conduit for hepatocyte-synthesised bile, excretes enzymes and mucins and modulates bile water content and composition.
- The *hepatic parenchima*, the bulk of the liver mass that encases the biliary tree. It is supplied by partially deoxygenated, low-pressure portal venous blood, rich in intestinal bacterial products and pancreatic hormones, and feeds into a unique sinusoidal bed. Sinusoids constitute a microvasculature, lined by liver sinusoidal endothelial cells (LSECs) and Kupffer cells (KC) which scavenge particulates/antigens and regulate immune responses.

The liver receives, from the enterohepatic circulation (portal circulation), all products coming from the intestinal metabolism (after intestinal digestion and absorption) such as amino acids, monosaccharides and vitamins and, through the hepatic artery, all substances coming from other organs and tissues; it is able to select substances for their different use and to eliminate the toxins.

The elementary structure is represented by the *hepatic lobule*, in which the hepatocytes are around the central vein, collecting the blood flow from the sinusoids; in parallel to the sinusoids, the biliary channels have an opposite flow, reaching the bile duct and finally the main biliary tree.

According to their position, the hepatocytes have different functions:

- Cells located in the periportal zone are mainly involved in oxidative metabolism (glycogen metabolism, gluconeogenesis, fatty acid β-oxidation, urea synthesis).
- Cells located in pericentral venule zone are more active in anaerobic glycolysis, lipogenesis and ketogenesis, lipoprotein synthesis and glutamine synthesis.

The cellular composition of the lobule is:

- 60–70%: Hepatocytes
- 30–40%: Non-parenchymal cells
  - Endothelial cells, lining the sinusoids: provided with 100 nm fenestrations favouring the molecules passage.
  - Kupffer cells: specialised macrophages with several functions—phagocytosis, immune defence, inflammatory response, cytokine release and hemocatheresis.
  - Stellate cells: 5–8% of hepatic cells; located in peri-sinusoidal spaces; they contain high amounts of lipids and vitamin A.
  - Natural killer cells/pit cells: cytotoxic lymphocytes, reacting against cancer cells and cells infected by viruses and bacteria.

The main role of the non-parenchymal cells is the recognition and degradation of foreign macromolecules reaching the liver; they can also degrade the lipoproteins, and they hydrolyse the cholesterol esters (scavenger cells), thus regulating the lipoproteins and cholesterol turnover [1, 4].

The liver structure and its main cellular components are represented in Figs. 2.1 and 2.2. A comprehensive overview of liver anatomy is provided in Chapter 3.

According to the different functions described in the next paragraphs, it is possible to identify the pathogenetic mechanisms for the diseases affecting or involving the liver, with specific attention to the paediatric age.

2.3 Glucose Metabolism

In the liver take place all the glucose metabolic pathways (glycogen-synthesis, glycogenolysis and gluconeogenesis).

The glucose metabolism starts with the entry of glucose through the GLUT2 transporter. After a meal, the level of glucose in the portal circulation is from 10 to 40 mMol, leading to a favourable gradient for the activity of GLUT2 and glucokinase. The enzyme glucokinase, induced by insulin, transforms glucose in glucose-6-P. Glucose 6-P is then converted to glucose-1-P, finally leading to the *glycogen synthesis*.

On the other hand, through the glucose-6-P phosphatase, the glucose-6-P is hydrolysed to glucose and inorganic P, leading to the possibility of releasing glucose in the bloodstream, for the metabolism in other organs.

The liver is also able to convert to glucose other monosaccharides (fructose, galactose). Fructose coming from the bowel to the liver is partly converted to fructose-6-P (from exokinases) and mainly converted to fructose-1-P (from fructokinases); the latter, leading to the glycolytic process, is present only in the liver.

2 Basic Principles of Liver Physiology

Fig. 2.1 The structure of the hepatic lobule

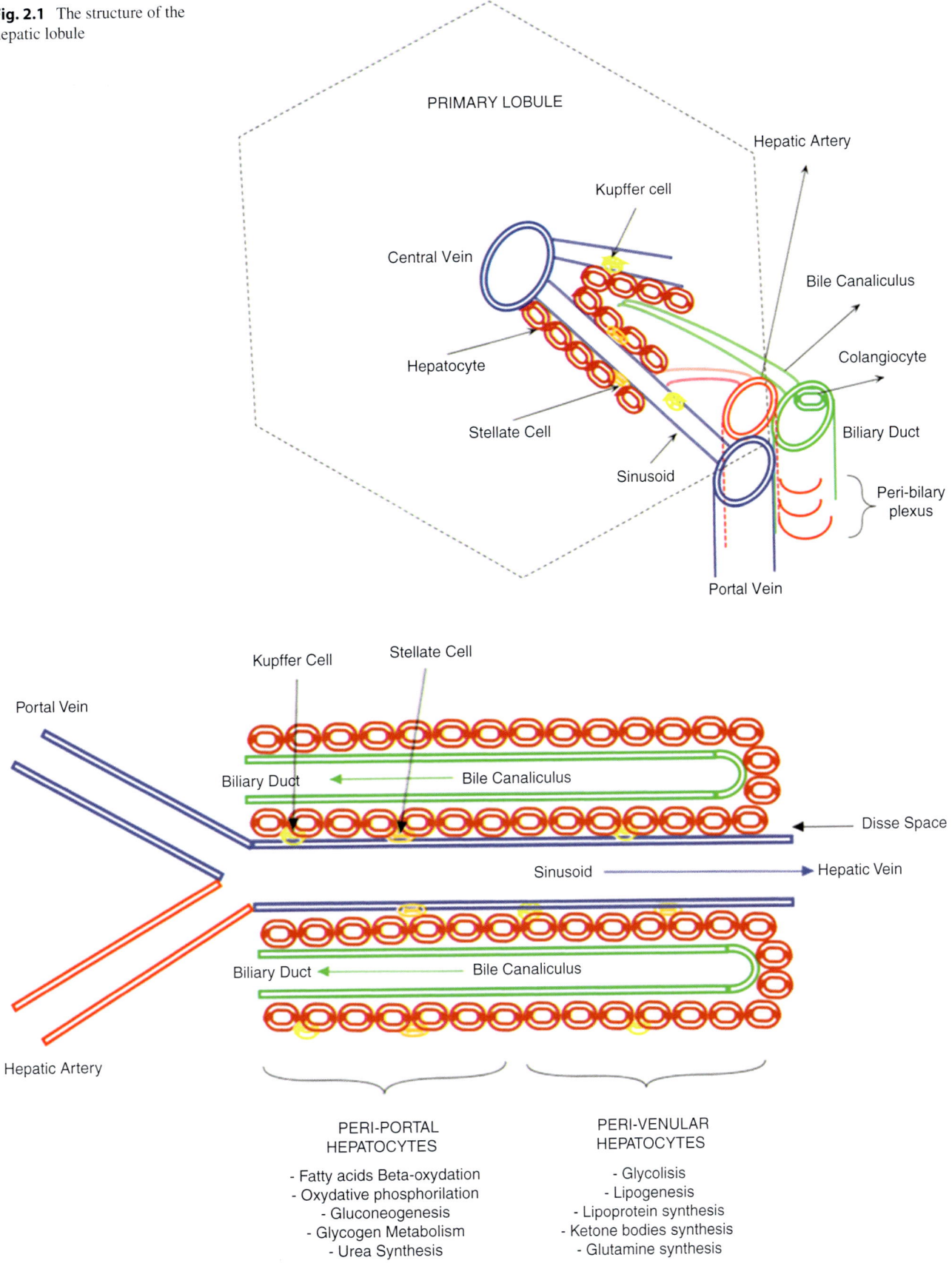

Fig. 2.2 The functional distribution of hepatocytes in the hepatic lobule

Through the *glycolysis* pathway, glucose is converted into pyruvate and then transformed to Acetyl-CoA, entering the Krebs cycle for further energy production.

Moreover, the liver is the site of *gluconeogenesis*, having the role of maintaining adequate glucose levels during fasting.

The substrates for this process are:

- *Lactic acid:* mainly coming from the muscle (anaerobic glycolysis); the *CORI cycle* in the liver transforms lactic acid into pyruvate and then to glucose.
- *Glucogenic amino acids:* mainly coming from muscles or kidneys. The process of transamination to pyruvate *(CAHILL cycle)*, oxaloacetate and alpha-ketoglutarate in the liver is the way to the gluconeogenesis.
- *Glycerol:* coming from triglycerides and phospholipids, glycerol in the liver is converted to 3-P-glycerol and then to glucose. This way is particularly active when glucose intake is low and lipids are abundant.

Thirty percent of glucose in the liver is metabolised in the *pentose phosphate pathway*, leading to the production of reducing equivalents (NADPH) required for several processes: fatty acid synthesis, cholesterol and bile acid synthesis and phase 1 reactions of detoxification (cytochrome p450).

During the foetal development, glucose accounts for 50–80% of the foetus energy consumption, with a mechanism completely dependent upon the mother (continuous glucose transfer across the placenta). Near term, the foetal liver contains an amount of glycogen 2–3 times higher than in the adult liver; these stores are important for maintenance of blood glucose levels during the perinatal period, before other sources become available and before the onset of hepatic gluconeogenesis.

At birth, the neonate must rapidly translate to independent control of glucose homeostasis. After birth and before the onset of suckling, the glucose is scarce, and ketone bodies are not available; the newborn is supplied with lactate; gluconeogenesis from lactate and pyruvate (30%) is established by 4–6 h after birth.

After the initiation of suckling, plasma insulin levels fall and glucagon and catecholamines rise, inducing glycogenolysis. When liver stores of glycogen are spent (12 h), gluconeogenesis is required.

Reaccumulation of glycogen stores occurs in the second postnatal week, and adult glycogen level is reached at 3 weeks.

Deficiency of different enzymes involved in glucose metabolism may lead to different metabolic diseases involving the liver, in particular galactosaemia, fructosaemia and different forms of glycogenosis, as shown in Figs. 2.3 and 2.4 [1, 3].

2.4 Amino Acid Metabolism

In the foetus, amino acids are a significant source of energy (40%), with glutamine as the most important. The foetal liver is in fact the primary site for glutamate production, which is released and taken up by the placenta and for the most part rapidly oxidised; the remaining glutamine is used by the foetal tissues for growth.

Most of the enzymes required for regulation of amino acid metabolism are expressed at birth.

The liver receives from the portal vein the intestinal absorbed amino acids and from the hepatic artery the amino acids coming from extrahepatic tissue protein degradation (in particular muscle tissue).

Amino acids from both sources are utilised by the liver for different functions, after the transamination process: gluconeogenesis, hepatic protein synthesis and plasmatic protein synthesis.

The main proteins that the liver produces are:

- Albumin
- Transport proteins (alpha and beta globulins)
- Coagulation proteins
- Apoproteins (APO-B100, APO A1)
- Protease inhibitors (alpha-1-antitrypsin)
- Complement proteins
- Acute-phase proteins
- HEME, purine and pyrimidine

Aspartate, glutamate and glutamine are used as energy substrate at intestinal level; the liver receives their products, in particular citrulline, arginine and ammonium, which enter in the *urea cycle*.

Through the urea cycle, the liver is able to eliminate the nitrogen produced in the whole body.

Abnormalities in the pathways of protein metabolism can lead to different diseases, such as tyrosinaemia and urea cycle defects, as shown in Fig. 2.5 [1, 2].

2.5 Lipid Metabolism

The liver has a central role in lipid metabolism, since it defines the final destinations of lipids coming from the circulation: ketone bodies, triglycerides, phospholipids or cholesterol.

The fat that accumulates in the foetal liver is mobilised soon after birth; the oxidation of fat results in significant generation of ATP for energy and ketone body formation for use by peripheral tissues. There is a marked increase in plasma-free fatty acid concentration after birth in infants.

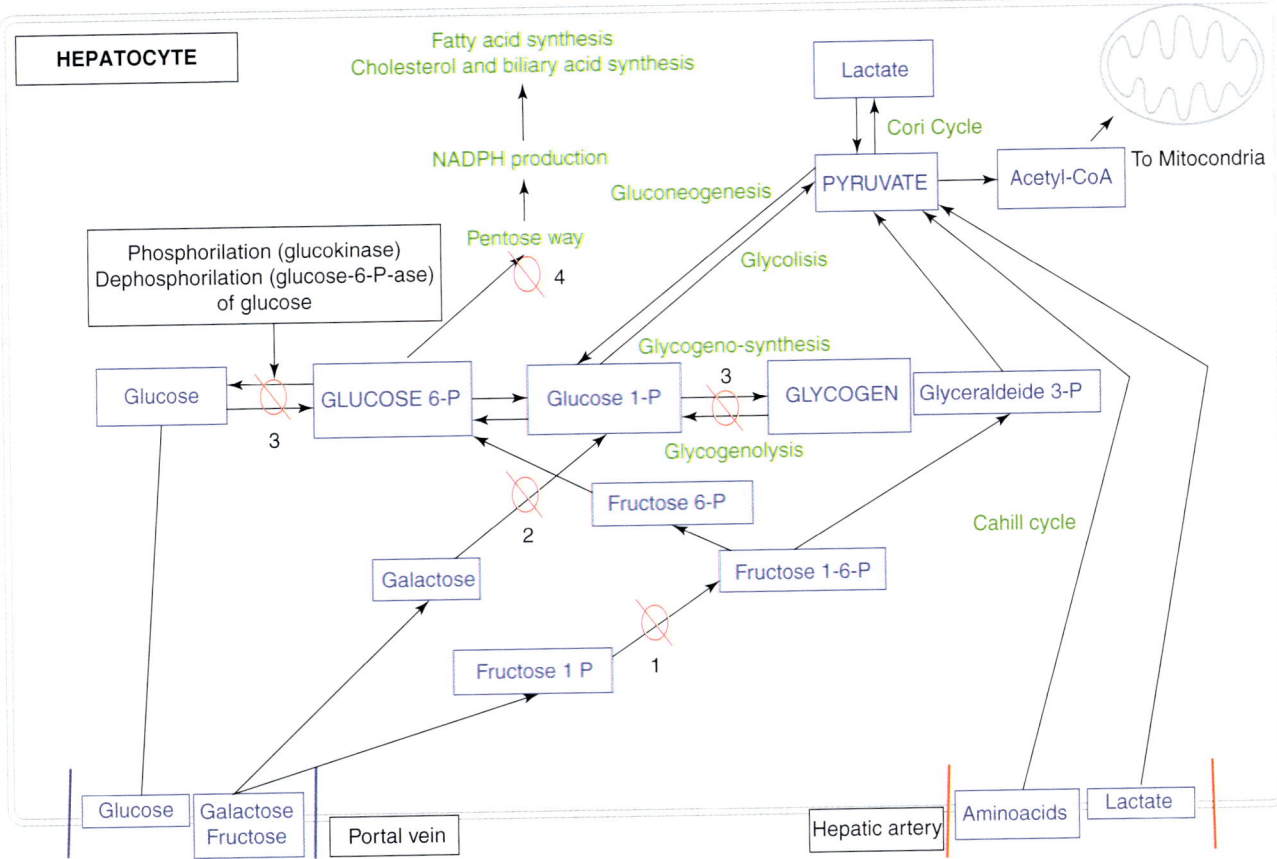

Fig. 2.3 Carbohydrate metabolic pathways and abnormalities associated with liver diseases. (1) Fructosaemia—aldolase deficiency. (2) Galactosaemia—galactose uridyl transferase deficiency. (3) Glycogenosis with liver involvement (type I, Gluc-6-P-ase deficiency (abnormal dephosphorylation of glucose); type III, deficiency in glycogen debranching enzyme activity; type IV, deficiency in glycogen branching enzyme activity; type VI, deficiency in glycogen phosphorylase; type IX, deficiency in glycogen phosphorylase B kinase). (4) Transaldolase deficiency (TALDO): inborn error of the pentose phosphate pathway

Rapid maturation of the ability of the liver to oxidise fatty acids occurs during the first days of life. The postnatal increase in hepatic fatty acid oxidation is critically important for the hepatic gluconeogenesis, supported by the exclusive milk feeding (high-fat, low-carbohydrate diet).

At weaning, the lipogenic capacity of the liver increases in response to high-carbohydrate diet.

Four different forms of fatty acids (FAs) are recognised:

- The *short-chain FAs* represent local growth factors in the intestine.
- The *medium-chain FAs* are relevant for the neonate, since they are present as triglycerides in human milk; they reach the liver and are converted to Acyl-CoA by specific enzymes.
- The *long-chain FAs* are the main metabolic substrates for the liver, coming from the adipose tissue as non-esterified fatty acids (NEFAs) and activated by Acyl-CoA. After the transfer to mitochondria, mediated by carnitine, NEFAs enter the beta-oxidation process. This pathway leads to the formation of Acetyl-CoA and H+, entering the Krebs cycle and the oxidative phosphorylation, finally resulting in ATP production, the energy source for all cellular functions.
- The *very-long-chain fatty acids (VLCFAs)* are structural components of the membranes; they are metabolised at peroxisomal level by the peroxisomal-beta oxidation, and then the oxidation proceeds at mitochondrial level.

2.6 Lipoprotein Synthesis

The synthesis of VLDL and HDL lipoprotein takes place in the liver. VLDLs have triglycerides and cholesterol as the main components; through these lipoproteins, the liver exports fat to other tissues; in HDL, the main components are phospholipids.

The lipoprotein synthesis starts in the endoplasmic reticulum (production of apolipoproteins), and then the lipid and glycidic parts are added. Any reduced production of lipoproteins, due to the deficiency in phospholipids or apolipoproteins, may lead to liver steatosis.

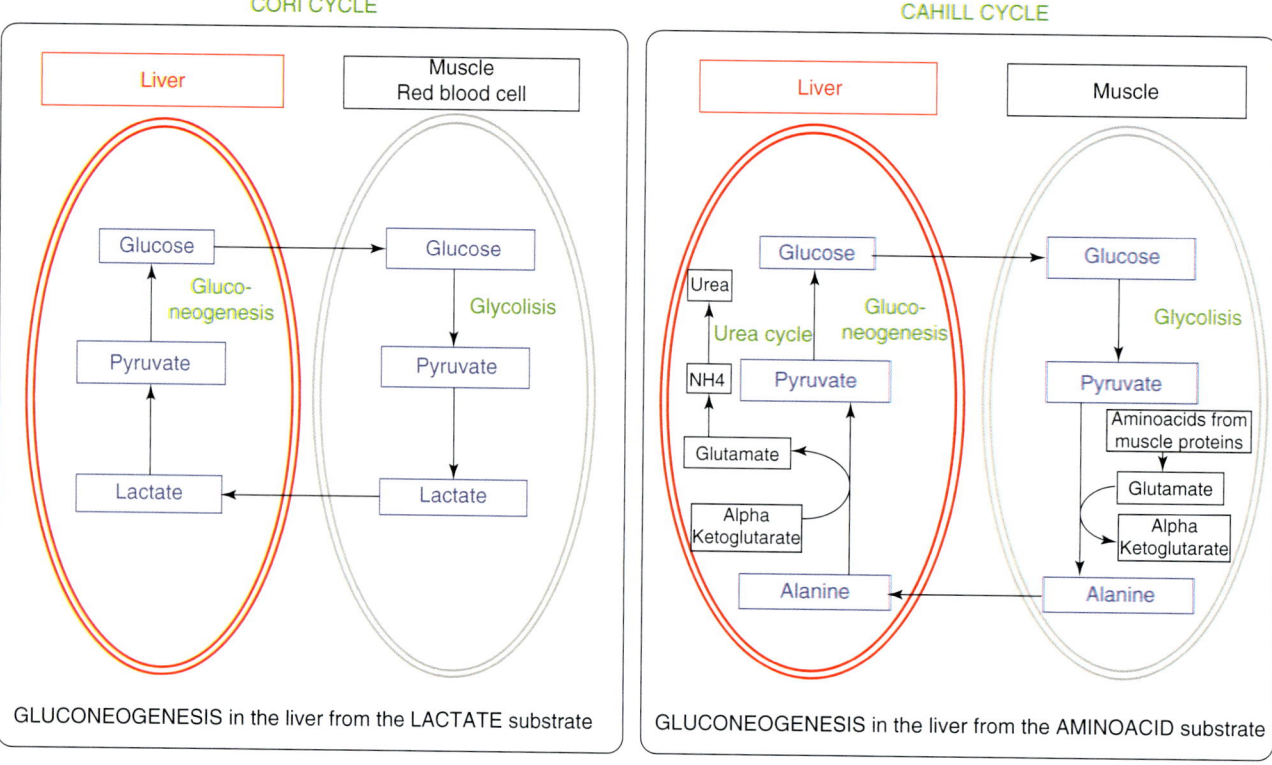

Fig. 2.4 Cori and Cahill cycles

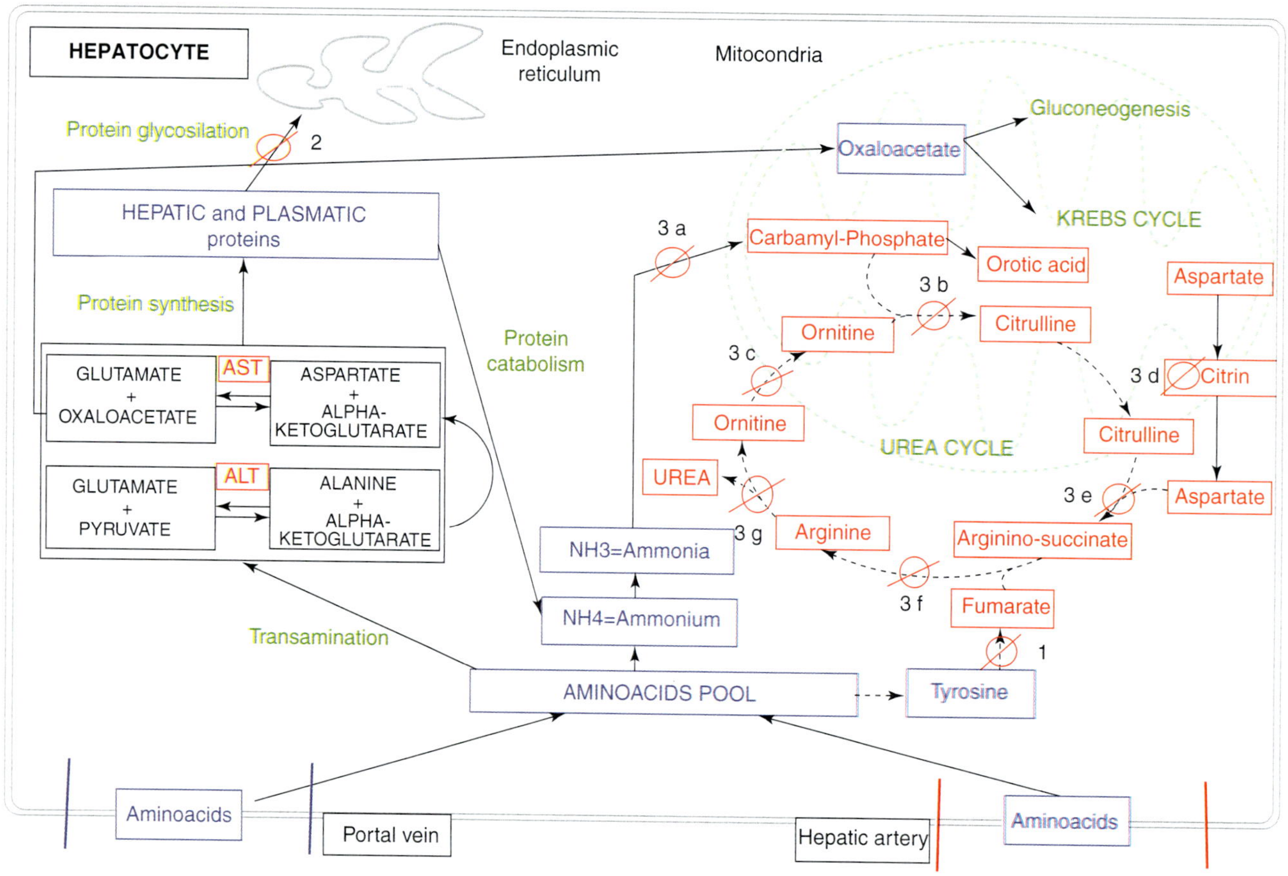

Fig. 2.5 Amino acid metabolism in the liver and associated diseases. *AST* aspartate aminotransferase, *ALT* alanine aminotransferase. (1) Tyrosinaemia: fumarylacetoacetate hydrolase deficiency. (2) CGD, congenital disorders of glycosylation. (3) Urea cycle of disorders: (3a) carbamyl-phosphate synthetase deficiency (CPS-I); (3b) ornithine transcarbamylase deficiency (OCT); (3c) ornithine translocase deficiency (ORNT1-HHH); (3d) citrin deficiency (citrullinaemia II); (3e) argininosuccinate synthetase deficiency (*ASS*, citrullinaemia I); (3f) argininosuccinate lyase deficiency (*ASL* argininosuccinic aciduria); (3g) arginase 1 deficiency (*ARG1* argininaemia)

2.7 Ketogenesis

The hepatic mitochondria are the main site for ketone body production; ketogenesis is activated when the Acyl-CoA production through the beta-oxidation process exceeds the amount that can enter the Krebs cycle.

During fasting, the energy requirement is provided by triglyceride metabolism from adipose tissue; the amount of NEFA to the liver is increased, and in turn the ketogenesis is activated.

Excessive increase of NEFA may be due to prolonged fasting, diabetes and excessive introduction of lipids with the diet; all these conditions lead to excess of triglycerides, and then of fatty acids, finally inducing liver steatosis. Abnormalities in the processes of lipid metabolism and storage can lead to different diseases involving the liver, as shown in Fig. 2.6 [1, 2]. The main conditions are:

1. Mitochondrial carnitine metabolism and beta-oxidation disorders:
   - Carnitine metabolism disorders: CPT1 deficiency, CAT deficiency and CPT2 deficiency
   - Mitochondrial beta-oxidation disorders: VLCAD, MCAD, SCAD and trifunctional protein deficiency
2. Peroxisomal disorders:
   - Disorders of peroxisome biogenesis: Zellweger syndrome, adrenoleukodystrophy and infantile Refsum disease
   - Isolated peroxisomal enzyme deficiency: D-bifunctional protein deficiency and primary hyperoxaluria type I
3. Lysosomal storage diseases:
   - Gaucher disease: deficient activity in lysosomal hydrolase, acid beta glucosidase → accumulation of undergraded glycolipid substrates, particularly glucosylceramide, in reticuloendothelial system

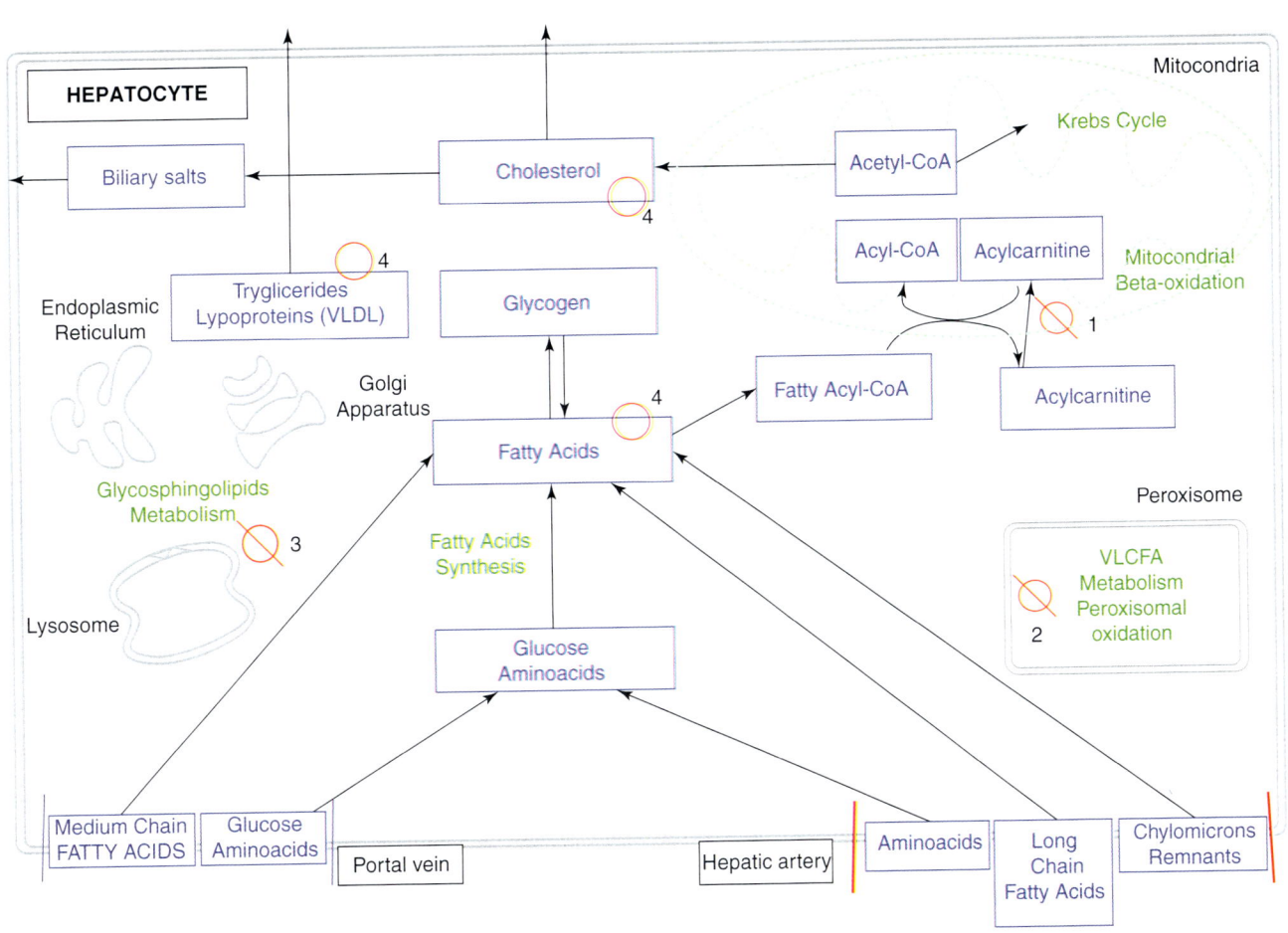

Fig. 2.6 Lipid metabolism in the liver and associated diseases with liver involvement. (1) Mitochondrial carnitine metabolism; (2) peroxisomal disorders; (3) lysosomal storage disorders; (4) abnormal accumulation of fatty acids

- Niemann-Pick (A and B): deficient activity of lysosomal enzyme sphingomyelinase → pathologic accumulation of sphingomyelin in the monocyte-macrophage system
- Niemann-Pick type C: abnormal lipid trafficking → accumulation of sphingomyelin and cholesterol in lysosomes
- Wolman disease/CESD (cholesteryl ester storage disease): deficiency in lysosomal acid lipase → accumulation of cholesteryl esters, triglycerides and other lipids in histiocytic foam cells of most of the visceral organs
4. Abnormal/excessive accumulation of FA, triglycerides and cholesterol → NAFLD; NASH

2.8 The Role of Mitochondria

Mitochondria are double-membrane intracellular organelles containing a soluble matrix and their own unique genome; they are the main source of the high-energy phosphate molecule adenosine triphosphate (ATP), produced through the Krebs cycle, which is pivotal for all active intracellular processes.

Because the metabolically active liver requires continuous synthesis of ATP, hepatocytes contain a relatively high density of mitochondria compared with other cells. This is why mitochondrial disorders are generally highly expressed in the liver.

ATP is produced by the respiratory chain on the inner mitochondrial membrane by the oxidative phosphorylation (OXPHOS). In this process, reduced cofactors (nicotinamide adenine dinucleotide [NADH], flavin adenine dinucleotide [FADH$_2$] and electron transfer flavoprotein [ETF]) generated from the intermediary metabolism of carbohydrates (glycolysis), proteins (tricarboxylic acid cycle) and lipids (fatty acid oxidation) donate electrons to complexes I and II and ubiquinone, which then flow down an electrochemical gradient to complexes III, to cytochrome c and finally to complex IV, resulting in the active translocation of protons (H+) out of the mitochondrial matrix into the intermembrane space, which establishes an electrochemical gradient. At complex V, protons flow back into the mitochondrial matrix, and the released energy is used to synthesise ATP (Fig. 2.7).

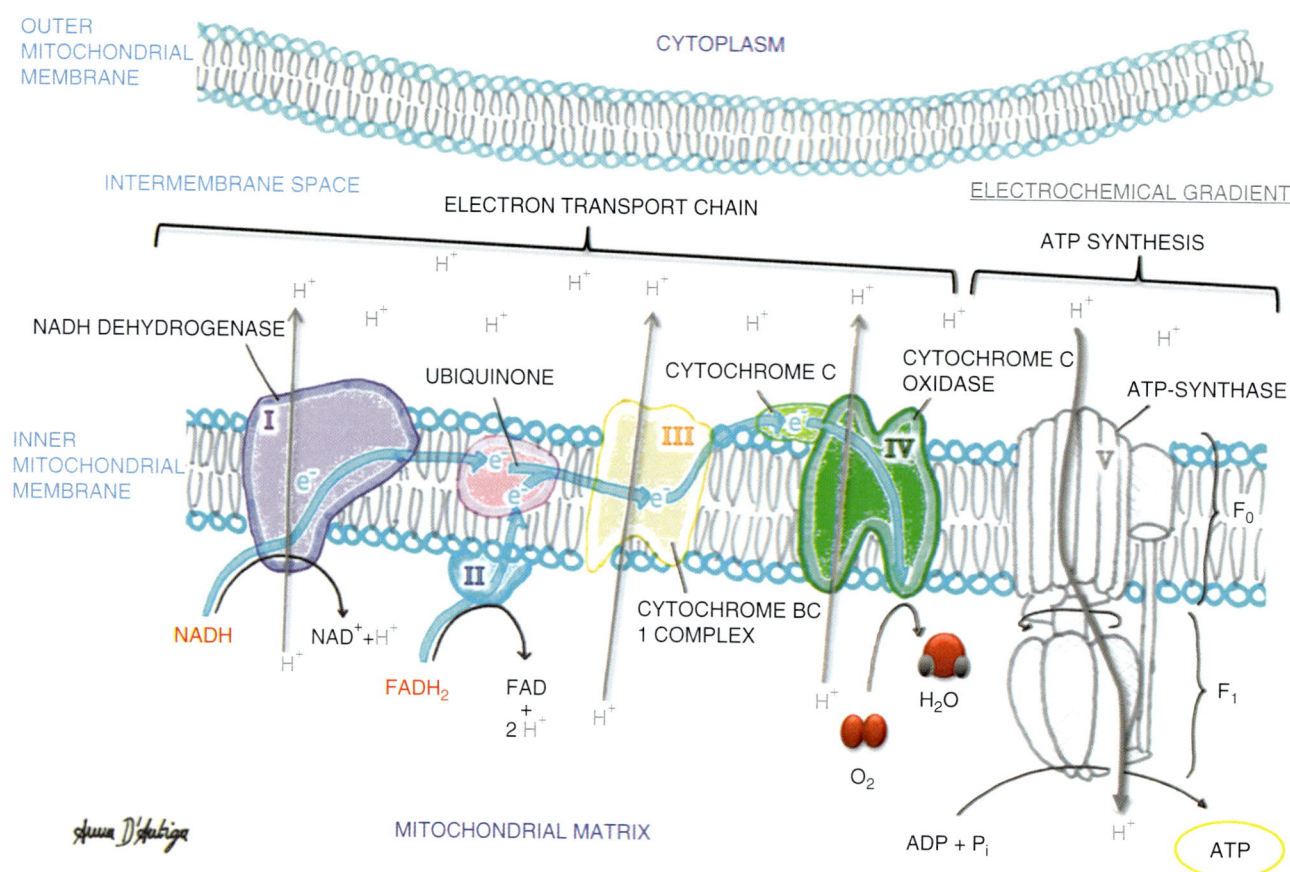

Fig. 2.7 Mitochondrial respiratory chain. I: complex I; II: complex II; III: complex III; IV: complex IV; V: complex V. Courtesy of Anna D'Antiga

A unique feature of mitochondria in mammalian cells is the presence of a distinct genome, mitochondrial DNA (mtDNA), which is independent from that of the nucleus. A typical hepatocyte contains ~1000 copies of mtDNA; both nuclear and mtDNA genes encode for respiratory chain components.

Thirteen essential polypeptides are synthesised from the mtDNA. In contrast, nuclear genes encode more than 70 respiratory chain subunits, and an array of enzymes and cofactors required to maintain mtDNA. These genes include DNA polymerase-γ (*POLG*), inner mitochondrial membrane protein (*MPV17*) and deoxyguanosine kinase (*DGUOK*), known to be associated with liver disease from mitochondrial depletion.

Disorders affecting mitochondrial oxidative phosphorylation (OXPHOS) and hepatocellular metabolism directly influence fatty acid oxidation, resulting in impaired bile flow and steatosis, cell death and fibrogenesis. In fact, hepatic manifestations of mitochondrial disorders range from hepatic steatosis, cholestasis and chronic liver disease with insidious onset to neonatal liver failure, frequently associated with neuromuscular symptoms.

Mitochondrial diseases can be distinguished as *primary disorders*, in which the mitochondrial defect is the primary cause of the liver disorder, and *secondary disorders*, in which a secondary insult to mitochondria is caused either by a genetic defect that affects non-mitochondrial proteins or by an acquired (exogenous) injury to mitochondria [5].

A summary of different metabolic pathways, the role of mitochondria and mitochondrial diseases involving the liver are represented in Figure 2.8.

Primary mitochondrial disorders involving the liver are mainly due to electron transport (respiratory chain) defects, because of different mutations in both nuclear and mitochondrial DNA. We can distinguish: (1) neonatal acute liver failure due to specific or multiple complex deficiency; (2) mitochondrial DNA depletion syndrome (tissue-specific reduction in mtDNA copy number): DGUOK mutation, POLG mutation (Alpers-Huttenlocher syndrome), MPV17 mutation (Navajo neurohepatopathy);

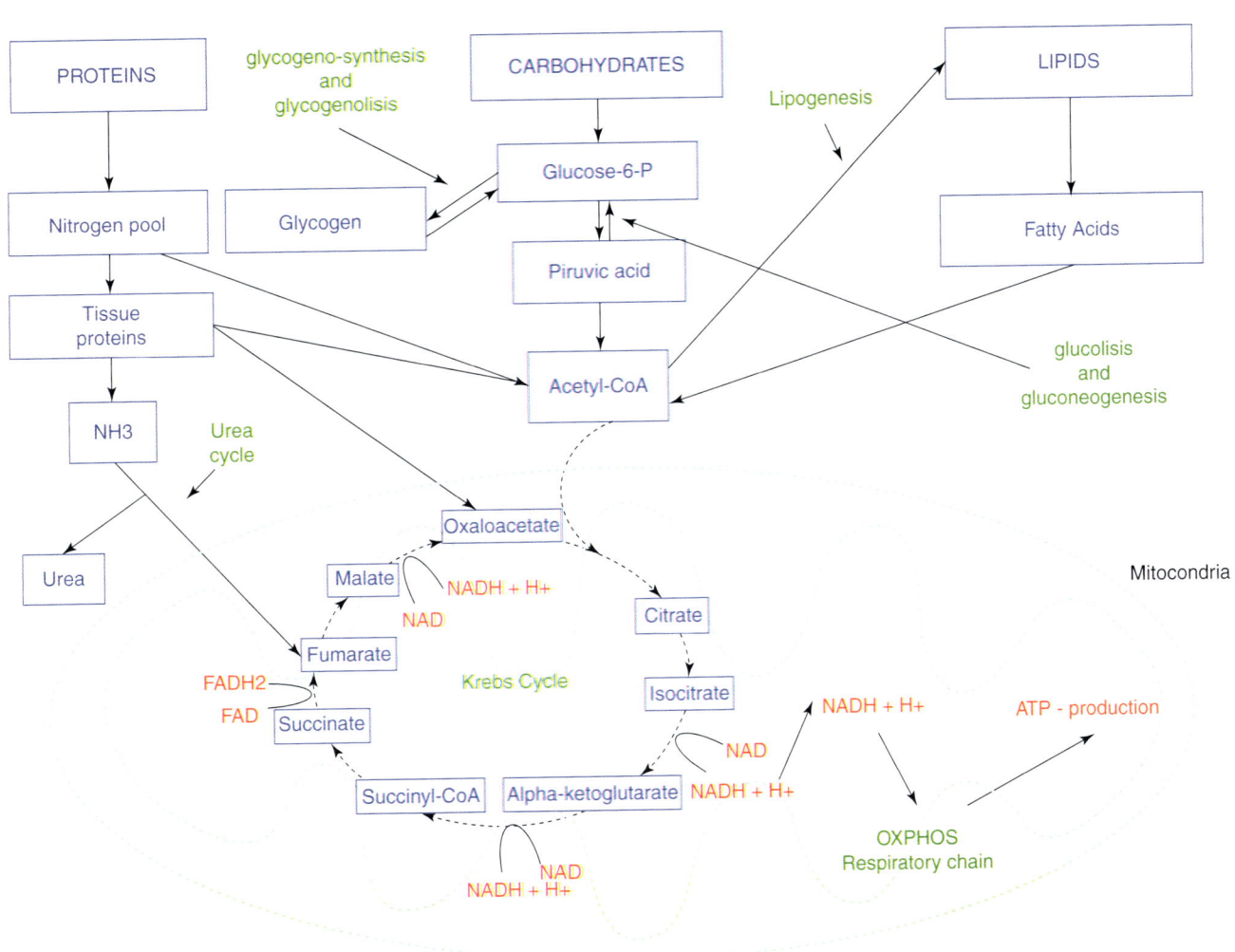

Fig. 2.8 Metabolism summary and pivotal role of the Krebs cycle in the mitochondria

(3) mtDNA deletion: Pearson's marrow-pancreas syndrome (associated with liver steatosis and cirrhosis).

2.9 The Hepatobiliary Function

As already described, the liver has a huge number of metabolic functions, some shared by other organs and others unique. One of the latter is the formation of bile.

Bile is an aqueous fluid produced by a number of interweaving processes, molecules and pathways that engage intracellular and membrane protein functions in both hepatocytes and cholangiocytes.

The bile has the following composition:

- Bile salts (or bile acids) (61%) needed for fat emulsification/absorption
- Fatty acids (12%)
- Cholesterol (9%)
- Phospholipids (3%)
- Bilirubin (3%)
- Proteins (7%) and other endogenous and exogenous compounds, including biotransformed drugs

Bile secretion starts at low concentrations at the beginning of the fourth month of gestation in humans; the bile is secreted into the gut and colours its content (meconium).

After birth, the conjugates of the primary bile acids cholate and chenodeoxycholate increase progressively in the serum to reach concentrations during the first week of life that are significantly higher than in normal older children and adults and similar to patients with cholestatic liver diseases. A gradual decline to adult levels occurs after 6 months of life. The level of serum bile acids is determined not only by the hepatic uptake but also by the intestinal absorption; since these processes are immature in infancy, a physiologic, mild cholestasis/hypercholanaemia is common.

Bile acid synthesis, bile acid pool size, intraluminal bile acid concentrations and presumably bile secretion increase gradually during the first year of life in humans.

The production and secretion of bile are regulated by the intestinal paracrine hormones cholecystokinin and secretin.

Bile acids are required for absorption of fats, steroids and lipid-soluble vitamins in the intestine and are signalling molecules that activate nuclear and membrane bile acid receptors to modulate hepatic lipid, glucose and energy metabolism.

The bile acid pool is defined as the total bile acids circulating in the enterohepatic circulation, including bile acids in the liver (<1%), intestine (~85–90%) and gallbladder (~10–15%).

In the liver, the conversion of cholesterol into bile acids is the major pathway for catabolism of cholesterol; the liver synthesises approximately 0.5 g bile acids per day, stored in the gallbladder. After a meal, cholecystokinin (CCK), released by the pancreas, stimulates gallbladder contraction to excrete the bile, and therefore the bile acids, into the gastrointestinal tract via the common bile ducts.

Some bile acids are passively absorbed in the upper intestine, but most are reabsorbed in the ileum and colon by an active transport system represented by an apical Na+-dependent bile salt transporter (ASBT).

The enterohepatic circulation of bile acids reabsorbs bile acids from the intestine and controls bile acid synthesis in the liver by a negative feedback mechanism; this maintains a constant bile acid pool.

This *enterohepatic circulation* is highly efficient, reuptaking about 95% of bile acids of the pool. The quote that is not reabsorbed (5% of the pool) undergoes deconjugation and dehydroxylation by intestinal flora (bacterial 7α-dehydroxylase activity) to form secondary bile acids, excreted in faeces. This small amount of bile acid lost in faeces (0.5 g/day) is replenished by de novo synthesis in the liver. A small amount (0.5 mg/day) of bile acid spillover into systemic circulation is cleared in urine (Fig. 2.9).

The entire enterohepatic recirculation of bile acids occurs on average of 6–8 times a day, to maintain a constant bile acid pool size of approximately 3 g.

Bile acids are involved in the regulation of more complex processes including bile production and glucose and lipid metabolism and in the modulation of immune response [1, 6–8].

In humans, the bile acid pool consists mainly of cholic acid (CA, ~40%) and chenodeoxycholic acid (CDCA, ~40%), the *primary* bile acids, that are produced in the liver and subsequently modified by gut bacteria in the small intestine to produce *secondary* bile acids, deoxycholic acid (DCA, ~20%) and lithocholic acid (LCA).

The liver is the only organ that has all the enzymes required for bile acid synthesis. There are two pathways in the liver, the *classic* or neutral pathway and the *alternative* or acidic pathway, leading to the synthesis of primary bile acids from cholesterol in hepatic microsomes.

The "classic pathway" of bile acid synthesis is initiated by the rate-limiting enzyme cholesterol 7α-hydroxylase (CYP7A1) to specifically hydroxylate cholesterol forming 7α-hydroxycholesterol, which is converted to 7α-hydroxy-4-cholesten-3-one (named C4) by 3β-hydroxy-Δ5-C27-steroid dehydrogenase (HSD3B7). C4 is the common precursor of cholic acid (CA) and chenodeoxycholic acid (CDCA).

The alternative bile acid pathway ("acidic pathway"), which forms less than 10% of total BA, is initiated by mitochondrial sterol 27-hydroxylase (CYP27A1), which converts cholesterol to 27-hydroxycholesterol and then to 3β-hydroxy-5-cholestenoic acid; these intermediates feed into pathways leading to the formation of CDCA (Fig. 2.10) [6–8].

Bile acids are then conjugated with glycine or taurine in the liver *peroxisomes* to produce the amphipathic structure

Fig. 2.9 The enterohepatic circulation of bile acids

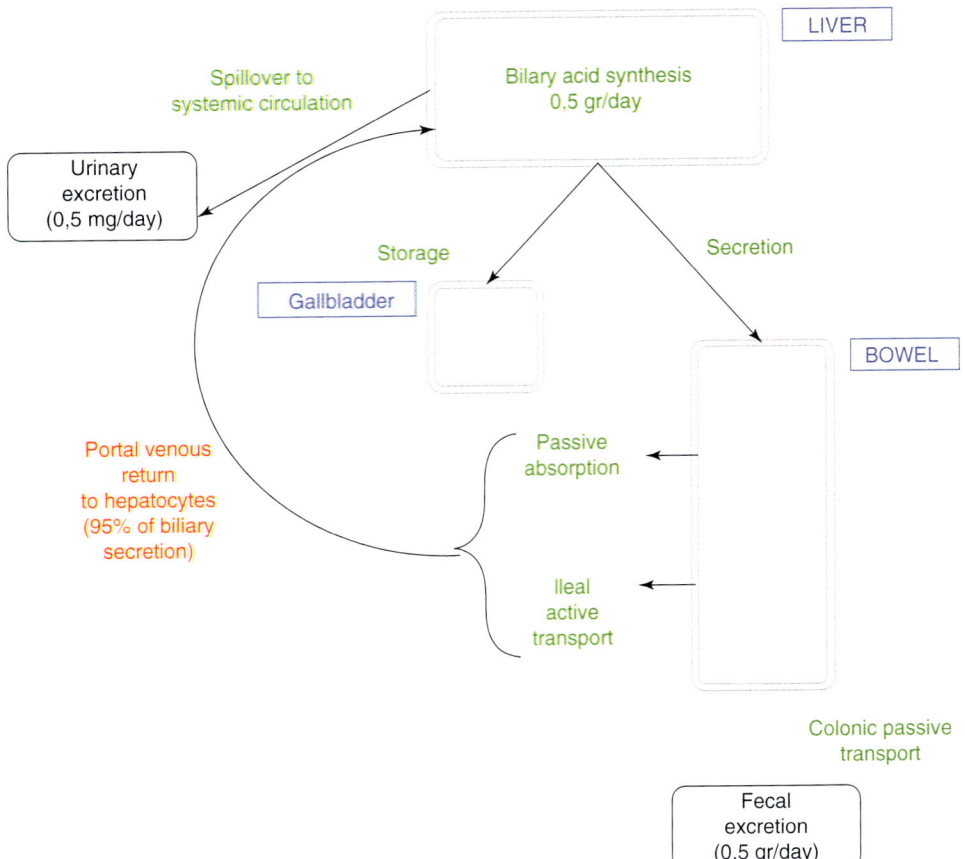

that contains both hydrophobic (lipid-soluble) and polar (hydrophilic) regions. The cholesterol portion of a bile acid is hydrophobic, and the amino acid conjugate is polar and hydrophilic. The polar BAs surround fat molecules and can present the hydrophobic fat molecules (which are insoluble in the aqueous phase) to the brush border membrane of the small intestine for digestion and absorption.

The polar nature of these bile salts (anionic detergents), which is essential for their function in fat digestion, makes them toxic to cell membranes of liver and gut cells.

The polarised hepatocyte is the primary structure responsible for the synthesis and transport of bile acids and thus is the most likely to be damaged by bile acid retention when bile flow is reduced.

In the normal liver, toxicity is moderated by the formation of mixed micelles (with bilirubin, cholesterol, phospholipid proteins), bile hydration, conjugation, alkalinisation, the presence of mucin and the regular outflow of the bile towards the gut.

The highest concentration of bile acids is in the canalicular lumen; the intracellular retention of bile acids appears to be the most important disease-producing consequences of cholestasis. The overall effect of cholestasis can be ascribed to the effects of retained bile acids, since the hepatocyte responds treating them as dangerous foreign compounds.

The downstream bile flow can be obstructed, because of the absence of a normal biliary tract or because of paucity of bile ducts; this is the case of biliary atresia and Alagille syndrome, respectively.

But cholestasis can occur without frank ductal obstruction, in the event of impaired function of the proteins necessary for the bile formation. When the bile flow is obstructed right at the canalicular membrane, bile acid concentration will rise within hepatocytes; prolonged retention of bile acids within the liver leads to activation of Kupffer cells, stellate cells and myofibroblasts, with consequent increased production of cytokines and matrix and with progression of fibrosis.

Several proteins are involved in the transport and metabolism of bile acids. To be excreted and reach the gastrointestinal tract, bile acids are actively transported across the canalicular (apical) membrane of hepatocytes by an ATP-dependent transporter, the bile salt export pump (BSEP), a protein encoded by ABCB11 gene. When this transporter is mutated, bile acid flow is reduced, and bile acids are retained within the hepatocytes, leading to PFIC type II. Once in the canalicular space, bile acids form mixed micelles with other lipids, in particular phosphatidylcholine (PC). The entry of PC into the bile is dependent upon another ATP-binding cassette (ABC) transporter called MDR3, encoded by ABCB4 gene; the presence

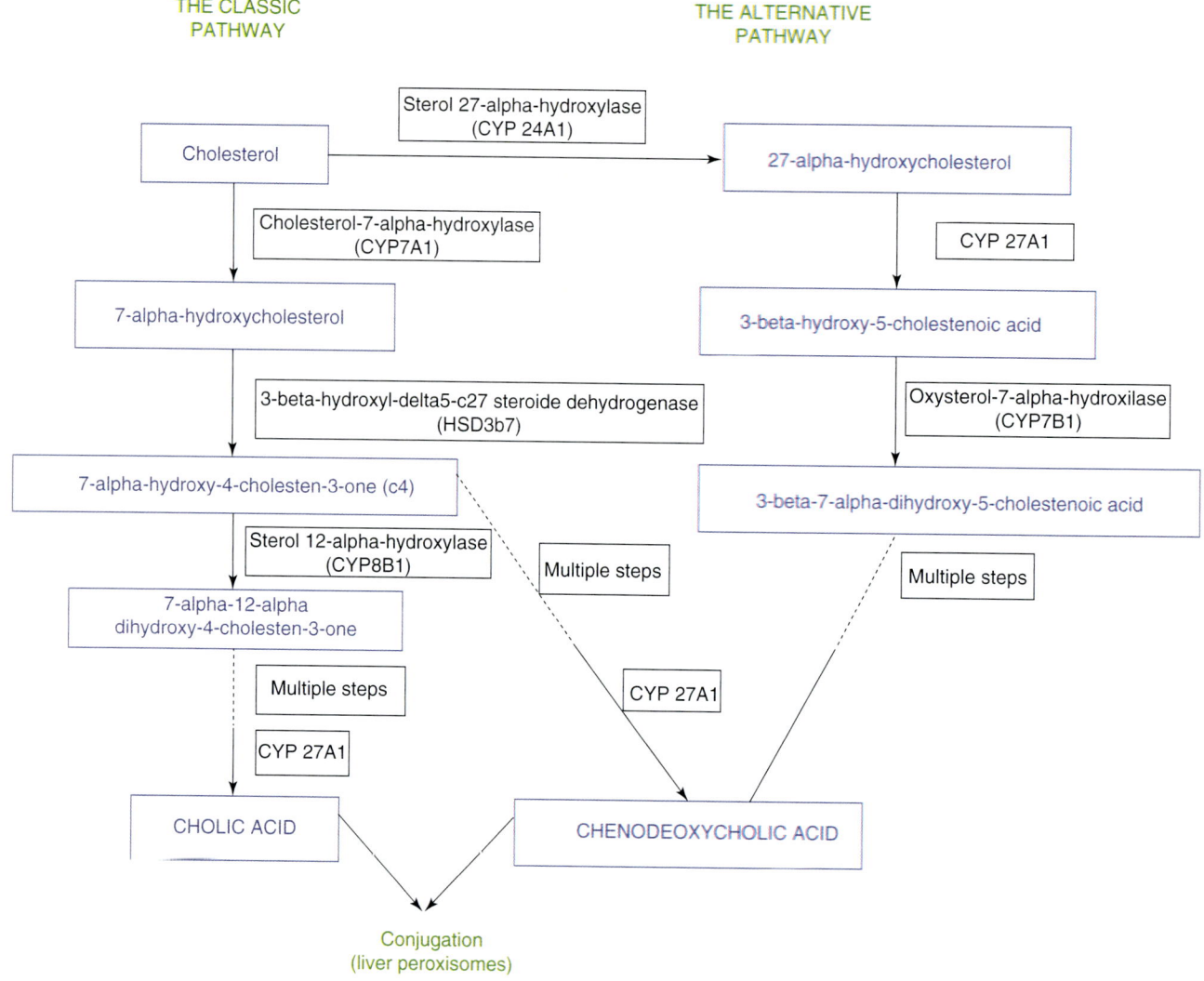

Fig. 2.10 The pathway of BA synthesis in the liver

of MDR3 allows the production of mixed micelles, significantly reducing the detergent effect. When ABCB4 is mutated, the PFIC type III occurs. During bile acid and phospholipid transport, aminophospholipids are flopped spontaneously into the biliary lumen surface, changing the composition of the plasma membrane and leading to higher susceptibility to the detergent effects of bile. P-Type ATPase, present in the canalicular membrane, is responsible for maintaining the non-random distribution of aminophospholipids (AL) across the membrane bilayer. Encoded by ATP8B1, the protein is called FIC1; in case of mutation of this protein, PFIC type I occurs.

More recently, the tight junction protein 2 gene was identified (TJP2), encoding tight junction protein-2, which is not a transporter but is involved in the organization of epithelial and endothelial intercellular junctions that, in the liver, separate the bile from the plasma. In TJP2 mutation, the characteristic compactness of the tight junctions is impaired, leading to a leakage of the biliary components through the paracellular space into the liver parenchyma. TJP2 dysfunction was found to be associated with low-GGT PFIC; this disease is now referred to as PFIC type IV.

Profound cholestasis and progressive liver failure can also occur in infants with inherited defects of the pathways synthesising bile acids. In these disorders the lack of primary bile acids, critical for generating canalicular bile flow, and the toxicity of abnormal bile acid precursors leads to cholestasis and progressive liver injury (Fig. 2.11).

Bile formation is dependent upon ion flux in both hepatocytes and cholangiocytes. Up to 40% of bile formation is derived from bile ducts, and a main determinant of bile flow is the secretion of chloride, determined by the apical positioning of CFTR in cholangiocytes. The origin of the pathogenic liver lesion in cystic fibrosis is focal hepatic biliary fibrosis due to impaired secretion of chloride into bile, which typically progresses slowly and unpredictably during childhood and adolescence.

2 Basic Principles of Liver Physiology

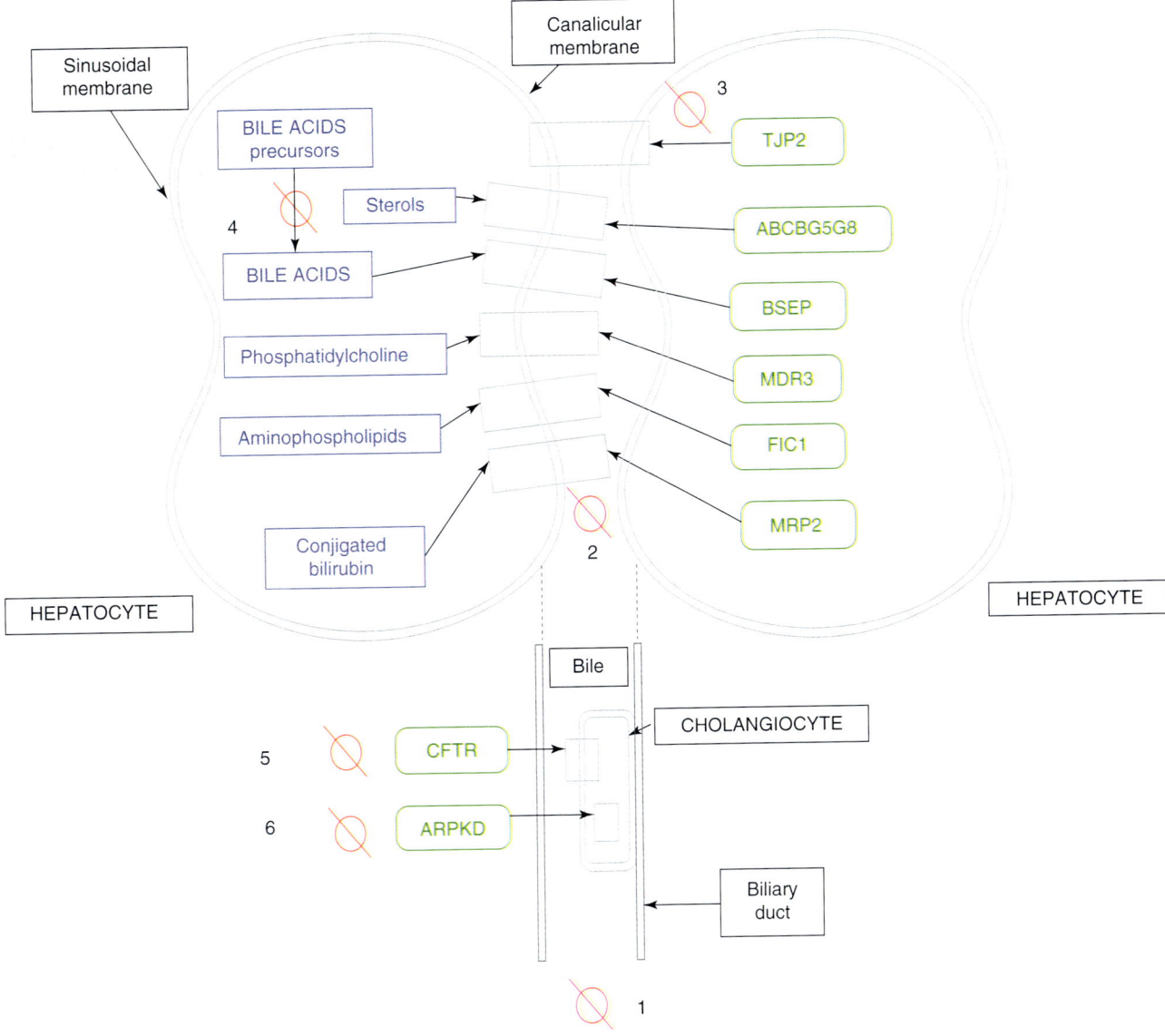

Fig. 2.11 Liver diseases associated with biliary tract development and bile salt transport abnormalities. (1) Biliary tree abnormal anatomy: biliary atresia and Alagille syndrome; (2) abnormalities in hepatic transporters involved in bile formation: PFIC1 (FIC1, ATP8B1), PFIC2 (BSEP, ABCB11), PFIC3 (MDR3, ABCB4), Dubin-Johnson Syndrome (MPR2, ABCC2), sitosterolaemia (ABCG5G8); (3) PFIC4 (TJP2; hepatobiliary integrity disruption); (4) bile acid synthesis defect; (5) Cystic fibrosis (CFTR mutation); (6) congenital hepatic fibrosis (ARPKD mutation → bile duct dilatation)

In addition to the single gene defects that can lead to cholestasis, it is possible that other multifactorial mechanisms can induce it.

Cholestasis can be observed as drug-induced effect, or as a consequence of sepsis, in particular Gram negative infections, or parenteral nutrition. Moreover, increased biliary sludge formation and gallstone in neonates may be a reflection of immature hepatic excretory function.

The final result in paediatric cholestatic liver diseases is the bile acid accumulation, leading to the activation of pro-inflammatory cytokine production, hepatocyte cell death, damage and rupture of the bile ducts and activation of hepatic stellate cells, the main sources of fibrotic tissue in the liver [2, 6–10].

2.10 The Role of Nuclear Receptors in Liver Physiopathology

Nuclear receptors (NRs) are a superfamily of transcription factors that respond to natural and/or synthetic ligands including endogenous compounds (such as steroid hormones, fatty acids, bile acids, vitamins and cholesterol) or exogenous ligands including various drugs and toxins.

The NR family is the largest group of transcriptional regulators in humans and consists of 48 family members.

NRs control a large variety of metabolic pathways, including hepatic lipid and glucose metabolism, bile acid homeostasis, as well as embryonic development, reproduction, inflammation, cell differentiation, various aspects of tissue repair including liver regeneration, fibrosis and finally tumour formation.

2.10.1 Nuclear Receptors and Bile Acid Metabolism

Bile acids (BA) activate in particular three members of NR superfamily: CAR, PXR and FXR (farnesoid X receptor). Most of these NRs are highly expressed in tissues exposed to high levels of BA, like the liver and the intestine. NRs play a central role in the regulation of BA synthesis, metabolism and transport. The physiological role of interaction of BA with NRs is probably to decrease the production of toxic hydrophobic BA and to increase their metabolic turnover towards polar and hydrophilic BA, to increase their excretion and thus to decrease their toxicity in the hepatocytes. Under cholestatic conditions with high intracellular bile acid load, NRs mediate a coordinated response aimed at protecting hepatocytes from toxic bile acids.

In particular, the *farnesoid X receptor (FXR)* is classically described to be the master regulator of bile acid synthesis. More recently, its role has been expanded to include regulation of the gut-liver axis in the fed state. FXR is mainly found in hepatocytes and enterocytes and acts as a sensor in the enterohepatic system regulating BA homeostasis (Fig. 2.12).

Cytochrome P7A1 (CYP7A1 or cholesterol 7a-hydroxylase) is the rate-limiting step in the conversion of cholesterol to bile acids in hepatocytes; in the normal liver, this enzyme is regulated by the interaction of FXR with bile acids. Intestinal FXR activation induces epithelial expression of FGF19, transported via the portal circulation to the liver, where it binds the fibroblast growth factor receptor 4 (FGFR4)-β-Klotho complex; the activation of this complex suppresses bile acid synthesis mainly by inhibiting cholesterol 7α-hydroxylase (CYP7A1), the rate-limiting enzyme of the bile acid synthesis.

In the bowel, the presence of intestinal microbial flora results in deconjugation and dehydroxylation of the primary BAs to produce secondary BAs, which then activate FXR in the ileal enterocyte, to produce FGF-15. FGF-15 reaches the liver via the portal circulation and reduces the hepatocyte BA synthesis, again by inhibiting the enzyme CYP7A1.

In patients with cholestatic liver disease, the presence of excess bile acids results in the concomitant upregulation of FXR. FXR agonists have been shown to protect against inflammation in cholestasis and cirrhosis.

Bile acids, as endogenous signalling molecules, can also activate other nuclear receptors, in particular:

- *Vitamin D receptor (VDR):* Despite hepatocytes do not express VDR, high levels are found in non-parenchymal liver cells such as Kupffer cells or sinusoidal endothelial cells. Stimulation of VDR induces production of the antimicrobial peptide cathelicidin in the bile duct epithelial cells, which may help maintaining biliary tract sterility.
- *Pregnane X Receptor (PXR):* PXR acts mainly as a xenobiotic sensor. It is activated by glucocorticoids, steroids, macrolide antibiotics, antifungals and some herbal extracts. Its main role is to form a barrier protecting the inner environment from xenobiotics. Therefore, its highest expression is found within the liver (not only in hepatocytes but also in stellate and Kupffer cells) and the intestine.
- *Constitutive androstane receptor (CAR):* CAR is closely related to PXR; this NR acts similarly as xenobiotic sen-

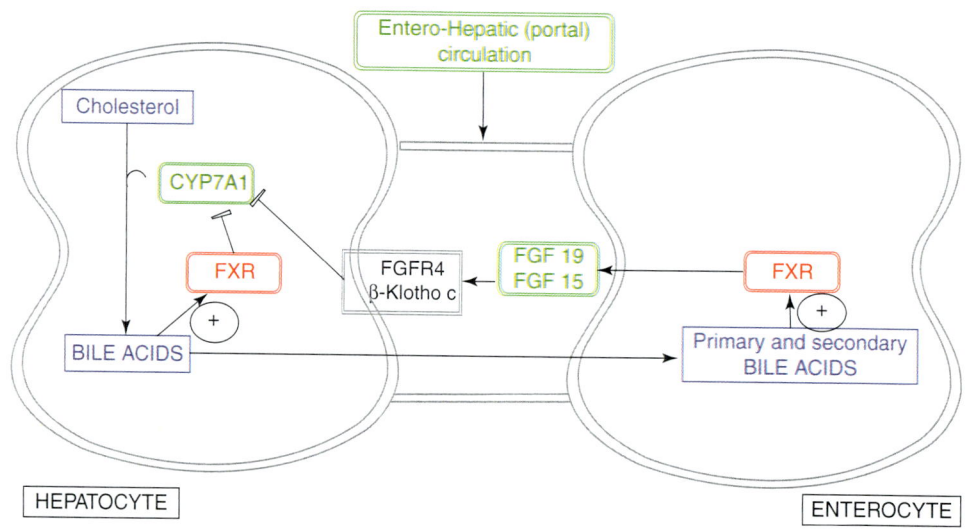

Fig. 2.12 The role of FXR nuclear receptor in bile acid metabolism. Elevated levels of bile acids (occurring in cholestatic disorders) lead to the upregulation of FXR, which in turn decreases bile acid synthesis and absorption from hepatocytes and increases bile salt secretion and detoxification. *FXR* farnesoid X receptor, *FGF19* fibroblast growth factor 19, *FGF 15* fibroblast growth factor 15, *FGFR4* fibroblast growth factor receptor 4 (FGFR4)-β-Klotho complex, *CYP7A1* cholesterol 7-alpha-hydroxylase

sor which regulates the expression of genes significant for biotransformation and excretion of exogenous compounds.
- Membrane G-protein-coupled receptors *Takeda G-Protein receptor 5 (TGR5)*: The activation of this receptor has been shown to protect the liver from bile acid overload during liver regeneration.

2.10.2 Nuclear Receptors and Energy Metabolism

Several nuclear receptors are involved in energy metabolism, and they may have a role in the pathogenesis of liver inflammation and fibrosis (Fig. 2.13).

In particular:

- *FXR:* Apart from its central role in bile acid metabolism, the activation of farnesoid X receptor regulates the expression of various genes crucial for lipid, glucose and lipoprotein metabolism. Hepatic FXR regulates lipid homeostasis by multiple mechanisms including decreased fatty acid synthesis, increased β-oxidation and decreased fatty acid uptake. Moreover, FXR has a crucial role in controlling the intestinal microbiome, intestinal epithelial permeability, hepatic inflammation and fibrogenesis.
- *Peroxisome proliferator-activated receptors α, β/δ and γ (PPAR):* This receptor subfamily acts as major regulator of lipid metabolism in many cell types, in particular for the gut-liver-adipose axis. PPARα is the major regulator in the hepatic processes of fatty acid uptake, mitochondrial and peroxisomal β-oxidation, ketogenesis, triglyceride turnover and bile acid synthesis.
- *Liver X receptor alpha (LXR):* This nuclear receptor can be found in tissues with high metabolic activity, such as the liver and small intestine. Its known endogenous ligands are oxysterols, and its physiologic role is the regulation of cholesterol, fatty acid and glucose homeostasis. LXR act as "cholesterol sensors" lowering cholesterol levels by way of increased expression of genes associated with reverse cholesterol transport, cholesterol conversion to bile acids and intestinal cholesterol absorption. LXR inhibits genes involved in the innate immune response and simultaneously induces genes involved in lipid metabolism, thus providing a molecular link between lipid metabolism and inflammation. LXR agonists reduce inflammatory processes in chronic inflammatory liver diseases such as nonalcoholic fatty liver disease.
- *Constitutive androstane receptor (CAR):* Apart from the role in xenobiotics metabolism, this nuclear receptor plays a central role in carbohydrate/lipid metabolism and even inflammation. CAR is believed to have a protective role during metabolic stress; more specifically, it protects the liver in the fed state and decreases hepatic steatosis and inflammation while also reducing obesity, insulin resistance and hypercholesterolemia; CAR activation diminishes liver gluconeogenesis and improves insulin sensitivity.
- *PXR:* Besides its role as xenobiotic sensor, PXR has anti-inflammatory properties and may reduce hepatic fibrogenesis. PXR activation has been associated with increased hepatic fatty acid and fatty acid precursor uptake, lipogenesis and decreased β-oxidation.
- *TGR5:* TGR5 is involved in energy metabolism, protecting the liver and intestine from inflammation and steatosis and improving insulin sensitivity.

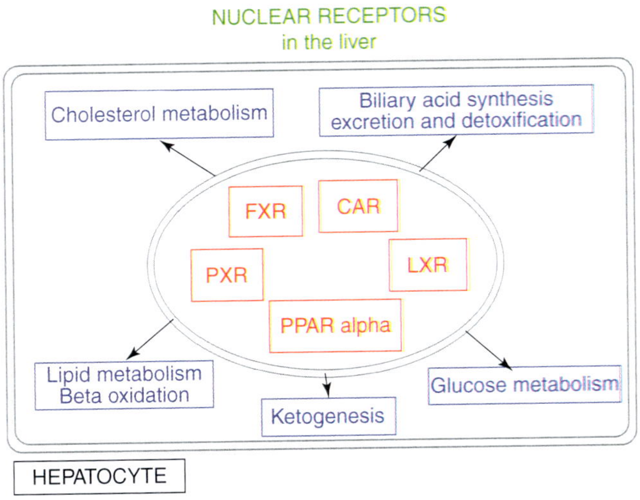

In summary, NRs play a key role in the transcriptional control of several pivotal aspects of liver function and metabolism.

For example, NRs control fatty acid flux from peripheral white adipose tissue to the liver and regulate several critical metabolic steps involved in the pathogenesis of NAFLD, including fat storage, lipolysis, export, uptake and oxidation. As gatekeepers of fatty acid flux from adipose tissue to the liver and key regulators of hepatic metabolism, inflammation and fibrosis, NRs play a central role in the progression from NAFLD to more aggressive NASH.

Understanding of NR biology is relevant for explaining the pathophysiology of a wide range of liver diseases. Moreover, NRs may represent valid therapeutic targets for these disorders. Specific targeting of individual NRs may

Fig. 2.13 Hepatocyte nuclear receptors involved in different metabolic pathways. *FXR* farnesoid X receptor, *PXR* pregnane X receptor, *PPAR* peroxisome proliferator-activated receptor, *LXR* liver X receptor, *CAR* constitutive androstane receptor

represent an effective way to treat diseases by readjusting deregulated NR-mediated pathways, leading to an individualised medicine in hepatology [11–13].

2.11 Ontogeny of Drug-Metabolizing Enzymes and Liver Injury in the Paediatric Population

The liver is the main organ where detoxification processes of endogenous (ammonium and bilirubin) or exogenous (xenobiotics: drugs, poisons, pollutants) products take place. The aim is to convert these substances to water-soluble products that can be easily eliminated (urine).

Appreciating the relevance of the ontogeny of metabolizing enzymes in the newborn liver is of paramount importance to understand the pathophysiology of liver disease in children. In fact, in paediatric age, most liver diseases occur early in life, including those related to environmental toxins, such as Gram-bacterial infections, parenteral nutrition and drugs. This noxae would not harm relevantly the liver of a toddler or older child, whereas have a relevant impact on newborn and infantile age groups.

Hepatic blood flow, plasma protein binding and intrinsic clearance constitute the physiological determinants of hepatic clearance.

Each of these determinants undergoes significant postnatal changes, and their maturation results in an enhanced capacity for hepatic elimination of compounds with advancing postnatal age.

The biotransformation of prescription or non-prescription medications, supplements and herbals into compounds that can be safely metabolised and excreted is not always possible in a safe and convenient way, leading to drug-induced liver injury (DILI) through a variety of mechanisms.

In adults, DILI occurs in about 14 cases per 100,000 people annually, while in the paediatric population, the incidence is unknown. We may speculate that the paediatric incidence is likely to be lower, because children take fewer medications, are less frequently prescribed medications commonly associated with DILI and metabolise drugs differently.

This means that infants and children may be more or less vulnerable to toxic liver injury than adults; the immaturity of pathways responsible for biotransformation may prevent the efficient degradation and elimination of a toxic compound; in other circumstances, the same immaturity may limit the formation of a reactive metabolite. All these conditions may confer some degree of protection.

The liver metabolises and excretes medications using three general steps:

- Phase 1 (Activation): production of reactive sites (oxydrilic groups). The most frequent reaction is hydroxylation, in which there is an insertion of one oxygen atom in the compound, creating an OH group.

The main complex involved in this process is the cytochrome P450 monooxygenases; the CYP enzymes represent a superfamily of heme-containing enzymes, which are cytochrome P450 dependent. CYP enzymes are found in the liver. The newborn has a limited capacity for hepatic biotransformation, and, in general, CYP enzyme-mediated metabolism improves with postnatal age, approaching the adult levels only after the first year of life.

The CYP3A subfamily is the most abundant and clinically important of the CYP enzymes in the liver and small intestine, being responsible for the metabolism of about 50% of the most commonly used drugs.

- Phase 2 (Detoxification): The conjugating enzymes modifies the metabolites that passed through the phase 1 or the original compound, increasing its water solubility and neutralising its toxicity. This happens through different conjugation reactions with hydrophilic substances that allow the transformation of the substance in a hydrophilic molecule, excreted with the urine. The possible phase 2 processes are glucuronidation, sulphation, acetylation and glutathione conjugation. These reactions are catalysed by a variety of enzymes, the activity of which appears to be associated with the human development.

For example, an important group of conjugation reactions are catalysed by the UGTs (UDP glucuronosyltransferase), involved in glucuronidation of many hydrophobic drugs (morphine, acetaminophen) but also in biotransformation of important endogenous substrates, including bilirubin.

Mutations of UGT1A protein can lead to Crigler-Najjar (absent or reduced enzyme activity) or Gilbert syndrome (mutation in the promoter region of the UGT1 gene, leading to a milder form of congenital unconjugated hyperbilirubinaemia).

Postnatal changes in the efficiency of phase 1 and 2 reactions, differences in their pattern of development and changes in the hepatocellular distribution and expression of phase 1 and 2 enzymes may produce many of the age-associated changes in the absorption, distribution, metabolism and excretion of drugs that culminate in altered pharmacokinetics and thus serve as the determinant of age-specific dose requirements.

- Phase 3 (Excretion): The water-soluble product is transported into the canalicular space and secreted with bile.

Once liberated from the uterine environment, the neonate is instantly exposed to a wide range of new macromolecules in the form of byproducts of cellular metabolism, dietary constituents, environmental toxins and pharmacologic agents, until the full liver maturation is achieved (Fig. 2.14). The rapid and efficient biotransformation of these compounds by phase 1 and phase 2 drug-metabolizing enzymes is an essential process to avoid the accumulation of reactive compounds that could produce cellular injury or tissue dysfunction.

The three phases of xenobiotics metabolism are under the control of different nuclear receptors, such as PXR and CAR. Prescription drugs activating these NRs can either lead to increased clearance and decreased therapeutic efficacy of other drugs or can induce drug bioactivation with formation of reactive intermediate metabolite causing hepatotoxicity (Fig. 2.15).

DILI is most often caused by accumulation of phase 1 metabolites, following one of the two patterns, intrinsic hepatotoxicity and idiosyncratic hepatotoxicity, respectively, reflecting a dominant role of drug toxicity (dose dependent) vs. host factors (no dose dependence) in liver injury.

The ability to solubilize and subsequently absorb lipophilic drugs can be influenced by age-dependent changes in pancreatic and biliary function. Moreover, age-dependent changes in body composition alter the physiologic spaces into which a drug may be distributed, with a relatively larger extracellular and total body water spaces in neonates and young infants as compared with adults.

Changes in composition and amount of circulating plasma proteins (such as albumin and α_1-acid glycoprotein) can also influence the distribution of highly bound drugs. A reduction in the quantity of total plasma proteins (including albumin) in the neonate and young infant increases the free fraction of drug, thereby influencing the availability of the active moiety.

The reported incidence and severity of DILI vary among drugs, suggesting that drug properties have a role in DILI risk determination. Conversely, drugs cause liver injury only in a small portion of patients, indicating that host factors play a major role in DILI development.

The host and drug interaction may lead to different phenotypes of DILI (i.e. cholestasis, hepatocellular, steatosis); the type of liver injury differs with age, with younger patients presenting more frequently hepatocellular damage as compared to cholestatic/mixed injury seen in the older.

The gut-liver axis plays a role in DILI, since the increased intestinal permeability due to damaged intestinal mucosal barrier increases hepatic endotoxin influx, which in turn activates Kupffer cells and the production of pro-inflammatory cytokines. Finally, pre-existing chronic liver diseases enhance the risk of hepatotoxicity [14–19].

2.12 The Pathophysiology of Hepatic Fibrosis in Chronic Liver Diseases

Chronic liver disease (CLD) is defined as a progressive destruction and regeneration of liver parenchyma leading to fibrosis and cirrhosis. CLD results from hepatic injury leading to the abnormal liver function, with impaired synthesis of serum proteins and clotting factors, compromised glycaemic control and ammonia metabolism, abnormal bile secretion and cholestasis [20].

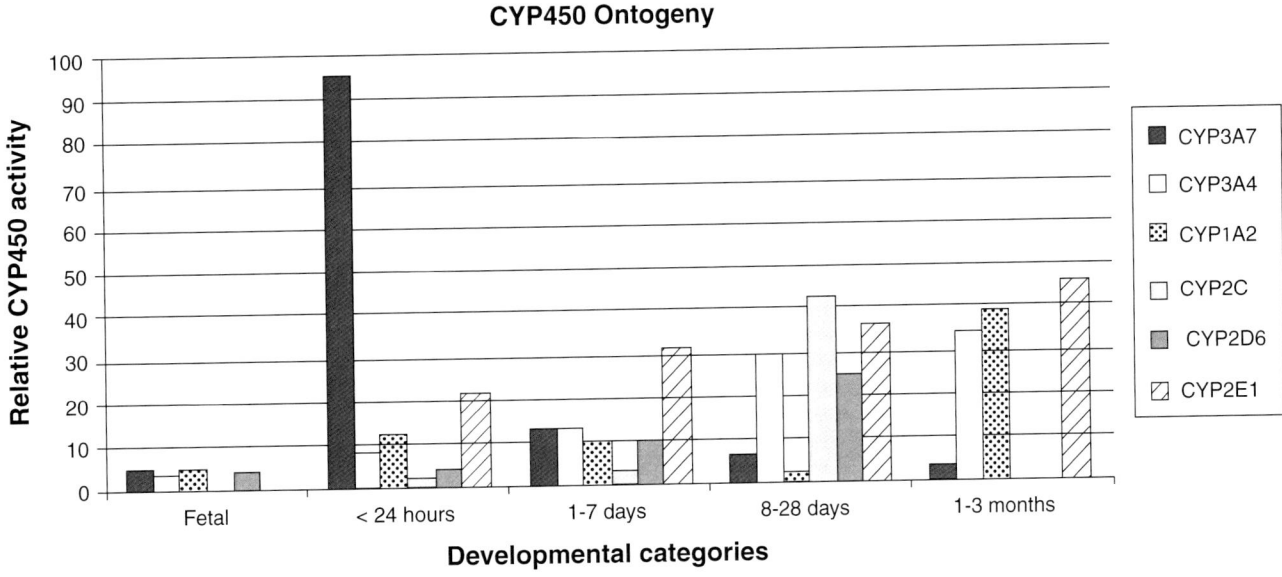

Fig. 2.14 Ontogeny of phase 1 liver enzymes at different pre- and postnatal ages. The activity of most CYP450s is very low at birth, increases during the first few weeks of life, but reaches full expression only after the sixth month of life (Reprinted with permission from [14])

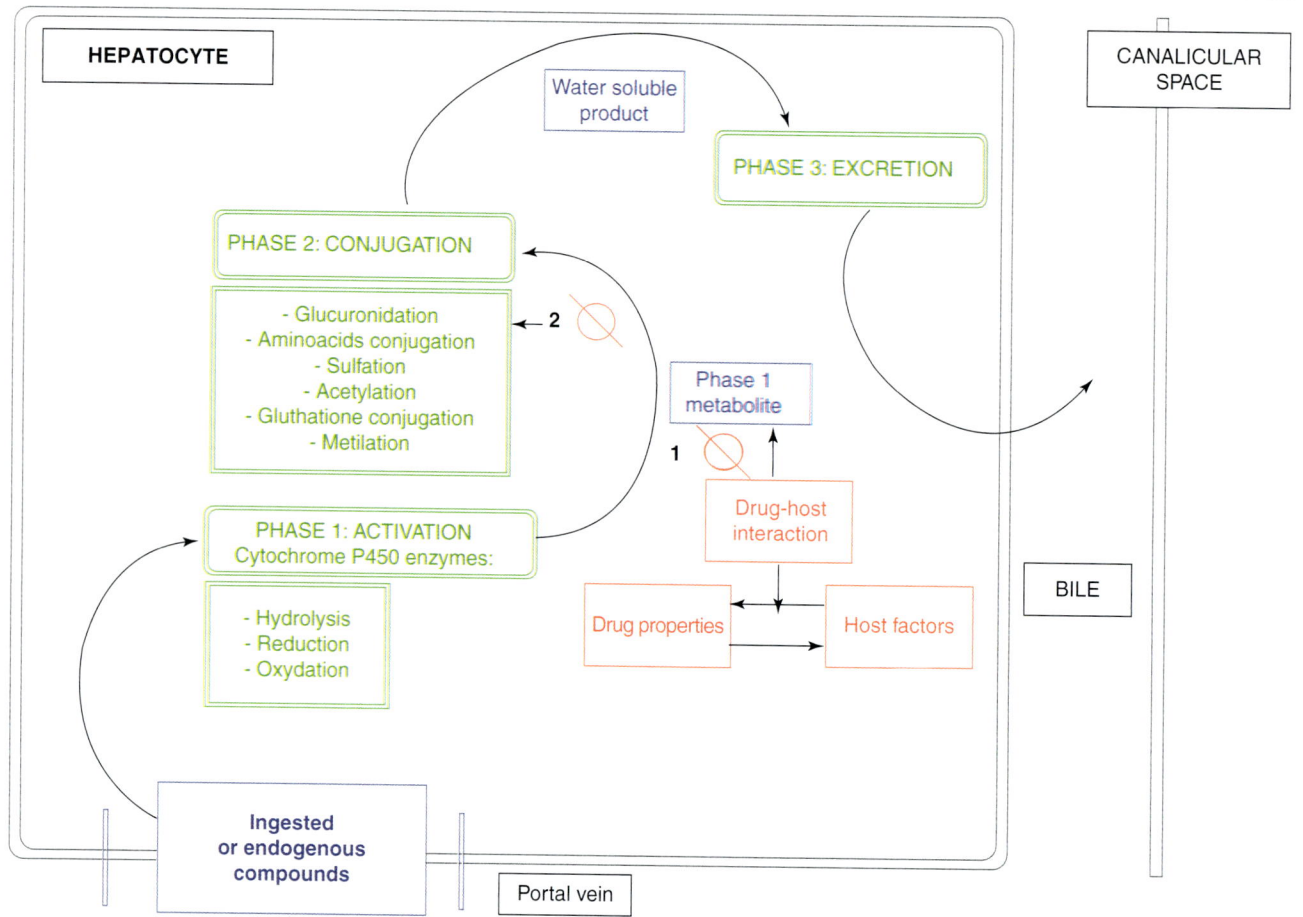

Fig. 2.15 Metabolism of drugs or endogenous compounds and mechanism of DILI (drug-induced liver injury). (1) DILI is usually due to phase 1 metabolite accumulation, secondary to intrinsic (drug toxicity) or idiosyncratic (host-dependent) hepatotoxicity. (2) An example of phase 2 metabolism is the bilirubin glucuronidation from UGT1A (UDP glucuronosyltransferase). Liver diseases associated with UGT1A mutations are Gilbert syndrome and Crigler-Najjar syndrome

In chronic cholestatic diseases, the toxic effects of bile acids induce hepatocellular apoptosis, which in turn plays a role in the activation of hepatic stellate cells (HSCs) into myofibroblasts.

Hepatic stellate cells inhabit the peri-sinusoidal space between hepatocytes and sinusoidal endothelial cells and in the normal liver are responsible for maintaining the basal membrane.

Apoptosis (or programmed cell death) is a process that occurs in the normal liver, aimed at removing unwanted, senescent or damaged cells, but in cholestasis apoptosis is increased and deregulated.

The bile acid-induced hepatocellular injury, whether due to liver cell apoptosis or to the release of soluble factors such as cytokines (oxidative stress-mediated pathway), results in the activation of HSC from a quiescent to a myofibroblastic phenotype (Fig. 2.16).

Moreover in this condition, several nuclear receptors (RAR, RXR, PPAR and FXR) modulate HSC activity.

Fibrosis represents the final response of the liver to chronic non-resolving injury; it is the result of a continuous remodelling process, in which various components of the extracellular matrix (ECM), growth factors, proteases and cytokines interact in a complex mechanism, finally producing fibrosis and cirrhosis.

Liver fibrosis, which is characterised by the excessive deposition of ECM proteins, involves both parenchymal and non-parenchymal hepatic cells and infiltrating immune cells.

Liver fibrosis was once deemed irreversible; however, early liver fibrosis is now managed by clinical treatment, and advanced fibrosis is also likely to be reversible, once the injurious trigger is removed.

Since HSCs are the primary mediators of liver pathology in this process, several molecules required for HSC activation are considered potential therapeutic targets [9, 21].

Recently, microRNAs (miRNAs) have been found to play multifaceted roles in hepatic fibrosis, including in HSC activation and proliferation and production of ECM proteins. miRNA concentration is stable in the circulation and is both disease- and tissue-specific, making them attractive circulatory biomarkers.

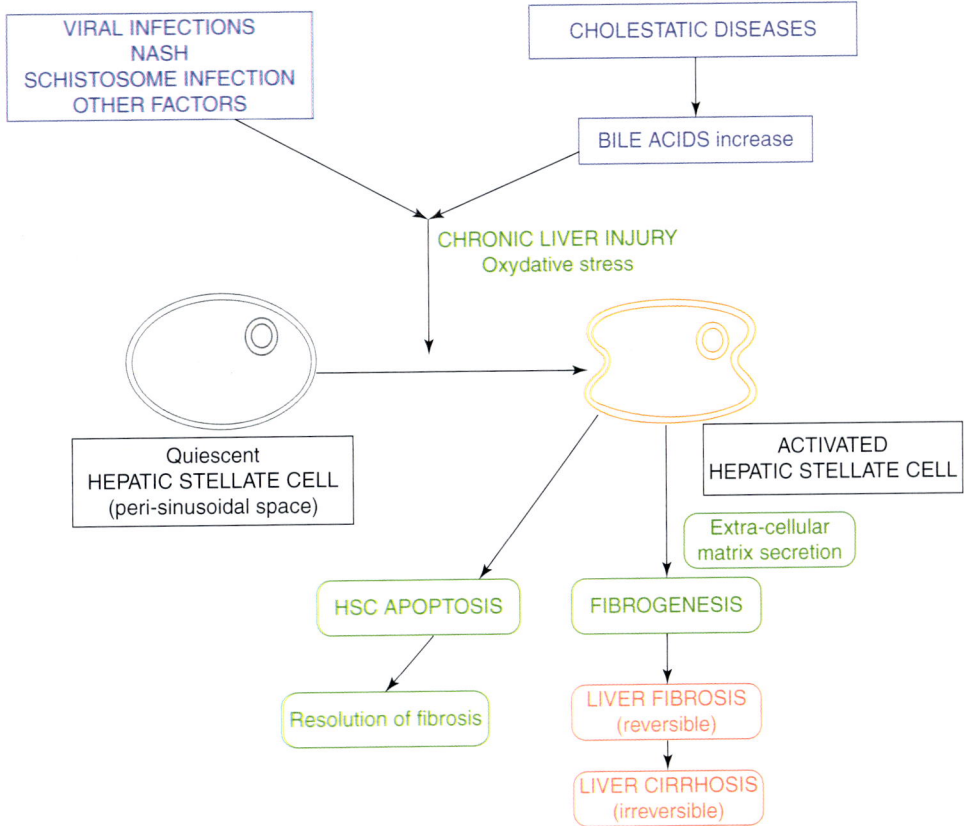

Fig. 2.16 The pathogenesis of liver fibrosis. *HSC* hepatic stellate cell

miRNAs are involved in the regulation of all biological and pathological processes in every cell type, including liver cells. Altered expression of miRNAs correlates with different liver aetiologies or is involved in the broader fibrogenic response to liver damage. The expression profiles of miRNAs also seem to be specific when compared between liver diseases of different aetiologies [22].

References

1. Riboni L, Guliani A. Liver biochemistry. Chapter 25. In: Siliprandi N, Tettamanti G, editors. Medical biochemistry. 4th ed. Padova, Italy: Piccin Nuova Libraria S. p. A.; 2011. p. 753–73.
2. Suchy F. Functional development of the liver. Chapter 2. In: Suchy FJ, Sokol RJ, Balistreri WF, editors. Liver disease in children. 4th ed. Cambridge: Cambridge University Press; 2016. p. 10–23.
3. Verhoeven NM, Huck JHJ, Roos B, Struys EA, et al. Transaldolase deficiency: liver cirrhosis associated with a new inborn error in the pentose phosphate pathway. Hum Genet. 2001;68:1086–92.
4. Demetris AJ, et al. Functional immune anatomy of the liver—as an allograft. Am J Transplant. 2016;16:1653–80.
5. Lee WS, Sokol RJ. Liver disease in mitochondrial disorders. Semin Liver Dis. 2007;27(3):259–73.
6. Camilleri M, Gores GJ. Therapeutic targeting of bile acids. Am J Physiol Gastrointest Liver Physiol. 2015;309(4):G209–15.
7. Chiang JYL, Ferrel JM. Bile acid metabolism in liver pathobiology. Gene Expr. 2018;18(2):71–87.
8. Gupta N. Mechanisms of bile formation and cholestasis. Chapter 3. In: Suchy FJ, Sokol RJ, Balistreri WF, editors. Liver disease in children. 4th ed. Cambridge: Cambridge University Press; 2016. p. 24–31.
9. Pereira TN, et al. Paediatric cholestatic liver disease: diagnosis, assessment of disease progression and mechanisms of fibrogenesis. World J Gastrointest Pathophysiol. 2010;1(2):69–84.
10. Sambrotta M, Thompson RJ. Mutations in TJP2, encoding zonula occludens 2, and liver disease. Tissue Barriers. 2015;3(3):e1026537.
11. Jurica J, et al. Bile acids, nuclear receptors and cyt ochrome P450. Physiol Res. 2016;65(Suppl. 4):S427–40.
12. Wagner M, et al. Nuclear receptors in liver disease. Hepatology. 2011;53:1023–34.
13. Cave MC, et al. Nuclear receptors and nonalcoholic fatty liver disease. Biochim Biophys Acta. 2016;1859(9):1083–99. https://doi.org/10.1016/j.bbagrm.2016.03.002.
14. Blake MJ, et al. Ontogeny of drug metabolizing enzymes in the neonate. Adv Drug Deliv Rev. 2006;58:4–14.
15. Hines RN. The ontogeny of drug metabolism enzymes and implications for adverse drug events. Pharmacol Ther. 2008;118:250–67.
16. Kearns GL, et al. Developmental pharmacology — drug disposition, action, and therapy in infants and children. N Engl J Med. 2003;349:1157–67.
17. Alcorna J, McNamarab PJ. Pharmacokinetics in the newborn. Adv Drug Deliv Rev. 2003;55:667–86.
18. Chen M, et al. Drug-induced liver injury: Interactions between drug properties and host factors. J Hepatol. 2015;63:503–14.
19. Mansi DA. Drug-induced liver injury in children. Curr Opin Pediatr. 2015;27:625–33.
20. Yang CH, et al. Nutritional needs and support for children with chronic liver disease. Nutrients. 2017;9:1127. https://doi.org/10.3390/nu9101127.
21. Zhang CY, et al. Liver fibrosis and hepatic stellate cells: etiology, pathological hallmarks and therapeutic targets. World J Gastroenterol. 2016;22(48):10512–22.
22. Calvopina DA, et al. Function and regulation of microRNAs and their potential as biomarkers in paediatric liver disease. Int J Mol Sci. 2016;17:1795. https://doi.org/10.3390/ijms17111795.

The Anatomy and Histology of the Liver and Biliary Tract

Maria Guido, Samantha Sarcognato, Diana Sacchi, and Kathrin Ludwig

Key Points

- Liver is one of the first organs to develop and arises as hepatic diverticulum from the endodermal layer of the most distal portion of the foregut during the 3rd to 4th week of gestation.
- During embryonal development, the liver is a site of hematopoiesis, which starts between weeks 6 and 7 and is intense in the mid-trimester. By 36 weeks, only scattered islands of hematopoiesis remain in the hepatic parenchyma.
- In children, the hepatocytes have a bilayered architecture and show numerous glycogenated nuclei until the age of 5–6 years. After this age, liver microanatomy becomes similar to the adult one.
- The knowledge of normal liver parenchyma provides the basis for the interpretation of pathological conditions.

3.1 Liver Development

3.1.1 Introduction

Liver develops as a tissue bud deriving from a diverticulum of the ventral foregut endoderm, which, subsequently, mingles with proliferating mesenchyme of the septum transversum to give rise to all the structures of the adult liver, the gallbladder, and the extrahepatic bile ducts (Fig. 3.1). Hepatocytes and cholangiocytes (the epithelial components of the liver) originate from the cranial portion of the hepatic diverticulum, while its caudal portion, which does not take part in the invasion of the septum transversum, gives rise to the extrahepatic biliary tree and other structures of the gastrointestinal tract [1–7].

The hepatic connective tissue framework and its stromal cells, where the endoderm elements grow, have a mesoderm origin and arise from both the septum transversum and the cellular elements lining the coelomic cavity [1–7].

3.1.2 Endodermal Specification

The first evidence of the embryonic liver can be seen during the 4th week of gestation; it is made of a focal thickening of the endoderm lining the ventral wall of the distal foregut. In this area (called *hepatic primordium*), the proliferation of cells gives origin to the *hepatic diverticulum*, budding from the ventral wall of the foregut. At this stage, the endodermal cells lining the hepatic diverticulum are called *hepatoblasts*. They organize in cords around the developing sinusoids in response to signals arising from the adjacent mesodermal cells. Subsequently they acquire a columnar shape and migrate through the *septum transversum* mesenchyme (which is located between the pericardial and peritoneal cavities) to form the *liver bud* [1–7] (Fig. 3.1).

Hepatoblasts are bipotential cells, expressing cytokeratin (CK) 8, CK18, and CK19 (Fig. 3.2), and, under the control of

---

This chapter is dedicated to a dear friend and colleague, **Flavia Bortolotti**, who has broadened our horizons on the fascinating world of pediatric liver.

M. Guido (✉) · S. Sarcognato · D. Sacchi
Department of Medicine—DIMED, Anatomic Pathology Unit, University of Padova, Padova, Italy
e-mail: mguido@unipd.it

K. Ludwig
Department of Medicine—DIMED, Unit of Pathology and Cytopathology, University Hospital of Padova, Padova, Italy

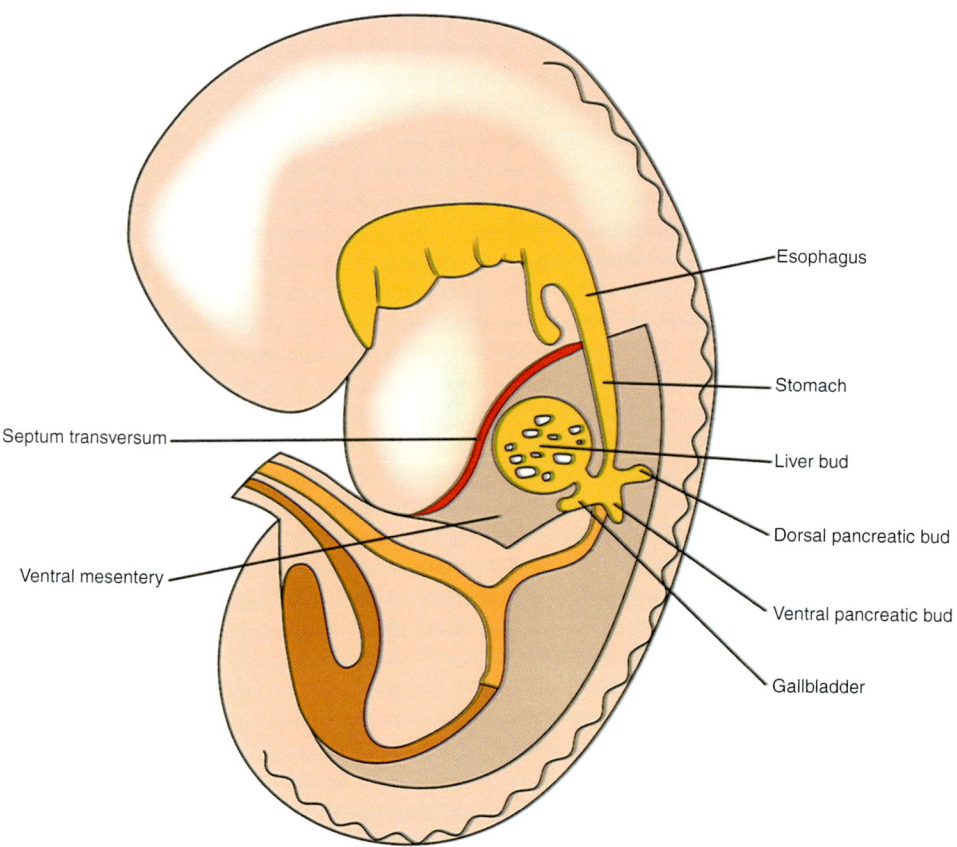

Fig. 3.1 A schematic representation of the embryo at 30 days after conception

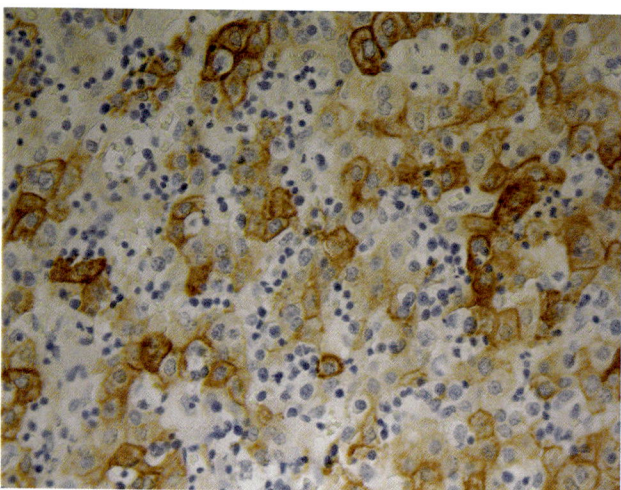

Fig. 3.2 (Immunohistochemistry; antibody to CK19). A strong expression of CK19 is visible in hepatoblasts at the 10th week of gestation. CK19 is no longer expressed after the 14th week, when the hepatoblasts are committed to hepatocytes

numerous and complex molecular mechanisms, they are committed to either the hepatocytic or cholangiocytic lineage [1–9]. Hepatoblast differentiation into hepatocytes begins soon after the mesenchymal invasion. Over the last few years, it has been shown that the balance between the two cell types depends on numerous and complex signaling—and transcriptional—networks, such as Jagged-Notch, hepatocyte growth factor, Oncostatin M, and others [1, 10–14]. The hepatoblasts, which are committed to become hepatocytes, gradually lose CK19, and, starting from the 14th week of gestation, the future hepatic parenchymal cells become immunoreactive only for CKs 8 and 18, the CK pair expressed in normal liver parenchymal cells [8, 9, 15].

Hepatocytes are the major parenchymal cell type in the liver [16]. They interact with other cell types (cholangiocytes, endothelial cells, sinusoidal endothelial cells, etc.) and are organized in a polarized fashion at the interface between the endothelial sinusoids and the bile ducts. Once committed to one specific cell lineage, they progressively change their morphology and functional phenotype until after birth [12, 13, 17]. The hepatocellular synthesis of α-fetoprotein begins around the 25th–30th day after conception and continues until birth [9] (Fig. 3.3). At about 8 weeks, glycogen starts to be present and progressively becomes plentiful in fetal hepatocytes and remains so until birth. Hemosiderin deposition in the hepatocytes is usually seen early during the intrauterine development, especially in the periportal ones (Fig. 3.4). Hepatocellular bile acid synthesis begins at the 5th to 9th week of gestation and bile secretion around the 12th week. However, the canalicular transport and the hepatic excretory function are physiologically and metabolically immature until the 4th to 6th week after birth [7, 9, 18].

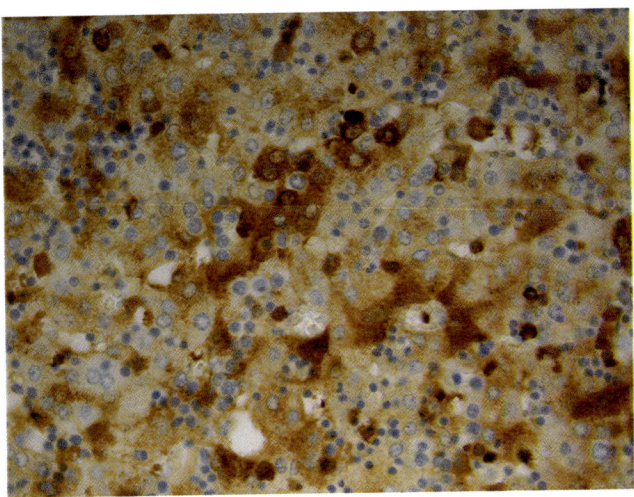

Fig. 3.3 (Immunohistochemistry; antibody to α-fetoprotein). α-fetoprotein expression in embryonic hepatoblasts at the 22nd week of gestation. Its synthesis begins around 25–30 days after conception and continues until birth

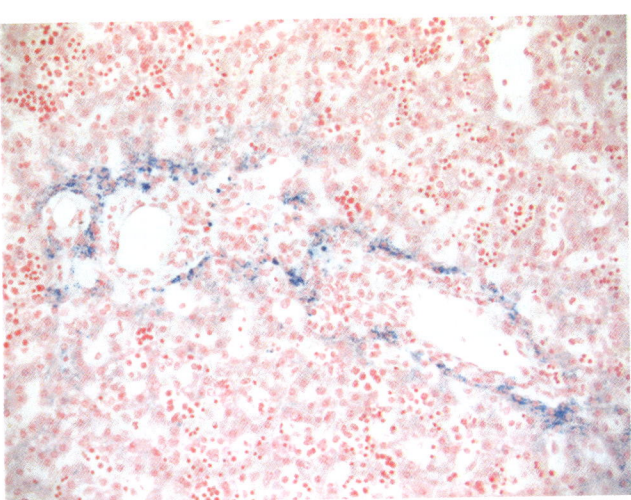

Fig. 3.4 (Perls iron stain). Hemosiderin deposition (blue granules) is seen early during the liver development, especially in periportal hepatocytes, as shown in this tissue slide obtained from a fetal liver at the 14th week of gestation

3.1.2.1 Development of the Biliary Tract

One of the major tasks of liver is to excrete bile in the small intestine, where it helps to break down fats during digestion by emulsification. The bile is produced by the apical portion of the hepatocytes, and it is transported through a network of initially intrahepatic—and, subsequently, extrahepatic—bile ducts [7].

The development of the intrahepatic biliary structures starts between the 5th and the 9th week of gestation, and the earliest sign of biliary differentiation seems to be the expression of Sox9 [18, 19].

The development of intrahepatic bile ducts begins with the *ductal plate* formation [15]. This structure is a single-layered ring (Fig. 3.5a) composed of hepatoblasts, which surround the mesenchyme of primordial portal tracts (PTs) after the acquisition of the biliary phenotype [15, 19, 20].

Around the 12th week, a remodeling occurs on the ductal plate leading to the formation of a bilayered (but discontinuous) structure called *double-layered ductal plate* (Fig. 3.5b). This gives subsequently rise to tubular structures with a circular cross section (Fig. 3.5c). Gradually, they are incorporated into the mesenchyme of the initial PT (*incorporating bile duct*). Once incorporated, the immature tubules are remodeled in single bile ducts, which progressively migrate to the center of the PT [15, 19, 20] (Fig. 3.5d). It is still a matter of controversy whether an eventual excess of not-incorporated epithelial elements in the ductal plate would gradually be deleted by apoptosis or undergo differentiation into hepatocytes [21, 22]. However, a failure in differentiation and/or in resorption during the fetal life is known to produce *ductal plate malformation* [21], and a destruction or agenesis of the ductal plate is thought to play a role in the development of intrahepatic biliary atresia [22–24] [see Chap. 5].

It has been recently shown that a phase of *transient asymmetry* occurs during tubulogenesis. The concept of asymmetry is based on the fact that the initial structure is lined by cholangiocytes (positive for Sox9 and CK19) on its portal side, and by cells resembling hepatoblasts, positive for the hepatocyte nuclear factor (HNF) 4 and the transforming growth factor receptor type-II, on its parenchymal side [15, 18, 19, 25]. Notch pathway has been shown to play an important role in the differentiation of hepatoblasts into cholangiocytes and in biliary tubulogenesis [19, 26, 27]. Its inactivation/failure has been associated with a defective biliary development beyond the monolayered ductal plate, determining, for instance, the bile duct paucity in Alagille syndrome [1, 20, 24, 26, 28, 29] [see Chap. 11]. The transforming growth factor-β and other hepatic transcription factors, such as HNF6 and HNF1β, are other factors involved in the intrahepatic biliary development [19, 20].

While the terminal bile ducts are maturing and incorporated into the PT, the connections with the hepatic parenchyma are allowed through the *bile ductules*, which are entirely lined by cholangiocytes [30, 31]. The bile ductules open into the *canals of Hering*, which is the anatomic and physiological hepato-biliary interface between the intralobular canalicular system and the biliary tree [30–32] (Fig. 3.5d).

The remodeling of the ductal plate, which continues throughout all the fetal life, begins in the PTs of the hepatic hilum and gradually extends toward the periphery [33]. During the active phase of portal myelopoiesis (around the 20th to 32nd week), the remodeling slows down, but it does not end until the first month after birth, when the CK7 expression is completely acquired [19, 34].

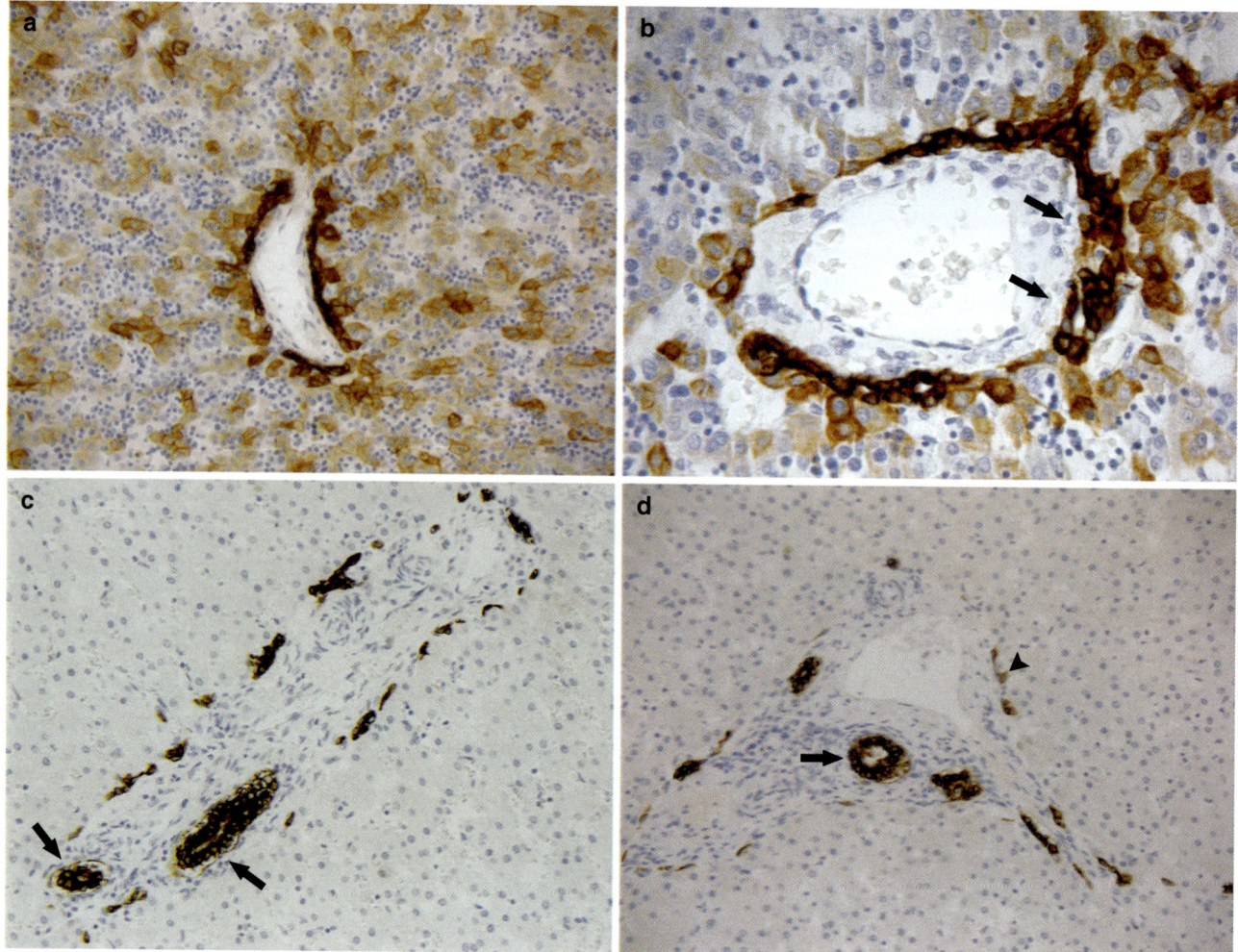

Fig. 3.5 (Immunohistochemistry; antibody to CK19). (**a**) A continuous single-layered rim of hepatoblasts surrounds the primordial portal tract in the embryo at 9 weeks of gestation. This represents the ductal plate. Hepatoblasts are committed to biliary cells, and they strongly express CK19. (**b**) Around the 12th week, the ductal plate becomes bilayered (arrows), and then (**c**) it gives rise to tubular structures (arrows) (**d**) which, subsequently, migrates from the periphery to the center of the portal tract (arrow). Canals of Hering are visible at the border of the portal tract (arrowhead)

Therefore, two important considerations have to be taken into account when examining perinatal/prenatal liver biopsies. Firstly, the maturity of the biliary structures on histological examination depends on the region one is focusing on: they are more mature in the perihilar regions compared to those at the periphery. Secondly, the bile duct/PT ratio is physiologically lower in premature babies than in full-term ones.

3.1.2.2 The Extrahepatic Bile Duct System

The extrahepatic bile ducts develop quicker than their intrahepatic counterparts, and they arise from the caudal part of the hepatic diverticulum, which is located caudally to the liver bud and closed to the ventral pancreatic bud [19, 33]. The intrahepatic and extrahepatic bile duct systems merge at the hepatic hilum.

The cystic duct and gallbladder become visible as a small outgrowth on the hepatic diverticulum by the 4th week of gestation. By the 5th week, all the extrahepatic bile duct elements (gallbladder, cystic duct, hepatic duct, common bile duct, pancreatic duct) are clearly evident; by the 11th week, the major bile ducts at the *porta hepatis* are fully formed, in concomitance with the saccular dilatation of the initially tubular gallbladder [19, 33]. The epithelial lining of the extrahepatic bile ducts, which has been recently suggested to be a continuous hollow structure, merges caudally with the duodenal epithelium and cranially with the primitive hepatic sheets [19, 33]. This would support the hypothesis that the biliary atresia [see Chap. 5] results from a failure of "canalization" [22, 32].

The development of the extrahepatic biliary tract relies on an appropriate function of both cholangiocyte epithelium and adjacent mesenchyme.

When compared to the intrahepatic biliary tract, little is known about the molecular mechanisms that control the development of the extrahepatic biliary structures. However, in murine models defective for different transcription factors (Hairy And Enhancer Of Split 1, HNF6, HNF1β, and Forkhead-Related Transcription Factor 1), alterations of the gallbladder and the common bile duct have been reported, suggesting their role in normal extrahepatic biliary structure development [19].

3.1.3 Mesodermal Specification

3.1.3.1 Development of the Hepatic Vasculature
The development of the hepatic vasculature is a multistep process combining angiogenesis, vasculogenesis, and vascular differentiation, regulated by specific growth and differentiation factors, including the vascular endothelial growth factor [35–37]. The hepatic vasculature is unique because the liver receives both a venous blood supply for its functional circulation (deriving from the intestines, pancreas, and spleen via the portal vein) and an arterial supply for nutritional purposes, provided by the hepatic artery.

3.1.3.2 Venous Vasculature
At the end of the 3rd week of gestation, the embryo comprises three major venous systems: the *vitelline veins*, the *umbilical veins*, and the *cardinal veins* [35, 37, 38]. Soon after the emergence of the liver bud (during the 4th week of gestation), the paired vitelline veins are connected by four anastomoses. Three of them are located in the prehepatic segment (*inferior* and *middle intervitelline anastomosis* and *superior or subhepatic anastomosis*), and one is immediately below the *sinus venosus* and above the hepatic primordium (*subdiaphragmatic anastomosis*) [35, 37, 39]. The developing hepatic parenchyma interrupts the venous structures lying in between the subhepatic and subdiaphragmatic anastomoses, consequently designing a network of small vessels that are all connected with sinusoids. The most marginal parts of this specific vitelline segment are not affected by the previous modification and give rise to the *venae advehentes* (where blood flows from the subhepatic anastomosis to the sinusoidal plexus) and the *venae revehentes* (where blood flows from the sinusoidal plexus to the subdiaphragmatic anastomosis) [35, 37].

Synchronously, the umbilical vein system (comprising one vein which directly drains into the liver parenchyma, and one which drains into the *sinus venosus* bypassing the liver) begins its modifications by the collapse of all except the prehepatic segment of the right umbilical vein [35, 37]. Besides, the posthepatic segment of the left umbilical vein collapses; the only exception is its intrahepatic portion, which progressively grows and eventually makes a connection with the left angle of the subhepatic intervitelline anastomosis, whereby the umbilical circulation is completely conveyed to the liver [35, 37–39]. Subsequently, from the beginning of the 5th week until the end of the 6th week of gestation, the portal vein takes origin from the anastomotic channels derived from the vitelline veins, and the ductus venosus develops from the umbilical system, so a continuous connection between the portal and the umbilical systems is finally established. This conjunction is termed *sinus intermedius* or *portal sinus* [35, 37].

The results of all these changes are two, unpaired and interconnected, venous vessels, which are present until birth. For this reason, this period is called *asymmetrical* stage [35, 37].

Studies on hemodynamics during the intrauterine life have shown the umbilical vein is the predominant afferent vessel of the left hepatic lobe, while the right one is mainly supplied by the portal vein [35].

At the time of birth, relevant changes occur in both the umbilical circulation and the intrahepatic portal system, leading to a persistence of the portal vein as the only afferent venous system of the liver. This modification leads to the establishment of the ultimate hepatic vascular architecture. A decrease in total blood flow determines the collapse of the *ductus venosus* and its subsequent obliteration by fibrous tissue, leading to the formation of the *ligamentum venosum*. On the other hand, the collapsed umbilical vein becomes the *ligamentum teres hepatis* [35].

These fibrous structures can maintain a vascular patency with potential repermeabilization in case of portal hypertension [35] [see Chap. 17].

3.1.3.3 Arterial Vasculature
The arterial development occurs later than the venous one, beginning at the 8th week of gestation. The first branch of the hepatic artery derives from the celiac trunk and becomes evident near the extrahepatic portal vein in the hepatic hilum.

The development of the intrahepatic arterial radicles firstly takes place along the large branches of the intrahepatic portal vein, and, subsequently, it extends toward the periphery of liver, following the smaller twigs of the portal vessels [35, 36]. It completely reaches the hepatic periphery around the 15th week of gestation [35, 36]. The hepatic arterial development is also closely associated with the intrahepatic biliary system formation. This is supported by the observation that the appearance of the first arterial radicles is temporarily related to the emergence of the ductal plate [21, 35].

3.1.3.4 Sinusoidal Differentiation
The precursors of hepatic sinusoids are recognizable in the cords of hepatoblasts, which invade the septum transversum around the 4th week of gestation. Two major hypotheses have been brought forward in order to explain the origin of hepatic sinusoids, and they both suggest hepatic sinusoids derived from preexisting vessels. The first hypothesis

assumes an origin from preexisting capillary vessels of the septum transversum, while the second one suggests a possible origin from a disruption of pre-existing vitelline veins due to a quick expansion of the hepatic primordium [35].

More recently, the sinusoidal differentiation has been divided into three main stages [35]. During the first stage (from the 4th to the 12th week of gestation), the main change of the capillary vessels lying between the hepatocyte cords is the loss of components in the organized basement membranes [35, 40] and the appearance of incompletely fenestrated sinusoids [41]. The second stage (from the 12th to the 20th week of gestation) is characterized by a progressive expression of specific sinusoidal endothelial markers, such as CD4 and CD14 [35, 40]. Little is known about the third stage of differentiation in humans. Rat studies have shown that the final structural endothelial differentiation of the sinusoids is reached during the perinatal period. In fact, at this time, a progressive disappearance of the large endothelial fenestrae, better adapted to the transmural migration of mature blood cells, and a marked increase in the number of small fenestrae, better adapted for macromolecular transport, are observed [35, 42].

3.1.4 Hematopoiesis

Extramedullary hepatic hematopoiesis starts between the 6th and the 7th week of gestation, and it is particularly intense during the second trimester, when liver is the main hematopoietic organ of the fetal body [43] (Fig. 3.6). Hematopoietic cells not only play the obvious mission of maintaining the homeostasis of the peripheral blood elements, but they are essential for hepatocyte maturation by the secretion of Oncostatin [43, 44]. Hematopoiesis has a zonal distribution, and it occurs in well-defined areas of the hepatic lobule. Erythropoiesis mainly occurs in the sinusoids; the erythroid cells are sometimes organized in small clusters around central macrophages, which is thought to be essential for the erythroid maturation. This histological organization is called *Bessis islands* [45]. On the contrary, myelopoiesis occurs in the PTs, mainly around the vascular structures [45].

As the fetus comes into the 3rd trimester, the hepatic hematopoiesis progressively decreases. At the 32nd week of gestation, hematopoiesis is very scanty in the liver. During the last weeks of gestation and the first postnatal period, few scattered islands of residual hematopoiesis or isolated erythroid cells could be visible [45]. After the first few months of life, a significant persistence of hepatic hematopoiesis should be regarded as a pathological finding [45].

3.2 Gross Anatomy

Even if liver is an abdominal organ, it lies deeply under the right lower ribs. In children, the highly elastic ribs offer a minimal protection from impacts. The adult liver weighs around 1400–1600 g, comprising 2.5% of the body weight. The newborn liver comprises 4% of the total body weight, and at puberty it increases ten times more [46, 47]. Along the midclavicular line, the liver is detected below the costal margins for approximately 2 cm in the newborn, 1–1.5 cm below until the first year, and 1 cm below from 18 months to 6 years. At 6–7 years, the liver is rarely palpable except in pathological cases [46–48]. The liver surface is covered by a thin connective tissue capsule, which is called *Glisson's capsule*. It lies just beneath a layer of flat peritoneal mesothelial cells. Most of the liver surface is covered by peritoneum, except for the attachment site of the gallbladder and a small area on the posterior surface, called *area nuda*, which adheres firmly to the diaphragm. A peritoneal fold forms the *falciform ligament* that divides the diaphragmatic surface of the liver into a right and left lobe. Anteriorly, on the inferior surface of the right liver lobe, the quadrangular *quadrate lobe* is visible, while the medial posterior part of the right liver lobe represents the *lobus caudatus (caudate lobe)*, separated from the quadrate lobe by the *porta hepatis*. The porta hepatis is the area where the portal vein and the hepatic artery come into the hepatic parenchyma, and the bile ducts leave it [24, 49, 50] (Fig. 3.7a, b).

Liver is subdivided into eight functional segments, and each of them is characterized by its own vascular inflow, outflow, and biliary drainage. This segmental division is important in surgical settings [24, 46–50].

Liver has a dual blood supply: the *hepatic artery* (a branch of the celiac axis) and the *portal vein* (formed by

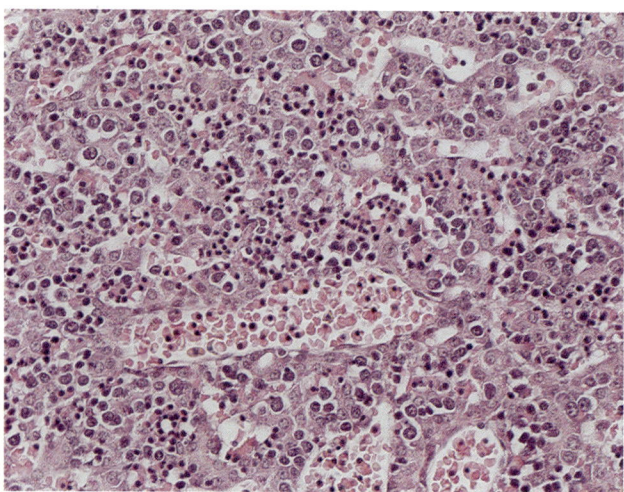

Fig. 3.6 (Hematoxylin-eosin). Sinusoids are plenty of hematopoietic cells in the embryo at the 14th week of gestation. At this time, liver is the main hematopoietic organ. Few foci of hematopoietic cells can be seen even after birth

Fig. 3.7 A schematic representation of gross anatomy of the liver: (**a**) front and (**b**) back vision

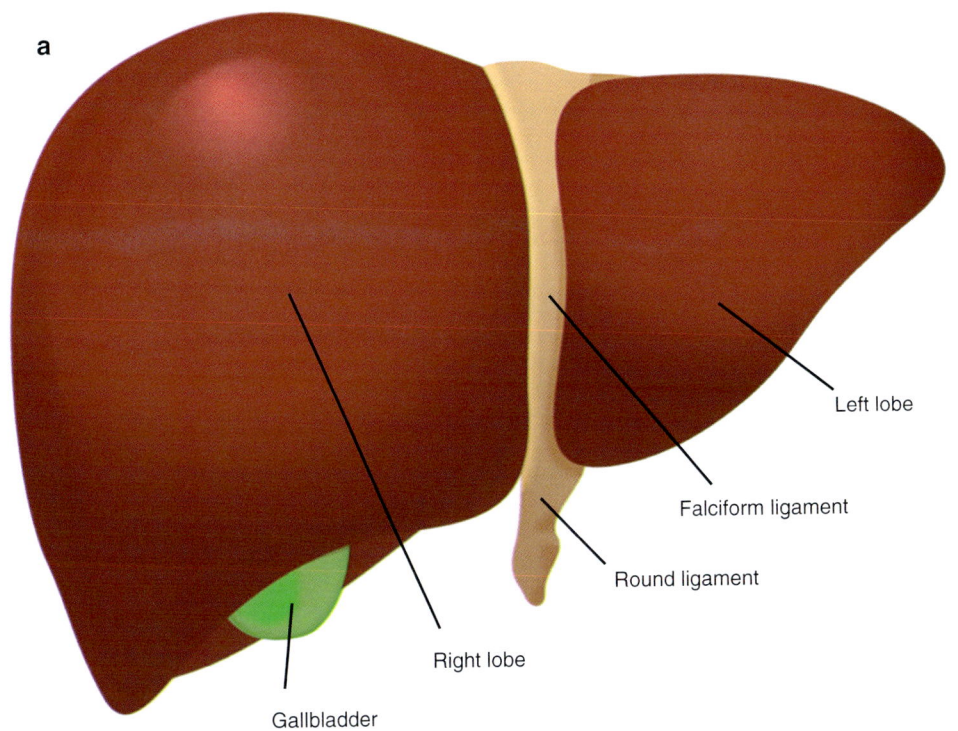

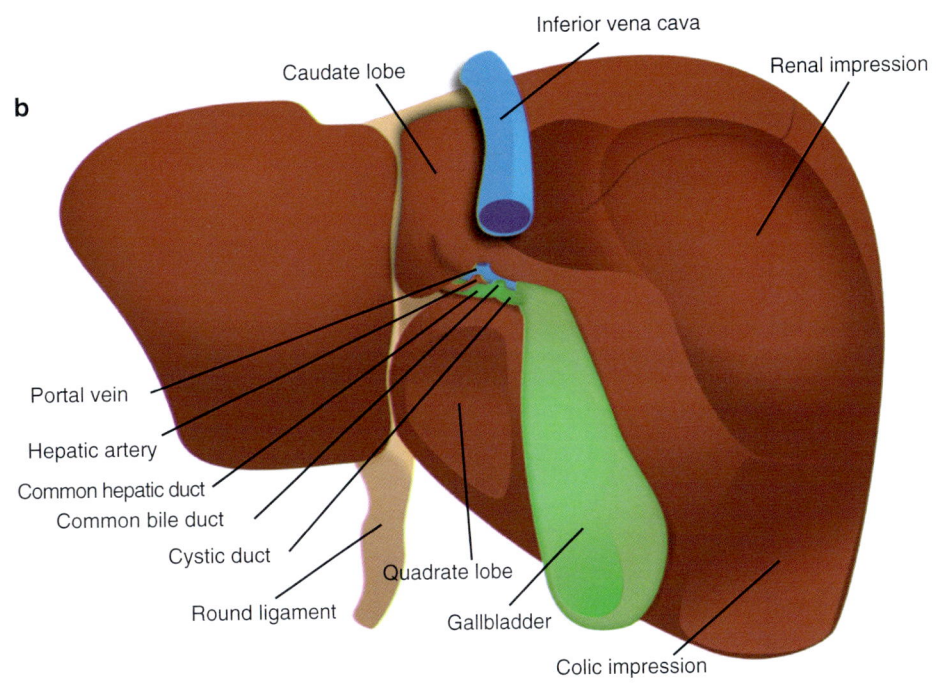

the splenic and the mesenteric superior veins). The efferent system—the *hepatic veins*—drains into the inferior vena cava, which is partly surrounded by the posterior surface of the liver (Fig. 3.7b). The portal vein is responsible for approximately 70% of the hepatic blood supply [49, 51]. Decrease in portal flow leads to a compensatory increase in hepatic arterial flow, which is termed hepatic arterial buffer response [52].

Hepatic lymphatic vessels mainly drain into the porta hepatis and the celiac lymph nodes. The liver is the largest source of lymph in the human body, producing about 15–20% of the overall total volume and 25–50% of thoracic duct flow [53].

3.3 Microanatomy

3.3.1 Structural Organization

The functional unit of the liver is defined as the smallest, structurally distinct, and "self-sufficient" unit that can independently carry out all the hepatic functions; however, its definition is still a matter of discussion [31]. Over the years, several models have been proposed.

Described by Kiernan in 1833 [54], the *classical lobule* still represents the standard way to refer to the hepatic microarchitecture in clinical practice. The lobule is a roughly hexagonal structure, and it consists of plates of hepatocytes lined by sinusoidal spaces, which radiate toward a central efferent vein (Fig. 3.8). The effluent hepatic vein is in the center of the lobule; thus its name is *central vein*. Each of the six hexagon corners is demarcated by a PT [50, 54].

Described by Rappaport in 1954, another model of the liver parenchyma organization is the *liver acinus* [55, 56]. In this three-dimensional, functional, and architectural structure, blood flows from the PT into the sinusoids, which subsequently drain into the *terminal hepatic vein* (i.e., the central vein) at the periphery of the acinus (Fig. 3.8). The acinus is divided into three different functional zones, each having different levels of oxygenation and metabolic function. The concept of liver acinus is very useful to understand the effects of ischemia and other pathological processes occurring in the hepatocytes. In *zone 1* (which is closest to the PT), the hepatocytes are the most highly oxygenated, whereas those in *zone 3* (which is close to the central veins) are less oxygenated [55–57]. Due to the difference in oxygenation, in zone 3 the hepatocytes are more severely and earlier damaged by ischemia and other insults [58]. The intermediate (midlobular) area is called *zone 2* [55–57]. In 1979, Matsumoto et al. proposed the concept of *primary lobule* as the functional unit of the liver, which was based on the vessel architecture and included the classic lobule as a secondary feature [59, 60]. Several alternative hepatic functional units have been proposed during the 1980s and 1990s, including the single sinusoidal, metabolic, zonal circulation, choleon, microcirculatory, and choleohepaton units [see MacSween's Pathology of the Liver, for review] [61], but the Matsumoto model remains the most widely accepted.

3.3.1.1 Hepatocytes

The hepatocytes are the major parenchymal cell type of the liver accounting for about 80% of its volume [16]. They are arranged in cords in a sponge-like fashion [31, 50, 54, 61]. During the intrauterine life, the initial hepatocyte cords are multilayered [6] (Fig. 3.9a). After birth, the cords progressively become thinner, and, at 5th month, they generally reach a bilayered architecture. At this time, the size of the hepatocytes is uniform. Subsequently, in adults and in children older than 5–6 years, the hepatocyte cords become only one cell thick (Fig. 3.9b), and their size is more variable [6]. The periportal hepatocytes are closely packed to each other and smaller than the others; they show a stronger nuclear staining and a more basophilic cytoplasm. The hepatocyte nucleus is centrally located, round, and contains one or more nucleoli. At birth, all but a few hepatocytes are mononuclear [31, 50, 54, 61]. The presence of *glycogenated nuclei*, which appear optically as empty vacuoles on H&E stain (Fig. 3.10), is a normal finding in childhood, mainly in periportal areas, and it may be seen even in young adults [6, 62]. Glycogenated nuclei are numerous in some metabolic conditions, such as in diabetes and in Wilson's disease, at any age [24, 61, 62]. The hepatocytes plasma membrane is well-defined and presents three specialized domains. Each domain has different molecular, chemical, and antigenic compositions and functions. The *sinusoidal domain* represents 70% of the total surface area and faces sinusoids; it is separated from the endothelial sinusoidal cells by the *space*

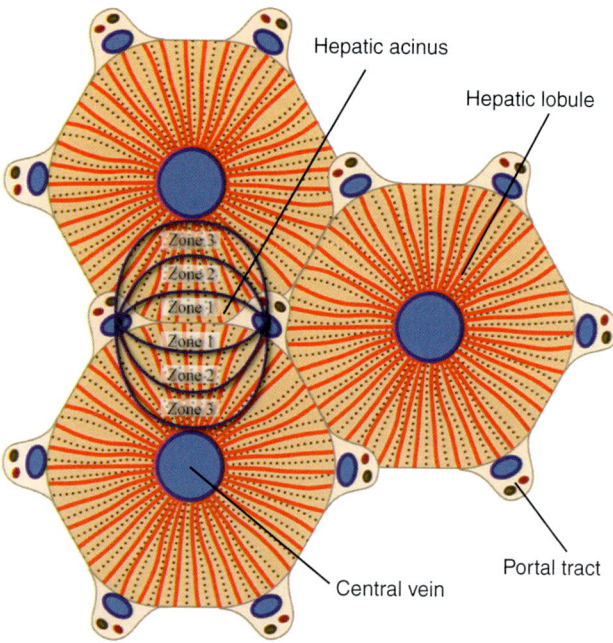

Fig. 3.8 A schematic representation of the classic hepatic lobule and the Rappaport acinus. The first one is a bidimensional lobular model which is currently used in clinical practice to describe the topography of the histological lesions. The lobule is a hexagon where the proximal part of the efferent venous system (the central vein) is centrally located, while the portal tracts are at its periphery. In this model, the hepatocyte cords seem to radiate from the center to the periphery. In contrast, the Rappaport acinus is a tridimensional structure where the central area is occupied by the portal tract and the peripheral one by the efferent vein. According to the proximity to the portal tract, three acinar zones are identified in accordance with a different metabolic function and a decreasing oxygenation: indeed, the periportal hepatocytes (zone 1) receive more oxygenated blood than the perivenular ones (zone 3). This model better explains the specific localization of the histological lesions, particularly in case of a toxic and/or ischemic injury

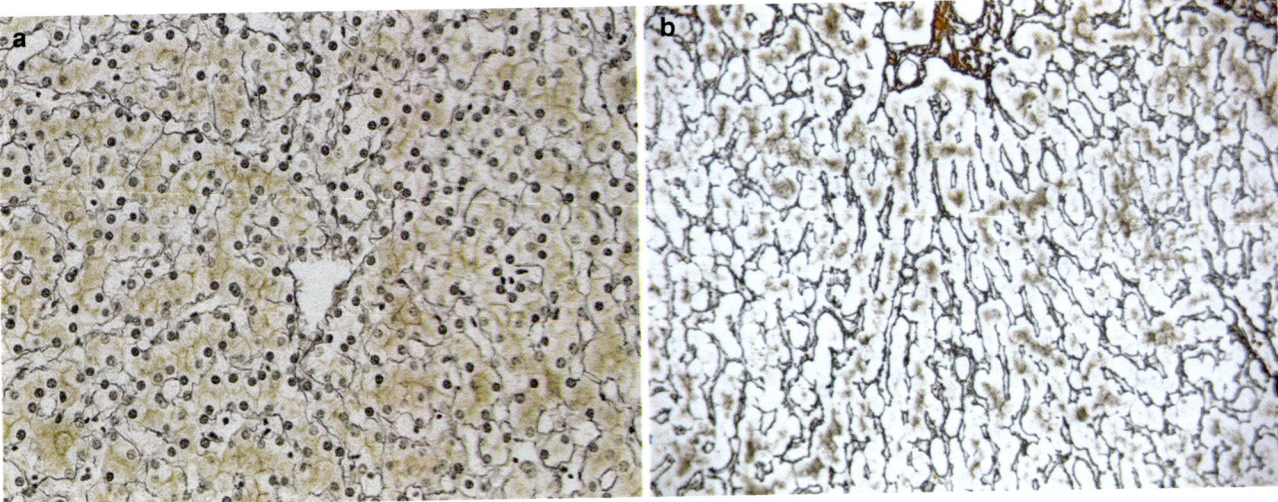

Fig. 3.9 (Reticulin stain). (**a**) At 32 weeks of gestation, fetal liver still shows a multilayered pattern of hepatocyte cords; (**b**) by the age of 5 years, the "mature" monolayered hepatocyte organization is fully developed

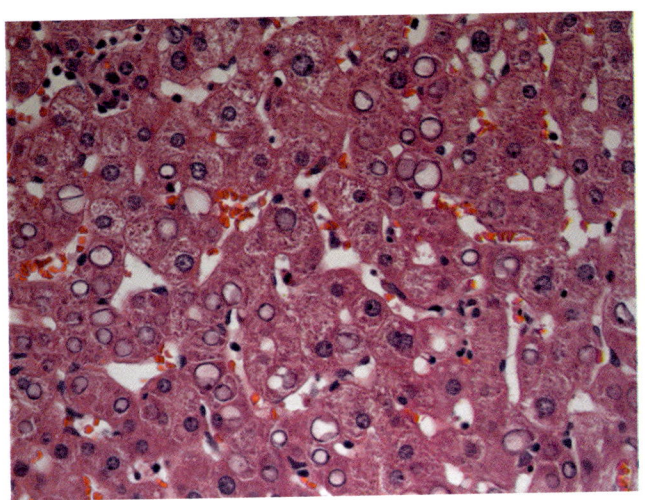

Fig. 3.10 (Hematoxylin-eosin). Glycogenated nuclei appear as optically empty vacuoles. They are numerous in the liver during the pediatric age and should not be confused as a sign of a metabolic disorder. They become progressively rare and even more rare in the adulthood. Glycogenated nuclei are also numerous in diabetes and Wilson's disease at any age

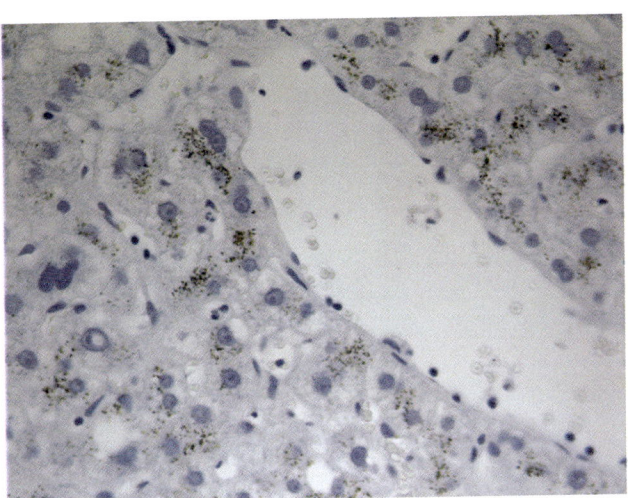

Fig. 3.11 (Timm's method). Copper (black dots) is detectable in the hepatocytes at birth

of Disse [31, 50, 61, 63]. The *bile canalicular domain* (15%) gives rise to the bile canaliculi, a collecting intercellular space, whose surface is characterized by the presence of microvilli. Different biliary proteins responsible for bile formation and flow are collected in the hepatocyte canalicular membrane [31, 50, 61]. Inherited defects in these proteins are responsible for heterogeneous intrahepatic cholestatic syndromes [23, 24] [see Chap. 11]. The *lateral domain* (15%) faces the rest of the intercellular space [31, 50, 61].

The hepatocyte functions (e.g., gene expression profiles and biochemical activities) are various, depending on their physical location in the hepatic lobule [17, 57, 58]. A pivotal recent study, based on a single-cell transcriptome analysis of the mouse liver, found that 50% of liver genes are zonated, including genes that are most significantly expressed in midlobular area (zone 2), which is an often overlooked zone in research [58, 64, 65]. This heterogeneous expression of some genes is very strong in fetal hepatocytes [14]. Metabolic zonation is dynamic, and all the functional zones are not anatomically rigid [66]. Their borders are related to feeding cycles and functional needs, and regulated by local nutritional factors, digestive hormones, and oxygen levels [57, 58]. The metabolic zonation of hepatocytes is likely to influence liver disease [58]. The livers of PiZ mice and human patients with α-1-antitrypsin deficiency have been recently found to have a severe perturbation of liver zonation [67].

The hepatocytes contain hemosiderin and copper at birth (Fig. 3.11). They gradually decrease and should disappear by

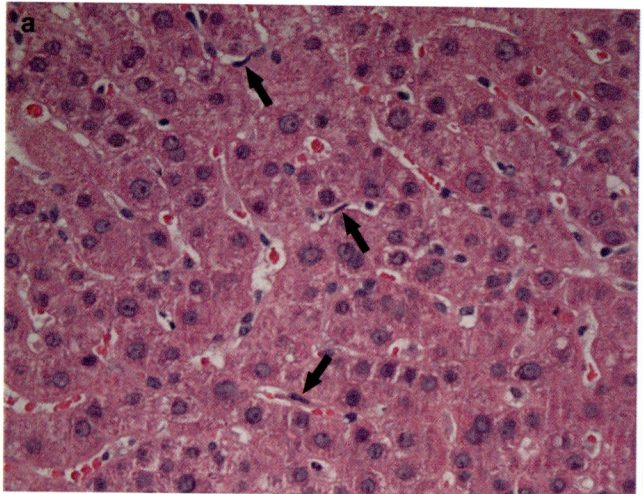

Fig. 3.12 (**a**) (Hematoxylin-eosin). The endothelial cells (arrows) show a thin and indistinct cytoplasm and a small, elongated, darkly stained nucleus without nucleoli. They are inconspicuous in normal liver; (**b**) (Immunohistochemistry; antibody to CD31). In normal liver, both the vascular and the sinusoidal endothelial cells express the vascular antigen CD31

6–9 months of age. In children, the hepatocyte cytoplasm is rich in glycogen but is devoid of lipofuscin, a finely granular, brown pigment representing oxidized lipids derived from cellular wear and tear. Lipofuscin accumulates around the nuclei of perivenular hepatocytes with age [6, 31, 61].

3.3.1.2 Sinusoids

Sinusoids are unique canals, which separate the plates of hepatocytes. This term was coined by Charles Sedgwick Minot (1852–1914), who distinguished sinusoids from the blood capillary with only the help of a light microscope (WAKE 2015) during the early 1900s [68]. The hepatic sinusoids are a complex system of canals to transport blood (a mixture of portal and arterial blood) through the hepatic parenchyma, from the porta hepatis to the inferior vena cava. The sinusoids are the principal vessels involved in the exchange between the bloodstream and the parenchymal cells [61, 69].

In healthy liver, sinusoids have a fairly uniform diameter and are barely visible. They appear as slit-like spaces that may contain few blood cells. The periportal sinusoids may be more tortuous than the perivenular ones. Hepatic sinusoids are lined by *fenestrated endothelial cells* and *Kupffer cells*, supported by reticulin fibers. In contrast to blood capillaries, hepatic sinusoids do not have a basement membrane, and the endothelial cells do not form junctions, but they are separated by several gaps, resulting in a sieve-like structure, which allows the free exchange between blood and hepatocytes [61, 69–71]. Under the microscope, the endothelial cells have a thin, indistinct cytoplasm and a small, elongated, darkly stained nucleus without nucleoli. They are rather inconspicuous in normal liver specimens [31, 61, 69, 72–74] but can be enlightened by the use of CD31 immunostaining, which identify a glycoprotein that is expressed at high levels on mature endothelial cells (Fig. 3.12a, b).

Kupffer cells (KCs) are the largest resident macrophage population, accounting for 20–35% of all non-parenchymal cells in the liver and 80–90% of tissue macrophages in the human body [16]. They are anchored to the luminal surface of the sinusoidal endothelium, and, thus, they are exposed to the bloodstream. KCs are important members of the innate and adaptive immune systems and play a role in the first line of defense against bacteria, microbial debris, and endotoxins derived from the gastrointestinal tract as well as from the systemic circulation [75, 76]. Moreover, KCs act as antigen-presenting cells and provide a bridge between the innate and the adaptive immune systems [75, 76].

KCs have an irregular stellate shape, not easily recognizable on H&E stained sections. At histology, they display a plump cytoplasm and a large bean-shaped nucleus (Fig. 3.13) and appear more numerous in the periportal area, suggesting that they may play an important role in the clearance of blood that comes into the liver through the portal vein and the hepatic artery. KCs can migrate along the sinusoids, both in the same or in the opposite direction of blood flow [31, 61, 75, 76].

The space of Disse is the virtual subendothelial space lying between the basolateral surface of the hepatocytes and the anti-luminal side of the sinusoidal endothelial cell layer. Firstly described by the German Joseph HV Disse in 1890 [63], this space contains plasma and a thin permeable connective tissue layer and allows the exchange of biomolecules between the portal blood flow, deriving from the gastrointestinal tract, and the hepatocytes [31, 61, 63]. *Hepatic stellate cells* (HSCs) (previously referred to as Ito cells, vitamin A-storing cells or fat-storing cells) reside within the space of

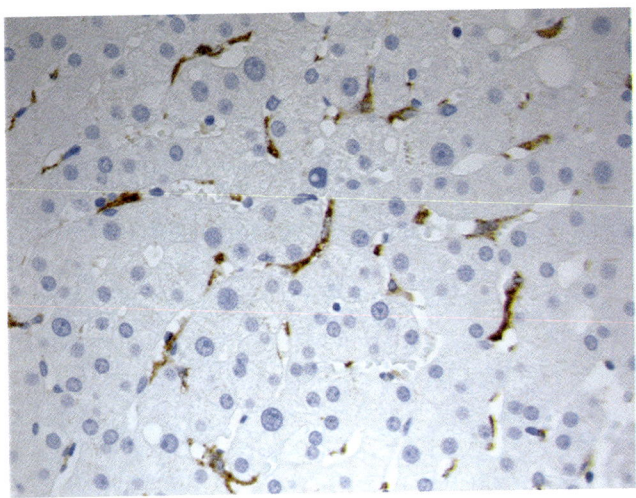

Fig. 3.13 (Immunohistochemistry; antibody to CD68). Kupffer cells are better recognizable by the use of immunostainings for histiocytic antigens, such as CD68

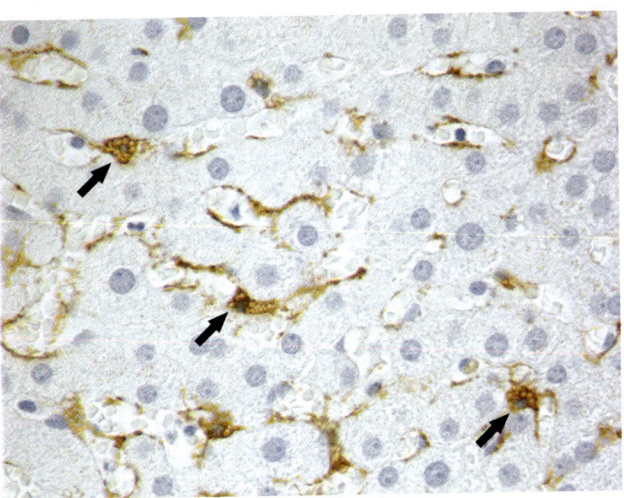

Fig. 3.14 (Immunohistochemistry; antibody to α-smooth muscle actin). Quiescent hepatic stellate cells are rarely visible in routine sections stained with hematoxylin-eosin. When activated to myofibroblasts under pathological stimuli, they lose their lipid droplets and, characteristically, express α-smooth muscle antigen. In this sample, lipid droplets are still evident in some of the activated hepatic stellate cells (arrows)

Disse [77–79]. They comprise approximately one-third of non-parenchymal cells and 15% of total resident cells in normal human liver [16, 77–79]. These cells are resident mesenchymal cells and retain features of the resident fibroblasts (embedded in normal stromal matrix) and the pericytes (attached to endothelial cells of capillaries) [77–79].

In healthy livers, HSCs are quiescent and contain numerous vitamin A lipid droplets, representing the largest reservoir of vitamin A in human body [77, 80]. They participate in several physiological processes, including vasoregulation through endothelial cell interactions, extracellular matrix homeostasis, drug detoxification, and immunotolerance [78–80]. Quiescent HSCs are not readily visualized on light microscopy in normal liver unless they become very numerous as in hypervitaminosis A [77–79]. During a liver injury, HSCs transform themselves into myofibroblasts, lose their lipid droplets, and start to produce excessive extracellular matrix [78–80]. Activated HSCs express α-smooth muscle actin and are readily identified by the use of immunohistochemical methods [78, 79] (Fig. 3.14). A key role of HSCs in liver fibrogenesis has been also demonstrated in children [81].

3.3.1.3 Liver-Associated Lymphocytes

Liver lymphocytes include cells of the adaptive and innate immune system. They are predominantly located within the PTs but are also found scattered throughout the parenchyma, where they are found in loose luminal contact with KCs or endothelial cells [82, 83]. Natural killer (NK) cells (first described as *pit cells* in the rat liver in the 1970s) [84], NK T cells, and unconventional T cells (γδ) [82–84] are up to 65% of all hepatic lymphocytes. Liver is the site in the human body where γδ T cells are more numerous. The lymphocyte populations can proliferate under certain experimental or pathological conditions [82, 83].

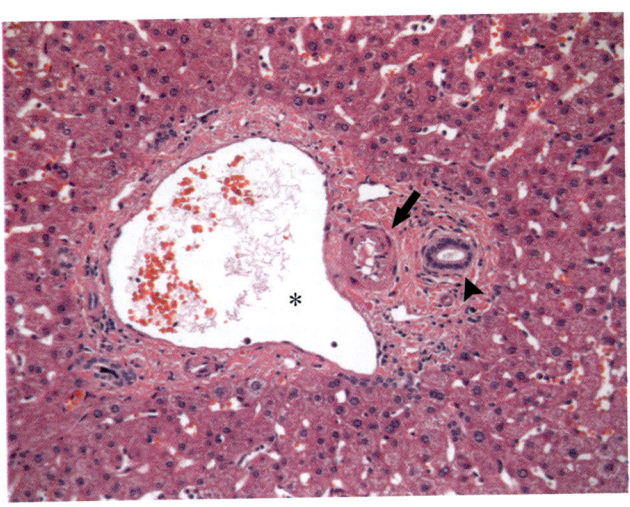

Fig. 3.15 A normal portal tract contains a branch of the portal vein (asterisk), a hepatic artery (arrow), and a bile duct (arrowhead)

3.3.1.4 Portal Tracts

The PT is a connective structure where a branch of the hepatic artery, the portal vein, and the bile duct are embedded (Fig. 3.15). A continuous *limiting plate* of hepatocytes surrounds them. Nerves and lymphatic vessels can be easily seen in large PTs [31, 61]. The amount of connective tissue and the size of the vascular and biliary structures depend on the level and plane of sectioning [31, 61]. On average, the size of a PT is three to four times the diameter of the hepatic artery branch. In a normal PT, hepatic arteries and bile ducts exhibit similar diameters. On average, the portal vein has a minimum diameter three times greater than the bile duct and can even be up to four times greater [31, 61]. In the most peripheral areas, *portal dyads* are commonly found; they contain only hepatic artery and bile duct profiles [85]. On the contrary, multiple ducts and vessels may be seen in larger PTs. Bile ducts are always associated with a hepatic artery, and, in normal liver, no more than 10% of unpaired arteries (artery without the bile duct) should be found [31, 61, 85]. In immature livers, ductal plate remnants can be found as a rim of biliary epithelium or ducts in the PTs [6, 31, 61]. Dilated and anastomosing ductal plate remnants embedded in fibrous stroma are a sign of ductal plate malformation [21]. Ductal plate remnants should not be confused with the *ductular reaction* (DR), which is a reactive process that arise at the interface between the portal (or septal) and parenchymal compartments in case of disease and injury [30, 86]. The term DR encompasses proliferating bile ductules, ductular hepatocytes, and intermediate hepatobiliary cells [30]. The proliferating bile ductules are always accompanied by an inflammatory cell infiltrate, mainly neutrophils [86]. DR is now recognized to occur ubiquitously in many acute and chronic liver diseases and not only in biliary disorders, although in bile duct obstructive conditions it may be extraordinarily prominent [86]. The origin of DR is still a matter of discussion. It may arise from proliferation of preexisting cholangiocytes or from progenitor cells and, rarely, from biliary metaplasia of hepatocytes [30, 86].

Normal PTs occasionally contain few and randomly distributed lymphocytes, while aggregates of lymphocytes or any amount of granulocytes and plasma cells should be regarded as an abnormal feature [31, 61].

Portal vein branches connect to sinusoids through the *inlet venules*. These are very short side branches, which have an endothelial lining with a basement membrane and scanty adventitial fibrous connective tissue but no smooth muscle in their walls. Inlet venules are usually not visible in normal conditions [31, 61].

3.3.1.5 The Biliary System

The intrahepatic biliary system begins with the *bile canaliculus*, which is formed by tight junctions between the canalicular membrane domains of adjacent hepatocytes. Bile canaliculi are barely visible under the light microscope, except when filled by bile [30, 34]. However, they could be revealed by immunohistochemical stains for antigens expressed on the canalicular membrane of hepatocytes (CD10; polyclonal carcinoembryonic antigen) [30, 34, 61] (Fig. 3.16). The bile canaliculi network is drained by the *canals of Hering*, which are lined on one side by hepatocytes and on the other by cholangiocytes [30, 87]. Under the light microscope, the canals of Hering are difficult to be recognized. They appear on an H&E stain as small groups or strings of cuboidal cells in the periportal regions and are better identified by immunohistochemical stains for the biliary CK7 and CK19 [30, 31, 34, 61, 87]. The canals of Hering are

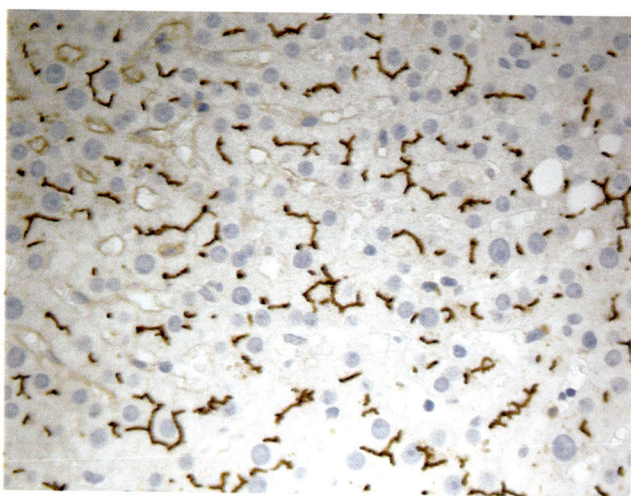

Fig. 3.16 (Immunohistochemistry; antibody to CD10). CD10 immunostaining is able to enlighten the twig-like structures of the bile canaliculi

thought to be the intra-organ stem or progenitor cell compartment of the liver, responsible for the ductular reaction [87]. The canals of Hering collect the bile and transport it to the edge of the PTs where they are connected to the *bile ductules* [87]. Bile ductules are located in the peripheral zone of the PTs and have a lumen diameter less than 20 μm. They, in turn, drain into the *interlobular bile ducts* [30]. Bile ductules and interlobular bile ducts are entirely lined by cuboidal or low columnar cholangiocytes. They have a basement membrane and a small amount of periductal connective tissue [30, 31, 61]. The interlobular bile ducts merge and form larger *septal ducts*. These are more than 100 μm in diameter and lined by a simple, tall, columnar epithelium with basal nuclei. The septal ducts further anastomose to each other to form the *intrahepatic bile ducts*, which give rise to the *main hepatic ducts* [30, 31, 61].

As many other cell types in human body, cholangiocytes have primary cilia, extending from the apical plasma membrane into the bile duct lumen. Cholangiocyte cilia regulate bile formation through mechanosensory, osmosensory, and chemosensory cues [31, 61, 88]. Defects in cholangiocyte ciliary structure and/or their integrated transducing function lead to a decrease in intracellular calcium and increase in cAMP, causing cholangiocyte hyperproliferation, abnormal cell matrix interactions, and altered fluid secretion/absorption, which can result in hepatic cystogenesis [88–90].

3.4 Technical Aspects of Liver Sampling

Liver biopsy (LB) samples may be obtained through different techniques: blind percutaneous needle biopsy (PNB) without imaging guidance, image-guided PLB, transjugular liver biopsy (TJLB), or surgical biopsy during laparoscopy or laparotomy [91]. Each technique has its own indications and advantages. The patient risk profile and the personal experience and practice of the medical operator mostly influence the choice of the LB technique [91]. Whatever method is chosen, a careful consideration is required on whether or not the specimen obtained is adequate for the intended purpose. A small specimen, obtained with a needle guided by ultrasound imaging, may be adequate for the diagnosis of neoplastic lesions, but not necessarily suitable for the histological evaluation of chronic hepatitis [85, 92]. In a non-neoplastic setting, the biopsy should be big enough to view a representative number of PTs, which is proportional to the bioptic specimen size. Based on experience in adults, most experts agree that an ideal biopsy size is 2–3 cm long after formalin fixation [93]. No specific rules for LB size in the pediatric setting are available.

In pediatric population, the percutaneous approach (with or without image guide) is used in most cases [94]. PLB is performed with aspiration devices (Menghini needle) [95] or a cutting needle (Tru-Cut biopsy) [91]. For diffuse liver diseases, a 16-gauge needle (internal diameter of cylinder: 1.2 mm) is typically preferred [91]. The use of fine needles (less than 18 or 16 gauge) is discouraged outside the setting of nodular lesions [93].

PLB is an invasive procedure with a range of adverse events [91, 96]. Minor complications comprise transient and moderate pain, while vasovagal episodes are infrequent. Severe complications such as hemoperitoneum, biliary peritonitis, and pneumothorax are rare [96]. In a study on pediatric outpatients, bleeding was reported in 1% of children, with clinical symptoms occurring within 4 h of LB [97]. As in the adult population, there is an increased risk of bleeding in patients with malignancies or after a bone marrow transplant [96, 98]. Three deaths (0.6%) have been reported in children who underwent LB: all of them had a history of malignancy or hematological disease [96].

The type of needle has been related to types of complications: a higher incidence of hemorrhage, pneumothorax, biliary leakage, and peritonitis has been reported using cutting needles, while puncturing of other internal organs and sepsis has been reported when Menghini needles are used. Whether the diameter of the needle is a factor predisposing to hemorrhage is still controversial [96, 97].

Plugged LB is a modification of percutaneous LB in which collagen, thrombin, or a similar material is injected as the needle is withdrawn. PLB with gelatin sponge pledget tract embolization is safe and effective for the diagnosis of hepatic disease in pediatric patients, even in the setting of coagulopathy [99]. Although a transvenous biopsy can be obtained in this subset of patients, the plugged approach is generally used when a larger specimen size is needed [99].

The transjugular route is indicated in subjects with significant coagulopathy and/or ascites. It requires considerable experience and has significant costs [100–102]. Furthermore, with this approach, liver samples are thinner and often fragmented [101, 102]. In a study of TJLB in children and adults, the complication rate was 2.4%, and the mortality rate was 0.25% [100].

Wedge biopsies, which are obtained intraoperatively, are a good way to assess focal hepatic lesions located at or just beneath the hepatic capsule; however, it is not indicated in case of clinical diffuse diseases. Indeed, capsular and subcapsular connective tissue may be quite prominent in wedge biopsies of normal liver, with a significant risk of overestimating the stage of fibrosis. Furthermore, tissue coagulation artifacts can completely hamper biopsy interpretation [91].

Once obtained, the liver specimen should be fixed as soon as possible in 10% neutral buffered formalin, which is adequate for subsequent application of most histochemical, immunohistochemical, and some molecular procedures [103, 104]. A core needle biopsy requires 2–4 h of fixation. This time can be shortened by the use of microwave processing [103, 104]. Operative wedge biopsies and larger specimens need longer fixation [103, 104]. In case of LB obtained in infants and children with jaundice, a snap-frozen section for molecular study and glutaraldehyde fixation for electron microscopy is required, due to the broad differential diagnosis which often includes inherited metabolic diseases [103, 104].

The stains routinely applied to liver biopsies depend on local custom. The minimum advised is hematoxylin and eosin and a reliable method for connective tissue. Routine staining for iron is helpful to screen for iron storage disease; the periodic acid-Schiff stain after diastase digestion provides a screening procedure for α-1-antitrypsin deficiency and highlights activated macrophages and bile duct basement membranes. Other methods are required in particular cases [103].

Liver biopsy does not always provide a final or complete diagnosis. In most cases, however, an adequate and properly processed biopsy will produce a clinically helpful report when interpreted on the light of full clinical, biochemical, immunological, and imaging data.

Acknowledgment The authors are grateful to Cristiano Frassetto for all the artworks.

References

1. Gordillo M, Evans T, Gouon-Evans V. Orchestrating liver development. Development. 2015;142:2094–108.
2. O'Rahilly R, Muller F, editors. Human embryology & teratology. 3rd ed. New York: Wiley-Liss; 2001.
3. Tremblay KD, Zaret KS. Distinct populations of endoderm cells converge to generate the embryonic liver bud and ventral foregut tissues. Dev Biol. 2005;280:87–99.
4. Deutsch G, Jung J, Zheng M, et al. A bipotential precursor population for pancreas and liver within the embryonic endoderm. Development. 2001;128:871–81.
5. Schoenwolf G, Bleyl S, Brauer P, Francis-West P, editors. Larsen's human embryology. 5th ed. Philadelphia: Churchill Livingstone; 2014.

6. Ober EA, Lemaigre FP. Development of the liver: insights into organ and tissue morphogenesis. J Hepatol. 2018;68:1049–62.
7. Si-Tayeb K, Lemaigre FP, Duncan SA. Organogenesis and development of the liver. Dev Cell. 2010;18:175–89.
8. Jung J, Zheng M, Goldfarb M, et al. Initiation of mammalian liver development from endoderm by fibroblast growth factors. Science. 1999;284:1998–2003.
9. Germain L, Blouin MJ, Marceau N. Biliary epithelial and hepatocytic cell lineage relationships in embryonic rat liver as determined by the differential expression of cytokeratins, alpha-fetoprotein, albumin, and cell surface-exposed components. Cancer Res. 1988;48:4909–18.
10. Lemaigre FP. Mechanisms of liver development: concepts for understanding liver disorders and design of novel therapies. Gastroenterology. 2009;137:62–79.
11. McLin VA, Zorn AM. Molecular control of liver development. Clin Liver Dis. 2006;10:1–25.
12. Kelley-Loughnane N, Sabla GE, Ley-Ebert C, et al. Independent and overlapping transcriptional activation during liver development and regeneration in mice. Hepatology. 2002;35:525–34.
13. Petkov PM, Zavadil J, Goetz D, et al. Gene expression pattern in hepatic stem/progenitor cells during rat fetal development using complementary DNA microarrays. Hepatology. 2004;39:617–27.
14. Spear BT, Jin L, Ramasamy S, et al. Transcriptional control in the mammalian liver: liver development, perinatal repression, and zonal gene regulation. Cell Mol Life Sci. 2006;63:2922–38.
15. Roskams T, Desmet V. Embryology of extra- and intrahepatic bile ducts, the ductal plate. Anat Rec (Hoboken). 2008;291:628–35.
16. Blouin A, Bolender RP, Weibel ER. Distribution of organelles and membranes between hepatocytes and nonhepatocytes in the rat liver parenchyma. A stereological study. J Cell Biol. 1977;72:441–55.
17. Jungermann K, Katz N. Functional specialization of different hepatocyte populations. Physiol Rev. 1989;69:708–64.
18. Antoniou A, Raynaud P, Cordi S, et al. Intrahepatic bile ducts develop according to a new mode of tubulogenesis regulated by the transcription factor SOX9. Gastroenterology. 2009;136:2325–33.
19. Strazzabosco M, Fabris L. Development of the bile ducts: essentials for the clinical hepatologist. J Hepatol. 2012;56:1159–70.
20. Raynaud P, Carpentier R, Antoniou A, et al. Biliary differentiation and bile duct morphogenesis in development and disease. Int J Biochem Cell Biol. 2011;43:245–56.
21. Desmet VJ. Congenital diseases of intrahepatic bile ducts: variations on the theme "ductal plate malformation". Hepatology. 1992;16:1069–83.
22. Vuković J, Grizelj R, Sprung J, et al. Ductal plate malformation in patients with biliary atresia. Eur J Pediatr. 2012;171:1799–804.
23. Gruppuso PA, Sanders JA. Regulation of liver development: implications for liver biology across the lifespan. J Mol Endocrinol. 2016;56:R115–25.
24. Dancygier H, editor. Clinical hepatology. Principles and practice of hepatobiliary diseases, vol. 1. 1st ed. Heidelberg: Springer; 2010.
25. Parviz F, Matullo C, Duncan SA. Hepatocyte nuclear factor 4alpha controls the development of a hepatic epithelium and liver morphogenesis. Nat Genet. 2003;34:292–6.
26. Zong Y, Panikkar A, Xu J, et al. Notch signaling controls liver development by regulating biliary differentiation. Development. 2009;136:1727–39.
27. Lemaigre FP. Notch signaling in bile duct development: new insights raise new questions. Hepatology. 2008;48:358–60.
28. McDaniell R, Warthen DM, Sanchez-Lara PA, et al. NOTCH2 mutations cause Alagille syndrome, a heterogeneous disorder of the notch signaling pathway. Am J Hum Genet. 2006;79:169–73.
29. Geisler F, Nagl F, Siveke JT, et al. Liver-specific inactivation of Notch2, but not Notch1, compromises intrahepatic bile duct development in mice. Hepatology. 2008;48:607–16.
30. Roskams TA, Theise ND, West AB, et al. Nomenclature of the finer branches of the biliary tree: canals, ductules, and ductular reactions in human livers. Hepatology. 2004;39:1739–45.
31. Saxena R, Theise ND, Crawford JM. Microanatomy of the human liver-exploring the hidden interfaces. Hepatology. 1999;30:1339–46.
32. Russo P, Ruchelli ED, Piccoli DA, editors. Pathology of pediatric gastrointestinal and liver disease. 2nd ed. Heidelberg: Springer; 2014.
33. Tan CE, Vijayan V. New clues for the developing human biliary system at the porta hepatis. J Hepatobiliary Pancreat Surg. 2001;8:295–302.
34. Nakanuma Y, Hoso M, Sasaki M, et al. Microstructure and development of the normal and pathologic biliary tract in humans, including blood supply. Microsc Res Tech. 1997;38:552–70.
35. Collardeau-Frachon S, Scoazec JY. Vascular development and differentiation during human liver organogenesis. Anat Rec (Hoboken). 2008;291:614–27.
36. Gouysse G, Couvelard A, Frachon S, et al. Relationship between vascular development and vascular differentiation during liver organogenesis in humans. J Hepatol. 2002;37:730–40.
37. Carlson BM, editor. Human embryology and developmental biology. 5th ed. Amsterdam: Elsevier; 2014.
38. Lassau JP, Bastian D. Organogenesis of the venous structures of the human liver: a hemodynamic theory. Anat Clin. 1983;5:97–102.
39. Dickson AD. The development of the ductus venosus in man and the goat. J Anat. 1957;91:358–68.
40. Couvelard A, Scoazec JY, Dauge MC, et al. Structural and functional differentiation of sinusoidal endothelial cells during liver organogenesis in humans. Blood. 1996;87:4568–80.
41. Enzan H, Himeno H, Hiroi M, et al. Development of hepatic sinusoidal structure with special reference to the Ito cells. Microsc Res Tech. 1997;39:336–49.
42. Barbera-Guillem E, Arrue JM, Vidal-Vanaclocha F, et al. Structural changes in endothelial cells of developing rat liver in the transition from fetal to postnatal life. J Ultrastruct Mol Struct Res. 1986;97:197–206.
43. Tavian M, Peault B. Embryonic development of the human hematopoietic system. Int J Dev Biol. 2005;49:243–50.
44. Khurana S, Jaiswal AK, Mukhopadhyay A. Hepatocyte nuclear factor-4alpha induces transdifferentiation of hematopoietic cells into hepatocytes. J Biol Chem. 2010;285:4725–31.
45. Timens W, Kamps WA. Hemopoiesis in human fetal and embryonic liver. Microsc Res Tech. 1997;39:387–97.
46. Watson EH, Lowrey GH. Growth and development of children. 5th ed. Chicago: Year Book Publishers; 1967.
47. Konus OL, Ozdemir A, Isik S, et al. Normal liver, spleen, and kidney dimensions in neonates, infants, and children: evaluation with sonography. AJR Am J Roentgenol. 1998;171:1693–8.
48. Huelke DF. An overview of anatomical considerations of infants and children in the adult world of automobile safety design. Annu Proc Assoc Adv Automot Med. 1998;42:93–113.
49. Reynolds JC, editor. The Netter collection of medical illustrations. Digestive system. Part III-liver, biliary tract, and pancreas. 2nd ed. Amsterdam: Elsevier; 2017.
50. Wanless IR. Physioanatomic considerations. In: Schiff ER, Sorrell MF, Maddrey WC, editors. Schiff's diseases of the liver. Philadelphia: Lippincott; 1999.
51. Hall JE, editor. Guyton and hall textbook of medical physiology. 13th ed. Amsterdam: Elsevier; 2015.
52. Rush N, Sun H, Saxena R, et al. Hepatic arterial buffer response: pathologic evidence in non-cirrhotic human liver with extrahepatic portal vein thrombosis. Mod Pathol. 2016;29:489–99.
53. Ohtani O, Ohtani Y. Lymph circulation in the liver. Anat Rec (Hoboken). 2008;29:643–52.
54. Kiernan F. The anatomy and physiology of the liver. Philos Trans R Soc Lond B Biol Sci Biol. 1833;123:711–70.

55. Rappaport AM, Borowy ZJ, Lotto WN, et al. Subdivision of hexagonal liver lobules into a structural and functional unit. Anat Rec. 1954;119:11–33.
56. Rappaport AM. The structural and functional unit in the human liver (liver acinus). Anat Rec. 1958;130:673–89.
57. Malarkey DE, Johnson K, Maronpot RR, et al. New insights into functional aspects of liver morphology. Toxicol Pathol. 2005;33:27–34.
58. Soto-Gutierrez A, Gough A, Monga SP, et al. Pre-clinical and clinical investigations of metabolic zonation in liver diseases: the potential of microphysiology systems. Exp Biol Med (Maywood). 2017;242:1605–16.
59. Matsumoto T, Komori R, Takasaki S, et al. A study on the normal structure of the human liver, with special reference to its angioarchitecture. Jikeikai Med J. 1979;26:1–40.
60. Matsumoto T, Kawakami M. The unit-concept of hepatic parenchyma–a re-examination based on angioarchitectural studies. Acta Pathol Jpn. 1982;32(Suppl 2):285–314.
61. Burt AD, Ferrell LD, Hubscher SG. MacSween's pathology of the liver. 7th ed. Philadelphia: Churchill Livingstone; 2018.
62. Levene AP, Goldin RD. Physiological hepatic nuclear vacuolation-how long does it persist? Histopathology. 2010;56:426–9.
63. Haubrich WS. Disse of the space of Disse. Gastroenterology. 2004;127:1684.
64. Bahar Halpern K, Shenhav R, Itzkovitz S, et al. Single-cell spatial reconstruction reveals global division of labour in the mammalian liver. Nature. 2017;542:352–6.
65. Benhamouche S, Decaens T, Colnot S, et al. Apc tumor suppressor gene is the "zonation-keeper" of mouse liver. Dev Cell. 2006;10:759–70.
66. Kaestner KH. In the zone: how a hepatocyte knows where it is. Gastroenterology. 2009;137:425–7.
67. Piccolo P, Annunziata P, Brunetti-Pierri N, et al. Down-regulation of hepatocyte nuclear factor-4α and defective zonation in livers expressing mutant Z α1-antitrypsin. Hepatology. 2017;66:124–35.
68. Minot CS. On a hitherto unrecognized form of blood circulation without capillaries in the organs of vertebrates. J Boston Soc Med Sci. 1900;4:133–4.
69. Wake K, Sato T. "The sinusoid" in the liver: lessons learned from the original definition by Charles Sedgwick Minot (1900). Anat Rec (Hoboken). 2015;298:2071–80.
70. Brunt EM, Gouw ASH, Wanless IR, et al. Pathology of the liver sinusoids. Histopathology. 2014;64:907–20.
71. McCuskey RS. The hepatic microvascular system in health and its response to toxicants. Anat Rec (Hoboken). 2008;291:661–71.
72. Lalor PF, Lai WK, Adams DH, et al. Human hepatic sinusoidal endothelial cells can be distinguished by expression of phenotypic markers related to their specialised functions in vivo. World J Gastroenterol. 2006;12:5429–39.
73. Poisson J, Lemoinne S, Rautou PE, et al. Liver sinusoidal endothelial cells: physiology and role in liver diseases. J Hepatol. 2017;66:212–27.
74. Elvevold K, Smedsrod B, Martinez I. The liver sinusoidal endothelial cell: a cell type of controversial and confusing identity. Am J Physiol Gastrointest Liver Physiol. 2008;294:G391–400.
75. Abdullah Z, Knolle PA. Liver macrophages in healthy and diseased liver. Pflugers Arch. 2017;469:553–60.
76. Li P, He Y, Gong J, et al. The role of Kupffer cells in hepatic diseases. Mol Immunol. 2017;85:222–9.
77. Senoo H, Mezaki Y, Fujiwara M. The stellate cell system (vitamin A-storing cell system). Anat Sci Int. 2017;92:387–455.
78. Yin C, Evason KJ, Stainier DYR, et al. Hepatic stellate cells in liver development, regeneration, and cancer. J Clin Invest. 2013;123:1902–10.
79. Friedman SL. Hepatic stellate cells: protean, multifunctional, and enigmatic cells of the liver. Physiol Rev. 2008;88:125–72.
80. Loo CK, Wu XJ. Origin of stellate cells from submesothelial cells in a developing human liver. Liver Int. 2008;28:1437–45.
81. Lotowska JM, Elzbieta Sobaniec-Lotowska M, Marek Lebensztejn D. Ultrastructural characteristics of the respective forms of hepatic stellate cells in chronic hepatitis B as an example of high fibroblastic cell plasticity. The first assessment in children. Adv Med Sci. 2018;63:127–33.
82. Freitas-Lopes MA, Mafra K, Menezes GB, et al. Differential location and distribution of hepatic immune cells. Cell. 2017;6:48–69.
83. Doherty DG, O'Farrelly C. Innate and adaptive lymphoid cells in the human liver. Immunol Rev. 2000;174:5–20.
84. Wisse E, Van't Noordende JM, Van der Meulen J, et al. The pit cell: description of a new type of cell occurring in rat liver sinusoids and peripheral blood. Cell Tissue Res. 1976;173:423–35.
85. Crawford AR, Lin XZ, Crawford JM. The normal adult human liver biopsy: a quantitative reference standard. Hepatology. 1998;28:323–31.
86. Gouw AS, Clouston AD, Theise ND. Ductular reactions in human liver: diversity at the interface. Hepatology. 2011;54:1853–63.
87. Theise ND, Saxena R, Crawford JM, et al. The Canals of Hering and hepatic stem cells in humans. Hepatology. 1999;30:1425–33.
88. Masyuk AI, Masyuk TV, LaRusso NF. Cholangiocyte primary cilia in liver health and disease. Dev Dyn. 2008;237:2007–12.
89. Waters AM, Beales PL. Ciliopathies: an expanding disease spectrum. Pediatr Nephrol. 2011;26:1039–56.
90. Masyuk T, Masyuk A, LaRusso N. Cholangiociliopathies: genetics, molecular mechanisms and potential therapies. Curr Opin Gastroenterol. 2009;25:265–71.
91. Dezsofi A, Baumann U, Knisely AS, et al. Liver biopsy in children: position paper of the ESPGHAN Hepatology Committee. J Pediatr Gastroenterol Nutr. 2015;60:408–20.
92. Lefkowitch J, editor. Scheuer's liver biopsy interpretation. 9th ed. Amsterdam: Elsevier; 2015.
93. Colloredo G, Guido M, Leandro G, et al. Impact of liver biopsy size on histological evaluation of chronic viral hepatitis: the smaller the sample, the milder the disease. J Hepatol. 2003;39:239–44.
94. Amaral JG, Schwartz J, Connolly B, et al. Sonographically guided percutaneous liver biopsy in infants: a retrospective review. AJR Am J Roentgenol. 2006;187:W644–9.
95. Menghini G. One-second biopsy of the liver–problems of its clinical application. N Engl J Med. 1970;283:582–5.
96. Cohen MB, A-Kader AK, Lambers D, et al. Complications of percutaneous liver biopsy in children. Gastroenterology. 1992;102:629–32.
97. Gonzalez-Vallina R, Alonso EM, Rand E, et al. Outpatient percutaneous liver biopsy in children. J Pediatr Gastroenterol Nutr. 1993;17:370–5.
98. Hoffer FA. Liver biopsy methods for pediatric oncology patients. Pediatr Radiol. 2000;30:481–8.
99. Tulin-Silver S, Obi C, Lungren M, et al. Comparison of transjugular liver biopsy and percutaneous liver biopsy with tract embolization in pediatric patients. J Pediatr Gastroenterol Nutr. 2018;67:180–4.
100. Smith TP, Presson TL, Heneghan MA, et al. Transjugular biopsy of the liver in pediatric and adult patients using an 18-gauge automated core biopsy needle: a retrospective review of 410 consecutive procedures. AJR Am J Roentgenol. 2003;180:167–72.
101. Dohan A, Guerrache Y, Soyer P, et al. Transjugular liver biopsy: indications, technique and results. Diagn Interv Imaging. 2014;95:11–5.
102. Behrens G, Ferral H. Transjugular liver biopsy. Semin Intervent Radiol. 2012;29:111–7.
103. Suriawinata AA, Thung SN. editors. Liver pathology. An atlas and concise guide. New York: Demos Medical Publishing; 2011.
104. Geller SA. Liver: tissue handling and evaluation. Methods Mol Biol. 2014;1180:303–21.

Laboratory Evaluation of Hepatobiliary Disease

Henrik Arnell and Björn Fischler

Key Points
- Biochemical tests to evaluate liver function are mainly AST, ALT, GGT, bilirubin, ALP, and INR, but they are non-liver-specific, since, during pediatric age, they can be raised because of other organs' injury or the use of medications.
- Chronic liver disease can develop subclinically even in patients with normal aminotransferases. Overall, there is no correlation between the level of aminotransferases and the severity of liver disease.
- Finding raised aminotransferases is quite common in children with any acute illness; therefore, this test needs to be repeated serially to suspect a liver disease deserving further investigations.
- Noninvasive tests revealing the type and the severity of liver disease are missing, and the diagnosis of hepatopathies often requires a high index of suspicion as well as the inputs from clinical, biochemical, and radiological findings.
- Liver histology remains the gold standard to make the diagnosis of a chronic liver disease.

Research Needed in the Field
- Normal reference values based on large population-based cohorts of entirely healthy children of all different ages and of both sexes are still lacking for several of the commonly used liver function tests described herein.
- There is still a further need for more refined evaluation of the synthetic function of the liver, i.e., tests that are even more specific than, for example, INR.
- There is also a need to develop tests for daily clinical practice to measure the capacity to metabolize drugs.

4.1 Introduction

Most of the biochemical tests used to screen for and characterize possible liver disease are not actual tests of the global liver function but merely reflecting an isolated aspect of the liver. Thus, biochemical testing for liver disease should be done by combining different analyses and thereby looking at the possible aberrations from different perspectives, collectively adding up to a full picture. By liver function tests, we often mean serum markers for hepatocyte turnover (primarily AST and ALT), for cholestasis (total and conjugated bilirubin, bile acids, GGT, ALP), for portal hypertension (platelets, leukocytes, and hemoglobin), for possible malignancy (AFP, CA-19), and finally for liver synthetic function (albumin, PK/INR, single coagulation factors).

4.2 Markers of Hepatocyte Turnover: AST and ALT

The most commonly used biochemical markers for liver disease are aspartate aminotransferase (AST) and alanine aminotransferase (ALT). These two aminotransferases were first demonstrated in human blood from healthy subjects and

H. Arnell (✉) · B. Fischler
Department of Paediatrics, Karolinska University Hospital and CLINTEC, Karolinska Institutet, Stockholm, Sweden
e-mail: henrik.arnell@sll.se; bjorn.fischler@sll.se

from patients with varying disease entities, proposing that these enzymes could serve as markers of ischemic heart disease [1]. ALT and AST, formerly known as serum glutamic-pyruvic transaminase (SGPT) and serum glutamic-oxaloacetic transaminase (SGOT), respectively, are nowadays most frequently used to detect liver damage. The terms transaminase and aminotransferase are interchangeable. Biochemically, they are both involved in the Krebs cycle, in transamination of amino groups from the amino acids alanine and aspartic acid, respectively. AST is found in the cytosol (cAST) and in the mitochondrion (mAST) in most cell types, whereas ALT is mainly cytosolic (cALT).

None of them are restricted solely to the hepatocyte and are found in large quantities in myocytes of the skeletal and heart muscle, in erythrocytes, and in renal tubular cells but also in pancreatic tissue, leukocytes, brain, and lung. Their half-life in blood differs depending on cellular localization and is approximately 48 h for cALT, 18 h for cAST, and >72 h for mAST [2, 3]. As with most serum markers, they are released into the blood stream from apoptotic cells and eliminated from the plasma at a relatively constant rate, thus keeping a stable plasma concentration. Enzyme activity of AST and ALT is often measured as units per mL (U/mL = μmol $\times$ min^{-1} $\times$ mL^{-1}), although the International System of Units (SI) recommends that catalytic activity of enzymes in serum should be expressed in the SI unit katal per liter (kat/L = mol $\times$ s^{-1} $\times$ L^{-1}) [4]. The conversion between the two units is as follows: 1 μkat/mL = 60 U/mL or 1 U/mL = 0.0167 μkat/mL.

When interpreting results of AST and ALT measurements, a few things must be remembered. First, think of extrahepatic causes; increased aminotransferase levels may be due to increased cellular turn-over in other tissues than the liver, most often myocyte degradation due to heavy exercise [5, 6] or underlying acute or chronic muscular disease. By testing for CK (creatinine kinase) or myoglobin, we can rule out damaged muscular tissue as the source. In addition to this, there is a plethora of other possible factors influencing the results, including day-to-day variations [7, 8], gender and age [9], specimen storage [10], and the rare presence of macroenzymemia including macro-AST [11, 12].

Second, the results must be put in a clinical context; normal aminotransferase levels do not rule out serious liver disease but merely reflect the actual number of damaged cells. Thus, in a liver with limited residual parenchyma, normal aminotransferase levels may be found. In fact, patients with end-stage liver disease with cirrhosis may have completely normal levels of aminotransferases. To this end, when end-stage disease could be suspected in a patient with completely or almost normal AST and ALT, the testing must also include markers of liver function, i.e., albumin and/or PK/INR.

Third, even slight elevations of AST and ALT should be noted and be reevaluated, as chronic liver disease in children may be very discrete and may reflect ongoing liver diseases, possibly progressing to end-stage liver disease, unless diagnosed and properly treated [13].

Looking closely at the dynamics of repeated aminotransferase analyses can often help us to understand the nature of the liver disease, including possible etiology, thereby guiding in differential diagnostics and predicting the natural course and prognosis of the liver disease, sometimes also aiding in evaluating effects of possible treatments. A steep rise of the aminotransferases followed by a quick decrease may hint toward a "one-hit etiology," such as temporary ischemia leading to liver damage, whereas a steep rise followed by a gradual decay of the liver enzymes instead would direct the clinician toward an ongoing process, such as a toxic or viral liver damage.

The ratio between ALT and AST in children may vary a lot. Increased AST/ALT ratios have been correlated with a less favorable outcome and may imply increased mitochondrial turnover or cirrhosis [14] or NAFLD [15]. Despite this, interpretations based on AST/ALT ratio should be done with caution.

Reference values in children have been published in several studies [16–23], and there are slight variations between age, gender, and race, but they should be interpreted with caution since the number of children especially in the youngest age groups often is too low for firm conclusions. It should be noted that the normal values in children are lower compared to adult normal values [24] and that AST activity in children and adolescents is somewhat higher than that of ALT [9].

4.2.1 Interpretation of Increased Levels of AST and ALT

Very high levels (>10 $\times$ ULN) are seen in acute liver disease—the highest levels in toxic and ischemic damage to the liver, sometimes also in acute viral hepatitis, less commonly in autoimmune hepatitis (AIH). These levels may also occur in Wilson's disease.

High levels (2–10 $\times$ ULN) are noted in all of the above and in metabolic liver disease including nonalcoholic fatty liver diseases (NAFLD) and autoimmune hepatobiliary diseases (including AIH and primary sclerosing cholangitis, PSC) but also in hereditary cholestatic liver diseases.

Slightly elevated liver enzymes (<2 $\times$ ULN) are commonly seen in all of the above but also in systemic and other GI diseases with liver involvement, alfa-1 antitrypsin disease, cystic fibrosis, celiac disease, and inflammatory bowel disease (Table 4.1).

Table 4.1 The aminotransferases AST and ALT markers of hepatocyte turnover

	AST activity	ALT activity	AST/ALT ratio	Weight (kg)	AST total	ALT total
Liver	7100	2850	2.5	1.5	10,650	4275
Kidney	4500	1200	3.8	0.25	1125	300
Heart	7800	450	17	0.3	2340	135
Muscle	5000	300	17	30	150,000	9000
Serum	1	1	1.0	3	3	3

Botros et al. [68]

4.3 Markers of Cholestasis

4.3.1 Alkaline Phosphatase (ALP)

The enzyme alkaline phosphatase (ALP), first described almost 100 years ago [25], with a half-life of approximately 7 days is abundant in many different human tissues including the sinusoidal membrane of the liver, intestine, kidney, bone, placenta, and white blood cells. It is represented by different isoenzymes, all catalyzing hydrolysis of phosphate esters in the different tissues, important in a number of basic physiologic mechanisms although still not exactly characterized [26, 27]. Despite its wide distribution, most ALP in humans emanates from bone tissue and from the hepatocyte, and increased levels are thus seen in bone disease and cholestatic liver disease. Although widely used as a reliable marker of obstructive cholangiopathy in adults, interpreting total ALP levels in growing children and adolescents with much higher osteoblast activity and turnover of bone tissue is therefore less straightforward. Thus, the value of total ALP activity as a marker of cholestatic liver disease in children and adolescents is limited as long as the exact origin of the isoenzyme is unknown. In other words, separating ALP into its isoenzymes and its isoforms would add value to the measurement of total enzyme activity. Increased levels of ALP activity are seen not only in bone and cholestatic liver disease but also in vitamin D deficiency, untreated celiac disease, and transient benign hyperphosphatasemia, where the serum levels of ALP may exceed 2000 U/L (or >30 μkat/L). The latter is not an uncommon entity in children less than 5 years of age, with no signs of bone or liver disease and ALP with isoforms of both bone and liver origin returning to normal levels within 4–6 months, and it is important to recognize to avoid misdiagnosis or unnecessary investigations [27–29]. Low serum levels of ALP in liver disease are found in patients with Wilson's disease, possibly due to the abundant copper ions competitively displacing zinc ions, a necessary cofactor of alkaline phosphatase, leading to low levels [30]. Low levels are seen in several non-hepatic diseases, including zinc deficiency, hypothyroidism, and congenital hypophosphatasia [26, 31].

4.3.2 Gamma-Glutamyltranspeptidase (GGT)

Gamma-glutamyltranspeptidase (GGT) belongs to a group of enzymes catalyzing the transfer of amino acids from one peptide to another amino acid or peptide. The main enzyme responsible for the transpeptidation of the gamma glutamyl group was initially studied in rat kidney tissue and named gamma-glutamyltranspeptidase [32].

GGT is abundant in renal, prostatic, pancreatic, and hepatobiliary tissue; smaller amounts are found in all other tissues except the muscle, and although liver tissue is the main source of serum GGT in humans, elevated GGT activity also occurs in patients with acute and chronic pancreatitis. Since the enzyme is found in as well the endoplasmic reticulum as in the canalicular membrane of the hepatocyte, increased activity indicates liver damage but does not perfectly discriminate between increased cell turnover and cholestasis [33].

Despite this, it is a valuable marker, especially in pediatric hepatology. Due to its tissue specificity, not found in bone or in muscle tissue, it adds valuable information when used in combination with less discriminate markers of cell turnover such as AST or ALT and those of cholestasis, such as ALP, with its low specificity in children and adolescents. Increased GGT activity is seen mainly in hepatobiliary disease, most often higher in cholestatic diseases than in non-cholestatic liver diseases, but elevated serum levels are also found in patients treated with certain enzyme-inducing drugs (antiepileptics) and in adult with alcohol overconsumption [34, 35]. In conclusion, GGT activity is a more useful marker of cholestasis than total ALP activity in children and adolescents due to their high bone tissue turnover. Despite this, there is a number of important cholestatic diseases including FIC1 deficiency, BSEP deficiency, and TJP2 deficiency, all characterized by decreased concentrations of biliary bile acids in the canaliculus, where GGT activity in serum remains low. Thus, in instances when infants or children present with clinical and biochemical signs of cholestasis, diseases of canalicular bile acid transport defects should be suspected [36].

4.3.3 Conjugated Serum Bilirubin

Bilirubin is a waste product from hemoglobin which undergoes conjugation in the liver. Conjugated bilirubin is secreted to the bile via the canalicular transporter multidrug resistance-associated protein 2 (MRP2). An elevated level of conjugated bilirubin in serum is considered one of the hallmarks of cholestasis in clinical practice. Using the SI unit system, a level of 30 µmol/L, corresponding to 1.75 mg/dL, or higher should definitely warrant further investigation, in particular if the conjugated fraction accounts for more than 20% of the total bilirubin level. In patients with isolated elevation of conjugated bilirubin but no other biochemical markers of cholestasis or hepatocellular injury, the alternative explanation of Dubin-Johnson syndrome may be considered. This benign state is caused by mutation in the gene encoding MRP2.

4.3.4 Serum Bile Acids

Bile acids are synthesized in the liver from cholesterol, excreted with the bile into the gut and very efficiently recirculated to the liver via the enterohepatic circulation. Under normal circumstances, the total bile acid levels in peripheral serum are therefore low, i.e., below 7 µmol/L. Cholestasis occurs if there is a blockage at any level of the enterohepatic circulation. This leads to a measurable increase of the bile acid levels in peripheral serum. While the occurrence of elevated levels, at least above 100 µmol/L, is a sensitive marker of cholestasis, it does not give any meaningful clue of the underlying cause. Thus, in a cholestatic infant, such levels can be seen both in biliary atresia and the different genetic cholestatic diseases, such as Alagille syndrome and the different types of progressive familial intrahepatic cholestasis. On the other hand, in cholestatic patients with inborn errors of bile acid synthesis, these levels, as analyzed by the hospital labs, are not elevated. The reason for this is that these routine methods measure only bile acids with a hydroxylation in the 3-alpha position, whereas the basic defect in these specific diseases causes accumulation of bile acids with hydroxylation in other positions of the molecule [37].

Mild elevations of bile acid levels in serum have been described in healthy infants below 6 months of age. This seems to be associated to an immature and therefore suboptimal transportation of bile acids at different points of the enterohepatic circulation and is denoted "physiologic cholestasis of the infant" [38].

Despite the limitations pointed out above, the bile acid level in peripheral serum is a useful biochemical marker of cholestasis, also in patients who are not obviously jaundiced, i.e., the serum levels of conjugated bilirubin may not be elevated.

4.4 Tumor Markers

4.4.1 α-Fetoprotein (AFP)

AFP is considered the most important binding protein in the fetus. During the first trimester, it is produced by the yolk sac; thereafter, the fetal liver is the main source of production. The steady fetal production results in high serum levels at birth, around 40,000 ng/mL. During the first year of life in a healthy infant, there is subsequently a logarithmic fall in the serum levels. However, the interindividual variation is large, and despite a half-life of 5–6 days, adult levels are not reached until 2 years of age. To assess single values obtained in infants, a nomogram should be used, and serial values are in fact strongly suggested [39, 40] (Fig. 4.1).

Elevated AFP is an important marker for germ cell tumors, hepatoblastoma (HB), and hepatocellular carcinoma. In HB, which is the most common hepatic malignancy in children, around 90% of the patients have elevated AFP. On the other hand, the minority with normal levels seem to have a poorer treatment outcome [41]. Repeated AFP testing is also useful, together with radiology, to estimate the effect of treatment with chemotherapy [42].

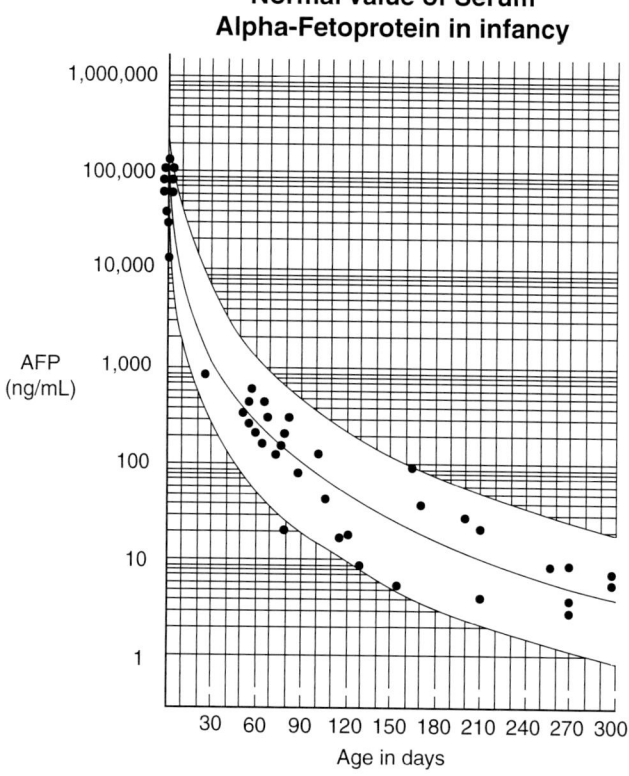

Fig. 4.1 Normal values of alpha-fetoprotein in infancy. Tsuchida et al. [69]

4.4.2 CA19-9

CA19-9 is a glycoprotein coated with sialylated blood group (carbohydrate) epitopes such as sialyl Lewis[a]. It is detected in low levels in healthy adult subjects, whereas pediatric data are scarce. Interestingly, Lewis-negative individuals, which are estimated to account for 7% of the population, have undetectable levels. Since the original descriptions in the late 1970s, CA19-9 has been suggested to be a marker for cholangiocarcinoma, for example, in adults with primary sclerosing cholangitis. However, the compiled results of several studies on this topic reveal a rather disappointing and diverging sensitivity of 38–89% and specificity of 50–98%. Other clinical situations than cholangiocarcinoma such as increasing cholestasis as well as bacterial cholangitis in patients with underlying hepatobiliary diseases will also cause an increase in the CA19-9 levels [43–45].

4.5 Markers of Synthetic Function

To make a relevant estimate of the remaining functional capacity in a patient with liver disease is complex. The different hepatic functions—for example, drug metabolism, excretion, and synthesis—may be more or less preserved in different types of diseases. To measure the synthesis or in fact the level of plasma proteins is therefore only one of several possible ways to assess this capacity. These analyses are extensively used, primarily because they are readily available to the clinician and the turnaround time at the laboratory is often relatively short.

4.5.1 Coagulation Factors

A majority of these proteins are produced in the liver, although it should be noted that coagulation factor 8 is also released from endothelial cells. If the functional liver cell mass is decreased, be it rapidly or over time, one would expect the production of coagulation factors to decrease.

The most widely used analysis is to measure prothrombin time. In recent years, the results obtained in this analysis have been standardized by comparison to reference tests, yielding the international normalized ratio (INR). However, the reference tests have for many years been based on samples from patients treated for thromboembolism with warfarin and not on patients with primary liver disease. Attempts have been made to standardize the results also in patients with liver disease [46, 47]. Furthermore, there are in fact two different laboratory methods available for prothrombin time, i.e., the Quick method which is dependent on the levels of factors 2, 7, and 10, which are vitamin K dependent, and on F5 and fibrinogen and on the other hand the Owren method which is only dependent on the levels of factors 2, 7, and 10 [47]. Finally, there are data both from adults and children with chronic liver disease that cholestasis may upregulate the synthesis of several coagulation factors. This can result in paradoxically high levels of certain coagulation factors despite progressive hepatic dysfunction, possibly making them less useful for evaluation of liver capacity in these patients [48, 49]. With the objections above in mind, it is still clear that INR is a widely used marker for synthetic function of the liver. For example, the definition of acute liver failure depends largely on the identification of an INR at or above 2.0 which does not improve on parenteral administration with vitamin K [50]. If the patient is encephalopathic, the corresponding INR level defining acute liver failure is set at 1.5. Since the half-life of the coagulation factors included in the analysis all varies between 6 and 48 h, repeated measurements of INR during the course of acute liver failure are often very relevant to predict the outcome [51].

Furthermore, INR is used as one of the parameters in several pediatric scoring systems, including PELD (pediatric end-stage liver disease) which several countries use for allocation of liver grafts for transplantation. PELD was primarily developed to assess short-term (i.e., 3 months) outcome in pediatric patients with severe chronic liver disease [52]. INR is also included in the King's College criteria for transplantation in acute liver failure [53], in the Wilson index for liver transplantation from the same institution [54], and also in the Liver Injury Unit scoring system suggested by the Pediatric Acute Liver Failure (PALF) Study Group [55].

Individual coagulation factors have for several decades also been used as prognostic markers in severe liver disease. The two main candidates have been factors 5 and 7, respectively.

For factor 5, there are several publications, mainly originating from French adult cohorts, suggesting it to be a useful predictor for outcome in patients with acute liver failure. In one of these, the authors assessed 115 patients above the age of 15 years with fulminant hepatitis B virus infection. In multivariate analysis, factor 5 levels, but not coma development, were found to predict outcome [56]. For comparison, in a British study of 110 patients above 13 years of age with fulminant liver failure, the positive predictive value (0.73) of low factor 5 levels was not as good as the previously mentioned King's College criteria (0.92) for the large subgroup of 88 patients with paracetamol intoxication as etiology. On the other hand, for the smaller subgroup with other etiologies (i.e., mainly viral hepatitis and unknown etiology), the positive predictive values of these two methods were close to 1 both for low factor 5 levels and for the King's College criteria [57].

The usefulness of determining coagulation factor 7 levels to predict outcome was suggested already in the 1970s, i.e., in the largely "pretransplant era." For example, based on a detailed investigation of 12 mainly adult patients with fulminant liver failure, of whom 6 survived and 6 died, it was noted that all patients with a factor 7 level above 9% of the normal survived. This is one of the few studies where both factors 5 and 7 were studied. Interestingly, neither the coma grade nor factor 5 levels could predict outcome as precisely as factor 7 levels [58]. In another report from a tertiary hepatology unit for adults on 68 consecutive patients with acute hepatitis and INR greater than 1.7, factor 7 at admission was a better predictor of outcome than factor 5. However, after 3 days of hospitalization, factor 5 did in fact perform better when predicting outcome, possibly suggesting that repeated measurements could be of value [59].

Other coagulation factors than those previously mentioned have also been suggested as good prognostic markers, for example, antithrombin and fibrinogen [58, 60]. The advantage of using these parameters, in contrast to coagulation factors 5 or 7, would be that the analyses are readily available in most hospital labs and that results can be obtained rapidly. Furthermore, the levels are not dependent on vitamin K levels. On the other hand, data to compare the use of antithrombin and/or fibrinogen with INR or factors 5 and/or 7 as prognostic markers seem very scarce.

It should be noted that the majority of studies published so far deal with adult patients who often have a different disease spectrum than children with liver disease. Furthermore, the levels of basically all coagulation factors have been shown to be different in children. Thus, newborns and infants have significantly lower levels which do increase to near-adult levels by the age of 6 months but do not reach fully adult levels until after puberty [61, 62].

4.5.2 Other Plasma Proteins

Albumin is the most abundantly detected plasma protein produced in the liver, and the levels are easily analyzed. It has therefore been widely used to estimate the synthetic function of the liver. However, the levels are subject to interference for several reasons. They will drop due to losses in patients with concomitant gastrointestinal disease, such as inflammatory bowel disease or celiac disease. Similarly, renal losses, ongoing inflammation, or poor nutritional status may yield lower levels and thereby obscure the interpretation of the results. Additionally, with a half-life of approximately 3 weeks, it is less likely to be of use in the short-term situation of acute liver failure.

With all these limitations in mind, there are still studies showing the importance of low levels of albumin as a prognostic marker, in particular in chronic liver disease [63] but possibly also in more acute situations [64].

Cholinesterase is another plasma protein produced mainly in the liver, and the levels are followed routinely in liver patients in some parts of the world. Although these levels may also be influenced by the nutritional status of the patient, they seem to be useful when predicting outcome, at least for chronic conditions, as shown in a few studies both in adults and children [65, 66]. Interestingly, its half-life is 12 days, i.e., somewhat shorter than that of albumin (Figs. 4.2 and 4.3) [67].

4 Laboratory Evaluation of Hepatobiliary Disease

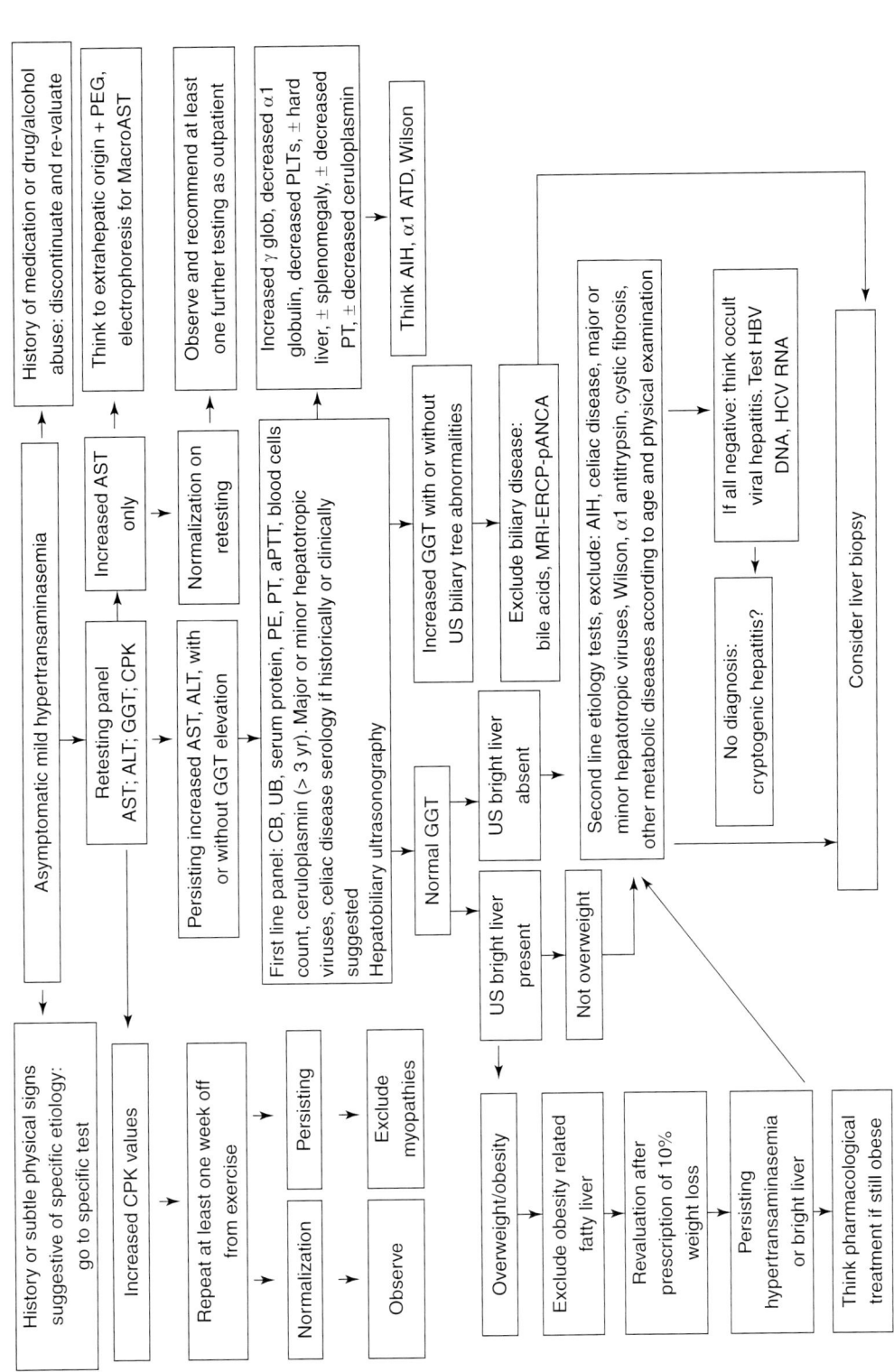

Fig. 4.2 Diagnostic algorithm for the diagnosis of pediatric mild chronic asymptomatic hypertransaminasemia. *ALT* alanine aminotransferase, *AST* aspartate aminotransferase, *CB* conjugated bilirubin, *UB* unconjugated bilirubin, *CPK* creatine kinase, *GGT* gamma-glutamyl transferase, *PE* pulmonary embolism, *PEG* polyethylene glycol, *PT* prothrombin time, *PTT* partial thromboplastin time, *US* ultrasound. *MRI* magnetic resonance imaging, *ERCP* endoscopic retrograde cholangiopancreatography, *pANCA* perinuclear anti-neutrophil cytoplasmic antibodies, *HBV* hepatitis B virus, *HCV* hepatitis V virus, *AIH* autoimmune hepatitis, *α1ATD* α1-antitrypsin deficiency. Suggested figure from Vajro P et al. [13]

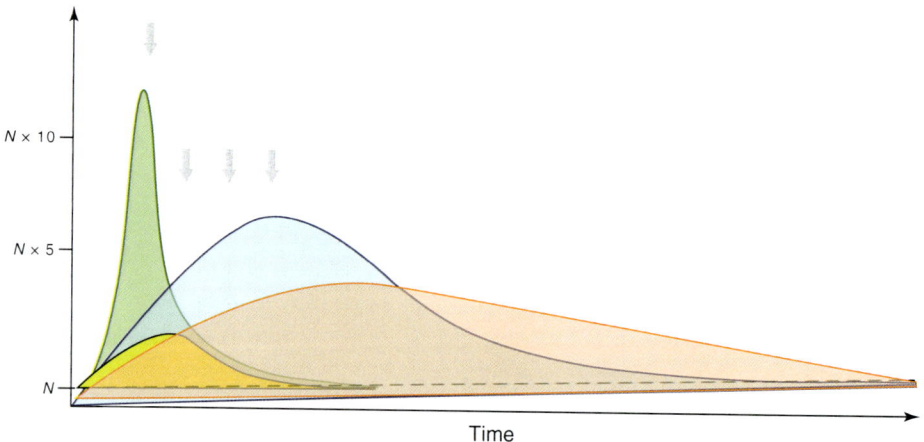

Fig. 4.3 Schematic representation of the rate of change of aminotransferase and bilirubin levels in a patient with acute ischemic hepatitis (green area, yellow area respectively) and acute viral hepatitis (blue area and orange area respectively). It is important to underscore that the pattern of enzyme alteration may vary and occasionally appear similar if a single observation point is taken into consideration (arrows) [70].

References

1. Karmen A, Wroblewski F, Ladue JS. Transaminase activity in human blood. J Clin Invest. 1955;34(1):126–31. PubMed PMID: 13221663; PubMed Central PMCID: PMC438594.
2. Panteghini M. Aspartate aminotransferase isoenzymes. Clin Biochem. 1990;23(4):311–9. Review. PubMed PMID: 2225456.
3. Price CP, Alberti KG. Biochemical assessment of liver function. In: Wright R, Alberti KGMM, Karran S, Millward-Sadler GH, editors. Liver and biliary disease—pathophysiology, diagnosis, management. London: WB Saunders; 1979. p. 381–416.
4. Dybkaer R. The tortuous road to the adoption of katal for the expression of catalytic activity by the General Conference on Weights and Measures. Clin Chem. 2002;48(3):586–90. PubMed PMID: 11861460.
5. Nuttall FQ, Jones B. Creatine kinase and glutamic oxalacetic transaminase activity in serum: kinetics of change with exercise and effect of physical conditioning. J Lab Clin Med. 1968;71(5):847–54. PubMed PMID: 5647686.
6. Pettersson J, Hindorf U, Persson P, Bengtsson T, Malmqvist U, Werkström V, Ekelund M. Muscular exercise can cause highly pathological liver function tests in healthy men. Br J Clin Pharmacol. 2008;65(2):253–9. PubMed PMID: 17764474.
7. Córdoba J, O'Riordan K, Dupuis J, Borensztajin J, Blei AT. Diurnal variation of serum alanine transaminase activity in chronic liver disease. Hepatology. 1998;28(6):1724–5. PubMed PMID: 9890798.
8. Rivera-Coll A, Fuentes-Arderiu X, Díez-Noguera A. Circadian rhythms of serum concentrations of 12 enzymes of clinical interest. Chronobiol Int. 1993;10(3):190–200. PubMed PMID: 8100488.
9. Rödöö P, Ridefelt P, Aldrimer M, Niklasson F, Gustafsson J, Hellberg D. Population-based pediatric reference intervals for HbA1c, bilirubin, albumin, CRP, myoglobin and serum enzymes. Scand J Clin Lab Invest. 2013;73(5):361–7. PubMed PMID: 23581477.
10. Williams KM, Williams AE, Kline LM, Dodd RY. Stability of serum alanine aminotransferase activity. Transfusion. 1987;27(5):431–3. PubMed PMID: 3629675.
11. Caropreso M, Fortunato G, Lenta S, Palmieri D, Esposito M, Vitale DF, Iorio R, Vajro P. Prevalence and long-term course of macro-aspartate aminotransferase in children. J Pediatr. 2009;154(5):744–8. https://doi.org/10.1016/j.jpeds.2008.11.010. Epub 2008 Dec 25. PubMed PMID: 19111320.
12. Moriyama T, Tamura S, Nakano K, Otsuka K, Shigemura M, Honma N. Laboratory and clinical features of abnormal macroenzymes found in human sera. Biochim Biophys Acta. 2015;1854(6):658–67.
13. Vajro P, Maddaluno S, Veropalumbo C. Persistent hypertransaminasemia in asymptomatic children: a stepwise approach. World J Gastroenterol. 2013;19(18):2740–51. Review. PubMed PMID: 23687411.
14. Rosenthal P, Haight M. Aminotransferase as a prognostic index in infants with liver disease. Clin Chem. 1990;36(2):346–8.
15. Lamireau T, McLin V, Nobili V, Vajro P. A practical approach to the child with abnormal liver tests. Clin Res Hepatol Gastroenterol. 2014;38:259–62.
16. Thierfelder N, Demuth I, Burghardt N, Schmelz K, Sperling K, Chrzanowska KH, Seemanova E, Digweed M. Extreme variation in apoptosis capacity amongst lymphoid cells of Nijmegen breakage syndrome patients. Eur J Cell Biol. 2008;87(2):111–21. Epub 2007 Oct 30. PubMed PMID: 17977616.
17. George J, Denney-Wilson E, Okely AD, Hardy LL, Aitken R. The population distributions, upper normal limits and correlations between liver tests among Australian adolescents. J Paediatr Child Health. 2008;44(10):579–85. PubMed PMID: 19012630.
18. England K, Thorne C, Pembrey L, Tovo PA, Newell ML. Age- and sex-related reference ranges of alanine aminotransferase levels in children: European paediatric HCV network. J Pediatr Gastroenterol Nutr. 2009;49(1):71–7. PubMed PMID: 19465871.
19. Lai DS, Chen SC, Chang YH, Chen CY, Lin JB, Lin YJ, Yang SF, Yang CC, Chen WK, Lin DB. Pediatric reference intervals for several biochemical analytes in school children in Central Taiwan. J Formos Med Assoc. 2009;108(12):957–63.
20. Southcott EK, Kerrigan JL, Potter JM, Telford RD, Waring P, Reynolds GJ, Lafferty AR, Hickman PE. Establishment of pediatric reference intervals on a large cohort of healthy children. Clin Chim Acta. 2010;411(19–20):1421–7. PubMed PMID: 20598674.
21. Colantonio DA, Kyriakopoulou L, Chan MK, Daly CH, Brinc D, Venner AA, Pasic MD, Armbruster D, Adeli K. Closing the gaps in pediatric laboratory reference intervals: a CALIPER database of 40 biochemical markers in a healthy and multiethnic population of children. Clin Chem. 2012;58(5):854–68. PubMed PMID: 22371482.

22. Hilsted L, Rustad P, Aksglæde L, Sørensen K, Juul A. Recommended Nordic paediatric reference intervals for 21 common biochemical properties. Scand J Clin Lab Invest. 2013;73(1):1–9. Epub 2012 Sep 26.
23. Bussler S, Vogel M, Pietzner D, Harms K, Buzek T, Penke M, Händel N, Körner A, Baumann U, Kiess W, Flemming G. New pediatric percentiles of liver enzyme serum levels (ALT, AST, GGT): Effects of age, sex, BMI and pubertal stage. Hepatology. 2018;68(4):1319–30. PubMed PMID: 28926121.
24. Schwimmer JB, Dunn W, Norman GJ, Pardee PE, Middleton MS, Kerkar N, Sirlin CB. SAFETY study: alanine aminotransferase cutoff values are set too high for reliable detection of pediatric chronic liver disease. Gastroenterology. 2010;138(4):1357–64, 1364. PubMed PMID: 20064512.
25. Robison R. The possible significance of hexosephosphoric esters in ossification. Biochem J. 1923;17(2):286–93. PubMed PMID: 16743183.
26. Van Hoof VO, De Broe ME. Interpretation and clinical significance of alkaline phosphatase isoenzyme patterns. Crit Rev Clin Lab Sci. 1994;31(3):197–293. Review. PubMed PMID: 7818774.
27. Sharma U, Pal D, Prasad R. Alkaline phosphatase: an overview. Indian J Clin Biochem. 2014;29(3):269–78. Review. PubMed PMID: 24966474.
28. Carroll AJ, Coakley JC. Transient hyperphosphatasaemia: an important condition to recognize. J Paediatr Child Health. 2001;37(4):359–62. PubMed PMID: 11532055.
29. Gualco G, Lava SA, Garzoni L, Simonetti GD, Bettinelli A, Milani GP, Provero MC, Bianchetti MG. Transient benign hyperphosphatasemia. J Pediatr Gastroenterol Nutr. 2013;57(2):167–71. PubMed PMID: 23539049.
30. Shaver WA, Bhatt H, Combes B. Low serum alkaline phosphatase activity in Wilson's disease. Hepatology. 1986;6(5):859–63.
31. Whyte MP. Hypophosphatasia and the role of alkaline phosphatase in skeletal mineralization. Endocr Rev. 1994;15(4):439–61. Review. PubMed PMID: 7988481.
32. Hanes CS, Hird FJ, Isherwood FA. Synthesis of peptides in enzymic reactions involving glutathione. Nature. 1950;166(4216):288–92. PubMed PMID: 15439292.
33. Goldberg DM. Structural, functional, and clinical aspects of gamma-glutamyltransferase. CRC Crit Rev Clin Lab Sci. 1980;12(1):1–58. Review. PubMed PMID: 6104563.
34. Vroon DH, Israili Z. Chapter 100. Alkaline phosphatase and gamma glutamyltransferase. In: Walker HK, Hall WD, Hurst JW, editors. Clinical methods: the history, physical, and laboratory examinations. 3rd ed. Boston: Butterworths; 1990. PubMed PMID: 21250047.
35. Cabrera-Abreu JC, Green A. Gamma-glutamyltransferase: value of its measurement in paediatrics. Ann Clin Biochem. 2002;39(Pt 1):22–5. Review. PubMed PMID: 11853185.
36. Wang NL, Li LT, Wu BB, Gong JY, Abuduxikuer K, Li G, Wang JS. The features of GGT in patients with ATP8B1 or ABCB11 deficiency improve the diagnostic efficiency. PLoS One. 2016;11(4):e0153114. PubMed PMID: 27050426.
37. Fischler B, Eggertsen G, Björkhem I. Genetic defects in synthesis and transport of bile acids. In: Pediatric endocrinology and metabolic diseases. 2017. p. 447–60.
38. Suchy FJ, Balistreri WF, Heubi JE, Searcy JE, Levin RS. Physiologic cholestasis: elevation of the primary serum bile acid concentrations in normal infants. Gastroenterology. 1981;80:1037–41.
39. Gitlin D, Perricelli A, Gitlin GM. Synthesis of α-fetoprotein by liver, yolk sac, and gastrointestinal tract of the human conceptus. Cancer Res. 1972;32:979–82.
40. Blohm ME, Vesterling-Hörner D, Calaminus G, et al. Alpha 1-fetoprotein (AFP) reference values in infants up to 2 years of age. Pediatr Hematol Oncol. 1998;15:135–42.
41. Murray MJ, Nicholson JC. α-Fetoprotein. Arch Dis Child Educ Pract Ed. 2011;96:141–7.
42. De Ioris M, Brugieres L, Zimmermann A, et al. Hepatoblastoma with a low serum alpha-fetoprotein level at diagnosis: the SIOPEL group experience. Eur J Cancer. 2008;44:545–50.
43. Koprowaski H, Steplewski Z, Mitchell K, et al. Colorectal carcinoma antigens detected by hybridoma antibodies. Somatic Cell Genet. 1979;5:957–72.
44. Nehls O, Gregor M, Klump B. Serum and bile markers for cholangiocarcinoma. Semin Liver Dis. 2004;24:139–54.
45. Lamerz R. Role of tumour markers, cytogenetics. Ann Oncol. 1999;10(Suppl. 4):S145–9.
46. Tripodi A, Chantarangkul V, Primignani M, Fabris F, Dell'Era A, Sei C, Mannucci PM. The international normalized ratio calibrated for cirrhosis (INR(liver)) normalizes prothrombin time results for model for end-stage liver disease calculation. Hepatology. 2007;46(2):520–7.
47. Magnusson M, Sten-Linder M, Bergquist A, et al. The international normalized ratio according to Owren in liver disease: interlaboratory assessment and determination of international sensitivity index. Thromb Res. 2013;132:346–51.
48. Cederblad G, Korsan-Bengtsen K, Olsson R. Observations of increased levels of blood coagulation factors and other plasma proteins in cholestatic liver disease. Scand J Gastroenterol. 1976;11:391–6.
49. Magnusson M, Fischler B, Svensson J, Petrini P, Schulman S, Németh A. Bile acids and coagulation factors: paradoxical association in children with chronic liver disease. Eur J Gastroenterol Hepatol. 2013;25:152–8.
50. Squires RH, Schneider BL, Bucuvalas J, et al. Acute liver failure in children: the first 348 patients in the Pediatric Acute Liver Failure Study Group. J Pediatr. 2006;148:652–8.
51. Franchini M, Lippi G. Prothrombin complex concentrates: an update. Blood Transfus. 2010;8(3):149–54.
52. McDiarmid SV, Anand R, Lindblad AS, Principal Investigators and Institutions of the Studies of Pediatric Liver Transplantation (SPLIT) Research Group. Development of a pediatric end-stage liver disease score to predict poor outcome in children awaiting liver transplantation. Transplantation. 2002;27:173–81.
53. O'Grady JG, Alexander GJ, Hayllar KM, Williams R. Early indicators of prognosis in fulminant hepatic failure. Gastroenterology. 1989;97:439–45.
54. Dhawan A, Taylor RM, Cheeseman P, et al. Wilson's disease in children: 37-year experience and revised King's score for liver transplantation. Liver Transpl. 2005;11:441–8.
55. Lu BR, Zhang S, Narkewicz MR, et al. Evaluation of the liver injury unit scoring system to predict survival in a multinational study of pediatric acute liver failure. J Pediatr. 2013;162:1010–6.
56. Bernuau J, Goudeau A, Poynard T, et al. Multivariate analysis of prognostic factors in fulminant hepatitis B. Hepatology. 1986;6:648–51.
57. Izumi S, Langley PG, Wendon J, et al. Coagulation factor V levels as a prognostic indicator in fulminant hepatic failure. Hepatology. 1996;23:1507–11.
58. Dymock IW, Tucker JS, Woolf IL, Poller L, Thomson JM. Coagulation studies as a prognostic index in acute liver failure. Br J Haematol. 1975;29:385–95.
59. Elinav E, Ben-Dov I, Hai-Am E, Ackerman Z, Ofran Y. The predictive value of admission and follow up factor V and VII levels in patients with acute hepatitis and coagulopathy. J Hepatol. 2005;42(1):82–6.
60. Rodzynek JJ, Preux C, Leautaud P, Abramovici J, Di Paolo A, Delcourt AA. Diagnostic value of antithrombin III and aminopyrine breath test in liver disease. Arch Intern Med. 1986;146:677–80.
61. Andrew M, Paes B, Milner R, et al. Development of the human coagulation system in the full-term infant. Blood. 1987;70:165–72.

62. Monagle P, Massicotte P. Developmental haemostasis: secondary haemostasis. Semin Fetal Neonatal Med. 2011;16:294–300.
63. Watanabe T. Short-term prognostic factors for primary sclerosing cholangitis. J Hepatobiliary Pancreat Sci. 2015;22:486–90.
64. Dabos KJ, Newsome PN, Parkinson JA, et al. Biochemical prognostic markers of outcome in non-paracetamol-induced fulminant hepatic failure. Transplantation. 2004;77:200–5.
65. Pferdmenges DC, Baumann U, Müller-Heine A, Framke T, Pfister ED. Prognostic marker for liver disease due to alpha1-antitrypsin deficiency. Klin Padiatr. 2013;225:257–62.
66. Abbas M, Abbas Z. Serum cholinesterase: a predictive biomarker of hepatic reserves in chronic hepatitis D. World J Hepatol. 2017;9:967–72.
67. Santarpia L, Grandone I, Contaldo F, Pasanisi F. Butyrylcholinesterase as a prognostic marker: a review of the literature. J Cachexia Sarcopenia Muscle. 2013;4(1):31–9.
68. Botros M, Sikaris KA. The de ritis ratio: the test of time. Clin Biochem Rev. 2013;34(3):117–30. Review. PubMed PMID: 24353357.
69. Tsuchida Y, Endo Y, Saito S, Kaneko M, Shiraki K, Ohmi K. Evaluation of alpha-fetoprotein in early infancy. J Pediatr Surg. 1978;13(2):155–62. PubMed PMID: 77324.
70. Giannini EG, et al. Liver enzyme alteration: a guide for clinicians. CMAJ. 2005;172(3):367–79.

Diagnostic and Interventional Radiology

R. Agazzi, P. Tessitore, and S. Sironi

Key Points
- Radiology plays a key role in the management of children with liver disease and transplant recipients.
- The main informations provided by radiology are the presence of anatomical variants, abnormal liver texture in chronic and storage disease, and focal lesions.
- Radiology evaluation of children requires special expertise in obtaining patient comfort and achieving knowledge on liver disease that are peculiar to the pediatric age.
- The availability of skilled interventional radiology is mandatory in pediatric liver transplantation centers, to allow prompt recognition of complications and treat them avoiding surgery.

Research Needed in the Field
- Improvement of MRI technique to reduce breathing artifacts and to refine spatial resolution of MRCP in very young children.
- Improvement of MRI sequences to gain not only a morphologic information but also functional data (e.g., T1 mapping of liver function, MRI as a marker of therapeutic response of malignant lesion after chemotherapy).
- Extend the use of contrast-enhanced ultrasound for liver transplant vascular complications avoiding the need for invasive imaging studies based on ionizing radiation and the use of iodinated or gadolinium contrast medium.
- Develop interventional devices tailored for children.

5.1 Introduction

The primary imaging modalities called upon to evaluate the pediatric liver are ultrasound (US), computed tomography (CT), and magnetic resonance imaging (MRI).

Ultrasound (with the combination of gray-scale and Doppler) is the initial imaging modality of choice for liver examination.

The advantages are it does not make use of ionizing radiation and may be repeated over and over again for follow-up studies, without any significant risks; it has real-time imaging capabilities; it can demonstrate the hepatic parenchyma, vessels, and bile ducts with a quite exquisite spatial resolution; it can be performed at the bedside; and it is less expensive than other modalities. This radiation-free modality is particularly attractive in children in which high-frequency linear array transducers are most commonly used providing excellent spatial resolution due to their reduced tissue thickness.

The limitations are as follows: the small acoustic window (bowel gas, obesity, and overlying bandaging) and the exam is operator dependent.

R. Agazzi
Interventional Radiology, Department of Diagnostic Radiology,
H Papa Giovanni XIII, Bergamo, BG, Italy
e-mail: ragazzi@asst-pg23.it

P. Tessitore
Department of Diagnostic Radiology,
H Papa Giovanni XIII, Bergamo, BG, Italy
e-mail: ptessitore@asst-pg23.it

S. Sironi (✉)
Department of Diagnostic Radiology,
H Papa Giovanni XIII, Bergamo, BG, Italy

Post-Graduate School of Radiology,
University of Milano-Bicocca, Monza, MB, Italy
e-mail: ssironi@asst-pg23.it

© Springer Nature Switzerland AG 2019
L. D'Antiga (ed.), *Pediatric Hepatology and Liver Transplantation*, https://doi.org/10.1007/978-3-319-96400-3_5

The conventional B-mode US gives information about liver volume, shape, and texture of parenchyma and biliary tree. Doppler US can measure hepatic blood flow and velocity, as well as evaluate indirect signs of portal venous hypertension and vascular complication after transplant. Ultrasound elastography techniques as transient elastography (FibroScan®), acoustic radiation force impulse imaging (ARFI), shear wave mode elastography, and strain elastography can be used to quantify liver stiffness as a marker of fibrosis and cirrhosis [1]. Ultrasound can also be integrated with contrast enhancement (CEUS) to characterize focal liver lesions. It needs to be underlined that US contrast agents registered in Europe are licensed only in adults for cardiac or, in the case of SonoVue®, liver, vascular [2], and breast applications. For the pediatric population, SonoVue® is recommended only for urinary tract, and the endovascular use is still off label. In cases in which US results are inconclusive, confirmation is required or clinical suspicion for a complication persists despite normal US results, CT or MRI imaging is performed. Conventional angiographic and cholangiographic studies should be reserved for nonsurgical treatment of some complications.

Computed Tomography (CT) should be used in case ultrasound does not provide an exhaustive evaluation and in emergency situations.

Advantages of CT scan are (a) rapidity that, especially with the most modern dual source tomographs, allows avoiding sedation in some cases, (b) reliability and reproducibility, and (c) availability of multi-planar cross-sectional imaging studies with an optimal anatomical spatial resolution. CT for liver investigation is performed with contrast medium that allows the detailed evaluation of parenchymatous organs, biliary tree, and arterial and venous structures. The disadvantage is ionizing radiation exposure. The increase of cancer risk is directly proportional to dose delivered. Risk factor for cancer induction in children is about ten times higher than in adults [3], and the risk of leukemia and brain cancer is three times higher with cumulative doses of 50 mGy and 60 mGy, respectively. Besides, children have longer life expectancy. Therefore, they have a greater potential for manifestation of possible harmful effects of radiations [4, 5].

Magnetic resonance imaging (MRI), as well as CT, has the capability of providing comprehensive morphologic evaluation of liver (parenchyma, biliary system, and vasculature), but the imaging characterization compared to normal hepatic parenchyma both before and following contrast enhancement is able to provide greater tissue differentiation than available with CT and US. The multi-planar competences permit anatomical localization similar to CT with the added advantage of not exposing the child to ionizing radiation. MRI is preferred over CT scan for most of the cross-sectional imaging workups in children. The major limitation of MRI is the time required to complete a comprehensive contrast study, which can take up to 1 h. As a result, young children often require sedation or even deep anesthesia [6]. In infants there might be the possibility of hyperthermia due to poorly developed thermoregulatory mechanisms in children, high basal temperatures, and relatively higher surface area to weight ratio [7–9]. The use of contrast medium must always be carefully evaluated due to recent evidences of Gadolinium-based contrast agent brain deposition and the concern about long-term effects of storage of contrast [10]. Furthermore, MRI contrast agents should be used with caution in children less than 1 year because of immature renal function. They should be carefully used even in the perioperative liver transplantation period and only following risk-benefit assessment due to the risk, rare but possible, of systemic nephrogenic fibrosis [11].

5.2 Focal Liver Lesions

The finding of a focal hepatic lesion in a child is not an uncommon event. This may represent a diagnostic challenge, since it requires the differential diagnosis between a neoplasm (benign, borderline, or malignant), a vascular malformation, and an infectious disease. In this section the benign and malignant tumor focal lesions will be discussed.

Hepatic liver tumor (HT) in the pediatric patients is rare, constituting about 5–6% of all pathological intra-abdominal masses [12]. As in adulthood, the most common neoplasm involving the liver in children is metastatic disease [13].

About two-thirds of most primary liver masses are malignant, and almost 70% of those are hepatocellular in origin, either hepatoblastomas or hepatocellular carcinomas [14]. Most benign focal liver lesions are inborn and may grow like the rest of the body, being either of mesenchymal or epithelial origin.

5.2.1 Benign Liver Lesions

The most common benign tumors are, in decreasing order of frequency, infantile hepatic hemangioendothelioma, mesenchymal hamartoma, focal nodular hyperplasia (FNH), and hepatocellular adenoma [15].

5.2.1.1 Infantile Hepatic Hemangioendothelioma
Infantile hemangioendothelioma, or infantile hepatic hemangioma (IHH), is the most common benign hepatic tumor of infancy, accounting 10–12% of all pediatric liver tumors. Female are more frequently affected than boys with incidence ratio 3:1 [2, 16]. About one-half of cases occur as solitary masses and one-half are multifocal [2]. The majority of IHHs, about 90% of cases, are usually diagnosed as an incidental finding in the first 6 months of life, rarely detected after the first year [17]. Screening for liver is requested when five or more cutaneous infantile hemangiomas are noticed [16]. Infantile hemangioma is traditionally considered a tumor of the microvasculature characterized by immature endothelial cells proliferation. Recent data suggest a putative origin in the embolism of placental chorionic villous mesenchymal core

cells during the first trimester, with subsequent proliferation and differentiation of a hemogenic endothelium [18]. The most common form of presentation is that of an abdominal mass due to hepatomegaly. IHHs are characterized by a rapid proliferative phase in the first 6–10 months, followed by a slow involution, which can last up to 10 years [18]. The biologic behavior is usually benign, but serious clinical complications may develop: congestive heart failure due to high-flow arteriovenous shunts (25% of cases); hypothyroidism may be caused by high levels of type III iodothyronine deiodinase activity produced by the tumor leading to cardiac dysfunction and mental retardation [19, 20]; rarely, trapping of platelets, resulting in thrombocytopenia due to intratumoral platelet sequestration (Kasabach-Merritt syndrome), may occur; and jaundice and rupture of a superficial IHH with hemoperitoneum are also possible complications [21]. Patients with multifocal liver lesions may have additional hemangiomas involving other sites: the skin, trachea, thorax, adrenal gland, and dura mater with a reported prevalence of up to 68%. However, larger series suggest that the prevalence is lower (10–15%) [17]. This is the reason why patients with multiple liver lesions should be evaluated with chest radiography and brain imaging [22]. IHH management is not standardized. It is a very vascularized tumor for which biopsy is a procedure that must be performed with great caution. If possible diagnosis can be made on the basis of typical imaging characteristic and the observation of involution over time. However, biopsy is a valid help to rule out histological type II lesions. In fact, imaging is not able to differentiate between different histological types (I and II). Type II IHH shows more immature cells and a more aggressive behavior than type I IHH. In our center, we managed 27 patients, and we found that 15% had poor prognosis, predicted by diffuse lesions, late presentation, cardiac failure, and type II histology; we concluded that these patients should be approached more aggressively (unpublished data). IHH typically presents in three different patterns: focal, multifocal, and diffuse lesions. Large focal lesions often show central hemorrhage, necrosis, fibrosis, and calcification. In the multifocal pattern, the lesions tend to be small and well defined and with uniform appearance. In diffuse disease, the lesions have poorly defined margins and an infiltrative growth with subversion of the hepatic parenchyma; the massive hepatomegaly can cause mass effect on adjacent organs and compression of the inferior vena cava [2, 17]. Sonographic and Doppler features are suggestive of IHH but not diagnostic. The main role of US is the initial detection of lesions and the follow-up. At US, multifocal and large IHH appear as well-demarcated masses that are hypoechoic or of mixed echogenicity (Fig. 5.1) with calcifications seen in up to 36% of cases. The hyperechoic pattern is uncommon. IHHs are high-flow lesion with a vascularization consisting of both arterial and venous hypertrophic vessels, both inside and perilesional (Fig. 5.2). There are several patterns of flow at color and spectral Doppler that can be detected within the lesion, depending on the various shunts that are created between the arterial and venous vessels: (a) arterial flow with little systolic-diastolic variation, (b) arterial and venous waveforms with high-frequency shifts, and (c) arterial and venous flow with low-frequency signals [17]. During the follow-up of the lesion will show not only the dimensional reduction but also the decrease of the arteriovenous shunts and inflow velocity. Findings at dynamic contrast-enhanced CT are often diagnostic, but this method is less used than MRI for the ionizing radiation exposure. At precontrast images, the lesion appears as hypodense and well defined; in the large masses, speckled calcifications are not uncommon. A typical lesion after contrast medium administration will show a peripheral nodular enhancement during arterial phase with progressive centripetal filling on portal venous and delayed phases. Large lesions can demonstrate a lesser homogeneity of structure due to central areas of necrosis and fibrosis that have no enhancement; instead small lesions can show an intense and uniform enhancement. The best diagnostic modality for a confident diagnosis of IHH is the MRI. On precontrast T1-weighted

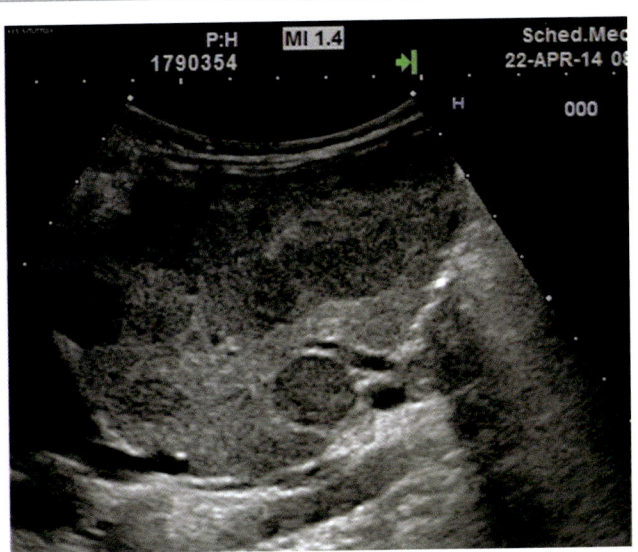

Fig. 5.1 Multifocal hypoechoic well-demarcated IHH

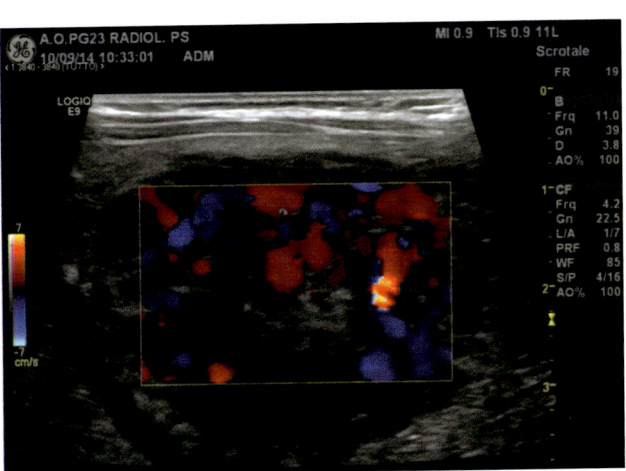

Fig. 5.2 Color US evaluation of IHH shows arterial (red color) and venous (blue color) hypertrophic intralesional vessels

images, IHHs are generally hypointense, sometimes with hyperintense foci of hemorrhage. On T2-weighted images, IHHs are markedly hyperintense. The enhancement pattern is similar to that seen on contrast-enhanced CT, with a centripetal filling pattern (Fig. 5.3) [17].

5.2.1.2 Mesenchymal Hamartoma

Mesenchymal hamartoma (MH) is the second most frequent benign liver lesion in children younger than 2 years, with 80% of lesions presenting within the two first years of life with male prevalence [17, 23]. In surgical series MH represent 8% of all pediatric hepatic tumors [2]. The clinical scenario can be that of a palpable mass, gastrointestinal symptoms, anorexia, and respiratory distress. A complete radical resection is the treatment of choice, with the possibility of local recurrence as an undifferentiated embryonic sarcoma [23]. Histologically, MA presents a disorganized proliferation of mesenchyme along periportal tracts containing bile ducts, normal hepatocyte cords, and cysts of different sizes. The fibromyxoid stroma is characterized by spindle cells in a porous mucopolysaccharide-rich matrix that permits the accumulation of fluid with tumor enlargement up to 30 cm [2, 17, 23]. In the younger pediatric population, the lesion is characterized by proliferating components represented by single or branching bile ducts, whereas the hepatocytes, which are compressed at the periphery of the mass, likely represent an inactive component. In older children, it has been described a more differentiated lesion with poor presence of ductular component, a prominent myxoid stroma, and absent cystic spaces [24]. The macroscopical appearance ranges from a prevalent cystic lesion content to prevalent solid component with small cysts, which constitutes a spectrum from a predominantly cystic mass to a predominantly solid mass containing a few small cysts. This wide spectrum influence imaging features. Cystic portions with thin or thick septa are avascular and solid portions are relatively hypovascular.

At US, the cystic portions have similar characteristics as other fluid-filled structures appearing anechoic or nearly anechoic with thin or thick echogenic septations. Low-level echoes may be seen within the fluid, presumably reflecting gelatinous content. The solid portions are echogenic. Color Doppler imaging shows relatively little blood flow, which is limited to solid portions and septa [2, 6, 17]. Imaging by CT is characterized by a heterogeneous cystic mass: cystic lesions show water attenuation and solid components that are hypodense. After contrast medium administration, enhancement will be demonstrated only in the internal septa and stromal portions. MRI signal is conditioned by complex hamartoma composition: cystic portions are hyperintense on T2-weighted images and show variable signal intensity on T1-weighted images (hypointensity or slightly hyperintensity) depending on the protein content of fluid. Solid portions are hypointense in T1- and T2-weighted images. As for the CT enhancement following contrast, this is mild and limited to septations and solid components [17].

5.2.1.3 Focal Nodular Hyperplasia

Focal nodular hyperplasia (FNH) is a benign epithelial liver tumor believed to originate from a hyperplastic response to a preexisting vascular anomaly or acquired vascular injury [25]. The gross appearance is of a solitary well-defined solid mass with a central stellate scar. Pediatric cases of FNH are unusual, accounting for only 2–7% of all pediatric hepatic tumors. There is a female predominance with age prevalence in 7–8-year-old children, although all pediatric age groups can be affected [2]. FNHs are seen with increased frequency in long-term survivors of childhood malignancies. In fact, it seems that acquired vascular injury by chemotherapy or radiotherapy with subsequent localized circulatory disturbances, such as thrombosis, high sinusoidal pressure, or increased flow, leads to the development of FNH long after completion of therapy. Histologically the lesion is characterized by a polyclonal proliferation of functioning hepatocytes, Kupffer cells, vascular structures, and biliary epithelium which forms ductules with no connection to biliary tree. The inner scar is constituted of a central artery and small veins in a centrifugal arrangement in a myxomatous stroma [17]. The appearance of FNH at imaging reflects both its histologic features and a preexisting history of malignancy. Towbin et al. demonstrated that patients without a history of malignancy usually had a single larger lesion and were more likely to have a central scar. Patients with a history of malignancy were more likely to have multiple smaller lesions and a lower frequency of a central scar (Fig. 5.4) [25, 26]. At US FNH can show a homogeneous isoechoic, hypoechoic, or hyperechoic lesion, sharply demarcated with a hyperechoic central scar. At color and power Doppler, the central scar shows an increased vascularity compared to the rest of the mass; the spectral analysis reveals an inner arterial flow. This feature allows distinguishing FNH from adenoma, the latter characterized by a venous inner flow. At unenhanced CT, FNH is typically well circumscribed and iso- to slightly hypoattenuated. After administration of contrast medium, FNH typically demonstrates uniform enhancement in the arterial phase, except for fibrous septa and central scars; CT angiography allows to demonstrate the central feeding artery with a "spoke-wheel" shape [27]. In the portal venous phase, FNH becomes isodense or hyperdense to the liver and isodense in delayed phases (Fig. 5.5). CT in the portal vein phase shows the vessels drain directly into the hepatic vein. The stellate scar typically shows a delayed enhancement to the remainder of the mass as contrast material diffuses into the myxomatous stroma. In the half of the lesions atypical features can be seen: lack of the central scar, rapid washout in the portal venous phase, lack of enhancement of the central scar on delayed images, early draining veins, and partial peripheral rim-like enhancement on delayed images [17, 27]. In this

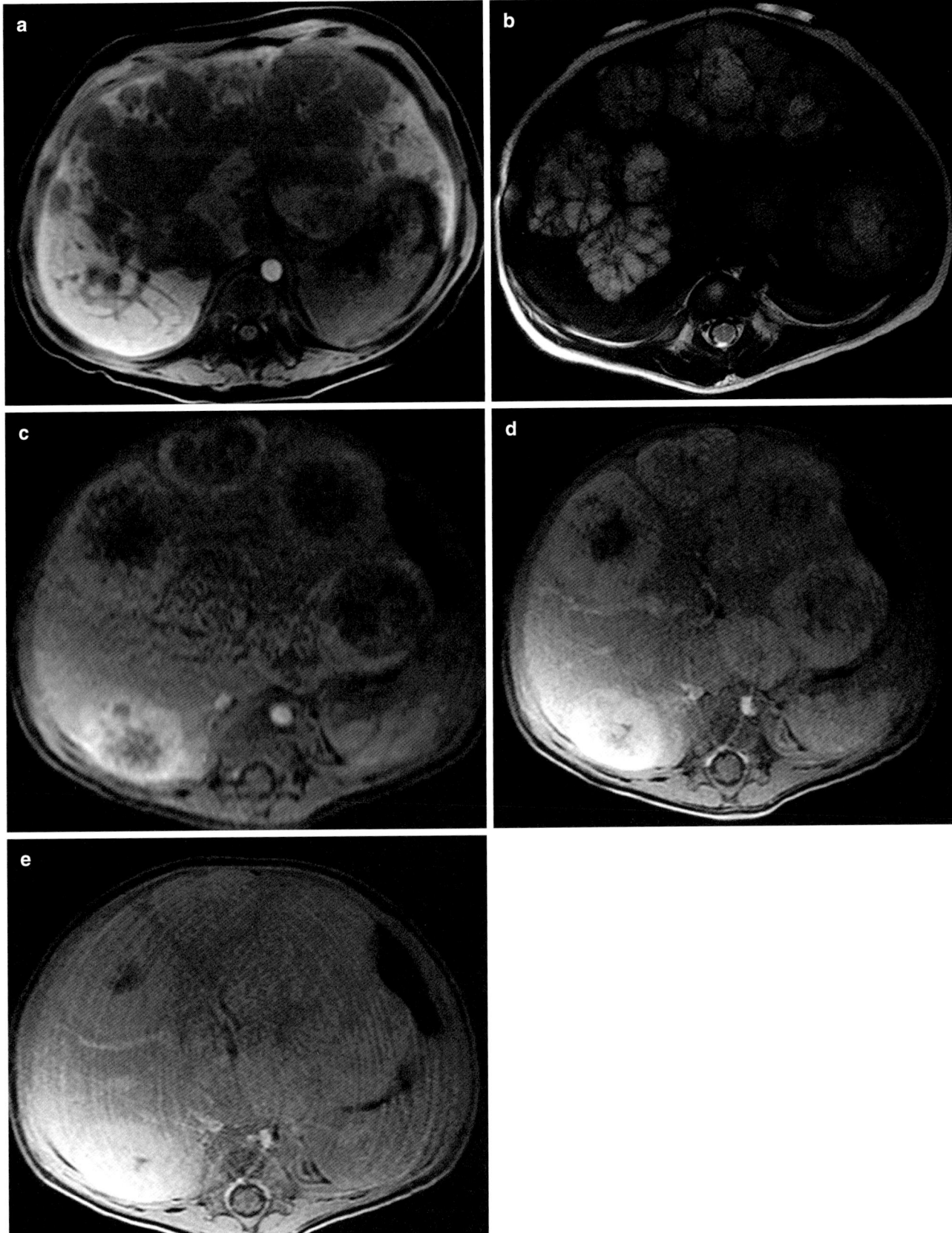

Fig. 5.3 MRI IHHs pre- and post-contrast enhancement. On precontrast T1-weighted image (**a**), IHHs are hypointense. On T2-weighted image (**b**), IHHs are markedly hyperintense. Post-contrast phases show a peripheral nodular enhancement during arterial phase (**c**) with progressive centripetal filling on portal venous (**d**) and delayed phases (**e**). These large lesions demonstrate a central area of necrosis and fibrosis that has no enhancement

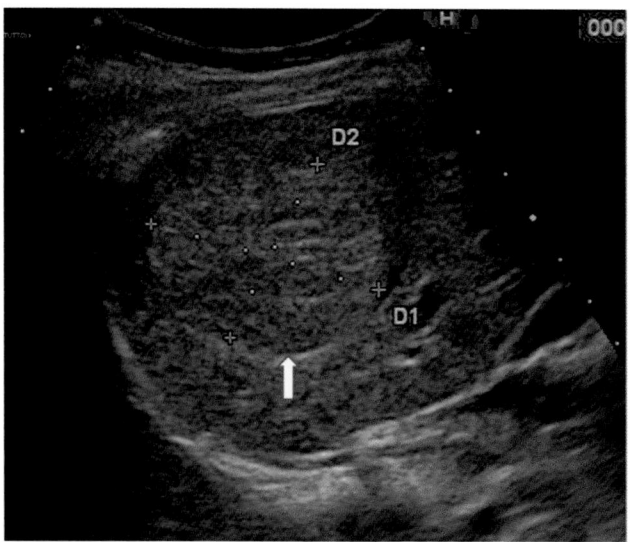

Fig. 5.4 B-mode US shows a homogeneous isoechoic sharply demarcated FNH without a recognizable central scar

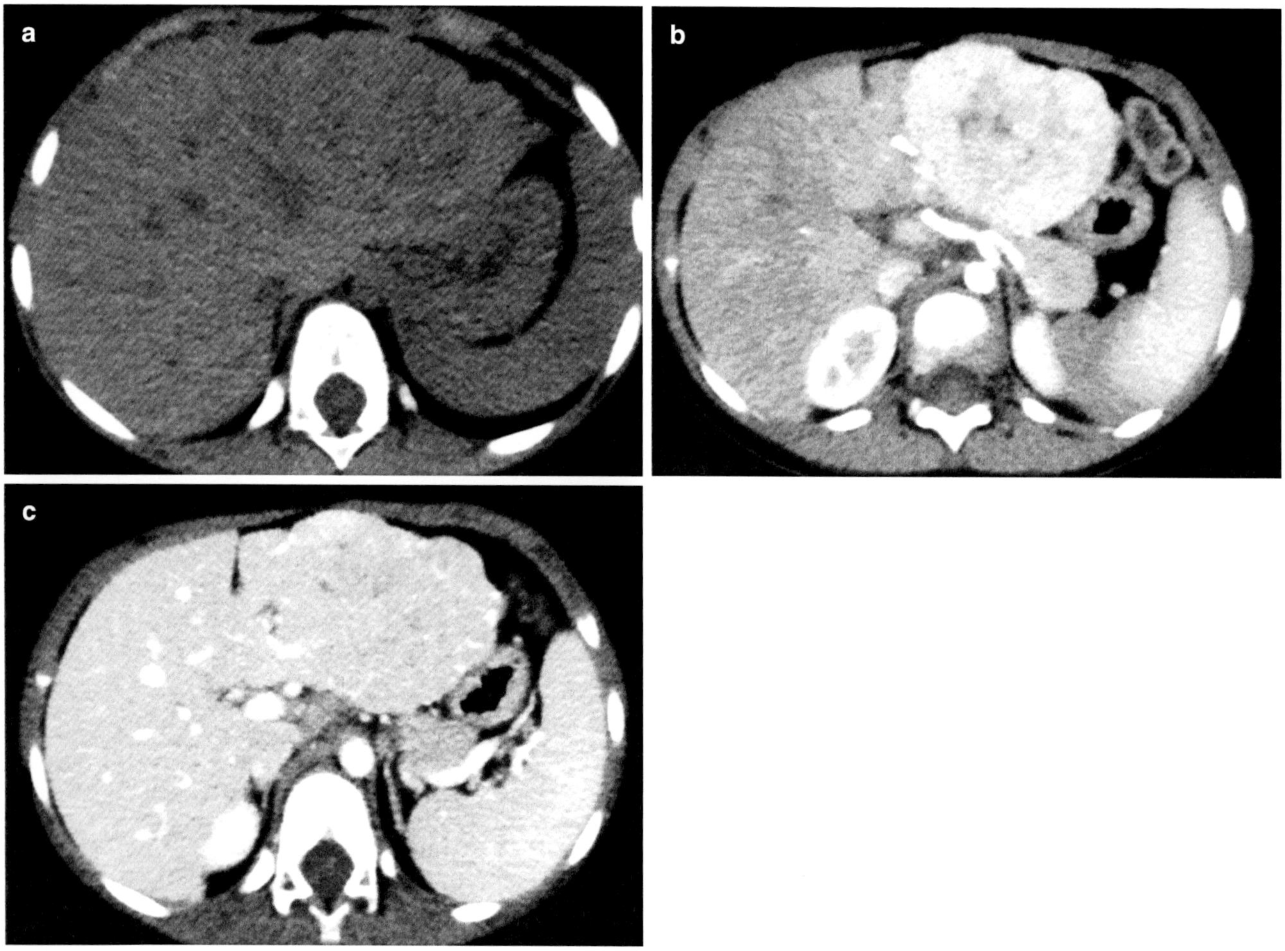

case the diagnosis is less certain. At precontrast MR imaging, FNH shows an homogeneous isointense to slightly hypointense signal on T1-weighted images and isointense to slightly hyperintense on T2-weighted images. The edema inside the central scar influences the signal hyperintensity on T2-weighted images (Fig. 5.6). After gadolinium administration FNH has the same features observed in CT examination: early uniform enhancement on the arterial phase with hyperintensity of the lesion and isointensity to slightly hyperintensity on portal phase. The central scar enhances in the delayed phase (Fig. 5.7) [17]. At single-photon emission computed tomography (SPECT) examination, most of FNHs show normal uptake of 99mTc sulfur colloid owing to the presence of Kupffer cells. Usually FNH is a slow growing tumor, and a conservative strategy is applied in asymptomatic children, but if the imaging features are atypical, further invasive investigations such as biopsy or surgical resection will be required [2, 17, 27].

Fig. 5.5 At unenhanced CT, FNH is well circumscribed and isoattenuating (**a**). After administration of contrast medium, FNH demonstrates uniform enhancement in the arterial phase, except for fibrous septa and central scars (**b**); in the portal venous phase, FNH becomes isodense to the liver (**c**)

5.2.1.4 Nodular Regenerative Hyperplasia

Nodular regenerative hyperplasia (NRH) is a lesion that can be seen in all ages, and it is rare in childhood. It consists of a compensatory hyperplasia of normal hepatocytes in the absence of significant fibrosis. The absence of intra- and perilesional fibrosis distinguishes NRH from the typical regeneration nodule in cirrhosis and from FNH, making it a histopathological distinctive entity [28]. The etiology is not well defined, but it is thought that there is a microvasculature damage, such as occlusive venopathy, functional or mechanical, which involves a reduced portal venous inflow. In hepatic regions in which vascular inflow is deficient, a cellular atrophy is observed, while adjacent areas of liver parenchyma with normal or increased blood supply result in hyperplasia [29, 30]. There are many diseases in which the coexistence of NRH is known: myelo- and lymphoproliferative disorders, autoimmune disorders, collagen vascular disease, Abernethy syndrome, the use of immunosuppressive drugs, and antineoplastic agents. The nodules may be asymptomatic when they are small and focal, while they may cause portal hypertension when confluent. NRH can vary from a few millimeters (1–3 mm) to a few centimeters. In the first case, micronodules may not be visible at imaging but may be incidentally found in liver biopsy. At US, if visible, the nodules may be usually hypoechoic or, less frequently, hyperechoic with an heterogeneous parenchymal texture. At CT scan, NRH appears hypodense or isodense, in the precontrast, arterial, and portal venous phases. At MRI, visible nodules usually are slightly hyperintense on T1-weighted images and variable on T2-weighted images. The content of intracellular fat induces decreased signal intensity on fat-suppressed T1-weighted. After contrast medium injection, the nodules may enhance in portal venous phase like normal liver parenchyma [17].

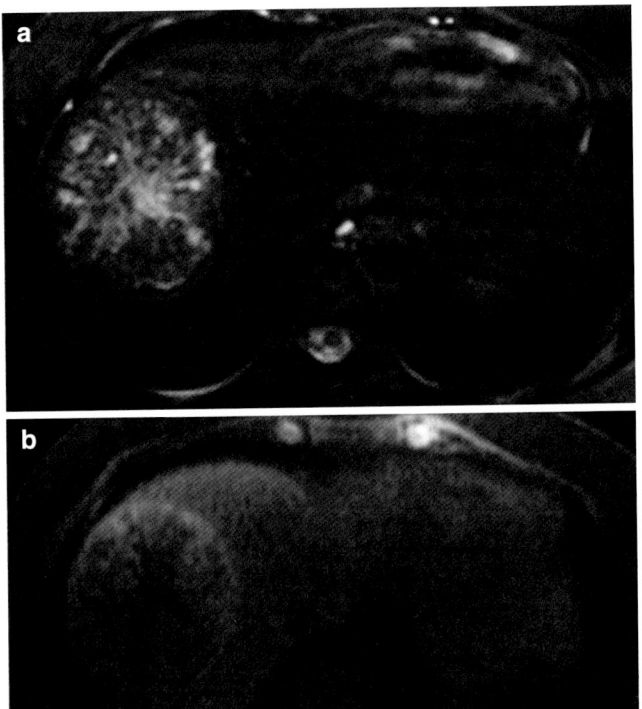

Fig. 5.6 Non-contrast MRI. On T2-weighted image, (**a**) central scar appears hyperintense due to myxomatous stroma. On T1-weighted image, (**b**) scar is hypointense

5.2.1.5 Adenoma

Hepatic adenomas (HA) are rare benign tumors of the liver. The majority of adenomas are solitary (80%) and typically occur in female patients [17]. Predisposing factors to adenoma formation include oral contraceptive use in female, anabolic steroid use in male patients, and glycogen storage disease. HAs have been reported in association also with galactosemia and

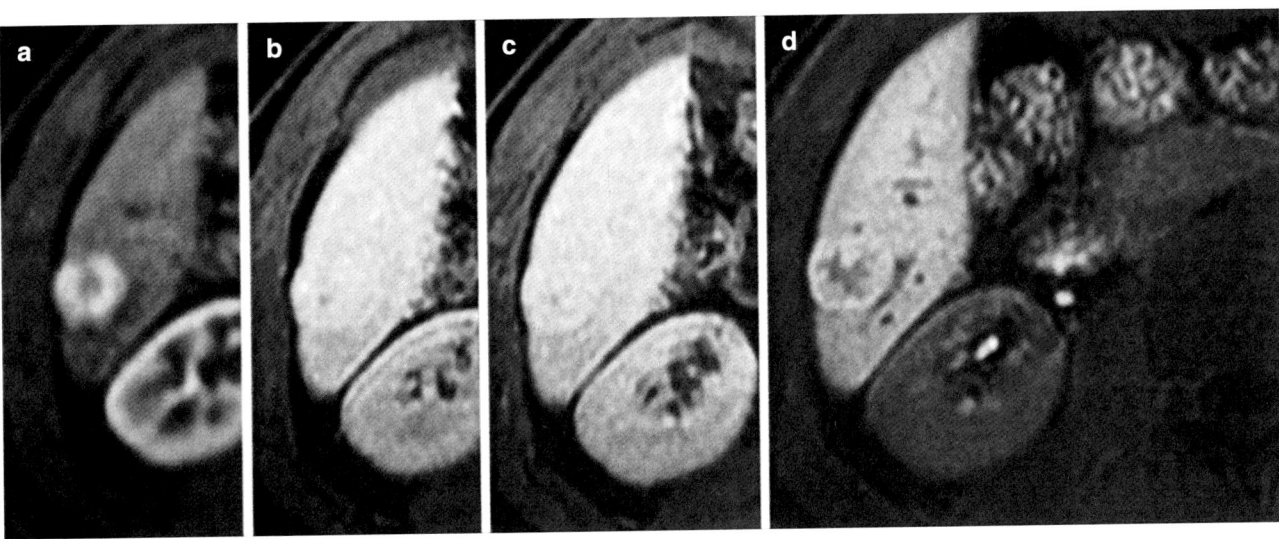

Fig. 5.7 Post-contrast MR imaging. FNH has early uniform enhancement on the arterial phase (**a**) with hyperintensity of the lesion and isointensity to slightly hyperintensity on portal venous phase images (**b, c**). Note the progressive enhancement of central scar. The hepatobiliary phase (**d**) shows very well the typical central scar

familial diabetes mellitus. There is furthermore an association with congenital and acquired abnormalities of the hepatic vasculature including portal vein absence or portal vein occlusion and hypervascular hepatic neoplasms such as adult hemangioma and FNH. Liver adenomatosis is a separate entity resulting of over ten adenomas per patient without underlying glycogen storage disease or steroid use [2, 17]. Patients are usually asymptomatic or present with an abdominal mass. However up to 10% adenomas can be complicated by intralesional hemorrhage with rupture and consequently intraperitoneal hemorrhage [17]. The adenoma is generally well-circumscribed lesion with variable degrees of hemorrhage, necrosis, fat, and calcification. On histopathological analysis, hepatic adenomas contain well-differentiated hepatocytes lacking bile ducts or portal tracts with the absence of connective tissue that predisposes to the intralesional hemorrhage [17, 31]. Imaging appearance depends on homogeneity or heterogeneity structure of the adenoma. At US, when adenomas are homogenous without hemorrhage, the appearance is similar to adjacent normal liver. Lesions with intratumoral hemorrhage or high lipid content (intracellular fat) may be hyperechoic to the surrounding liver; however, in the setting of glycogen storage disease or diffuse fatty infiltration of the liver, adenomas may be hypoechoic. Intratumoral vessels with a venous Doppler spectrum, associated with either pulsatile or continuous peripheral flow, were detected in the adenoma but not in FNH, which has predominant central arterial flow. The association of CEUS with color Doppler US can improve the diagnostic performance of focal nodular hyperplasia and hepatocellular adenoma [32, 33]. At non-contrast CT most adenomas are hypodense, although portions of hyperdensity are seen in case of hemorrhage. The presence of calcification and fat can contribute to the heterogeneity of the lesion. After contrast medium administration, adenoma shows homogeneous or heterogeneous enhancement (depending on the structure) with hyperdense pattern in arterial phase and isodense pattern during the portal venous and delayed phases. At MR imaging, most of the adenomas are T1- and T2-weighted hyperintense compared with the surrounding of the liver. T1-weighted findings are most likely caused by blood degeneration products or glycogen storage. T2-weighted hyperintensity is due to hemorrhage or areas of peliosis-like changes [17]. It is possible to highlight a perilesional pseudocapsule: this is not a true capsule but only the compressed adjacent liver tissue that appears hypointense on T1-weighted images and variable on T2-weighted images and may enhance after contrast administration. The pattern of the enhancement after contrast medium administration is similar to that of CT: hyperintense in arterial phase and isointense in portal venous and delayed phase.

5.2.2 Malignant Liver Lesions

As in adulthood the most common neoplasm involving the liver in children is metastatic disease. Primary hepatic tumors (HT) are therefore a further rare condition accounting for 1–2% of all childhood tumors [13]. The majority of primary HT are malignant and derived from the hepatocyte lineage. The most common are hepatoblastoma (HB), hepatocellular carcinoma (HCC), undifferentiated (embryonal) sarcoma (UES), angiosarcoma, and embryonal rhabdomyosarcoma [34]. The proper characterization and management of HT rely upon patients' age, clinical symptoms, alpha-fetoprotein (AFP), and diagnostic imaging. HT often appears as a palpable abdominal mass or pain and distension of abdomen, associated with low-grade fever or weight loss. Not all neoplasias of the liver produce AFP; however the presence of a liver mass and raising of AFP could exclude with a certain confidence the benign origin [35].

5.2.2.1 Hepatoblastoma (HB)

HB is the most common primary pediatric liver tumor, accounting for 91% of cases among children less than 5 years of age [36]. Its incidence is low, with 1.0–1.5 new cases per million children, yet slightly increasing, at least in Western countries. The peak incidence is at 1–2 years, with a median age of onset of 18 months. After 5 years of age, HB is rare although it may occur also during adolescence, and in this case its behavior is more aggressive [37, 38]. There is a prevalence in male in comparison to female (ratio 2:1) [21]. Ascertained risk factors are premature and low-weighted birth [39]. Other predisposing conditions include Beckwith-Wiedemann syndrome, hemihypertrophy, familial polyposis coli, Gardner's syndrome, fetal alcohol syndrome, and Wilms' tumor [12]. HB appears as a large, solitary or multifocal, liver mass well circumscribed by a capsule and with lobulated contours and internal septa. Multifocality characterizes 20% of cases. Histologically, hepatoblastoma is classified in epithelial type and mixed epithelial and mesenchymal type [40]. Patients with hepatoblastoma clinically manifest with enlarged abdomen and nonspecific symptoms such as weight loss and anorexia. Sometimes they can present with acute abdominal pain due to tumor rupture and hemorrhage. The liver function is usually well preserved. Hepatoblastoma frequently metastasizes to the lung (10–15% of cases) and to the lymph nodes, brain, and bone [15]. In the majority of cases AFP level is remarkably elevated and serves to monitor chemotherapy and to detect recurrence. Radiological characteristics of hepatoblastoma reflect its pathological and histological composition. At US epithelial type appears as a large lesion isoechoic to liver parenchyma, while the mixed type more often has a higher echoic signal compared to the surrounding liver (Fig. 5.8). This type can contain calcifications and anechoic foci representative of necrosis. Septa can be seen as hypoechoic linear structures [41]. On unenhanced CT scan hepatoblastoma appears as a low attenuating heterogeneous mass with calcifications seen in half of cases. After intravenous contrast agent injection, tumor enhances slightly but less than the liver parenchyma, so it will appear as hypodense in portal venous phase (Fig. 5.9). If an arterial phase is performed, capsule and septa may be observed as hyperenhancing. Thrombosis of portal vein and its branches can occur and easily detected during portal venous phase as an endoluminal filling defect [21]. On MRI hepatoblastoma appears differently according to the histological type. The epithelial type is hypointense on T1-weighted sequence and hyperintense on T2-weighted sequence, while the mixed type is more heterogeneous. Calcification and fibrotic septa are seen as hypointense both on T1-weighted and T2-weighted sequences, while hemorrhagic foci will appear as hyperintense on T1-weighted sequence. Post-contrast behavior is the same described for CT scan [42]. Overall survival rate for children with hepatoblastoma depends on the stage at presentation, AFP levels, vascular invasion, and resectability ranging from 45% for patients with metastatic disease to over 90% for patients suitable for surgery [43]. Liver resection is the curative treatment of choice. In fact total hepatectomy and orthotopic liver transplantation following epatectom is increasingly used with survival similar to patients undergoing partial hepatectomy [44].

5.2.2.2 Hepatocellular Carcinoma

Hepatocellular carcinoma is the second most common liver tumor in children. It has a prevalence of 0.5–1.0 cases per million children; however in endemic hepatitis B regions, such as South and East Asia, the prevalence is higher [45]. The peak incidence is at 10–14 years, and its presentation is rare in children <5 years. There is a slight prevalence in male patients with a male-to-female ratio of 2:1 [46]. All the diseases predisposing to liver cirrhosis are risk factors for HCC. These include biliary atresia, genetic cholestase, glycogen storage disease type I, alpha-1-antitrypsin deficiency, Wilson disease, and hepatitis B or C infection. A strong association is particularly described with tyrosinemia type I and BSEP deficiency (PFIC2). However, HCC can arise in a normal liver without predisposing liver disease. This form of "de novo" HCC is biologically completely different from HCC arising in a cirrhotic liver [47–49]. HCC can appear as single lesion, multinodular, or diffuse/infiltrative disease. Microvascular invasion of portal and hepatic veins is frequent. In case of solitary mass, a fibrous capsule can be present. Histologically, HCC cells can vary from well to poorly differentiated and usually grow with a trabecular pattern. Fat, glycogen and copper inclusions may be found [34]. Patients with HCC clinically present with vague abdominal pain, abdominal mass, hepatomegaly, and, in advanced cases, anorexia and weight loss. Extrahepatic metastases at presentation are frequent [50]. An elevation of AFP levels is present in over 70% of cases [45]. In pediatric patients the most common presentation of HCC not associated with chronic disease is a large tumor, due to the lack of screening programs. At US it appears as a large heterogeneous lesion, with hyperechoic area due to fat or hemorrhagic foci. The capsule can

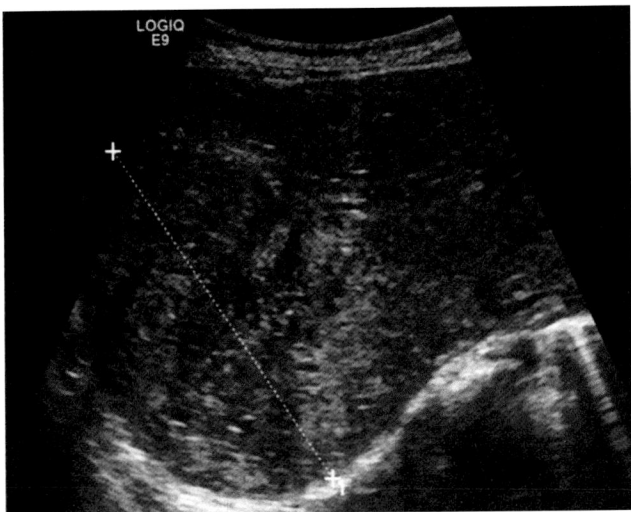

Fig. 5.8 At US hepatoblastoma appears as a large lesion isoechoic to liver parenchyma

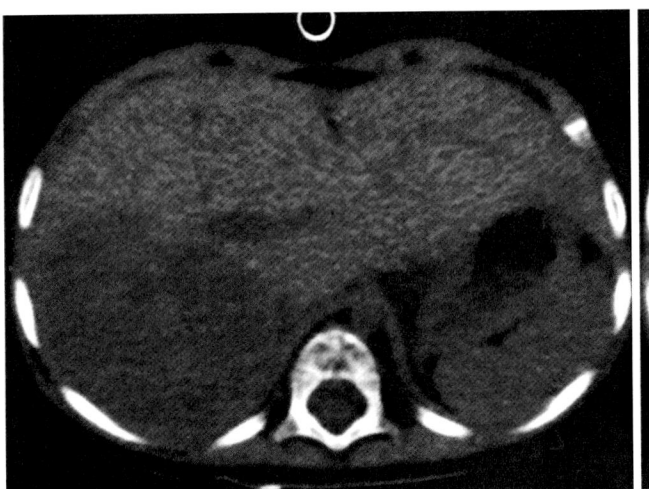 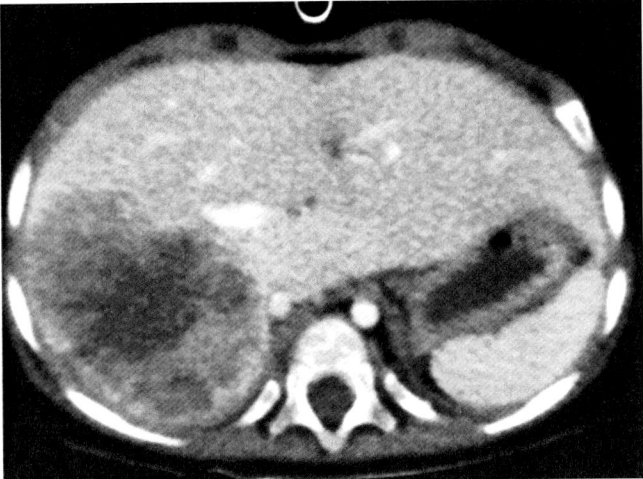

Fig. 5.9 At unenhanced CT scan hepatoblastoma is low attenuating heterogeneous mass. After intravenous contrast agent, tumor is heterogeneous hypodense lesion

be seen as a thin hypoechoic layer. This typical heterogeneous aspect is detected also at unenhanced examination, where HCC has a so-called mosaic pattern. During hepatocarcinogenesis intranodular arterial vascularity increases due to the appearance of unpaired arteries (capillarization), while portal blood supply progressively decreases. For this reason, HCC is hyperdense during arterial phase and hypodense, with rapid washout, during portal venous phase. Tumor capsule is seen as hypodense rim in precontrast CT and may enhance in the delayed phase [51]. At MRI HCC will be slightly hyperintense to normal liver on T2-w and iso-hypointense on T1-w. Larger lesions have a more heterogeneous signal intensity due to the possible presence of fat, necrosis, copper, and hemorrhagic foci. After injection of gadolinium-based contrast agent, HCC presents the classical wash-in and washout appearance [52]. Infiltrative HCC appears as disruption of normal liver parenchyma with retraction of liver capsule at all imaging techniques. The prognosis of pediatric patients with HCC not associated with chronic liver disease is very poor, ranging from 10 to 30%, due to the late diagnosis often when the tumor is already metastatic and unresectable. Liver resection is the only curative choice but unfortunately only a small proportion can benefit of it. Neoadjuvant chemotherapy is not so effective in this tumor and the role of liver transplantation is limited due to the advanced stage at diagnosis [45, 53–55].

5.2.2.3 Fibrolamellar Carcinoma

Fibrolamellar carcinoma (FLC) is a histological variant of HCC. It is more common in females and adolescents or young adults [56]. Nor cirrhosis neither other metabolic conditions predispose to FLC, which in fact develops in the setting of normal liver parenchyma. In over two-thirds of cases, FLC appears as a large, well defined but non-capsulated mass with a predilection for left liver lobe. In 60–70% of solitary FLC, a central scar, with calcification in some cases, may be seen. Other patterns of growth include an intrahepatic mass with satellite lesions (10–15%), a bilobar mass (5%), or multifocal masses (<1%) [57]. FLC shows vascular invasion in up to 35% of cases and spreading to local lymph nodes is frequent. Patients with FLC suffer of nonspecific abdominal pain and mass. AFP levels are not useful in monitoring treatment efficacy since they are usually normal. On US FLC often looks as a solitary mass with heterogeneous aspect and a hyperechoic central fibrous scar. On unenhanced CT scan, it is typically hypodense in comparison to the surrounding parenchyma and, after injection of contrast agent, is hyperdense in arterial phase and can be hyper-, iso-, or hypodense in portal venous phase. Central scar always appears hypodense. On MRI the lesion is slightly iso-hypointense on T1-w sequence and slightly iso-hyperintense on T2-w sequence. The fibrous central scar is hypointense both on T1-w and on T2-w sequences and does not enhance after contrast agent injection [57]. FLC prognosis is similar to that of HCC. Positive prognostic factors include resectability, younger age, lack of neoplastic thrombosis, and extrahepatic spread [58].

5.2.2.4 Undifferentiated Embryonal Sarcoma

Undifferentiated embryonal sarcoma (UES) is the third most common primary liver malignancy in pediatric patients. It presents in later childhood with a mean age at presentation of 6–10 years. There is a slight prevalence in male patients [59]. UES typically appears as a large, solid lesion well delineated by a fibrous pseudocapsule with areas of hemorrhage and cystic degeneration. It is a neoplasm of mesenchymal origin, and there is a documented conversion from mesenchymal hamartoma to UES [60]. Histologically it is composed of sarcomatous stellate or spindle-shaped cells with ill-defined borders [61]. Patients with UES present with vague pain and abdominal discomfort. Symptoms of acute abdomen may occur in case of rupture of the lesion. Metastases at diagnosis are common and involve the brain, bone, and lung. AFP levels are usually in the normal range. The characteristic of this tumor is the discrepancy in the imaging appearance between US and CT or MRI. In fact at US, it looks like the typical solid lesion with heterogeneous echoic signs due to the presence of cystic foci, which appear anechoic in the context of a lesion, iso- or hyperechoic relative to normal liver. By the contrary on CT and on MRI, UES appears as a cystic lesion. On unenhanced CT, it is hypodense, and after contrast agent injection, it shows no or just a tiny rim enhancement [62]. Also on MRI it has the typical aspect of fluid content that is hypointense on T1-w sequence and hyperintense on T2-w sequence. Hyperintense foci on T1-w sequence corresponding to hypointense foci on T2-weighted sequence may be seen and refer to hemorrhagic areas. After gadolinium-based contrast agent injection, the peripheral enhancement of pseudocapsule is observed [63].

UES is a very aggressive tumor and the prognosis is poor. The best outcome is achieved with tumor resection. Some unresectable patients could benefit of neoadjuvant chemotherapy [64]; however, 25–50% are resistant to chemotherapy. Promising results are expected with major hepatic resection and liver transplantation; however, there are still few data reported in literature [65].

5.2.2.5 Angiosarcoma

Angiosarcoma is a rare pediatric liver tumor. Few cases have been described in young female patients following the initial diagnosis of hemangioma [22]. Angiosarcoma commonly manifests as multinodular disease involving both the liver lobes. In some cases a single, large lesion or a dominant mass with multiple nodules can be found. It is a tumor of vascular origin, and its cells form a variety of vascular structures; the tumor forms anastomosing channels and cavernous spaces and invades preexisting normal vascular structures leading to hepatocytes' death. Patients with angiosarcoma suffer from vague abdominal pain, although acute symptoms, due to the rupture of the tumor, are not infrequent. Lung and spleen metastases at diagnosis are a common finding. On US it appears heterogeneous due to the presence of necrotic and hemorrhagic foci. On unenhanced CT multiple nodules are hypodense and after intravenous contrast agent injection show an early, central or ring enhancement and a persistent enhancement on delayed phase, without complete centripetal fill-in [66]. Angiosarcoma has a low signal intensity on T1-w sequence (with hyperintense hemorrhagic foci) and a slightly high signal intensity on T2-w sequence. After injection of gadolinium-based contrast agent, the tumor shows the typical delayed enhancement with incomplete centripetal fill-in [67]. Prognosis is poor, with an expectancy of life form diagnosis of 6–12 months [68].

5.2.2.6 Embryonal Rhabdomyosarcoma

Embryonal rhabdomyosarcoma (ER) is the most common soft tissue sarcoma in children. It can occur anywhere in the body, and in fewer cases, it arises at any level of the biliary tree. Biliary rhabdomyosarcoma (BR) is a rare tumor, accounting for <1% of malignancies in pediatric population. Mean age at presentation is 3 years [69]. BR is generally large (8–20 cm in diameter) and typically grows inside the extrahepatic bile ducts, although intrahepatic bile ducts' localization has been described. The pattern of growth is polypoid or grape-like. Cystic areas inside the lesion can be found [70]. Of the three histologic subtypes of rhabdomyosarcoma, only the embryonal subtype arises in the biliary tree. BR manifests with obstructive jaundice, which is the most common presenting symptom (60–80% of cases), accompanied by abdominal distention, fever, hepatomegaly, or nausea and vomiting. Laboratory tests reflects the mechanical tumor obstruction of biliary tree and so conjugated bilirubin and alkaline phosphatase are usually elevated while AFP levels are normal. Metastases at diagnosis can be present in 30% of patients [71]. At imaging BR will appear as a large mass growing within the bile ducts, often in the extrahepatic tract and for this reason localized near the porta hepatis. Dilatation of intra- and extrahepatic bile ducts is commonly seen. Foci of intralesional necrotic degeneration may be observed. At US, the tumor looks like a solitary hypoechoic mass with hyperechoic area or multiple hypoechoic nodules separated by septa. The CT scan shows a heterogeneous mass for the combining presence of hyperdense and hypodense areas. Contrast enhancement may be variable, ranging from hyperenhancing to nonenhancing. On MRI BR has low signal intensity on T1-w sequence and high signal intensity on T2-w sequence. MR cholangiography may be used to detect the intraductal growth of the lesion [70]. BR is often localized at diagnosis; however, complete surgical resection is possible only in 20–40% of cases due to the common hilar location. Fortunately these tumors are very chemotherapy and radiation therapy responsive, with a 5-year survival rate of 78% for patients with local disease [72].

5.3 Diffuse Liver Disease

The burden of diffuse liver disease in pediatric patients is still poorly investigated. It is estimated that the overall incidence is approximately 1/2500 live births in the USA with age-related differences in frequencies and diagnosis [73]. The causes of infant cholestasis are numerous and commonly classified as intrahepatic or extrahepatic. Biliary atresia is the most common cause of extrahepatic cholestasis. Intrahepatic group is commonly referred as neonatal hepatitis (NH). The most common causes of NH include alpha-1-antitrypsin (A1AT) deficiency, infection (bacterial and viral), inborn error of metabolism, and genetic cholestatic disorder (Alagille syndrome and familial intrahepatic cholestasis). When a clear cause is not identified, it is defined as idiopathic neonatal hepatitis [74].

In this setting, imaging techniques play a crucial role in the management of patients with suspected liver disease, due to the overlap of signs and symptoms among the different etiologies.

Liver ultrasound (US) is the first level imaging technique employed in the setting of diffuse liver disease. Normal liver echotexture is homogeneous and isoechoic or slightly hypoechoic relative to the renal cortex. The length of the right hepatic lobe should be 4–9.5 cm in terms of infants and should not exceed costal margin more than 1 cm (Table 5.1) [75]. In nonpathologic condition, intrahepatic bile ducts are not visualized during US examination, while the normal common bile duct (CBD) should be less than 1 mm in neonates, less than 2 mm in infants

Table 5.1 Right liver lobe length measured in midclavicular line (adapted from Konus OL, Ozdemir A, Akkaya A et al. Normal liver, spleen, and kidney dimensions in neonates, infants, and children: evaluation with sonography. Am J Roentgenol. 1998;171:1693–8) [75]

Liver (right lobe length, cm)		
Age (years)	Mean (sd)	Limits of normal
0–0.25	6.4 (1.0)	4.0–9.0
0.25–0.5	7.3 (1.1)	4.5–9.5
0.5–0.75	7.9 (0.8)	6.0–10.0
1–2.5	8.5 (1.0)	6.5–10.5
3–5	8.6 (1.2)	6.5–11.5
5–7	10.0 (1.4)	7.0–12.5
7–9	10.5 (1.1)	7.5–13.0
9–11	10.5 (1.2)	7.5–13.5
11–13	11.5 (1.4)	8.5–14.0
13—15	11.8 (1.5)	8.5–14.0
15–17	12.1 (1.2)	9.5–14.5

up to 1 year old, and less than 4 mm in older children. The normal gallbladder length is 1.5–3 cm in infants up to 1 year and 3–7 cm in older children [76]. Hepatic arteries, portal veins, and hepatic veins are visualized as hypoechoic tubular structure; the diameter of portal trunk in infants is 3–5 mm (Tables 5.2 and 5.3). Spleen size and texture also should be evaluated. Normal spleen length is up to 6 cm in infants 0–3 year old and up to 12 cm in children aged 12–15 years (Table 5.4). US should always be completed with color Doppler examination which allows to differentiate vessels form enlarged bile ducts [76]. Magnetic resonance is the second-level imaging technique of choice due to its high-contrast resolution and the lack of ionizing radiations. Specific neonatal MRI coils or head and extremity coils should be used. Anesthesia is required to guarantee high-quality imaging with breath holding.

Standard protocol comprises:

- Axial T1-weighted in-and-out-of-phase gradient echo sequences.
- Axial (and coronal) turbo spin echo T2-weighted sequences with and without fat saturation.
- Axial 3D T1-weighted fat-suppressed spoiled recalled-echo sequences before (and after) contrast agent injection.

If a disease of the biliary three is suspected, a MR cholangiography (MRCP) should be performed by using a volumetric three-dimensional T2-weighted sequences. The most frequent causes of diffuse liver disease and their relative imaging findings will be discussed.

5.3.1 Biliary Atresia

Biliary atresia (BA) is the most common cause of jaundice in the first 3 months of life and the most frequent indication for pediatric liver transplantation. Its incidence in USA and Europe is 1:12,000–18,000, and it is more common in female patients [77]. From a pathogenetic point of view, BA is characterized by progressive fibrosis with destruction of biliary tree, but its etiology is still unknown. These infants are asymptomatic at birth, and cholestatic-related signs and symptoms are late findings. In the group defined as biliary atresia with splenic malformation (BASM), accounting for 6% of cases, patients have one or more malformations (polysplenia, asplenia, preduodenal portal vein, the absence of the cava, genitourinary, or cardiac malformations), but no laterality defects. Patients with syndromic BA (10%) have laterality defects (i.e., situs inversus) and are symptomatic from birth [78]. Prompt diagnosis of BA and surgical correction with Kasai operation, a porto-entero anastomosis able to reestablish bile flow, is essential to avoid complications such as liver cirrhosis and death. Several sonographic parameters have been described in BA, to support its diagnosis. The most useful are the triangular cord sign, abnormal gallbladder morphology, lack of gallbladder contraction after oral feeding, absent common bile duct, and hepatic artery diameter. The triangular cord sign is defined as a hyperechoic area, tube-shaped, anterior to the porta hepatis, and it is thought to represent the fibrotic remnant of biliary tree (Fig. 5.10). This sign has a high specificity (96–100%) but a low sensitivity (62–73%). The accuracy increases if the thickness of the triangu-

Table 5.2 Diameter of common bile duct (adapted from Hernanz-Schulman M, Ambrosino MM, Freeman PC, et al. Common bile duct in children: sonographic dimensions. Radiology. 1995;195:193–5)

Common bile duct		
Age (years)	Mean (sd)	Diameter (mm)
0	0.2–1.6	0.7
1	0.2–1.7	1.2
2	0.3–1.8	1.0
3	0.3–1.9	1.3
4	0.4–2.0	1.1
5	0.5–2.1	0.8
6	0.5–2.2	1.2
7	0.6–2.3	1.3
8	0.6–2.4	1.5
9	0.7–2.5	1.9
10	0.7–2.6	1.7
11	0.8–2.7	1.7
12	0.8–2.8	1.9

Table 5.4 Spleen length in male children (adapted from Megremis SD, Vlachonikolis IG, Tsilimigaki AM. Spleen length in childhood with US: normal values based on age, sex, and somatometric parameters. Radiology. 2004;231:129–34)

Spleen length (cm)		
Age	Mean	SD
0–3 months	4.6	0.84
3–6 months	5.8	0.65
6–12 months	6.4	0.78
1–2 years	6.8	0.72
2–4 years	7.6	1.07
4–6 years	8.1	1.01
6–8 years	8.9	0.91
8–10 years	9.0	1.02
10–12 years	9.8	1.05
12–14 years	10.2	0.81
14–17 years	10.7	0.9

Table 5.3 Adapted from Gubernick J, Rosenberg H, Ilaslan H, Kessler A. US approach to jaundice in infants and children. Radiographics. 2000;20(1):173–95 [76]

Organ	Neonates	Infants–1 years old	Older children 2–12	Adolescents–adults 12–16
Gallbladder (length)	1.5–3 cm		3–7 cm	
Portal vein diameter		3–5 mm	8.5 mm (<10 years)	10 mm

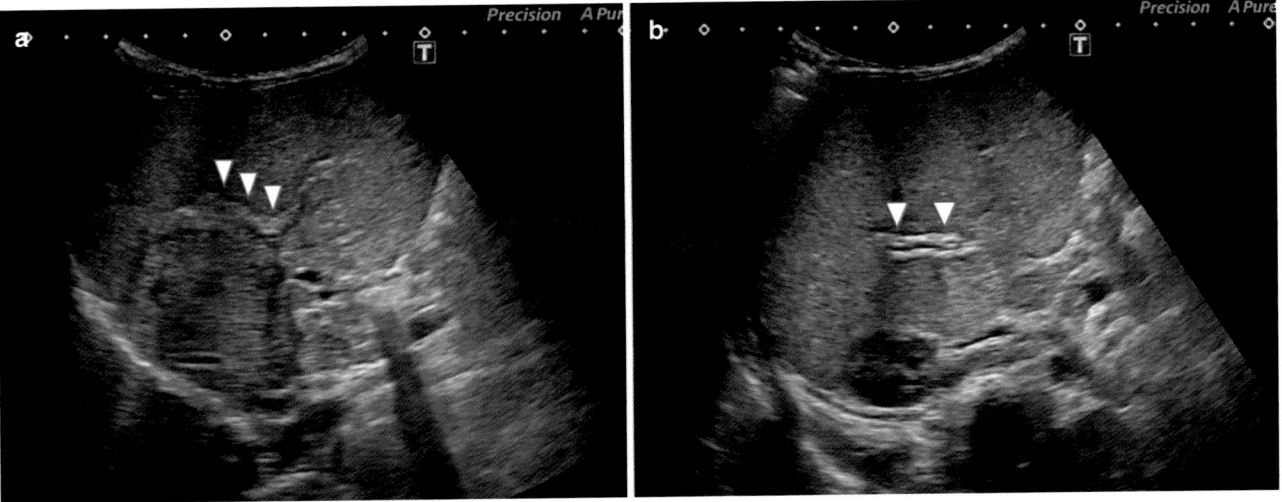

Fig. 5.10 The triangular cord sign is a hyperechoic area, tube-shaped, anterior to the porta hepatis (arrowheads) that represents the fibrotic residual of biliary tree

lar cord is >4 mm [79–81]. The absence or an abnormal shape of the gallbladder (i.e., irregular outline, irregularly thick walls, or sometimes a small lumen) is common finding in BA. Recently a classification of gallbladder abnormalities has been proposed: type I, gallbladder not detected; type II, gallbladder detected without (or with partial) lumen, but with the visualization of hyperechoic mucosa and thickened wall; type III, gallbladder detected with a fully filled lumen and lumen length equal to or less than 1.5 cm without wall thickening; and type IV, gallbladder detected with fully filled lumen and length greater than 1.5 cm without wall thickening. This classification had a high diagnostic accuracy in the detection of BA (sensitivity 86.8% and specificity 90.3%). An absent gallbladder and a gallbladder up to 1.5 cm had a positive predictive value of 100% and 95.1%, respectively, in the diagnosis of biliary atresia, while gallbladder without lumen or with lumen partially filled are more likely to occur in patients without BA [82]. Other suggestive findings are an absent common bile duct (sensitivity of 93% and specificity of 95%) and a hypertrophic hepatic artery. Color Doppler can be useful in detecting hepatic subcapsular flow which had a reported sensitivity, specificity, and positive and negative predictive values of 100%, 86%, 85%, and 100%, respectively [83]. All these signs combined together can raise the accuracy of US in the diagnosis of BA. However, US remains an operator-dependent technique, with a certain rate of false negatives. Hepatobiliary scintigraphy assesses the radiotracer extraction in small bowel. Despite its high sensitivity (99%), it has a low specificity (70–93%) [84]. In fact patients with idiopathic hepatitis and low birth weight and those on parenteral nutrition may also have a non-extracting scans [85]. Among the noninvasive diagnostic modalities, MRCP allows the visualization of intra- and extrahepatic biliary trees. High-quality images are difficult to obtain in children due to the small caliber of bile ducts and to motion artifacts; however, few studies investigated the accuracy of this technique in BA. The largest series recently published reported high sensitivity but very low specificity (99% and 36%, respectively). Invasive procedures such as percutaneous transhepatic cholangiography (PTC) and endoscopic retrograde cholangiopancreatography (ERCP) can be used in unsolved cases despite they require dedicated expertise, specific equipment, and, as in case of MRCP, general anesthesia. In 8% of cases BA manifests as a cystic dilatation of extrahepatic biliary tract, containing either cyst fluid or bile depending on whether communication with the intrahepatic biliary system persists. Intrahepatic bile ducts are obliterated. This form is the only one that could be detected prenatally, and it should be distinguished from choledochal cystic malformations. At US small, static, anechoic cysts and an irregular, elongated gallbladder are in favor of cystic BA. MR cholangiopancreatography can help in differential diagnosis through the atypical appearance of intrahepatic biliary tree [86].

5.3.2 Choledochal Cyst

Choledocal cyst (CC) represents a congenital, rare, disease. It is more frequent in female sex and in Asian population [87]. These lesions manifest as intra- and/or extrahepatic bile duct dilatation and can lead to cholangitis, perforation, liver failure, and malignancy. The pathogenesis is probably related to the presence of a long, common bilio-pancreatic channel (that should be no longer than 15 mm) which causes reflux of pancreatic secretions and subsequent chronic inflammation, bile duct wall damage, and cystic changes [88]. CCs are classified according to Todani classification in five types. Type I is a diffuse or focal dilatation of extrahepatic biliary duct which can involve the common hepatic duct or common biliary duct or cystic duct and account for the majority of cases (80–90%). Type II (2% of all CC) is a diverticular dilatation of extrahepatic bile duct. Type III (4% of all CC) also known as coledochocele is a dilatation of the intraduodenal tract of common bile duct. Type IV (15–20% of all CC) is represented by multiple bile duct cystic dilatations involving intra- and/or extrahepatic branches. It is further divided in type IV a (both intrahepatic and extrahepatic ductal dilatations) and type IV b (multiple, extrahepatic dilatations without intrahepatic involvement). Type V, also known as Caroli disease, consists of cystic dilatation of only intrahepatic branches. If this condition is associated with congenital hepatic fibrosis, it is called Caroli syndrome [89]. Type I and type IV have the highest risk of malignancies. CC typically manifests as abdominal pain and jaundice, caused by plugs and stones formed by refluxed biliary and pancreatic juices. Type I, II, and III CC appear at US examination as simple extrahepatic cyst in communication with the biliary ductal system. In Caroli disease, single or multiple intrahepatic cysts converged to the porta hepatis are commonly visualized. Common biliary duct could be enlarged, and hepatic fibrosis or cirrhosis, signs of portal hypertension, and polycystic kidneys could be associated. US is highly sensitive in the diagnosis of CC and can be sufficient if there is no evidence of intrahepatic bile ducts dilatation [90]. MRCP is more sensitive and specific (70–100% and 90–100%, respectively) in defining CC subtypes and the pancreatic-biliary duct anatomy [91] and should be performed in preoperative assessment of patients. As previously reported, differential diagnosis should be carried out with cystic BA which has completely different management. Cystic BA clinically presents earlier (<3 months of age), and their cysts are smaller with no dilatation of the intrahepatic biliary system. Moreover in cystic BA the gallbladder is atretic or elongated with irregular wall. Definitive treatment of CC is surgical and varies from the excision of the cysts to hepatectomy or even liver transplantation, depending on the extension of the disease.

5.3.3 Neonatal Hepatitis

Neonatal hepatitis (NH) occurs at 1–4 weeks of age, and it is more common in male. Differentiation of NH from BA or CC is of paramount importance because the last two disorders require a surgical approach. At ultrasound the liver could appear enlarged or normal sized with a hyperechoic parenchyma. The intrahepatic branches of portal vein are less detectable while gallbladder and biliary tree are commonly normal. In the first day of life, some infants can have a physiological reduction of biliary excretion, resulting in an underfilled gallbladder which can be misdiagnosed with BA. Hepatic artery enlargement is a useful sign to distinguish BA from NH [92]. Hepatobiliary scintigraphy can help in differential diagnosis, by demonstrating radiotracers excretion in small bowel [76]. As previously reported, there are several causes of NH, and the major causes are shown below.

5.3.3.1 Alagille Syndrome

Alagille syndrome (ALGS) is an autosomal dominant multisystemic disorder, due to defects in the Notch signalling pathway, the majority of which (97%) are caused by haploinsufficiency of the JAG1 gene; the remaining cases (1–3%) are caused by mutations in NOTCH2 [93]. It is a rare condition; its incidence in fact is reported to be 1:30,000 and the prevalence 1:70,000, but this data could be underestimated due to the reduced penetrance of the disease [94]. The diagnosis is made by the presence of intrahepatic bile duct paucity at liver biopsy, along with three of the following five clinical criteria: chronic cholestasis, congenital heart disease (most commonly peripheral pulmonary artery stenosis), characteristic facies, axial skeleton/vertebral anomalies (most common butterfly vertebra), eye/posterior embryotoxon (prominence of Schwalbe's ring at the junction of the iris and cornea) [95]. Although the diagnosis is mainly clinical, US and hepatobiliary scintigraphy can be used in the initial assessment of infants with cholestasis. Unfortunately imaging findings are not specific for AGLS due to the similarity with BA, including abnormal gallbladder shape and size and hypertrophic hepatic artery [96]. Moreover hepatobiliary scintigraphy is not specific for ALGS, since even in this condition no excretion of radiotracer may be observed, a finding that overlaps with BA. The final diagnosis is reached with genetic test and liver biopsy. ALGS presenting early in life may have favorable liver outcome. Liver transplantation (LT) is the treatment of choice in a minority of patients. Patients who are not candidate to LT should be routinely followed up due to the increased risk of developing HCC [97].

5.3.3.2 Progressive Familial Intrahepatic Cholestasis

Progressive familial intrahepatic cholestasis (PFIC) is a group of autosomal recessive diseases characterized by mutations in genes encoding proteins associated with transport systems of bile components from hepatocytes to biliary ducts. It is a rare disease with an estimated incidence of 1:50,000/100,000 without prevalence of gender nor race [98]. The gold standard for the diagnosis of the different forms of PFIC is genetic test. US is routinely performed in the initial evaluation of children with high level of conjugated bilirubin, but unfortunately in PFIC, the liver imaging is normal. In some cases of PFIC 2/3, the presence of cholelithiasis could be found. Other imaging techniques, such as MRCP, can help in excluding other causes of cholestasis.

5.3.3.3 Alpha-1-Antytripsin Deficiency

Alpha-1-antitrypsin deficiency (A1ATD) is the most common cause of inherited cholestasis. Infants present with severe cholestasis and high level of AST, ALT, GGT, and bilirubin. Imaging techniques are not useful for the early diagnosis of A1ATD which is currently made through genetic testing or immunophenotyping [99].

5.3.3.4 Inborn Errors of Metabolism

Inborn errors of metabolism (IEMs) are heterogeneous groups of genetic disorders caused by a defect in a metabolic pathway, leading to the accumulation of toxic intermediate metabolites [100]. Some of these IEMs can manifest with cholestasis. In many countries tyrosinemia and galactosemia are currently diagnosed early, thanks to prenatal screening tests. In the early phase, imaging is not useful for the diagnosis since no liver alterations will be detected. However, these conditions could evolve into chronic liver disease and cirrhosis and show the typical features of chronic liver damage. Moreover imaging follow-up is mandatory due to the increased risk of HCC in tyrosinemia [101, 102].

5.3.3.5 Viral Hepatitis

The widespread use of vaccination in infants and children/adolescents, the routine virological screening in pregnant women and in blood and organ products, and the progresses in drug treatment have dramatically reduced the prevalence of hepatitis B virus (HBV) and C virus (HCV) infection; however, in some subtropical regions and in the Far East, the prevalence is still high [103, 104]. In the acute phase of infection, the diagnosis is made through family, laboratory tests, and liver biopsy. Imaging is not useful in this phase because no specific changes occur. At US an enlarged and hyperechoic liver could be found, but in most cases, the exam is completely normal. The natural history of both virus B and virus C infections is generally favorable. It is estimated that 3–5% of HBV and 2% of HCV young infected patients will eventually develop cirrhosis [105, 106].

5.3.4 Diffuse Liver Disease in Older Children

5.3.4.1 Cirrhosis

Liver cirrhosis in pediatric patients is a very uncommon finding, although it can occur in case of viral infection, biliary atresia, congenital hepatic fibrosis, and metabolic disorders (Wilson disease, alpha-1-antitrypsin deficiency, etc.). The chronic damage leads to injury to hepatic parenchyma with fibrotic replacement and nodular regeneration. The liver surface is irregular and margins are rounded. The echotexture is coarse with nodular (micro or macro) aspects of the liver parenchyma. Regenerating nodules can appear as well-defined and hypoechoic lesions with a size that varies from a few millimeters to several centimeters. In the advanced phase of liver cirrhosis, portal hypertension (PH) can occur. Typical signs of PH on US and Doppler US are splenomegaly, collateral vessels, enlargement of portal vein, change in velocity and direction of portal vein flow (slower and hepatofugal), and ascites, although Doppler US cannot measure portal pressure but only flow velocity, providing only indirect hints to portal hypertension [76].

5.3.4.2 Nonalcoholic Fatty Liver Disease

Nonalcoholic fatty liver disease (NAFLD) is defined as the accumulation of triglycerides into the hepatocytes. This may induce hepatocyte dysfunction with various degrees of inflammation, known as nonalcoholic steatohepatitis (NASH) and fibrosis and eventually liver cirrhosis. The worldwide epidemic of obesity linked to the development of NAFLD, which is nowadays the leading cause of chronic liver disease in children and adolescents [107]. NAFLD is generally asymptomatic, and the diagnosis is made through the evidence of abnormal level of liver enzymes and the exclusion of all other causes of liver disease. At the US liver appears hyperechoic in comparison to kidney ("bright liver") due to the increased echogenicity of the liver parenchyma (Fig. 5.11), caused by intracellular accumulation of fat vacuoles. The evaluation of NAFLD on US is based on visual qualitative assessment of hepatic echogenicity and has a great intra- and inter-observer variability. Moreover US is unable to detect fat infiltration below 30% and cannot assess disease severity [108]. Transient elastography (TE) utilizes pulsed ultrasound waves to measure liver stiffness and may assess the degree of fibrosis in pediatric patients with NAFLD [109]. However, the presence of visceral fat and obesity is one of the known limits of TE. MRI, through several methods (i.e., chemical shift, fat saturation), has a high sensitivities and specificities in detecting histologic steatosis ≥5% (76.7%–90.0% and

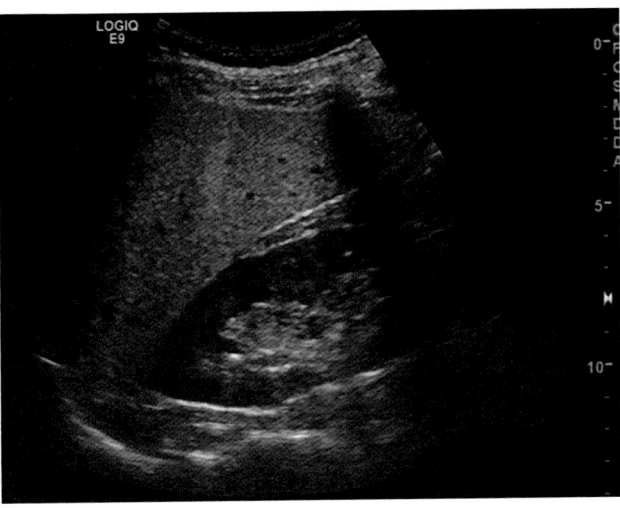

Fig. 5.11 Liver steatosis

87.1%–91%, respectively) [110]. Moreover recent algorithms (IDEAL—iterative decomposition of water and fat with echo asymmetry and least-squares estimation) allow the quantification of fat into the hepatocytes [111]. Unfortunately there are still insufficient data about the accuracy of MRI in staging liver steatosis and fibrosis and for this reason liver biopsy remains the gold standard.

5.3.5 Primary Sclerosing Cholangitis

Primary sclerosing cholangitis (PSC) rarely affect children and often in association to inflammatory bowel diseases or in an overlap syndrome with autoimmune hepatitis [112]. Clinical manifestations are anorexia, abdominal pain, pruritus, and fatigue. PSC has a chronic and a progressive course in children. Complications are portal hypertension, bacterial cholangitis, and cholangiocarcinoma (the last extremely rare). The median survival with native liver is 2.8–3.5 years [113]. The chronic inflammation cause irreversible damage of intrahepatic and extrahepatic bile ducts with obliterative fibrosis up to liver cirrhosis. ERCP is the standard for diagnosis. MRCP has a specificity and positive predictive value of 100% and an accuracy of 85% [114]. Findings are irregular bile duct walls, multifocal segmental strictures, intermittence between strictures and sacculations ("beaded" appearance), pseudodiverticula, and paucity of peripheral bile ducts completely obliterated ("pruned tree" appearance) [115].

5.4 Interventional Radiology

Interventional procedures are minimally invasive and image-guided procedures that allow diagnostic examinations or therapeutic maneuvers performed through percutaneous or vascular accesses under ultrasound, fluoroscopic, CT, and MRI guidance. Many diseases that once required surgical treatment can be treated nonsurgically by interventional radiologists with less risk, less pain, and faster recovery time. Interventional procedures are increasing in number, variety, and complexity, thanks to the development of new devices, even if not always dedicated to small patients, and thanks to the improvement of sedation techniques. Techniques used in newborns, infants, and children are borrowed from those for adults. However, it is more difficult to perform them considering the small size of the patient and anatomical structures, the greater risk of heat loss due to relatively larger body surface and immature thermoregulation [116]. IR is routinely used to perform biopsies and embolization, to place stents, drainage tubes, and peripherally inserted central catheters (PICCs). Vascular abnormalities, biliary pathologies, portal hypertension, trauma, and liver transplant complications are the main indications.

Finally, in the pediatric patient, the attitude may be more aggressive than in adult patients because the intent is more curative than palliative [116].

5.4.1 Interventional Radiology in the Native Liver

5.4.1.1 Liver Biopsy

Liver biopsy is performed to make a diagnosis and for staging liver diseases. Standard indications are changing, and they are becoming more individualized; the reason is that noninvasive techniques such as imaging and laboratory exams may substitute histological evaluation [117]. When biopsy is not proposed routinely, the aim is to exclude other diseases. It can be a targeted or nontargeted procedures, guided by US or fluoroscopy. The targeted biopsy is directed to sample focal liver lesions to make a differential diagnosis; the nontargeted biopsy is performed randomly obtaining hepatic tissue in suspected diffuse liver disease including cholestatic disorders and graft rejection in case of liver transplantation. There are two types of approach: percutaneous core needle biopsy (PCNB) and transjugular liver biopsy (TJLB). PCNB is performed by using needles from 21 to 16 gauge or with a coaxial technique (Menghini or Tru-cut needle) if more than one core is required; it usually presupposes a subxiphoid, subcostal, or intercostal approach. The major complications are hemoperitoneum, hematoma, hepatic arterial pseudoaneurysm, choleperitoneum, pneumothorax, local infection [118], hemobilia, and arterioportal fistula. TJLB is an alternative method in patients that cannot undergo a percutaneous biopsy because of uncorrectable coagulopathy, ascites, or both and if a concurrent procedure is requested (e.g., wedge hepatic vein pressure measurement) [116, 119]. However, TJLB can be challenging in very young patient because of unavailability of devices of appropriate size. When feasibility, US guidance is used for jugular venous access. Then, the middle or the right hepatic vein is selectively catheterized. A biopsy specimen is obtained by firing the outer cutting cannula over the stylet to acquire a core of tissue. The risk of hemorrhage is lower than PCNB because the needle insertion is through a branch of the hepatic vein and any bleeding from puncture site remains within the vascular space. Complications can be subcapsular hematoma, intraperitoneal bleeding, direct arterial injury such as pseudoaneurysm or AV fistula, and venous perforation of the inferior vena cava (IVC) or renal veins, pneumothorax, and hemothorax [120, 121].

5.4.1.2 Portal Hypertension

Portal hypertension is one of the fields of pediatric hepatology that involves interventional radiology. Interventional procedures have not only a diagnostic role with the assess-

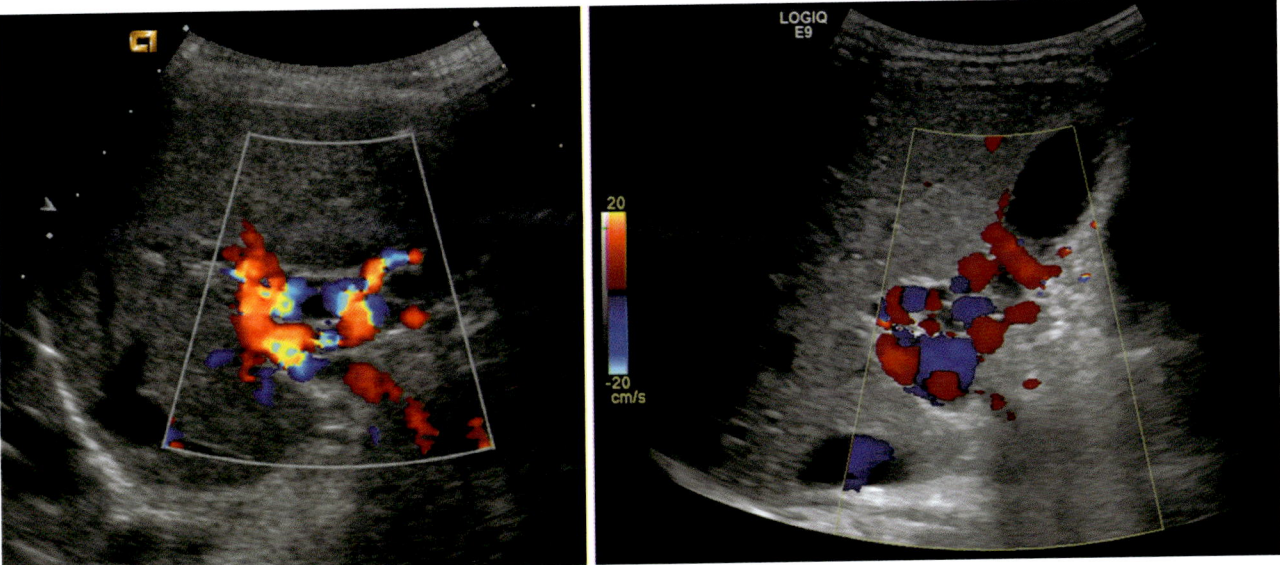

Fig. 5.12 Color Doppler US shows portal cavernoma with hepatopetal and hepatofugal veins; opposite collateral veins' flow direction is represented by red and blue colors

ment of pressure gradients but also therapeutic role in the treatment of portal hypertension complications. Portal hypertension may develop in both a cirrhotic and non-cirrhotic liver. The most frequent cause of non-cirrhotic portal hypertension in the pediatric age is represented by the extrahepatic portal vein obstruction (EHPVO). EHPVO refers to extrahepatic portal vein occlusion and subsequent development of hepatopetal and hepatofugal veins (cavernoma) (Fig. 5.12). Predisposing factors in neonates include umbilical venous catheterization with or without infection; for older children, liver transplantation, splenectomy, sepsis, dehydration, sickle cell disease, and congenital and acquired prothrombotic disorders have been associated to this condition [122]. Other causes of non-cirrhotic portal hypertension in children include congenital hepatic fibrosis, nonalcoholic fatty liver disease, nodular regenerative hyperplasia, sinusoidal obstruction syndrome, Budd-Chiari, and rarely metabolic diseases (Gaucher's and Zellweger syndrome), schistosomiasis, and hepatoportal sclerosis [123, 124]. At baseline conditions, the portal flow has a pressure of 7–10 mmHg, and the hepatic venous pressure gradient (HVPG), defined as the difference between the wedged hepatic veins pressure and the free hepatic venous pressure, has a value of 1–4 mmHg. In portal hypertension, the portal pressure is greater than 10 mmHg and the HVPG greater than 4 mmHg [125].

The first radiological approach to children with portal hypertension starts with US, both in gray-scale and Doppler mode, to assess liver parenchyma, low velocity, hepatofugal flow and patency of portal vein, revascularization of umbilical vein, varices, fistulous communications, and ascites. MRI and CT scan are useful to give a panoramic assessment of liver parenchyma and vasculature and to better evaluate the possible cavernomatous transformation in case of portal vein thrombosis.

The treatment of children with portal hypertension is conservative and aims to contain side effects, first of all variceal bleeding. Variceal bleeding is cured with endoscopic sclerotherapy and/or band ligation, but if varices are refractory to conservative treatment, the option of creating a meso-Rex surgical shunt or a portosystemic shunt (TIPS) should be considered. The Rex shunt restores physiologic, hepatopetal flow by bridging the superior mesenteric vein with the Rex recess of the left portal vein by an autologous graft [122]. TIPS instead creates a portosystemic shunt connecting the hepatic vein with portal vein by a stent. Before performing a shunt, it is essential to evaluate the patency of the two ends to be connected: porto-spleno-mesenteric and systemic venous side. The main indication of *wedged hepatic vein portography* is the preoperative assessment of patency of intrahepatic left portal vein (Rex recessus) and the communication between left and right portal veins in extrahepatic portal vein obstruction (EHPVO) with the aim to attempt a meso-portal bypass. In these case the wedged hepatic vein portography is performed by catheterization of the left hepatic vein via internal vein jugular approach. The portal system is opacified in a retrograde way obtaining retrograde opacification and visualization of portal branches through the hepatic sinusoids.

5.4.1.3 Transjugular Intrahepatic Portosystemic Shunt (TIPS)

TIPS is a standardized procedure in the adult population for the treatment of portal hypertension complications; on the other hand, studies about the use in pediatric population are still few and with short follow-ups [126]. However, the feasibility and efficacy of this procedure has already been demonstrated [126–128]. Patients eligible for TIPS are those with complications of portal hypertension such as ascites and variceal bleeding refractory to conservative medical and endoscopic treatment, both in native and transplanted as well as a bridge to transplantation. Furthermore, TIPS can be an option in patients with EHPVO who are not eligible for surgical meso-portal bypass. Absolute contraindications to TIPS placement include severe pulmonary hypertension, severe tricuspid regurgitation, congestive heart failure, severe liver failure, and polycystic liver disease or cholangitis. Other relative contraindications include recurrent HE, hepatocellular carcinoma and other liver tumors, and bile duct dilation [129]. TIPS is a procedure that creates a low-resistance intrahepatic tunnel that bridges the hepatic vein or the inferior vena cava to a portal vein branch (usually the right one) to obtain a portosystemic shunt. The intrahepatic tract remains patent, thanks to the release of an expandable covered stent (Fig. 5.13). The procedure is less invasive than the surgical operation because performed via transjugular access that allows the selective catheterization both of hepatic veins and portal vein (Fig. 5.14). If portal vein targeting is difficult, additional percutaneous access is required for catheterization of the portal vein. After the transjugular access and the catheterization of the hepatic vein, a wedged hepatic vein portography is performed. The wedged hepatic vein portography need to have a roadmap for the release of the stent. After portography the radiologist tries to puncture the portal vein with a dedicated needle; a second operator under ultrasound guide acts as a navigator allowing direct visualization of the needle respect into the portal vein branch, in order to reduce the procedural times and the radiation exposure. Subsequently, the venous pressure gradient is measured; if the portosystemic gradient is greater than 12 mmHg, the placement of shunt is indicated. A preventive dilation of the intraparenchymal tract previously created by the needle is performed after which the stent is placed. In the past only bare stents, with high risk of closure, were used [130]; currently expanded polytetrafluoroethylene (ePTFE)-covered stents are preferred. The first one was prone to allow intrastent neointimal proliferation, with the direct consequence of stent occlusion. The covered stents, instead, have shown a dramatically improvement of primary and secondary long-term patency [131]. However, the ePTFE-covered stents are available only in adult format, not tailored for children. In fact the only available caliper sizes are 8 and 10 mm too big to adapt to a very small child vessels. Following the stent positioning a venography and measurement of the pressures are performed to confirm the correct stent positioning and the reduction of pressure gradient. TIPS success is confirmed with reduction of the portosystemic gradient (PSG) to <12 mmHg or by >25% [126]. Choosing the correct stent diameter may be challenging. A too small or a too large stent caliper can lead to early thrombosis and liver encephalopathy, respectively. Procedural complications are intraperitoneal bleeding, intrahepatic hematoma, subcapsular hematoma, and hepatic infarction. US examination should be performed after 2–3 days after the procedure; the reason is that the PTFE contains a small amount of air between its meshes and the air generates US artifact soon after placement with an erratic evaluation of the flow inside the TIPS. After a few days the air of the PTFE is reabsorbed allowing the correct display of the TIPS. Doppler US shows the patency of the device through the measurement of maximal peak flow velocity and the evaluation of the direction of flow within the shunt and in the portal vein (Fig. 5.15). At Doppler US signs of TIPS stenosis or thrombosis are absent flow inside the shunt, low-peak flow velocity (<50 cm/s), high-peak shunt velocity (>180 cm/s), low mean portal vein velocity (<30 cm/s), and significant change in shunt velocity

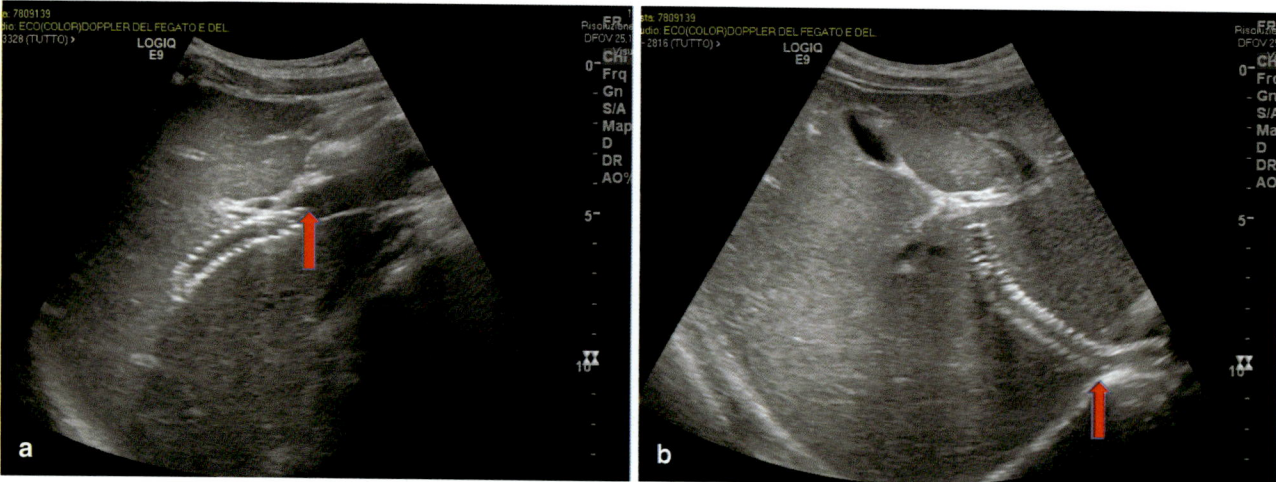

Fig. 5.13 B-mode US; (**a**) intercostal projection shows TIPS portal side (arrow); (**b**) subxiphoid projection shows TIPS hepatic vein side (arrow)

(>50 cm/s) compared with the immediate post-procedure. The procedure is long and not without technical difficulties due to the small size of children and anatomical structures. Although effective and feasible, TIPS involves a significant exposure to X-ray, and we believe it is mandatory to puncture the portal vein (the most time-consuming portion of the procedure) under ultrasound guidance in order to reduce exposure to ionizing radiation as much as possible. For these reasons TIPS should be performed by experts interventional radiologists.

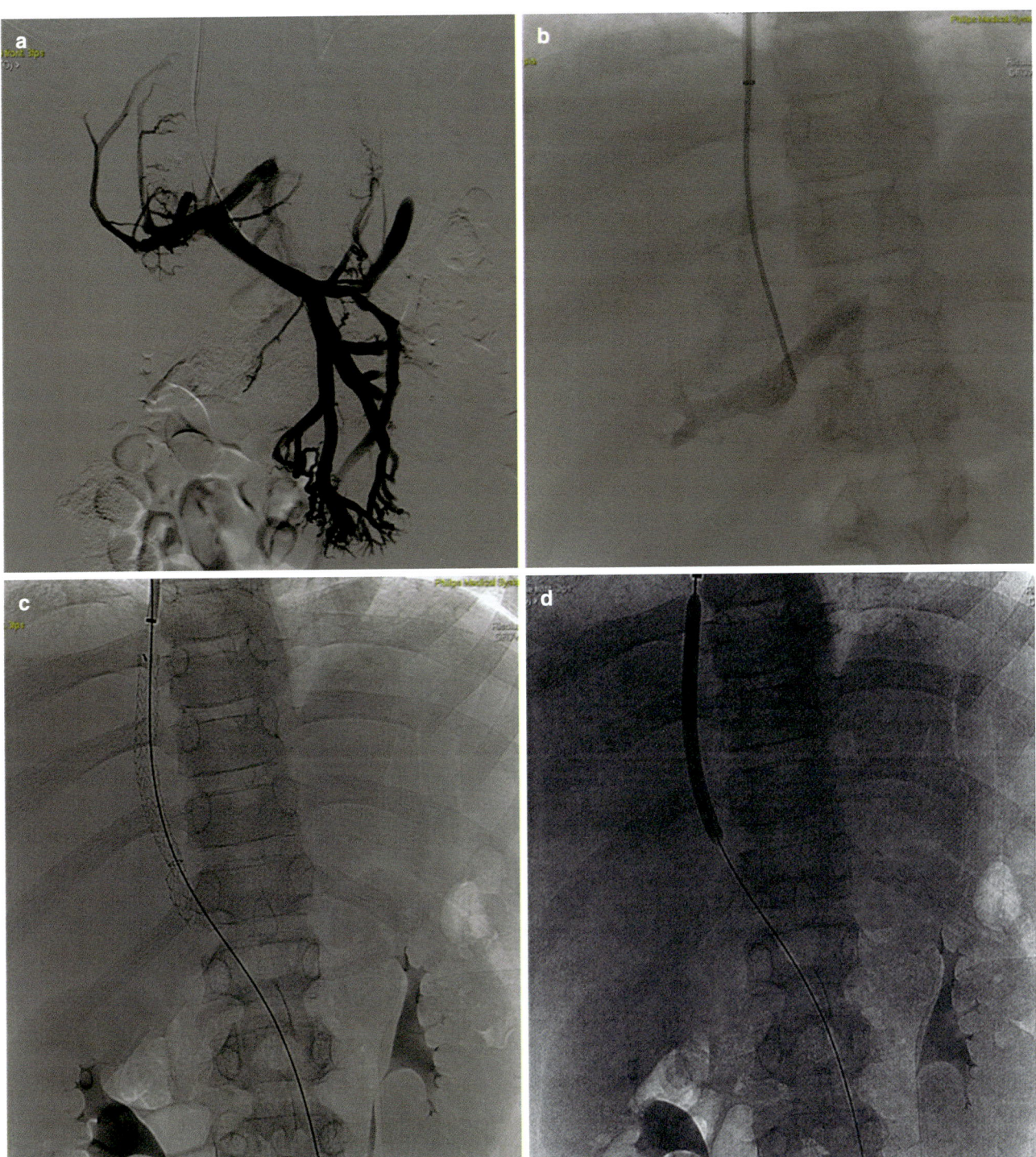

Fig. 5.14 TIPS placement: (**a**) portal preliminary catheterization; (**b**) creation of the intrahepatic tunnel that bridges the hepatic vein to portal vein branch; (**c**) placement of ePTFE-covered stents; (**d**) intrastent ballooning; (**e**) final step procedure with patent TIPS

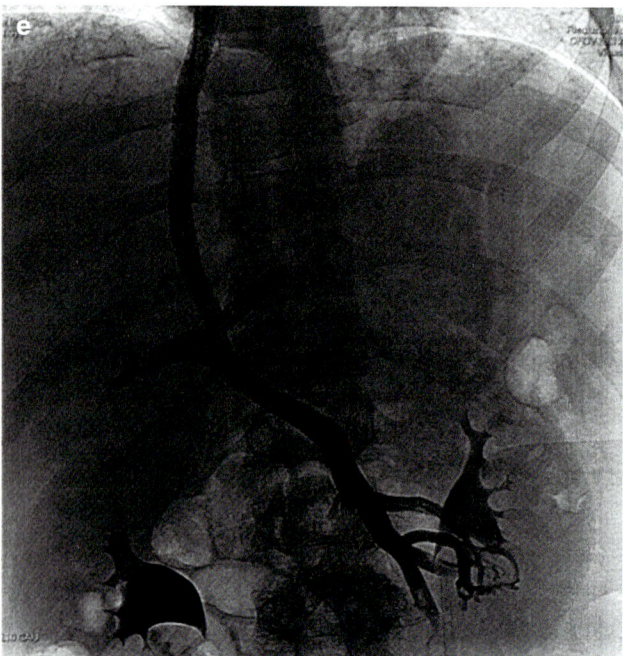

Fig. 5.14 (continued)

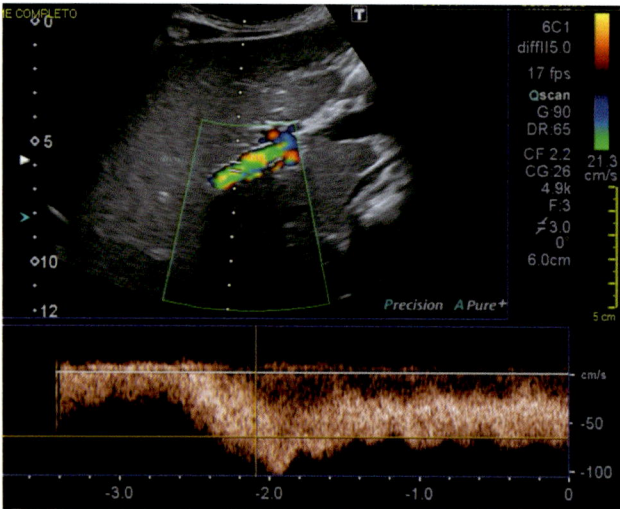

Fig. 5.15 Spectral color Doppler US shows TIPS patency with flow velocity (>50 cm/s)

5.4.1.4 Vascular Anomalies

According to the latest classification of International Society for the Study of Vascular Anomalies (ISSVA 2014), vascular anomalies are subdivided into vascular tumors and vascular malformations. The first group includes the neoplastic lesions with marked angioproliferative activity, divided into benign, locally aggressive or borderline, and malignant. The group of benign vascular tumors includes infant hepatic hemangiomas, which we have previously discussed. The group of vascular malformations is distinguished in simple vascular malformations (arteriovenous malformation (AVM), arteriovenous fistula, etc.) and combined malformations, those of major named vessels (e.g., Abernethy malformation) and those associated with other anomalies. Depending on vessels involved, we can distinguish high-flow connections (fistulae or arteriovenous malformations) and low-flow connections (venous and lymphatic malformations). Below we will discuss about the vascular anomalies of greater interventional radiology interest.

In the *infantile hepatic hemangioma*, there are multiple arteriovenous connections consisting of low-resistance tumor vessels with a large feeding artery and draining veins that create a high-flow shunt; the arteriovenous shunt is characterized by a hepatic artery enlargement with a low-resistance index (RI) and increased flow velocities in the hepatic veins that may show an arterialized spectral pattern. The high-flow that characterizes these shunts can cause high output heart failure. Asymptomatic patients undergo follow-up until regression of the lesion. Symptomatic patients undergo propranolol therapy with or without steroids as appropriate. Patients who are not responsive to medical treatment may benefit from endovascular treatment [132]. After femoral access it is performed a diagnostic arteriography to study both the arterial collaterals that supply the tumor and the venous collaterals (Fig. 5.16). The success of the endovascular embolization procedure can be affected by the presence of extrahepatic arterial collaterals and portal venous contribution. Embolization is performed by the delivery of coils or polyvinyl alcohol (PVA) particles or microspheres through a microcatheter. The most important complication is necrosis of the hepatic parenchyma following artery occlusion [133].

The *arterioportal fistula* may be extrahepatic or intrahepatic and congenital or acquired. Congenital forms are rare and may be associated with hereditary hemorrhagic telangi-

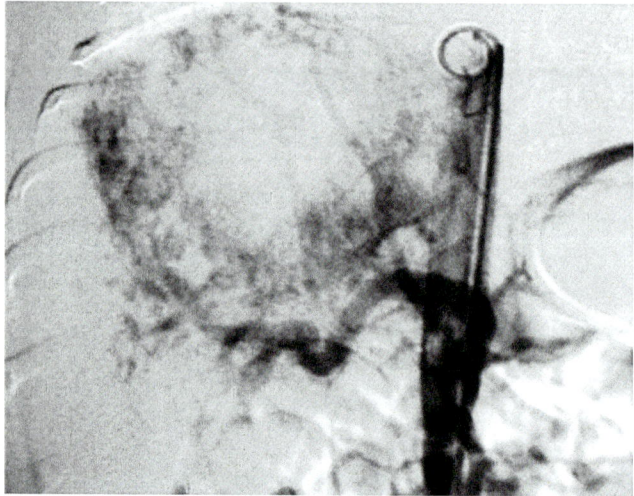

Fig. 5.16 Angiographic appearance of IHH with intra- and perilesional vascular collaterals

ectasia, Ehlers-Danlos syndrome. The acquired forms are usually the result of a trauma, iatrogenic or not, which causes direct communication between an arterial branch and a branch of the portal system. Major causes are percutaneous hepatic biopsy, endovascular cannulation, transhepatic cholangiography, and blunt or penetrating trauma. Some pathological diseases such as cirrhosis and liver tumors can also lead to arterial-portal connections. At the color Doppler examination, it is possible to visualize a dilatation of the segmental hepatic artery and portal branch involved and high-velocity and low-resistance arterial waveforms with arterialized portal venous flow. On CT and MRI, early enhancement of the portal vein is seen in the segmental portal venous branch close to the shunt during the arterial phase. It is possible to see a parenchymal transient wedge-shaped peripheral enhancement to the shunt as the result of transient perfusion alteration (named THAD on CT and THID on MRI). This is due to the regional increase in arterial inflow caused by the inverted portal flow or to the increase in portal vein inflow due to the shunt itself [133, 134]. Endovascular treatment is performed with selective catheterization of hepatic artery and embolization of the affected arterial segment with coils. Treatment of fistulas in patients with cirrhosis may be problematic because the liver becomes dependent on arterial inflow and the arterial embolization with coils can cause fatal hepatic necrosis. In transplanted patients, arterio-portal fistula is a frequent complication of repeated biopsies to exclude rejection; however, 90% undergo spontaneous regression within a week. In these patients, the management is controversial; in general it seems wise to treat only fistulae associated with signs of portal hypertension. Asymptomatic fistulae are monitored over time [135, 136].

5.5 Liver Transplantation

Orthotopic liver transplantation constitutes a validated therapeutic modality in patients with acute liver failure and with end-stage liver disease for which no other therapy is available.

The transplantation techniques performed in children include whole pediatric cadaveric organ grafting, reduced-size liver, split liver, and living related adult organ grafting [137]. In all transplantations, a series of anastomosis are created: donor hepatic artery and recipient hepatic artery in end-to-end fashion, portal venous anastomosis between the main portal veins of the donor and that of the recipient, vena cava that can be anastomosed to the recipient suprahepatic inferior vena cava or that can be preferred the piggyback variant, and biliary anastomosis end-to-end fashion or, more frequently, a biliary reconstruction performed in a hepatic jejunostomy. The main postsurgical complications may involve the vasculature, biliary ducts, liver parenchyma, and perihepatic space and can occur in the early postoperative period or during long-term follow-up. Imaging is crucial for early detection of complications because the clinical manifestations are frequently wide and nonspecific.

5.5.1 Imaging Point of View

The first imaging modality chosen for liver evaluation after transplantation is ultrasound since it can be performed at the bedside, is accurate and noninvasive, and can avoid ionizing radiation. The evaluation includes both B-mode and color Doppler US modalities. B-mode is used to visualize liver parenchyma and biliary tree. Color Doppler enables to estimate blood flow and measure the resistance index (RI) in the peripheral branches of hepatic artery. We routinely perform the first US examination 6–7 h after transplantation and every day while the patient is in the intensive care unit. When the patient is transferred to the pediatric ward, a control study is performed twice weekly. If US results are unsatisfactory or clinical suspicion for a complication arises, it is mandatory to perform a further investigation with CT or MRI. Conventional angiographic and cholangiographic studies are reserved for nonsurgical treatment of some complications. At US the normal hepatic artery spectral Doppler waveform is pulsatile and anterograde during the entire cardiac cycle and has a low-resistance pattern measured by the resistance index (RI). RI represents the ratio of peak systolic velocity – peak diastolic velocity/peak systolic velocity, and the normal range is between 0.5 and 0.7 (Fig. 5.17). The decrease of RI (<0.5) is a marker of complications such as hepatic artery stenosis and thrombosis. The elevation of RI (>0.7) is a nonspecific finding and can be observed in the postprandial state and in diffuse peripheral microvascular (arteriolar) alterations, as seen in chronic hepatocellular disease (including cirrhosis), hepatic venous congestion, cold

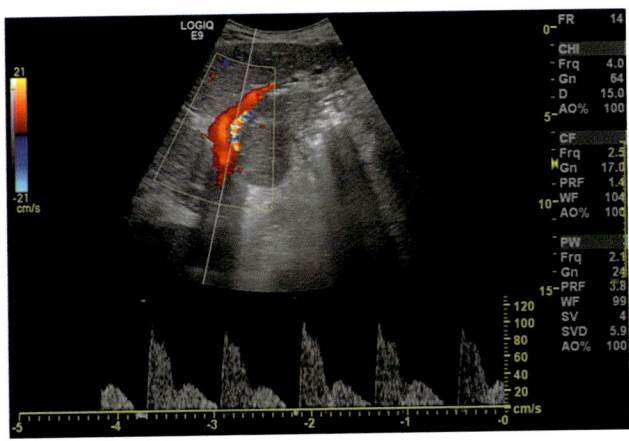

Fig. 5.17 Normal hepatic artery spectral Doppler waveform is pulsatile, anterograde during the entire cardiac cycle, and a low-resistance pattern

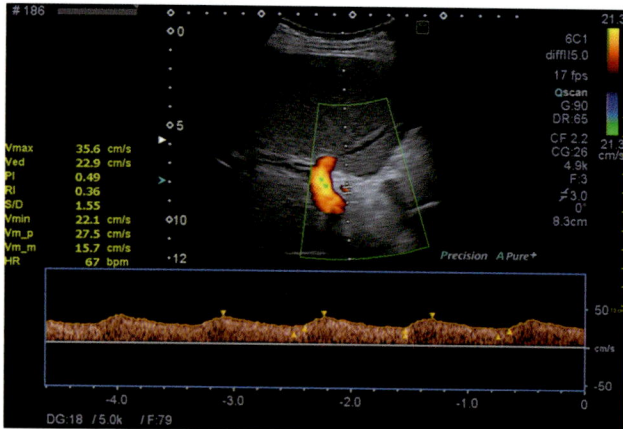

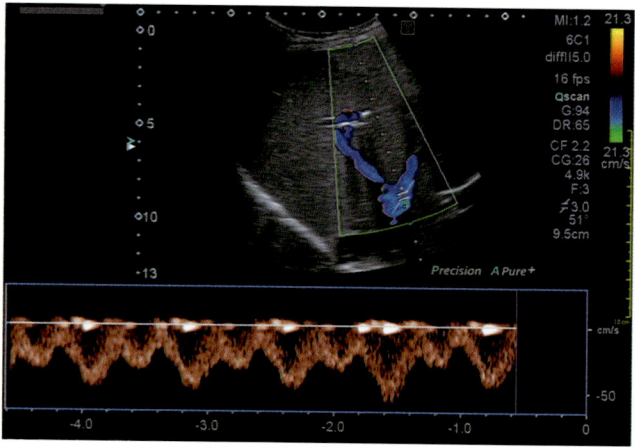

Fig. 5.18 The spectral color Doppler shows "tardus-parvus" arterial waveform, characterized by slowed systolic upstroke and reduced peak systolic velocity. Note the reduced RI of 0.36 in stenosis of hepatic artery

Fig. 5.20 The normal hepatic vein spectral Doppler waveform is tetraphasic, bidirectional, but predominantly antegrade; flow variations are created by pressure variations related to the cardiac cycle and respiratory motions

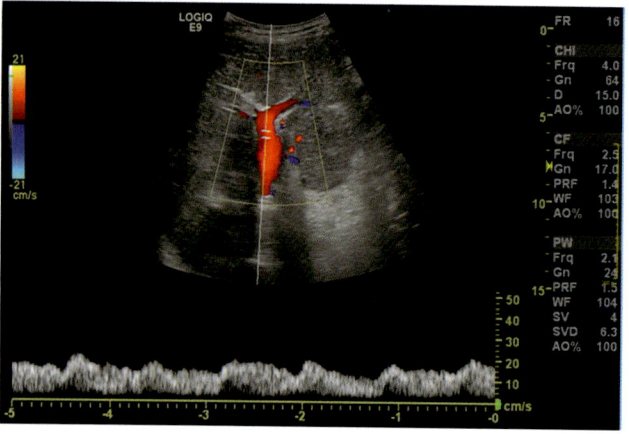

Fig. 5.19 The normal portal vein spectral Doppler waveform is phasic, with mild velocity variations, anterograde, and hepatopetal, and the flow velocity is relatively low

ischemia (posttransplantation), and any stage of transplant rejection. In case of reduced arterial flow it is possible to observe the "tardus-parvus" spectral waveform, characterized by slowed systolic upstroke and reduced peak systolic velocity (Fig. 5.18) [138]. Tardus-parvus waveform can be a sign of arterial stenosis or thrombosis.

The normal portal vein spectral Doppler waveform is phasic, with mild velocity variations, anterograde, and hepatopetal, and the flow velocity in this vessel is relatively low (16–40 cm/s) (Fig. 5.19). Indicators of a pathologic portal venous flow usually are increased pulsatility, slow portal venous flow (<16 cm/s), hepatofugal flow, and absent flow. The hepatic venous waveform is characterized by alternating antegrade-retrograde pressure or flow variations, which are in turn created by pressure variations related to the cardiac cycle and the respiratory variations (Fig. 5.20). Signs of pathologic hepatic venous flow may be increased pulsatility with dramatic fluctuations between abnormally tall retrograde waves and abnormally deep antegrade waves, decreased phasicity and spectral widening, and absent flow [139].

5.5.2 Vascular Complication

Vascular complications can occur early (within a month) or late (after a month) from transplantation and can affect hepatic artery, portal vein, hepatic vein, and inferior vena cava. In pediatric patients the complication rate is greater than that of adults for two main reasons: the small anatomical structures that make the anastomosis fashioning more difficult and the anatomical discrepancy between graft vessels (most from adult donors) and the recipient.

Hepatic artery complications include thrombosis, stenosis, kinks, pseudo aneurysms, dissection, and arterial steal syndrome. Portal vein and inferior vena cava complications include thrombosis and stenosis. The most important complications will be discussed.

The *hepatic artery stenosis* usually occurs within 3 months after transplantation in up to 14% of cases [140]; it can affect either the anastomotic site, due to surgical injury or small vascular caliper, or the nonanastomotic site due to graft rejection or necrosis. In hepatic artery stenosis, the spectral analysis depends on the site where the artery is sampled. At the narrowing site, the flow is characterized by a focal accelerated velocity greater than 200 cm/s, with associated turbulence distal to the stenosis. The stricture is difficult to find, and the diagnosis is usually made sampling flow in the arterial branches distal to the narrowing; in this case spectral analysis reveals tardus-parvus pattern with a prolonged acceleration time and decreased resistive index (inferior to 0.5). One must be careful because the isolated finding of tardus-parvus may represent a false-positive test; adding peak systolic velocity (PSV) cutoff of less than or equal to 48 cm/s greatly improves the predictive positive value and reduces the false-positive rate from 11 to 1% [141]. However, Doppler examination can be normal in the presence of mild degrees of artery stenosis, and if there is a high clinical suspicion, it is advisable to perform CT angiography or MRI [142]. Interventional arteriography is performed only when there is a high suspicion of stenosis or with interventional aims. Hepatic arteriography is usually performed by using a coronary angiography endovascular set (for the small size of the patient) with a transfemoral approach. The hepatic artery is catheterized, and the guidewire is lead through the stenosis to measure the trans-stenotic pressure gradient. If the stenosis is hemodynamically significant (pressure gradient >10 mmHg), an angioplasty is performed with ballooning of the stenotic tract. The placement of a stent is recommended only after angioplasty failure or after post-procedural complications (artery dissection or rupture).

Hepatic artery thrombosis is a real emergency often leading to graft loss, since the hepatic artery is the sole blood supply to biliary system of the graft. It is usually seen in less than 5% of cases, but in some series it has been described in up to 17% of patients [140]. In hepatic artery thrombosis, the Doppler US shows, in most cases, the complete absence of arterial flow in the proper hepatic and intrahepatic artery. However, the radiologist may raise the suspect early, if there are progressive changes of some parameters that enable to predict the subsequent thrombosis (syndrome of impending thrombosis): over 3–10 days, the Doppler US may show a progressive decrease in systolic and diastolic flow, followed by the absent diastolic component, the dampening of the systolic peak, and, finally, the total loss of hepatic waveform [143]. After the thrombosis has occurred, it is possible the development of arterial collateral vessel with subsequent presence of intrahepatic arterial flow. However, the intrahepatic arterial flow will display a tardus-parvus pattern and a RI lower than 0.5. False-positive diagnosis may occur in the setting of markedly diminished hepatic artery flow (massive hepatic necrosis, hepatic edema, or systemic hypotension). In this case CT or MRI can evaluate the arterial patency and identify patients requiring further treatment. Nowadays, the treatment options are urgent thrombectomy with revascularization or repeated transplantation, even if encouraging results begin to be reported for percutaneous revascularization after early detection of hepatic artery thrombosis [144]. This can be achieved through a selective thrombolysis via transfemoral approach followed by angioplasty. When effective, this interventional procedure allows to avoid retransplantation.

Portal vein stenosis (uncommon) usually occurs in 4–8% of pediatric liver transplants at the anastomotic site. The causes are the vein mismatch and the reduced length of native portal vein with the need for interposition grafts that characterizes reduced-size liver transplantation [116]. Color Doppler US shows focal color aliasing at the stenosis with more than a three- to fourfold increase in velocity at the prestenotic segment. A post-stenotic jet with a velocity between 1 and 3 m/s is a characteristic finding [140]. The diagnosis of portal vein stenosis must be done with caution to differentiate stenosis from pseudostenosis. The first one is hemodynamically significant and must be treated. The second one is not physiologically significant and related to difference in caliper between donor and recipient portal veins: this leads to increased velocity and turbulence at the anastomotic site at Doppler US, but this is increased less than three- to fourfold (Fig. 5.21). The treatment of choice is percutaneous transhepatic angioplasty with US-guided portal puncture. The technique allows to insert a catheter through the stenosis and ballooning the lesion. Before the balloon dilatation, an intravenous heparinization is administered. After the procedure a residual transtenotic gradient pressure >5 mmHg is an indication for stenting. Stenting is also required in recurrent or nonresponsive elastic stenosis. Procedural complications include intraperitoneal, gastrointestinal, and biliary tract bleeding and infections. Restenosis occurs in up to 5% of treated children [116].

Portal vein thrombosis usually occurs in main extrahepatic tract and in reduced-size liver transplantation. It is associated with surgical technique complications, the use of cryopreserved venous conduits, and all situations that can decrease portal vein inflow (prior portosystemic shunts, splenectomy, and vessel redundancy). US is characterized by an echogenic luminal thrombus with no detectable flow at color Doppler modality. Importantly, an acute thrombus may be anechoic and not visible on gray-scale US images, and the abnormality may become evident only at color Doppler analysis. Partial portal vein thrombosis can also appear as a narrowing vessel with a non-occlusive filling defect. Occasionally, in association with no flow signal in main portal vein, a reversed intrahepatic portal flow due to arterioportal shunts development may be detected. At CT and MRI, the thrombus appears as an occluding vascular defect after contrast medium administration. Portal vein thrombosis can be treated with surgical approach (thrombectomy or segmental vein resection) or interventional approach. The last includes mechanical thrombectomy and pharmacologic thrombolysis [145] with or without stent placement. Nowadays a more aggressive management is preferred, recanalizing also chronic thrombosis to prevent the formation of cavernoma and its complications related to portal hypertension, especially in view of future retransplantation.

Inferior vena cava and hepatic veins complications are rare but more common in the pediatric population than adults. This complication tends to be more frequent in the superior anastomosis and is often associated to technical difficulties that can involve also the hepatic vein anastomosis [120].

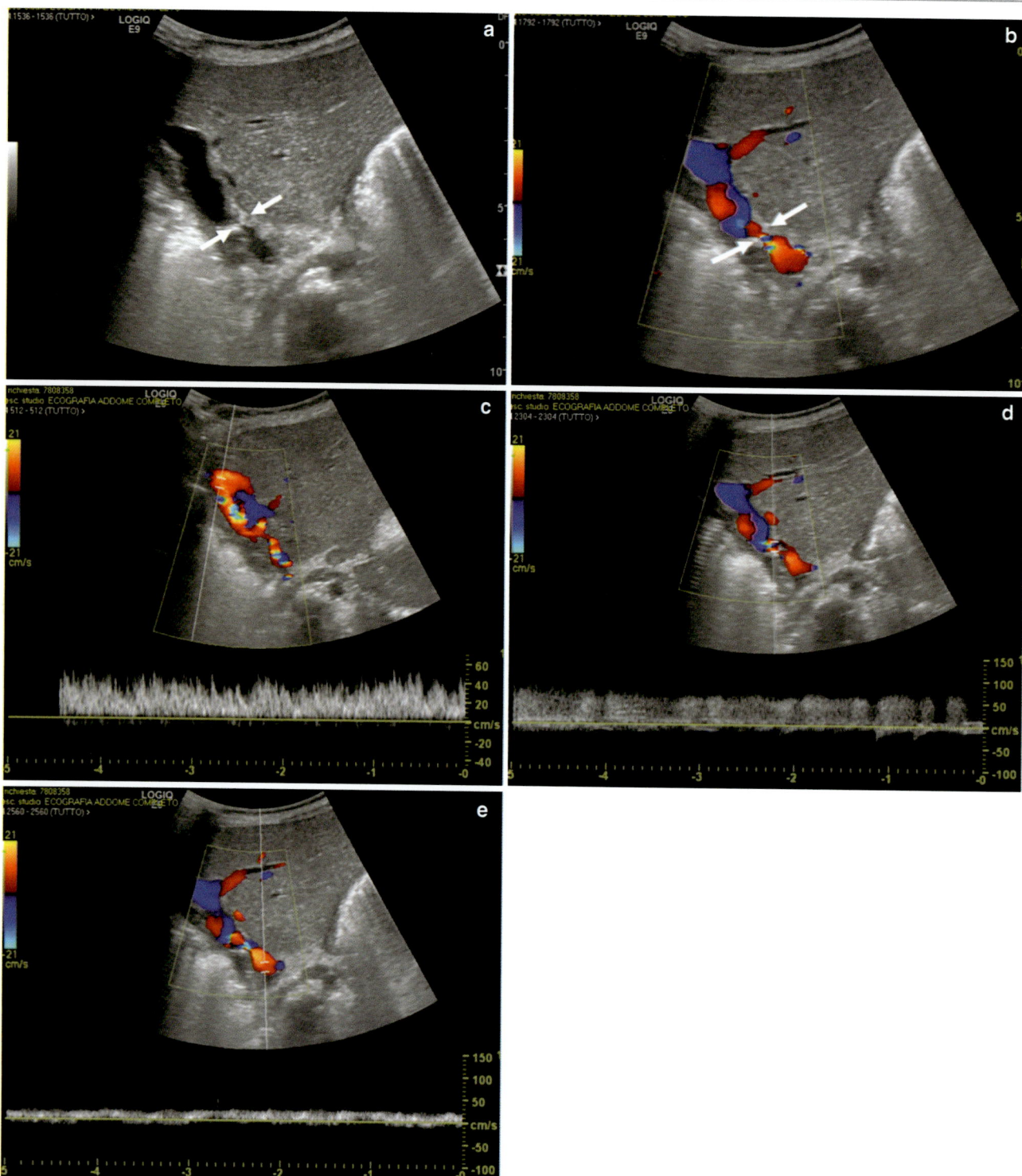

Fig. 5.21 Portal pseudostenosis. B-mode US and color US modalities (**a**, **b**) show difference in caliper between donor and recipient portal vein, but there is no significant increase in velocity flow sample in graft portal vein (**c**), pseudostenotic tract (**d**), and recipient portal tract (**e**)

Inferior vena cava stenosis occurs in up to 5% of cases and hepatic vein stenosis occurs in some 1% of pediatric liver transplant recipients. Early stenosis can be due to graft size discrepancy or kinking from organ rotation. Delayed stenosis is usually secondary to fibrosis, chronic thrombus, or neointimal hyperplasia. B-mode and Doppler US findings are narrowing at the site of anastomosis, three- to fourfold increase in velocity through the stenosis as compared with that at the prestenotic segment, and aliasing. A significant suprahepatic caval stenosis may result in reversed flow or the absence of phasicity in the hepatic veins. Pseudo-stenosis, instead, can be caused by graft growth and twisting and can be present or disappear depending on the patient's posture [140]. Cavography can aid to distinguish stenosis from pseudostenosis measuring the gradient pressure through the narrowing tract. Inferior vena cava and hepatic vein thrombosis can be detected at duplex ultrasound for the presence of echogenic intraluminal thrombus with the absence of flow. In case of stenosis, the first treatment is represented by angioplasty with transfemoral or transjugular approach. The balloon catheter is inserted in to the vein and is repetitively inflated and deflated to obtain a normalization of transluminal gradient pressure. Stenting is used in case of suboptimal results, with residual gradient pressure, or for restenosis.

5.5.3 Biliary Complications

Biliary complications are the most frequently observed postoperative complications due to a suboptimal peribiliary arterial supply at the cut surface of a segmental graft [146]; the majority of biliary strictures occur within the first 3–6 months after surgery [142]. Classification is based on the time of occurrence (early occur within 30-day posttransplant and late complications after 90-day posttransplant), localization (anastomotic or nonanastomotic), or etiology (surgical method of biliary reconstruction, prolonged cold ischemia time, immunologic reactions, hepatic artery thrombosis, ABO blood group system incompatibility). Complications include strictures, leaks, bilomas, stones or sludge, mucocele, and dysfunction of the sphincter of Oddi (in end-to-end anastomoses).

The rate of *biliary strictures incidence is estimated between 2 and 35%*, depending probability on the percentage of segmental grafts and the attitude to look for it. The anastomotic strictures are associated to technical problems and hypertrophy of the surgical scar and appear as dilatation of common bile ducts proximally to the anastomosis and intrahepatic ducts dilatation (Fig. 5.22). However, the graft stiffness may not always allow biliary dilatation, and some strictures might be suspected only on histological findings suggesting mechanical cholestasis. The nonanastomotic strictures can be the result of artery insufficiency or thrombosis and are often localized at the hepatic hilum and extend peripherally or may be intrahepatic and multiple; US shows focal segmental intrahepatic or hilar ductal dilatation without an obstructing mass or stone. In the most severe forms of nonanastomotic strictures (early hepatic artery thrombosis), the bile ducts are filled of epithelial cells due to the partial or complete biliary necrosis that forms sludge or biliary casts [146]. If clinical suspicion persists despite normal US, MR cholangiography can be a useful tool to delineate the anatomy and morphologic features of bile ducts and detect bili-

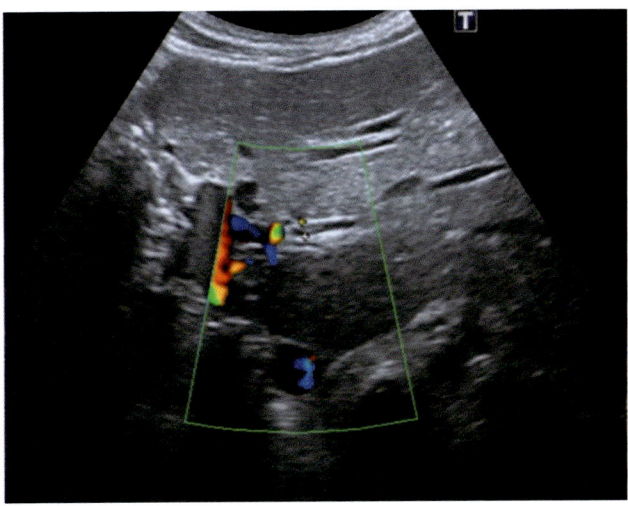

Fig. 5.22 Intrahepatic ductal dilatation in anastomotic biliary stricture in liver split II–III transplantation

ary strictures. The ultrasound examination has a low sensitivity in identifying the stenosis (24%), despite high specificity. The sensitivity and specificity in the evaluation of anastomotic stenosis are higher for cholangio-MR (90%), although the sensitivity is reduced in case of biliary-entero anastomosis [147, 148]. If cholangio-MR shows no biliary dilatation, percutaneous transhepatic cholangiography (PTC) should be performed, accomplishing diagnostic and interventional assessment. PTC plays a fundamental role and allows to treat strictures at biliary jejunostomy (not approachable by ERCP) avoiding surgery (Fig. 5.23). The first step involves a percutaneous subxiphoid or subcostal access in left segment liver transplantation or an intercostal access in whole liver and right split liver transplantation. The access to the biliary system is achieved by direct needle puncture of a segmentary bile duct, with the subsequent insertion of a guidewire and of a catheter. A first diagnostic cholangiography is performed. The diagnostic cholangiography enables to visualize the biliary stricture site and establish a roadmap to identify the biliary-entero anastomosis through which an internal-external biliary drainage catheter (IEBDC) can be positioned. The next step is dilation of stricture site with simple balloon catheter or cutting balloon catheter in cases of resistant stenosis. There is no literature agreement about when to perform balloon dilation of biliary strictures. Some authors prefer to leave in site the biliary drainage catheter to decompress the biliary system for a week and then to begin the first dilatation session. This choice is dictated by reducing the risk of cholangitis. In our experience, if it is possible to immediately overcome the stenosis, we prefer to drain and dilate in a single session to reduce x-ray exposure. One or two dilations are performed for 30–60 s. The drainage is left in place on average of 1 month after which a diagnostic PTC is carried out, and if a residual stenosis is demonstrated, a

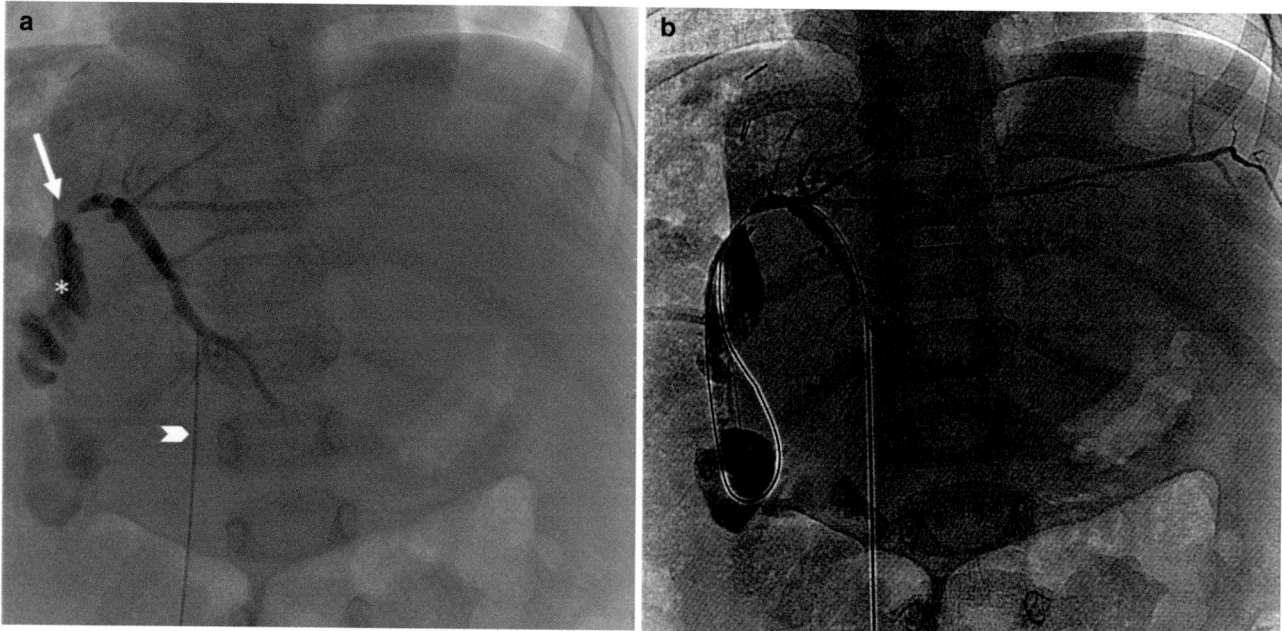

Fig. 5.23 At PTC, stricture of biliary-entero anastomosis: (**a**) a guide wire (short arrow) is inserted through the stricture (arrow) up to jejunal loop (asterisks) (**b**). Ballooning (arrow) with dilatation of stricture (**c**). After bilioplasty (**d**), a biliary drainage catheter (IEBDC) is left inside, with an external side (short arrow) and an internal side (curved arrow)

new session of dilatation is performed, after which the drainage catheter is placed again and left in site for another month. Recurrence rate is high, with up to 66% of treated patients having a restenosis within a median follow-up of 4.4 years. In the largest study reported in the literature the greatest risk is for intrahepatic stenosis (90%) and in patients presenting with both anastomotic and intrahepatic stenosis, with recurrence rate of 100% [149]. Biliary strictures that do not respond to dilatation and stenting will require surgical repair or even retransplantation. PTC procedural complications are hemobilia, hematoma, and cholangitis.

Bile leaks may occur at the anastomosis, at the T-tube site insertion, at the cystic duct, or along the cut surface of partial liver grafts (Fig. 5.24) [146]. The bile can form intrahepatic fluid collection or a contained perihepatic fluid collection (biloma) and can leak into the peritoneal cavity, where it is detectable with US. In addition to anastomotic bile leaks, nonanastomotic leaks can also be observed, although less frequently. A nonanastomotic leak is a sign of serious complication caused by diffuse necrosis of the bile ducts as a result of hepatic artery thrombosis or stenosis or vasculitis. At US, CT and MRI bile leakage can appear as nonspecific perihepatic fluid collection. Cholangiography can show contrast medium leakage from the biliary tree [135]. Biloma can be treated with placement, under US guidance, of a percutaneous drainage; anastomotic leakage is managed with insertion of IEBDC. In transplant recipients the alteration in bile composition may be a predisposing factor in biliary stone and sludge formation. *Bile duct stones* at US appear as biliary filling

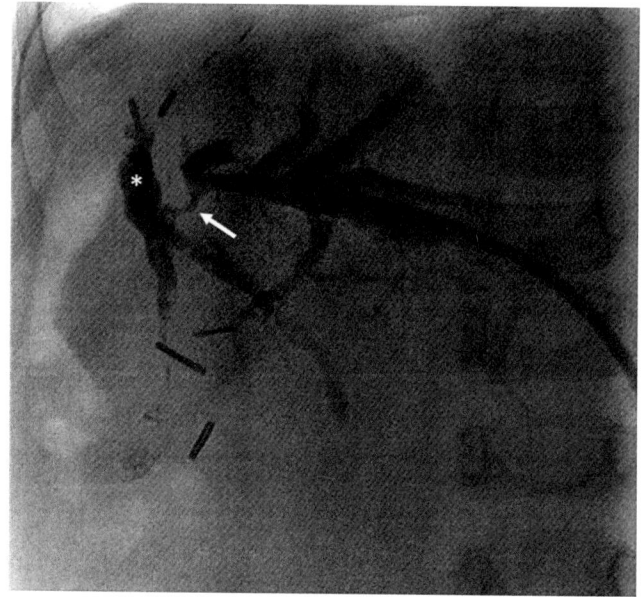

Fig. 5.24 Stenosis of biliary ductal anastomosis (arrow) associated to biliary fistula (asterisks)

echogenic structures with distal acoustic shadowing (Fig. 5.25). At MRCP the stones appear as intraluminal, well-defined margin defect that helps distinguishing them from casts, sludge, or debris. Mucocele is a distended cystic duct remnant of the donor, containing mucus that can compress the common bile duct. At US it appears as rounded fluid collection near the porta hepatis. *Sphincter of Oddi dysfunction*

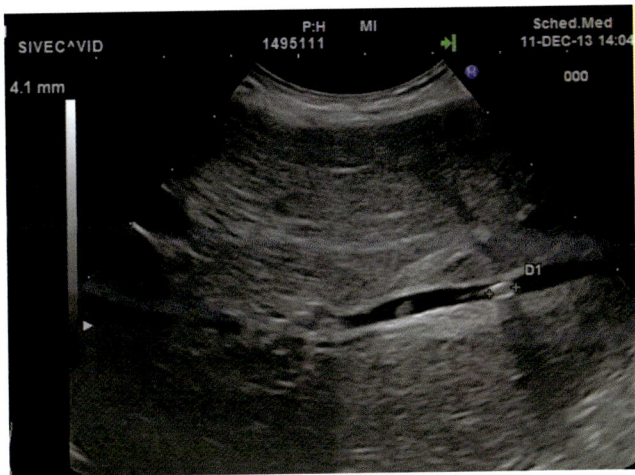

Fig. 5.25 B-mode US shows intrahepatic bile duct stones (echogenic) with characteristic posterior shadow

(in end-to-end anastomoses) is probably secondary to devascularization or denervation of the ampulla of Vater. US shows dilatation of the bile duct (both the extrahepatic donor duct and the native duct) without anastomotic stenosis [150].

5.5.4 Liver Parenchyma Complications

Infarct is an avascular areas of parenchyma that can appear as a round or geographic lesion with central areas of necrosis. At US it shows as a hypoechoic lesion, and it is possible to find a small amount of gas within the infarcted area, visible as small echogenic speckles with dirty acoustic shadowing posteriorly, secondary to reverberation artifact [150]. At CT the infarct shows an irregular or wedge-shaped lesion located peripherally to the liver or as irregular-shaped lesion along the course of bile ducts. The infarct does not have enhancement after contrast medium administration. *Biloma* can appear as round intrahepatic bile collection following an ischemic break in the wall of bile ducts, usually due to hepatic artery thrombosis or stenosis. At US biloma appears as an hypo- to anechoic lesion with posterior acoustic enhancement. At CT it shows a hypoattenuated area. At MRI the pattern is that of a fluid lesion: hypointense on T1-weighted images and hyperintense on T2-weighted images. A severe and wide bile duct necrosis can look like a biloma extended along the periportal spaces and appears as periportal cuffing mimicking edema [140, 151]. An *abscess* is a parenchymal hypoechoic lesion characterized by irregularly thick wall and a central anechoic liquefied area that may contain gas; it can arise from infarcted areas or from infected bilomas. At CT, the abscess is characterized by lower attenuation than the adjacent liver parenchyma, both before and after contrast medium administration. Sometimes it can show a peripheral enhancement that corresponds to perilesional granulation tissue. At MR imaging, abscesses show pattern of fluid lesion, although sometimes on unenhanced T1-weighted images, they may appear hyperintense for the high protein composition. *Acute rejection* does not have a specific appearance, and often the only identifiable pattern is heterogeneity of the liver parenchyma [140]. The diagnosis is made with graft biopsy. Imaging can exclude other possible causes that may mimic clinical signs and symptoms of acute cellular rejection.

5.5.5 Fluid Collections

Perihepatic fluid collections are common and are differentiated into serous, blood, lymphatic, and biliary collections. They are usually found at the anastomotic site; in the lesser sac, surrounding the ligamentum teres hepatis; and in peri- and right subhepatic spaces (the bare part of the liver results by the removal of the peritoneal reflections). Fluid collections become visible within a few days from the intervention and usually regress spontaneously within a few weeks. The ultrasound has a good sensitivity but does not allow to discriminate between the different fluid collections, since bile, blood, lymph, and pus can all present as homogeneous anechoic collections. Hematomas and pus over the time become particulate nonhomogeneous anechoic fluids, due to echogenic layers and spots that correspond to corpuscular material. At non-contrast CT, the blood collections are hyperdense and can be characterized by fluid-fluid levels for declive arrangement of corpuscular portions of the blood. Whenever collections do not regress spontaneously or become superinfected, they should be treated with percutaneous drainage [140].

References

1. Gerstenmaier J, Gibson R. Ultrasound in chronic liver disease. Insights Imaging. 2014;5(4):441–55.
2. Chiorean L, Cui XW, Tannapfel A, Franke D, Stenzel M, Kosiak W, et al. Benign liver tumors in pediatric patients—review with emphasis on imaging features. World J Gastroenterol. 2015;21:8541–61.
3. Hall EJ. Lessons we have learned from our children: cancer risks from diagnostic radiology. Pediatr Radiol. 2002;32:700–6.
4. Pearce M, Salotti J, Little M, McHugh K, Lee C, Kim K, et al. Radiation exposure from CT scans in childhood and subsequent risk of leukemia and brain tumors: a retrospective cohort study. Lancet. 2012;4:499–505.
5. Mathews J, Forsythe A, Brady Z, Butler M, Goergen S, Byrnes G, et al. Cancer risk in 680,000 people exposed to computed tomography scans in childhood or adolescence: data linkage study of 11 million Australians. BMJ. 2013;21:f2360.
6. Vo N, Shet N. Radiology of the liver in children. In: Murray K, Horslen S, editors. Diseases of the liver in children. New York: Springer; 2014.

7. Machata AM, Willschke H, Kabon B, Prayer D, Marhofer P. Effect of brain MRI on body core temperature in sedated infants and children. Br J Anaesth. 2009;102:385–9.
8. Isaacson L, Yanosky J, Jones A, Dennehy N, Spandorfer P, Baxter L. Effect of MRI strength and propofol sedation on pediatric core temperature change. J Magn Reson Imaging. 2011;33:950–6.
9. Subaar C, Amoako J, Owusu A, Fletcher JJ, Suurbaar J. Numerical studies of radiofrequency of the electromagnetic radiation power absorption in paediatrics undergoing brain magnetic resonance imaging. J Radiat Res Appl Sci. 2017;10:188–93.
10. Blumfield E, Moore M, Drake K, Goodman TR, Lewis N, Meyer T, et al. Survey of gadolinium-based contrast agent utilization among the members of the Society for Pediatric Radiology: a Quality and Safety Committee report. Pediatr Radiol. 2017;47(6):665–73.
11. Nardone B, Saddleton E, Laumann AE, Edwards BJ, Raisch DW, McKoy JM, et al. Pediatric nephrogenic systemic fibrosis is rarely reported: a RADAR report. Pediatr Radiol. 2014;44(2):173–80.
12. Jha P, Chawla SC, Tavri S, Patel C, Gooding C, Daldrup-Link H. Pediatric liver tumors—a pictorial review. Eur Radiol. 2009;19(1):209–19.
13. Meyers RL. Tumors of the liver in children. Surg Oncol. 2007;16(3):195–203.
14. López-Terrada D, Alaggio R, de Dávila MT, Czauderna P, Hiyama E, Katzenstein H, et al. Towards an international pediatric liver tumor consensus classification: proceedings of the Los Angeles COG liver tumors symposium. Mod Pathol. 2014;27:472–91.
15. Stocker JT. Hepatic tumors in children. Clin Liver Dis. 2001;5(1):259–81.
16. Gnarra M, Behr G, Kitajewski A, Wu JK, Anupindi SA, Shawber CJ, et al. History of the infantile hepatic hemangioma: From imaging to generating a differential diagnosis. World J Clin Pediatr. 2016;5(3):273–80.
17. Chung M, Cube R, Lewis B, Conran M. From the archives of the AFIP. Pediatric liver masses: radiologic-pathologic correlation part 1. Benign tumors. Radiographics. 2010;30:801–26.
18. Itinteang T, Withers AH, Davis F, Tan ST. Biology of infantile hemangioma. Front Surg. 2014;1:38.
19. Christison-Lagay ER, Burrows PE, Alomari A, Dubois J, Kozakewich HP, Lane TS, et al. Hepatic hemangiomas: subtype classification and development of a clinical practice algorithm and registry. J Pediatr Surg. 2007;42(1):62–8.
20. Huang A, Tu M, Harney W, Venihaki M, Butte J, Kozakewich PW, et al. Severe hypothyroidism caused by type 3 iodothyronine deiodinase in infantile hemangiomas. N Engl J Med. 2000;343:185–9.
21. Helmberger TK, Ros PR, Mergo PJ, Tomczak R, Reiser MF. Pediatric liver neoplasms: a radiologic-pathologic correlation. Eur Radiol. 1999;9:1339–47.
22. Burrows P, Dubois J, Kassarjian A. Pediatric hepatic vascular anomalies. Pediatr Radiol. 2001;31(8):B533–45.
23. Arrunategui M, Caicedo LA, Thomas S, Botero V, García O, Carrascal E, et al. Giant mesenchymal hamartoma in pediatric patients: a new indication for liver transplantation. J Pediatr Surg Case Rep. 2017;21:1–3.
24. Virgone C, Cecchetto G, Dall'Igna P, Zanon G, Cillo U, Alaggio R. Mesenchymal hamartoma of the liver in older children: an adult variant or a different entity? Report of a case with review of the literature. Appl Immunohistochem Mol Morphol. 2015;23(9):667–73.
25. Cha DI, Yoo SY, Kim JH, Jeon TY, Eo H. Clinical and imaging features of focal nodular hyperplasia in children. Am J Roentgenol. 2014;202:960–5.
26. Towbin AJ, Luo GG, Yin H, Mo JQ. Focal nodular hyperplasia in children, adolescents, and young adults. Pediatr Radiol. 2011;41:341–9.
27. Liu QY, Zhang WD, Lai DM, Ou-Yang Y, Gao M, Lin XF. Hepatic focal nodular hyperplasia in children: imaging features on multi-slice computed tomography. World J Gastroenterol. 2012;18(47):7048–55.
28. Wanless I. Micronodular transformation (nodular regenerative hyperplasia) of the liver: a report of 64 cases among 2,500 autopsies and a new classification of benign hepatocellular nodules. Hepatology. 1990;11:787–97.
29. Reshamwala PA, Kleiner DE, Heller T. Nodular regenerative hyperplasia: not all nodules are created equal. Hepatology. 2006;44(1):7–14.
30. Hartleb M, Gutkowski K, Milkiewicz P. Nodular regenerative hyperplasia: evolving concepts on underdiagnosed cause of portal hypertension. World J Gastroenterol. 2011;17(11):1400–9.
31. Campos JT, Sirlin B, Choi JY. Focal hepatic lesions in Gd-EOB-DTPA enhanced MRI: the atlas. Insights Imaging. 2012;3:451–74.
32. Bartolozzi C, Lencioni R, Paolicchi A, Moretti M, Armillotta N, Pinto F. Differentiation of hepatocellular adenoma and focal nodular hyperplasia of the liver: comparison of power Doppler imaging and conventional color Doppler sonography. Eur Radiol. 1997;7:1410–5.
33. Kong WT, Wang WP, Huang BJ, Ding H, Mao F, Si Q. Contrast-enhanced ultrasound in combination with color Doppler ultrasound can improve the diagnostic performance of focal nodular hyperplasia and hepatocellular adenoma. Ultrasound Med Biol. 2015;41:944–51.
34. Ishak K, Goodman Z, Stocker J. Tumors of the liver and intrahepatic bile ducts. Washington, DC: Armed Forces Institute of Pathology; 2001.
35. Schneider D, Calaminus G, Göbel U. Diagnostic value of alpha 1-fetoprotein and beta-human chorionic gonadotropin in infancy and childhood. Pediatr Hematol Oncol. 2001;18:11–26.
36. Darbari A, Sabin K, Shapiro C, Schwarz K. Epidemiology of primary hepatic malignancies in U.S. children. Hepatology. 2003;38:560–6.
37. Czaudernaa P, Haeberle B, Hiyama E, Rangaswami A, Krailo M, Maibach R, et al. The Children's Hepatic tumors International Collaboration (CHIC): novel global rare tumor database yields new prognostic factors in hepatoblastoma and becomes a research model. Eur J Cancer. 2016;52:92–101.
38. Saettini F, Conter V, Provenzi M, Rota M, Giraldi E, Foglia C, et al. Is multifocality a prognostic factor in childhood hepatoblastoma? Pediatr Blood Cancer. 2014;61(9):1593–7.
39. Maruyama K, Ikeda H, Koizumi T, Tsuchida Y, Tanimura M, Nishida H, et al. Case-control study of perinatal factors and hepatoblastoma in children with an extremely low birthweight. Pediatr Int. 2000;42:492–8.
40. Stocker J, Schmidt D. Hepatoblastoma. In: Hamilton S, Aatonen L, editors. Pathology and genetics of tumours of the digestive system. Lyon: IARC Press; 2000. p. 184–9.
41. Chung M, Lattin E, Cube R, Lewis B, Marichal-Hernández C, Shawhan R, et al. From the archives of the AFIP pediatric liver masses: radiologic- pathologic correlation part 2. Malignant tumors. Radiographics. 2011;31(2):483–507.
42. Powers C, Ros PR, Stoupis C, Johnson W, Segel K. Primary liver neoplasms: MR imaging with pathologic correlation. Radiographics. 1994;14(3):459–82.
43. Katzenstein H. COG clinical trials for children with liver cancer. In: Presented at the International Pediatric Liver Tumors Symposium. Texas Medical Center, Houston, TX, 25–26 Feburary; 2016.
44. Otte J, Pritchard J, Aronson D, Brown J, Czauderna P, Maibach R, et al. Liver transplantation for hepatoblastoma: results from the International Society of Pediatric Oncology (SIOP) Study SIOPEL-1 and review of the world experience. Pediatr Blood Cancer. 2004;42:74–83.
45. Yu S, Kim H, Eo H, Won J, Jung S, Park K, et al. Clinical characteristics and prognosis of pediatric hepatocellular carcinoma. World J Surg. 2006;30(1):43–50.

46. Katzenstein H, Krailo M, Malogolowkin M, et al. Hepatocellular carcinoma in children and adolescents: results from the Pediatric Oncology Group and the Children's Cancer Group Intergroup Study. J Clin Oncol. 2002;20:2789–97.
47. Aronson D, Meyers R. Malignant tumors of the liver in children. Semin Pediatr Surg. 2016;25(5):265–75.
48. Ravà M, D'Andrea A, Doni M, Kress T, Ostuni R, Bianchi V, et al. Mutual epithelium-macrophage dependency in liver carcinogenesis mediated by ST18. Hepatology. 2017;65(5):1708–19.
49. Iannelli F, Collino A, Sinha S, Radaelli E, Nicoli P, D'Antiga L, et al. Corrigendum: massive gene amplification drives paediatric hepatocellular carcinoma caused by bile salt export pump deficiency. Nat Commun. 2015;2(6):7456.
50. Ni Y, Chang M, Hsu H, et al. Hepatocellular carcinoma in childhood. Clinical manifestations and prognosis. Cancer. 1991;68:1737–41.
51. Yu S, Yeung D, So N. Imaging features of hepatocellular carcinoma. Clin Radiol. 2004;59(2):145–56.
52. Hussain S, Zondervan P, IJzermans J, Schalm S, de Man R, Krestin G. Benign versus malignant hepatic nodules: MR imaging findings with pathologic correlation. Radiographics. 2002;22(5):1023–39.
53. Murawski M, Weeda V, Maibach R, Morland B, Roebuck D. Hepatocellular carcinoma in children: does modified platinum- and doxorubicin-based chemotherapy increase tumor resectability and change outcome? Lessons learned from the SIOPEL 2 and 3 studies. J Clin Oncol. 2016;34(10):1050–6.
54. Baumann U, Adam R, Duvoux C, Mikolajczyk R, Karam V, D'Antiga L, et al. Survival of children after liver transplantation for hepatocellular carcinoma. Liver Transpl. 2018;24(2):246–55.
55. Romano F, et al. Favorable outcome of primary liver transplantation in children with cirrhosis and hepatocellular carcinoma. Pediatr Transplant. 2011;15(6):573–9.
56. Torbenson M, et al. Review of the clinicopathologic features of fibrolamellar carcinoma. Adv Anat Pathol. 2007;14(3):217–23.
57. McLarney J, Rucker P, Bender G, Goodman Z, Kashitani N, Ros P. Fibrolamellar carcinoma of the liver: radiologic-pathologic correlation. Radiographics. 1999;19(2):453–71.
58. Liu S, Chan K, Wang B, Qiao L. Fibrolamellar hepatocellular carcinoma. Am J Gastroenterol. 2009;104(10):2617–25.
59. Lack E, Schloo B, Azumi N, Travis W, Grier HE, Kozakewich HP. Undifferentiated (embryonal) sarcoma of the liver: clinical and pathologic study of 16 cases with emphasis on immunohistochemical features. Am J Surg Pathol. 1991;15(1):1–16.
60. O'Sullivan M, Swanson P, Knoll J, et al. Undifferentiated embryonal sarcoma with unusual features arising within mesenchymal hamartoma of the liver: report of a case and review of the literature. Pediatr Dev Pathol. 2001;4:482–9.
61. Zheng J, Tao X, Xu A, Chen X, Wu M, Zhang S. Primary and recurrent embryonal sarcoma of the liver: clinicopathological and immunohistochemical analysis. Histopathology. 2007;51(2):195–203.
62. Kim M, Tireno B, Slanetz P. Undifferentiated embryonal sarcoma of the liver. Am J Roentgenol. 2008;190(4):W261–2.
63. Yoon W, Kim J, Kang HK. Hepatic undifferentiated embryonal sarcoma: MR findings. J Comput Assist Tomogr. 1997;21:100–2.
64. Merli L, Mussini C, Gabor F, et al. Pitfalls in the surgical management of undifferentiated sarcoma of the liver and benefits of preoperative chemotherapy. Eur J Pediatr Surg. 2015;25(1):132–7.
65. Plant A, Busuttil R, Rana A, et al. A single—institution retrospective case series of childhood undifferentiated embryonal liver sarcoma (UELS): success of combined therapy and the use of orthotopic liver transplant. Pediatr Hematol Oncol. 2013;35(6):451–5.
66. Park Y, Kim J, Kim K, Lee I, Yoon H, Ko G, et al. Primary hepatic angiosarcoma: imaging findings and palliative treatment with transcatheter arterial chemoembolization or embolization. Clin Radiol. 2009;64(8):779–85.
67. Koyama T, Fletcher J, Johnson C, Kuo M, Notohara K, Burgart L. Primary hepatic angiosarcoma: findings at CT and MR imaging. Radiology. 2002;222(3):667–73.
68. Ishak K, Anthony P, Niederau C, Nakanuma Y. Mesenchymal tumours of the liver. In: Hamilton S, Aatonen L, editors. Pathology and genetics of tumours of the digestive system. Lyon: IARC Press; 2000.
69. Malkan A, Fernandez-Pineda I. The evolution of diagnosis and management of pediatric biliary tract rhabdomyosarcoma. Curr Pediatr Rev. 2016;12(3):190–198(9).
70. Roebuck D, Yang W, Lam W. Stanley. Hepatobiliary rhabdomyosarcoma in children: diagnostic radiology. Pediatr Radiol. 1998;28(2):101–8.
71. Ruymann F, Raney RJ, Crist W, Lawrence WJ, Lindberg R, Soule E. Rhabdomyosarcoma of the biliary tree in childhood: a report from the Intergroup Rhabdomyosarcoma Study. Cancer. 1985;56(3):575–81.
72. Spunt S, Lobe T, Pappo A, et al. Aggressive surgery is unwarranted for biliary tract rhabdomyosarcoma. J Pediatr Surg. 2000;35(2):309–16.
73. Balistreri W. Liver disease in infancy and childhood. In: Schiff E, Sorrell M, Maddrey W, editors. Schiff's diseases of the liver. 8th ed. Philadelphia: Lippincott, Williams & Wilkins; 1998.
74. Fischler B, Lamireau T. Cholestasis in the newborn and infant. Clin Res Hepatol Gastroenterol. 2014;38(3):263–7.
75. Konuş O, Ozdemir A, Akkaya A, Erbaş G, Celik H, Işik S. Normal liver, spleen, and kidney dimensions in neonates, infants, and children: evaluation with sonography. Am J Roentgenol. 1998;171(6):1693–8.
76. Gubernick J, Rosenberg H, Ilaslan H, Kessler A. US approach to jaundice in infants and children. Radiographics. 2000;20(1):173–95.
77. Feldman A, Mack CL. Biliary atresia: clinical lessons learned. J Pediatr Gastroenterol Nutr. 2015;61(2):167–75.
78. Schwarz K, Haber B, Rosenthal P, et al. Extrahepatic anomalies in infants with biliary atresia: results of a large prospective North American multicenter study. Hepatology. 2013;58:1724–31.
79. Humphrey T, Stringer MD. Biliary atresia: US diagnosis. Radiology. 2007;244(3):845–51.
80. Choi S, Park W, Lee H, Woo S. 'Triangular cord': a sonographic finding applicable in the diagnosis of biliary atresia. J Pediatr Surg. 1996;31(3):363–6.
81. Kanegawa K, Akasaka Y, Kitamura E, Nishiyama S, Muraji T, Nishijima E, et al. Sonographic diagnosis of biliary atresia in pediatric patients using the triangular cord sign versus gallbladder length and contraction. Am J Roentgenol. 2003;181(5):1387–90.
82. Zhou L, Wang W, Shan Q, Liu B, Zheng Y, Xu Z, et al. Optimizing the US diagnosis of biliary atresia with a modified triangular cord thickness and gallbladder classification. Radiology. 2015;277(1):181–91.
83. Lee M, Kim M, Lee M, Yoon C, Han S, Oh J, et al. Biliary atresia: color Doppler US findings in neonates and infants. Radiology. 2009;252(1):282–9.
84. Kianifar H, Tehranian S, Shojaei P, et al. Accuracy of hepatobiliary scintigraphy for differentiation of neonatal hepatitis from biliary atresia: systematic review and meta-analysis of the literature. Pediatr Radiol. 2013;43(8):905–19.
85. Gilmour S, Hershkop M, Reifen R, et al. Outcome of hepatobiliary scanning in neonatal hepatitis syndrome. J Nucl Med. 1997;38:1279–82.
86. Caponcelli E, Knisely A, Davenport M. Cystic biliary atresia: an etiologic and prognostic subgroup. J Pediatr Surg. 2008;43(9):1619–24.

87. Soares K, Arnaoutakis D, Kamel I, Rastegar N, Anders R, Maithel S, et al. Choledochal cysts: presentation, clinical differentiation, and management. J Am Coll Surg. 2014;219(6):1167–80.
88. Wiedmeyer D, Stewart E, Dodds WJ, Geenen J, Vennes J, Taylor A. Choledochal cyst: findings on cholangiopancreatography with emphasis on ectasia of the common channel. Am J Roentgenol. 1989;153(5):969–72.
89. Todani T, Watanabe Y, Narusue M, Tabuchi K, Okajima K. Congenital bile duct cysts: classification, operative procedures, and review of thirty-seven cases including cancer arising from choledochal cyst. Am J Surg. 1977;134(2):263–9.
90. Murphy A, Axt J, Crapp S, Martin C, Crane G. Lovvorn H3. Concordance of imaging modalities and cost minimization in the diagnosis of pediatric choledochal cysts. Pediatr Surg Int. 2012;28(6):615–21.
91. Tipnis N, Werlin SL. The use of magnetic resonance cholangiopancreatography in children. Curr Gastroenterol Rep. 2007;9(3):225–9.
92. Kim W, Cheon J, Youn B, et al. Hepatic arterial diameter measured with US: adjunct for US diagnosis of biliary atresia. Radiology. 2007;245(2):549–55.
93. Hartley J, Gissen P, Kelly D. Alagille syndrome and other hereditary causes of cholestasis. Clin Liver Dis. 2013;17:279–300.
94. Turnpenny P, Ellard S. Alagille syndrome: pathogenesis, diagnosis and management. Eur J Hum Genet. 2012;20(3):251–7.
95. Alagille D, Estrada A, Hadchouel M, Gautier M, Odièvre M, Dommergues J. Syndromic paucity of interlobular bile ducts (Alagille syndrome or arteriohepatic dysplasia): review of 80 cases. J Pediatr. 1987;110:195–200.
96. Cho H, Kim W, Choi Y, et al. Ultrasonography evaluation of infants with Alagille syndrome: in comparison with biliary atresia and neonatal hepatitis. Eur J Radiol. 2016;85(6):1045–52.
97. Kamath B, Loomes K, Piccoli DA. Medical management of Alagille syndrome. J Pediatr Gastroenterol Nutr. 2010;50(6):580–6.
98. Jacquemin E. Progressive familial intrahepatic cholestasis. Clin Res Hepatol Gastroenterol. 2012;36(suppl 1):S26–35.
99. Pittschieler K, Massi G. Liver involvement in infants with PiSZ phenotype of alpha 1-antitrypsin deficiency. J Pediatr Gastroenterol Nutr. 1992;15:315–8.
100. Mak C, Lee H, Chan A, et al. Inborn errors of metabolism and expanded newborn screening: review and update. Crit Rev Clin Lab Sci. 2013;50:142–62.
101. van Ginkel W, Pennings J, van Spronsen F. Liver cancer in Tyrosinemia Type 1. Adv Exp Med Biol. 2017;959:101–9.
102. Pfeiffenberger J, Mogler C, Gotthardt D, Schulze-Bergkamen H, Litwin T, Reuner U, et al. Hepatobiliary malignancies in Wilson disease. Liver Int. 2015;35(5):1615–22.
103. World Health Organization. WHO website [online]. 2013.
104. Lavanchy D. The global burden of hepatitis C. Liver Int. 2009;29:74–81.
105. Chang M, Hsu H, Hsu H, et al. The significance of spontaneous hepatitis B e antigen seroconversion in childhood: with special emphasis on the clearance of hepatitis B e antigen before 3 years of age. Hepatology. 1995;22:1387–92.
106. Bortolotti F, Verucchi G, Camma C, et al. Long-term course of chronic hepatitis C in children: from viral clearance to end-stage liver disease. Gastroenterology. 2008;134:1900–7.
107. Vajro P, Lenta S, Socha P, Dhawan MKP, Baumann U, et al. Diagnosis of nonalcoholic fatty liver disease in children and adolescents: position paper of the ESPGHAN Hepatology Committee. J Pediatr Gastroenterol Nutr. 2012;54(5):700–13.
108. Lee S, Park S. Radiologic evaluation of nonalcoholic fatty liver disease. World J Gastroenterol. 2014;20(23):7392–402.
109. Nobili V, et al. Accuracy and reproducibility of transient elastography for the diagnosis of fibrosis in pediatric nonalcoholic steatohepatitis. Hepatology. 2008;48:442–8.
110. van Werven J, Marsman H, Nederveen A, Smits N, ten Kate F, van Gulik T, et al. Assessment of hepatic steatosis in patients undergoing liver resection: comparison of US, CT, T1-weighted dual-echo MR imaging, and point-resolved 1H MR spectroscopy. Radiology. 2010;256(1):159–68.
111. Chiang H, Lin L, Li C, Lin C, Chiang H, Huang T, et al. Magnetic resonance fat quantification in living donor liver transplantation. Transplant Proc. 2014;46(3):666–8.
112. Molla-Hosseini D, Mack CL. Pediatric primary sclerosing cholangitis. In: Forman LM, editor. Primary sclerosing cholangitis. Cham: Springer; 2017.
113. Deneau MR, El-Matary W, Valentiino PL. The natural history of primary sclerosing cholangitis in 781 children: a multicenter, international collaboration. Hepatology. 2017;66(2):518–27.
114. Chavhan GB, Babyn PS, Manson D, Vidarsson L. Pediatric MR cholangiopancreatography: principles, technique, and clinical applications. Radiographics. 2008;28:1951–62.
115. Vitellas K, Keogan M, Freed K, Enns R, Spritzer C, Baillie J, et al. Radiologic manifestations of sclerosing cholangitis with emphasis on MR cholangiopancreatography. Radiographics. 2000;20(4):959–75.
116. Franchi-Abella S, Cahill AM, Barnacle M, Pariente D, Roebuck DJ. Hepatobiliary intervention in children. Cardiovasc Intervent Radiol. 2014;37:37–54.
117. Dezsöf A, Baumann U, Dhawan A, Durmaz O, Fischler B, Hadzic N, et al. Liver biopsy in children: position paper of the ESPGHAN Hepatology Committee. J Pediatr Gastroenterol Nutr. 2015;60(3):408–20.
118. Hatfield MK, Beres RA, Sane SS, Zaleski GX. Percutaneous imaging-guided solid organ core needle biopsy: coaxial versus noncoaxial method. AJR. 2008;190:413–7.
119. Kalambokis G, Manousou P, Vibhakorn S, Marelli L, Cholongitas E, Senzolo M, et al. Transjugular liver biopsy—Indications, adequacy, quality of specimens, and complications—a systematic review. J Hepatol. 2007;47:284–94.
120. Miraglia R, Maruzzelli L, Caruso S, Marrone G, Carollo V, Spada M, et al. Interventional radiology procedures in pediatric patient with complication after liver transplantation. Radiographics. 2009;29:567–84.
121. Navuluri R, Ahmed O. Complications of transjugular biopsies. Semin Interv Radiol. 2015;32:42–8.
122. Cárdenas M, Epelman M, Darge K, Rand EB, Anupindi SA. Pre- and postoperative imaging of the rex shunt in children: what radiologists should know. AJR. 2012;198:1032–7.
123. Deganello A, Sellars MEK. Diagnostic procedures in pediatric hepatology. In: Guandalini S, Dhawan A, Branski D, editors. Textbook of pediatric gastroenterology, hepatology and nutrition. Cham: Springer International; 2016.
124. Feldman AG, Sokol RJ. Noncirrhotic portal hypertension in the pediatric population. Clin Liver Dis. 2015;5(5):116–9.
125. Gugig R, Rosenthal P. Management of portal hypertension in children. World J Gastroenterol. 2012;18(11):1176–84.
126. Yong L, Chuangye H, Wengang G, Zhanxin Y, Jianhong W, Bojing Z, et al. Transjugular intrahepatic portosystemic shunt for extrahepatic portal venous obstruction in children. J Pediatr Gastroenterol Nutr. 2016;62(2):233–41.
127. Di Giorgio A, Agazzi R, Alberti D, et al. Feasibility and efficacy of transjugular intrahepatic portosystemic shunt (TIPS) in children. J Pediatr Gastroenterol Nutr. 2012;54:594–600.
128. Zurera L, Espejo J, Lombardo S, et al. Safety and efficacy of expanded polytetrafluoroethylene-covered transjugular intrahepatic portosystemic shunts in children with acute or recurring upper gastrointestinal bleeding. Pediatr Radiol. 2015;45:422–9.
129. Copelan A, Kapoor B, Sands M. Transjugular intrahepatic portosystemic shunt: indications, contraindications, and patient work-up. Semin Intervent Radiol. 2014;31:235–42.

130. Richter G, Noeldge G, Palmaz J, et al. The transjugular intrahepatic portosystemic stent-shunt (TIPSS): results of a pilot study. Cardiovasc Intervent Radiol. 1990;13:200–7.
131. Xingshun Q, Yulong T, Wei Z, Zhiping Y, Xiaozhong G. Covered versus bare stents for transjugular intrahepatic portosystemic shunt: an updated meta-analysis of randomized controlled trials. Ther Adv Gastroenterol. 2017;10(1):32–41.
132. Merrow AC, Gupta A, Patel MN, Adams DM. 2014 Revised Classification of vascular lesions from the International Society for the Study of Vascular Anomalies: radiologic-pathologic update. Radiographics. 2016;36:1494–516.
133. Gallego C, Miralles M, Marìn C, Muyor P, González G, Garcìa-Hidalgo E. Congenital hepatic shunts. Radiographics. 2004;24:755–72.
134. Bhargava P, Vaidya S, Kolokythas O, et al. Hepatic vascular shunts: embryology and imaging appearances. Br J Radiol. 2011;84:1142–52.
135. Drudi FM, Pagliara E, Cantisani V, Arduini F, D'Ambrosio U, Alfano G. Post-transplant hepatic complications: imaging findings. J Ultrasound. 2007;10:53–8.
136. Girometti R, Como G, Bazzocchi M, Zuiani C. Post-operative imaging in liver transplantation: state-of-the-art and future perspectives. World J Gastroenterol. 2014;20(20):6180–200.
137. Kim J, Broering D, Tustas R, et al. Split liver transplantation: past, present and future. Pediatr Transplant. 2004;8:644–8.
138. Platt J, Yutzy G, Bude R, Ellis J, Rubin J. Use of Doppler sonography for revealing hepatic artery stenosis in liver transplant recipients. Am J Roentgenol. 1997;168:473–6.
139. McNaughton DA, Abu-Yousef MM. Doppler US of the liver made simple. Radiographics. 2011;31:161–88.
140. Berrocal T, Parrón M, Alvarez-Luque A, Prieto C, Santamaria ML. Pediatric liver transplantation: a pictorial essay of early and late complications. Radiographics. 2006;26:1187–209.
141. Park YS, Kim KW, Lee SJ, Lee J, Jung DH, Song GW, et al. Hepatic arterial stenosis assessed with Doppler US after liver transplantation: frequent false-positive diagnoses with Tardus Parvus waveform and value of adding optimal peak systolic velocity cutoff. Radiology. 2011;260(3):884–91.
142. Crossin JD, Muradali D, Wilson SR. US of liver transplants: normal and abnormal. Radiographics. 2003;23:1093–114.
143. Nolten A, Sproat IA. Hepatic artery thrombosis after liver transplantation: temporal accuracy of diagnosis with duplex US and the syndrome of impending thrombosis. Radiology. 1996;198:553–9.
144. Jeon GS, Won JH, Wang HJ, Kim BW, Lee BM. Endovascular treatment of acute arterial complications after living-donor liver transplantation. Clin Radiol. 2008;63:1099–105.
145. Rossi C, Zambruni A, Ansaloni F, et al. Combined mechanical and pharmacologic thrombolysis for portal vein thrombosis in liver-graft recipients and in candidates for liver transplantation. Transplantation. 2004;78:938–40.
146. Seehofer D, Eurich D, Veltzke-Schlieker W, Neuhaus P. Biliary complications after liver transplantation: old problems and new challenges. Am J Transplant. 2013;13:253–65.
147. Zemel G, Zajko A, Skolnick M, et al. The role of sonography and transhepatic cholangiography in the diagnosis of biliary complications after liver transplantation. Am J Roentgenol. 1988;151:943–6.
148. Feier FH, da Fonseca EA, Seda-Neto J, Chapchap P. Biliary complications after pediatric liver transplantation: risk factors, diagnosis and management. World J Hepatol. 2015;7(18):2162–70.
149. Sunku B, Salvalaggio PRO, Donaldson JS, Rigsby CK, Neighbors K, Superina RA, et al. Outcomes and risk factors for failure of radiologic treatment of biliary strictures in pediatric liver transplantation recipients. Liver Transpl. 2006;12:821–6.
150. Bhargava P, Vaidya S, Dick AAS, Dighe M. Imaging of orthotopic liver transplantation: review. Am J Roentgenol. 2011;196:WS15–25.
151. Camacho JC, Coursey-Moreno C, Telleria JC, Aguirre DA, Torres WE, Mittal PK. Nonvascular post–liver transplantation complications: from US screening to cross-sectional and interventional imaging. Radiographics. 2015;35:87–104.

Practical Approach to the Jaundiced Infant

Ekkehard Sturm and Steffen Hartleif

Key Points
- Jaundice in a neonate older than 14 days requires further investigations for liver disease.
- Coagulopathy should be ruled out in any infant presenting with conjugated hyperbilirubinemia.
- Biliary atresia should be excluded in any infant presenting with conjugated hyperbilirubinemia and pale stools.
- Optimization of nutrition with sufficient energy uptake using middle-chain triglycerides and fat-soluble vitamins is an important treatment element of infants with direct hyperbilirubinemia.
- The prevalence of many cholestatic diseases in infancy is rare, but they are responsible for the majority of indications for liver transplantation at pediatric age.

Research Needed in the Field
- Novel genetic causes of childhood cholestatic liver diseases are increasingly being identified, which also has helped to better understand the normal physiology.
- Which strategies can enhance earlier recognition of neonatal cholestatic disease and its specific etiologies?
- What are accepted prognostic parameters for long-term success of Kasai portoenterostomy?
- Which strategies following the Kasai portoenterostomy (KPE) may delay or prevent the need for liver transplantation?
- Is centralized care essential for improving prognosis in neonatal liver disease?
- How can the transition from pediatric to adult care be facilitated through the acquisition of self-responsibility and self-management?

6.1 The Jaundiced Infant

Jaundice is very common in babies, with physiological jaundice occurring in up to 60% of infants in the first days of life. Although jaundice at 2 weeks of age is a relatively common finding, which is observed in up to 15% of newborns, it should alert healthcare professionals to the possibility of cholestasis [1]. Therefore, all infants who are jaundiced after this time require investigations to identify conjugated hyperbilirubinemia and liver disease.

6.1.1 Unconjugated Hyperbilirubinemia

In most cases, unconjugated hyperbilirubinemia is benign and does not require specific treatment. However, occasionally, rare diseases have to be taken into account (Table 6.1) requiring

E. Sturm (✉) · S. Hartleif
University Children's Hospital Tübingen, Tübingen, Germany
e-mail: ekkehard.sturm@med.uni-tuebingen.de;
steffen.hartleif@med.uni-tuebingen.de

Table 6.1 Causes of unconjugated hyperbilirubinemia in infancy

Conditions	Frequency	Features/clinical presentation
Physiological jaundice	Very common (up to 60%)	– Usually benign – 8–20% of infants may have serum bilirubin >300 μmol/L requiring temporary phototherapy – Stools are always pigmented
Hemolytic jaundice	Common	– AB0 and Rh incompatibilities – Glucose-6-phosphate dehydrogenase (G6PD) deficiency – Erythrocyte membrane defects
Breast milk jaundice	Common	– High levels of maternal hormones within the milk – Intestinal deconjugation – Overlap with physiological jaundice, may continue for up to 3 months – Stools are always pigmented – Does not require any phototherapy
Systemic infection/sepsis	Common	Sick infants with neonatal infections (sepsis, pneumonia, urinary tract infection, or meningitis)
Hypothyroidism	Common	Thyroid function test (TSH/fT4)
Gilbert syndrome	Common, 10–15% of healthy population	– Frequent cause of unconjugated hyperbilirubinemia, benign condition – Polymorphism of the 5′ end of the promoter of the UGT1A1 gene
Crigler-Najjar syndrome type 1	Rare	– Autosomal recessive, mutations in the UGT1A1 gene resulting in either truncated nonfunctional enzyme or nonrecognition of the substrate bilirubin – High risk of kernicterus
Crigler-Najjar syndrome type 2	Rare	– Autosomal recessive, mutations in the UGT1A1 gene – Clinically less severe than type 1 disease – Responsive to phenobarbital therapy

additional investigations [2]. One of these diseases is Crigler-Najjar syndrome (CNS). CNS and the milder Gilbert's syndrome develop due to variants of different impact the *UGT1A1* gene encoding the protein uridine diphosphate glucuronosyltransferase (UDPGT). This protein catalyzes the conversion of bilirubin to bilirubin monoglucuronides and then diglucuronides. The severity of the clinical symptoms correlates with the degree of residual function of UDPGT. While UDPGT is only mildly affected in Gilbert's syndrome, CNS type 1 leads to complete loss of function of the enzyme with bilirubin levels rising to 400–750 μmol/L and an increased risk for kernicterus. The aim of treatment is to keep bilirubin <150 μmol/L by phototherapy. Liver transplantation may be necessary to prevent neurological damage in the long term. Gene therapy has been successfully tested in an animal model [3] and is currently evaluated in clinical trials in CNS type 1 patients. Rare syndromes of bilirubin transport include Dubin-Johnson and Rotor syndrome. Both syndromes do not require treatment in most cases.

6.1.2 Conjugated Hyperbilirubinemia

Conjugated hyperbilirubinemia affects proximately 1 in every 2,500 term infants. The most common cause is biliary atresia in up to 40% of infants with conjugated hyperbilirubinemia [4]. It is very important to identify or exclude biliary atresia early, as adequate timing of the operative intervention is associated with survival with native liver [5].

6.1.3 Clinical History and Physical Examination

First, obtaining a detailed prenatal and infant history is fundamental. History should include occurrence of perinatal infections, any medications the infant has received, and details of the neonatal screening. History should focus on detailed information on the onset of jaundice, changes in stool pigmentation, and urine color. Parents and healthcare professionals often assess stool pigmentation subjectively, and pale stools are frequently misinterpreted. Therefore, stool color cards may be helpful to identify acholic stools [6, 7]. To date, except from regional initiatives, stool cards have not been systematically implemented in Europe or the United States.

Details in the family history including previous and current pregnancy and information on miscarriages, pruritus, or liver dysfunction in maternal history or other family members should be noted. History of infections or medication taken during pregnancy is important. Further, the family history on hemolytic diseases and/or cardiac anomalies may be relevant.

On physical examination, all organ systems should be evaluated with special focus on extrahepatic manifestation of liver disease. Apart from assessing hepatomegaly and splenomegaly, the clinician should also consider dysmorphic features, growth, and nutritional status, as well as dermatologic, neurologic, or pulmonary symptoms. Cardiac auscultation may reveal a murmur suggesting pulmonary artery stenosis in Alagille syndrome or cardiac anomalies associated with biliary atresia (e.g., septal defects).

6.2 Diagnostic Evaluation

6.2.1 General Approach

After clinical assessment of the jaundiced infant, a basic work-up can help to identify treatable disorders as well as to estimate the severity of the liver involvement [4]. This includes basic laboratory tests as full blood count, liver function parameters including gamma-GT, albumin and INR, blood glucose, blood lactate, bile acid levels in selected patients, alpha-1-antitrypsin level/phenotype, TSH, and fT4. The results of the newborn screening should be checked for metabolic disorders including galactosemia. In addition, urinalysis and culture can identify urinary tract infections, which can present with cholestasis in the neonatal period [8]. Consider bacterial cultures of blood, urine, and, depending on the clinical symptoms, cerebrospinal fluid especially if the infant appears to be critically ill or septic.

The other basic investigation in all children with suspected neonatal cholestasis is an abdominal sonography, preferably a fasting ultrasound (see below).

Thereafter, further diagnostic work-up can be stratified and extended in a stepwise manner (compare Fig. 6.1 for diagnostic algorithm). The following questions can help to direct the subsequent procedures:

- Is the infant acutely ill?
  - *Rule out sepsis/severe systemic infection.*
  - *Rule out acute liver failure/metabolic crisis/mitochondrial disorder.*
- Coagulopathy persisting after substitution with vitamin K.
  - *Work-up for acute neonatal liver failure (compare Chap. 10; [9]).*
- Pigmentation of stool: Is the feces acholic?
  - *Rule out biliary atresia.*

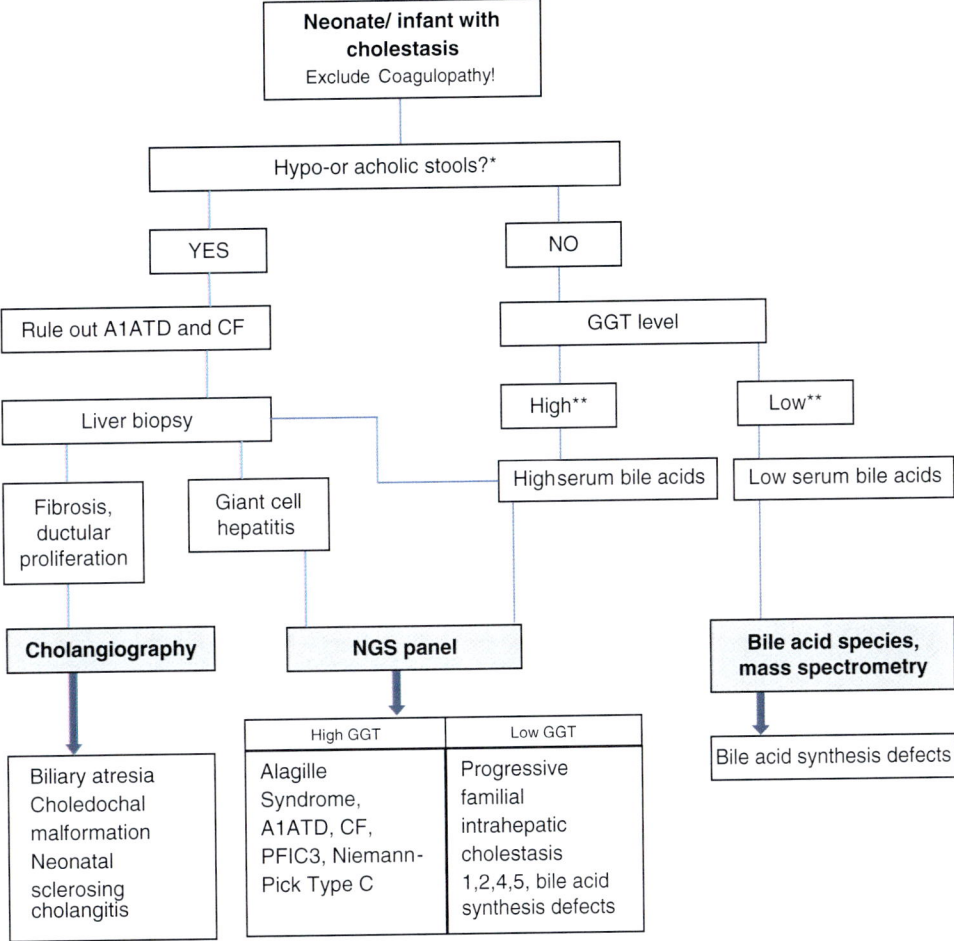

Fig. 6.1 Algorithm to the diagnostic approach to neonatal jaundice focused on the main differential diagnosis. A1ATD should be quantified early in infants with acholic stools before proceeding to invasive diagnostic procedures or Kasai portoenterostomy. *Ultrasonography* may be used in the primary work-up of infants with neonatal cholestasis with focus on morphology of bile ducts and gallbladder, echogenicity of liver parenchyma, and organomegaly. **Work-up at that stage may include infectious disease screening, thyroid function tests, galactosemia, and further metabolic screening

- Is gamma-GT elevated?
  - *Rule out biliary atresia.*
- Is gamma-GT activity normal in cholestatic infants?
  - *Rule out FIC1 and BSEP deficiency (PFIC type 1 and 2), bile acid synthesis defects.*

The aim is to identify infants with conditions requiring further specific therapy such as biliary atresia, gestational alloimmune liver disease (GALD), or tyrosinemia early on in the course (see specific sections). In biliary atresia, early diagnosis and timely Kasai portoenterostomy are associated with favorable outcome and longer survival with native liver [5]. In cases of persisting unexplained neonatal cholestasis with a suspected hereditary background, further diagnostics including next-generation sequencing can help to establish a diagnosis [10].

6.2.2 Specific Evaluations

6.2.2.1 Infectious Disease Work-Up
- Cytomegalovirus (CMV) may cause cholestatic liver disease in infants by congenital infection in term or postnatal infection after virus shedding in breast milk in preterm infants [11]. The diagnosis of CMV infection is confirmed by culture or detection of DNA in blood or urine soon after birth. CMV serology testing is of limited value and not recommended for routine testing in infants.
- Early tests for viral hepatitis A, B, and C in the evaluation of neonatal cholestasis are generally unwarranted unless a specific history points to an exposure to hepatitis viruses.
- Other infections such as syphilis, rubella, toxoplasmosis, enterovirus, and herpesvirus can present with neonatal cholestasis, coagulopathy, and failure to thrive. Check maternal history for risk factors including screening results during pregnancy.

6.2.2.2 Metabolic/Endocrine Work-Up
- Basic metabolic screening including plasma level of amino acids, urine excretion of organic acids, and plasma carnitine and acyl carnitine profile.
- Assess lactate and ammonia for acute metabolic disease in conjunction with blood gas analysis.
- Test for TSH, total and free T4, early-morning cortisol level, and IGF-1 [12]. Thyroid disorders and panhypopituitarism may present with neonatal cholestasis [13].
- On suspicion of lysosomal storage disorders, bone marrow aspirate and liver tissue should be evaluated for storage cells. Additional lysosomal enzyme studies can be performed in fibroblast culture. Determination of serum activity of chitotriosidase can serve as screening marker for lysosomal storage diseases [14].
- If bile acid synthesis errors are suspected, analysis of bile acid composition in serum and urine by mass spectroscopy may reveal a high concentration of intermediate metabolites. Detection of gene variants in determinants of bile acid synthesis may become the preferred diagnostic tool.

6.2.3 Diagnostic Imaging

Several imaging studies have been established for evaluation of the jaundiced infant. Prior stratification in context of the clinical picture is essential to apply the most helpful tool.

The abdominal ultrasound is an easy and noninvasive first diagnostic imaging tool to assess for visible obstructing lesions of the biliary tree or to identify a choledochal cyst and to assess for signs of advanced liver disease or vascular and/or splenic abnormalities. Several hepatic sonographic parameters, such as the triangular cord sign, abnormal gallbladder morphology, gallbladder contraction after oral feeding, the presence and diameter of the common bile duct, liver size and echotexture, spleen size, caliber of the right branch of the hepatic artery, and caliber of the right branch of the portal vein, have been described as sonographic markers of biliary atresia, yet they lack sensitivity and specificity [15]. Further, it is important to remember that a normal gallbladder does not exclude biliary atresia [16]. In addition, findings such as abdominal heterotaxy, polysplenia, asplenia, and preduodenal portal vein point to a potential association with biliary atresia as part of a malformation syndrome.

The primary goal of diagnostic evaluations in cholestatic infants is the determination of patency of the extrahepatic biliary tree in order to rule out biliary atresia. For this purpose, the contribution of endoscopic retrograde cholangiopancreatography (ERCP) in the work-up for BA has been significant [17–19]. While the routine or selective use of ERCP intervention is discussed controversially, the procedure has an excellent risk-benefit ratio, in particular when used to exclude BA by demonstrating bile duct patency (see Fig. 6.2a, b). The procedure, however, requires an experienced endoscopist and appropriate infant endoscopy equipment.

6.2.3.1 Magnetic Resonance Cholangiopancreatography

Magnetic resonance cholangiopancreatography (MRCP) is a useful tool for evaluating a wide variety of disorders of the intra- and extrahepatic biliary system in pediatric patients [20]. The diagnostic value of three-dimensional MRCP for diagnosing BA is of limited specificity and therefore should not generally be used for this indication [21]. However, MRCP may help to assess other disease of biliary tract, e.g., choledochal cysts, and MRI can assess tumor masses and signs of advanced liver disease and/or vascular abnormalities.

6.2.3.2 Percutaneous Transhepatic Cholangiography

As an alternative to ERCP, percutaneous transhepatic cholangiography (PTC) offers the possibility of visualization of bile ducts. The bile duct (if dilated), or the gallbladder, is

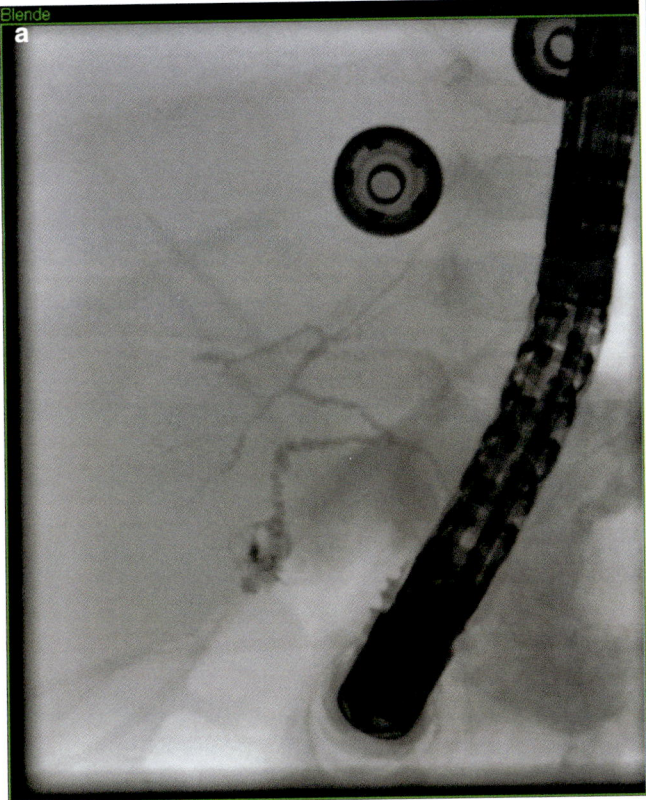
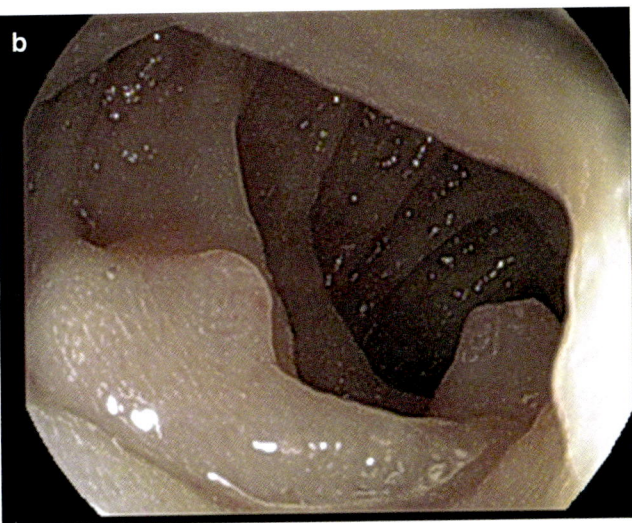

Fig. 6.2 (**a**) demonstration of bile duct patency in an infant with acholic stools. Contrast media is shown in both right and left main ducts, the cystic duct, and the gallbladder. (**b**) anatomy of major and minor papilla before cannulation (Courtesy of Prof. M Goetz, University Hospital Tuebingen)

punctured, and radiographic contrast medium is injected. In addition, this technique allows interventions such as dilation of strictures or external biliary drainage [22]. PTC has been largely replaced by MRCP as diagnostic tool for disease of the biliary tree.

6.2.3.3 Hepatobiliary Scintigraphy

Soluble radioisotopes such as technetium trimethyl 1-bromoiminodiacetic acid (TEBIDA), which are taken up well by hepatocytes despite elevated bilirubin levels, have been used to demonstrate either hepatic uptake or biliary excretion. Pretreatment with phenobarbital (5 mg/kg) for 3–5 days prior to the scintigraphy may improve hepatic uptake of the tracer. Radioisotope scanning has been used to assess biliary excretion and to confirm biliary tract patency. However, this technique is limited by its low specificity (range 68.5–72.2%) [23]. Thus, limited etiologic interpretation of negative tracer excretion hampers its use and offers little advantage over visual monitoring of stool pigment excretion [24]. Therefore, this technique should be used selectively, and results of hepatobiliary scanning require cautious interpretation.

6.2.3.4 Histopathology

If the initial noninvasive tests and ultrasound cannot verify the cause of cholestasis, the liver biopsy remains the cornerstone of the diagnostic work-up of infants with cholestatic jaundice. The interpretation of liver biopsy by an experienced pathologist can provide the correct diagnosis in about 79–98% of cases and help to avoid unnecessary surgery in patients with intrahepatic disease [25].

Histopathological investigations enable assessment of the following questions:

- Integrity of hepatocytes or signs of ballooning and cellular stress? Giant cells?
- Inflammatory infiltrates?
- Signs of biliary obstruction? Bile plugs? Bile duct proliferation?
- Extent and pattern of liver fibrosis?
- Storage cells?

Most centers apply aspiration technique, using a Menghini needle. Sonography-guided percutaneous core liver biopsy is a very safe and effective procedure in children. There are a number of complications of percutaneous liver biopsy such as pain, infection, organ perforation, or biliary leak, but bleeding is the most relevant [26]. Clinically significant bleeding events requiring blood transfusion were reported in 2.8% of 469 children after percutaneous liver biopsy and increased with malignancies or after bone marrow transplant [27]. Patients with acute liver failure, coagulopathy, and ascites are at increased risk for major bleeding. Percutaneous liver biopsy is not universally recommended [26]. For these cases of elevated risk for bleeding, a transjugular liver biopsy, where the liver is biopsied through a special catheter passed from the internal jugular vein into one of the hepatic veins [28], is possible in many centers. Although this procedure has been described for children weighing as little as 3 kg [29], it remain technically challenging in small children.

The classic histologic features of biliary obstruction are bile duct proliferation, bile plugs, portal or perilobular fibrosis, and edema, with preservation of the basic hepatic lobular architecture. Unspecific giant cell transformation can be seen in 20–50% of patients with BA also early in the course. The histologic pattern of biliary obstruction, however, develops with time. Earliest histologic changes of BA may be relatively non-specific, and biopsies performed too early in the course of the disease may result in a falsely negative diagnosis. Therefore, serial biopsies can help to determine the underlying disease [30].

In comparison, hepatocyte ballooning, lobular disarray, and inflammatory cells seen within the portal areas are the dominating picture in neonatal hepatitis [31]. Here, the bile ductules show little or no alteration. Disorders that can mimic BA histologically are parenteral nutrition-associated cholestasis, cystic fibrosis, and alpha-1-antitrypsin deficiency. All these conditions may show variable ductular reaction, and it may be impossible to distinguish them from BA without clinical, imaging, or laboratory data [25, 31].

Immunohistochemistry with biliary cytokeratins 7 and 19 can help to confirm paucity of bile ducts (loss of CK19 expression) and ductular transformation such as duct proliferations (high expression of CK17) MDR3 and BSEP immunostaining are helpful in supporting the phenotypic diagnosis of familial cholestasis syndromes and in differentiating from other causes of neonatal cholestasis [32]. However, expression of BSEP or MDR3 protein does not exclude loss of function mutations (see Fig. 6.3a, b).

6.2.3.5 Genetic Tests

Etiology of neonatal conjugated hyperbilirubinemia or cholestasis may remain unclear after excluding relevant diagnoses, e.g., BA and infections, by conventional means. Formerly these cases were often termed "idiopathic neonatal hepatitis". Next-generation sequencing has contributed to identification of a genetic etiology in many of these cases presenting with conjugated jaundice so this term is used significantly less frequently now [10]. High-throughput, or next-generation, sequencing methodology allows analyzing millions of different DNA fragments in one assay. After DNA amplification, clusters of DNA sequences are read and captured for bioinformatics analysis. The high-throughput sequencing allows parallel analysis of causative gene panels as well as whole exome or genome analyses [33]. The decision between panel diagnostics and exome analysis depends on the clinical question: If the clinical phenotype points to a certain group of causatives genes, the technical restriction to a defined gene panel offers the advantage of highest sensitivity for diagnostics in these predetermined genes. However, in the case of non-specific phenotypes, the exome analysis could be an alternative to extend the diagnostic approach to a number of genes outside a designated panel for liver disease. Interpretation of sequencing results may be difficult in some cases, as many variants of genes in these rare liver diseases have not been yet described and in silico prediction of variant pathogenicity is unclear [34].

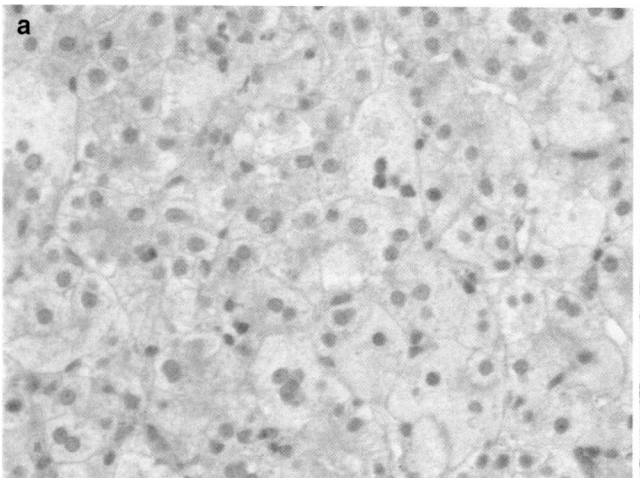
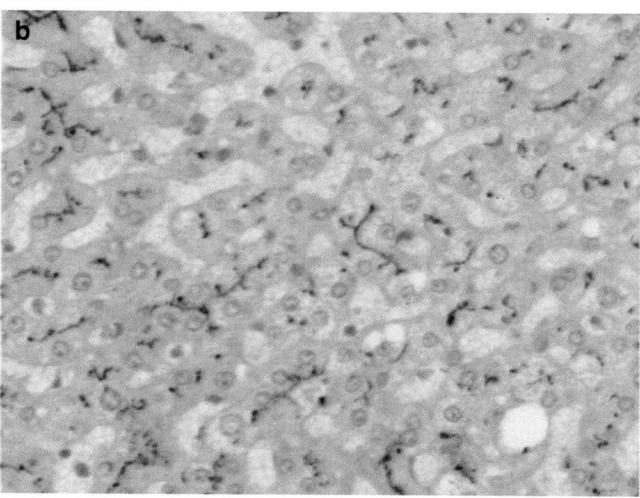

Fig. 6.3 Immunohistochemical examination in liver tissue of a 3-month-old infant with BSEP deficiency. (**a**) Neonatal giant cell hepatitis with cholestasis. In contrast to control (**b**), no chicken wire staining of the BSEP protein (Courtesy of Prof. Sipos, University Hospital Tuebingen, anti-BSEP antibody, biotin reaction/hematoxylin, 200-fold)

6.2.3.6 Risk-Adapted Diagnostic Algorithm

First, all infants should receive basic diagnostic work-up including detailed history, physical examination, basic laboratory work-up (compare Fig. 6.1), and abdominal ultrasound. The typical pictures of biliary obstruction as a cause of neonatal cholestasis are icterus, acholic stools, and elevated gamma-GT. Ultrasound can show gallbladder abnormalities or can be normal. In this constellation, there is a high suspicion for BA. Timely investigations are needed to confirm the diagnosis of BA and to proceed to Kasai portoenterostomy. In the sequence of diagnostic procedures, early investigations should exclude alpha-1-antitrypsin deficiency and cystic fibrosis. A biopsy should be performed which may show signs of biliary obstruction or unspecific giant cell hepatitis. In order to exclude biliary atresia, ERCP may be the next step to assess patency of biliary tree. If bile ducts are patent and GGT is increased, Alagille syndrome may be a differential diagnosis. With normal GGT, the patient should be evaluated for PFIC types 1 or 2 (for differential diagnoses, see Table 6.2). In these cases, early genetic panel diagnostic can be helpful to determine genetic cholestasis syndromes.

Table 6.2 Overview: causes of neonatal cholestasis and differential diagnosis of biliary atresia

Differential diagnosis	Investigation
Infections	
Viral: Adenovirus, cytomegalovirus, echovirus, enterovirus, herpes simplex virus, human immunodeficiency virus, parvovirus B19, rubella	Virus PCRs
Bacterial: Urinary tract infection, sepsis, syphilis	Blood culture, urine culture, serology
Protozoal: Toxoplasma	Maternal and fetal serology
Primary diseases of the hepatocyte	
Familial cholestatic diseases (ATP8B1, ABCB11, ABCB4, MYO5B)	– Gamma-GGT to distinguish subtypes – Liver biopsy including BSEP and MDR3 staining – DNA for mutations

Disorders of bile acid synthesis
    3β-Hydroxy-Δ5-C27-steroid dehydrogenase deficiency
    Δ4-3-oxosteroid-5β-reductase deficiency
    Oxysterol 7-α-hydroxylase deficiency
    Bile acid conjugation defects (BAAT and BAL)
    Zellweger syndrome
	– Gamma-GT ↓
	– Serum concentration of bile acids
	– Analysis of bile acid composition in serum and urine by mass spectroscopy
	– Genetic panel

ARC syndrome (arthrogryposis-renal dysfunction-cholestasis)	– Gamma-GT ↓ – Clinical features of joint dysplasia – Renal and/or cardia disease
Metabolic disease	
Alpha-1-antitrypsin deficiency	– Alpha-1 antitrypsin level – PiZ phenotype
Citrin deficiency	– Plasma and urine amino acids – Genetic
Cystic fibrosis liver disease	– Sweat test – Genetic testing for CFTR mutations
Disorders of lipid metabolism	
Wolman disease (infantile-onset LAL-D)	– Enzyme activity of lysosomal acid lipase (dried blood spot or leukocytes) – Genetic
Niemann-Pick type C	– Splenomegaly at presentation – Elevated oxysterols in plasma (cholestane-3β,5α,6β-triol, 7-ketocholesterol) – Serum level of chitotriosidase as screening test for lysosomal diseases – Filipin stain in fibroblasts – Genetic testing
Gaucher disease	– Serum level of chitotriosidase as screening test for lysosomal diseases – Cerebrosid-β-glucosidase activity in leukocytes or cultured fibroblasts
Diseases of the diseases of the cholangiocyte and bile ducts	
Alagille syndrome	– Echocardiogram – Thoracic vertebrae X-ray – Slit lamp examination – DNA for mutations in JAG1 or NOTCH2

(continued)

Table 6.2 (continued)

Differential diagnosis	Investigation
Choledochal malformation	Sonography, MRCP
Inspissated bile/mucous plug	– Ultrasound – Hemolysis – Rule out CF: Sweat test, CFTR genetic
Cholelithiasis or biliary sludge	Sonography
Tumors/masses (intrinsic and extrinsic)	Sonography, MRI
Neonatal sclerosing cholangitis	Mutations TJP2 on chromosome 9q21.11
Spontaneous perforation of the bile ducts	Sonography, MRCP
Endocrine	
Hypopituitarism (septo-optic dysplasia)	– TSH, fT4 – Morning cortisol (low) – Cerebral MRI
Hypothyroidism	TSH, fT4
Acute neonatal liver failure	
Mitochondrial disorders	– Serum lactate levels ↑ – Hypoglycemia – Genetic panel for mitochondrial disorders
Gestational alloimmune liver disease	– Ferritin serum level ↑↑ – Extrahepatic iron storage (MRI or buccal biopsy)
Hemophagocytic lymphohistiocytosis	– Fever, hepatosplenomegaly and pancytopenia – Ferritin ↑↑, triglycerides ↑, interleukin-2 receptor ↑↑, fibrinogen ↓
Tyrosinemia	– Amino acids in plasma – Organic acids in urine (elevated succinylacetone)
Galactosemia	– Urine-reducing substances – Plasma Gal-1-Put
Toxic	
Drugs	– Patient's history – Antibiotics recently administered
Parenteral nutrition	– Preterm infant? – Type of lipid emulsions?
Extrahepatic	
Shock/hypoperfusion	– Clinical assessment – Echocardiography
Intestinal obstruction	– Intestinal failure associated liver disease – Sonography – Contrast study

6.3 Differential Diagnosis

6.3.1 Infections

Cholestasis is functionally defined as an impairment of bile flow and clinically characterized by elevated plasma concentrations of biliary constituents, resulting in jaundice and liver damage. Cholestatic disorders in hepatocytes can arise from gene mutations or from acquired diseases, e.g., viral, bacterial, or toxic injury. Infections may lead to inflammation-induced cholestasis. In sepsis, for instance, mediators from the non-parenchymal liver cells initiate the hepatic "acute phase" of the inflammatory response. In the neonatal period, hepatobiliary dysfunction secondary to sepsis is common: this condition may occur in particular with gram-negative bacteria but also with gram-positive bacterial strains as well as viruses [35]. Hyperbilirubinemia tends to rise early in the disease course and persist well beyond the end of the clinical inflammatory response, up to period of 60 days. Long-term complications of inflammation-associated cholestasis are rare [36], but can occur in specific infections. In the following, features of some selected congenital infections will be discussed in detail.

6.3.1.1 Cytomegalovirus

CMV is the most common cause of congenital infection affecting 1–2% of newborns, most of whom are asymptomatic but may lead to sensorineural hearing loss and neurodevelopmental sequelae [37]. Primary maternal infection in the second or third trimester is associated with more severe fetal disease. Cytomegalovirus (CMV) is reactivated in the lactating breast in up to 96% of CMV-seropositive mothers. The onset, the dynamics, and the end of virus shedding into breast milk are variable [38].

Clinical Features

Sepsis-like symptoms (SLS) have been described in association with postnatal CMV infection in VLBW preterm infants, comprising apnea and bradycardia, hepatosplenomegaly, hepatitis, gray pallor, distending bowels, thrombocytopenia, neutropenia, and elevated liver enzymes [39]. Other signs may include intrauterine growth retardation, jaundice, petechial rash, hepatosplenomegaly, and central nervous system involvement (e.g., microcephaly intracranial calcification and chorioretinitis). Manifestation of postnatal infection may be milder or inapparent in term infants. Congenital infection may also present with hepatosplenomegaly and altered liver function; however, CNS manifestation is frequent. CMV has also been found in unspecific neonatal cholestatic disease and in association with biliary atresia [40].

Investigations

CMV PCR and culture from the urine can be used to detect the virus. CMV IgM may be found but does not help to differentiate between congenital and acquired disease. Liver biopsy may show giant cell hepatitis and bile duct paucity in selected cases.

Management and Prognosis

Most cases resolve without hepatic sequelae. Occasionally signs of chronic liver disease such as hepatic fibrosis and portal hypertension have been reported. Treatment with ganciclovir or valganciclovir improves long-term neurological and hearing function as well as survival [41].

6.3.1.2 Herpes and Enteric Viral Sepsis

Herpes simplex viruses (HSV) types 1 and 2 as well as echovirus, coxsackievirus, and adenovirus can cause severe liver failure and multiorgan failure in the first weeks of life.

Clinical Features

HSV usually occurs in the first 2 weeks of life with or without vesicles. HSV type 2 infection may be acquired from genital infection. Enteroviruses may lead to vertical infection around the time of birth with peaks in the summer months or early fall. All viruses cause a non-specific syndrome with severe hepatitis, hyperbilirubinemia, and coagulopathy in association with non-hepatic organ failure, e.g., the heart in coxsackievirus infection. HSV causes serious multiorgan disease with high mortality. Early diagnosis and treatment are mandatory.

Investigations

Viruses can be detected by blood PCR or in samplings from vesicles (HSV), in cerebrospinal fluid, in stool culture, or in throat swabs. Liver histology shows areas of necrosis and in some cases viral inclusions.

Management

Early treatment with acyclovir may modify the clinical course in HSV disease. Antivirals such as pleconaril and cidofovir may also improve enterovirus disease depending on the specific virus. However, overall mortality is high. Liver transplantation may be successful in controlled extrahepatic disease [42].

6.3.1.3 Other Viruses

Varicella infection occurs in infants acquired in the context of peripartal maternal disease. It may lead to severe manifestation, particularly in premature infants, affecting the liver and the lungs and presenting with extensive skin involvement. Treatment with acyclovir may be curative. The hepatotropic viruses A–E rarely lead to neonatal liver disease. Hepatitis B vertical infection is subclinical but should prompt simultaneous vaccination with vaccine and hepatitis B immunoglobulins. Failure to vaccinate increases the risk of developing a chronic carrier state or, rarely, acute and severe hepatitis following an incubation period. Human herpesvirus type 6 has been shown to cause acute liver failure in rare instances. Respiratory syncytial virus (RSV) can lead to severe giant cell hepatitis in neonates and fulminant organ failure, particularly in older children. RSV hepatitis may lead to a chronic form of liver disease requiring transplantation.

6.3.1.4 Bacterial Infection

Congenital infection with *Listeria monocytogenes* typically involves the liver. In most cases meningitis and pneumonia are clinically dominant; however, infants may have hepatosplenomegaly and jaundice. The organism may be isolated from blood, cerebrospinal fluid, or liver tissue. Penicillin is used for treatment.

Congenital tuberculosis is rare. Affected infants may present with hepatosplenomegaly and jaundice and in rare cases with progressive liver failure [43]. Presentation may be atypical, and a high level of suspicion is needed. Liver tissue may show caseating granuloma, and investigations of the placenta or maternal genital organs show tuberculous infection. Timely administration of antituberculosis therapy leads to a better outcome [44].

6.3.2 Primary Diseases of the Hepatocyte

6.3.2.1 Genetic Cholestatic Disease

Progressive familial intrahepatic cholestasis (PFIC) is a group of rare disorders caused by transport defects in the hepatocyte (see below for details) with an estimated incidence of 1:25,000–1:100,000. The spectrum of genetic cholestatic syndromes also includes ultra-rare diseases such as the *arthrogryposis-renal dysfunction-cholestasis*

(ARC) syndrome. This disorder is caused by mutations in the *VPS33B* gene and is inherited in an autosomal-recessive trait; many patients are from consanguineous families [45]. Similar to other genetic cholestatic diseases, infants may have extrahepatic features. In ARC these are arthrogryposis, renal and cardiac defects, and a biochemical pattern with normal GGT activity in spite of severe cholestasis. However, a unique and important feature of ARC syndrome is a bleeding tendency, and patients undergoing liver biopsy often experience severe hemorrhage. Thus, although biopsy contributes to diagnosis of other familial cholestatic diseases, in ARC syndrome the diagnosis should be made by mutation analysis, and organ biopsy should be avoided. Details on other genetic cholestatic syndromes are discussed in the following underlining similarities which can used in the diagnostic approach and specifics of subtypes which are important for management.

Progressive Familial Intrahepatic Cholestasis

Under physiological circumstances, the canalicular membrane of the hepatocyte plays a key role in the elimination of bile components. For this purpose specialized transport proteins are located on the canalicular domain, contributing directly or indirectly to transport of different substrates into bile. The bile salt export pump protein (BSEP, *ABCB11*) transports bile acids. Phospholipid transport is performed by the MDR3 P-glycoprotein (*ABCB4*), and the FIC1 protein ("familial intrahepatic cholestasis 1," *ATP8B1*) stabilizes the structure and thereby functional capacity of the canalicular membrane. Variants in the *ATP8B1*/FIC1, *ABCB11*/BSEP, and *ABCB4*/MDR3 genes are responsible for clinically different forms of progressive familial intrahepatic cholestasis. Further genes have been identified that lead to PFIC phenotypes or hypercholanemia: *MYO5B*, *TJP2*, and *BAAT*. Bile acid synthesis defects are also familial cholestasis disorders and are discussed (see Table 6.3 for overview). PFIC diseases are rare or ultra-rare with an incidence of 1 in 25,000 to 1 in 100,000,000. High-impact mutations may lead to an early manifestation of disease in infants and young children, whereas low-impact mutations manifest later, sometimes in adult age. Other proteins in the enterohepatic circulation may act as disease modifiers or are potential targets for novel therapies for these rare disorders (Table 6.3).

Clinical Features

PFIC types 1 and 2 both frequently lead to jaundice or cholestasis in the first months of life in many cases combined with unrelenting pruritus. *ATP8B1* is also expressed in extrahepatic tissue which may lead to clinical features such as pancreatitis, diarrhea, sensorineural deafness, and short stature. Fat-soluble vitamin K deficiency may lead to coag-

Table 6.3 Familial intrahepatic cholestasis disease - overview of genetic diseases affecting transport and metabolism of bile acids and other biliary constituents

Disease	Synonym	Gene	Phenotype	Treatment
FIC-1 deficiency	PFIC 1	ATP8B1 (FIC1) Aminophospholipid translocator	May occur periodically, cholestasis and jaundice, pruritus. Extrahepatic manifestation: diarrhea, pancreatitis, hearing impairment. Normal γGT activity	Ursodeoxycholic acid, partial external or internal diversion (liver transplantation, risk of adverse effects: steatosis and diarrhea)
BSEP deficiency	PFIC 2	ABCB11 Bile salt export pump	Neonatal hepatitis, progressive cholestasis, pruritus, failure to thrive, fibrosis. BSEP protein not detectable on IHC, normal γGT activity	Ursodeoxycholic acid, partial external or internal diversion, liver transplantation (risk of recurrence)
MDR3 deficiency	PFIC 3	ABCB4 P-glycoprotein 3; phospholipid translocator	Cholestasis, portal hypertension, bile duct proliferation and fibrosis, MDR3 not detectable on IHC, γGT activity increased	Ursodeoxycholic acid, partial external or internal diversion, liver transplantation
MYO5B deficiency	PFIC 4	MYO5B, myosin 5B	Resembles PFIC types 1 and 2, may occur with diarrhea (microvillus-inclusion disease) or without	See PFIC and 1 + 2
FXR deficiency	PFIC 5	NR1H4, farnesoid-x receptor	Resembles PFIC type 2	See PFIC 2
Hypercholanemia		EPHX1, TJP2 (synonym ZO2), BAAT, BAL, SLC10A1	Elevated serum bile acid concentrations, itching, and fat malabsorption	Treat fat and vitamin malabsorption; *progressive forms of TJP2 deficiency* may require a treatment similar to PFIC including transplantation
Bile acid synthesis defects	BASD	Δ4-3-oxosteroid-5β reductase 3β-Hydroxy C_{27}steroid dehydrogenase/isomerase 24,25-Dihydroxy-cholanoic cleavage enzyme	Cholestasis and neonatal hepatitis, γGT and serum bile acids normal in majority of cases depending on subtype	Cholic-, chenodeoxycholic acid, single or combined treatment with ursodeoxycholic acid

NOTE: TJP2 and FXR deficiency are infrequently termed PFIC 4 and PFIC 5.

ulopathy. Patients affected by high-impact *ABCB11* mutations have an increased risk for hepatocellular carcinoma [46] and should be followed in specialized centers with AFP and ultrasound monitoring in regular intervals. PFIC 3 presents with cholestasis in younger children or later in child- or even adulthood. Pruritus is often less severe than in PFIC 1 and 2, and portal hypertension is a dominant feature in later life. Cholelithiasis may occur in PFIC 3 and lead to symptoms occasionally persisting after cholecystectomy. Adult manifestation of low-impact mutations may lead to cholestasis of pregnancy or drug-induced liver disease, e.g., triggered by the contraceptive pill. Other genes encoding determinants of biliary transport may cause phenotypes similar to PFIC or limited to hypercholanemia (see Table 6.3).

Diagnosis
Liver function analysis shows increased aminotransferases and bile acids, while GGT activity remains low in PFIC 1 and 2 but is elevated in PFIC type 3. Coagulopathy and bleeding may occur in early presentation due to vitamin K deficiency. In general terms, the degree of hepatic dysfunction is often more pronounced in ABCB11 than in ATP8B1 deficiency, so that clinical differentiation of these subtypes is possible to some degree [47]. Ultrasound does not detect specific findings but is useful to exclude biliary obstruction and focal neoplasia.

Histology
While PFIC 1 shows bland cholestasis with no bile duct proliferation and minimal inflammation, PFIC 2 shows features of canalicular cholestasis, hepatocellular ballooning, necrosis, and giant cell transformation. Bile duct hypoplasia can be a feature. In high-impact mutations, immunohistochemical staining shows lack of BSEP expression (see Fig. 6.3). In PFIC 3 disease, liver biopsy shows portal fibrosis and ductular proliferation with a mixed inflammatory infiltrate. In progressive disease, older patients may present with biliary cirrhosis.

Genetics
It is estimated that 10% of all diseases presenting with neonatal cholestasis belong to the group of PFIC disorders. Therefore, next-generation sequencing has a growing impact also in detection of variants in relevant genes that are correlated with different PFIC phenotypes [10]. To maximize interpretive potential of sequencing results, the use of an algorithm to combine use of standard diagnostic tools with NGS technology may strongly improve the power to discriminate between etiologies of infantile cholestatic diseases. It is important that parental DNA is available to confirm biallelic variants in autosomal-recessively inherited diseases. NGS has largely replaced single-gene sequencing, which may still be used to confirm variants detected in NGS in other family members.

Management
Depending on the disease subtype, UDCA may be effective in improving the disease phenotype, e.g., to enhance biliary secretion of phospholipids in PFIC 3 disease. It rarely offers benefit in treatment of cholestatic pruritus. Managing cholestatic pruritus in PFIC remains a challenge. Different means to interrupt the enterohepatic circulation in PFIC have been tested. Bile absorptive resins such as cholestyramine are not sufficiently effective and are unpalatable. Interventionally or surgically created interruptions of the enterohepatic circulation have been more successful in subgroup of patients by nasobiliary drainage and, most frequently, by partial external and internal biliary diversion [48, 49]. A novel approach includes the use of IBAT (ileal bile acid transporter, synonym ASBT, apical sodium dependent bile acid transporter) inhibitors which target the main intestinal bile acid uptake protein and is currently tested in clinical trials [50]. Nutritional support to enhance growth and development in spite of chronic cholestasis is essential as well as supplementation of fat-soluble vitamins. Many patients will need liver transplantation for progressive disease when supportive, medical, and surgical therapy do not lead to amelioration of symptoms and/or control of liver failure. However, in PFIC 1 extrahepatic manifestations of diarrhea and graft steatosis may severely impact posttransplant outcome. Recurrence of PFIC 2 disease in grafts due to immunological activation against the BSEP as an alloantigen in the graft has been reported.

Bile Acid Synthesis Defects
There are nine known defects of bile acid synthesis, including oxysterol 7α-hydroxylase deficiency (*CYP7B*), Δ4-3-oxosteroid-5β-reductase deficiency (*AKR1D1*, *SRD5B1*), 3β-hydroxy-Δ5-C27-steroid dehydrogenase deficiency (*HSD3B7*), cerebrotendinous xanthomatosis (also known as sterol 27-hydroxylase deficiency, *CYP27A1*), α-methylacyl-CoA racemase deficiency (*AMACR*), and Zellweger syndrome (also known as cerebrohepatorenal syndrome, *PEX*). These are rare genetic disorders which are characterized by a failure to produce normal bile acids and an accumulation of unusual bile acids and bile acid intermediaries [51].

Failure to diagnose any of these conditions can result in liver failure or progressive chronic liver disease. If recognized early, many patients can have a remarkable clinical response to oral bile acid therapy.

Clinical Features
Inborn errors of bile acid synthesis can present as neonatal cholestasis, neurologic disease, or fat-soluble vitamin deficiencies. Jaundice is common, but failure to thrive without jaundice may occur. Poor growth is a frequent symptom. Coagulopathy and ascites may be found. Patient may present with cataracts in some subgroups.

3β-Hydroxy-Δ5-C27-steroid dehydrogenase deficiency (3βHSD) may present in the neonatal period with neonatal hepatitis, cholestasis, and acholic stools. Milder cases are not jaundiced and present with failure to thrive and fat-soluble vitamin deficiency.

Δ4-3-Oxosteroid-5β-reductase deficiency is heterogeneous regarding the clinical presentation, similar to *3βHSD*. Cholestasis may be severe in infancy, and chronic liver disease may be noted in later childhood.

Cerebrotendinous xanthomatosis is also known as *sterol 27-hydroxylase deficiency, CTX*. In this condition, cholestasis in infancy is highly variable, and cases may not become apparent until later childhood when cataracts and diarrhea develop. A progressive neurological dysfunction is noted in the second to third decades.

Zellweger syndrome presents with craniofacial abnormalities and neuronal migration defects, polycystic kidneys, chronic liver disease, and bony abnormalities.

Bile acid conjugation defects (*BAAT* and *BAL*) have been identified in children with neonatal cholestasis and severe failure to thrive and fat-soluble vitamin deficiencies.

Investigations
Individuals with inborn errors of bile acid synthesis generally present with the hallmark features of normal or low serum bile acid concentrations, normal γ-glutamyl transpeptidase (GGT) concentrations, and the absence of pruritus. GGT is low in the majority of cases, and fat-soluble vitamin deficiency can be profound. Abnormal bile acid composition can be found in serum and urine, and high concentrations of intermediary metabolites can be measured. This analysis is done frequently by fast atom bombardment mass spectroscopy (FAB-MS) of urine which is time consuming. Histology may show neonatal cholestasis but also signs of steatosis and iron overload. Next-generation or exome sequencing may become the fastest way to confirm the disease by detecting pathologic variants in genes that are crucial in the bile acid pathway.

Management
Replacement of primary bile acids reduces the formation of intermediary metabolites. Cholic acid (15 mg/kg once daily) alone and in some cases in combination with ursodeoxycholic acid (15 mg/kg twice daily) is beneficial. Glycocholic acid ameliorates fat malabsorption in bile acid amidation defects but is presently only available for clinical trials [52]. In Zellweger syndrome bile acid therapy can only lead to transient improvement. The peroxisomal defect is a multisystem disease with high mortality.

6.3.3 Metabolic Disease

6.3.3.1 Alpha-1-Antitrypsin Deficiency
Alpha-1-antitrypsin deficiency (A1AT deficiency) is inherited as an autosomal-recessive trait with an estimated incidence of 1 in 2500. It is the most common inherited metabolic disorder causing liver disease in infants. Mutations in the *SERPINA1* gene cause abnormal folding of the protein leading to the PiZ or PiS subtypes, leading to a pathological structure of the protein, which is retained in the endoplasmic reticulum. Only part of the homozygous carriers of PiZ develops liver disease, so cofactors must play a role.

6.3.3.2 Clinical Features
The clinical picture is very similar to that of the biliary atresia; therefore, accurate differentiation is important. The liver disease may present at any age, but manifestation in the neonatal period with conjugated hyperbilirubinemia is common. Stools may be pale or pigmented. Hepatomegaly may be noted; splenomegaly in early stages of the disease is rare. It may present in older children together with other signs of portal hypertension. As in biliary atresia, vitamin K deficiency with complicating cerebral hemorrhage may occur; correction with parenteral vitamin K administration is therefore important.

6.3.3.3 Investigations
The diagnosis is made by the detection of a reduced serum A1AT concentration and the analysis of the A1AT protease inhibitor (Pi) phenotype or the detection of the *SERPINA1* mutation. A1AT is an acute phase reactant which may cause unreliability of the serum level as a disease marker. The Pi phenotype (M, S, or Z) is assessed by isoelectric focusing. PiMM is the most common normal phenotype, whereas PiZZ is the most common form leading to disease. PiMZ does not cause liver disease but may be a cofactor for pathogenesis of other liver diseases, e.g., cystic fibrosis-associated liver disease.

Histopathology may show acute hepatitis of varying severity and resemble the findings typical for biliary atresia, e.g., ductular reaction with varying degrees of fibrosis. Predominantly in later stages, PAS-positive diastase-resistant granules are positive in hepatocytes, corresponding to amorphous material in the endoplasmic reticulum.

6.3.3.4 Management and Prognosis
In most children, the liver disease is benign, with eventual regeneration of the liver function with supportive treatment. An optimal nutritional regime is important. Patients should be followed in specialized centers to detect deteriorating liver function early and initiate interventions for control of portal hypertension or evaluation for liver transplantation. Persistent liver dysfunction with signs of advanced fibrosis and bile duct proliferation are poor prognostic signs. Antisense oligonucleotides, carbamazepine as a stimulant for autophagy, and therapeutic genome editing with CRISPR/Cas9 in the treatment of A1AT liver disease in animal models are being tested [53, 54].

6.3.3.5 Cystic Fibrosis Liver Disease

The incidence of liver disease in children with cystic fibrosis (CF) is 27–35% [55]. Cholestasis in infants is an uncommon condition in CF affecting only 5.7% of the screened newborn CF population. The greatest risk factor for developing cholestasis is the presence of meconium ileus (MI). However, the presence of MI appears not to be associated with the development of CF liver disease [56].

Clinical Features
The presenting features are variable. Hepatomegaly may be present. Some infants have neonatal giant cell hepatitis, paucity of bile ducts, or severe steatosis without jaundice. Others may present with extrahepatic bile duct obstruction or lesions resembling biliary atresia requiring portoenterostomy to restore bile flow.

Investigations
For CF diagnosis sweat chloride analysis and genetic screening for CFTR mutations are most frequently used (see chapter 15). Determination of fecal pancreatic elastase activity detects exocrine pancreatic insufficiency. Imaging of the bile ducts by ERCP or MRCP is needed to plan the optimal approach to therapy in patients with suspected biliary obstruction.

Management
Multidisciplinary management of patients with CF liver disease is crucial. This includes treatment of complications such as meconium ileus, maintenance of pulmonary function, and improving nutritional status. The objective of UDCA treatment is to delay the progression of the disease. Therefore treatment should be started as soon as the diagnosis of CF liver disease is made. However, there is no data on long-term outcomes such as death or need for liver transplantation. A daily dose of 20 mg/kg is initially recommended. A therapeutic schedule based on multiple divided doses (at least twice/day) seems to be more effective because of incomplete intestinal absorption [57].

6.3.3.6 Citrin Deficiency

Citrin deficiency (neonatal-onset type 2 citrullinemia) is caused by a mutation of the *SLC25A13* gene. Lack of citrin leads to specific dysfunction of argininosuccinate synthetase. This enzyme is important for disposition of nicotinamide adenine dinucleotide [NADPH] which is critical in aerobic glycolysis. The adult form presents with fatty liver, hyperammonemia, neurological symptoms, and iron accumulation. The infant form has also been termed "neonatal intrahepatic cholestasis with citrin deficiency."

Clinical Features and Investigations
Infants with citrin deficiency have transient intrahepatic cholestasis, diffuse fatty liver, and parenchymal cellular infiltration associated with hepatic fibrosis, low birth weight, and growth retardation. Citrin deficiency as a cause of neonatal intrahepatic cholestasis occurs predominantly in Asian infants [58]. Liver function may be abnormal: hypoproteinemia, decreased concentrations of coagulation factors, and/or hypoglycemia may occur. Plasma levels of citrulline, tyrosine, threonine, arginine, and methionine are elevated.

Management
Symptoms remit with fat-soluble vitamin supplementation and the use of lactose-free formula or formulas containing medium-chain triglycerides. Later in life, some of these patients may develop adult-onset citrullinemia type 2. Occasionally the liver disease is progressive and may require liver transplantation.

6.3.4 Endocrine Disorders

6.3.4.1 Hypothyroidism
Hypo- or hyperthyroidism may lead to hyperbilirubinemia, both indirect and direct, and cholestasis. In liver biopsy neonatal hepatitis may be detected. Thyroxin may play a role in altering bile flow [59].

6.3.4.2 Hypopituitarism
These patients typically present with failure to thrive, hypoglycemia, and jaundice. In males a micropenis may be detected [13]. Septo-optic dysplasia is frequently found.

6.3.4.3 Investigations
Analysis of pituitary hormones will reveal low levels. The aminotransferases may be mildly elevated and can be normal. In the majority of cases, GGT activity is normal. In histology canalicular cholestasis and eosinophilic infiltrates predominate. Imaging should focus on septo-optic dysplasia which is associated with absent corpus callosum, septum pellucidum, and hypoplasia of the optic nerves.

6.3.4.4 Management
The cholestasis is thought to be due to the central adrenal insufficiency and may improve spontaneously. Hormone replacement may accelerate regeneration of liver function. Cirrhosis may develop if no hormone replacement is initiated.

6.3.5 Acute Neonatal Liver Failure

Acute liver failure in infants usually presents with multisystem involvement. Diagnosis may be difficult as jaundice may be a late feature. Infants may be small for gestational age or have intrauterine growth retardation. Clinical features may include hypotonia, hypoglycemia, hypotension, and coagulopathy.

Ammonia may be elevated. Encephalopathy may be difficult to recognize. Lactic acidosis or renal tubular acidosis is common. Maintaining glucose homeostasis is crucial in management. The focus in treatment should be on antibacterial, antiviral, and antimycotic therapy and correction of coagulopathy if necessary and exchange transfusions if indicated (see section on GALD). Galactosemia should be excluded in any case of infantile acute liver failure. Unless there is signs or irreversible multiorgan disease, patients without response to conventional therapy or potential of liver regeneration should be assessed for liver transplantation.

6.3.5.1 Gestational Alloimmune Liver Disease (GALD, Neonatal Hemochromatosis)

Gestational alloimmune liver disease (GALD), previously known as neonatal hemochromatosis or neonatal iron storage disease, is a disorder characterized by hepatic failure and hepatic and extrahepatic iron accumulation (hemosiderosis) during the neonatal period. The new term reflects the alloimmune mechanism that is responsible for the disorder, as described below [60]. The term "neonatal hemochromatosis" is misleading because the disorder is unrelated to hereditary hemochromatosis. Hepatic iron deposition may also be seen in some inborn errors of metabolism, including tyrosinemia type 1 and inborn errors of bile acid synthesis. The iron deposition is a consequence, rather than a cause, of the liver injury. GALD has been shown to be the result of maternal alloimmune injury [61]. Like other gestational alloimmune diseases, the disorder is caused by transplacental passage of specific reactive immunoglobulin G. The maternal alloantibody activates fetal complement cascade to produce a membrane attack complex and fetal liver injury. The target protein of the maternal immune response has not been identified.

Clinical Features and Investigations

The onset of GALD is intrauterine, and newborns present with signs of severe liver failure, including coagulopathy, ascites, and hypoalbuminemia. The liver may appear cirrhotic. Hyperbilirubinemia typically is both conjugated and unconjugated, although conjugated bilirubin levels may be only modestly elevated. Hepatic cirrhosis is common, underscoring the antenatal timing of the hepatic insult [62]. The diagnosis may be suspected on the basis of the iron studies. Traditionally, demonstration of extrahepatic (or extra reticuloendothelial) iron was required for the diagnosis. However, now that the alloimmune mechanism has been recognized, cases may be identified by the characteristic immunohistologic features of alloimmune disease that are present, specifically the antihuman C5b-9 complex [60] (see Fig. 6.4). Cases with these immunohistochemical findings and with either mild or severe disease or no iron overload have been reported [63]. Thus, the new understanding of the pathogenesis encompasses a spectrum of different phenotypes of GALD, mild and severe forms requiring early identification and treatment.

Management

The combination of exchange transfusion and intravenous immunoglobulin (IVIG) is the current treatment of choice for neonates with GALD [64]. Liver transplantation remains an option for infants who do not respond to IVIG treatment. With high-dose IVIG treatment, usually given in combination

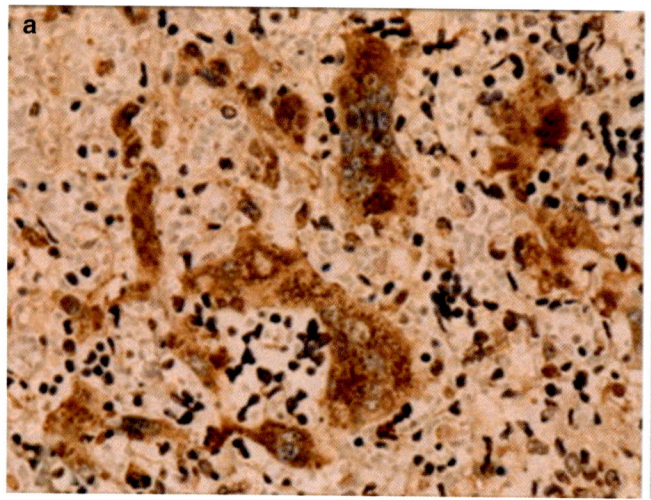
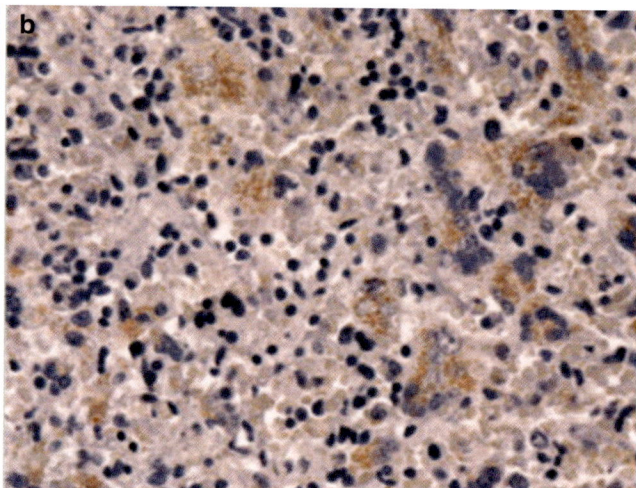

Fig. 6.4 Sections were immunostained with antihuman C5b-9 complex, the terminal complement cascade neoantigen formed in the assembly of membrane attack complex. (**a**) The liver from a GALD case for which immunohistochemistry was performed with the specific anti-C5b-9 monoclonal antibody. The warm brown color produced in a true-positive immunoperoxidase reaction could be seen in all the hepatocytes. Scattered nonhepatocytes are also stained. The shapes and sizes of these cells suggest that they were macrophages/Kupffer cells, endothelial cells, and oval cells. (**b**) Same field of the same liver with the primary antibody omitted. Hemosiderin, predominantly in hepatocytes, retained a rust-brown color that did not have the same tone as the product of the immunoperoxidase reaction (Reprinted with permission (modified) [60])

with exchange transfusion, transplant-free survival was reported up to 79% [65]. Liver transplantation can be curative, but transplantation is difficult in this age group due to lack of appropriate donors and the increased risk of vascular and infectious complications. Thus, early referral is important. For pregnant women with a previous pregnancy that resulted in an infant with GALD, gestational therapy (prenatal treatment) with high-dose IVIG dramatically reduces the risk for recurrence of disease [66].

6.3.5.2 Mitochondrial Disorders

This group of disorders present with acute liver failure, multiorgan disease, and Alpers syndrome. Clinical phenotypes and mode of inheritance may be variable. Clinical features are a consequence of adenosine triphosphate deficiency and impaired fat oxidation as well as generation of toxic free radicals. Mitochondrial DNA (mtDNA) is a separate genome of maternal origin encoding RNA subtypes and 13 subunits of the respiratory chain. Nuclear DNA encodes most subunits of the respiratory chain and all complex 2 subunits, as well as proteins required to maintain DNA [67]. In primary mitochondrial hepatopathies, liver involvement is often part of multiorgan manifestations. In acute liver failure of infancy, three entities are relevant: isolated deficiencies of the electron transport chain enzymes, mtDNA depletion syndromes, and Alpers syndrome.

Deficiencies of the Electron Transport Chain Enzymes

Nuclear genes coding for respiratory chain assembly factors can cause hepatopathy. Lactic acidosis, liver involvement, and Fanconi-type renal tubulopathy are common when the complex III assembly factor gene *BCS1L* harbors mutations. The most severe form is the GRACILE syndrome (growth restriction, aminoaciduria, cholestasis, iron overload, lactic acidosis, and early death). Complex IV deficiency leads to severe acidosis, hypotonia, hypoglycemia, enlarged liver, and liver failure with hepatic steatosis [67]. Mutations in nuclear translation factor genes (*TRMU*, *EFG1*, and *EFTu*) of the respiratory chain enzyme complexes have been linked to neonatal liver failure or dysfunction and chronic liver disease.

Mitochondrial DNA Depletion Syndrome

Pathogenic mutations in at least four genes lead to mtDNA depletion syndrome and liver disease: *DGUOK*, *POLG*, *MPV17*, and *Twinkle*. Depletion of mtDNA is caused by a number of nuclear genes that, when affected by mutations, will lead to altered replication of mtDNA.

Alpers Syndrome

POLG1 mutations are a common cause of mtDNA depletion, resulting in low concentrations of respiratory chain complexes I, III, and IV and presenting as Alpers-Huttenlocher syndrome or neonatal liver failure. Liver transplantation (LT) is generally contraindicated because of its systemic nature and the inevitable progression of severe central nervous system lesions and symptoms despite LT. Treatment of complex seizures in patients with Alpers-Huttenlocher syndrome with valproic acid may precipitate ALF. In these patients, the respiratory chain enzyme activities and mtDNA content in skeletal muscle may be normal; thus, liver tissue analysis or genotyping is necessary to establish the diagnosis [68].

Clinical Presentation

Approximately 12% of the affected infants were born preterm, and another 30% had intrauterine growth retardation [69]. Onset may occur within the first weeks to months of life and may manifest as mild hepatic dysfunction that progresses to liver failure. Vomiting, poor feeding, hypotonia, seizures, and lethargy may occur. In these patients, laboratory investigations generally reveal an elevated serum lactate level (>2.5 mmol/L), increased lactate/pyruvate molar ratio (>25 mol/mol), hypoglycemia, prolonged prothrombin time, hyperammonemia, and variably elevated aminotransferase and bilirubin concentrations [67].

Investigations

A structured diagnostic evaluation is required to diagnose mitochondrial liver disorders. Persistent lactic acidemia is a strong indicator for a mitochondriopathy. Definitive diagnosis is by genetic testing via new-generation sequencing technology. More common mutations can be found in *POLG*, *DGUOK*, *MPV17*, and *TRMU*. Additional tests may include free fatty acids, carnitine and acylcarnitine, plasma amino acids, CK levels, organic acids in urine, lactate and protein in cerebrospinal fluid, echocardiography and electrocardiogram, and electroencephalogram. If no pathogenic mutations are detected, function of electron transport chain needs to be analyzed in the affected tissue, or reduced mtDNA copy number needs to be shown. Demonstration of extrahepatic manifestation will in most cases preclude liver transplantation as a cure. Liver biopsy will show steatosis with hepatocyte degeneration and cirrhosis in some cases. Electron chain transport analysis in liver tissue may be difficult to interpret due to the secondary alterations of chronic liver damage. Liver electron microscopy will demonstrate dysmorphology of the mitochondria. Cranial MR and spectroscopy may be useful in confirming CNS involvement. However, CNS lactate may be elevated when levels are high in the plasma compartment so the findings are not specific.

Management and Prognosis

In neonatal ALF due to mitochondrial disease, supportive therapy includes prevention of hypoglycemia and correction of acidosis and hyperammonemia. In children with chronic liver disease, management includes feeding a formula enriched with medium-chain triglycerides, providing a diet with 30–40% of energy as fat, preventing hypoglycemia, and providing adequate fat-soluble vitamin supplementation. Various pharmacologic therapies have been advocated for mitochondrial disorders. However, a recent Cochrane systemic review examining the efficacies of coenzyme Q10, dichloroacetate, creatine monohydrate, and a whey-based, dietary supplement failed to show any clear evidence supporting their use in treating mitochondrial disorders [70]. Nonetheless, some disorders appear to respond to treatment, such as coenzyme Q deficiency.

The role of liver transplantation (LT) in treating mitochondrial hepatopathies remains controversial. In many mitochondrial diseases, post-LT progression of neuromuscular, cardiac, or other symptomatology may prove fatal despite excellent results of the LT procedure, and thus the outcomes after LT have not been encouraging. However, there is a subset of patients who do not exhibit progression of respiratory chain dysfunction in other organs after LT. It is hoped that with vigilant pre-LT evaluation and selection to exclude neurologic and extrahepatic involvement, post-LT deterioration and death can be avoided in most, if not all, patients. However, it should be emphasized that in infants with acute liver failure (ALF), even thorough evaluation might not detect extrahepatic involvement, early manifestation usually is predictive of poor outcome, and thus an indication for transplantation should be considered with caution. Outcome of LT in patients with *DGUOK* disease without significant neurologic involvement may be better than that in patients with other forms of mitochondrial hepatopathy [71]. In this disease nystagmus is a negative prognostic indicator and should alert clinicians to CNS involvement precluding LT [72]. LT is usually contraindicated in patients with mitochondrial disease caused by mutations in *POLG* and *MPV17*. In patients undergoing LT, family members should be counseled about the possibility of other organ involvement after LT that may be potentially devastating and fatal. The most difficult cases are those in which a young child presents in ALF without definable extrahepatic involvement and with a previously normal history. Ideally, a thorough evaluation with magnetic resonance imaging/magnetic resonance spectroscopy (and possibly electroencephalography) of the brain, echocardiography, retinal examination, cerebrospinal fluid analysis, respiratory chain testing of muscle and/or liver, and genotyping for the likely genetic defects should be performed if time permits.

6.3.5.3 Tyrosinemia

Hereditary tyrosinemia type 1 (HT1), also known as hepatorenal tyrosinemia, is the most severe disorder of tyrosine metabolism. HT1 occurs in 1 in 12,000 to 1 in 100,000 individuals of Northern European descent. HT1 is caused by deficiency of fumarylacetoacetate hydrolase (FAH), the last enzyme in the pathway of tyrosine catabolism (see Fig. 6.5). Fumarylacetoacetate (FAA), the substrate for FAH in the tyrosine pathway, accumulates in FAH-deficient hepatocytes and proximal renal tubular cells, resulting in liver and kidney damage. The oxidative and DNA damage caused by FAA leads to either cell death or a profound perturbation of gene expression, especially in the liver [73]. As a result, many metabolic processes, including gluconeogenesis, detoxification of ammonia, and synthesis of secreted proteins, are impaired. Tyrosine itself is not toxic to the liver or kidney but causes dermatologic, ophthalmologic, and possibly neurodevelopmental problems. The principal metabolites of FAA, succinylacetoacetate (SAA) and succinylacetone (SA), are released into the circulation and can be measured for diagnosis. The mode of inheritance for hereditary tyrosinemia type 1 (HT1) is autosomal recessive.

Clinical Features

Hereditary tyrosinemia type 1 (HT1) is characterized by severe, progressive liver disease and renal tubular dysfunction. The latter typically is manifest as the Fanconi syndrome with renal tubular acidosis, aminoaciduria, and hypophosphatemia (due to phosphate wasting). Features of rickets often are present. Most patients present in early infancy with failure to thrive and hepatomegaly. Some develop conjugated hyperbilirubinemia. An often marked elevation in serum alpha-fetoprotein (AFP) is common in HT1. Liver disease may begin prenatally, leading to finding of nodularity or cirrhosis in affected neonates. Progression of the liver disease can be chronic or acute, with rapid deterioration and early death. Liver dysfunction commonly results in hypoglycemia and coagulation abnormalities. Serum aminotransferase levels typically are only mildly elevated and often disproportionately low compared with the marked degree of coagulopathy. Complications of liver failure, including jaundice, ascites, and hemorrhage, often develop.

The chronic form consists of a mixed micronodular and macronodular cirrhosis. The risk of hepatocellular cancer formation is high in this group and is thought to be caused by the mutagenicity of FAA.

In older patients, severe neurologic manifestations resembling neuropathic porphyrias are common in poorly controlled HT1 and contribute to morbidity and mortality. Cardiomyopathy may be a feature which is reversible with nitisinone therapy [74].

Investigations

The most important diagnostic test for HT1 is the measurement of SA either in urine or in blood. Many newborn screening programs perform sensitive SA measurements on dried blood spots and confirmatory testing. Elevation of SA is pathognomonic for the disorder. Molecular testing for disease-causing mutations is available through multiple

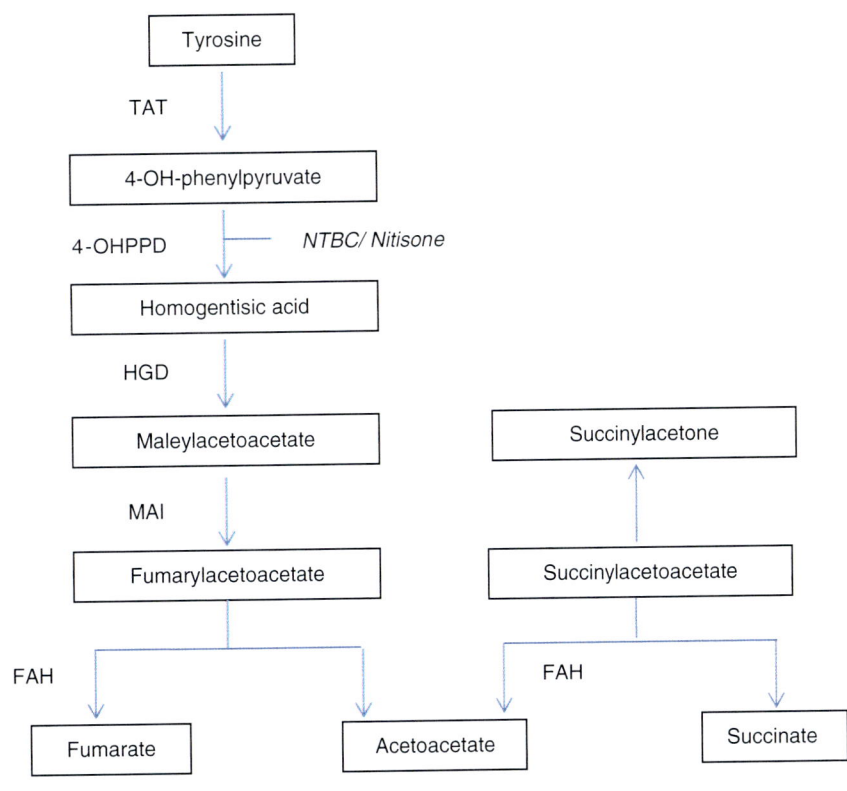

Fig. 6.5 Tyrosine degradation. In tyrosinemia type 1, FAH is deficient. Deficiencies of the other enzymes in the pathway are involved in other types of tyrosinemia (e.g., TAT in tyrosinemia type 2 or HGD in alkaptonuria). *TAT* tyrosine aminotransferase; *4-OHPPD* 4-hydroxy phenylpyruvate dioxygenase; *HGD* homogentisic acid dioxygenase; *MAI* maleylacetoacetate isomerase; *FAH* fumarylacetoacetate hydrolase

laboratories, but treatment should not be delayed until molecular confirmation is available. Affected patients usually also have elevated plasma concentrations of AFP, tyrosine, and methionine and excrete tyrosyl compounds in the urine.

Management

Dietary treatment, consisting of foods with low or absent phenylalanine and tyrosine and restriction of natural protein, results in decreased tyrosine plasma levels. However, this approach does not stop the production of SA or prevent the progression of liver or renal disease. The medical treatment of choice is nitisinone, formerly known as NTBC, which inhibits 4-OH phenylpyruvate dioxygenase (HPD), an early step in the tyrosine degradation pathway. This treatment reduces metabolic flow through the pathway and limits formation of the toxic compounds FAA and SA (Fig. 6.5). Nitisinone should be started as early as possible (i.e., immediately after diagnosis of HT1 by blood or urine measurement of SA).

Nitisinone is effective with the approximately 90 percent of treated patients improving clinically [75]. Treatment started at an early age reduces the risk of early development of hepatocellular carcinoma, although longer follow-up is needed to determine if the effect persists throughout life. Therapy with nitisinone also decreases the need for orthotopic liver transplantation (OLT), particularly when started in early infancy.

The long-term risk of developing neurologic problems on nitisinone therapy is unknown. There is a concern of neurologic complications as cognitive impairment may occur in up to a third of patients [75]. It is not known whether this phenotype is related to elevated tyrosine, phenylalanine deficiency, or caused by other factors. Nitisinone is typically started with 1 mg/kg per day, divided into a morning and evening dose and given orally. Because nitisinone increases plasma tyrosine levels, patients should have a protein-restricted diet that is low in phenylalanine and tyrosine. The dietary protein intake is adapted to keep the plasma tyrosine level <500 μmol/L. The dose of nitisinone should be adjusted to completely suppress excretion of SA. The maximal dose of 2 mg/kg/day may be needed, especially in infants. A general target for blood level of nitisinone is 50–60 μmol/L. Monitoring of the blood levels is recommended for dose adjustment and also for monitoring compliance. Metabolic monitoring includes the measurement of plasma amino acids, blood or urinary SA, liver function tests, complete blood count (CBC) with differential, nitisinone levels, and serum AFP (which increases further with hepatocellular carcinoma). Ophthalmologic examination and hepatic imaging (magnetic resonance imaging is preferred) should be performed annually. Liver transplantation is performed in patients with persistent liver failure who do not respond to nitisinone therapy or have hepatic malignancy.

6.3.6 Diseases of the Bile Ducts

6.3.6.1 Biliary Atresia

About one quarter of infants with progressive liver dysfunction are diagnosed with biliary atresia (BA). BA is characterized by an inflammatory, fibrosing cholangiopathy leading to bile duct obliteration. It is actually a common phenotype of several etiologically different conditions (see Chap. 7 for details). BA may be associated with cardiac, vascular, and intra-abdominal malformations as well as with chromosomal aberrations; thus, these cases may be termed syndromic (BASM). Cystic BA involves extrahepatic cyst development. The precise etiology of BA remains unknown. Immune dysregulation is one of the main hypotheses for etiology [76]. Other contributing factors may include infections, maternal microchimerism, a genetic predisposition, and environmental factors. When direct and conjugated bilirubin were measured in newborn babies, the ratios of both values were found to be elevated in newborns ultimately diagnosed with biliary atresia. This suggests that some cases of BA involve a process established prior to birth and are not a consequence of a postnatal event [77].

Diagnosis

The survival rate with native liver is higher in children undergoing palliative surgery (Kasai portoenterostomy) within 46 days of birth [5]. Therefore, early diagnosis is important because the likelihood of successful Kasai portoenterostomy decreases as the disease progresses [76]. Biliary atresia occurs in eutrophic, mature newborns, but premature infants may also be affected. More frequently associated malformations in syndromic cases include splenic malformations, situs inversus, preduodenal or hypoplastic portal vein, intestinal malrotation, or cardiac anomalies. Symptoms include jaundice, frequently in the first 4 weeks of life, in combination with discolored or barely colored stools and, less often noticed, dark urine. Importantly, cerebral bleeding complications may be among the first symptoms to occur requiring immediate parenteral vitamin K administration [78]. Hepatomegaly with a firm consistency, failure to thrive despite adequate nutrition and coagulopathy may also be noted. Later, splenomegaly and ascites also occur. Blood tests will reveal conjugated hyperbilirubinemia, likely increased γ-GT, and aminotransferase activity, as well as signs of coagulopathy. For an algorithm on diagnostic procedures, see also Fig. 6.1. Ultrasound plays an important role in imaging, where abnormalities in the morphology of the biliary tract (infrequently dilations, cysts) and the gallbladder (dysplasia, scarring) (Fig. 6.6) as well as possible associations with vascular or splenic malformations can be detected. However, 20% of patients have normal sonographic

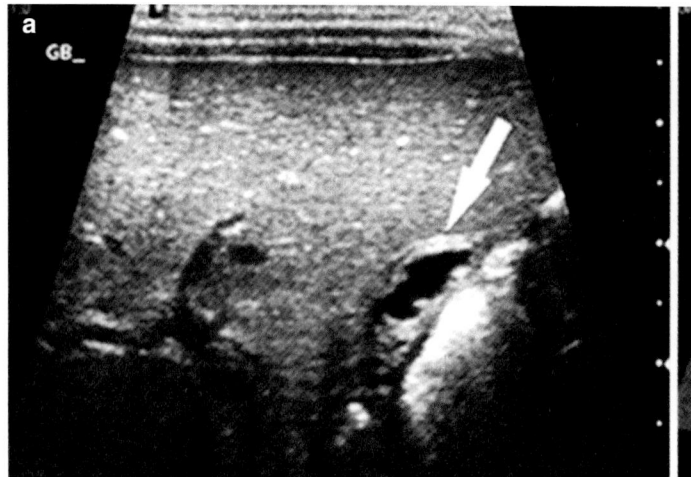
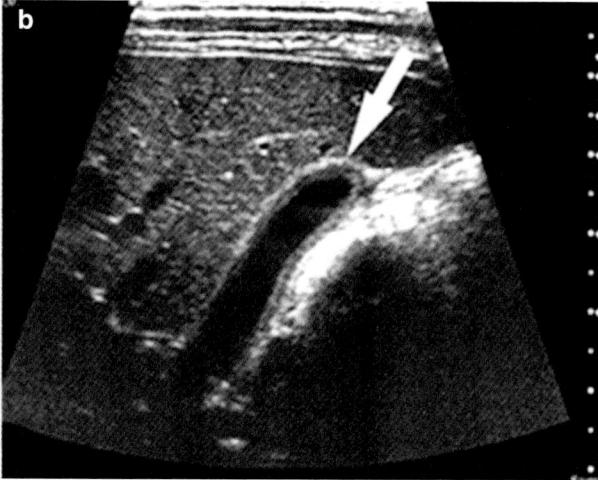

Fig. 6.6 Liver sonography in a patient with biliary atresia. (**a**) Scarred, dysplastic gallbladder, the liver parenchyma shows altered echogenicity. (**b**) Sonogram of a normal gallbladder in the infant in comparison (Courtesy of Prof. P. Haber, University Children's Hospital Tübingen) (Reprinted with permission [133])

findings. Further imaging allows a more detailed study of the affected structure, i.e., the biliary tree. Depending on technical equipment and expertise, this can be carried out through endoscopic retrograde cholangiopancreatography (ERCP) [79], magnetic resonance cholangiopancreatography (MRCP) [76, 80], or percutaneous transhepatic cholangiography (PTC) [81]. The findings of the radioisotope excretion scan (HIDA) are non-specific as other cholestatic diseases of hepatocellular origin may also prevent tracer secretion [24]. ERCP in particular may be useful in unclear cases to demonstrate patency of the bile ducts and exclude biliary atresia. The liver biopsy provides information on biliary obstruction with ductular proliferation and bile plugs, fibrosis, and edema yielding high diagnostic specificity. However, the earlier the biopsy is performed, the more unspecific the histological changes may be. It may be useful to repeat the liver biopsy at a later time point [30]. The gold standard for confirming the diagnosis and definitive test is still the intraoperative cholangiography. After confirming atresia of the biliary tree intraoperatively, the Kasai hepatoportoenterostomy is performed (Fig. 6.7).

Upon suspected biliary atresia, the infant should receive fat-soluble vitamins and high-calorie MCT-based feeding. Ursodeoxycholic acid at a dose of 20 mg/kg/day may be started to stimulate bile flow; however, it confers a risk of increasing biliary pressure and subsequent liver damage in patients with complete blockade of bile drainage [82]. Prior to the operative procedures, luminal antibiotics may be used to decrease the bacterial intestinal load. The benefit of steroids in the postoperative treatment after Kasai procedure is still debated; a meta-analysis has shown improved clearance of jaundice in particular in infants less affected by early liver scarring [83, 84]. To prevent cholangitis many centers use prophylactic antibiotic therapy, e.g., amoxicillin and trimethoprim.

Complications include cholangitis, fat-soluble vitamin deficiency, and failure to thrive, which should be treated aggressively. Despite restoration of bile flow and clearance of jaundice, the inflammatory process continues and frequently leads to portal hypertension with splenomegaly and/or hypersplenism. In the course of the disease, the majority of children will need to be evaluated for complications of increased portal pressure such as varices.

A large multicenter North American study following patients after a successful Kasai procedure showed that 75% had normal synthetic liver function; however, only 2% had no liver disease with no signs of portal hypertension. The majority of patients reported a beneficial health-related quality of life assessment [85]. In patients with unsuccessful Kasai procedure, recurrent cholangitis, malnutrition, increasing risk for variceal bleeding, and ascites not responding to medical treatment, the indication for liver transplantation needs to be evaluated.

6.3.6.2 Alagille Syndrome

Alagille syndrome (AGS) is a multisystem genetic disorder characterized by bile duct paucity in combination with extrahepatic abnormalities and a characteristic facial appearance. AGS is a dominant genetic disorder, but its expressivity varies greatly, with members of the same family having different features. The finding of patients with deletions on the short arm of chromosome 20 led to the localization and, subsequently, positional cloning of the disease gene, Jagged1 (JAG1). The estimated incidence of AGS in Western Europe is about 1:123,000 [86] but may be underestimated due to the high variability of expression. The high variability suggests the presence of modifying factors which are currently unknown in humans.

Genetics of AGS

AGS is caused by mutations of *JAG1* [87, 88]. JAG1 is a cell surface protein that functions as a ligand for the Notch transmembrane receptors. These receptor-ligand pairs are part of the evolutionarily conserved Notch signaling pathway. This pathway is important in the development of the organ systems affected, i.e., the liver, heart, skeleton, eye, face, and kidney. The molecular outcome of the initiation of Notch signaling is the transcription of Notch-sensitive genes, which then act to regulate cellular differentiation, specifically in cardiac and bile duct development [89–91]. JAG1 mutations have been detected in approximately 70% of AGS patients. In AGS patients without JAG1 mutations, Notch2 mutations have been identified [92]. Expression of AGS is variable with a wide range of clinical effects. Signs and symptoms may be subclinical or severe with complex heart disease being the only reliable indicator for mortality.

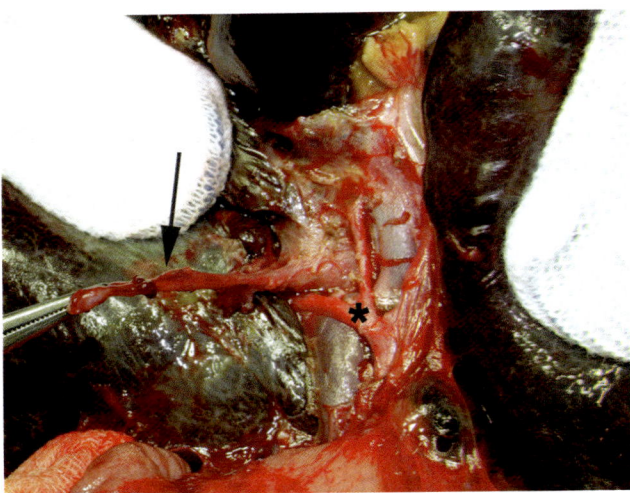

Fig. 6.7 Preparation of the scarred choledochal duct (arrow) in a patient with biliary atresia during a Kasai procedure (* scarred portal area) (Courtesy of Prof. J. Fuchs, University Children's Hospital Tübingen) (Reprinted with permission [133])

In patients suffering from AGS-associated liver disease, it is impossible to predict progression to terminal liver failure although in young children laboratory markers may indicate a worse outcome in later life [93].

Histopathology of the Liver in AGS

In his original description, Alagille based the diagnosis of bile duct hypoplasia on a bile duct-to-portal tract ratio of less than 0.5 [94]. However, the presence of bile duct paucity varies with patient age at biopsy [95, 96]. The number of bile ducts may at first be normal in infants ultimately shown to have AGS. Longitudinal studies and cross-sectional analysis documenting the biopsy changes at different ages have demonstrated that in infants less than 6 months of age, adequate numbers of bile ducts may be present in AGS, resting the diagnosis completely on clinical manifestations [95, 97–99]. Early histologic changes in these cases may be non-specific, consisting of cholestasis with giant cell formation and variable signs of bile duct injury. Bile duct proliferation has been reported infrequently in patients with documented AGS [96, 98, 100]. This finding makes the differentiation from biliary atresia difficult. Due to the challenge posed by making the diagnosis of AGS in infants, patients have undergone a Kasai procedure, adversely affecting outcome and with early need for liver transplantation [101, 102]. Paucity of bile ducts is seen more frequently in later infancy or childhood [95, 96, 98, 100]. Late histologic changes include portal expansion and fibrosis with bridging occurring in approximately 50% of patients. It is important to note that cirrhosis, however, occurs in only about 20% of AGS patients. Of interest is that biochemical cholestasis may improve with time despite the lack of histological bile duct reappearance.

Clinical Manifestations of AGS

Hepatic Manifestations

Jaundice is present in most symptomatic patients, and conjugated hyperbilirubinemia is found during the neonatal period which sometimes resolves in later childhood. As stated above, it is particularly important but also difficult to distinguish AGS from biliary atresia. Cholestasis is a very prominent feature of AGS. Pruritus is among the most severe of all chronic liver disease in childhood, markedly reducing the quality of life of children with AGS [103]. Pruritus is usually the most debilitating symptom, leading to cutaneous mutilation, loss of sleep, poor attention and impaired school performance, and occasionally suicide. Due to persistent cholestasis and hypercholesterolemia, disfiguring xanthomata may form. Hepatomegaly is recognized in nearly all patients at early age, whereas splenomegaly is rare in infancy but develops later in life [104].

The most common laboratory abnormalities include extreme elevations of bile acids, conjugated bilirubin, alkaline phosphatase, gamma-glutamyl transpeptidase, and, in the majority of patients, profoundly higher serum cholesterol than commonly found in cholestatic conditions. Abnormalities in hepatic metabolism or synthesis are less pronounced. Usually hepatic synthetic function stays stable over long periods in spite of persistent significant elevations of aminotransferases. Approximately 20% of patients progress to cirrhosis and hepatic failure. Cholestasis leads to ineffective absorption of dietary lipids, essential fatty acids, and fat-soluble vitamins. Hypercholesterolemia is almost always present in AGS. Hepatic synthetic and detoxification function is frequently well preserved. Serum albumin and ammonia are typically normal, as is the prothrombin time (with adequate vitamin K supplementation). Total bilirubin >6.5 mg/dL, conjugated bilirubin >4.5 mg/dL, and cholesterol >520 mg/dL in children younger than 5 years of age are likely to be associated with severe liver disease in later life. These data represent cutoff values below which a child is likely to have a benign outcome and above which more aggressive therapy may be warranted and can thus be used to guide management [93].

Malnutrition and Growth Failure

Growth failure, malnutrition, and delayed pubertal development are common in children with AGS [105]. The etiology of growth failure is unknown, but insufficient caloric intake, steatorrhea from liver disease, and the primary defect of JAG may play a role. In patients undergoing liver transplantation, poorer catch-up growth is observed than patients with other cholestatic liver diseases. On this basis, a genetic etiology for poor growth in AGS has been discussed [106]. However, as significant cardiovascular or renal disease may be present, growth failure is most likely multifactorial. Endocrine dysregulation, caloric deprivation from fat malabsorption, poor nutrient and vitamin intake, and intrinsic skeletal abnormalities are likely to be contributors.

Cardiovascular Malformations

A wide range of cardiovascular abnormalities has been reported in patients with syndromic paucity of bile ducts [107]. An audible murmur is present at some time in 97% of patients. The most common lesions are pulmonary artery stenoses at various sites in the proximal and distal tree, commonly at bifurcations (Fig. 6.8). The entire pulmonary vascular tree may be hypoplastic, either alone or in association with other cardiovascular lesions. Among these, tetralogy of Fallot (TOF) is the most common. Intracranial vessel abnormalities are found in AGS among other vascular anomalies including involvement of the aorta and renal, celiac, superior mesenteric, and subclavian arteries. Studies showed that predominantly cardiac and not hepatic disease predicted increased mortality in AGS patients [95]. Thorough evaluation of AGS individuals with symptoms of concern or before operative procedures such as liver transplantation and close monitoring of cardiovascular function during operative procedures and intensive care are indicated.

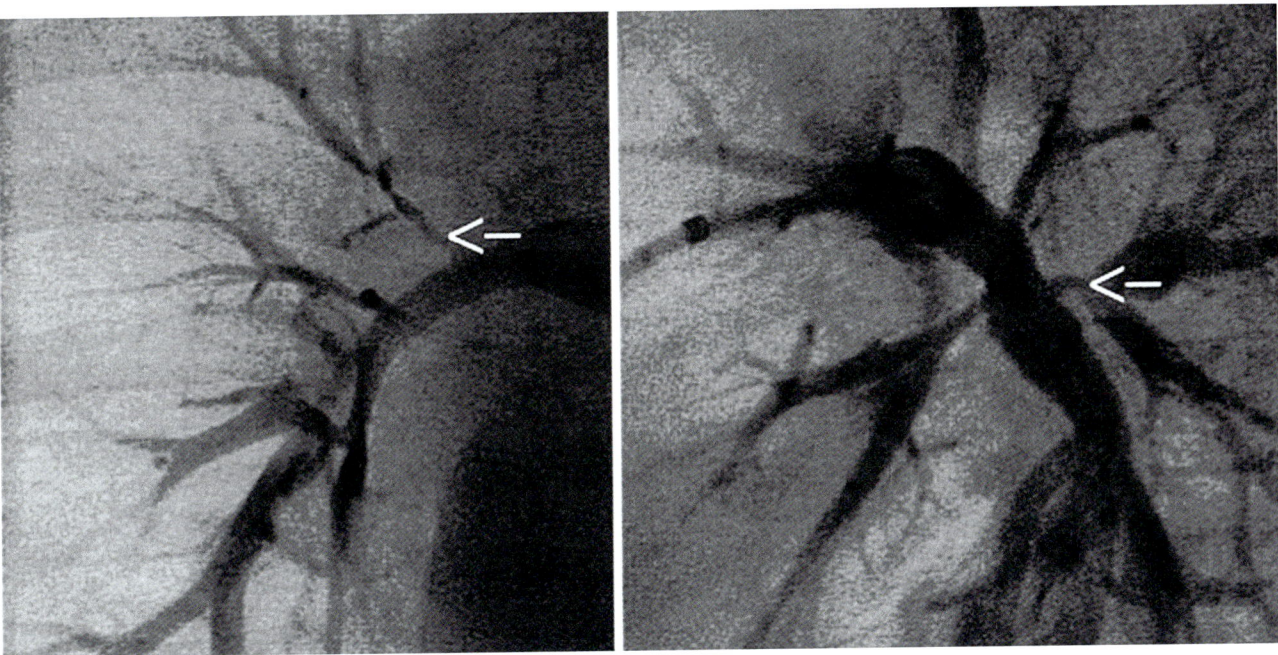

Fig. 6.8 Peripheral bilateral pulmonary stenoses in a toddler with Alagille syndrome (see arrows; courtesy of Dr. M. Talsma, Beatrix Children's Hospital, Groningen, the Netherlands) (Reprinted with permission [134])

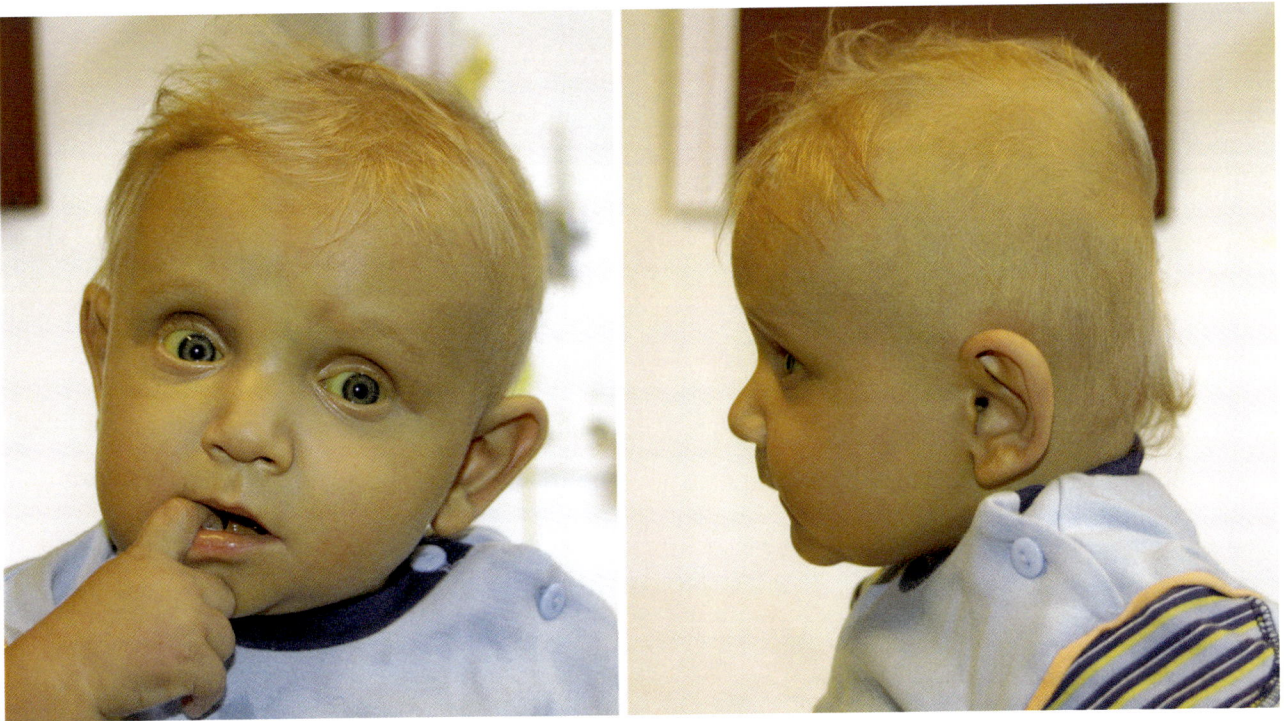

Fig. 6.9 Patient with Alagille syndrome and typical facies: wide forehead, low-lying eyes, hypertelorism (Reprinted with permission [133])

Characteristic Facies

Characteristic facial features were described in the original reports of bile duct paucity. These include a prominent forehead, deep-set eyes with moderate hypertelorism, a pointed chin, and a saddle or straight nose with a bulbous tip. The combination of these features gives the face a triangular appearance (Fig. 6.9). The facies may be present in infancy but becomes more prominent with increasing age.

Vertebral and Musculoskeletal Abnormalities

The most characteristic musculoskeletal finding in AGS patients is the sagittal cleft or butterfly vertebrae. The affected vertebral bodies are split sagittally into two hemivertebrae (Fig. 6.10). This anomaly is asymptomatic, has no structural significance, and can be found in normal individuals. Other abnormalities such as phalangeal or ulnar shortening, decreased bone mineral density, and pathological

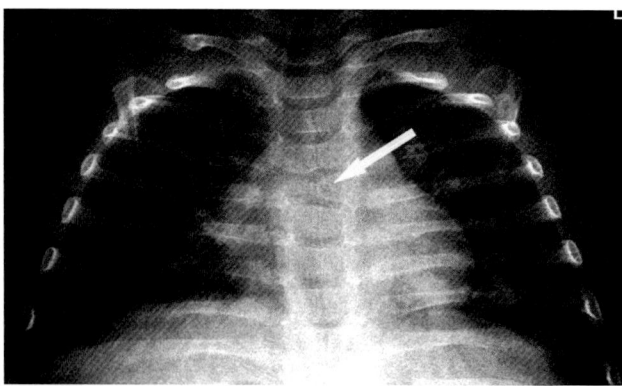

Fig. 6.10 Butterfly vertebra (marked by arrow) in a patient with Alagille syndrome (Reprinted with permission [133])

fractures, particularly of the lower extremities, may occur. Malabsorption of fat, calcium, and vitamin D as well as malnutrition may contribute to this complication.

Further Abnormalities

The cornea, iris, retina, and optic disc may be affected in AGS patients. One study in 23 patients reported posterior embryotoxon (95%), iris abnormalities (45%), diffuse fundus hypopigmentation (57%), speckling of the retinal pigment epithelium (33%), and optic disc anomalies (76%) as well as myelinated retinal nerve fibers [108, 109]. The posterior embryotoxon is diagnostically most important. It is a prominent, centrally positioned Schwalbe line at the point where the corneal epithelium and the uveal trabecular meshwork join (Fig. 6.11). It is not pathognomonic as it occurs in 8–15% of normal persons. Glaucoma, uni- or bilateral optic disc drusen, visual loss, and idiopathic intracranial hypertension [110–112] have been reported in AGS. Mental retardation has been a prominent feature in early reports of AGS. However, earlier recognition, improved nutritional therapy, and vitamin supplementation may have contributed to a significant decrease in frequency of this feature in AGS patients [95]. Clearly, nutritional factors and vitamin deficiency, specifically for vitamin E, play an important role in prevention of neurological deficits in patients with AGS and other cholestatic diseases [113, 114]. Patients with AGS are at significant risk of intracranial bleeding [115] and other bleeding complications. Frequently, it is not associated with significant coagulopathy, and the bleeding tendency may thus be genetically determined. A generalized cerebral vasculopathy may be part of AGS [116, 117]. Thus, cerebral magnetic resonance imaging may have a valuable role in screening for treatable lesions, in particular when evaluating a patient before liver transplantation.

Coagulopathy should be corrected, and observation after head trauma is critical.

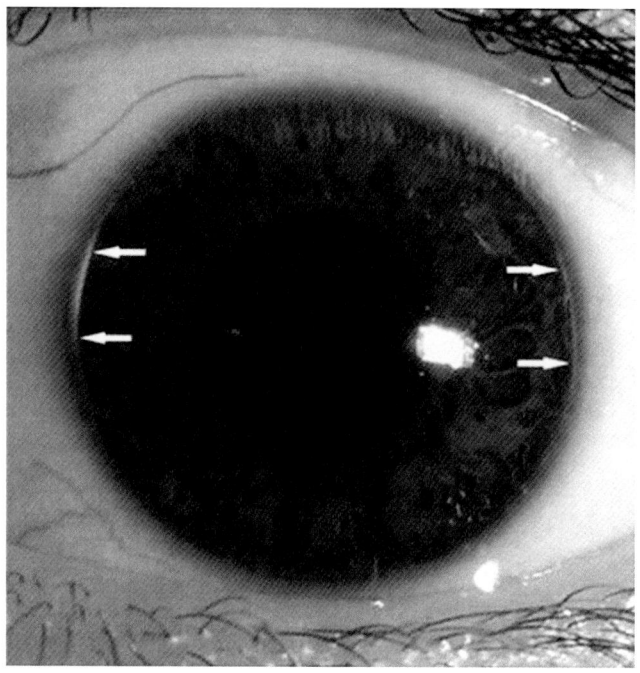

Fig. 6.11 Posterior embryotoxon (arrows), a common finding in patients with Alagille syndrome (Reprinted with permission [109])

Clinical Diagnosis

In principle, the diagnosis of AGS is based on clinicopathological criteria: compatible histopathology, cardiac and vertebral abnormalities, chronic cholestasis, posterior embryotoxon, and the characteristic facies. In patients with isolated cardiac disease or apparently non-syndromic paucity of bile ducts, molecular testing can reveal whether JAG1 or Notch2 abnormalities are present. DNA analysis may also help to identify other oligosymptomatic family members.

In most patients, the hepatic manifestations of the disease dominate the clinical picture. Patients may present with jaundice, pruritus, cholestasis, and signs and symptoms of cardiac disease or may be identified as asymptomatic siblings (or parents). The syndrome must be distinguished from neonatal cholestasis of other etiologies and in particular from biliary atresia as described below. The usual evaluation will include an initial laboratory screen for infectious or metabolic etiologies. An abdominal ultrasound, a liver biopsy, and possibly an operative cholangiogram may contribute to differential diagnosis. An infant with AGS will usually have an elevated conjugated bilirubin and moderately elevated levels of the aminotransferases. The gamma-glutamyl transpeptidase and alkaline phosphatase serum activities as well as levels of serum bile acids and cholesterol may be dramatically elevated, but none of these findings aids in the discrimination of syndromic bile duct paucity from biliary atresia or other causes of extrahepatic obstruction.

Differentiation from biliary atresia can be difficult [95, 118]. Reliable diagnostic tools to demonstrate patency of the extrahepatic biliary tree include endoscopic retrograde and intraoperative cholangiography. Improvements in magnetic resonance cholangiography may make this a more important tool for this purpose in the future. The liver biopsy is the most useful preoperative study for the discrimination of syndromic bile duct paucity from extrahepatic biliary atresia. However, difficulties in histologic diagnosis may arise early in infancy because bile duct proliferation may obscure duct paucity or because some ducts may, in fact, be present early in life. If laparotomy is undertaken, a wedge biopsy of liver should be obtained. An intraoperative cholangiogram performed by an experienced surgeon must be attempted and carefully interpreted prior to the construction of a portoenterostomy. The extrahepatic bile ducts are anatomically normal and patent in AGS but may be so narrow that operative cholangiography will fail to identify a patent system. A careful preoperative search must be performed for the syndromic features of AGS. Hepatoportoenterostomy is inappropriate in AGS and may increase morbidity [118]. The diagnosis is also important for its genetic implications.

Treatment
The aims of therapy for AGS-related liver disease are optimization of nutrition, supplementation of fat-soluble vitamins, amelioration of symptoms, and, when indicated, liver transplantation in patients with terminal liver failure or uncontrollable symptoms and poor quality of life. Most patients with chronic cholestasis suffer from fat malabsorption. Therefore MCT supplementation of nutrition for children should be considered. Supplementation of fat-soluble vitamins is important as most patients with chronic cholestasis are deficient to different degrees. Vitamin K supplementation should be closely monitored to decrease the risk of bleeding in AGS. Vitamin D standard supplementation doses may not be sufficient, and absorption may be enhanced by co-administration of d-alpha-tocopherol polyethylene glycol-1000 succinate (TPGS) [119]. The TPGS preparation of vitamin E is more effective than the standard supplementation and reverses symptoms. Pruritus is the predominant and most troubling symptom in patients with AGS. The pruritus frequently is unrelenting and debilitating and interferes with daytime activities and sleep. Medical therapy for pruritus is often unsuccessful although preliminary results in a small clinical trial with inhibitors of IBAT (ileal bile acid transporter) have been promising [50]. Most cases do not respond to topical therapy, ursodeoxycholic acid (UDCA), or cholestyramine as a bile salt-binding resin. Some patients experience relief with rifampicin, which facilitates bile salt metabolism. Successful treatment by partial external biliary diversion or ileal exclusion has been reported [120]. When evaluated for liver transplantation, many candidates do not suffer from terminal liver failure but from an unacceptable quality of life due to intractable pruritus [121]. Cardiovascular disease may be a limiting factor for suitability for this procedure. Transplant evaluation and monitoring during and after the transplant procedure should be directed at limiting the risk of complications through vascular malformations and increased tendency for bleeding. Caution should be taken when considering relatives as potential donors for living-related transplant because unsuspected disease in the parent has thwarted donation [122].

Prognosis
The prognosis of liver disease is worse in patients presenting with neonatal cholestasis. However, the general outcome of AGS is highly variable and is most directly related to the severity of the hepatic and the cardiovascular lesions. It is important to understand that AGS confers an increased risk for hepatocellular carcinoma. Variable outcome has been reported after liver transplantation, with patient survival ranging from 45 to 100% [123]. Of particular concern is a clustering of posttransplant deaths short term after the procedure focusing on the risk of vascular anomalies in AGS.

6.3.6.3 Congenital Choledochal Malformations

Choledochal malformation or biliary cysts are cystic dilations that may occur singly or in multiples throughout the biliary tree. They were originally termed choledochal cysts due to their involvement of the extrahepatic bile duct. For details on congenital choledochal malformations, see Chap. 7.

6.3.7 Diseases of the Non-Parenchymal Cells

6.3.7.1 Lysosomal Storage Disorders

Many metabolic diseases are associated with liver dysfunction in children. Jaundice is not generally a presenting symptom. However, it is frequently present in infants presenting with lysosomal storage disorders. Two of these disorders will be discussed in the following.

Niemann-Pick Diseases
Niemann-Pick disease (NPD) is divided into certain subtypes. NPD type A is a deficiency of sphingomyelinase deficiency. Clinical features include hepatosplenomegaly, failure to thrive, and progressive neurological deterioration. Some patients will develop ascites; jaundice, however, is rare.

Niemann-Pick Disease Type C
Niemann-Pick disease type C (NP-C) is a rare neurovisceral lysosomal disorder caused by autosomal-recessive mutations in *NPC1* or *NPC2* (95% and ~4% of patients) [124]. Pathological variants in these genes lead to abnormal intracellular trafficking of lipids and therefore accumulation of

cholesterol and glycophospholipids in multiple organs (brain, liver, and spleen). The clinical presentation is highly variable as the neurological signs arise at different ages, from neonatal period to adulthood.

Clinical Features

NP-C should be considered in the differential diagnosis of children with visceral symptoms such as hepatosplenomegaly, isolated splenomegaly, prolonged unexplained neonatal jaundice lasting >2 weeks with conjugated hyperbilirubinemia, and acute neonatal liver failure. Other symptoms preceding the onset of neurological symptoms may include fetal hydrops and ascites. Those surviving liver disease in early infancy may develop chronic liver disease and neurological manifestations including muscular hypotonia, motor developmental delay, cerebellar signs, dystonia, abnormal vertical and horizontal eye movements with eventual supranuclear gaze palsy, and psychiatric symptoms in adults.

Investigations

Apart from a rigorous clinical work-up, biochemical markers are important for diagnosing NP-C. Aminotransferases may be slightly elevated, and LDL-C and HDL-C may be decreased, while triglycerides are elevated. Oxysterols (cholesterol oxidation products) are the most established, accessible, and widely used biomarkers, with the largest evidence base to support their reliability and sensitivity for NP-C [125]. Cholestane-3β,5α,6β-triol (C-triol) and 7-ketocholesterol (7-KC) were shown to be elevated in plasma from patients with NP-C. Chitotriosidase is used as a screening tool for lysosomal diseases and may be positive in NP-C but is unspecific. The filipin stain (see Fig. 6.12) in fibroblasts demonstrates impaired cellular cholesterol transport and, if positive, supports the genetic findings of two pathogenic alleles in NPC1 or NPC2 which will confirm the diagnosis [125]. Liver histology shows severe neonatal hepatitis, fibrosis, and pseudoacinar formation. The PAS-D-resistant foam in Kupffer cells may be visualized. Foam cells may also be demonstrated in the bone marrow.

Management

Miglustat is a competitive inhibitor for the enzyme glucosylceramide synthase which catalyzes the first step in glycosphingolipid synthesis. It has been used for late-onset neurological disease and cognitive or psychiatric disease manifestations. Data is limited on infant neurological manifestations. Aside from seizures, hypotonia, dysphagia, and feeding difficulties (onset: 5–12 months of age) have been observed. Earliest reported miglustat therapy is 7 months of age [126, 127]. Diarrhea which may require dietary and pharmacologic management and growth reductions, both weight and height, has been reported in pediatric patients with NP-C on miglustat. Miglustat therapy does not seem to prevent early-onset neurological deterioration in NP-C [126].

Lysosomal Acid Lipase Deficiency (LAL-D)

Lysosomal acid lipase deficiency (LAL-D) is an autosomal-recessive disease caused by pathogenic variants of the *LIPA* gene leading to absent or decreased activity of LAL enzyme, which results in a progressive lysosomal accumulation of cholesteryl esters (CE) in hepatocytes, adrenal glands, intestines, and macrophage-monocyte cells [128].

Diseases secondary to LAL-D are a continuum, classically divided into the complete LAL deficiency, causing

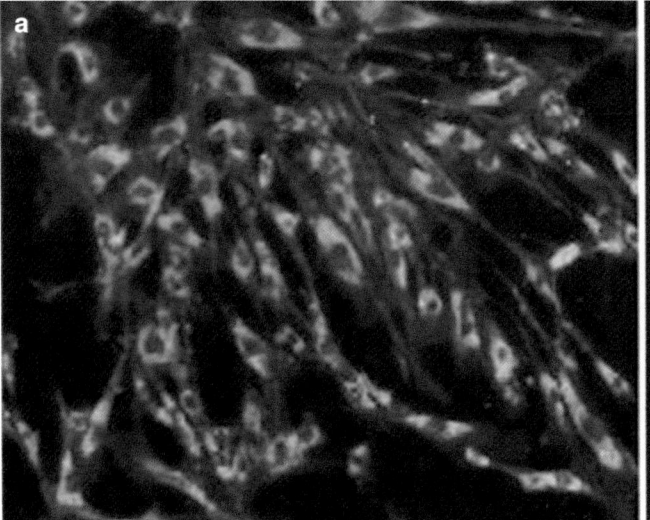

Fig. 6.12 Infantile Niemann-Pick disease type C. (**a**), positive filipin test in cultured fibroblasts: light courts around the dark nuclei correspond to cholesterol-storing lysosomes. (**b**), material of a healthy control person (Courtesy of Prof. Harzer, Prof. Krägeloh-Mann, University Children's Hospital Tübingen, magnification 200×) (Reprinted with permission [135])

infantile-onset LAL-D (formerly known as Wolman disease, WD), and the LAL deficiency with residual enzymatic activity leading to a childhood/adult-onset form (formerly known as cholesteryl ester storage disease, CESD).

Clinical Features
WD has its onset in the first month of life, and it is characterized by a progressive course frequently leading to death before 1 year of age [128, 129]. Hepatosplenomegaly, steatorrhea, abdominal distension, severe malabsorption with resultant malnutrition, and adrenal insufficiency with adrenal calcification are the cardinal features of WD [129].

CESD has a less severe clinical course; isolated hepatomegaly or hepatosplenomegaly, increased plasma transaminases, type 2a or 2b hypercholesterolemia, and hypoalphalipoproteinemia are the more common initial presentations. Hepatic fibrosis with unpredictable progression to micronodular cirrhosis, as well as premature atherosclerosis, can occur [130]. Intermediate clinical presentations are also reported, as well as prenatal forms characterized by nonimmune fetal hydrops [129] and asymptomatic elderly forms.

Investigations
Diagnosis of LAL deficiency is suspected in individuals with characteristic clinical findings such as hepatomegaly, elevated transaminases, and a typical serum lipid profile: high total serum concentrations of cholesterol, low-density lipoprotein, and triglycerides and low serum concentration of high-density lipoprotein. The diagnosis is confirmed by identification of either biallelic pathogenic variants in *LIPA* or deficient LAL enzyme activity in peripheral blood leukocytes, fibroblasts, or dried blood spots [128].

Management
When Wolman disease and CESD become manifest, enzyme replacement therapy with sebelipase alfa administered at a dose of 1 mg/kg body weight every other week can be life-saving for those with severe Wolman syndrome and life-improving with prolonged survival in those who have CESD [131]. Liver transplantation may be indicated when liver disease progresses to cirrhosis and liver failure. In Wolman disease, consultation with a nutrition team to limit malnutrition if possible, including use of parenteral nutrition and corticosteroid and mineralocorticoid replacement in the presence of adrenal insufficiency, may be indicated.

6.3.7.2 HLH
HLH is a clinical syndrome, caused by severe hypercytokinemia due to a highly stimulated but ineffective immune response. HLH is not a disease by its own; it has to be viewed as the consequence of an inherited or acquired inability of the immune system to cope with a trigger [132]. HLH may present as a life-threatening condition with severe liver dysfunction or acute liver failure in infants. Genetic disease may predispose to HLH. Acquired forms are more frequent and occur with infections, particularly with viral disease caused by viruses from the herpes family.

Clinical Features and Investigations
Cardinal symptoms of HLH are prolonged fever, hepatosplenomegaly, and pancytopenia. Characteristic laboratory values include increased ferritin, triglycerides, transaminases, bilirubin, lactate dehydrogenase, soluble interleukin-2 receptor α-chain, and decreased fibrinogen. Hepatosplenomegaly and the frequently observed skin rash occur due to infiltration with lymphocytes and histiocytes. Hemophagocytosis may be found in bone marrow or lymph nodes. Natural killer cell activity may be low or absent. Genetic testing (i.e., identification of an HLH gene mutation) is indicated in all patients that meet the HLH diagnostic criteria and in those with a high likelihood of HLH based on the initial evaluation.

Management
Without treatment HLH is a fatal condition; thus early initiation of therapy is important. Regimens include steroids, ciclosporin, and etoposide. Hematopoietic stem cell transplantation may be lifesaving in subtypes.

References

1. Kelly DA, Stanton A. Jaundice in babies: implications for community screening for biliary atresia. BMJ. 1995;310(6988):1172–3.
2. Erlinger S, Arias IM, Dhumeaux D. Inherited disorders of bilirubin transport and conjugation: new insights into molecular mechanisms and consequences. Gastroenterology. 2014;146(7):1625–38.
3. Greig JA, Nordin JML, Draper C, Bell P, Wilson JM. AAV8 gene therapy rescues the newborn phenotype of a mouse model of Crigler-Najjar. Hum Gene Ther. 2018.
4. Fawaz R, Baumann U, Ekong U, Fischler B, Hadzic N, Mack CL, et al. Guideline for the evaluation of cholestatic jaundice in infants: joint recommendations of the north American Society for Pediatric Gastroenterology, Hepatology, and Nutrition and the European Society for Pediatric Gastroenterology, Hepatology, and Nutrition. J Pediatr Gastroenterol Nutr. 2017;64(1):154–68.
5. Serinet MO, Wildhaber BE, Broue P, Lachaux A, Sarles J, Jacquemin E, et al. Impact of age at Kasai operation on its results in late childhood and adolescence: a rational basis for biliary atresia screening. Pediatrics. 2009;123(5):1280–6.
6. Chen SM, Chang MH, Du JC, Lin CC, Chen AC, Lee HC, et al. Screening for biliary atresia by infant stool color card in Taiwan. Pediatrics. 2006;117(4):1147–54.
7. Wildhaber BE. Screening for biliary atresia: Swiss stool color card. Hepatology. 2011;54(1):367–8. author reply 9.
8. Seeler RA, Hahn K. Jaundice in urinary tract infection in infancy. Am J Dis Child. 1969;118(4):553–8.
9. Shanmugam NP, Bansal S, Greenough A, Verma A, Dhawan A. Neonatal liver failure: aetiologies and management—state of the art. Eur J Pediatr. 2011;170(5):573–81.
10. Nicastro E, D'Antiga L. Next generation sequencing in pediatric hepatology and liver transplantation. Liver Transpl. 2018;24(2):282–93.

11. Dreher AM, Arora N, Fowler KB, Novak Z, Britt WJ, Boppana SB, et al. Spectrum of disease and outcome in children with symptomatic congenital cytomegalovirus infection. J Pediatr. 2014;164(4):855–9.
12. Mitchell ML, Hsu HW, Sahai I. Changing perspectives in screening for congenital hypothyroidism and congenital adrenal hyperplasia. Curr Opin Endocrinol Diabetes Obes. 2014;21(1):39–44.
13. Binder G, Martin DD, Kanther I, Schwarze CP, Ranke MB. The course of neonatal cholestasis in congenital combined pituitary hormone deficiency. J Pediatr Endocrinol Metab. 2007;20(6):695–702.
14. Hollak CE, van Weely S, van Oers MH, Aerts JM. Marked elevation of plasma chitotriosidase activity. A novel hallmark of Gaucher disease. J Clin Invest. 1994;93(3):1288–92.
15. Mittal V, Saxena AK, Sodhi KS, Thapa BR, Rao KL, Das A, et al. Role of abdominal sonography in the preoperative diagnosis of extrahepatic biliary atresia in infants younger than 90 days. Am J Roentgenol. 2011;196(4):W438–45.
16. Farrant P, Meire HB, Mieli-Vergani G. Ultrasound features of the gall bladder in infants presenting with conjugated hyperbilirubinaemia. Br J Radiol. 2000;73(875):1154–8.
17. Negm AA, Petersen C, Markowski A, Luettig B, Ringe KI, Lankisch TO, et al. The role of endoscopic retrograde cholangiopancreatography in the diagnosis of biliary atresia: 14 years' experience. Eur J Pediatr Surg. 2018;28(3):261–7.
18. Shanmugam NP, Harrison PM, Devlin J, Peddu P, Knisely AS, Davenport M, et al. Selective use of endoscopic retrograde cholangiopancreatography in the diagnosis of biliary atresia in infants younger than 100 days. J Pediatr Gastroenterol Nutr. 2009;49(4):435–41.
19. Felux J, Sturm E, Busch A, Zerabruck E, Graepler F, Stuker D, et al. ERCP in infants, children and adolescents is feasible and safe: results from a tertiary care center. United European Gastroenterol J. 2017;5(7):1024–9.
20. Metreweli C, So NM, Chu WC, Lam WW. Magnetic resonance cholangiography in children. Br J Radiol. 2004;77(924):1059–64.
21. Liu B, Cai J, Xu Y, Peng X, Zheng H, Huang K, et al. Three-dimensional magnetic resonance cholangiopancreatography for the diagnosis of biliary atresia in infants and neonates. PLoS One. 2014;9(2):e88268.
22. Perisic V. Role of percutaneous transhepatic cholangiography and endoscopic cholangiopancreatography in the diagnostic imaging of hepatobiliary system in infants and children. J Pediatr Gastroenterol Nutr. 1985;4(5):846–7.
23. Kianifar HR, Tehranian S, Shojaei P, Adinehpoor Z, Sadeghi R, Kakhki VR, et al. Accuracy of hepatobiliary scintigraphy for differentiation of neonatal hepatitis from biliary atresia: systematic review and meta-analysis of the literature. Pediatr Radiol. 2013;43(8):905–19.
24. Gilmour SM, Hershkop M, Reifen R, Gilday D, Roberts EA. Outcome of hepatobiliary scanning in neonatal hepatitis syndrome. J Nucl Med. 1997;38(8):1279–82.
25. Russo P, Magee JC, Boitnott J, Bove KE, Raghunathan T, Finegold M, et al. Design and validation of the biliary atresia research consortium histologic assessment system for cholestasis in infancy. Clin Gastroenterol Hepatol. 2011;9(4):357–62e2.
26. Dezsofi A, Baumann U, Dhawan A, Durmaz O, Fischler B, Hadzic N, et al. Liver biopsy in children: position paper of the ESPGHAN Hepatology Committee. J Pediatr Gastroenterol Nutr. 2015;60(3):408–20.
27. Cohen MB, Kader HH, Lambers D, Heubi JE. Complications of percutaneous liver biopsy in children. Gastroenterology. 1992;102(2):629–32.
28. Furuya KN, Burrows PE, Phillips MJ, Roberts EA. Transjugular liver biopsy in children. Hepatology. 1992;15(6):1036–42.
29. Habdank K, Restrepo R, Ng V, Connolly BL, Temple MJ, Amaral J, et al. Combined sonographic and fluoroscopic guidance during transjugular hepatic biopsies performed in children: a retrospective study of 74 biopsies. Am J Roentgenol. 2003;180(5):1393–8.
30. Azar G, Beneck D, Lane B, Markowitz J, Daum F, Kahn E. Atypical morphologic presentation of biliary atresia and value of serial liver biopsies. J Pediatr Gastroenterol Nutr. 2002;34(2):212–5.
31. Morotti RA, Jain D. Pediatric cholestatic disorders: approach to pathologic diagnosis. Surg Pathol Clin. 2013;6(2):205–25.
32. El-Guindi MA, Sira MM, Hussein MH, Ehsan NA, Elsheikh NM. Hepatic immunohistochemistry of bile transporters in progressive familial intrahepatic cholestasis. Ann Hepatol. 2016;15(2):222–9.
33. Biesecker LG, Green RC. Diagnostic clinical genome and exome sequencing. N Engl J Med. 2014;371(12):1170.
34. Togawa T, Sugiura T, Ito K, Endo T, Aoyama K, Ohashi K, et al. Molecular genetic dissection and neonatal/infantile intrahepatic cholestasis using targeted next-generation sequencing. J Pediatr. 2016;171:171–7e1-4.
35. Bernstein J, Brown AK. Sepsis and jaundice in early infancy. Pediatrics. 1962;29:873–82.
36. Khalil S, Shah D, Faridi MM, Kumar A, Mishra K. Prevalence and outcome of hepatobiliary dysfunction in neonatal septicaemia. J Pediatr Gastroenterol Nutr. 2012;54(2):218–22.
37. Goelz R, Meisner C, Bevot A, Hamprecht K, Kraegeloh-Mann I, Poets CF. Long-term cognitive and neurological outcome of preterm infants with postnatally acquired CMV infection through breast milk. Arch Dis Child Fetal Neonatal Ed. 2013;98(5):F430–3.
38. Hamprecht K, Goelz R. Postnatal cytomegalovirus infection through human milk in preterm infants: transmission, clinical presentation, and prevention. Clin Perinatol. 2017;44(1):121–30.
39. Neuberger P, Hamprecht K, Vochem M, Maschmann J, Speer CP, Jahn G, et al. Case-control study of symptoms and neonatal outcome of human milk-transmitted cytomegalovirus infection in premature infants. J Pediatr. 2006;148(3):326–31.
40. Goel A, Chaudhari S, Sutar J, Bhonde G, Bhatnagar S, Patel V, et al. Detection of cytomegalovirus in liver tissue by PCR in infants with neonatal cholestasis. Pediatr Infect Dis J. 2018.
41. Josephson CD, Caliendo AM, Easley KA, Knezevic A, Shenvi N, Hinkes MT, et al. Blood transfusion and breast milk transmission of cytomegalovirus in very low-birth-weight infants: a prospective cohort study. JAMA Pediatr. 2014;168(11):1054–62.
42. Sundaram SS, Alonso EM, Narkewicz MR, Zhang S, Squires RH, Pediatric Acute Liver Failure Study Group. Characterization and outcomes of young infants with acute liver failure. J Pediatr. 2011;159(5):813–e1.
43. Berk DR, Sylvester KG. Congenital tuberculosis presenting as progressive liver dysfunction. Pediatr Infect Dis J. 2004;23(1):78–80.
44. Pediatrics AAO. Tuberculosis. In: Kimberlin DW, Brady MT, Jackson MA, Long SS, editors. Red Book: 2015 Report of the Committee on infectious diseases. Elk Groove Village. IL: American Academy of Pediatrics; 2015.
45. Gissen P, Tee L, Johnson CA, Genin E, Caliebe A, Chitayat D, et al. Clinical and molecular genetic features of ARC syndrome. Hum Genet. 2006;120(3):396–409.
46. Iannelli F, Collino A, Sinha S, Radaelli E, Nicoli P, D'Antiga L, et al. Massive gene amplification drives paediatric hepatocellular carcinoma caused by bile salt export pump deficiency. Nat Commun. 2014;5:3850. https://doi.org/10.1038/ncomms4850.3850.
47. Pawlikowska L, Strautnieks S, Jankowska I, Czubkowski P, Emerick K, Antoniou A, et al. Differences in presentation and progression between severe FIC1 and BSEP deficiencies. J Hepatol. 2010;53(1):170–8.
48. Lemoine C, Bhardwaj T, Bass LM, Superina RA. Outcomes following partial external biliary diversion in patients with

progressive familial intrahepatic cholestasis. J Pediatr Surg. 2017;52(2):268–72.
49. Ramachandran P, Shanmugam NP, Sinani SA, Shanmugam V, Srinivas S, Sathiyasekaran M, et al. Outcome of partial internal biliary diversion for intractable pruritus in children with cholestatic liver disease. Pediatr Surg Int. 2014;30(10):1045–9.
50. Sturm E, Baumann U, Lacaille F, Gonzales E, Arnell H, Fischler B, et al. The ileal bile acid transport inhibitor A4250 reduced pruritus and serum bile acid levels in children with cholestatic liver disease and pruritus: final results from a multiple-dose, open-label, multinational study. Hepatology. 2017;66:646A–7A.
51. Sundaram SS, Bove KE, Lovell MA, Sokol RJ. Mechanisms of disease: inborn errors of bile acid synthesis. Nat Clin Pract Gastroenterol Hepatol. 2008;5(8):456–68.
52. Heubi JE, Setchell KD, Jha P, Buckley D, Zhang W, Rosenthal P, et al. Treatment of bile acid amidation defects with glycocholic acid. Hepatology. 2015;61(1):268–74.
53. Hidvegi T, Ewing M, Hale P, Dippold C, Beckett C, Kemp C, et al. An autophagy-enhancing drug promotes degradation of mutant alpha1-antitrypsin Z and reduces hepatic fibrosis. Science. 2010;329(5988):229–32.
54. Bjursell M, Porritt MJ, Ericson E, Taheri-Ghahfarokhi A, Clausen M, Magnusson L, et al. Therapeutic genome editing with CRISPR/Cas9 in a humanized mouse model ameliorates alpha1-antitrypsin deficiency phenotype. EBioMedicine. 2018.
55. Debray D, Narkewicz MR, Bodewes F, Colombo C, Housset C, de Jonge HR, et al. Cystic fibrosis-related liver disease: research challenges and future perspectives. J Pediatr Gastroenterol Nutr. 2017;65(4):443–8.
56. Leeuwen L, Magoffin AK, Fitzgerald DA, Cipolli M, Gaskin KJ. Cholestasis and meconium ileus in infants with cystic fibrosis and their clinical outcomes. Arch Dis Child. 2014;99(5):443–7.
57. Debray D, Kelly D, Houwen R, Strandvik B, Colombo C. Best practice guidance for the diagnosis and management of cystic fibrosis-associated liver disease. J Cyst Fibros. 2011;10(Suppl 2):S29–36.
58. Yeh JN, Jeng YM, Chen HL, Ni YH, Hwu WL, Chang MH. Hepatic steatosis and neonatal intrahepatic cholestasis caused by citrin deficiency (NICCD) in Taiwanese infants. J Pediatr. 2006;148(5):642–6.
59. Laukkarinen J, Sand J, Saaristo R, Salmi J, Turjanmaa V, Vehkalahti P, et al. Is bile flow reduced in patients with hypothyroidism? Surgery. 2003;133(3):288–93.
60. Pan X, Kelly S, Melin-Aldana H, Malladi P, Whitington PF. Novel mechanism of fetal hepatocyte injury in congenital alloimmune hepatitis involves the terminal complement cascade. Hepatology. 2010;51(6):2061–8.
61. Whitington PF. Neonatal hemochromatosis: a congenital alloimmune hepatitis. Semin Liver Dis. 2007;27(3):243–50.
62. Ekong UD, Melin-Aldana H, Whitington PF. Regression of severe fibrotic liver disease in 2 children with neonatal hemochromatosis. J Pediatr Gastroenterol Nutr. 2008;46(3):329–33.
63. Debray FG, de Halleux V, Guidi O, Detrembleur N, Gaillez S, Rausin L, et al. Neonatal liver cirrhosis without iron overload caused by gestational alloimmune liver disease. Pediatrics. 2012;129(4):e1076–9.
64. Rand EB, Karpen SJ, Kelly S, Mack CL, Malatack JJ, Sokol RJ, et al. Treatment of neonatal hemochromatosis with exchange transfusion and intravenous immunoglobulin. J Pediatr. 2009;155(4):566–71.
65. Whitington PF. Gestational alloimmune liver disease and neonatal hemochromatosis. Semin Liver Dis. 2012;32(4):325–32.
66. Whitington PF, Kelly S, Taylor SA, Nobrega S, Schreiber RA, Sokal EM, et al. Antenatal treatment with intravenous immunoglobulin to prevent gestational Alloimmune liver disease: comparative effectiveness of 14-week versus 18-week initiation. Fetal Diagn Ther. 2017.
67. Lee WS, Sokol RJ. Mitochondrial hepatopathies: advances in genetics, therapeutic approaches, and outcomes. J Pediatr. 2013;163(4):942–8.
68. Rahman S. Gastrointestinal and hepatic manifestations of mitochondrial disorders. J Inherit Metab Dis. 2013;36(4):659–73.
69. Gibson K, Halliday JL, Kirby DM, Yaplito-Lee J, Thorburn DR, Boneh A. Mitochondrial oxidative phosphorylation disorders presenting in neonates: clinical manifestations and enzymatic and molecular diagnoses. Pediatrics. 2008;122(5):1003–8.
70. Pfeffer G, Majamaa K, Turnbull DM, Thorburn D, Chinnery PF. Treatment for mitochondrial disorders. Cochrane Database Syst Rev. 2012;4:CD004426.
71. Nobre S, Grazina M, Silva F, Pinto C, Goncalves I, Diogo L. Neonatal liver failure due to deoxyguanosine kinase deficiency. BMJ Case Rep. 2012;2012.
72. Dimmock DP, Dunn JK, Feigenbaum A, Rupar A, Horvath R, Freisinger P, et al. Abnormal neurological features predict poor survival and should preclude liver transplantation in patients with deoxyguanosine kinase deficiency. Liver Transpl. 2008;14(10):1480–5.
73. Grompe M, al-Dhalimy M, Finegold M, Ou CN, Burlingame T, Kennaway NG, et al. Loss of fumarylacetoacetate hydrolase is responsible for the neonatal hepatic dysfunction phenotype of lethal albino mice. Genes Dev. 1993;7(12A):2298–307.
74. Arora N, Stumper O, Wright J, Kelly DA, McKiernan PJ. Cardiomyopathy in tyrosinaemia type I is common but usually benign. J Inherit Metab Dis. 2006;29(1):54–7.
75. Masurel-Paulet A, Poggi-Bach J, Rolland MO, Bernard O, Guffon N, Dobbelaere D, et al. NTBC treatment in tyrosinaemia type I: long-term outcome in French patients. J Inherit Metab Dis. 2008;31(1):81–7.
76. Hartley JL, Davenport M, Kelly DA. Biliary atresia. Lancet. 2009;374(9702):1704–13.
77. Harpavat S, Finegold MJ, Karpen SJ. Patients with biliary atresia have elevated direct/conjugated bilirubin levels shortly after birth. Pediatrics. 2011;128(6):e1428–33.
78. van Hasselt PM, de Koning TJ, Kvist N, de Vries E, Lundin CR, Berger R, et al. Prevention of vitamin K deficiency bleeding in breastfed infants: lessons from the Dutch and Danish biliary atresia registries. Pediatrics. 2008;121(4):e857–e63.
79. Petersen C, Meier PN, Schneider A, Turowski C, Pfister ED, Manns MP, et al. Endoscopic retrograde cholangiopancreaticography prior to explorative laparotomy avoids unnecessary surgery in patients suspected for biliary atresia. J Hepatol. 2009;51(6):1055–60.
80. Takaya J, Nakano S, Imai Y, Fujii Y, Kaneko K. Usefulness of magnetic resonance cholangiopancreatography in biliary structures in infants: a four-case report. Eur J Pediatr. 2007;166(3):211–4.
81. Jensen MK, Biank VF, Moe DC, Simpson PM, Li SH, Telega GW. HIDA, percutaneous transhepatic cholecysto-cholangiography and liver biopsy in infants with persistent jaundice: can a combination of PTCC and liver biopsy reduce unnecessary laparotomy? Pediatr Radiol. 2012;42(1):32–9.
82. Fickert P, Pollheimer MJ, Silbert D, Moustafa T, Halilbasic E, Krones E, et al. Differential effects of norUDCA and UDCA in obstructive cholestasis in mice. J Hepatol. 2013;58(6):1201–8.
83. Chen Y, Nah SA, Chiang L, Krishnaswamy G, Low Y. Postoperative steroid therapy for biliary atresia: systematic review and meta-analysis. J Pediatr Surg. 2015;50(9):1590–4.
84. Davenport M. Adjuvant therapy in biliary atresia: hopelessly optimistic or potential for change? Pediatr Surg Int. 2017;33(12):1263–73.
85. Ng VL, Haber BH, Magee JC, Miethke A, Murray KF, Michail S, et al. Medical status of 219 children with biliary atresia surviving long-term with their native livers: results from a north American multicenter consortium. J Pediatr. 2014;165(3):539–46e2.

86. Danks DM, Campbell PE, Jack I, Rogers J, Smith AL. Studies of the aetiology of neonatal hepatitis and biliary atresia. Arch Dis Child. 1977;52(5):360–7.
87. Li L, Krantz ID, Deng Y, Genin A, Banta AB, Collins CC, et al. Alagille syndrome is caused by mutations in human Jagged1, which encodes a ligand for Notch1. Nat Genet. 1997;16(3):243–51.
88. Oda T, Elkahloun AG, Pike BL, Okajima K, Krantz ID, Genin A, et al. Mutations in the human Jagged1 gene are responsible for Alagille syndrome. Nat Genet. 1997;16(3):235–42.
89. Niessen K, Karsan A. Notch signaling in cardiac development. Circ Res. 2008;102(10):1169–81.
90. Sparks EE, Perrien DS, Huppert KA, Peterson TE, Huppert SS. Defects in hepatic Notch signaling result in disruption of the communicating intrahepatic bile duct network in mice. Dis Model Mech. 2011;4(3):359–67.
91. Tchorz JS, Kinter J, Muller M, Tornillo L, Heim MH, Bettler B. Notch2 signaling promotes biliary epithelial cell fate specification and tubulogenesis during bile duct development in mice. Hepatology. 2009;50(3):871–9.
92. Kamath BM, Bauer RC, Loomes KM, Chao G, Gerfen J, Hutchinson A, et al. NOTCH2 mutations in Alagille syndrome. J Med Genet. 2012;49(2):138–44.
93. Kamath BM, Munoz PS, Bab N, Baker A, Chen Z, Spinner NB, et al. A longitudinal study to identify laboratory predictors of liver disease outcome in Alagille syndrome. J Pediatr Gastroenterol Nutr. 2010;50(5):526–30.
94. Alagille D, Estrada A, Hadchouel M, Gautier M, Odievre M, Dommergues JP. Syndromic paucity of interlobular bile ducts (Alagille syndrome or arteriohepatic dysplasia): review of 80 cases. J Pediatr. 1987;110(2):195–200.
95. Emerick KM, Rand EB, Goldmuntz E, Krantz ID, Spinner NB, Piccoli DA. Features of Alagille syndrome in 92 patients: frequency and relation to prognosis. Hepatology. 1999;29(3):822–9.
96. Hashida Y, Yunis EJ. Syndromatic paucity of interlobular bile ducts: hepatic histopathology of the early and endstage liver. Pediatr Pathol. 1988;8(1):1–15.
97. Hashida Y, Gaffney PC, Yunis EJ. Acute hemorrhagic cystitis of childhood and papovavirus-like particles. J Pediatr. 1976;89(1):85–7.
98. Dahms BB, Petrelli M, Wyllie R, Henoch MS, Halpin TC, Morrison S, et al. Arteriohepatic dysplasia in infancy and childhood: a longitudinal study of six patients. Hepatology. 1982;2(3):350–8.
99. Kahn E. Paucity of interlobular bile ducts. Arteriohepatic dysplasia and nonsyndromic duct paucity. Perspect Pediatr Pathol. 1991;14:168–215.
100. Kahn E, Daum F, Markowitz J, Teichberg S, Duffy L, Harper R, et al. Nonsyndromatic paucity of interlobular bile ducts: light and electron microscopic evaluation of sequential liver biopsies in early childhood. Hepatology. 1986;6(5):890–901.
101. Quiros-Tejeira RE, Ament ME, Heyman MB, Martin MG, Rosenthal P, Hall TR, et al. Variable morbidity in Alagille syndrome: a review of 43 cases. J Pediatr Gastroenterol Nutr. 1999;29(4):431–7.
102. Kaye AJ, Rand EB, Munoz PS, Spinner NB, Flake AW, Kamath BM. Effect of Kasai procedure on hepatic outcome in Alagille syndrome. J Pediatr Gastroenterol Nutr. 2010;51(3):319–21.
103. Lykavieris P, Hadchouel M, Chardot C, Bernard O. Outcome of liver disease in children with Alagille syndrome: a study of 163 patients. Gut. 2001;49(3):431–5.
104. Deprettere A, Portmann B, Mowat AP. Syndromic paucity of the intrahepatic bile ducts: diagnostic difficulty; severe morbidity throughout early childhood. J Pediatr Gastroenterol Nutr. 1987;6(6):865–71.
105. Wasserman D, Zemel BS, Mulberg AE, John HA, Emerick KM, Barden EM, et al. Growth, nutritional status, body composition, and energy expenditure in prepubertal children with Alagille syndrome. J Pediatr. 1999;134(2):172–7.
106. Quiros-Tejeira RE, Ament ME, Heyman MB, Martin MG, Rosenthal P, Gornbein JA, et al. Does liver transplantation affect growth pattern in Alagille syndrome? Liver Transpl. 2000;6(5):582–7.
107. McElhinney DB, Krantz ID, Bason L, Piccoli DA, Emerick KM, Spinner NB, et al. Analysis of cardiovascular phenotype and genotype-phenotype correlation in individuals with a JAG1 mutation and/or Alagille syndrome. Circulation. 2002;106(20):2567–74.
108. Hingorani M, Nischal KK, Davies A, Bentley C, Vivian A, Baker AJ, et al. Ocular abnormalities in Alagille syndrome. Ophthalmology. 1999;106(2):330–7.
109. Voykov B, Guenova E, Sturm E, Deuter C. Alagille syndrome associated with myelinated retinal nerve fibers. Ophthalmologica. 2009;223(5):348–50.
110. Potamitis T, Fielder AR. Angle closure glaucoma in Alagille syndrome. A case report. Ophthalmic Paediatr Genet. 1993;14(2):101–4.
111. Nischal KK, Hingorani M, Bentley CR, Vivian AJ, Bird AC, Baker AJ, et al. Ocular ultrasound in Alagille syndrome: a new sign. Ophthalmology. 1997;104(1):79–85.
112. Narula P, Gifford J, Steggall MA, Lloyd C, Van Mourik ID, McKiernan PJ, et al. Visual loss and idiopathic intracranial hypertension in children with Alagille syndrome. J Pediatr Gastroenterol Nutr. 2006;43(3):348–52.
113. Sokol RJ, Guggenheim MA, Heubi JE, Iannaccone ST, Butler-Simon N, Jackson V, et al. Frequency and clinical progression of the vitamin E deficiency neurologic disorder in children with prolonged neonatal cholestasis. Am J Dis Child. 1985;139(12):1211–5.
114. Sokol RJ, Guggenheim MA, Iannaccone ST, Barkhaus PE, Miller C, Silverman A, et al. Improved neurologic function after long-term correction of vitamin E deficiency in children with chronic cholestasis. N Engl J Med. 1985;313(25):1580–6.
115. Kamath BM, Spinner NB, Emerick KM, Chudley AE, Booth C, Piccoli DA, et al. Vascular anomalies in Alagille syndrome: a significant cause of morbidity and mortality. Circulation. 2004;109(11):1354–8.
116. Lykavieris P, Crosnier C, Trichet C, Meunier-Rotival M, Hadchouel M. Bleeding tendency in children with Alagille syndrome. Pediatrics. 2003;111(1):167–70.
117. Emerick KM, Krantz ID, Kamath BM, Darling C, Burrowes DM, Spinner NB, et al. Intracranial vascular abnormalities in patients with Alagille syndrome. J Pediatr Gastroenterol Nutr. 2005;41(1):99–107.
118. Markowitz J, Daum F, Kahn EI, Schneider KM, So HB, Altman RP, et al. Arteriohepatic dysplasia. I. Pitfalls in diagnosis and management. Hepatology. 1983;3(1):74–6.
119. Argao EA, Heubi JE, Hollis BW, Tsang RC. D-alpha-tocopheryl polyethylene glycol-1000 succinate enhances the absorption of vitamin D in chronic cholestatic liver disease of infancy and childhood. Pediatr Res. 1992;31(2):146–50.
120. Yang H, Porte RJ, Verkade HJ, De Langen ZJ, Hulscher JB. Partial external biliary diversion in children with progressive familial intrahepatic cholestasis and Alagille disease. J Pediatr Gastroenterol Nutr. 2009;49(2):216–21.
121. Englert C, Grabhorn E, Burdelski M, Ganschow R. Liver transplantation in children with Alagille syndrome: indications and outcome. Pediatr Transplant. 2006;10(2):154–8.
122. Gurkan A, Emre S, Fishbein TM, Brady L, Millis M, Birnbaum A, et al. Unsuspected bile duct paucity in donors for living-related liver transplantation: two case reports. Transplantation. 1999;67(3):416–8.

123. Kamath BM, Schwarz KB, Hadzic N. Alagille syndrome and liver transplantation. J Pediatr Gastroenterol Nutr. 2010;50(1):11–5.
124. Vanier MT. Niemann-Pick disease type C. Orphanet J Rare Dis. 2010;5:16.
125. Vanier MT, Gissen P, Bauer P, Coll MJ, Burlina A, Hendriksz CJ, et al. Diagnostic tests for Niemann-Pick disease type C (NP-C): a critical review. Mol Genet Metab. 2016;118(4):244–54.
126. Di Rocco M, Barone R, Madeo A, Fiumara A. Miglustat does not prevent neurological involvement in Niemann Pick C disease. Pediatr Neurol. 2015;53(4):e15.
127. Di Rocco M, Dardis A, Madeo A, Barone R, Fiumara A. Early miglustat therapy in infantile Niemann-Pick disease type C. Pediatr Neurol. 2012;47(1):40–3.
128. Hoffman EP, Barr ML, Giovanni MA, Murray MF. Lysosomal acid lipase deficiency. In: Adam MP, Ardinger HH, Pagon RA, Wallace SE, LJH B, Stephens K, et al., editors. . Seattle, WA: GeneReviews (R); 1993.
129. Jones SA, Valayannopoulos V, Schneider E, Eckert S, Banikazemi M, Bialer M, et al. Rapid progression and mortality of lysosomal acid lipase deficiency presenting in infants. Genet Med. 2016;18(5):452–8.
130. Aldenhoven M, Wynn RF, Orchard PJ, O'Meara A, Veys P, Fischer A, et al. Long-term outcome of Hurler syndrome patients after hematopoietic cell transplantation: an international multicenter study. Blood. 2015;125(13):2164–72.
131. Erwin AL. The role of sebelipase alfa in the treatment of lysosomal acid lipase deficiency. Ther Adv Gastroenterol. 2017;10(7):553–62.
132. Janka GE, Lehmberg K. Hemophagocytic syndromes—an update. Blood Rev. 2014;28(4):135–42.
133. Sturm E. Lebererkrankungen des Säuglings. Monatsschr Kinderheilk. 2010;158:1086–94.
134. Sturm E, Verkade HJ. Disorders of the Intraheptic Bile Ducts. In: Kleinman RE, Sanderson IR, Goulet O, Sherman PM, Mieli-Vergani G, Shneider B, editors. Pediatric gastrointestinal disease. 6th Shelton: People's Medical Publishing House; 2016.
135. Sturm E, Hortnagel K. Genetic diagnostics of liver diseases in childhood. Monatsschr Kinderh. 2016;164(6):448–54.

Biliary Atresia and Other Congenital Disorders of the Extrahepatic Biliary Tree

Pietro Betalli and Mark Davenport

Key Points
- Biliary atresia, congenital choledochal malformations and spontaneous bile duct perforations are the usual surgical causes of obstructive jaundice in infancy.
- Novel mechanisms (immune dysregulation, genetic aspects, viral infections) have been considered in the pathophysiology of biliary atresia.
- The diagnosis of biliary atresia is made with imaging, laboratory tests and (usually) liver biopsy. Infants should be evaluated as soon as possible because the success rate of Kasai operation diminishes with an older age at surgery.
- The treatment of biliary atresia and congenital choledochal malformations always involves surgical correction.
- Biliary atresia is a rare disease, but it is responsible for the highest proportion of liver transplantations performed in children and young persons.

Research Required in the Field
- National databases with rigorous follow-up on cases of biliary atresia to assess national outcomes with this disease and facilitate collaborative multi-centre studies and frame future research initiatives.
- Utilization of next-generation screening of genome of syndromic forms of biliary atresia.
- Evaluation of effectiveness and safety of corticosteroids after Kasai operation.
- Exploration of new therapeutic strategies (e.g. antiviral therapy, anti-fibrotic therapy, stem cell therapy).

7.1 Part I: Biliary atresia

7.1.1 Introduction

The most frequent cause of surgical jaundice in infants is biliary atresia (BA) and dates from the time of birth in the vast majority of cases with presentation in the first few weeks of life. It is the end result of a destructive sometimes inflammatory process with unclear origins affecting intra- and extrahepatic bile ducts.

The earliest reference to what was probably an infant with BA was reported in 1817 by Dr. John Burns as an "incurable state of the biliary apparatus" [1]. Towards the end of the nineteenth century, John Thompson in 1892 made the first accurate description of the clinical features and post-mortem findings in an infant who appeared to have no common hepatic duct [2].

Treatment is entirely surgical being an attempt to restore bile flow from the native liver in the first instance and is known as a Kasai portoenterostomy (KPE), reserving liver transplantation for those where this approach is unsuccessful. The first surgical successes were probably described by the Boston surgeon William E. Ladd in 1935 in a series of patients with congenital biliary obstruction [3]. Typically he anastomosed dilated proximal parts of the obstructed biliary tree with the intestines so restoring some kind of continuity [3]. It, however, became clear that in most infants recognized to have BA, there was no proximal dilated remnant to find irrespective of how high one dissected into the porta hepatis. These were described as having "uncorrectable" BA. This dire situation really did not change until the work of Morio Kasai became more widely appreciated outside of Japan [4, 5]. In the late 1950s, Morio Kasai first began simply to transect high in the porta hepatis and join this up to a mobilized Roux loop even if there were no visible ducts present. In a proportion this enabled restoration of bile flow and clearance of jaundice.

7.1.2 Epidemiology

There is a marked variation in geographical incidence of BA ranging from about 1 in 5–10,000 live births in Japan, China and Taiwan [6] to about 1 in 15–20,000 in Europe [7], England and Wales [8] and North America [9]. There is a female preponderance in those considered to have a "developmental" origin but is near to equality in the majority with isolated BA [10, 11]. The incidence of biliary atresia splenic malformation syndrome (BASM) is rarely reported in Asian series but accounts for about 10% of European and North American series [12–14].

7.1.3 Aetiology and Pathogenesis

BA should be thought of as a number of diseases with a similar appearance by the time of presentation (Fig. 7.1). There appears to be a number of different aetiological mechanisms and phenotypes, and at least four different variants of BA can be distinguished based on clinical or laboratory features [15, 16].

1. Associated with other congenital anomalies and typically **BASM.**
2. **Cystic BA,** i.e. extrahepatic cyst development within an otherwise obliterated biliary tree.
3. Viral-associated BA—Particularly **CMV-associated (IgM-positive) BA.**
4. **Isolated BA,** i.e. no features of the above.

It is highly likely that BA with other congenital anomalies and cystic BA have in utero origins and can be regarded as "developmental" variants. BASM is associated with extrahepatic abnormalities such as polysplenia or asplenia; cardiovascular anomalies; situs inversus, malrotation or non-rotation; pre-duodenal portal vein; and absence of the inferior vena cava with azygous continuation. About 1/3 have situs inversus and have been quoted as examples of "laterality defects", strongly suggesting their origin within the early embryonic phase of development.

Given this it also seems probable that there is a genetic or epigenetic aetiology [10, 11, 17]. Genetic mouse models exist with defects of laterality and failure to form normal bile ducts, though as yet the putative gene defects themselves (*CFC-1, INV* et al.) have yet to be identified in humans. Our own series identified maternal diabetes as a key clinical association possibly acting in an epigenetic manner. Other variants include an association with other major congenital malformations such as oesophageal or jejunal atresia but without any sign of laterality defects (<2% overall) [18].

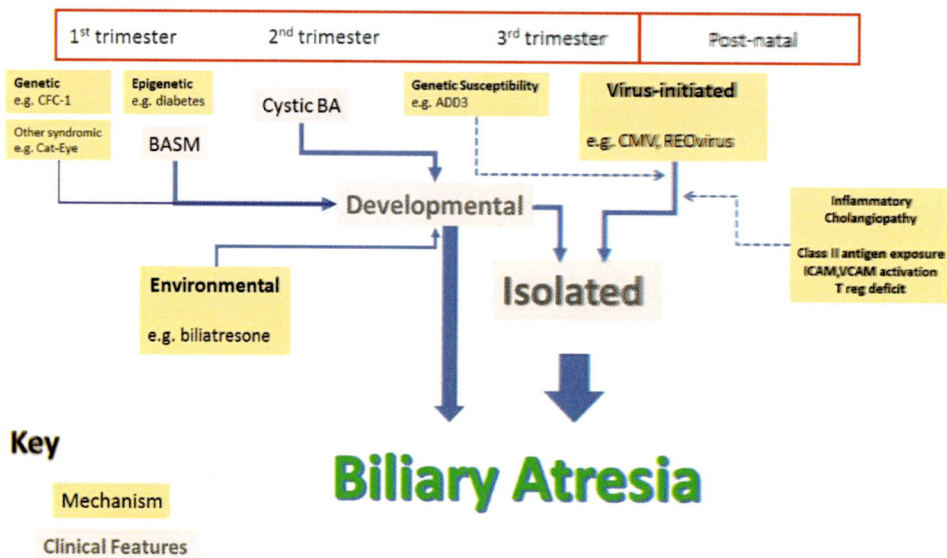

Fig. 7.1 Schematic illustration of possible pathophysiology of biliary atresia

Cystic biliary atresia (Fig. 7.2) is seen in about 5–10% of most large series, whatever the geographic origins. The cyst may contain bile or mucus implying in the former case onset after establishment of continuity between intra- and extrahepatic bile ducts [16]. Redkar et al. [19] showed that many examples of cystic BA can be detected by ultrasound during prenatal scanning and that they have a good prognosis post-surgery.

Most infants with BA will simply appear as isolated anomalies with a negative serological profile for common hepatotropic viruses for which we have no evidence of a specific cause. It is controversial whether infants born with a normal biliary tree can be damaged secondarily after birth, although much experimental research with animal models is based on this assumption. Harpavat et al. from Texas, USA, retrospectively analysed blood obtained from their BA series on day 1 or 2 of life and showed that all had elevated levels of conjugated bilirubin at this point implying that all had biliary obstruction at the time of birth [20].

Still, there have been many theories regarding pathogenesis of isolated BA. The viral-induced, immune or autoimmune-mediated inflammatory obstruction of the biliary tree has been the most commonly accepted theory but is most entirely based on experimental laboratory observations in mice. We have described infants with a different clinical and laboratory phenotype (later presentation, an inflammatory appearance in liver histology and a Th1-dominant T cell infiltrate) in our clinical series associated with CMV-associated (IgM-positive) serology [14–21], but that doesn't automatically mean cause and effect.

BA is as an occlusive pan-ductular cholangiopathy affecting both intra- and extrahepatic bile ducts. The most common pathological classification divides biliary atresia into three types based on the most proximal level of occlusion of the extrahepatic biliary tree (Fig. 7.3).

In Type 1, a biliary lumen exists from the liver to the common bile duct which is atretic, and many are associated with cystic change; in Type 2, the biliary lumen extends to the common hepatic duct which is atretic. In both types there is a degree of preservation of structure in the intrahepatic bile ducts, but they are still irregular although not dilated (a key distinction from congenital choledochal malformation). Type 3 is the most common (>95% of all cases) in which there is no apparent connection and a "solid" proximal bile duct remnant at the level of the porta hepatis. Type 3 intrahepatic bile ducts are inevitably grossly abnormal with myriad small ductules coalescing at the porta hepatis, which can be accessed at KPE. Sometimes this can be visualized radiographically as a "cloud".

Extrahepatic cyst formation may also be evident containing clear mucus or bile and therefore may be described as Type 3 or 1 (CBA), respectively.

Liver histology shows features suggestive of "large duct obstruction" with oedematous expansion of the portal areas, ductular proliferation and the appearance of bile plugs. There is in some a marked inflammatory aspect with infiltration of activated mononuclear cells, such as CD4+ T cells and NK cells. As the disease progresses, monocytes/macrophages also appear prominent with progressive bridging fibrosis between portal areas. The extrahepatic remnant in Type 3 BA is characterized by a multiplicity of microscopic bile ductules embedded within a fibro-inflammatory stroma—most evident at the level of the porta hepatis. Even in these the gallbladder and distal common bile duct may look completely normal, though the former contains clear "mucus".

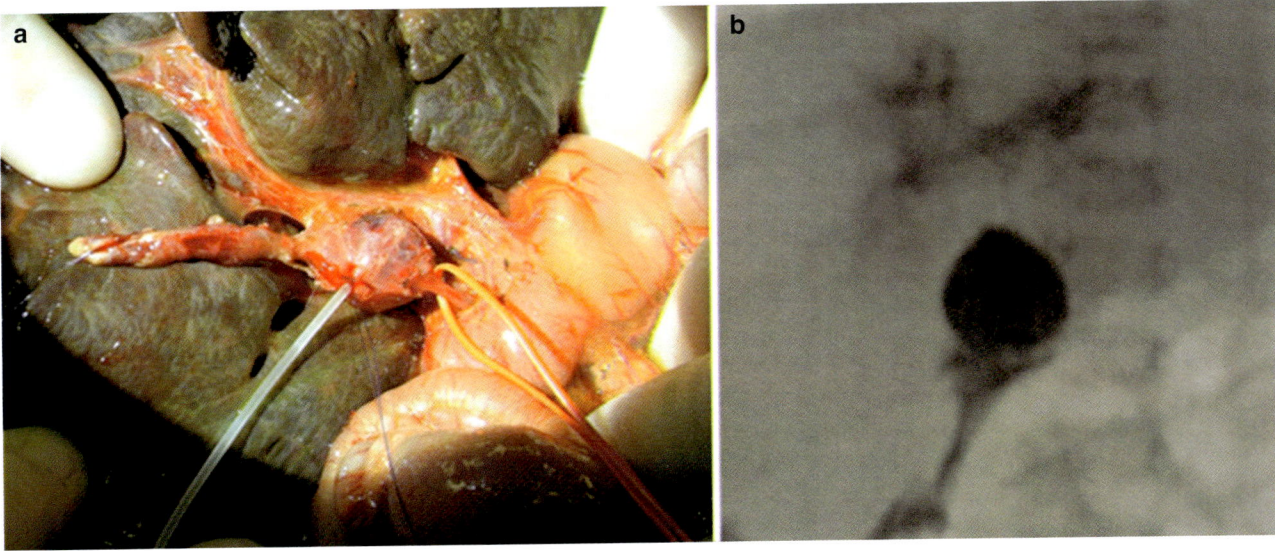

Fig. 7.2 Cystic biliary atresia: 10-mm-diameter bile-containing antenatally detected cyst and cholangiogram showing presence of and communication with primitive, disorganized ("cloud-like") intrahepatic duct system

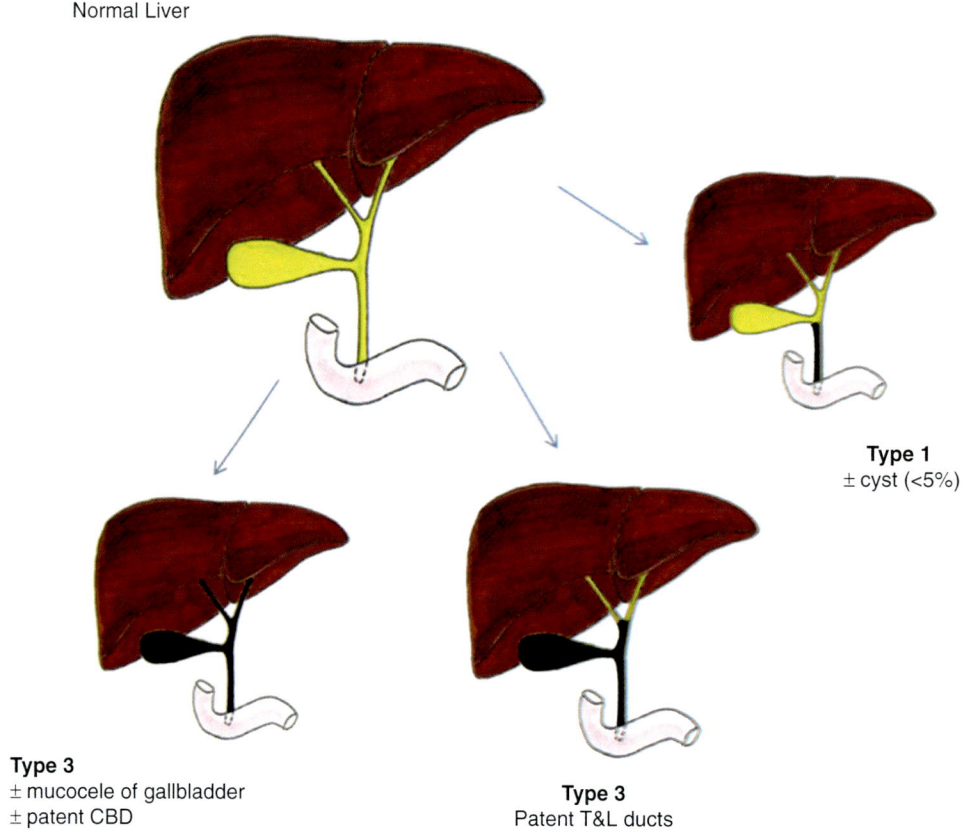

Fig. 7.3 Pathological classification of biliary atresia (NB atretic bile ducts shown in black)

A pro-inflammatory molecular profile was reported in a large-scale gene expression analysis of liver biopsies from infants with BA. This study suggested a genetic footprint in which genes involved in the Th1 helper cell response were activated at an early stage, with simultaneous but transient suppression of markers of humoral immunity [22].

A novel mechanism of immune damage has been suggested by Muraji et al. [23] based on the observation that male BA infants have a threefold increase in maternal origin cells in their livers. These were later shown to be maternal origin chimeric CD8+ T cells and CD45 NK cells and certainly appear capable of initiating immune cholangiolar damage. This has been termed *maternal microchimerism*, and it may explain why the destructive process seems time-limited and most potent shortly after birth.

Recently an intriguing explanation of outbreaks of biliary atresia in animals has been advanced demonstrating a possible environmental cause which may have human implications. Sheep farms around the Burrinjuck Dam, New South Wales, Australia, reported [24] recurrent outbreaks of biliary atresia in lambs where their pregnant mothers had been allowed to graze on the foreshores of the dam which had become exposed to drought conditions. It appeared that a particular weed known as the red crumbweed (*Dysphania glomulifera* subsp. *glomulifera*) in these conditions had proliferated and was the major source of maternal nutrition. In later years whenever the exact combination of exposed foreshore, weed proliferation and grazing pregnant livestock occurred then affected offspring were born.

This concept was further developed in the laboratory using the popular zebrafish model. In this the genome can be manipulated; organ development can be tracked in vivo because the larvae are transparent and furthermore they have a short lifespan and a fully developed biliary system by 5 days postfertilization. Potential hepatotoxic compounds derived from the various isoflavonoids found in the red crumbweed were tested in this zebrafish model. One, now known as **biliatresone**, caused biliary maldevelopment [25] and provided a chemical environmental explanation to the Burrinjuck conundrum.

Is this possible in humans? It appears highly unlikely that it results from maternal exposure to this particular weed although there may be similar compounds or metabolism of non-toxic precursors such as beta-vulgarin found in more common plant foods such as sugar beet, beetroot and chard [26].

In conclusion, the aetiology and pathogenesis of BA remain a land ripe for discovery with several intriguing possibilities for the different clinical phenotypes on show.

7.1.4 Clinical Features and Diagnosis

Conjugated jaundice is the key feature of BA. This together with pale stools and dark urine in an otherwise healthy infant should really set alarm bells ringing (Fig. 7.4).

Such infants despite the absence of gastrointestinal bile usually thrive initially, masking the serious underlying cause of what is after all a common observation in neonatal life, jaundice, and deceiving the child's medical advisers. Recognition that jaundice persisting after 2 weeks in a term infant is not normal should encourage suspicion and further examination of stool and urine. The latter at this age should be colourless and should not stain the nappy [27].

Screening programmes have been developed in countries such as Taiwan and parts of Japan and, nearer to home, in parts of Switzerland and the Netherlands. These rely on stool colour observation by the parents and return of a completed stool colour card distributed to all mothers. They have reported a remarkable improvement in the time it takes to diagnosis BA where there had been delays. Some European countries such as Switzerland or regions such as North Netherlands are also practising screening though the results have not been published.

In all other countries, late presentation of infants with established cirrhosis is still common, beset by diagnostic inertia and confusion particularly with breast-fed jaundice.

The physical signs, apart from jaundice, in the first weeks of life may be minimal and consist only of soft hepatomegaly. Late signs include failure to thrive, ascites and cutaneous signs of chronic liver disease with splenomegaly. In some infants, the actual presenting feature is fat-soluble vitamin K deficiency leading to coagulopathy and bleeding. Sometimes this is innocuous gastrointestinal haemorrhage but in some can be catastrophic and intracranial.

The biochemical characteristics of BA include conjugated (direct) hyperbilirubinaemia, raised hepatocellular enzymes, raised alkaline phosphatase and γ-glutamyl transpeptidase, but there is a significant overlap with many other causes of neonatal conjugated jaundice, and no test is specific.

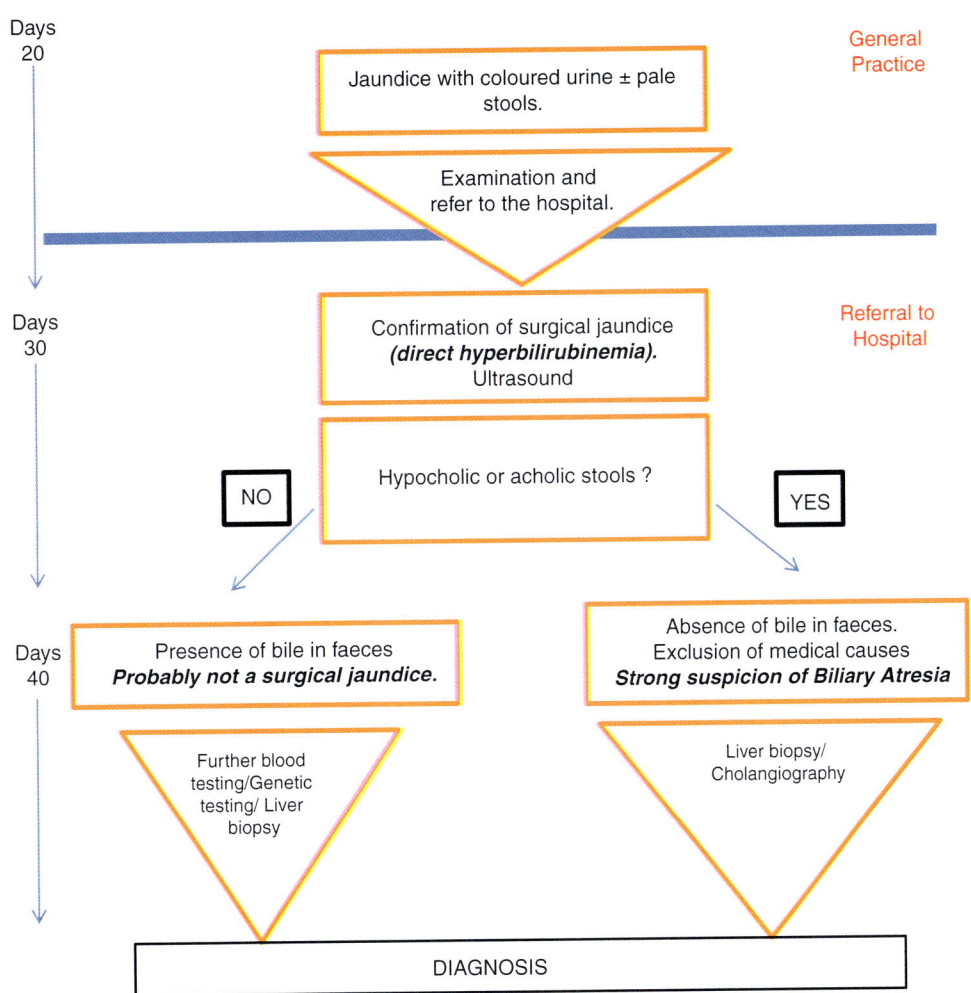

Fig. 7.4 Flow chart for diagnosis of biliary atresia

Ultrasonography (USS) is usually the next step. This typically shows absence of biliary tract dilatation with non-visualization of the gallbladder. One feature that has been suggested as specific is the so-called triangular cord sign illustrating the cone-shaped periportal fibrous mass cranial to the bifurcation of the portal vein [28].

There is no single pathognomonic preoperative finding of BA, but reasonable suspicion necessitates progression to more invasive tests. In our practice percutaneous liver biopsy after exclusion of medical causes of cholestatic jaundice (e.g. α-1-antitrypsin deficiency, Alagille's syndrome and neonatal hepatitis) is then indicated. Negative USS and positive histology results establish the correct preoperative diagnosis in more than 85% of cases of BA [29]. Key histological features might include bile duct proliferation, a small cell infiltrate, portal fibrosis and absence of sinusoidal fibrosis [30].

A 24-h duodenal aspiration and analysis for bile have been used for diagnosis in some Asian centres, but its accuracy has never been published. Other non-invasive tests such as radionuclide scans using a variety of technetium-labelled imino-diacetic acid derivatives are now less commonly used because discrimination between medical and surgical causes can be poor. The use of endoscopic retrograde cholangiopancreatography (ERCP) is possible in infants but is currently confined to highly specialized centres [31]. In our experience, infants with equivocal biopsy results undergo ERCP, although it should be noted that this diagnosis depends crucially on failure to show a biliary tree, and hence appropriate experience and judgement are essential. Furthermore there is currently a dearth of appropriately sized endoscopes available with manufacturers pulling out of production, and this doesn't bode well for being able to continue with this method in the future.

Operative visualization of biliary tree at laparotomy or laparoscopy with on-table cholangiography remains "the last resort" when all non-invasive methods have finished.

7.1.5 Treatment

In most centres and in most infants, the usual management of BA is a surgical attempt to restore bile flow using the Kasai portoenterostomy (KPE) technique [4, 5]. If this fails for one reason or another and if facilities are available, then liver transplantation should be considered. The aim of KPE is to restore, albeit imperfectly, the residual intrahepatic biliary system with the gastrointestinal tract and abbreviate any ongoing tendency to liver fibrosis.

The preoperative management includes correcting the coagulopathy and maybe an antibacterial bowel preparation. Perioperative antibiotics should be effective against aerobic and anaerobic flora.

Initially, the diagnosis is confirmed through a limited right upper quadrant muscle-cutting incision, allowing access to the gallbladder. A cholangiogram may need to be done, but as the first thing one usually sees is an atrophic gallbladder with no lumen, then this may be actually impossible, and the appearance in itself should be regarded as enough of a positive sign to proceed further. This may not be possible in some simply because the gallbladder has no lumen—but this, in itself, is indicative of BA and allows progression. Neonatal sclerosing cholangitis or various hypoplastic biliary appearances (typically seen with Alagille's syndrome) can be seen in some cholangiograms showing patency with proximal intrahepatic ducts. Little more can be done in these circumstances and surgery may be terminated.

Although visible bile-containing ducts may be evident in Type 1 or 2 BA and a hepaticojejunostomy performed, it is probably better that further proximal tissue is resected completely leading to the need of a portoenterostomy. Sometimes on-table evidence of cirrhosis and variceal change may seem to make a portoenterostomy futile. However this is rarely absolutely predictable, and there are insufficient criteria to confidently decide when a late KPE is too late. Late KPE has been variably defined as age >90, 100 or 120 days, and the reported survival with native liver in these patients is 42% at 2 years, 23–45% at 4–5 years, 15–40% at 10 years and <10% at 20 years. The decision to perform KPE after day 100 may be relevant, as KPE in infants with cirrhosis and ascites may precipitate hepatic decompensation, and the procedure is associated with an increased risk for bowel perforations and biliary complications at the time of LT.

Some authors have found that higher stages of fibrosis, a ductal plate configuration and a moderate to marked bile duct injury at KPE were independently associated with a higher risk of transplantation. Nevertheless there is uncertainty on whether liver histology can predict outcome after surgery as the key determinant is restoration of bile flow, something that is only evident after surgery.

A reasonable working rule might be that in infants older than 100 days primary LT may be considered more judicious (obviously where it is available) particularly if there is clinical and USS evidence of nodularity on the liver substance and moderate to severe ascites [32–34].

If the BA diagnosis is confirmed, we believe that the most consistent and efficient dissection of the porta hepatis is facilitated by mobilization of the liver (Fig. 7.5). This need not involve division of all the suspensory ligaments and can be limited to just the falciform and the left triangular, but this still allows the entire organ to be everted onto the anterior abdominal cavity. The fibrotic remnant of the extrahepatic bile ducts is dissected free, dividing first the common bile duct to allow it to be tracked back to the porta hepatis. It is then transected at the level of the liver capsule. This transected portal plate is then anastomosed to a retrocolic 40 cm jejunal Roux loop to restore biliary continuity. A liver biopsy is performed at the conclusion of the operation in order to document hepatic histology. The goals of the operation are to restore the bile flow to the intestine, reduce jaundice and halt ongoing liver damage.

Almost 15 years has now passed since Esteves et al. [35] reported the first laparoscopic KPE. Further reports have been published though none has shown any significant advantage over open KPE and in one German study it worsened the outlook [36]. This laparoscopic approach has still not been taken up by the larger centres in Japan, Europe and North America.

The use of steroids is controversial but appealing given the possible role of inflammation in the aetiology of BA. Davenport et al. [37] in the first randomized placebo-controlled trial of oral prednisolone (2 then 1 mg/kg/day in first month) reported definite improvements in early clearance of jaundice but a lack of real effect on final results and need for transplant. The same authors followed this using an open-label trial structure and a higher dose (starting at 5 mg/kg/day) which showed a statistically significant 15% increase in clearance of jaundice compared to control and placebo in those <70 days at KPE [38]. In 2014, Bezerra et al. [39] studied the effects of a 13-week course of steroids on clearance of jaundice with the native liver at 6 months after Kasai. This was multicentre and had an older population than the UK trials, and though the difference between active and placebo groups was also 12–15% because of their lower numbers in the comparison groups, they declared that there was no statistical difference. Nonetheless subsequent meta-analysis has shown statistically significant evidence of benefit of high-dose steroid regimens (Fig. 7.6) [40].

Ursodeoxycholic acid (UDCA) is widely thought to be beneficial but only if surgery has already restored bile flow to reasonable levels. UDCA "enriches" bile and has a choleretic effect, increasing hepatic clearance of supposedly toxic endogenous bile acids and may confer a cytoprotective effect on hepatocytes.

7.1.6 Complications

Ascending cholangitis is the more frequent complication after Kasai portoenterostomy especially in the first postoperative year and is probably due to the restoration of direct communications between intrahepatic bile ducts and the small bowel. Clinical presentation of cholangitis is with fever, jaundice and abdominal pain. Acholic stool and a deterioration in liver function tests should also be present. Early diagnosis is very important to prevent the loss of remaining

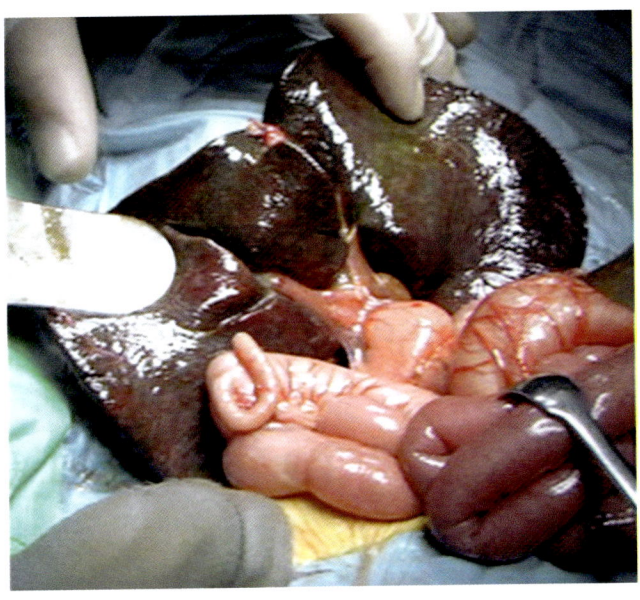

Fig. 7.5 Mobilization of the liver to facilitate porta hepatis dissection in Kasai portoenterostomy

Study or subgroup	Steroid Events	Total	Control Events	Total	Weight	Odds Ratio M–H, Random, 95% CI
Bezerra 2014	41	70	34	70	24.4%	1.50 [0.77, 2.92]
Chung 2008	7	13	8	17	8.5%	1.31 [0.31, 5.58]
Davenport 2007	16	34	18	37	16.5%	0.94 [0.37, 2.38]
Davenport 2013	29	44	36	72	20.7%	1.93 [0.89, 4.20]
Meyers 2003	11	14	3	14	5.8%	13.44 [2.21, 81.77]
Petersen 2008	6	20	11	29	11.3%	0.70 [0.21, 2.36]
Vejchapipat 2007	20	33	10	20	12.7%	1.54 [0.50, 4.72]
Total (95% CI)		228		259	100.0%	1.51 [0.95, 2.41]
Total events	130		120			

Heterogeneity: Tau^2 = 0.12; Chi^2 = 8.60, df = 6 (P = 0.20); I^2 = 30%
Test for overall effect: Z = 1.75 (P = 0.08)

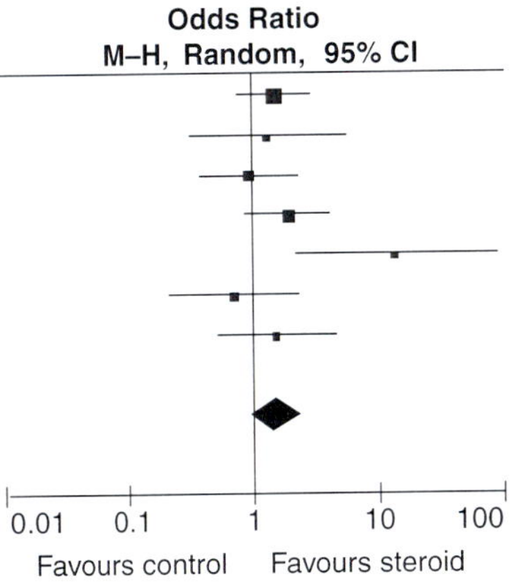

Fig. 7.6 Meta-analysis of steroids in biliary atresia. Forest plot showing improved clearance of jaundice with steroids (reproduced with permission from [24])

patent bile ducts and to preserve the native liver function. Percutaneous liver biopsy may be done to identify the causative organism, but this is uncommon. Cholangitis should be treated aggressively with intravenous antibiotics against Gram-negative organisms.

A prophylactic regimen with oral antibiotics such as amoxicillin, trimethoprim and cephalexin might be considered in all children who have undergone KPE in order to prevent cholangitis. In cases of children with recurrent cholangitis, following clearance of jaundice, liver scintigraphy may detect a Roux loop obstruction. This is important as it is surgically correctable.

Portal hypertension and oesophageal varices are two serious complications after KPE, and they are due to the progressive liver fibrosis causing sustained elevation of portal venous pressure. Progressive hepatosplenomegaly, gastrointestinal bleeding, ascites, encephalopathy and portopulmonary syndrome may all be signs of portal hypertension. Among adult survivors with native liver, the incidence of portal hypertension varies from 50 to 90% [41].

Portal venous pressure is often already high before surgery. Some studies have shown that infants with this early high level of portal venous pressure have worse outcomes in terms of native liver survival and risk for varices and variceal bleeding. Duche et al. also showed that the presence of ascites, serum bilirubin concentration >20 μmol/L, prothrombin ratio <80% and portal vein diameter >5 mm are significant risk factors for bleeding [42]. Although bleeding is unusual before 9 months, each child should probably undergo periodic endoscopic surveillance and endoscopic variceal ligation or injection sclerotherapy if necessary. Sometimes primary prophylaxis as prevention of variceal bleeding may be warranted. Occasionally, emergency treatment of bleeding varices using a Sengstaken tube is necessary. There is a wide variation in estimation of the complications of portal hypertension—from 10 to 60% of patients' transplant-free survival present with at least one episode of gastrointestinal bleeding during 5 years of follow-up [43]. Developing fibrosis and cirrhotic nodules are the natural progression of the liver affected by biliary atresia. Perhaps, one of the most dangerous complications of cirrhosis is the development of hepatocellular carcinoma. Fortunately it seems that only a small percentage of children with BA develop this kind of neoplasm and, in absence of the extrahepatic involvement, liver transplantation is the effective treatment [44].

7.1.7 Prognosis

Several factors may influence the outcome of infants with biliary atresia. Age at surgical intervention remains a critical

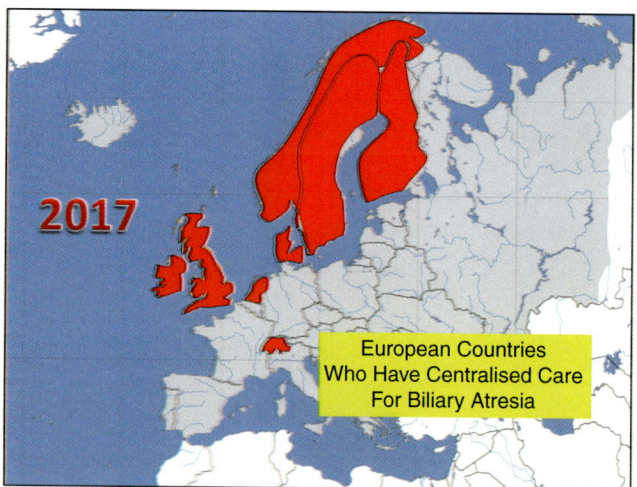

Fig. 7.7 Centralization of biliary atresia centres in Europe

issue, and it is widely accepted that late age at surgery contributes to a worse outcome in the long term. The age at surgery also reflects on the effectiveness of the referring primary care system and efficacy of the diagnostic process. The current accepted standard in Europe and North America is to perform KPE at the earliest possible age and carried out by an experienced biliary surgeon. The experience of the centre performing the operation also appears as a major prognostic factor. Centralization of hepatobiliary services occurred in England and Wales at the end of the 1990s, and results following this showed significant improvement on national outcome for this disease [45–47] and have been followed by a similar policy shift at least in Northern European countries (Fig. 7.7).

7.1.8 Implications for Liver Transplantation

BA is the most common indication for liver transplantation (LT) in the paediatric population accounting for about half. Optimal timing is crucial to achieve a successful outcome and avoid deaths on the waiting list. The main factor affecting indication and timing of LT is the success of KPE. Children not achieving clearance of jaundice in the first few months after surgery are usually transplanted by 2 years of age. If jaundice has resolved by 3 months after KPE, the 10-year transplant-free survival rate has been shown to range from 75 to 90%, whereas if jaundice persists after KPE, the 3-year transplant-free survival rate is only 20% [48]. In a recent North American study of the Childhood Liver Disease Research Network (ChiLDReN), infants with bilirubin >2 mg/dL (≈34 μmol/L) at 3 months from KPE had diminished weight gain and greater probability of developing ascites, hypoalbuminaemia and coagulopathy and were more likely to die or require LT [49]. Thus, children who do not demonstrate good bile flow and clearance of jaundice by 3 months after KPE should be evaluated early for transplantation, ideally by 6–9 months of age [50].

Infectious complications may sometimes threaten the life of a child with BA who had a successful KPE. Repeated episodes of ascending cholangitis were associated with a threefold increased risk for early failure after KPE. This complication should prompt listing to LT in case of recurrent episodes despite aggressive antibiotic therapy, multiresistant bacterial organisms, episodes of life-threatening sepsis or severely impaired quality of life due to frequent hospitalizations [51].

Portal hypertension (PH) accompanies the rapid progression of end-stage liver disease in children with a failed KPE, raising the issue of surveillance endoscopy of these patients while awaiting LT. However in most patients, the risk of bleeding starts after the first year of life [52]. Considering that varix treatment is difficult in infants (due to the lack of a suitable banding device), that variceal bleed is rarely associated with death and that in most centres LT is performed by 12–18 months of age, a conservative approach to PH based only on clinical observation in these patients seems reasonable. Despite a much slower course, PH develops almost invariably even after a successful KPE. A study from the USA, analysing 163 children with BA who survived with their native liver to a mean age of 9.2 years, showed that PH could be identified in 67%. Variceal bleeding had occurred in 20% of subjects, although the majority (62%) had only one episode [53]. In Canada and Europe, up to 96% of adult patients with BA had features of PH, with 65% having evidence of varices, 91% splenomegaly and 14% ascites. A French study showed that 99% of BA survivors with their native liver into adulthood had evidence of cirrhosis and 70% had significant PH [41, 54]. Extrahepatic complications of portal hypertension, such as spontaneous bacterial peritonitis, hepatopulmonary syndrome, porto-pulmonary hypertension and spontaneous bacterial peritonitis, represent a clear indication to promptly place the patient on the transplant list [55].

Deciding the best timing to list for LT in a BA patient who had a failed Kasai may be challenging and probably depends more on the transplant programme setting rather than on an individual patient's features. A tool validated in children with chronic liver disease is the paediatric end-stage liver disease (PELD) score. PELD score is calculated based on the age, growth failure, albumin, international normalized ratio and total bilirubin level and is an excellent predictor for the outcome of paediatric LT patients. However, it has been reported that the PELD score in BA patients does not accurately represent the true mortality risk associated with complications of portal hypertension, variceal bleeding, refractory ascites and hepatopulmonary syndrome. The US experience showed that

Table 7.1 Indications for liver transplantation in biliary atresia

• Failure of Kasai portoenterostomy
–Persistent jaundice
–Recurrence of jaundice
• Late diagnosis: Primary LT
• Failure to thrive despite aggressive nutritional support
• Recurrent/life-threatening bacterial cholangitis
• Recurrent hospitalizations impairing quality of life
• Refractory variceal bleeding
• Hepatopulmonary syndrome
• Porto-pulmonary hypertension
• Significant ascites and episodes of spontaneous bacterial peritonitis
• Hepato-renal syndrome
• Hepatic malignancy

BA patients have a median wait time on the list of 90 days and a median calculated PELD score of 15 at the time of transplant (UNOS data); 15% of children with chronic liver disease have either died on the waiting list or been removed because they were too ill to transplant. These figures are probably related to the fact that in the US network, only approximately 10% of eligible donor livers are split, missing an opportunity to expand access to transplant for BA patients and leading to a high mortality on the list in children younger than 2 years of age [56–58]. This is not the case in countries, such as Italy, where the split technique is widely adopted; thus many left lateral segment grafts are offered to the centres, and the mortality on the list of recipients below 2 years of age is close to 0% [59] (Table 7.1).

7.2 Part II: Congenital Choledochal Malformation

7.2.1 Introduction

Congenital choledochal malformation (CCM) is a term used to describe biliary malformation where the distinguishing feature is dilatation of some part. Usually and typically these are not actually obstructed to discriminate from situations of biliary dilatation due to intraluminal stones, for instance.

Many CCM are associated with an abnormal union between the pancreatic and distal common bile duct (Fig. 7.8). An example was first described by Abraham Vater in 1723, but there is much about its aetiology and pathophysiology which can still be debated. CCM may cause symptoms at any age but typically present with obstructive jaundice in infants and recurrent abdominal pain often due to pancreatitis in children. Other recognized complications include cholangitis, cholelithiasis and malignant degeneration though this is only really found in adults.

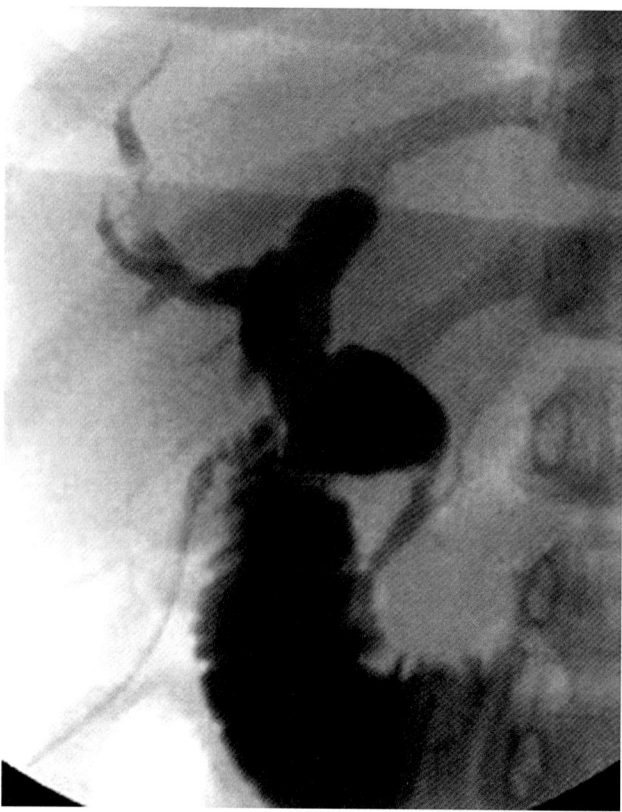

Fig. 7.8 Congenital choledochal malformation with abnormal pancreatobiliary junction (common channel)

7.2.2 Epidemiology

CCM are rare malformations with an incidence in the Western population of anywhere between 1 in 100,000–150,000 births though this is entirely guesswork [60]. It is known to be remarkably higher in Asian populations though the reason is still unclear. There is also a female-male preponderance of up to 4:1, and more than two-thirds of cases are diagnosed in children <10 years of age.

Alonso Lej et al. [60] proposed the first classification for CCM in 1959, describing three types of bile duct dilatation. In 1977, Todani [61] expanded this classification to include intrahepatic and multiple cysts. Our own version of this is a little simpler and is as follows (Fig. 7.9):

- **Type 1** (75%)—extrahepatic dilatation.
  - Predominantly **cystic** dilatation (**1C**), with distinct demarcation at the top and bottom.
  - Predominately **fusiform** dilatation (**1F**), less dilated and more indistinct.
- **Type 2** (<1%)—extrahepatic **supraduodenal diverticulum** of the bile duct.
- **Type 3** (< 1%)—**choledochocele**, a localized dilatation of the intramural duodenal bile duct.
- **Type 4** (20%)—combination of type 1C/F and intrahepatic dilatation.
- **Type 5** (4%)—intrahepatic biliary dilatation.
  - **Caroli's disease:** genetic origin, R and L lobes, liver fibrosis and renal disease (cysts or fibrosis).
  - Isolated intrahepatic dilatation, usually peripheral.

7.2.3 Aetiology and Pathogenesis

The aetiology of CCM, particularly Types 1 (C&F) and 4, is still unclear, although many theories have been proposed. Two deserve wider explanation. The first and oldest would suggest that there is a congenital distal bile duct stenosis which causes increased proximal intrabiliary pressure and dilatation. This is a common scenario in many congenital atresias such as jejunal and oesophageal atresia. The alternative, first suggested by Donald Babbitt, an American radiologist, on the basis of noticing that there was reflux from the bile ducts into the pancreatic duct via the common channel at the time of on-table cholangiography. He surmised that this could go the other way and activated proteolytic pancreatic juice could damage the wall of the bile duct causing weakness and dilatation [62].

Clinical research at King's tends to refute this as an aetiological theory [63–65]. Thus, we have routinely measured choledochal pressure and bile amylase levels (as a surrogate of pancreatic reflux into the biliary tree) at the time of surgery and first showed an inverse relationship between the pressure within the choledochal malformation and bile amylase levels [64, 65]. Most recently, we looked at the histological appearance of the biliary lining in 73 patients with CCM and correlated it with their pressures and bile amylase levels [65]. This showed that those with the most damaged and abnormal epithelium were those with the highest pressures and the *lowest levels of bile amylase* (and by extension other pancreatic enzymes) (Fig. 7.10). These observations strongly suggest that Babbitt's aetiological speculations are invalid.

7.2.4 Clinical Features and Diagnosis

The majority (80%) of CCM are diagnosed in childhood. Some may be detected at routine prenatal USS examination as early as 15 weeks' gestation and may be confused with duodenal atresia, ovarian cysts or intestinal duplication [19]. The CCM antenatally diagnosed are typically and almost exclusively Type 1C lesions (Fig. 7.11).

Clinical presentation of CC varies depending on age of patient. The classic triad of jaundice, abdominal pain and right upper quadrant mass is uncommon and seen mainly in children. Abdominal pain is a more prominent symp-

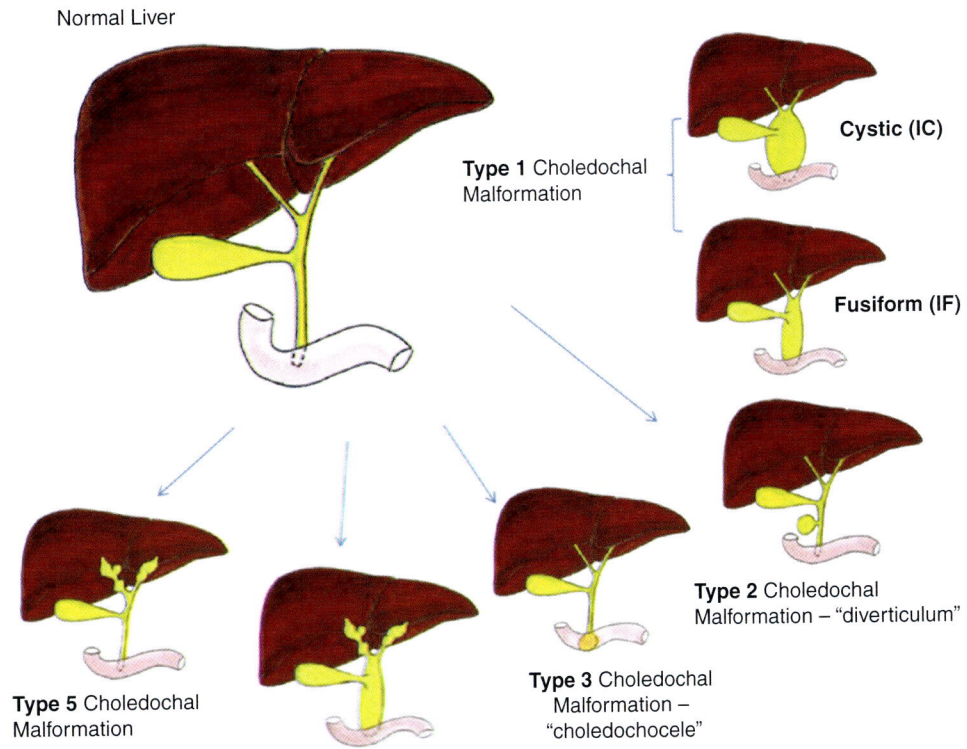

Fig. 7.9 Schematic version of King's College Hospital classification of congenital choledochal malformation

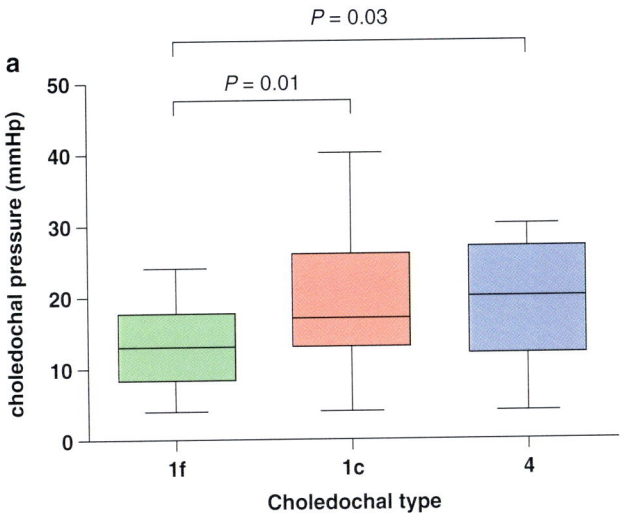
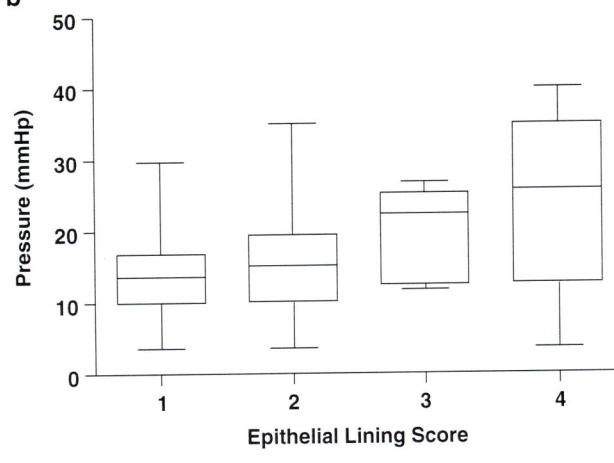

Fig. 7.10 Choledochal pressure: morphology and epithelial consequences. (**a**) Choledochal pressure (mmHg) in relation to the type of choledochal malformation in 47 patients (20 Type 1f, 20 Type 1c and 7 Type 4). (**b**) Choledochal pressure (mmHg) vs. epithelial lining score where 1 = normal and 4 = epithelial necrosis and bile impregnation. Modified from [65]

tom in older children and jaundice in the young. Biliary amylase levels may be elevated and correlate with an initial clinical presentation with acute pancreatitis [63]. Caroli's disease typically presents with cholangitis and stone formation.

Infants are most likely to present with painless, obstructive jaundice. Vomiting, failure to thrive and an abdominal mass also may be noted. Even in the presence of the concomitant common channel, hyperamylasaemia may not be found in infants as its concentration in pancreatic juice at birth and after is low only reaching significant levels at about 1–2 years of age [63]. An incidental presentation is perhaps less common in the paediatric population but seen in nearly one-third of adult CCM patients [66].

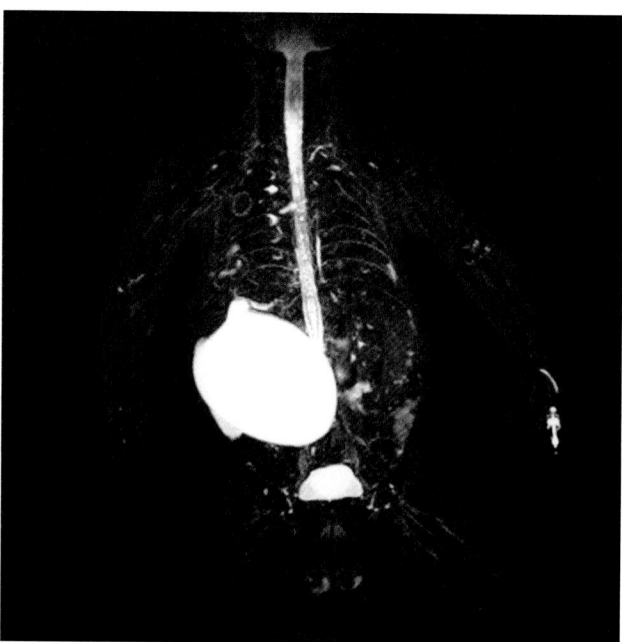

Fig. 7.11 MRCP of huge cystic choledochal malformation (Type 1C)—antenatally diagnosed

Biliary peritonitis secondary to rupture of a CCM is uncommon and described in <2% of cases [67]. They are usually children (only about 20–30% present as adults) with the classic triad of palpable abdominal mass, pain in right upper quadrant and jaundice. Perforations may be single or multiple, and there is no apparent relationship between cyst size and rupture.

Irwin and Morrison [68] reported the first CCM-associated malignancy in 1944. The mechanism remains unclear; however, pancreatic reflux, biliary stasis and formation of mutagenic secondary biliary acids are thought to play a role. Although a malignancy may develop anywhere within the biliary tree, over 50% of tumours develop within the cyst itself. In a review of 5780 CCM cases in the literature, Sastry et al. reported that 7% of patients had cancer—cholangiocarcinoma (70%) and gallbladder cancer (23%). The incidence of malignancy at <18 was 0.42 versus 11% in adults [69]. We looked at two possible contributory factors in order to try and identify those children who might be susceptible to later development of malignant change after resection of the extrahepatic portion during childhood [70]. These were levels of CA 19-9, a known biomarker of pancreatic and hepatobiliary malignancy, in bile at the time of surgery, and the histological expression of MIB-1 on resected choledochal mucosa, which is regarded as marker of epithelial instability. Both proved surprisingly uninformative. High levels of CA 19-9 (>10,000 iu/L) were found unexpectedly in bile, completely independently of bile amylase, and later staining showed that it was expressed in all parts of normal biliary mucosa. Furthermore there were 8 infants and children (of 43 patients) with moderate and high levels of MIB-1 expression without any kind of unifying factor or explanation.

The diagnosis of CCM is typically suspected using USS and can allow an accurate evaluation of size, contour and position of the biliary malformation. Uncommon complications such as cholelithiasis, perforation or even ascites may be noted. Diagnosis requires demonstration of continuity of the cyst with the biliary tree so that it can be differentiated from other intra-abdominal cysts such as pancreatic pseudocysts, echinococcal cysts or hepatic cysts. Technetium-99 HIDA scans may also be used to show bile content of cysts and then degree of obstruction and drainage. This scan will show an initial area of photopenia at the cyst, with consequent filling and then, usually, delayed empting into the bowel [71].

Cross-sectional imaging may be used including MRI, to derive an MRCP (magnetic retrograde cholangiopancreatogram). This is now considered to be the standard to diagnose CCM and can create images by differential signal intensity of stagnant pancreatic fluid and bile compared with surrounding structures [72]. CT with contrast clearly shows any cyst and dilated intrahepatic bile ducts and may be useful in those with acute pancreatitis and perhaps where an associated malignancy is suspected. Currently, endoscopic retrograde cholangiopancreatography (ERCP) and percutaneous transhepatic cholangiography (PTC) are best reserved because of their invasive nature but may be used to decompress an obstructed bile duct or define more complex pancreatic duct arrangement in the setting of recurrent pancreatitis.

7.2.5 Treatment

Primary excision of the dilated part of the extrahepatic biliary system should be performed soon after diagnosis. Early surgery provides the opportunity to exclude cystic biliary atresia in infants and hepatic complications such as fibrosis while reducing the risk of cholangitis and perforation.

Intraoperative cholangiography should always be done prior to any dissection and provides key anatomical details of biliary variation. Excision and hepaticojejunostomy are the treatment of choice in virtually all circumstances. Extrahepatic duct excision should extend proximally to the confluence of the right and the left, leaving a single ring to anastomose. Choledochoscopy performed after duct excision helps to identify intrahepatic bile ducts, stenosis and stone formation and can also be done in the dilated common channel to confirm absence of obstruction and debris. While there are flexible dedicated cholangioscopes, a small flexible ureteroscope or bronchoscope should suffice.

A long (40 cm) Roux-en-Y hepaticojejunostomy is the preferred method of enteric bile drainage and has an excellent long-term outcome. If cyst excision of the distal portion proves difficult due to recurrent inflammation and scarring, removal of just the mucosa is acceptable, in order to avoid damage to the underlying pancreatic duct and portal vein. A liver biopsy is performed at the conclusion of the operation in order to document hepatic histology.

Excision of the diverticulum of a Type 2 CCM should be relatively straightforward leaving the common bile duct intact.

Large choledochoceles, often only a problem in adulthood, can be removed transduodenally in those with Type 3 CCM, and smaller ones can be treated by sphincteroplasty or endoscopic sphincterotomy [73–75].

There is an increasing experience throughout the world with laparoscopic excision and reconstruction though it has to be said that most proponents with anything like decent series are in the Far East. Liem et al. [76] from Hanoi in Vietnam have reported their experience with an almost unbelievable 400 cases of laparoscopic cyst excision and hepaticoduodenostomy or HJ reconstruction for CCM. Anastomotic leaks occurred in <5%, and conversion to open surgery was only required in two children. This experience will never be repeated in Western Europe or North America because the cases are just not there. They were able to show good results with low conversion rate and outcomes similar to those with open surgery [77].

One way of making the most difficult and challenging part of the procedure, the hepaticojejunostomy, easier is to do it robotically. The team from Leeds, UK, has reported an experience of 27 children of which 22 were successfully completed robotically with extracorporeal jejunal anastomosis. The conversions were for anatomical concerns or technical reasons, and one was for a bile leak [78]. Of course you have to spend up to two million dollars to buy yourself a robot so it can never be cost-effective in any realistic paediatric environment.

7.2.6 Complications

Surgical treatment of CCM achieves consistently good results, even in small infants. Early postoperative complications such as anastomotic leakage, bleeding, pancreatitis and intestinal occlusion are uncommon. The long-term complication rate in the literature ranges between 5 and 15%, and reoperation rates range between 1 and 20%. Cholangitis occurs in 1–9% of the patients, stricture of the biliary anastomosis occurs in up to 9% of the patients, and there is a reoperation rate of 1–20% [79, 80].

7.2.7 Liver Transplantation and Caroli's Disease

Caroli's disease (CD) is a rare autosomal recessive inherited disorder characterized by macroscopic saccular or segmental ectasias of the intrahepatic bile ducts. CD is frequently associated with congenital hepatic fibrosis and autosomal recessive polycystic kidney disease, and the clinical course is determined by the extent of underlying pathologic abnormalities. Biliary cystic dilatation and narrowing lead to cholestasis and cholangitis. CD may also be complicated with the formation of extra- and intrahepatic bile duct stones with development of hepatic abscess and portal hypertension [81]. The surgical treatment of CD consists in drainage of biliary obstruction and/or abscess, partial hepatic resection in case of localized lobar disease and the liver transplantation in case of diffuse, bi-lobar symptomatic disease and of concomitant portal hypertension due to hepatic fibrosis. Excellent survival rates [82] are reported regarding liver transplantation in those patients with Caroli's disease that are principally complicated by recurrent cholangitis and concomitant renal disease.

7.3 Part III: Spontaneous Bile Duct Perforation

SBP in infancy was first described by Dijkstra in 1932 [83], and small series of affected infants have been reported [84] since, with the largest being that of Chardot et al. [85] from Paris who described 11 infants seen over a 22-year period. Spontaneous biliary perforation (SBP), together with inspissated bile syndrome, and after biliary atresia are other possible causes of surgical jaundice in early infancy [29]. Perforation may occur more commonly in the anterior part of the duct where the cyst meets the common hepatic duct but also has been reported at the back adjacent to portal vein [86]. Anomalous entry of the CBD into the duodenum, bile duct stenosis or intraluminal obstruction with bile plugs may predispose to a sudden rise in duct pressure leading to "blowout". Anterior perforations lead to bile ascites and may be obvious in boys by causing bile discolouration of hydroceles and hernias. Posterior perforations leak around the tissues supporting the portal vein and spill into the lesser sac being much more constrained [29]. As a consequence diagnosis may be difficult. Late portal vein thrombosis is a late complication of this posterior perforation [86].

Liver function tests may be normal, though jaundice is usual, and serum alkaline phosphatase and γ-glutamyl transferase levels are mildly raised. Ultrasound is abnormal showing some kind of paraductal mass and varying degrees of bile ascites. Posterior perforations may show more a complex echogenic mass around the duct into the lesser sac. The differential diagnosis must include perforation in a pre-existing usually cystic choledochal malformation. Radionuclide hepatobiliary scanning shows zones of persistent radioactivity around the common bile duct, as well as generalized abdominal radioactivity caused by leakage of bile into the general peritoneal cavity.

The current management of SBP is still laparotomy in the absence of sufficiently small ERCP stents. Simple drainage of the peritoneal cavity is reasonable outside of specialist centres, following cholangiography through the gallbladder. More invasive surgery should be left to experts and might include primary duct repair, T-tube insertion, choledocojejunostomy or cholecystojejunostomy [84, 85].

7.4 Part IV: Ciliated Hepatic Foregut Cyst

Although congenital cysts of the liver are uncommon, with the widespread use of US, particularly during prenatal period, their prevalence appears to be increasing [87]. Ciliated hepatic foregut cyst (CHFC) is a rare cystic malformation of the liver described first by Wheeler and Edmonson in 1984 [88]. The histogenesis is still unclear, but most authors think that CHFC probably arises from the remnants of embryonic foregut, similar to that of bronchial and oesophageal cysts. CHFC has been reported in about 60 patients, but only a small proportion are children despite its supposed congenital origin [89–91]. The differential diagnosis in childhood includes choledochal malformations and cystic neoplasm, but detailed imaging investigations (US and MRCP) are usually able to establish the correct diagnosis (Fig. 7.12). Increasing cyst size and sign and symptoms of biliary drainage obstruction remain recognized indications for surgery [91].

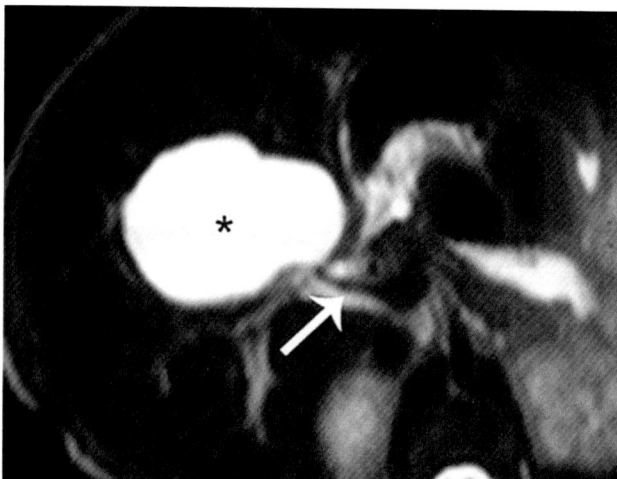

Fig. 7.12 MRI of ciliated hepatic foregut cyst (*asterisk*). NB No communication with the normal biliary tree (arrow)

References

1. Burns J. Principles of midwifery, including the diseases of women and children. London: Longman; 1817.
2. Thomson J. On congenital obliteration of the bile ducts. Edinb Med J. 1891;37:523–31.
3. Ladd WE. Congenital obstruction of the bile ducts. Ann Surg. 1935;102:742–51.
4. Kasai M, Kimura S, Asakura Y, Suzuki H, Taira Y, Ohashi E. Surgical treatment of biliary atresia. J Pediatr Surg. 1968;3:665–75.
5. Kasai M, Watanabe I, Ohi R. Follow-up studies of long term survivors after hepatic portoenterostomy for "noncorrectable" biliary atresia. J Pediatr Surg. 1975;10:173–82.
6. Wada H, Muraji T, Yokoi A, Okamoto T, Sato S, Takamizawa S, et al. Insignificant seasonal and geographical variation in incidence of biliary atresia in Japan: a regional survey of over 20 years. J Pediatr Surg. 2007;42:2090–2.
7. Chardot C, Carton M, Spire-Bendelac N, Le Pommelet C, Golmard JL, Auvert B. Epidemiology of biliary atresia in France: a national study 1986-96. J Hepatol. 1999;31:1006–13.
8. Livesey E, Cortina Borja M, Sharif K, Alizai N, McClean P, et al. Epidemiology of biliary atresia in England and Wales (1999-2006). Arch Dis Child Fetal Neonatal Ed. 2009;94:451–5.
9. Schreiber RA, Barker CC, Roberts EA, Martin SR, Canadian Pediatric Hepatology Research Group. Biliary atresia in Canada: the effect of centre caseload experience on outcome. J Pediatr Gastroenterol Nutr. 2010;51:61–5.
10. Davenport M, Savage M, Mowat AP, Howard ER. The biliary atresia splenic malformation syndrome. Surgery. 1993;113:662–8.
11. Davenport M, Tizzard SA, Underhill J, Mieli-Vergani G, Portmann B, Hadzić N. The biliary atresia splenic malformation syndrome: a 28-year single-center retrospective study. J Pediatr. 2006;149:393–400.
12. Fischler B, Ehrnst A, Forsgren C, Orvell C, Nemeth A. The viral association of neonatal cholestasis in Sweden: a possible link between cytomegalovirus infection and extrahepatic biliary atresia. J Pediatr Gastroenterol Nutr. 1998;27:57–64.
13. Rauschenfels S, Krassmann M, Al-Masri AN, Verhagen W, Leonhardt J, Kuebler JF, et al. Incidence of hepatotropic viruses in biliary atresia. Eur J Pediatr. 2009;168:469–76.
14. Zani A, Quaglia A, Hadzić N, Zuckerman M, Davenport M. Cytomegalovirus-associated biliary atresia: an aetiological and prognostic subgroup. J Pediatr Surg. 2015;50:1739–45.
15. Davenport M. Biliary atresia: clinical aspects. Semin Pediatr Surg. 2012;21:175–84.
16. Lakshminarayanan B, Davenport M. Biliary atresia: a comprehensive review. J Autoimmun. 2016;76:1–9.
17. Asai A, Miethke A, Bezzerra JA. Pathogenesis of biliary atresia: defining biology to understand clinical phenotypes. Nat Rev Gastroenterol Hepatol. 2015;12:342–52.
18. Verkade HJ, Bezerra AJ, Davenport M, Schreiber RA, Mieli-Vergani G, Hulscher JB, et al. Biliary atresia and other cholestatic childhood diseases: advances and future challenges. J Hepatol. 2016;65:631–42.
19. Redkar R, Davenport M, Howard ER. Antenatal diagnosis of congenital anomalies of biliary tract. J Pediatr Surg. 1998;33:700–4.
20. Harpavat S, Finegold MJ, Karpen SJ. Patients with biliary atresia have elevated direct/conjugated bilirubin levels shortly after birth. Pediatrics. 2011;128:1428–33.
21. Hill R, Quaglia A, Hussain M, Hadzic N, Mieli-Vergani G, Vergani D, et al. Th-17 cells infiltrate the liver in human biliary atresia and are related to surgical outcome. J Pediatr Surg. 2015;50:1297–303.
22. Bezzerra JA, Tiao G, Ryckman FC, Alonso M, Sabla GE, Shneider B, et al. Genetic induction of proinflammatory immunity in children with biliary atresia. Lancet. 2002;360:1563–659.

23. Muraji T, Hosaka N, Irie N, Yoshida M, Imai Y, Tanaka K, et al. Maternal microchimerism in underlying pathogenesis of biliary atresia: quantification and phenotypes of maternal cells in the liver. Pediatrics. 2008;121:517–21.
24. Harper P, Plant JW, Unger DB. Congenital biliary atresia and jaundice in lambs and calves. Aust Vet J. 1990;67:18–22.
25. Lorent K, Gong W, Koo KA, Waisbourd-Zinman O, Karjoo S, Zhao X, et al. Identification of a plant isoflavonoid that causes biliary atresia. Sci Transl Med. 2015;7(286):286ra267.
26. Davenport M. Biliary atresia: from Australia to the zebrafish. J Pediatr Surg. 2016;51:200–5.
27. Hussein M, Howard ER, Mieli-Vergani G, Mowat AP. Jaundice at 14 days: exclude biliary atresia. Arch Dis Child. 1991;66:1177–9.
28. Imanieh MH, Dehghani SM, Bagheri MH, Emad V, Haghighat M, Zahmatkeshan M, et al. Triangular cord sign in detection of biliary atresia: is it valuable sign? Dig Dis Sci. 2010;55:172–5.
29. Davenport M, Betalli P, D'Antiga L, Cheeseman P, Mieli-Vergani G, Howard ER. The spectrum of surgical jaundice in infancy. J Pediatr Surg. 2003;38:1471–9.
30. Russo P, Magee JC, Boitnott KE, Bove T, Raghunathan T, Finegold M, et al. Design and validation of the biliary atresia research consortium histologic assessment system for cholestasis in infancy. Clin Gastroenterol Hepatol. 2011;9:357–62.
31. Shanmugam NP, Harrison PM, Devlin P, Peddu P, Knisely AS, Davenport M, et al. Selective use of endoscopic retrograde cholangiopancreatography in the diagnosis of biliary atresia in infants younger than 100 days. J Pediatr Gastroenterol Nutr. 2009;46:1689–94.
32. Davenport M, Puricelli V, Farrant P, Hadzic M, Mieli-Vergani G, Portmann B, et al. The outcome of the older (>100 days) infant with biliary atresia. J Pediatr Surg. 2004;39:575–81.
33. Neto JS, Feier FH, Bierrenbach AL, Toscano CM, Fonseca EA, Pugliese R, et al. Impact of Kasai portoenterostomy on liver transplantation outcomes: a retrospective cohort study of 347 children with biliary atresia. Liver Transpl. 2015;21:922–7.
34. Russo P, Magee JC, Anders RA, Bove KE, Chung C, Cummings OW, et al. Childhood Liver Disease Research Network (ChiLDReN). Key histopathologic features of liver biopsies that distinguish biliary atresia from other causes of infantile cholestasis and their correlation with outcome: a multicenter study. Am J Surg Pathol. 2016;40:1601–15.
35. Esteves E, Clemente Neto E, Ottaiano Neto M, Devanir J Jr, Esteves PR. Laparoscopic Kasai portoenterostomy for biliary atresia. Pediatr Surg Int. 2002;18:737–40.
36. Ure BM, Kuebler JF, Schukfeh N, Engelmann C, Dingemann J, Petersen C. Survival with the native liver after laparoscopic versus conventional Kasai portoenterostomy in infants with biliary atresia: a prospective trial. Ann Surg. 2011;253:826–30.
37. Davenport M, Stringer MD, Tizzard SA, McClean P, Mieli-Vergani G, Hadzic N. Randomized, double-blind, placebo-controlled trial of corticosteroids after Kasai portoenterostomy for biliary atresia. Hepatology. 2007;46:1821–7.
38. Davenport M, Tizzard SA, Parsons C, Hadzic N. Single surgeon, single centre: experience with steroids in biliary atresia. J Hepatol. 2013;59:1054–8.
39. Bezerra JA, Spino C, Magee JC, Schneider BL, Rosenthal P, Wang KS, et al. Use of corticosteroids after hepatoportoenterostomy for bile drainage in infants with biliary atresia: the START randomized clinical trial. JAMA. 2014;311:1750–9.
40. Chen Y, Nah SA, Chiang L, Krishnaswamy G, Low Y. Postoperative steroid therapy for biliary atresia: systematic review and meta-analysis. J Pediatr Surg. 2015;50:1590–4.
41. Lykavieris P, Chardot C, Sokhn M, Gauthier F, Valayer J, Bernard O. Outcome in adulthood of biliary atresia: a study of 63 patients who survived for over 20 years with their native liver. Hepatology. 2005;41(2):366–71.
42. Duche M, Ducot B, Tournay E, Fabre M, Cohen J, Jacquemin E, Bernard O. Prognostic value of endoscopy in children with biliary atresia at risk for early development of varices and bleeding. Gastroenterology. 2010;139:1952–60.
43. Miga D, Sokol RJ, Mackenzie T. Survival after first esophageal variceal hemorrhage in patients with biliary atresia. J Pediatr. 2001;139:291–6.
44. Hadzic N, Quaglia A, Portmann B, Paramalingam S, Heaton ND, Rela M, Mieli-Vergani G, Davenport M. Hepatocellular carcinoma in biliary atresia: King's college hospital experience. J Pediatr. 2011;159:617–22.
45. Davenport M, De Ville de Goyet J, Stringer MD, Mieli-Vergani G, Kelly DA, McClean P, et al. Seamless management of biliary atresia in England and Wales (1999-2002). Lancet. 2004;363:1354–7.
46. Davenport M, Ong E, Sharif K, Alizai N, McClean P, Hadzic N, et al. Biliary atresia in England and Wales: results of centralization and new benchmark. J Pediatr Surg. 2011;46:1689–94.
47. Durkin N, Davenport M. Centralization of pediatric surgical procedures in the United Kingdom. Eur J Pediatr Surg. 2017;27(5):416–21.
48. Shneider BL, Brown MB, Haber B, Whitington PF, Schwarz K, Squires R, et al. Biliary Atresia Research Consortium. A multicenter study of the outcome of biliary atresia in the United States, 1997 to 2000. J Pediatr. 2006;148:467–74.
49. Shneider BL, Magee JC, Karpen SJ, Rand EB, Narkewicz MR, Bass LM, et al. Childhood Liver Disease Research Network (ChiLDReN). Total serum bilirubin within 3 months of hepatoportoenterostomy predicts short-term outcomes in biliary atresia. J Pediatr. 2016;170:211–7.
50. Nightingale S, Stormon MO, O'Loughlin EV, Shun A, Thomas G, et al. Early post-hepatoportoenterostomy predictors of native liver survival in biliary atresia. J Pediatr Gastroenterol Nutr. 2017;64:203–9.
51. Qiao G, Li L, Cheng W, Zhang Z, Ge J, Wang C. Conditional probability of survival in patients with biliary atresia after Kasai portoenterostomy: a Chinese population-based study. J Pediatr Surg. 2015;50:1310–5.
52. Duché M, Ducot B, Ackermann O, Baujard C, Chevret L, Frank-Soltysiak M, et al. Experience with endoscopic management of high-risk gastroesophageal varices, with and without bleeding, in children with biliary atresia. Gastroenterology. 2013;145:801–7.
53. Sundaram SS, Mack CL, Feldman AG, Sokol RJ. Biliary atresia: indications and timing of liver transplantation and optimization of pretransplant care. Liver Transplant. 2017;23(1):96–109.
54. Kumagi T, Drenth JP, Guttman O, Ng V, Lilly L, Therapondos G, et al. Biliary atresia and survival into adulthood without transplantation: a collaborative multicentre clinic review. Liver Int. 2012;32:510–8.
55. Di Giorgio A, D'Antiga L. Portal hypertension in children. Textbook of pediatric gastroenterology, hepatology and nutrition. Basel: Springer; 2016. p. 791–817.
56. Arnon R, Leshno M, Annunziato R, Florman S, Iyer K. What is the optimal timing of liver transplantation for children with biliary atresia? A Markov model simulation analysis. J Pediatr Gastroenterol Nutr. 2014;59:398–402.
57. Utterson EC, Sheperd RW, Sokol RJ, Bucuvalas J, Magee JC, McDiarmid SV, et al. Biliary atresia: clinical, profiles, risk factors, and outcomes of 755 patients listed for liver transplantation. J Pediatr. 2005;147:180–5.
58. Barshes NR, Lee TC, Udell IW, O'Mahoney CA, Karpen SJ, Carter BA, et al. The pediatric end-stage liver disease (PELD) model as a predictor of survival benefit and posttransplant survival in pediatric liver transplant recipients. Liver Transpl. 2006;12:475–80.
59. Gridelli B, Spada M, Petz W, Bertani A, Lucianetti A, Colledan M, et al. Split-liver transplantation eliminates the need for living-donor

liver transplantation in children with end-stage cholestatic liver disease. Transplantation. 2003;75:1197–203.
60. Alonso-Lej F, Rever WB, Pessagno DJ. Congenital choledochal cyst with a report of 2, and an analysis of 94 cases. Int Abstr Surg. 1959;108:1–30.
61. Todani W, Watanabe Y, Narusue M, Tabuchi K, Okajima K. Classification, operative procedures and review of 37 cases including cancer arising from choledochal cyst. Am J Surg. 1977;134:263–9.
62. Babbitt DP. Congenital choledochal cyst: new etiological concept based on anomalous relationships of the common bile duct and pancreatic bulb. Ann Radiol. 1969;12:231–40.
63. Davenport M, Stringer MD, Howard ER. Biliary amylase and congenital choledochal dilatation. J Pediatr Surg. 1995;30(3):474–7.
64. Davenport M, Basu R. Under pressure: choledochal malformation manometry. J Pediatr Surg. 2005;40:331–5.
65. Turowski C, Knisely AS, Davenport M. Role of pressure and pancreatic reflux in the aetiology of choledochal malformation. Br J Surg. 2011;98:1319–26.
66. Soares KC, Arnaoutakis DJ, Kamel I, Rastegar N, Anders R, Maithel S, et al. Choledochal cysts: presentation, clinical differentiation, and management. J Am Coll Surg. 2014;219:1167–80.
67. Ando K, Miyano T, Kohno S, Takamizawa S, Lane G. Spontaneous perforation of choledochal cyst: a study of 13 case. Eur J Pediatr Surg. 1998;8:23–5.
68. Irwin ST, Morison JE. Congenital cyst of the common bile duct containing stones and undergoing cancerous change. Br J Surg. 1944;32:319–21.
69. Sastry AV, Abbadessa B, Wayne MG, Steele JG, Cooperman AM. What is the incidence of biliary carcinoma in choledochal cysts, when do they develop, and how should it affect management? World J Surg. 2015;39(2):487–92.
70. La Pergola E, Zen Y, Davenport M. Congenital choledochal malformation: search for a marker of epithelial instability. J Pediatr Surg. 2016;51:1445–9.
71. Atkinson JJ, Davenport M. Controversies in choledochal malformation. S Afr Med J. 2014;104:816–9.
72. Kim MJ, Han SJ, Yoon CS, Kim JH, Oh JT, Chung KS, et al. Using MR cholangiopancreatography to reveal anomalous pancreaticobiliary ductal union in infants and children with choledochal cysts. Am J Roentgenol. 2002;179:209–14.
73. Huang SP, Wang HP, Chen JH, Wu MS, Shun CT, Lin JT. Clinical application of EUS and peroral cholangioscopy in choledochocele with choledocholithiasis. Gastrointest Endosc. 1999;50:568–71.
74. Ziegler KM, Pitt HA, Zyromski NJ, Chauhan A, Sherman S, Moffatt D, et al. Choledochoceles: are they choledochal cysts? Ann Surg. 2010;252:683–90.
75. Dohmoto M, Kamiya T, Hunerbein M, Valdez H, Ibanegaray J, Prado J. Endoscopic treatment of a choledochocele in a 2-year-old child. Surg Endosc. 1996;10:1016–8.
76. Liem NT, Pham HD, Dung le A, Son TN, Vu HM. Early and intermediate outcomes of laparoscopic surgery for choledochal cysts with 400 patients. J Laparoendosc Adv Surg Tech A. 2012;22:599–603.
77. Powell CS, Sawyers JL, Reynolds VH. Management of adult choledochal cysts. Ann Surg. 1981;193:666–76.
78. Alizai NK, Dawrant MJ, Najmaldin AS. Robot-assisted resection of choledochal cysts and hepaticojejunostomy in children. Pediatr Surg Int. 2014;30(3):291–4.
79. Urushihara N, Fukumoto K, Fukuzawa H, Mitsunaga M, Watanabe K, Aoba T, et al. Long-term outcomes after excision of choledochal cysts in a single institution: operative procedures and late complications. J Pediatr Surg. 2012;47(12):2169–74.
80. Ohtsuka H, Fukase K, Yoshida H, Motoi F, Hayashi H, Morikawa T, et al. Long-term outcomes after extrahepatic excision of congenital choladocal cysts: 30 years of experience at a single center. Hepato-Gastroenterology. 2013;62(137):1–5.
81. Lai Q, Lerut J. Proposal for an algorithm for liver transplantation in Caroli's disease and syndrome: putting an uncommon effort into a common task. Clin Transpl. 2016;30:3–9.
82. Kassahun WT, Khan T, Wittekind C, Mossner J, Caca K, Hauss J, et al. Caroli's disease: liver resection and liver transplantation: experience in 33 patients. Surgery. 2005;138:888.
83. Dijkstra CH. Graluistorting in de buikholte bij een zuigeling. Maandschr Kindegeneeskd. 1932;1:409–14.
84. Davenport M, Heaton ND, Howard ER. Spontaneous perforation of the bile duct in infancy. Br J Surg. 1991;78:1068–70.
85. Chardot C, Iskandarani F, De Dreuzy O, Dusquesne B, Pariente D, Bernard O, et al. Spontaneous perforation of the biliary tract in infancy: a series of 11 cases. Eur J Pediatr Surg. 1996;6:41–6.
86. Livesey E, Davenport M. Spontaneous perforation of the biliary tract and portal vein thrombosis in infancy. Pediatr Surg Int. 2008;24:357–9.
87. Charlesworth P, Ade-Ajayi N, Davenport M. Natural history and long-term follow-up of antenatally detected liver cysts. J Pediatr Surg. 2007;42:494–9.
88. Wheeler DA, Edmonson HA. Ciliated hepatic foregut cyst. Am J Surg Pathol. 1984;8:467–70.
89. Stringer M, Jones MO, Woodley H, Wyatt J. Ciliated hepatic foregut cyst. J Pediatr Surg. 2006;41:1180–3.
90. Carnicer J, Duran C, Donoso L, Saez A, Lopez A. Ciliated hepatic foregut cyst. J Pediatr Gastroenterol Nutr. 1996;23:191–3.
91. Betalli P, Gobbi D, Talenti E, Alaggio R, Gamba PG, Zanon GF. Ciliated hepatic foregut cyst: from antenatal diagnosis to surgery. Pediatr Radiol. 2008;38:230–2.

Acute Liver Failure in Children

Naresh Shanmugam and Anil Dhawan

Key Points
- Encephalopathy is not essential in the diagnosis of ALF in children.
- Coagulopathy is being used as a prognostic marker in paediatric ALF.
- Role of liver assist devices and hepatocyte transplant is still limited.
- Auxiliary liver transplantation if feasible should be offered where indicated as it provides a chance for native liver regeneration.

Research Needed in the Field
- Surrogate markers of prognosis in ALF
- Defining liver transplant criteria with improved sensitivity and specificity
- Clinical trials in human hepatocyte transplantation

8.1 Definition

Trey and Davidson coined the term "fulminant liver failure" 40 years ago to define onset of altered mental status within 8 weeks of initial symptoms of liver dysfunction in an otherwise healthy individual with no previous history of liver disease [1]. This definition was difficult to apply in children with ALF as the disease process could start in utero and time quantification might not be possible and, also, encephalopathy might be difficult to diagnose. Trying to address this issue, Bhaduri and Vergani defined ALF in children as "a rare multisystem disorder in which severe impairment of liver function, with or without encephalopathy, occurs in association with hepatocellular necrosis in a patient with no recognized underlying chronic liver disease" [2]. This newer definition for children failed to differentiate between acute hepatitis and ALF as "severe impairment of liver function" is very subjective and can vary from person to person.

Paediatric Acute Liver Failure (PALF) study group has come up with practical definition to select cases for their multicentre study. They used the following criteria to define acute liver failure (ALF) in children: (1) hepatic-based coagulopathy defined as a prothrombin time (PT) $\geq$ 15 s or international normalized ratio (INR) $\geq$ 1.5 not corrected by vitamin K in the presence of clinical hepatic encephalopathy (HE) or a PT $\geq$ 20 s or INR $\geq$ 2.0 regardless of the presence or absence of clinical hepatic encephalopathy (HE), (2) biochemical evidence of acute liver injury and (3) no known evidence of chronic liver disease [3]. Due to its simplicity and objectivity, PALF definition is widely used in children.

8.1.1 Coagulopathy

PALF has used INR as a surrogate marker to denote overall liver synthetic inadequacy and an impending multiorgan failure. Coagulopathy is not only a key criterion in diagnosing paediatric ALF but also helps as prognostic marker. Due to short half of several liver-based clotting factors, PT/INR functions as a dynamic marker of synthetic inadequacy due to loss of functioning hepatocytes in ALF. Factors II, VII, IX and X depend on vitamin K for carboxylation of terminal glutamic acid residues to convert them into active form (Fig. 8.1). Correction of coagulopathy by intravenous vitamin K differentiates between vitamin K deficiency due to decreased absorption and synthetic liver failure. Isolated prolonged APTR is not due to liver disease, as factor VII in extrinsic pathway (Fig. 8.1) has the shortest half-life of the

N. Shanmugam
Institute of Advanced Paediatrics, Dr. Rela Institute and Medical Centre, Chennai, India
e-mail: naresh.s@relainstitute.com

A. Dhawan (✉)
Paediatric Liver GI and Nutrition Center and Mowat Labs, King's College Hospital, London, UK
e-mail: anil.dhawan@nhs.net

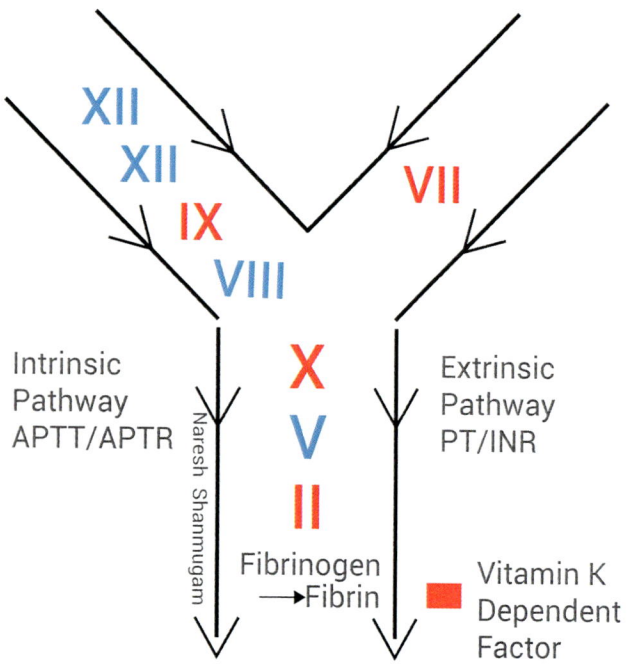

Fig. 8.1 The liver is the major site for synthesis of clotting factors, except for von Willebrand factor and tissue plasminogen activator. Factors V and VII are theoretically more sensitive markers than INR (Reproduced with permission from Shanmugam et al., Coagulopathy in liver disease, manual of paediatric liver intensive care) (Springer publication in print)

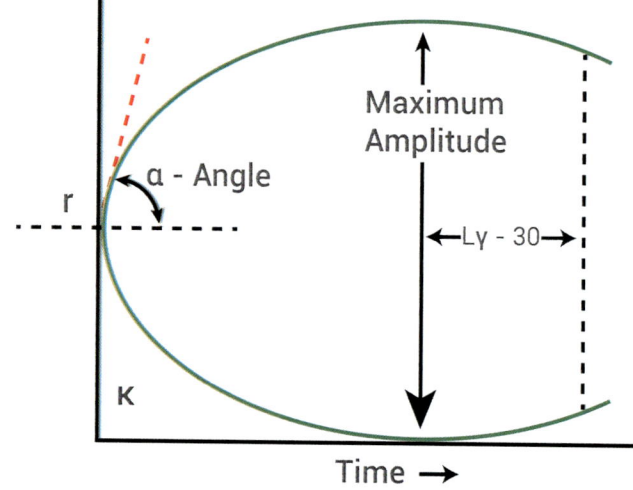

Fig. 8.2 Figure showing standard TEG in a normal person. Reaction time in minutes (r), time between beginning of the clotting cascade to the initial formation of fibrin; kinetic time in minutes (k), time between initial fibrin formation to reach a specific clot firmness; α-angle in degrees, deals with kinetics of clot formation, rate of fibrin formation and crosslinking of platelets. Maximum amplitude in mm, measures the maximum clot strength; clot lysis at 30 min (Ly-30; in percentage), percentage of clot dissolution within 30 min of maximum amplitude (Reproduced with permission from Shanmugam et al., Coagulopathy in liver disease, manual of paediatric liver intensive care) (Springer publication in print)

vitamin K-dependent factors; therefore, it is the first factor depleted in ALF and invariably affects INR. Due to defective synthesis and impaired clearance of procoagulant/anticoagulant factors, inflammatory mediators, infection, etc., there could be a degree of intravascular coagulation (IC) that invariably exists in ALF which can progress to fulminant disseminated intravascular coagulation. Haemostasis in liver disease is best assessed using thromboelastography (TEG). TEG is a point-of-care assay using a specialized machine that assesses clot formation in whole blood, including plasmatic and cellular components. TEG provides a graphical representation (Fig. 8.2) of assembly of a clot in whole blood and provides an assessment of overall haemostasis.

8.2 Aetiology

The causes of ALF vary with the age and geographical location. Infectious aetiology predominates as a cause of ALF in children in the developing countries, while drug-induced ALF predominates in adults and is indeterminate in children in Europe and North America [4]. Table 8.1 shows aetiology of 215 consecutive children with ALF, at King's College Hospital, London. ALF occurring during neonatal period differs from the rest of the age group by means of aetiology and prognosis [5]. Though exact frequency of ALF in the paediatric age group is unknown, overall annual incidence of ALF in the USA was around 5.5 million population among all ages [6]. Investigation of ALF in children is outlined in Table 8.2.

8.3 Drugs and Toxins

In developed countries drugs and toxins have become the most common identifiable cause of drug-induced acute liver failure in adults and children. Drug-induced liver injury (DILI) can be a dose-dependent response, an idiosyncratic reaction or a synergistic reaction when two medications are given together. It is essential to enquire about any indigenous/herbal medicine intake as some are potentially hepatotoxic [7]. Acetaminophen is the most common drug associated with ALF and is normally a dose-dependent hepatotoxic agent. Acetaminophen is detoxified mainly by glucuronidation (40%), sulphation (20–40%) and N-hydroxylation (15%). A small fraction is metabolized via cytochrome P450 to yield N-acetyl-para-benzoquinone-imide (NAPQI), a toxic intermediate compound which irreversibly conjugates with the sulphhydryl group of glutathione and causes hepatocyte necrosis [8]. NAPQI forms acetaminophen-protein adducts, which acts as a specific biomarker for chronic acetaminophen-related toxicity. In acute acetaminophen poisoning, serum levels after 4 h of ingestion are useful in identifying high-risk patients. Genetic polymorphism of cytochrome P450 isoenzymes could predispose affected

Table 8.1 Aetiological evaluation in paediatric liver failure

Aetiology	Investigations
Infective	
Hepatitis A	Anti-HAV IgM antibody
Hepatitis B	HBsAg, HBcAb(IgM), HBcAg
Hepatitis C	Anti-hep C antibody, hep C PCR
Hepatitis D	Anti-hep D antibody
Hepatitis E	Anti-HEV antibody(IgM)
Herpes simplex virus (neonates)	PCR
Cytomegalovirus, Epstein-Barr virus	PCR
Measles/varicella/adenovirus/echovirus	Serology/PCR (if needed)
Dengue/malaria/scrub typhus	Serology/microscopy in tropical countries
Blood, urine, stool, throat swab, sputum, skin lesion if present, ascitic fluid if present	Culture
Metabolic	
Galactosaemia	Galactose-1-phosphate uridyl transferase
Tyrosinaemia	Urinary succinylacetone
Fructose intolerance	Quantitative enzyme assay, q22.3 band mutation in chr 9
Mitochondrial disorders	Quantitative mitochondrial DNA assay, mutation analysis, lactate, lactate/pyruvate ratio, CK
Congenital disorders of glycosylation	Transferrin isoelectrophoresis
MCAD deficiency	Plasma acylcarnitine
Urea cycle defects	Ammonia, serum amino acid profile
Wilson's disease	Serum copper and ceruloplasmin 24-h urinary copper pre- and post-penicillamine
Autoimmune	Immunoglobulins Antinuclear antibodies Smooth muscle antibody Liver cytosol antibodies Soluble liver antigen Liver kidney microsomal antibody Antineutrophil cytoplasmic antibodies
Haematological malignancy	Bone marrow examination Ascitic or cerebrospinal fluid cytospin Genetics for HLH
Neonatal haemochromatosis	Serum ferritin MR of liver, pancreas Lip biopsy
Budd-Chiari syndrome	Ultrasound, echocardiography, computed tomography
Drugs and toxins	**History, drug levels**

(Reproduced with permission from Shanmugam et al., Acute liver failure in children: Management Protocol, manual of paediatric liver intensive care) (Springer publication in print)

HAV hepatitis A virus, *HEV* hepatitis E virus, *HBcAg* hepatitis B core antigen, *HBsAg* hepatitis B surface antigen, *HLH* haemophagocytic lymphohistiocytosis, *IgM* immunoglobulin M, *MR* magnetic resonance

Table 8.2 Aetiological evaluation in paediatric liver

Specific therapies for ALF
Autoimmune hepatitis: steroids (methylprednisolone 2 mg/kg/day, Max 60 mg/day)
Acetaminophen toxicity: *N*-acetylcysteine (100 mg/kg/day) until INR is normal
Mushroom poisoning: benzylpenicillin (1,000,000 U/kg/day) or thioctic acid (300 mg/kg/day)
Galactosaemia/hereditary fructose intolerance: elimination diet
Hereditary tyrosinaemia: NTBC (0.5 mg/kg bd) + elimination diet
Haemophagocytic lymphohistiocytosis: Chemotherapy ± haematopoietic stem cell transplantation (familial/genetically verified and persistent/reactivation of secondary HLH)
Neonatal haemochromatosis: Double volume exchange transfusion and intravenous immunoglobulin (1 g/kg)

(Reproduced with permission from Shanmugam et al., Acute liver failure in children: Management protocol, manual of paediatric liver intensive care) (Springer publication in print)

people to acetaminophen toxicity. Anti-tuberculosis drugs, particularly isoniazid, are associated with drug-induced ALF. The mechanism of toxicity is similar to acetaminophen; oxidation via cytochrome P450 pathway results in toxic metabolites.

The true incidence of idiosyncratic drug-induced liver injury (DILI) is unknown; reports have suggested to up to 14 new cases/100,000/year [9]. Around 8% of idiosyncratic DILI developed ALF [10]. DILI is unpredictable, but genetic susceptibility of an individual to certain drugs and underlying mitochondrial cytopathies are proposed causes [11]. The Councils for International Organizations of Medical Sciences/Roussel Uclaf Causality Assessment Method (CIOMS/RUCAM) scale is helpful in establishing causal relationship between offending drug and liver damage. Using the scoring system, suspected drug could be categorized into "definite or highly probable" (score > 8), "probable" (score 6–8), "possible" (score 3–5), "unlikely" (score 1–2) and "excluded" (score $\leq$ 0) [12]. This scale is helpful in identifying drug-induced hepatotoxicity even in newly marketed drugs and for a previously unreported older drug. Chemotherapy drugs are known to produce veno-occlusive disease leading on to ALF due to endothelial damage. Few of the common drugs that cause ALF are outlined in Table 8.2.

8.3.1 Viral Hepatitis

Water-borne viral hepatitis (hepatitis A and E) is the most common cause of ALF in developing countries with poor sanitation facilities. Following infection with hepatitis A virus, the risk of developing liver failure is 0.1–0.4%, and this further increases with underlying chronic liver disease. Usually the disease runs a benign course with spontaneous recovery, but some might require liver transplantation [13]. With hepatitis E infection, the risk of developing ALF in adults is 0.6–2.8% [14]. Recent evidence suggests that case fatality due to hepatitis E-induced ALF in pregnancy is similar to that of age-matched general population [15]. The ALF due to hepatitis B virus (HBV) can occur at the time of acute infection, reactivation of chronic HBV infection or seroconversion from a hepatitis B e antigen-positive to a hepatitis B e antibody (HBeAb)-positive state. Superinfection or co-infection of HBV-infected patients with hepatitis delta virus (HDV) can cause liver failure.

Hepatitis C virus (HCV) infection has not been reported as a cause of ALF, and herpes simplex virus can cause ALF, of which herpes simplex virus 1 and 2 (HSV) is the predominant cause of viral-induced ALF during the first month of life.

Babies presenting with fever, rash, lethargy, poor feeding and raised transaminase (in thousands) are usually suggestive of HSV hepatitis. Disseminated neonatal herpes with liver failure carries high mortality. In stable neonates with ALF due to HSV, liver transplantation has been successful. Treatment with high-dose acyclovir should be initiated in all neonates with ALF, until serology results are known. Other members of herpes virus family such as cytomegalovirus, Epstein-Barr virus and varicella-zoster virus can cause ALF. Dengue virus causing ALF is common in tropical countries, which was thought to be multifactorial due to direct viral injury, dysregulated immune response, hypoxic/ischemic injury secondary to shock, etc. [16].

8.4 Neonatal Haemochromatosis

Neonatal haemochromatosis (NH) is the single most common cause of ALF during the first month of life, due to massive iron deposition in the liver and extrahepatic tissues with sparing of the reticuloendothelial system. NH presents with jaundice, coagulopathy, moderately elevated alanine aminotransferase, high ferritin and raised iron saturation levels. The disease varies in severity; at one end of spectrum, it is associated with foetal death, while at the other end, spontaneous recovery is reported.

The pattern of iron overloading is similar to hereditary haemochromatosis, but NH is entirely different condition affecting newborn, and so far no specific genetic mutation has been identified [17]. Current hypothesis suggests NH to be an alloimmune process where maternal antibody is directed towards foetal liver cells resulting in hepatocyte loss [18, 19]. This hypothesis is supported by successful prevention of severe disease by antenatal and postnatal treatment with intravenous immunoglobulin. High serum ferritin is a non-specific marker and elevated in other causes of ALF and so should not be used a marker for diagnosis. The diagnosis could be safely confirmed by labial salivary gland biopsy, showing extrahepatic iron deposits with reticuloendothelial system sparing [20].

8.5 Metabolic Disorders

Metabolic disorders are important cause of ALF in paediatric population particularly during infancy. Galactosaemia, tyrosinaemia type I and fructosaemia are few of the metabolic disorders that could present as ALF. Tyrosinaemia type I is an inborn error of amino acid metabolism, due to absence of enzyme fumarylacetoacetase, the last enzyme in a series of five enzymes needed to break down tyrosine. This results in formation of intermediate compounds, maleylacetoacetic acid and fumarylacetoacetic acid, which is converted to succinylacetone, a toxin that damages the liver and kidneys. Oral NTBC (nitro-4-trifluoromethylbenzoyl-1,3-cyclohexanedione) and phenylalanine- and tyrosine-free diet could help liver recovery, but some children might require LT. Galactosaemia type 1 is autosomal recessive disorder with mutation in galactose-1-phosphate uridyl transferase (GALT) gene located on chromosome 9p13. Lactose-free diet should be started in any infant presenting with ALF or hepatitis until the quantitative GALT activity is available. Galactose-free diet and supportive treatment may allow recovery of ALF. Rarely inborn errors of bile acid synthesis can present as ALF.

Mitochondrial disorders are group of spontaneous or inherited disorders of mitochondrial proteins resulting in defective oxidative phosphorylation, fatty acid oxidation, urea cycle and other mitochondrial pathways [21]. Deficiencies of complexes I, III and IV, multiple complex deficiencies and mitochondrial DNA (mtDNA) depletion syndrome are associated with liver failure. Diagnosis might be difficult due to particularly (mtDNA) depletion syndrome where there is tissue-specific mitochondrial enzyme deficiency. These infants usually present with hypotonia, hypoglycaemia, feeding difficulties, seizures and deranged liver function. Liver transplantation could be done in isolated liver-based mitochondrial disorders, and it is usually contradicted in multisystemic involvement [22]. Sasaki et al. have reported 78% survival in a cohort of nine children with mitochondrial respiratory chain disorder, which included children with extrahepatic manifestation such as developmental delay and failure to thrive [23].

Medium-chain acyl-coenzyme A dehydrogenases (MCAD) are group of enzymes involved in β-oxidation of 6–12 carbon chain fatty acids in mitochondria. Affected children could present with hypoketotic hypoglycaemia and recurrent liver failure, precipitated by otherwise minor illness. Unless treated with dextrose supplementation, these episodes may quickly progress to coma and death.

Wilson's disease, an autosomal recessive disorder, could present as ALF. The acute hepatic presentation is usually characterized by the presence of liver failure, Coombs-negative haemolytic anaemia and low serum alkaline phosphatase. Diagnosis might be difficult in acute presentation as blood test might show weakly positive autoantibodies, and tissue copper estimation might not be possible due to coagulopathy. New Wilson index proposed by Dhawan et al. used five parameters such as serum bilirubin, serum albumin, international normalized ratio, aspartate aminotransferase (AST) and white cell count (WCC) at presentation. Based on serum levels, each parameter is graded from 0 to 4, with a total maximum score of 20. They identified a cutoff score of more than 11 for death without transplantation and proved to be 93% sensitive and 98% specific, with a positive predictive value of 88% [24].

8.6 Malignancies

Haemophagocytic lymphohistiocytosis (HLH) is a type of haematological malignancy that could present as ALF in children. HLH is due to paradoxical overactivation of natural killer cells and of CD8+ T-cell lymphocytes resulting in destruction of own haemopoietic cells. It could be familial (inherited) or acquired. Familial HLH usually presents during infancy, while secondary HLH usually occurs after systemic infection or immunodeficiency, which can affect people at any age. Familial HLH is an autosomal recessive disease resulting in reduced or defective production of cytoplasmic granules such as perforin in cytotoxic cells resulting in paradoxical overactivation. HLH presents with fever, cutaneous rash, hepatosplenomegaly, pancytopenia and, in severe cases, ALF [25]. Though rare, leukaemia or lymphoma could present with ALF [26].

Other causes: Autoimmune hepatitis (AIH), particularly type 2 (positive liver-kidney microsomal (LKM) antibody), can present with ALF. ALF due to AIH with encephalopathy usually does not respond to any form of immunosuppression and needs urgent liver transplant [27]. In spite of extensive investigation, the diagnosis could not be found in some of the children (indeterminate). There is centre-to-centre variation in incidence of indeterminate ALF, probably due to incomplete investigations, which has been highlighted by Narkewicz et al. [28].

8.7 Investigations

General investigation should include liver function tests, serum electrolytes, uric acid, lactate, cholesterol/triglyceride, amylase, serum amino acids, blood gas analysis, blood glucose levels, full blood count, blood grouping, Coombs test coagulation studies (INR), urinary amino/organic acids and toxicology screen along with surveillance blood and urine cultures. In liver function tests, coagulation should be checked on regular basis that helps in monitoring the progression of disease. Investigations to establish the underlying aetiology are listed in Table 8.2. Detailed clinical history and physical examination give valuable clue of underlying diagnosis. This would provide guidance in choosing appropriate investigations.

8.8 Prognosis

Transplant-free survival is aetiology dependent. Age of patient was not associated with outcome in adults [29], while in children, neonates have worst prognosis (Fig. 8.2), probably due to predominance of certain aetiology in different age groups. Prognostic scoring helps in predicting mortality and helps in listing appropriate patients for transplantation.

For non-acetaminophen ALF, several prognostic scoring systems are available for adults, but in children there are no universally accepted criteria for listing. To date, INR and factor V concentration remain the best indicators of mortality without transplantation in paediatric ALF. Bhaduri and Mieli-Vergani showed that the maximum INR reached during the course of illness was the most sensitive predictor of the outcome, with 73% of children with an INR less than 4 surviving compared with only 4 of 24 (16.6%) with an INR greater than 4 [2]. In children, a factor V concentration of less than 25% of normal suggests a poor outcome. A prognostic score incorporating serum bilirubin, serum albumin, international normalized ratio, aspartate aminotransferase (AST) and white cell count (WCC) is available predicting the outcome of decompensated Wilson's disease [24]. In acetaminophen overdose adult criteria of INR > 6.5, creatinine > 300 μmol/L and hyperphosphatemia or metabolic acidosis arterial pH less than 7.3, after the second day of overdose in adequately hydrated patients, is used to list children for liver transplantation [30].

8.9 Management

Management of ALF and its complications still remains a challenge. Early diagnosis helps in initiation of investigation and safe transfer to a specialist centre. Diagnostic algorithm for any child with abnormal liver function test is outlined in Fig. 8.3.

8.10 General Measures

All children with ALF should be closely monitored in a quiet setting. Vital parameters such as oxygen saturation, pulse, blood pressure and neurologic observations should be done on regular basis. Prophylactic broad-spectrum antibiotics and antifungals should be started in all children, and acyclovir should be added in infants and neonates. Hypoglycaemia should be avoided either by parenteral glucose or adequate enteral feeds. Children with encephalopathy or an INR > 4 (regardless of encephalopathy) should be admitted to an intensive care unit for continuous monitoring. Prophylactic histamine 2 blockers or proton-pump inhibitors should be started to all patients requiring mechanical ventilation [31]. Coagulopathy is corrected only if the patient is already listed for transplant or prior to an invasive procedure. To correct coagulopathy, fresh frozen plasma could be given at a dose of 10 mL/kg and cryoprecipitate at 5 mL/kg (if fibrinogen is <1 g/L). Factor VII concentrates improve the coagulopathy for a short period. Platelet count should be maintained above 50×10^9/dL, as thrombocytopenia is an important risk factor for haemorrhage.

N-acetylcysteine (NAC) is being increasingly used as a part of general supportive measure in non-acetaminophen-induced ALF, as it enhances circulation and improves oxygen delivery. In a prospective, double-blind trial in adults with non-acetaminophen ALF, NAC usage is associated with significant improvement in transplant-free survival in patients with early (stage I–II) coma [32]. A similar study in children failed to show any benefit, and Paediatric Acute Liver Failure study group does not recommend routine use of

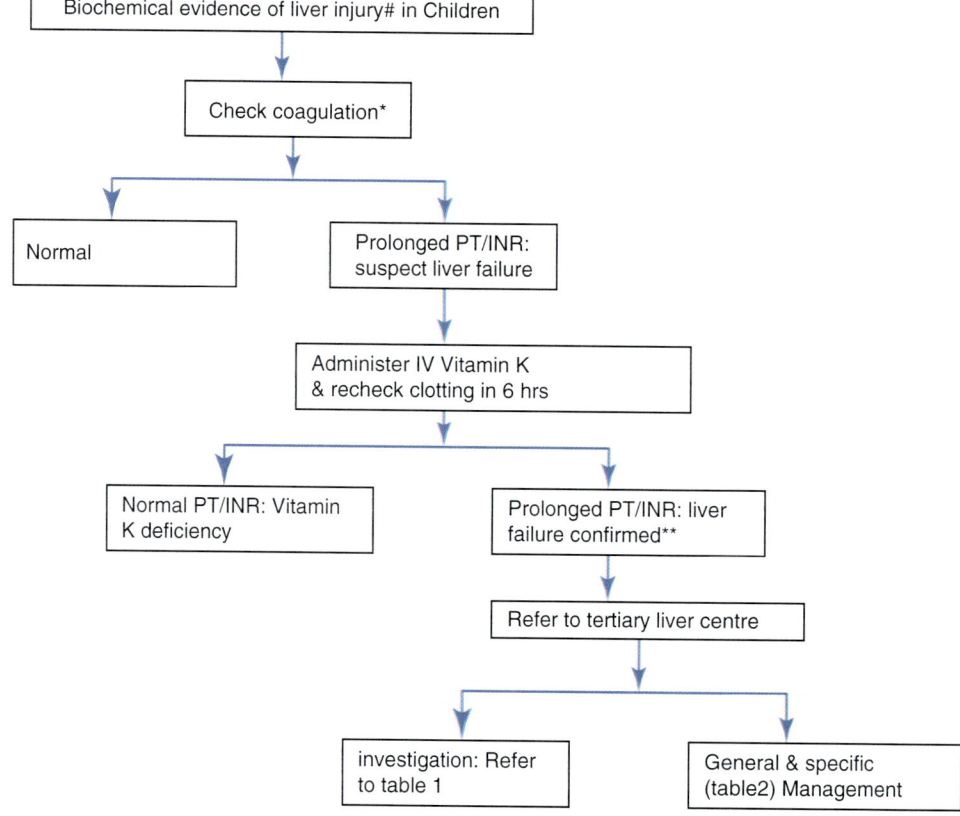

Fig. 8.3 Approach to children with biochemical evidence of liver injury (Reproduced with permission from Shanmugam et al., Neonatal liver failure: aetiologies and management state of the art. Eur J Pediatr. 2011 May; 170(5):573–81). # Raised alanine aminotransferase (ALT), bilirubin, gamma-glutamyltransferase (GGT). *Check prothrombin time (PT)/international normalized ratio (INR), activated partial thromboplastin ratio (APTR), fibrinogen and d-dimers. Isolated prolonged APTR is not due to liver disease. In disseminated intravascular coagulopathy (DIC), there will be low fibrinogen levels and increased d-dimers. **INR ≥ 1.5 with encephalopathy or INR ≥ 2.0 regardless of the presence or absence of encephalopathy

NAC in non-acetaminophen-induced ALF in children [33]. Bowel cleansing agents and benzodiazepine antagonists are of no proven benefit [34].

8.11 Airway and Ventilation

Elective intubation and mechanical ventilation should be considered for patients with grade 3/4 encephalopathy. Apart from providing secure airway, sedation and controlled ventilation help in reducing sudden variation of intracranial pressure (ICP). Induction using suxamethonium and fentanyl and combination of morphine or fentanyl with a hypnotic such as midazolam for sedation is usually safe in children. Normocapnia is to be maintained, as hypercapnia causes vasodilatation and increases cerebral congestion, while hypocapnia causes vasoconstriction and thus decreased blood flow to the brain.

8.12 Fluid Management and Renal Failure

Intravenous fluids should be restricted to two-thirds maintenance, with the idea of decreasing the possibility of development of cerebral oedema. Ultrasonic cardiac output monitor (USCOM), which is a non-invasive method to measure cardiac parameters, helps in decision-making regarding appropriate fluid regimens/inotropes even in small infants. In the presence of persistent hypotension, noradrenaline is the inotropic agent of choice. Continuous filtration or dialysis systems should be considered when the urine output is less than 1 mL/kg/h to prevent acidosis and volume overload.

8.13 Neurologic Complications

The most serious complications of ALF are cerebral oedema with resultant encephalopathy and intracranial hypertension, progressively leading on to brain herniation and death. Systemic hypertension, bradycardia, hypertonia, hyperreflexia and in extreme cases decerebrate or decorticate posturing are clinical features of raised ICP. Ammonia-lowering measures such as dietary protein restriction, bowel decontamination or lactulose are of limited or no value in rapidly advancing encephalopathy. Mannitol is an osmotic diuretic commonly used to treat intracranial hypertension. A rapid bolus of 0.5 g/kg as a 20% solution over a 15-min period is recommended, and the dose can be repeated if the serum osmolarity is less than 320 mOsm/L. Hypertonic saline could be also used in emergency situation, where there is impending brainstem herniation. Studies have shown mild cerebral hypothermia (32–35 °C), sodium thiopental and hypernatremia (serum sodium > 145 mmol/L) improves cerebral perfusion.

8.14 Disease-Specific Management

Disease-specific management is outlined in Table 8.2. Intravenous immunoglobulin (IVIG) at a dose of 1 g/kg body weight given weekly from the 18th week until the end of gestation as antenatal prophylaxis to mothers whose previous pregnancy/child was affected with NH has been associated with milder phenotypic expression of the disease and 100% survival of babies [35]. Evidence is accumulating towards the usefulness of high-dose IVIG (1 g/kg), in combination with exchange transfusion resulting in significant decrease in the need for liver transplantation in NH. Dietary intervention with restriction of phenylalanine and tyrosine together with oral medication, 2(2-nitro-4-trifluoromethylbenzoyl)-1,3-cyclohexenedione (NTBC), helps in normalization of liver function, but doesn't prevent long-term risk for development of hepatocellular carcinoma in children started beyond infancy.

8.15 Plasmapheresis/Plasma Exchange in ALF

Plasmapheresis is the removal or exchange of blood plasma. Therapeutic plasmapheresis and therapeutic plasma exchange (TPE) are terms that are often used synonymously. TPE has been increasingly used over the past decade as a first-line and lifesaving treatment for various conditions classified by the American Society for Apheresis (ASFA). In acute fulminant Wilson's disease, it can rapidly remove significant amount of copper and, thereby, reduce haemolysis, prevent progression to renal failure and provide clinical stabilization. It has been reported to be used as a bridge to LT or can lead to elimination of the need for urgent LT. TPE is also helpful in stabilizing ALF due to viral hepatitis, drug-induced hepatitis, etc. by removing albumin-bound toxins, large molecular weight toxins, aromatic amino acids, ammonia, endotoxin, indols, mercaptans, phenols, etc.

8.16 Liver Assist Devices

Simple liver assist devices detoxify blood by simple osmotic diffusion, while bioartificial liver support system which contains human or animal liver cells could perform complex synthetic function and detoxifying and detoxification. These devices have shown to decrease the toxins (ammonia, bilirubin, cytokines, etc.) but have no effect on mortality. Successful use of these devices in children with ALF as a bridge therapy, supporting liver function while the native liver regenerates, is not recommended outside research setting.

8.17 Liver Transplantation

Liver transplant remains the only proven treatment that has improved the outcome of ALF. Appropriate patient selection and timing of transplantation are essential for graft and patient survival. Several surgical techniques such split liver grafts, reduced grafts and auxiliary liver transplants are practiced, depending upon patient size, organ availability and surgical expertise available. Auxiliary liver transplant is a surgical technique where the donor liver is placed alongside of native liver and the allograft supports the entire liver function, while the native liver regenerates. Either left lateral segment or right lobe allograft could be used, based on recipient weight. Once native liver regeneration is optimal [36], then immunosuppression could be weaned and eventually stopped. In a series from King's College Hospital, of the 20 children who received auxiliary liver transplantation for ALF, immunosuppression was withdrawn successfully in 11 patients at a median time of 23 months after transplantation [37]. This would be an ideal option in ALF due to indeterminate aetiology, as spontaneous regeneration of native liver remains a possibility.

Liver transplantation is indicated in ALF due to liver-based disorders while contraindicated in haematological malignancies, uncontrolled sepsis, systemic mitochondrial/metabolic disorders and severe respiratory failure (ARDS) [38]. Relative contraindications are increasing inotropic requirements, infection under treatment, cerebral perfusion pressure of less than 40 mmHg for more than 2 h and a history of progressive or severe neurologic problems.

Hepatocyte transplantation, where hepatocytes are infused intraportally into the patient's liver, has been tried with variable success in certain liver-based metabolic disorders [39]. Research is underway to use alginate-encapsulated hepatocytes, which could be injected intraperitoneally. This could act as a bridge until native liver regenerates. Hepatocyte transplantation is not recommended outside research setting.

8.18 Conclusion

Improved intensive care management has greatly increased the ALF survival. When compared to adult ALF, the spectrum of underlying aetiology, management and outcome varies in paediatric ALF. Acyclovir should be started in all neonates with ALF along with prophylactic antibiotics, until viral cultures are negative. Liver transplantation is the only definitive treatment that improves survival in paediatric ALF. Wilson's disease and autoimmune liver disease presenting as ALF usually do not respond to medical management and warrant liver transplantation. Liver assist devices and hepatocyte transplantation are potential emerging therapies in paediatric ALF.

References

1. Trey C, Davidson CS. The management of fulminant hepatic failure. Prog Liver Dis. 1970;3:282–98.
2. Bhaduri BR, Mieli-Vergani G. Fulminant hepatic failure: pediatric aspects. Semin Liver Dis. 1996;16(4):349–55.
3. Squires RH Jr, et al. Acute liver failure in children: the first 348 patients in the pediatric acute liver failure study group. J Pediatr. 2006;148(5):652–8.
4. Alam S, et al. Profile and outcome of first 109 cases of paediatric acute liver failure at a specialized paediatric liver unit in India. Liver Int. 2017;37(10):1508–14.
5. Shanmugam NP, et al. Neonatal liver failure: aetiologies and management—state of the art. Eur J Pediatr. 2011;170(5):573–81.
6. Bower WA, et al. Population-based surveillance for acute liver failure. Am J Gastroenterol. 2007;102(11):2459–63.
7. Larrey D. [Hepatotoxicity of drugs and chemicals]. Gastroenterol Clin Biol. 2009;33(12):1136–46.
8. Davis M. Protective agents for acetaminophen overdose. Semin Liver Dis. 1986;6(2):138–47.
9. Bjornsson E. Review article: drug-induced liver injury in clinical practice. Aliment Pharmacol Ther. 2010;32(1):3–13.
10. Idilman R, et al. The characteristics and clinical outcome of drug-induced liver injury: a single-center experience. J Clin Gastroenterol. 2010;44(6):e128–32.
11. Ghabril M, Chalasani N, Bjornsson E. Drug-induced liver injury: a clinical update. Curr Opin Gastroenterol. 2010;26(3):222–6.
12. Andrade RJ, et al. Assessment of drug-induced hepatotoxicity in clinical practice: a challenge for gastroenterologists. World J Gastroenterol. 2007;13(3):329–40.
13. Ciocca M, et al. Prognostic factors in paediatric acute liver failure. Arch Dis Child. 2008;93(1):48–51.
14. Krawczynski K, Kamili S, Aggarwal R. Global epidemiology and medical aspects of hepatitis E. Forum (Genova). 2001;11(2):166–79.
15. Bhatia V, et al. A 20-year single-center experience with acute liver failure during pregnancy: is the prognosis really worse? Hepatology. 2008;48(5):1577–85.
16. Samanta J, Sharma V. Dengue and its effects on liver. World J Clin Cases. 2015;3(2):125–31.
17. Hardy L, et al. Neonatal hemochromatosis. Genetic analysis of transferrin-receptor, H-apoferritin, and L-apoferritin loci and of the human leukocyte antigen class I region. Am J Pathol. 1990;137(1):149–53.
18. Whitington PF, Malladi P. Neonatal hemochromatosis: is it an alloimmune disease? J Pediatr Gastroenterol Nutr. 2005;40(5):544–9.
19. Pan X, et al. Novel mechanism of fetal hepatocyte injury in congenital alloimmune hepatitis involves the terminal complement cascade. Hepatology. 2010;51(6):2061–8.
20. Smith SR, et al. Minor salivary gland biopsy in neonatal hemochromatosis. Arch Otolaryngol Head Neck Surg. 2004;130(6):760–3.
21. Treem WR, Sokol RJ. Disorders of the mitochondria. Semin Liver Dis. 1998;18(3):237–53.
22. Dhawan A, Mieli-Vergani G. Liver transplantation for mitochondrial respiratory chain disorders: to be or not to be? Transplantation. 2001;71(5):596–8.
23. Sasaki K, et al. Liver transplantation for mitochondrial respiratory chain disorder: a single-center experience and excellent marker of differential diagnosis. Transplant Proc. 2017;49(5):1097–102.
24. Dhawan A, et al. Wilson's disease in children: 37-year experience and revised King's score for liver transplantation. Liver Transpl. 2005;11(4):441–8.
25. Henter JI, et al. HLH-2004: diagnostic and therapeutic guidelines for hemophagocytic lymphohistiocytosis. Pediatr Blood Cancer. 2007;48(2):124–31.
26. Kader A, et al. Leukaemia presenting with fulminant hepatic failure in a child. Eur J Pediatr. 2004;163(10):628–9.

27. Mieli-Vergani G, Vergani D. Autoimmune paediatric liver disease. World J Gastroenterol. 2008;14(21):3360–7.
28. Narkewicz MR, et al. Pattern of diagnostic evaluation for the causes of pediatric acute liver failure: an opportunity for quality improvement. J Pediatr. 2009;155(6):801–6.e1.
29. Ostapowicz G, et al. Results of a prospective study of acute liver failure at 17 tertiary care centers in the United States. Ann Intern Med. 2002;137(12):947–54.
30. O'Grady JG, et al. Early indicators of prognosis in fulminant hepatic failure. Gastroenterology. 1989;97(2):439–45.
31. Polson J, Lee WM. AASLD position paper: the management of acute liver failure. Hepatology. 2005;41(5):1179–97.
32. Koch A, Trautwein C. N-acetylcysteine on its way to a broader application in patients with acute liver failure. Hepatology. 2010;51(1):338–40.
33. Squires RH, et al. Intravenous N-acetylcysteine in pediatric patients with nonacetaminophen acute liver failure: a placebo-controlled clinical trial. Hepatology. 2013;57(4):1542–9.
34. Cochran JB, Losek JD. Acute liver failure in children. Pediatr Emerg Care. 2007;23(2):129–35.
35. Whitington PF, Hibbard JU. High-dose immunoglobulin during pregnancy for recurrent neonatal haemochromatosis. Lancet. 2004;364(9446):1690–8.
36. Dhawan A. Clinical human hepatocyte transplantation: current status and challenges. Liver Transpl. 2015;21(Suppl 1):S39–44.
37. Faraj W, et al. Auxiliary liver transplantation for acute liver failure in children. Ann Surg. 2010;251(2):351–6.
38. Strom SC, et al. Hepatocyte transplantation as a bridge to orthotopic liver transplantation in terminal liver failure. Transplantation. 1997;63(4):559–69.
39. Forbes SJ, Gupta S, Dhawan A. Cell therapy for liver disease: from liver transplantation to cell factory. J Hepatol. 2015;62(1 Suppl):S157–69.

Chronic Viral Hepatitis

Giuseppe Indolfi and Lorenzo D'Antiga

Key Points

HBV
- HBV infection acquired in childhood is often a chronic infection.
- Regular monitoring of liver function tests, serological tests and HBV deoxyribonucleic acid level is mandatory to evaluate the possible evolution of the infection.
- The therapies currently available for treatment of chronic HBV infection in children can obtain effective long-term suppression of viral replication but are largely ineffective towards obtaining virological cure and elimination of the infection.

HCV
- Direct-acting antivirals active against HCV can efficiently cure the infection after a short course of treatment (8–12 weeks).
- The fixed-dose combination of ledipasvir/sofosbuvir has been approved by the Food and Drug Administration and the European Medicines Agency for treatment of children older than 12 years of age and infected by HCV genotype 1, 4 and 5.
- The combination of sofosbuvir and ribavirin has been approved by the Food and Drug Administration and the European Medicines Agency for treatment of children older than 12 years of age and infected by HCV genotype 2 and 3.
- Interferon-based treatments are no longer recommended for treatment of children with chronic HCV infection.

Research Needed in the Field
- Up-to-date prevalence of HBsAg and HCV antibodies in children according to different age cohorts and world regions
- Establish a consensus on when to start treatment in HBV-infected children
- Development of new HBV curative treatment strategies to eliminate all replicative forms, including covalently closed circular DNA form in the nucleus
- Evaluation of effectiveness and safety of long-term use of nucleos(t)ide analogues regimens in different paediatric populations
- Development of direct-acting antivirals in children across all paediatric ages

9.1 Hepatitis B Virus

9.1.1 Epidemiology

9.1.1.1 Burden of Hepatitis B Virus Infection

According to the World Health Organization (WHO), globally, in 2015, 257 million people were living with chronic hepatitis B virus (HBV) infection [1, 2]. Prevalence of HBV infection (as measured by HBsAg positivity) in the general population varies by geographical region being highest (>6%) in the WHO Western Pacific and African regions, followed by intermediate prevalence (2–3.5%) in Southeast Asia and East Mediterranean regions and by lower prevalence in Europe and the Americas [2]. Chronic HBV infection (CHB) is associated with significant morbidity and mortality. Around 20–30% of the people with CHB will develop complications such as cirrhosis and hepatocellular carcinoma (HCC). More than half of all liver cancers are the consequence of HBV infection. Worldwide, it is estimated that around 890,000 people die each year from the complications of CHB [2].

To my Family

G. Indolfi (✉)
Meyer Children's University Hospital, Firenze, Italy
e-mail: giuseppe.indolfi@meyer.it

L. D'Antiga
Paediatric Hepatology, Gastroenterology and Transplantation, Hospital Papa Giovanni XXIII, Bergamo, Italy
e-mail: ldantiga@asst-pg23.it

© Springer Nature Switzerland AG 2019
L. D'Antiga (ed.), *Pediatric Hepatology and Liver Transplantation*, https://doi.org/10.1007/978-3-319-96400-3_9

The only paediatric estimation of the prevalence of HBV infection is available for children under 5 years of age, and it was about 1.3% in 2015 [2]. Data for older paediatric age cohorts are missing. Geographical distribution for children is similar to adults with the highest prevalence in the African region. In high-income countries where adult seroprevalence is below 2%, HBsAg positivity in patients under 18 years of age is rare [1, 2] due to the widespread use of infant vaccination [2] although in these settings there is experience of an increasing number of infected children migrating from countries with high prevalence of the infection [3, 4].

9.1.1.2 Routes of Transmission

Routes of transmission of HBV infection are summarized in Table 9.1. Worldwide and especially in high prevalence regions, mother-to-child transmission (MTCT) and horizontal transmission during early childhood are the main mechanisms by which HBV is transmitted [1, 5–7]. In countries where prevention of MTCT through infant vaccination has been implemented, the infection is acquired mainly in adulthood. Adults at high risk of acquiring the infection are unvaccinated persons injecting drug use, men who have sex with men, sex workers and unvaccinated persons with multiple sex partners [1, 8–10]. In these countries, only a minority of vaccinated children could get the infection as a consequence of intrauterine transmission or of immunoprophylaxis regimen failure [11]. Since the introduction of donor screening and blood testing for blood-borne pathogens in most countries worldwide, the incidence of post-transfusion hepatitis B is very low (1 in 500,000 per unit exposure) [12]. The extent of horizontal transmission which includes transmissions due to traditional practices and transmission due to poor injection safety during medical and surgical procedures is uncertain.

9.1.1.3 Prevention of MTCT

The risk of vertical transmission, in the absence of any intervention, has been estimated to be 10–40% from HBsAg-positive, HBeAg-negative mothers and 70–90% for HBsAg- and HBeAg-positive mothers [13]. The administration of monovalent hepatitis B vaccine within 24 hours of birth followed by completion of the HBV vaccine series with two more doses within 6–12 months has been demonstrated to be 90–95% effective in preventing the infection [11, 14,

Table 9.1 Routes of transmission of hepatitis B virus infection

Vertical
Mother-to-child transmission
Horizontal transmission among unvaccinated persons
Sexual with higher risk for people with multiple sexual partners and men who have sex with men
Unsafe injections
Unscreened or inadequately screened transfusions or dialysis
Traditional practices

15]. Including a dose of hepatitis B immune globulin (HBIG) at birth to infants can further reduce the risk of transmission to less than 5% [16].

Despite active-passive immunization (vaccine + HBIG), residual transmission may occur from HBV-infected mothers [17] due to transplacental/intrauterine infection or immunoprophylaxis regimen failure [17, 18]. HBeAg-positive mothers with high circulating concentrations of HBV DNA (>10^6 IU/m) are at highest risk of MTCT of HBV [17, 19]. The use of lamivudine, telbivudine or tenofovir [20–22] during third trimester of pregnancy in highly viraemic, HBeAg-positive mothers in combination with standard active-passive immunization to the infant was demonstrated to be effective in further preventing MTCT of HBV with over 70% reductions in the rates of infant HBsAg and HBV deoxyribonucleic acid (DNA) positivity at 6–12 months postpartum [18–22]. In a recent meta-analysis of 26 studies that enrolled 3622 pregnant women, antiviral therapy reduced MTCT when defined as infant HBsAg seropositivity by a risk ratio of 0.3 (95% confidence interval 0.2–0.4) and when defined as infant HBV DNA seropositivity by a risk ratio of 0.3 (95% confidence interval 0.2–0.5) at 6–12 months [22].

9.1.2 Aetiology

HBV is a double-stranded DNA virus, member of the *Hepadnaviridae* family, of the genus *Orthohepadnavirus*. The genetic variability of HBV is very high. There are at least eight major genotypes of HBV labelled A through H. Genotypes are divided into sub-genotypes with distinct virological and epidemiological properties.

9.1.3 Pathophysiology

The pathogenesis and clinical manifestations of HBV infection are due to the interaction of the virus and the host immune system. The immune system attacks HBV and causes liver injury that is the result of an immunologic reaction when activated CD4+ and CD8+ lymphocytes recognize various HBV-derived peptides on the surface of the hepatocytes. Impaired immune reactions (e.g. cytokine release, antibody production) or a relatively tolerant immune status results in chronic hepatitis. Age is a key factor in determining the risk of chronic infection. This is because the immune response to the virus of neonates, infants and children younger than 5 years is physiologically weaker than adults [23]. Young children, being more immune-tolerant, are more likely to develop chronic infection [24–27]. Chronicity rate has been estimated to be 90% for neonates born to HBeAg-positive mothers, 25–30% for children under the age of 5 and less than 5% for adolescents and adults [26–28] (Fig. 9.1).

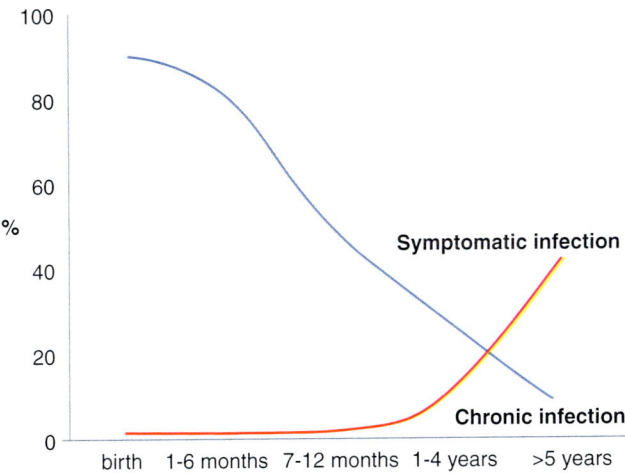

Fig. 9.1 Outcomes of hepatitis B virus infection by age at infection (modified from [71])

Basing on the result of the interplay between the virus and the immune system, HBV can cause acute and chronic infection ranging from asymptomatic infection or mild disease to severe or fulminant hepatitis. The natural history of CHB is dynamic and progresses non-linearly through several recognizable phases of variable duration, which are not necessarily sequential [26, 29]. Historically, the terms "immune-tolerant", "immune-active", "immune-control" and "immune-escape" have been used to describe these different phases, but it is increasingly recognized that these descriptions are not fully supported by immunological data and do not always relate directly to criteria and indications for antiviral therapy. The new accepted nomenclature is now based on the description of infection (characterized by normal aminotransferase) or hepatitis (with raised aminotransferases) and on HBeAg status of the patient. Table 9.2 summarises the revised definitions of the phases of CHB [30].

9.1.3.1 Natural History of Hepatitis B in Children

When hepatitis B is acquired in infancy and childhood, it is likely to lead to chronic asymptomatic infection [25, 31–42]. Only 5–10% of the children develop and resolve acute infection that, although can be associated with severe symptoms in adults [43], is usually asymptomatic in vertically infected children [25, 44]. Children with CHB are expected to be asymptomatic with no clinically detectable sign of liver disease although CHB may lead to progressive liver disease and development of cirrhosis and HCC.

The natural history of CHB in children has been depicted by few large and long-term prospective studies [25, 31–36, 45] with additional data from smaller prospective and retrospective studies [37–42]. Children acquiring HBV infection vertically usually experience a high replicative, low inflammatory phase of long duration. The exact duration of this phase is unpredictable, but it is affected by the route of HBV infection acquisition (it lasts longer in subjects who acquired HBV vertically than in those infected horizontally), by environmental factors such as nutritional status and by viral genotype (HBV genotype C infection is associated with delayed spontaneous seroconversion). In the 29-year longitudinal study from Italy, 89 of the 91 HBeAg-positive children underwent HBeAg seroconversion (i.e. the loss of HBeAg with the appearance of anti-HBe), and the median age of onset of the HBeAg-positive hepatitis phase after vertical infection was 30 years [25]. Overall, across different studies around 90% of children less than 15 years of age are still HBeAg positive, and only a minority of the children infected vertically presents HBeAg seroconversion spontaneously before puberty. In the HBeAg-positive hepatitis phase, aminotransferases are elevated and HBV DNA levels start to decrease. It is noteworthy that in this phase, active inflammation can be found in the liver with necrosis of the parenchyma that can develop into fibrosis over time.

Spontaneous HBeAg/anti-HBe seroconversion leads to the entry in the HBeAg-negative infection phase that is characterized by normalization of aminotransferases, absent or low viral replication, with low (<2000 IU/mL or <10^4 copies/mL) or undetectable HBV DNA and inactive liver histology. Regression of liver fibrosis has been described in this phase, and, in the long term, around 15% of the patients in this phase became anti-HBs positive marking the resolution of HBV infection. In these patients the overall prognosis is good if cirrhosis has not developed before anti-e and anti-s seroconversion.

Low-level HBV replication with detectable HBV DNA in the liver may persist in patients who became anti-HBs positive. Few patients (5%) in the HBeAg-negative infection phase can experience the selection of precore mutants leading to HBeAg-negative hepatitis with persistent viral replication and abnormal aminotransferases that is histologically active. The precore mutation, a G3A mutation at codon 1896 that results in the occurrence of a stop codon, makes the virus unable to encode for HBeAg leading to HBV replication uncontrolled by the host's immune system. There is overwhelming evidence from different studies that basal core promoter mutations are independent risk factors for the development of active liver disease and HCC. Finally, in patients in the HBeAg-negative infection phase who undergoes immune-suppression phase reactivations characterized by a rise in HBV DNA, high aminotransferases and hepatic necroinflammatory changes on liver biopsies with or without reverse seroconversion to HBeAg and HBsAg positivity are possible. HBV reactivation may be explained by the persistence of low-level HBV replication in the liver and/or by the presence of covalently closed circular DNA in the nucleus of infected hepatocytes.

Overall, the development of cirrhosis during childhood has been described in 1–5% of HBeAg-positive children

Table 9.2 Phases in natural history of chronic hepatitis B virus infection [30]

Old terminology	New terminology	Characteristics	Notes
Immune-tolerant phase	HBeAg-positive infection	**HBsAg**: high **Aminotransferases**: normal **HBV DNA**: >10⁷ IU/mL **Liver disease**[a]: none/minimal **Progression to cirrhosis**: none or slow **Treatment**: not generally indicated	Stage seen in most of the children infected at birth (90%) or in the first few 5 years of life (20–60%); young adults infected in the perinatal or early childhood period are in this phase
Immune-active phase	HBeAg-positive hepatitis	**HBsAg**: high **Aminotransferases**: elevated **HBV DNA**: >2000 IU/mL (constantly raised or fluctuating) **Liver disease**: moderate to severe **Progression to cirrhosis**: possible **Treatment**: may be indicated	This phase correlates strictly with treatment in paediatric guidelines; may develop anti-HBe with normalization of ALT leading to "immune-control" phase
Inactive carrier/immune-control phase	HBeAg-negative infection	**HBsAg**: low **Aminotransferases**: normal **HBV DNA**: <2000 IU/mL **Liver disease**: none **Progression to cirrhosis**: none **Treatment**: not indicated	Anti-HBe positive; risk of cirrhosis and HCC reduced; may develop HBeAg-negative hepatitis; monitoring required for reactivation and HCC; the rate of spontaneous seroconversion to anti-HBe is <2% per year in children younger than 3 years of age and 8% and during puberty; the rate of spontaneous seroconversion to anti-HBe is 12% per year in adults
Immune-escape phase	HBeAg-negative hepatitis	**HBsAg**: intermediate **Aminotransferases**: elevated **HBV DNA**: >2000 IU/mL **Liver disease**: moderate to severe **Progression to cirrhosis**: more rapid than in other phases **Treatment**: may be indicated	HBeAg-negative chronic hepatitis progresses slowly in children. The overall annual incidence of HBeAg-negative hepatitis was 0.37% (95% CI 0.35–0.39) in spontaneous HBeAg seroconverters. HBeAg seroconversion during childhood predicts a lower risk of HBeAg-negative hepatitis in later life [45] According to the old terminology "reactivation" or "acute-on-chronic hepatitis" (characterized by HBeAg-positive or HBeAg-negative hepatitis, moderate to high levels of HBV DNA, seroreversion to HBeAg positivity if HBeAg negative, with high risk of decompensation in presence of cirrhosis) is now classified as HBeAg-positive or HBeAg-negative hepatitis. Reactivation can occur spontaneously or be precipitated by immunosuppression (chemo- or immunosuppressive therapy, human immunodeficiency infection or transplantation), development of antiviral resistance or withdrawal of antiviral therapy
Occult HBV infection	HBsAg-negative infection	**HBV DNA**: undetectable **Aminotransferases**: normal **Liver disease**: none **Progression to cirrhosis**: none **Treatment**: not indicated	Anti-HBc positive, anti-HBs positive or negative

[a]Necroinflammatory changes

[25, 37, 38] and of HCC in 2–5% [25, 31]. HBeAg seroconversion before the age of 3 years and a longer duration of the HBeAg-positive hepatitis phase [25, 31, 46] have been identified as risk factors for development of cirrhosis in children. HCC is more common in males and cirrhotic children [25, 31, 38]. Long-term risk of HCC is correlated to viral replication and serum HBV DNA levels [47], while seroconversion to anti-HBe reduces the overall risk of developing HCC [48]. Cirrhosis or HCC can occur anytime during childhood or later in adult life. Vertically acquired HBV can cause significant morbidity and mortality beyond the paediatric age. The annual incidence of HCC in HBeAg-negative adults has been estimated to be 0.2% that is 1.6% of asymptomatic HBsAg carriers [48]. In Taiwan, before the start of the universal HBV vaccination program, the estimated incidence of HCC in children with CHB was 0.52–0.60 per 100,000 person-year. HCC incidence in Taiwan was significantly impacted by vaccination and the preventive effect of vaccination extended from childhood to early adulthood confirming that the morbidity related to vertical acquisition of HBV extends beyond the paediatric age [49].

CHB has been associated in children with extrahepatic manifestations such as kidney disease (nephrotic syndrome, non-nephrotic membranous glomerulonephritis, end-stage renal disease and acute kidney injury) [50–52].

9.1.4 Diagnosis

9.1.4.1 Serological Diagnosis

The diagnosis of CHB is usually based on a serological assay to detect HBsAg in two different serum samples taken 6 months apart. In HBsAg-positive children, testing of anti-HBV antibodies and quantification of HBV DNA levels could confirm and define the phase of the infection. Testing of infants born to HBV-infected mothers is problematic because of the presence of maternal antibodies passively transferred during pregnancy. Maternal antibodies usually persist in the child's blood for less than 12 months, but it is generally recommended to test exposed infants for HBsAg and anti-HBV antibodies after 12 months of age to limit the possibility of false positive results [53].

9.1.4.2 Staging of Liver Disease

Staging of liver fibrosis using non-invasive tests (NIT) is the new standard of care in adults. Liver biopsy is no longer used routinely to make treatment decisions in most adults with CHB [7, 29, 30, 54, 55]. Among NIT transient elastography (TE) and serum biomarker-based tests such as fibrosis-4 (FIB-4), aspartate aminotransferase-to-platelet ratio index (APRI) and FibroTest have been validated and are now widely used to assess stage of liver disease and diagnosis of cirrhosis in adults [56–58]. In contrast to adults, only few studies exploring the role of NITs in children with CHB are available [59–65]. The diagnostic and prognostic value of NIT in children with CHB has not yet been well established. Liver biopsy is still the gold standard in children to assess the degree of liver inflammation and stage of fibrosis and indication for treatment [53, 66]. The procedure, although invasive, is associated with a low rate of complications when performed by trained operators [66]. The European Society for Pediatric Gastroenterology, Hepatology and Nutrition (ESPGHAN) recommends liver biopsy in children with CHB presenting elevated serum aminotransferase levels for at least 6 months before considering treatment [53]. In these children, histological assessment of the degree of inflammation and of the stage of fibrosis is crucial [24, 53] as response to treatment with currently available therapies is more likely when at least moderate necroinflammation or moderate fibrosis is present [24, 67].

9.1.4.3 Monitoring

Monitoring of children not yet on antiviral therapy depends on the patient's serological profile (HBeAg positive or negative) and aminotransferases and HBV DNA levels. The evidence base is limited and the optimal timing is not well established. The ESPGHAN guidance to treatment of children with CHB suggested monitoring of aminotransferases and HBV DNA levels every 3–4 months for at least 1 year in HBeAg-positive and HBeAg-negative children with increased aminotransferase levels to evaluate the indication for treatment and to rule out HBeAg-negative active disease [53]. Monitoring every 6 months was recommended in HBeAg-positive children with normal aminotransferase level.

For children receiving treatment, as well after discontinuation of treatment, there are no specific recommendations, and frequency of monitoring for safety, adherence and efficacy should be determined on an individual basis [53].

9.1.5 Treatment

9.1.5.1 Goals of Treatment

The goals of antiviral treatment for patients with CHB are described in Table 9.3 and are usually achieved through effective and sustained suppression of HBV replication [7, 29, 53, 54, 68] that is associated with normalization of serum aminotransferases, loss of HBeAg with or without seroconversion to anti-HBe and improvement in liver histology [69]. Attainment of HBsAg loss and seroconversion to anti-HBs status is achieved in less than 1% of patients using currently available nucleos(t)ide analogues (NA) therapy although the longer is the treatment, the higher are the rates of HBsAg seroconversion [70].

Table 9.3 Goals of antiviral treatment for children with chronic hepatitis B virus infection

Reduce or reverse necroinflammatory change and hepatic fibrosis
Long-term clinical outcomes:
Decrease the risk of disease progression to cirrhosis
Decrease the risk of HCC
Decrease the risk of HBV-related morbidity and mortality
Surrogate measures of long-term treatment outcomes used to assess efficacy
Biochemical measures: normalization of serum aminotransferases as a surrogate measure for the resolution of necroinflammation in the liver
Virological markers: reduction in HBV DNA to undetectable levels by PCR; HBeAg loss or seroconversion to anti-HBe status; HBsAg loss and seroconversion to anti-HBs status

Table 9.4 Antiviral drugs approved for children with chronic hepatitis B virus infection

Drug	Use in children	Dose	Formulation
Adefovir	≥12 years	10 mg daily	Tablets (10 mg)
Entecavir	≥2 years	10–30 kg: 0.015 mg/kg daily (max 0.5 mg)	Oral solution (0.05 mg/mL) Tablets (0.5 mg and 1 mg)
Interferon-α-2b	≥1 year	6 million IU/m^2 3 times a week	Subcutaneous injections
Lamivudine	≥2 years	3 mg/kg daily (max 100 mg)	Oral solution (5 mg/mL) Tablets (100 mg)
Pegylated-interferon-α-2a	≥3 year	180 μg once a week	Subcutaneous injections
Tenofovir alafenamide[a]	≥12 years	25 mg daily	Tablets (25 mg)
Tenofovir disoproxil fumarate	≥12 years	300 mg daily	Oral powder (40 mg per 1 g) Tablets (150, 200, 250 and 300 mg)

[a]Data available for children with human immunodeficiency virus infection

9.1.5.2 Indications for Treatment

According to the guidance to treatment by the ESPGHAN and the American Association for the Study of Liver Disease (AASLD) [53, 54], the decision to start treatment for children with CHB is based on a combined assessment of stage of liver disease, HBV DNA viral load and alanine aminotransferase (ALT) levels, HBeAg, as well as other considerations such as family of history of HCC and/or co-existence of other liver disease [7, 30, 53, 54, 71].

The European paediatric guideline recommends treatment when ALT is persistently elevated for at least 6 months in HBeAg-positive children and for 12 months in HBeAg-negative children. Liver biopsy should demonstrate in these children the presence of moderate to severe inflammation and fibrosis [53]. The AASLD guidelines recommend treatment in HBeAg-positive children with both elevated ALT and measurable HBV DNA levels [54], with no specific duration of ALT elevation (though most studies were based on those with an ALT elevation >1.3 times upper limit of normal for at least 6 months). A family history of HCC was reported as an additional factor to support treatment initiation [53]. AASLD guidelines also recommended deferral of therapy when the HBV DNA level is <10^4 IU/mL, until spontaneous HBeAg seroconversion is excluded [54].

9.1.5.3 Antiviral Treatment

Currently, eight HBV antiviral agents are approved and licensed for the treatment of CHB in adults: four nucleoside (entecavir, lamivudine, emtricitabine and telbivudine) and two nucleotide analogues (adefovir dipivoxil, TDF/tenofovir alafenamide [TAF]), of which four are also approved for children with age-specific limitations (Table 9.4), as well as standard interferon (IFN) and pegylated (PEG) IFN α-2b.

IFN and PEG IFN are immune-stimulators and can be administered in non-cirrhotic patients for a predefined duration to inducing an immune-mediated control of HBV infection and to achieve long-lasting suppression of viral replication off-treatment [7, 30, 53, 54, 71]. IFN therapy has been associated with possibly higher rates of HBsAg loss when compared to NA [70] but cannot be used in infants and in pregnant women and is contraindicated in persons with autoimmune disease, uncontrolled psychiatric disease, cytopenia, severe cardiac disease, uncontrolled seizures and decompensated cirrhosis.

The NA are used as oral monotherapy for long-term treatment to suppress viral replication or for treatment of finite duration (with or without IFN) to obtain sustained off-treatment virological response [7, 30, 53, 54, 71]. The risk of resistance is the main concern with the use of these drugs. Entecavir and tenofovir are potent HBV inhibitors with high barriers to resistance, while telbivudine, adefovir and lamivudine have lower genetic barrier to resistance.

A recent systematic review and meta-analysis showed that in children with CHB, antivirals compared to no antiviral therapy improved attainment of HBV DNA suppression (124/256, 48.4% and 50/180, 27.7%, respectively; relative risk = 1.4, 95% confidence intervals 1.1–1.8), ALT normalization (106/133, 79.7% and 40/69, 57.9%, respectively; relative risk = 1.4, 95% confidence intervals 1.1–1.7) and HBeAg seroconversion (57/180, 31.7% and 14/110, 12.7%, respectively; relative risk = 2.1, 95% confidence intervals 1.3–3.5) [70].

9.1.5.4 Recommended Drugs

IFN, entecavir and TDF are recommended for treatment of CHB in children by ESPGHAN and AASLD [7, 53, 54]. TDF and adefovir are currently approved by the Food and Drug Administration (FDA) and European Medicines

Agency (EMA) for children 12 and older and entecavir and lamivudine from age 2 and 3 years, respectively. EMA recently approved the use of TAF for children aged 12 years and older and weighing >35 kg. IFN α is approved for use in children older than 1 year, while, only recently, in September 2017, PEG IFN α-2b has been approved by EMA for use in children older than 3 years. Advantages of IFN and PEG IFN for use in children are the absence of viral resistance and the predictable finite duration of treatment [53, 54]. However, use of IFN and PEG IFN is difficult for children as it requires subcutaneous injections three times and once per week, respectively, and is associated with a high risk of adverse events [30, 53, 54]. The AASLD guideline suggests that providers consider use of PEG IFN α-2a as it has the advantage of once weekly administration for children older than 5 years with chronic HBV [54].

Overall, IFN α-2b, lamivudine, adefovir, TDF and entecavir for children with CHB were approved based on the results of five randomized placebo-controlled trials (Table 9.5) [72–76]. A placebo-controlled randomized controlled trial of TDF in adolescents showed a high virological response (89%) and normalization of serum ALT at 72 weeks of treatment, and no observed resistance [72] although HBeAg seroconversion was rare. A placebo-controlled trial of entecavir in children demonstrated the superiority of entecavir at reducing HBV DNA levels to <50 IU/mL (49.2% vs 3.3%; $p < 0.0001$), inducing HBeAg seroconversion (24.2% [29 of 120] vs 10.0% [6 of 60]; $p = 0.0210$) after 48 weeks of treatment (24% vs 2%) and normalizing serum ALT levels (67% vs 23.3%; $p < 0.0001$) [73]. Overall, a good treatment response (defined by the reduction of serum HBV DNA to undetectable levels, by the loss of serum HBeAg and/or by the normalization of aminotransferases) was associated with greater baseline disease activity (i.e. high baseline histology activity index score and aminotransferase levels) and lower baseline HBV DNA levels.

Although for both children and adults in the HBeAg-positive infection phase (the immune-tolerant phase according to the old nomenclature) a conservative approach is warranted, results of two pilot studies in children were highly promising. In the first study, the 23 children enrolled received 8 weeks of lamivudine followed by 44 weeks of combined lamivudine and IFN-α treatment [77]. Seventy-eight percent of the children treated became HBV DNA negative at the end of treatment (62 weeks), five (22%) seroconverted to anti-HBe, and four (17%) of these became persistently HBsAg negative and anti-HBs positive. No YMDD mutation was found [77]. On the basis of this study, two controlled trials in children in the HBeAg-positive infection phase are currently being conducted in the United States (entecavir/PEG IFN-α; NCT01368497) and United Kingdom (lamivudine/PEG IFN-α NCT02263079). A second, recent randomized controlled study have explored the efficacy of IFN-α monotherapy for 12 weeks followed by the combination therapy of IFN-α and lamivudine up to week 72 and subsequently lamivudine alone till week 96 in treatment-naïve chronically HBV-infected Chinese children aged 1–16 years. Of the 46 patients in the treatment group, 73.9% had undetectable serum HBV DNA, 32.6% achieved HBeAg seroconversion and 21.7% lost HBsAg at treatment week 96, confirming the efficacy of the combine therapy in children in the HBeAg-positive infection phase [78]. No lamivudine resistance emerged during the treatment [78].

9.1.5.5 Balancing the Knowledge of the Natural History of CHB with the Effectiveness of the Anti-HBV Drugs That Are Currently Available

HBV infection acquired in infancy or in early childhood is often a chronic infection. In uncomplicated CHB cases, the few and clinically irrelevant symptoms do not represent a

Table 9.5 Main results of therapeutic trials with anti-hepatitis B drugs in children

	Interferon-α-2b [74]	Lamivudine [75]	Adefovir [76]	Tenofovir DF [72]	Entecavir [73]
Virological response (HBeAg negative; HBV DNA negative) (% treated versus placebo)	26% (vs 11%)	23% (vs 13%)	10.6% (vs 0)	21.2% (vs 0)	24.2% (vs 3.3%)
HBsAg negative (% treated versus placebo)	10% (vs 1%)	2% (vs 0)	0.8% (vs 0)	1.9% (vs 0)	5.8% (vs 0)
Number treated	144	191	173	52	120
Duration of treatment (weeks)	24	52	48	72	48
Dose	6 MU/m² thrice weekly	3 mg/kg daily (max 100 mg)	2–7 years: 0.3 mg/kg daily >7–12 years: 0.25 mg/kg >12–18 years: 10 mg	300 mg daily	0.015 mg/kg daily (max 0.5 mg)

HBeAg hepatitis B e antigen, *HBV DNA* hepatitis B virus deoxyribonucleic acid, *HBsAg* hepatitis B s antigen

correct and valid indication for starting treatment. Histologically, liver damage (i.e. inflammation and progressive fibrosis) is low in the HBeAg-positive infection phase, while it starts progressing in the HBeAg-positive hepatitis phase. Few children, around 10% of those younger than 15 years, progress to this phase. Continuous monitoring is crucial to identifying children with possible histological progression and treating them according to the indications provided by the major scientific societies described above. In these children, IFN and PEG IFN accelerate spontaneous clearance of the virus but with no major advantage as compared with the natural history of the infection [79]. At the same time, IFN and PEG IFN improve the rate of HBsAg loss that is the current goal of the available therapies. HBsAg loss rate is unsatisfactory as it could be achieved only around 10% of the children treated at the cost of a long therapy with significant side effects. NAs are safe and highly effective in obtaining control of viral replication that results in turn in reduction of the inflammation in the liver, but the duration of treatment is unpredictable and possibly lifelong. Neither IFN nor NA are actually able to cure the infection eradicating the virus and its replicative forms including covalently closed circular DNA form in the nucleus. In the future, the ideal treatment should be aimed at eradicating the virus and preventing the histological progression and therefore should be started in the HBeAg-positive infection phase. The preliminary experience with combined treatments with IFN and NA in HBeAg and highly viraemic patients are promising but far to achieve satisfactory high rates of virological and immunological response and, again, at the cost of significant IFN-based side effects.

9.2 Hepatitis C Virus

9.2.1 Epidemiology

9.2.1.1 Burden of Hepatitis C Virus Infection

The exact prevalence of HCV infection in children is unknown. According to the latest WHO estimation, in 2015, about 71 million persons (1% of the world population) were living with HCV infection in the world with the highest prevalence in the Eastern Mediterranean Region followed by the European and African Regions (1%) [2]. Paediatric epidemiological global data are limited. Based on studies from 102 countries approximately 3.5 million children younger than 19 years of age were estimated to be infected with HCV worldwide [80]. Higher rates of infection have been reported in special groups such as children treated in hospital for renal failure and malignancy or those who had undergone surgical procedures or haemodialysis [81].

9.2.1.2 Routes of Transmission

Vertical transmission of HCV from the mother to the child is actually the main route of acquisition of the infection worldwide [82]. Before the introduction in the early nineties of universal blood supply screening for HCV, parenteral transmission through unscreened or inadequately screened blood transfusions was the major route of transmission of HCV in children [83].

The rate of vertical transmission from mothers positive for anti-HCV antibodies irrespective of HCV ribonucleic acid (RNA) status is <2% [84]. The risk is higher (10.8%; 95% confidence intervals, 7.6–15.2%) when the mother is HCV RNA positive and co-infected with human immunodeficiency virus and is 5.8% (95% confidence intervals, 4.2–7.8%) from HCV RNA positive, human immunodeficiency virus-negative women [85]. Vertical transmission from the HCV-infected mother to the foetus or to the child can occur during pregnancy or in the perinatal period [86] although its exact timing is unknown. Only few children who acquire the infection vertically are HCV RNA positive in the first days of life [87, 88] suggesting early intrauterine infection. The majority (more than two third) of the children who are vertically infected presents detectable HCV RNA levels several weeks after delivery, suggesting late intrauterine or intrapartum transmission [88–90]. Maternal viraemia, independently of HCV genotype, is the major risk factor and the limiting condition for vertical transmission of HCV [91]. A higher concentration of maternal serum HCV RNA has been associated with a higher risk of vertical transmission in few studies although significant overlap of viraemia levels between transmitting and non-transmitting mothers has been reported [92, 93]. All the conditions favouring the contact between maternal infected blood and the child can theoretically increase the risk of vertical transmission. Some reports showed an increased risk of transmission related to invasive internal foetal monitoring [94, 95] and to prolonged (>6 hours) duration of the rupture of membranes [94]. On the other side, large studies comparing vaginal delivery, which exposes the child to the contact with maternal blood, with elective or emergent caesarean section did not find any difference in the risk of vertical transmission of the virus [96]. Breastfeeding was not associated with an increased risk of vertical transmission of HCV [89, 97]. Table 9.6 summarizes the factors that have not been associated with an increased risk of vertical transmission of HCV.

Table 9.6 Factors not associated with vertical transmission of HCV

Mode of delivery
Breastfeeding
HCV genotype
Previous delivering of a child infected perinatally with HCV
Mother–child HLA class I concordance
Single nucleotide polymorphisms of *interferon λ3*

In high-income countries, horizontal transmission through injection drug use has been described as an emerging and concerning route of acquisition of HCV in adolescents [98]. On the other side, in low-income countries, iatrogenic transmission and transmission through traditional practices such as scarification and circumcision are still relevant and could account for the higher prevalence of the infection in these settings [99].

9.2.1.3 Prevention of Mother-to-child transmission (MTCT)

A hepatitis C vaccine, capable of protecting against hepatitis C, is not available. Most vaccines work through inducing an antibody response that targets the outer surfaces of viruses. However, the HCV is highly variable among strains and rapidly mutating, making an effective vaccine very difficult to develop. The major preventive measures for HCV infection therefore stand on improvement of injection safety, with adoption of nonreusable syringes and on policies to reduce unnecessary injections [100, 101]. With regard to MTCT, caesarean section is not recommended to reduce the risk of vertical transmission of HCV [96], and breastfeeding from HCV-infected mothers is not contraindicated.

The parents of the HCV-infected child should be informed of the possibility of transmission of the infection to others. Household contacts should avoid sharing toothbrush, shaving, equipment, nail clippers, tweezers, glucometers or other personal items that may be contaminated with blood [102]. Parents should not be forced to disclose the child's infection status, and restriction from any routine childhood activity is not recommended [102]. HCV is not transmitted by casual contact (e.g. kissing, hugging, holding hands), and the infected child does not pose a risk to other children [102]. He can participate in all regular childhood activities (school, sports and athletic activities) without restrictions [102]. Parents should be informed that universal precautions should be followed at school and at any place as well as at home. Moreover, the child should be educated to minimize the risk of HCV transmission and avoid any blood exposure by using gloves and dilute bleach to clean up blood [102]. Adolescents with HCV infection should be aware that the risk of sexual transmission is low, but barrier precautions are nevertheless recommended [102].

9.2.2 Aetiology

HCV is a small (55–65 nm in size), enveloped, positive-sense single-stranded RNA virus, member of the *Flaviviridae* family, of the genus *Hepacivirus* [103]. Seven major viral genotypes of the virus have been identified in different regions of the world [104], and each genotype comprehends several subtypes. Among the different genotypes, genotype 1 is the most prevalent. Genotypes and subtypes have different geographic distribution.

HCV virions consist of a core of genetic material (RNA), surrounded by an icosahedral protective shell of protein, and further enveloped in a lipid bilayer in which two glycoproteins (E1 and E2) are anchored. HCV has a positive sense single-stranded RNA genome of approximately 9.6 kb with a single open reading frame translated in a single polyprotein of approximately 3000 amino acids [105]. The polyprotein is processed by host signal peptidases encoding structural proteins (E1 and E2) and nonstructural proteins (p7, NS2, NS3, NS4A, NS4B, NS5A and NS5B) [105, 106]. Viral replication is mediated by HCV RNA polymerase together with nonstructural proteins. New direct-acting antivirals (DAA) active against HCV inhibit viral replication targeting nonstructural proteins of the virus.

9.2.3 Pathophysiology

HCV is a non-cytopathic virus that enters the liver cell and undergoes replication simultaneously causing cell necrosis by several mechanisms including immune-mediated cytolysis. Innate immunity presents a first-line defence for the control of HCV infection as it does for several other viral infections, while successful clearance of HCV during acute HCV infection depends on the rise, strength and persistence of the adaptive, Th1-mediated immune response. Following HCV infection around one third of the infected adults and children present viral clearance and a self-limited disease course, while the remaining develop chronic infection.

9.2.3.1 Natural History of Hepatitis C in Children

Following MTCT of HCV, spontaneous clearance of the virus has been described in approximately 20% of the infected children usually in the first 4 years of life. Spontaneous clearance is an unpredictable phenomenon. Children with HCV genotype 3 infection and raised aminotransferase levels in the first year of life are more likely to present spontaneous clearance [107]. Recently, the single nucleotide polymorphism rs12979860 of the *interferon λ3* gene and altered natural killer cells number and phenotypes were associated with spontaneous clearance of HCV in children, suggesting a primary role of the innate immunity [108–110].

In patients who do not clear the virus (about 80% of the vertically infected), chronic HCV infection (CHC) persists into adulthood. CHC is usually asymptomatic in children [83, 111]. Only few cases of severe hepatitis have been described [112, 113]. According to the results of a multicentre, European, prospective study on 266 children born to HCV-infected mothers, hepatomegaly was the only clinical finding reported in 10% of the children, usually in the first year of life [114]. In the same study, persistently raised alanine aminotransferase levels were described in almost half of the children during follow-up [83, 114]. There is limited amount of information concerning liver disease progression in children with CHC [115]. Liver fibrosis usually progresses slowly [111, 116–125]. The majority of children presents minimal changes at liver histology after more than two decades of CHC [116, 117, 119, 125], although very young children with advanced liver disease have been described [83, 116]. Liver fibrosis increases with the patient's age [111, 117, 118, 122], the duration of the infection [117–119] and the severity of histological necroinflammation [116, 122–124]. Overall, in large cohorts of selected children afferent to highly specialized centres, cirrhosis has been described in 1–4% of children with chronic hepatitis C, while bridging fibrosis and severe inflammation is reported in about 15% of them [83, 111, 114, 116]. Comorbidities such as obesity, alcohol consumption, malignancy, haematological diseases with iron overload and viral co-infections (human immunodeficiency virus and HBV) accelerate the development of liver disease [116, 117]. Only few cases of hepatocellular carcinoma in children with HCV infection have been described [126, 127].

HCV infection is not confined to hepatocytes, but it involves also other cells such as thyrocytes [128], lymphocytes [129] and endothelial cells of the blood–brain barrier [130]. The direct and the indirect involvement of organs other than liver is thought to contribute to the development of extrahepatic manifestations of CHC. Extrahepatic manifestations of the infection are common and potentially severe in adults [131] and are considered rare in children [132]. The most common extrahepatic manifestation of the infection in children is the appearance of non-organ-specific autoantibodies (NOSA) which include smooth muscle autoantibody (SMA), antinuclear antibody (ANA) and liver kidney microsomal type-1 (LKM-1) [133–136]. The production of NOSA is probably due to the interaction between HCV and B lymphocytes and to the ability of HCV to trigger an autoimmune response via a molecular mimicry mechanism [136]. HCV can induce cellular injury allowing the exposure of "self" antigens, which are normally protected from the immune system and eliciting an autoimmune response [137, 138]. The clinical significance of NOSA production is still not well defined. NOSAs production could be considered a simple consequence of hepatocellular damage without pathogenic significance. Children presenting with NOSA generally do not show increased transaminases and other features of autoimmunity such as increased IgG levels [133–135]. On the other hand, some studies reported that LKM-1-positive HCV-infected children seem to have a more advanced liver disease when compared with LKM-1-negative peers, suggesting that NOSA may have a possible negative impact on the course of the chronic infection [137].

Subclinical hypothyroidism and autoimmune thyroiditis have been described in 11% and 5.6% of HCV-infected children, respectively [139]. Membranoproliferative glomerulonephritis, the most frequently observed HCV-related renal disease in adults [140], is extremely rare in children with only few cases described [141–143]. Other extrahepatic manifestations such as inflammatory myopathy and opsoclonus-myoclonus syndrome are anecdotal [136].

9.2.4 Diagnosis

9.2.4.1 Serological Diagnosis

Diagnosis of HCV infection is based on the detection of anti-HCV antibodies and on the identification of HCV RNA by polymerase chain reaction (PCR) assays [144]. The detection of immunoglobulin (Ig) M against HCV is not useful to discriminate between acute and chronic infection, because some patients with chronic infection produce specific IgM intermittently and not all patients respond to acute HCV infection by producing specific IgM [145]. When vertical transmission of HCV is suspected, testing the child for HCV-specific antibodies is not informative up to 18 months of age, due to the persistence of maternal antibodies in the child's blood. Before 18 months of age, PCR for HCV RNA is the only useful test for identification of the infection. Different criteria are available to diagnose vertical transmission of HCV. A practical and widely acceptable recommendation is to consider children born to anti-HCV-positive mothers infected as with HCV when HCV RNA is detected in at least two serum samples at least 3 months apart during the first year of life and/or when testing of antibodies against HCV is positive after 18 months of age [146]. A practical diagnostic algorithm for diagnosis and management of children born to HCV-infected mothers is provided in Fig. 9.2.

9.2.4.2 Staging of Liver Disease

NITs using serological markers (APRI, FIB-4, FibroTest) and TE have now replaced in adults with CHC liver biopsy as reference methods for grading the necroinflammatory activity and staging of fibrosis [147]. So far, there has been limited evaluation and validation of these non-invasive methods for staging of liver fibrosis in children. Only few studies have evaluated the role of TE in children with CHC [63, 132, 148, 149], and only in a minority of cases, the results of TE have been compared with liver biopsy results [63, 149]. The use of non-invasive methods in routine clinical practice in children is not yet recommended [66] but can be considered while the performance characteristics are being evaluated.

9.2.4.3 Monitoring

The North American Society for Pediatric Gastroenterology, Hepatology and Nutrition suggests annual monitoring of serum aminotransferases, bilirubin, albumin, HCV RNA levels, complete blood count and prothrombin time/international normalized ratio in children with CHC not receiving antiviral therapy [102]. A proposed algorithm for monitoring of children undergoing treatment with DAA is summarized in Fig. 9.3 [150]. Following treatment, a single viral load measurement at 12 weeks following discontinuation of treatment is recommended, i.e. in both adults and children, to document treatment success. Continued follow-up of those with cirrhosis is recommended, since complications can occur even after successful HCV eradication.

9.2.5 Treatment

Treatment of CHC for adults and children has changed radically with the discovery of new highly effective DAA drugs active against HCV. Since 2011, ten different oral regimens have been licensed by the EMA and the US FDA for treatment of adults with CHC. Each of these regimens has been demonstrated to be highly effective and safe, independently of viral genotype, staging of liver disease and co-infection with human immunodeficiency virus. Between April and July 2017, the first two DAA regimens have been licensed for adolescents with age- and weight-specific limitations (Table 9.7).

9.2.5.1 Goals of Treatment

The main goal of treatment of CHC in children is to cure the infection aiming to prevent the progression of liver disease and its possible complications. Although the risk of HCV-related hepatic and extrahepatic complications such as liver

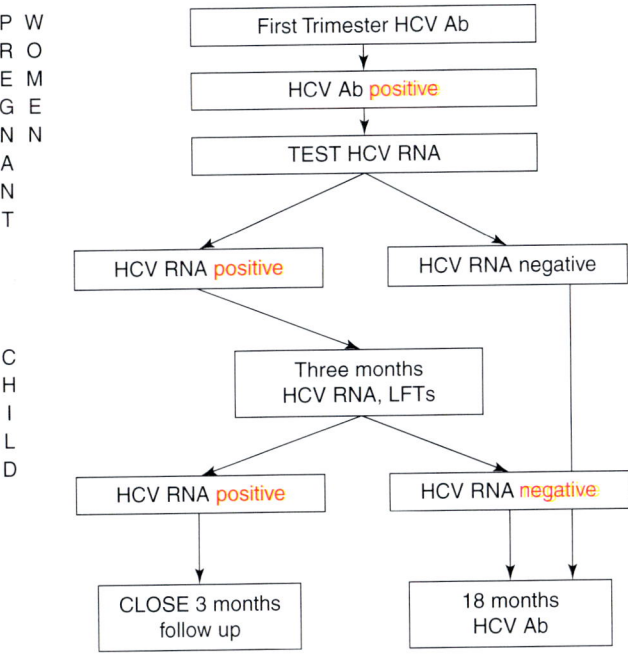

Fig. 9.2 Diagnostic algorithm for children born to hepatitis C virus-infected mothers

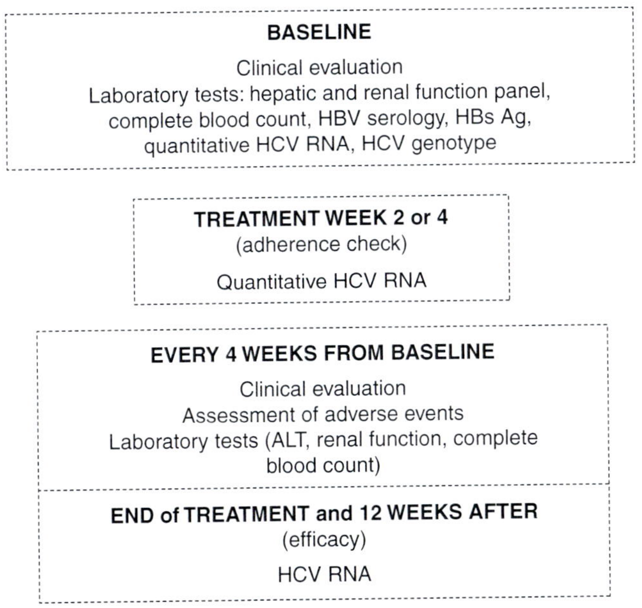

Fig. 9.3 Proposed algorithm for monitoring of children undergoing treatment with direct-acting antivirals (modified from [150])

BASELINE
Clinical evaluation
Laboratory tests: hepatic and renal function panel, complete blood count, HBV serology, HBs Ag, quantitative HCV RNA, HCV genotype

TREATMENT WEEK 2 or 4
(adherence check)
Quantitative HCV RNA

EVERY 4 WEEKS FROM BASELINE
Clinical evaluation
Assessment of adverse events
Laboratory tests (ALT, renal function, complete blood count)

END of TREATMENT and 12 WEEKS AFTER
(efficacy)
HCV RNA

Table 9.7 Direct-acting antiviral regimens approved by the Food and Drug Administration and European Medicines Agency for children with chronic hepatitis C virus infection with age- and weight-specific limitations

Ledipasvir/sofosbuvir	
Hepatitis C Virus Genotypes	1, 4, 5, 6
Age of the patient	12–18 years (only for the Food and Drug Administration, independently of age, if weight >35 kg)
Dose	– 12–17 years: fixed-dose combination sofosbuvir 400 mg/ledipasvir 90 mg
Treatment duration	– 12 weeks: treatment-naïve or -experienced with or without cirrhosis – 24 weeks: treatment-experienced patients (pegylated-interferon + ribavirin ± protease inhibitor) with genotype 1 infection and cirrhosis
Sofosbuvir and ribavirin	
Hepatitis C Virus genotypes	2, 3
Age of the patient	12–18 years (only for the Food and Drug Administration, independently of age, if weight > 35 kg)
Dose	– 12–17 years: sofosbuvir 400 mg; ribavirin 15 mg/kg in two doses (maximum <75 kg = 1000 mg and ≥75 kg = 1200 mg; with food)
Treatment duration	– Genotype 2: 12 weeks – Genotype 3: 24 weeks

fibrosis, cirrhosis and hepatocellular carcinoma in children is low and lower than for adults [120], the clinical course of CHC in childhood is unpredictable, and the long-term outcome of vertically infected children into adulthood is uncertain [83, 111, 116, 124]. The endpoint of anti-HCV therapy is sustained virological response (SVR). SVR is obtained when HCV RNA is undetectable in the blood of patients by using sensitive molecular method with a lower limit of detection (<15 IU/mL). SVR at 12 weeks (SVR12) and/or 24 weeks (SVR24) after the end of treatment are conventionally used as endpoints in studies on CHC therapy.

9.2.5.2 Indications for Treatment

Treatment is recommended for all adults with CHC independently of treatment history (both for treatment-naïve and -experienced) and of liver disease severity (compensated or decompensated HCV-related chronic liver disease) [68, 147, 151, 152]. The rationale for treatment in adults is valid also for children [151, 153].

IFN-based treatments were generally deferred in children with CHC because of the burdensome safety profile and the low efficacy of PEG IFN and ribavirin together with the overall benign course of the infection [154, 155]. However, the clinical course of CHC in children and the progression to advanced liver disease sometimes are rapid and unpredictable [117, 124, 126]. The availability of the new effective, safe, all-oral, DAA therapies changes the treatment perspective. Early treatment, i.e. treatment of children older than 4 years (the threshold age up to the child can still present spontaneous clearance of the infection), can prevent the unlikely but unpredictable progression of the infection and all its indirect consequences. Studies assessing the physical and psychosocial health and cognitive functioning of asymptomatic children with CHC, for example, showed a significant reduction in performances compared to children without HCV [156, 157]. From another point of view, the medical costs of the management of infected children in the long term could be significant, and therapy, despite the costs of drugs, could have a positive economic impact [158]. Moreover, the treatment of young children could reduce the possibility as adolescents and young adults of vertical and horizontal transmission of the infection by injecting drug use and sexual transmission.

9.2.5.3 IFN-Based Therapies

Up to December 2018, the combination of PEG IFN and ribavirin is the only treatment option available for children aged less than 12 years. Basing on the results of registration trials [115, 159–162], the combination of PEG IFN α-2a and ribavirin has been approved by EMA in December 2009 and by FDA in December 2008. PEG IFN α-2b and ribavirin have been approved by EMA in March 2013 and by FDA in December 2009. The standard duration of treatment with PEG IFN and ribavirin is 48 weeks for children with HCV genotypes 1 or 4 infection and 24 weeks for children with genotype 2 or 3 [115, 159–162]. Less than 50% of the children with genotype 1 or 4 infection and 90% of those with genotype 2 or 3 achieve SVR24 when treated with PEG IFN and ribavirin [161, 162]. Although the efficacy of PEG IFN and ribavirin is good for HCV genotype 2 and 3, the safety of this combination is poor. The more common adverse effects related to PEG IFN and ribavirin include flu-like symptoms, myalgia and neutropoenia [163]. Anaemia, thrombocytopenia, thyroid disease and alopecia are less frequently observed [163, 164]. PEG IFN therapy is also associated with neuropsychiatric manifestations ranging from mood alterations, irritability and agitation to aggressive behaviour, depression, anxiety and suicidal ideation [154, 165]. Weight loss and decrease in growth velocity are other two major issues in children with CHC treated with PEG IFN and ribavirin. While compensatory weight gain generally occurs following the end of therapy [160, 162], growth velocity does not appear to be fully compensatory. The long-term evaluation of height in children treated led to controversial results with some studies showing the complete recovery of height growth velocity [161] and others, the failure to return to the baseline height-for-age scores after 2 years of observation [162, 166].

Given the low efficacy of IFN-based therapy for HCV genotype 1 and 4 infection, the burdensome safety profile and the availability of new highly effective all-oral, DAA therapies, the updated ESPGHAN [153] and the AASLD [151] guidance for treatment of CHC in children no longer recommend PEG IFN and ribavirin for treatment of children younger (and older) than 12 years [153]. In age cohorts and countries where PEG IFN and ribavirin are the only treatment available, therapy can be generally postponed until the expected extension to the existing age indication for DAAs is granted [151, 153]. Therapy with PEG IFN plus ribavirin may be warranted in the rare situation in which liver biopsy shows significant fibrosis and DAAs are not available. In this case, the decision to administer PEG IFN and ribavirin should take in consideration HCV genotype, severity of the disease, potential side effects, presence of comorbidities and the likelihood of response [153] and should be balanced against the possible risk of deferring treatment or with the possible off-label use of DAAs.

9.2.5.4 DAA

The discovery of DAA changed the history of treatment of CHC. DAAs target viral enzymes responsible for crucial steps of the life cycle of HCV [167] and have different molecular targets: HCV NS5B polymerase inhibitors, HCV NS3/4A protease inhibitors and HCV NS5A inhibitors [167]. Up to December 2018, EMA and FDA have approved two different IFN-free treatment regimens based on DAA combinations in children: the fixed-dose combination of ledipasvir/sofosbuvir and sofosbuvir and ribavirin. Thus far, both regimens can be administered to children older than 12 years or, according to FDA, with a body weight of at least of 35 kg. Ledipasvir, a NS5A inhibitor, in the fixed-dose combination with sofosbuvir (90 and 400 mg daily in a single dose) is approved for treatment of children infected with HCV genotype 1 or 4. Treatment duration for sofosbuvir/ledipasvir is 12 weeks for all children except for those treatment-experienced with HCV genotype 1 infection who should receive 24 weeks of treatment. Sofosbuvir (400 mg daily in a single dose), a NS5B polymerase inhibitor, used with ribavirin (15 mg/kg per day in two divided doses) is approved for treatment of children infected with HCV genotype 2 for 12 weeks and genotype 3 for 24 weeks. The approval of the new treatment regimens has been based on the results of the registration trials [168, 169]. The efficacy and safety of the combination of sofosbuvir/ledipasvir have been evaluated in 100 adolescents with HCV genotype 1 infection [168]. The efficacy of the combination was high (SVR12 98%, intention to treat analysis). Of the 100 patients who started the treatment, 99 completed and 1 discontinued the treatment, while 1 did not attend the post-treatment follow-up visits after having achieved end of treatment response. No patients had virologic non-response, breakthrough or relapse. The efficacy was similar among treatment-naïve (78/80, SVR12 98%; 95% CI 91–100%) and treatment-experienced patients (20/20, SVR12 100%; 95% CI 83–99%). The only patient with cirrhosis was treatment-naïve, received 12 weeks of therapy and achieved SVR12 [168]. The efficacy and safety of the association sofosbuvir and ribavirin have been evaluated in 52 adolescents (75% genotype 3 and 25% genotype 2). Fifty-one of them (95% CI 90–100%, intention to treat analysis) achieved SVR12 (100% for genotype 2, 95% CI 75–100%, and 97% for genotype 3, 95% CI 87–100%). Nine children were treatment-experienced and achieved SVR12 (100%; 95% CI 66–100%). The single patient, who did not achieve SVR12, achieved end of treatment response and SVR4 (HCV RNA negative 4 weeks after the end of treatment) and then was lost to follow up. No patients had virologic non-response, breakthrough or relapse [169]. The two regimens showed an excellent safety profile. No treatment discontinuation due to adverse events has been reported [168, 169]. The most commonly reported adverse events during treatment with ledipasvir/sofosbuvir have been headache (27%), diarrhoea (14%) and fatigue (13%) [168], nausea (27%) and headache (23%) with the association of sofosbuvir plus ribavirin [169].

IFN-free regimens are the recommended options for treatment of adolescents older than 12 years of age or weighing more than 35 kg. According to the recent ESPGHAN and AASLD-ISDA guidance for treatment of CHC in children, PEG IFN plus ribavirin are no longer recommended [151, 153]. Indications for treatment in patient with co-infections (human immunodeficiency virus and HBV), comorbidities and patients who did not achieve SVR with DAA are still lacking, but also in these special groups of patients, IFN-free therapies will be the best option, since new regimens based on DAA will be available soon.

9.2.5.5 Other DAA Regimens

Preliminary results of new combinations of DAA already approved for treatment of CHC in adults are available for children. The ZIRCON trial is an open-label, multicentre study exploring the safety and efficacy of the combination of ombitasvir (NS5A inhibitor)/paritaprevir (NS3/4A protease inhibitor)/ritonavir with or without dasabuvir (NS5B polymerase inhibitor), with or without ribavirin in treatment-naïve and treatment-experienced children, aged 3–17 years, with HCV genotype 1 or 4 infection and with or without compensated cirrhosis [170]. In this study the fixed-dose combination of ombitasvir/paritaprevir/ritonavir has been used with dasabuvir for patients with genotype 1 infection and with ribavirin for those with genotype 1a and 4 infection. The duration of treatment has been 12 weeks for all the patients enrolled except for those with genotype 1a infection or with compensated cirrhosis who have been treated for 24 weeks. Preliminary results have been recently presented for the 12–17 age cohort [170]. Thirty-eight adolescents have been enrolled, and the combination showed excellent efficacy and a good safety profile. SVR12 was 100%, independently of genotype, treatment history and stage of liver disease [170]. Moreover, no adverse event led to discontinuation of the study drugs [170].

The preliminary results of a trial on the efficacy and safety of the combination of sofosbuvir plus daclatasvir with or without ribavirin have been recently presented [171]. Thirteen adolescents aged between 15 and 17 years with HCV genotype 4 infection received 24 weeks of treatment [171]. Ribavirin was added for four patients with cirrhosis [171]. SVR12 was 100% [171]. No serious adverse event has been reported, but mild adverse events were noted in the form of mild headache, dizziness, itching and ribavirin-induced haemoglobin reduction [171]. Interestingly, a recent pilot study explored the efficacy of a shortened 8-week duration of sofosbuvir and daclatasvir in a cohort of ten consecutive adolescents. All patients (10/10; 100% CI, 72.25–100%) achieved sustained virologic response at week 12 post-treatment (SVR12) with good tolerability and no serious adverse events [172].

New treatment perspectives will be offered in the near future by the pangenotypic combinations glecaprevir (NS3/4A protease inhibitor)/pibrentasvir (NS5A inhibitor) and sofosbuvir/velpatasvir (NS5A inhibitor) which have become recently available for adults and are being studied in children. The pangenotypic efficacy will make genotype identification no more necessary, and these DAA regimens will be a reliable option for treatment of CHC also in low-income countries, where HCV genotyping is often not available. Furthermore, these new-generation DAA regimens have the advantage of a shorter treatment duration (8 weeks).

9.2.6 Implications for Liver Transplantation

HBV and HCV infections in children without any comorbidity lead only in a minority of cases to end-stage liver disease and liver transplantation. For children with CHB who present decompensated cirrhosis as a consequence of HBV infection or due to the co-existence of other chronic liver disease, adults' guidelines suggest the use of NA with high barrier to resistance (i.e. entecavir or tenofovir) irrespective of the level of HBV replication while being assessed for liver transplantation. PEG IFN is contraindicated in patients with decompensated cirrhosis. Antiviral therapy could modify the natural history of decompensated cirrhosis, improving liver function and increasing survival. In patients with CHB who undergo liver transplantation, the combination of HBIG and NA is recommended after liver transplantation for the prevention of HBV recurrence. The same approach should be used for noninfected recipients (HBsAg negative) receiving livers from donors with evidence of past HBV infection (anti-HBc positive) who are at risk of HBV recurrence and should receive antiviral prophylaxis with a NA [30].

For children with CHC, isolated experiences with young children undergoing liver transplantation or with cirrhosis who were treated with DAA are available [173, 174]. In adults with CHC and decompensated cirrhosis without HCC, awaiting liver transplantation, the suggested approach is to initiate treatment with DAA as soon as possible in order to complete a full treatment course before transplantation [68, 151]. The positive effect of viral clearance on liver function may lead to delisting selected cases. When the patient is listed for liver transplantation and the expected waiting time is shorter than the duration of the full DAA treatment course, there is indication to make the transplant first and treat for HCV promptly after transplantation [68, 151]. In adults with HCV, recurrence after liver transplantation treatment with DAA is considered without delay [68, 151]. Similar approaches seem reasonable for children with decompensated cirrhosis without HCC awaiting or having undergone liver transplantation.

References

1. Schweitzer A, Horn J, Mikolajczyk RT, Krause G, Ott JJ. Estimations of worldwide prevalence of chronic hepatitis B virus infection: a systematic review of data published between 1965 and 2013. Lancet. 2015;386(10003):1546–55.
2. WHO. Global Hepatitis Report 2017. Geneva: World Health Organization; 2017. World Health Organization, 2017 Contract No.: Licence: CC BY-NC-SA 3.0 IGO.
3. Liu HF, Sokal E, Goubau P. Wide variety of genotypes and geographic origins of hepatitis B virus in Belgian children. J Pediatr Gastroenterol Nutr. 2001;32(3):274–7.
4. Belhassen-Garcia M, Perez Del Villar L, Pardo-Lledias J, Gutierrez Zufiaurre MN, Velasco-Tirado V, Cordero-Sanchez M, et al. Imported transmissible diseases in minors coming to Spain from low-income areas. Clin Microbiol Infect. 2015;21(4):370.e5–8.
5. Ott JJ, Stevens GA, Groeger J, Wiersma ST. Global epidemiology of hepatitis B virus infection: new estimates of age-specific HBsAg seroprevalence and endemicity. Vaccine. 2012;30(12):2212–9.
6. Yi P, Chen R, Huang Y, Zhou RR, Fan XG. Management of mother-to-child transmission of hepatitis B virus: propositions and challenges. J Clin Virol. 2016;77:32–9.
7. Sarin SK, Kumar M, Lau GK, Abbas Z, Chan HL, Chen CJ, et al. Asian-Pacific clinical practice guidelines on the management of hepatitis B: a 2015 update. Hepatol Int. 2016;10(1):1–98.
8. Nelson PK, Mathers BM, Cowie B, Hagan H, Des Jarlais D, Horyniak D, et al. Global epidemiology of hepatitis B and hepatitis C in people who inject drugs: results of systematic reviews. Lancet. 2011;378(9791):571–83.
9. Diamond C, Thiede H, Perdue T, Secura GM, Valleroy L, Mackellar D, et al. Viral hepatitis among young men who have sex with men: prevalence of infection, risk behaviors, and vaccination. Sex Transm Dis. 2003;30(5):425–32.
10. Hope VD, Eramova I, Capurro D, Donoghoe MC. Prevalence and estimation of hepatitis B and C infections in the WHO European Region: a review of data focusing on the countries outside the European Union and the European Free Trade Association. Epidemiol Infect. 2014;142(2):270–86.
11. Hepatitis B vaccines: WHO position paper—July 2017. Wkly Epidemiol Rec. 2017;92(27):369–92.
12. Zou S, Stramer SL, Notari EP, Kuhns MC, Krysztof D, Musavi F, et al. Current incidence and residual risk of hepatitis B infection among blood donors in the United States. Transfusion. 2009;49(8):1609–20.
13. Thio CL, Guo N, Xie C, Nelson KE, Ehrhardt S. Global elimination of mother-to-child transmission of hepatitis B: revisiting the current strategy. Lancet Infect Dis. 2015;15(8):981–5.
14. Zhang L, Xu A, Yan B, Song L, Li M, Xiao Z, et al. A significant reduction in hepatitis B virus infection among the children of Shandong Province, China: the effect of 15 years of universal infant hepatitis B vaccination. Int J Infect Dis. 2010;14(6):e483–8.
15. Ni YH, Huang LM, Chang MH, Yen CJ, Lu CY, You SL, et al. Two decades of universal hepatitis B vaccination in Taiwan: impact and implication for future strategies. Gastroenterology. 2007;132(4):1287–93.
16. Lee C, Gong Y, Brok J, Boxall EH, Gluud C. Hepatitis B immunisation for newborn infants of hepatitis B surface antigen-positive mothers. Cochrane Database Syst Rev. 2006;(2):Cd004790.
17. Lin X, Guo Y, Zhou A, Zhang Y, Cao J, Yang M, et al. Immunoprophylaxis failure against vertical transmission of hepatitis B virus in the Chinese population: a hospital-based study and a meta-analysis. Pediatr Infect Dis J. 2014;33(9):897–903.
18. Chen HL, Lin LH, Hu FC, Lee JT, Lin WT, Yang YJ, et al. Effects of maternal screening and universal immunization to prevent mother-to-infant transmission of HBV. Gastroenterology. 2012;142(4):773–81.e2.
19. Wen WH, Chang MH, Zhao LL, Ni YH, Hsu HY, Wu JF, et al. Mother-to-infant transmission of hepatitis B virus infection: significance of maternal viral load and strategies for intervention. J Hepatol. 2013;59(1):24–30.

20. Pan CQ, Duan Z, Dai E, Zhang S, Han G, Wang Y, et al. Tenofovir to prevent hepatitis B transmission in mothers with high viral load. N Engl J Med. 2016;374(24):2324–34.
21. Zhang H, Pan CQ, Pang Q, Tian R, Yan M, Liu X. Telbivudine or lamivudine use in late pregnancy safely reduces perinatal transmission of hepatitis B virus in real-life practice. Hepatology. 2014;60(2):468–76.
22. Brown RS Jr, McMahon BJ, Lok AS, Wong JB, Ahmed AT, Mouchli MA, et al. Antiviral therapy in chronic hepatitis B viral infection during pregnancy: a systematic review and meta-analysis. Hepatology (Baltimore, Md). 2016;63(1):319–33.
23. Prendergast AJ, Klenerman P, Goulder PJ. The impact of differential antiviral immunity in children and adults. Nat Rev Immunol. 2012;12(9):636–48.
24. McMahon BJ, Holck P, Bulkow L, Snowball M. Serologic and clinical outcomes of 1536 Alaska Natives chronically infected with hepatitis B virus. Ann Intern Med. 2001;135(9):759–68.
25. Bortolotti F, Guido M, Bartolacci S, Cadrobbi P, Crivellaro C, Noventa F, et al. Chronic hepatitis B in children after e antigen seroclearance: final report of a 29-year longitudinal study. Hepatology. 2006;43(3):556–62.
26. McMahon BJ. The natural history of chronic hepatitis B virus infection. Semin Liver Dis. 2004;24(Suppl 1):17–21.
27. McMahon BJ, Alward WL, Hall DB, Heyward WL, Bender TR, Francis DP, et al. Acute hepatitis B virus infection: relation of age to the clinical expression of disease and subsequent development of the carrier state. J Infect Dis. 1985;151(4):599–603.
28. Shimakawa Y, Toure-Kane C, Mendy M, Thursz M, Lemoine M. Mother-to-child transmission of hepatitis B in sub-Saharan Africa. Lancet Infect Dis. 2016;16(1):19–20.
29. World Health Organization. Guidelines for the prevention, care and treatment of persons with chronic hepatitis B infection. WHO Guidelines Approved by the Guidelines Review Committee. Geneva; 2015.
30. EASL. EASL 2017 Clinical Practice Guidelines on the management of hepatitis B virus infection. J Hepatol. 2017;67(2):370–98.
31. Wen WH, Chang MH, Hsu HY, Ni YH, Chen HL. The development of hepatocellular carcinoma among prospectively followed children with chronic hepatitis B virus infection. J Pediatr. 2004;144(3):397–9.
32. Marx G, Martin SR, Chicoine JF, Alvarez F. Long-term follow-up of chronic hepatitis B virus infection in children of different ethnic origins. J Infect Dis. 2002;186(3):295–301.
33. Wu JF, Su YR, Chen CH, Chen HL, Ni YH, Hsu HY, et al. Predictive effect of serial serum alanine aminotransferase levels on spontaneous HBeAg seroconversion in chronic genotype B and C HBV-infected children. J Pediatr Gastroenterol Nutr. 2012;54(1):97–100.
34. Ni YH, Chang MH, Wang KJ, Hsu HY, Chen HL, Kao JH, et al. Clinical relevance of hepatitis B virus genotype in children with chronic infection and hepatocellular carcinoma. Gastroenterology. 2004;127(6):1733–8.
35. Roushan MR, Bijani A, Ramzaninejad S, Roushan MH, Amiri MJ, Baiani M. HBeAg seroconversion in children infected during early childhood with hepatitis B virus. J Clin Virol. 2012;55(1):30–3.
36. Tseng YR, Wu JF, Ni YH, Chen HL, Chen CC, Wen WH, et al. Long-term effect of maternal HBeAg on delayed HBeAg seroconversion in offspring with chronic hepatitis B infection. Liver Int. 2011;31(9):1373–80.
37. Chang MH, Hsu HY, Hsu HC, Ni YH, Chen JS, Chen DS. The significance of spontaneous hepatitis B e antigen seroconversion in childhood: with special emphasis on the clearance of hepatitis B e antigen before 3 years of age. Hepatology. 1995;22(5):1387–92.
38. Iorio R, Giannattasio A, Cirillo F, D'Alessandro L, Vegnente A. Long-term outcome in children with chronic hepatitis B: a 24-year observation period. Clin Infect Dis. 2007;45(8):943–9.
39. Fujisawa T, Komatsu H, Inui A, Sogo T, Miyagawa Y, Fujitsuka S, et al. Long-term outcome of chronic hepatitis B in adolescents or young adults in follow-up from childhood. J Pediatr Gastroenterol Nutr. 2000;30(2):201–6.
40. Ni YH, Chang MH, Chen PJ, Tsai KS, Hsu HY, Chen HL, et al. Viremia profiles in children with chronic hepatitis B virus infection and spontaneous e antigen seroconversion. Gastroenterology. 2007;132(7):2340–5.
41. Ruiz-Moreno M, Otero M, Millan A, Castillo I, Cabrerizo M, Jimenez FJ, et al. Clinical and histological outcome after hepatitis B e antigen to antibody seroconversion in children with chronic hepatitis B. Hepatology. 1999;29(2):572–5.
42. Popalis C, Yeung LT, Ling SC, Ng V, Roberts EA. Chronic hepatitis B virus (HBV) infection in children: 25 years' experience. J Viral Hepat. 2013;20(4):e20–6.
43. Wai CT, Fontana RJ, Polson J, Hussain M, Shakil AO, Han SH, et al. Clinical outcome and virological characteristics of hepatitis B-related acute liver failure in the United States. J Viral Hepat. 2005;12(2):192–8.
44. Tseng YR, Wu JF, Kong MS, Hu FC, Yang YJ, Yeung CY, et al. Infantile hepatitis B in immunized children: risk for fulminant hepatitis and long-term outcomes. PLoS One. 2014;9(11):e111825.
45. Wu JF, Chiu YC, Chang KC, Chen HL, Ni YH, Hsu HY, et al. Predictors of hepatitis B e antigen-negative hepatitis in chronic hepatitis B virus-infected patients from childhood to adulthood. Hepatology (Baltimore, Md). 2016;63(1):74–82.
46. Iloeje UH, Yang HI, Su J, Jen CL, You SL, Chen CJ. Predicting cirrhosis risk based on the level of circulating hepatitis B viral load. Gastroenterology. 2006;130(3):678–86.
47. Chen CJ, Yang HI, Su J, Jen CL, You SL, Lu SN, et al. Risk of hepatocellular carcinoma across a biological gradient of serum hepatitis B virus DNA level. JAMA. 2006;295(1):65–73.
48. Hsu YS, Chien RN, Yeh CT, Sheen IS, Chiou HY, Chu CM, et al. Long-term outcome after spontaneous HBeAg seroconversion in patients with chronic hepatitis B. Hepatology (Baltimore, Md). 2002;35(6):1522–7.
49. Chang MH, You SL, Chen CJ, Liu CJ, Lee CM, Lin SM, et al. Decreased incidence of hepatocellular carcinoma in hepatitis B vaccines: a 20-year follow-up study. J Natl Cancer Inst. 2009;101(19):1348–55.
50. Gooden M, Miller M, Shah D, Soyibo AK, Williams J, Barton EN. Clinicopathological features of atypical nephrotic syndrome in Jamaican children. West Indian Med J. 2010;59(3):319–24.
51. Ozdamar SO, Gucer S, Tinaztepe K. Hepatitis-B virus associated nephropathies: a clinicopathological study in 14 children. Pediatr Nephrol (Berlin, Germany). 2003;18(1):23–8.
52. Slusarczyk J, Michalak T, Nazarewicz-de Mezer T, Krawczynski K, Nowoslawski A. Membranous glomerulopathy associated with hepatitis B core antigen immune complexes in children. Am J Pathol. 1980;98(1):29–43.
53. Sokal EM, Paganelli M, Wirth S, Socha P, Vajro P, Lacaille F, et al. Management of chronic hepatitis B in childhood: ESPGHAN clinical practice guidelines: consensus of an expert panel on behalf of the European Society of Pediatric Gastroenterology, Hepatology and Nutrition. J Hepatol. 2013;59(4):814–29.
54. Terrault NA, Bzowej NH, Chang KM, Hwang JP, Jonas MM, Murad MH. AASLD guidelines for treatment of chronic hepatitis B. Hepatology (Baltimore, Md). 2016;63(1):261–83.
55. EASL clinical practice guidelines: management of chronic hepatitis B virus infection. J Hepatol. 2012;57(1):167–85.
56. Castera L. Noninvasive methods to assess liver disease in patients with hepatitis B or C. Gastroenterology. 2012;142(6):1293–302.e4.

57. Park SH, Kim CH, Kim DJ, Suk KT, Cheong JY, Cho SW, et al. Usefulness of multiple biomarkers for the prediction of significant fibrosis in chronic hepatitis B. J Clin Gastroenterol. 2011;45(4):361–5.
58. Zhang YG, Wang BE, Wang TL, Ou XJ. Assessment of hepatic fibrosis by transient elastography in patients with chronic hepatitis B. Pathol Int. 2010;60(4):284–90.
59. Tokuhara D, Cho Y, Shintaku H. Transient elastography-based liver stiffness age-dependently increases in children. PLoS One. 2016;11(11):e0166683.
60. Jalal Z, Iriart X, De Ledinghen V, Barnetche T, Hiriart JB, Vergniol J, et al. Liver stiffness measurements for evaluation of central venous pressure in congenital heart diseases. Heart (British Cardiac Society). 2015;101(18):1499–504.
61. Lee CK, Perez-Atayde AR, Mitchell PD, Raza R, Afdhal NH, Jonas MM. Serum biomarkers and transient elastography as predictors of advanced liver fibrosis in a United States cohort: the Boston children's hospital experience. J Pediatr. 2013;163(4):1058–64.e2.
62. Goldschmidt I, Streckenbach C, Dingemann C, Pfister ED, di Nanni A, Zapf A, et al. Application and limitations of transient liver elastography in children. J Pediatr Gastroenterol Nutr. 2013;57(1):109–13.
63. Fitzpatrick E, Quaglia A, Vimalesvaran S, Basso MS, Dhawan A. Transient elastography is a useful noninvasive tool for the evaluation of fibrosis in paediatric chronic liver disease. J Pediatr Gastroenterol Nutr. 2013;56(1):72–6.
64. Engelmann G, Gebhardt C, Wenning D, Wuhl E, Hoffmann GF, Selmi B, et al. Feasibility study and control values of transient elastography in healthy children. Eur J Pediatr. 2012;171(2):353–60.
65. de Ledinghen V, Le Bail B, Rebouissoux L, Fournier C, Foucher J, Miette V, et al. Liver stiffness measurement in children using FibroScan: feasibility study and comparison with Fibrotest, aspartate transaminase to platelets ratio index, and liver biopsy. J Pediatr Gastroenterol Nutr. 2007;45(4):443–50.
66. Dezsofi A, Baumann U, Dhawan A, Durmaz O, Fischler B, Hadzic N, et al. Liver biopsy in children: position paper of the ESPGHAN Hepatology Committee. J Pediatr Gastroenterol Nutr. 2015;60(3):408–20.
67. Hom X, Little NR, Gardner SD, Jonas MM. Predictors of virologic response to Lamivudine treatment in children with chronic hepatitis B infection. Pediatr Infect Dis J. 2004;23(5):441–5.
68. EASL. EASL recommendations on treatment of hepatitis C 2016. J Hepatol. 2017;66(1):153–94.
69. Chang TT, Liaw YF, Wu SS, Schiff E, Han KH, Lai CL, et al. Long-term entecavir therapy results in the reversal of fibrosis/cirrhosis and continued histological improvement in patients with chronic hepatitis B. Hepatology. 2010;52(3):886–93.
70. Jonas MM, Lok AS, McMahon BJ, Brown RS Jr, Wong JB, Ahmed AT, et al. Antiviral therapy in management of chronic hepatitis B viral infection in children: a systematic review and meta-analysis. Hepatology (Baltimore, Md). 2016;63(1):307–18.
71. World Health Organization. Guidelines for the prevention, care and treatment of persons with chronic hepatitis B infection. Geneva: WHO Library Cataloguing-in-Publication Data; 2015.
72. Murray KF, Szenborn L, Wysocki J, Rossi S, Corsa AC, Dinh P, et al. Randomized, placebo-controlled trial of tenofovir disoproxil fumarate in adolescents with chronic hepatitis B. Hepatology. 2012;56(6):2018–26.
73. Jonas MM, Chang MH, Sokal E, Schwarz KB, Kelly D, Kim KM, et al. Randomized, controlled trial of entecavir versus placebo in children with hepatitis B envelope antigen-positive chronic hepatitis B. Hepatology (Baltimore, Md). 2016;63(2):377–87.
74. Sokal EM, Conjeevaram HS, Roberts EA, Alvarez F, Bern EM, Goyens P, et al. Interferon alfa therapy for chronic hepatitis B in children: a multinational randomized controlled trial. Gastroenterology. 1998;114(5):988–95.
75. Jonas MM, Mizerski J, Badia IB, Areias JA, Schwarz KB, Little NR, et al. Clinical trial of lamivudine in children with chronic hepatitis B. N Engl J Med. 2002;346(22):1706–13.
76. Jonas MM, Kelly D, Pollack H, Mizerski J, Sorbel J, Frederick D, et al. Safety, efficacy, and pharmacokinetics of adefovir dipivoxil in children and adolescents (age 2 to <18 years) with chronic hepatitis B. Hepatology. 2008;47(6):1863–71.
77. D'Antiga L, Aw M, Atkins M, Moorat A, Vergani D, Mieli-Vergani G. Combined lamivudine/interferon-alpha treatment in "immunotolerant" children perinatally infected with hepatitis B: a pilot study. J Pediatr. 2006;148(2):228–33.
78. Zhu S, Zhang H, Dong Y, Wang L, Xu Z, Liu W, et al. Antiviral therapy in hepatitis B virus-infected children with immune-tolerant characters: a pilot open-label randomized study. J Hepatol. 2018;68(6):1123–8.
79. Bortolotti F, Jara P, Barbera C, Gregorio GV, Vegnente A, Zancan L, et al. Long term effect of alpha interferon in children with chronic hepatitis B. Gut. 2000;46(5):715–8.
80. El-Sayed MH, Razavi H. P1263: global estimate of HCV infection in the pediatric and adolescent population. J Hepatol. 2015;62:S831–2.
81. Thursz M, Fontanet A. HCV transmission in industrialized countries and resource-constrained areas. Nat Rev Gastroenterol Hepatol. 2014;11(1):28–35.
82. Bortolotti F, Iorio R, Resti M, Camma C, Marcellini M, Giacchino R, et al. Epidemiological profile of 806 Italian children with hepatitis C virus infection over a 15-year period. J Hepatol. 2007;46(5):783–90.
83. Bortolotti F, Verucchi G, Cammà C, Cabibbo G, Zancan L, Indolfi G, et al. Long-term course of chronic hepatitis C in children: from viral clearance to end-stage liver disease. Gastroenterology. 2008;134(7):1900–7.
84. Yeung LT, King SM, Roberts EA. Mother-to-infant transmission of hepatitis C virus. Hepatology. 2001;34(2):223–9.
85. Benova L, Mohamoud YA, Calvert C, Abu-Raddad LJ. Vertical transmission of hepatitis C virus: systematic review and meta-analysis. Clin Infect Dis. 2014;59(6):765–73.
86. Indolfi G, Resti M. Perinatal transmission of hepatitis C virus infection. J Med Virol. 2009;81(5):836–43.
87. Mok J, Pembrey L, Tovo PA, Newell ML. When does mother to child transmission of hepatitis C virus occur? Arch Dis Child Fetal Neonatal Ed. 2005;90(2):F156–60.
88. Resti M, Azzari C, Mannelli F, Moriondo M, Novembre E, de Martino M, et al. Mother to child transmission of hepatitis C virus: prospective study of risk factors and timing of infection in children born to women seronegative for HIV-1. Tuscany Study Group on Hepatitis C Virus Infection. BMJ. 1998;317(7156):437–41.
89. Gibb DM, Goodall RL, Dunn DT, Healy M, Neave P, Cafferkey M, et al. Mother-to-child transmission of hepatitis C virus: evidence for preventable peripartum transmission. Lancet. 2000;356(9233):904–7.
90. Effects of mode of delivery and infant feeding on the risk of mother-to-child transmission of hepatitis C virus. European Paediatric Hepatitis C Virus Network. BJOG. 2001;108(4):371–7.
91. Indolfi G, Azzari C, Resti M. Perinatal transmission of hepatitis C virus. J Pediatr. 2013;163(6):1549–52.e1.
92. Okamoto M, Nagata I, Murakami J, Kaji S, Iitsuka T, Hoshika T, et al. Prospective reevaluation of risk factors in mother-to-child transmission of hepatitis C virus: high virus load, vaginal delivery, and negative anti-NS4 antibody. J Infect Dis. 2000;182(5):1511–4.
93. Ceci O, Margiotta M, Marello F, Francavilla R, Loizzi P, Francavilla A, et al. Vertical transmission of hepatitis C virus in a cohort of 2,447 HIV-seronegative pregnant women: a 24-month prospective study. J Pediatr Gastroenterol Nutr. 2001;33(5):570–5.
94. Mast EE, Hwang LY, Seto DS, Nolte FS, Nainan OV, Wurtzel H, et al. Risk factors for perinatal transmission of hepatitis C virus

(HCV) and the natural history of HCV infection acquired in infancy. J Infect Dis. 2005;192(11):1880–9.
95. Steininger C, Kundi M, Jatzko G, Kiss H, Lischka A, Holzmann H. Increased risk of mother-to-infant transmission of hepatitis C virus by intrapartum infantile exposure to maternal blood. J Infect Dis. 2003;187(3):345–51.
96. Cottrell EB, Chou R, Wasson N, Rahman B, Guise JM. Reducing risk for mother-to-infant transmission of hepatitis C virus: a systematic review for the U.S. Preventive Services Task Force. Ann Intern Med. 2013;158(2):109–13.
97. Conte D, Fraquelli M, Prati D, Colucci A, Minola E. Prevalence and clinical course of chronic hepatitis C virus (HCV) infection and rate of HCV vertical transmission in a cohort of 15,250 pregnant women. Hepatology. 2000;31(3):751–5.
98. Hepatitis C virus infection among adolescents and young adults:Massachusetts, 2002-2009. MMWR Morb Mortal Wkly Rep. 2011;60(17):537–41.
99. Layden JE, Phillips RO, Owusu-Ofori S, Sarfo FS, Kliethermes S, Mora N, et al. High frequency of active HCV infection among seropositive cases in west Africa and evidence for multiple transmission pathways. Clin Infect Dis. 2015;60(7):1033–41.
100. World Health Organization. Injection safety policy and global campaign 2015. http://www.who.int/injection_safety/global-campaign/en/.
101. World Health Organization. WHO guideline on the use of safety-engineered syringes for intramuscular, intradermal and subcutaneous injections in health care settings 2016. http://www.who.int/infection-prevention/publications/is_guidelines/en/.
102. Mack CL, Gonzalez-Peralta RP, Gupta N, Leung D, Narkewicz MR, Roberts EA, et al. NASPGHAN practice guidelines: diagnosis and management of hepatitis C infection in infants, children, and adolescents. J Pediatr Gastroenterol Nutr. 2012;54(6):838–55.
103. Choo QL, Kuo G, Weiner AJ, Overby LR, Bradley DW, Houghton M. Isolation of a cDNA clone derived from a blood-borne non-A, non-B viral hepatitis genome. Science. 1989;244(4902):359–62.
104. Murphy DG, Sablon E, Chamberland J, Fournier E, Dandavino R, Tremblay CL. Hepatitis C virus genotype 7, a new genotype originating from central Africa. J Clin Microbiol. 2015;53(3):967–72.
105. Penin F, Dubuisson J, Rey FA, Moradpour D, Pawlotsky JM. Structural biology of hepatitis C virus. Hepatology. 2004;39(1):5–19.
106. Kanda T, Steele R, Ray R, Ray RB. Small interfering RNA targeted to hepatitis C virus 5′ nontranslated region exerts potent antiviral effect. J Virol. 2007;81(2):669–76.
107. Resti M, Jara P, Hierro L, Azzari C, Giacchino R, Zuin G, et al. Clinical features and progression of perinatally acquired hepatitis C virus infection. J Med Virol. 2003;70(3):373–7.
108. Indolfi G, Mangone G, Bartolini E, Nebbia G, Calvo PL, Moriondo M, et al. Comparative analysis of rs12979860 SNP of the IFNL3 gene in children with hepatitis C and ethnic matched controls using 1000 Genomes Project data. PLoS One. 2014;9(1):e85899.
109. Indolfi G, Mangone G, Calvo PL, Bartolini E, Regoli M, Serranti D, et al. Interleukin 28B rs12979860 single-nucleotide polymorphism predicts spontaneous clearance of hepatitis C virus in children. J Pediatr Gastroenterol Nutr. 2014;58(5):666–8.
110. Indolfi G, Mangone G, Moriondo M, Serranti D, Bartolini E, Azzari C, et al. Altered natural killer cells subsets distribution in children with hepatitis C following vertical transmission. Aliment Pharmacol Ther. 2016;43(1):125–33.
111. Jara P, Resti M, Hierro L, Giacchino R, Barbera C, Zancan L, et al. Chronic hepatitis C virus infection in childhood: clinical patterns and evolution in 224 white children. Clin Infect Dis. 2003;36(3):275–80.
112. Kumar RM, Frossad PM, Hughes PF. Seroprevalence and mother-to-infant transmission of hepatitis C in asymptomatic Egyptian women. Eur J Obstet Gynecol Reprod Biol. 1997;75(2):177–82.
113. Kong MS, Chung JL. Fatal hepatitis C in an infant born to a hepatitis C positive mother. J Pediatr Gastroenterol Nutr. 1994;19(4):460–3.
114. European Paediatric Hepatitis C Virus Network. Three broad modalities in the natural history of vertically acquired hepatitis C virus infection. Clin Infect Dis. 2005;41(1):45–51.
115. Indolfi G, Guido M, Azzari C, Resti M. Histopathology of hepatitis C in children, a systematic review: implications for treatment. Expert Rev Anti Infect Ther. 2015;13(10):1225–35.
116. Goodman ZD, Makhlouf HR, Liu L, Balistreri W, Gonzalez-Peralta RP, Haber B, et al. Pathology of chronic hepatitis C in children: liver biopsy findings in the Peds-C Trial. Hepatology. 2008;47(3):836–43.
117. Guido M, Bortolotti F, Leandro G, Jara P, Hierro L, Larrauri J, et al. Fibrosis in chronic hepatitis C acquired in infancy: is it only a matter of time? Am J Gastroenterol. 2003;98(3):660–3.
118. Badizadegan K, Jonas MM, Ott MJ, Nelson SP, Perez-Atayde AR. Histopathology of the liver in children with chronic hepatitis C viral infection. Hepatology. 1998;28(5):1416–23.
119. Castellino S, Lensing S, Riely C, Rai SN, Davila R, Hayden RT, et al. The epidemiology of chronic hepatitis C infection in survivors of childhood cancer: an update of the St Jude Children's Research Hospital hepatitis C seropositive cohort. Blood. 2004;103(7):2460–6.
120. García-Monzón C, Jara P, Fernández-Bermejo M, Hierro L, Frauca E, Camarena C, et al. Chronic hepatitis C in children: a clinical and immunohistochemical comparative study with adult patients. Hepatology. 1998;28(6):1696–701.
121. Guido M, Bortolotti F, Jara P, Giacomelli L, Fassan M, Hierro L, et al. Liver steatosis in children with chronic hepatitis C. Am J Gastroenterol. 2006;101(11):2611–5.
122. Harris HE, Mieli-Vergani G, Kelly D, Davison S, Gibb DM, Ramsay ME, et al. A national sample of individuals who acquired hepatitis C virus infections in childhood or adolescence: risk factors for advanced disease. J Pediatr Gastroenterol Nutr. 2007;45(3):335–41.
123. Kage M, Fujisawa T, Shiraki K, Tanaka T, Fujisawa T, Kimura A, et al. Pathology of chronic hepatitis C in children. Child Liver Study Group of Japan. Hepatology. 1997;26(3):771–5.
124. Mohan P, Barton BA, Narkewicz MR, Molleston JP, Gonzalez-Peralta RP, Rosenthal P, et al. Evaluating progression of liver disease from repeat liver biopsies in children with chronic hepatitis C: a retrospective study. Hepatology. 2013;58(5):1580–6.
125. Vogt M, Lang T, Frösner G, Klingler C, Sendl AF, Zeller A, et al. Prevalence and clinical outcome of hepatitis C infection in children who underwent cardiac surgery before the implementation of blood-donor screening. N Engl J Med. 1999;341(12):866–70.
126. Gonzalez-Peralta RP, Langham MR Jr, Andres JM, Mohan P, Colombani PM, Alford MK, et al. Hepatocellular carcinoma in 2 young adolescents with chronic hepatitis C. J Pediatr Gastroenterol Nutr. 2009;48(5):630–5.
127. Strickland DK, Jenkins JJ, Hudson MM. Hepatitis C infection and hepatocellular carcinoma after treatment of childhood cancer. J Pediatr Hematol Oncol. 2001;23(8):527–9.
128. Antonelli A, Ferri C, Fallahi P, Ferrari SM, Ghinoi A, Rotondi M, et al. Thyroid disorders in chronic hepatitis C virus infection. Thyroid. 2006;16(6):563–72.
129. Zignego AL, Giannini C, Gragnani L. HCV and lymphoproliferation. Clin Dev Immunol. 2012;2012:980942.
130. Fletcher NF, Wilson GK, Murray J, Hu K, Lewis A, Reynolds GM, et al. Hepatitis C virus infects the endothelial cells of the blood-brain barrier. Gastroenterology. 2012;142(3):634–43.e6.
131. Cacoub P, Gragnani L, Comarmond C, Zignego AL. Extrahepatic manifestations of chronic hepatitis C virus infection. Dig Liver Dis. 2014;46(Suppl 5):S165–73.

132. Garazzino S, Calitri C, Versace A, Alfarano A, Scolfaro C, Bertaina C, et al. Natural history of vertically acquired HCV infection and associated autoimmune phenomena. Eur J Pediatr. 2014;173(8):1025–31.
133. Bortolotti F, Vajro P, Balli F, Giacchino R, Crivellaro C, Barbera C, et al. Non-organ specific autoantibodies in children with chronic hepatitis C. J Hepatol. 1996;25(5):614–20.
134. Gregorio GV, Pensati P, Iorio R, Vegnente A, Mieli-Vergani G, Vergani D. Autoantibody prevalence in children with liver disease due to chronic hepatitis C virus (HCV) infection. Clin Exp Immunol. 1998;112(3):471–6.
135. Muratori P, Muratori L, Verucchi G, Attard L, Bianchi FB, Lenzi M. Non-organ-specific autoantibodies in children with chronic hepatitis C: clinical significance and impact on interferon treatment. Clin Infect Dis. 2003;37(10):1320–6.
136. Indolfi G, Bartolini E, Olivito B, Azzari C, Resti M. Autoimmunity and extrahepatic manifestations in treatment-naive children with chronic hepatitis C virus infection. Clin Dev Immunol. 2012;2012:785627.
137. Bogdanos DP, Mieli-Vergani G, Vergani D. Virus, liver and autoimmunity. Dig Liver Dis. 2000;32(5):440–6.
138. Maecker HT, Do MS, Levy S. CD81 on B cells promotes interleukin 4 secretion and antibody production during T helper type 2 immune responses. Proc Natl Acad Sci U S A. 1998;95(5):2458–62.
139. Indolfi G, Stagi S, Bartolini E, Salti R, de Martino M, Azzari C, et al. Thyroid function and anti-thyroid autoantibodies in untreated children with vertically acquired chronic hepatitis C virus infection. Clin Endocrinol (Oxf). 2008;68(1):117–21.
140. Zignego AL, Ferri C, Pileri SA, Caini P, Bianchi FB. Extrahepatic manifestations of Hepatitis C Virus infection: a general overview and guidelines for a clinical approach. Dig Liver Dis. 2007;39(1):2–17.
141. Sugiura T, Yamada T, Kimpara Y, Fujita N, Goto K, Koyama N. Effects of pegylated interferon alpha-2a on hepatitis-C-virus-associated glomerulonephritis. Pediatr Nephrol (Berlin, Germany). 2009;24(1):199–202.
142. Matsumoto S, Nakajima S, Nakamura K, Etani Y, Hirai H, Shimizu N, et al. Interferon treatment on glomerulonephritis associated with hepatitis C virus. Pediatr Nephrol (Berlin, Germany). 2000;15(3–4):271–3.
143. Romas E, Power DA, Machet D, Powell H, d'Apice AJ. Membranous glomerulonephritis associated with hepatitis C virus infection in an adolescent. Pathology. 1994;26(4):399–402.
144. Ghany MG, Strader DB, Thomas DL, Seeff LB. Diagnosis, management, and treatment of hepatitis C: an update. Hepatology. 2009;49(4):1335–74.
145. de Leuw P, Sarrazin C, Zeuzem S. How to use virological tools for the optimal management of chronic hepatitis C. Liver Int. 2011;31(Suppl 1):3–12.
146. Resti M, Bortolotti F, Vajro P, Maggiore G, Committee of Hepatology of the Italian Society of Pediatric Gastroenterology and Hepatology. Guidelines for the screening and follow-up of infants born to anti-HCV positive mothers. Dig Liver Dis. 2003;35(7):453–7.
147. WHO. Guidelines for the screening, care and treatment of persons with chronic hepatitis C infection 2016. http://www.who.int/hepatitis/publications/hepatitis-c-guidelines-2016/en/.
148. El-Asrar MA, Elbarbary NS, Ismail EA, Elshenity AM. Serum YKL-40 in young patients with beta-thalassemia major: relation to hepatitis C virus infection, liver stiffness by transient elastography and cardiovascular complications. Blood Cells Mol Dis. 2016;56(1):1–8.
149. Awad Mel D, Shiha GE, Sallam FA, Mohamed A, El Tawab A. Evaluation of liver stiffness measurement by fibroscan as compared to liver biopsy for assessment of hepatic fibrosis in children with chronic hepatitis C. J Egypt Soc Parasitol. 2013;43(3):805–19.
150. Indolfi G, Serranti D, Resti M. Direct-acting antivirals for adolescents with chronic hepatitis C. Lancet Child Adolesc Health. 2018;2(4):298–304.
151. AASLD-IDSA. Recommendations for testing, managing, and treating hepatitis C. http://www.hcvguidelines.org. Accessed Dec 2018.
152. Omata M, Kanda T, Wei L, Yu ML, Chuang WL, Ibrahim A, et al. APASL consensus statements and recommendation on treatment of hepatitis C. Hepatology Int. 2016;10:702–26.
153. Indolfi G, Hierro L, Dezsofi A, Janel J, Debray D, Hadzich N, et al. Treatment of chronic hepatitis C virus infection in children. A Position Paper by the Hepatology Committee of ESPGHAN. J Pediatr Gastroenterol Nutr. 2018;66(3):505–15.
154. Granot E, Sokal EM. Hepatitis C virus in children: deferring treatment in expectation of direct-acting antiviral agents. Isr Med Assoc J. 2015;17(11):707–11.
155. Lee CK, Jonas MM. Hepatitis C: issues in children. Gastroenterol Clin N Am. 2015;44(4):901–9.
156. Nydegger A, Srivastava A, Wake M, Smith AL, Hardikar W. Health-related quality of life in children with hepatitis C acquired in the first year of life. J Gastroenterol Hepatol. 2008;23(2):226–30.
157. Rodrigue JR, Balistreri W, Haber B, Jonas MM, Mohan P, Molleston JP, et al. Impact of hepatitis C virus infection on children and their caregivers: quality of life, cognitive, and emotional outcomes. J Pediatr Gastroenterol Nutr. 2009;48(3):341–7.
158. Jhaveri R, Grant W, Kauf TL, McHutchison J. The burden of hepatitis C virus infection in children: estimated direct medical costs over a 10-year period. J Pediatr. 2006;148(3):353–8.
159. Wirth S, Pieper-Boustani H, Lang T, Ballauff A, Kullmer U, Gerner P, et al. Peginterferon alfa-2b plus ribavirin treatment in children and adolescents with chronic hepatitis C. Hepatology. 2005;41(5):1013–8.
160. Jara P, Hierro L, de la Vega A, Díaz C, Camarena C, Frauca E, et al. Efficacy and safety of peginterferon-alpha2b and ribavirin combination therapy in children with chronic hepatitis C infection. Pediatr Infect Dis J. 2008;27(2):142–8.
161. Sokal EM, Bourgois A, Stéphenne X, Silveira T, Porta G, Gardovska D, et al. Peginterferon alfa-2a plus ribavirin for chronic hepatitis C virus infection in children and adolescents. J Hepatol. 2010;52(6):827–31.
162. Wirth S, Ribes-Koninckx C, Calzado MA, Bortolotti F, Zancan L, Jara P, et al. High sustained virologic response rates in children with chronic hepatitis C receiving peginterferon alfa-2b plus ribavirin. J Hepatol. 2010;52(4):501–7.
163. Karnsakul W, Schwarz KB. Hepatitis B and C. Pediatr Clin North Am. 2017;64(3):641–58.
164. Serranti D, Indolfi G, Nebbia G, Cananzi M, D'Antiga L, Ricci S, et al. Transient hypothyroidism and autoimmune thyroiditis in children with chronic hepatitis C treated with pegylated-interferon-alpha-2b and ribavirin. Pediatr Infect Dis J. 2018;37(4):287–91.
165. Schwarz KB, Gonzalez-Peralta RP, Murray KF, Molleston JP, Haber BA, Jonas MM, et al. The combination of ribavirin and peginterferon is superior to peginterferon and placebo for children and adolescents with chronic hepatitis C. Gastroenterology. 2011;140(2):450–8.e1.
166. Jonas MM, Balistreri W, Gonzalez-Peralta RP, Haber B, Lobritto S, Mohan P, et al. Pegylated interferon for chronic hepatitis C in children affects growth and body composition: results from the pediatric study of hepatitis C (PEDS-C) trial. Hepatology. 2012;56(2):523–31.
167. Serranti D, Indolfi G, Resti M. New treatments for chronic hepatitis C: an overview for paediatricians. World J Gastroenterol. 2014;20(43):15965–74.

168. Balistreri WF, Murray KF, Rosenthal P, Bansal S, Lin CH, Kersey K, et al. The safety and effectiveness of ledipasvir-sofosbuvir in adolescents 12-17 years old with hepatitis C virus genotype 1 infection. Hepatology. 2017;66(2):371–8.
169. Wirth S, Rosenthal P, Gonzalez-Peralta RP, Jonas MM, Balistreri WF, Lin CH, et al. Sofosbuvir and ribavirin in adolescents 12-17 years old with hepatitis C virus genotype 2 or 3 infection. Hepatology. 2017;66(4):1102–10.
170. Leung DH, Wirth S, Yao BB, Viani RM, Gonzalez-Peralta RP, Jonas MM, Lobritto SJ, Narkewicz MR, Sokal E, Fortuny C, Hsu EK, Del Valle-Segarra A, Zha J, Larsen L, Liu L, Shuster DL, Cohen DE, Rosenthal P. Ombitasvir/paritaprevir/ritonavir with or without dasabuvir and with or without ribavirin for adolescents with HCV genotype 1 or 4. Hepatol Commun. 2018;2(11):1311–9.
171. El-Sayed M, Hassany M, Asem N. THU-412—a pilot study for safety and efficacy of 12 weeks sofosbuvir plus daclatasvir with or without ribavirin in Egyptian adolescents with chronic hepatitis C virus Infection. J Hepatol. 2017;66(1 Suppl):S178.
172. El-Shabrawi M, Abdo AM, El-Khayat H, Yakoot M. Shortened 8 weeks course of dual sofosbuvir/daclatasvir therapy in adolescent patients, with chronic hepatitis C infection. J Pediatr Gastroenterol Nutr. 2018;66(3):425–7.
173. Psaros-Einberg A, Fischler B. Successful treatment of paediatric hepatitis C with direct acting antivirals in selected cases. J Pediatr Gastroenterol Nutr. 2018;64(S1):636.
174. Huysentruyt K, Stephenne X, Varma S, Scheers I, Leclercq G, Smets F, et al. Sofosbuvir/ledipasvir and ribavirin tolerability and efficacy in pediatric liver transplant recipients. Liver Transpl. 2017;23(4):552–3.

Autoimmune Liver Disease

Giorgina Mieli-Vergani and Diego Vergani

Juvenile autoimmune liver disease has been recognized only recently in the history of medicine. Autoimmune hepatitis in young women was first described in the 1950s, juvenile autoimmune sclerosing cholangitis in the 1980s and de novo autoimmune hepatitis after liver transplantation in the 1990s. This chapter explores the peculiarities of autoimmune liver disease in children and adolescents, their possible pathogenic mechanisms, their management and their outcome.

Key Points
- There are three forms of juvenile liver disease with an autoimmune component to their pathogenesis: autoimmune hepatitis (AIH), autoimmune sclerosing cholangitis (ASC) and de novo autoimmune hepatitis (de novo AIH) after liver transplantation (LT).
- AIH is in turn divided into two types: AIH-1, positive for anti-nuclear (ANA) and/or anti-smooth muscle (SMA) autoantibodies, and AIH-2, positive for anti-liver-kidney microsomal type 1 (anti-LKM1) and/or anti-liver cytosol type 1 (anti-LC1) autoantibodies.
- The typical histological feature, common to AIH, ASC and de novo AIH after LT, is interface hepatitis.
- ASC is serologically (ANA/SMA) and histologically similar to AIH-1 but in addition has bile duct damage demonstrable by cholangiography usually already at presentation.
- The International Autoimmune Hepatitis Group (IAIHG) scoring systems do not allow differentiation between AIH and ASC; a scoring system specific for juvenile autoimmune liver disease has been proposed by an ESPGHAN Hepatology Committee Position Statement.
- Both in AIH and ASC, the parenchymal inflammation responds satisfactorily to standard immunosuppressive treatment with steroids ± azathioprine, but in ASC the bile duct disease progresses in about 50% of cases, leading to LT.
- ASC is more frequently associated with inflammatory bowel disease than AIH, and deterioration of liver disease, as well as the risk of ASC recurrence after transplant, is correlated to the activity of the gut disease.
- Those patients with AIH or ASC, who do not respond to standard treatment, or who relapse frequently should be offered alternative immunosuppression in specialized centres (including in order of priority mycophenolate mofetil, calcineurin inhibitors, rituximab, anti-TNF-α).
- Relapse occurs in about 40% of patients while on treatment and is frequently due to drug non-adherence, particularly in adolescents.
- Both AIH and ASC can recur after LT, recurrence being more common in ASC than AIH.
- In both AIH and ASC, regulatory T cells defective in number and/or function are likely to play a major role in the loss of tolerance that leads to autoimmune liver damage.
- De novo AIH after LT for non-autoimmune conditions responds to the classical treatment of AIH, but not to standard antirejection treatment.

Research Needed in the Field
- New specific biomarkers for the diagnosis and the monitoring of autoimmune liver disease.
- Understanding T cells, B cells and innate immunity interplays in the causation of the autoimmune damage.
- Understanding the role of the gut-liver axis and of the microbiome in the pathogenesis of liver disease.
- Randomized controlled studies to identify the most effective second-line treatments in children who fail standard therapy.

G. Mieli-Vergani (✉)
MowatLabs, Paediatric Liver, GI and Nutrition Centre,
King's College Hospital, London, UK
e-mail: giorgina.vergani@kcl.ac.uk

D. Vergani
MowatLabs, Institute of Liver Studies,
King's College Hospital, London, UK
e-mail: diego.vergani@kcl.ac.uk

10.1 Definition

Autoimmune liver diseases are inflammatory liver disorders characterized histologically by a dense mononuclear cell infiltrate in the portal tract (interface hepatitis; Fig. 10.1a) and serologically by high transaminase and immunoglobulin G (IgG) levels and positive autoantibodies. All other known causes of liver disease must be excluded. Autoimmune liver diseases typically respond to immunosuppressive treatment, which should be instituted as soon as the diagnosis is made [1].

In paediatrics, there are three liver disorders in which liver damage is deemed to arise from an autoimmune attack: autoimmune hepatitis (AIH), autoimmune sclerosing cholangitis (ASC) and de novo autoimmune hepatitis after liver transplantation (de novo AIH).

10.2 Autoimmune Hepatitis

AIH affects mainly girls and is divided into two main types according to the autoantibody profile: AIH type 1 (AIH-1) is positive for anti-nuclear (ANA) and/or anti-smooth muscle (SMA) antibodies and AIH type 2 (AIH-2) is positive for anti-liver-kidney microsomal antibody type 1 (anti-LKM-1) and/or anti-liver cytosol type 1 (anti-LC-1) antibodies.

10.2.1 Epidemiology

AIH occurs worldwide, but its prevalence is unknown. Initial epidemiological information including adult and juvenile AIH was obtained for AIH-1 before the introduction of the IAIHG diagnostic scoring system [2, 3], therefore without standard criteria for patient inclusion. Early prevalence reports range from 1.9 cases/100,000 in Norway [4] and 1/200,000 in the US general population [5] to 20/100,000 in females over 14 years of age referred to a tertiary centre in Spain [6]. A study from a UK secondary referral centre reported an AIH annual incidence of 3.5/100,000 [7]. Two studies using standardized criteria for the diagnosis of AIH published in 2002 and 2010 report a point prevalence of 24.5/100,000 in New Zealand [8] and of 34.5/100,000 in Alaskan natives [9]. Though AIH prevalence and incidence are reported to be lower in the Asia-Pacific area than in Europe and America [10], a better awareness of its clinical characteristics has led to an increased frequency in the diagnosis of AIH in China, where this condition was considered very rare [11]. Also in Japan the incidence and prevalence of AIH may be higher than previously thought [12]. Studies on the largest patient cohorts come from Northern Europe. A population-based investigation in Denmark reports an incidence rate of 1.68 per 100,000 populations per year, which doubled during the 1994–2012 period of observation [13]. In a large Swedish cohort, AIH point prevalence was reported as 17.3/100,000 inhabitants in 2009, with a yearly incidence of 1.2/100,000 inhabitants between 1990 and 2009 [14]. A large Dutch study reports an AIH prevalence of 18.3 per 100,000 [15].

All these epidemiological figures are likely to be underestimates, since AIH, particularly in adults, may remain undiagnosed for several years and present eventually with decompensated liver disease attributed to 'cryptogenic' cirrhosis.

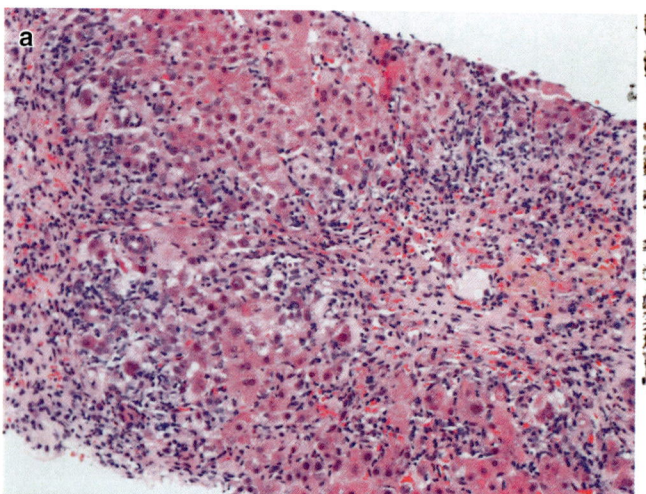 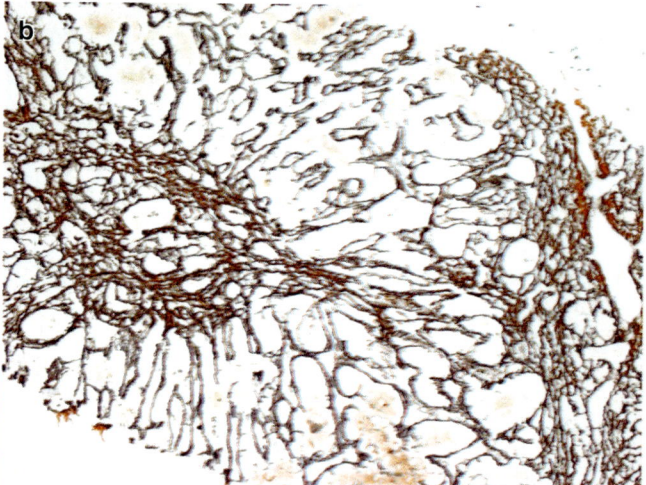

Fig. 10.1 Autoimmune hepatitis presenting acutely: (**a**) Portal and periportal lymphocyte and plasma cell infiltrate, disrupting the limiting plate (interface hepatitis) and extending into the parenchyma. Swollen hepatocytes, pyknotic necrosis and acinar inflammation are present (haematoxylin-eosin, original magnification 40×); (**b**) Reticulin staining showing connective-tissue collapse resulting from hepatocyte death and expanding from the portal area into the lobule (Images kindly provided by Dr. Alberto Quaglia)

The prevalence of AIH-2, which affects mainly children and young adults, is unknown, also because the diagnosis is probably often overlooked. Intriguingly AIH-2 has been reported more frequently in Europe that in the United States [16], possibly because of the under-testing for anti-LKM-1 antibodies in the latter, due to the unsubstantiated belief that AIH-2 is rare in Northern America and therefore that testing for anti-LKM-1 antibodies is not cost-effective [17]. In a study in Canada including 159 children/adolescents with AIH the annual incidence was 0.23 per 100,000 children, AIH-1 being diagnosed 5.5 times more frequently than AIH-2 [18].

Data collected at the King's College Hospital Paediatric Hepatology tertiary referral centre show a sixfold increase in the yearly incidence of juvenile AIH between the 1990s and 2000s [19], and a large study in Denmark shows a twofold increase in the incidence of adult AIH in the same period of time [13], suggesting either a better awareness of this condition, leading to an increased referral rate and diagnosis, or a real increase in the incidence of autoimmune liver disease.

10.2.2 Aetiology and Pathogenesis

The aetiology of AIH is unknown, although both genetic and environmental factors are involved in its expression [20].

Genetics. AIH is a 'complex-trait' disease—i.e. a condition not inherited in a Mendelian autosomal dominant, autosomal recessive or sex-linked fashion. The mode of inheritance of a complex-trait disorder is unknown and involves one or more genes operating alone or in concert to increase or reduce the risk of the trait and interacting with environmental factors [21].

Susceptibility to AIH is imparted by genes in the histocompatibility leukocyte antigen (HLA) region on the short arm of chromosome 6, especially those encoding DRB1 alleles. These class II major histocompatibility complex (MHC) molecules are involved in peptide antigen presentation to CD4 T cells, suggesting the involvement of MHC class II antigen presentation and T-cell activation in the pathogenesis of AIH. The prominent predisposing role of genes encoded in the HLA region has been confirmed in the largest genome-wide association study performed to date in AIH [22].

In Europe and North America, susceptibility to AIH-1 in adults is conferred by the possession of HLA DR3 (*DRB1*0301*) and DR4 (*DRB1*0401*), both heterodimers containing a lysine residue at position 71 of the DRB1 polypeptide and the hexameric amino acid sequence LLEQKR at positions 67–72 [23, 24]. In Japan, Argentina and Mexico, susceptibility is linked to *DRB1*0405* and *DRB1*0404*, alleles encoding arginine rather than lysine at position 71, but sharing the motif LLEQ-R with *DRB1*0401* and *DRB1*0301* [25]. Thus, K or R at position 71 in the context of LLEQ-R may be critical for susceptibility to AIH, favouring the binding of autoantigenic peptides, complementary to this hexameric sequence.

The lysine-71 and other models for AIH-1 cannot explain the disease completely, since in European and North American patients, for example, the presence of lysine-71 is associated with a severe and mainly juvenile disease in those who are positive for *DRB1*0301*, but to a mild and adult onset disease in those who are positive for *DRB1*0401*. Other genes inside and/or outside the MHC are therefore likely to be involved in determining the phenotype. The cytotoxic T lymphocyte antigen-4 (CTLA-4) [26], the tumour necrosis factor-alpha (TNF-α) gene promoter [27] and Fas [28] are notable examples.

A possible other candidate is the MHC-encoded complement gene, mapping to the class III MHC region, as patients with AIH, whether positive for anti-LKM-1 or ANA/SMA, have isolated partial deficiency of the HLA class III complement component C4, which is genetically determined [29].

In Northern Europe, paediatric AIH-1, similar to adult AIH, is associated with the possession of the human leukocyte antigen (HLA) *DRB1*03*. In contrast to adult patients, possession of *DRB1*04* does not predispose to AIH in childhood and can even exert a protective role [30]. Susceptibility to AIH-2 is conferred by the possession of HLA DR7 (*DRB1*0701*) and, in DR7 negative patients, with possession of DR3 (*DRB1*0301*), those patients positive for *DRB1*0701* having a more aggressive disease and a more severe prognosis [31]. In Egypt AIH-2 appears to be associated also with possession of *HLA-DRB1*15* [32]. In Brazil and in Egypt, the primary susceptibility allele for AIH-1 is *DRB1*1301*, but a secondary association with *DRB1*0301* has also been identified [32, 33]. Interestingly, in South America, possession of the HLA *DRB1*1301* allele not only predisposes to paediatric AIH-1 but is also associated with persistent infection with the endemic hepatitis A virus [34, 35]. Homozygosity for DR3 plays a major role in the predisposition to juvenile autoimmune liver disease [36]. The combination of HLA DRB1*1301 and a specific functional form of the killer cell immunoglobulin-like receptor (KIR2DS4-FL) imparts a strong predisposition to paediatric AIH-1 in South America [37]. Susceptibility to, and severity of, AIH-2 has been linked to alleles encoding the DRB1*0301 and DRB1*0701 molecules in the United Kingdom and Brazil. Allelic variation within HLA-DRB1 has been linked to differences in the autoantibody seropositivity profiles of AIH-2 patients [38].

A form of AIH serologically resembling AIH-2 affects some 20% of patients with autoimmune polyendocrinopathy-candidiasis-ectodermal dystrophy (APECED). APECED is a monogenic autosomal recessive disorder caused by homozygous mutations in the AIRE1 gene and characterized by a variety of organ-specific autoimmune diseases, the most common of which are hypoparathyroidism and primary adrenocortical failure, accompanied by chronic mucocutaneous candidiasis [39, 40]. Interestingly there are neutralizing autoantibodies to type 1 interferons, perhaps accounting for the associated immune deficiencies. APECED has a high level of variability in symptoms, especially between populations. Carriers of a single AIRE1 mutation (heterozygotes) do not develop APECED. However, although the inheritance pattern of APECED indicates a strictly recessive disorder, there are anecdotal data of mutations in a single copy of AIRE1 being associated with human autoimmunity of a less severe form than classically defined APECED [39, 40].

The role of the AIRE1 heterozygote state in the development of AIH-2 remains to be established, though heterozygous AIRE1 mutations have been reported in three children with severe AIH-2 and extrahepatic autoimmune manifestations [41].

Immune mechanisms [42]. Immunohistochemical studies have shown that the majority of the cells infiltrating the portal tract and invading the parenchyma in the typical AIH histological picture of interface hepatitis are T lymphocytes mounting the α/β T-cell receptor. Among the T cells, the majority are positive for the CD4 helper/inducer phenotype, and a sizable minority are positive for the CD8 cytotoxic phenotype. Lymphocytes of non-T-cell lineage are fewer and include (in decreasing order of frequency) natural killer cells (CD16/CD56-positive), macrophages and B lymphocytes. Natural killer T cells, which simultaneously express markers of both natural killer (CD56) and T cells (CD3), appear to be involved in liver damage in an animal model of autoimmune hepatitis.

Powerful stimuli must lead to the formation of the massive inflammatory cell infiltrate that is present at diagnosis in both AIH and ASC. Whatever the initial trigger, it is most probable that such a high number of activated inflammatory cells cause liver damage.

There are different possible pathways that an autoimmune attack can follow to inflict damage on hepatocytes (Fig. 10.2). Liver damage is probably orchestrated by CD4 T lymphocytes recognizing a self-antigenic liver peptide. To trigger an autoimmune response, the peptide has to be embraced by an HLA class II molecule and presented to uncommitted (naïve) CD4+ T-helper (Th0) cells by professional antigen-presenting cells (APC), such as dendritic cells (DCs), macrophages and B lymphocytes. The liver is home to several specialized APC

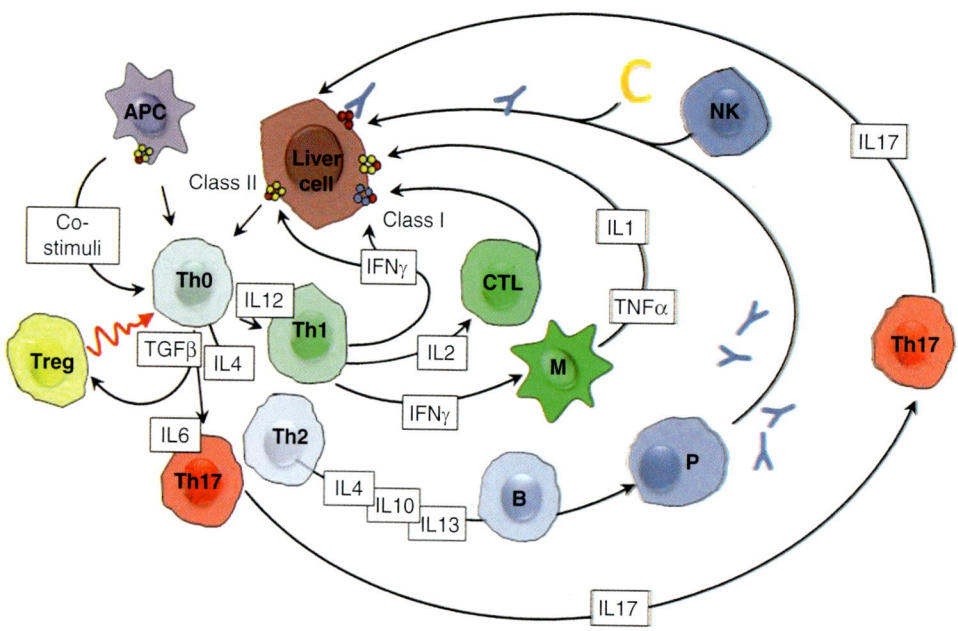

Fig. 10.2 Autoimmune attack to the hepatocyte: An autoantigen is presented to uncommitted T-helper (Th0) lymphocytes within the HLA class II molecule of an antigen-presenting cell (APC) either in the regional lymph nodes or within the liver itself. Activated Th0 cells differentiate into Th1 or Th2 cells in the presence of interleukin (IL)-12 or IL-4, respectively, and according to the nature of the antigen. This triggers a series of immune reactions determined by the cytokines they produce. Th1 cells secrete IL-2 and interferon (IFN)-γ, which are cytokines that stimulate cytotoxic T lymphocytes (CTL), enhance expression of class I HLA molecules, induce expression of class II HLA molecules on the liver cells and activate macrophages. Macrophages (M) release IL-1 and tumour necrosis factor (TNF). TH2 cells secrete mainly IL-4, IL-10 and IL-13 and stimulate autoantibody production by B lymphocytes. Regulatory T cells (T-reg) are derived from Th0 in the presence of transforming growth factor (TGF)-β. In the presence of defective T-reg, hepatocyte destruction ensues from the engagement of damaging effector mechanisms, including CTL, cytokines released by Th1 and by activated macrophages, complement activation or adhesion of natural killer (NK) cells to autoantibody-coated hepatocytes through their Fc receptors. Th17 cells produce the inflammatory cytokine IL-17 and derive from Th0 cells in the presence of TGF-β and IL-6. They are the focus of current investigations

populations, including liver sinusoidal endothelial cells (LSECs), Kupffer cells and DCs, where antigen presentation to both CD4 and CD8 effector T cells can occur in situ, perhaps averting the need for trafficking to the regional lymphoid tissues [43, 44]. CD4$^+$ T-cell activation is promoted by interaction of two ligands, CD28 on Th0 cells and CD80 on APC. Th0 cells then become activated and differentiate into functional phenotypes according to the cytokines prevailing in the microenvironment and the nature of the antigen and initiate a cascade of immune reactions determined by the cytokines these activated T cells produce. Th1 cells, arising in the presence of the macrophage-produced interleukin 12 (IL-12), secrete mainly IL-2 and interferon gamma (IFN-γ), which activate macrophages, enhance expression of HLA class I (increasing liver cell vulnerability to a CD8 T-cell cytotoxic attack) and induce expression of HLA class II molecules on hepatocytes. Th2 cells, which differentiate from Th0 if the microenvironment is rich in IL-4, mainly produce IL-4, IL-10 and IL-13, which favour autoantibody production by B lymphocytes. Physiologically, Th1 and Th2 antagonize each other. Th17 cells arise in the presence of transforming growth factor-β (TGF-β) and IL-6 and have an important effector role in inflammation and autoimmunity. The process of autoantigen recognition is strictly controlled by regulatory mechanisms, such as those exerted by CD4$^+$CD25$^+$FOXP3$^+$CD127$^-$ regulatory T cells, which are derived from Th0 in the presence of TGF-β but in the absence of IL-6. If regulatory mechanisms fail, the autoimmune attack develops and persists.

Various aspects of the above pathogenic scenario have been investigated during the last 40 years:

- *Regulatory T cells* [45]. Autoimmunity arises against a background of defective immunoregulation, and this has been repeatedly reported in AIH. Early studies showed that patients with AIH have low levels of circulating T cells expressing the CD8 marker and impaired suppressor cell function, which segregates with the possession of the disease-predisposing HLA haplotype *B*08/DRB1*03* and is correctable by therapeutic doses of corticosteroids. It is possible, although not formally tested, that these early characterized CD8 T cells with a suppressor function represent the later described CD8$^+$CD28$^-$ suppressor T cells. Furthermore, patients with AIH have been shown to have a defect in a subpopulation of T cells controlling the immune response to liver-specific membrane antigens. More recent experimental evidence confirms an impairment of the immunoregulatory function in AIH. Among T-cell subsets with potential immunoregulatory function, CD4 cells constitutively expressing the IL-2 receptor alpha chain (CD25) (T-regulatory cells, T-regs) represent the dominant one. These cells, constituting 5–10% of all peripheral CD4 cells in health, control innate and adaptive immune responses by limiting the proliferation and effector function of autoreactive T cells. They act by direct contact with the target cells and, to a lesser extent, by releasing immunoregulatory cytokines, such as IL-10 and tissue growth factor beta 1. Besides CD25, which is also present on T cells undergoing activation, T-regs express additional markers, including the glucocorticoid-induced tumour necrosis factor receptor, CD62L, CTLA4 and the forkhead/winged-helix transcription factor FOXP3, whose expression has been associated with the acquisition of regulatory properties. Importantly, they express little or no CD127, the IL-7 receptor. In children with AIH, T-regs are defective in number and function in comparison with normal controls, and this impairment relates to the stage of disease, being more evident at diagnosis than during drug-induced remission. The percentage of T-regs inversely correlates with markers of disease severity, such as anti-soluble liver antigen (anti-SLA) and anti-LKM-1 autoantibody titres, suggesting that a reduction in regulatory T cells favours the serological expression of autoimmune liver disease. Importantly, several studies show that T-regs from AIH patients at diagnosis are impaired in their ability to control the proliferation of CD4 and CD8 effector cells compared to T-regs isolated from AIH patients at remission or from healthy subjects. Effector CD4 T cells isolated from patients with AIH are less susceptible to the regulatory control exerted by T-regs. This defect is linked to reduced expression of the inhibitory receptor T-cell-immunoglobulin-and-mucin-domain-containing-molecule-3 (Tim-3), which upon ligation of galectin-9 present on T-regs induces effector cell death. If loss of immunoregulation is central to the pathogenesis of AIH, treatment should concentrate on restoring the T-regs' ability to expand, with a consequent increase in their number and function. This is at least partially achieved by standard immunosuppression, since numbers of T-regs increase during remission.
- *Autoreactive T cells* [42]. As mentioned above, to trigger an autoimmune response, a peptide embraced by an HLA class II molecule has to be presented to uncommitted T-helper (Th0) cells by professional APCs (Fig. 10.2). Given the impaired regulatory function described above, it is suspected that in AIH, an autoantigenic peptide is indeed presented to the helper/inducer T cells, leading to their sustained activation.

Major advances in the study of T cells have occurred in AIH-2, since the main autoantigenic target of anti-LKM-1 has been identified as cytochrome P4502D6 (CYP2D6), making it possible to characterize both CD4 and CD8 T cells targeting this cytochrome. One study has shown that CD4 T cells from patients with AIH-2 who are positive for the predisposing HLA allele *DRB1*0701* recognize seven regions of CYP2D6, five of which have later been shown to be also recognized by CD8 T cells. High numbers of antigen-specific interferon gamma-producing CD4 and CD8 T cells are associated with biochemical evidence of liver damage, suggesting a combined cellular immune attack.

What triggers the immune system to react to an autoantigen is unknown. A lesson may be learned by the study of humoral autoimmune responses during viral infections. Thus, studies aimed at determining the specificity of the LKM-1 antibody—present in both the juvenile form of AIH and in some patients with chronic hepatitis C virus (HCV) infection—have shown a high amino acid sequence homology between the HCV polyprotein and CYP2D6, implicating a mechanism of molecular mimicry as a trigger for the production of anti-LKM-1 in HCV infection. It is therefore conceivable that an as yet unknown viral infection may be at the origin of the autoimmune attack in AIH.

The possible role of Th17 cells in the pathogenesis of AIH is under investigation. Th17 cells contribute to autoimmunity by producing the pro-inflammatory cytokines IL-17, IL-22 and TNF-α and inducing hepatocytes to secrete IL-6 [46], which further enhances Th17 activation. An elevated level of Th17 cells has been reported in both blood and liver of patients with AIH [46, 47].

10.2.3 Clinical Features (Table 10.1)

As mentioned above, AIH is divided into two forms according to its autoantibody profile: AIH-1 is positive for ANA and/or SMA and AIH-2 for anti-LKM-1 and/or anti-LC-1. Three quarters of patients with either type of AIH are female. AIH-1 affects all ages, with two peaks, one in childhood/adolescence and the other in adulthood around the age of 40 years. AIH-2 affects mainly children and young adults, being rare, though not absent, in older individuals. In paediatrics, AIH-1 accounts for at least two-thirds of the cases and presents usually during adolescence, while AIH-2 presents at a younger age, including infancy. IgG are usually raised at onset in both types, though 15% of children with AIH-1 and 25% of those with AIH-2 have levels within the normal range, particularly when the disease presents acutely, [1]. Interestingly, also these children with IgG within the normal range experience a reduction in levels during treatment. Partial IgA deficiency is common in AIH-2, affecting some 40% of patients [30, 48]. While most adult patients with AIH-1 have a chronic disease course with non-specific symptoms such as fatigue, nausea, abdominal pain and arthralgia [49], juvenile AIH has a more aggressive phenotype. The clinical course has been mainly described in patients of European origin [30, 50, 51–56], individuals from other ethnic groups being considered rarely affected by this condition. AIH, however, is being increasingly reported in children and adolescents of non-Caucasoid descent, probably because the diagnosis of autoimmune liver disease was previously overlooked in view of the presence of epidemic viral hepatitis B and/or C. Reports from India [57, 58], Malaysia [59], Pakistan [60], Bahrain [61], Iran [62], Egypt [63], Jamaica [64], and Mexico [65] on cohorts including between 5 and 181 (median 34) patients indicate a clinical presentation and response to immunosuppressive treatment similar to those described in Caucasoid patients, but an overall worse response to treatment and outcome, possibly related to delay in referral to specialized centres and diagnosis.

The mode of presentation of AIH in childhood is variable (Table 10.2), and the disease should be suspected and excluded in all children presenting with symptoms and signs of prolonged or severe liver disease. Acute hepatitis episodes

Table 10.1 Comparison between autoimmune hepatitis type 1, autoimmune hepatitis type 2 and autoimmune sclerosing cholangitis

Variable		AIH-1	AIH-2	ASC
Female sex		80%	80%	50%
Male sex		20%	20%	50%
ANA or SMA[a]	≥1:20	++	+/−	++
Anti-LKM-1[a]	≥1:10	−	++	+/−
Anti-LC-1	Positive	−	++	−
Anti-SLA	Positive	+	+	+
pANNA	Positive	+	−	++
IgG	>Upper limit of normal	++	+	++
	>1.20 times upper limit of normal	++	+	++
Liver histology	Compatible with AIH	+	+	+
	Typical of AIH	+	+	+
Viral hepatitis (A, B, C, E, EBV), NASH, Wilson disease and drug exposure		−	−	−
Presence of extrahepatic autoimmunity		+	+	+
Family history of autoimmune disease		+	+	+
Cholangiography	Normal	+	+	−
	Abnormal	−	−	+
Biochemical and immunological response to steroid treatment	Yes	+	+	+
	No	−	−	−

AIH-1 autoimmune hepatitis type 1, *AIH-2* autoimmune hepatitis type 2, *ASC* autoimmune sclerosing cholangitis, *ANA* anti-nuclear antibody, *SMA* anti-smooth muscle antibody, *anti-LKM-1* anti-liver-kidney microsomal antibody type 1, *anti-LC-1* anti-liver cytosol type 1, *anti-SLA* anti-soluble liver antigen, *IgG* immunoglobulin G, *NASH* non-alcoholic steatohepatitis

[a]Antibodies measured by indirect immunofluorescence on a composite rodent substrate (kidney, liver, stomach)

Table 10.2 Modes of presentation of juvenile autoimmune hepatitis

Mode of presentation	Clinical features
Acute	Non-specific symptoms similar to viral hepatitis: malaise, nausea/vomiting, anorexia, joint and abdominal pain, followed by jaundice, dark urine, and pale stools (40–50% of patients); transaminase levels can fluctuate
Fulminant hepatic failure	Grade II to IV hepatic encephalopathy developing 2 weeks to 2 months after the onset of symptoms (~3% of patients with AIH-1 and ~20% of patients with AIH-2)
Insidious onset	Non-specific symptoms (progressive fatigue, relapsing jaundice, amenorrhea, headache, anorexia, joint and abdominal pain, diarrhoea, weight loss), lasting from months to a few years before diagnosis (~40% of patients with AIH-1 and ~25% of patients with AIH-2)
Complications of cirrhosis and portal hypertension	Haematemesis from oesophageal/gastric varices, bleeding diathesis, splenomegaly, without previous history of jaundice or liver disease (~10 of both AIH types)
Asymptomatic	Incidental finding of raised aminotransferases, without any symptoms or signs (rare in large series but real prevalence unknown)

alternating with spontaneous clinical and biochemical improvement are not uncommon, a relapsing pattern that often leads to a dangerous delay in diagnosis and treatment. Hence AIH should always be suspected when known causes of acute hepatitis are excluded.

At least one-third of patients with AIH have cirrhosis at diagnosis, irrespective of the mode of presentation [1], indicating that the disease process is long-standing. AIH patients presenting acutely have often advanced fibrosis or cirrhosis on liver biopsy.

Severity of disease is similar in the two AIH types. AIH-2, however, has a higher tendency to present as acute liver failure (ALF) and is more refractory to eventual treatment withdrawal [30, 63, 65]. In both types a family history of autoimmune disease is frequent (~40%), and some 20% of patients have associated autoimmune disorders either present at diagnosis or developing during follow-up, including thyroiditis, inflammatory bowel disease (IBD), haemolytic anaemia, vitiligo, coeliac disease, insulin-dependent diabetes, Behçet disease, Sjögren syndrome, glomerulonephritis, idiopathic thrombocytopenia, urticaria pigmentosa, hypoparathyroidism, and Addison disease (the latter mainly in AIH-2) [30, 66]. These conditions should be actively sought for prompt treatment [67]. In this context diagnoses of particular importance are thyroiditis with hypothyroidism that affects 8–23% [30, 66], coeliac disease that affects between 5 and 10% [68–71] and IBD that affects ~18% of patients [50]. Interestingly patients with AIH and coeliac disease have been reported to achieve treatment-free sustained remission in a significantly higher proportion of cases, when compared with patients with AIH without coeliac disease, suggesting a possible long-term adjuvant effect of the gluten-free diet [72].

As mentioned above, AIH-2 responsive to immunosuppressive treatment has been described in 20–30% of patients with APECED syndrome [73–75].

10.2.4 Diagnostic Criteria

The diagnosis of AIH is based on a combination of clinical, biochemical, immunological and histological features and the exclusion of other known causes of liver disease that may share serological and histological features with AIH (e.g. hepatitis B, C and E, Epstein-Barr virus infection, Wilson disease, non-alcoholic steatohepatitis [NASH] and drug-induced liver disease). Liver biopsy is needed to confirm the diagnosis and to evaluate the severity of liver damage [76, 77]. In the absence of a single diagnostic test for AIH, the International Autoimmune Hepatitis Group (IAIHG) has devised a diagnostic system for comparative and research purposes, which includes several positive and negative scores, the sum of which gives a value indicative of probable or definite AIH [2, 3]. A simplified IAIHG scoring system published more recently is better suited to clinical application [78]. However, neither scoring system is applicable to the juvenile form of the disease [79], in particular in the context of fulminant hepatic failure [80, 81]. Moreover, diagnostically relevant autoantibodies in paediatrics often have titres lower than the cut-off value considered positive in adults [82] and neither IAIHG system allows distinction between AIH and ASC (see below) [50, 83], which can only be differentiated if a cholangiogram is performed at presentation. A recent European Society of Paediatric Gastroenterology Hepatology and Nutrition (ESPGHAN) Hepatology Committee Position Statement proposes a scoring system for juvenile autoimmune liver disease to differentiate between AIH and ASC [1] (Table 10.3).

10.2.5 Laboratory Findings

Characteristic laboratory findings are elevated serum transaminase and IgG/γ-globulin levels and presence of autoantibodies (ANA and/or SMA in AIH-1, anti-LKM-1 and/or anti-LC-1 in AIH-2) [82, 84]. International normalized prothrombin ratio (INR) and bilirubin and albumin levels are variably abnormal, depending on the severity and chronicity of the disease. Alkaline phosphatase and gammaglutamyl transferase (GGT) levels can vary from normal to moderately elevated. Anti-LKM-1-positive patients tend to have higher levels of bilirubin and transaminases at presentation than those who are ANA/SMA-positive, reflecting the higher incidence of acute presentation in AIH-2.

Table 10.3 Proposed scoring criteria for the diagnosis of juvenile autoimmune liver disease

Variable	Cut-off	Points AIH	Points ASC
ANA and/or SMA[a]	≥1:20[b]	1	1
	≥1:80	2	2
Anti-LKM-1[a] or	≥1:10[b]	1	1
	≥1:80	2	1
Anti-LC-1	Positive[b]	2	1
Anti-SLA	Positive[b]	2	2
pANNA	Positive	1	2
IgG	>ULN	1	1
	>1.20 ULN	2	2
Liver histology	Compatible with AIH	1	1
	Typical of AIH	2	2
Absence of viral hepatitis (A, B, E, EBV), NASH, Wilson disease and drug exposure	Yes	2	2
Presence of extrahepatic autoimmunity	Yes	1	1
Family history of autoimmune disease	Yes	1	1
Cholangiography	Normal	2	−2
	Abnormal	−2	2

Score ≥ 7, probable AIH; ≥8, definite AIH
Score ≥ 7, probable ASC; ≥8, definite ASC
AIH autoimmune hepatitis, *ASC* autoimmune sclerosing cholangitis, *ANA* anti-nuclear antibody, *SMA* anti-smooth muscle antibody, *anti-LKM-1* anti-liver-kidney microsomal antibody type 1, *anti-LC-1* anti-liver cytosol type 1, *anti-SLA* anti-soluble liver antigen, *IgG* immunoglobulin G, *EBV* Epstein-Barr virus, *NASH* non-alcoholic steatohepatitis, *ULN* upper limit of normal
[a]Antibodies measured by indirect immunofluorescence on a composite rodent substrate (kidney, liver, stomach)
[b]Addition of points achieved for ANA, SMA, anti-LKM-1, anti-LC-1 and anti-SLA autoantibodies cannot exceed a maximum of 2 points

10.2.6 Immunoglobulins

The majority (80%) of patients has increased levels of IgG, but some 20% have serum IgG levels within the normal range for age, particularly those presenting with acute hepatic failure, indicating that normal IgG values do not exclude the diagnosis of AIH. Measurement of IgG levels is particularly useful in monitoring disease activity and response to treatment [85]. Partial IgA deficiency is common in AIH-2 (~40%).

10.2.7 Autoantibodies

Key to the diagnosis of AIH is positivity for circulating autoantibodies [2, 3, 78, 82] (Table 10.4) though autoantibodies can be present in other liver disorders and are not diagnostic in isolation. Their detection by indirect immunofluorescence on a rodent substrate not only assists in the diagnosis but also allows differentiation into the two forms of AIH. ANA and SMA characterize AIH-1; anti-LKM-1 and anti-LC1 define AIH-2 [82, 86]. The two autoantibody profiles can occur simultaneously, but not frequently. As interpretation of the immunofluorescence patterns can be difficult, guidelines have been provided by the IAIHG regarding methodology and interpretation of liver autoimmune serology [82]. A major advantage of testing for autoantibodies by indirect immunofluorescence on a freshly prepared rodent substrate that includes the kidney, liver and stomach is that it allows the concurrent detection of several autoreactivities relevant to AIH. These include ANA, SMA, anti-LKM-1 and

Table 10.4 Diagnostic autoantibodies and their targets in juvenile autoimmune liver disease

Autoantibody	Target antigen(s)	Liver disease	Conventional method of detection	Molecular-based assays
ANA	Chromatin Histones Centromeres Cyclin A Ribonucleoproteins Double-stranded DNA Single-stranded DNA Unknown	AIH-1 and ASC	IIF	ELISA, IB, LIA
SMA	Microfilaments (Filamentous actin) Intermediate filaments (Vimentin, desmin)	AIH-1 and ASC	IIF	ELISA
Anti-LKM-1	Cytochrome P4502D6	AIH-2	IIF	ELISA, IB, LIA, RIA
Anti-LC-1	Forminino-transferase cyclodeaminase	AIH-2	IIF, DID, CIE	ELISA, LIA, RIA
Anti-SLA	tRNP(Ser)Sec	AIH-1, AIH-2, ASC Prognostic of severe disease, relapse and treatment dependence	Inhibition ELISA	ELISA, IB, RIA
pANNA	Nuclear lamina Proteins	ASC and AIH-1	IIF	N/A

ANA anti-nuclear antibodies, *SMA* anti-smooth muscle antibodies, *anti-LKM-1* anti-liver-kidney microsomal antibody type 1, *anti-LC-1* anti-liver cytosol antibody type 1, *SLA* soluble liver antigens, *pANNA* peripheral anti-nuclear neutrophil antibodies, also known as atypical pANCA, *AIH* autoimmune hepatitis, *ASC* autoimmune sclerosing cholangitis, *IIF* indirect immunofluorescence, *DID* double-dimension immune-diffusion, *CIE* counter-immune-electrophoresis, *ELISA* enzyme-linked immunosorbent assay, *IB* immunoblot, *LIA* line-immuno-assay, *RIA* radio-immune-precipitation assay, *N/A* not applicable

anti-LC1, as well as anti-mitochondrial antibody (AMA), the serological hallmark of primary biliary cholangitis (PBC), the presence of which weighs against the diagnosis of AIH [2, 3, 78, 82], though rare cases of AMA-positive AIH have been reported, including in children [87–90].

Autoantibodies are considered positive when present at a dilution ≥1:40 in adults, while in children, who are rarely positive for autoantibodies in health, positivity at a dilution ≥1:20 for ANA and SMA or ≥1:10 for anti-LKM-1 is clinically significant [82]. Both in adults and children autoantibodies may be present at a low titre or even be negative at disease onset, particularly during acute or fulminant presentations, to become detectable during follow-up.

ANA is detectable on all rodent tissues and in AIH usually has a homogeneous pattern. For a clearer definition of the pattern, HEp2 cells that have prominent nuclei are used, but these cells are not recommended for screening purposes, because of a high positivity rate in the normal population [82, 91, 92] and in the presence of infection, particularly in children [93].

There are no ANA molecular targets specific for AIH. Though ANA reactivities similar to those found in lupus erythematosus (nuclear chromatin, histones, centromere, single–/double-stranded DNA, ribonucleoproteins) have been reported [94, 95], some 30% of AIH patients positive for ANA by immunofluorescence do not react with known nuclear targets [94]. Immunofluorescence remains therefore the gold standard for ANA testing.

The immunofluorescent staining of SMA is detected in the arterial walls of rodent kidney, liver and stomach. In the kidney, SMA can have three patterns: V (vessels), G (glomeruli) and T (tubules) [82]. The V pattern is present in non-autoimmune inflammatory liver disease, in autoimmune diseases not affecting the liver and in viral infections, but the VG and VGT patterns are indicative of AIH. The VGT pattern corresponds to the 'F actin' or microfilament (MF) pattern observed using cultured fibroblasts as substrate. The molecular target of the microfilament reactivity remains to be identified. Though anti-actin reactivity is strongly associated with AIH, some 20% of AIH-1 patients do not possess anti-actin antibodies [82].

The anti-LKM-1 pattern is characterized by bright staining of the hepatocyte cytoplasm and of the P3 portion of the renal tubules. Anti-LKM-1 can be confused with AMA, as both autoantibodies stain the liver and kidney, though AMA, in contrast to anti-LKM-1, also stains gastric parietal cells. The identification of the molecular targets of anti-LKM-1, cytochrome P4502D6, and of AMA, enzymes of the 2-oxo-acid dehydrogenase complexes, has allowed the establishment of immuno-assays using recombinant or purified antigens [82], which can be used to resolve doubtful cases.

Anti-LC1, an additional marker for AIH-2, can be present on its own but frequently occurs in association with anti-LKM-1 and targets formimino-transferase cyclodeaminase (FTCD) [96]. Anti-FTCD antibody can be detected by commercial ELISA [82].

Other autoantibodies less commonly tested, but of diagnostic importance, include anti-soluble liver antigen (anti-SLA) and anti-perinuclear neutrophil cytoplasm (pANCA) antibodies.

Anti-SLA is highly specific for the diagnosis of autoimmune liver disease [94, 95], and its presence identifies patients with more severe disease and worse outcome [97]. At variance with standard diagnostic autoantibodies, anti-SLA is not detectable by immunofluorescence. The discovery of the molecular target of anti-SLA as Sep (O-phosphoserine) tRNA:Sec (selenocysteine) tRNA synthase (SEPSECS) [98] and its cloning has led to the availability of molecularly based diagnostic assays.

In AIH-1, akin to ASC and IBD, pANCA are frequently detected, but they are atypical, since they react with peripheral nuclear membrane components, and are therefore also termed peripheral anti-nuclear neutrophil antibodies (pANNA). In contrast to AIH-1, pANNA are virtually absent in AIH-2 [82].

A seronegative form of AIH responsive to steroid treatment has been reported in paediatric retrospective studies, at times associated with the development of aplastic anaemia [60, 62, 99]. In these reports, however, autoantibody testing has not been performed according to IAIHG guidelines. The true prevalence of AIH negative for all the autoantibodies listed above can only be established with a rigorous prospective study.

10.2.8 Histology

Liver biopsy is necessary to establish the diagnosis (Table 10.5). The typical histological feature of AIH is interface hepatitis (Fig. 10.1a), which is however not exclusive to this condition [100]. Interface hepatitis is characterized by a dense inflammatory infiltrate composed of lymphocytes and

Table 10.5 Histological features of autoimmune hepatitis

Feature	Description
Inflammation	Dense mononuclear and plasma cell infiltration of the portal areas
Interface hepatitis	Erosion of the limiting plate and invasion of the parenchyma by plasma cell-rich mononuclear cells that surround damaged hepatocytes
Bridging collapse	Connective-tissue collapse resulting from hepatocyte death and expanding from the portal area into the lobule
Rosette formation	Hepatic regeneration with liver cells forming clusters resembling 'rosettes'
Emperipolesis	Mononuclear cells within hepatocytes
Hyaline droplets	Hyaline droplets in Kupffer cells containing IgG
Fibrosis/Cirrhosis	New collagen deposition eventually disrupting the liver architecture

plasma cells, which crosses the limiting plate and invades the surrounding parenchyma. Hepatocytes surrounded by inflammatory cells are swollen and undergo pyknotic necrosis. Though plasma cells are characteristically abundant at the interface and within the lobule, their presence in low number does not exclude the diagnosis of AIH. When AIH presents acutely, and during episodes of relapse, a common histological finding is panlobular hepatitis with connective-tissue collapse resulting from hepatocyte death expanding from the portal area into the lobule (bridging necrosis) (Fig. 10.1b). Other features that point to the diagnosis of AIH are emperipolesis and hepatocyte rosetting [101]. These findings, however, are not present in all patients. A recent paper in a paediatric AIH cohort suggests that the finding of hyaline droplets in Kupffer cells is a useful diagnostic marker to distinguish AIH from other forms of chronic hepatitis. The hyaline droplets occur specifically in AIH regardless of the type and are positive for IgG by immunohistochemistry, correlating with a >2-fold increase in serum level of IgG [102].

Histology is also the gold standard for evaluating the extent of fibrosis and helps in identifying overlap syndromes as well as the possible presence of concomitant diseases, such as NASH [103]. Though inflammatory changes surrounding the bile ducts are present also in a small proportion of patients with classical AIH, when conspicuous they suggest an overlap with sclerosing cholangitis [50].

In contrast to patients with an insidious course, those presenting with acute liver failure (ALF) show histological damage predominantly in the centrilobular area [104] often with massive necrosis and multilobular collapse indistinguishable from other forms of acute liver failure [105]. In one paediatric study, histology did not allow distinguishing autoimmune ALF from indeterminate ALF [106]. In the presence of coagulopathy, liver biopsy should be performed by the transjugular route, which is not without risk. If transjugular biopsy is technically not available, the absence of histology should not preclude prompt initiation of immunosuppressive treatment, but liver biopsy should be performed as soon as coagulation indices permit.

10.2.9 Treatment

10.2.9.1 Definition of Remission/Relapse

In paediatric age, remission of AIH has been long defined as complete clinical recovery with transaminase levels within the normal range and is achieved in 60–90% of patients [18, 30, 57, 62, 63], the rapidity and degree of the response to treatment depending on the disease severity at presentation. In more recent years, three more criteria have been added to the definition of remission: normalization of IgG levels, negative or very low titer autoantibodies and histological resolution of inflammation [1]. The histological response, however, lags behind the biochemical response [107–109], and clinical/biochemical/immunological remission does not always reflect histological resolution, though 95% of patients have a marked histological improvement after a mean duration of 4 years of effective treatment [107]. As liver biopsy cannot be repeated frequently, for clinical purposes remission is considered complete when transaminase and IgG levels are normal, ANA and SMA are negative or low titre (<1:20) and anti-LKM-1 and anti-LC1 are negative.

Relapse is characterized by increase of serum aminotransferase levels after remission has been achieved. Relapse during treatment is frequent, occurring in about 40% of patients and requiring a temporary increase in the steroid dose. An important element in relapse is played by non-adherence, which is common, particularly in adolescents [59, 110]. In more aggressive cases, the risk of relapse is higher if steroids are administered on an alternate-day schedule, which is often instituted in the assumption that may have a less negative effect on the child's growth. Small daily doses, however, are more effective in maintaining disease control and minimize the need for high-dose steroid pulses during relapses (with consequent more severe side effects) and do not affect final height [111].

10.2.9.2 When to Treat

AIH should be suspected and sought in all children with evidence of liver disease after exclusion of infectious and metabolic aetiologies. AIH is exquisitely responsive to immunosuppression, and treatment should be initiated promptly to avoid progression of disease. The goal of treatment is to reduce or eliminate liver inflammation, induce remission, improve symptoms and quality of life and prolong life expectancy [1, 112]. Although cirrhosis is present in between 44% and 80% of children at the time at diagnosis [30, 54, 107, 112], mortality within childhood/adolescence is low, and most patients remain clinically stable and well on long-term treatment.

10.2.9.3 How to Treat

With the exception of a fulminant presentation with encephalopathy (see below), AIH responds satisfactorily to immunosuppressive treatment whatever the degree of liver impairment, with a reported remission rate of up to 90% [18, 30, 50, 58].

Standard treatment (Table 10.6)—Conventional treatment of AIH consists of prednisolone (or prednisone) 2 mg/kg/day (maximum 60 mg/day), which is gradually decreased over a period of 4–8 weeks, in parallel to the decline of transaminase levels, to a maintenance dose of 2.5–5 mg/day [1, 76, 77, 113, 114]. In most patients an 80% decrease of the transaminase levels is achieved in the first 2 months, but their complete normalization may take several months [105, 113]. During the first 6–8 weeks of treatment, liver function

10 Autoimmune Liver Disease

Table 10.6 Immunosuppressive treatment regimens for juvenile autoimmune liver disease

	Initial regimen		Maintenance			Definition of remission	Treatment length	Before attempting treatment withdrawal
			Predniso(lo)ne 0.1–0.2 mg/kg/day or 5 mg/day	**Azathioprine** 1–2 mg/kg/day if required	**Azathioprine monotherapy (in AIH-1)** 1.2–1.6 mg/kg/day			
AIH	**Predniso(lo)ne** 2 mg/kg/day (up to 60 mg/daily) decreased weekly in parallel to transaminase levels decrease to a minimum maintenance dose of 2.5–5 mg daily	**Azathioprine** 1–2 mg/kg/day added gradually if transaminase levels plateau or increase Alternatively, added in all patients after 2 weeks of predniso(lo)ne treatment				– Normal transaminase and IgG levels – Negative or low titre (<1:20) ANA/SMA – Negative anti-LKM-1/anti-LC-1	3 years before considering suspension	Remission for at least 3 years + follow-up liver biopsy showing no inflammatory changes
ASC	**Predniso(lo)ne ± azathioprine** as above, plus **ursodeoxycholic acid** 15 mg/kg/day		**Predniso(lo)ne ± azathioprine** as above, plus **ursodeoxycholic acid** 15 mg/kg/day			As above	As above	As above

AIH autoimmune hepatitis, *ASC* autoimmune sclerosing cholangitis

tests should be checked weekly to allow frequent dose adjustments, avoiding severe steroid side effects. The timing for the addition of azathioprine as a steroid sparing agent varies according to the protocols used in different centres. In some, azathioprine is added only in the presence of serious steroid side effects or if the transaminase levels stop decreasing on steroid treatment alone, at a starting dose of 0.5 mg/kg/day. In the absence of signs of toxicity, the dose is increased up to a maximum of 2.0–2.5 mg/kg/day until biochemical control is achieved. In other centres azathioprine is added at a dose of 0.5–2 mg/kg/day after a few weeks (usually 2 weeks) of steroid treatment. Whatever the protocol, 85% of the patients eventually require the addition of azathioprine. Some centres use a combination of steroids and azathioprine from the beginning [56], but caution is recommended with this approach because azathioprine can be hepatotoxic, particularly in cirrhotic and severely jaundiced patients [77]. A recent retrospective analysis of patients treated with a combination of azathioprine and prednisolone from diagnosis reports more side effects (93%) and a higher relapse rate (67%) [115] than what observed in AIH children treated with steroid induction followed by azathioprine addition only when indicated (relapse rate 33–36%; side effects 18–38%) [30, 50].

Measurement of thiopurine methyltransferase (TPMT) activity level before initiating azathioprine therapy has been proposed as a predictor of drug metabolism and toxicity [105] though, at least in adult patients, advanced fibrosis, but not TPMT genotype or activity, was able to predict azathioprine toxicity in AIH [116]. Measurement of the azathioprine metabolites 6-thioguanine (6-TGN) and 6-methylmercaptopurine has been reported to help in identifying drug toxicity and non-adherence and in achieving a level of 6-TGN considered therapeutic for IBD [117], though an ideal therapeutic level for AIH has not been determined. In a recent retrospective review, 87% of 66 children with AIH were reported to maintain sustained biochemical remission (normal transaminase levels) in association with low 6-TGN levels ranging from 50 to 250 pmol on an azathioprine dose of 1.2–1.6 mg/kg/day [118]. Moreover, the same report shows that remission can be maintained on monotherapy with this dose of azathioprine in AIH-1 [118].

Alternative treatments (Table 10.7)—Alternative AIH treatments have been proposed (a) to induce remission at disease onset in an attempt to decrease steroid side effects and (b) to treat refractory patients, i.e. those intolerant of or unresponsive to standard immunosuppression, often referred to as 'difficult-to-treat'.

(a) **For induction of remission**—An attractive drug for the induction and maintenance of remission in AIH is budesonide, a drug with hepatic first-pass clearance of >90% of the oral dose and fewer side effects than predniso(lo)ne, representing an ideal 'topical' liver treatment, more acceptable to patients [119]. A drawback is that it cannot be used in the presence of cirrhosis, which affects at least one-third of AIH patients. In a large European trial, comprising 160 adult and 46 paediatric patients, a combination of budesonide and azathioprine was compared with a combination of prednisone and azathioprine [120]. Remission was defined as normal transaminase levels without steroid side effects. The effect of budesonide at a dose of 3 mg three times daily, decreased upon response, was compared with that of prednisone 40 mg once daily reduced per protocol, irrespective of response, for 6 months; and then budesonide was given to all patients for further 6 months. The results among the children recruited into the study were disappointing, with a similarly low remission rate of 16% for budesonide/azathioprine and 15% for prednisone/azathioprine after 6 months of treatment and of 50% and 42%, respectively, after 12 months of treatment, with similar steroid side effects in both groups, apart from a higher frequency of weight gain in children on prednisone [121]. As these remission rates are much poorer than

Table 10.7 Alternative treatments for juvenile autoimmune liver disease

Agent	Pros	Cons
Mycophenolate mofetil	Favourable toxicity profile Experience as transplant immunosuppressant	Contradictory reports regarding its efficacy Teratogenicity
Tacrolimus	Potent immunosuppressant Experience in the transplant setting	Anecdotal experience Unclear efficacy Renal toxicity
Cyclosporine	Potent immunosuppressant Experience in the transplant setting	Unclear benefit over standard treatment Cosmetic effects Renal toxicity
Budesonide	High first-pass metabolism in the liver Less side effects than prednisolone	Ineffective in cirrhotic patients Less effective as first line treatment compared to standard treatment
Rituximab	Relatively favourable toxicity profile	Infectious complications Anecdotal experience Unclear efficacy
Infliximab	Potent immunomodulatory properties Effective in inflammatory bowel disease	Unclear efficacy in liver disease Infectious complications Paradoxical development of AIH
Ursodeoxycholic acid	Putative immunomodulatory capacities Choleretic	Efficacy yet to be demonstrated

those achieved with the standard treatment schedule, caution is advisable in using budesonide to induce remission in juvenile AIH [19]. A controlled trial in a larger number of treatment-naïve paediatric AIH patients, using a study design that includes strict diagnostic criteria and drug schedules appropriate for the juvenile disease, is needed to establish whether budesonide has a role in the treatment of this condition. Nevertheless, budesonide could be considered as an alternative treatment in selected non-cirrhotic patients who are at risk of adverse effects from steroids.

Induction of remission has been obtained in treatment-naïve children using cyclosporine A alone for 6 months, followed by the addition of prednisone and azathioprine; 1 month later the cyclosporine was discontinued [122, 123]. Cyclosporine was used at the dose of 4 mg/kg/day in three divided doses, increased if necessary every 2–3 days to achieve a whole blood concentration of 250 ± 50 ng/mL for 3 months. If there was clinical and biochemical response in the first months, cyclosporine was reduced to achieve a concentration of 200 ± 50 ng/mL for the following 3 months, before discontinuing it. Whether this mode of induction has any advantage over the standard treatment has yet to be evaluated in controlled studies. Tacrolimus, a more potent immunosuppressive agent than cyclosporine with similar drug class toxicity, has anecdotally been used to induce remission in adults with AIH. Its use in the juvenile form of the disease is limited to one report [124], where tacrolimus was administered to 17 children with newly diagnosed AIH with or without the addition of prednisolone and/or azathioprine and to 3 children who had failed conventional therapy. Target tacrolimus trough levels were relatively low (2.5–5 ng/mL) and similar to those used in the maintenance of successful liver transplant. Though the study shows that monotherapy with tacrolimus is not sufficient to achieve complete remission in most cases, the calcineurin inhibitor is reported to allow reduction of the dose of prednisolone and azathioprine, avoiding their side effects.

(b) **For refractory cases** (Table 10.7)—A promising drug for difficult-to-treat patients is mycophenolate mofetil (MMF), the prodrug of mycophenolic acid. In juvenile AIH patients in whom standard immunosuppression is unable to induce stable remission, or who are intolerant to azathioprine, MMF at a dose of 20 mg/kg twice daily, together with prednisolone, has been used successfully [125]. A recent meta-analysis, including data from several small, even anecdotal, studies of second-line treatments in children refractory to standard therapy suggests that calcineurin inhibitors might have the highest response rate at 6 months but also have the highest rate of adverse events; MMF was the second most effective drug with a low side effect profile, supporting the notion that MMF should be the primary choice for second-line therapy in AIH children refractory to standard treatment [126]. If there is a persistent absence of response or if there is intolerance to MMF (headache, diarrhoea, nausea, dizziness, hair loss and neutropaenia), the use of calcineurin inhibitors should be considered.

Anecdotal experience with successful use of the anti-B lymphocytes monoclonal antibody rituximab in two children with refractory AIH has been reported [127]. However, despite the relatively low adverse event profile of this drug, its use has been associated with a 2.4% rate of sepsis in children with autoimmune diseases [128].

Infliximab has been reported to be effective in the treatment of refractory AIH, including in a paediatric case [129–131]. However, its use as a rescue treatment should be carefully evaluated in view of the potential serious side effects, including infections and hepatotoxicity [129]. Moreover, anti-TNF-α-induced AIH has been reported in adults and children treated for IBD or other autoimmune conditions [132, 133]. Better understanding of the role of TNF-α in the pathogenesis of AIH is needed before recommending its use.

As patients with AIH have a defect in immunoregulation, sirolimus, a drug that selectively expands regulatory T cells in vivo and in vitro [134] has been used in four patients with refractory AIH, with short-term beneficial effect in two of them [135].

Interestingly, a recent survey on management of juvenile AIH commissioned by the IAIHG [136] has shown that within the paediatric IAIHG community there is considerable more experience with second-line therapeutic agents, than among the IAIHG adult hepatologists [137].

Fulminant hepatic failure management—The management of AIH presenting with fulminant hepatic failure (FHF), i.e. with hepatic encephalopathy, is controversial. In adults, corticosteroid therapy is reported to be of little benefit in AIH FHF and to favour septic complications [138]. In a recent paediatric cohort, prednisone treatment has led to the recovery of four out of nine children with AIH FHF referred to a transplant centre, the other five requiring liver transplant despite steroids [106]. In that paper AIH was diagnosed on the basis of positivity for autoantibodies and raised immunoglobulin G. Though liver histology was also obtained, it did not differentiate AIH FHF from cryptogenic FHF, highlighting that fact that liver biopsy in FHF is not only dangerous, because of severe coagulopathy, but also does not provide diagnostic information. Similarly good results with steroid therapy are reported in a paper from India, where 10 out of 13 patients with severe acute presentation of AIH, including encephalopathy in 6, were rescued by prednisone treatment [58].

10.2.10 When and How to Stop Treatment

In paediatric AIH, current recommendation is to treat children for at least 3 years and to attempt withdrawal of treatment only if transaminase and IgG levels have been normal and autoantibody negative (or at maximum titre of 1:20 by immunofluorescence on rodent tissue for ANA/SMA) for at least a year. A liver biopsy is advisable before deciding to attempt treatment cessation, as residual inflammatory changes, even with normal blood tests, herald relapse [1, 76, 77]. Following this protocol, successful long-term complete withdrawal of treatment was possible in 20% of patients with AIH-1, but not in AIH-2, relapse while attempting withdrawal affecting 45% [50]. A recent retrospective review, which includes also a fair proportion (21.4%) of children with AIH/sclerosing cholangitis overlap (who have a different response to treatment, see below), reports successful withdrawal of immunosuppression in some 40% of patients with AIH-1 in whom withdrawal was attempted. Failure to suspend immunosuppression successfully was associated with elevated international normalized ratio (INR), positivity for ANCA, cirrhosis and presence of non-hepatic autoimmune disorders [52]. These encouraging results in juvenile AIH contrast with reports in the adult population [139] possibly because of lack of strict criteria before attempting treatment withdrawal in the latter.

10.3 Autoimmune Sclerosing Cholangitis

Sclerosing cholangitis is a chronic inflammatory disorder that affects the intrahepatic and/or extrahepatic biliary tree leading to bile duct and liver fibrosis. The diagnosis is based on typical bile duct lesions being visualized on cholangiography. With the growing use of non-invasive biliary imaging, sclerosing cholangitis, hitherto considered rare in children, is diagnosed with increasing frequency in paediatric age. It is an important cause of morbidity and mortality, accounting for approximately 2% of the paediatric liver transplants in the United States between 1988 and 2008 [United Network for Organ Sharing (UNOS) Data Report—October 2009. http://www.unos.org/data/].

Sclerosing cholangitis in children/adolescents is widely referred to as primary sclerosing cholangitis (PSC), borrowing the adult definition. However, there are important differences between adult PSC and juvenile sclerosing cholangitis [140].

'Primary' denotes ignorance about aetiology and pathogenesis, while in paediatrics there are well-defined forms of sclerosing cholangitis, including biliary atresia and autosomal recessive neonatal sclerosing cholangitis. Other inherited conditions, e.g. mild to moderate defects in the *ABCB4* (MDR3) gene, are being increasingly recognized as a possible cause of small duct sclerosing cholangitis in both children and adults [141]. Sclerosing cholangitis may also complicate a wide variety of disorders, including primary and secondary immunodeficiencies, Langerhans cell histiocytosis, psoriasis, cystic fibrosis, reticulum cell sarcoma and sickle cell anaemia. An overlap syndrome between AIH and sclerosing cholangitis (autoimmune sclerosing cholangitis, ASC) is more common in children than in adults. Though the name ASC is not universally accepted, it is becoming increasingly more used by both the paediatric and adult hepatology community. Only in those paediatric patients in whom sclerosing cholangitis occurs without any of the above defining features the name of 'primary' would be appropriate.

The only published prospective study aiming at defining the prevalence of ASC versus AIH in children has shown that when cholangiographic studies are performed at presentation, ASC is as prevalent as AIH-1 [50]. This study shows that, in contrast to AIH, ASC affects equally males and females (Table 10.1) and that almost all patients with ASC have autoimmune serology and histological characteristics similar to AIH-1 (Fig. 10.3). The differential diagnosis between AIH and ASC is achieved only by cholangiographic studies, which show evidence of bile duct disease, usually from disease onset (Fig. 10.4). Of note, alkaline phosphatase and GGT levels—usually elevated in cholestatic disease—are often normal or only mildly increased in the early disease stages of ASC, though the alkaline phosphatase/AST ratio is significantly higher in ASC than AIH. A quarter of the children with ASC, despite abnormal cholangiograms, have no histological features suggesting bile duct involvement; conversely, 27% of the patients with AIH have some biliary features on histology (including bile duct damage, acute and/or chronic cholangitis, biliary periportal hepatitis) [50, 142]. The pathognomonic feature of adult sclerosing cholangitis—i.e. fibrous obliterative cholangitis with periductular fibrosis ('onion skin fibrosis')—is rarely seen at presentation in ASC and is a sign of advanced disease.

As mentioned above, neither the original nor the simplified IAIHG scoring systems [2, 3, 78] discriminate between AIH and ASC, as they do not include cholangiographic studies at disease onset. ASC is therefore frequently diagnosed and treated as AIH-1, and the presence of sclerosing cholangitis may be discovered during follow-up, after the appearance of an overt cholestatic biochemical profile. Hence, the ESPGHAN Hepatology Committee Position Statement proposes a new scoring system for juvenile autoimmune liver disease [1] (Table 10.3). The prospective study mentioned above shows that if treatment is started early, the parenchymal liver damage in ASC responds well in terms of normalization of biochemical and immunological parameters to the same immunosuppressive treatment used for AIH, with good medium to long-term survival. However, the bile duct disease progresses in about 50% of patients despite treatment

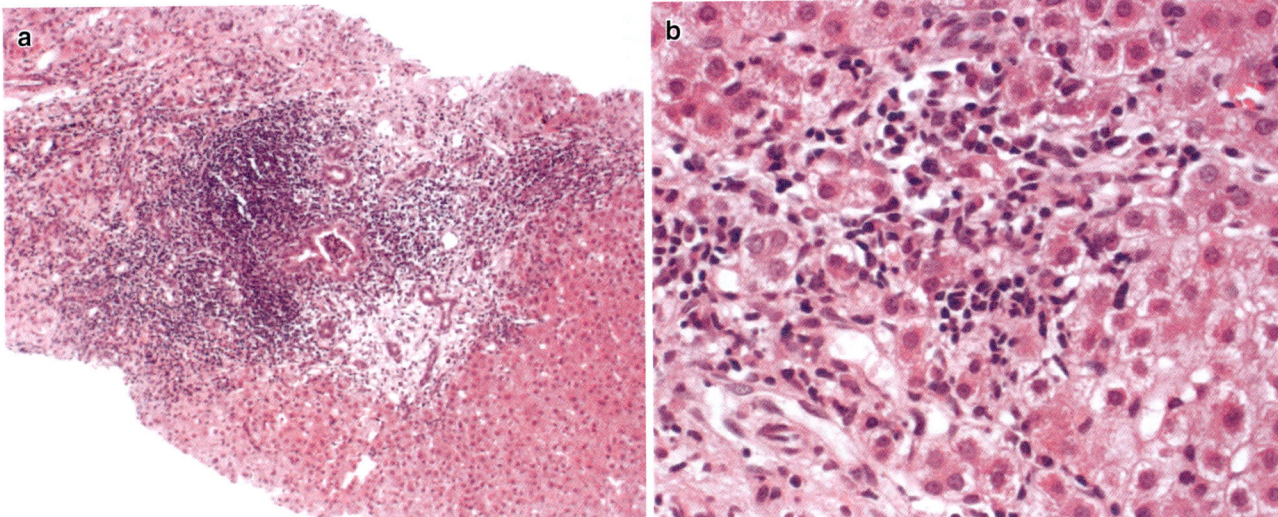

Fig. 10.3 Autoimmune sclerosing cholangitis: (**a**) Portal and periportal lymphocyte and plasma cell infiltrate, disrupting the limiting plate (interface hepatitis) and extending into the parenchyma. The picture is similar to what observed in autoimmune hepatitis; in addition in this case bile duct reduplication and cholangiolitis are observed (haematoxylin-eosin, original magnification 40×); (**b**) Higher magnification (100×) showing inflammatory infiltration with numerous plasma cells (Images kindly provided by Dr. Yoh Zen)

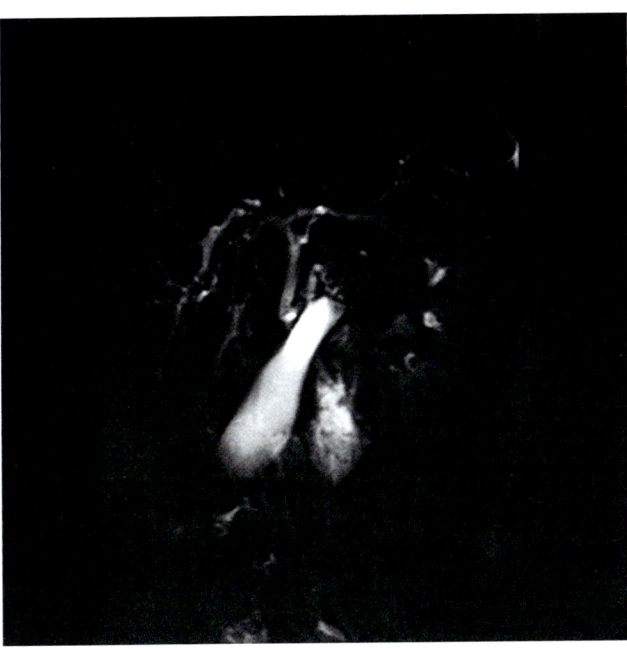

Fig. 10.4 Autoimmune sclerosing cholangitis: Magnetic resonance imaging showing diffuse cholangiopathy with ductal changes in both liver lobes

[50], particularly in those with associated difficult-to-control IBD. In a retrospective study aiming at comparing the response to treatment and outcome of children with AIH and ASC, no difference is reported between the two groups of patients, with a good response to prednisolone ± azathioprine in both [143]. However, in contrast to the prospective study, in this paper the diagnosis of ASC was only made in those patients developing cholestatic manifestations during follow-up, no cholangiographic studies having been performed at presentation, making the comparison between the two studies impossible.

Ursodeoxycholic acid (UDCA) treatment was added to immunosuppression in the prospective study [50], but whether it has any role in arresting the progression of the bile duct disease remains to be established. In adults with PSC, high-dose UDCA was reported as more beneficial than standard doses [144], but a randomized double-blind controlled study shows that high-dose UDCA has a negative long-term effect [145]. It is prudent, therefore, to use doses not higher than 15 mg/kg/day.

Most of the other published series of paediatric sclerosing cholangitis are retrospective studies from single centres, based on small patient numbers, with the exception of a recently published retrospective multicentre large cohort of juvenile sclerosing cholangitis [146]. In these reports the incidence of the various clinical forms of sclerosing cholangitis differs depending upon the year of publication and the centre where the study was conducted, reflecting different study designs, patterns of referral and diagnostic protocols. In all these retrospective series, cholangiographic studies were prompted by biochemical and/or histological features of cholestatic disease. In all, boys are more affected than girls; 20–40% of patients have intrahepatic cholangiopathy with normal extrahepatic bile ducts, and there is a strong association with IBD, which is described in 60–90% of cases according to study design. More than two-thirds of the patients have ulcerative colitis, the others having indeterminate colitis or Crohn disease. IBD can precede the diagnosis of liver disease by many years, be diagnosed at the same time or develop during follow-up.

In all retrospective studies, a variable proportion of patients have ASC, but while in some this condition is reported to respond favourably to treatment with immunosuppression, having a better prognosis than PSC [53, 147–149], in others the prognosis of ASC is reported to be severe and not ameliorated by immunosuppressive treatment [150] or similar to that of PSC irrespective of treatment [146, 151–153]. Major limitations of all these retrospective studies are uneven diagnostic protocols and lack of accurate information on the treatment of IBD before the diagnosis of sclerosing cholangitis, as immunosuppression for IBD has an effect also on the presentation and course of the liver disease. Thus, as shown by the prospective study, which is often cited negatively to support a worse prognosis for ASC compared to AIH, immunosuppressive treatment is effective in controlling both parenchymal and biliary disease in 50% of ASC cases [50], suggesting that the real prognosis of ASC compared to PSC cannot be adequately established in retrospective cohorts with variable diagnostic approaches and treatment protocols.

Recently, it has been suggested that the chronic IBD associated with ASC may represent a distinct nosologic entity, different from classic ulcerative colitis and Crohn disease, being characterized by right-sided colitis with frequent rectal sparing, and small bowel mucosal breaks on capsule enteroscopy [154].

Multicentre prospective studies are needed for defining hepatic and intestinal phenotype of ASC, for establishing diagnostic criteria and for exploring pathogenic mechanisms with the aim of devising more effective forms of treatment.

10.4 Outcome

10.4.1 Autoimmune Hepatitis

Once remission is achieved, the medium- to long-term prognosis of AIH is good. Frequent relapses herald progression of disease. Evolution to cirrhosis is more common in AIH-1 than in AIH-2 [30]. A more severe disease and a higher tendency to relapse are associated with the possession of antibodies to soluble liver antigen (SLA), which are present in about half of patients with either type of AIH at diagnosis [97].

A recent study on 30 children with autoimmune liver disease (AIH, PSC and ASC) reports a decreased health-related quality of life score in patients compared to healthy controls, the worse scores being found in those with complications of chronic liver disease, in particular ascites [155]. In this study, however, 73% of the 30 patients investigated had advanced liver disease. It would be interesting to assess a larger and more representative cohort, including a higher proportion of those patients on long-term immunosuppression without liver-related complications, who represent the majority.

Overall, pregnancy and childbirth appear to be safe for both child and mother, even in women with compensated liver cirrhosis, without the need to withdraw azathioprine [156–160]. For women who are concerned about the use of azathioprine in pregnancy, treatment with steroids alone can be considered. One large series from Sweden reports an increased risk of gestational diabetes, preterm birth and low-birth-weight infants compared with the general population [161]. Clinical improvement and disease exacerbation have been observed in relation to pregnancy, the latter particularly in the post-partum period [159], indicating that high-quality antenatal and postnatal care is essential for women with AIH and their infants.

Despite the efficacy of standard immunosuppressive treatment, severe hepatic decompensation in patients with AIH may develop even after many years of apparently good biochemical control, leading to transplantation 10–15 years after diagnosis in 10% of the patients [30].

10.4.2 Autoimmune Sclerosing Cholangitis

The medium- to long-term prognosis of ASC is worse than that of AIH because of progression of bile duct disease despite treatment in some 50% of patients, with 20% eventually requiring liver transplantation. Reactivation of the liver disease often follows flares of the intestinal disease in patients with IBD. It is therefore essential to control the bowel pathology to avoid progression of liver disease. A beneficial effect of oral vancomycin (500 mg tds) has been reported in patients with sclerosing cholangitis and IBD [162]. All patients showed improvement of liver function tests and erythrocyte sedimentation rate, which was more marked in those without cirrhosis. These results await confirmation in a larger number of patients. Whether vancomycin acts through its antibiotic, choleretic or immunomodulatory properties remains to be elucidated.

Fat-soluble vitamin supplements are required if cholestasis develops. As in AIH, measurement of autoantibody titres and IgG levels is useful in monitoring disease activity and the response to treatment [85]. Evolution from AIH to ASC has been documented, suggesting that AIH and ASC may be part of the same pathogenic process [50].

10.4.3 Neoplasia

Long-term immunosuppressive treatment could be associated with the development of malignancies since extrahepatic cancers, including non-Hodgkin lymphoma and skin cancer, are reported to be more frequent in patients with AIH than in age-matched and sex-matched normal populations [163–166]. The risk of developing primary hepatocellular carcinoma (HCC) in AIH is associated with the presence of cirrhosis, akin to other chronic liver diseases [164, 165, 167–169]. Both the American Association for the Study of Liver Disease (AASLD) and European Association for the Study of the Liver (EASL) Autoimmune Hepatitis Guidelines recommend active surveillance for HCC [76, 77].

Cholangiocarcinoma (CC) is a very rare complication of paediatric sclerosing cholangitis. While in adult patients with PSC, the incidence and prevalence of CC are reportedly between 5–36% and 0.6% per year, respectively [170]; in paediatrics, there are only three cases of CC described in patients with PSC, two by Deneau et al. [53] and one by Ross et al. [171]. The three patients were 17.9, 18 and 14 years of age at the time of CC diagnosis, all had ulcerative colitis and developed CC 6, 4.2 years and 14 months after the diagnosis of PSC, respectively. None of the patients with ASC enrolled in the prospective study mentioned above [50] has developed CC over an observation period of 30 years. Long-term follow-up of cases identified in paediatric age is needed to establish the incidence and prevalence of CC in juvenile sclerosing cholangitis.

10.5 Implications for Liver Transplantation

Liver transplantation (LT) is a treatment option for AIH and ASC patients with end-stage chronic liver disease, hepatic malignancy or intractable symptoms, as well as for AIH patients presenting with severe acute liver failure unresponsive to steroid treatment.

AIH accounts for 2–5% of paediatric LTs performed in Europe and the United States [76, 172]. The transplant rate for AIH is variable, ranging from 9 to 55%, the interval between presentation and transplantation being as short as days in case of fulminant onset to several years after diagnosis [30, 51, 53, 173]. These different transplant rates depend on several factors: expertise of the reporting centre (primarily transplant or hepatology unit), type of survey (single centre or population based), late referral/treatment, missed diagnosis of ASC and different ethnic background. The reported 5-year survival rate after LT for AIH is excellent, being 80–90% [174].

Sclerosing cholangitis accounts for 2–3% of LTs performed in paediatric-aged patients [175] (United Network for Organ Sharing (UNOS) Data Report—October 2009. http://www.unos.org/data/) only some of whom have ASC [140]. Overall, LT rate for sclerosing cholangitis ranges between 15% and 45%, and the interval between diagnosis and LT ranges from 6 to 12 years [53, 150–152, 176]. In the King's College Hospital prospective study, 4 out of 27 patients with ASC underwent LT during the 16-year study period [50], though it is likely that the rate of LT will increase when the long-term outcome and transition into adulthood data will be analysed [177].

10.5.1 Recurrence of AIH After Liver Transplant

Notwithstanding the good outcome of transplantation for AIH, the disease can recur in the allograft despite immunosuppression [178–182]. The reported recurrence rate is variable and depends on the criteria used for diagnosis, the immunosuppressive regimen, length of follow-up and performance of 'per protocol' biopsies. Mean time from LT to recurrence is 5 years [76, 183], and recurrence rate increases with the post-surgery interval, but it may occur as early as 35 days after LT [184]. The reported recurrence rates in children transplanted for AIH vary from 38 to 83% [51, 173, 185].

The recurrence of AIH after LT can be readily explained. The recipient's immune system is sensitized to species-specific antigens and has a pool of memory cells, which are restimulated and re-expanded when the target antigens, 'autoantigens', are presented to the recipient's immune system either by the recipient's APC repopulating the grafted liver or by the donor's APC sharing histocompatibility antigens with the recipient.

The diagnosis of recurrent AIH is based on the reappearance of clinical symptoms and signs, elevation of transaminases and IgG levels, autoantibodies and interface hepatitis, along with response to prednisolone and azathioprine [76, 186].

Features reported to be associated with recurrence of AIH after LT are possession of either HLA-DR3 or HLA-DR4 by the recipient [187, 188]; discontinuation of corticosteroids after LT [189–191]—therefore caution should be exercised in weaning patients off immunosuppression; and the severity of necroinflammatory activity in the native liver at the time of LT [184, 192]. Most transplant recipients with recurrent AIH respond to reintroduction or an increase in the dose of corticosteroids and azathioprine, which should be implemented as soon as the diagnosis is made. In the case of treatment failure, alternatives include addition of MMF in lieu of azathioprine to the standard therapeutic regimen, replacement of tacrolimus with cyclosporine [193] and replacement of calcineurin inhibitors with sirolimus.

Recurrent disease, particularly if not diagnosed and not treated promptly, may have serious consequences on graft function. In the first paediatric report, out of the five patients who developed recurrent AIH, three progressed to end-stage liver disease requiring re-transplantation [185]. In a series from Birmingham, UK, none of the patients with AIH-1 who developed recurrence progressed to graft failure, while 80% of patients originally transplanted for AIH-2 required re-transplantation [51]. Further support to the negative impact of disease recurrence on allograft survival comes from a United Network for Organ Sharing database; out of 174 children with AIH transplanted between 2002 and 2012, 19%

lost the graft due to recurrent disease [194]. Successful management of recurrent AIH relies greatly on its early diagnosis and prompt treatment. Because histologic evidence can precede clinical evidence of recurrence, it might be useful to include a follow-up liver biopsy in the protocol for the management of patients transplanted for AIH [183, 195].

10.5.2 Recurrence of Sclerosing Cholangitis After Liver Transplant

Recurrence of sclerosing cholangitis after paediatric LT has been reported in between 10% and 50% of recipients without distinction of the form of sclerosing cholangitis leading to transplantation [151, 152, 177, 196], the wide range depending on the length of follow-up, as the risk for recurrence increases over time.

The diagnosis of recurrent sclerosing cholangitis is suggested by histological and/or cholangiographic findings of bile duct disease. Indicative histological findings include fibrous cholangitis, fibro-obliterative lesions with or without ductopaenia, fibrosis or cirrhosis and/or interface hepatitis, whereas the cholangiography generally shows diffuse biliary stricturing [197]. Other causes of non-anastomotic biliary strictures in the graft should be carefully excluded, including ischemic biliary insults (e.g. as consequence of hepatic artery thrombosis), ABO incompatibility between donor and recipient, bacterial or fungal cholangitis and chronic ductopaenic rejection [198]. No consistent risk factors have been reported in association to the development of recurrent sclerosing cholangitis. Some paediatric studies point to an association between active IBD after LT and the development of recurrent disease [152, 177]. Similarly, a study in adult patients transplanted for PSC shows that persistent ulcerative colitis is associated with an increased risk of developing recurrent disease in the graft, whereas colectomy before or during LT conferred protection against the development of recurrent disease [199].

There is no established treatment for recurrent sclerosing cholangitis after paediatric LT. If dominant strictures are present, they should be dilated by interventional cholangiographic means whenever possible [200].

Ursodeoxycholic acid treatment has been advocated in the setting of transplanted adult PSC patients because it seems to improve biochemical indices of liver disease, but it remains unknown whether it has an impact on outcomes [200].

While in adults the impact of recurrence of sclerosing cholangitis on graft survival is controversial, in paediatrics recurrent disease, particularly in the context of ASC, is associated with seriously compromised graft survival: in the King's College Hospital prospective study, two-thirds of patients who experienced recurrent disease eventually required re-transplantation [177].

10.5.3 De Novo Autoimmune Hepatitis After Liver Transplant

De novo AIH after LT affects patients transplanted for disorders other than autoimmune liver disease. While non-specific development of autoantibodies over time after LT is common, affecting over 70% of recipients [178, 201], the prevalence of de novo AIH in children ranges from 2 to 6% [179, 180, 202–206]. The condition was first reported in a paediatric cohort, affecting 4% of children transplanted in a single centre for various non-autoimmune conditions [202]. The patients developed a form of graft dysfunction with features identical to those of classical AIH, namely, high transaminase levels, hypergammaglobulinemia, positivity for autoantibodies—ANA, SMA and typical and atypical anti-LKM-1 (i.e. staining renal tubules only)—and histological features of chronic hepatitis with portal/periportal inflammation and centrilobular necrosis. Other causes of post-LT graft dysfunction, like rejection, infection and hepatic artery thrombosis, were excluded. Patients with de novo AIH did not respond to conventional antirejection treatment but only to the classical treatment of AIH. None of the children had undergone transplantation for autoimmune conditions, and all had serum concentration of calcineurin inhibitor within therapeutic antirejection levels at the time of de novo AIH diagnosis. Since the original observation, several other groups have reported the occurrence of de novo AIH after both paediatric and adult LT. De novo AIH has been described also as a complication in living-donor LT [207]. In the largest study published to date in children, describing 41 (5.2%) patients—out of 788 LTs performed in a single centre—who developed de novo AIH, rejection and steroid dependence were identified as factors predisposing to this complication [206]. In adults, it has been suggested that a histological pattern of centrilobular injury characterized by necroinflammatory activity with plasma cell infiltration might predict the development of this condition [208]. In a paediatric series, the most common early histological feature of de novo AIH was lobular hepatitis, often without interface necroinflammatory activity or prominent plasma cell infiltrates [209].

Awareness that treatment with prednisolone alone or in combination with azathioprine or MMF is successful in de novo AIH has led to excellent graft and patient survival [210]. Akin to the treatment for classical AIH, children should be given a starting dose of 1–2 mg/kg/day of predniso(lo)ne, without exceeding a daily dose of 60 mg, in combination with azathioprine (1–2 mg/kg/day); the steroids should then be tapered over 4–8 weeks, to reach a maintenance dose of 5–10 mg/day. In the absence of response, azathioprine should be replaced by MMF [210]. The importance of maintenance therapy with steroids in de novo AIH was shown in a study comparing treatment with and without steroids: whereas all steroid-untreated patients developed cirrhosis and either died or required re-transplantation, none of the steroid-treated patients had progressive disease [211].

Akin to autoimmune liver disease outside the context of transplantation, the pathogenesis of post-LT de novo AIH remains to be defined. There are several possible explanations, which are not mutually exclusive. In addition to the release of autoantigens from damaged tissue, one possible mechanism is molecular mimicry, in which exposure to viruses that share amino acid sequences with autoantigens leads to cross-reactive immunity [212]. Viral infections, which are frequent after LT, may also lead to autoimmunity through other mechanisms, including polyclonal stimulation, enhancement and induction of membrane expression of MHC class I and II antigens and/or interference with immunoregulatory cells. Another possible mechanism documented in experimental animals is linked to the use of calcineurin inhibitors, which predispose to autoimmunity and autoimmune disease, possibly by interfering with the maturation of T lymphocytes and the function of T-regs, with consequent emergence and activation of auto-aggressive T-cell clones. Another proposed mechanism stems from observation that patients with de novo AIH often have an antibody directed to glutathione-S-transferase T1 (GSTT1) [213]. Since the gene encoding this protein is defective in a fifth of Caucasoid individuals and the encoded enzyme was absent in patients experiencing de novo AIH, the authors speculated that graft dysfunction resulted from the recognition as foreign of GSTT1 acquired with the graft. However, we have been unable to confirm this observation, having investigated reactivity against GSTT1 sequentially on 60 occasions in 20 patients with post-transplantation de novo AIH.

In murine models of heart allograft, heart transplantation from an allogeneic donor results not only in rejection but also in the production of antibodies and CD4 T cells directed against cardiac myosin in the recipient [214]. The relative importance of autoantigenic and allogeneic stimuli in the development of de novo AIH after liver transplantation remains to be elucidated.

10.6 Conclusions

Autoimmunity is an important cause of liver disease in childhood. The prognosis with immunosuppressive treatment is excellent, with symptom-free long-term survival in the majority of patients with AIH and in some 50% of those with ASC. However, a failure to diagnose and promptly treat these conditions has severe consequences, including progression to cirrhosis, end-stage liver disease, transplantation or death. During the past 40 years, several pathogenic aspects of liver autoimmunity have been elucidated, including predisposing genetic factors and disease-specific humoral and cellular immune responses. Research tasks for the future include further elucidation of the pathogenesis, and the establishment of novel treatments aimed at specifically arresting liver auto-aggression or, ideally, at reinstating tolerance to liver antigens.

References

1. Mieli-Vergani G*, Vergani D* (*contributed equally), Baumann U, Czubkowski P, Debray D, Dezsofi A, Fischler B, Gupte G, Hierro L, Indolfi G, Jahnel J, Smets F, Verkade HJ, Hadzic N. Diagnosis and management of pediatric autoimmune liver disease: ESPGHAN Hepatology Committee Position Statement. J Pediatr Gastroenterol Nutr. 2018;66:345–60.
2. Johnson PJ, McFarlane IG. Meeting report: International Autoimmune Hepatitis Group. Hepatology. 1993;18(4):998–1005.
3. Alvarez F, Berg PA, Bianchi FB, Bianchi L, Burroughs AK, Cancado EL, et al. International Autoimmune Hepatitis Group Report: review of criteria for diagnosis of autoimmune hepatitis. J Hepatol. 1999;31(5):929–38.
4. Boberg KM, Aadland E, Jahnsen J, Raknerud N, Stiris M, Bell H. Incidence and prevalence of primary biliary cirrhosis, primary sclerosing cholangitis, and autoimmune hepatitis in a Norwegian population. Scand J Gastroenterol. 1998;33(1):99–103.
5. Manns MP, Luttig B, Obermayer-Straub P. Autoimmune hepatitis. In: Rose NR, Mackay IR, editors. The autoimmune diseases. 3rd ed. San Diego: Academic Press; 1998. p. 511–25.
6. Primo J, Merino C, Fernandez J, Moles JR, Llorca P, Hinojosa J. Incidence and prevalence of autoimmune hepatitis in the area of the Hospital de Sagunto (Spain). Gastroenterol Hepatol. 2004;27(4):239–43.
7. Whalley S, Puvanachandra P, Desai A, Kennedy H. Hepatology outpatient service provision in secondary care: a study of liver disease incidence and resource costs. Clin Med. 2007;7(2):119–24.
8. Ngu JH, Bechly K, Chapman BA, Burt MJ, Barclay ML, Gearry RB, et al. Population-based epidemiology study of autoimmune hepatitis: a disease of older women? J Gastroenterol Hepatol. 2010;25(10):1681–6.
9. Hurlburt KJ, McMahon BJ, Deubner H, Hsu-Trawinski B, Williams JL, Kowdley KV. Prevalence of autoimmune liver disease in Alaska Natives. Am J Gastroenterol. 2002;97(9):2402–7.
10. Yang F, Wang Q, Bian Z, Ren LL, Jia J, Ma X. Autoimmune hepatitis: East meets West. J Gastroenterol Hepatol. 2015;30(8):1230–6.
11. Qiu D, Wang Q, Wang H, Xie Q, Zang G, Jiang H, et al. Validation of the simplified criteria for diagnosis of autoimmune hepatitis in Chinese patients. J Hepatol. 2011;54(2):340–7.
12. Yoshizawa K, Joshita S, Matsumoto A, Umemura T, Tanaka E, Morita S, et al. Incidence and prevalence of autoimmune hepatitis in the Ueda area. Japan Hepatol Res. 2016;46(9):878–83.
13. Gronbaek L, Vilstrup H, Jepsen P. Autoimmune hepatitis in Denmark: incidence, prevalence, prognosis, and causes of death. A nationwide registry-based cohort study. J Hepatol. 2014;60(3):612–7.
14. Danielsson Borssen A, Marschall HU, Bergquist A, Rorsman F, Weiland O, Kechagias S, et al. Epidemiology and causes of death in a Swedish cohort of patients with autoimmune hepatitis. Scand J Gastroenterol. 2017;52(9):1022–8.
15. van Gerven NM, Verwer BJ, Witte BI, van Erpecum KJ, van Buuren HR, Maijers I, et al. Epidemiology and clinical characteristics of autoimmune hepatitis in the Netherlands. Scand J Gastroenterol. 2014;49(10):1245–54.
16. Czaja AJ, Freese DK. Diagnosis and treatment of autoimmune hepatitis. Hepatology. 2002;36(2):479–97.

17. Duchini A, McHutchison JG, Pockros PJ. LKM-positive autoimmune hepatitis in the western United States: a case series. Am J Gastroenterol. 2000;95(11):3238–41.
18. Jimenez-Rivera C, Ling SC, Ahmed N, Yap J, Aglipay M, Barrowman N, et al. Incidence and characteristics of autoimmune hepatitis. Pediatrics. 2015;136(5):e1237–48.
19. Mieli-Vergani G, Vergani D. Budesonide for juvenile autoimmune hepatitis? Not yet. J Pediatr. 2013;163(5):1246–8.
20. Liberal R, Krawitt EL, Vierling JM, Manns MPL, Mieli-Vergani G, Vergani D. Cutting edge issues in autoimmune hepatitis. J Autoimmun. 2016;75:6–19.
21. Mann DA. Epigenetics in liver disease. Hepatology. 2014;60(4):1418–25.
22. de Boer YS, van Gerven NM, Zwiers A, Verwer BJ, van Hoek B, van Erpecum KJ, et al. Genome-wide association study identifies variants associated with autoimmune hepatitis type 1. Gastroenterology. 2014;147(2):443–52.e5.
23. Donaldson P. Genetics in autoimmune hepatitis. Semin Liver Dis. 2002;22(4):353–64.
24. Donaldson PT. Genetics of liver disease: immunogenetics and disease pathogenesis. Gut. 2004;53(4):599–608.
25. Czaja AJ, Donaldson PT. Genetic susceptibilities for immune expression and liver cell injury in autoimmune hepatitis. Immunol Rev. 2000;174:250–9.
26. Agarwal K, Czaja AJ, Jones DE, Donaldson PT. Cytotoxic T lymphocyte antigen-4 (CTLA-4) gene polymorphisms and susceptibility to type 1 autoimmune hepatitis. Hepatology. 2000;31(1):49–53.
27. Cookson S, Constantini PK, Clare M, Underhill JA, Bernal W, Czaja AJ, et al. Frequency and nature of cytokine gene polymorphisms in type 1 autoimmune hepatitis. Hepatology. 1999;30(4):851–6.
28. Agarwal K, Czaja AJ, Donaldson PT. A functional Fas promoter polymorphism is associated with a severe phenotype in type 1 autoimmune hepatitis characterized by early development of cirrhosis. Tissue Antigens. 2007;69(3):227–35.
29. Doherty DG, Underhill JA, Donaldson PT, Manabe K, Mieli-Vergani G, Eddleston AL, et al. Polymorphism in the human complement C4 genes and genetic susceptibility to autoimmune hepatitis. Autoimmunity. 1994;18(4):243–9.
30. Gregorio GV, Portmann B, Reid F, Donaldson PT, Doherty DG, McCartney M, et al. Autoimmune hepatitis in childhood: a 20-year experience. Hepatology. 1997;25(3):541–7.
31. Ma Y, Bogdanos DP, Hussain MJ, Underhill J, Bansal S, Longhi MS, et al. Polyclonal T-cell responses to cytochrome P450IID6 are associated with disease activity in autoimmune hepatitis type 2. Gastroenterology. 2006;130(3):868–82.
32. Elfaramawy AA, Elhossiny RM, Abbas AA, Aziz HM. HLA-DRB1 as a risk factor in children with autoimmune hepatitis and its relation to hepatitis A infection. Ital J Pediatr. 2010;36:73.
33. Oliveira LC, Porta G, Marin ML, Bittencourt PL, Kalil J, Goldberg AC. Autoimmune hepatitis, HLA and extended haplotypes. Autoimmun Rev. 2011;10(4):189–93.
34. Pando M, Larriba J, Fernandez GC, Fainboim H, Ciocca M, Ramonet M, et al. Pediatric and adult forms of type I autoimmune hepatitis in Argentina: evidence for differential genetic predisposition. Hepatology. 1999;30(6):1374–80.
35. Fainboim L, Canero Velasco MC, Marcos CY, Ciocca M, Roy A, Theiler G, et al. Protracted, but not acute, hepatitis A virus infection is strongly associated with HLA-DRB*1301, a marker for pediatric autoimmune hepatitis. Hepatology. 2001;33(6):1512–7.
36. Wang P, Su H, Underhill J, Blackmore LJ, Longhi MS, Grammatikopoulos T, et al. Autoantibody and human leukocyte antigen profiles in children with autoimmune liver disease and their first-degree relatives. J Pediatr Gastroenterol Nutr. 2014;58(4):457–62.
37. Podhorzer A, Paladino N, Cuarterolo ML, Fainboim HA, Paz S, Theiler G, et al. The early onset of type 1 autoimmune hepatitis has a strong genetic influence: role of HLA and KIR genes. Genes Immun. 2016;17(3):187–92.
38. Djilali-Saiah I, Fakhfakh A, Louafi H, Caillat-Zucman S, Debray D, Alvarez F. HLA class II influences humoral autoimmunity in patients with type 2 autoimmune hepatitis. J Hepatol. 2006;45(6):844–50.
39. Simmonds MJ, Gough SC. Genetic insights into disease mechanisms of autoimmunity. Br Med Bull. 2004;71:93–113.
40. Liston A, Lesage S, Gray DH, Boyd RL, Goodnow CC. Genetic lesions in T-cell tolerance and thresholds for autoimmunity. Immunol Rev. 2005;204:87–101.
41. Lankisch TO, Strassburg CP, Debray D, Manns MP, Jacquemin E. Detection of autoimmune regulator gene mutations in children with type 2 autoimmune hepatitis and extrahepatic immune-mediated diseases. J Pediatr. 2005;146(6):839–42.
42. Liberal R, Longhi MS, Mieli-Vergani G, Vergani D. Pathogenesis of autoimmune hepatitis. Best Pract Res Clin Gastroenterol. 2011;25(6):653–64.
43. Crispe IN. Liver antigen-presenting cells. J Hepatol. 2011;54(2):357–65.
44. Ebrahimkhani MR, Mohar I, Crispe IN. Cross-presentation of antigen by diverse subsets of murine liver cells. Hepatology. 2011;54(4):1379–87.
45. Liberal R, Grant CR, Longhi MS, Mieli-Vergani G, Vergani D. Regulatory T cells: mechanisms of suppression and impairment in autoimmune liver disease. IUBMB Life. 2015;67(2):88–97.
46. Zhao L, Tang Y, You Z, Wang Q, Liang S, Han X, et al. Interleukin-17 contributes to the pathogenesis of autoimmune hepatitis through inducing hepatic interleukin-6 expression. PLoS One. 2011;6(4):e18909.
47. Thomas-Dupont P, Remes-Troche JM, Izaguirre-Hernandez IY, Sanchez-Vargas LA, Maldonado-Renteria Mde J, Hernandez-Flores KG, et al. Elevated circulating levels of IL-21 and IL-22 define a cytokine signature profile in type 2 autoimmune hepatitis patients. Ann Hepatol. 2016;15(4):550–8.
48. Oettinger R, Brunnberg A, Gerner P, Wintermeyer P, Jenke A, Wirth S. Clinical features and biochemical data of Caucasian children at diagnosis of autoimmune hepatitis. J Autoimmun. 2005;24(1):79–84.
49. Al-Chalabi T, Underhill JA, Portmann BC, McFarlane IG, Heneghan MA. Impact of gender on the long-term outcome and survival of patients with autoimmune hepatitis. J Hepatol. 2008;48(1):140–7.
50. Gregorio GV, Portmann B, Karani J, Harrison P, Donaldson PT, Vergani D, et al. Autoimmune hepatitis/sclerosing cholangitis overlap syndrome in childhood: a 16-year prospective study. Hepatology. 2001;33(3):544–53.
51. Chai PF, Lee WS, Brown RM, McPartland JL, Foster K, McKiernan PJ, et al. Childhood autoimmune liver disease: indications and outcome of liver transplantation. J Pediatr Gastroenterol Nutr. 2010;50(3):295–302.
52. Deneau M, Book LS, Guthery SL, Jensen MK. Outcome after discontinuation of immunosuppression in children with autoimmune hepatitis: a population-based study. J Pediatr. 2014;164(4):714–9.e2.
53. Deneau M, Jensen MK, Holmen J, Williams MS, Book LS, Guthery SL. Primary sclerosing cholangitis, autoimmune hepatitis, and overlap in Utah children: epidemiology and natural history. Hepatology. 2013;58(4):1392–400.
54. Saadah OI, Smith AL, Hardikar W. Long-term outcome of autoimmune hepatitis in children. J Gastroenterol Hepatol. 2001;16(11):1297–302.
55. Radhakrishnan KR, Alkhouri N, Worley S, Arrigain S, Hupertz V, Kay M, et al. Autoimmune hepatitis in children—impact of cir-

56. Vitfell-Pedersen J, Jorgensen MH, Muller K, Heilmann C. Autoimmune hepatitis in children in Eastern Denmark. J Pediatr Gastroenterol Nutr. 2012;55(4):376–9.
57. Amarapurkar D, Dharod M, Amarapurkar A. Autoimmune hepatitis in India: single tertiary referral centre experience. Trop Gastroenterol. 2015;36(1):36–45.
58. Ramachandran J, Sajith KG, Pal S, Rasak JV, Prakash JA, Ramakrishna B. Clinicopathological profile and management of severe autoimmune hepatitis. Trop Gastroenterol. 2014;35(1):25–31.
59. Lee WS, Lum SH, Lim CB, Chong SY, Khoh KM, Ng RT, et al. Characteristics and outcome of autoimmune liver disease in Asian children. Hepatol Int. 2015;9(2):292–302.
60. Hassan N, Siddiqui AR, Abbas Z, Hassan SM, Soomro GB, Mubarak M, et al. Clinical profile and HLA typing of autoimmune hepatitis from Pakistan. Hepat Mon. 2013;13(12):e13598.
61. Farid E, Isa HM, Al Nasef M, Mohamed R, Jamsheer H. Childhood autoimmune hepatitis in Bahrain: a tertiary center experience. Iran J Immunol. 2015;12(2):141–8.
62. Dehghani SM, Haghighat M, Imanieh MH, Honar N, Negarestani AM, Malekpour A, et al. Autoimmune hepatitis in children: experiences in a tertiary center. Iran J Pediatr. 2013;23(3):302–8.
63. Abu Faddan NH, Abdel-Baky L, Aly SA, Rashed HA. Clinico-laboratory study on children with auto-immune hepatitis in Upper Egypt. Arab J Gastroenterol. 2011;12(4):178–83.
64. Roye-Green K, Willis R, Mc Morris N, Dawson J, Whittle D, Barton E, et al. Autoimmune hepatitis in a Jamaican cohort spanning 40 years. Hum Antibodies. 2013;22(3–4):87–93.
65. Nares-Cisneros J, Jaramillo-Rodriguez Y. Autoimmune hepatitis in children: progression of 20 cases in northern Mexico. Rev Gastroenterol Mex. 2014;79(4):238–43.
66. Wong GW, Heneghan MA. Association of extrahepatic manifestations with autoimmune hepatitis. Dig Dis. 2015;33(Suppl 2):25–35.
67. Guo L, Zhou L, Zhang N, Deng B, Wang B. Extrahepatic autoimmune diseases in patients with autoimmune liver diseases: a phenomenon neglected by gastroenterologists. Gastroenterol Res Pract. 2017;2017:2376231.
68. Francavilla R, Castellaneta S, Davis T, Tung J, Hadzic N, Mieli-Vergani G. Serological markers of coeliac disease in children with autoimmune hepatitis. Acta Endoscopia. 2001;3:281–2.
69. Najafi M, Sadjadei N, Eftekhari K, Khodadad A, Motamed F, Fallahi GH, et al. Prevalence of celiac disease in children with autoimmune hepatitis and vice versa. Iran J Pediatr. 2014;24(6):723–8.
70. Anania C, De Luca E, De Castro G, Chiesa C, Pacifico L. Liver involvement in pediatric celiac disease. World J Gastroenterol. 2015;21(19):5813–22.
71. Vajro P, Paolella G, Maggiore G, Giordano G. Pediatric celiac disease, cryptogenic hypertransaminasemia, and autoimmune hepatitis. J Pediatr Gastroenterol Nutr. 2013;56(6):663–70.
72. Nastasio S, Sciveres M, Riva S, Filippeschi IP, Vajro P, Maggiore G. Celiac disease-associated autoimmune hepatitis in childhood: long-term response to treatment. J Pediatr Gastroenterol Nutr. 2013;56(6):671–4.
73. Ahonen P, Myllarniemi S, Sipila I, Perheentupa J. Clinical variation of autoimmune polyendocrinopathy-candidiasis-ectodermal dystrophy (APECED) in a series of 68 patients. N Engl J Med. 1990;322(26):1829–36.
74. Meloni A, Willcox N, Meager A, Atzeni M, Wolff AS, Husebye ES, et al. Autoimmune polyendocrine syndrome type 1: an extensive longitudinal study in Sardinian patients. J Clin Endocrinol Metab. 2012;97(4):1114–24.
75. Ferre EM, Rose SR, Rosenzweig SD, Burbelo PD, Romito KR, Niemela JE, et al. Redefined clinical features and diagnostic criteria in autoimmune polyendocrinopathy-candidiasis-ectodermal dystrophy. JCI Insight. 2016;1(13).
76. Manns MP, Czaja AJ, Gorham JD, Krawitt EL, Mieli-Vergani G, Vergani D, et al. Diagnosis and management of autoimmune hepatitis. Hepatology. 2010;51(6):2193–213.
77. European Association for the Study of the Liver. EASL clinical practice guidelines: autoimmune hepatitis. J Hepatol. 2015;63(4):971–1004.
78. Hennes EM, Zeniya M, Czaja AJ, Pares A, Dalekos GN, Krawitt EL, et al. Simplified criteria for the diagnosis of autoimmune hepatitis. Hepatology. 2008;48(1):169–76.
79. Ebbeson RL, Schreiber RA. Diagnosing autoimmune hepatitis in children: is the International Autoimmune Hepatitis Group scoring system useful? Clin Gastroenterol Hepatol. 2004;2(10):935–40.
80. Ferri PM, Ferreira AR, Miranda DM, Simoes ESAC. Diagnostic criteria for autoimmune hepatitis in children: a challenge for pediatric hepatologists. World J Gastroenterol. 2012;18(33):4470–3.
81. Mileti E, Rosenthal P, Peters MG. Validation and modification of simplified diagnostic criteria for autoimmune hepatitis in children. Clin Gastroenterol Hepatol. 2012;10(4):417–21.e1–2.
82. Vergani D, Alvarez F, Bianchi FB, Cancado EL, Mackay IR, Manns MP, et al. Liver autoimmune serology: a consensus statement from the committee for autoimmune serology of the International Autoimmune Hepatitis Group. J Hepatol. 2004;41(4):677–83.
83. Hiejima E, Komatsu H, Sogo T, Inui A, Fujisawa T. Utility of simplified criteria for the diagnosis of autoimmune hepatitis in children. J Pediatr Gastroenterol Nutr. 2011;52(4):470–3.
84. Liberal R, Grant CR, Longhi MS, Mieli-Vergani G, Vergani D. Diagnostic criteria of autoimmune hepatitis. Autoimmun Rev. 2014;13(4–5):435–40.
85. Gregorio GV, McFarlane B, Bracken P, Vergani D, Mieli-Vergani G. Organ and non-organ specific autoantibody titres and IgG levels as markers of disease activity: a longitudinal study in childhood autoimmune liver disease. Autoimmunity. 2002;35(8):515–9.
86. Villalta D, Girolami E, Alessio MG, Sorrentino MC, Tampoia M, Brusca I, et al. Autoantibody profiling in a cohort of pediatric and adult patients with autoimmune hepatitis. J Clin Lab Anal. 2016;30(1):41–6.
87. Gregorio GV, Portmann B, Mowat AP, Vergani D, Mieli-Vergani G. A 12-year-old girl with antimitochondrial antibody-positive autoimmune hepatitis. J Hepatol. 1997;27(4):751–4.
88. Invernizzi P, Alessio MG, Smyk DS, Lleo A, Sonzogni A, Fabris L, et al. Autoimmune hepatitis type 2 associated with an unexpected and transient presence of primary biliary cirrhosis-specific antimitochondrial antibodies: a case study and review of the literature. BMC Gastroenterol. 2012;12:92.
89. Saadah OI, Bokhary RY. Anti-mitochondrial antibody positive autoimmune hepatitis triggered by EBV infection in a young girl. Arab J Gastroenterol. 2013;14(3):130–2.
90. Bailloud R, Bertin D, Roquelaure B, Roman C, Ballot E, Johanet C, et al. Anti-mitochondrial-2 antibodies (anti-PDC-E2): a marker for autoimmune hepatitis of children? Clin Res Hepatol Gastroenterol. 2012;36(4):e57–9.
91. Tan EM, Feltkamp TE, Smolen JS, Butcher B, Dawkins R, Fritzler MJ, et al. Range of antinuclear antibodies in "healthy" individuals. Arthritis Rheum. 1997;40(9):1601–11.
92. Hilario MO, Len CA, Roja SC, Terreri MT, Almeida G, Andrade LE. Frequency of antinuclear antibodies in healthy children and adolescents. Clin Pediatr (Phila). 2004;43(7):637–42.
93. Litwin CM, Binder SR. ANA testing in the presence of acute and chronic infections. J Immunoassay Immunochem. 2016;37(5):439–52.
94. Bogdanos DP, Mieli-Vergani G, Vergani D. Autoantibodies and their antigens in autoimmune hepatitis. Semin Liver Dis. 2009;29(3):241–53.

95. Liberal R, Mieli-Vergani G, Vergani D. Clinical significance of autoantibodies in autoimmune hepatitis. J Autoimmun. 2013;46:17–24.
96. Lapierre P, Hajoui O, Homberg JC, Alvarez F. Formiminotransferase cyclodeaminase is an organ-specific autoantigen recognized by sera of patients with autoimmune hepatitis. Gastroenterology. 1999;116(3):643–9.
97. Ma Y, Okamoto M, Thomas MG, Bogdanos DP, Lopes AR, Portmann B, et al. Antibodies to conformational epitopes of soluble liver antigen define a severe form of autoimmune liver disease. Hepatology. 2002;35(3):658–64.
98. Palioura S, Sherrer RL, Steitz TA, Soll D, Simonovic M. The human SepSecS-tRNASec complex reveals the mechanism of selenocysteine formation. Science. 2009;325(5938):321–5.
99. Maggiore G, Socie G, Sciveres M, Roque-Afonso AM, Nastasio S, Johanet C, et al. Seronegative autoimmune hepatitis in children: spectrum of disorders. Dig Liver Dis. 2016;48(7):785–91.
100. Czaja AJ, Carpenter HA. Autoimmune hepatitis. In: Macsween RNM, Burt AD, Portmann BC, editors. Pathology of the liver. 4th ed. New York: Churchill Livingstone; 2001. p. 415–34.
101. Miao Q, Bian Z, Tang R, Zhang H, Wang Q, Huang S, et al. Emperipolesis mediated by CD8 T cells is a characteristic histopathologic feature of autoimmune hepatitis. Clin Rev Allergy Immunol. 2015;48(2–3):226–35.
102. Tucker SM, Jonas MM, Perez-Atayde AR. Hyaline droplets in Kupffer cells: a novel diagnostic clue for autoimmune hepatitis. Am J Surg Pathol. 2015;39(6):772–8.
103. Tiniakos DG, Brain JG, Bury YA. Role of histopathology in autoimmune hepatitis. Dig Dis. 2015;33(Suppl 2):53–64.
104. Stravitz RT, Lefkowitch JH, Fontana RJ, Gershwin ME, Leung PS, Sterling RK, et al. Autoimmune acute liver failure: proposed clinical and histological criteria. Hepatology. 2011;53(2):517–26.
105. Krawitt EL. Autoimmune hepatitis. N Engl J Med. 2006;354(1):54–66.
106. Di Giorgio A, Bravi M, Bonanomi E, Alessio G, Sonzogni A, Zen Y, et al. Fulminant hepatic failure of autoimmune aetiology in children. J Pediatr Gastroenterol Nutr. 2015;60(2):159–64.
107. Ferreira AR, Roquete ML, Toppa NH, de Castro LP, Fagundes ED, Penna FJ. Effect of treatment of hepatic histopathology in children and adolescents with autoimmune hepatitis. J Pediatr Gastroenterol Nutr. 2008;46(1):65–70.
108. Sogo T, Fujisawa T, Inui A, Komatsu H, Etani Y, Tajiri H, et al. Intravenous methylprednisolone pulse therapy for children with autoimmune hepatitis. Hepatol Res. 2006;34(3):187–92.
109. Al-Chalabi T, Heneghan MA. Remission in autoimmune hepatitis: what is it, and can it ever be achieved? Am J Gastroenterol. 2007;102(5):1013–5.
110. Kerkar N, Annunziato RA, Foley L, Schmeidler J, Rumbo C, Emre S, et al. Prospective analysis of nonadherence in autoimmune hepatitis: a common problem. J Pediatr Gastroenterol Nutr. 2006;43(5):629–34.
111. Samaroo B, Samyn M, Buchanan C, Mieli-Vergani G. Long-term daily oral treatment with prednisolone in children with autoimmune liver disease does not affect final adult height. Hepatology. 2006;44:438A.
112. Alvarez F. Autoimmune hepatitis and primary sclerosing cholangitis. Clin Liver Dis. 2006;10(1):89–107, vi.
113. Floreani A, Liberal R, Vergani D, Mieli-Vergani G. Autoimmune hepatitis: contrasts and comparisons in children and adults—a comprehensive review. J Autoimmun. 2013;46:7–16.
114. Czaja AJ, Bianchi FB, Carpenter HA, Krawitt EL, Lohse AW, Manns MP, et al. Treatment challenges and investigational opportunities in autoimmune hepatitis. Hepatology. 2005;41(1):207–15.
115. Pniewska A, Sobolewska-Pilarczyk M, Pawlowska M. Evaluation of the effectiveness of treatment with prednisone and azathioprine of autoimmune hepatitis in children. Prz Gastroenterol. 2016;11(1):18–23.
116. Heneghan MA, Allan ML, Bornstein JD, Muir AJ, Tendler DA. Utility of thiopurine methyltransferase genotyping and phenotyping, and measurement of azathioprine metabolites in the management of patients with autoimmune hepatitis. J Hepatol. 2006;45(4):584–91.
117. Rumbo C, Emerick KM, Emre S, Shneider BL. Azathioprine metabolite measurements in the treatment of autoimmune hepatitis in pediatric patients: a preliminary report. J Pediatr Gastroenterol Nutr. 2002;35(3):391–8.
118. Sheiko MA, Sundaram SS, Capocelli KE, Pan Z, McCoy AM, Mack CL. Outcomes in pediatric autoimmune hepatitis and significance of azathioprine metabolites. J Pediatr Gastroenterol Nutr. 2017;65(1):80–5.
119. Mohammad S. Budesonide as first-line therapy for non-cirrhotic autoimmune hepatitis in children: a decision analysis. Scand J Gastroenterol. 2016;51(6):753–62.
120. Manns MP, Woynarowski M, Kreisel W, Lurie Y, Rust C, Zuckerman E, et al. Budesonide induces remission more effectively than prednisone in a controlled trial of patients with autoimmune hepatitis. Gastroenterology. 2010;139(4):1198–206.
121. Woynarowski M, Nemeth A, Baruch Y, Koletzko S, Melter M, Rodeck B, et al. Budesonide versus prednisone with azathioprine for the treatment of autoimmune hepatitis in children and adolescents. J Pediatr. 2013;163(5):1347–53 e1.
122. Alvarez F, Ciocca M, Canero-Velasco C, Ramonet M, de Davila MT, Cuarterolo M, et al. Short-term cyclosporine induces a remission of autoimmune hepatitis in children. J Hepatol. 1999;30(2):222–7.
123. Cuarterolo M, Ciocca M, Velasco CC, Ramonet M, Gonzalez T, Lopez S, et al. Follow-up of children with autoimmune hepatitis treated with cyclosporine. J Pediatr Gastroenterol Nutr. 2006;43(5):635–9.
124. Marlaka JR, Papadogiannakis N, Fischler B, Casswall TH, Beijer E, Nemeth A. Tacrolimus without or with the addition of conventional immunosuppressive treatment in juvenile autoimmune hepatitis. Acta Paediatr. 2012;101(9):993–9.
125. Aw MM, Dhawan A, Samyn M, Bargiota A, Mieli-Vergani G. Mycophenolate mofetil as rescue treatment for autoimmune liver disease in children: a 5-year follow-up. J Hepatol. 2009;51(1):156–60.
126. Zizzo AN, Valentino PL, Shah PS, Kamath BM. Second-line agents in pediatric patients with autoimmune hepatitis: a systematic review and meta-analysis. J Pediatr Gastroenterol Nutr. 2017;65(1):6–15.
127. D'Agostino D, Costaguta A, Alvarez F. Successful treatment of refractory autoimmune hepatitis with rituximab. Pediatrics. 2013;132(2):e526–30.
128. Kavcic M, Fisher BT, Seif AE, Li Y, Huang YS, Walker D, et al. Leveraging administrative data to monitor rituximab use in 2875 patients at 42 freestanding children's hospitals across the United States. J Pediatr. 2013;162(6):1252–8.e1.
129. Weiler-Normann C, Schramm C, Quaas A, Wiegard C, Glaubke C, Pannicke N, et al. Infliximab as a rescue treatment in difficult-to-treat autoimmune hepatitis. J Hepatol. 2013;58(3):529–34.
130. Rajanayagam J, Lewindon PJ. Infliximab as rescue therapy in paediatric autoimmune hepatitis. J Hepatol. 2013;59(4):908–9.
131. Nedelkopoulou N, Vadamalayan B, Vergani D, Mieli-Vergani G. Anti-TNFalpha treatment in children and adolescents with combined inflammatory bowel disease and autoimmune liver disease. J Pediatr Gastroenterol Nutr. 2018;66(1):100–5.
132. Rodrigues S, Lopes S, Magro F, Cardoso H, Horta e Vale AM, Marques M, et al. Autoimmune hepatitis and anti-tumor necrosis factor alpha therapy: a single center report of 8 cases. World J Gastroenterol. 2015;21(24):7584–8.

133. Mostamand S, Schroeder S, Schenkein J, Miloh T. Infliximab-associated immunomediated hepatitis in children with inflammatory bowel disease. J Pediatr Gastroenterol Nutr. 2016;63(1):94–7.
134. Battaglia M, Stabilini A, Roncarolo MG. Rapamycin selectively expands CD4+CD25+FoxP3+ regulatory T cells. Blood. 2005;105(12):4743–8.
135. Kurowski J, Melin-Aldana H, Bass L, Alonso EM, Ekong UD. Sirolimus as rescue therapy in pediatric autoimmune hepatitis. J Pediatr Gastroenterol Nutr. 2014;58(1):e4–6.
136. de Boer YS, Liberal R, Vergani D, Mieli-Vergani G, International Autoimmune Hepatitis Group. Real world management of juvenile autoimmune liver disease. J Hepatol. 2017;66(S550).
137. Liberal R, de Boer YS, Andrade RJ, Bouma G, Dalekos GN, Floreani A, et al. Expert clinical management of autoimmune hepatitis in the real world. Aliment Pharmacol Ther. 2017;45(5):723–32.
138. Ichai P, Duclos-Vallee JC, Guettier C, Hamida SB, Antonini T, Delvart V, et al. Usefulness of corticosteroids for the treatment of severe and fulminant forms of autoimmune hepatitis. Liver Transpl. 2007;13(7):996–1003.
139. van Gerven NM, Verwer BJ, Witte BI, van Hoek B, Coenraad MJ, van Erpecum KJ, et al. Relapse is almost universal after withdrawal of immunosuppressive medication in patients with autoimmune hepatitis in remission. J Hepatol. 2013;58(1):141–7.
140. Mieli-Vergani G, Vergani D. Sclerosing cholangitis in children and adolescents. Clin Liver Dis. 2016;20(1):99–111.
141. Ziol M, Barbu V, Rosmorduc O, Frassati-Biaggi A, Barget N, Hermelin B, et al. ABCB4 heterozygous gene mutations associated with fibrosing cholestatic liver disease in adults. Gastroenterology. 2008;135(1):131–41.
142. Rojas CP, Bodicharla R, Campuzano-Zuluaga G, Hernandez L, Rodriguez MM. Autoimmune hepatitis and primary sclerosing cholangitis in children and adolescents. Fetal Pediatr Pathol. 2014;33(4):202–9.
143. Rodrigues AT, Liu PM, Fagundes ED, Queiroz TC, de Souza Haueisen Barbosa P, Silva SL, et al. Clinical characteristics and prognosis in children and adolescents with autoimmune hepatitis and overlap syndrome. J Pediatr Gastroenterol Nutr. 2016;63(1):76–81.
144. Mitchell SA, Bansi DS, Hunt N, Von Bergmann K, Fleming KA, Chapman RW. A preliminary trial of high-dose ursodeoxycholic acid in primary sclerosing cholangitis. Gastroenterology. 2001;121(4):900–7.
145. Lindor KD, Kowdley KV, Luketic VA, Harrison ME, McCashland T, Befeler AS, et al. High-dose ursodeoxycholic acid for the treatment of primary sclerosing cholangitis. Hepatology. 2009;50(3):808–14.
146. Deneau MR, El-Matary W, Valentino PL, Abdou R, Alqoaer K, Amin M, et al. The natural history of primary sclerosing cholangitis in 781 children: a multicenter, international collaboration. Hepatology. 2017;66(2):518–27.
147. Debray D, Pariente D, Urvoas E, Hadchouel M, Bernard O. Sclerosing cholangitis in children. J Pediatr. 1994;124(1):49–56.
148. Smolka V, Karaskova E, Tkachyk O, Aiglova K, Ehrmann J, Michalkova K, et al. Long-term follow-up of children and adolescents with primary sclerosing cholangitis and autoimmune sclerosing cholangitis. Hepatobiliary Pancreat Dis Int. 2016;15(4):412–8.
149. Tenca A, Farkkila M, Arola J, Jaakkola T, Penagini R, Kolho KL. Clinical course and prognosis of pediatric-onset primary sclerosing cholangitis. United European Gastroenterol J. 2016;4(4):562–9.
150. Wilschanski M, Chait P, Wade JA, Davis L, Corey M, St Louis P, et al. Primary sclerosing cholangitis in 32 children: clinical, laboratory, and radiographic features, with survival analysis. Hepatology. 1995;22(5):1415–22.
151. Feldstein AE, Perrault J, El-Youssif M, Lindor KD, Freese DK, Angulo P. Primary sclerosing cholangitis in children: a long-term follow-up study. Hepatology. 2003;38(1):210–7.
152. Miloh T, Arnon R, Shneider B, Suchy F, Kerkar N. A retrospective single-center review of primary sclerosing cholangitis in children. Clin Gastroenterol Hepatol. 2009;7(2):239–45.
153. Valentino PL, Wiggins S, Harney S, Raza R, Lee CK, Jonas MM. The natural history of primary sclerosing cholangitis in children: a large single-center longitudinal cohort study. J Pediatr Gastroenterol Nutr. 2016;63(6):603–9.
154. Bjarnason I, Hayee B, Pavlidis P, Kvasnovsky C, Scalori A, Sisson G, et al. Contrasting pattern of chronic inflammatory bowel disease in primary and autoimmune sclerosing cholangitis. EBioMedicine. 2015;2(10):1523–7.
155. Gulati R, Radhakrishnan KR, Hupertz V, Wyllie R, Alkhouri N, Worley S, et al. Health-related quality of life in children with autoimmune liver disease. J Pediatr Gastroenterol Nutr. 2013;57(4):444–50.
156. Heneghan MA, Norris SM, O'Grady JG, Harrison PM, McFarlane IG. Management and outcome of pregnancy in autoimmune hepatitis. Gut. 2001;48(1):97–102.
157. Candia L, Marquez J, Espinoza LR. Autoimmune hepatitis and pregnancy: a rheumatologist's dilemma. Semin Arthritis Rheum. 2005;35(1):49–56.
158. Terrabuio DR, Abrantes-Lemos CP, Carrilho FJ, Cancado EL. Follow-up of pregnant women with autoimmune hepatitis: the disease behavior along with maternal and fetal outcomes. J Clin Gastroenterol. 2009;43(4):350–6.
159. Braga AC, Vasconcelos C, Braga J. Pregnancy with autoimmune hepatitis. Gastroenterol Hepatol Bed Bench. 2016;9(3):220–4.
160. Danielsson Borssen A, Wallerstedt S, Nyhlin N, Bergquist A, Lindgren S, Almer S, et al. Pregnancy and childbirth in women with autoimmune hepatitis is safe, even in compensated cirrhosis. Scand J Gastroenterol. 2016;51(4):479–85.
161. Stokkeland K, Ludvigsson JF, Hultcrantz R, Ekbom A, Hoijer J, Bottai M, et al. Increased risk of preterm birth in women with autoimmune hepatitis—a nationwide cohort study. Liver Int. 2016;36(1):76–83.
162. Davies YK, Cox KM, Abdullah BA, Safta A, Terry AB, Cox KL. Long-term treatment of primary sclerosing cholangitis in children with oral vancomycin: an immunomodulating antibiotic. J Pediatr Gastroenterol Nutr. 2008;47(1):61–7.
163. Wang KK, Czaja AJ, Beaver SJ, Go VL. Extrahepatic malignancy following long-term immunosuppressive therapy of severe hepatitis B surface antigen-negative chronic active hepatitis. Hepatology. 1989;10(1):39–43.
164. Werner M, Almer S, Prytz H, Lindgren S, Wallerstedt S, Bjornsson E, et al. Hepatic and extrahepatic malignancies in autoimmune hepatitis. A long-term follow-up in 473 Swedish patients. J Hepatol. 2009;50(2):388–93.
165. Danielsson Borssen A, Almer S, Prytz H, Wallerstedt S, Friis-Liby IL, Bergquist A, et al. Hepatocellular and extrahepatic cancer in patients with autoimmune hepatitis—a long-term follow-up study in 634 Swedish patients. Scand J Gastroenterol. 2015;50(2):217–23.
166. Arinaga-Hino T, Ide T, Miyajima I, Ogata K, Kuwahara R, Amano K, et al. Risk of malignancies in autoimmune hepatitis type 1 patients with a long-term follow-up in Japan. Hepatol Res. 2018;48(3):E222–31.
167. Yeoman AD, Al-Chalabi T, Karani JB, Quaglia A, Devlin J, Mieli-Vergani G, et al. Evaluation of risk factors in the development of hepatocellular carcinoma in autoimmune hepatitis: implications for follow-up and screening. Hepatology. 2008;48(3):863–70.
168. Wong RJ, Gish R, Frederick T, Bzowej N, Frenette C. Development of hepatocellular carcinoma in autoimmune hepatitis patients: a case series. Dig Dis Sci. 2011;56(2):578–85.
169. Tansel A, Katz LH, El-Serag HB, Thrift AP, Parepally M, Shakhatreh MH, et al. Incidence and determinants of hepatocellular carcinoma in autoimmune hepatitis: a systematic

review and meta-analysis. Clin Gastroenterol Hepatol. 2017;15(8):1207–17 e4.
170. Burak K, Angulo P, Pasha TM, Egan K, Petz J, Lindor KD. Incidence and risk factors for cholangiocarcinoma in primary sclerosing cholangitis. Am J Gastroenterol. 2004;99(3):523–6.
171. Ross AM IV, Anupindi SA, Balis UJ. Case records of the Massachusetts General Hospital. Weekly clinicopathological exercises. Case 11-2003. A 14-year-old boy with ulcerative colitis, primary sclerosing cholangitis, and partial duodenal obstruction. N Engl J Med. 2003;348(15):1464–76.
172. Martin SR, Alvarez F, Anand R, Song C, Yin W, Group SR. Outcomes in children who underwent transplantation for autoimmune hepatitis. Liver Transpl. 2011;17(4):393–401.
173. Bahar RJ, Yanni GS, Martin MG, McDiarmid SV, Vargas JH, Gershman GB, et al. Orthotopic liver transplantation for autoimmune hepatitis and cryptogenic chronic hepatitis in children. Transplantation. 2001;72(5):829–33.
174. Vergani D, Mieli-Vergani G. Autoimmunity after liver transplantation. Hepatology. 2002;36(2):271–6.
175. Miloh T, Anand R, Yin W, Vos M, Kerkar N, Alonso E, et al. Pediatric liver transplantation for primary sclerosing cholangitis. Liver Transpl. 2011;17(8):925–33.
176. Squires RH, Ng V, Romero R, Ekong U, Hardikar W, Emre S, et al. Evaluation of the pediatric patient for liver transplantation: 2014 practice guideline by the American Association for the Study of Liver Diseases, American Society of Transplantation and the North American Society for Pediatric Gastroenterology. Hepatology. 2014;60(1):362–98.
177. Scalori A, Heneghan MA, Hadzic D, Vergani D, Mieli-Vergani G. Outcome and survival in childhood onset autoimmune sclerosing cholangitis and autoimmune hepatitis: a13-year follow up study. Hepatology. 2007;46S:555A.
178. Liberal R, Zen Y, Mieli-Vergani G, Vergani D. Liver transplantation and autoimmune liver diseases. Liver Transpl. 2013;19(10):1065–77.
179. Edmunds C, Ekong UD. Autoimmune liver disease post-liver transplantation: a summary and proposed areas for future research. Transplantation. 2016;100(3):515–24.
180. Kerkar N, Yanni G. 'De novo' and 'recurrent' autoimmune hepatitis after liver transplantation: a comprehensive review. J Autoimmun. 2016;66:17–24.
181. Liberal R, Vergani D, Mieli-Vergani G. Recurrence of autoimmune liver disease and inflammatory bowel disease after pediatric liver transplantation. Liver Transpl. 2016;22(9):1275–83.
182. Montano-Loza AJ, Bhanji RA, Wasilenko S, Mason AL. Systematic review: recurrent autoimmune liver diseases after liver transplantation. Aliment Pharmacol Ther. 2017;45(4):485–500.
183. Puustinen L, Boyd S, Arkkila P, Isoniemi H, Arola J, Farkkila M. Histologic surveillance after liver transplantation due to autoimmune hepatitis. Clin Transpl. 2017; https://doi.org/10.1111/ctr.12936.
184. Ayata G, Gordon FD, Lewis WD, Pomfret E, Pomposelli JJ, Jenkins RL, et al. Liver transplantation for autoimmune hepatitis: a long-term pathologic study. Hepatology. 2000;32(2):185–92.
185. Birnbaum AH, Benkov KJ, Pittman NS, McFarlane-Ferreira Y, Rosh JR, LeLeiko NS. Recurrence of autoimmune hepatitis in children after liver transplantation. J Pediatr Gastroenterol Nutr. 1997;25(1):20–5.
186. Banff Working Group, Demetris AJ, Adeyi O, Bellamy CO, Clouston A, Charlotte F, et al. Liver biopsy interpretation for causes of late liver allograft dysfunction. Hepatology. 2006;44(2):489–501.
187. Wright HL, Bou-Abboud CF, Hassanein T, Block GD, Demetris AJ, Starzl TE, et al. Disease recurrence and rejection following liver transplantation for autoimmune chronic active liver disease. Transplantation. 1992;53(1):136–9.

188. Gonzalez-Koch A, Czaja AJ, Carpenter HA, Roberts SK, Charlton MR, Porayko MK, et al. Recurrent autoimmune hepatitis after orthotopic liver transplantation. Liver Transpl. 2001;7(4):302–10.
189. Prados E, Cuervas-Mons V, de la Mata M, Fraga E, Rimola A, Prieto M, et al. Outcome of autoimmune hepatitis after liver transplantation. Transplantation. 1998;66(12):1645–50.
190. Sempoux C, Horsmans Y, Lerut J, Rahier J, Geubel A. Acute lobular hepatitis as the first manifestation of recurrent autoimmune hepatitis after orthotopic liver transplantation. Liver. 1997;17(6):311–5.
191. Czaja AJ. The immunoreactive propensity of autoimmune hepatitis: is it corticosteroid-dependent after liver transplantation? Liver Transpl Surg. 1999;5(5):460–3.
192. Montano-Loza AJ, Mason AL, Ma M, Bastiampillai RJ, Bain VG, Tandon P. Risk factors for recurrence of autoimmune hepatitis after liver transplantation. Liver Transpl. 2009;15(10):1254–61.
193. Hurtova M, Duclos-Vallee JC, Johanet C, Emile JF, Roque-Afonso AM, Feray C, et al. Successful tacrolimus therapy for a severe recurrence of type 1 autoimmune hepatitis in a liver graft recipient. Liver Transpl. 2001;7(6):556–8.
194. Jossen J, Annunziato R, Kim HS, Chu J, Arnon R. Liver transplantation for children with primary sclerosing cholangitis and autoimmune hepatitis: UNOS database analysis. J Pediatr Gastroenterol Nutr. 2017;64(4):e83–e7.
195. Duclos-Vallee JC, Sebagh M, Rifai K, Johanet C, Ballot E, Guettier C, et al. A 10 year follow up study of patients transplanted for autoimmune hepatitis: histological recurrence precedes clinical and biochemical recurrence. Gut. 2003;52(6):893–7.
196. Venkat VL, Ranganathan S, Mazariegos GV, Sun Q, Sindhi R. Recurrence of primary sclerosing cholangitis in pediatric liver transplant recipients. Liver Transpl. 2014;20(6):679–86.
197. Graziadei IW, Wiesner RH, Batts KP, Marotta PJ, LaRusso NF, Porayko MK, et al. Recurrence of primary sclerosing cholangitis following liver transplantation. Hepatology. 1999;29(4):1050–6.
198. Graziadei IW. Recurrence of primary sclerosing cholangitis after liver transplantation. Liver Transpl. 2002;8(7):575–81.
199. Alabraba E, Nightingale P, Gunson B, Hubscher S, Olliff S, Mirza D, et al. A re-evaluation of the risk factors for the recurrence of primary sclerosing cholangitis in liver allografts. Liver Transpl. 2009;15(3):330–40.
200. Carbone M, Neuberger J. Liver transplantation in PBC and PSC: indications and disease recurrence. Clin Res Hepatol Gastroenterol. 2011;35(6–7):446–54.
201. Chen CY, Ho MC, Wu JF, Jeng YM, Chen HL, Chang MH, et al. Development of autoantibodies after pediatric liver transplantation. Pediatr Transplant. 2013;17(2):144–8.
202. Kerkar N, Hadzic N, Davies ET, Portmann B, Donaldson PT, Rela M, et al. De-novo autoimmune hepatitis after liver transplantation. Lancet. 1998;351(9100):409–13.
203. Hernandez HM, Kovarik P, Whitington PF, Alonso EM. Autoimmune hepatitis as a late complication of liver transplantation. J Pediatr Gastroenterol Nutr. 2001;32(2):131–6.
204. Gupta P, Hart J, Millis JM, Cronin D, Brady L. De novo hepatitis with autoimmune antibodies and atypical histology: a rare cause of late graft dysfunction after pediatric liver transplantation. Transplantation. 2001;71(5):664–8.
205. Andries S, Casamayou L, Sempoux C, Burlet M, Reding R, Bernard Otte J, et al. Posttransplant immune hepatitis in pediatric liver transplant recipients: incidence and maintenance therapy with azathioprine. Transplantation. 2001;72(2):267–72.
206. Venick RS, McDiarmid SV, Farmer DG, Gornbein J, Martin MG, Vargas JH, et al. Rejection and steroid dependence: unique risk factors in the development of pediatric post-transplant de novo autoimmune hepatitis. Am J Transplant. 2007;7(4):955–63.
207. Miyagawa-Hayashino A, Haga H, Egawa H, Hayashino Y, Sakurai T, Minamiguchi S, et al. Outcome and risk factors of de

novo autoimmune hepatitis in living-donor liver transplantation. Transplantation. 2004;78(1):128–35.
208. Sebagh M, Castillo-Rama M, Azoulay D, Coilly A, Delvart V, Allard MA, et al. Histologic findings predictive of a diagnosis of de novo autoimmune hepatitis after liver transplantation in adults. Transplantation. 2013;96(7):670–8.
209. Pongpaibul A, Venick RS, McDiarmid SV, Lassman CR. Histopathology of de novo autoimmune hepatitis. Liver Transpl. 2012;18(7):811–8.
210. Liberal R, Longhi MS, Grant CR, Mieli-Vergani G, Vergani D. Autoimmune hepatitis after liver transplantation. Clin Gastroenterol Hepatol. 2012;10(4):346–53.
211. Salcedo M, Vaquero J, Banares R, Rodriguez-Mahou M, Alvarez E, Vicario JL, et al. Response to steroids in de novo autoimmune hepatitis after liver transplantation. Hepatology. 2002;35(2):349–56.
212. Vergani D, Choudhuri K, Bogdanos DP, Mieli-Vergani G. Pathogenesis of autoimmune hepatitis. Clin Liver Dis. 2002;6(3):439–49.
213. Aguilera I, Sousa JM, Gavilan F, Bernardos A, Wichmann I, Nunez-Roldan A. Glutathione S-transferase T1 mismatch constitutes a risk factor for de novo immune hepatitis after liver transplantation. Liver Transpl. 2004;10(9):1166–72.
214. Fedoseyeva EV, Zhang F, Orr PL, Levin D, Buncke HJ, Benichou G. De novo autoimmunity to cardiac myosin after heart transplantation and its contribution to the rejection process. J Immunol. 1999;162(11):6836–42.

Fibrocystic Liver Disease

Laura Cristoferi, Giovanni Morana, Mario Strazzabosco, and Luca Fabris

Key Points
- Fibro(poly)cystic liver disease (PLD) is a group of congenital and rare diseases, the so-called ciliopathies, secondary to an altered development of the 'ductal plate' leading to biliary dysgenesis.
- The main causative gene mutated in PLD is *PKHD1* encoding for fibrocystin, a ciliary protein involved in intracellular signalling for several processes, from cell differentiation and proliferation to interactions with the extracellular matrix.
- Congenital hepatic fibrosis is characterized by progressive portal fibrosis developing in close proximity to dysgenetic bile ducts and consequent portal hypertension. It is often associated with dilation of intrahepatic bile ducts (Caroli syndrome) and autosomal recessive polycystic kidney disease.
- Dilation involving intra- and extrahepatic bile ducts such as Caroli disease and choledochal cysts has a later onset and clinical features related to bile stasis.
- The most feared and not rarely life-threatening complications of these diseases are related to portal hypertension (acute gastrointestinal bleeding), infections (acute cholangitis) and malignant evolution (cholangiocarcinoma).
- Radiological imaging is the gold standard for the diagnosis, allowing also evaluation of the concurrent renal disease; in particular, magnetic resonance with cholangiopancreatography is essential for the diagnosis of CD and CCs.
- Medical therapy is not currently available, but interventional radiology and surgical approaches and, eventually, liver transplantation are used in selected cases.

Research Needed in This Field
- To clarify the molecular mechanisms of fibrogenesis to identify targets for therapeutic intervention.
- To develop screening protocols for the early diagnosis of cholangiocarcinoma in paediatric population.
- To assess the clinical outcomes to optimize indications and timing of liver transplantation.

L. Cristoferi
Division of Gastroenterology, Department of Medicine and Surgery, University of Milan-Bicocca, Milan, Italy

International Center for Digestive Health, University of Milan-Bicocca, Milan, Italy
e-mail: laura.cristoferi@unimi.it

G. Morana
Division of Radiology, Treviso Regional Hospital, Treviso, Italy
e-mail: gmorana@ulss.tv.it

M. Strazzabosco (✉)
Division of Gastroenterology, Department of Medicine and Surgery, University of Milan-Bicocca, Milan, Italy

International Center for Digestive Health, University of Milan-Bicocca, Milan, Italy

Digestive Disease Section, Yale University, New Haven, CT, USA
e-mail: mario.strazzabosco@yale.edu

L. Fabris
International Center for Digestive Health, University of Milan-Bicocca, Milan, Italy

Digestive Disease Section, Yale University, New Haven, CT, USA

Department of Molecular Medicine, University of Padua, Padua, Italy
e-mail: luca.fabris@unipd.it

11.1 Introduction and Epidemiology

Fibrocystic liver diseases include a number of liver conditions characterized by the presence of liver cysts, in the liver alone or in conjunction with cystic disease of other organ. It is clinically, genetically, morphologically and pathophysiologically appropriate to separate polycystic liver disease (PLD) (either alone or in combination with adult dominant polycystic kidney disease—PLD-ADPKD) from the rarer and more severe fibrocystic liver diseases. Fibro(poly)cystic liver disease is a collective definition given to a group of unique diseases of the biliary tree, of congenital origin, epidemiologically rare, deriving from an altered development of the embryonic ductal plate, i.e. the foetal structure that originates the intrahepatic biliary epithelium.

This group includes congenital hepatic fibrosis (CHF), biliary hamartomas, Caroli disease (CD), choledochal cysts (CCs). The common theme of these diseases is the dysgenesis of the biliary tree at multiple levels, leading to the development of biliary microhamartomas when the small intrahepatic bile ducts are affected (CHF) and to segmental dilatations if the larger intrahepatic bile ducts are targeted (CD/CS). CD is the disease condition characterized by ectasia of the larger intrahepatic ducts, which is less common than CS, where biliary ectasia coexists with malformations of the small intrahepatic bile ducts (CHF). In CD/CS biliary dilations may be diffuse or segmental and often are limited to one lobe of the liver, more commonly the left lobe.

Together with fibrocystic renal disease, they are often part of the multisystemic hepatorenal fibrocystic diseases, in which dysgenesis of the biliary structures is associated with the fibrocystic degeneration of the kidneys. Renal and hepatic involvement frequently coexists in various combinations, and different liver disease conditions can overlap in the same subject, suggesting common underlying genetic mechanisms.

This chapter will focus on diseases of paediatric interest, such as CHF and its association with autosomal recessive polycystic kidney disease (ARPKD), including also CD, which however is more frequently diagnosed during adulthood, and choledochal cysts (CC). Given their rarity, the estimated prevalence of these conditions is not completely known. Although no firm prevalence data have been specifically published for CHF, it is estimated that 1/10,000–20,000 subjects may suffer from it based on the prevalence of the different conditions associated with CHF. CD is even rarer, with an estimated prevalence of about 1/1,000,000 subjects.

11.2 Aetiology

11.2.1 Ciliopathies

Defects in ciliary proteins represent a major cause of diseases presenting with hepatic fibrocystic phenotype. The central role of cilia dysfunction has led to this group of disorders being designated as 'ciliopathies', laying the basis to our understanding of the common pathophysiological mechanisms of this spectrum of diseases [1–3].

There are two types of cilia: motile and non-motile. The motile cilia are present in respiratory epithelium, fallopian tube epithelium, ependymal cells and sperm, and their function is to transport fluid along the epithelial surface with concerted movement. Dysfunctional motile cilia cause primary ciliary dyskinesia with symptoms of bronchiectasis, situs inversus and infertility [4, 5].

Non-motile cilia are sensory organelles extending outward from the cell surface and they act as a signal transducer between the extracellular and intracellular milieu [6]. Most polarized, eukaryotic cells express primary cilia, among which cholangiocytes and renal tubular epithelial cells are the most frequently targeted by genetic defects in humans. Primary non-motile cilia abnormalities cause ciliopathies. These are a very diverse group of diseases often associated with the development of cystic lesions.

For example, in the kidney, an organ most often affected by ciliopathies, disease manifestations related to ciliary dysfunction range from urinary concentration defects in normal-appearing kidneys to frankly abnormal kidneys. While autosomal dominant polycystic kidney disease (ADPKD) and ARPKD represent the most common ciliopathies, nephronophthisis, cystic dysplastic kidneys, medullary sponge kidney and several overlap syndromes contribute to the wide spectrum of kidney diseases observed in ciliopathies [3].

Cilia are a very 'popular' location for proteins that mediate cell interactions with other cells and the microenvironment, so it remains unclear if the pathophysiological mechanism is a failure of cyst function or of a protein (or group of protein) that happen to be in the cilia.

However, clinical phenotypes of 'ciliopathies' are highly variable and can involve several systems under the control of numerous genetic modifiers regulating ciliary proteins [4]. Furthermore, in addition to their role as signal transducers, primary cilia exert multiple functions during development, tissue morphogenesis and homeostasis [4]. Defective ciliary function during embryogenesis explains the clinical and histological findings in human ciliopathies associated with early onset [7].

11.2.2 Embryology

Ductal plate malformation (DPM) is the key pathological feature of liver disease in ciliopathies. To understand the pathophysiological aspects of DPM is therefore important to summarize the fundamental mechanisms of biliary embryogenesis. The biliary tree develops from the endodermal

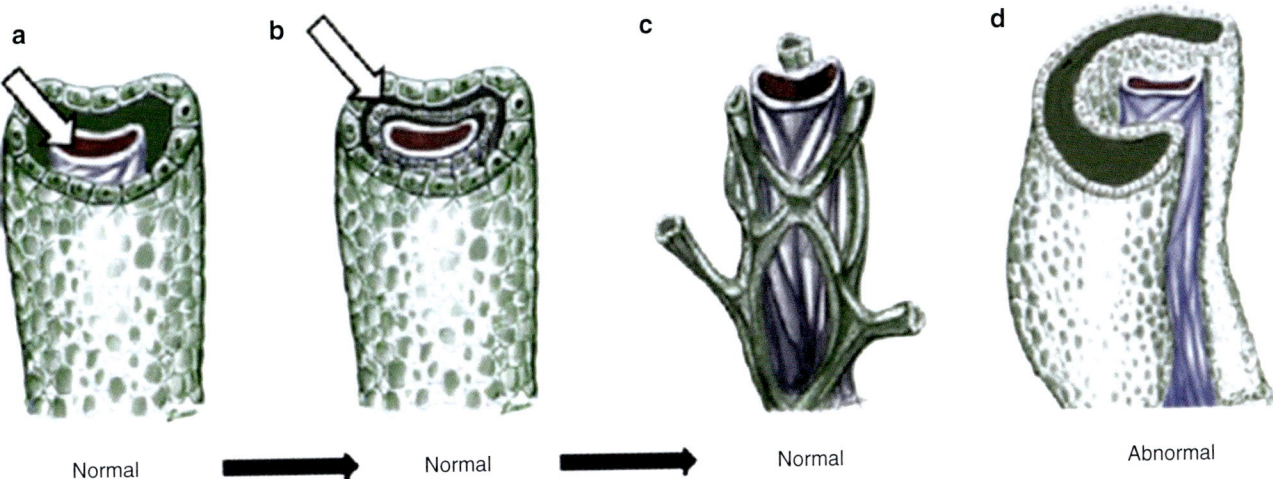

Fig. 11.1 Schematic of ductal plate development. Progression from (**a**) a single-layer ductal plate surrounding the portal vein (arrow) to (**b**) a double-layer ductal plate with slit-like bile duct lumen (arrow) to (**c**) resorption of the primitive bile duct. (**d**) Insufficient resorption leads to dysmorphic bile ducts/fibrocystic liver diseases (reprinted with permission from Marchal GJ et al.) [65]

hepatic diverticulum of the ventral foregut endoderm, which extends into the septum transversum, an intermediate structure located between the pericardial and peritoneal cavities [8, 9]. Two parts originate from the ventral foregut endoderm, the cranial part, leading to the intrahepatic bile duct epithelium, and the caudal part, which generates the extrahepatic bile ducts.

The biliary system starts to develop at the 8th week of gestation with the formation of a single layer of hepatoblasts surrounding the portal mesenchyme, the so-called ductal plate. Ductal plate cells ultimately differentiate into periportal hepatocytes and hepatic progenitor cells. Studies performed in mouse embryos have shown that nascent tubules are formed by ductal plate cells with a dual epithelial identity, resembling cholangiocytes on the side facing the portal tract and hepatocytes on the opposite parenchymal side [10]. Duplication of ductal plate cells forms a double layer where hepatoblasts are replaced by cholangiocytes, with a progressive dilation of the structure acquiring a tubular morphology, which identifies the primitive bile duct (Fig. 11.1).

Once the lumen is formed, the nascent bile duct matures along both cross-sectional and cranio-caudal axis, extending from the hilum to the periphery until the 30th week of gestation. The progressive elongation of bile ducts is coordinated by a critical mechanism that orientates mitosis along the right axis and maintains the tubular architecture within the ductal plane, the so-called planar cell polarity.

This mechanism is finely orchestrated by mutual interactions between the ductal plate and mesenchymal cells regulated by a huge number of growth and transcription factors, stimulating cell migration and cholangiocyte differentiation in a coordinated fashion, that when defective, leads to abnormal dilated or disconnected bile ducts, resulting in biliary cystic structures.

11.2.3 Genetics

Ciliopathies belong to a large spectrum of pathologies with similar clinical features, despite very different genetic defects. The main causative gene mutated in fibrocystic liver diseases, such as CHF/CD and ARPKD, is *PKHD1*, a 500 kb gene located on chromosome 6p21.1p12 encoding for fibrocystin. This is a large membrane, receptor-like protein located in the basal body of cilia and centromeres predominantly expressed by collecting ducts and thick ascending loops in kidneys and by ductal epithelia of the liver and pancreas. Although fibrocystin functions are mostly unknown, it seems to be involved in several processes, from cell proliferation to secretion, terminal differentiation, tubulogenesis and interactions with the extracellular matrix [9, 11]. Recent evidences indicate that fibrocystin is also involved in the control of 'planar cell polarity', where it likely acts in concert with the β-catenin signalling independently of Wnt activation.

In the last decade, several studies have analysed the genetic structure and mutations of *PKHD1*, finding more than 300 mutations, with a detection rate varying between 42 and 87% [12]. Despite the advances at the molecular level, the factors that modulate disease expression have yet to be defined. The rates of progression of hepatic and renal disease may vary, even among patients with the same *PKHD1* mutation, indicating the involvement of modifier genes to determine the different clinical phenotypes of the disease. Ultimately, current mutation analysis is not necessarily predictive of outcome [13].

Recent studies have shown that defective function of fibrocystin (the gene product of the PKHD 1 gene) is associated with important changes in intracellular signalling (increased signalling from PKA and beta-catenin) leading to secretin of cyto-/chemokines able to attract macrophages

Table 11.1 Hepatorenal fibrocystic disease

Disease	Gene(s)	Renal disease	Hepatic disease	Associated features
ARPDK	PDHD1	Collecting duct dilation	CHF; CD	Growth retardation
ADPDK	PDK1, PDK2	Cysts along entire nephron	Biliary cysts; CHF	Pancreatic, arachnoid membrane and seminal vesicles cysts
NPHP	NPHP1-NPHP15	Tubulo-interstitial fibrosis Cysts at the corticomedullary junction	CHF	Tapetoretinal degeneration Situs inversus
Joubert syndrome	JBTS1-JBTS20	Cystic dysplasia; NPHP	CHF, CD	Cerebellar vermis hypo-/aplasia with episodic hyperpnoea, abnormal eye movements, intellectual disability
Bardet-Biedl syndrome	BBS1-BBS15	Cystic dysplasia; NPHP	CHF	Retinal degeneration, obesity, postaxial polydactyly, hypogonadism in males, intellectual disability
Meckel-Gruber syndrome	MKS1-MKS10	Cystic dysplasia	CHF	Occipital encephalocele, polydactyly
Oral-facial-digital syndrome type I	OFD1	Glomerular cysts	CHF (rare)	Malformation of the face, oral cavity and digits
Jeune syndrome (asphyxiating thoracic dystrophy)	IFT80 (ATD2), DYNC2H1 (ATD3), ADT1, ADT4, ADT5	Cystic dysplasia	CHF; CD	Short stature, skeletal dysplasia, small thorax, short limbs, polydactyly, hypoplastic pelvis

Genetics and clinical features. Adapted with permission from Hartung EA et al. [19]

and mesenchymal cells and ultimately leading to pericystic collagen deposition [14, 15]. These mechanisms could in principle be targeted at several levels, raising hopes for future therapeutic strategies.

Besides *PKDH1*, other genes are involved in the pathogenesis of CHF and CD, as shown in Table 11.1. Among them, in rodent models, mutations in the gene *IFT88/Polaris*, a component of the intraflagellar transport essential for ciliogenesis and for the regulation of the cell cycle, generate a liver phenotype with strong similarities to fibrocystin deficiency [16].

11.3 Pathophysiology, Clinical Presentation and Diagnosis

As noted above, pathogenesis of PLD is associated with DPM. Since DPM may affect the intrahepatic biliary tree at any level, the affected anatomic level determines a specific clinical entity in this group of liver disease [17]. Based on this assumption, and very schematically, herein we report the anatomic level affected by DPM and the resulting disease condition:

- **Small intralobular bile ducts (<20 μm)**: von Meyenburg complex
- **Interlobular and septal bile ducts (20–50 μm)**: congenital hepatic fibrosis
- **Larger intrahepatic bile ducts (> 50 μm)**: Caroli disease
- **Extrahepatic bile ducts**: choledochal cysts

However, this phenotypic distinction has some limitations. In fact, depending on the stage of the maturation arrest, either the small interlobular bile ducts or the larger intrahepatic ducts may be affected.

11.3.1 Congenital Hepatic Fibrosis

CHF is characterized by ductal plate malformation of the interlobular bile ducts, which is associated with progressive peribiliary fibrosis, leading to portal hypertension and its feared complications. CHF is a rare autosomal recessive disorder with a variable course and clinical manifestations, whose severity however is strictly related to the renal function. In fact, more commonly, CHF is associated with a renal disease such as ARPKD and others.

The clinical manifestations of CHF are often non-specific, making the diagnosis of this disease difficult. Although clinical onset is highly variable, spanning from early childhood to the sixth decade of life, CHF is most frequently diagnosed during adolescence or young adulthood [18]. Most patients are asymptomatic, but mild right upper quadrant pain may be present. Physical examination reveals hepatomegaly, splenomegaly and nephromegaly, when associated to polycystic renal disease [19]. Notably, splenomegaly may not be detectable in early childhood, because portal fibrosis and portal hypertension develop slowly and progress with age.

Liver function is often well preserved at the laboratory tests, and only mild elevation in liver enzymes can be appreciated. Marked cholestasis may be detected in patients with

Table 11.2 Clinical phenotypes of CHF

Clinical phenotypes	Frequency	Signs and symptoms	Laboratory
Portal hypertension predominant	Frequent	– Hepatomegaly – Splenomegaly – Gastrointestinal bleeding	Normal LFTs Thrombocytopaenia Normal prothrombin time Normal serum ammonium
Cholestatic form (most often in association with CD)	Frequent	– Abdominal pain – Pruritus – Recurrent cholangitis	– Cholestasis tests increased
Mixed form	Rare		
Latent disease	Rare	Isolated hepatomegaly	

Adapted from Rock et al. [7]

cholangitic forms, although these are more frequent in patients with CS. Furthermore, renal function should always be tested, regardless of the presence of renal disease. According to the dominating symptoms, four clinical phenotypes can be distinguished [18]:

1. *Portal hypertension predominant*, which is the most common form. In this form, variceal bleeding is often the first clinical manifestation.
2. *Cholestatic forms with recurrent acute cholangitis* of infectious origin (most often in association with CS).
3. *Mixed forms*.
4. *Latent disease with late-onset presentation*.

Clinical feature of CHF are summarized in Table 11.2.

11.3.2 Caroli Syndrome and Caroli Disease

CS and CD are rare congenital diseases characterized by ductal plate malformation of interlobular and larger bile ducts resulting in intrahepatic bile ducts ectasia. It may involve the entire biliary tree (bi-lobar disease) or a segmental part such as a single lobe, more commonly the left one. CD is sporadic, less common than CS with a prevalence of 1:1,000,000 inhabitants and congenital hepatic impairment is limited to development of cystic dilation. CS is autosomal recessive disease, frequently associated with kidney polycystic disease, in which malformation of bile ducts is associated with CHF.

CD has no pathognomonic symptoms or signs. It may remain asymptomatic or experiences infrequent and non-specific symptoms throughout life [20]. Onset is usually during childhood or adolescence, but it may be also diagnosed in adulthood [17, 20, 21]. Patients who present with symptoms of CD before the age of 40 years are more likely to have concomitant CHF considering the earlier onset of portal hypertension complications. When symptomatic, patients with CD may present with right upper quadrant pain, fever and jaundice as a consequence of bile's stasis which may lead to stone's formation and predispose to cholangitis [17, 20]. Patients may also present with anorexia and fatigue, often accompanied by severe infections such as abscesses or septicaemia. Recurrent episodes of cholangitis in turn increase the risk of lithiasis worsening bile stasis that may evolve in secondary biliary cirrhosis.

CS is characterized by both features of CD associated with signs and symptoms secondary to portal hypertension such as splenomegaly, ascites, peripheral oedema, coagulation disorders and oesophageal varices.

11.3.3 Complications

The most relevant complication of CHF/CS is portal hypertension and its related manifestations, recurrent acute cholangitis and the increased risk of development of cholangiocarcinoma. All of them may also represent indication to liver transplantation in the paediatric population. Moreover, the clinical approach should always take into consideration the renal function and eventually, the rate of progression of renal failure, which is often associated with liver disease and may influence prognosis and response to therapies.

- **Portal hypertension** in CHF/CS is a major clinical problem, more often associated with the presence of gastro-oesophageal varices and splenomegaly, with thrombocytopenia. Other complications of portal hypertension are rare in these patients. Indeed, development of ascites is quite uncommon, and when detected, other underlying causes, such as portal vein thrombosis (PVT) or recurrent peritonitis, in patients undergoing peritoneal dialysis, must be carefully considered. PVT and the subsequent progression to portal vein cavernoma may represent an intrinsic feature of the disorder. Doppler ultrasound examination should be routinely performed in CHF patients with PH to exclude PVT or even, in the context of a known ARPKD, to evaluate whether it is associated with CHF [22].
- As mentioned above, variceal bleeding can be the first manifestation of CHF, occurring at any age; however, significant

PH takes time to develop, and most commonly, it affects older children or young adults. The management of acute variceal bleeding as well as the primary and secondary prophylaxis should follow the standard guidelines reported for children with PH from other causes [22] and outline in specific chapter of this book.

- **Cholangitis** is more common of CD but is a feared complication also in CHF, especially because it is difficult to diagnose and because of the high risk of sepsis. The classical triad of fever, jaundice and right upper quadrant pain is rarely observed in children, and more common causes of fever in childhood must be considered first if CHF is not known. Of note, fever can be the only sign of acute cholangitis in CHF, as it can occur in the absence of intra- or extrahepatic biliary radiological findings or significant liver biochemistry alterations, making the diagnosis even more difficult. Notably, the risk of sepsis-related mortality increases if antibiotic treatment is delayed. Indeed, this potential life-threatening complication has to be suspected in case of any unexplained fever in patients with diagnosis of CHF/CS or of ARPKD without known association with liver disease. In ARPKD patients, this suspicion should be even higher after renal transplantation with immunosuppressive therapy. Recent studies reported acute cholangitis in 152 out of 1230 patients with CHF (12%), with a lethal outcome in 3 out of 23 patients undergoing renal transplantation [23]. In the management of ARPKD patients with at least one episode of cholangitis, antibiotic prophylaxis for 6–12 weeks is recommended when enhanced immunosuppression is required or immediately following renal transplantation, though routine antibiotic prophylaxis is not indicated [22].
- **Cholangiocarcinoma** (CCA) is the most dreadful complication in patients with PLD. The incidence of CCA in CD and CS ranges from 2.5 to 16% [24] with a median age of 58.8 years at diagnosis (range 33–75). In a large study of 1230 patients with CHF, CD and CS, most of CCAs were detected incidentally at the time of lobe resection. In this series, the majority of CCA (53%) arose on CD/CS, but the 37% had isolated CHF [23]. However, the incidence of CCA on isolated CHF could be overestimated by the lack of MRI studies for most of these cases during the time of observation. In fact, the recent improvements in radiological techniques often allow to avoid histological confirm. MRI is the most useful single investigation and is the imaging modality of choice for intrahepatic CCA (iCCA) with accuracy rate close to 90% [25]. Positron emission tomography with fluorodeoxyglucose (PET-FDG) is a valid associate imaging study for detection of small iCCA with sensitivity ranging between 85 and 91% but in case of inflammation, frequent in these disease, could provide false-positive results [25].
- Even if, despite dreaded event, there are not surveillance guidelines for CCA in paediatric age, radiological technique for the diagnosis are improving the accuracy in the recent years [23, 26–28].

11.3.4 Associated Disease and Syndromes

CHF, CS and CD occur in association with a range of both inherited and non-inherited disorders. The most common association is with renal disease, collectively referred to as the hepatorenal fibrocystic disease (HRFCD), as reported in Table 11.1.

However, despite the presence of some distinctive features, some overlap of clinical findings and associated genes exists in several of them. The common manifestations, presented singularly or variably grouped in syndromes, which are shared by HRFCD, include:

- Cystic dysplastic kidney degeneration
- Polydactyly
- Mid- and hindbrain abnormalities
- Retinal degeneration
- Iris or retinal colobomas
- Pancreatic cystic lesions

The most common associated renal disease is ARPKD. It is the most common childhood-onset ciliopathy, with a prevalence of 1 in 20,000 live births [29–31]. ARPDK patients have non-obstructive fusiform dilations of the renal-collecting ducts, which lead to progressive renal insufficiency with associated DPM of the liver, as discussed above. In the majority of cases, mutations in the *PDKHD1* gene are reported, as in CHF/CS, often accompanying ARPDK.

Differing from ADPDK, in ARPDK, renal involvement is already detectable at birth. Kidneys are symmetrically enlarged due to dilated collecting ducts and retain their reniform conformation. Whereas most of collecting ducts though dilated still produce urine flow, some dilated ducts become closed cysts disconnected from the urinary tract as child grows. This led to US finding of macrocysts on the background of a diffuse hyper-echogenicity.

Approximately 30% of the affected infants die in the neonatal period or within the first year of life mainly due to respiratory insufficiency and/or pulmonary infections. However, the constant progresses in neonatal respiratory support and renal replacement therapy led to a significant amelioration of the 10-year survival beyond 80%. Therefore, liver disease complications related to CHF and CS are becoming more prominent and may dominate the clinical picture in adolescents and adults [31, 32]. In neonatal survivors, the severity of liver involvement has the strongest effect on ARPKD prognosis, and almost a half will be developing portal hypertension over time [33]. Moreover, most of the pre- or post-transplant problems that may affect the clinical outcome depends upon the liver disease [34]. Notably, combined renal and hepatobiliary involvement is present in about 40% of patients with ARPDK, but whether severity of both diseases does correlate is at present uncertain. In a recent study, splenomegaly did not correlate with kidney involvement, rather it correlated with glomerular filtration rate, likely reflecting a temporal progression of both renal and liver conditions [35].

11.3.5 Choledochal Cysts or Bile Duct Cysts

Choledochal cysts (CCs) are congenital lesions deriving from the ductal plate malformation targeting the largest intra- or extrahepatic bile ducts. They have a low prevalence (from 1:13,000 to 1:200,000 live births), which is higher in Asiatic countries, particularly in Japan, where 33–50% of cases are found [36, 37]. A certain female predominance has been widely reported (F/M = 3:1) [38].

Typically, CC is diagnosed in childhood, in 25% of cases within the first year of life, and only in 20% in adulthood [38]. Increased prevalence has been reported in the last decades due to the improved sensibility and wide use of the non-invasive radiological studies [39].

11.3.5.1 Classification

CCs are categorized according to the site (extrahepatic and/or intrahepatic), extent (segmental or complete) and shape (cystic or saccular, fusiform) of the biliary involvement.

According to Todani, five types of CCs are classically distinguished (Fig. 11.2) [39, 40]:

- **Type I** is characterized by dilation of the common bile duct and is the most common (70–90%). Morphologically, it is subdivided into three subtypes: I-A for cystic, I-B for segmental and I-C for fusiform dilation.
- **Type II** is localized in the supraduodenal area, appearing as a common bile duct diverticulum (2%).
- **Type III** (also known as choledochocele) is the dilation of the common bile duct within the duodenal wall (4%).
- **Type IVa** is characterized by multiple dilations affecting the intrahepatic as well as the extrahepatic bile tree ducts. Although second in frequency (10–20%), it is the most prevalent in adults, thus suggesting it likely develops later in life or progresses with age.
- **Type IVb** consists of multiple and segmental dilations of the extrahepatic biliary tree.
- **Type V (or Caroli disease)** is the ductal dilation limited to the intrahepatic biliary system, without extrahepatic involvement (1%). Dilations are more often confined to one single hepatic lobe (80%), especially the left lobe, though the disease may diffusely involve the entire intrahepatic biliary tree.

11.3.5.2 Pathophysiology

The pathophysiology of CC is controversial. Depending upon Todani categories, different theories have been proposed. As aforementioned, unlike CS, in CD, DPM is limited to the largest intrahepatic bile ducts preserving the smaller interlobular bile ducts.

The classical pathogenetic viewpoints to the role of a defective bilio-pancreatic junction (ABPJ), derived from a common channel with pancreatico-biliary junction upstream to the sphincter of Oddi [41]. This common channel may allow reflux of pancreatic juice into the biliary tree, which increases the intra-ductal pressure and relatively inflammation, ultimately leading to secondary ductal dilatation [42]. This is supported by the high incidence of ABPJ, which ranges from 96 to 100%, in children affected by CC [38, 43]. Consistent with this hypothesis, in these patients, bile sample analysis shows a high concentration of pancreatic enzymes.

Another hypothesis highlights the importance of an anatomical or functional obstruction of the distal part of the extrahepatic biliary tree. The inadequate autonomic innervation owed to oligogangliosis of the distal part of the common bile duct may result in dysmotility and functional obstruction that could be responsible for or worsen the duct lumen dilation as seen in oesophageal achalasia or in *Hirschsprung* disease of the colon [44].

11.3.5.3 Clinical Presentation and Complications

Generally, CC remains asymptomatic for years, and the diagnosis is incidental on imaging studies performed for unrelated reasons. Clinical presentation can occur at any time, but 80% of patients present overt manifestations before 10 years. In these cases, at least two symptoms of the classic triad, jaundice, right upper quadrant abdominal pain and palpable abdominal mass, are present in 85% of children. These symptoms are less frequent in adults, who usually present with abdominal pain, pancreatitis or a history of cholecystectomy for presumed biliary stones.

Symptoms associated with all types of CCs are usually related to ascending acute cholangitis and acute pancreatitis [36, 45–47]. These complications are due to bile stasis and secondary stone formation, leading to recurrent biliary infections, chronic inflammation, ductal strictures and cyst dilations [36, 48, 49].

Moreover, protein plug formation in the bile associated with chronic inflammation and bile lithiasis in the distal portions of the common bile duct and of the pancreatic duct can favour the development of acute pancreatitis [50–52]. Since eradication of cystic lesions is difficult, these complications often evolve chronically harbouring the risk of liver abscesses and life-threatening sepsis [53]. The endpoint of the alternate sequence of recurrent cholangitis and chronic biliary obstruction may lead to secondary biliary cirrhosis in 40–50% of patients, especially those with intrahepatic involvement. In these patients, signs of portal hypertension may develop

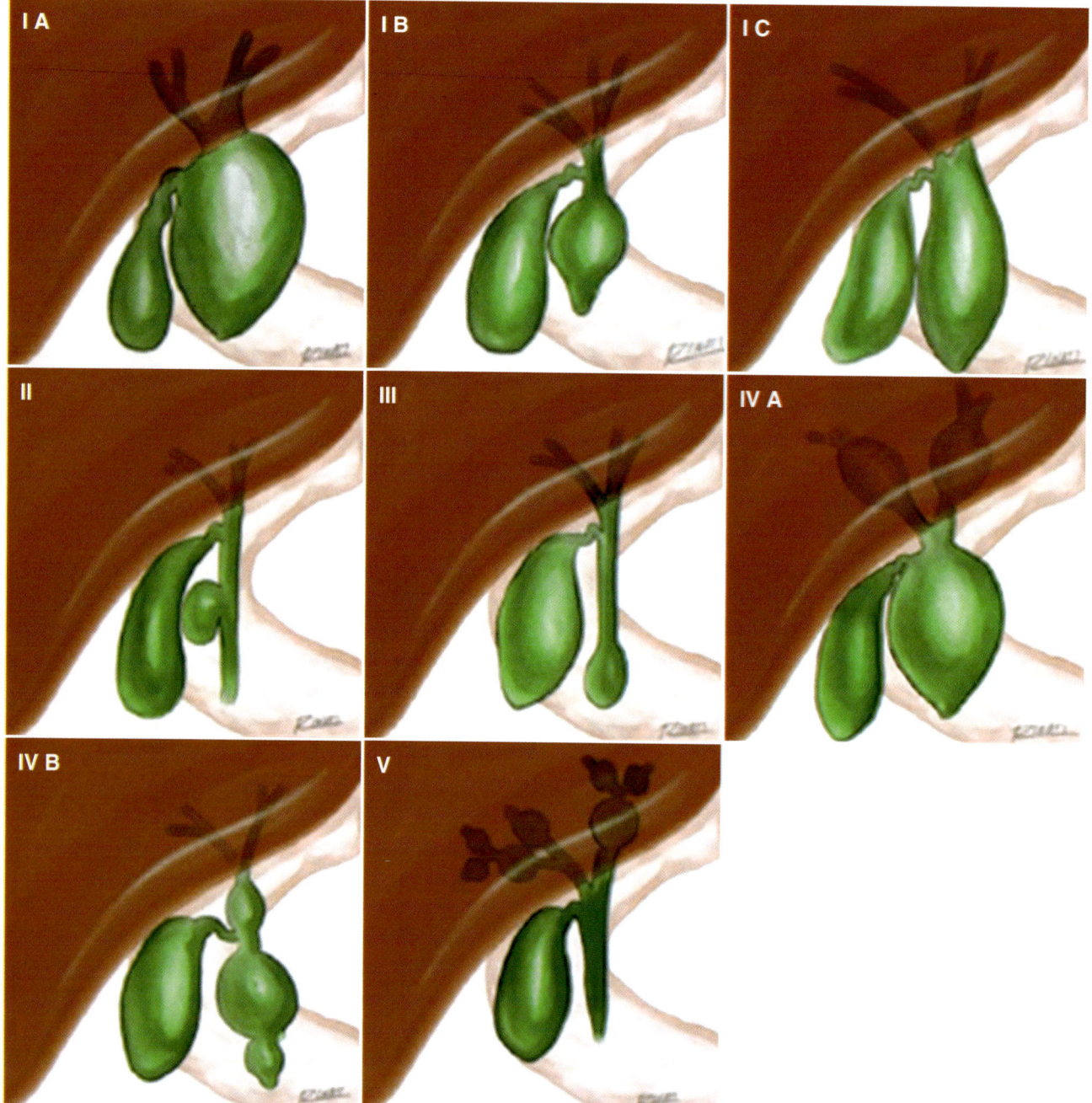

Fig. 11.2 Classification of choledochal cysts. Reprinted with permission of Todani et al. [40]

in adulthood [54], even though portal hypertension can occur even without cirrhosis, if the cyst exerts mechanic compression on the portal vein [55, 56].

In addition to portal vein, gastric outlet can be also affected by *ab extrinseco* compression of biliary cysts, in particular type III lesions, which may also favour intestinal wall intussusception [57].

Another feared complication of CCs is the rupture of the biliary cysts, which occurs spontaneously and represents the first manifestation of the disease in about 1–12% of patients. It is clinically characterized by abdominal pain, sepsis and biliary peritonitis [58, 59]. Diagnosis is based on the detection of bile-stained ascites generally intraoperatively. Sometimes, cyst's decompression secondary to rupture may mislead a diagnosis made through US showing an apparently normal biliary tree. The spontaneous rupture depends on the ductal fragility induced by chronic inflammation that, coupled with the increased ductal pressure derived from distal obstruction and with conditions of increased abdominal pressure (i.e. pregnancy), places cystic lesions to an increased risk of biliary leak [60]. The site of rupture most commonly involved is the confluence between the common bile duct and the cystic duct [61].

11.3.5.4 Malignant Evolution of CCs

There is a known association between CCs and risk of malignancy of the hepatobiliopancreatic area, which increases with age. CCA is the most frequent oncologic association, but liver parenchymal or pancreatic malignancies have been also reported.

In a large report from 73 Japanese institutions, incidence of CCA was 17.5% in patients with CCs, much higher than the 0.01–0.38% reported in large autopsy series of normal population [39], thereby accounting for a 20- to 30-fold higher risk of developing CCA [62]. The increased risk of malignancy is age-related, but unfortunately, it is present since childhood, from 0.7% in the first decade of life up to 14.3% after 20 years [63]. Impact of CC-associated CCA is relevant, because the mean age of diagnosis is 32 years, about two decades earlier than the more conventional form of CCA [62].

Interestingly, the risk of malignant transformation of the biliary epithelium extends beyond the cystic area, and CCA may arise in either the remnant tissue or not dilated segments [40, 64]. Although all types of CC may develop CCA, type I and especially type IV-A CCs show the greatest incidence. Cyst-enteric drainage procedures are a further risk factor as shown in a large Todani's series (241 cases), with 18.6% cases of CCA following such type of intervention. In that series, the mean interval between the biliary bypass procedure and the detection of CCA was 10 years. Based on these findings, elective excision of CC should be always considered even in asymptomatic patients, if previously treated by cyst enterostomy [62].

11.4 Diagnosis

11.4.1 Congenital Hepatic Fibrosis, Caroli Syndrome and Caroli Disease

Ultrasonography (US) is generally the first-line diagnostic approach, given its ability in detecting fine bile duct and liver parenchymal alterations [65]. In addition, its unique capability of detecting either liver or renal involvement contributes to its fundamental role as gold standard in the diagnostic workup of CHF.

Typical US findings include:

- Increased or heterogeneous echogenicity of the liver with hyperechoic portal triad and periportal thickening.
- Hypertrophy of the left lateral and caudate segment and normal or hypertrophic left medial segment and atrophic right lobe.
- Hepatosplenomegaly.
- Dilated intrahepatic bile ducts with duct stones when CD coexists.

Furthermore, Doppler US studies are useful to evaluate further the patency of the portal vasculature and to assess vascular complications, such as portal thrombosis or cavernous transformation from liver cirrhosis and portal hypertension.

As compared with US, computed tomography (CT) scan provides a better visualization of the liver vasculature and detects periportal cuffing as sign of fibrosis development. In the initial approach of CHF, a brain CT is crucial for the differential diagnosis of syndromes with cerebral involvement associated with the disease.

On the other hand, magnetic resonance imaging (MRI) is an alternative tool for a thorough evaluation of the biliary abnormalities (MR cholangiopancreatography), in particular to assess their connection with the ductal system. Moreover, alternatively to CT, brain MRI allows identification of cerebellar malformations associated with CHF-related disorders, such as the Joubert and COACH syndromes. Since the radiological findings are highly suggestive, particularly if fibrocystic renal involvement is also present, liver biopsy is not required [3], though in uncertain cases, it allows unequivocal diagnosis of CHF (Fig. 11.3). The classical histological findings are

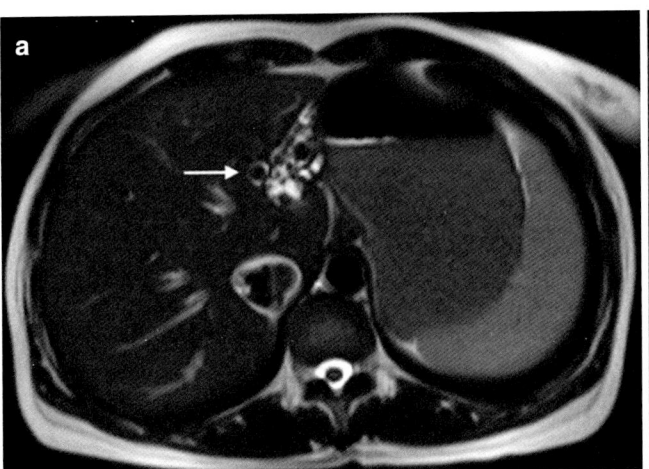
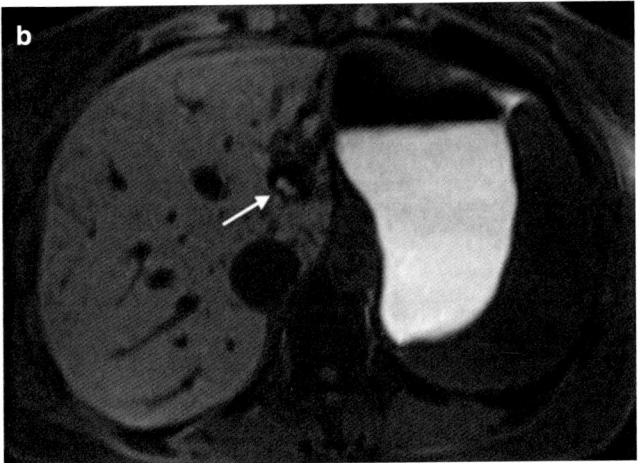

Fig. 11.3 (a–c) Caroli's disease. F, 35-year-old. A dilatation of the biliary ducts in the left lobe can be appreciated with small defects within due to calculi (arrow), which appear hypointense on T2w (a) and hyperintense on T1w (b). At MRCP (c) a significant dilatation of the biliary ducts is well appreciated

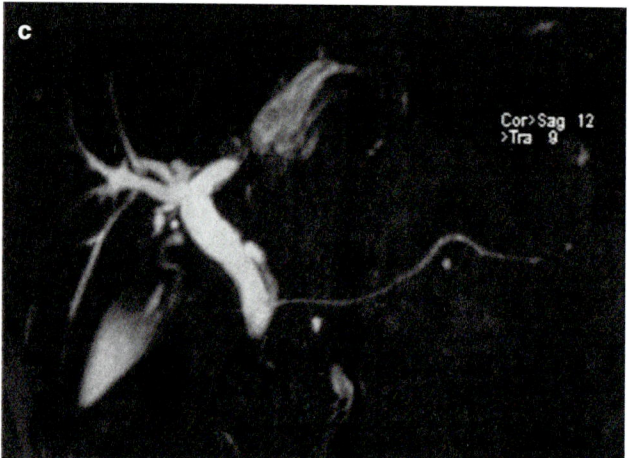

Fig. 11.3 (continued)

varying degrees of peribiliary fibrosis centred on dysgenetic bile ducts retaining a DPM configuration, eventually leading to cystic dilations when CD coexists. Biliary fibrosis may progress to nodular formation, which may become extensive. However, the porto-portal bridging of fibrotic tissue deposition, in absence of portal to central bridging, is a distinctive feature of CHF from cirrhosis. Moreover, abnormal branching of the portal vein (i.e. hypoplasia) along with an increased number of the hepatic artery branches accompanying the dysgenetic biliary structures (described as 'pollard willow' pattern) is a typical finding of conditions associated with DPM (Fig. 11.4).

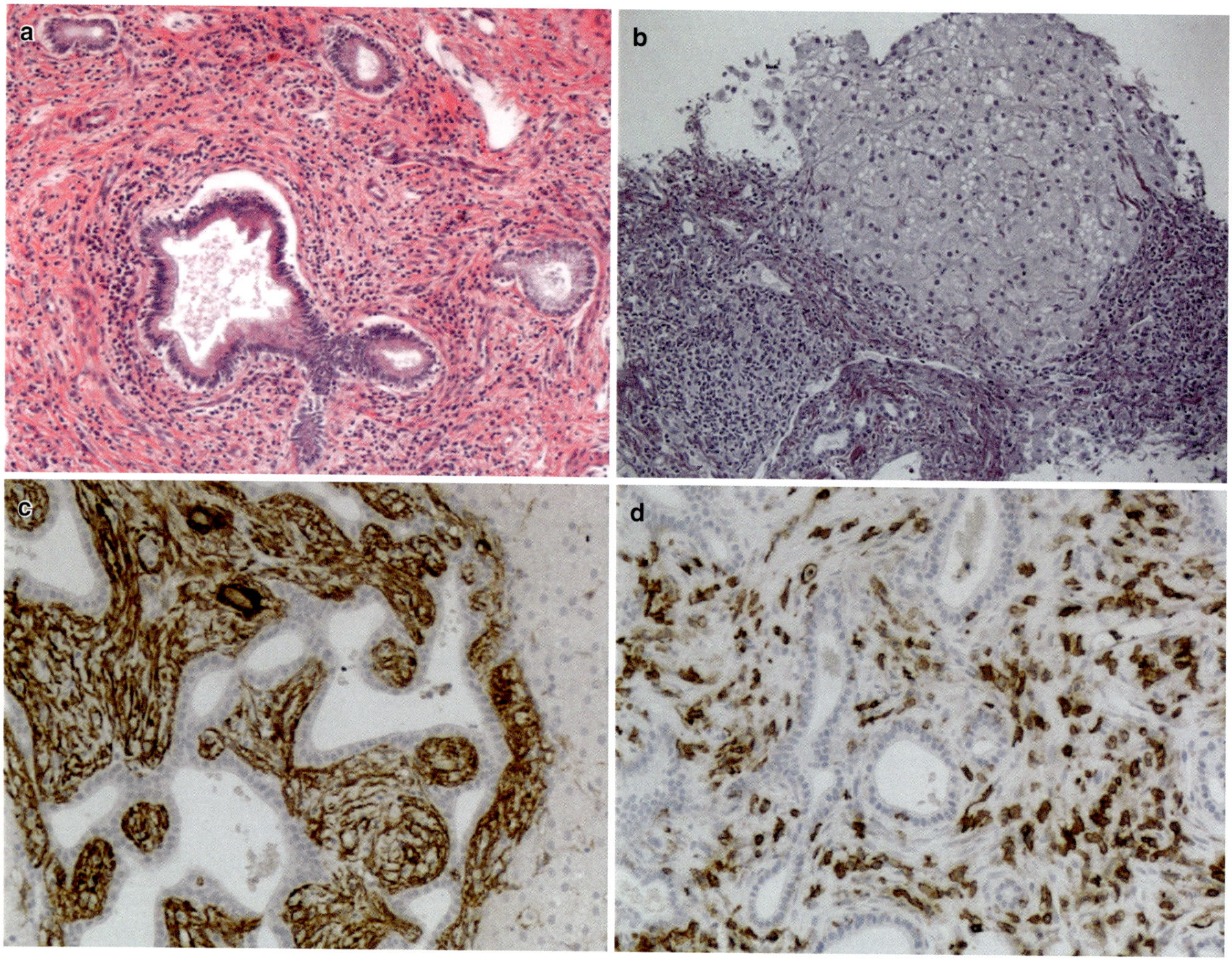

Fig. 11.4 Liver histology from a patient with CHF showing biliary microhamartomas developing in conjunction with peribiliary fibrosis and mild inflammation. (**a**) H&E ($M = 20\times$), (**b**) Masson trichrome ($M = 10\times$), (**c**) Immunohistochemistry for alpha-SMA, decorating portal myofibroblasts aligning with the external profile of the dysgenetic bile ducts ($M = 40\times$), (**d**) Immunohistochemistry for CD45, decorating inflammatory cells (mainly macrophages) recruited within the portal space ($M = 40\times$)

11.4.2 Choledochal Cysts

The 'gold standard' for diagnosis and staging CC is magnetic resonance coupled with cholangiopancreatography (MRCP) (Figs. 11.5 and 11.6) [38]. This non-invasive diagnostic technique permits to assess cyst anatomy and size and to define precisely the presence and the extent of the intrahepatic ductal involvement. Furthermore, it is useful in detecting presence of anomalies in BPJ with 100% of accuracy without feared risk of pancreatitis or cholangitis sometimes encountered with endoscopic retrograde cholangiopancreatography (ERCP) [66, 67]. However, when MRCP and conventional CT and MRI fail to determine extension of disease and to delineate the anatomy of the lesion and the surrounding structures, they should be supplemented by the addition of percutaneous transhepatic cholangiography (PTC) or ERCP which have sensitivity up to 100% [68]. These methods should be preferred in case of suspected associated biliary tract anomalies and diseases such as hepatolithiasis, ductal stricture or carcinoma for which a concomitant endoscopic treatment may be necessary.

Finally, recently also the role of endoscopic ultrasonography (EUS) appears to have the potential to differentiate between choledochal and pancreatic cysts, particularly in patients with type II choledochal cysts [69]. In case of equivocal radiological imaging EUS demonstrated to be more precise for the definition of the anatomical confines of adjacent structures and to discriminate more precisely the different cysts with the help of EUS-guided fluid aspiration [69].

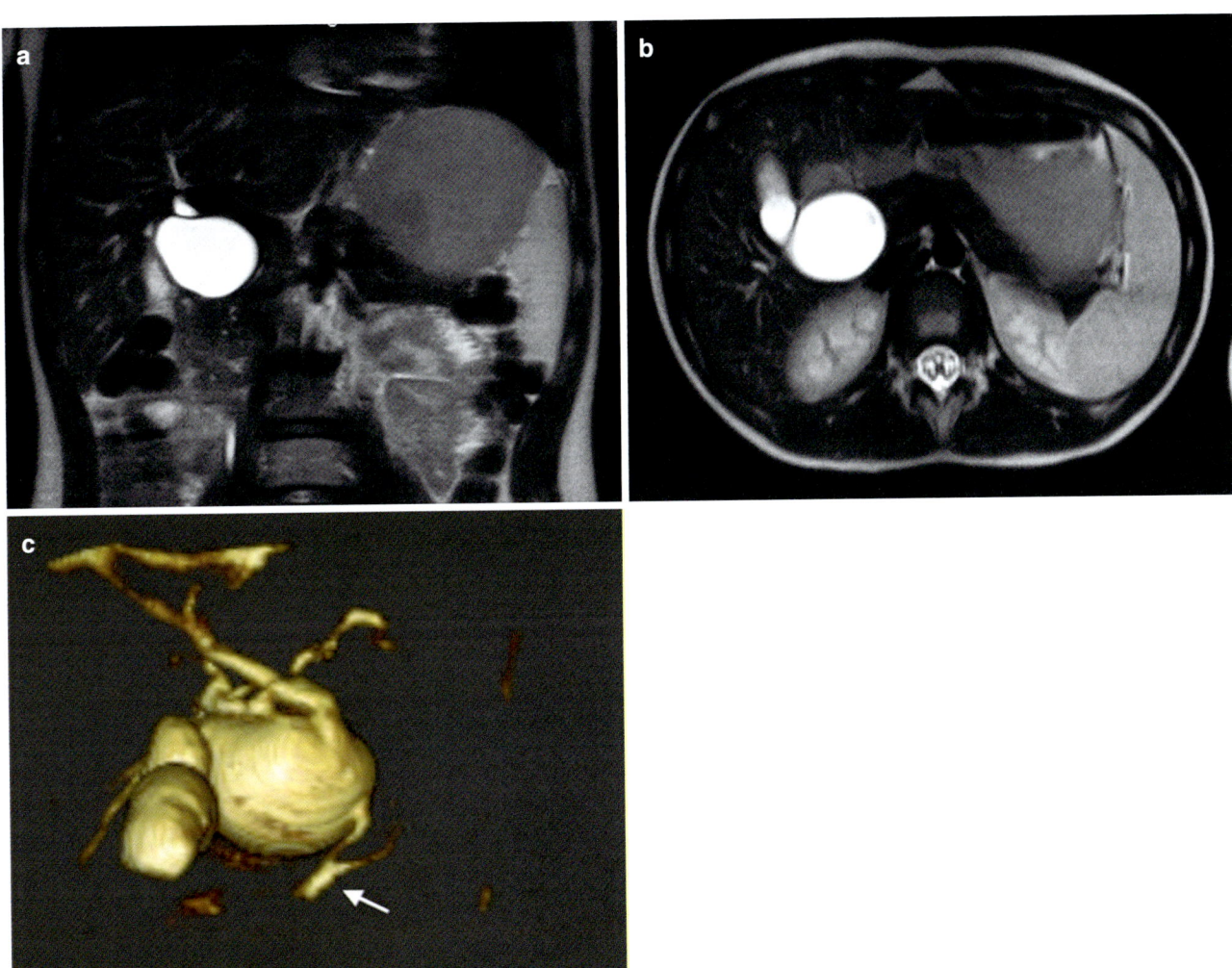

Fig. 11.5 (a–c) Type II choledochal cyst. F, 12-year-old. Admitted at ED for abdominal pain and increase in hepatic and pancreatic enzymes. At US (not shown) a large cyst between the liver and the pancreas is observed. At T2w MRI (coronal and axial scan: **a**, **b**) the cyst is confirmed. At MRCP (**c**) a large diverticulum in the pre-pancreatic portion of choledochus can be seen. A long common tract of bilio-pancreatic junction can be appreciated (arrow)

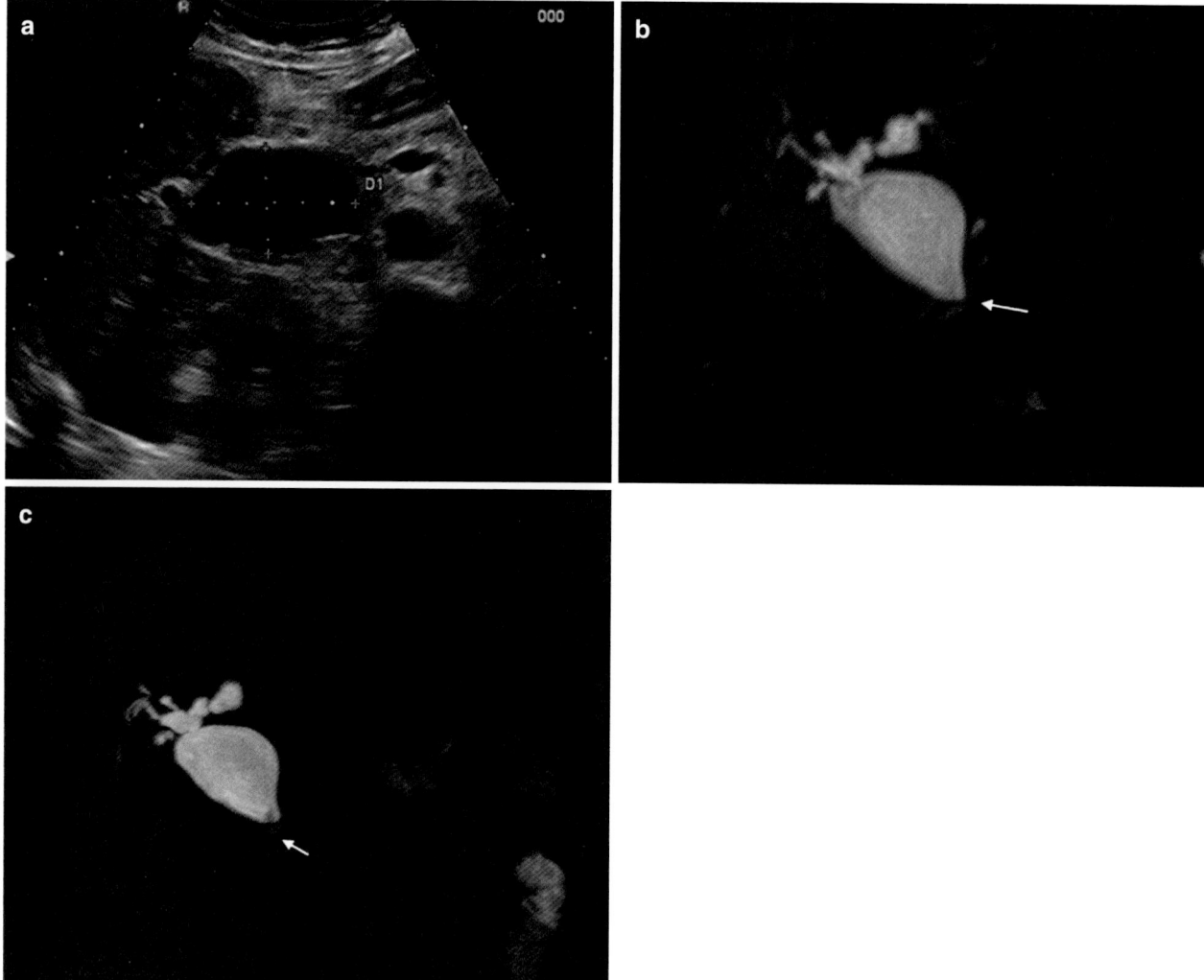

Fig. 11.6 (a–c) Type IVa choledochal cyst. F, 72-year-old. At US (a) a large cyst between the liver and the pancreas is appreciated. At T2w MRCP (b) a uniform and fusiform dilatation of the choledochus is shown, with involvement of the left biliary duct. An abnormal communication can be appreciated between the choledochus and the Wirsung's duct (arrow). At T1w MRCP, obtained after administration of hepatobiliary contrast agent (Gadobenate dimeglumine, Multihance™, Bracco, Milan, Italy) the choledochus appears hyperintense due to the contrast agent in the bile. The Wirsung's duct is visible (arrow) due to the abnormal passage of bile in the pancreatic duct

11.5 Treatment of Fibrocystic Liver Disease and Implications for Liver Transplantation

Clinical decision-making in the treatment of fibrocystic liver disease is complex and not well established in literature. Liver and renal diseases, when associated, advance at independent rates, and manifestations from either organ system have the potential to influence the outcome of organ-specific intervention.

The major liver-related issues in fibrocystic liver disease are portal hypertension complications, cholangitis, hepatolithiasis and the increased risk of development of cholangiocarcinoma. Along with these liver issues, the therapeutic approach has to take into account the state and rate of progress of potential associated renal insufficiency.

11.5.1 Congenital Hepatic Fibrosis, Caroli Syndrome and Caroli Disease

As yet, no treatment modality has been shown to actually stop or even reverse the pathological process in CHF. Instead, as noted above, for CHF treatment is directed at the management of its complication.

Management of portal hypertension complications, such as variceal bleeding, is better outlined in a specific chapter of this book.

Oesophageal endoscopic band ligation (EBL) is a very low complication rate procedure and is recommended in patients with active bleeding. In isolated varices, use of cyanoacrylate glue is not contraindicated in children, but there aren't studies about CHF/CS paediatric population. On the contrary, sclerotherapy is unfrequently used as gold standard therapy for acute bleeding because of its higher complication rate. Further studies are needed to define the use of unselective β-blockade in CHF/CS paediatric population that are currently not recommended [34, 70]. In patients with recurrent variceal bleeding, there is lack of information also on the utilization of portal decompressive surgical shunts that are uncommon in paediatric patients and are currently not frequently performed. In fact, the success of surgical shunt is largely associated with the technical skill of the surgeon, the type of shunt performed and the size of the patient. In patients without end-stage liver disease with preserved hepatic synthesis, surgical portosystemic shunting may be effective [71]. Moreover, the use of shunts in ARPKD/CHF population isn't common [23] and should be considered with caution in patients with associated end-stage renal disease for reported risk of terminal encephalopathy [72] and the increased surgical complexity for future potential kidney transplantation [34].

As already noted above, fibrocystic liver disease predisposes to biliary stasis, resulting in intrahepatic lithiasis and septic complications including recurrent episodes of cholangitis, liver abscess and septicaemia [73]. However, there is no correlation between the severity of biliary abnormalities and the risk of cholangitis, and it should be considered in every patient with fever and fibrocystic liver disease [22]. In symptomatic patients, septic complications can be rapidly life-threatening and should be rapidly diagnosed and treated with wide broad-spectrum antibiotics or a specific one chosen on the basis of susceptibility testing on blood cultures when available [74]. Antibiotic prophylaxis is indicated for 6–12 weeks after a cholangitis episode immediately following transplantation or in the context of enhanced immunosuppression. The use of ursodeoxycholic acid has been shown to have limited efficacy in reducing the risk of development of cholangitis and hepatolithiasis and, for this reason, is not routinely recommended in primary and secondary prophylaxis [75].

Along with septic complications, morbidity and mortality are related to the risk of development of oncological complications such as intrahepatic cholangiocarcinoma with a 100-fold increase risk in these patients [76].

Thus, several factors should be considered in the treatment of patients with Caroli disease and recurrent cholangitis:

- Extension of the lesion in the liver: bi-lobar, lobar or segmental
- Associated symptoms
- Presence and severity of septic complications
- Concomitant CHF and grade of complications related to portal hypertension
- Presence and severity of renal disease
- Synchronous CCA or potential malignant degeneration over time

The treatment of CD and CS is multidisciplinary and must include hepatologists, endoscopists, interventional radiologists and surgeons.

Nowadays, the use of radiological, endoscopic and surgical drainage of septic abscess and clearance of lithiasis complications is getting relevant due to the continuous progress in these fields. However, it doesn't halt the progression of the disease leading sometimes to further morbidity and mortality rate especially because of infectious complications [77]. Furthermore, few studies have been published about paediatric population.

Before surgery, the extension of disease should be carefully evaluated. In symptomatic patients with localized mono-lobar disease, partial hepatic resection represents an excellent therapeutic option [78]. Liver resection (LR) leads to excellent long-term results for localized forms without underlying chronic liver disease when the impaired intrahepatic bile ducts have been completely resected. The largest series of LR for polycystic liver disease (n = 111; almost 90% in left lobe) reports a zero mortality and good long-term results (median follow-up 25 months) [73]. Before surgery, in patients with mono-lobar disease, it is important to evaluate the real extension of liver disease; in fact, incomplete resection is associated with poor long-term results [78].

Liver transplantation (LT) remains the only therapeutic approach in patients with bi-lobar extension or with underlying chronic liver disease such as in CS. In fact, LT enables a complete resection of diffuse disease, the treatment of the underlying concomitant liver fibrosis in CHF and CS, the prevention of recurrence of septic complications and the treatment and prevention of the risk of development of CCA. Unfortunately, as a consequence of the heterogeneity and rarity of these diseases, the place of LT in the treatment of these conditions is still and therefore not well standardized.

LT induces almost 10% of perioperative mortality and exposes recipients to complications related to immunosuppressive therapy [73]. For this reason, LT should be recommended as the treatment of choice only in symptomatic patients with bi-lobar disease complicated by recurrent episodes of cholangitis and in those with cirrhosis and complications correlated to portal hypertension [79–81]. In the largest published series [77, 81], based on the European Liver Transplant Registry (ELTR) and on the United Network for Organ Sharing (UNOS) data, survival rate at 1, 5 and 10 years are 89%, 86% and 76% and 88.5%, 80.9% and 77.8%, respectively. Older age, concomitant CHF and superinfection at the time of LT are correlated with worst outcomes in other series [79]. Patients with preoperative superinfection should be considered for LT in a timely fashion. Some authors reported few recommendations to limits postoperative septic complications that should be followed mostly in patients under immunosuppressive therapy that are about to undergo LT [78, 80]. In essence, it is recommended to avoid performance of preoperative invasive biliary procedure, to perform LT only after biliary sepsis has been controlled and to perform prolonged antibiotics therapy after LT.

In case of simultaneous involvement of kidney and liver, therapeutic approach changes considering the stage of both diseases. As already noted above, end-stage disease is unlikely to affect both liver and kidney in patients with PLD. Patients usually have more severe involvement in only one organ, and both diseases progress at independent rate without any genotype-phenotype association [1]. However, a small subset of patients requires transplantation in both organs, either sequentially or in combination. In this small population of patients, the clinician faces the question of whether double transplantation is really indicated and which type of approach would be the best for patients (sequential or simultaneous).

In a large series of patients with fibrocystic liver and kidney disease (n 716), receiving a liver and/or kidney transplant (KT) from 1990 to 2010, the majority received KT (86%), while just a small number received LT (10%) or simultaneous liver/kidney transplantation (SLK) (6%). Furthermore, in this cohort a relatively small proportion of subjects required transplantation in alternate organ (7% of LT recipients and 5% of KT recipients). Interestingly, the mortality rate after LT was higher (23%) than after KT (10%) and after simultaneous liver/kidney transplant (12%) [82]. These data support the concept of isolated or sequential organ transplant when necessary rather than simultaneous liver/kidney transplant with pre-emptive purposes, giving the low number of patients requiring transplantation of the alternate organ. However, it has been demonstrated that transplanting one organ has potential side effects on the other organ involved. In fact, a decline in renal function was noticed in children after LT, which may be caused by the use of nephrotoxic immunosuppressive drugs in patients with pre-existing renal disease [83]. To protect the kidney after LT, calcineurin inhibitor levels should be kept as low as possible [84].

On the other hand, immunosuppression and pancytopenia in patients receiving KT with concomitant liver disease such as CS may contribute to the later development of ascending cholangitis. Giving this, in patients with end-stage renal disease candidate to KT, combined liver/kidney transplantation should be considered in case of recurrent cholangitis or refractory complication of portal hypertension and might also be considered in cases of single episode of cholangitis (or unexplained fever) or in case of marked abnormalities in the biliary system [85].

Conversely, another consideration about SLK is the potential immunological advantage for the kidney when a liver is transplanted at the same time. Even in individuals who are highly sensitized and/or cross-matched positive, simultaneous liver/kidney transplantation may provide better outcomes in both kidney and graft rejection and graft survival both in adults and children [86, 87]. Liver protective effect leads to significant improvement in the late kidney graft survival in SLK compared with isolated KT decreasing episodes of antibody-mediated rejections [88].

In patients with diagnosis of CCA, surgical resection is the treatment of choice. However, prognosis is poor with 1-year survival rate of only 33% [73]. LT is frequently contraindicated in patients with diagnosed invasive preoperatively CCA [89, 90] in consideration of high rate of recurrence under immunosuppressive therapy with survival rate far below the survival rate of those who underwent LT for other causes [91].

In patients with diffuse bi-lobar disease, further studies are needed to assess the indication of prophylactic LT in asymptomatic patients without diagnosis of CCA. When LT is considered for benign liver disease, the decision about the type of graft, low risk standard or no standard extended criteria (EC) is always difficult. If the patient has developed a malignant complication such as CCA, a LT with extended criteria graft supersedes the risk of death without LT; however LT in patients with CCA is offered only in highly selected cases. In other cases, not complicated by CCA, the difficulty of the choice is complicated by the usually low MELD and PELD score of these patients. In fact, the main indications for LT in patients with CD or CS are cholangitis and in the case of CHF refractory complications of portal hypertension rather than end-stage cirrhosis frequently not expressed through high MELD scores [78]. The problem of lower priority on waiting list could be improved by living donor LT (LDLT) that has been recently performed for these conditions [92] with good outcomes. In these cases perspective donors should be investigated for subclinical manifestations of the disease.

11.5.2 Choledochal Cysts

Cyst excision is the definitive treatment for CCs. This has become the preferred management strategy instead of drainage procedures such as choledochocystoduodenostomy or choledochocystojejunostomy which were attempted in the past with high morbidity rate [93, 94]. Furthermore, a complete resection of cyst reduces completely the risk of malignant degeneration, a critical point in paediatric patients with a long life expectance.

The specific approach depends on cyst type, but the common goal is cyst's full exeresis and restoration of enteric biliary drainage either into the duodenum or via Roux-en-Y hepaticojejunostomy. Surgical intervention should be elective, and patients should be medically optimized prior to operative intervention.

In type I and type IVb cysts, the treatment comprises resection of extrahepatic biliary tree with hepaticoenterostomy and cholecystectomy.

Type II cysts are typically managed with diverticulectomy or simple cyst excision. Closure can be performed primarily or over a T-tube, and occasionally RYHJ reconstruction is required if there is significant luminal narrowing.

In type III cysts, also known as choledococele, the treatment of choice is endoscopic sphincterotomy without excising the cyst. Various reports report good symptom control with this approach [95, 96], but long-term follow-up is lacking. Whether endoscopic treatment is not possible, lateral duodenotomy with sphincteroplasty and unroofing or marsupialization of the cavity may be performed.

The surgical management of IVa cysts is more complex because of both extrahepatic and intrahepatic involvement. The intrahepatic extension of the disease determines the surgical type of intervention. The correct classification of the cyst is of foremost importance and necessary to distinguish a real dilation of intrahepatic bile duct by an upstream ductal dilation secondary to biliary stasis and functional obstruction that may be seen in type I cysts [39]. If anatomic intrahepatic cystic dilation is confirmed, partial hepatectomy may be allowed due to the risk of malignant transformation in intrahepatic biliary system [97]. If the imaging is not conclusive and there is a doubt of upstream dilation, treatment in a type I cyst with a strict follow-up of intrahepatic ducts is suggested [98]. In fact, in some reported cases, the intrahepatic dilation has resolved in 3–6 months following adequate drainage [99]. In adults, to determine whether the dilation is primary or secondary to obstruction, preoperative percutaneous biliary drainage to decompress the intrahepatic biliary ductal system should be performed.

Surgery for CC disease can be either open or laparoscopically depending on patient characteristics and on surgeon experience. Laparoscopic cyst excision with reconstruction has been performed in children as young as 3 months [100] and as small as 6 kg [101]. Laparoscopy is associated with longer operative time but shorter hospital stay [102–104] and outcome largely comparable [105]. Hepaticoduodenostomy and RYHJ are the two most commonly utilized techniques of reconstruction; however, in most series, hepaticoduodenostomy seems to be more associated with bile reflux compared with RYHJ [106], which is the most common technique used.

Symptoms are a strong indication for surgery at any age. In asymptomatic patients the classic recommendation was to perfume surgery with reconstruction by age 6 months [107], though there is some evidence for repair as early as the first month of life in asymptomatic neonates [108].

Early postoperative complications are anastomotic leak, postoperative bleeding, wound infection, acute pancreatitis and pancreatic or biliary fistula [109, 110] whether late complications include anastomotic stricture with consequent cholangitis, hepatolithiasis, biliary cirrhosis and malignancy. Benign anastomotic stricture with recurrent cholangitis is less common than in adults but is still seen in as many as 10–25% of patients and can be associated with both intrahepatic and bile duct stone formation [111, 112].

A strictly long-term follow-up is suggested because of the risk of biliary carcinoma, most often CCA that remains more elevated compared to the general population even after CC excision [113, 114] with a rate up to 14% [46, 112]. In fact, cancer is the most frequent cause of late mortality in paediatric CC series.

References

1. Guay-Woodford LM. Renal cystic diseases: diverse phenotypes converge on the cilium/centrosome complex. Pediatr Nephrol. 2006;21(10):1369–76.
2. Gascue C, Katsanis N, Badano JL. Cystic diseases of the kidney: ciliary dysfunction and cystogenic mechanisms. Pediatr Nephrol. 2011;26(8):1181–95.
3. Gunay-Aygun M. Liver and kidney disease in ciliopathies. Am J Med Genet C Semin Med Genet. 2009;151C(4):296–306.
4. Fliegauf M, Benzing T, Omran H. When cilia go bad: cilia defects and ciliopathies. Nat Rev Mol Cell Biol. 2007;8(11):880–93.
5. Avidor-Reiss T, Maer AM, Koundakjian E, Polyanovsky A, Keil T, Subramaniam S, et al. Decoding cilia function: defining specialized genes required for compartmentalized cilia biogenesis. Cell. 2004;117(4):527–39.
6. Mahjoub MR. The importance of a single primary cilium. Organogenesis. 2013;9(2):61–9.
7. Rock N, McLin V. Liver involvement in children with ciliopathies. Clin Res Hepatol Gastroenterol. 2014;38(4):407–14.
8. Roskams T, Desmet V. Embryology of extra- and intrahepatic bile ducts, the ductal plate. Anat Rec. 2008;291(6):628–35.
9. Strazzabosco M, Fabris L. Development of the bile ducts: essentials for the clinical hepatologist. J Hepatol. 2012;56(5):1159–70.
10. Furuyama K, Kawaguchi Y, Akiyama H, Horiguchi M, Kodama S, Kuhara T, et al. Continuous cell supply from a Sox9-expressing progenitor zone in adult liver, exocrine pancreas and intestine. Nat Genet. 2011;43(1):34–41.
11. Mai W, Chen D, Ding T, Kim I, Park S, Cho S, et al. Inhibition of Pkhd1 impairs tubulomorphogenesis of cultured IMCD cells. Mol Biol Cell. 2005;16(9):4398–409.
12. Adeva M, El-Youssef M, Rossetti S, Kamath PS, Kubly V, Consugar MB, et al. Clinical and molecular characterization defines a broadened spectrum of autosomal recessive polycystic kidney disease (ARPKD). Medicine. 2006;85(1):1–21.
13. Rawat D, Kelly DA, Milford DV, Sharif K, Lloyd C, McKiernan PJ. Phenotypic variation and long-term outcome in children with congenital hepatic fibrosis. J Pediatr Gastroenterol Nutr. 2013;57(2):161–6.
14. Locatelli L, Cadamuro M, Spirli C, Fiorotto R, Lecchi S, Morell CM, et al. Macrophage recruitment by fibrocystin-defective biliary epithelial cells promotes portal fibrosis in congenital hepatic fibrosis. Hepatology. 2016;63(3):965.

15. Kaffe E, Fiorotto R, Pellegrino F, Mariotti V, Amenduni M, Cadamuro M, et al. β-catenin and IL-1β dependent CXCL10 production drives progression of disease in a mouse model of congenital hepatic fibrosis. Hepatology. 2018;67(5):1903–19.
16. Cano DA, Murcia NS, Pazour GJ, Hebrok M. Orpk mouse model of polycystic kidney disease reveals essential role of primary cilia in pancreatic tissue organization. Development. 2004;131(14):3457–67.
17. Desmet VJ. Ludwig symposium on biliary disorders—part I. Pathogenesis of ductal plate abnormalities. Mayo Clin Proc. 1998;73(1):80–9.
18. Di Bisceglie AM, Befeler AS. Cystic and nodular diseases on the liver. In: Schiff's diseases of the liver. 10th ed. Philadelphia: Wiley; 2012. p. 1231–51.
19. Hartung EA, Guay-Woodford LM. Autosomal recessive polycystic kidney disease: a hepatorenal fibrocystic disorder with pleiotropic effects. Pediatrics. 2014;134(3):e833–45.
20. Wu KL, Changchien CS, Kuo CM, Chuah SK, Chiu YC, Kuo CH. Caroli's disease—a report of two siblings. Eur J Gastroenterol Hepatol. 2002;14(12):1397–9.
21. Alves De Tommaso AM, Moreira Santos DS, Hessel G. Caroli's disease: 6 case studies. Acta Gastroenterol Latinoam. 2003;33(1):47–51.
22. Guay-Woodford LM, Bissler JJ, Braun MC, Bockenhauer D, Cadnapaphornchai MA, Dell KM, et al. Consensus expert recommendations for the diagnosis and management of autosomal recessive polycystic kidney disease: report of an international conference. J Pediatr. 2014;165(3):611–7.
23. Srinath A, Shneider BL. Congenital hepatic fibrosis and autosomal recessive polycystic kidney disease. J Pediatr Gastroenterol Nutr. 2012;54(5):580–7.
24. Bayraktar Y. Novel variant syndrome associated with congenital hepatic fibrosis. World J Clin Cases. 2015;3(10):904.
25. Bridgewater J, Galle PR, Khan SA, Llovet JM, Park J-W, Patel T, et al. Guidelines for the diagnosis and management of intrahepatic cholangiocarcinoma. J Hepatol. 2014;60:1268–89.
26. Nehls O, Gregor M, Klump B. Serum and bile markers for cholangiocarcinoma. Semin Liver Dis. 2004;24(2):139–54.
27. Albert MB, Steinberg WM, Henry JP. Elevated serum levels of tumor marker CA19-9 in acute cholangitis. Dig Dis Sci. 1988;33(10):1223–5.
28. Ong SL, Sachdeva A, Garcea G, Gravante G, Metcalfe MS, Lloyd DM, et al. Elevation of carbohydrate antigen 19.9 in benign hepatobiliary conditions and its correlation with serum bilirubin concentration. Dig Dis Sci. 2008;53(12):3213–7.
29. Zerres K, Rudnik-Schöneborn S, Deget F, Holtkamp U, Brodehl J, Geisert J, et al. Autosomal recessive polycystic kidney disease in 115 children: clinical presentation, course and influence of gender. Arbeitsgemeinschaft für Pädiatrische, Nephrologie. Acta Paediatr. 1996;85(4):437–45.
30. Roy S, Dillon MJ, Trompeter RS, Barratt TM. Autosomal recessive polycystic kidney disease: long-term outcome of neonatal survivors. Pediatr Nephrol. 1997;11(3):302–6.
31. Guay-Woodford LM, Desmond RA. Autosomal recessive polycystic kidney disease: the clinical experience in North America. Pediatrics. 2003;111(5 Pt 1):1072–80.
32. Fonck C, Chauveau D, Gagnadoux MF, Pirson Y, Grünfeld JP. Autosomal recessive polycystic kidney disease in adulthood. Nephrol Dial Transplant. 2001;16(8):1648–52.
33. Bergmann C, Senderek J, Windelen E, Küpper F, Middeldorf I, Schneider F, et al. Clinical consequences of PKHD1 mutations in 164 patients with autosomal-recessive polycystic kidney disease (ARPKD). Kidney Int. 2005;67(3):829–48.
34. Telega G, Cronin D, Avner ED. New approaches to the autosomal recessive polycystic kidney disease patient with dual kidney-liver complications. Pediatr Transplant. 2013;17(4):328–35.
35. Gunay-Aygun M, Font-Montgomery E, Lukose L, Tuchman Gerstein M, Piwnica-Worms K, Choyke P, et al. Characteristics of congenital hepatic fibrosis in a large cohort of patients with autosomal recessive polycystic kidney disease. Gastroenterology. 2013;144(1):112–121.e2.
36. Wiseman K, Buczkowski AK, Chung SW, Francoeur J, Schaeffer D, Scudamore CH. Epidemiology, presentation, diagnosis, and outcomes of choledochal cysts in adults in an urban environment. Am J Surg. 2005;189(5):527–31; discussion 531.
37. Yamaguchi M. Congenital choledochal cyst. Analysis of 1,433 patients in the Japanese literature. Am J Surg. 1980;140(5):653–7.
38. Söreide K, Körner H, Havnen J, Söreide JA. Bile duct cysts in adults. Br J Surg. 2004;91(12):1538–48.
39. Todani T, Watanabe Y, Toki A, Morotomi Y. Classification of congenital biliary cystic disease: special reference to type Ic and IVA cysts with primary ductal stricture. J Hepato-Biliary-Pancreat Surg. 2003;10(5):340–4.
40. Todani T, Watanabe Y, Narusue M, Tabuchi K, Okajima K. Congenital bile duct cysts: classification, operative procedures, and review of thirty-seven cases including cancer arising from choledochal cyst. Am J Surg. 1977;134(2):263–9.
41. Babbitt DP. Congenital choledochal cysts: new etiological concept based on anomalous relationships of the common bile duct and pancreatic bulb. Ann Radiol. 1969;12(3):231–40.
42. Han SJ, Hwang EH, Chung KS, Kim MJ, Kim H. Acquired choledochal cyst from anomalous pancreatobiliary duct union. J Pediatr Surg. 1997;32(12):1735–8.
43. Nagorney DM. Bile duct cysts in adults. In: Blumbert LH, Fong Y, editors. Surgery of the liver and biliary tract. 3rd ed. London: Saunders; 2000. p. 1229–44.
44. Davenport M, Basu R. Under pressure: choledochal malformation manometry. J Pediatr Surg. 2005;40(2):331–5.
45. Nicholl M, Pitt HA, Wolf P, Cooney J, Kalayoglu M, Shilyansky J, et al. Choledochal cysts in western adults: complexities compared to children. J Gastrointest Surg. 2004;8(3):245–52.
46. de Vries JS, de Vries S, Aronson DC, Bosman DK, Rauws EAJ, Bosma A, et al. Choledochal cysts: age of presentation, symptoms, and late complications related to Todani's classification. J Pediatr Surg. 2002;37(11):1568–73.
47. Sela-Herman S, Scharschmidt BF. Choledochal cyst, a disease for all ages. Lancet. 1996;347(9004):779.
48. Hewitt PM, Krige JE, Bornman PC, Terblanche J. Choledochal cysts in adults. Br J Surg. 1995;82(3):382–5.
49. Postema RR, Hazebroek FW. Choledochal cysts in children: a review of 28 years of treatment in a Dutch children's hospital. Eur J Surg. 1999;165(12):1159–61.
50. Hiramatsu K, Paye F, Kianmanesh AR, Sauvanet A, Terris B, Belghiti J. Choledochal cyst and benign stenosis of the main pancreatic duct. J Hepato-Biliary-Pancreat Surg. 2001;8(1):92–4.
51. Swisher SG, Cates JA, Hunt KK, Robert ME, Bennion RS, Thompson JE, et al. Pancreatitis associated with adult choledochal cysts. Pancreas. 1994;9(5):633–7.
52. Ochiai K, Kaneko K, Kitagawa M, Ando H, Hayakawa T. Activated pancreatic enzyme and pancreatic stone protein (PSP/reg) in bile of patients with pancreaticobiliary maljunction/choledochal cysts. Dig Dis Sci. 2004;49(11–12):1953–6.
53. Li M-J, Feng J-X, Jin Q-F. Early complications after excision with hepaticoenterostomy for infants and children with choledochal cysts. Hepatobiliary Pancreat Dis Int. 2002;1(2):281–4.
54. Rao KLN, Chowdhary SK, Kumar D. Choledochal cyst associated with portal hypertension. Pediatr Surg Int. 2003;19(11):729–32.
55. Martin LW, Rowe GA. Portal hypertension secondary to choledochal cyst. Ann Surg. 1979;190(5):638–9.
56. Furugaki K, Yoshida J, Hashizume M, Ota M, Tanaka M. The development of extrahepatic portal obstruction after undergoing

multiple operations for a congenital dilatation of the bile duct: report of a case. Surg Today. 1998;28(3):355–8.
57. Ramos A, Castelló J, Pinto I. Intestinal intussusception as a presenting feature of choledochocele. Gastrointest Radiol. 1990;15(1):211–4.
58. Kiresi DA, Karabacakoğlu A, Dilsiz A, Karaköse S. Spontaneous rupture of choledochal cyst presenting in childhood. Turk J Pediatr. 2005;47(3):283–6.
59. Fumino S, Iwai N, Deguchi E, Ono S, Shimadera S, Iwabuchi T, et al. Spontaneous rupture of choledochal cyst with pseudocyst formation-report on 2 cases and literature review. J Pediatr Surg. 2006;41(6):e19–21.
60. Moss RL, Musemeche CA. Successful management of ruptured choledochal cyst by primary cyst excision and biliary reconstruction. J Pediatr Surg. 1997;32(10):1490–1.
61. Arda IS, Tuzun M, Aliefendioglu D, Hicsonmez A. Spontaneous rupture of extrahepatic choledochal cyst: two pediatric cases and literature review. Eur J Pediatr Surg. 2005;15(5):361–3.
62. Stain SC, Guthrie CR, Yellin AE, Donovan AJ. Choledochal cyst in the adult. Ann Surg. 1995;222(2):128–33.
63. Chaudhary A, Dhar P, Sachdev A, Kumar N, Vij JC, Sarin SK, et al. Choledochal cysts—differences in children and adults. Br J Surg. 1996;83(2):186–8.
64. Sugiyama M, Atomi Y, Kuroda A. Pancreatic disorders associated with anomalous pancreaticobiliary junction. Surgery. 1999;126(3):492–7.
65. Marchal GJ, Desmet VJ, Proesmans WC, Moerman PL, Van Roost WW, Van Holsbeeck MT, et al. Caroli disease: high-frequency US and pathologic findings. Radiology. 1986;158(2):507–11.
66. Fitoz S, Erden A, Boruban S. Magnetic resonance cholangiopancreatography of biliary system abnormalities in children. Clin Imaging. 2007;31(2):93–101.
67. Kim SH, Lim JH, Yoon H-K, Han BK, Lee SK, Kim YI. Choledochal cyst: comparison of MR and conventional cholangiography. Clin Radiol. 2000;55(5):378–83.
68. Nagi B, Kochhar R, Bhasin D, Singh K. Endoscopic retrograde cholangiopancreatography in the evaluation of anomalous junction of the pancreaticobiliary duct and related disorders. Abdom Imaging. 2003;28(6):847–52.
69. Oduyebo I, Law JK, Zaheer A, Weiss MJ, Wolfgang C, Lennon AM. Choledochal or pancreatic cyst? Role of endoscopic ultrasound as an adjunct for diagnosis: a case series. Surg Endosc. 2015;29(9):2832–6.
70. Büscher R, Büscher AK, Weber S, Mohr J, Hegen B, Vester U, et al. Clinical manifestations of autosomal recessive polycystic kidney disease (ARPKD): kidney-related and non-kidney-related phenotypes. Pediatr Nephrol. 2014;29(10):1915–25.
71. Shneider BL, Bosch J, de Franchis R, Emre SH, Groszmann RJ, Ling SC, et al. Portal hypertension in children: expert pediatric opinion on the report of the Baveno V consensus workshop on methodology of diagnosis and therapy in portal hypertension. Pediatr Transplant. 2012;16(5):426–37.
72. Tsimaratos M, Cloarec S, Roquelaure B, Retornaz K, Picon G, Chabrol B, et al. Chronic renal failure and portal hypertension—is portosystemic shunt indicated? Pediatr Nephrol. 2000;14(8–9):856–8.
73. Mabrut J, Kianmanesh R, Nuzzo G, Castaing D, Boudjema K, Létoublon C, et al. Surgical management of congenital intrahepatic bile duct dilation, Caroli's disease and syndrome. Ann Surg. 2013;258:713–21.
74. Tsuchida Y, Sato T, Sanjo K, Etoh T, Hata K, Terawaki K, et al. Evaluation of long-term results of Caroli's disease: 21 years' observation of a family with autosomal "dominant" inheritance, and review of the literature. Hepato-Gastroenterology. 1995;42(2):175–81.
75. Ros E, Navarro S, Bru C, Gilabert R, Bianchi L, Bruguera M. Ursodeoxycholic acid treatment of primary hepatolithiasis in Caroli's syndrome. Lancet. 1993;342(8868):404–6.
76. Dayton MT, Longmire WP, Tompkins RK. Caroli's Disease: a premalignant condition? Am J Surg. 1983;145(1):41–8.
77. De Kerckhove L, De Meyer M, Verbaandert C, Mourad M, Sokal E, Goffette P, et al. The place of liver transplantation in Caroli's disease and syndrome. Transpl Int. 2006;19(5):381–8.
78. Mabrut J-Y, Partensky C, Jaeck D, Oussoultzoglou E, Baulieux J, Boillot O, et al. Congenital intrahepatic bile duct dilatation is a potentially curable disease. Ann Surg. 2007;246(2):236–45.
79. Habib S, Shakil O, Couto OF, Demetris AJ, Fung JJ, Marcos A, et al. Caroli's disease and orthotopic liver transplantation. Liver Transpl. 2006;12(3):416–21.
80. Hori T, Oike F, Ogura Y, Ogawa K, Hata K, Yonekawa Y, et al. Liver transplantation for congenital biliary dilatation: a single-center experience. Dig Surg. 2010;27(6):492–501.
81. Harring TR, Nguyen NTT, Liu H, Goss JA, O'Mahony CA. Caroli disease patients have excellent survival after liver transplant. J Surg Res. 2012;177(2):365–72.
82. Wen JW, Furth SL, Ruebner RL. Kidney and liver transplantation in children with fibrocystic liver-kidney disease: data from the US Scientific Registry of Transplant Recipients: 1990-2010. Pediatr Transplant. 2014;18(7):726–32.
83. Ko JS, Yi N-J, Suh KS, Seo JK. Pediatric liver transplantation for fibrocystic liver disease. Pediatr Transplant. 2012;16(2):195–200.
84. Meier C, Deutscher J, Müller S, Haluany K, Fangmann J, Siekmeyer W, et al. Successful liver transplantation in a child with Caroli's disease. Pediatr Transplant. 2008;12(4):483–6.
85. Shneider BL, Magid MS. Liver disease in autosomal recessive polycystic kidney disease. Pediatr Transplant. 2005;9(5):634–9.
86. Rogers J, Bueno J, Shapiro R, Scantlebury V, Mazariegos G, Fung J, et al. Results of simultaneous and sequential pediatric liver and kidney transplantation. Transplantation. 2001;72(10):1666–70.
87. Gutiérrez A, Crespo M, Mila J, Torregrosa JV, Martorell J, Oppenheimer F. Outcome of simultaneous liver-kidney transplantation in highly sensitized, crossmatch-positive patients. Transplant Proc. 2003;35(5):1861–2.
88. De La Cerda F, Jimenez WA, Gjertson DW, Venick R, Tsai E, Ettenger R. Renal graft outcome after combined liver and kidney transplantation in children: UCLA and UNOS experience. Pediatr Transplant. 2010;14(4):459–64.
89. Balsells J, Margarit C, Murio E, Lazaro JL, Charco R, Vidal MT, et al. Adenocarcinoma in Caroli's disease treated by liver transplantation. HPB Surg. 1993;7(1):81–6; discussion 86–7.
90. Takatsuki M, Uemoto S, Inomata Y, Egawa H, Kiuchi T, Hayashi M, et al. Living-donor liver transplantation for Caroli's disease with intrahepatic adenocarcinoma. J Hepato-Biliary-Pancreat Surg. 2001;8(3):284–6.
91. Meyer CG, Penn I, James L. Liver transplantation for cholangiocarcinoma: results in 207 patients. Transplantation. 2000;69(8):1633–7.
92. Sapisochin G, Rodríguez de Lope C, Gastaca M, Ortiz de Urbina J, Suarez MA, Santoyo J, et al. "Very early" intrahepatic cholangiocarcinoma in cirrhotic patients: should liver transplantation be reconsidered in these patients? Am J Transplant. 2014;14(3):660–7.
93. Schier F, Clausen M, Kouki M, Gdanietz K, Waldschmidt J. Late results in the management of choledochal cysts. Eur J Pediatr Surg. 1994;4(3):141–4.
94. Todani T, Watanabe Y, Toki A, Urushihara N, Sato Y. Reoperation for congenital choledochal cyst. Ann Surg. 1988;207(2):142–7.
95. Saeki I, Takahashi Y, Matsuura T, Takahata S, Tanaka M, Taguchi T. Successful endoscopic unroofing for a pediatric choledochocele. J Pediatr Surg. 2009;44(8):1643–5.

96. Dohmoto M, Kamiya T, Hünerbein M, Valdez H, Ibanegaray J, Prado J. Endoscopic treatment of a choledochocele in a 2-year-old child. Surg Endosc. 1996;10(10):1016–8.
97. He X-D, Wang L, Liu W, Liu Q, Qu Q, Li B-L, et al. The risk of carcinogenesis in congenital choledochal cyst patients: an analysis of 214 cases. Ann Hepatol. 2014;13(6):819–26.
98. Acker SN, Bruny JL, Narkewicz MR, Roach JP, Rogers A, Karrer FM. Preoperative imaging does not predict intrahepatic involvement in choledochal cysts. J Pediatr Surg. 2013;48(12):2378–82.
99. Joseph VT. Surgical techniques and long-term results in the treatment of choledochal cyst. J Pediatr Surg. 1990;25(7):782–7.
100. Le DM, Woo RK, Sylvester K, Krummel TM, Albanese CT. Laparoscopic resection of type 1 choledochal cysts in pediatric patients. Surg Endosc. 2006;20(2):249–51.
101. Lee J-H, Kim S-H, Kim H-Y, Choi YH, Jung S-E, Park K-W. Early experience of laparoscopic choledochal cyst excision in children. J Korean Surg Soc. 2013;85(5):225.
102. Liuming H, Hongwu Z, Gang L, Jun J, Wenying H, Wong KKY, et al. The effect of laparoscopic excision vs open excision in children with choledochal cyst: a midterm follow-up study. J Pediatr Surg. 2011;46(4):662–5.
103. Zhen C, Xia Z, Long L, Lishuang M, Pu Y, Wenjuan Z, et al. Laparoscopic excision versus open excision for the treatment of choledochal cysts: a systematic review and meta-analysis. Int Surg. 2015;100(1):115–22.
104. Nguyen Thanh L, Hien PD, Dung LA, Son TN. Laparoscopic repair for choledochal cyst: lessons learned from 190 cases. J Pediatr Surg. 2010;45(3):540–4.
105. Ure BM, Nustede R, Becker H. Laparoscopic resection of congenital choledochal cyst, hepaticojejunostomy, and externally made Roux-en-Y anastomosis. J Pediatr Surg. 2005;40(4):728–30.
106. Shimotakahara A, Yamataka A, Yanai T, Kobayashi H, Okazaki T, Lane GJ, et al. Roux-en-Y hepaticojejunostomy or hepaticoduodenostomy for biliary reconstruction during the surgical treatment of choledochal cyst: which is better? Pediatr Surg Int. 2005;21(1):5–7.
107. Okada T, Sasaki F, Ueki S, Hirokata G, Okuyama K, Cho K, et al. Postnatal management for prenatally diagnosed choledochal cysts. J Pediatr Surg. 2004;39(7):1055–8.
108. Diao M, Li L, Cheng W. Timing of surgery for prenatally diagnosed asymptomatic choledochal cysts: a prospective randomized study. J Pediatr Surg. 2012;47(3):506–12.
109. Fujishiro J, Masumoto K, Urita Y, Shinkai T, Gotoh C. Pancreatic complications in pediatric choledochal cysts. J Pediatr Surg. 2013;48(9):1897–902.
110. Ono S, Maeda K, Baba K, Usui Y, Tsuji Y, Yano T, et al. The efficacy of double-balloon enteroscopy for intrahepatic bile duct stones after Roux-en-Y hepaticojejunostomy for choledochal cysts. Pediatr Surg Int. 2013;29(11):1103–7.
111. Miyano T, Yamataka A, Kato Y, Segawa O, Lane G, Takamizawa S, et al. Hepaticoenterostomy after excision of choledochal cyst in children: a 30-year experience with 180 cases. J Pediatr Surg. 1996;31(10):1417–21.
112. Todani T, Watanabe Y, Urushihara N, Noda T, Morotomi Y. Biliary complications after excisional procedure for choledochal cyst. J Pediatr Surg. 1995;30(3):478–81.
113. Benjamin IS. Biliary cystic disease: the risk of cancer. J Hepato-Biliary-Pancreat Surg. 2003;10(5):335–9.
114. Soares KC, Kim Y, Spolverato G, Maithel S, Bauer TW, Marques H, et al. Presentation and clinical outcomes of choledochal cysts in children and adults: a multi-institutional analysis. JAMA Surg. 2015;150(6):577–84.

Gallstone Disease

Fabiola Di Dato, Giusy Ranucci, and Raffaele Iorio

Key Points

- Ultrasonography is the method of choice for gallstone detection.
- There are no guidelines for the management of cholelithiasis in children.
- Spontaneous resolution of cholelithiasis is typical of foetus, infants, and patients with pseudolithiasis due to ceftriaxone.
- In symptomatic patients with gallstones, laparoscopic cholecystectomy is indicated.
- Asymptomatic patients can be monitored with periodical clinical and ultrasonoghraphic controls.
- Ursodeoxycholic acid (UDCA) should not be used to treat paediatric gallstones, except in cases of symptomatic children with contraindications to surgery or when cholecystectomy must be deferred for other reasons.

Research Needed in the Field

- Prevalence studies should be conducted to assess the real prevalence of gallstone disease in childhood.
- Prospective studies are necessary to assess the natural history of gallstone disease in children.
- Paediatric guidelines on gallstone disease management would be desirable.

12.1 Introduction

Gallstones are crystallized deposits containing cholesterol and/or bilirubin that form most commonly in the gallbladder. Gallstone disease is defined as the presence of gallstones accompanied by symptoms attributable to their presence (biliary colic) or complications such as acute cholecystitis, acute cholangitis, gallstone pancreatitis, choledocholithiasis and obstructive jaundice. About 15% of adults in Europe and the United States present gallstones, and the prevalence varies worldwide because of both genetic and environmental factors [1, 2]. In recent years, gallbladder disease, mainly in the form of cholelithiasis, is increasing among children, not only for the extensive use of ultrasound but also for the concomitant increase in childhood of obesity and metabolic syndrome. Furthermore, following the routine use of ultrasound examination during pregnancy, foetal gallstones also are progressively increasing. Gallstone disease may be observed in different categories of children: patients with haemolytic disorders in whom cholelithiasis is systematically expected; patients with underlying conditions such as chronic liver disease, cystic fibrosis and total parenteral nutrition in whom cholelithiasis can easily occur; and otherwise healthy subjects, commonly obese, in whom cholelithiasis is sporadically observed. Although paediatric gallbladder disease is less prevalent than in adults, clinicians caring for children need to be aware of this problem and know the manifestations of biliary disease in the paediatric population [3].

Symptoms and complications of gallstones have been known for centuries, but the natural history, the associations between gallstones and related diseases and the risks and benefits of surgical and medical interventions are not fully elucidated [1].

12.2 Epidemiology

Gallstone disease is a frequent disorder in the Western world with a prevalence of 10–20% in adults [4]. Cholelithiasis is one of the commonest diseases in adults with gastrointestinal disorders but is still considered an uncommon disease in children. The prevalence of gallstones in the paediatric population has been reported infrequently; an ultrasonographic survey, carried out on 1570 Italian children (ages 6–19 years), showed an overall prevalence of gallstone disease of 0.13% (0.27% in female subjects) [5]. During childhood, cases of gallstones tend to increase with age, and after puberty the frequency of cholelithiasis is significantly greater in females than in males and becomes comparable to the adult ratio, with a 4:1 female predominance.

Despite the remarkable number of foetal scans performed annually worldwide, foetal cholelithiasis is uncommon, with an incidence of anomalies of the gallbladder, including sludge and gallstones, of about 0.40%, with a slightly greater male predominance [6].

Table 12.1 Conditions associated with cholelithiasis

Paediatric disease
– Haemolytic disease (sickle cells, thalassemia, spherocytosis)
– Gilbert syndrome
– Liver cirrhosis
– Anatomic biliary disease
– Cystic fibrosis
– Obesity, insulin resistance, dyslipidaemia
– Bowel resection
– Biliary dyskinesia
– Progressive familial intrahepatic cholestasis
– Celiac disease
– Wilson disease
– Sepsis
– Crohn's disease
– Stem cell transplantation
– Down's syndrome
– IgA deficiency
Risk factors
– Prematurity
– Total parenteral nutrition
– Familiarity
– Abdominal and cardiac surgery
– Rapid weight loss
– Drugs: ceftriaxone, furosemide, cyclosporine
– Sedentary lifestyle
– Prolonged fasting

12.3 Aetiology and Pathophysiology

Gallstones are usually formed from bile stasis. When bile is not fully drained from the gallbladder, it can precipitate as sludge and subsequently evolve into stones.

There are different types of gallstones developing in the gallbladder and bile ducts, distinguished by their chemical composition into [7, 8]:

1. *Cholesterol stones*: radiolucent, yellow or green, round or faceted, smooth or mammillated, multiple or solitary and variable in diameter, composed between 70% and 100% of cholesterol.
2. *Black pigment stones*: radiopaque, usually black, small, multiple and with irregular surface, composed of calcium bilirubinate and associated with haemolysis and total parenteral nutrition (TPN).
3. *Mixed cholesterol stones*: they contain cholesterol, protein, bilirubin and carbonate.
4. *Brown pigment stones*: they have a rough surface and contain large amounts of fatty acid and calcium bilirubinate; they are formed when bacterial enzymes deconjugate bilirubin from glucuronic acid and hydrolyse phospholipids, so that excess bilirubin and free fatty acids precipitate with calcium. They are associated with bile duct dilatation, bile stasis and bacterial infections.

This classification has an academic value, because in the majority of cases, especially during the initial diagnostic evaluation of the patient, the real composition of gallstones may be only presumed on the basis of risk factors and presence or absence of radiopacity. Furthermore, nowadays, this classification does not even have a direct impact on management of paediatric patients with cholelithiasis, because bile acid dissolution therapy with UDCA, indicated for radiolucent stones, has overall a low rate of efficacy. Therefore, in many centres X-ray evaluation is no longer performed.

Many risk factors for paediatric cholelithiasis have been identified (Table 12.1). **Familiarity for cholelithiasis, obesity** and **haemolytic disorders** seem to be the predominant risk factors in children with gallstones [9]. In adolescents, obesity represents an important risk factor, especially in Western countries, because of its influence on most pathogenic mechanisms for gallstone formation: supersaturation of bile with cholesterol, increased propensity to cholesterol crystallization, stone aggregation and defective gallbladder emptying. Less prominent risk factors include acute renal failure, prolonged fasting, low-calorie diet and rapid weight loss. **Genetic conditions**, such as **progressive familial intrahepatic cholestasis type 3 and Gilbert syndrome**, can also predispose to gallstone formation. **Defects in the *ABCB4*** gene have been increasingly recognized in both adults and children with recurrent cholestasis and cholesterol gallstones. This condition can induce gallstones, intrahepatic sludge and microlithiasis that develop before the age of 40, with biliary symptoms that can recur after cholecystectomy.

In the majority of cases, there is a genetic background determining an individual predisposition to develop cholesterol gallstones in response to environmental factors. Several pathogenic mechanisms influencing cholesterol homeostasis have been linked to cholesterol gallstones (hepatic hypersecretion of cholesterol resulting in supersaturated bile, hypomotile gallbladder, increased absorption of cholesterol from the intestine). Genetic elements are considered a major risk factor; they are estimated to account for approximately 25% of the overall gallstone risk by the analysis on a large population of twins [10].

In Western adult populations, cholesterol gallstones represent the 90–95% of all gallstones; mixed or pigment stones are more frequent in developing nations and Asia. Black pigment stones are the major stone type in patients with chronic haemolytic disorders or cirrhosis, even if these risk factors can be absent in most patients. Cholesterol and black pigment stones are usually detectable in the gallbladder, whereas brown pigment stones develop primarily in the main bile duct [11].

Pigment stones are the commonest type of gallstones in childhood, without recognizable predisposing factors in infants, secondary to a predisposing condition such as chronic haemolysis and ileal disease in older children. In adolescents, idiopathic cholesterol gallstones accounts for the majority of cases, such as in adults. Increased BMI and female gender are definitive risk factors for gallstone growth, and the first is also associated with higher frequency of symptomatic gallstone disease. For this reason, healthy diet and lifestyle, regular physical activity and maintenance of an ideal body weight might prevent cholesterol and symptomatic gallbladder stones. Observational studies have identified an association between low vitamin C consumption and risk of gallstones/gallbladder disease or cholecystectomy [11].

Gallstone prevalence is associated not only with obesity but also with diabetes and insulin resistance, and the association between gallstones and increased cardiovascular disease incidence may simply reflect the presence of these shared risk factors. Besides, gallstone-associated abnormalities in the pathways of the farnesoid X receptor (FXR) and liver X receptor (LXR) may also be involved in metabolic regulation. Similar considerations apply for the association between gallstones and non-alcoholic fatty liver disease [1, 12].

Common bile duct stones (CBDS) easily lead to biliary complications such as obstruction, secondary cholangitis, pancreatitis and obstructive jaundice, seldom causing life-threatening events. Therefore, CBDS needs timely treatment once diagnosed. Recurrence of choledocholithiasis after bile duct stone clearance may be related to different factors such as infections, biliary strictures, endoscopic and surgical treatment [13].

Biliary sludge was first described in the 1970s. It is defined as a mixture of particulate matter precipitated from bile. The sediment composition varies, but usually it consists

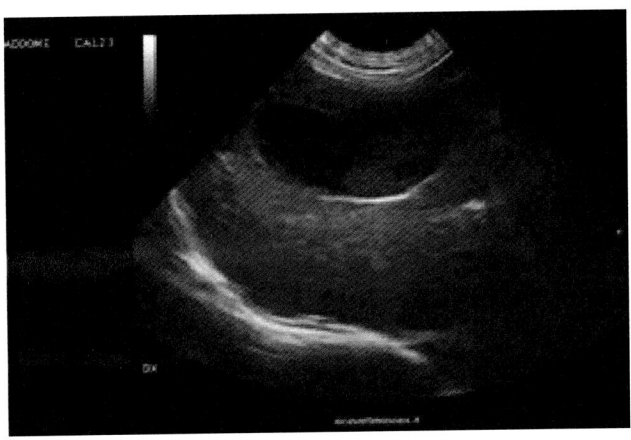

Fig. 12.1 Biliary sludge in gallbladder

of cholesterol crystals, calcium bilirubinate pigment and other calcium salts. Biliary sludge is a non-shadowing, echogenic sediment present in the gallbladder lumen and is generally considered a dynamic condition not necessarily evolving into gallstones (Fig. 12.1). Biliary sludge is more commonly observed in patients on parenteral nutrition, critically ill patients (sepsis, abdominal surgery, cardiac surgery, etc.), patients with diabetes, people who were very overweight and lost weight very quickly and recipients of organ transplants. Biliary sludge is often found in conditions of increased gallbladder stasis and/or concurrent change of biliary composition, e.g. prolonged fasting [11, 14].

Ceftriaxone-related gallbladder pseudolithiasis was firstly reported in children in 1986. The terms biliary pseudolithiasis, reversible cholelithiasis and apparent pseudolithiasis are commonly used to describe this complication of ceftriaxone. Biliary sludge has been reported to form after a mean duration of 9 days of ceftriaxone therapy, and it generally resolves with discontinuation of the drug. Like bilirubin, ceftriaxone can precipitate with calcium and with small amounts of cholesterol crystals and bilirubinate crystal, so that long-term therapy predisposes patients to sludge or gallstone formation. These precipitations present similarly to gallstones on ultrasound examination. With increasing ceftriaxone dosages, the saturation index for calcium-ceftriaxone in human bile increases; this corresponds to a decrease in solubility. Once-daily dosage of ceftriaxone instead of two-daily dosage is currently recommended because of the observed lower incidence of ceftriaxone-related pseudolithiasis [14, 15].

Foetal gallstones. Many maternal and foetal condition can be associated with gallstones in the foetal population, such as maternal placental abruption, diabetes of any type, pharmacological treatment (ceftriaxone, furosemide, prostaglandin E2), foetal rhesus or ABO blood group incompatibility, genetic anomalies (trisomy 21), chromosomal aberrations and growth restriction. Foetal stones and sludge are more commonly identified in the foetal gallbladder during the third trimester, maybe because of an abnormal production, composition and mode of transportation of bile in the biliary tract [6].

12.4 Clinical Presentation

Cholelithiasis primarily affects the gallbladder and may cause irritation of the gallbladder mucosa resulting in chronic calculous cholecystitis and symptoms of biliary colic. The complications of cholelithiasis in children are similar to those in adults. If a gallstone obstructs the cystic duct, acute cholecystitis can occur, with distension of the gallbladder wall and possible necrosis and spillage of bile. If gallstones migrate from the gallbladder into the cystic duct and main biliary ductal system, further complications can occur, such as choledocholithiasis, biliary obstruction with or without cholangitis and gallstone pancreatitis.

As in adults, also in children cholelithiasis can be asymptomatic in most cases, and gallstones are often diagnosed accidentally on ultrasound examination carried out for reasons unrelated to cholelithiasis. Colicky pain and jaundice, often associated with nausea and vomiting, can occur in symptomatic children; acholic stools and dark urine are present in the case of severe obstruction. Biliary colic is the term used for gallbladder pain experienced by a person with gallstones, in absence of an overt infection of the gallbladder [16]. Colicky pain is described as suddenly developing pain and intermittent cramping, usually located in the right upper quadrant or in the epigastrium, which may radiate to the back or right shoulder. A Murphy sign (inspiratory arrest during right upper quadrant palpation) is considered pathognomonic of cholelithiasis. Commonly, symptomatic children complain of recurrent, non-specific postprandial abdominal pain, sometimes epigastric pain, associated with nausea, vomiting and food intolerance, particularly with fatty foods. Rarely, cholelithiasis can present with complications such as cholecystitis, choledocholithiasis, acute pancreatitis and cholangitis. Acute cholecystitis is characterized by fever, pain in the right upper quadrant and often a palpable mass. Spontaneous perforation of the gallbladder with acute abdomen is extremely rare but relatively more common in immunodeficient children [8, 17].

Foetal and infant cholelithiasis most commonly resolves in absence of clinical manifestations; the complications are rare and not well documented for foetal gallstones. As for biliary sludge, the clinical course varies from complete resolution to possible progression to gallstones; it is often asymptomatic, but complications such as biliary colic, acute cholecystitis and acute pancreatitis may arise [14].

An estimated 4–25% of adults and 8–46% of children who receive ceftriaxone develop biliary sludge, which is typically asymptomatic and reversible; complete resolution occurs within 2–63 days after discontinuation of ceftriaxone. Only in rare cases ceftriaxone-induced biliary sludge is symptomatic. It is uncommon for ceftriaxone to cause increases in laboratory indexes, such as bilirubin levels. Clinicians need to be aware of the association of ceftriaxone and biliary pseudolithiasis and monitor it accordingly [14, 18].

Common bile duct stones are unusual in children, occurring in 2–6% of cases with cholelithiasis, often in association with obstructive jaundice and pancreatitis. There is no consensus on indications to perform an operative cholangiography at the time of cholecystectomy to detect unsuspected common duct calculi [17].

Some 80% of adult gallstone carriers are asymptomatic. It has been estimated that symptoms develop with a rate of 1–4% per year, 20% become symptomatic within 20 years from diagnosis and complications occur with a rate of 1–3% per year after the first colic episode and 0.1–0.3% in asymptomatic patients. In about 50% of patients, the pain episodes recur after a first biliary attack. In childhood, complications of gallstones are less frequent in asymptomatic than in symptomatic patients (5% vs 28%). While the natural history of asymptomatic adults with gallstones is well known and suggests that most remain asymptomatic throughout life, there are not similar data in paediatric age [11, 19].

A clinical entity that has to be distinguished from cholelithiasis is **biliary dyskinesia** (BD). BD is defined, according to Rome IV adult diagnostic criteria, as patients having episodes of recurrent severe epigastric or right upper quadrant abdominal pain that interrupts daily activities and is not related to bowel movements and not relieved by postural change or acid suppression. Additionally, pain cannot be explained by any other structural disease, and gallstones are absent on ultrasound. An abnormal gallbladder ejection fraction on scintigraphy and normal liver and pancreatic enzymes are supportive criteria for the diagnosis. Biliary dyskinesia is increasingly being diagnosed in children even if, in literature, there is no consensus concerning its definition and diagnostic criteria used. Although laparoscopic cholecystectomy is a possible treatment for patients with BD, a significant fraction of patients do not report long-term relief of symptoms after cholecystectomy. On the other hand, it has been reported a symptom resolution rate of 75% in patients with BD managed conservatively for a 2-year follow-up. For this reason it could be recommended a trial of observation and medication before surgical management, since biliary dyskinesia is not a life-threatening disorder and has no serious complications [20–22].

12.5 Diagnosis

Diagnosis of cholelithiasis is usually performed on the basis of clinical history, physical examination and ultrasonography. When a child with suspected or documented cholelithiasis is evaluated, the following parameters should be looked for: scleral jaundice, jaundice, pale stools and dark urine, pallor, obesity, hepatomegaly, splenomegaly, fever, abdominal mass, Murphy sign, signs of pancreatitis and signs of acute abdomen.

Abdominal X-ray, suggested by recent adult guidelines, may reveal opaque calculi but is no longer performed in the common paediatric clinical practice because it has little impact on management and exposes to X-ray.

Ultrasound scan (USS) is the most accurate and useful diagnostic test for the diagnosis of cholelithiasis. In all patients with a recent history of biliary pain, abdominal ultrasound should be performed. USS allows the recognition of echogenic foci and acoustic shadows with mobility in the gallbladder, as well as the assessment of gallbladder size and wall thickness and of the diameter of the common bile duct (Fig. 12.2). The patients should be examined in different positions such as supine and left lateral decubitus to differentiate stones from polyps through the ability to move. Ultrasound also allows the diagnosis of biliary sludge that is based on the presence of a non-shadowing, echogenic, intraluminal sediment [11].

Laboratory tests are usually normal in children with asymptomatic gallstones. In case of biliary obstruction, an increase in conjugated bilirubin, transaminases, gamma-glutamyl transpeptidase and alkaline phosphatase serum levels may be observed. Leucocytosis and increase of C-reactive protein can also be present in case of complications. Amylase and lipase serum levels should be tested in order to exclude a pancreatic involvement induced by gallstone disease but also to distinguish between biliary and pancreatic pain. In addition, the laboratory evaluation allows finding the presence of gallstone predisposing factors such as haemolytic disorders, hyperlipidaemia, IgA deficiency and Gilbert syndrome.

Cholecystography has become obsolete, while magnetic resonance cholangiopancreatography (MRCP) is nowadays recognized as an accurate, non-invasive diagnostic tool for investigating the biliary and pancreatic ducts. It provides excellent anatomic details with a sensitivity of 85–87% and a specificity of 93–95% for detecting choledocholithiasis [8, 23]. When common bile duct stones are found, a choledocal cyst with anomalous pancreatobiliary duct junction needs to be excluded; in this case, magnetic resonance cholangiopancreatography should be performed as first line.

Endoscopic ultrasound (EUS) has a sensitivity of 94–98% to detect cholecystolithiasis in patients with biliary pain but normal abdominal ultrasound. The procedure might be particularly helpful in patients with unexplained acute and acute recurrent pancreatitis, which might be caused by biliary sludge. Both EUS and MRCP have high diagnostic accuracy for detection of common bile duct stones, and the choice of which test to use depends on the availability and contraindications to each test. Patients with positive EUS or MRCP should undergo endoscopic or surgical extraction of common bile duct stones, whereas those with negative EUS or MRCP usually do not need further investigations. In patients with asymptomatic gallstone disease or symptomatic patients without CBD dilatation and biochemical alterations, MRCP and EUS are not routinely recommended. In case of strong clinical suspicion of gallbladder stones or CBDS and negative abdominal ultrasound, endoscopic ultrasound (or magnetic resonance imaging) may be performed. There is insufficient evidence to evaluate if the benefits of EUS outweigh its procedural risks, especially in children where adequate equipment is necessary [11, 23, 24]. Computed tomography (CT) is less useful for the diagnosis of gallbladder stones.

Endoscopic retrograde cholangiopancreatography (ERCP) can also be a useful tool in preoperative diagnosis and in the management of choledocholithiasis. It has the advantage of providing a therapeutic option when gallstones are identified, but complications related to the procedure may arise, such as pancreatitis, cholangitis, perforation of the duodenum or bile duct and bleeding.

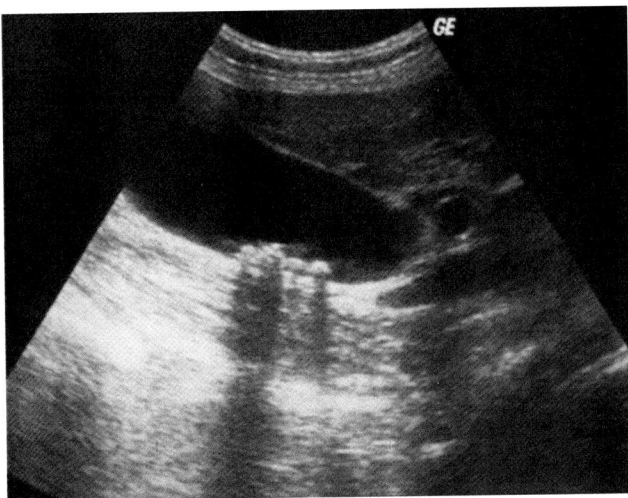

Fig. 12.2 Gallstones in gallbladder

12.6 Treatment

There are no guidelines for the management of cholelithiasis in children, while they are available for adulthood [11, 24, 25]. In the past few decades, paediatric biliary disease had a marked rise in incidence as well as in cholecystectomy rates, perhaps related to the parallel rise in paediatric obesity and improved survival of critically ill patients, but little is known about natural history of cholelithiasis in childhood, especially in asymptomatic subjects [26]. As for prevention of gallstone disease, healthy diet and lifestyle, regular physical activity and maintenance of an ideal body weight might prevent cholesterol gallbladder stones and symptomatic gallstones. In children with gallstone disease, the aim of treatment is to provide long-term relief from the symptoms and to minimize the possibility of complications and recurrence.

Spontaneous resolution of cholelithiasis is more commonly observed in infants; sometimes it is possible to observe spontaneous elimination of stones in faeces [19, 27].

The prognosis of foetal gallstones is very good, and complete spontaneous resolution between 1 and 12 months after birth is generally observed. Complications are very rare. For all these reasons, the best recommended practice is to reassure parents of children with foetal gallstones, monitoring the clinical evolution with periodic abdominal ultrasound and avoiding any treatment [6].

Ceftriaxone-associated biliary pseudolithiasis is a benign condition, usually asymptomatic, that resolves spontaneously. Ceftriaxone should be discontinued if possible and the patient managed conservatively. Also when this reversible complication becomes symptomatic, unnecessary cholecystectomy should be avoided, but if more serious complications occur, laparoscopic or open cholecystectomy should be considered. Knowledge of this condition is important in order to avoid unnecessary surgical treatment [14, 15, 28].

Children with gallstones should be divided into two groups: asymptomatic or symptomatic.

Considering the low rate of complications of asymptomatic gallstones, a nonaggressive management with periodical clinical and ultrasonographic controls is recommended. Routine treatment with UDCA is not recommended in adult patients with asymptomatic gallbladder stones. It is noteworthy that life expectancy of asymptomatic patients is not increased by surgical treatment, because the risk of surgery should be balanced with the probability of gallstone complications. Furthermore, monitoring patients with asymptomatic gallstones costs less than performing prophylactic cholecystectomy [11, 24]. Although similar data are not available for children, on the basis of what recommended in adults, it is advisable to manage children likewise.

For children with symptomatic gallstones or complicated disease, a surgical approach with laparoscopic cholecystectomy is indicated. In both paediatric patients and adults, laparoscopic cholecystectomy has become the procedure of choice to remove the gallbladder and the best standard procedure to treat cholelithiasis and prevent its recurrence. This procedure is safe, effective and well tolerated. It results in a short hospital stay, early return to activity and reduced hospital costs. There is currently no evidence that laboratory tests are mandatory before surgery, but we believe that blood count, liver function test and coagulation parameters should be sought. Preoperative evaluation should include verification of gallstones by ultrasound; in young patients both ECG and chest X-ray may not be required except in selected cases with high risk of complications. The rate of postoperative complications and post-cholecystectomy syndrome is low. Intraoperative complications of laparoscopic cholecystectomy include bile duct damage, bleeding and damage to other organs. Postoperative complications include haemorrhage, bile spillage, wound infection, shoulder pain and subcutaneous emphysema. It is important to keep in mind that the gallbladder wall of infants is thinner than in adults, so that perforations are more frequent in children, while bile duct injuries, often reported in adults, are rare in childhood. Besides, paediatric patients may have biliary tree anomalies, such as gallbladder duplication, ductal abnormalities, accessory bile ducts or accessory cystic arteries to which surgeon has to pay attention [8, 11, 25].

In case of symptomatic patients with cholelithiasis and severe clinical conditions (liver disease, severe obesity, cystic fibrosis, cardiomyopathy, etc.), the surgical risk of cholecystectomy has to be carefully considered and the risks/benefits ratio accurately evaluated.

Ursodeoxycholic acid (UDCA) should not be used to treat paediatric gallstones, except in cases of symptomatic children with contraindications to surgery or when cholecystectomy must be deferred for other reasons.

In brief, cholecystectomy is not indicated for silent gallstones, except in children with a predisposing disease such as chronic haemolysis. In patients with chronic haemolysis or ileal disease, cholecystectomy can be carried out at the same time as another surgical procedure. Cholecystectomy should be considered in asymptomatic gallstones patients with hereditary spherocytosis and sickle cell disease at the time of splenectomy. In patients with sickle cell disease and asymptomatic gallstones, an additional reason for prophylactic cholecystectomy during other abdominal surgery is to avoid diagnostic uncertainty in case of sickle cell crises.

Asymptomatic patients with porcelain gallbladder should undergo cholecystectomy.

In case of uncomplicated biliary colic or acute cholecystitis, early laparoscopic cholecystectomy is recommended within 24 h or 72 h, respectively to avoid the onset of complications and reduce hospital stay. Also in case of patients with mild biliary acute pancreatitis, who frequently do not undergo surgery during their initial hospitalization, early cholecystectomy appears to be safe and does not increase complications [1, 11, 24–26].

In patients with simultaneous gallbladder and bile duct stones, early laparoscopic cholecystectomy should be performed within 72 h after preoperative ERCP for choledocholithiasis.

Treatment of common bile duct stones includes interventional radiologic, endoscopic or surgical procedures. Stone extraction may be performed at endoscopic retrograde cholangiopancreatography with or without sphincterotomy, combined with laparoscopic cholecystectomy. Currently, preoperative ERCP and laparoscopic cholecystectomy are the preferred option, even if recent metanalysis showed that single-stage management for cholecysto-choledocholithiasis is better in terms of stone clearance, hospital stay and total operative time. In children without a predisposing disease or no residual gallstones indicating a cholecystectomy, conservative management (percutaneous cholangiography with biliary drainage) may be proposed in specialized centres, especially for infants. A hepaticojejunostomy is indicated in cases of choledocal cyst with anomalous pancreatobiliary duct junctions. No general recommendation can be given for pharmacological prevention of recurrent bile duct stones [11, 26, 29].

Patients with asymptomatic choledocholithiasis must be treated because of the high risk of developing complications. For them, endoscopic or surgical removal of common bile duct stones is indicated [11, 24, 26]. In patients with gallstones in common bile duct that cannot be cleared with ERCP, it is indicated a biliary stenting to achieve biliary drainage as a temporary measure until definitive endoscopic or surgical clearance is in place. These patients should avoid food and drink that triggers their symptoms until they have their gallbladder or gallstones removed [24].

Percutaneous cholecystostomy is indicated to manage gallbladder empyema when surgery is contraindicated at presentation and conservative management is unsuccessful. For these patients, laparoscopic cholecystectomy must be reconsidered once they are well enough to undergo surgery [24].

In all cases in which surgery is deferred for any reason, parents should be counselled about symptoms consistent with cholecystitis or obstruction of the common bile duct, because in presence of these complications, patients should be promptly hospitalized.

12.6.1 Medical Treatment

The pharmacological approach to paediatric cholelithiasis is based on the use of ursodeoxycholic acid (UDCA). The rationale is to interfere with the supersaturation of bile, the major factor responsible for the formation of cholesterol gallstones. This therapy was commonly indicated in patients with radiolucent floating stones, less than 15 mm in diameter by ultrasonography, and with normal gallbladder function, but on the basis of the available data, UDCA has shown to be ineffective for the dissolution of gallstones in most children, with a high rate of recurrence. However, UDCA had a positive effect on abdominal discomfort in a subset of symptomatic patients, regardless of the type of gallstones. Nonsurgical treatment with UDCA has been reported to significantly reduce the risk of biliary tract pain, surgery and acute cholecystitis even in symptomatic patients. On the other hand, it is to note that symptomatic children with cholelithiasis must be candidate to surgery. Therefore, the use of UDCA therapy in this subset of patients should be limited to subjects who, for various reasons, cannot undergo surgery.

The optimal dosage and administration regimen of bile acid formulations differ between the published report. In patients with cholelithiasis, UDCA is commonly used at 8–10 mg/kg body weight/day. Higher doses do not seem to offer a major efficacy. Little information is available about the optimal doses in paediatric patients.

Ursodeoxycholic acid and cholecystokinin have undergone preliminary investigation for prevention of biliary sludge; however, at this time point, they cannot be recommended for routine clinical use, even in high-risk patients.

Recent studies have suggested a role for ezetimibe, which inhibits intestinal absorption of cholesterol, in the prevention and treatment of cholesterol gallstones, but further investigations are necessary.

There are no indication to use UDCA for the prevention of gallstones in the general population, but in adult patients with rapid weight loss (e.g. very low-calorie diet, bariatric surgery), temporary ursodeoxycholic acid may be recommended [11]. Similar data are not available for children. The pharmacological prophylaxis of gallstone recurrence should be restricted to very high-risk subgroups or to patients not fitting the criteria for cholecystectomy. A few studies have suggested that long-term prophylactic therapy with UDCA should be initiated in patients with heterozygous mutation of the gene ABCB4.

Litholysis with extracorporeal shock wave lithotripsy is not recommended for gallbladder stones. In adulthood, evidence from randomized controlled trials, systematic reviews and cohort studies shows that extracorporeal shock wave lithotripsy (ESWL), similar to bile acid dissolution therapy with UDCA alone, has a low rate of cure and a high rate of recurrence.

12.6.2 Management of Biliary Colic

Scant information is available for children. In adults, biliary colic should be treated with nonsteroidal anti-inflammatory drugs (e.g. diclofenac, indomethacin). In addition, spasmolytics (e.g. butylscopolamine) and, for severe symptoms, opioids (e.g. buprenorphine) may be indicated. Nonsteroid anti-inflammatory drugs (NSAIDs) may decrease the frequency of short-term complications, such as mild form of acute cholecystitis, jaundice, cholangitis and acute pancreatitis. They may also increase the occurrence of possibly life-threatening adverse events such as gastrointestinal bleeding, renal function impairment, cardiovascular events or minor events such as abdominal pain, drowsiness, headache, dizziness or cutaneous manifestations. Their beneficial effect on pain relief has been confirmed. When compared to placebo and spasmolytic drugs, NSAIDs significantly reduced biliary pain. NSAIDs, compared to spasmolytics, seem to have a lower risk of complications such as acute cholecystitis, acute pancreatitis, jaundice, cholangitis. No significant difference has been demonstrated between NSAIDs and opioids [11, 16]. There is no evidence for the management of biliary colic in children. Paracetamol used at high dose (30 mg/Kg as load dose and then 15 mg/Kg as maintenance dose) is the first choice in case of mild-moderate pain. NSAIDs or opioids can also be used in case of severe pain, but attention has to be paid to the possible side effects.

References

1. Tiderington E, Lee SP, Ko CW. Gallstones: new insights into an old story [version 1; referees: 3 approved]. F1000Res. 2016;5(F1000 Faculty Rev):1817. https://doi.org/10.12688/f1000research.8874.1.
2. Portincasa P, Moschetta A, Palasciano G. Cholesterol gallstone disease. Lancet. 2006;368:230–9. https://doi.org/10.1016/S0140-6736(06)69044-2.
3. Poffenberger CM, Gausche-Hill M, Ngai S, Myers A, Renslo R. Cholelithiasis and its complications in children and adolescents: update and case discussion. Pediatr Emerg Care. 2012;28:68–76. https://doi.org/10.1097/PEC.0b013e31823f5b1e.
4. van Dijk AH, de Reuver PR, Besselink MG, van Laarhoven KJ, Harrison EM, Wigmore SJ, Hugh TJ, Boermeester MA. Assessment of available evidence in the management of gallbladder and bile duct stones: a systematic review of international guidelines. HPB (Oxford). 2017;19:297–309. https://doi.org/10.1016/j.hpb.2016.12.011.
5. Palasciano G, Portincasa P, Vinciguerra V, Velardi A, Tardi S, Baldassarre G, Albano O. Gallstone prevalence and gallbladder volume in children and adolescents: an epidemiological ultrasonographic survey and relationship to body mass index. Am J Gastroenterol. 1989;84:1378–82.
6. Triunfo S, Rosati P, Ferrara P, Gatto A, Scambia G. Fetal cholelithiasis: a diagnostic update and a literature review. Clin Med Insights Case Rep. 2013;6:153–8. https://doi.org/10.4137/CCRep.S12273.
7. Jones MW, Ghassemzadeh S. Gallbladder, gallstones (calculi). StatPearls [Internet]. Treasure Island (FL): StatPearls Publishing; 2018–2017 Oct 6.
8. Esposito C, De Marco M, Della Corte C, Iorio R, Vajro P, Settimi A. Chapter 31 Biliary lithiasis in children. In: Biliary lithiasis. Basic science, current diagnostic and therapeutic approaches. Cordiano, Borzellino: Springer; 2008.
9. Della Corte C, Falchetti D, Nebbia G, Calacoci M, Pastore M, Francavilla R, Marcellini M, Vajro P, Iorio R. Management of cholelithiasis in Italian children: a national multicenter study. World J Gastroenterol. 2008;14:1383–8.
10. Katsika D, Grjibovski A, Einarsson C, Lammert F, Lichtenstein P, Marschall HU. Genetic and environmental influences on symptomatic gallstone disease: a Swedish study of 43,141 twin pairs. Hepatology. 2005;41:1138–43. https://doi.org/10.1002/hep.20654.
11. European Association for the Study of the Liver (EASL). EASL Clinical Practice Guidelines on the prevention, diagnosis and treatment of gallstones. J Hepatol. 2016;65:146–81. https://doi.org/10.1016/j.jhep.2016.03.005.
12. Moschetta A, Bookout AL, Mangelsdorf DJ. Prevention of cholesterol gallstone disease by FXR agonists in a mouse model. Nat Med. 2004;10:1352–8. https://doi.org/10.1038/nm1138.
13. Cai JS, Qiang S, Bao-Bing Y. Advances of recurrent risk factors and management of choledocholithiasis. Scand J Gastroenterol. 2017;52:34–43. https://doi.org/10.1080/00365521.2016.1224382.
14. Bickford CL, Spencer AP. Biliary sludge and hyperbilirubinemia associated with ceftriaxone in an adult: case report and review of the literature. Pharmacotherapy. 2005;25:1389–95. https://doi.org/10.1592/phco.2005.25.10.1389.
15. Onlen Y, Gali E, Incecik F, Deviren MU, Savas L. Ceftriaxone-associated biliary sludge and pseudolithiasis in children. Infect Dis Clin Pract. 2007;15:167–70.
16. Fraquelli M, Casazza G, Conte D, Colli A. Non-steroid anti-inflammatory drugs for biliary colic. Cochrane Database Syst Rev. 2016;9:CD006390. https://doi.org/10.1002/14651858.CD006390.pub2.
17. Frederick JS. Chapter 366 Diseases of the gallbladder. In: Nelson textbook of paediatrics. 20 ed. 2016.
18. Schaad UB, Wedgewood-Krucko J, Tschaeppeler H. Reversible ceftriaxone-associated biliary pseudolithiasis in children. Lancet. 1988;2:1411–3.
19. Bogue CO, Murphy AJ, Gerstle JT, Moineddin R, Daneman A. Risk factors, complications, and outcomes of gallstones in children: a single-center review. J Pediatr Gastroenterol Nutr. 2010;50:303–8.
20. Cotton PB, Elta GH, Carter RC, Pasricha PJ, Corazziari ES. Gallbladder and sphincter of oddi disorders. Gastroenterology. 2016;150:1420–9. https://doi.org/10.1053/j.gastro.2016.02.033.
21. Santucci NR, Hyman PE, Harmon CM, Schiavo JH, Hussain SZ. Biliary dyskinesia in children: a systematic review. J Pediatr Gastroenterol Nutr. 2017;64:186–93. https://doi.org/10.1097/MPG.0000000000001357.
22. Scott Nelson R, Kolts R, Park R, Heikenen J. A comparison of cholecystectomy and observation in children with biliary dyskinesia. J Pediatr Surg. 2006;41:1894–8. https://doi.org/10.1016/j.jpedsurg.2006.06.018.
23. Giljaca V, Gurusamy KS, Takwoingi Y, Higgie D, Poropat G, Štimac D, Davidson BR. Endoscopic ultrasound versus magnetic resonance cholangiopancreatography for common bile duct stones. Cochrane Database System Rev. 2015;(2):CD011549.
24. Gallstone disease issued. NICE clinical guideline. 2014. p. 188.
25. Tazuma S, Unno M, Igarashi Y, Inui K, Uchiyama K, et al. Evidence-based clinical practice guidelines for cholelithiasis 2016. J Gastroenterol. 2017;52:276–300. https://doi.org/10.1007/s00535-016-1289-7.
26. Rothstein DH, Harmon CM. Gallbladder disease in children. Semin Pediatr Surg. 2016;25:225–31. https://doi.org/10.1053/j.sempedsurg.2016.05.005.
27. Pernas Gómez P, Gómez López L, Moreno Hernando J. Spontaneous elimination of a gallstone in an infant. An Pediatr (Barc). 2008;68:73–5.
28. Biner B, Oner N, Celtik C, Bostancıoğlu M, Tunçbilek N, Güzel A, Karasalihoğlu S. Ceftriaxone-associated biliary pseudolithiasis in children. J Clin Ultrasound. 2006;34:217–22. https://doi.org/10.1002/jcu.20228.
29. Zhu HY, Xu M, Shen HJ, Yang C, Li F, Li KW, Shi WJ, Ji F. A meta-analysis of single-stage versus two-stage management for concomitant gallstones and common bile duct stones. Clin Res Hepatol Gastroenterol. 2015;39:584–93. https://doi.org/10.1016/j.clinre.2015.02.002.

Genetic Cholestatic Disorders

13

Emanuele Nicastro and Lorenzo D'Antiga

Key Points
- A large proportion of cholestatic disorders are caused by monogenic defects affecting the hepatocellular or biliary functions responsible for bile formation.
- Several genetic diseases can cause transient or permanent cholestasis, including canalicular transport and tight junction defects, bile acid synthesis defects, biliary developmental defects and metabolic disorders.
- In an infant with conjugated jaundice, once biliary atresia is ruled out, the most likely aetiology is a monogenic defect, nowadays recognisable by next-generation sequencing.
- In the last decade, several new defects causing intrahepatic cholestasis have been discovered, such as TJP2 deficiency, FXR deficiency and MYO5B deficiency.
- Although the diagnostic yield in this scenario is remarkably improved, no effective treatment is available for most genetic cholestatic disorders, making them candidates to some 20% of all liver transplants performed in children.

Research Needed in the Field
- To improve the diagnostic yield of genetic testing for cholestatic diseases through widely adopted next-generation sequencing panels and protocols
- To develop strategies able to modify the phenotype of these disorders, by gene therapy/editing, cell therapy, RNA interference, chaperones, etc., to avoid the progression to end-stage liver disease
- To test different forms of medical and surgical biliary diversion, especially in conditions that are only partially corrected by liver transplantation, such as PFIC1

13.1 Introduction

Neonatal and infantile cholestatic liver diseases are a group of diverse hepatobiliary disorders characterised by the retention of bile components into hepatocytes and/or bile ducts, ultimately flowing back to the bloodstream. Excluding the extrahepatic causes, represented by biliary atresia or other biliary obstructive diseases, the knowledge about the underlying aetiology of the so-called "intrahepatic" cholestasis has been rapidly expanding in the last four decades. The great advances in molecular genetics have clarified that the vast majority of these conditions are monogenic liver disorders. Here the different genetic causes of cholestasis will be described and classified on the basis of the pathogenesis and of the clinical context in which they occur.

E. Nicastro (✉) · L. D'Antiga
Paediatric Hepatology, Gastroenterology and Transplantation,
Hospital Papa Giovanni XXIII, Bergamo, Italy
e-mail: enicastro@asst-pg23.it; ldantiga@asst-pg23.it

13.2 Genetic Cholestatic Disorders

13.2.1 Defects of the Biliary Canalicular Transport

Progressive familial intrahepatic cholestasis (PFIC) is a group of heterogeneous autosomal recessive disorders causing hepatocellular cholestasis often presenting in the neonatal age or in the first year of life [1, 2]. With an incidence roughly comprised between 1:50,000 and 1:100,000, they represent about 9–12% of the causes of infantile cholestasis and a major indication for LT in children [3, 4]. Beyond the classically recognised PFIC1 (Byler disease), PFIC2 [Bile Salt Export Pump (BSEP) deficiency] and PFIC3 (MDR3 deficiency), high-throughput sequencing studies have recently identified new gene mutations associated with previously unexplained cases, thus expanding the disease spectrum to the so-called PFIC4 (*TJP2* deficiency), PFIC5 (related to *NR1H4*) and *MYO5B*-associated cholestasis [5–7]. The different proteins and their role in canalicular transport are illustrated in Fig. 13.1.

13.2.1.1 Clinical Presentation

All these disorders usually present in the first months of life, with recurrent episodes of cholestatic jaundice that eventually become permanent [8–11]. Pruritus is common, often intractable, representing one of the indications to LT in later childhood. It has been reported that 15% of patients with PFIC1 and 44% of those affected by PFIC2 present by the first month of age [8]. All these entities invariably show progression to fibrosis and cirrhosis, but in the case of PFIC2, cholestasis is more severe, and the course of the disease appears to be more aggressive. Another feature of PFIC2 is the possible occurrence of early (in the first year of age) hepatocellular carcinoma (HCC) and, less commonly, cholangiocarcinoma.

Unlike the other forms, PFIC3 is usually diagnosed later in infancy and can also be identified during childhood or even in young adult age. In PFIC3 the main clinical feature is portal hypertension. Remarkably, since commonly these patients are not jaundiced and have milder pruritus, cirrhosis and its complications may not be overlooked until the age of 3 [9, 12].

In addition to cholestasis, PFIC1 is associated with other organ involvement, such as enteropathy, pancreatitis, elevated sweat electrolyte concentration, short stature and sensorineural deafness, underscoring the importance of evaluating the expression of FIC1 protein outside the liver, especially when it comes to listing to LT [13, 14].

Interestingly, milder mutations in PFIC1-PFIC2 genes (*ATP8B1* and *ABCB11*) have been also associated with relapsing episodes of jaundice or pruritus called benign recurrent intrahepatic cholestasis (BRIC1-BRIC2) or with cholestasis of pregnancy [15].

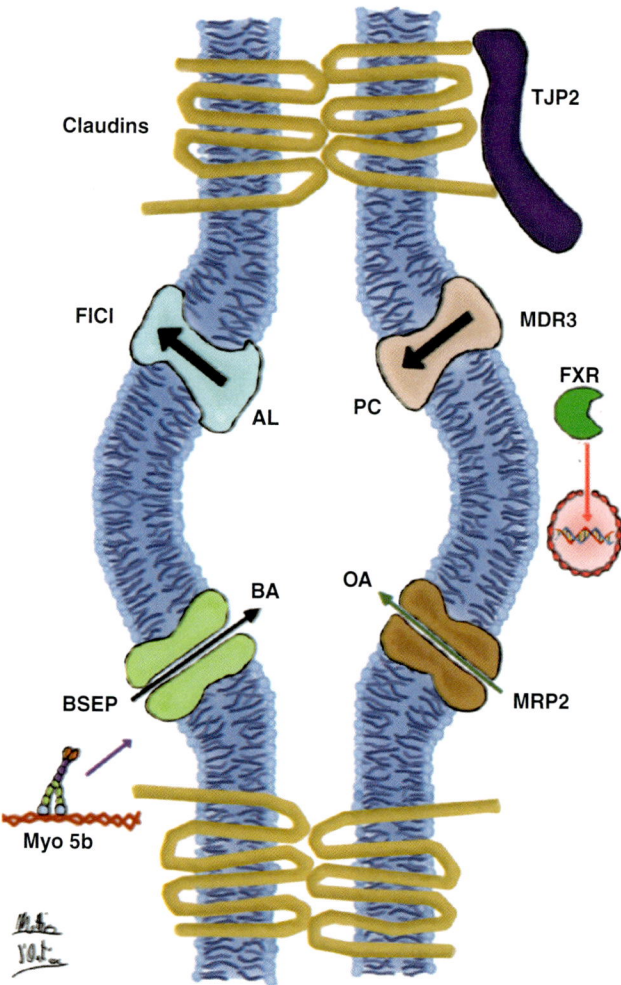

Fig. 13.1 Simplified view of the most important transporters of the biliary canaliculus. BSEP (encoded by *ABCB11*) provides high concentration of bile acids against gradient across the biliary pole plasma membrane; FIC1 (encoded by *ATP8B1*) is a flippase responsible for the aminophospholipid enrichment of the outer leaflet, protecting hepatocyte from the detergent action of bile acids; MDR3 (encoded by ABCB4) is the major phospholipid transporter, essential for bile micellar balance; TJP2 represent a connection between transmembrane claudins and actin cytoskeleton; MRP2 is a transporter for the organic anions, including conjugated bilirubin; FXR is a bile acid-sensitive nuclear receptor that enhances the expression of multiple genes including ABCB11; Myosin 5b is a cytoskeletal component directly involved in recycling BSEP-containing endosomes to the membrane maintaining polarity. *Myo 5b* myosin 5b, *AL* aminophospholipids, *PC* phosphatidylcholine, *OA* organic anions, *BA* bile acids. Courtesy of Mattia D'Antiga

13.2.1.2 Laboratory and Histological Findings

Typically, many PFICs show cholestasis with very high serum bile acids but normal GGT activity, while serum cholesterol is usually normal. PFIC2 is characterised by higher serum transaminases and alpha-fetoprotein. On the other hand, the biochemical features of the patients with PFIC3 are

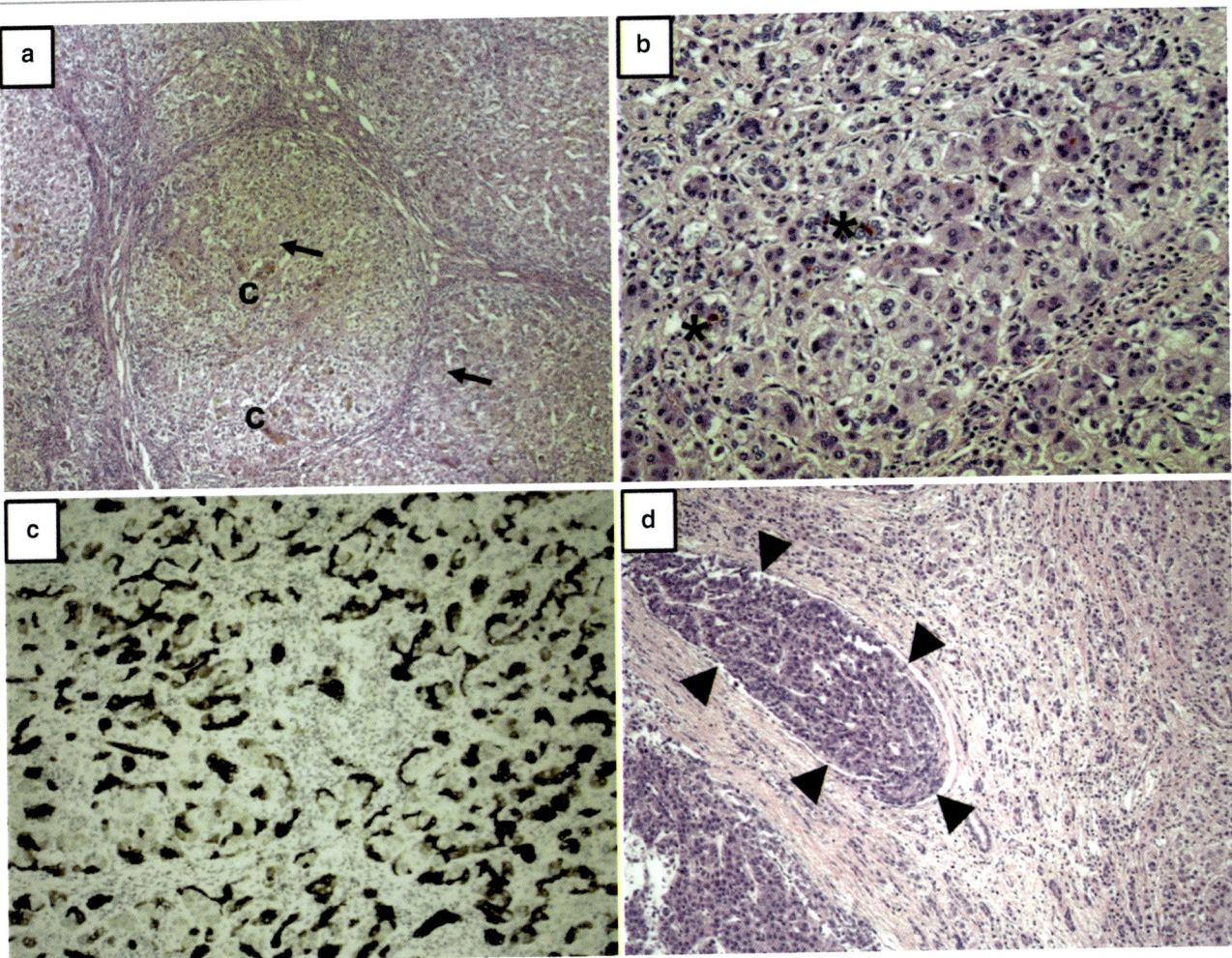

Fig. 13.2 Histological features of PFIC2. (**a**) Cirrhotic architecture with canalicular cholestasis (c) and focal giant cell transformation (arrows); (**b**) higher magnification showing pseudo-glandular arrangement or rosetting (*); (**c**) immunohistochemistry for cytokeratin 7 identifying biliary metaplasia of the hepatocytes; (**d**) nodule of hepatocellular carcinoma on cirrhosis in a PFIC2 patient at hepatectomy invading a blood vessel (arrowheads). Courtesy of Aurelio Sonzogni

quite different: GGT is invariably elevated, and serum bile acids are moderately increased [16].

Liver biopsies from PFIC patients show almost invariably canalicular cholestasis and giant cell transformation, while ductular proliferation is generally absent or mild. Focal biliary metaplasia of the hepatocytes can be seen in periportal areas (Fig. 13.2a–c). Steatosis is occasionally noted in PFIC1 patients. Noteworthy, in PFIC2, the pronounced abnormalities of liver function tests are reflected by a more disrupted parenchymal structure, with lobular inflammation and early portal fibrosis. Also from the histologic point of view, PFIC3 behaves quite differently from the other familial cholestasis: ductular proliferation is seen at onset, and portal fibrosis is a feature, while giant cell transformation is mild. Other specific features of the different aetiologies are shown in Table 13.1.

13.2.2 Aetiology and Specific Features

13.2.2.1 PFIC1

PFIC1, also referred to as "Byler disease", is caused by mutations in *ATP8B1*, encoding FIC1, a P-type ATPase acting as a "flippase", responsible for the maintenance of the phosphatidylserine and phosphatidylethanolamine abundance of the inner leaflet of the plasma membrane. Such composition is crucial for the integrity of the canalicular membranes in presence of concentrated bile acids [17]. However, the definite pathogenesis of cholestasis in PFIC1 is unclear, and several mechanisms have been advocated. The abnormal plasma membrane structure is thought to indirectly determine an impairment in bile acids excretion, as witnessed by the very low primary bile acids that can be measured in the duodenal

Table 13.1 Clinical, laboratory, and histologic features of the most frequent genetic cholestatic diseases

	Pruritus	Accompanying symptoms/features	Laboratory findings	Histology	Gene	Treatment
Canalicular BA transport			All: ↑ Bil, AST/ALT, sBA	All: GCT, canalicular cholestasis		All: UDCA, cholestyramine, PEBD, EBD
PFIC1	++	Diarrhoea, pancreatitis, short stature, deafness; post-LT allograft steatohepatitis	↓ GGT; +/− ↑ sweat chloride	+/− steatosis	ATP8B1	
PFIC2	+++	—	↓ GGT, ↑↑ AST/ALT, ↑ AFP	↑ parenchymal disruption, ↓ BSEP staining	ABCB11	
PFIC3	+	Possible later onset	↑ GGT	+/− ductular proliferation, periductal fibrosis	ABCB4	
FXR deficiency (PFIC5)	+/−	—	↓ GGT, ↑ PT INR, ↑ AFP at onset	↓ BSEP staining	NR1H4	
MYO5B cholestasis	+	+/− microvillus inclusion disease	↓ GGT	+/− steatosis, ↓ BSEP staining	MYO5B	
Tight junction defects			All: ↑ Bil, AST/ALT, sBA			
TJP2 deficiency	++	—	↓ GGT	GCT, canalicular cholestasis, ↓ Claudin-1 staining	TJP2	UDCA, cholestyramine, PEBD
NISCH syndrome	+++	Ichthyosis, alopecia, enamel abnormalities and hypodontia, irregular biliary tree	↑ GGT	Canalicular cholestasis, portal fibrosis, ductular proliferation	CLDN1	UDCA
Bile acid synthesis defects			All: ↑ Bil, AST/ALT, ↓ sBA			
3β-HSD-oxidoreductase deficiency	−	Fat-soluble vitamins malabsorption	↓ GGT, ↑ 3β-hydroxy-Δ⁵ BA	GCT, canalicular cholestasis	HSD3B7	CA, CDCA
Δ4-3-oxosteroid 5β-reductase deficiency	−	Early presentation with predominant coagulopathy	↑ GGT, ↑ PT INR, ↑ 3-oxo-7α-OH-4-CA, 3-oxo-7α,12α-diOH-4-CA	GCT, parenchymal disruption, hepatocellular cholestasis, absent canaliculi	AKR1D1	CA, UDCA
Cerebrotendinous xanthomatosis	−	Rarely present with neonatal cholestasis	↑ cholesterol, ↑ cholestanol, ↓/↑ GGT, ↓/↑ sBA	GCT, canalicular cholestasis, scant steatosis	CYP27A1	CA, CDCA
BACL deficiency[a]	−	Fat-soluble vitamins malabsorption	↓ GGT, absent glycol- and tauro-conjugate BA	GCT, canalicular cholestasis	SLC27A5	GCA (investigational)
BAAT deficiency[a]	−	Fat-soluble vitamins malabsorption	↓ GGT, ↑ PT INR, absent glycol- and tauro-conjugate BA	GCT, canalicular cholestasis	BAAT	GCA (investigational)
2-methylacil-CoA racemase deficiency[a]	−	Fat-soluble vitamins malabsorption	↓ GGT, ↑ cholestanoic (C27) acids	GCT, canalicular cholestasis	AMACR	CA, CDCA
Oxisterol-7α-hydroxylase deficiency	−	Early cirrhosis	↓ GGT, ↑ 3β-monohydroxy-Δ⁵ BA	GCT, canalicular cholestasis, portal fibrosis, ductular proliferation	CYP7B1	−

Trafficking/canalicular targeting defects						
ARC syndrome	+++	Arthrogryposis, renal tubular acidosis, platelet dysfunction, cardiac defects	↑ Bil, AST/ALT, sBA, ↓ GGT	GCT, canalicular cholestasis, portal fibrosis	VPS33B VIPAR	UDCA
Biliary developmental defects						
Alagille syndrome	+++	Triangular facies, butterfly vertebrae, embriotoxon, pulmonary stenosis, renal tubular dysfunction, short stature, aneurysms	↑ Bil, AST/ALT, sBA, GGT, ↑↑ cholesterol	Ductopenia, ductular reaction in early cases	JAG1[b], NOTCH2[b]	UDCA
DCDC2-NSC	+	Irregular biliary tree	↑ Bil, AST/ALT, sBA, GGT	Ductular proliferation, portal fibrosis, bile plugs	DCDC2	UDCA
Metabolic diseases						
Galactosemia	+/−	Hepatomegaly, E. Coli sepsis	↑↑ AST/ALT, ↑ Bil, sBA, GGT	Steatosis, rosettes, fibrosis, bile plugs	GALT	Galactose-free diet
Transaldolase deficiency	+/−	Hepatomegaly, peculiar facies, cutis laxa, cardiac defects, renal tubular dysfunction, thrombocytopenia, large clitoris	↑↑ AST/ALT, ↑ Bil, sBA, GGT	Steatosis, fibrosis, bile plugs	TALDO1	UDCA, NAC
CDGs	+/−	Hepatomegaly, dysmorphisms, neurological impairment, epilepsy, sensorineural deafness	↑ AST/ALT, ↑ Bil, sBA, ↑/N GGT, abnormal transferrin IEF	Steatosis, fibrosis	~120 different defects	Dietary monosaccharides in some disorders
Tyrosinemia	+/−	Hepatomegaly, renal tubular dysfunction	↑↑ AST/ALT, ↑ Bil, sBA, GGT, ↑ Tyr, ↑ SAC	Steatosis, fibrosis, cirrhosis, dysplastic changes	FAH	Tyrosine/Alanine restriction, NTBC
NICCD	+/−	Hepatomegaly, failure to thrive	↑ Bil, AST/ALT, sBA, GGT, hypoglycemia, ↑ Cit, Arg	Steatosis	SLC25A13	Carbohydrate-restricted diet, arginine
Mitochondrial depletion syndromes	−	Hepatomegaly, neurodevelopmental delay, hypotonia, myoclonus, sensorineural impairment, leukoencephalopathy at imaging	↑ Bil, AST/ALT, sBA, GGT, hypoglycemia, lactic acidosis	Steatosis, fibrosis, ductular proliferation, lobular collapse	POLG1, DGUOK, MPV17	Nutritional modulation, cofactor administration
Alpha-1 antitrypsin deficiency	+/−	Hepatomegaly, acholic stools	↑ Bil, AST/ALT, sBA, GGT, ↓ serum A1AT	GCT, ductular proliferation, PAS + diastase-resistant inclusions	SERPINA1	UDCA

Bil conjugated bilirubin, *sBA* total serum bile acids, *GCT* giant cell transformation, *UDCA* ursodeoxycholic acid, *GCA* glycocholic acid, *(PJEBD)* (partial) external biliary diversion, *AFP* alpha-fetoprotein, *CA* cholic acid, *CDCA* chenodeoxycholic acid, *IEF* isoelectrofocusing, *Tyr* tyrosine, *SAC* succinylacetone, *NTBC* nitisinone, *Cit* citrulline, *Arg* arginine, *A1AT* alpha-1 antitrypsin

[a]Peroxisomal enzymes
[b]Autosomal dominant inheritance

fluid after duodenal aspiration. This can be due to a different degree of downregulation of the farnesoid X receptor (FXR), which in turn is responsible for a reduced expression of BSEP and for a steady upregulation of the intestinal apical sodium bile salt transporter (ASBT) [18, 19]. Intriguingly, ATB8B1-deficient cells have an impaired apical localisation of the cystic fibrosis transmembrane conductance regulator (CFTR) that could contribute to the bile components retention and also account for some cystic fibrosis-like features of PFIC1. In fact, some extrahepatic manifestations include pancreatitis, abnormal chloride sweat content and even lung infections [1, 20]. ATP8B1 is widely expressed in the liver, pancreas, kidney and small intestine, where it can cause chronic diarrhoea through the alteration of the enterohepatic cycling of bile acids and where it may play a central role in the post-transplant PFIC1 allograft steatohepatitis and related metabolic complications [13]. Other extrahepatic features of the disease are short stature and sensorineural deafness [1, 21].

13.2.2.2 PFIC2

BSEP, encoded by the gene *ABCB11*, is the most important canalicular transporter, able to concentrate bile acids against extreme gradients. Its absence or reduced function can lead to bile acids retention and hepatocellular cholestasis [22]. BSEP disease spectrum is variable from BRIC to severe cholestasis with rapidly progressing chronic liver disease and possible risk of HCC (Fig. 13.2d). A genotype-phenotype correlation exists and explains part of the disease variability [23]. For instance, the two most common PFIC2-causing missense mutations of BSEP (D482G and E297G) exhibit a higher degree of impairment of the enzymatic activity and of the protein trafficking compared to those associated with a BRIC phenotype (such as A570T and R1050C). Alternatively, PFIC2-causing mutations may lead to milder, late-onset diseases if carried in compound heterozygosity with polymorphisms such as V444A. On the other hand, frameshift or protein-truncating mutations severely disrupt BSEP transport function and lead to the poorest membrane expression, and, consistently, they are associated with a poorer outcome and the highest risk of HCC [24, 25]. However, if protein-truncating mutations are likely to cause negative BSEP staining at liver biopsy, detectable BSEP expression does not preclude functional BSEP deficiency, whereas undetectable BSEP is seen also in other non-BSEP familial cholestasis, so that genetics has largely replaced immunohistochemistry for both diagnostic and prognostic purposes.

13.2.2.3 PFIC3

At the concentrations occurring in intrahepatic bile, bile acids could theoretically damage the apical membrane of the hepatocytes, but this is effectively counteracted by an enhanced cholesterol and phospholipid transport in the canalicular lumen [26]. The class III multidrug resistance of P-glycoprotein (MDR3, encoded by *ABCB4*) is the major phospholipid translocator enriching bile in phosphatidylcholine at the canalicular membrane. Loss of function of MDR3 results in inadequate phospholipid content with subsequent extracellular (canalicular) bile acid toxic effect. In addition, the imbalanced phosphatidylcholine content leads to unstable mixed micelles, favouring the cholesterol nucleation and the formation of gallstones. The result of these two phenomena is a cholangitis that represents the mechanism of liver damage in the PFIC3 [2]. PFIC3 could present with very different pictures, from neonatal cholestasis to cirrhosis in young adults. Histologically, it can mimic sclerosing cholangitis, since signs of biliary obstruction can be seen at liver biopsy and cholangiography may show abnormalities of the biliary tree [16].

13.2.2.4 FXR Deficiency (*NR1H4*-Associated Cholestasis, PFIC5)

The farnesoid X receptor (FXR, encoded by *NR1H4*) is a hepatocyte bile acid-sensitive nuclear receptor, involved in several hepatocyte metabolic pathways, especially biliary homeostasis. In response to high bile acids concentration, FXR suppresses bile acids biosynthesis and uptake and increases their export [27, 28]. Homozygous mutations in *NR1H4* causing loss of functions of FXR have been described in a few patients presenting with low-GGT cholestasis very early in life, usually in the first month after birth or at birth with ascites, pleural effusion and coagulopathy, very high alpha-fetoprotein (trending down with time) and rapid progression to liver failure [6]. The hallmark of FXR deficiency is coagulopathy that is invariably present and is disproportionate to the liver injury. This can be explained by the fact that FXR directly regulates coagulation and complement factors. Since also BSEP expression is regulated by FXR, it is not surprising that BSEP staining was negative in all the described patients. Interestingly, some patients displayed post-transplant graft dysfunction and steatosis that could be related to the decreased production of FGF19, an intestinal growth factor that in normal conditions sends a negative feedback to the bile acid synthesis in the liver.

13.2.2.5 *MYO5B*-Associated Cholestasis

Myosin 5b (encoded by *MYO5B*) is a protein involved in plasma membrane recycling and transcytosis through its protein-to-protein interaction with Rab8a and Rab11a, essential for the polarisation of different epithelial cells and for the targeting of some transmembrane transporters, including CFTR and BSEP [29–32]. Until recently, the genetic defect in human pathology was known for its role as the cause of an enterocyte structural defect causing microvillous inclusion disease, an autosomal recessive disorder characterised by congenital diarrhoea often leading to intestinal failure and need for long-term parenteral nutrition. These children tend to develop cholestasis with unexpectedly low GGT and intractable pruritus, occurring before or even after intestinal transplantation, with negative BSEP staining at histology [33]. Recently, it has been clarified that mutations in *MYO5B* can cause isolated cholestasis, accounting for up to 20% of the neonatal cholestasis of previously indeterminate aetiology. Although the disease seems to invariably present in the first year of age, cholestasis can be transient, recurrent or persistent and progressive. Clinical features are similar to other low-GGT PFICs, with elevated serum bile acids, mild to moderate transaminases elevation and very low primary bile acids in duodenal aspiration, while BSEP and MDR staining can be absent or displaced to cytoplasm [7, 34]. These features overlap with those of PFIC2, but alpha-fetoprotein has been described as normal in these patients. *MYO5B* mutations causing isolated cholestasis are usually single nucleotide variants causing a single amino acid change, whereas those causing microvillous inclusion disease are commonly protein-truncating or disrupting the binding with Rab11a [7].

13.2.3 Tight Junction Defects

Tight junctions are the most apical cell junction complexes that determine cell polarity and create a barrier preventing and regulating the paracellular diffusion of water or small proteins. These complexes are made of transmembrane components (claudins, occludins and junction adhesion molecules) and cytosolic components such as tight junction proteins that act binding transmembrane proteins to the actin cytoskeleton [35] (Fig. 13.1). Since the tight junction system is redundant in humans, the loss of function of one of its components is critical only in unusually hostile environment, such as the canalicular membranes, which face high concentrations of detergent bile acids [36].

13.2.3.1 *TJP2* Deficiency (PFIC4)

Homozygous mutations in TJP2 abolishing protein translation cause isolated, low-GGT, intrahepatic cholestasis that is indistinguishable from the classical PFICs on clinical ground [5]. The patients affected by this new entity present with cholestatic jaundice by the third month of life and almost invariably progress to cirrhosis needing LT; only a few of those described so far remained with stable cholestatic liver disease. Histology is similar to other forms of intrahepatic cholestasis, BSEP staining is maintained, while Claudin-1 (the major transmembrane protein binding TJP2) fails to localise at the canalicular membrane, although its expression is normal. Abnormal tight junctions can be observed at electron microscopy. Interestingly, missense *TJP2* mutations were previously known to be associated with familial Amish hypercholanemia (a disorder characterised by pruritus and fat-soluble vitamins malabsorption) in a supposed oligogenic inheritance with coexistent homozygous BAAT missense mutations [37] and with autosomal dominant non-syndromic hearing loss in Korean families [38].

13.2.3.2 NISCH Syndrome

Neonatal sclerosing cholangitis is a severe cholangiopathy that presents early in life with a picture mimicking biliary atresia but with patent, although abnormal, bile ducts. In the very few cases described, this picture results from a rare autosomal recessive condition associated with neonatal ichthyosis (neonatal ichthyosis and sclerosing cholangitis, (NISCH)), caused by mutations in *CLDN1* encoding Claudin-1. The majority of the families described are of Moroccan origin. Cholestasis usually presents in the first months of life with increased GGT, and dermatologic features are better appreciated later in life (Fig. 13.3a, b). Disproportionate pruritus,

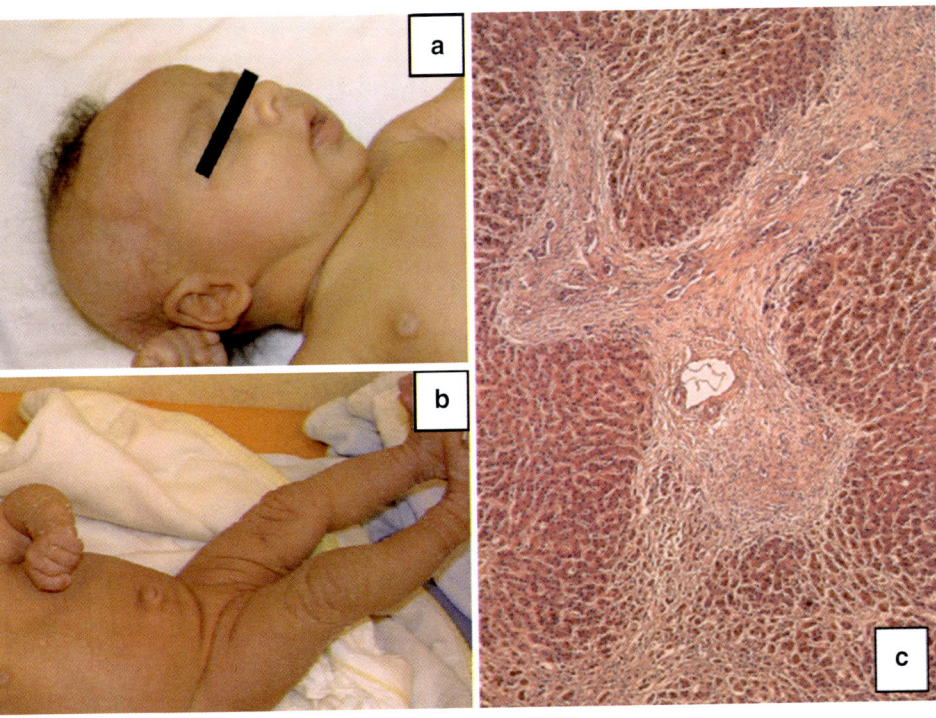

Fig. 13.3 (a) Alopecia and (b) ichthyosis in a 6-month-old NISCH patient; (c) liver histology with interlobular septa, moderate inflammatory infiltrate and absence of interlobular bile ducts. *NISCH* neonatal ichthyosis sclerosing cholangitis. Courtesy of Massimiliano Paganelli

alopecia/hypotrichosis and ichthyosis are almost invariably present, and enamel abnormalities and hypodontia can be adjunctive features. Hepatocellular and canalicular cholestasis can be accompanied by a variable degree of portal fibrosis and ductular proliferation at liver biopsy (Fig. 13.3c). Cholangiography shows patent but abnormal biliary tree [39].

13.2.4 Bile Acid Synthesis Defects (BASD)

Synthesis of bile acids from cholesterol involves at least 14 enzymatic reactions. The mechanism of disease consists not only in a reduced bile flow but also in the lack of negative feedback operated by cholic and chenodeoxycholic acid on the FXR, so that hepatocytes continue to metabolise cholesterol leading to the accumulation of abnormal and toxic intermediates, ultimately determining cholestasis, fat-soluble vitamin malabsorption and, in some subtypes, neurological impairment. BASDs account for only 1–2% of all paediatric liver diseases, with a prevalence in Europe of 1–9/1,000,000, but their identification is compelling due to the availability of medical treatment [40, 41].

Of note, when BASDs present in infancy, generally with low-GGT cholestasis, pruritus is nearly absent, since there are no circulating primary bile acids. However these disorders can be diagnosed in older children or young adults presenting with neurological symptoms due to fat-soluble vitamin malabsorption. Their biochemical hallmark is the cholestasis with low serum bile acids, since standard assays detect primary bile acids (cholic and chenodeoxycholic acid) but not bile acids precursors and sterols. The detection of metabolites characterising BASDs relies on mass spectrometry. The metabolic pathway leading to endogenous primary bile acid synthesis is illustrated in Fig. 13.4.

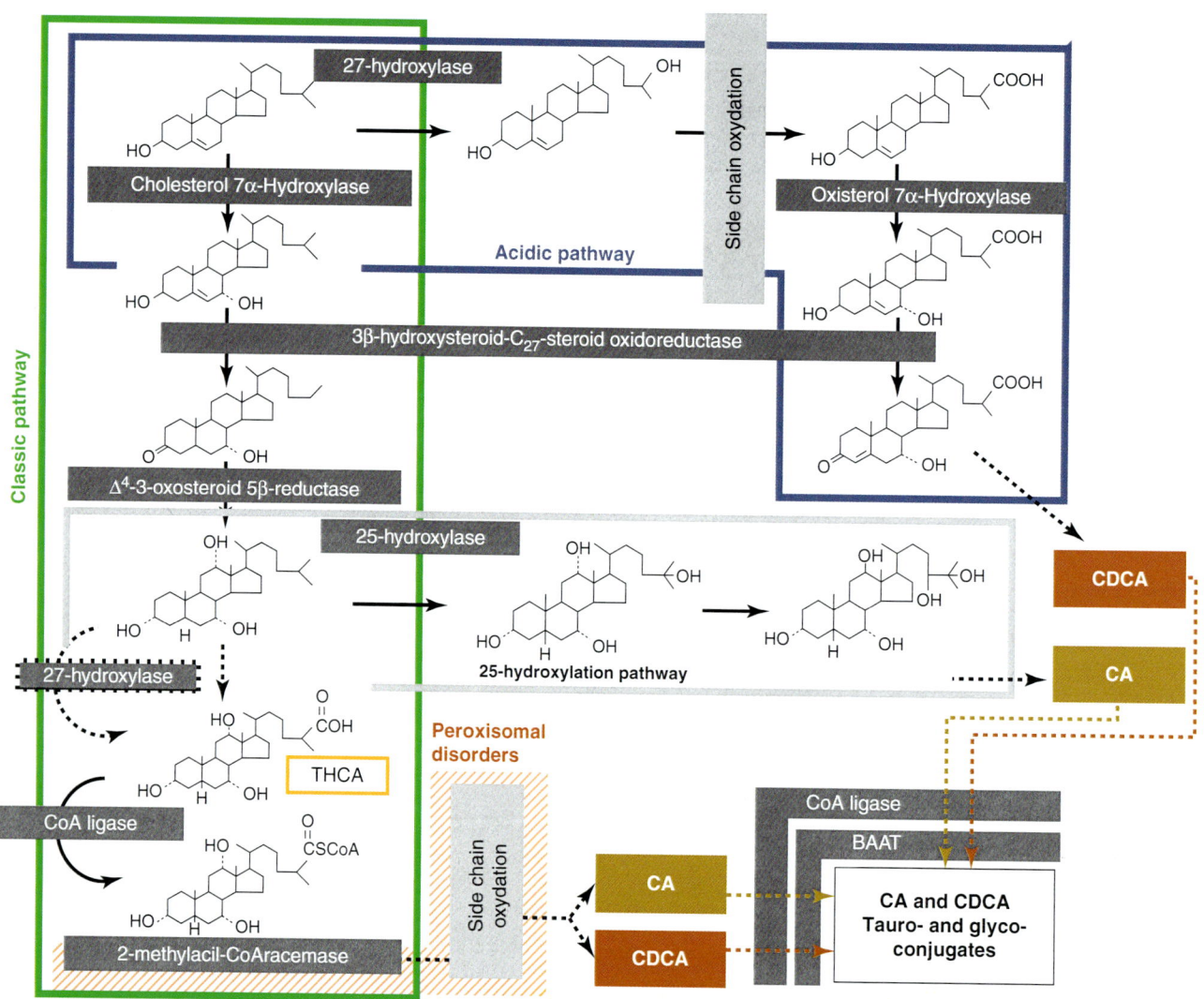

Fig. 13.4 Schematic representation of the endogenous primary bile acid synthesis. The classical pathway is represented in green, while the alternative acidic and 25-hydroxylase pathways are shown in blue and grey, respectively. In the grey boxes, the enzymes whose loss of function is associated with bile acid synthesis defects (BASDs) are indicated. The hatched red area indicates enzymatic activities requiring peroxisomal integrity. *CA* cholic acid, *CDCA* chenodeoxycholic acid, *THCA* $3\alpha,7\alpha,12\alpha$-trihydroxy-5β-cholestanoic acid

13.2.5 Aetiology and Specific Features

13.2.5.1 3β-Hydroxysteroid-C_{27}-Steroid Oxidoreductase Deficiency (3β-HSD Deficiency)

This is the most frequent BASD, caused by the impairment of the conversion of 7α-hydroxycholesterol to 7α-hydroxy-4-cholesten-3-one. The onset is in neonatal age with low-GGT cholestasis, hypertransaminasemia, hepatomegaly with or without splenomegaly and fat-soluble vitamin malabsorption [42]. Liver biopsy is characterised by hepatocellular cholestasis and giant cell transformation. The phenotype is very heterogeneous: while the majority of the affected infants show progression to cirrhosis in absence of treatment, some of the patients transiently resolve their jaundice to present later on with a more severe derangement. Nowadays, some cases are identified investigating chronic cholestasis or cirrhosis of indeterminate aetiology.

The signature of the defect is the presence of sulphate and glycosulfate conjugates of the 3β-hydroxy-Δ^5 bile acids at urine or blood mass spectrometry, while genetic testing can find mutations in the *HSD3B7* gene (Fig. 13.5).

13.2.5.2 Δ^4-3-Oxosteroid 5β-Reductase Deficiency

This enzymatic defect causes the loss of conversion of the intermediates 7α-hydroxy-4-cholesten-3-one and 7α,12α dihydroxy-4-cholesten-3-one to the corresponding 3-oxo-5β(H) intermediates. Clinically it is very similar to 3β-HSD deficiency, but it presents at a younger age and is characterised by a more severe course [Clayton 1988]. Of note, GGT is elevated, while cytolysis and jaundice are remarkable. Coagulopathy is often a feature, in some cases resembling neonatal hemochromatosis [43]. Histology reveals a substantial parenchymal disturbance, with giant cell transformation, hepatocellular cholestasis and, uniquely, absent or slit-like biliary canaliculi [44]. The latter feature is thought to be a consequence of the toxicity of the relatively insoluble Δ^4-3-oxo bile acids that represent the main pointer to the diagnosis when detected by urine mass spectrometry. The diagnosis can be genetically confirmed by sequencing of *AKR1D1*.

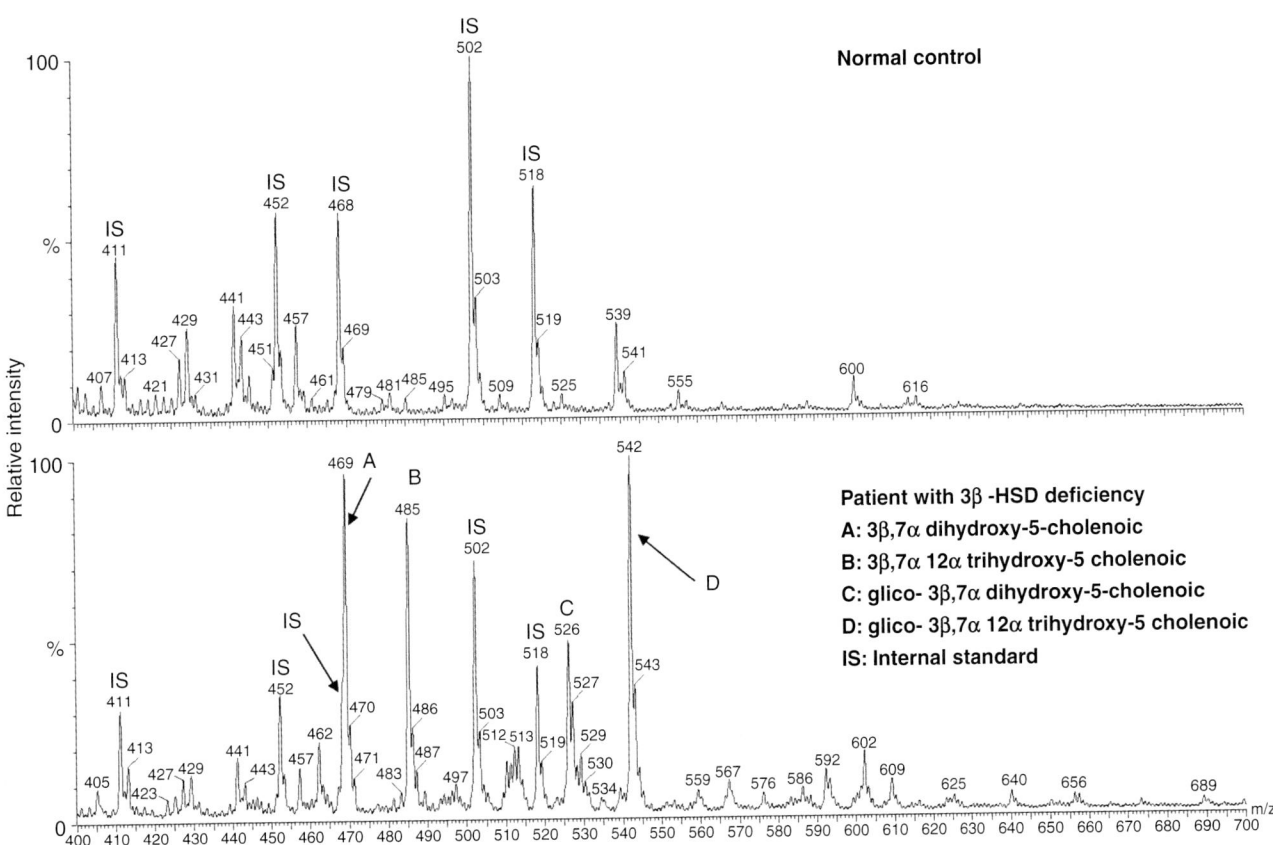

Fig. 13.5 Liquid chromatography-tandem mass spectrometry spectra of full scan obtained from a patient with bile acid synthesis defect at the time of diagnosis, compared with spectra obtained from the urine of a normal control. Peaks A–D correspond to metabolites diagnostic for 3β-HSD deficiency. Adapted from [91]

13.2.5.3 Cerebrotendinous Xanthomatosis (27-Hydroxylase Deficiency)

The name of this condition immediately evokes the presentation in adulthood, characterised by xanthomas of the brain and the tendons and by cognitive deterioration, with ataxia and, sometimes, cataracts. With the refinement of the diagnostic techniques, it has been clarified that this condition, caused by the loss of 27-sterol-hydroxylase activity (i.e. the entry step of the classical bile acid synthetic pathway), can present with a picture of neonatal cholestasis that can progress to liver failure or alternatively resolve, even spontaneously [45–48]. Since primary bile acids, especially cholic acid, can be synthesised via the alternative 25-hydroxylase pathway, total serum bile acids can be quite elevated and GGT not as low as in other BASDs. As a result of the enzymatic defect and of the increased cholesterol biosynthesis in presence of an impairment of the side chain oxidation, several bile acid glucuronides and 5α-cholestan-3β-ol (cholestanol) accumulate and can be detected by mass spectrometry.

13.2.5.4 Bile Acid Amidation Defects (BACL and BAAT Deficiency)

Two defects are responsible for the lack of bile acid conjugation with the amino acids glycine and taurine: bile acid-CoA ligase (BACL) deficiency and bile acid-CoA:amino acid N-acyltransferase (BAAT) deficiency. Both defects can present with low-GGT and mild cholestasis of neonatal onset [49] and almost invariably show marked fat-soluble vitamin malabsorption, but patients with BAAT deficiency have been also described to present with marked coagulopathy and no jaundice. The detected spectrum on urine mass spectrometry invariably shows the lack of conjugated primary bile acids. Recently, the treatment with glycocholic acid has been reported as safe and effective to control cholestasis and improve malabsorption of amidation defects [50].

13.2.5.5 2-Methylacil-CoA Racemase Deficiency

Only few patients have been described with this defect that allows the critical step of formation of the 25S-enantiomer of the 13α,7α,12α-trihydroxy-5β-cholestanoic acid (THCA). Such patients have been identified in adult age because of fat-soluble vitamin malabsorption or in infancy for cholestatic liver disease. The hallmark metabolites are the cholestanoic acids that cannot enter the peroxisomal oxidation.

13.2.5.6 Oxisterol-7α-Hydroxylase Deficiency

This defect has been described in only two children [51, 52]. The enzyme belongs to the alternative acidic bile acid synthesis pathway that seems to be important early in life. Of note, liver biopsy, in addition to the features commonly observed in BASDs, shows portal fibrosis and ductular proliferation. Typically, 3β-monohydroxy-Δ^5 bile acids are observed in urine and blood by mass spectrometry.

13.2.5.7 Secondary BASDs

In peroxisomal disorders—classically presenting at different ages with dysmorphic feature, neurological abnormalities and other organ involvement—the phenotype includes also a variable degree of liver disease due to the disruption of the organelle environment in which the transformation of the THCA into cholic acid takes place. Zellweger syndrome, infantile Refsum disease and neonatal adrenoleukodystrophy show substantial trihydroxycoprostanoic and dihydroxycoprostanoic acid amounts in urine [53–55].

Another disorder which typically presents in neonatal age with cholestasis due to impaired bile acid biosynthesis is Smith-Lemli-Opitz syndrome (SLOS) [56]. Due to the loss of function of 7-dehydrocholesterol Δ_7-reductase catalysing the last step of cholesterol synthesis, SLOS patients lack the substrate for bile acid formation, since Δ_7-sterols are poorly 7α-hydroxylated. The consequent cholestasis complicates a multi-organ picture with a poor prognosis characterised by dysmorphisms; microcephaly; failure to thrive; limb, cardiac, renal and endocrine abnormalities; cataracts; and mental retardation.

13.2.6 Trafficking and Canalicular Targeting Defects

13.2.6.1 Arthrogryposis-Renal Dysfunction-Cholestasis (ARC) Syndrome

ARC syndrome is a rare autosomal recessive multisystem disorder, characterised by the presence of arthrogryposis, renal tubular acidosis and neonatal cholestatic jaundice [1]. Other possible accompanying features can be ichthyosis (~50%), platelet anomalies (~25%), agenesis of the corpus callosum (>20%), congenital cardiovascular anomalies (~10%), deafness and recurrent infections [57]. Two genes are involved in its pathogenesis, *VPS33B* and the one encoding its interacting protein *VIPAR* [58]. VPS33B protein is involved in vacuolar sorting and in the intracellular vesicular trafficking pathways, including vesicular exocytosis, synaptic transmission and general secretion. Its loss of function causes abnormal localisation or accumulation of plasma proteins in polarised cells [59]. VIPAR interacts with VPS33B and is essential to maintain polarity and apical membrane protein restriction [60]. In these newborns, cholestasis is characterised by low GGT and slightly increased transaminases, but jaundice and pruritus are marked. Treatment is supportive and the prognosis is generally poor.

13.2.7 Biliary Developmental Defects

13.2.7.1 Alagille Syndrome

Alagille syndrome (AS) is the most common monogenic cause of neonatal cholestasis, with an estimated incidence of 1:30,000. AS is an autosomal dominant multisystem disorder caused by the loss of Notch2 signalling that is crucial for developmental processes of many organs and tissues, specifically caused by mutations in *JAG1* or *NOTCH2* (~94% and ~2% of the cases, respectively) [61]. The syndrome is defined by a paucity of intrahepatic bile ducts associated with at least three of the following: cholestasis, cardiac disease (most commonly peripheral pulmonary artery stenosis), skeletal abnormalities ("butterfly vertebras"), ocular abnormalities (embriotoxon) and peculiar facial features (triangular face, pointed chin, prominent forehead, hypertelorism) [62]. Beyond these diagnostic criteria, affected children usually have short stature [63] and may present brain vascular anomalies at risk of bleeding or stroke (including "moyamoya" disease) [64], as well as renal dysfunction in up to 40% (Fig. 13.6) [65]. Cholestasis arises from bile duct paucity. Whatever the gene involved, the pathogenesis of ductopenia has been eminently reviewed in a recent article [66]: Jag1 protein expression in the embryo portal vein mesenchyme initiates the bile duct development, interacting with Notch2 to induce the expression of Hes1, HNF1β and Sox9, which in turn promote and regulate ductal plate and intrahepatic bile duct morphogenesis [67–69]. Interestingly, Notch2 is essential for prenatal but not for secondary bile duct formation, which could explain the partial recovery of cholestasis during infancy of some patients [70, 71]. Hepatic manifestations are conjugated hyperbilirubinemia with high GGT, increased serum bile acids and striking elevation in serum cholesterol and triglycerides, with early development of xanthomas. Additional features are failure to thrive and malabsorption. Cholestatic pruritus is often the main problem in children with AS, and, if intractable, it may represent an indication for LT. Histology classically shows intrahepatic bile duct paucity, but in biopsies taken in the first few months of life, ductal proliferation may be the dominant feature, leading to a possible misdiagnosis of biliary atresia. The diagnosis of AS is clinical and histological and nowadays requires genetic confirmation. Genetic testing has an important role in incomplete phenotypes that are very common in this condition and easily overlooked. Cholestasis is unremitting and progresses to cirrhosis and liver insufficiency in about 15–20% of infants, who then require LT early in life. A multi-organ evaluation is needed before listing these patients for LT, in order to assess the risk related to cardiac, renal and vascular abnormalities [72].

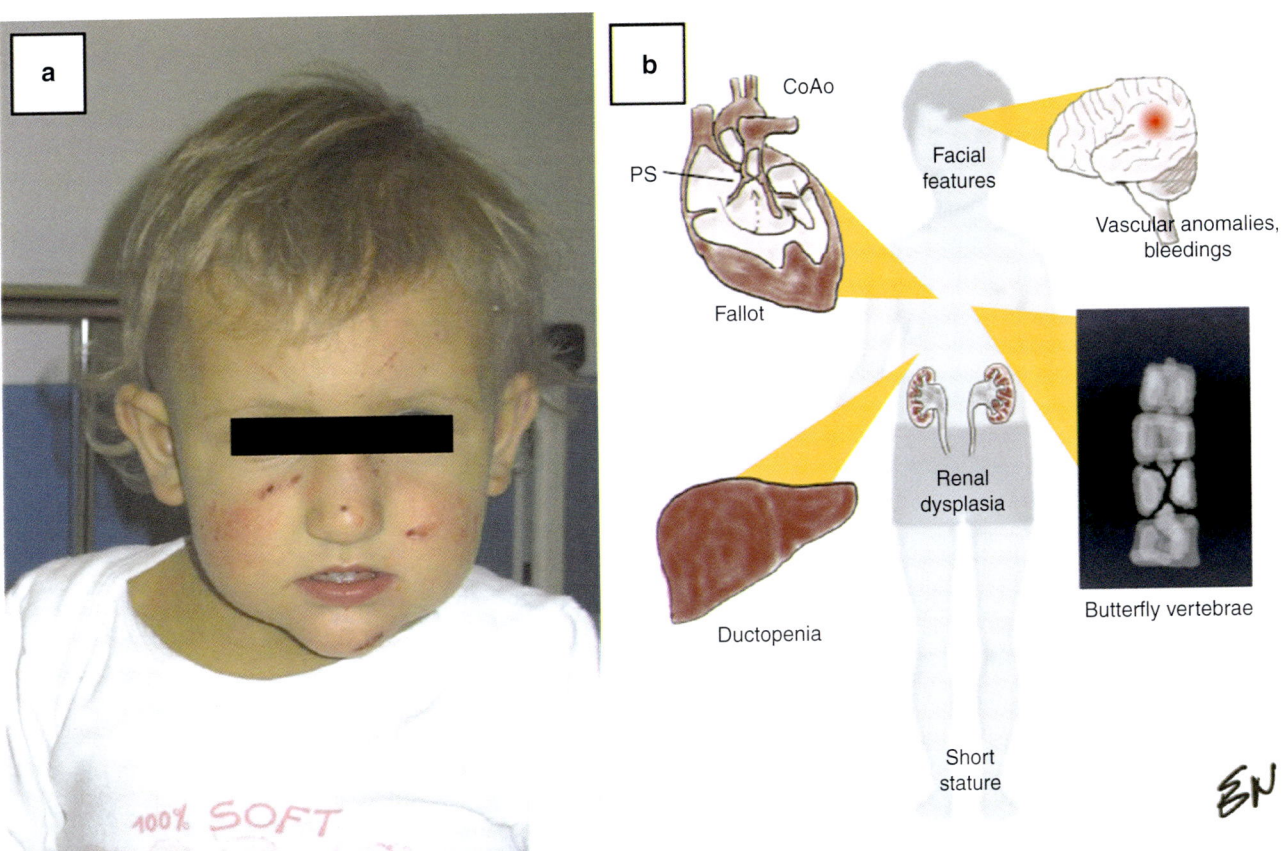

Fig. 13.6 (**a**) Facial and (**b**) body features of Alagille syndrome. *PS* pulmonary stenosis, *CoAo* aortic coarctation

13.2.7.2 Neonatal Sclerosing Cholangitis Related to *DCDC2*

In 2016 *DCDC2* (encoding the Doublecortin domain-containing protein 2) was found to cause a proportion of cases of neonatal sclerosing cholangitis that had no mutations in *CLDN1* [73, 74]. The encoded protein is highly expressed as a component of cholangiocyte primary cilia, which, in affected children, fails to localise in this structure but is found in the cytoplasm. This change is supposed to cause liver disease by modifying the bile composition and/or reducing the protection of the epithelium against the bile and by disrupting the microtubular structure of the biliocyte. From the point of view of the pathogenesis, this entity should be classified as a ciliopathy, but, due to the peculiar presentation, *DCDC2* disease should be considered a monogenic cholestatic disorder rather than a type of fibrocystic disease of the liver. Affected children present with cholestatic jaundice and pale stools, hepatomegaly and high GGT. The liver biopsy shows features consistent with biliary atresia such as ductular reaction and portal fibrosis, but cholangiography reveals an irregular but patent biliary tract. No specific treatment exists for these children, and LT is the only option.

13.2.8 Metabolic Diseases Secondarily Causing Cholestasis

13.2.8.1 Carbohydrate Metabolism Defects

Some defects of the carbohydrate metabolism can affect the liver early in life and are briefly treated in this chapter because, even if they do not directly impair bile components production and transport, they can present in neonatal or infantile period with cholestasis. Most of them are addressed in the chapter addressing the "practical approach to the jaundiced infant".

Galactosemia nowadays is often diagnosed in asymptomatic children, in countries that implemented the universal newborn metabolic screening. The undiagnosed patient with a classical phenotype (related to *GALT* mutations that almost completely abolish the GALT enzyme activity) presents after the introduction of galactose in the diet with signs of hepatocellular damage, raised transaminases, jaundice (70%), hepatomegaly (40%) and coagulopathy, accompanied by vomiting, failure to thrive and frequent bacterial infections, typically *Escherichia coli* sepsis. If a galactose-free diet is not rapidly established, liver failure rapidly ensues.

Transaldolase deficiency (TALDO) is a rare disorder of the pentose phosphate pathway identified in 2001, caused by mutations in *TALDO1* [75]. The lack of enzymatic activity leads to the accumulation of sugar phosphates and abnormal polyols (erythritol, D-arabitol and ribitol) in several tissues. The sugar phosphates are thought to be responsible for liver injury that can present in newborns but also with unexplained cirrhosis by 3 years of age. Hepatomegaly is almost invariably present, sometimes accompanied by splenomegaly, while liver function tests show elevated transaminases and hyperbilirubinemia in about 60% and 36% of the patients, respectively. At diagnosis, a synthetic derangement can be present in about a half of the children, and progression to cirrhosis and HCC or liver failure has been described. The systemic nature of the disease is revealed by the presence of other symptoms: dysmorphism (cutis laxa, triangular face, low-set ears, thin lips), congenital cardiac defects (aortic coarctation, bicuspid aortic valve, ventricular or atrial septum defects), renal tubular dysfunction and hematologic abnormalities such as thrombocytopenia, developmental delay and gonadal dysfunction. Treatment is supportive, while N-acetylcysteine has been used to counteract the depletion of NADP. LT is an option in advanced disease or HCC.

Congenital disorders of glycosylation (CDGs) are a group of metabolic diseases caused by abnormal protein or lipid glycosylation. Over the last 10 years, the number of CGDs has increased from about 40 to over 125 different entities, following the advent of next-generation DNA sequencing and especially with the use of whole exome sequencing [76]. CDGs are of difficult identification, since they have varied multisystem involvement. Liver involvement in CDGs occurs in approximately 20% of the known defects, and its severity is very variable. For the purposes of this chapter, only the forms with isolated or predominant liver involvement will be mentioned. *MPI-CDG* is caused by the lack of function of mannose phosphate isomerase, a cytosolic enzyme that catalyses the isomerisation of fructose-6-phosphate to mannose-6-phosphate as first step of the N-glycosylation [77]. Affected children present often in the postneonatal age with signs of liver dysfunction commonly associated with enteropathy, vomiting and failure to thrive. However, the picture is dominated by hepatomegaly and elevated transaminases rather than cholestasis, and liver fibrosis develops early and progressively unless mannose treatment is started promptly. Some cases present developmental abnormalities of the ductal plate, with a picture overlapping that of congenital hepatic fibrosis. *CCDC115-CDG* can present in the first months of life with cholestatic jaundice and hepatomegaly, failure to thrive, redundant skin, developmental delay and epilepsy. Transaminases are increased, GGT is not as elevated as alkaline phosphatase, ceruloplasmin is low when tested, and patients exhibit a type 2 CDG transferrin isoelectrofocusing profile [78]. The X-linked ATP6AP1 deficiency can present with neonatal jaundice, hepatomegaly and immunodeficiency with hypogammaglobulinemia, epilepsy, mild developmental delay and sensorineural deafness. In *PMM2-CDG* several dysmorphisms can be observed, including the hint of inverted nipples, and liver involvement is variable, ranging from mild hepatomegaly and hypertransaminasemia to severe disease leading to cirrhosis by the fourth month of age. *COG-CDGs* also can present with unremitting cholestasis and diverse degree of liver disease, with variably severe neurological involvement, as well as other organ involvement, and growth retardation of intrauterine onset.

13.2.8.2 Amino Acid Metabolism Defects

These diseases are more extensively treated in the Chap. 16. Here the conditions presenting predominantly with cholestasis will be briefly addressed.

Tyrosinemia type 1 (incidence 1:100,000) is caused by an impairment of the aromatic amino acid tyrosine (that is metabolised only in hepatocytes and proximal renal tubular cells) due to loss of the fumarylacetoacetate hydrolase activity (encoded by the *FAH* gene) [79]. The tissue damage is caused by the accumulation of the toxic intermediates fumarylacetoacetate (that is highly mutagenic) and succinylacetone (mitochondrial toxicity, hepatotoxicity), the latter being the major toxic and also a biochemical hallmark of the disease, easily found in the urine of the affected patients [80]. The disease course varies from acute to subacute and chronic forms, with jaundice, cytolysis, hepatomegaly and synthetic derangement, features predominantly characterising the neonatal presentation. Renal tubular dysfunction can be present. In the absence of treatment, the disease leads to cirrhosis and HCC. The diagnosis is easily made, if suspected, by the serum amino acid profile showing elevated tyrosine and methionine and by the urinary organic acid profile revealing high succinylacetone excretion. Low phenylalanine end tyrosine restriction diet is insufficient to prevent liver disease progression, while nitisinone, a compound inhibiting the upward step by the hydroxyphenylpyruvate dioxygenase, dramatically reduces, even though not completely, the metabolite toxicity and the oncogenic risk, especially if introduced before the sixth month of life. LT, required if HCC arises, is curative.

Neonatal intrahepatic cholestasis caused by citrin deficiency (NICCD) is the neonatal phenotype caused by the loss of function of the gene *SLC25A13* encoding citrin, a mitochondrial aspartate glutamate carrier important for aerobic glycolysis and gluconeogenesis. The disease is more common in Eastern Asia. The picture is typically characterised by cholestasis (generally transient), aminoacidaemia (notably increased citrulline but also tyrosine, threonine, arginine and methionine) and galactosuria [81]. Hypoglycemia and failure to thrive coexist in most of the cases described, and evidence of clotting derangement can be present. This rare entity generally improves and completely resolves even spontaneously, but these patients may present later in young adulthood with neurological deterioration due to the secondary urea cycle defect or suddenly with hyperammonemic coma or hypoglycaemia. In these cases chronic liver dysfunction with steatosis may become evident [82]. A prompt diagnosis allows the initiation of a low-carbohydrate diet and helps in preventing the delayed complications.

13.2.9 Defects of the Cellular Energy Production

Mitochondrial disorders (MDSs) are mainly related to mutations in genes involved in the respiratory chain and have heterogeneous phenotypes, most commonly characterised by a defect of cellular energy production. Those presenting with predominant liver involvement are related to nuclear gene products (inherited with autosomal recessive pattern in 90% and autosomal dominant and X-linked pattern in 10%), responsible for mitochondrial DNA replication (*POLG1*), maintenance of deoxyribonucleoside triphosphate (dNTP) pools (*DGUOK*) and membrane mitochondrial integrity (*MPV17*) [83, 84]. Mutations in these genes cause mitochondrial DNA depletion syndromes, characterised by hepatocerebral phenotypes, unlike those of maternal inheritance characterised by predominant neurological involvement. In addition to liver dysfunction, these children present variable degrees of hypotonia, severe developmental delay and failure to thrive; myoclonus and nystagmus are often present. Hypoglycemia, lactic acidosis and plasma amino acid profile consistent with a blocked energy production metabolism are clues to the diagnosis. In *Alpers syndrome* (due to mutations in *POLG1*) sodium valproate administered because of intractable seizures often triggers acute liver decompensation and death. The histological changes on liver biopsy include fatty degeneration, bile duct proliferation, fibrosis and lobular collapse. LT is contraindicated because of the irreversible neurological involvement [85].

13.2.10 Storage Diseases

The hepatic phenotype of *alpha-1 antitrypsin (A1AT) deficiency* is caused by homozygous mutations in the *SERPINA1* gene, modifying the aggregation properties of the protein, so that loop-sheet polymers accumulate in the hepatocytes causing fibrosis and cirrhosis. Some affected children can present early in life with completely acholic stools and histological features mimicking biliary atresia. In most patients, a borderline or frankly low serum A1AT level is a good pointer to the diagnosis, although, since A1AT is an acute phase reactant, during inflammation its serum level can be found in the normal range, and the condition may be overlooked. At liver biopsy, characteristic PAS-positive, diastase-resistant hepatocyte inclusions suggest the aetiology, although these vacuoles tend to develop beyond the first few months of life, resulting an unreliable marker for an early diagnosis.

Lysosomal storage diseases (such as *Niemann-Pick type C*, *Gaucher* and *Wolman disease*) can present with neonatal cholestasis diseases, but hepatosplenomegaly is predominant. In particular, in neonatal/infantile cholestasis, the very early development of splenomegaly (when portal hypertension is very unlikely to be already established) should raise the suspicion of a lysosomal storage disease [86].

13.3 Diagnosis

In a child with neonatal/infantile cholestasis, the surgical causes (biliary atresia, choledochal cyst) should be sought first. If biliary atresia is ruled out, the picture is most likely related to a monogenic liver disease.

Careful physical examination may point out valuable features and symptoms, which might not be obvious in very young patients. Dysmorphisms are quite evident in ARC syndrome and in Zellweger disease spectrum. Triangular-shaped face, prominent forehead, pointed chin and thin hair suggest Alagille syndrome. Transaldolase deficiency, although rare, could be easily recognised by low hair implantation, hirsutism, cutis laxa, low-set ears and clitoridomegaly.

The serum GGT activity is a good discriminant to guide initial evaluation, unravelling at least part of the diagnostic conundrum. In a child with low or normal GGT for age, serum bile acids can point to a diagnosis of PFIC (when elevated) or to a much rarer BASD (if low). In case of a low-GGT PFICs (PFIC1, PFIC2, PFIC4 or TJP2 deficiency, PFIC5 or FXR deficiency, MYO5B deficiency) genetic testing is needed to reach a definite diagnosis. If a BASD is suspected, a screening procedure through urine tandem gas chromatography-mass spectrometry is preferred to characterise the type of defect, and a trio genetic testing can be used for confirmation and for counselling purposes.

In all the other cases, in which GGT is high, the differential diagnosis is rather wide. Serum A1AT is a useful screening for A1AT deficiency, and the diagnosis is confirmed looking for the *SERPINA1* Z-allele mutations. A metabolic screening with urinary galactose, plasma amino acid profile, urinary succinylacetone and organic acids, lactic acid and blood gas analysis can rule out the most common metabolic causes.

When there are no clear pointers to a metabolic and genetic defect, or to confirm a suspected diagnosis, physical or virtual gene panels by next-generation sequencing are the best method to achieve a definite diagnosis in this setting [87].

In Fig. 13.7 we report a diagnostic algorithm that implements the use of genetic testing in such scenario.

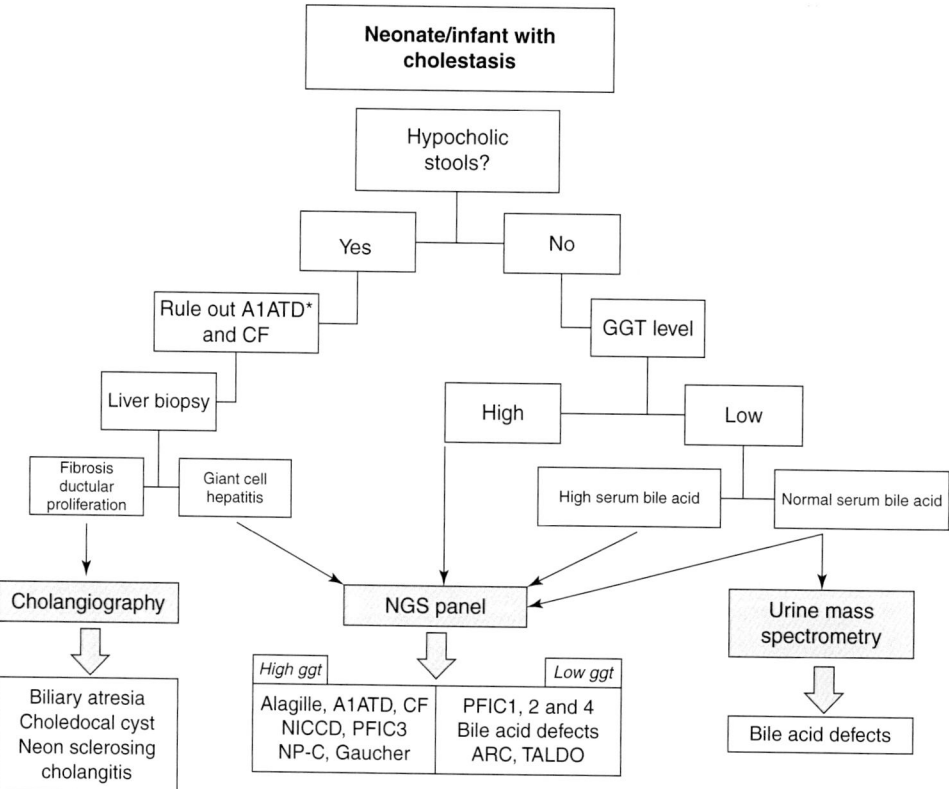

Fig. 13.7 Proposed algorithm for the diagnostic workup of cholestatic infants. *A1ATD* alpha-1 antitrypsin deficiency, *CF* cystic fibrosis, *GGT* gamma-glutamyl transpeptidase, *NICCD* neonatal idiopathic cholestasis due to citrin deficiency, *PFIC* progressive familial intrahepatic cholestasis, *NP-C* Niemann-Pick type C disease, *ARC* arthrogryposis renal dysfunction and cholestasis syndrome, *TALDO* transaldolase deficiency, *In infants with acholic stools, A1AT should be tested in serum before Kasai portoenterostomy, whereas its genetic testing is included in the NGS panel we use in children with cholic stools

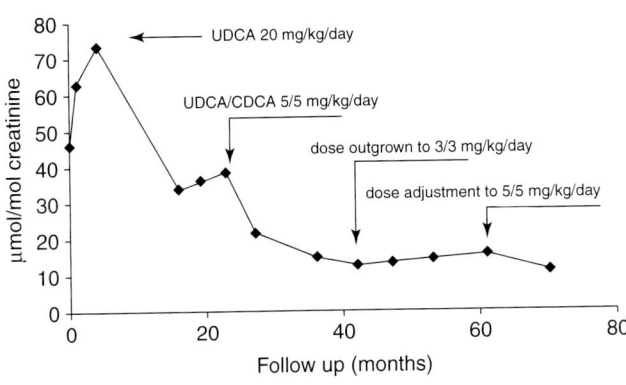

Fig. 13.8 Titration of bile acid supplements based on the level of the toxic metabolite 3β,7α-dihydroxy-5-cholenoic acid (3β-D-OH-5C) in the urine of two patients affected by 3βHSD. UDCA reduces but does not normalise the level of toxic metabolites, whereas CDCA (and cholic acid) does. *CDCA* chenodeoxycholic acid, *UDCA* ursodeoxycholic acid. Adapted from [91]

13.4 Treatment

The primary goal for the treatment of familial/genetic cholestatic diseases is the control of pruritus and possibly of the cholestasis itself. The currently available standard medical treatment is based on UDCA, which replaces the more toxic endogenous bile acids and has choleretic properties increasing the bile flow. Treatment of pruritus is based on symptomatic drugs, such as rifampicin, naloxone/naltrexone and cholestyramine, and antihistaminic drugs. Nutritional support includes fat-soluble vitamin and MCT supplementation.

In case of medical treatment failure, in patients with preserved liver synthetic function and without substantial fibrosis, surgical biliary diversion becomes the first choice. Biliary diversion can be total or partial, external (cholecysto-jejunostomy, button cholecystostomy, less frequently cholecysto-appendicostomy) and internal (generally isoperistaltic jejunal loop connecting the gallbladder and colon; ileal bypass). Whatever the type of surgery, the mechanism of action is based on the reduction of circulating bile acid pool. The overall success rate of these interventions mainly depends on the patients' selection. Patients with PFIC1 have the greatest benefit, while those with PFIC2 should be stratified according to the genotype: patients with at least one mild mutation (p.D482G and p.E297G) are most likely to respond and bear less risk to develop hepatocellular carcinoma. With these cautions, the event-free survival of PFIC patients under biliary diversion increases from 40% to more than 80% [10, 88, 89].

Patients with Alagille syndrome have also been treated with biliary diversion, but the benefit has been much lower than in PFICs, since the progression of fibrosis in presence of uncontrolled cholestasis is the rule [90].

Coming to the new drugs, two bile acid reuptake inhibitors are in the pipeline. Both products (inhibiting the ileal bile acid transporter and the apical sodium-dependent bile acid transporter, respectively) are being tested in phase 3 studies in PFIC1-PFIC2 patients, with the rationale of realising a "medical biliary diversion", depleting the bile acid circulating pool.

Patients with BASDs usually benefit from the administration of primary bile acids, and the specific treatment is described in Table 13.1. Of note, administered primary bile acids bear potential toxic effects; therefore they should be given at the minimum dose sufficient to produce a negative feedback to bile acid synthesis. The required dose of primary bile acid (usually much lower than that used in other cholestatic disorders) can be titrated monitoring the abnormal intermediates in the urine by mass spectrometry [91] (Fig. 13.8).

13.5 Implications for Liver Transplantation

The following situations represent an indication to list the patients affected by genetic cholestatic disorders to LT: the uncontrolled cholestasis in presence of severe fibrosis and cirrhosis, the suspected or confirmed hepatocellular carcinoma and the failure of previous surgical biliary diversion. Overall, PFICs and Alagille syndrome account for some 20% of paediatric LT (http://www.eltr.org/Pediatric-transplantation.html), with overall excellent outcomes. However, specific transplant-related issues must be addressed.

In patients transplanted for PFIC1, the liver allograft can become affected by severe steatosis possibly progressing to steatohepatitis and cirrhosis with graft failure [92, 93]. Since this happens almost invariably in correspondence of exacerbation of diarrhoea, it is very likely that the allograft disease be the result of the interaction between the native bowel and the liver graft by diverse mechanisms. In fact, biliary diversion has been success-

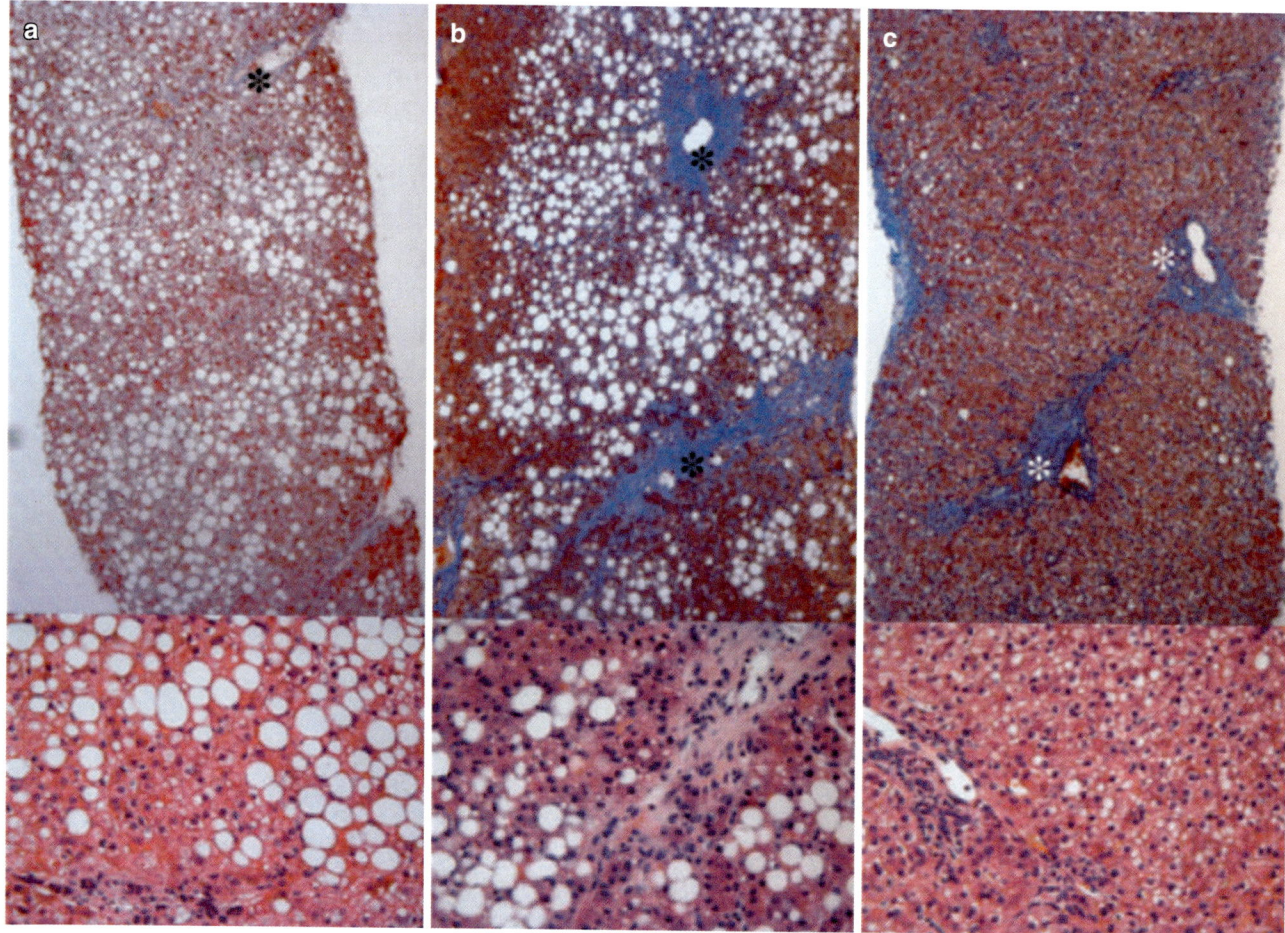

Fig. 13.9 Liver biopsies of a PFIC1 patient developing graft steatohepatitis 6 (**a**) and 24 months (**b**) after LT and 6 months after EBD (30 months after LT; **c**). Both upper and lower pictures show the diffuse macrovacuolar steatosis and the worsening fibrosis beginning from the portal tracts (*) (**a**, **b**). Six months after EBD, a dramatic improvement of the steatosis can be observed (**c**). *LT* liver transplantation, *EBD* external biliary diversion. Adapted from [94]

fully used to treat diarrhoea in these patients, permanently improving graft steatofibrosis and function [94] (Fig. 13.9). The severity of post-LT steatohepatitis is a further reason to consider these patients for a primary biliary diversion before listing them for LT or at the time of LT.

A recurrent post-LT BSEP deficiency, due to the development of anti-BSEP antibodies, has been well described in PFIC2 patients [95]. Such condition has been proved to be complement-mediated, associated with C4d deposition detectable at liver histology, and to improve under rituximab treatment [96].

In Alagille syndrome patients, the pre-LT checklist should routinely encompass a careful cardiological evaluation and a brain angio-MR. In fact, pulmonary obstruction due to stenosis and possible right ventricular dysfunction, as well as the described brain vascular abnormalities, accounts for not negligible transplant morbidity and mortality.

References

1. Davit-Spraul A, Gonzales E, Baussan C, Jacquemin E. Progressive familial intrahepatic cholestasis. Orphanet J Rare Dis. 2009;4(1):1. BioMed Central.
2. Jacquemin E. Progressive familial intrahepatic cholestasis. Clin Res Hepatol Gastroenterol. 2012;36(Suppl 1):S26–35.
3. Fischler B, Papadogiannakis N, Nemeth A. Aetiological factors in neonatal cholestasis. Acta Paediatr. 2007;90(1):88–92. Wiley/Blackwell (10.1111).
4. Kamath BM, Chen Z, Romero R, Fredericks EM, Alonso EM, Arnon R, et al. Quality of life and its determinants in a multicenter cohort of children with Alagille syndrome. J Pediatr. 2015;167(2):390–3.
5. Sambrotta M, Strautnieks S, Papouli E, Rushton P, Clark BE, Parry DA, et al. Mutations in TJP2 cause progressive cholestatic liver disease. Nat Genet. 2014;46(4):326–8.
6. Gomez-Ospina N, Potter CJ, Xiao R, Manickam K, Kim M-S, Kim KH, et al. Mutations in the nuclear bile acid receptor FXR cause progressive familial intrahepatic cholestasis. Nat Commun. 2016;7:10713. Nature Publishing Group.
7. Qiu Y-L, Gong J-Y, Feng J-Y, Wang R-X, Han J, Liu T, et al. Defects in myosin VB are associated with a spectrum of previously

7. undiagnosed low γ-glutamyltransferase cholestasis. Hepatology. 2017;65(5):1655–69.
8. Davit-Spraul A, Fabre M, Branchereau S, Baussan C, Gonzales E, Stieger B, et al. ATP8B1 and ABCB11 analysis in 62 children with normal gamma-glutamyl transferase progressive familial intrahepatic cholestasis (PFIC): phenotypic differences between PFIC1 and PFIC2 and natural history. Hepatology. 2010;51(5):1645–55.
9. Mehaidib Al A, Shahrani Al A. 1381 progressive familial intrahepatic cholestasis in ARABS. J Hepatol. 2013;58:S555–6.
10. Englert C, Grabhorn E, Richter A, Rogiers X, Burdelski M, Ganschow R. Liver transplantation in children with progressive familial intrahepatic cholestasis. Transplantation. 2007;84(10):1361–3.
11. Wanty C, Joomye R, Van Hoorebeek N, Paul K, Otte JB, Reding R, et al. Fifteen years single center experience in the management of progressive familial intrahepatic cholestasis of infancy. Acta Gastroenterol Belg. 2004;67(4):313–9.
12. Jacquemin E. Role of multidrug resistance 3 deficiency in pediatric and adult liver disease: one gene for three diseases. Semin Liver Dis. 2001;21(4):551–62. Copyright © 2001 by Thieme Medical Publishers, Inc., 333 Seventh Avenue, New York, NY 10001, USA. Tel.: +1(212) 584-4662.
13. Lykavieris P, van Mil S, Cresteil D, Fabre M, Hadchouel M, Klomp L, et al. Progressive familial intrahepatic cholestasis type 1 and extrahepatic features: no catch-up of stature growth, exacerbation of diarrhea, and appearance of liver steatosis after liver transplantation. J Hepatol. 2003;39(3):447–52.
14. Demeilliers C, Jacquemin E, Barbu V, Mergey M, Paye F, Fouassier L, et al. Altered hepatobiliary gene expressions in PFIC1: ATP8B1 gene defect is associated with CFTR downregulation. Hepatology. 2006;43(5):1125–34. Wiley-Blackwell.
15. Pauli-Magnus C, Meier PJ. Hepatobiliary transporters and drug-induced cholestasis. Hepatology. 2006;44(4):778–87. Wiley-Blackwell.
16. Davit-Spraul A, Gonzales E, Baussan C, Jacquemin E. The spectrum of liver diseases related to ABCB4Gene mutations: pathophysiology and clinical aspects. Semin Liver Dis. 2010;30(2):134–46. © Thieme Medical Publishers.
17. Paulusma CC, Groen A, Kunne C, Ho-Mok KS, Spijkerboer AL, Rudi de Waart D, et al. Atp8b1 deficiency in mice reduces resistance of the canalicular membrane to hydrophobic bile salts and impairs bile salt transport. Hepatology. 2006;44(1):195–204. Wiley-Blackwell.
18. Chen F, Ananthanarayanan M, Emre S, Neimark E, Bull LN, Knisely AS, et al. Progressive familial intrahepatic cholestasis, type 1, is associated with decreased farnesoid X receptor activity. Gastroenterology. 2004;126(3):756–64.
19. Alvarez L, Jara P, Sánchez-Sabaté E, Hierro L, Larrauri J, Diaz MC, et al. Reduced hepatic expression of farnesoid X receptor in hereditary cholestasis associated to mutation in ATP8B1. Hum Mol Genet. 2004;13(20):2451–60.
20. van der Mark VA, de Jonge HR, Chang J-C, Ho-Mok KS, Duijst S, Vidović D, et al. The phospholipid flippase ATP8B1 mediates apical localization of the cystic fibrosis transmembrane regulator. Biochim Biophys Acta. 2016;1863(9):2280–8.
21. Egawa H, Yorifuji T, Sumazaki R, Kimura A, Hasegawa M, Tanaka K. Intractable diarrhea after liver transplantation for Byler's disease: successful treatment with bile adsorptive resin. Liver Transpl. 2002;8(8):714–6.
22. Strautnieks SS, Byrne JA, Pawlikowska L, Cebecauerová D, Rayner A, Dutton L, et al. Severe bile salt export pump deficiency: 82 different ABCB11 mutations in 109 families. Gastroenterology. 2008;134(4):1203–14.
23. Thompson R, Strautnieks S. BSEP: function and role in progressive familial intrahepatic cholestasis. Semin Liver Dis. 2001;21(4):545–50. Copyright © 2001 by Thieme Medical Publishers, Inc., 333 Seventh Avenue, New York, NY 10001, USA. Tel.: +1(212) 584-4662.
24. Kagawa T, Watanabe N, Mochizuki K, Numari A, Ikeno Y, Itoh J, et al. Phenotypic differences in PFIC2 and BRIC2 correlate with protein stability of mutant Bsep and impaired taurocholate secretion in MDCK II cells. Am J Physiol Gastrointest Liver Physiol. 2008;294(1):G58–67. American Physiological Society.
25. Lam P, Pearson CL, Soroka CJ, Xu S, Mennone A, Boyer JL. Levels of plasma membrane expression in progressive and benign mutations of the bile salt export pump (Bsep/Abcb11) correlate with severity of cholestatic diseases. Am J Physiol Cell Physiol. 2007;293(5):C1709–16. American Physiological Society.
26. Amigo L, Mendoza H, Zanlungo S, Miquel JF, Rigotti A, González S, et al. Enrichment of canalicular membrane with cholesterol and sphingomyelin prevents bile salt-induced hepatic damage. J Lipid Res. 1999;40(3):533–42.
27. Matsubara T, Li F, Gonzalez FJ. FXR signaling in the enterohepatic system. Mol Cell Endocrinol. 2013;368(1–2):17–29.
28. Kuipers F, Bloks VW, Groen AK. Beyond intestinal soap—bile acids in metabolic control. Nat Rev Endocrinol. 2014;10(8):488–98. Nature Publishing Group.
29. Lapierre LA, Kumar R, Hales CM, Navarre J, Bhartur SG, Burnette JO, et al. Myosin Vb is associated with plasma membrane recycling systems. Guidotti G, editor. Mol Biol Cell. 2001;12(6):1843–57.
30. Roland JT, Kenworthy AK, Peranen J, Caplan S, Goldenring JR. Myosin Vb interacts with Rab8a on a tubular network containing EHD1 and EHD3. Brennwald P, editor. Molecular Biology of the Cell. 2007;18(7):2828–37.
31. Swiatecka-Urban A, Talebian L, Kanno E, Moreau-Marquis S, Coutermarsh B, Hansen K, et al. Myosin Vb is required for trafficking of the cystic fibrosis transmembrane conductance regulator in Rab11a-specific apical recycling endosomes in polarized human airway epithelial cells. J Biol Chem. 2007;282(32):23725–36. American Society for Biochemistry and Molecular Biology.
32. Wakabayashi Y, Dutt P, Lippincott-Schwartz J, Arias IM. Rab11a and myosin Vb are required for bile canalicular formation in WIF-B9 cells. Proc Natl Acad Sci U S A. 2005;102(42):15087–92.
33. Girard M, Lacaille F, Verkarre V, Mategot R, Feldmann G, Grodet A, et al. MYO5B and bile salt export pump contribute to cholestatic liver disorder in microvillous inclusion disease. Hepatology. 2014;60(1):301–10. Wiley-Blackwell.
34. Gonzales E, Taylor SA, Davit-Spraul A, Thébaut A, Thomassin N, Guettier C, et al. MYO5B mutations cause cholestasis with normal serum gamma-glutamyl transferase activity in children without microvillous inclusion disease. Hepatology. 2017;65(1):164–73.
35. Sawada N. Tight junction-related human diseases. Pathol Int. 2013;63(1):1–12. Wiley/Blackwell (10.1111).
36. Grosse B, Cassio D, Yousef N, Bernardo C, Jacquemin E, Gonzales E. Claudin-1 involved in neonatal ichthyosis sclerosing cholangitis syndrome regulates hepatic paracellular permeability. Hepatology. 2012;55(4):1249–59. Wiley-Blackwell.
37. Carlton VEH, Harris BZ, Puffenberger EG, Batta AK, Knisely AS, Robinson DL, et al. Complex inheritance of familial hypercholanemia with associated mutations in TJP2 and BAAT. Nat Genet. 2003;34(1):91–6. Nature Publishing Group.
38. Kim M-A, Kim Y-R, Sagong B, Cho H-J, Bae JW, Kim J, et al. Genetic analysis of genes related to tight junction function in the Korean population with non-syndromic hearing loss. Weber CR, editor. PLoS One. 2014;9(4):e95646. Public Library of Science.
39. Paganelli M, Stéphenne X, Gilis A, Jacquemin E, Henrion-Caude A, Girard M, et al. Neonatal ichtyosis and sclerosing cholangitis

syndrome: extremely variable liver disease severity from claudin-1 deficiency. J Pediatr Gastroenterol Nutr. 2011;53(3):350–4.
40. Setchell KDR, Heubi JE. Defects in bile acid biosynthesis-diagnosis and treatment. J Pediatr Gastroenterol Nutr. 2006;43(Suppl 1):S17–22.
41. Heubi J, Setchell K, Bove K. Inborn errors of bile acid metabolism. Semin Liver Dis. 2007;27(3):282–94.
42. Jacquemin E, Setchell KDR, O'Connell NC, Bernard O. A new cause of progressive intrahepatic cholestasis: 3β-Hydroxy-C27-steroid dehydrogenase/isomerase deficiency. J Pediatr. 1994;125(3):379–84.
43. Shneider BL, Setchell KDR, Whitington PF, Neilson KA, Suchy FJ. Δ4-3-Oxosteroid 5β-reductase deficiency causing neonatal liver failure and hemochromatosis. J Pediatr. 1994;124(2):234–8.
44. Daugherty CC, Setchell KD, Heubi JE, Balistreri WF. Resolution of liver biopsy alterations in three siblings with bile acid treatment of an inborn error of bile acid metabolism (delta 4-3-oxosteroid 5 beta-reductase deficiency). Hepatology. 1993;18(5):1096–101.
45. Pierre G, Setchell K, Blyth J, Preece MA, Chakrapani A, McKiernan P. Prospective treatment of cerebrotendinous xanthomatosis with cholic acid therapy. J Inherit Metab Dis. 2008;31(S2):241–5.
46. Vaz FM, Bootsma AH, Kulik W, Verrips A, Wevers RA, Schielen PC, et al. A newborn screening method for cerebrotendinous xanthomatosis using bile alcohol glucuronides and metabolite ratios. J Lipid Res. 2017;58(5):1002–7. American Society for Biochemistry and Molecular Biology.
47. Clayton PT, Verrips A, Sistermans E, Mann A, Mieli-Vergani G, Wevers R. Mutations in the sterol 27-hydroxylase gene (CYP27A) cause hepatitis of infancy as well as cerebrotendinous xanthomatosis. J Inherit Metab Dis. 2002;25(6):501–13.
48. Gong J-Y, Setchell KDR, Zhao J, Zhang W, Wolfe B, Lu Y, et al. Severe neonatal cholestasis in cerebrotendinous xanthomatosis: genetics, immunostaining, mass spectrometry. J Pediatr Gastroenterol Nutr. 2017;65(5):561–8.
49. Heubi J, Setchell K, Bove K. Inborn errors of bile acid metabolism. Semin Liver Dis. 2007;27(3):282–94. Copyright © 2007 by Thieme Medical Publishers, Inc., 333 Seventh Avenue, New York, NY 10001, USA.
50. Heubi JE, Setchell KDR, Jha P, Buckley D, Zhang W, Rosenthal P, et al. Treatment of bile acid amidation defects with glycocholic acid. Hepatology. 2015;61(1):268–74. 1st ed. Wiley-Blackwell.
51. Setchell KD, Schwarz M, O'Connell NC, Lund EG, Davis DL, Lathe R, et al. Identification of a new inborn error in bile acid synthesis: mutation of the oxysterol 7alpha-hydroxylase gene causes severe neonatal liver disease. J Clin Invest. 1998;102(9):1690–703. American Society for Clinical Investigation.
52. Ueki I, Kimura A, Nishiyori A, Chen H-L, Takei H, Nittono H, et al. Neonatal cholestatic liver disease in an Asian patient with a homozygous mutation in the oxysterol 7α-hydroxylase gene. J Pediatr Gastroenterol Nutr. 2008;46(4):465–9.
53. Goldfischer S, Moore CL, Johnson AB, Spiro AJ, Valsamis MP, Wisniewski HK, et al. Peroxisomal and mitochondrial defects in the cerebro-hepato-renal syndrome. Science. 1973;182(4107):62–4.
54. Poll-The BT, Saudubray JM, Ogier H, Schutgens RB, Wanders RJ, Schrakamp G, et al. Infantile Refsum's disease: biochemical findings suggesting multiple peroxisomal dysfunction. J Inherit Metab Dis. 1986;9(2):169–74.
55. Goldfischer S, Collins J, Rapin I, Coltoff-Schiller B, Chang CH, Nigro M, et al. Peroxisomal defects in neonatal-onset and X-linked adrenoleukodystrophies. Science. 1985;227(4682):67–70.
56. Smith DW, Lemli L, Opitz JM. A newly recognized syndrome of multiple congenital anomalies. J Pediatr. 1964;64(2):210–7.
57. Zhou Y, Zhang J. Arthrogryposis–renal dysfunction–cholestasis (ARC) syndrome: from molecular genetics to clinical features. Ital J Pediatr. 2014;40(1):1. BioMed Central.
58. Gissen P, Tee L, Johnson CA, Genin E, Caliebe A, Chitayat D, et al. Clinical and molecular genetic features of ARC syndrome. Hum Genet. 2006;120(3):396–409.
59. Peterson MR, Emr SD. The class C Vps complex functions at multiple stages of the vacuolar transport pathway. Traffic. 2001;2(7):476–86. Wiley/Blackwell (10.1111).
60. Cullinane AR, Straatman-Iwanowska A, Zaucker A, Wakabayashi Y, Bruce CK, Luo G, et al. Mutations in VIPAR cause an arthrogryposis, renal dysfunction and cholestasis syndrome phenotype with defects in epithelial polarization. Nat Genet. 2010;42(4):303–12. Nature Publishing Group.
61. Saleh M, Kamath BM, Chitayat D. Alagille syndrome: clinical perspectives. Appl Clin Genet. 2016;9:75–82. Dove Press.
62. Danks DM, Campbell PE, Jack I, Rogers J, Smith AL. Studies of the aetiology of neonatal hepatitis and biliary atresia. Arch Dis Child. 1977;52(5):360–7.
63. Emerick KM, Rand EB, Goldmuntz E, Krantz ID, Spinner NB, Piccoli DA. Features of Alagille syndrome in 92 patients: frequency and relation to prognosis. Hepatology. 1999;29(3):822–9. Wiley-Blackwell.
64. Kamath BM, Spinner NB, Emerick KM, Chudley AE, Booth C, Piccoli DA, et al. Vascular anomalies in Alagille syndrome: a significant cause of morbidity and mortality. Circulation. 2004;109(11):1354–8. American Heart Association, Inc.
65. Kamath BM, Spinner NB, Rosenblum ND. Renal involvement and the role of Notch signalling in Alagille syndrome. Nat Rev Nephrol. 2013;9(7):409–18.
66. Mašek J, Andersson ER. The developmental biology of genetic Notch disorders. Development. 2017;144(10):1743–63. Oxford University Press for the Company of Biologists Limited.
67. Antoniou A, Raynaud P, Cordi S, Zong Y, Tronche F, Stanger BZ, et al. Intrahepatic bile ducts develop according to a new mode of tubulogenesis regulated by the transcription factor SOX9. Gastroenterology. 2009;136(7):2325–33.
68. Geisler F, Nagl F, Mazur PK, Lee M, Zimber-Strobl U, Strobl LJ, et al. Liver-specific inactivation of Notch2, but not Notch1, compromises intrahepatic bile duct development in mice. Hepatology. 2008;48(2):607–16. Wiley-Blackwell.
69. Kodama Y, Hijikata M, Kageyama R, Shimotohno K, Chiba T. The role of notch signaling in the development of intrahepatic bile ducts. Gastroenterology. 2004;127(6):1775–86.
70. Walter TJ, Vanderpool C, Cast AE, Huppert SS. Intrahepatic bile duct regeneration in mice does not require Hnf6 or notch signaling through Rbpj. Am J Pathol. 2014;184(5):1479–88.
71. Riely CA. Arteriohepatic dysplasia: a benign syndrome of intrahepatic cholestasis with multiple organ involvement. Ann Intern Med. 1979;91(4):520–7. American College of Physicians.
72. Pavanello M, Severino M, D'Antiga L, Castellan L, Calvi A, Colledan M, et al. Pretransplant management of basilar artery aneurysm and moyamoya disease in a child with Alagille syndrome. Liver Transpl. 2015;21(9):1227–30. Wiley-Blackwell.
73. Grammatikopoulos T, Sambrotta M, Strautnieks S, Foskett P, Knisely AS, Wagner B, et al. Mutations in DCDC2 (doublecortin domain containing protein 2) in neonatal sclerosing cholangitis. J Hepatol. 2016;65(6):1179–87.
74. Girard M, Bizet AA, Lachaux A, Gonzales E, Filhol E, Collardeau-Frachon S, et al. DCDC2 mutations cause neonatal sclerosing cholangitis. Hum Mutat. 2016;37(10):1025–9. Wiley-Blackwell.
75. Verhoeven NM, Huck JHJ, Roos B, Struys EA, Salomons GS, Douwes AC, et al. Transaldolase deficiency: liver cirrhosis associated with a new inborn error in the pentose phosphate pathway. Am J Hum Genet. 2001;68(5):1086–92.
76. Ng BG, Freeze HH. Perspectives on glycosylation and its congenital disorders. Trends Genet. 2018;34(6):466–76.
77. Marques-da-Silva D, Reis Ferreira dos V, Monticelli M, Janeiro P, Videira PA, Witters P, et al. Liver involvement in congenital dis-

orders of glycosylation (CDG). A systematic review of the literature. J Inherit Metab Dis. 2017;40(2):195–207. 6th ed. Springer Netherlands.
78. Jansen JC, Cirak S, van Scherpenzeel M, Timal S, Reunert J, Rust S, et al. CCDC115 deficiency causes a disorder of Golgi homeostasis with abnormal protein glycosylation. Am J Hum Genet. 2016;98(2):310–21.
79. Morrow G, Tanguay RM. Biochemical and clinical aspects of hereditary tyrosinemia type 1. Adv Exp Med Biol. 2017;959(11):9–21. 8th ed. Cham: Springer International Publishing.
80. Grompe M. The pathophysiology and treatment of hereditary tyrosinemia type 1. Semin Liver Dis. 2001;21(4):563–71. Copyright © 2001 by Thieme Medical Publishers, Inc., 333 Seventh Avenue, New York, NY 10001, USA. Tel.: +1(212) 584-4662.
81. Dimmock D, Kobayashi K, Iijima M, Tabata A, Wong LJ, Saheki T, et al. Citrin deficiency: a novel cause of failure to thrive that responds to a high-protein, low-carbohydrate diet. Pediatrics. 2007;119(3):e773–7.
82. Fiermonte G, Soon D, Chaudhuri A, Paradies E, Lee PJ, Krywawych S, et al. An adult with type 2 citrullinemia presenting in Europe. N Engl J Med. 2008;358(13):1408–9.
83. Cui H, Li F, Chen D, Wang G, Truong CK, Enns GM, et al. Comprehensive next-generation sequence analyses of the entire mitochondrial genome reveal new insights into the molecular diagnosis of mitochondrial DNA disorders. Genet Med. 2013;15(5):388–94. Springer Nature.
84. Dames S, Chou L-S, Xiao Y, Wayman T, Stocks J, Singleton M, et al. The development of next-generation sequencing assays for the mitochondrial genome and 108 nuclear genes associated with mitochondrial disorders. J Mol Diagn. 2013;15(4):526–34. Elsevier.
85. Spinazzola A, Invernizzi F, Carrara F, Lamantea E, Donati A, Dirocco M, et al. Clinical and molecular features of mitochondrial DNA depletion syndromes. J Inherit Metab Dis. 2008;32(2):143–58. Springer Netherlands.
86. Gotti G, Marseglia A, De Giacomo C, Iascone M, Sonzogni A, D'Antiga L. Neonatal Jaundice with splenomegaly: not a common pick. Fetal Pediatr Pathol. 2016;35(2):108–11.
87. Nicastro E, D'Antiga L. Next generation sequencing in pediatric hepatology and liver transplantation. Liver Transpl. 2018;24(2):282–93. Wiley-Blackwell.
88. Arnell H, Papadogiannakis N, Zemack H, Knisely AS, Nemeth A, Fischler B. Follow-up in children with progressive familial intrahepatic cholestasis after partial external biliary diversion. J Pediatr Gastroenterol Nutr. 2010;51(4):494–9.
89. Davit-Spraul A, Fabre M, Branchereau S, Baussan C, Gonzales E, Stieger B, et al. ATP8B1 and ABCB11 analysis in 62 children with normal gamma-glutamyl transferase progressive familial intrahepatic cholestasis (PFIC): phenotypic differences between PFIC1 and PFIC2 and natural history. Hepatology. 2010;51(5):1645–55. Wiley-Blackwell.
90. Emerick KM, Elias MS, Melin-Aldana H, Strautnieks S, Thompson RJ, Bull LN, et al. Bile composition in Alagille syndrome and PFIC patients having partial external biliary diversion. BMC Gastroenterol. 2008;8:47.
91. Riello L, D'Antiga L, Guido M, Alaggio R, Giordano G, Zancan L. Titration of bile acid supplements in 3beta-hydroxy-Delta 5-C27-steroid dehydrogenase/isomerase deficiency. J Pediatr Gastroenterol Nutr. 2010;50(6):655–60.
92. Miyagawa-Hayashino A, Egawa H, Yorifuji T, Hasegawa M, Haga H, Tsuruyama T, et al. Allograft steatohepatitis in progressive familial intrahepatic cholestasis type 1 after living donor liver transplantation. Liver Transpl. 2009;15(6):610–8. Wiley-Blackwell.
93. Usui M, Isaji S, Das BC, Kobayashi M, Osawa I, Iida T, et al. Liver retransplantation with external biliary diversion for progressive familial intrahepatic cholestasis type 1: a case report. Pediatr Transplant. 2009;13(5):611–4. Wiley/Blackwell (10.1111).
94. Nicastro E, Stéphenne X, Smets F, Fusaro F, de Magnée C, Reding R, et al. Recovery of graft steatosis and protein-losing enteropathy after biliary diversion in a PFIC 1 liver transplanted child. Pediatr Transplant. 2012;16(5):E177–82.
95. Jara P, Hierro L, Martínez-Fernández P, Alvarez-Doforno R, Yánez F, Diaz MC, et al. Recurrence of bile salt export pump deficiency after liver transplantation. N Engl J Med. 2009;361(14):1359–67. Massachusetts Medical Society.
96. Patel KR, Harpavat S, Finegold M, Eldin K, Hicks J, Firan M, et al. Post-transplant recurrent bile salt export pump disease: a form of antibody-mediated graft dysfunction and utilization of C4d. J Pediatr Gastroenterol Nutr. 2017;65(4):364–9.

Wilson's Disease

Piotr Socha and Wojciech Janczyk

Key Points
- Wilson's disease should be considered in children older than 1 year with any symptoms of liver disease.
- Diagnosis of WD should be made based on combination of liver tests, copper metabolism markers, and ATP7B gene molecular analysis.
- Quick diagnosis of Wilson's disease is essential in acute liver failure.
- In a long term, effect of therapy is mainly dependent on compliance.
- The King's College index should be applied in acute liver failure to make decisions on liver transplantation in WD patients.

Research Needed in the Field
- To explain variable course of WD (gene modifiers? environmental factors?)
- To explain pathophysiology and progression of organ injury in WD
- To develop noninvasive markers of liver injury in WD
- To test new drugs and gene therapy

14.1 Introduction

Wilson's disease (WD) is an autosomal recessive genetic disorder of copper metabolism leading to liver or brain injury. The estimated prevalence is around 1:30,000 but WD seems to be underdiagnosed [1]. It is caused by mutations in the *ATP7B* gene encoding a copper transporting P-type ATPase—which is responsible for copper binding with ceruloplasmin and is required for copper excretion into the bile. ATPase dysfunction leads to progressive accumulation of copper in the liver from infancy and consequently in other organs, mainly in the nervous system and corneas but also in kidneys and the heart [2].

Recently, the European expert group published a position statement on diagnosis and treatment of Wilson's disease in children on behalf of the European Society for Pediatric Gastroenterology, Hepatology, and Nutrition which gives important clinical recommendations [3].

14.2 Copper Metabolism and WD

Copper is carried in portal blood as Cu^{2+}, as the hepatocyte basolateral membrane is reduced to Cu^+, by a metalloreductase, and is presented to the high-affinity copper uptake transporter, Ctr1. Within the hepatocyte, copper is chaperoned to its various sites of action so is always protein bound [4] (Fig. 14.1). Copper transport protein antioxidant 1, or atox1, presents Cu to the six similar N-terminal Cu-binding sequences of ATP7B. APT7B is essential for further trafficking of copper—which includes excretion to the bile and binding with ceruloplasmin (Cp). Most serum copper is in Cp. Non-Cp copper includes a fraction bound to albumin and to a high molecular weight carrier, transcuprein. Cp is a marker of WD, but has no direct pathologic significance. Low plasma ceruloplasmin concentrations are found in WD and heterozygotes; Menkes syndrome; copper deficiency; some congenital disorders of glycosylation; and a recently described MEDNIK disorder of mental retardation, enteropathy, deafness, neuropathy, ichthyosis, and keratodermia caused by AP1S1 gene mutations [5].

ATP7B-ase mutations cause Wilson's disease by disturbing copper metabolism-decreased trafficking to bile, and decreased binding to ceruloplasmin leads to copper accumulation in the liver and other tissues (Fig. 14.1). Given the extreme clinical variability of WD, it would be prognostically very useful if

P. Socha (✉) · W. Janczyk
The Children's Memorial Health Institute, Warsaw, Poland
e-mail: P.Socha@IPCZD.PL; w.janczyk@ipczd.pl

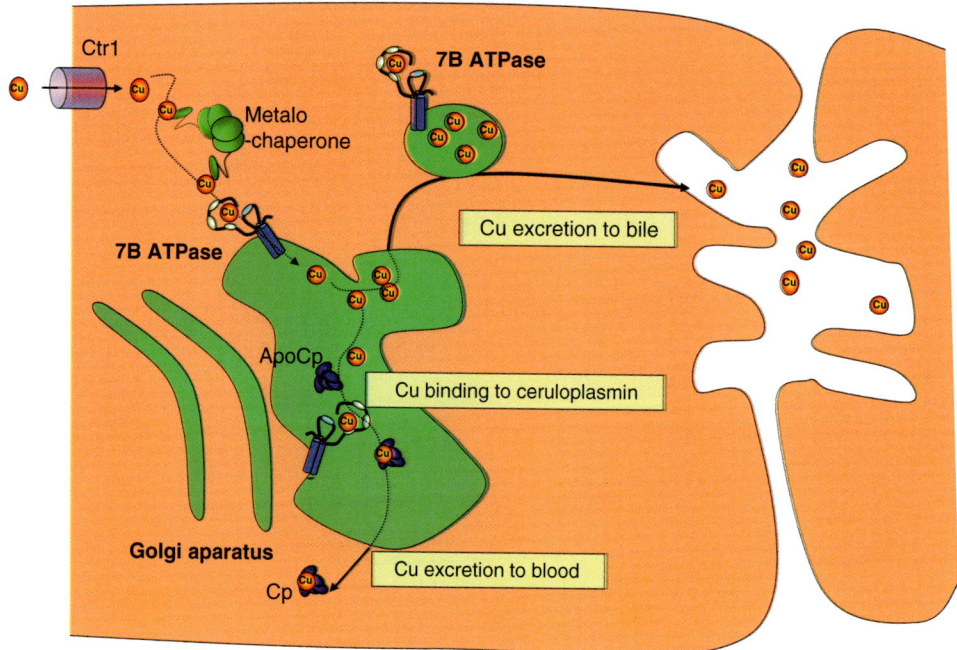

Fig. 14.1 Copper metabolism under physiological conditions

there was a clear mutation/phenotype relationship. Still, many studies were not able to find a clear relationship between clinical symptoms and mutations. However, patients homozygous for H1069Q tend to present later and with neurological disease. It was also suggested that fulminant hepatic failure is more likely in patients with truncating mutations.

14.3 Clinical Presentation

Children present mainly with liver disease—the most frequent are incidentally detected increased serum transaminases—which may be combined with hepatomegaly, hyperechogenic liver on ultrasound, or severe cause of liver disease as acute liver failure (ALF) or cirrhosis. The presenting symptoms can be complications of liver cirrhosis like portal hypertension with esophageal varices, splenomegaly, low platelet count, or decompensated cirrhosis with ascites [6]. WD was described in children from over 2 years of age but is rarely symptomatic before 5 years of age [7].

Differential diagnosis should include viral hepatitis, non-alcoholic fatty liver disease (NAFLD), autoimmune hepatitis (AIH), and metabolic liver diseases [8]. AIH can be confused with WD as low-titre autoantibodies can be found in WD. It should be advised to exclude Wilson disease before making diagnosis of AIH or when AIH poorly responds to treatment.

Neurological symptoms are rarely seen in childhood and usually do not occur before the age of 10 years. Kayser-Fleischer (K-F) ring, caused by copper deposition on Descemet's membrane, may appear mainly in neurological presentation of WD but is very rare in children. Still, the slit lamp examination should be performed in children as this is a typical feature of WD. Other symptoms that may be observed are acute hemolysis and psychiatric problems (like depression) [9].

14.4 Diagnosis of WD

Diagnosis of WD can be a challenge as it cannot be based on single test and especially young asymptomatic children may have normal ceruloplasmin levels and urinary copper excretion.

Wilson disease can be diagnosed based on clinical symptoms and laboratory tests. Neurological symptoms are relatively typical for WD, but liver symptoms are not specific enough and require wide laboratory testing.

Therefore, the Ferenci scoring system should be applied to children for diagnosis of WD, which combines laboratory and clinical findings (Table 14.1). It was agreed in 2001 at an international expert meeting [10]. Mutation analysis of the ATPB7 gene is included in the scoring system, and determination of two disease-causing mutations can finally establish the diagnosis.

In children, the Ferenci score provided a relatively high sensitivity and specificity for the diagnosis of WD in children—98.14% and 96.59%, respectively, in one study and 90% and 91.6%, respectively, in the other. In this latest study, considering 40 μg/24 h instead of 100 μg/24 h as the urinary copper excretion, cutoff increased the sensitivity of the scoring system to 93% with no change in the specificity [11].

Ceruloplasmin is one of the major laboratory tests used for diagnosis of WD. It is responsible for transportation of the circulating copper and can be decreased when copper-

Table 14.1 Diagnostic Ferenci score for Wilson's disease, agreed at a consensus meeting [10]

Score	−1	0	1	2	4
Kayser-Fleischer rings		Absent		Present	
Neuropsychiatric symptoms suggestive of WD (or typical brain MRI)		Absent		Present	
Coombs-negative hemolytic anemia + high serum copper		Absent	Present		
Urinary copper (in the absence of acute hepatitis)		Normal	1–2 × ULN	>2 × ULN or normal but >5 × ULN 1 day after challenge with 2 × 0.5 g d-penicillamine	
Liver copper quantitative	Normal		<5 × ULN (<250 μg/g)	>5 × ULN (>250 μg/g)	
Rhodanine staining for copper of liver biopsy (only if quantitative Cu measurement is not available)		Absent	Present		
Serum ceruloplasmin concentration (nephelometric assay)		>0.2 g/L	0.1–0.2 g/L	<0.1 g/L	
Disease-causing mutations detected		None	1		2
Diagnosis of Wilson's disease is					
0–1: unlikely		**2–3: probable**		**4 or more: highly likely**	

Abbreviations: *ULN* upper limit of normal

binding capacity decreases with low ATP7B activity. Serum ceruloplasmin concentration is low in neonates, and standard normal levels can not be applied at this age. Typically in WD, ceruloplasmin is reduced below 20 mg/dL (Table 14.2) but can be normal in about 20% patients [12]. Heterozygotes can also present with decreased serum ceruloplasmin levels, which can be also found in liver failure, glycosylation disorders, Menkes disease, nephrotic syndrome, protein-losing enteropathy, and hereditary aceruloplasminemia.

There are different methods to measure ceruloplasmin—the enzymatic assay measuring oxidase activity is more accurate, while the immunological-nephelometric assay which measures both ceruloplasmin and the biologically inactive apo-form may give slightly increased levels.

Total serum copper had been also used for diagnosis of WD, but finally it is not included in the diagnostic set as it may be decreased with the decreased serum ceruloplasmin or may increase. The serum-free copper (non-ceruloplasmin-bound copper) concentration usually increases in WD, but as this is not the direct measurement—estimated from the serum copper and serum ceruloplasmin levels—it is not highly accurate for diagnosis.

Urinary copper excretion can be regarded a basic diagnostic test for WD, which should be performed with ceruloplasmin determination. In young children or in asymptomatic children, urinary copper values are often normal. The basal urinary copper diagnostic cutoff value is 40 μg/24 h (0.65 μmol/24 h), but the cutoff values of 100 μg/24 h (Table 14.2) are regarded to be specific for WD [11]. The penicillamine challenge test (i.e., 0.5 g d-penicillamine given at the beginning of the 24-h urine collection and 12 h later) is not commonly used in children because of its low sensitivity—especially in asymptomatic children.

Table 14.2 Copper metabolism tests in diagnosis of Wilson's disease

	Normal values	Suspicion of Wilson's disease
Serum ceruloplasmin	20–40 mg/dL	<20 mg/dL (high suspicion when <10 mg/dL)
24-h urinary copper excretion	<40 μg (<0.65 μmol)	>100 μg (1.6 μmol)
Liver copper content	<50 μg/g dry weight	>250 μg/g dry weight (>4 μmol/g dry weight)

Sensitivity depends on the cutoff values which can be 12% for 1575 μg/24 h (25 μmol/24 h), or increase to 88% with lowering the cutoff to five times the upper normal limit of basal urinary copper excretion (200 μg/24 h, 3.2 μmol/24 h) increased the sensitivity to 88% but with a considerable loss in specificity (24.1%) [13]. There is a high risk of contamination of urine sample with copper—patient should be advised about the procedure and use plastic or acid-washed glass containers.

Mutation analysis can finally confirm diagnosis. There are more than 500 ATP7B gene mutations—mostly identified as compound heterozygotes [14]. High frequency of some mutations was reported for specific populations like H1069Q mutations which are very frequent in Eastern Europe and Met645Arg which is common in Spain and c-441_427del15 in Sardinia and 229insC and Arg778Leu in Japan. Some caution when reading the molecular results is needed—mainly when new mutation/variants are identified with unknown functionality—but also some molecular defects outside the coding regions and small deletions can be missed. Still, the availability of next-generation sequencing (NGS) makes the diagnosis of Wilson's disease much easier [15].

Copper estimation in the liver tissue could be helpful in children where the diagnosis is uncertain. Liver biopsy is usually performed for differential diagnosis or to assess liver damage—in this case, liver sample should be preserved for estimation of copper (preferably >1 cm long, min. 0.5 cm, in a dry plastic copper-free container). The diagnostic value of WD is copper content greater than 250 μg/g dry weight (normal <50 μg/g dry weight). The test is relatively specific but liver copper can also increase in cholestatic patients, mainly in PSC. Lower concentrations were also described in WD which could be related to sampling error. In an adult large cohort (178 patients with WD), a high proportion (47.8%) of patients with primary biliary cirrhosis or primary sclerosing cholangitis also had liver copper values ≥250 μg/g dry weight [16]. Nicastro et al. in a pediatric study reported an increase in liver copper >250 μg/g dry weight in 28 of 30 WD children with mild liver disease [11].

Liver histology does not allow to establish the diagnosis of WD. Various features of liver injury can be described including inflammation, portal fibrosis, microvesicular and macrovesicular steatosis, or cirrhosis [17]. Copper deposition may be demonstrable by rhodanine, orcein, or rubeanic acid staining but has limited diagnostic value and should not replace direct copper measurement (Fig. 14.2).

Some other tests can be also used for diagnosis of WD, but are not commonly available and are not well validated. These include the measurement of the incorporation of radiolabeled copper into ceruloplasmin and the measurement of serum exchangeable copper. Exchangeable copper (CuEXC) corresponds to the labile fraction of copper in the serum complexed to albumin and other peptides and has been reported to provide 100% sensitivity and 100% specificity for the diagnosis of WD in adults [18].

Liver function tests may help to raise suspicion of WD but do not allow to establish diagnosis. In acute presentation of WD with liver failure, high total bilirubin levels (>300 μmol/L, >17.5 mg/dL) combined with relatively low serum transaminase levels (100–500 IU/L) and low serum alkaline phosphatase level (due to zinc deficiency) presenting with a low alkaline phosphatase (IU/L) to total bilirubin (mg/dL) ratio <1 can be observed [19].

14.5 Genetic Counseling and Family Screening

Genetic counseling is essential for families of WD patients to assess the risks of the disease in the family. All siblings of any patient newly diagnosed with WD should be screened for WD because the chance of being a homozygote and developing clinical disease is 25%. This should include serum ceruloplasmin, liver function tests, and molecular testing for ATP7B mutations in all children above 2 years of age [3]. It seems reasonable to screen also an offspring of an affected parent as the occurrence of WD in two consecutive generations has been reported in apparently nonconsanguineous families. Taking into account late onset of WD, parents of a child newly diagnosed with WD should also be screened by performing liver tests, ceruloplasmin, urinary copper excretion, and suitable genetic testing [20].

14.6 Treatment

Pharmacological treatment in Wilson's disease aims to remove excess of copper by inhibition of intestinal copper absorption (zinc salts) or by chelating agents such as

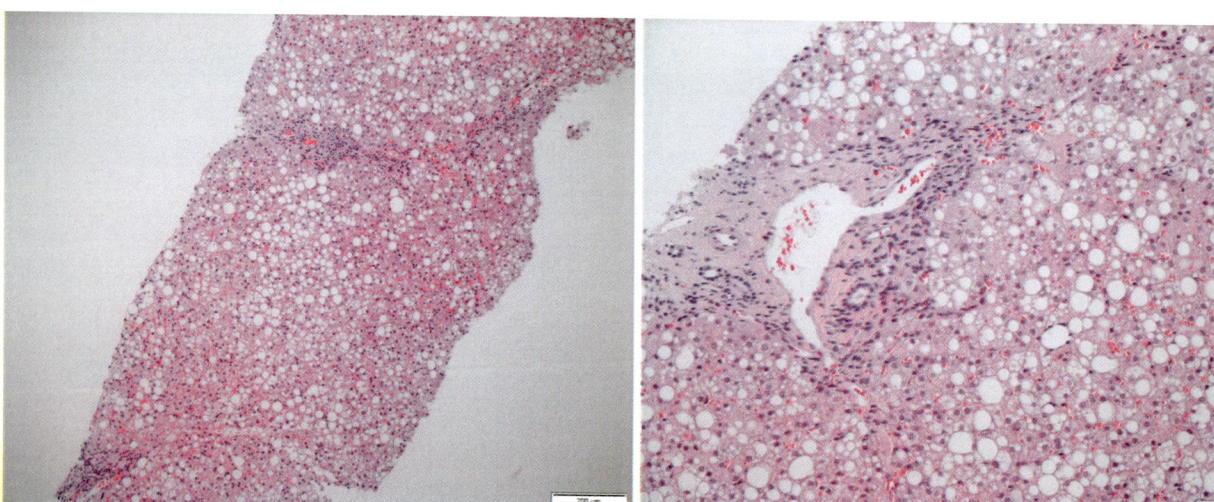

Fig. 14.2 Histopathology of the liver biopsy in a patient with Wilson's disease-massive steatosis, periportal and lobular inflammation, and moderate fibrosis (from Maciej Pronicki, Department of Pathology, The Children's Memorial Health Institute)

Table 14.3 Dosage and monitoring of therapy in WD

	Zinc acetate/sulfate	D-Penicillamine	Trientine
Dosage	**Per elemental zinc** • Age >16 years and body weight >50 kg: 150 mg/day in three divided doses • Age 6–16 years and body weight <50 kg: 75 mg/day in three divided doses • Under 6 years of age: 50 mg/day in two divided doses	• Starting dose: 150–300 mg/day, gradually increasing once a week up to 20 mg/kg/day given in two or three divided doses or 1000 mg (max 1500 mg) in young adults given in two or four divided doses • Maintenance dose: 10–20 mg/kg/day up to 750–1000 mg/day in two divided doses	• Starting dose: 20 mg/kg/day or 1000 mg (max 1500 mg) in young adults given in two or three divided doses • Maintenance dose: 900–1500 mg/day in two or three divided doses
Administration	1 h before meal or 2 h after meal	1 h before meal or 2 h after meal	1 h before meal or 3 h after meal
Adequacy of treatment parameters	• Urinary copper excretion: 30–75 µg (0.5–1.2 µM)/24 h on maintenance treatment • Serum zinc level >125 µg/dL • Urinary zinc >2 mg/24 h on maintenance treatment	• Urinary copper excretion: 200–500 µg (3–8 µM)/24 h on maintenance treatment	• Urinary copper excretion: 200–500 µg (3–8 µM)/24 h on maintenance treatment
Liver function improvement	Usually 2–6 months, ALT normalization up to 1 year	Up to 6 months	Up to 6 months
Indication for a drug change	• Persistent ALT >3x upper limit of normal and/or INR >1.5 • Poor tolerance or side effects, e.g., abdominal pain	Poor tolerance or side effects	Poor tolerance or side effects

d-penicillamine and trientine. Copper-rich food (e.g., shellfish, nuts, chocolate, mushrooms, and organ meats) should be avoided; however, its restriction does not necessary prevent copper accumulation [21]. Treatment should be started immediately after diagnosis in symptomatic children to prevent further progression of liver and/or neurological disease. Pre-symptomatic children diagnosed by family screening should receive treatment no later than at 3 years of age. There is no high-quality evidence for the optimal first-line treatment choice in WD.

14.7 D-Penicillamine

D-Penicillamine chelates copper and enhances its excretion into urine. Additionally, it induces the endogenous hepatic metallothionein—a cytosolic metal-binding protein which sequesters copper and prevents liver from its toxic effects.

D-Penicillamine has been shown to efficiently prevent the progression of disease in children with WD. It improved liver symptoms in over 80% of symptomatic children within a mean time of 16 months [22], including those presenting with liver failure but no hepatic encephalopathy.

Adverse effects due to d-penicillamine resulted in drug withdrawal in up to 30% of cases in children or adults [23, 24]. Worsening of neurologic symptoms also occurred [25]. Early adverse effects include sensitivity reactions, e.g., fever, cutaneous eruptions, neutropenia thrombocytopenia, lymphadenopathy, and proteinuria. There are reports of d-penicillamine-related lupus-like syndrome, bone marrow toxicity with severe thrombocytopenia or aplasia, and skin changes as *elastosis perforans serpiginosa*, *cutis laxa*, pemphigus, *lichen planus*, and aphthous stomatitis [26].

The dose of d-penicillamine should be gradually increased to 20 mg/kg/day given in two or three doses with close follow-up for the occurrence of adverse events mentioned above. Drug should be administered 1 h before or 2 h after meals (Table 14.3).

14.8 Trientine

Triethylene tetramine hydrochloride (trientine) was originally introduced as a second-line chelating agent in patients with WD who developed adverse events related to d-penicillamine [27]. Adverse effects to trientine seem to be less frequent than d-penicillamine but may include allergic reactions, arthralgias, muscle cramps, and sideroblastic anemia [28].

The therapeutic efficacy of trientine is similar to d-penicillamine which was shown a cohort of adults with liver symptoms [29]. Interestingly trientine, when compared to d-penicillamine, had a higher risk of neurologic worsening in patients with neurologic manifestation of WD. In a pediatric study, trientine, used as second-line therapy after d-penicillamine intolerance, improved liver function but did not alleviate accompanying neurological or psychiatric symptoms [28].

The dose of trientine in children is 20 mg/kg/day given in 2–3 doses. During therapy, patients should avoid concomitant iron supplementation. Tablets must be kept refrigerated and given 1 h before or 2–3 h after food for optimal absorption (Table 14.3).

14.9 Zinc

Zinc induces metallothionein in enterocytes, and subsequently copper is sequestered in enterocytes which at the end of their life cycle carry copper into the lumen. Zinc also has impact on hepatocyte metallothionein and may have additional copper detoxifying effect.

Zinc salts are usually used as first-line treatment of asymptomatic or pre-symptomatic patients and for maintenance therapy after initial de-coppering with d-penicillamine. Zinc monotherapy in symptomatic patients with liver disease has been questioned [30]. Zinc as first-line monotherapy showed a better tolerance profile than d-penicillamine in various presentations of WD [31, 32]. However, treatment failure was reported in symptomatic children with liver disease. Furthermore, patients who relapsed on zinc improved after reintroduction of chelating agents [33, 34]. As in other treatment modalities, zinc salts also present risk of neurological deterioration [35].

There are several formulations of zinc salts available: zinc sulfate, zinc acetate, and zinc gluconate. Zinc sulfate is associated with gastrointestinal problems, such as nausea, vomiting, epigastric pain, and gastric/duodenal mucosal ulceration that may lead to poor adherence [36]. They usually resolve when switching to zinc acetate. Other less common adverse reactions include anemia and increase of serum amylase and lipase levels without clinical and radiological features of pancreatitis.

The recommended dose of zinc is 25 mg of elemental zinc in children under 5 years of age, 75 mg/day (<50 kg of body weight) or 150 mg/day (if body weight >50 kg) in 2–3 divided doses (3, 92, 94). Zinc should not be taken with food because it interferes with its absorption (Table 14.3).

14.10 Treatment Considerations in Wilson's Disease

Pharmacological treatment in children with WD should be individually tailored according to the patient's clinical condition, type, and severity of organ involvement. Noncompliance and underdosage are the main risk factors for an unfavorable clinical outcome. Prognosis is excellent provided that patients adhere to a lifelong pharmacological treatment.

So far, due to the lack of high-quality clinical studies, there have been various therapeutic approaches for children with WD among pediatric hepatologists. Recent ESPGHAN Hepatology Committee Position Paper on Wilson's Disease in Children addressed the issue of treatment in WD [3]. Following the experts' statement, zinc salts are recommended for pre-symptomatic children or as maintenance therapy in patients with normal serum transaminases. Copper-chelating agents (d-penicillamine or trientine) should be used in case of significant liver disease, such as cirrhosis or abnormal INR. All patients should be monitored following initiation of therapy: every 1–3 months and then 3–6 months for treatment efficacy and compliance. Basic checkups include physical examination, biochemical tests (i.e., blood cell count, liver function tests, urea, creatinine, proteinuria), serum copper, serum zinc, and 24-h urinary copper or/and zinc excretion (Table 14.3). Drug change might be necessary in selected cases if adverse effects occur or transaminases relapse despite treatment. Poor compliance or low pharmacological efficacy should be suspected any time. Children with acute liver failure should be managed in pediatric liver transplantation centers.

14.11 Liver Transplantation in Children with WD

Liver transplantation may be indicated in WD in the stage of ALF or progression of liver dysfunction despite drug therapy [37]. Excellent post-LT outcomes were reported. In French studies of children and adults patient, survival rates were 87% at 5, 10, and 15 years in patients transplanted between 1985 and 2009 for ALF (53%), decompensated cirrhosis (41%), or severe neurological disease (6%) [38]. In another study analyzing the United Network for Organ Sharing (UNOS) database including 170 WD children who underwent LT between 1987 and 2008, 1- and 5-year survival were 90.1% and 89%, respectively [39]. In both studies, patients transplanted for end-stage chronic liver disease had better long-term survival than patients transplanted for ALF. Extracorporeal liver support systems as a bridge to LT may improve the outcome [40]. Neurological and especially psychiatric involvement may show limited improvement after LT.

Table 14.4 Wilson's disease scoring system to predict the outcome of children with hepatic decompensation (King's College index) by Dhawan et al.

Score	Bilirubin (μmol/L)	INR	AST	Leukocytes (10⁹/L)	Albumin (g/L)
0	0–100	0–1.29	0–100	0–6.7	>45
1	101–150	1.3–1.6	101–150	6.8–8.3	34–44
2	151–200	1.7–1.9	151–200	8.4–10.3	25–33
3	201–300	2.0–2.4	201–300	10.4–15.3	21–24
4	>300	>2.5	>300	>15.3	0–20

If over 11 points → urgent listing for LT

Chelation therapy may be successful in some children with decompensated liver cirrhosis with liver failure but no hepatic encephalopathy; however, response to medical treatment may take time with improvement of PT after a minimum of 1 month and normalization within 3 months to 1 year [41]. Close follow-up and monitoring of clinical status is vital to timely list a child for LT. In 1986, Nazer et al. devised a scoring system to predict the outcome of patients including adults and children with hepatic decompensation in adults with WD [42]. In 2005, the score was reassessed in the pediatric population by Dhawan et al. who proposed a new scoring system (King's College index (CI)) that had a better positive predictive value for mortality without transplantation (Table 14.4) [43]. The CI is reported to be 93% sensitive and 98% specific, with a positive predictive value of 93%, and should be applied for prognostic assessment and decision for liver transplantation in these children.

References

1. Reilly M, Daly L, Hutchinson M. An epidemiological study of Wilson's disease in the Republic of Ireland. J Neurol Neurosurg Psychiatry. 1993;56:298–300.
2. Bandmann O, Weiss KH, Kaler SG. Wilson's disease and other neurological copper disorders. Lancet Neurol. 2015;14:103–13.
3. Socha P, Janczyk W, Dhawan A, Baumann U, D'Antiga L, Tanner S, et al. Wilson's disease in children: a position paper by the Hepatology Committee of the European Society for paediatric gastroenterology, hepatology and nutrition. J Pediatr Gastroenterol Nutr. 2018;66(2):334–44.
4. Moore SD, Helmle KE, Prat LM, Cox DW. Tissue localization of the copper chaperone ATOX1 and its potential role in disease. Mamm Genome. 2002;13(10):563–8.
5. Tanzi RE, Petrukhin K, Chernov I, et al. The Wilson disease gene is a copper transporting ATPase with homology to the Menkes disease gene. Nat Genet. 1993;5(4):344–50.
6. Dhawan A, Taylor RM, Cheeseman P, et al. Wilson's disease in children: 37-year experience and revised King's score for liver transplantation. Liver Transpl. 2005;11:441–8.
7. Wilson DC, Phillips MJ, Cox DW, et al. Severe hepatic Wilson's disease in preschool-aged children. J Pediatr. 2000;137:719–22.
8. Iorio R, Sepe A, Giannattasio A, et al. Hypertransaminasemia in childhood as a marker of genetic liver disorders. J Gastroenterol. 2005;40:820–6.
9. Lin LJ, Wang DX, Ding NN, et al. Comprehensive analysis on clinical features of Wilson's disease: an experience over 28 years with 133 cases. Neurol Res. 2014;36:157–63.
10. Ferenci P, Caca K, Loudianos G, et al. Diagnosis and phenotypic classification of Wilson disease. Liver Int. 2003;23:139–42.
11. Nicastro E, Ranucci G, Vajro P, et al. Re-evaluation of the diagnostic criteria for Wilson disease in children with mild liver disease. Hepatology. 2010;52:1948–56.
12. Mak CM, Lam CW, Tam S. Diagnostic accuracy of serum ceruloplasmin in Wilson disease: determination of sensitivity and specificity by ROC curve analysis among ATP7B-genotyped subjects. Clin Chem. 2008;54:1356–62.
13. Muller T, Koppikar S, Taylor RM, Carragher F, Schlenck B, Heinz-Erian P, Kronenberg F, et al. Re-evaluation of the penicillamine challenge test in the diagnosis of Wilson's disease in children. J Hepatol. 2007;47:270–6.
14. Kenney SM, Cox DW. Sequence variation database for the Wilson disease copper transporter, ATP7B. Hum Mutat. 2007;28:1171–7.
15. Glenn TC. Field guide to next-generation DNA sequencers. Mol Ecol Resour. 2011;11:759–69.
16. Yang X, Tang XP, Zhang YH, et al. Prospective evaluation of the diagnostic accuracy of hepatic copper content, as determined using the entire core of a liver biopsy sample. Hepatology. 2015;62:1731–41.
17. Johncilla M, Mitchell KA. Pathology of the liver in copper overload. Semin Liver Dis. 2011;31:239–44.
18. Trocello JM, El Balkhi S, Woimant F, Girardot-Tinant N, Chappuis P, Lloyd C, Poupon J. Relative exchangeable copper: a promising tool for family screening in Wilson disease. Mov Disord. 2014;29:558–62.
19. Tissieres P, Chevret L, Debray D, Devictor D. Fulminant Wilson's disease in children: appraisal of a critical diagnosis. Pediatr Crit Care Med. 2003;4:338–43.
20. Brunet AS, Marotte S, Guillaud O, Lachaux A. Familial screening in Wilson's disease: think at the previous generation! J Hepatol. 2012;57:1394–5.
21. Roberts EA, Schilsky ML. Diagnosis and treatment of Wilson disease: an update. Hepatology. 2008;47:2089–111.
22. Manolaki N, Nikolopoulou G, Daikos GL, Panagiotakaki E, Tzetis M, Roma E, Kanavakis E, et al. Wilson disease in children: analysis of 57 cases. J Pediatr Gastroenterol Nutr. 2009;48:72–7.
23. Wiggelinkhuizen M, Tilanus ME, Bollen CW, Houwen RH. Systematic review: clinical efficacy of chelator agents and zinc in the initial treatment of Wilson disease. Aliment Pharmacol Ther. 2009;29:947–58.
24. Czlonkowska A, Litwin T, Karlinski M, Dziezyc K, Chabik G, Czerska M. D-penicillamine versus zinc sulfate as first-line therapy for Wilson's disease. Eur J Neurol. 2014;21:599–606.
25. Kalita J, Kumar V, Chandra S, Kumar B, Misra UK. Worsening of Wilson disease following penicillamine therapy. Eur Neurol. 2014;71:126–31.
26. Ranucci G, Di Dato F, Leone F, Vajro P, Spagnuolo MI, Iorio R. Penicillamine-induced elastosis perforans serpiginosa in Wilson's disease: is useful switching to zinc? J Pediatr Gastroenterol Nutr. 2017;64(3):e72–3.
27. Walshe JM. Treatment of Wilson's disease with trientine (triethylene tetramine) dihydrochloride. Lancet. 1982;1:643–7.
28. Taylor RM, Chen Y, Dhawan A. Triethylene tetramine dihydrochloride (trientine) in children with Wilson disease: experience at King's College Hospital and review of the literature. Eur J Pediatr. 2009;168:1061–8.
29. Weiss KH, Thurik F, Gotthardt DN, Schafer M, Teufel U, Wiegand F, Merle U, et al. Efficacy and safety of oral chelators in treatment of patients with Wilson disease. Clin Gastroenterol Hepatol. 2013;11:1028–1035 e1021–1022.
30. Mizuochi T, Kimura A, Shimizu N, Nishiura H, Matsushita M, Yoshino M. Zinc monotherapy from time of diagnosis for young pediatric patients with presymptomatic Wilson disease. J Pediatr Gastroenterol Nutr. 2011;53:365–7.
31. Ranucci G, Di Dato F, Spagnuolo MI, Vajro P, Iorio R. Zinc monotherapy is effective in Wilson's disease patients with mild liver disease diagnosed in childhood: a retrospective study. Orphanet J Rare Dis. 2014;9:41.
32. Marcellini M, Di Ciommo V, Callea F, Devito R, Comparcola D, Sartorelli MR, Carelli G, et al. Treatment of Wilson's disease with zinc from the time of diagnosis in pediatric patients: a single-hospital, 10-year follow-up study. J Lab Clin Med. 2005;145:139–43.
33. Weiss KH, Gotthardt DN, Klemm D, Merle U, Ferenci-Foerster D, Schaefer M, Ferenci P, et al. Zinc monotherapy is not as effective as chelating agents in treatment of Wilson disease. Gastroenterology. 2011;140:1189–1198 e1181.

34. Santiago R, Gottrand F, Debray D, Bridoux L, Lachaux A, Morali A, Lapeyre D, et al. Zinc therapy for Wilson disease in children in French pediatric centers. J Pediatr Gastroenterol Nutr. 2015;61:613–8.
35. Litwin T, Dziezyc K, Karlinski M, Chabik G, Czepiel W, Czlonkowska A. Early neurological worsening in patients with Wilson's disease. J Neurol Sci. 2015;355:162–7.
36. Wiernicka A, Janczyk W, Dadalski M, Avsar Y, Schmidt H, Socha P. Gastrointestinal side effects in children with Wilson's disease treated with zinc sulphate. World J Gastroenterol. 2013;19:4356–62.
37. Fischer RT, Soltys KA, Squires RH Jr, Jaffe R, Mazariegos GV, Shneider BL. Prognostic scoring indices in Wilson disease: a case series and cautionary tale. J Pediatr Gastroenterol Nutr. 2011;52:466–9.
38. Guillaud O, Dumortier J, Sobesky R, Debray D, Wolf P, Vanlemmens C, Durand F, et al. Long term results of liver transplantation for Wilson's disease: experience in France. J Hepatol. 2014;60:579–89.
39. Arnon R, Annunziato R, Schilsky M, Miloh T, Willis A, Sturdevant M, Sakworawich A, et al. Liver transplantation for children with Wilson disease: comparison of outcomes between children and adults. Clin Transpl. 2011;25:E52–60.
40. Rustom N, Bost M, Cour-Andlauer F, Lachaux A, Brunet AS, Boillot O, Bordet F, et al. Effect of molecular adsorbents recirculating system treatment in children with acute liver failure caused by Wilson disease. J Pediatr Gastroenterol Nutr. 2014;58:160–4.
41. Santos Silva EE, Sarles J, Buts JP, Sokal EM. Successful medical treatment of severely decompensated Wilson disease. J Pediatr. 1996;128:285–7.
42. Nazer H, Ede RJ, Mowat AP, Williams R. Wilson's disease: clinical presentation and use of prognostic index. Gut. 1986;27:1377–81.
43. Dhawan A, Taylor RM, Cheeseman P, De Silva P, Katsiyiannakis L, Mieli-Vergani G. Wilson's disease in children: 37-year experience and revised King's score for liver transplantation. Liver Transpl. 2005;11:441–8.

Liver Disease in Cystic Fibrosis

Dominique Debray

Key Points
- Focal biliary cirrhosis is the most clinically relevant cystic fibrosis-associated liver disease, as extension of the focal fibrogenic process may lead to multilobular biliary cirrhosis, portal hypertension, and related complications in 5–10% of patients.
- CF-associated liver diseasv(CFLD) develops during the first decade and is usually asymptomatic until cirrhosis and portal hypertension develop.
- All patients with CF should receive yearly screening for evidence of liver involvement with physical examination by a gastro-hepatologist, liver ultrasound, and liver biochemical tests.
- MR cholangiography is indicated if there are symptoms suggestive of biliary colic, cholangitis, or large bile duct dilatation on ultrasound.
- There is no clear evidence of benefit for the use of ursodeoxycholic acid (UDCA) in CF patients with liver disease even in those who have bile duct strictures (i.e., sclerosing cholangitis).
- The main complications associated with cirrhosis are those related to the development of portal hypertension, i.e., variceal bleeding, ascites, hepatopulmonary syndrome, portopulmonary hypertension, and malnutrition. Liver failure is a rare and late event.
- Extreme care should be taken not to underestimate the degree of portal hypertension even if there is little evidence of liver disease clinically or on imaging, as portal hypertension related to obliterative portal venopathy without cirrhosis (i.e., non-cirrhotic portal hypertension) may occur.
- Most centers propose screening for upper gastrointestinal endoscopy to evaluate the risk of bleeding, although primary prophylaxis with band ligation remains controversial as evidence of its safety and efficacy in CF patients is still lacking.
- Indications for liver transplantation in CF include cirrhosis with evidence for hepatic decompensation (hypoalbuminemia (<3 g/dL and declining), persistent hypoglycemia, and/or worsening coagulopathy (INR > 1.5) that is not corrected by administration of intravenous vitamin K, ascites, and jaundice), uncontrollable variceal bleeding that cannot be managed by a portosystemic shunt, and hepatopulmonary and portopulmonary syndromes.
- Early liver transplantation may be considered for children with deteriorating nutritional status and lung function as there is evidence that liver transplantation may prevent further decline.

Research Required in This Field
- Use of consistent definitions for CFLD across all CF centers which is essential for addressing epidemiology, and natural disease course, and for assessing effects of novel therapeutic strategies on CFLD.
- Elucidate relevant mechanisms of disease to optimize future therapeutic options.
- Investigate the role of elastography in the characterization of fibrosis in CF as an ancillary tool for epidemiology.
- Develop endpoints short of cirrhosis that correlate with the development of cirrhosis.

D. Debray (✉)
Pediatric Liver Unit, Reference Center for Biliary Atresia and Genetic Cholestatic Diseases, Hôpital Necker-Enfants Malades, Paris, France
e-mail: dominique.debray@aphp.fr

Cystic fibrosis is the most common autosomal recessive disease of the Caucasian population, with an incidence of approximately 1 in every 3000 live births worldwide [1]. It is a multiorgan disease caused by mutations in the cystic fibrosis transmembrane conductance receptor (*CFTR*), affecting mostly the lungs, pancreas, sweat glands, and in males the Wolffian ducts. Other clinically relevant manifestations include intestinal obstruction in the neonatal period (meconium ileus) or later in life (distal intestinal obstructive syndrome) and hepatobiliary disease.

In 1989, the discovery of the gene responsible for CF led to recognition of the key role of the encoded protein—the cystic fibrosis transmembrane regulator (*CFTR*)—a low-conductance cyclic adenosine monophosphate (cAMP)-dependent chloride channel expressed at the apical membrane of epithelial cells, where it promotes transmembrane efflux of chloride ions [2]. Therefore, the CF secretory defect leads to a decrease luminal hydration of ducts, resulting in physicochemical abnormalities of secretions and duct obstruction.

To date, more than 1500 different disease-causing mutations have been identified (www.genet.sickkids.on.ca/cftr/app). Mutations are grouped into six classes according to the known or presumed molecular mechanisms of dysfunction of the *CFTR* protein and the corresponding residual activity at the apical membrane of epithelial cells. Class I, II, and III mutations (i.e., severe mutations) result in complete loss of the chloride channel function; in contrast, class IV, V, and VI mutations (i.e., mild mutations) are associated with altered conductance properties, reduced synthesis, or defective stability of normal *CFTR*, but some residual *CFTR* membrane activity [1]. Using this classification, class I, II, and III mutations have been associated with the highest mortality [3].

Presently, median survival is over 40 years. Lung disease is the primary cause of morbidity and mortality. Improvement in the outcome of the disease is expected, thanks to the development of drugs aimed at enhancing synthesis or function of the protein, acting as *CFTR* potentiator and *CFTR* corrector [4].

Unlike pulmonary and pancreatic diseases that affect the majority of CF patients, liver disease develops in no more than one-third of patients and may progress to cirrhosis and portal hypertension in a minority of patients (5–10%) [5–7]. In 2014, CF-associated liver disease (CFLD) was the third most common cause of mortality after cardiorespiratory and transplant-related causes, responsible for approximately 2.8% of deaths [8].

15.1 Epidemiology

15.1.1 Prevalence of Liver Disease

There are marked differences in the reported prevalence of CF-associated liver disease (CFLD), which may be explained by differences in the definition and diagnostic criteria of CFLD and in the populations studied [9]. The lack of a uniform definition of CF-associated liver disease increases the risk of important aspects of this disease being ignored or that minor transaminase abnormalities are overinterpreted.

With its frequently asymptomatic presentation and wide spectrum of manifestations, liver disease can be very difficult to diagnose in the early phases of development. The highest figures have been provided by autopsy studies, which documented a prevalence of liver disease of 10% in infants [10] increasing to more than 70% in adults [11].

Prevalence of CFLD reported in retrospective clinical studies range between 4.2 and 17%, but prospective long-term follow-up studies of cohorts of CF patients demonstrated a cumulative incidence of liver disease increasing through childhood and reaching a plateau in mid-adolescence ranging between 27 and 41%, without incident cases after the age of 18 years [5–7].

15.1.2 Spectrum of Liver Involvement in CF

The spectrum of liver involvement in CF and the reported prevalence are shown in Table 15.1 [12]. Liver disease ascribable to the underlying *CFTR* defect at the hepatobiliary level should be distinguished from lesions of iatrogenic origin or related to extrahepatic manifestations of CF [13].

- Focal biliary cirrhosis is the classic histological lesion of CF-associated liver disease ascribed to the *CFTR* defect in biliary epithelial cells (i.e., cholangiocytes) and results from biliary obstruction by inspissated secretions (Fig. 15.1a) and progressive periportal fibrosis (Fig. 15.1b). It has been reported in up to 70% in autopsy studies of CF patients [11]. This is the most clinically relevant CF-associated hepatic lesion, since extension of the initially focal fibrogenic process may lead to multilobular biliary cirrhosis (Fig. 15.1c, d), portal hypertension, and related complications [14]. Multilobular cirrhosis is an early event generally diagnosed by the end of the second decade of life which most commonly manifests as complications of portal hypertension such as hypersplenism and variceal bleeding [15, 16]. In the largest series of 561 CF patients with cirrhosis and portal hypertension, 90% is presented by 18 years of age with a mean of 10 years [15].
- The development of liver cirrhosis does not seem to be a prerequisite for portal hypertension [17–19]. Indeed, obliterative portal venopathy (OPV) has been recently recognized in a subset of CF patients with portal hypertension without cirrhosis, i.e., non-cirrhotic portal hypertension (NCPH) [20, 21]. The prevalence of OPV in CF patients remains unknown, and the cause of this portal branch venopathy remains obscure. It could be due to spillover of inflammatory infiltrate of the bile ducts, to microthrombosis from platelet activation, or to endothelial injury related to the *CFTR* defect.

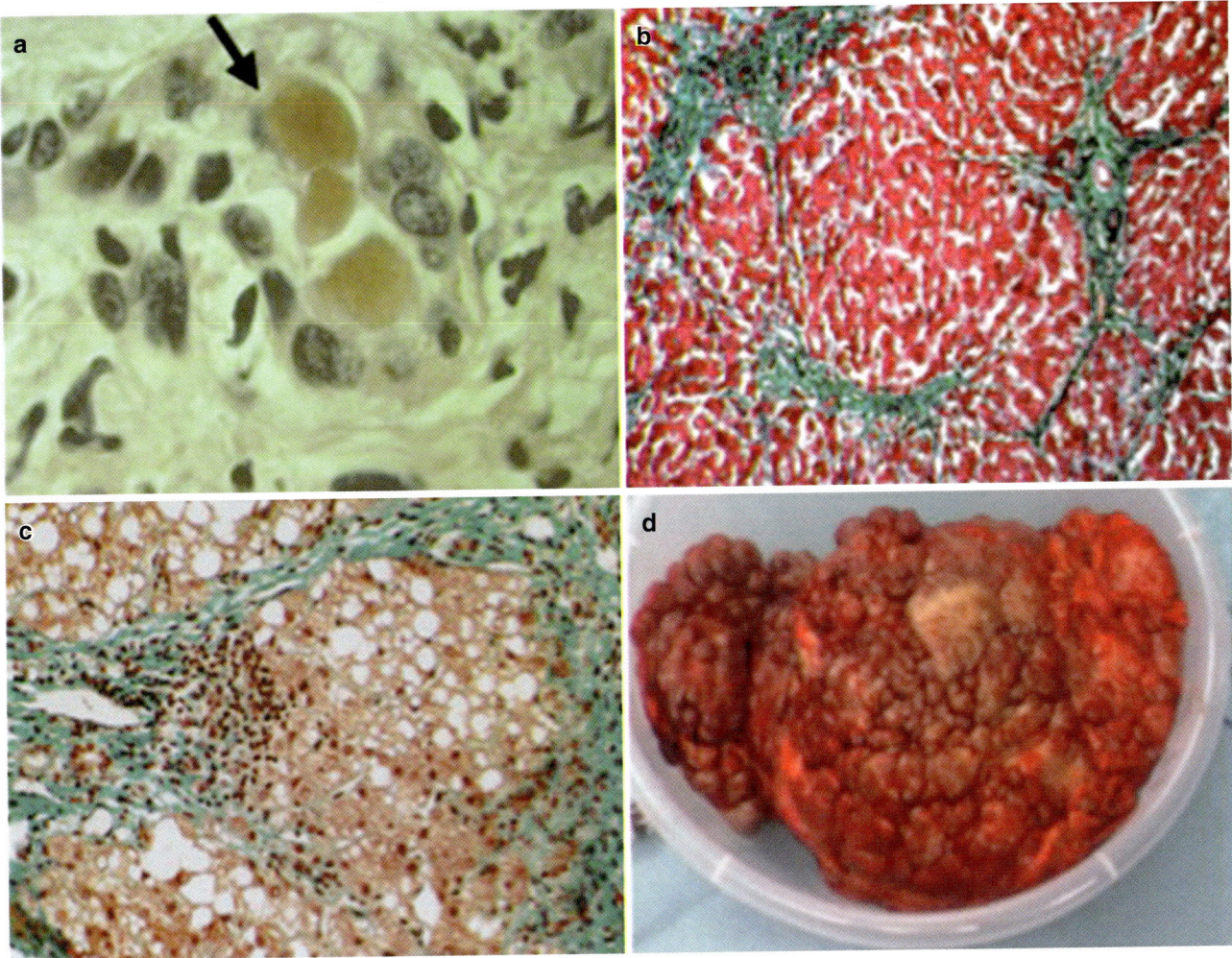

Fig. 15.1 Histopathological feature of hepatobiliary disease in CF. (**a**) Obstruction of bile duct by inspissated secretions. (**b**) Focal biliary cirrhosis. (**c**) Multilobular cirrhosis associated with steatosis. (**d**) Liver explant: multilobular biliary cirrhosis in a 13-year-old boy with cystic fibrosis

Table 15.1 Spectrum of liver involvement in CF and reported prevalence

Type of lesion	Clinical manifestation and possible causes	Frequency
Related to the underlying *CFTR* defect in cholangiocytes	Neonatal cholestasis	<1% (usually associated with meconium ileus)
	Hepatomegaly/abnormal liver tests	
	– Focal biliary cirrhosis	10–70% (at autopsy)
	– Multilobular biliary cirrhosis	5–10%
	– Cholangiopathy/sclerosing cholangitis	frequent in adults, often silent
	Portal hypertension	2–5% (with or without signs of liver disease)
	Gallbladder abnormalities at ultrasonography	
	– Micro-gallbladder	10–40%
	– Gallbladder dysfunction (hypokinesia)	50%
	– Cholelithiasis (pigmented stones)	0.6–15% (increases with age)
Lesions of iatrogenic origin	Abnormal liver tests (often isolated)	
	– Hepatic steatosis	20–70%
	– Drug hepatotoxicity	Unknown
Related to extrahepatic manifestations of CF	Hepatomegaly	
	– Hepatic congestion	Rare (advanced CF)

- Other biliary manifestations of CF include micro-gallbladder, biliary dyskinesia, cholelithiasis, large duct biliary strictures, and intrahepatic sclerosing cholangitis [22]. These manifestations are not well reported with a subsequent wide range of prevalence. Gallbladder abnormalities are frequent, including asymptomatic gallstones (20–30% of patients), micro-gallbladder (10–40% of patients), and gallbladder dysfunction (i.e., impaired emptying) (>50% of patients) [22–24]. Submucosal cysts, septate gallbladders, and adenomyomas have been also described [11]. Symptomatic cholelithiasis is uncommon. A large study reported that 3.6% of 670 patients with CF developed symptomatic gallbladder disease, the majority of whom were adults with obstructive cholelithiasis or cholecystitis [25]. The Cystic Fibrosis Foundation Patient Registry reported in 2014 that 0.6% of all registry participants had gallstones, while 0.8% required cholecystectomy or other intervention, with a slightly increased burden of gallbladder disease in adults as compared to children and adolescents [8]. Overall, symptomatic gallbladder disease requiring consideration for cholecystectomy may occur in up to 4% of patients [22]. Gallstones are generally "black" pigmented stones (i.e., calcium bilirubinate), thought to result from abnormal acidification of the bile [22, 26, 27]. In addition, bile stasis due to gallbladder hypokinesia and abnormalities in the biliary mucus may serve as a nidus for stone formation. Intrahepatic biliary strictures have been reported in children and adults with CF [22, 28–32]. The pattern and appearance of these strictures are often similar to that found in patients with primary sclerosing cholangitis (PSC). Indeed, these strictures reflect ongoing inflammation and fibrosis in the biliary tree and may be further complicated in CF by the accumulation of thick, inspissated mucus or intra-biliary cholelithiasis. Using ERCP, sclerosing cholangitis of the larger intrahepatic bile ducts was initially reported in adult CF patients with a frequency of 3.9%, sometimes in association with inflammatory bowel disease [32]. Using magnetic resonance cholangiography (MRCP), typical cholangiographic abnormalities of the intrahepatic bile ducts have been reported in the majority of adult CF patients with liver disease but also in 50% of CF patients without clinically apparent liver disease [30]. CF patients also have a high likelihood of presenting with large duct strictures. Stenosis of the intrapancreatic portion of the common bile duct has also been reported. In one controversial study, 96% of patients with liver disease had evidence of biliary tract obstruction at hepatobiliary scans, related to a stricture of the distal common bile duct [33]. At least one subsequent study using ERCP evaluation for stricture assessment did not reveal distal common bile duct strictures in patients with CF [28]. Additionally, there are multiple case reports of adult patients with CF and biliary disease who developed cholangiocarcinoma, including cases that occurred following lung transplantation [34–37]. An increased risk of gallbladder cancer has also been recently reported from registry data [38], suggesting that the absence of *CFTR* throughout the biliary epithelia contributes to a chronic inflammatory state that increases the risk of epithelial dysplasia.
- Steatosis, notably mild steatosis, is detected in CF patients of all ages with a wide range of reported frequencies (20–70%), but does not seem to be directly related to the CF basic defect [13, 39, 40]. It has been associated with selective nutritional deficiencies including essential fatty acids, carnitine, and choline and with altered phospholipid metabolism, diabetes, or long-term antibiotic therapy [6, 41]. Massive steatosis, once frequently observed in newly diagnosed patients with pancreatic insufficiency and severe malnutrition, is now infrequent due to earlier diagnosis and better nutritional care. Although considered benign in CF and without a proven relationship to developing cirrhosis, recent data on the progression of nonalcoholic steatohepatitis to cirrhosis in children such as in adults may change this view.
- Finally, hepatic congestion from right-side heart failure may occur in older patients with advanced CF.

15.2 Pathophysiology of Hepatobiliary Disease in CF

The pathogenesis remains not well understood. The progression from cholestasis to focal biliary cirrhosis and multilobular cirrhosis is a slow process that could be viewed as a continuum [42].

Cholangiocyte injury with periductular collagen deposition has for long been described in CF patients, even in those without clinical evidence of liver disease [43]. This suggests that damage to the bile duct epithelium is likely to represent the primary event in the development of periportal fibrosis.

CFTR expression is restricted to the apical membrane of cholangiocytes of both intrahepatic and extrahepatic biliary epithelia and the gallbladder epithelia where it drives fluid and bicarbonate secretion primarily increasing bile acid-independent bile flow [44]. Therefore, the primary hypothesis for the development of CF-associated liver disease is based on decreased or absent *CFTR* function in cholangiocytes leading to decreased chloride, bicarbonate, and osmotically coupled water transport to the bile resulting in plugging of intrahepatic bile ducts by inspissated secretions and retention of endogenous hydrophobic bile acids (Fig. 15.1a). Abnormalities in mucin secretion may also contribute to increased bile viscosity. This in turn causes inflammation and collagen deposition around the bile ducts and portal tracts, leading to focal portal biliary fibrosis (Fig. 15.1b) [42].

The importance of *CFTR* in maintaining homeostasis in the biliary tree through a bicarbonate balance has been highlighted in the "bicarbonate umbrella" hypothesis, in which a proper alkaline balance is critical to prevent cholangiocyte damage by hydrophobic bile acids [45]. Therefore, loss of *CFTR* function may contribute to pH dysregulation resulting in injury of the biliary tree. Activated hepatic stellate cells (HSC) are held responsible for the production of this collagen matrix [17, 40, 46, 47]. The possible role of portal myofibroblasts distinct from HSCs has been recently underlined [9].

There is evidence of the importance of *CFTR* in bile acid homeostasis [9], but no strong indication that increased hydrophobicity and/or cytotoxicity of bile in CF is important for the pathophysiology of CFLD. Studies in children with CF and CF mouse models detected increased loss of bile acids in the feces, suggesting a defect in ileal bile acid reabsorption [48–52]. This is compensated by increased hepatic synthesis of the primary bile acids, cholic and chenodeoxycholic acid, leading to higher hydrophobicity of the bile [51, 53, 54]. However bile cytotoxicity in a CF mouse model with hepatobiliary pathology was unaltered suggesting this does not impact development of CFLD [52]. A study from Strandvik et al. suggested that well-nourished adult patients with CF had normal bile acid concentrations and bile acid pool compared to controls [55]. A recent study in *CFTR*-deficient and F508del mice without liver disease revealed disruption of the enterohepatic circulation of bile acids and downregulation of primary bile acid synthesis resulting from impaired emptying of the gallbladder and cycling of bile acids to the liver by a cholecystohepatic shunt, thus decreasing the exposure of the liver to toxic (i.e., secondary) bile acids [56]. In CF, this mechanism may, with pancreatic defects, contribute to fat malabsorption.

Recent investigations have identified another mechanism by which the loss of *CFTR* in the biliary epithelium may lead to biliary disease in CF. It has been shown in mouse models of CF that *CFTR* deficiency results in increased vulnerability to bacterial endotoxin, which results in a pathologic innate immune response with secretion of inflammatory cytokines within biliary cells [57]. Experimental studies in the CF mouse have generated a hypothesis whereby small intestinal bacterial overgrowth (SIBO), impaired intestinal motility, and aberrant gut microbiota (i.e., gut dysbiosis) in CF induce inflammation with increased intestinal permeability, endotoxinemia, and significant biliary injury [58, 59]. *CFTR*-deficient mice harbor a defect in the nuclear receptor peroxisome proliferator-activated receptor gamma (PPARγ) signaling, known to repress transcriptional activation of inflammatory response genes in mouse macrophages [60]. Stimulation of the synthetic PPARγ ligand rosiglitazone significantly attenuated biliary damage and inflammation in Cftr knockout mice with induced portal endotoxinemia [61, 62]. Therefore, loss of *CFTR* may make the biliary tree more sensitive to inflammation from bacterial products from the intestine, which can lead to chronic damage and eventual fibrosis of the biliary tree. Several factors may predispose CF patients to dysbiosis (prolonged small bowel transit, frequent antibiotic exposure, small bowel bacterial overgrowth, etc.). A link between gut dysbiosis, intestinal inflammation, and cirrhosis was also reported in CF patients [63]. From a clinical perspective, multicenter longitudinal microbiome studies in CF patients at higher risk for developing liver disease are needed.

15.2.1 Risk Factors for CFLD

The reasons why only one-third of CF patients develop liver disease and why liver disease shows a great degree of variability in terms of severity remain poorly understood. Additional genetic factors (termed "modifier genes") and/or extrinsic factors (environmental, therapeutic, and iatrogenic) are probably important in determining disease heterogeneity.

Age does not appear to correlate with the severity of pathological changes [39], and in the only study looking at serial biopsies in CFLD patients, lesions did not progress over time [6]. The development of liver disease appears to be restricted to patients with severe genotypes (i.e., class I, II, or III mutations on both alleles), but no specific *CFTR* mutation has been associated with the presence and severity of liver disease [5]. The poor concordance of liver disease in sibling pairs excludes a major role for environmental factors. On the other hand, discordance for liver expression in CF siblings suggests that genetic factors inherited independently from the *CFTR* gene, i.e., modifier genes could modulate the clinical expression and severity of liver disease in CF. To date, *SERPINA-1* is the only reported modifier gene, whereby the heterozygous Z allele mutation of α1-antitrypsin is overrepresented in children with CFLD and portal hypertension over those without CFLD [16].

The preponderance of male subjects among CF patients with liver disease has been consistently reported, suggesting the possible role of endocrine factors in the development of this complication [5, 15, 64].

Although still controversial [65], a few studies have reported a significantly higher incidence of liver disease in CF patients with a positive history of meconium ileus [5, 7, 64, 66, 67].

15.3 Clinical Features

Liver disease associated with CF usually develops before puberty, is often asymptomatic, and is slowly progressive. The clinical spectrum ranges from neonatal cholestasis to cirrhosis and portal hypertension (Table 15.1).

- *Neonatal cholestasis*, caused by the obstruction of extrahepatic bile ducts by viscous biliary secretions, may be the presenting symptom of CF and may mimic biliary atresia. Infants with meconium ileus are at greater risk, particularly those with another risk of cholestasis, i.e., total parenteral nutrition or abdominal surgery. Cholestasis generally resolves spontaneously over the first months of life, perhaps because of resolution of physiological cholestasis and maturation of biliary secretion. Serum cholesterol concentrations are generally low or normal. Whether these infants are at higher risk of developing cirrhosis remains uncertain [68].
- *Hepatomegaly* is the most common clinical finding that may be associated with abnormalities in liver biochemistry. Hepatomegaly may be due to steatosis, to fibrosis, or to right-side heart failure (i.e., hepatic congestion) in older patients with advanced CF.
- *Splenomegaly* may develop and suggests portal hypertension associated with or without cirrhosis. Splenomegaly is often asymptomatic, but hypersplenism may develop, with thrombocytopenia and leucopenia. Massive splenic enlargement may cause abdominal discomfort or pain.
- *Signs* such as jaundice, palmar erythema, and spider nevi, ascites, and encephalopathy are rarely present and are limited to patients with end-stage liver disease.
- *Abdominal pain* and right upper quadrant pain with or without jaundice may reveal a biliary complication such as cholelithiasis, cholecystitis, or motor abnormalities of the extrahepatic biliary tree (dyskinesia, often associated with gallbladder distension) although uncommon [22]. Other causes of biliary pain or bacterial cholangitis include intrahepatic stones and large duct biliary strictures [25, 29]. Notably, there is a frequent lack of association between liver test abnormalities and the presence of biliary strictures [29]. One recent study described a small cohort of adults with CF and large duct strictures who developed recurrent pyogenic cholangitis, several of which ultimately required hepatobiliary surgery for refractory biliary disease [69].

15.4 Diagnosis of Cystic Fibrosis-Associated Liver Disease

15.4.1 Assessment of Liver Disease

Evidence of liver disease in CF patients is usually subclinical, with normal or mild abnormalities of biochemical liver function tests; therefore it is often underdiagnosed unless regular screening is implemented. The diagnosis of liver disease is based on clinical examination and a combination of biochemical tests and imaging techniques [12, 14]. The goal is to detect CFLD prior to the development of cirrhosis and to distinguish CFLD from other CF liver abnormalities such as steatosis and exclude other causes of liver disease (Table 15.2). Relevant biomarkers to identify patients at risk of bile duct injury, fibrosis development, or portal hypertension and to assess the effects of novel therapies are still lacking but under investigation [9].

Annual screening for CFLD is recommended for all children with CF (<18 years of age) and should include physical examination by a gastro-hepatologist, liver biochemistry, and abdominal ultrasonography [12, 14].

Table 15.2 Other causes of liver disease to be excluded in CF patients showing hepatic abnormalities

Disease	Investigations
Acute/chronic viral hepatitis	Serology for HAV[a], HBV[a], HCV, EBV, CMV, adenovirus, HHV 6, parvovirus
α1 antitrypsin deficiency	Serum α1 antitrypsin level, including phenotype
Autoimmune hepatitis	Non-organ-specific autoantibodies (SMA, anti-LKM1, LC1)
Celiac disease	Total IgA, IgA anti-tissue transglutaminase
Wilson disease	Ceruloplasmin, serum copper, 24-h urinary copper, slit lamp examination (Kayser-Fleischer rings)
Genetic hemochromatosis (adults)	Iron, ferritin, transferrin-binding capacity
Other causes of steatosis	Malnutrition, optimization of pancreatic enzyme supplementation, diabetes, obesity, metabolic disease (such as lysosomal acid lipase deficiency)

HAV hepatitis A virus, *HBV* hepatitis B virus, *HCV* hepatitis C virus, *EBV* Epstein Barr virus, *CMV* cytomegalovirus, *HHV6* herpes hominis virus type 6, *SMA* smooth muscle antibody, *LKM1* liver kidney microsomal type 1, *LC1* liver cytosol type 1
[a]If negative, vaccination is recommended

15.4.2 Physical Examination

Regular clinical examination is essential for the detection of hepatomegaly and signs of portal hypertension. The liver may be firm and nodular and its enlargement may be limited to the right or, more often, to the left lobe that protrudes centrally. Since the liver is often pushed down as a result of pulmonary disease, it is important to measure the liver span at the right mid-clavicular line through percussion and palpation. However, hepatomegaly may be absent in cases of cirrhosis with atrophic liver. Splenomegaly is the first sign of portal hypertension and requires close monitoring at every follow-up visit. Attention should also be paid to the presence of jaundice, spider nevi, palmar erythema, distension of abdominal wall veins, and ascites. Extreme care should be taken not to underestimate the degree of portal hypertension, even if there is little evidence of liver disease clinically or at ultrasonography suggesting obliterative portal venopathy (i.e., non-cirrhotic portal hypertension) [20, 21].

15.4.3 Liver Biochemistry

Liver enzyme abnormalities are frequently mild or intermittently present and lack specificity and sensitivity [39, 70]. While abnormal liver enzymes (aspartate aminotransferase (AST), alanine aminotransferase (ALT), and γ-glutamyl transpeptidase (GGT)) are common in CF, data are conflicting as to whether this correlates with the presence or severity of CFLD [71]. Increased liver enzymes (AST, ALT) have been documented in more than 50% of infants with CF with complete normalization in most cases by 2–3 years of age and no impact on future development of liver disease [6]. Persisting increased serum levels of GGT are reported in those with more serious liver disease, and appear to be an early marker of CFLD, with increasing specificity at higher cutoffs and high negative predictive values [70, 72].

Not infrequently, CF patients with multilobular biliary cirrhosis have normal liver biochemistry [15, 40].

On the other hand, biochemical abnormalities may result from drug hepatotoxicity, infection, steatosis, or any other cause of concomitant acute or chronic liver disease that needs to be excluded (Table 15.2) [14].

15.4.4 Ultrasonography

Ultrasonography is the most suitable initial method of investigation for assessment of abnormalities of the liver parenchyma and of the gallbladder in patients with CF. Ultrasonography (Fig. 15.2a, b) reliably distinguishes normal parenchyma, steatosis, fibrosis, and cirrhosis and can easily evaluate large intrahepatic or extrahepatic bile duct dilatation, gallbladder abnormalities, and signs of portal hypertension such as splenomegaly and decreased portal venous flow velocities or reversal of flow (hepatofugal) in the portal vein at Doppler ultrasound. Abnormal echogenicity may precede clinical manifestations of liver disease and may identify patients at risk of progressive disease suggesting that routine ultrasonography is a valuable marker of early liver disease in CF (Fig. 15.2a) [73–75]. However, ultrasonography is associated with substantial intra- and interobserver variability, and the positive predictive value of a normal ultrasound can be as low as 33% with 57% sensitivity [18].

15.4.5 Other Imaging Techniques [14]

- Hepatobiliary scintigraphy has been used to screen for gallbladder and biliary tract disease in CF patients [22, 24, 76]. Nowadays, magnetic resonance cholangiography is more commonly used.
- Computed tomography has once been helpful in confirming the presence of multilobular biliary cirrhosis and portal hypertension, but it lacks both specificity and sensitivity in diagnosing focal biliary cirrhosis.
- Percutaneous transhepatic cholangiography and endoscopic retrograde cholangiography (ERCP) are invasive procedures but may be useful for the investigation and therapy of patients with choledocholithiasis or a dominant large duct stricture or distal stenosis of the common bile duct.
- Magnetic resonance cholangiography imaging of the biliary tree has become the best modality for the assessment of the biliary tree, demonstrating variable dilation of the bile ducts. MRCP has revealed intrahepatic or large duct strictures in patients with or without clinically apparent liver disease or liver test abnormalities suggesting that it may be employed for early detection of intrahepatic biliary tract involvement [29, 30]. Magnetic resonance imaging is also a valuable method to quantify and assess the severity of steatosis [77].

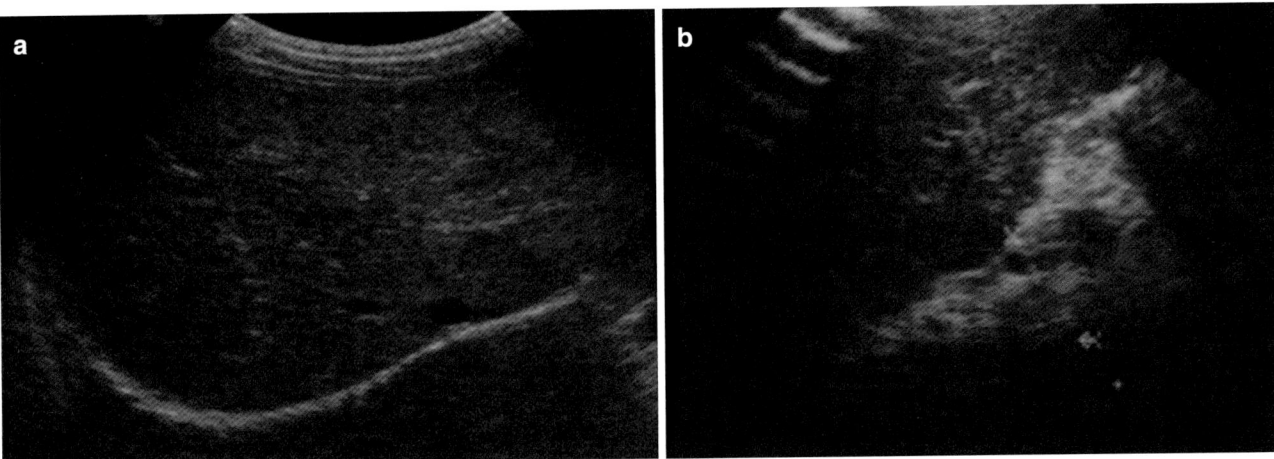

Fig. 15.2 Ultrasound examination may demonstrate a heterogenous liver texture (**a**) or signs of cirrhosis and portal hypertension (**b**). Note the irregular contours of the liver and the increased size of the small omentum

15.4.6 Liver Pathology

Histological assessment is the gold standard in the diagnostic work-up of many chronic liver diseases but remains controversial in CF patients because of the patchy distribution of lesions leading to a potential risk of sampling error and underrepresentation of the extent of the disease. Using a dual-pass needle core liver biopsy increases the sensitivity of the detection of hepatic fibrosis by 22% compared with a single-pass liver biopsy [40].

Although liver biopsy is not a routine investigation in many centers, it may provide important information on the type of lesion (steatosis or focal biliary cirrhosis) and the extent of portal fibrosis, but it carries a risk of complications limiting its usefulness in evaluating liver disease progression. It may also be helpful for select cases, indications whom the diagnosis of CFLD is confounded, particularly those suspected of having a concomitant liver disease (i.e., hepatitis C, alpha-1-antitrypsin deficiency, drug toxicity, or autoimmune hepatitis).

The histological hallmark of CF-associated liver disease is the deposition of inspissated bile (appearing as eosinophilic material with variable degrees of periodic acid-Schiff-positive reaction) in dilated cholangioles although infrequently seen beyond infancy (Fig. 15.1a) [10, 39]. Signs of focal periportal obstructive disease with bile duct proliferation and cholangitis inflammation around the portal tracts and various degrees of portal fibrosis extending intralobularly are usually seen (Fig. 15.1b). Mild steatosis (hepatocyte vacuolization with micro- and macrodroplet steatosis) is often associated (Fig. 15.1c). Particular attention should be paid to portal vein branches (obliteration, absence of portal veins), suggesting obliterative portal venopathy [20].

15.4.7 Noninvasive Assessment of Hepatic Fibrosis

Several methods have shown promise for the detection of clinically silent fibrosis and are being evaluated among the CF population.

15.4.7.1 Biomarkers

Identification of serum markers of liver fibrosis would be useful for the early detection of patients with CFLD. The AST to platelet ratio index (APRI) and FIB-4 (Fibrosis-4) that incorporate standard laboratory data (i.e., AST, ALT, platelet count, age) show a good correlation with severe fibrosis, but not for differentiating fibrosis at earlier stages [12, 15, 78]. A recent study suggests that serum-based miRNA analyses could be used as diagnostic biomarkers with potential to predict early hepatic fibrosis, although sensitivity needs to be improved [79].

15.4.7.2 Elastography

Several clinical ultrasonographic systems, such as transient elastography, acoustic radiation force impulse (ARFI), point shear wave elastography, supersonic shear wave elastography (SSWE), and magnetic resonance elastography (MRE) [80], are currently available for quantitative elastography measurements in clinical practice, but better-quality studies and further validation are still needed particularly for the diagnosis of mild to moderate fibrosis [12, 80–86]. Indeed, in a recent prospective study evaluating TE and ARFI simultaneously in 55 adult CF patients, both TE and ARFI did not significantly discriminate between non-cirrhotic CFLD and CF without liver disease but only discriminated between CF patients with liver cirrhosis and earlier stages of CFLD [80]. SSWE may be more accurate for assessing early stages of fibrosis but warrant further investigations in the CF population [83]. Importantly, hepatic steatosis and necroinflammatory activity may be confounding factors for liver stiffness assessments. MRE is a new technology to detect earlier stages of liver fibrosis, under investigation in the CF population [87].

15.4.8 Hemodynamic Measurements of Hepatic Venous Pressure Gradient

Hepatic venography is indicated in patients with portal hypertension without evidence of cirrhosis to measure the hepatic venous pressure gradient (HVPG). Intrahepatic presinusoidal (non-cirrhotic) portal hypertension is indicated if the HVPG is normal (≤5 mmHg) or only slightly increased (5–10 mmHg) [20].

15.4.9 Diagnosis of CF-Associated Liver Disease

A diagnosis of progressive CFLD is made if two or more of the following findings are present [12, 14]:

- Hepatomegaly (e.g., liver edge palpable more than 2 cm below the costal margin) and/or splenomegaly, confirmed by ultrasonography
- Abnormalities of ALT, AST, and GGT above the laboratory upper limits of normal for >6 months, after excluding steatosis and other causes of liver disease
- Ultrasonographic evidence of coarseness, nodularity, heterogenous echogenicity, or portal hypertension, as described above
- Liver biopsy showing focal biliary cirrhosis or multilobular cirrhosis (if performed)

15.5 Outcome of Liver Disease

The accumulating successes in therapeutic management of CF have moved CFLD from a primarily pediatric disease to an adult disease [88].

15.5.1 Hepatic Outcome

In most cases, liver involvement in CF remains asymptomatic. However, multilobular biliary cirrhosis may develop in a minority of patients during the first decade of life impacting clinical outcomes [5, 12, 15, 64]. The progression of liver disease to liver failure remains unpredictable, but hepatic function remains usually well preserved for a long time [64, 67]. In contrast, early development of portal hypertension is common in the pediatric age group [12, 64, 89]. Signs of portal hypertension may develop in patients without signs suggesting cirrhosis (i.e., NCPH) related to obliterative portal venopathy [20, 21]. Extreme care should therefore be taken not to underestimate the degree of portal hypertension, even if there is little evidence of liver disease clinically or on imaging.

Esophageal varices develop in a high percentage of CF patients with cirrhosis [12, 64, 67]. Although hemorrhage is relatively rare in terms of bleeds per patient years, it is often associated with significant morbidity (ascites and infections) [5, 7, 64, 67]. In a recent large study including 943 participants (41% females, mean age 18.1 years) with reported cirrhosis in the CF Foundation Patient Registry from 2003 to 2012, 10-year cumulative variceal bleeding, liver transplantation, and liver death rates were 6.6%, 9.9%, and 6.9% respectively, with an all-cause mortality (ACM) of 39.2% [89]. Seventy-three subjects had reported variceal bleeding: 38 with first variceal bleeding and new cirrhosis reported simultaneously and 35 with variceal bleeding after cirrhosis report. ACM was not increased in subjects with variceal bleeding compared to those without. CF-related diabetes and variceal bleeding were associated with higher liver transplantation risk, whereas only worse lung function was associated with increased liver death in multivariate analysis [89].

Rarer complications of portal hypertension include ascites, hepatopulmonary syndrome, and hepatopulmonary hypertension that should trigger an evaluation for liver transplantation [12, 14].

Additionally, there are multiple case reports of adult patients with CF and biliary disease who developed cholangiocarcinoma, including cases that occurred following lung transplantation [34–37]. An increased risk of gallbladder cancer has also been recently reported from registry data [38], suggesting that the absence of *CFTR* throughout the biliary epithelia contributes to a chronic inflammatory state that increases the risk of epithelial dysplasia.

15.5.2 Extrahepatic Outcomes

It has been reported that CF children with liver disease may have a better pulmonary prognosis than those without liver disease in longitudinal studies [5, 7, 90], while in CF adults, cirrhosis is independently associated with mortality and lung transplantation risks [67]. Large multicenter prospective studies are needed to describe the long-term outcome of CFLD in adulthood and define the respective indication for liver, lung, or lung-liver transplantation in the presence of CFLD [9].

Malnutrition, a common complication of CF, may be exacerbated by the development of advanced liver disease with an increase in resting energy expenditure, fat malabsorption (due to the combined effect of cholestasis and pancreatic insufficiency), abnormal metabolism of nutrients, and protein wasting. In addition, advanced liver disease may induce insulin resistance and increase the risk of developing CF-related diabetes [91].

15.6 Follow-Up of Liver Disease

European guidelines recommend annual screening for liver involvement with abdominal examination by a gastro-hepatologist, biochemical evaluation (AST, ALT, GGT, ALP, prothrombin time, platelets), and ultrasonography and MR imaging if concern exists about biliary tract involvement (such as sclerosing cholangitis) [14].

The main complications associated with cirrhosis are those related to the development of portal hypertension, i.e., variceal bleeding, ascites, and malnutrition [64, 89].

Upper gastrointestinal endoscopy remains the most accurate and reliable test to detect the presence of esophageal varices and portal hypertensive gastropathy. Most centers offer endoscopic screening and treatment of large varices [9]. An important consideration is the safety of repeated general anesthesia. Although safe and well tolerated, esophageal capsule endoscopy for the evaluation of esophageal or small bowel varices would be useful, particularly in the CF population to avoid deleterious repeated general anesthesia, but requires further evaluation particularly in the pediatric population [92, 93]. Elastography of the liver or spleen may improve bleeding prediction [94]. Children at risk of variceal bleeding may be identified according to a predictive score based on noninvasive biomarkers such as platelet counts and spleen size [95, 96].

In patients with portal hypertension, screening for hepatopulmonary syndrome and portopulmonary syndrome is mandatory, especially when considering a portosystemic shunting procedure to prevent variceal bleeding [12, 14]. Hepatopulmonary syndrome results from dilatation of intrapulmonary capillaries leading to a functional right-to-left shunt and hypoxemia. Oxygen saturation should be monitored in the supine and upright position: a significant decrease in oxygen saturation (>5%) when the patient moves from a supine to an upright position (called orthodeoxia) is suggestive of the diagnosis. Proof of intrapulmonary capillary dilatation may be obtained by means of contrast-enhanced (bubble) echocardiography or technetium 99-labeled macro aggregated albumin scintigraphy. Pulmonary arterial hypertension (i.e., portopulmonary syndrome) is easily detected by echocardiography.

Prothrombin time and coagulation factors should be measured at least once a year to detect early signs of liver failure. A prominent decrease in coagulation factor V compared to other cofactors is often noted in patients with a large splenomegaly, possibly as a result of intrasplenic consumption. An isolated decrease in cofactors VII, X, and II suggests that vitamin K deficiency should be corrected with oral or intramuscular vitamin K supplementation. Liver failure should be considered if PT and coagulation cofactors VII, X, and II remain decreased despite vitamin K supplementation [14].

Finally, in patients with cirrhosis, α-fetoprotein levels should be measured annually to monitor the possible development of hepatocellular carcinoma [97, 98]. Since an increased risk of biliary tract cancer has been reported in CF patients, attention should be paid to the occurrence of jaundice, bile duct strictures, and gallbladder polyps [38].

15.7 Treatment Options for Cystic Fibrosis-Associated Liver Disease

15.7.1 Bile Acid Therapy

The only medical therapy currently used for CFLD is the natural hydrophilic bile acid, ursodeoxycholic acid (UDCA), a secretagogue stimulating hepatocellular and cholangiocellular bile secretion, aimed at reducing bile viscosity, improving biliary secretion and bile acid composition, and ultimately slowing liver fibrosis. UDCA may also have a direct cytoprotective effect on cell membranes and a protective effect against apoptosis induced by endogenous hydrophobic bile acids. Beneficial effects on different aspects of CFLD (clinical, biochemical, imaging) have led to its widespread use, despite the lack of long-term randomized controlled trials and of proven long-term efficacy [99]. A recent Cochrane review, which analyzed its reported use for all variants of CF-associated liver disease, concluded that there is insufficient evidence to justify its routine use in CF [100]. As with the management of large duct PSC [101], there is no clear evidence of benefit for the use of ursodeoxycholic acid (UDCA) in patients with CF who have duct strictures. Expert opinion differs regarding UDCA use for all patients with CFLD [12, 14].

Concerns were raised about the risk of adverse events when high doses were given to PSC patients (28–30 mg/kg/day), thought to be due to the possible biotransformation of UDCA in toxic bile acids. Analysis of the serum bile acid composition in CF patients on long-term UDCA treatment did not show significantly greater concentrations of potentially toxic bile acids in CF patients [102]. The recommended dosage for patients with CF-associated liver disease is 15–20 mg/kg/day [14].

15.7.2 Nutritional Support

Most children with CFLD need high-energy diets with pancreatic enzyme supplements to prevent as possible malabsorption and malnutrition [103].

The following dietary management is recommended [14]:

- An increase in energy intake of 150% is the estimated average requirement. Diet can be supplemented by high-energy carbohydrate and protein drinks.
- Increasing the proportion of fat to 40–50% of the energy content or a diet with special attention to increase supplementation of polyunsaturated fatty acids.
- Providing protein supplements to ensure an intake of 3 g/kg/day.
- Ensuring that sufficient pancreatic enzymes are prescribed to allow optimal absorption of long-chain triglycerides and essential fatty acids.
- Fat-soluble vitamin (A, D, E, K) supplementation as needed [103]. Plasma levels and prothrombin time should be monitored. Bone density scans should be considered.

In children in whom anorexia is a problem, enteral nasogastric or gastrostomy feeding may be required to ensure adequate caloric intake. Gastrostomy feeding is not recommended in children with advanced liver disease, varices, or portal gastropathy because of the risk of gastric hemorrhage.

15.7.3 Treatment of Biliary Complications [22]

- In cases of symptomatic gallbladder disease, the indication for cholecystectomy has to be weighed against the risk of complications including worsening of pulmonary function postanesthesia, postoperative pulmonary infections, weight loss, and distal intestinal obstruction syndrome due to bowel inactivity and the use of pain medications. Multidisciplinary evaluation by the pulmonologist and anesthesiologist should be pursued to assess surgical risk. On the basis of a proper surgical timing and adequate preoperative physiotherapy, laparoscopic cholecystectomy appears a safe procedure in patients with cystic fibrosis indicated in cases of symptomatic cholelithiasis [104]. In CF patients with advanced lung disease, conservative management with symptom control may be best. Gallstones in CF are not responsive to therapy with UDCA, because their main component is not cholesterol bile [22, 26, 27].

- In cases of partial or complete bile duct obstruction, MR cholangiography should be performed to look for dominant strictures that could benefit from endoscopic intervention with ERCP for balloon dilation and or stenting.

15.7.4 Treatment of Portal Hypertension and End-Stage Liver Disease

The management of CF patients with advanced liver disease, severe portal hypertension, and hypersplenism is similar to that for other patients.

Salicylic acid and nonsteroidal antiinflammatory drugs are contraindicated to prevent bleeding from portal hypertensive gastropathy and GI varices. Vaccination against hepatitis A and B is recommended.

There is no available evidence of the benefit of primary prophylaxis (before first variceal bleed) in terms of safety, efficacy, and survival outcomes. CF patients with severe portal hypertension may remain stable for years, and long-term survival has been reported even after variceal bleeding [89, 105]. Despite this, it is offered to selected patients in most centers for detection and treatment of large varices with red wale signs (grade 2 and more) to prevent bleeding [14].

Esophageal band ligation is the preferred method for primary prophylaxis. It is generally preferred over nonselective beta-blockers due to concerns of poor tolerance of the latter.

Esophageal band ligation should be repeated until varices are eradicated which has implications for CF patients who require intensive physiotherapy and intravenous antibiotics before anesthesia.

Although endoscopic treatment is successful in most cases, in some patients gastric or rectal variceal bleeding or portal hypertensive gastropathy develops and may require additional therapeutic interventions. Options include a transjugular intrahepatic portosystemic shunt (TIPSS), a surgical portosystemic shunt, or liver transplantation. Studies are lacking to identify the most beneficial and least risky therapeutic option and the appropriate timing of intervention. In view of the good hepatic synthetic function, management of patients with CF who have NCPH should probably seek the alleviation of this portal hypertension by shunting procedures rather than referring these patients for liver transplantation. TIPSS has been successfully employed for portal decompression in CF patients with recurrent bleeding, both as a long-term therapy for portal hypertension and as a bridge for liver transplantation [106]. Elective surgical portosystemic shunts represent a more definitive treatment option for refractory bleeding in patients with preserved liver function and without severe pulmonary disease, allowing prolonged postoperative survival [64].

Splenectomy has been performed, alone or in association with a splenorenal shunt, in CF patients with hypersplenism showing an accelerated decline in lung function and/or variceal bleeding. These procedures are presently not recommended [14].

15.7.5 Liver Transplantation

Liver transplantation is an effective therapeutic option for CF patients developing end-stage liver failure. The agreed indications for liver transplant in CF include cirrhosis with evidence for hepatic decompensation (hypoalbuminemia (<3 g/dL and declining), persistent hypoglycemia, and/or worsening coagulopathy (INR > 1.5) that is not corrected by administration of intravenous vitamin K, ascites, and jaundice), uncontrollable variceal bleeding that cannot be managed by a portosystemic shunt, and hepatopulmonary syndrome [14].

Selection criteria and timing have not been clearly established, and whether severe malnutrition unresponsive to intensive nutritional support, or related deteriorating quality of life, severe portal hypertension should indicate LT is questionable. Assessment should include pulmonary and cardiac function to establish whether liver transplantation alone or a combined heart/lung/liver transplant is more appropriate [107]. Combined lung/liver should be considered for young adults with severe lung disease (<50% FEV1) and liver failure [108].

Opinions vary between those who feel transplantation should be performed early to prevent progression of pulmonary disease and malnutrition and those who feel transplantation is only indicated if there is clear evidence of liver failure [109–111]. There is evidence that poor growth and nutritional status are associated with deteriorating lung function and increased posttransplant mortality, and stabilization of lung function posttransplantation is reported [109]. A poll among European CF and transplant centers on current practice and outcome for liver transplant in CF patients in Europe revealed that in the majority of cases, the decision to transplant was based on the complications of portal hypertension, and often transplantation was performed before the development of end-stage liver disease [112].

Median 1-year and 10-year survival after LT is approximately 90% and 80%, respectively [109, 113], but long-term outcome is dependent on the other CF manifestations, late mortality being generally related to progression of pulmonary disease. Notably, renal impairment is a frequent complication [109]. Survival data for combined liver/lung transplantation are comparable to those observed in other groups of patients receiving lung transplants, with reported 1- and 5-year actuarial survival rates of 85% and 64% [109].

Preoperative management should include treatment of lung disease such as vigorous physiotherapy, control of infection, and mucus-dissolving agents. It is essential to plan appropriate postoperative antibiotic therapy by ensuring that regular sputum cultures are performed to identify the antibiotic sensitivity of colonized organisms.

The place of pancreas transplantation in CF, either in isolation or combined with other solid organ transplantation, is yet to be clearly established. Pancreatic insufficiency is present in 70–90% of CF patients, becoming clinically evident in 90% of cases within the first year of life and resulting in malnutrition when inadequately managed. CF-related diabetes is a serious CF complication, with 35–50% of patients developing insulin-dependent diabetes mellitus before the age of 30 years.

The increased risk of diabetes in this population, particularly after liver transplantation, supports implementation of combined liver-pancreas transplantation. However, an analysis of United Network for Organ Sharing data from 1987 to 2014 showed low rates of pancreas transplants in the CF population, despite generally encouraging outcomes [114]. Among 4600 CF patients, only 28 (<1%) had undergone pancreas transplants (with or without liver, lung, and kidney transplants). Two-year posttransplant survival was 88% in the 17 liver-pancreas transplant patients. Posttransplant diabetes developed in 7% of CF pancreas transplant recipients versus 24% of CF liver and 29% of CF lung recipients.

Several reasons can potentially account for the underutilization of pancreatic transplantation; there are few experienced surgeons to perform this technically difficult procedure, and it may be associated with significant posttransplant complications. On the other hand, given the availability of enzyme replacement therapy and insulin, it is not considered lifesaving. In a recent poll of 50 pediatric transplantation centers, 94% reported that they would consider combined liver/pancreas transplantation for CFLD and diabetes, 50% for CFLD and glucose intolerance, and 24% for CFLD and pancreatic insufficiency [115].

15.7.6 Future Treatment Options

– With better knowledge of mechanisms involved in the pathogenesis of CF-associated liver disease, there is potential for several therapeutic strategies. A number of investigational CFLD drug candidates targeting different aspects of liver disease are being explored including NorUDCA, a side chain-shortened homologue of UDCA, farnesoid X receptor (FXR) analogs, PPARγ agonist such as FGF1, and vitamin D receptor (VDR) agonist [9].
– Pharmacological correction of the CF ion transport defect by targeting the mutant *CFTR* gene (with correctors and/or potentiators) is presently an area of intensive investigation and may prove to be an effective therapeutic approach for CF-associated liver disease in the near future. With the development of ivacaftor, which corrects the gating defect of the CF transmembrane regulator channel, there is a potential new therapy available for this subgroup of the CF patient population [116, 117].

References

1. Rowe SM, Miller S, Sorscher EJ. Cystic fibrosis. N Engl J Med. 2005;352:1992–2001.
2. Riordan JR, Rommens JM, Kerem B, Alon N, Rozmahel R, Grzelczak Z, Zielenski J, et al. Identification of the cystic fibrosis gene: cloning and characterization of complementary DNA. Science. 1989;245:1066–73.
3. McKone EF, Emerson SS, Edwards KL, Aitken ML. Effect of genotype on phenotype and mortality in cystic fibrosis: a retrospective cohort study. Lancet. 2003;361:1671–6.
4. Amaral MD. Novel personalized therapies for cystic fibrosis: treating the basic defect in all patients. J Intern Med. 2015;277:155–66.
5. Colombo C, Battezzati PM, Crosignani A, Morabito A, Costantini D, Padoan R, Giunta A. Liver disease in cystic fibrosis: a prospective study on incidence, risk factors, and outcome. Hepatology. 2002;36:1374–82.
6. Lindblad A, Glaumann H, Strandvik B. Natural history of liver disease in cystic fibrosis. Hepatology. 1999;30:1151–8.
7. Lamireau T, Monnereau S, Martin S, Marcotte JE, Winnock M, Alvarez F. Epidemiology of liver disease in cystic fibrosis: a longitudinal study. J Hepatol. 2004;41:920–5.
8. Cystic Fibrosis Foundation Patient Registry ADRttCD, Bethesda. p. 73. https://www.cff.org/2014-Annual-Data-Report.pdf.
9. Debray D, Narkewicz MR, Bodewes F, Colombo C, Housset C, de Jonge HR, Jonker JW, et al. Cystic fibrosis-related liver disease: research challenges and future perspectives. J Pediatr Gastroenterol Nutr. 2017;65:443–8.
10. Oppenheimer EH, Esterly JR. Hepatic changes in young infants with cystic fibrosis: possible relation to focal biliary cirrhosis. J Pediatr. 1975;86:683–9.
11. Vawter GF, Shwachman H. Cystic fibrosis in adults: an autopsy study. Pathol Annu. 1979;14(Pt 2):357–82.
12. Leung DH, Narkewicz MR. Cystic fibrosis-related cirrhosis. J Cyst Fibros. 2017;16(Suppl 2):S50–61.
13. Colombo C, Battezzati PM. Liver involvement in cystic fibrosis: primary organ damage or innocent bystander? J Hepatol. 2004;41:1041–4.
14. Debray D, Kelly D, Houwen R, Strandvik B, Colombo C. Best practice guidance for the diagnosis and management of cystic fibrosis-associated liver disease. J Cyst Fibros. 2011;10(Suppl 2):S29–36.
15. Stonebraker JR, Ooi CY, Pace RG, Corvol H, Knowles MR, Durie PR, Ling SC. Features of severe liver disease with portal hypertension in patients with cystic fibrosis. Clin Gastroenterol Hepatol. 2016;14:1207–1215.e3.
16. Bartlett JR, Friedman KJ, Ling SC, Pace RG, Bell SC, Bourke B, Castaldo G, et al. Genetic modifiers of liver disease in cystic fibrosis. JAMA. 2009;302:1076–83.

17. Lewindon PJ, Pereira TN, Hoskins AC, Bridle KR, Williamson RM, Shepherd RW, Ramm GA. The role of hepatic stellate cells and transforming growth factor-beta(1) in cystic fibrosis liver disease. Am J Pathol. 2002;160:1705–15.
18. Mueller-Abt PR, Frawley KJ, Greer RM, Lewindon PJ. Comparison of ultrasound and biopsy findings in children with cystic fibrosis related liver disease. J Cyst Fibros. 2008;7:215–21.
19. Pereira TN, Lewindon PJ, Greer RM, Hoskins AC, Williamson RM, Shepherd RW, Ramm GA. Transcriptional basis for hepatic fibrosis in cystic fibrosis-associated liver disease. J Pediatr Gastroenterol Nutr. 2012;54:328–35.
20. Witters P, Libbrecht L, Roskams T, De Boeck K, Dupont L, Proesmans M, Vermeulen F, et al. Liver disease in cystic fibrosis presents as non-cirrhotic portal hypertension. J Cyst Fibros. 2017;16:e11–3.
21. Hillaire S, Cazals-Hatem D, Bruno O, de Miranda S, Grenet D, Pote N, Soubrane O, et al. Liver transplantation in adult cystic fibrosis: clinical, imaging, and pathological evidence of obliterative portal venopathy. Liver Transpl. 2017;23:1342–7.
22. Assis DN, Debray D. Gallbladder and bile duct disease in cystic fibrosis. J Cyst Fibros. 2017;16(Suppl 2):S62–9.
23. Santamaria F, Vajro P, Oggero V, Greco L, Angelillo M, Carrillo F, De Ritis G. Volume and emptying of the gallbladder in patients with cystic fibrosis. J Pediatr Gastroenterol Nutr. 1990;10:303–6.
24. O'Connor PJ, Southern KW, Bowler IM, Irving HC, Robinson PJ, Littlewood JM. The role of hepatobiliary scintigraphy in cystic fibrosis. Hepatology. 1996;23:281–7.
25. Stern RC, Rothstein FC, Doershuk CF. Treatment and prognosis of symptomatic gallbladder disease in patients with cystic fibrosis. J Pediatr Gastroenterol Nutr. 1986;5:35–40.
26. Angelico M, Gandin C, Canuzzi P, Bertasi S, Cantafora A, De Santis A, Quattrucci S, et al. Gallstones in cystic fibrosis: a critical reappraisal. Hepatology. 1991;14:768–75.
27. Colombo C, Bertolini E, Assaisso ML, Bettinardi N, Giunta A, Podda M. Failure of ursodeoxycholic acid to dissolve radiolucent gallstones in patients with cystic fibrosis. Acta Paediatr. 1993;82:562–5.
28. O'Brien S, Keogan M, Casey M, Duffy G, McErlean D, Fitzgerald MX, Hegarty JE. Biliary complications of cystic fibrosis. Gut. 1992;33:387–91.
29. Nagel RA, Westaby D, Javaid A, Kavani J, Meire HB, Lombard MG, Wise A, et al. Liver disease and bile duct abnormalities in adults with cystic fibrosis. Lancet. 1989;2:1422–5.
30. Durieu I, Pellet O, Simonot L, Durupt S, Bellon G, Durand DV, Minh VA. Sclerosing cholangitis in adults with cystic fibrosis: a magnetic resonance cholangiographic prospective study. J Hepatol. 1999;30:1052–6.
31. Waters DL, Dorney SF, Gruca MA, Martin HC, Howman-Giles R, Kan AE, De Silva M, et al. Hepatobiliary disease in cystic fibrosis patients with pancreatic sufficiency. Hepatology. 1995;21:963–9.
32. Strandvik B, Hjelte L, Gabrielsson N, Glaumann H. Sclerosing cholangitis in cystic fibrosis. Scand J Gastroenterol Suppl. 1988;143:121–4.
33. Gaskin KJ, Waters DL, Howman-Giles R, de Silva M, Earl JW, Martin HC, Kan AE, et al. Liver disease and common-bile-duct stenosis in cystic fibrosis. N Engl J Med. 1988;318:340–6.
34. Abdul-Karim FW, King TA, Dahms BB, Gauderer MW, Boat TF. Carcinoma of extrahepatic biliary system in an adult with cystic fibrosis. Gastroenterology. 1982;82:758–62.
35. Tesluk H, McCauley K, Kurland G, Ruebner BH. Cholangiocarcinoma in an adult with cystic fibrosis. J Clin Gastroenterol. 1991;13:485–7.
36. Perdue DG, Cass OW, Milla C, Dunitz J, Jessurun J, Sharp HL, Schwarzenberg SJ. Hepatolithiasis and cholangiocarcinoma in cystic fibrosis: a case series and review of the literature. Dig Dis Sci. 2007;52:2638–42.
37. Naderi AS, Farsian FN, Lee WM. Cholangiocarcinoma after lung transplantation in a patient with cystic fibrosis. Eur J Gastroenterol Hepatol. 2008;20:1115–7.
38. Maisonneuve P, Marshall BC, Knapp EA, Lowenfels AB. Cancer risk in cystic fibrosis: a 20-year nationwide study from the United States. J Natl Cancer Inst. 2013;105:122–9.
39. Potter CJ, Fishbein M, Hammond S, McCoy K, Qualman S. Can the histologic changes of cystic fibrosis-associated hepatobiliary disease be predicted by clinical criteria? J Pediatr Gastroenterol Nutr. 1997;25:32–6.
40. Lewindon PJ, Shepherd RW, Walsh MJ, Greer RM, Williamson R, Pereira TN, Frawley K, et al. Importance of hepatic fibrosis in cystic fibrosis and the predictive value of liver biopsy. Hepatology. 2011;53:193–201.
41. Chen AH, Innis SM, Davidson AG, James SJ. Phosphatidylcholine and lysophosphatidylcholine excretion is increased in children with cystic fibrosis and is associated with plasma homocysteine, S-adenosylhomocysteine, and S-adenosylmethionine. Am J Clin Nutr. 2005;81:686–91.
42. Feranchak AP, Sokol RJ. Cholangiocyte biology and cystic fibrosis liver disease. Semin Liver Dis. 2001;21:471–88.
43. Lindblad A, Hultcrantz R, Strandvik B. Bile-duct destruction and collagen deposition: a prominent ultrastructural feature of the liver in cystic fibrosis. Hepatology. 1992;16:372–81.
44. Cohn JA, Strong TV, Picciotto MR, Nairn AC, Collins FS, Fitz JG. Localization of the cystic fibrosis transmembrane conductance regulator in human bile duct epithelial cells. Gastroenterology. 1993;105:1857–64.
45. Beuers U, Hohenester S, de Buy Wenniger LJ, Kremer AE, Jansen PL, Elferink RP. The biliary HCO(3)(−) umbrella: a unifying hypothesis on pathogenetic and therapeutic aspects of fibrosing cholangiopathies. Hepatology. 2010;52:1489–96.
46. Hultcrantz R, Mengarelli S, Strandvik B. Morphological findings in the liver of children with cystic fibrosis: a light and electron microscopical study. Hepatology. 1986;6:881–9.
47. Kinnman N, Lindblad A, Housset C, Buentke E, Scheynius A, Strandvik B, Hultcrantz R. Expression of cystic fibrosis transmembrane conductance regulator in liver tissue from patients with cystic fibrosis. Hepatology. 2000;32:334–40.
48. Goodchild MC, Murphy GM, Howell AM, Nutter SA, Anderson CM. Aspects of bile acid metabolism in cystic fibrosis. Arch Dis Child. 1975;50:769–78.
49. Watkins JB, Tercyak AM, Szczepanik P, Klein PD. Bile salt kinetics in cystic fibrosis: influence of pancreatic enzyme replacement. Gastroenterology. 1977;73:1023–8.
50. O'Brien S, Mulcahy H, Fenlon H, O'Broin A, Casey M, Burke A, FitzGerald MX, et al. Intestinal bile acid malabsorption in cystic fibrosis. Gut. 1993;34:1137–41.
51. Bijvelds MJ, Jorna H, Verkade HJ, Bot AG, Hofmann F, Agellon LB, Sinaasappel M, et al. Activation of CFTR by ASBT-mediated bile salt absorption. Am J Physiol Gastrointest Liver Physiol. 2005;289:G870–9.
52. Bodewes FA, van der Wulp MY, Beharry S, Doktorova M, Havinga R, Boverhof R, James Phillips M, et al. Altered intestinal bile salt biotransformation in a cystic fibrosis (Cftr−/−) mouse model with hepato-biliary pathology. J Cyst Fibros. 2015;14:440–6.
53. Bijvelds MJ, de Jonge HR, Verkade HJ. Bile acid handling in cystic fibrosis: marked phenotypic differences between mouse models. Gastroenterology. 2012;143:e19–20; author reply e20.
54. Bodewes FA, Wouthuyzen-Bakker M, Bijvelds MJ, Havinga R, de Jonge HR, Verkade HJ. Ursodeoxycholate modulates bile flow and bile salt pool independently from the cystic fibrosis transmembrane regulator (Cftr) in mice. Am J Physiol Gastrointest Liver Physiol. 2012;302:G1035–42.

55. Strandvik B, Einarsson K, Lindblad A, Angelin B. Bile acid kinetics and biliary lipid composition in cystic fibrosis. J Hepatol. 1996;25:43–8.
56. Debray D, Rainteau D, Barbu V, Rouahi M, El Mourabit H, Lerondel S, Rey C, et al. Defects in gallbladder emptying and bile acid homeostasis in mice with cystic fibrosis transmembrane conductance regulator deficiencies. Gastroenterology. 2012;142:1581–1591.e6.
57. Fiorotto R, Scirpo R, Trauner M, Fabris L, Hoque R, Spirli C, Strazzabosco M. Loss of CFTR affects biliary epithelium innate immunity and causes TLR4-NF-kappaB-mediated inflammatory response in mice. Gastroenterology. 2011;141:1498–508, 1508 e1491–1495.
58. Fiorotto R, Villani A, Kourtidis A, Scirpo R, Amenduni M, Geibel PJ, Cadamuro M, et al. The cystic fibrosis transmembrane conductance regulator controls biliary epithelial inflammation and permeability by regulating Src tyrosine kinase activity. Hepatology. 2016;64:2118–34.
59. Blanco PG, Zaman MM, Junaidi O, Sheth S, Yantiss RK, Nasser IA, Freedman SD. Induction of colitis in cftr−/− mice results in bile duct injury. Am J Physiol Gastrointest Liver Physiol. 2004;287:G491–6.
60. Pascual G, Fong AL, Ogawa S, Gamliel A, Li AC, Perissi V, Rose DW, et al. A SUMOylation-dependent pathway mediates transrepression of inflammatory response genes by PPAR-gamma. Nature. 2005;437:759–63.
61. Scirpo R, Fiorotto R, Villani A, Amenduni M, Spirli C, Strazzabosco M. Stimulation of nuclear receptor peroxisome proliferator-activated receptor-gamma limits NF-kappaB-dependent inflammation in mouse cystic fibrosis biliary epithelium. Hepatology. 2015;62:1551–62.
62. Harmon GS, Dumlao DS, Ng DT, Barrett KE, Dennis EA, Dong H, Glass CK. Pharmacological correction of a defect in PPAR-gamma signaling ameliorates disease severity in Cftr-deficient mice. Nat Med. 2010;16:313–8.
63. Flass T, Tong S, Frank DN, Wagner BD, Robertson CE, Kotter CV, Sokol RJ, et al. Intestinal lesions are associated with altered intestinal microbiome and are more frequent in children and young adults with cystic fibrosis and cirrhosis. PLoS One. 2015;10:e0116967.
64. Debray D, Lykavieris P, Gauthier F, Dousset B, Sardet A, Munck A, Laselve H, et al. Outcome of cystic fibrosis-associated liver cirrhosis: management of portal hypertension. J Hepatol. 1999;31:77–83.
65. Leeuwen L, Magoffin AK, Fitzgerald DA, Cipolli M, Gaskin KJ. Cholestasis and meconium ileus in infants with cystic fibrosis and their clinical outcomes. Arch Dis Child. 2014;99:443–7.
66. Maurage C, Lenaerts C, Weber A, Brochu P, Yousef I, Roy CC. Meconium ileus and its equivalent as a risk factor for the development of cirrhosis: an autopsy study in cystic fibrosis. J Pediatr Gastroenterol Nutr. 1989;9:17–20.
67. Chryssostalis A, Hubert D, Coste J, Kanaan R, Burgel PR, Desmazes-Dufeu N, Soubrane O, et al. Liver disease in adult patients with cystic fibrosis: a frequent and independent prognostic factor associated with death or lung transplantation. J Hepatol. 2011;55:1377–82.
68. Lykavieris P, Bernard O, Hadchouel M. Neonatal cholestasis as the presenting feature in cystic fibrosis. Arch Dis Child. 1996;75:67–70.
69. Buxbaum J, Nguyen N, Kulkarni S, Palmer S, Rao A, Selby R. Multidisciplinary treatment of cystic fibrosis-related recurrent pyogenic cholangitis (CF-RPC). Dig Dis Sci. 2015;60:1801–4.
70. Woodruff SA, Sontag MK, Accurso FJ, Sokol RJ, Narkewicz MR. Prevalence of elevated liver enzymes in children with cystic fibrosis diagnosed by newborn screen. J Cyst Fibros. 2017;16:139–45.
71. Mayer-Hamblett N, Kloster M, Ramsey BW, Narkewicz MR, Saiman L, Goss CH. Incidence and clinical significance of elevated liver function tests in cystic fibrosis clinical trials. Contemp Clin Trials. 2013;34:232–8.
72. Bodewes FA, van der Doef HP, Houwen RH, Verkade HJ. Increase of serum gamma-Glutamyltransferase associated with development of cirrhotic cystic fibrosis liver disease. J Pediatr Gastroenterol Nutr. 2015;61:113–8.
73. Lenaerts C, Lapierre C, Patriquin H, Bureau N, Lepage G, Harel F, Marcotte J, et al. Surveillance for cystic fibrosis-associated hepatobiliary disease: early ultrasound changes and predisposing factors. J Pediatr. 2003;143:343–50.
74. Williams SM, Goodman R, Thomson A, McHugh K, Lindsell DR. Ultrasound evaluation of liver disease in cystic fibrosis as part of an annual assessment clinic: a 9-year review. Clin Radiol. 2002;57:365–70.
75. Leung DH, Ye W, Molleston JP, Weymann A, Ling S, Paranjape SM, Romero R, et al. Baseline ultrasound and clinical correlates in children with cystic fibrosis. J Pediatr. 2015;167:862–868.e2.
76. Colombo C, Castellani MR, Balistreri WF, Seregni E, Assaisso ML, Giunta A. Scintigraphic documentation of an improvement in hepatobiliary excretory function after treatment with ursodeoxycholic acid in patients with cystic fibrosis and associated liver disease. Hepatology. 1992;15:677–84.
77. Reeder SB, Cruite I, Hamilton G, Sirlin CB. Quantitative assessment of liver fat with magnetic resonance imaging and spectroscopy. J Magn Reson Imaging. 2011;34:729–49.
78. Leung DH, Khan M, Minard CG, Guffey D, Ramm LE, Clouston AD, Miller G, et al. Aspartate aminotransferase to platelet ratio and fibrosis-4 as biomarkers in biopsy-validated pediatric cystic fibrosis liver disease. Hepatology. 2015;62:1576–83.
79. Cook NL, Pereira TN, Lewindon PJ, Shepherd RW, Ramm GA. Circulating microRNAs as noninvasive diagnostic biomarkers of liver disease in children with cystic fibrosis. J Pediatr Gastroenterol Nutr. 2015;60:247–54.
80. Karlas T, Neuschulz M, Oltmanns A, Guttler A, Petroff D, Wirtz H, Mainz JG, et al. Non-invasive evaluation of cystic fibrosis related liver disease in adults with ARFI, transient elastography and different fibrosis scores. PLoS One. 2012;7:e42139.
81. Manco M, Zupone CL, Alghisi F, D'Andrea ML, Lucidi V, Monti L. Pilot study on the use of acoustic radiation force impulse imaging in the staging of cystic fibrosis associated liver disease. J Cyst Fibros. 2012;11:427–32.
82. Gominon AL, Frison E, Hiriart JB, Vergniol J, Clouzeau H, Enaud R, Bui S, et al. Assessment of liver disease progression in cystic fibrosis using transient elastography. J Pediatr Gastroenterol Nutr. 2018;66:455–60.
83. Franchi-Abella S, Corno L, Gonzales E, Antoni G, Fabre M, Ducot B, Pariente D, et al. Feasibility and diagnostic accuracy of supersonic shear-wave elastography for the assessment of liver stiffness and liver fibrosis in children: a pilot study of 96 patients. Radiology. 2016;278:554–62.
84. Witters P, De Boeck K, Dupont L, Proesmans M, Vermeulen F, Servaes R, Verslype C, et al. Non-invasive liver elastography (Fibroscan) for detection of cystic fibrosis-associated liver disease. J Cyst Fibros. 2009;8:392–9.
85. Menten R, Leonard A, Clapuyt P, Vincke P, Nicolae AC, Lebecque P. Transient elastography in patients with cystic fibrosis. Pediatr Radiol. 2010;40:1231–5.
86. Aqul A, Jonas MM, Harney S, Raza R, Sawicki GS, Mitchell PD, Fawaz R. Correlation of transient elastography with severity of cystic fibrosis-related liver disease. J Pediatr Gastroenterol Nutr. 2017;64:505–11.

87. Tang A, Cloutier G, Szeverenyi NM, Sirlin CB. Ultrasound elastography and MR elastography for assessing liver fibrosis: part 2, diagnostic performance, confounders, and future directions. AJR Am J Roentgenol. 2015;205:33–40.
88. Burgel PR, Bellis G, Olesen HV, Viviani L, Zolin A, Blasi F, Elborn JS. Future trends in cystic fibrosis demography in 34 European countries. Eur Respir J. 2015;46:133–41.
89. Ye W, Narkewicz MR, Leung DH, Karnsakul W, Murray KF, Alonso EM, Magee JC, et al. Variceal hemorrhage and adverse liver outcomes in patients with cystic fibrosis cirrhosis. J Pediatr Gastroenterol Nutr. 2018;66:122–7.
90. Slieker MG, van der Doef HP, Deckers-Kocken JM, van der Ent CK, Houwen RH. Pulmonary prognosis in cystic fibrosis patients with liver disease. J Pediatr. 2006;149:144; author reply 144–145.
91. Pencharz PB, Durie PR. Pathogenesis of malnutrition in cystic fibrosis, and its treatment. Clin Nutr. 2000;19:387–94.
92. Sacher-Huvelin S, Cales P, Bureau C, Valla D, Vinel JP, Duburque C, Attar A, et al. Screening of esophageal varices by esophageal capsule endoscopy: results of a French multicenter prospective study. Endoscopy. 2015;47:486–92.
93. McCarty TR, Afinogenova Y, Njei B. Use of wireless capsule endoscopy for the diagnosis and grading of esophageal varices in patients with portal hypertension: a systematic review and meta-analysis. J Clin Gastroenterol. 2017;51:174–82.
94. Goldschmidt I, Brauch C, Poynard T, Baumann U. Spleen stiffness measurement by transient elastography to diagnose portal hypertension in children. J Pediatr Gastroenterol Nutr. 2014;59:197–203.
95. Gana JC, Turner D, Mieli-Vergani G, Davenport M, Miloh T, Avitzur Y, Yap J, et al. A clinical prediction rule and platelet count predict esophageal varices in children. Gastroenterology. 2011;141:2009–16.
96. Isted A, Grammatikopoulos T, Davenport M. Prediction of esophageal varices in biliary atresia: derivation of the "varices prediction rule", a novel noninvasive predictor. J Pediatr Surg. 2015;50:1734–8.
97. Kelleher T, Staunton M, O'Mahony S, McCormick PA. Advanced hepatocellular carcinoma associated with cystic fibrosis. Eur J Gastroenterol Hepatol. 2005;17:1123–4.
98. McKeon D, Day A, Parmar J, Alexander G, Bilton D. Hepatocellular carcinoma in association with cirrhosis in a patient with cystic fibrosis. J Cyst Fibros. 2004;3:193–5.
99. Colombo C, Battezzati PM, Podda M, Bettinardi N, Giunta A. Ursodeoxycholic acid for liver disease associated with cystic fibrosis: a double-blind multicenter trial. The Italian Group for the Study of Ursodeoxycholic acid in cystic fibrosis. Hepatology. 1996;23:1484–90.
100. Cheng K, Ashby D, Smyth RL. Ursodeoxycholic acid for cystic fibrosis-related liver disease. Cochrane Database Syst Rev. 2017;9:CD000222.
101. Eaton JE, Talwalkar JA, Lazaridis KN, Gores GJ, Lindor KD. Pathogenesis of primary sclerosing cholangitis and advances in diagnosis and management. Gastroenterology. 2013;145:521–36.
102. Colombo C, Crosignani A, Alicandro G, Zhang W, Biffi A, Motta V, Corti F, et al. Long-term ursodeoxycholic acid therapy does not alter lithocholic acid levels in patients with cystic fibrosis with associated liver disease. J Pediatr. 2016;177:59–65.e51.
103. Dodge JA, Turck D. Cystic fibrosis: nutritional consequences and management. Best Pract Res Clin Gastroenterol. 2006;20:531–46.
104. Cogliandolo A, Patania M, Curro G, Chille G, Magazzu G, Navarra G. Postoperative outcomes and quality of life in patients with cystic fibrosis undergoing laparoscopic cholecystectomy: a retrospective study. Surg Laparosc Endosc Percutan Tech. 2011;21:179–83.
105. Gooding I, Dondos V, Gyi KM, Hodson M, Westaby D. Variceal hemorrhage and cystic fibrosis: outcomes and implications for liver transplantation. Liver Transpl. 2005;11:1522–6.
106. Pozler O, Krajina A, Vanicek H, Hulek P, Zizka J, Michl A, Elias P. Transjugular intrahepatic portosystemic shunt in five children with cystic fibrosis: long-term results. Hepatogastroenterology. 2003;50:1111–4.
107. Arnon R, Annunziato RA, Miloh T, Padilla M, Sogawa H, Batemarco L, Willis A, et al. Liver and combined lung and liver transplantation for cystic fibrosis: analysis of the UNOS database. Pediatr Transplant. 2011;15:254–64.
108. Desai CS, Gruessner A, Habib S, Gruessner R, Khan KM. Survival of cystic fibrosis patients undergoing liver and liver-lung transplantations. Transplant Proc. 2013;45:290–2.
109. Dowman JK, Watson D, Loganathan S, Gunson BK, Hodson J, Mirza DF, Clarke J, et al. Long-term impact of liver transplantation on respiratory function and nutritional status in children and adults with cystic fibrosis. Am J Transplant. 2012;12:954–64.
110. Fridell JA, Bond GJ, Mazariegos GV, Orenstein DM, Jain A, Sindhi R, Finder JD, et al. Liver transplantation in children with cystic fibrosis: a long-term longitudinal review of a single center's experience. J Pediatr Surg. 2003;38:1152–6.
111. Milkiewicz P, Skiba G, Kelly D, Weller P, Bonser R, Gur U, Mirza D, et al. Transplantation for cystic fibrosis: outcome following early liver transplantation. J Gastroenterol Hepatol. 2002;17:208–13.
112. Melzi ML, Kelly DA, Colombo C, Jara P, Manzanares J, Colledan M, Strazzabosco M, et al. Liver transplant in cystic fibrosis: a poll among European centers. A study from the European Liver Transplant Registry. Transpl Int. 2006;19:726–31.
113. Mendizabal M, Reddy KR, Cassuto J, Olthoff KM, Faust TW, Makar GA, Rand EB, et al. Liver transplantation in patients with cystic fibrosis: analysis of united network for organ sharing data. Liver Transpl. 2011;17:243–50.
114. Usatin DJ, Perito ER, Posselt AM, Rosenthal P. Under utilization of pancreas transplants in cystic fibrosis recipients in the united network organ sharing (UNOS) data 1987–2014. Am J Transplant. 2016;16:1620–5.
115. Bandsma RH, Bozic MA, Fridell JA, Crull MH, Molleston J, Avitzur Y, Mozer-Glassberg Y, et al. Simultaneous liver-pancreas transplantation for cystic fibrosis-related liver disease: a multicenter experience. J Cyst Fibros. 2014;13:471–7.
116. Hayes D Jr, Warren PS, McCoy KS, Sheikh SI. Improvement of hepatic steatosis in cystic fibrosis with ivacaftor therapy. J Pediatr Gastroenterol Nutr. 2015;60:578–9.
117. Colombo C. Mutation-targeted personalised medicine for cystic fibrosis. Lancet Respir Med. 2014;2:863–5.

Inherited Metabolic Disorders

Nedim Hadzic and Roshni Vara

Key Points
- IMDs are increasingly considered as indications for LT.
- Short-term results are comparable to other elective indications for LT.
- Neurodevelopmental delay usually stabilised, but does not reverse.
- LT, in the majority of IMDs, improves the phenotype rather than correcting completely the disease.

Research Needed in the Field
- Better definition of genotype/phenotype correlations in IMDs.
- Establish which conditions are good candidates for LT.
- Evaluate the medium-to-long-term outcome for LT in IMDs.

Table 16.1 Clinical presentations of inherited metabolic disease

Acute liver failure syndrome (coagulopathy, conjugated jaundice, hepatocellular cytolysis, hypoglycaemia, ascites, oedema)
Galactosaemia
GALD/neonatal haemochromatosis
Mitochondrial cytopathies (*POLG, DGUOK, TRMU, MPV17*)
Tyrosinaemia type I
Hereditary fructose intolerance
GRACILE syndrome
Citrin deficiency
Niemann-Pick type C disease
Cholestatic jaundice (with failure to thrive)
PiZ alpha-1-antitrypsin deficiency
PFIC syndrome
Niemann-Pick type C disease
Inborn errors of bile acid metabolism
Congenital glycosylation disorders
Peroxisomal disorders
Cholesterol biosynthesis defects
Hypoglycaemia (with hepatomegaly/seizures)
Glycogen storage disease (types I and III)
Severe hyperinsulinism
Gluconeogenesis defects
Hepatosplenomegaly
Lysosomal storage disorders
Cystic fibrosis
with Chronic liver disease/cirrhosis:
Cholesterol ester storage disease
Transaldolase deficiency
GSD Type IV
with Fatty liver disease:
Cholesterol ester storage disease
Mitochondrial cytopathies
with Hyperammonaemia:
Urea cycle defects
Fatty acid oxidation defects
Organic acidaemias

Inherited metabolic disorders (IMDs) are relatively rare monogenic conditions, requiring specific lifelong management. They are usually acquired in autosomal recessive manner, exceptions being some forms of urea cycle disorders or glycogen storage diseases, where X-linked inheritance is observed. Paediatric hepatologists encounter IMDs either in early infancy, when they typically present, or later when these patients are considered for liver transplantation (LT). Their initial manifestations may often be similar to clinical features of chronic liver disease (Table 16.1). Consanguinity, previous miscarriages or unexplained early infantile deaths increase the suspicion of an underlying metabolic problem. Of note, they are not frequently associated with prematurity or dysmorphism

N. Hadzic (✉)
Kings College Hospital, London, UK
e-mail: nedim.hadzic@kcl.ac.uk

R. Vara
Paediatric Inherited Metabolic Disease,
Evelina Children's Hospital, London, UK
e-mail: roshni.vara@gstt.nhs.uk

[1]. Clinical symptoms are rather nonspecific and could include lethargy, poor feeding, vomiting, hypoglycaemia with convulsions or abnormal movements, which could often be interpreted as sepsis-related. However, persistently elevated serum lactate in the absence of obvious infection or tissue hypoperfusion should always be taken as a serious pointer to IMD.

History of problems originating during pregnancy could occasionally be noted in some of the IMDs. Examples include Niemann-Pick disease, or long-chain 3-hydroxyacyl-CoA dehydrogenase (LCHAD), which could be associated with foetal hydrops [1]. Babies with GRACILE syndrome (foetal growth retardation, lactic acidosis, failure to thrive, hyperaminoaciduria, very high serum ferritin, liver haemosiderosis and early death) are born with severe intrauterine growth retardation [2]. Dysmorphic features such as microcephaly and facial dysmorphism could be observed in peroxisomal disorders; micrognathia and ambiguous genitalia in Smith-Lemli-Opitz syndrome, or inverted nipples and abnormal fat distribution in carbohydrate glycoprotein deficiency type 1a [1, 4]. Unusual urine odour could suggest some of the organic acidaemias, including maple syrup urine disease (MSUD), while trichorrhexis nodosa could be seen in argininosuccinate lyase deficiency. Physical signs associated with infantile liver disease have been recently reviewed [5].

A diagnostic approach is not simple and includes first-line metabolic investigations such as serum lactate, ammonia, acylcarnitine profile, plasma amino acids and urine organic acids. Mass spectrometry detection of acylcarnitines, following their esterification from carnitine with attached specific metabolites produced secondarily in IMDs, represents a biochemical basis for this valuable screening test [6]. Abnormalities in these tests could offer further direction to more specific biochemical investigations. Some of the blood spot screening tests, such as the ones for medium-chain acyl-coenzyme A deficiency (MCAD), galactosaemia or cystic fibrosis—to name a few—are often included in the national neonatal screening programmes. Nowadays, there is an increasing use of set panels for prolonged neonatal cholestasis ("jaundice chips") where some of the IMDs are increasingly included. Early contact with metabolic specialists is strongly advised as some of the clinical and biochemical features could overlap or may just be secondary to primary liver injury or immature enzymatic systems of a newborn child. Immediate treatment can vary, but it is always prudent to initially remove galactose from the diet, correct hypoglycaemia, attempt improving coagulopathy with vitamin K and cover infectious causes with antibiotics and antivirals until more information is available. It is strongly recommended to store the urine, blood and skin biopsy samples at presentation with suspected metabolic conditions, particularly in clinically unwell children.

Pathophysiological mechanisms leading to the liver impairment in IMDs could be quite diverse. For example, defective energy metabolism is the main problem in mitochondrial cytopathies, fatty acid oxidation (FAO) disorders or congenital lactic acidaemia. Retention of pathological substances in the organelles of the hepatocytes in lysosomal storage conditions, glycogen storage diseases or PiZ alpha-1-antitrypsin deficiency could activate cellular inflammatory responses and lead to their progressive structural damage. Finally, some of the aberrant metabolites could be directly toxic to the liver cells, such as in tyrosinaemia type 1 or in primary bile acid synthesis disorders. Of note, many IMDs will not damage hepatic microarchitecture as enzymatic defect remains at a functional level, and the liver biopsy could appear completely normal, which can be seen in organic acidaemias [7], maple syrup urine disease (MSUD), urea cycle defects or FAO disorders between the symptomatic episodes.

16.1 Inherited Metabolic Disorders Considered for Liver Transplantation

16.1.1 Urea Cycle Disorders

The complete urea cycle is expressed in the liver and is the main pathway for ammonia detoxification. Defects in the urea cycle are inherited in an autosomal recessive manner with the exception of ornithine transcarbamylase (OTC) deficiency, which is X-linked. Deficiencies in the more proximal steps [i.e. *N*-acetyl glutamate synthase (NAGS), carbamyl phosphate synthase 1 (CPS1), OTC and argininosuccinate synthase (ASS)] tend to present in the first few days of life with significant hyperammonaemia, poor feeding, encephalopathy and often coma. The more distal enzymatic steps [argininosuccinate lyase (ASL) and arginase] tend to present later with mild hyperammonaemia and neurological symptoms but can also present with neonatal hyperammonaemia. Urea cycle disorders are diagnosed on plasma amino acid and urine organic acid findings with genetic confirmation and/or enzymology studies. Long-term medical therapy includes a protein-restricted diet, ammonia-lowering medications, essential amino acid supplementation and carbohydrate emergency regimens for "sick days" [8]. There is ongoing risk of hyperammonaemic episodes and neurological injury, particularly in more severe cases, e.g. neonatal male-onset OTC deficiency or severe NAGS or CPS1 deficiency, where LT is often indicated within the first year of life [9, 10]. There are increasing reports of long-term neurological deficit and developmental delay despite medical management. The indication for LT is less clear in ASS and ASL deficiency and reserved for those with frequent metabolic decompensations or development of decompensated chronic liver injury seen in ASL deficiency [11, 12]. Survival rates following LT in urea cycle defects are excellent, and it should be considered as a management option in selected cases [13].

16.1.2 Classical Maple Syrup Urine Disease (MSUD)

Classical MSUD is an organic acidaemia caused by severe deficiency of branched-chain alpha-ketoacid dehydrogenase complex (BCKDH) resulting in the inability to breakdown leucine, isoleucine and leucine. Leucine is extremely neurotoxic and leads to clinical presentation in the first few days of life with poor feeding, lethargy, encephalopathy, cerebral oedema and seizures. Long-term medical management includes a protein-restricted diet, branched-chain amino acid formula, regular blood spot monitoring and supervised emergency plans. Some newborn screening programmes include MSUD, and early intervention has shown good neurological outcomes with medical management [14]. LT has been shown to be a successful treatment option for classical MSUD and reduces the burden of specialised diet, removes the risk of significant metabolic decompensation and improves quality of life [15]. LT is essentially curative and has been shown to replace sufficient enzyme activity, but there is also a significant extrahepatic expression of BCKDH in the muscle, kidneys and central nervous system. MSUD livers have been successfully used in domino transplantation with normal branched-chain amino acid metabolism subsequently demonstrated in the recipients [16].

16.1.3 Propionic Acidaemia (PA) and Methylmalonic Acidaemia (MMA)

PA and MMA are organic acidaemias caused by enzyme defects in the catabolic pathway of branched-chain amino acids (isoleucine, valine, methionine and threonine), odd chain fatty acids and cholesterol. Propionyl-CoA carboxylase is deficient in PA and encoded by the PCCA and PCCB genes. Classical MMA is due to methylmalonyl-CoA mutase deficiency, and severe cases tend to have little or no activity (mut0). The clinical presentation of severe forms is in the first few days of life with poor feeding, encephalopathy, ketoacidosis, hyperammonaemia and coma. Long-term treatment includes a protein-restricted diet with or without specialised supplements, ammonia-lowering agents, if required, and emergency management plans [17]. There is significant extrahepatic enzyme expression for PA and MMA and considerable multisystem involvement (cardiac, renal, central nervous system, pancreatitis, optic atrophy). Despite maximal medical therapy, neurocognitive outcomes for PA and MMA remain suboptimal [18]. LT has been shown to be successful in some cases, but remains uncertain, particularly in MMA [19, 20]. LT is usually considered in cases with frequent decompensations and severe disease and/or to improve quality of life. Management perioperatively and postoperatively requires a multispecialty team and the availability of metabolic expertise [21, 22]. LT provides only a partial cure in PA and MMA and has been shown to achieve a milder metabolic phenotype with reduction in metabolic decompensations and potentially extrahepatic complications.

16.1.4 Glycogen Storage Disorders (GSD)

Disorders of glycogen metabolism considered for LT encompass type I, III and IV. GSD type Ia is due to deficiency of glucose-6-phosphatase, and GSD type Ib is due to defects in the glucose-6-phosphatase translocase enzyme. GSD type I presents in early infancy with hepatomegaly, hypoglycaemia, lactic acidosis, hyperlipidaemia, hyperuricaemia and neutropenia (type 1b).

GSD type III is due to deficiency of glycogen-branching enzyme and presents in infancy with hepatomegaly, hypoglycaemia, hyperlipidaemia and risk of myopathy and cardiomyopathy in later life. GSD types I and III are also associated with the development of hepatic adenoma in later life. The medical treatment is avoidance of fasting and correction of hypoglycaemia and lactic acidosis with a closely supervised metabolic diet [23, 24]. GSD type IV is rare with variable phenotype and is due to glycogen-debranching enzyme deficiency, which results in an abnormal glycogen (amylopectin), leading to liver fibrosis, cirrhosis, cardiomyopathy and myopathy in some. The progressive hepatic form tends to result in decompensated liver requiring LT before 5 years, and the nonprogressive form results in stable liver disease, requiring surveillance [25]. Medical treatment for GSD types I and III is successful; however LT has been reported in the presence of a poor metabolic control to improve quality of life and when hepatocellular neoplasms could develop. Neutropenia and hyperuricaemia may persist in GSD 1a following LT [26].

16.1.5 Mitochondrial Disease

Mitochondria are ubiquitous in cells and hence their disorders can present at any age with any symptom. Oxidative phosphorylation and generation of adenosine triphosphate via the respiratory chain complex, fatty acid oxidation, the urea cycle and other pathways within the mitochondria can be affected. Primary mitochondrial hepatopathies are inherited disorders, usually nuclear DNA defects, which affect the structure or function of mitochondria. The mitochondrial

DNA (mtDNA) depletion syndrome, which often leads to liver failure and neurologic abnormalities, is caused by a nuclear gene defects that control mtDNA replication or stability. Hepatic presentations of mitochondrial disease with acute liver failure, recurrent acute liver failure, fatty liver disease and chronic liver disease are increasingly recognised with the emergence of rapid genetic testing. The hepatocerebral form of mitochondrial DNA depletion syndrome is usually due to mutations in *POLG, DGUOK, MPV17, SUCLG1 and Twinkle* genes. Biochemical investigations such as plasma lactate, plasma amino acids, urine organic acids, acylcarnitines, CSF lactate and MRI brain scan can be helpful but may not be diagnostic. Muscle biopsy is often contraindicated in the acute situation due to coagulopathy. LT in mitochondrial disease is a difficult decision, particularly if the diagnosis cannot be confirmed promptly. LT remains controversial, and it is imperative to attempt to make a genetic diagnosis and exclude extrahepatic involvement when considering this option [27, 28].

16.2 Management

Basic management principles for IMDs include (a) long-term specific dietary restrictions to minimise the traffic through defective pathway and the accumulation of toxic metabolites, (b) the use of cofactors to enhance the residual activity of residual enzyme, (c) supplementation of downstream products beyond the metabolic defect, (d) preventing catabolism with emergency regimens in specific conditions and (e) disposal of toxic metabolites, where possible. Therapeutic improvements in different IMDs are variable, but unfortunately frequently result only in a limited overall biochemical control and medical stabilisation with sometimes suboptimal neurocognitive outcomes despite medical therapy.

The development of hepatocellular carcinoma (HCC) is a rare but well-recognised complication of some IMDs, including tyrosinaemia type 1, bile salt export pump (BSEP) deficiency, mitochondrial cytopathies and PiZ alpha-1-antitrypsin deficiency. Adenomas often develop in glycogen storage disease types I and III, but usually not before the second or third decade of life. They also may progress to HCC. Mechanisms responsible for the neoplastic proliferation are not completely understood, but are likely to be multifactorial, albeit driven by the abnormal metabolites. Therefore, HCC surveillance with regular liver ultrasonography and serum alpha-fetoprotein measurement is mandatory in the majority of IMDs.

It is becoming increasingly clear that many children with IMDs, despite medical treatment, will continue to require hospital admission due to metabolic decompensations and suboptimal chronic metabolic control, resulting in missed milestones, developmental delay, social and learning difficulties and poor education [6, 17]. This disappointing scenario, now confirmed after decades of expert follow-up for IMDs, has prompted increasing consideration for the liver replacement, where effective provision of a normal enzymatic supply could potentially be achieved [10].

16.3 Inherited Metabolic Disorders and Liver Transplantation

Liver transplantation (LT) is now the widely established mode of clinical management for many cholestatic, anatomical, neoplastic and toxic conditions. The standardisation of surgical methods, the introduction of tailor-made immune suppression and effective anti-infectious regimes have reduced mortality risks for elective indications to less than 5% in most of the large specialist centres [29]. LT has therefore emerged as one of the management options for IMDs due to ongoing issues with their conventional treatment, including very restricted metabolic diets, lifelong use of potentially toxic medications, frequent requirements for hospital admissions in metabolic crises and, most importantly, unsatisfactory neurological and intellectual outcome medium term [6, 30]. Worldwide, IMDs currently represent approximately 15–25% of the primary indications for LT [9, 31, 32].

Selection for LT is always a complex undertaking, but in this particular setting, it is even more challenging as risks of this complex surgico-medical intervention need to be carefully counterbalanced by potential benefits of the effective metabolic correction. This can only be achieved by a close collaboration between metabolic physicians and LT team during each phase of the process. Due to their relative rarity, clinical experiences with particular IMDs will never be extensive in any single centre. Table 16.2 is an attempt to summarise present clinical indications for LT among IMDs, but it is by no means definite (Table 16.2).

The benefits of LT depend on the provision of the defective enzyme provided by the liver graft cells and re-establishment of the physiological metabolic pathway. This reparatory process could be difficult to anticipate and is variably effective, depending on the biology of the underlying IMD. In addition, the clinical manifestations could be diverse even within the same condition (e.g. infantile vs. juvenile types) or even within the same family (e.g. Wilson disease or PiZ alpha-1-antitrypsin deficiency). Another unsolved question is about the quantity of missing enzyme required to achieve a clinical modification of the phenotype, which is known for only a handful of IMDs. This could be a relevant clinical point if the liver graft function becomes suboptimal for whatever postoperative complication, but also during donor selection process. Living-related donor

Table 16.2 Metabolic conditions of childhood potentially treatable by liver transplantation

Curable by liver transplantation
Wilson disease
Alpha-1-antitrypsin PiZ deficiency
Tyrosinaemia type 1
Bile salt export pump (BSEP) deficiency
Multiple drug resistance 3 (MDR3) deficiency
Double domain-containing protein 2 (DCDC2) deficiency
Urea cycle disorders
Ornithine transcarbamylase (OTC) deficiency
Carbamoyl phosphate synthetase 1 (CPS1) deficiency
Citrullinaemia
Argininosuccinate lyase (ASL) deficiency
Argininaemia
Familial hypercholesterolaemia
Organic acidaemias
Maple syrup urine disease (MSUD)
Coagulation disorders
Haemophilia A and B
Factor VII deficiency
Protein C and S deficiencies
Acute intermittent porphyria
Complement factor H and I deficiency
Afibrinogenaemia
Hereditary haemochromatosis
Partially treated by liver transplantation
FIC-1 disease
TJP2 deficiency
Organic acidaemias
Propionic acidaemia
Methylmalonic acidaemia
Cystic fibrosis
Glycogen disease type III and IV
Familial amyloidosis
Experimental
Mitochondrial hepatopathies
Mitochondrial DNA depletion (POLG1, MPV17, DGUOK)
Erythropoietic protoporphyria
Cholesterol-esterase storage disease
Gaucher disease
Phenylketonuria
Citrin deficiency
Relative contraindications
Niemann-Pick type C disease
Peroxisomal disorders
Alpers syndrome

options, involving typically one of the parents, are increasingly exploited in paediatric liver centres and contribute to reducing waiting times and ameliorating chronic donor shortages. In IMDs, living donation is less desirable as parents are expected to be phenotypically unaffected carriers. However, effects of the major surgery on their metabolic control and long-term complications and viability of the heterozygous graft are generally incompletely understood [33, 34]. In OTC deficiency, inherited in an X-linked manner, it is preferable to investigate the father as a prospective living donor, as the carrier mothers could have a different enzymatic expression, and formal assessment to measure the levels in the liver tissue may be necessary. Large experience from Japan, where the living liver donation is predominant, is overall encouraging [35], but many other centres still prefer avoiding obligate carriers as donors for IMD indications and obtain the organs from unrelated anonymous sources. However, routine LT criteria for conventional indications in paediatric hepatology (coagulopathy, serum bilirubin, albumin, platelet count, etc.) usually do not apply to IMDs, and transplant centres tend to develop their own internal policies for these conditions. These scoring tasks are not simple as they must account for different biology of distinct IMDs, but also their increasing referrals for LT consideration, which should not jeopardise expected standard waiting times for the routine life-threatening transplant indications in other children.

One potential attractive option in LT for IMDs is using the auxiliary grafting, where only a part of the native liver is replaced during the operation, providing the missing enzymatic supply [36]. The remaining native liver could still represent a reliable backup option should the graft function becomes seriously deranged for whatever reason during follow-up. Furthermore, auxiliary LT leaves a possibility of genetic manipulation or genetic material transfer open for the future. Auxiliary LT, in children usually with the left segmental graft, is more technically challenging but should be considered in conditions where extrahepatic expression of the missing enzyme is limited, requirements for correction are known, and the clinical effects are easily monitored (e.g. serum bilirubin in Crigler-Najjar syndrome type 1, or ammonia, ketones and metabolic acidosis in organic acidaemias). Preferential surgical redistribution of the portal flow by partial banding between the auxiliary and native liver may be required in order to increase the blood supply and improve desired enzymatic activity [37]. Overall, elective auxiliary LT should be considered in the presence of sufficient local surgical expertise for indications where gene transfer therapy will not be imminently available.

On a positive side, patients with IMDs will only exceptionally have evidence of chronic liver disease, portal hypertension or previous abdominal surgeries, which could make LT technically more straightforward [29]. However, some of the previous long-term dietary restrictions, for example, in protein intake, may affect postoperative healing process and recovery. It is also possible that some of the IMDs may render children procoagulant [38] or having mild immune deficiency (like in propionic acidaemia) [39]. If the explanted liver or its part is histopathologically unaffected, it could be potentially considered for domino grafting in patients affected by unrelated conditions [40, 41]. This concept has been well-documented in LT for MSUD, where the missing branched-chain amino acid enzyme from the explanted liver graft was counterbalanced by the normal extrahepatic metabolic pathways of the domino recipient [42].

16.4 Perioperative Management

Children with IMDs were noted to be prone to more significant metabolic derangements during the surgery. One study has described higher levels of oxidative stress, transforming growth factor-β1 and complement activity during LT for IMDs in comparison to children with biliary atresia [43]. In preparation for LT, many centres try to minimise preoperative fasting, ensure steady intravenous supply of a glucose infusion rate of at least 6–8 mg/kg/min (to avoid hypoglycaemia and catabolic state) and strictly control fluid and electrolyte balance [42, 44]. Administering short-term parenteral nutrition may occasionally be necessary. From experience with levels of the branched-chain amino acids in MSUD, the metabolic correction can be achieved within 6 h after LT [42, 44], but strict observation for several more postoperative days—until normal enteral intake is established—appears prudent.

If LT genuinely represents a good long-term management option for some IMDs, then the timing of this intervention becomes critically important. It is conceivable that earlier LT could reduce the risk of neurological and developmental damage in children who remain at risk due to brittle clinical course of their underlying IMDs. After the first 3 months of life, surgical issues become less challenging, while immunological aspects could actually be favourable for an early LT. Of note, it has also been hypothesised that rapid growth and development in the first year of life, with increased utilisation of nitrogen, could reduce retention of potentially toxic compounds such as ammonia in urea cycle disorders and presumably protect from detrimental neurodevelopmental effects until the growth relatively slows down after 2 or 3 years of age [10]. This "honeymoon" period should then offer an optimal opportunity window for the LT. In any case, there are increasing trends of working up the infants with IMDs for the surgery in the first year of life to minimise the impact of the suboptimal metabolic control on the developing brain of young children. However, given the overall rarity of IMDs, phenotypic differences, lack of reliable markers of metabolic control and difficulties in consistent neurodevelopmental assessment and follow-up, each decision about benefits/risks of LT must be carefully balanced and strictly individualised. In that context, comprehensive family education and the early use of elective accelerated immunisation schedules are very important. Novel methods such as hepatocyte transplantation may offer some palliative measures of metabolic control ("bridging") until the small neonate or young infant becomes physically fit for LT as a definite corrective intervention. At the present time, medium-term viability of the cell transplantation has not been yet established, but attempts of its expansion are ongoing.

16.5 Management After Liver Transplantation

There is emerging evidence that in patients with IMDs, a good graft function after LT provides a stable clinical phenotype with no metabolic crises and a much improved quality of life [19, 45]. Reported 5- and 10-year patient and graft survival are around 90 and 80%, respectively, with ever-improving trends [29, 32]. The effects of successful LT to neurological, cognitive and intellectual aspects are much more difficult to ascertain due to individual differences and the lack of consistent psychometric and neurodevelopmental quantitative monitoring [19, 45].

Strict dietary restrictions are usually completely removed after LT in disorders where the defect is corrected, e.g. urea cycle defects; however, some restriction may be required in organic acidaemias where the correction is incomplete. Some children, who had been showing aversion to certain food, for example, protein, may start showing renewed interest after the surgery, resulting in improved growth and development. There is no evidence whether the dietary restrictions should not be lifted in living-related LT or where graft function may have been suboptimal.

It is unclear yet whether the effective LT arrests development of all extrahepatic complications, such as cardiac, renal or ophthalmic. In propionic acidaemia, there is some evidence that hypertrophic cardiomyopathy could be reverted following effective LT [46]. Some children post LT for tyrosinaemia type 1 continue excreting succinylacetone in urine with low normal activity of the enzyme porphobilinogen (PBG) synthase, which could indicate the ongoing activity of the aberrant tyrosinaemia pathway [47]. It is therefore arguable whether there are potential benefits of using metabolic modifier nitisinone after LT in order to completely abolish the production of succinylacetone and minimise long-term renal toxicity due to both the original disease and anti-rejection therapy with calcineurin inhibitors. There is no present consensus on that, but further research into whether some forms of adjunct metabolic management, particularly for IMDs with known extrahepatic features, are still required.

In conclusion, LT offers a viable management option for many IMDs. With careful selection, benefits often outweigh the long-term risks associated with LT. After the surgery the clinical phenotype becomes stable with only exceptional occurrence of metabolic derangements or life-threatening metabolic crises. The standard measures of quality of life for the child and family usually dramatically improve. However, one has to offer realistic expectations about the neurocognitive outcome, which usually does not deteriorate, but also does not get better with the established metabolic control. Pre-existing neurological changes usually do not revert. Given the increasing confidence and acceptable safety profile of elective LT, the overall intuitive approach is to consider this procedure much earlier in the infancy. The role of auxiliary and living-related LT is not optimally defined and may well need to be individualised for different conditions. Clinical indications for LT in IMDs will continue to change, dependent on the further success of transplantation options, including stem and mesenchymal cell transfer techniques, better understanding of natural history and long-term complications of individual IMDs, the general impact of the metabolic defect on neurodevelopment and the quality of life for the child and the family and whether any new superior therapeutic modalities will become available in the foreseeable future.

References

1. Saudubray JM, Nassogne MC, de Lonlay P, Touati G. Clinical approach to inherited metabolic disorders in neonates: an overview. Semin Neonatol. 2002;7:3–15.
2. Fellman V, Rapola J, Pihko H, et al. Iron-overload disease in infants involving fetal growth retardation, lactic acidosis, liver haemosiderosis, and amino aciduria. Lancet. 1998;351:490–3.
3. Jaeken J, Matthijs G, Saudubray JM, et al. Phosphomannomutase isomerase deficiency: a carbohydrate-deficient glycoprotein syndrome with hepatic-intestinal presentation. Am J Hum Genet. 1998;62:1535–9.
4. Hadzic N, Verkade HJ. The changing spectrum of neonatal hepatitis. J Pediatr Gastroenterol Nutr. 2016;63:316–9.
5. Santra S, Hendriksz C. How to use acylcarnitine profiles to help diagnose inborn errors of metabolism. Arch Dis Child Educ Pract Ed. 2010;95:151–6. https://doi.org/10.1136/adc.2009.174342.2010.
6. Oishi K, Arnon R, Wasserstein MP, Diaz GA. Liver transplantation for pediatric inherited metabolic disorders: considerations for indications, complications, perioperative management. Pediatr Transplant. 2016;20:756–69. https://doi.org/10.1111/petr.12741.
7. Imbard A, Garcia Segarra N, Tardieu M, Broué P, Bouchereau J, Pichard S, de Baulny HO, Slama A, Mussini C, Touati G, Danjoux M, Gaignard P, Vogel H, Labarthe F, Schiff M, Benoist JF. Long-term liver disease in methylmalonic and propionic acidemias. Mol Genet Metab. 2018;123(4):433–40.
8. Häberle J, Boddaert N, Burlina A, Chakrapani A, Dixon M, Huemer M, Karall D, Martinelli D, Crespo PS, Santer R, Servais A, Valayannopoulos V, Lindner M, Rubio V, Dionisi-Vici C. Suggested guidelines for the diagnosis and management of urea cycle disorders. Orphanet J Rare Dis. 2012;7:32.
9. Yu L, Rayhill SC, Hsu EK, Landis CS. Liver transplantation for urea cycle disorders: analysis of the united network for organ sharing database. Transplant Proc. 2015;47(8):2413–8.
10. Ah Mew N, Krivitzky L, McCarter R, Batshaw M, Tuchman M. Clinical outcomes of neonatal onset proximal versus distal urea cycle disorders do not differ. J Pediatr. 2013;162:324–9.e1. https://doi.org/10.1016/j.jpeds.2012.06.065.
11. Yankol Y, Mecit N, Kanmaz T, Acarli K, Kalayoglu M. Argininosuccinic aciduria—a rare indication for liver transplant: report of two cases. Exp Clin Transplant. 2017;15(5):581–4.
12. Robberecht E, Maesen S, Jonckheere A, Van Biervliet S, Carton D. Successful liver transplantation for argininosuccinate lyase deficiency (ASLD). J Inherit Metab Dis. 2006;29(1):184–5.
13. Kido J, Matsumoto S, Momosaki K, Sakamoto R, Mitsubuchi H, Endo F, Nakamura K. Liver transplantation may prevent neurodevelopmental deterioration in high-risk patients with urea cycle disorders. Pediatr Transplant. 2017;21(6).
14. Morton DH, Strauss KA, Robinson DL, Puffenberger EG, Kelley RI. Diagnosis and treatment of maple syrup disease: a study of 36 patients. Pediatrics. 2002;109(6):999–1008.
15. Díaz VM, Camarena C, de la Vega Á, Martínez-Pardo M, Díaz C, López M, Hernández F, Andrés A, Jara P. Liver transplantation for classical maple syrup urine disease: long-term follow-up. J Pediatr Gastroenterol Nutr. 2014;59(5):636–9.
16. Celik N, Squires RH, Vockley J, Sindhi R, Mazariegos G. Liver transplantation for maple syrup urine disease: a global domino effect. Pediatr Transplant. 2016;20(3):350–1.
17. Fraser JL, Venditti CP. Methylmalonic and propionic acidemias: clinical management update. Curr Opin Pediatr. 2016;28:682–93.
18. Kölker S, Valayannopoulos V, Burlina AB, Sykut-Cegielska J, Wijburg FA, Teles EL, Zeman J, Dionisi-Vici C, Barić I, Karall D, Arnoux JB, Avram P, Baumgartner MR, Blasco-Alonso J, Boy SP, Rasmussen MB, Burgard P, Chabrol B, Chakrapani A, Chapman K, Cortès I Saladelafont E, Couce ML, de Meirleir L, Dobbelaere D, Furlan F, Gleich F, González MJ, Gradowska W, Grünewald S, Honzik T, Hörster F, Ioannou H, Jalan A, Häberle J, Haege G, Langereis E, de Lonlay P, Martinelli D, Matsumoto S, Mühlhausen C, Murphy E, de Baulny HO, Ortez C, Pedrón CC, Pintos-Morell G, Pena-Quintana L, Ramadža DP, Rodrigues E, Scholl-Bürgi S, Sokal E, Summar ML, Thompson N, Vara R, Pinera IV, Walter JH, Williams M, Lund AM, Garcia-Cazorla A. The phenotypic spectrum of organic acidurias and urea cycle disorders. Part 2: the evolving clinical phenotype. J Inherit Metab Dis. 2015;38(6):1059–74.
19. Vara R, Turner C, Mundy H, Heaton ND, Rela M, Mieli-Vergani G, Champion M, Hadzic N. Liver transplantation for propionic acidaemia in children. Liver Transpl. 2011;17:661–7.
20. Niemi AK, Kim IK, Krueger CE, Cowan TM, Baugh N, Farrell R, Bonham CA, Concepcion W, Esquivel CO, Enns GM. Treatment of methylmalonic acidemia by liver or combined liver-kidney transplantation. J Pediatr. 2015;166(6):1455–61.
21. Rajakumar A, Kaliamoorthy I, Reddy MS, Rela M. Anaesthetic considerations for liver transplantation in propionic acidemia. Indian J Anaesth. 2016;60(1):50–4.
22. Sloan JL, Manoli I, Venditti CP. Liver or combined liver-kidney transplantation for patients with isolated methylmalonic acidemia: who and when? J Pediatr. 2015;166(6):1346–50.
23. Weinstein DA, Steuerwald U, De Souza CFM, Derks TGJ. Inborn errors of metabolism with hypoglycemia: glycogen storage diseases and inherited disorders of gluconeogenesis. Pediatr Clin North Am. 2018;65(2):247–65.
24. Bhattacharya K. Investigation and management of the hepatic glycogen storage diseases. Transl Pediatr. 2015;4(3):240–8.
25. Szymańska E, Szymańska S, Truszkowska G, Ciara E, Pronicki M, Shin YS, Podskarbi T, Kępka A, Śpiewak M, Płoski R, Bilińska ZT, Rokicki D. Variable clinical presentation of glycogen storage

disease type IV: from severe hepatosplenomegaly to cardiac insufficiency. Some discrepancies in genetic and biochemical abnormalities. Arch Med Sci. 2018;14(1):237–47.
26. Davis MK, Weinstein DA. Liver transplantation in children with glycogen storage disease: controversies and evaluation of the risk/benefit of this procedure. Pediatr Transplant. 2008;12(2):137–45.
27. De Greef E, Christodoulou J, Alexander IE, Shun A, O'Loughlin EV, Thorburn DR, Jermyn V, Stormon MO. Mitochondrial respiratory chain hepatopathies: role of liver transplantation. A case series of five patients. JIMD Rep. 2012;4:5–11.
28. Dubern B, Broue P, Dubuisson C, Cormier-Daire V, Habes D, Chardot C, Devictor D, Munnich A, Bernard O. Orthotopic liver transplantation for mitochondrial respiratory chain disorders: a study of 5 children. Transplantation. 2001;71(5):633–7.
29. Mazariegos G, Shneider B, Burton B, Fox IJ, Hadzic N, Kishnani P, Morton DH, McIntire S, Sokol RJ, Summar M, White D, Chavanon V, Vockley J. Liver transplantation for pediatric metabolic disease. Mol Genet Metab. 2014;111:418–27. https://doi.org/10.1016/j.ymgme.
30. McKiernan PJ. Liver transplantation and cell therapies for inborn errors of metabolism. J Inherit Metab Dis. 2013;36:675–80. https://doi.org/10.1007/s10545-012-9581-z.
31. Fagiuoli S, Daina E, D'Antiga L, Coledan M, Remuzzi G. Monogenic diseases that can be cured by liver transplantation. J Hepatol. 2013;59:595–612.
32. Arnon R, Kerkar N, Davis MK, Anand R, Yin W, González-Peralta RP, SPLIT Research Group. Liver transplantation in children with metabolic diseases: the studies of pediatric liver transplantation experience. Pediatr Transplant. 2010;14:796–805. https://doi.org/10.1111/j.1399-3046.2010.01339.x.
33. Rahayatri TH, Uchida H, Sasaki K, et al. Hyperammonemia in ornithine transcarbamylase-deficient recipients following living donor liver transplantation from heterozygous carrier donors. Pediatr Transplant. 2017;21:e12848. https://doi.org/10.1111/petr.12848.
34. Feier F, Schwartz IV, Benkert AR, Seda Neto J, Miura I, Chapchap P, da Fonseca EA, Vieira S, Zanotelli ML, Pinto e Vairo F, Camelo JS Jr, Margutti AV, Mazariegos GV, Puffenberger EG, Strauss KA. Living related versus deceased donor liver transplantation for maple syrup urine disease. Mol Genet Metab. 2016;117:336–43. https://doi.org/10.1016/j.ymgme.2016.01.005. Epub 2016 Jan 12.
35. Kasahara M, Sakamoto S, Horikawa R, et al. Living donor liver transplantation for pediatric patients with metabolic disorders: the Japanese multicenter registry. Pediatr Transplant. 2014;18:6–15.
36. Reddy MS, Rajalingam R, Rela M. Revisiting APOLT for metabolic liver disease: a new look at an old idea. Transplantation. 2017;101:260–6. https://doi.org/10.1097/TP.0000000000001472.
37. Rela M, Bharathan A, Palaniappan K, Cherian PT, Reddy MS. Portal flow modulation in auxiliary partial orthotopic liver transplantation. Pediatr Transplant. 2015;19:255–60. https://doi.org/10.1111/petr.12436.
38. Dowman JK, Gunson BK, Mirza DF, Bramhall SR, Badminton MN, Newsome PN, UK Liver Selection and Allocation Working Party. Liver transplantation for acute intermittent porphyria is complicated by a high rate of hepatic artery thrombosis. Liver Transpl. 2012;18:195–200. https://doi.org/10.1002/lt.22345.
39. Raby RB, Ward JC, Herrod HG. Propionic acidaemia and immunodeficiency. J Inherit Metab Dis. 1994;17:250–1.
40. Chen CY, Liu C, Lin NC, Tsai HL, Loong CC, Hsia CY. Exchange of partial liver transplantation between children with different non-cirrhotic metabolic liver diseases: how do we arrive there? Ann Transplant. 2016;21:525–30.
41. Govil S, Shanmugam NP, Reddy MS, Narasimhan G, Rela M. A metabolic chimera: two defective genotypes make a normal phenotype. Liver Transpl. 2015;21:1453–4. https://doi.org/10.1002/lt.24202.
42. Mazariegos GV, Morton DH, Sindhi R, Soltys K, Nayyar N, Bond G, Shellmer D, Shneider B, Vockley J, Strauss KA. Liver transplantation for classical maple syrup urine disease: long-term follow-up in 37 patients and comparative United Network for Organ Sharing experience. J Pediatr. 2012;160:116–21.e1. https://doi.org/10.1016/j.jpeds.2011.06.033.
43. Hussein MH, Hashimoto T, Suzuki T, Daoud GA, Goto T, Nakajima Y, Kato T, Hibi M, Tomishige H, Hara F, Kato S, Kakita H, Kamei M, Ito T, Kato I, Sugioka A, Togari H. Children undergoing liver transplantation for treatment of inherited metabolic diseases are prone to higher oxidative stress, complement activity and transforming growth factor-β1. Ann Transplant. 2013;18:63–8. https://doi.org/10.12659/AOT.883820.
44. Strauss KA, Mazariegos GV, Sindhi R, Squires R, Finegold DN, Vockley G, Robinson DL, Hendrickson C, Virji M, Cropcho L, Puffenberger EG, McGhee W, Seward LM, Morton DH. Elective liver transplantation for the treatment of classical maple syrup urine disease. Am J Transplant. 2006;6:557–64.
45. Shellmer DA, DeVito Dabbs A, Dew MA, Noll RB, Feldman H, Strauss KA, Morton DH, Vockley J, Mazariegos GV. Cognitive and adaptive functioning after liver transplantation for maple syrup urine disease: a case series. Pediatr Transplant. 2011;15:58–64. https://doi.org/10.1111/j.1399-3046.2010.01411.x.
46. Romano S, Valayannopoulos V, Touati G, Jais JP, Rabier D, de Keyzer Y, Bonnet D, de Lonlay P. Cardiomyopathies in propionic aciduria are reversible after liver transplantation. J Pediatr. 2010;156:128–34. https://doi.org/10.1016/j.jpeds.2009.07.002.
47. Bartlett DC, Preece MA, Holme E, Lloyd C, Newsome PN, McKiernan PJ. Plasma succinylacetone is persistently raised after liver transplantation in tyrosinaemia type 1. J Inherit Metab Dis. 2013;36:15–20. https://doi.org/10.1007/s10545-012-9482-1. Epub 2012 Mar 29.

Nonalcoholic Fatty Liver Disease and Steatohepatitis in Children

Antonella Mosca, Silvio Veraldi, Andrea Dellostrologo, Mariateresa Sanseviero, and Valerio Nobili

Key Points
- NAFLD is the most common liver disease in children and adolescents.
- Obese and selected overweight children should be routinely screened for NAFLD.
- Liver biopsy is still the reference standard for diagnosis NAFLD, but it should not be performed in all patients.
- NAFLD can be associated with other features of metabolic syndrome.
- Weight loss is the cornerstone of NAFLD therapy.

Research Needed in the Field
- Deepening of our knowledge of pathophysiology of the disease, mainly about gut-liver interactions.
- Identify a reliable, noninvasive diagnostic tool to diagnose and stage NAFLD/NASH.
- Evaluate safety and effectiveness of the new pharmacologic treatments.

Professor Valerio Nobili suddenly passed away on March 15, 2019, at the age of 52. The editor and the authors of this book wish to honor the memory of the pediatric hepatologist who brought to light the importance of hepatic steatosis in children's liver disease, an inspired and passionate scientist, and a dear friend.

–Lorenzo D'Antiga

A. Mosca (✉) · S. Veraldi · A. Dellostrologo · M. Sanseviero
Hepatology, Gastroenterology and Nutrition Unit, "Bambino Gesù" Children's Hospital, Rome, Italy
e-mail: antonella.mosca@opbg.net

V. Nobili (deceased)
Hepatology, Gastroenterology and Nutrition Unit, "Bambino Gesù" Children's Hospital, Rome, Italy

Department of Pediatrics, Facoltà di Medicina e Psicologia, Sapienza University of Rome, Rome, Italy

17.1 Introduction

NAFLD represents the most common cause of chronic liver disease in children and adolescents; it is characterized by accumulation of fat in the hepatocytes (5%) in the absence of other causes of liver steatosis, such as Wilson's disease, deficiency of alpha-1-antitripsin, celiac disease, autoimmune hepatitis, HCV infection, metabolic disorders, and alcohol or drug consumption [1].

The simple hepatic steatosis is usually a benign condition, but in some cases, it progresses to more advanced forms of liver injury, characterized by the presence of inflammation and various degrees of fibrosis up to cirrhosis, predisposing to liver failure and/or hepatocellular carcinoma (HCC) [2].

NAFLD is closely associated with insulin resistance; obesity and metabolic syndrome are common underlying factors [3].

From the first studies, it emerged that the main cause of the accumulation of liver fat is visceral adipose tissue. In fact, the adipose tissue fulfils important endocrine functions, producing pro-inflammatory adipocytokines, such as tumor necrosis factor-α (TNF-α), interleukin 6 (IL-6), leptin, and adiponectin, which are implicated in the clinical manifestation of NAFLD and its progression to NASH and cirrhosis [4]. However, in the last years, other several causes of NAFLD were showed, such as gut-liver axis derangements. In this chapter the epidemiology, pathogenesis, and clinical, diagnostic, and therapeutic strategies of NAFLD currently known will be discussed.

17.2 Epidemiology

The exact prevalence of pediatric NAFLD is actually unknown, but available data report a prevalence ranging from 3 to 12% in the general pediatric population, with peaks of 70% in obese children. Clinical series of NAFLD children demonstrate the predominance of boys versus girls, with a male to female ratio of 2:1 [5]. In addition to gender, race and ethnicity also play an important role in the development of NAFLD. Fatty liver is more prevalent in children and adolescents of Hispanic ethnicity and less prevalent among black children and adolescents [6]. Ethnic differences may be related to genetic, environmental, or sociocultural factors as well as differences in body composition, insulin sensitivity, and adipocytokine profile. In Western countries, the NAFLD prevalence is estimated to be around 20–46%, while in Asian children, the prevalence is 5–18%. In Asia and Pacific islands, significant difference is reported between urban and rural populations with a prevalence of 16–32% in urban areas versus 9% in rural populations for the prevalence of NAFLD. Obesity-related NAFLD was reported in 77% of Chinese children. In Australia, the prevalence of pediatric NAFLD was estimated to be approximately 10% in the total population and 27.6% among overweight and obese children.

Age is another striking factor: one postmortem study in the USA showed that 17% of teenagers had NAFLD compared to 0.7% of 2–4-year-olds, owing both to a longer period to accumulate steatosis and an increased incidence in adolescents. Despite the diversity of diagnostic criteria used in population-based studies, obesity is the main risk factor for pediatric NAFLD [7]. In fact, the prevalence of NAFLD in obese children increases up to 80% in several obesogenic countries, including the USA, Europe, and Japan. Recent studies reported that in a population of schoolchildren aged 6–12 years, the rates of NAFLD were 3% in the normal weight range, 25% in the overweight range, and 76% in obese children.

NAFLD in children represents a metabolic condition, which is strongly associated with other metabolic features, such as waist circumference >95th percentile, hypertension and insulin resistance increasing the risk of developing type 2 diabetes mellitus, metabolic syndrome, and cardiovascular disease at a young age.

17.3 Pathophysiology

17.3.1 Multiple-Hit Hypothesis

Several mechanisms may lead to steatosis: dietary habits, environmental and genetic factors, development of insulin resistance, obesity with adipocyte proliferation, and changes in the composition of intestinal microbiota.

Adipose tissue is a metabolically active endocrine organ that causes the release of proinflammatory cytokines, such as TNF-α and IL-6, whereas beneficial adipokines are suppressed. This situation leads to the development of peripheral insulin resistance and hyperinsulinemia and increased fatty acid delivery to the hepatocyte. The disruption of normal insulin signaling in the hepatocyte and increased abundance of fatty acids leads to disordered lipid metabolism, characterized by the over-activation of de novo lipogenesis (DNL) transcriptional factors, causing more fatty acid and glucose products to be shunted into these lypogenetic pathways. Beta-oxidation in the mitochondria is also inhibited, as well as very-low-density lipoprotein (VLDL) packaging and export, leading to buildup of triglycerides in the hepatocytes. Gluconeogenesis is not suppressed despite hyperinsulinemia in the insulin-resistant hepatocyte, and increased glucose levels provide more substrate for DNL in a positive feedback loop [8].

The role of intestinal microbiota has been recently considered within this metabolic dysregulation. A bad diet (rich in fats and lipids) and increase of intestinal bacteria products (i.e., endotoxins, proteins, metabolites, lipopolysaccharides (LPS)) with the subsequent activation of the Toll-like receptor pathway (TLR) may act as inductors of inflammation and progression of hepatic steatosis to NASH and fibrosis. This process seems also be aggravated by the increased intestinal permeability that has been demonstrated in subjects with liver disease, where the gut seems to go through a tight junction disruption process that could be reversed by changes in the microbiota [9].

17.3.2 Lipogenesis and Lipotoxicity

The role of DNL in the development of hepatic steatosis is a common element in patients with metabolic syndrome and with high consumption of fatty acid. Specific dietary compositions may have different effects. The carbohydrates in the diet will positively influence the amount of DNL in the liver. Simple sugars are converted to fatty acids more easily than complex carbohydrates, and fructose is a more potent inducer of DNL than glucose [10]. Diets rich in saturated fat stimulate DNL by upregulating SREBP-1 (sterol-responsive element-binding protein-1), a key regulator of the lipogenic genes in the liver. Moreover, not all individuals with hepatic steatosis had increased DNL nor upregulated expression of SREBP-1; in fact paradoxical dissociation between hepatic DNL and hepatic fat content due to the PNPLA3 148M allele has been proved [11].

In the pathogenesis of NASH, multiple mechanisms are operative to produce hepatic damage by short-chain fatty acids (SFAs) and free cholesterol from de novo synthesis. The long-chain saturated fatty acids (LCFAs) are transported to mitochondria for β-oxidation or to be esterified for either excretion in the form of VLDL (very low density lipoproteins) or storage as lipid droplets. Free cholesterol accumulation causes liver injury due to activation of intracellular signaling pathways in Kupffer cells (KCs), hepatic stellate cells (HSCs), and hepatocytes. The activation of KCs and HSCs promotes inflammation and fibrogenesis.

Moreover, free cholesterol and SFAs can activate a variety of intracellular responses that causes mitochondrial death pathway activation, resulting in lipotoxic stress in the endoplasmic reticulum and mitochondria. The Toll-like receptor 4 (TLR4) is a receptor that activates a proinflammatory signaling pathway in response to excessive SFAs. This pathway is initiated by recruiting adaptor molecules such as toll/IL-1 receptor domain containing adaptor protein (TIRAP) and myeloid differentiation factor 88(MyD88) that ultimately lead to activation of nuclear factor κB with production of TNF-α [12].

Insulin Resistance. Studies have highlighted the fact that insulin resistance is a characteristic feature of NAFLD and is caused by a variety of factors, including release of soluble mediators derived from immune cells and/or adipose tissue, such as TNF-α and IL-6 [2].

Insulin-resistant subjects with NAFLD show reduced insulin sensitivity mainly in the muscles, liver, and adipose tissue, which can lead to a far more complex metabolic disorder. Serine phosphorylation of insulin receptor substrates by inflammatory signal transducers such as c-jun N-terminal protein kinase 1 (JNK1) or inhibitor of nuclear factor-κB kinase-β (IKK-β) is considered one of the key aspects that disrupt insulin signaling [13]. It is worth noting that insulin resistance is characterized not only by increased circulating insulin levels but also by increased hepatic gluconeogenesis, impaired glucose uptake by the muscle, and increased release of free fatty acids (FFAs) and inflammatory cytokines from peripheral adipose tissues, which are the key factors promoting accumulation of liver fat and progression of hepatic steatosis.

17.3.3 Oxidative Stress

In the presence of high concentrations of FFAs in hepatocytes, oxidative stress is due to lipid peroxidation and high levels of reactive oxygen/nitrogen species (ROS/RNS) that are generated during the metabolism of FFAs in microsomes, peroxisomes, and mitochondria [14]. Peroxidation of plasma and intracellular membranes causes direct cell necrosis or apoptosis, while ROS-induced expression of Fas ligand on hepatocytes may induce fratricidal cell death. Recent studies support the idea that oxidative stress may be a primary cause of liver fat accumulation and subsequent liver damage, and ROS may play a part even in fibrosis development. Importantly, these species can initiate lipid peroxidation by targeting polyunsaturated fatty acids (PUFAs), resulting in the formation of highly reactive aldehyde products. These reactive lipid derivatives have the potential to amplify intracellular damage by mediating the diffusion of ROS/RNS into the extracellular space, thus causing tissue injury [15].

17.3.4 Gut Microbiota

The data of the close connection between the liver and the intestine has been known for a long time. In the intestine occurs the absorption of the nutrients ingested with the diet (vitamins, proteins, carbohydrates, and lipids). These elements reach the liver, through the portal vein and the hepatic artery, where they are metabolized in order to guarantee the main cellular and metabolic functions. Other nutrients such as fats, fat-soluble vitamins, and trace elements (copper, zinc, etc.) need the presence of bile to be absorbed. Finally, the intestine secretes a series of hormones, neuropeptides, and growth factors that influence hepatic functions. The liver receives more than 70% of its blood supply from the intestine, via the portal vein and hepatic artery; therefore, it is the main organ exposed to toxic factors of intestinal origin [16].

In the interaction between the intestine and the liver, a key role is played by the microbiota. A "dysmicrobiosis" or bacterial overgrowth influences the absorption of nutrients and alters the structure of the intestinal walls, compromising their permeability. This favors the passage of macromolecules, bacteria, and bacterial products in the portal and systemic circulation. Probably increased intestinal permeability is the principal pathogenic step in the alteration of the intestinal liver axis, thus favoring the onset or progression of liver diseases [17].

Recent studies have suggested that the intestinal microbiota is responsible for the synthesis of various hepatotoxic bacterial substances (i.e., ammonia, phenols, and ethanol). The main bacterial product involved in the pathogenesis of NASH/NAFLD is lipopolysaccharide (LPS), an active component of bacterial endotoxin. The endogenous production of LPS due to bacterial death induces its translocation through the intestinal capillaries thanks to the TLR4-dependent mechanism [18]. The LPS, through a complex process of association with LPS-binding protein and CD14, activates TLR-4 located on different inflammatory cells, increasing the expression of target genes involved in the synthesis of inflammatory cytokines such as TNF-α and interleukins 1 and 6, promoting thus insulin resistance, hepatic steatosis, hepatic inflammation, and fibrogenesis. In fact, it is now known that TNF-α and tumor growth factor-b1 (TGF-b1) are strongly linked to the progression of NAFLD. The hepatic expression of TNF-α is significantly increased in children with NASH. At the same time, the TGF-b1 concentrations correlate with HSC activation, promoting TLR-4-mediated fibrogenesis. In one of the first pediatric studies, it was shown that the permeability (measured by the lactulose/mannitol ratio) is increased in children with NAFLD compared to healthy controls. This association between increased permeability and NAFLD suggests that bacterial translocation expounds the liver to endotoxins that influence the development of NAFLD and progression in NASH [19, 20].

On the other hand, the microbiota is influenced by many other factors, including bile acids and diet (choline, fructose, etc.). It is possible that changes to the microflora composition alter the intestinal barrier, allowing the intestinal contents to enter in the liver, influencing the development of steatosis and its progression to NASH.

17.3.5 Bile Acid

Bile acids are synthesized in hepatocytes from cholesterol through enzymatic pathways and then conjugated with glycine or taurine before secretion into bile and release into the small intestine. In the small intestine, conjugated bile acids are not only involved in lipid absorption and transport but have also been increasingly recognized to function as nuclear receptor binders and to have a role in function of microbiota. Bacteria within the intestine can also chemically modify bile acids and thereby alter the composition of the bile acid [21]. Besides the classic role as detergents to facilitate fat absorption, bile acids have also been recognized as important cell signaling molecules regulating lipid and carbohydrate metabolism and inflammatory response. These molecular functions are mediated through their binding and activation of the nuclear hormone receptor, farnesoid X receptor (FXR), and the G protein-coupled cell surface receptor TGR5. Intestinal FXR activity upregulates endocrine FGF19 expression, which inhibits hepatic bile acid synthesis via CYP7A1 signaling [22]. Recently, it was showed that hepatic FXR protein content and plasma FGF19 concentrations in children and adolescents with NASH were decreased compared to levels in children with "simple" NAFLD. Hepatic FXR protein level was positively correlated with serum FGF-19 concentrations, and both FXR and FGF19 concentrations were inversely and independently associated with NASH. This suggests that further studies are needed on the role of FXR in NAFLD [23].

17.3.6 Genetic

Single nucleotide polymorphisms (SNPs) in the genes involved in lipid metabolism (Lipin 1 (LPIN1), patatin-like phospholipase domain containing protein 3 (PNPLA3)), oxidative stress (superoxide dismutase 2 (SOD2)), insulin signaling (insulin receptor substrate 1 (IRS-1)), and fibrogenesis (Kruppel-like factor 6 (KLF6)) have been associated with the severity of liver damage in NAFLD patients. Moreover, an interesting interaction has recently been reported between genetic risk factors (PNPLA3 I148M), dietary components, and the severity of steatosis [24].

The PNPLA3, also known as adiponectin, is a member of the patatin-like phospholipase family. The rs738409 C>G single-nucleotide polymorphism (SNP), encoding the Ile 148Met variant protein of PNPLA3, is described as genetic determinant of hepatic steatosis. Several studies have established a strong link between PNPLA3 and the development of NAFLD. PNPLA3 is associated with an increased risk of advanced fibrosis among patients with a variety of liver diseases and is an independent risk factor for hepatocellular carcinoma among patients with NASH [25]. Moreover, the polymorphism rs738409 is not only associated with NASH but also with the severity of necroinflammatory changes independent of metabolic factors. NASH was more frequently observed in GG than CC homozygous; in fact rs738409 GG genotype versus the CC genotype was associated with a 28% increase in serum ALT levels and had 3.24-fold greater risk of higher necroinflammatory scores and 3.2-fold greater risk of developing fibrosis compared to CC homozygous [26].

Recently, additional SNPs of genes implicated in NASH pathogenesis have been shown to influence liver damage and fibrosis progression in patients. These include genetic variants regulating insulin receptor activity, ectoenzyme nucleotide pyrophosphate phosphodiesterase 1 (ENPP1), and the insulin receptor substrate-1 (IRS-1), thus underscoring the causal role of IR in the progression of liver damage in NAFLD. The manganese superoxide dismutase (SOD2), regulating SOD2 mitochondrial import and antioxidant activity, and the Kruppel-like factor 6 (KLF6), regulating alternative splicing isoforms of the transcription factor KLF6, are involved in the regulation of metabolism in hepatocytes and fibrogenesis in hepatic stellate cells [11].

The investigation of relevant genetic variants associated with pediatric NAFLD can be useful for the disease both in childhood and in adulthood to better understand their role in the pathogenesis of NAFLD.

17.4 Diagnosis

NAFLD is the most common liver disease in children, so it is essential to identify it as soon as possible in order to intervene promptly, changing the natural evolution of the disease and preventing complications.

The main problem in the diagnostic approach to the disease is represented by the poverty of suggestive clinical signs. In fact, diagnosis of NAFLD is often posed following the occasional finding of hypertransaminasemia and/or ultrasound abnormalities when these exams are performed for other reasons.

The categories most at risk of developing NAFLD are:

- Obese (BMI > 95th percentile) or overweight (BMI > 85th percentile) children
- Children with cardiometabolic risk factors (insulin-resistance, hypertension, dyslipidemia, cardiac and respiratory complications, and elevated waist circumference)
- Children with familiarity for NAFLD

Table 17.1 Causes of hepatic steatosis in pediatrics

Systemic diseases	Genetic or metabolic disease	Drugs	Toxics
Protein energy malnutrition	Cystic fibrosis	Nifedipine	Ethanol
Total parenteral nutrition	Wilson disease	Diltiazem	Ecstasy
Rapid weight loss	α1-Antitrypsin deficiency	Estrogens	Cocaine
Anorexia nervosa	HFE (hemochromatosis)	Corticosteroids Amiodarone	Solvents
Cachexia	Bile acids synthesis defects	Tamoxifen	Pesticides
Metabolic syndrome	Organic acidosis	Methotrexate	
Polycystic ovary syndrome	Citrin deficiency	Valproate	
Inflammatory bowel disease	Galactosemia	Vitamin A	
Celiac disease	Fructosemia	L-asparaginase	
Hepatitis C	Tyrosinemia type 1	Zidovudine	
Nephrotic syndrome	Cholesteryl ester storage disease	Acetaminophen	
Type 1 diabetes mellitus	Glycogenosis		
Thyroid disorders	Madelung lipomatosis Lipodystrophies		
Hypothalamic-pituitary disorders	Familial hyperlipoproteinemias		
	A- or hypo-betalipoproteinemia		
	ß-oxidation defects		
	Porphyria		
	Homocystinuria		
	Congenital disorders of glycosylation		
	Dorfman-Chanarin syndrome		
	Turner syndrome		
	Alström syndrome		
	Bardet-Biedl syndrome		
	Prader-Willi syndrome		
	Cohen syndrome		
	Weber-Christian disease		

In literature, there is a lack of uniformity on what screening tool is more effective to identify the pathology in subjects at risk. The European Society of Pediatric Gastroenterology Hepatology and Nutrition (ESPGHAN) suggests using both the measurement of serum alanine aminotransferase (ALT) concentration and liver ultrasound (US) as a screening method; the North American Society of Pediatric Gastroenterology Hepatology and Nutrition (NASPGHAN) indicates the use of ALT and not US. The National Institute for Health and Care Excellence (NICE) suggests using US and not ALT. Regardless of the method used, the finding of ALT > 30–40 IU/L or a US score ≥2 guarantees a specificity ≥90%, but the sensitivity of these tests, individually, does not exceed 50%, with an intrinsic risk of false negatives. It is also useful to remember that these methods do not provide any information on the degree of inflammation and liver fibrosis. Screening should be initiated between 9 and 11 years of age in obese or overweight children with a cardiometabolic risk factor and repeated every 2–3 years if the risk factors remain unchanged [1, 27, 28].

Hepatic steatosis is not synonymous for NAFLD: there are other pathologies that can lead to an increase in liver fat content (Table 17.1). The differential diagnosis of these conditions must take into account the patient's anamnestic and clinical characteristics, as well as the outcome of laboratory tests, imaging studies, and liver biopsy.

17.5 Clinical Features

Diagnostic work-up starts with the evaluation of patient's *medical history* followed by *physical examination*.

Medical History. A complete collection of data on the patient's past and present clinical history is required. Two aspects need to be focused:

– Familiar history of NAFLD or other liver diseases, metabolic syndrome, and obesity.
– Evaluation of patient's dietary habits, physical activity, lifestyle, and drug consumption.

Physical Examination. As previously stated, specific signs and symptoms do not characterize NAFLD, but it is possible to look for signs of comorbidity.

– Measurement of waist circumference and calculation of BMI permit diagnosis and staging of overweight/obesity.
– Blood pressure should be measured in all children and compared with age and sex-matched centiles.
– The presence of striae rubrae or striae albae (atrophic purple or white linear bands of skin) is common in obese patients. Acanthosis nigricans is a hyperpigmentation of the flexural areas of the body (mainly cervical, axillary, and inguinal) suggesting of insulin resistance.
– Hepatomegaly (palpable liver edge 2 cm below the right costal margin) is a common feature in patients with

NAFLD, while signs of chronic hepatic disease (e.g., spider nevi, ascites, and splenomegaly) are rare in pediatric NAFLD. Some children with NAFLD suffer from fatigue or discomfort in the right upper abdomen quadrant.

17.6 Laboratory Tests

In the laboratory assessment of children with suspected NAFLD/NASH, it is possible to identify two test categories:

- *Routine laboratory test*: widespread and accessible tests that allow an initial assessment and exclusion of other major liver disease
- *Novel biomarkers*: second-level tests that allow, once diagnosed with NAFLD, a noninvasive estimation of the severity of the disease

Routine Laboratory Test:
- *Liver function*: alanine transaminase (ALT), aspartate transaminase (AST), and gamma-glutamyltransferase (GGT). Increase in transaminases or GGT should be considered a warning sign for hepatic disease, but it is noteworthy that advanced liver fibrosis may have normal or mild elevation of these enzymes. Moreover, they do not correlate with NAFLD severity. Measurement of blood albumin, INR, and coagulation tests should be included in liver evaluation.
- *Glucose metabolism*: fasting insulin and glucose should be assessed in all children. HOMA-IR is an index of insulin resistance and can be calculated as follows: fasting insulin (mU/L) × fasting glucose (µmol/L)/22.5. A value ≥2.5 is suggestive of insulin resistance. In selected patients (obese, presence of acanthosis nigricans, abnormal fasting insulin or glucose), oral glucose tolerance test (OGTT) and hemoglobin A1c dosage should be considered.
- *Lipid metabolism*: triglycerides; total, LDL-, and HDL-cholesterol; and lipoproteins should be performed. The severity of liver disease is associated with a more atherogenic lipid profile.
- *Uric acid*: a diet rich in fructose may increase uric acid concentrations. Hyperuricemia (UA ≥5.9 mg/dL) is an independent factor associated with a higher risk to develop NASH in NAFLD patients.
- *Others*: blood counts, urea, electrolytes, thyroid function tests, and morning cortisol.
- *Differential diagnosis*: depending on history and clinical information, it is possible to request specific test for possible causes of hepatic steatosis/hypertransaminasemia other than NAFLD (Table 17.2).

Table 17.2 Causes of hypertransaminasemia other than NAFLD and diagnostic tests

Differential diagnosis	Test
Cystic fibrosis	Sweat test
Hemocromatosis	Iron, ferritin
Wilson disease	Serum copper, ceruloplasmin levels, 24-h urinary copper
Alpha-1 antitrypsin deficiency	α1-Antitrypsin levels
Viral hepatitis	Specific serology
Autoimmune hepatitis	ANA, ASMA, LKM1, LC-1
Screening for metabolic diseases	Amino and organic acids. Plasma-free fatty acids and acyl carnitine profile

Novel Biomarkers. Once the diagnosis of NAFLD is made, one of the most difficult challenges is to estimate the severity of the disease in a noninvasive manner. Higher levels of C-reactive protein and proinflammatory cytokines, such as TNF-α, IL-1, and IL-6, have been associated with evolution from NAFLD to NASH, while two adipokines (adiponectin and retinol-binding protein 4) have been inversely correlated to the degree of liver damage; however all these markers lack of specificity for NAFLD.

Recently Citokeratin-18 (a marker of hepatocyte apoptosis) fragment levels and Cathepsin-D (a lysosomal protease) were identified as reliable markers of NASH. In fact, it has been demonstrated that Cathepsin-D has a high diagnostic value to distinguish pediatric patients with hepatic inflammation from children with steatosis, while Citokeratin-18 correlates significantly with hepatic fibrosis and with NAFLD severity. Actually, the main limitation of these markers is the applicability in community-based practices [29, 30].

17.7 Imaging Techniques

17.7.1 Ultrasonography

Because of its availability, security, and relatively low cost, ultrasound (US) is the most common imaging technique used to diagnose NAFLD. Hepatic steatosis is characterized by a liver echotexture more reflective (hyperechoic) when compared to that of the right kidney ("bright liver"); moreover the liver may appear increased in size. The assessment of hepatic echogenicity and liver vessels and diaphragm visualization allow the US grading of steatosis (Table 17.3).

US has some limitations: it is unable to distinguish NAFLD from NASH and to detect liver fibrosis. Moreover, it may be unreliable in evaluating severely obese patients (BMI ≥ 40 kg/m^2) or when liver fatty liver infiltration is <30%. Finally, US is an operator- and machine-dependent technique, so its results may change depending on the operator's experience and training [31].

Table 17.3 US-based grading of NAFLD

Grading	US image
No steatosis—grade 0	Normal hepatic echogenicity, liver vessels, and diaphragm visualization
Mild steatosis—grade 1	Slightly increased echogenicity with normal liver vessels and diaphragm visualization
Moderate steatosis—grade 2	Markedly increased echogenicity of liver parenchyma with reduction of liver vessel and diaphragm visualization
Severe steatosis—grade 3	Severely increased echogenicity of liver parenchyma, with poor or no visualization of diaphragm and intrahepatic vessels

17.7.2 Elastography

The term elastography refers to a series of imaging techniques that allow the estimation of liver tissue rigidity by measuring the propagation of specific elastic waves (shear waves, S-waves) emitted by the probe.

Elastography imaging can be US-based (e.g., transient elastography, FibroScan®) or magnetic resonance-based (magnetic resonance elastography, MRE).

These methods have proven to be effective in distinguishing NAFLD from NASH and in highlighting the presence and severity of fibrotic infiltration in the liver, especially in studies conducted in the adult population. The absence of certain cutoff values and the relatively poor diffusion of the equipment currently limit their use. Moreover, MRE is an expensive exam, and to date its application is limited mainly for clinical research purposes.

17.7.3 Other Imaging Techniques

Computed tomography (CT) should not be routinely used for the assessment of NAFLD in pediatrics because it has a nonacceptable cost-effectiveness ratio due to unjustified exposure to ionizing radiation in relation to information that can be obtained. Moreover, CT is unable to identify mild steatosis (sensitivity for steatosis detection estimated between 46 and 72%).

Magnetic resonance imaging (MRI) is actually considered the most accurate imaging technique to assess liver fat storage in NAFLD patients because it can differentiate tissues containing only water from those containing both fat and water.

MR spectroscopy (MRS) is a novel variant of classical MRI which quantifies triglycerides accumulation within hepatocyte through the measurement of acyl groups within the selected liver region of interest. MRS can discriminate healthy patients from those with NAFLD with a sensitivity of 92.6% and a specificity of 95.7% [32].

In younger children the correct execution of MR requires sedation of the patient. This element, associated with relatively high cost and the need of specific expertise for MRS, limits the application of MRI in everyday clinical practice.

17.8 Liver Biopsy

Liver biopsy (LB) is actually considered the gold standard for NAFLD diagnosis as it is the only method which can distinguish NAFLD from NASH and provide a reliable scoring system designed to estimate the severity of the disease. In addition, it may help in the differential diagnosis work-up and in detecting coexisting liver diseases. LB should not be performed in all children. In 2015 the ESPGHAN Hepatology Committee defined indications for LB in NAFLD pediatric patients (Fig. 17.1): it is important to highlight that LB should not be considered a screening method [33].

Before performing LB, a careful coagulation study is required because abnormal coagulation and/or thrombocytopenia may preclude LB execution. Furthermore, LB is contraindicated in case of ascites, biliary dilatation, peliosis, hemangioma, and anatomic variation such as abdominal situs inversus.

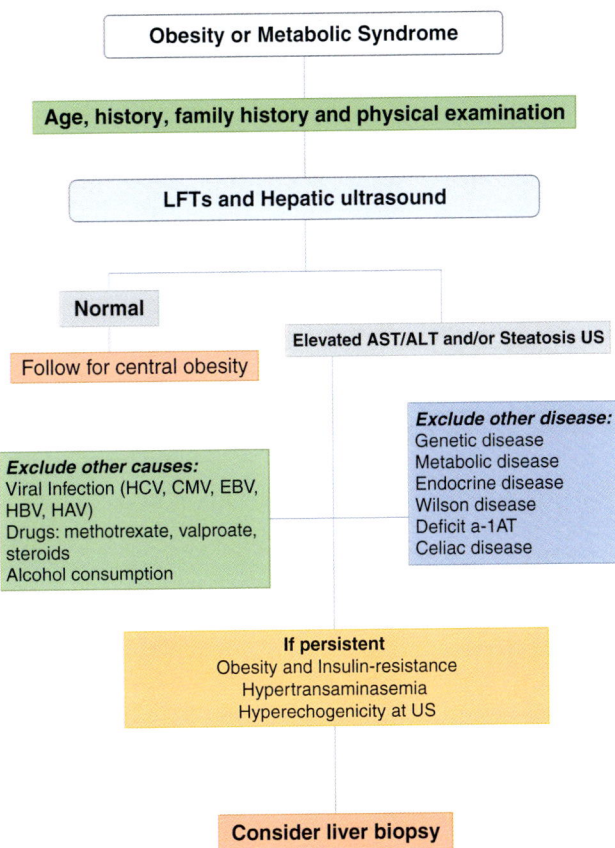

Fig. 17.1 Diagnostic work-up of patient's with NAFLD

LB is burdened with some limitations: it is an invasive technique with minor and major complication risks. Pain and bleeding are the most common complications (84% and 2.8%, respectively); other reported complications are infections, visceral perforation, arteriovenous fistula, pneumothorax, hemothorax, and death (0.6%). Another limitation of LB is represented by sampling errors; in fact biopsy specimen could not be representative of whole-liver status. Finally, LB is an operator-dependent technique.

Due to limitations and invasiveness in recent years, new research strands have been developed to identify safe and equally effective methods for diagnosing and staging NAFLD, but to date the biopsy remains the "imperfect reference standard."

17.9 Histopathology

By definition, NAFLD is characterized by the presence of hepatic steatosis in at least 5% of hepatocytes.

In relation to the histological features, NASH can be classified into three subtypes [34]:

- Type 1: steatosis with ballooning degeneration and/or perisinusoidal fibrosis, without
- portal involvement
- Type 2: steatosis with portal inflammation and/or fibrosis, in the absence of ballooning degeneration or perisinusoidal involvement
- Overlap type: coexisting elements from both type 1 and 2

17.9.1 Steatosis

In children, steatosis is most prominent in the zone 1 (periportal zone) of the hepatic acinus, with a decreasing trend of fatty hepatocyte presence from zone 1 to zone 3. In adolescents and adults, the steatosis pattern is opposite. In NAFLD hepatocellular steatosis is mainly macrovesicular (single fat lipid droplet in the cytoplasm shifting the nucleus to periphery) rather than microvesicular (multiple small drops not-displacing nucleus), but mixed macro-microvesicular steatosis is often observed [35].

17.9.2 Ballooning

Ballooning degeneration of the hepatocyte is the histological lesion indicatives of cell damage due to fat droplet accumulation, cytoskeletal injury, and intracellular fluid retention. Cells lose their original polygonal shape and become enlarged; cytoplasm is vacuolated and Mallory-Denk bodies (MDB) could be found. MDB are intracellular protein aggregates (mainly intermediate filaments) which are a typical feature of NASH even if they may be present in other chronic liver diseases (e.g., alcoholic steatohepatitis, Wilson disease, chronic cholestasis, and metabolic disorders) [36].

17.9.3 Inflammation

Inflammation in NAFLD, when present, is usually mild. Evidence of severe, confluent inflammation should raise suspicion for other liver diseases. The major type of inflammation highlighted in NASH is lobular inflammation; portal inflammation may be present and represents the stigma of type 2 NASH. Cells mainly involved in the inflammatory process are lymphocytes, histiocytes, and PMN leukocytes. These last can surround ballooned hepatocytes containing MDB, forming a complex known as satellitosis. Histiocytes instead are responsible for the formation of lipogranulomas [35].

17.9.4 Fibrosis

Fibrosis is the result of collagen and other extracellular matrix fiber depositions due to hepatic stellate cell activation. Fibrosis distribution pattern varies with age: in adults and older adolescents, onset of fibrosis is typically observed in acinar zone 3 (perisinusoidal/pericellular fibrosis), and as NASH progresses, portal areas are involved. In advanced diseases, bridging fibrosis and cirrhosis may develop [37]. On the other hand, in children and younger adolescents, fibrosis may begin from the acinar zone 1 with bridging fibrosis connecting portal areas [35]. Cirrhosis is rarely observed in pediatric subset, and when it's present, it is most commonly macronodular or mixed. At the cirrhotic stage, the whole hepatic architecture may be subverted.

Other microscopic findings can be found in NAFLD as megamitochondria, acidophilic bodies, and vacuolated glycogen-filled nuclei, but they are nonspecific elements with little diagnostic significance.

17.9.5 Scoring Systems

In recent years, in parallel with the rise of pediatric obesity, an exponential increase in NAFLD frequency was observed in children, and consequently a greater number of LBs have been performed. This has imposed the need to design a standardized approach for assessing the severity of the disease; three principal scoring systems are used in clinical and research activities: the Brunt system, the NASH Clinical Research Network (CRN) system, and the Pediatric NAFLD Histological Score (PNHS). The Brunt system was described for the first time in 1999 and takes account of steatosis, ballooning, lobular and portal inflammation, and cell infiltrates to classify NAFLD in three categories (mild or grade 1, moderate or grade 2, severe or grade 3) [38].

The NASH CRN validated a histological score (NAFLD Activity Score or NAS) based on the evaluation of three parameters each of which is assigned a score (steatosis, 0–3; lobular inflammation, 0–3; and ballooning, 0–2). NAS results from the unweighted sum of these parameters for a total score ranging from 0 to 8. A NAS ≥ 5 is suggestive of NASH, while a NAS ≤ 2 excludes NASH [39].

PNHS was designed with the aim of developing a new scoring system that included portal inflammation. PNHS results from the weighted sum of steatosis, ballooning, and lobular and portal inflammation scores; a PNHS value of 85 has a sensitivity of 77% and a specificity of 98% for the prediction of NASH [40] (Fig. 17.2).

17.9.6 Genetic Tests

Genetic screening tests are now available: they are easy to perform and have a low cost and can assess the risk of the subject of developing severe forms of NAFLD. Currently, a simple oral swab that searches for mutations in a combination of four genes (KLF6, PNPLA3, SOD2, LPIN1), each of which is related to NAFLD, is able to estimate the risk of severe hepatopathy [41].

17.10 Therapy

The main objective of the NAFLD therapy is to halt the progression of liver damage and possibly restore the hepatic original histology, with the ultimate goal of improving the patient's quality of life and reducing NAFLD-related morbidity and mortality. The cornerstone of therapy is represented by lifestyle changes, with hypocaloric diet and regular physical exercise, aimed at weight loss although this approach is burdened with a high failure rate due to poor adherence often associated with a low perception of disease. Pharmacological approaches for treating NAFLD are limited by the small number of randomized, controlled trials conducted in pediatric population, but recent studies have shown promising results.

17.11 Non-pharmacological Treatment

The first step in the treatment of pediatric NAFLD is lifestyle intervention, based on a healthy and balanced diet and physical activity.

In literature, no specific dietary regimens are described for children with NAFLD; however intervention must always take into account the state of health, comorbidity, and degree of activity of the child. As a general rule, caloric intake should be around 25–30 kcal/kg/day for overweight/obese patients and 40–45 kcal/kg/day for normal weight patients

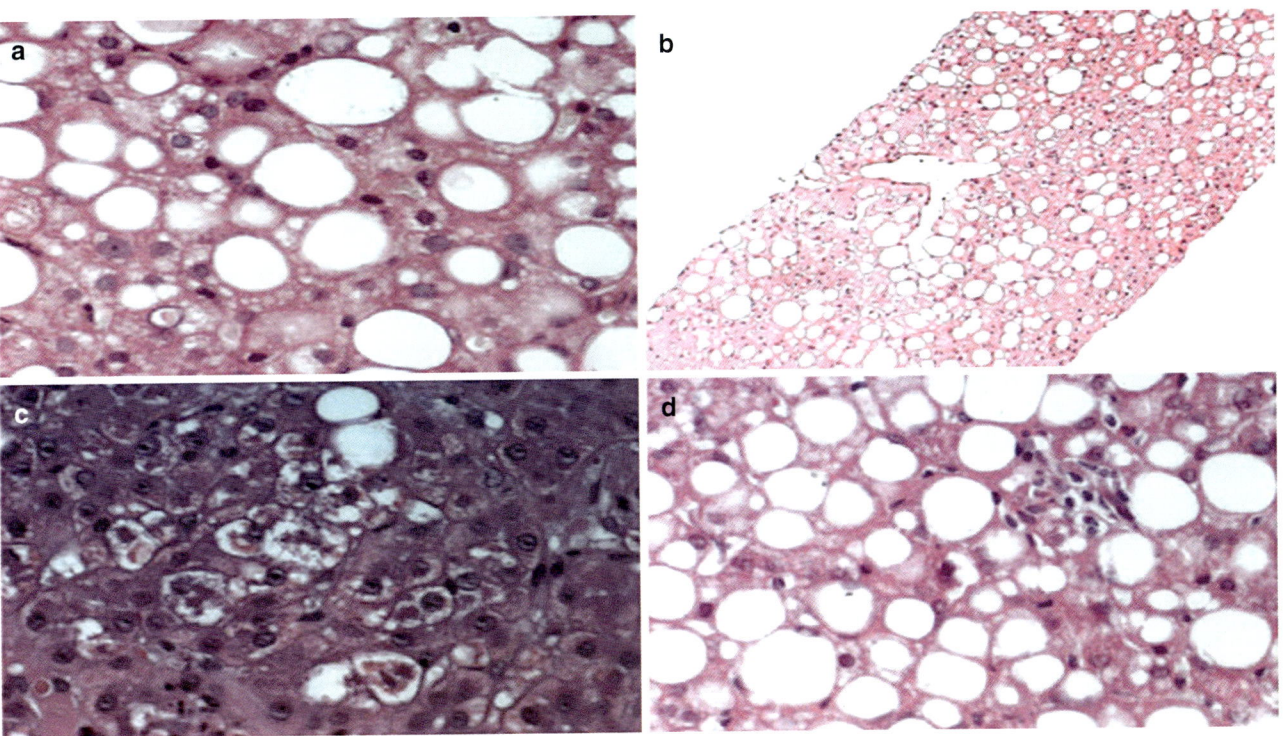

Fig. 17.2 The histological features of NAFLD/NASH in children (Histological features of pediatric NAFLD/NASH. Steatosis is evident in (**a**) (40× magnification; EE (eosin hematoxylin)) and (**b**) (10× EE); ballooning and lipogranulomas are present in (**c**) and (**d**), respectively (40× EE))

with macroelements respecting the following proportions: 50–60% carbohydrates, 25–30% fat, and 15–20% protein. Unsaturated fatty acids (ideally 2/3 of total lipid intake) should be preferred than saturated fatty acids (1/3 of total lipid intake), with a ω3–ω6 ratio equal to 1:4. The dietary program should encourage consumption of food with low glycemic index, in order to improve insulin sensitivity; it is therefore necessary to reduce the quantity of simple sugars, white rice, and white bread in favor of fruit, vegetables, and legumes.

As previously stated, fructose may play a central role in NAFLD pathogenesis, so it is crucial to avoid foods and beverages with high fructose content including soft drinks and energy drinks.

The dietary regimen should be accompanied with an active lifestyle, with regular physical activity preferring aerobic exercise, and restriction of time spent in front of the screens (TV, PC, smartphone, and tablet).

In patients with NAFLD, a gradual loss of weight is desirable since a rapid weight loss may be associated with a paradoxical effect resulting in worsening of the liver damage and increase in metabolic comorbidities. For these reasons, a weight reduction not exceeding 10% in 6 months is recommended.

LS intervention can improve liver histology, mainly steatosis, and other metabolic features as insulin resistance and dyslipidemia, but it is limited by the high failure rate, due to the poor and non-lasting compliance of patients and their families with a success rate estimated <10% 2 years after the onset of treatment [42].

Bariatric surgery (BS) and nonsurgical obesity treatments based on minimally invasive intragastric balloons are emerging as therapeutic alternatives to be carefully considered in obese children with NAFLD, mostly in patients with numerous, unsuccessful weight loss attempts. In 2015 a position paper of ESPGHAN has established eligibility criteria for BS in pediatrics: selected obese patients with BMI >40 kg/m^2 and severe comorbidities (including NASH with advanced fibrosis) or with BMI more than 50 kg/m^2 and mild comorbidities (including NASH) [43].

In a recent pediatric trial, laparoscopic sleeve gastrectomy (a restrictive intervention consisting in the removal of the gastric fundus) has proved to be more effective than lifestyle approach, even when combined with intragastric devices, in reducing NASH and fibrosis in obese patients after 1 year of treatment and in improving dyslipidemia, sleep apnea, and hypertension [44]. Despite encouraging results, BS should not be considered as a first-line therapy, and a careful evaluation of the patient, considering emotional, psychological, and clinical features, should be performed before performing surgery. Moreover, further studies are needed in order to evaluate long-term efficacy and safety of these procedures.

17.11.1 Pharmacological Treatment

In recent years, numerous studies have contributed to elucidate new aspects of the pathogenesis of NAFLD, which remains partially unknown. Understanding the pathogenic mechanisms is crucial to identify molecular targets in order to change the natural history of the disease. Limited knowledge of the pathogenesis and the low number of uniform RCTs available in pediatrics currently limit the use of pharmacological approaches in NAFLD.

17.11.2 Insulin Sensitizers

Insulin resistance is a common feature in obese patients with NAFLD. *Metformin* is a biguanide that acts both on lipid metabolism (inhibition of lipogenesis) and on glucose metabolism (reduction of gluconeogenesis and improvement of insulin sensitivity). The TONIC trial, conducted in 173 children with biopsy-proven NAFLD, showed that metformin (500 mg twice daily) was not superior to placebo in decreasing ALT level and/or in improving any histological lesion but ballooning degeneration [45]. To date metformin is not recommended for treating NAFLD in nondiabetic children.

Thiazolidinediones are agonists of peroxisome proliferator-activated receptors-gamma (PPAR-G), a group of nuclear receptors that improves insulin sensitivity and reduce hepatic fat content. Although promising results in adult studies, their applicability in pediatrics is limited by the risk of cardiotoxicity associated with the use of these drugs.

17.11.3 Antioxidants

Oxidative stress is implicated in NAFLD pathogenesis and acts a key role in the progression from steatosis to steatohepatitis mainly through the release of ROS (reactive oxygen species) from mitochondria. *Vitamin E* is the most studied antioxidant agent, but its real therapeutic value has not been fully clarified. In the TONIC trial, an arm of patients was treated with vitamin E (400 UI/day), but this group did not benefit from the treatment. Recently, other antioxidants, such as polyphenols (e.g., resveratrol, silymarin, epigallocatechin gallate, anthocyanin, curcumin, and quercetin), have been studied, but despite encouraging findings observed on murine models, human studies have not provided solid results and therefore require further investigations.

17.11.4 Ursodeoxycholic Acid

Ursodeoxycholic acid (UDCA) is a secondary bile acid, endogenously produced by the gut microbiota, which regulates cholesterol absorption, and it is largely used in biliary diseases in order to prevent formation of cholesterol gallstones. Recently UDCA was speculated to be involved in several other mechanisms, as glutathione synthesis and activation of glucocorticoid receptor, contributing to the antioxidant and anti-inflammatory pathways. Despite these effects, administration of UDCA does not result in concrete benefits in treating NAFLD [46].

17.11.5 Omega-3 Fatty Acids

Omega-3 fatty acids are a variety PUFAs. The most studied omega-3 in humans are eicosapentaenoic acid (EPA) and docosahexaenoic acid (DHA) which can be found in fish, algae, and fish oil. Omega-3 are modulators of the transcription of genes regulating lipid metabolism and provide anti-inflammatory and insulin-sensitizing systemic activity.

Several trials evaluated the efficacy of omega-3 supplementation, alone or in combination with other compounds (e.g., vitamin D, Colin, and vitamin E), in improving the biochemical and histological parameters of NAFLD. DHA is effective in reducing liver steatosis, and, when combined with vitamin D, it ameliorates insulin resistance and lipid profile [47].

17.11.6 Probiotics

Considering the recent findings regarding the central role of intestinal dysbiosis in the pathogenesis of NAFLD through the so-called gut-liver axis, probiotics have been suggested as a possible therapeutic option for the treatment of the disease. In 2016, a triple-blind trial, conducted among 64 obese children with sonographic NAFLD, who were randomly allocated to receive probiotic capsule (containing *Lactobacillus acidophilus*, *Bifidobacterium lactis*, *B. bifidum*, and *L. rhamnosus*) or placebo for 12 weeks, showed that the probiotic group improved their lipid profile and waist circumference, decreased levels of AST and ALT, and had a higher percentage of subjects with remission of steatosis to US evaluation compared to placebo group [48].

17.11.7 Vitamin D

Vitamin D deficiency is frequently reported in obese patients with NAFLD: it is estimated that about 80% of children with steatosis present with Vitamin D insufficiency (≤20 ng/mL) or deficiency (≤10 ng/mL). Vitamin D is not only responsible for the calcium-phosphorus metabolism but is involved in different immunoregulatory processes (pleiotropic action). The combination of DHA and Vitamin D has proved to be effective in reducing the activation of hepatic stellate cells (involved in fibrotic accumulation) and fibrillary collagen deposit with the prospect of being able to revert the already existing fibrotic lesions [47].

17.11.8 Novel Treatments

The increase in the prevalence of NAFLD, associated with the absence of effective pharmacological treatments, has led to the study of new molecules to counteract NAFLD.

The farnesoid X receptor (FXR) is a nuclear receptor, expressed primarily in the liver and intestine, which binds to bile acids. When activated, FXR migrates into the cell nucleus and modulates the transcription of specific genes involved in the regulation of inflammation and glucose and lipid metabolism. Numerous studies, mostly based on animal models, have shown that the use of FXR-agonists (e.g., obeticholic acid) could improve hepatic steatosis and steatohepatitis [49].

Liraglutide is an analogue of glucagone-like peptide 1 (GLP-1), a gut-derived incretin hormone that induces weight loss and insulin sensitivity. In 2016, the LEAN study, conducted on 52 adult patients with NASH, showed that liraglutide led to histological resolution of steatohepatitis. The treatment was safe and well tolerated by the patients [50].

Among the various molecules under investigation, cysteamine bitartrate (an antioxidant) and pentoxifylline (PTX, a xanthine derivative with anti-inflammatory effects) are showing promising results, but further studies are needed to assess their efficacy and safety in pediatrics.

17.12 Implication for Liver Transplantation

NAFLD is often perceived by the patients as a "minor" disease compared to other liver conditions, but recent studies stated that fibrotic potential of NAFLD is as severe as that of chronic hepatitis C, with an average interval time of transition from NASH to cirrhosis estimated around 8–10 years [51]. Prevalence data have decreed NAFLD as the most widespread liver disease in Western countries. 30–40% and 3–5% of adult US population are affected by NAFLD and NASH, respectively: this reflects the risk for millions of people to develop, over the years, end-stage liver disease potentially requiring liver transplantation (LT). Over the past 25 years, in the USA, the number of LTs performed for NASH cirrhosis has doubled from 5.5 to 11% of all reported LTs, and to date NAFLD is the third cause of LT preceded only by alcoholic liver disease and hepatitis C virus. Considering the prevalence trend of NAFLD, the delay of diagnosis due to the absence of noninvasive diagnostic tool, the absence of effective treatments, and new antiviral drugs for HCV infections, NASH cirrhosis is expected to become the main indication for LT by 2030 [52].

Because of its natural history, LT for NASH cirrhosis is a rare occurrence in the pediatric context; in fact the average age of transplantation is around 58.5 ± 8 years old [53].

According to data extracted from the Scientific Registry of Transplant Recipients (SRTR) and United Network for Organ Sharing (UNOS) databases, the survival outcomes of NASH recipients at 1, 3, and 5 years after transplant were similar to LTs performed for other causes and were 87.6%, 82.2%, and 76.7%, respectively [54]. The principal cause of death after LT for NASH cirrhosis is attributable to sepsis and cardiovascular events. The latter account for 11% of death at 1 year in LT recipients, and it's important to highlight that NAFLD patients have, per se, a higher cardiovascular risk because they often suffer from comorbidities such as insulin resistance, dyslipidemia, and high blood pressure. In fact, a BMI ≥ 40 kg/m^2 and/or the diagnosis of diabetes mellitus type 2 are considered the principal risk factors for increased mortality after LT. In this perspective, a careful stratification of patients' risk before transplantation is essential to predict the possibility of cardiovascular complications and to implement specific precautions.

A pathological entity that may occur in the follow-up of LT is posttransplant NAFLD, which may be a recurrence of disease or a first manifestation in patients previously not affected by NAFLD (de novo NAFLD). The posttransplant NAFLD is caused by the coexistence of both host and graft risk factors. In patients with NASH-related LT, the risk of recurrence is also due to the fact that transplantation does not improve the metabolic alterations (e.g., insulin resistance, dyslipidemia, intestinal dysbiosis) which predispose to NAFLD and can act on transplanted organ. Moreover, there are genetic factors that increase the odds of recurrence (e.g., the presence of specific polymorphisms of the PNPLA3 gene) which is why these patients should be identified before transplantation and subjected to more stringent controls over time.

Another issue regarding LT and NAFLD is the impact of NAFLD on liver donors. The decreasing liver quality could compromise LT volume; in fact a recent analysis has hypothesized that liver utilization could fall from 78 to 44% by 2030 because of NAFLD [55].

To date, there are no standardized protocols for the assessment of donor liver. A liver with a fat content <30% can be safely used for transplantation, while if the percentage is >60%, the organ cannot be used because of high risk of primary nonfunctioning due to the intrinsic reduced tolerance to ischemic stress and the greater possibility of reperfusion injury. To date, there are no univocal approaches when the steatosis is between 30 and 60% [56].

NAFLD is a pathology of public interest with health and economic implications. Actually the main obstacles in clinical practice are represented by the absence of a noninvasive method capable of diagnosing and staging the disease and the need to identify an effective treatment in reversing the natural history of the disease. Epidemiological data and projections on the future are not reassuring, so much so that NAFLD is expected to become the first cause of liver transplantation in the next 15 years.

Considering all these elements, it is essential to undertake national and international prevention policies in order to halt the "NAFLD epidemic" and to protect the health of children and adolescents.

References

1. Vajro P, Lenta S, Socha P, et al. Diagnosis of nonalcoholic fatty liver disease in children and adolescents: position paper of the ESPGHAN Hepatology Committee. J Pediatr Gastroenterol Nutr. 2012;54:700–13.
2. Nobili V, Svegliati-Baroni G, Alisi A, Miele L, Valenti L, Vajro P. A 360-degree overview of paediatric NAFLD: recent insights. J Hepatol. 2013;58:1218–29.
3. Yki-Jarvinen H. Non-alcoholic fatty liver disease as a cause and a consequence of metabolic syndrome. Lancet Diabetes Endocrinol. 2014;2:901–10.
4. Sayin O, Tokgoz Y, Arslan N. Investigation of adropin and leptin levels in pediatric obesity-related nonalcoholic fatty liver disease. J Pediatr Endocrinol Metab. 2014;27:479–84.
5. Brunt EM. Pathology of nonalcoholic fatty liver disease. Nat Rev Gastroenterol Hepatol. 2010;7:195–203.
6. Feldstein AE, Charatcharoenwitthaya P, Treeprasertsuk S, et al. The natural history of non-alcoholic fatty liver disease in children: a follow-up study for up to 20 years. Gut. 2009;58:1538–44.
7. Brunt EM, Wong VW, Nobili V, et al. Nonalcoholic fatty liver disease. Nat Rev Dis Primers. 2015;1:15080.
8. Brunt EM, Kleiner DE, Wilson LA, et al. Nonalcoholic fatty liver disease (NAFLD) activity score and the histopathologic diagnosis in NAFLD: distinct clinicopathologic meanings. Hepatology. 2011;53(3):810–20.
9. Nobili V, Putignani L, Mosca A, et al. Bifidobacteria and lactobacilli in the gut microbiome of children with non-alcoholic fatty liver disease: which strains act as health players? Arch Med Sci. 2018;14(1):81–7.
10. Li ZZ, Berk M, McIntyre TM, et al. Hepatic lipid partitioning and liver damage in nonalcoholic fatty liver disease: role of stearoyl-CoA desaturase. J Biol Chem. 2009;284(9):5637–44.
11. Lin YC, Chang PF, Chang MH, et al. Genetic variants in GCKR and PNPLA3 confer susceptibility to nonalcoholic fatty liver disease in obese individuals. Am J Clin Nutr. 2014;99:869–74.
12. Fessler MB, Rudel LL, Brown JM. Toll-like receptor signaling links dietary fatty acids to the metabolic syndrome. Curr Opin Lipidol. 2009;20(5):379–85.
13. Pappachan JM, Babu S, Krishnan B, et al. Non-alcoholic fatty liver disease: a clinical update. J Clin Transl Hepatol. 2017;5(4):384–93.
14. Selvakumar PKC, Kabbany MN, Nobili V, et al. Nonalcoholic fatty liver disease in children: hepatic and Extrahepatic complications. Pediatr Clin N Am. 2017;64(3):659–75.
15. Mann JP, Raponi M, Nobili V. Clinical implications of understanding the association between oxidative stress and pediatric NAFLD. Expert Rev Gastroenterol Hepatol. 2017;11(4):371–82.
16. Doulberis M, Kotronis G, Gialamprinou D, et al. Non-alcoholic fatty liver disease: an update with special focus on the role of gut microbiota. Metabolism. 2017;71:182–97.

17. Poeta M, Pierri L, Vajro P. Gut-liver axis derangement in non-alcoholic fatty liver disease. Children (Basel). 2017;4(8).
18. Silva Figueiredo P, Carla Inada A, Marcelino G, et al. Fatty acids consumption: the role metabolic aspects involved in obesity and its associated disorders. Nutrients 2017;9(10).
19. Del Chierico F, Nobili V, Vernocchi P, et al. Gut microbiota profiling of pediatric nonalcoholic fatty liver disease and obese patients unveiled by an integrated meta-omics-based approach. Hepatology. 2017;65(2):451–64.
20. Della Corte C, Vajro P, Socha P, Nobili V. Pediatric non-alcoholic fatty liver disease: recent advances. Clin Res Hepatol Gastroenterol. 2014;38(4):419–22.
21. Ramírez-Pérez O, Cruz-Ramón V, Chinchilla-López P, Méndez-Sánchez N. The role of the gut microbiota in bile acid metabolism. Ann Hepatol. 2017;16(Suppl. 1: s3-105):s15–20. https://doi.org/10.5604/01.3001.0010.5494.
22. Molinaro A, Wahlström A, Marschall HU. Role of bile acids in metabolic control. Trends Endocrinol Metab. 2018;29(1):31–41.
23. Nobili V, Alisi A, Mosca A, et al. Hepatic farnesoid X receptor protein level and circulating fibroblast growth factor 19 concentration in children with NAFLD. Liver Int. 2018;38(2):342–9.
24. Carpino G, Pastori D, Baratta F, et al. PNPLA3 variant and portal/periportal histological pattern in patients with biopsy-proven non-alcoholic fatty liver disease: a possible role for oxidative stress. Sci Rep. 2017;7(1):15756.
25. Nobili V, Bedogni G, Donati B, et al. The I148M variant of PNPLA3 reduces the response to docosahexaenoic acid in children with non-alcoholic fatty liver disease. J Med Food. 2013;16:957–60.
26. Mangge H, Baumgartner BG, Zelzer S, et al. Patatin-like phospholipase 3 (rs738409) gene polymorphism is associated with increased liver enzymes in obese adolescents and metabolic syndrome in all ages. Aliment Pharmacol Ther. 2015;42:99–105.
27. Vos MB, Abrams SH, Barlow SE, et al. NASPGHAN clinical practice guideline for the diagnosis and treatment of nonalcoholic fatty liver disease in children: recommendations from the Expert Committee on NAFLD (ECON) and the North American Society of Pediatric Gastroenterology, Hepatology and Nutrition (NASPGHAN). J Pediatr Gastroenterol Nutr. 2017;64(2):319–34.
28. Glen J, Floros L, Day C, et al. Non-alcoholic fatty liver disease (NAFLD): summary of NICE guidance. BMJ. 2016;354:i4428.
29. Mandelia C, Collyer E, Mansoor S, et al. Plasma cytokeratin-18 level as a novel biomarker for liver fibrosis in children with nonalcoholic fatty liver disease. J Pediatr Gastroenterol Nutr. 2016;63(2):181–7.
30. Walenbergh SM, Houben T, Hendrikx T, et al. Plasma cathepsin D levels: a novel tool to predict pediatric hepatic inflammation. Am J Gastroenterol. 2015;110(3):462–70.
31. Di Martino M, Koryukova K, Bezzi M. Imaging features of non-alcoholic fatty liver disease in children and adolescents. Children (Basel). 2017;4(8).
32. Di Martino M, Pacifico L, Bezzi M, et al. Comparison of magnetic resonance spectroscopy, proton density fat fraction and histological analysis in the quantification of liver steatosis in children and adolescents. World J Gastroenterol. 2016;22(39):8812–9.
33. Dezsőfi A, Baumann U, Dhawan A, et al. Liver biopsy in children: position paper of the ESPGHAN Hepatology Committee. J Pediatr Gastroenterol Nutr. 2015;60(3):408–20.
34. Mann JP, De Vito R, Mosca A, et al. Portal inflammation is independently associated with fibrosis and metabolic syndrome in pediatric nonalcoholic fatty liver disease. Hepatology. 2016;63(3):745–53.
35. Kleiner DE, Makhlouf HR. Histology of NAFLD and NASH in adults and children. Clin Liver Dis. 2016;20(2):293–312.
36. Strnad P, Zatloukal K, Stumptner C, et al. Mallory-Denk-bodies: lessons from keratin-containing hepatic inclusion bodies. Biochim Biophys Acta. 2008;1782(12):764–74.
37. Brunt EM, Tiniakos DG. Histopathology of nonalcoholic fatty liver disease. World J Gastroenterol. 2010;16(42):5286–96.
38. Brunt EM, Janney CG, Di Bisceglie AM, et al. Nonalcoholic steatohepatitis: a proposal for grading and staging the histological lesions. Am J Gastroenterol. 1999;94(9):2467–74.
39. Kleiner DE, Brunt EM, Van Natta M. Design and validation of a histological scoring system for nonalcoholic fatty liver disease. Hepatology. 2005;41(6):1313–21.
40. Alkhouri N, De Vito R, Alisi A, et al. Development and validation of a new histological score for pediatric non-alcoholic fatty liver disease. J Hepatol. 2012;57(6):1312–8.
41. Nobili V, Donati B, Panera N, et al. A 4-polymorphism risk score predicts steatohepatitis in children with nonalcoholic fatty liver disease. J Pediatr Gastroenterol Nutr. 2014;58(5):632–6.
42. Nobili V, Marcellini M, Devito R, et al. NAFLD in children: a prospective clinical-pathological study and effect of lifestyle advice. Hepatology. 2006;44(2):458–65.
43. Nobili V, Vajro P, Dezsofi A, et al. Indications and limitations of bariatric intervention in severely obese children and adolescents with and without nonalcoholic steatohepatitis: ESPGHAN Hepatology Committee Position Statement. J Pediatr Gastroenterol Nutr. 2015;60(4):550–61.
44. Manco M, Mosca A, De Peppo F, et al. The benefit of sleeve gastrectomy in obese adolescents on nonalcoholic steatohepatitis and hepatic fibrosis. J Pediatr. 2017;180:31–37.e2.
45. Lavine JE, Schwimmer JB, Van Natta ML, et al. Effect of vitamin E or metformin for treatment of nonalcoholic fatty liver disease in children and adolescents: the TONIC randomized controlled trial. JAMA. 2011;305:1659–68.
46. Vajro P, Franzese A, Valerio G, et al. Lack of efficacy of ursodeoxycholic acid for the treatment of liver abnormalities in obese children. J Pediatr. 2000;136:739–43.
47. Della Corte C, Carpino G, De Vito R, et al. Docosahexanoic acid plus vitamin D treatment improves features of NAFLD in children with serum vitamin D deficiency: results from a single centre trial. PLoS One. 2016;11(12):e0168216.
48. Famouri F, Shariat Z, Hashemipour M, et al. Effects of probiotics on non-alcoholic fatty liver disease in obese children and adolescents: a randomized clinical trial. J Pediatr Gastroenterol Nutr. 2017;64:413–7.
49. Kim S-G, Kim B-K, Kim K, et al. Bile acid nuclear receptor Farnesoid X receptor: therapeutic target for nonalcoholic fatty liver disease. Endocrinol Metab (Seoul). 2016;31(4):500–4.
50. Armstrong MJ, Gaunt P, Aithal GP, et al. Liraglutide safety and efficacy in patients with non-alcoholic steatohepatitis (LEAN): a multicentre, double-blind, randomised, placebo-controlled phase 2 study. Lancet. 2016;387(10019):679–90.
51. Charlotte F, Le Naour G, Bernhardt C, et al. A comparison of the fibrotic potential of nonalcoholic fatty liver disease and chronic hepatitis C. Hum Pathol. 2010;41(8):1178–85.
52. Shaker M, Tabbaa A, Albeldawi M, et al. Liver transplantation for nonalcoholic fatty liver disease: new challenges and new opportunities. World J Gastroenterol. 2014;20(18):5320–30.
53. Alkhouri N, Hanouneh IA, Zein NN, et al. Liver transplantation for nonalcoholic steatohepatitis in young patients. Transpl Int. 2016;29(4):418–24.
54. Zezos P, Renner EL. Liver transplantation and non-alcoholic fatty liver disease. World J Gastroenterol. 2014;20(42):15532–8.
55. Orman ES, Mayorga ME, Wheeler SB, et al. Declining liver graft quality threatens the future of liver transplantation in the United States. Liver Transpl. 2015;21(8):1040–50.
56. Pais R, Barritt AS, Calmus Y, et al. NAFLD and liver transplantation: current burden and expected challenges. J Hepatol. 2016;65(6):1245–57.

Complications of Liver Cirrhosis

A. Holvast and H. J. Verkade

Key Points

- There are several tools to support the suspicion of cirrhosis: physical examination, ultrasound, elastography, and CT/MRI scan. However the gold standard for the diagnosis remains histology, obtained via a liver biopsy.
- Clinically it is important to distinguish compensated from decompensated cirrhosis.
- Even compensated cirrhosis carries serious complications which warrant aggressive treatment, such as hepatocellular carcinoma, hepatopulmonary syndrome, or portopulmonary hypertension.

Research Needed in the Field

- Elucidation of the molecular mechanism(s) underlying hepatopulmonary syndrome, portopulmonary hypertension, and hepatorenal syndrome
- Development of tailored preventive and therapeutic strategies for these complications
- Successful targeting of liver fibrogenesis, in order to prevent, mitigate, or even reverse liver fibrosis in the different forms of liver disease

18.1 Cirrhosis

18.1.1 Pathophysiology

Liver cirrhosis is characterized by severe hepatic fibrosis and nodular replacement of normal liver architecture. It is a final common pathway for many chronic liver diseases. It is caused by the deposition of a matrix containing fibronectin and collagen, produced by activated hepatic stellate cells (transformed into myofibroblasts) and portal fibroblasts (transformed into another myofibroblast phenotype) [1]. Progressive fibrosis leads to portal hypertension and an increasing risk of disturbances of liver function.

Up to a certain point, fibrosis is reversible upon successful treatment of the underlying condition. Also medication interfering with fibrogenic signals may reverse fibrosis, as has been demonstrated in animal models, but this is not yet available for clinical practice in children.

18.1.2 Clinical Presentation and Diagnosis

Clinical signs associated with liver cirrhosis are rather aspecific, such as anorexia, weight loss, weakness, and fatigue. Physical examination may reveal [2]:

- Signs of portal hypertension: splenomegaly, prominent abdominal veins/caput medusae, ascites.
- Jaundice.
- Palmar erythema.
- Spider angiomata.
- Nail changes, presumably by effects of hypoalbuminemia.
- Digital clubbing.
- Note: a cirrhotic liver is not necessarily small but may (still) be normal sized or even enlarged.

A. Holvast · H. J. Verkade (✉)
Pediatric Hepatology, Beatrix Children's Hospital-UMCG, University of Groningen, Groningen, The Netherlands
e-mail: h.j.verkade@umcg.nl

Liver cirrhosis can be suspected clinically based on findings during physical examination. There are several imaging tools to support the suspicion of cirrhosis: ultrasound, elastography, and CT/MRI scan. The gold standard for the diagnosis, however, remains histology, obtained via a liver biopsy. Histology allows staging of fibrosis, for which several scoring systems can be used, of which METAVIR is the most commonly used [3]. Histology based on liver biopsy does carry the risk of sampling error, which is inherent to a condition with an inhomogeneous distribution.

18.1.3 Compensated and Decompensated Cirrhosis

During the course of fibrosis progressing to cirrhosis, the liver function usually remains quite stable for a prolonged time. Liver function encompasses the integrated functions of synthesis (i.e., coagulation factors, albumin), detoxification (i.e., ammonia), excretion (i.e., bilirubin), and storage (glycogen), as well as filtering of blood from portal vein-drained viscera. Even in the cirrhotic stage, liver function can be maintained reasonably well. However, the more progressive the liver disease, the more prone the patient is for what is called decompensated cirrhosis. In decompensated cirrhosis, liver function starts failing in one or more of its functions, and/or complications of cirrhosis become manifest. Signs and symptoms of hepatic decompensation can be jaundice, pruritus, signs of upper gastrointestinal bleeding, abdominal distension from ascites, confusion due to hepatic encephalopathy, or spontaneous bacterial peritonitis. Decompensation can develop slowly, as part of a gradual development toward manifest liver failure in end-stage liver disease. Decompensation can also be triggered more acutely, e.g., by infections, disturbances of fluid balance, trauma, or operative procedures.

18.2 Complications of Cirrhosis

18.2.1 Cardiorespiratory Complications: Hepatopulmonary Syndrome

18.2.1.1 Epidemiology and Pathophysiology

Liver cirrhosis in children may be complicated by hepatopulmonary syndrome (HPS). Although physiological signs can be found in up to 40% of patients, clinically relevant HPS is more rare (estimated 5–10%). HPS is characterized by intrapulmonary dilatation of the small pulmonary vessels, which leads to arteriovenous shunting and ventilation perfusion mismatch. This leads to an increased alveolar-arterial oxygen gradient and arterial hypoxemia that is rather unresponsive to increasing oxygen content of the inhaled air. The cause of intrapulmonary vascular dilatation has not been fully elucidated. It may partly result from downstream effects of liver injury, as was shown that in animals, endothelin 1 release leads to increasing production of nitric oxide by pulmonary endothelial cells. Partly it may be caused through other mechanisms than liver injury, as HPS may also occur in case of portal hypertension without liver dysfunction, such as extrahepatic portal vein obstruction, though HPS is less frequent in this population. One hypothesis is that intestine-derived vasoactive compounds are not filtered by the liver in case of portosystemic shunting. Therefore, portosystemic shunting of blood in itself is a contributing factor to the development of HPS, and cirrhosis by itself is not a prerequisite for HPS to develop [4].

18.2.1.2 Presentation and Diagnosis

One of the first (sub)clinical symptoms of HPS is frequently a decrease in exercise tolerance, due to shortage of breath. This may stay unnoticed until a more advanced stage, with permanent hypoxemia. Chronic hypoxemia may lead to clubbing and cyanosis. Using pulse oximetry to detect arterial hypoxemia can be misleading, as pulse oximetry may not detect mild to moderate hepatopulmonary syndrome in which pulse oximetry values are usually normal (>98%) [5]. Suspicion should be raised upon a lower pulse oximetry values in upright versus supine position ("orthodeoxia"). The presently conventional method to demonstrate the existence of HPS is by contrast-enhanced echocardiography, in which, in the absence of intracardiac shunts, air bubbles appear in the left atrium between the third and eighth cardiac cycle after they first appear in the right atrium.

HPS is categorized as:

- Mild: $PaO_2 \geq 80$ mmHg and $PAaO_2 \geq 15$ mmHg
- Moderate: PaO_2 60–80 mmHg and $PAaO_2 \geq 15$ mmHg
- Severe: $PaO_2 < 60$ mmHg and $PAaO_2 \geq 15$ mmHg

18.2.1.3 Management and Outcome

There is no curative treatment other than liver transplantation. Of note, pretransplant mortality is increased in HPS and advanced, and long-term HPS may complicate the oxygenation of the donor organ, shortly after transplantation. Supportive care is limited. Oxygen can be suppleted, either continuously or during exercise, but the objective benefit is doubtful. Following liver transplantation, HPS resolves within months, though it may persist up to a year. Survival posttransplant is comparable to patients receiving liver transplantation without HPS.

18.2.2 Cardiorespiratory Complications: Portopulmonary Hypertension

18.2.2.1 Epidemiology and Pathophysiology
Liver cirrhosis may be complicated by the development of portopulmonary hypertension (PPH) in a small group of patients (1–2%). It is hypothesized to result from increased cardiac output in portosystemic shunting due to portal hypertension, leading to mechanic stress in the pulmonary vasculature. This may induce increased pulmonary vascular resistance due to vasoconstriction and may result in structural changes due to remodeling of endothelial cells and smooth muscle cells.

18.2.2.2 Presentation and Diagnosis
Clinical presentation may be insidious with slowly developing dyspnea and hypoxemia. PPH may be suspected based on Doppler echocardiography with signs of right ventricular hypertrophy and increased pulmonary artery systolic pressure. Gold standard is a catheterization, with diagnostic criteria being a mean pulmonary artery pressure >25 mmHg, pulmonary vascular resistance index >3 Woods units m^2, and pulmonary capillary wedge pressure <15 mmHg.

18.2.2.3 Management and Outcome
If cirrhosis is the basis of PPH, the only curative treatment is liver transplantation. It is important to detect PPH early, as with increasing mean pulmonary artery pressure, there is an increase in the risk of right-sided heart failure prior to and following liver transplantation with associated mortality. In adults a mean pulmonary artery pressure >45 mmHg is a contraindication for transplantation. Supportive care is given by oxygen supplementation, and preoperative vasodilator therapy may be considered [6].

18.2.3 Cardiorespiratory Complications: Cirrhotic Cardiomyopathy

Liver cirrhosis may lead to cirrhotic cardiomyopathy, which is a spectrum of cardiac dysfunction which may include conduction abnormalities, diastolic dysfunction, and systolic dysfunction. Its pathophysiology is not well understood. Data on prevalence cirrhotic cardiomyopathy are limited. It has been reported that 18% of children with portal hypertension develop latent cirrhotic cardiomyopathy and that 2% of patients may develop manifest cirrhotic cardiomyopathy. Diagnostic criteria are modified from adult guidelines. Supportive care can be given, but liver transplantation is the only curative treatment [7].

18.2.4 Hepatorenal Syndrome (HRS)

18.2.4.1 Epidemiology and Pathophysiology
In patients with chronic cirrhotic liver disease, hepatorenal syndrome (HRS) can develop. It is estimated that 5% of children with cirrhosis develop HRS. Pathophysiologically, portal hypertension leads to splanchnic vasodilatation due to nitric oxide. This is detected by renal baroreceptors as decrease in effective circulating volume, which activates the renin-angiotensin-aldosterone system and leads to renal vasoconstriction. As a result, renal hypoperfusion and impairment develop.

18.2.4.2 Presentation and Diagnosis
HRS is divided into two subtypes. Type 1 HRS is an acute renal impairment, often triggered by an intercurrent event. In HRS 2 the course is more chronic, with a slow rise in serum creatinine and coinciding with a progressive course of end-stage liver disease and refractory ascites.

In adults, cutoff values of serum creatinine have been established to diagnose HRS (serum creatinine >1 mg/dL/133 μmol/L). In children, however, due to lower baseline creatinine levels, cutoff values are not well defined. It is suggested that a twofold increase in baseline creatinine is a useful diagnostic criterion.

18.2.4.3 Management and Outcome
With regard to treatment of HRS, the only definitive treatment is liver transplantation. To bridge this period, supportive care should be given, and diuretics should be discontinued. In HRS 1, vasopressive treatment and albumin supplementation can be given. Vasopressins that can be used are terlipressin, norepinephrine, or the combination of octreotide/midodrine. In HRS 2, there is insufficient evidence to support the use of vasopressins and albumin. Furthermore, TIPS (transjugular intrahepatic portosystemic shunt) can be considered as a palliating therapy. Patients with HRS have a lower survival rate following liver transplantation. However, in a successful course, renal function has a good recovery in the vast majority of patients [8].

18.2.5 Bacterial Infectious Complications, Including Spontaneous Bacterial Peritonitis (SBP)

18.2.5.1 Epidemiology and Pathophysiology
Patients with liver cirrhosis are at increased risk of a bacterial infection, both in general and more specific such as spontaneous bacterial peritonitis (SBP). This increased risk is a result of a decrease in several aspects of the immune response, intestinal bacterial overgrowth, and increased risk of bacterial translocation across the intestine.

With regard to a diminished immune response, several factors are involved. In many patients with advanced cirrhosis, serum levels of complement factors (C3, C4) are markedly decreased. In addition, there are defects of cellular immune aspects such as in neutrophil, monocyte, and T-cell function [9].

Intestinal bacterial overgrowth is partly a result of a decrease in bile acids in the small bowel, in case of cholestasis. Intestinal bacterial translocation results from both immune deficiency, bacterial overgrowth, and other factors such as intestinal barrier dysfunction due to inflammation and portal hypertension [10]. In adults, a higher Child-Pugh class has been associated with increased intestinal bacterial translocation, to up to 30% in Child-Pugh C patients.

In SBP, ascites is spontaneously infected, supposedly through bacterial translocation. In SBP there is no gross intra-abdominal cause such as a bowel perforation. SBP is typically caused by a single microbe, whereas a perforation usually results in a mixture of microbes. The immunodeficiency in end-stage liver disease adds to the risk of SBP. Its occurrence may be decreased by preventive measures. First, vaccination protocols are of influence. *Streptococcus pneumonia* was a frequent cause of SBP, but its occurrence has declined since pneumococcal vaccination. Presently, gram-negative bacteria appear to be most prevalent [11]. Another preventive measure may be antibiotic prophylaxis, which is usually started following a first episode of SBP. Trimethoprim/sulfamethoxazole is a frequent first choice in children.

18.2.5.2 Presentation and Diagnosis

The clinical presentation SBP is often not very specific. SPB should be suspected in case of any combination of fever of unknown origin and ascites. Suggestive symptoms can be new onset or worsening of ascites, abdominal tenderness, and rebound tenderness. Other potential accompanying signs include encephalopathy, renal insufficiency, and deterioration of liver function tests. CRP can be increased but is sometimes misleadingly low [12]. Renal insufficiency may be present at presentation but may also develop later during an SBP and deteriorate into hepatorenal syndrome type 1.

The key diagnostic test is analysis of ascites via ascites puncture. Analysis of ascites should include a leukocyte count and differentiation, albumin, as well as an ascites culture. A general cutoff for the diagnosis of SBP is >250 polymorphonuclear (PMN) cells/mm^3 and a positive ascitic fluid culture. Bacterial ascites is defined as a positive culture with less than 250 PMN cells/mm^3.

18.2.5.3 Management and Outcome

In general, in suspected SBP, a broad-spectrum non-nephrotic third-generation cephalosporin is recommended. As said, close monitoring of kidney function is warranted because of the increased risk on subsequent hepatorenal syndrome type 1.

18.2.6 Oncologic: Hepatocellular Carcinoma

18.2.6.1 Epidemiology and Pathophysiology

In liver cirrhosis, there is a clear increased risk in developing hepatocellular carcinoma (HCC). However, the majority of children in whom HCC is diagnosed (60–70%) does not have an underlying cirrhosis. Risk of HCC is increased in patients with Alagille syndrome, progressive familial intrahepatic cholestasis (bile salt export pump deficiency), alpha-1 antitrypsin deficiency, tyrosinemia, Wilson's disease, glycogen storage disease, and chronic hepatitis B or C infection.

18.2.6.2 Presentation and Diagnosis

HCC is often insidious in its clinical presentation. To screen patients at risk, including children with cirrhosis of the liver, alpha-fetoprotein (AFP) and liver ultrasounds can be used. CT or MRI should be used for further diagnostic evaluation in case of suspected HCC.

18.2.6.3 Management and Outcome

HCC is poorly responsive to chemotherapy. Curation depends on complete tumor resection, which may require liver transplantation. Chemotherapy may have a place as an adjuvant therapy. Radiofrequency ablation and transarterial chemoembolization may have a place in the therapeutic approach, particularly in adults, but mostly these modalities are limited as a bridge to curative surgical approaches, such as liver transplantation.

18.2.7 Endocrine Dysfunction

In chronic and advanced liver cirrhosis in children, several endocrine problems frequently occur.

18.2.7.1 Growth Restriction

The cause of growth restriction is multifactorial, including increased resting energy expenditure, decreased nutrient intake, nutrient malabsorption, abnormal nitrogen balance, and alterations of the growth hormone axis. Growth restriction appears to be about −0.5 SD [13].

18.2.7.2 Osteoporosis

Bone mass density is reduced in chronic liver cirrhosis, also after correcting for confounding variables (weight, height, and pubertal stage). Possible mechanisms are chronic cholestasis, poor nutrition, deficiencies in calcium and vitamin D, poor muscle mass and low body mass index, immobility, hypogonadism and other hormonal abnormalities, and medications [14].

18.2.7.3 Delayed Puberty

Puberty can be markedly delayed in children with liver cirrhosis. After successful liver transplantation, puberty will catch up, though posttransplant children can be significantly later in reaching puberty milestones [13].

18.2.7.4 Adrenal Dysfunction

In children with severe end-stage liver disease who had to be admitted to the ICU, prior to liver transplantation, adrenal dysfunction was found to be present in about 80% of children. Support is given symptomatically, with liver transplantation being the only therapeutic solution [15].

18.2.8 Other Complications of Liver Cirrhosis

In addition to the complications discussed above, there are several other complications discussed in detail elsewhere in the book.

First, liver cirrhosis gives rise to *portal hypertension and its complications*, including varices, hypersplenism, hyperammonemia, and ascites. See chapter "Cirrhotic and Noncirrhotic Portal Hypertension."

Second, achieving an acceptable *nutritional status* in liver cirrhosis is challenging. Malabsorption, decreased intake, and *metabolic derangements* play a role. See chapter "Nutrition and Liver Disease."

References

1. Lee UE, Friedman SL. Mechanisms of hepatic fibrogenesis. Best Pract Res Clin Gastroenterol. 2011;25(2):195–206.
2. Heidelbaugh JJ, Bruderly M. Cirrhosis and chronic liver failure: part I. Diagnosis and evaluation. Am Fam Physician. 2006;74(5):756–62.
3. Goodman ZD. Grading and staging systems for inflammation and fibrosis in chronic liver diseases. J Hepatol. 2007;47(4):598–607.
4. Borkar VV, Poddar U, Kapoor A, Ns S, Srivastava A, Yachha SK. Hepatopulmonary syndrome in children: a comparative study of non-cirrhotic vs. cirrhotic portal hypertension. Liver Int. 2015;35(6):1665–72.
5. Hoerning A, Raub S, Neudorf U, Muntjes C, Kathemann S, Lainka E, et al. Pulse oximetry is insufficient for timely diagnosis of hepatopulmonary syndrome in children with liver cirrhosis. J Pediatr. 2014;164(3):2.
6. Karrer FM, Wallace BJ, Estrada AE. Late complications of biliary atresia: hepatopulmonary syndrome and portopulmonary hypertension. Pediatr Surg Int. 2017;33(12):1335–40.
7. Celtik C, Durmaz O, Oner N, Yavuz T, Gokce S, Aydogan A, et al. Investigation of cardiomyopathy in children with cirrhotic and noncirrhotic portal hypertension. J Pediatr Gastroenterol Nutr. 2015;60(2):177–81.
8. Elizabeth Parsons C, Nelson R, Book LS, Kyle Jensen M. Renal replacement therapy in infants and children with hepatorenal syndrome awaiting liver transplantation: a case-control study. Liver Transpl. 2014;20(12):1468–74.
9. Leonis MA, Balistreri WF. Evaluation and management of end-stage liver disease in children. Gastroenterology. 2008;134(6):1741–51.
10. Papp M, Norman GL, Vitalis Z, Tornai I, Altorjay I, Foldi I, et al. Presence of anti-microbial antibodies in liver cirrhosis—a tell-tale sign of compromised immunity? PLoS One. 2010;5(9):e12957.
11. Vieira SM, Matte U, Kieling CO, Barth AL, Ferreira CT, Souza AF, et al. Infected and noninfected ascites in pediatric patients. J Pediatr Gastroenterol Nutr. 2005;40(3):289–94.
12. Preto-Zamperlini M, Farhat SC, Perondi MB, Pestana AP, Cunha PS, Pugliese RP, et al. Elevated C-reactive protein and spontaneous bacterial peritonitis in children with chronic liver disease and ascites. J Pediatr Gastroenterol Nutr. 2014;58(1):96–8.
13. Mohammad S, Grimberg A, Rand E, Anand R, Yin W, Alonso EM, et al. Long-term linear growth and puberty in pediatric liver transplant recipients. J Pediatr. 2013;163(5):7.
14. Uslu N, Saltik-Temizel IN, Demir H, Usta Y, Ozen H, Gurakan F, et al. Bone mineral density in children with cirrhosis. J Gastroenterol. 2006;41(9):873–7.
15. Hauser GJ, Brotzman HM, Kaufman SS. Hepatoadrenal syndrome in pediatric patients with end-stage liver disease. Pediatr Crit Care Med. 2012;13(3):145.

Portal Hypertension

Angelo Di Giorgio and Lorenzo D'Antiga

Key Points
- Portal hypertension is defined as a portal pressure greater than 10 mmHg or as elevation of the hepatic venous pressure gradient to >4 mmHg.
- The most important pathogenetic factors for the development of PH are an increased portal vascular resistance and an increased portal blood flow.
- A significant proportion of children with acute and chronic liver diseases develop PH and its complications including bleeding from intestinal varices, ascites, splenomegaly with hypersplenism, hepatic encephalopathy and pulmonary complications. Unlike in adults, in children variceal bleeding is a major contributor to morbidity but a rare cause of mortality.
- The hyperdynamic syndrome is a late consequence of portal hypertension, and it is characterized by haemodynamic changes including high cardiac output, increased heart rate and total blood volume and reduced total systemic vascular resistance.
- The management of non-cirrhotic portal vein thrombosis is mainly directed to the treatment of complications of portal hypertension, through medical and endoscopic means, and to restore, if feasible, a hepatopetal flow by surgery and interventional radiology.

Portal hypertension (PH) is a common complication in adults and children with chronic liver disease. It usually accompanies advanced liver disease, leading to severe complications such as bleeding from oesophageal varices, ascites, hepatopulmonary syndrome and hepatic encephalopathy [1]. It is estimated that approximately 50% of paediatric patients with chronic liver disease and 90% of those with extrahepatic portal vein obstruction (EHPVO) will experience gastrointestinal bleeding [2, 3]. In children, the mortality rate from variceal bleeding is much lower compared to adults; however haematemesis is a frightening event, giving the impression of impending death and contributing to great fear and anxiety in patients and carers [2, 3].

There are further several differences between children and adults with PH. In adults, the largest cohort of patients has 'cirrhotic PH'. In fact, because of organ scarcity, these patients remain in follow-up care for many years before undergoing liver transplantation (LT). Consequently, in adults the literature is rich of prospective studies providing evidence on the management of PH in cirrhotic patients. On the contrary, in paediatrics, the largest cohort of children with cirrhotic PH is affected by biliary atresia and is commonly transplanted in the first few years of life. Therefore the paediatric patients remaining with long-standing PH are those with 'non-cirrhotic PH', such as those with portal vein thrombosis and fibrocystic liver disease, usually having normal liver function and thus not requiring LT. This difference is more pronounced by the relatively larger availability of segmental organ donation, allowing to resolve PH by LT much sooner compared to the adult population. The fact that the length of the follow-up of children with severe cirrhotic PH is short has hampered the accomplishment of large prospective trials on features and management of this condition during the paediatric age. As a consequence, unlike adults, in paediatrics there are neither published prospective studies nor guidelines on the management of PH complications. The Baveno conference, which is held every 5 years, and representing the most relevant meeting and consensus on PH in adults, has recently involved a panel of paediatric experts with the aim to provide best practice recommendations for the management of PH in children [4–8]. In the absence of standardized guidelines, the management of paediatric PH differs remarkably worldwide, depending on local facilities and centre experience.

A. Di Giorgio (✉) · L. D'Antiga
Paediatric Hepatology, Gastroenterology and Transplantation, Hospital Papa Giovanni XXIII, Bergamo, Italy
e-mail: adigiorgio@asst-pg23.it; ldantiga@asst-pg23.it

19.1 Anatomy of the Portal Venous System

The liver has the most complicated circulation of any organ. Blood flow to the liver is unique in that it receives both oxygenated and deoxygenated blood from two main vessels. The first vessel is the proper hepatic artery, which is a branch of the common hepatic artery arising from celiac trunk. It supplies oxygenated blood accounting for 25% of the blood entering the liver. The second important vessel is represented by the portal vein (PV), which drains deoxygenated blood from the gastrointestinal tract, accounting for 75% of liver blood flow. The portal system lies between two capillary beds, being therefore difficult to be accessed for diagnostic and interventional procedures. Despite the liver mass represents only 2.5% of the total body weight, this organ receives nearly 25% of the cardiac output, therefore total hepatic blood flow ranges between 800 and 1200 mL/min, which is equivalent to approximately 100 mL/min per 100 g of wet liver.

Portal venous flow across the liver is given by a minute pressure gradient between the portal inflow and the hepatic venous outflow which is usually no more than 5 mmHg. The resistance to blood flow through the portal vein is so low because of the unique hepatic vasculature, with conducting blood vessels terminating in each of the microvascular units of the acinus and flowing past only approximately 20 hepatocytes before exiting into the wide hepatic venules. Thus at least 50% of the entire blood content of the liver can be expelled without adding significant vascular resistance [1]. The portal venous system refers to the vessels involved in the drainage of the capillary beds of the gastrointestinal tract (including bowel, pancreas and gallbladder) and spleen into the capillary bed of the liver up to reach the heart (Fig. 19.1). The most important vessel of the portal venous system is the PV which is formed by the union of the splenic vein (SV) and the superior mesenteric vein (SMV). It conveys blood from viscera and ramifies like an artery at the liver parenchyma, ending at the sinusoids. Immediately before entering the liver, the portal vein divides into right and left branches which then enter the liver separately. Tributaries of the PV, which make up the portal venous system, are the splenic, superior mesenteric (SMV), inferior mesenteric (IMV), left gastric, right gastric, paraumbilical and cystic veins. The SMV is formed by tributaries from the small intestine, colon and head of the pancreas and irregularly from the stomach via the right gastroepiploic vein. The SV is formed by several veins that drain the spleen at the hilum. It travels posterior to the body and tail of the pancreas, joins the inferior mesenteric vein and then merges with SMV vein to form the portal vein. The IMV drains blood away from the descending colon, rectum and sigmoid, which are all parts of the large intestine, and reaches the splenic vein in its medial third. Anatomical variations include the IMV draining in the SMV or into the confluence of the SMV and the splenic vein.

After reaching the liver, the portal vein splits to form the right and left branches, each supplying about half of the liver. Then it ramifies further, forming smaller venous branches and ultimately the portal venules, which run alongside a hepatic arteriole to constitute the vascular components of the

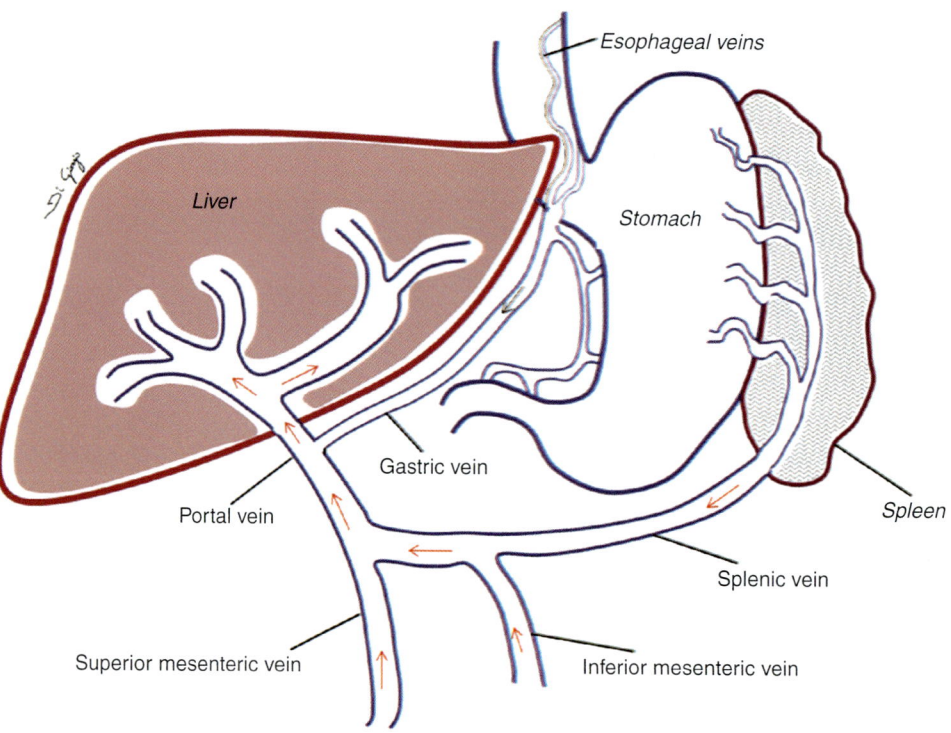

Fig. 19.1 Anatomy of the portal system

portal triad. These vessels ultimately merge into the hepatic sinusoids to supply blood to the liver. Three hepatic veins (right, middle and left) drain deoxygenated blood from the liver into the inferior vena cava (IVC) (Fig. 19.1) [2].

19.2 Pathophysiology

19.2.1 Etiopathogenetic Factors of Portal Hypertension

The major concepts in the pathophysiology of portal hypertension have been the 'backward' and the 'forward' flow theories. The former postulates that all consequences of PH result from obstruction to portal venous flow. The latter postulates that increased inflow to the portal venous system causes the changes that lead to the clinical findings of portal hypertension. As explained later, current evidences show that both theories contribute to the pathophysiology of PH [2, 3].

Haemodynamic factors play a central role in PH because of the cardinal relationship between portal venous resistance and portal venous blood flow in maintaining an elevated portal pressure. Studies on animal models and eventually clinical studies in humans have provided interesting data to understand haemodynamic alterations and molecular mechanisms involved in this syndrome [3–5].

Portal hypertension occurs when there is increased portal vascular resistance and/or an increased portal blood flow. According to Ohm's law ($AP = Q \times R$), portal venous pressure is directly proportional to blood flow and resistance: AP is the change in portal pressure along the vessel, Q is portal blood flow and R is the resistance to flow. According to Poiseuille's equation, vessel resistance (R) is directly proportional to the length (L) of the vessel and inversely proportional to the radius to the fourth power (r^4). Therefore, a small decrease in the vessel diameter produces a large increase in the portal vascular resistance and, in turn, in portal blood pressure. In the normal liver, intrahepatic resistance changes with variations in portal blood flow, thereby keeping portal pressure within normal limits [2, 3].

The portal venous system has a low baseline portal pressure of 5–10 mmHg and the hepatic venous pressure gradient (HVPG) ranges from 1 to 4 mmHg. Portal hypertension is defined as a portal pressure greater than 10 mmHg or as elevation of the hepatic venous pressure gradient to >4 mmHg. In adults, a portal pressure above 10 mmHg is associated with the occurrence of portal hypertension complications, including the occurrence of gastrointestinal varices and ascites, as well as variceal bleeding if above 12 mmHg [6, 7].

Increased vascular resistance: It represents the most important pathogenetic factor in the development of PH. Depending on the site in which it occurs, PH can be classified into two main groups: extrahepatic and intrahepatic. The former group may be further subclassified into two forms (prehepatic and posthepatic) while the latter group into three forms including presinusoidal (portal venules), sinusoidal (sinusoids) and postsinusoidal (terminal hepatic venules, central veins) (Table 19.1). In extrahepatic PH (e.g. portal vein or hepatic vein obstruction), the pathogenic mechanism to explain an increased vascular resistance is quite obvious. The pathogenesis is more complicated in intrahepatic PH (e.g. in cirrhosis), in which many factors, both mechanical and dynamic, may occur simultaneously [7]. The factors playing a relevant role in the increase of hepatic vascular resistance are illustrated in Fig. 19.2.

Increased portal blood flow: It represents the second factor contributing to the development and mainly to the maintenance of PH. This is due to the production of vasodilatory factors which cause arterial vasodilation of the splanchnic circulation, leading to an increase in blood flow into the portal venous system. Several factors have been cited as possible mediators of splanchnic vasodilation, including nitric oxide (NO), glucagon and endothelin (activated by the vasoactive intestinal peptide), as well as the activation of the sympathetic and the renin-angiotensin systems. These biochemical mediators cause sodium and water retention, hypervolemia, renal hypoperfusion and increase in cardiac output and in splanch-

Table 19.1 Classification and Aetiology of Portal Hypertension

Prehepatic	Peliosis hepatis
Portal vein thrombosis	Rendu-Osler-Weber syndrome
Congenital stenosis or extrinsic compression of the portal vein	Chronic hepatitis
	Intrahepatic sinusoidal
Splenic vein thrombosis	Liver cirrhosis (independent of cause)
Arteriovenous fistulae	
Intrahepatic presinusoidal	Wilson's disease
Congenital hepatic fibrosis	Haemochromatosis
Chronic viral hepatitis (HBV and HCV)	Storage diseases (fatty liver, glycogenosis type III, Niemann-Pick disease, α1-antitrypsin deficiency)
Primary biliary cirrhosis	
Myeloproliferative diseases (Hodgkin's disease, leukaemia)	Acute hepatitis (viral and autoimmune)
Focal nodular hyperplasia	Hypervitaminosis A
Idiopathic portal hypertension (IPH)/non-cirrhotic portal fibrosis (NCFP)/hepatoportal sclerosis	**Intrahepatic postsinusoidal**
	Veno-occlusive disease (VOD)
	Hepatic vein thrombosis (Budd-Chiari syndrome)
Granulomatous diseases (schistosomiasis, sarcoidosis, tuberculosis)	**Posthepatic**
	Inferior vena cava obstruction (thrombosis, neoplasms)
Amyloidosis	
Gaucher's disease	Right heart failure
Polycystic liver disease	Constrictive pericarditis
Infiltration of liver hilum (independent of cause)	Tricuspid valve diseases
Benign and malignant neoplasms	
Toxins and drugs (arsenic, vinyl chloride monomer poisoning, methotrexate, 6-mercaptopurine)	

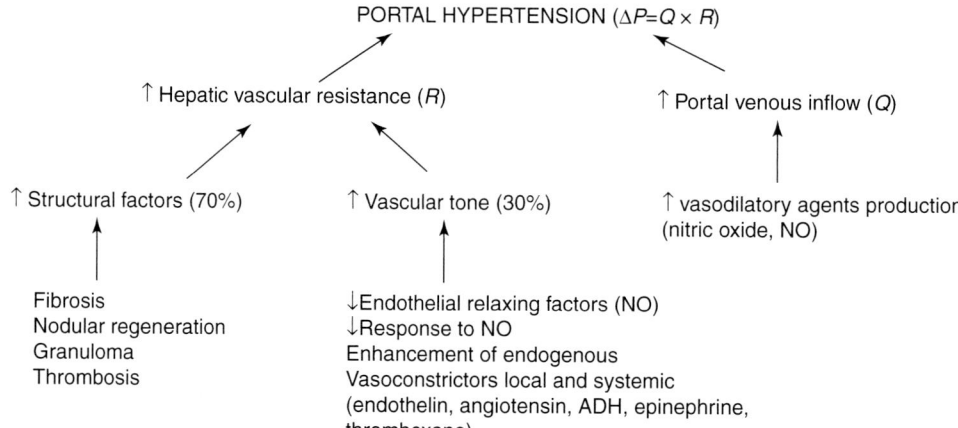

Fig. 19.2 Portal hypertension development according to Ohm's law

nic blood inflow, resulting in a hyperdynamic vascular status which characterizes the advanced stages of PH (Fig. 19.2). This may explain why, despite the formation of a significant collateral network, PH persists as a result of increased cardiac output and decreased splanchnic arteriolar tone.

19.2.2 Hyperdynamic Syndrome in Portal Hypertension

The hyperdynamic syndrome is a condition characterized by a decrease in systemic vascular resistance and increase in cardiac output and heart rate. This syndrome was first described in the 1950s, when some physicians observed that patients with cirrhosis often showed 'warm extremities, cutaneous vascular spiders, wide pulse pressure and capillary pulsations in the nail beds'. In 1953 Kowalski and Abelmann published the first study in which demonstrated an increase in cardiac output and a decrease in peripheral vascular resistance in patients with alcohol-induced cirrhosis [8]. These haemodynamic changes explained the symptoms described in cirrhotic patients. For many years the dominant theory explaining portal hypertension in cirrhosis was the 'backward flow' theory, which postulated that increased portal vascular resistance was the only cause for the increase in portal pressure. However, some years later, the researchers showed that there was also a secondary phenomenon which lead to splanchnic and systemic arterial vasodilation, contributing to increased splanchnic blood flow to the liver and increased portal pressure despite collateral formation [9]. Therefore, the hyperdynamic syndrome should be better called 'progressive vasodilatory syndrome', because the vasodilation is the main factor that brings about all the vascular changes and finally the multiorgan involvement seen in cirrhosis [10]. In the 1990s, researchers discovered that nitric oxide (NO) was responsible for the vasodilation and in turn of the multiple organ malfunctions characterizing the hyperdynamic circulation (Fig. 19.2) [11]. The hyperdynamic circulation should not be considered a complication of cirrhosis but a complication of PH. In fact, it was observed also in non-cirrhotic subjects and confirmed in different experimental models of PH [9, 11].

Splanchnic Circulation. The hyperdynamic splanchnic circulation is central to the development of the hyperdynamic syndrome. The vasodilation of the splanchnic circulation is a process mediated by humoral vasodilatory agents, and it is probably the initial signal triggering the hyperdynamic systemic circulation. Splanchnic vasodilation makes a proportion of circulating blood volume to remain confined to the splanchnic system, with a subsequent reduction of central blood volume. The result is an increased portal venous blood inflow, contributing to the maintenance and the aggravation of PH [9, 12]. This process is called the 'forward flow' theory, and it provides a rationale for the use of vasoconstrictors in patients with portal hypertension [4].

Systemic Circulation. Haemodynamic changes include an increased cardiac output and heart rate and decreased systemic vascular resistance with low arterial blood pressure. It leads to abnormalities in the cardiovascular system and several regional vascular beds [13]. Compensatory mechanisms include the activation of baroreceptor and volume receptors as well as the production of neurohormonal substances leading to sodium and water retention, with plasma volume expansion and increase in cardiac output [14]. The cardiac response is directly related to splanchnic vasodilation and plasma volume expansion, together with an increased venous return that is mostly due to the formation of portosystemic shunts. Although vasodilation is essential as the initiating factor, no hyperdynamic circulation occurs without expansion of the plasma volume and portosystemic shunting [15]. Creation of portosystemic shunting is caused by the increase in resistance to outflow from the portal venous system and is characterized by opening of collateral circulation through the reperfusion and dilation of pre-existing vessels, as well as the generation of new vessels (called collateral vessels). These veins directly connect the portal blood vessels to veins that divert the blood away from the liver into the systemic circulation, in an attempt to decompress the portal venous system. The main collateral network is the gastroepiploic system, responsible for the formation of gastro-oesophageal varices, which, together with thrombocytopenia caused by hypersplenism, are the clinical hallmarks of PH. Other collateral vessels may develop on the abdominal wall and in the rectum. These vessels are prone to rupture, leading to gastrointestinal bleeding.

A drawback of this compensatory process is that substances (such as ammonia and toxins) that are normally removed from the blood by the liver, pass directly into the systemic circulation and have adverse effects in other organs [16].

Lung Circulation. Intrapulmonary vascular abnormalities consisting of pulmonary vascular dilation, intrapulmonary shunting and a low pulmonary vascular resistance have been described in patients with portal hypertension and liver shunting. The major pulmonary vascular consequences of chronic liver disease are hepatopulmonary syndrome (HPS) and portopulmonary hypertension (PPH); these conditions are characterized by hypoxia due to pulmonary arteriovenous shunts and pulmonary hypertension, respectively [17]. The pathogenic mechanism of these complications is not fully understood. However, it is thought to be mainly related to the effect of multiple vasoactive substances including NO and carbon monoxide [18, 19]. HPS and PPS are described in detail in Chap. 17.

Renal Circulation. Renal circulation is affected indirectly by the hyperdynamic state. Progressive vasodilation induces a state of 'relative hypovolaemia' which results from an increase of the vascular compartment caused by vasodilation, leading to a reduction in central blood volume, and activation of vasoconstrictive and volume-retaining neurohumoral mechanisms that perpetuate the sodium and water retentive state [20]. To balance the progressive systemic vasodilation and respond to a perceived hypovolaemia, the kidney activates compensatory mechanisms including the activation of renin-angiotensin-aldosterone system and antidiuretic hormone secretion with the aim to retain sodium and water.

In the early stage of the disease, the intravascular volume and the cardiac output increase to maintain the arterial perfusion pressure [21]. Eventually, with the progression of the disease, the cardiac response is not enough to maintain perfusion pressure, and therefore the renal blood flow drops and renal failure develops, in a condition known as hepatorenal syndrome (HRS) [22, 23]. HRS is described in detail in Chap. 17.

19.3 Aetiology

19.3.1 Extrahepatic Causes of PH

Prehepatic causes. They are due to the obstruction of the splenic vein and/or the portal vein (congenital atresia or stenosis, extrinsic compression by tumours and thrombosis). In these disorders the obstruction in the prehepatic portal venous system leads to an increased portal venous pressure [24].

Left-sided portal hypertension (LSPH). This condition is due to isolated obstruction of the splenic vein and can cause lienal hypertension that, although rare, may cause severe episodes of upper gastrointestinal bleeding. The incidence of LSPH has increased over the past three decades due to increased awareness of the entity and advances in diagnostic approaches. Since most patients are asymptomatic and experience no complications, its exact incidence is unknown. Following obstruction of the splenic vein, splenic blood drains through the short gastric veins to the stomach. In the gastric wall veins of the fundus, blood flow and pressure increase and submucosal structures consequently dilate, producing isolated gastric varices. The most common causes of splenic vein occlusion are pancreatic diseases, such as pancreatic cancer, pancreatitis or a pseudocyst. This disease is quite rare in children though it should be suspected in the presence of isolated gastric bleeding with normal liver function and unexplained splenomegaly. The diagnosis may be difficult and splenectomy represents the treatment of choice in symptomatic patients.

Portal vein thrombosis (PVT). This disease refers to an obstruction in the main trunk of the portal vein. In adults, it is frequent in advanced liver cirrhosis, often associated with hepatocellular carcinoma; it is less frequent in compensated cirrhosis and is a relatively rare condition in patients with a previously healthy liver. Conversely, in children PVT is the most common cause of non-cirrhotic PH.

The most frequent aetiological factors which can cause the thrombosis of the PV are umbilical vein catheterization, omphalitis/umbilical sepsis, thrombophilia (acquired, hereditary), myeloproliferative disorders, surgery (splenectomy, liver transplantation), dehydration and multiple exchange transfusions in the neonatal period. However, previous studies demonstrated that in around 50% of cases the aetiology remains unknown [25–27].

A multicentre Italian study on 187 children with PVT showed that it is commonly associated with a neonatal disorder. Results showed the mean age at diagnosis was 4 years, 59% were born preterm, 65% had a history of umbilical catheterization and 82% had associated illnesses such as complications of prematurity and cardiac malformations. The patients were diagnosed upon detection of splenomegaly (39.5%), after an episode of gastrointestinal bleeding (36.6%), because of hypersplenism (5.2%), by chance in the context of other investigations (16.3%). The 10-year survival rate was 98.8% (personal data, unpublished).

The pathophysiology of PH is related to the occlusion of the PV by a thrombus which causes an increased vascular resistance in the portal venous system. Initially the occlusion is followed by compensatory vasodilation of the hepatic artery buffering the need for blood supply to the liver. As the portal vein thrombosis evolves, fibroblasts transform the clot into a firm, collagenous plug in which tortuous venous channels develop. This transformation called portal cavernoma begins within days of the acute thrombosis and continues to evolve over weeks to months. Part of these collaterals may reperfuse the liver, whereas the majority contributes to the portosystemic shunting developing at various levels in the portal system. Since there is no ongoing parenchymal damage (a part from mild ischemia leading eventually to liver hypotrophy), liver function tests are usually normal.

The management of PVT is mainly directed to the treatment of PH complications, through medical and endoscopic means, and to restore, if feasible, a hepatopetal flow or at least a normal pressure in the portal venous system. Endoscopic treatment is effective in obliterating oesophageal varices and reducing the risk of GI bleeding, although it remains a palliative procedure, moving the problem to other districts (such as portal hypertensive gastropathy) and to later complications (related to increased portosystemic shunting). The main surgical option for PVT is represented by the meso-Rex bypass, which consists of placing a vascular autograft (usually the patient's own internal jugular vein) between the SMV and the left branch of the portal vein, if patent, in order to decompress the portal venous system and restore a physiological intrahepatic venous flow. The meso-Rex bypass should be considered in the primary prophylaxis of bleeding in paediatric PVT, and all patients should be screened for its feasibility. Surgical portosystemic shunts, to be considered if the meso-Rex bypass is unfeasible, may normalize the portal venous pressure but are at risk of obstruction from thrombotic events; besides, not restoring the physiological portal venous flow, they increase the complications of portosystemic shunting. In cases not amenable to meso-Rex bypass, the indications for surgical portosystemic shunting include acute variceal bleeding not controlled by endoscopic means, persistent oesophageal varices formation, massive symptomatic splenomegaly, growth retardation and complicated portal hypertensive biliopathy [28, 29]. In the hands of experienced radiologists, a proportion of cases of PVT may be managed by transjugular intrahepatic portosystemic shunts, replacing the more invasive surgical shunts [2]. The clinical features and management of portal vein thrombosis are also discussed in Chap. 19.

Posthepatic causes of PH are uncommon. They can result from increased resistance to blood flow in the major hepatic veins, caudal vena cava or right heart. Major causes are the thrombosis/stenosis of the hepatic veins or the atriocaval junction and the conditions increasing the right atrial pressure such as constrictive pericarditis and right-sided cardiac failure. The postsurgical status of some congenital cardiac malformations, such as the Fontan circulation, can result in increased central venous pressure and increased resistance to liver outflow [30]. In posthepatic PH the liver blood stagnation may compromise the liver function leading to cirrhosis [31].

Budd-Chiari syndrome (BCS). It is one of the most common causes of posthepatic PH both in adults and children. It is a rare and potentially life-threatening disorder characterized by obstruction of the hepatic outflow tract at any level between the junction of the inferior vena cava with the right atrium and the small hepatic veins. Irrespective of the cause of hepatic venous outflow obstruction, increased hepatic sinusoidal pressure and portal hypertension quickly ensue, resulting in venous congestion and ischemic damage to the surrounding sinusoidal hepatocytes [32]. A wide variety of predisposing factors may cause this disease including congenital or acquired thrombotic, inflammatory or neoplastic processes.

Overall, BCS is a rare cause of liver disease in children in the western world. In studies including patients younger than 10 years, the percentage of cases of paediatric BCS accounted for 1–7% of all, although in some areas such as Africa, India and China, the rate of paediatric BCS may raise up to 16% of all children with liver disease [33, 34].

The presentation can be acute, chronic or fulminant. The acute or fulminant form is uncommon and presents with abdominal pain, hepatomegaly, ascites and rapidly progressive hepatic failure. Conversely, the chronic form may be asymptomatic and accompanied by normal liver tests until the persistent hepatic venous outflow obstruction leads to hepatic dysfunction and symptoms of PH such as ascites and hepatosplenomegaly. Different therapeutic modalities for the management of BCS patients include palliative medical treatment (anticoagulation, thrombolytic therapy), percutaneous radiological interventions (angioplasty, stenting, TIPS), surgical portosystemic shunting and LT [45]. The stage of the disease at diagnosis influences the management strategy and an early diagnosis offers the best chance of cure without major surgery [35].

19.3.2 Intrahepatic Causes of PH

Based on the relation with the sinusoidal bed involved, the intrahepatic causes of PH can be divided into three subgroups: presinusoidal, sinusoidal and postsinusoidal (Table 19.1).

Presinusoidal obstruction. It accounts for 10–15% of cases of portal hypertension and may occur in the intra- or extrahepatic parts of the portal system. Remarkably, the increased portal pressure cannot be detected by the hepatic vein catheter study because the wedge hepatic venous pressure (WHVP) measurement reflects the venous pressure of the sinusoids that are distal to the lesion and therefore have

Table 19.2 Hepatic venous pressure gradient measurements according to the pathophysiology of portal hypertension

Aetiology of PH		ISP	PVP	RAP	WHVP	FHVP	HVPG
Prehepatic		↑↑	↑↑	N	N	N	N
Intrahepatic	Presinusoidal	↑↑	↑↑	N	N or ↑	N	N or ↑
	Sinusoidal	↑↑	↑↑	N	↑↑	N	↑↑
	Postsinusoidal	↑↑	↑↑	N	↑↑	N	↑↑
Posthepatic		↑↑	↑↑	N or ↑	↑↑	↑↑	N or ↑

ISP intrasplenic pressure, *PVP* portal vein pressure, *RAP* right atrial pressure, *WHVP* wedged hepatic venous pressure, *FHVP* free hepatic venous pressure, *HVPG* hepatic venous pressure gradient (difference between WHVP and FHVP), *N* normal
↑↑ severe increase, ↑ mild increase

normal blood pressure in these conditions. Therefore, only the direct measurement of portal venous pressure can provide data on the real degree of presinusoidal PH (Table 19.2).

Schistosoma infection is one of the most important causes of non-cirrhotic portal hypertension in Latin America, Africa and Asia. All schistosomiasis can induce hepatic disease, consequence of the eggs embolization of the terminal vessels of the portal system. However, only Schistosoma mansoni and Asian bilharziasis, mainly the *Schistosoma japonicum*, are the cause of severe fibrosis responsible of prehepatic portal hypertension [36]. Liver injury results from a granulomatous inflammatory reaction around trapped *Schistosoma* eggs in the presinusoidal periportal spaces. In early phases of infection, a predominantly hypercellular nonfibrotic granuloma response produces liver dysfunction that is not clinically detectable. Eventually, chronic granulomatous inflammation, consequence of parasitic infection, leads to hepatic fibrosis and, in 4–8% of cases, presinusoidal PH. The natural history of PH in this condition is closely related to the number of eggs deposited in the liver [37, 38].

Sinusoidal obstruction. It occurs in cirrhosis and is characterized by an increase in intrahepatic vascular resistance at the level of the hepatic microcirculation (sinusoids). A secondary event, the increase in portal blood flow (*F*), plays a key role to maintain and worsen the increased portal pressure, giving rise to the hyperdynamic circulation syndrome. In cirrhotic portal hypertension, the measurement of the degree of portal pressure is characterized by an increase of hepatic venous pressure gradient (HVPG), normal free hepatic venous pressure (FHVP) and raised wedge hepatic venous pressure (WHVP) (Table 19.2) [39, 40].

In cirrhosis the pathogenetic mechanisms are based on two main factors: *structural factor* and *dynamic factor*.

The *structural factor* accounts for around 70% of the intrahepatic resistance in cirrhosis; it results from hepatic architectural derangement and is characterized by hepatocyte swelling, hyperplasia, portal tract inflammation and fibrosis in response to liver injury. Besides collagen deposition in the space of Disse may contribute to increased intrahepatic resistance [41]. Although it is not acutely modifiable, disease stabilization (e.g. treatment of chronic viral hepatitis) can improve fibrosis and the mechanical component of PH.

The *dynamic factor*, potentially modifiable, is represented by the active contraction of myofibroblasts and vascular smooth muscle cells of the intrahepatic veins in response to endogenous molecules and pharmacological agents resulting in changes of the intrahepatic vascular resistance. It is an important target for future therapy. Endogenic factors such as endothelin-1 (ET-1), alpha-adrenergic stimulus and angiotensin II can increase the hepatic vascular resistance, while other agents including nitric oxide (NO), prostacyclin and vasodilating drugs (e.g. organic nitrates, adrenolytics, calcium channel blockers) can decrease hepatic vascular resistance [7, 42, 43].

In cirrhosis, an increased production of vasoconstrictors and a deficient release of vasodilators in combination to an exaggerate response to vasoconstrictors and an impaired vasodilatory response of the hepatic vascular bed are the main mechanisms responsible for the increased dynamic component of intrahepatic resistance. A key role is played by two agents, ET-1 and NO. The former is a powerful vasoconstrictor synthesized by sinusoidal endothelial cells, which is implicated in the increased hepatic vascular resistance and in the development of liver fibrosis. The latter is a powerful vasodilator substance that is also synthesized by sinusoidal endothelial cells. In cirrhotic PH the production of NO is decreased whereas that of ET-1 is increased. The result of these changes is an evident vasoconstrictive effect that, in cirrhosis, accounts for approximately 20–30% of the increased intrahepatic resistance [44–46].

Hepatic stellate cells (HSCs) can also influence the dynamic factor leading to an increase of intrahepatic vascular resistance. They are located in the perisinusoidal space of Disse beneath the endothelial barrier. In normal liver, they have the capacity to contract or relax in response to vasoactive mediators such as ET-1 and NO, therefore having a crucial role in controlling intrahepatic vascular resistance and blood flow at sinusoidal level [57]. Following acute or chronic liver injury, HSCs are activated and undergo a process of transdifferentiation leading to a myofibroblastic phenotype. During HSCs activation their production of extracellular matrix changes qualitatively and quantitatively leading to an increase of intravascular resistance [57].

Postsinusoidal obstruction. It comprises different disorders such as the right-sided heart failure, the inferior vena cava obstruction, the small venules Budd-Chiari syndrome and the sinusoidal obstruction syndrome (SOS). Here, the measurement of HVPG shows an elevated WHVP, whereas HVPG and free hepatic venous pressure (FHVP) can be either normal or elevated, depending on the site of obstruction, intrahepatic, postsinusoidal or posthepatic, respectively (Table 19.2) [58–60].

Hepatic sinusoidal obstruction syndrome (SOS), previously known as veno-occlusive disease (VOD), is a distinctive and potentially fatal form of obliterative venulitis of the terminal hepatic venules. It may occur in patients undergoing haematopoietic stem cell transplantation (HSCT) and less commonly following the use of chemotherapeutic agents in non-transplant settings, ingestion of alkaloid toxins, after high-dose radiation therapy or liver transplantation. The clinical presentation includes jaundice, development of right-upper quadrant pain and tender hepatomegaly, ascites and unexplained weight gain. Its incidence in the paediatric HSCT population is between 22 and 28%, with an associated mortality of up to 47% [47, 48]. Endothelial injury seems to be the initiating step in the cascade of events leading to the hepatic changes and clinical manifestation of SOS. The pathologic injury initiates in zone 3 of the liver acinum with subendothelial oedema of hepatic venules, fibrin deposition, microthrombosis, venular narrowing and sclerosis, followed by hepatocyte necrosis [49]. The result is a postsinusoidal increased resistance to hepatic venous outflow resulting in acute PH and, in some cases, multiorgan failure [50–52].

19.3.3 Uncommon Aetiologies of Portal Hypertension

Obliterative portal venopathy (OPV). OPV is a disorder characterized by lesions of the intrahepatic branches of the portal vein that lead to the occlusion or the obliteration of the small portal branches resulting in non-cirrhotic portal hypertension. This disorder has received various denominations including hepatoportal sclerosis, idiopathic portal hypertension, idiopathic non-cirrhotic portal hypertension and non-cirrhotic portal fibrosis that somehow correspond to various stages of the disease. The mainstay of the diagnosis is the histology which is characterized by portal fibrosis, phlebosclerosis or thickened smooth muscle wall of the portal veins, presence of numerous dilated vascular channels in or around the portal tracts, nodular/lobular regenerative activity and sinusoidal dilation [68]. The literature in this setting is poor; therefore the characteristics of this disease and the patients' outcome have not been well characterized. In a study on 48 children diagnosed with OVP, the authors reported that the disease can present at any age in childhood, and presenting features are gastrointestinal (GI) bleeding (9 patients) or the fortuitous finding of an enlarged spleen (21 patients), raised serum alanine aminotransferase activity (6 patients), thrombocytopenia (6 patients), hepatomegaly (3 patients) and abnormal liver on ultrasonography (2 patients) [68]. Despite several factors have been suspected as cause of OVP, including immunological and haematological mechanisms, chemical or drug toxicity, infection and thrombophilia, in most cases no aetiology can be established. A possible genetic cause has been demonstrated by French authors who performed whole exome sequencing in two families including six patients with OPV. In each family they identified a heterozygous mutation in a novel gene located on chromosome 4 that they called FOPV (familial obliterative portal venopathy), possibly inherited in an autosomal dominant fashion with incomplete penetrance [53].

Artero-portal fistula (APF). APF is a rare cause of non-cirrhotic portal hypertension in which there is a communication between the splanchnic arteries and the portal venous system. It can be congenital or acquired as consequence of surgery, trauma, transhepatic intervention or biopsy or ruptured hepatic artery aneurysms. Clinically it may progress silently for many years but at diagnosis is usually life-threatening since long-standing APF can cause an overflow in the portal venous system leading to arterialization of the portal vein, reversal of the portal flow and thickening/narrowing of the extrahepatic portal vein. The haemodynamic consequences are generally the development of arterialised portal hypertension, with severe intestinal bleeding, oesophageal varices and ascites.

If there is evidence of portal hypertension, the closure of the fistula is essential. This may be performed by interventional radiology, which aims to close the arteriovenous fistula and restores a normal portal vein flow, although often the fistulae recur and liver transplantation may become the only therapeutic option [54].

Banti's syndrome. This is a disorder characterized by portal hypertension (varices and portosystemic collateral vessels), splenomegaly and anaemia (hypersplenism) in the absence of haematological and liver disease. It is an eponymous disease as it was first described by Guido Banti, an Italian physician in the year 1898. He described it as a condition characterized by splenomegaly, portal hypertension and anaemia with normal liver histology. No aetiology was found to explain the development of splenomegaly and hypersplenism, leading to consider it as a form of PH due to a primary splenic cause. The actual existence of this condition is still matter of debate [67].

19.4 Clinical Manifestations

Several clinical manifestations are associated with PH in children including gastrointestinal haemorrhage, ascites and splenomegaly with hypersplenism and, in a minority of patients, hepatic encephalopathy, pulmonary vascular disorders and kidney disease [55] (Table 19.3).

19.4.1 Gastrointestinal Haemorrhage (GIH)

Gastrointestinal haemorrhage (GIH), also known as gastrointestinal bleeding, is defined as all forms of bleeding in the gastrointestinal tract. Depending on the site of bleeding, it can be classified as proximal or distal, acute or chronic. Bleeding from the upper digestive tract (oesophagus, stomach and upper portion of the small bowel) causes haematemesis and melena, whereas bleeding from the lower digestive tract (lower portion of the small intestine, large intestine and rectum) causes dark blood or bright red blood mixed with stools, depending on the proximity to the anal sphincter [71].

In children with PH, GH is usually related to bleeding from upper varices (oesophagus and stomach) and, less frequently, from portal hypertensive gastropathy, gastric antral vascular ectasia or gastric, duodenal, peristomal or rectal varices (Fig. 19.3). The size of the varices and their tendency to bleed are directly related to the portal pressure [56].

Acute GIH is often the first symptom of a long-standing silent liver disease (such as portal vein thrombosis), and therefore it is a frightening event for patients and carers, giving the impression of impending death.

Bleeding can be predicted in patients with large varices, associated red signs, presence of gastric varices and portal hypertensive gastropathy. Although the mortality from gastrointestinal bleeding in children is lower than in adults, acute GIH remains a major source of morbidity and life-threatening events and requires prompt medical intervention. Conversely, symptoms as refractory iron-deficiency anaemia and positive faecal occult blood test are a consequence of an underlying chronic GI bleeding that, in absence of large varices, can be managed by oral iron supplementation [71, 72].

Several conditions may potentially contribute to rupture and bleeding from varices including an episode of upper respiratory tract infection, an increased abdominal pressure during coughing or sneezing, the increased cardiac output due to fever, the erosive effect of nonsteroidal anti-inflammatory drugs used to treat the fever as well as gastro-oesophageal reflux which contributes to erosion and rupture of oesophageal varices [57–59].

Haematemesis and melena are the most common presenting symptoms in children with both intrahepatic and extrahepatic PH. The sentinel bleeding episode in children may occur in a wide range of ages, starting as early as 2 months of age [27, 60–63]. The age at the first bleeding episode is related to the

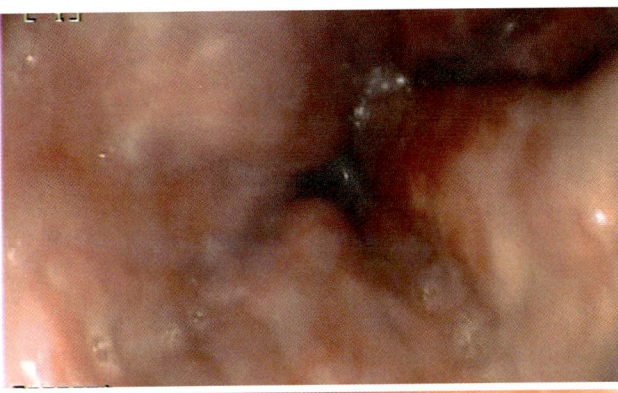
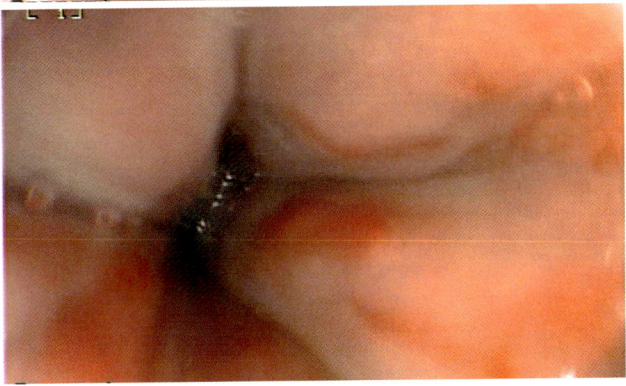

Fig. 19.3 Endoscopic appearance of large oesophageal varices with red signs in two children with portal hypertension. Reprinted with permission from [103]

Table 19.3 Clinical evaluation and investigations useful to recognize patients with suspected portal hypertension

Step	Aim
Clinical history	Ask for neonatal umbilical catheterization, episodes of gastrointestinal bleeding, results of previous blood tests, investigations for an undefined splenomegaly
Physical examination	Assess liver size and consistency, look for splenomegaly, abdominal venous patterning (site and direction of venous flow), spider naevi and telangiectasias, palmar erythema, ascites, limbs oedema
Liver function tests	Assess liver function and full blood count for hypersplenism
Ultrasonography and Doppler of the liver	Evaluate liver parenchyma, patency of portal vein and direction of venous blood flow, hepatic veins patency, venous anatomical abnormalities, hepatic artery (patency and abnormalities), portal-systemic shunts, ascites, splenomegaly, renal abnormalities
Upper endoscopy	Assess varices and hypertensive gastropathy
CT scan of the abdomen	Assess liver parenchyma, biliary tree conformation, vascular anatomy, Rex recessus patency and signs of portal hypertensive biliopathy
Measure portal venous pressure (HVPG, WHVP, FHVP)	Evaluate the degree of portal hypertension. Diagnose prehepatic, intrahepatic, posthepatic causes
Liver biopsy	Assess fibrosis/cirrhosis, inflammation, histological pattern

underlying aetiology. In children with biliary atresia, the first bleed was variably described but most commonly between 1 and 3 years of age, while in children with cystic fibrosis-related PH, it occurred at an average age of 11.5 years [56, 64].

In a study on 225 children with biliary atresia, it was demonstrated that high total serum bilirubin concentration, young age and high number/grade of oesophageal varices at the first endoscopy were significantly related to the emergence of high-risk varices. The probability of the appearance of high-risk signs was higher and these signs appeared faster in infants 12 months of age or younger and when the first endoscopic examination had displayed >1 grade 1 or grade 2 varices [80].

The previous hypothesis that variceal bleeding decreased in adolescence due to the development of spontaneous porto-systemic collaterals is not supported by recent data [81]. In a study carried out in Bergamo on 65 children with extrahepatic portal vein obstruction (EHPVO), 32 (49%) patients presented with bleeding at a median age of 3.8 years and 43 (66%) had at least one bleeding during a median follow-up period of 8.4 years [60]. Similar results were reported by Triger et al. who followed 44 children with EHPVO for a mean follow-up of 8 years [65]. The bleeding rate was 49% at age 16 years and 76% at 24 years of age, but if the child bled before 12 years of age, the probability of bleeding was higher than in those who had not bled before age 12. Furthermore, there was no evidence of variceal regression over time.

Non-selective β-blockers, endoscopic treatment of varices and surgical and radiological procedures represent the main valuable therapeutic options for the management of bleeding in children with PH. They will be discussed in the following session.

19.4.2 Splenomegaly

Splenomegaly indicates an enlargement of the spleen usually associated to a splenic overactivity, defined as hypersplenism, which leads to premature destruction of blood cells.

Splenomegaly is the most common finding in children with PH along with GI bleeding; therefore the association between GI bleeding and splenomegaly should be suggestive of PH until disproven [56].

Splenomegaly is due to PH which causes at the beginning only spleen congestion and eventually tissue hyperplasia and fibrosis.

Usually, an enlarged spleen is first discovered on routine physical examination, and in the clinical practice, an extensive haematological evaluation, including bone marrow biopsies, may be undertaken before portal hypertension is considered. Sometimes splenomegaly due to PH is misdiagnosed as infectious mononucleosis, if the child comes to the medical attention during a viral illness.

The increase in spleen size is commonly followed by an increase in splenic blood flow, which actively participates in PH causing congestion of the portal system [66]. Despite that, splenic size alone does not correlate well with portal pressure. Liver function tests and a Doppler ultrasound are mandatory in healthy children with splenomegaly and hypersplenism to exclude the presence of EHPVO and avoid worthless procedures [56, 67]. Some studies have tried to identify the best non-invasive method to diagnose the presence of oesophageal varices (OV) in children with PH. Platelet count and splenomegaly are usually considered the most reliable parameter to predict the presence of OV. The clinical prediction rule proposed by Gana has high predictive value (area under the ROC curve 0.80) and is calculated according to the following formula: (0.75 × platelets)/ (spleen Z score + 5) + 2.5 × albumin [68].

Different results were reported in a study on 89 children with cirrhosis in which the authors demonstrated that the platelet count (PC) to spleen diameter (SD) ratio was inappropriate for detecting EV in children with cirrhosis [84]. These results demonstrate there are no strong evidences to replace the endoscopic surveillance with non-invasive methods for diagnosing oesophageal varices in children with PH. Table 19.4 shows some scores reported to have a good prognostic values on the presence of oesophageal varices.

Table 19.4 Scores previously reported as predictors of portal hypertension and oesophageal varices

Author	Score name	Patients	End point	Sensitivity (%)	Specificity (%)	AUROC
Park et al.	Risk score [14.2−7.1 × log(10) (platelet) + 4.2 × log (10)(bilirubin)]	61 treatment naïve adults with liver fibrosis	EV	82	86	0.8
Gana et al.	Clinical prediction rule (0.75 × platelets/ SAZ + 5) + (2.5 × albumin)	108 children with intra/extra hepatic PH	EV	81	73	0.8
Gana et al.	Clinical prediction rule (0.75 × platelets/ SAZ + 5) + (2.5 × albumin)	51 children with intra/extra hepatic PH	EV	94	81	0.9
Witters et al.	Kings variceal prediction score (3 × albumin) − (2 × equivalent adult spleen size)	124 children with chronic liver disease	CSV	72	73	0.7
Isted et al.	Variceal prediction score (albumin × platelets/1000)	195 infants with biliary atresia	CSV	78	73	0.8

AUROC area under the receiver operating characteristic curve, *OV* oesophageal varices, *CSV* clinically significant varices, *PH* portal hypertension

Usually, there is no indication for treating an isolated splenomegaly, with or without hypersplenism, unless other complications of PH (ascites and GI bleeding) occur. Once LTX or portosystemic shunting is performed, splenomegaly and hypersplenism may improve significantly, but sometimes they persist for long, depending on the grade of splenic hyperplasia and fibrosis developed over time [69, 70].

19.4.3 Ascites

Ascites describes the condition of pathologic fluid collection within the abdominal cavity. It is usually seen in patients with PH due to cirrhosis, and it is the presenting sign of portal hypertension in 7–21% of children [71]. It appears when the hydrostatic pressure goes above the osmotic pressure within the hepatic and mesenteric capillaries, and the transfer of fluids from blood vessels to lymphatics overcomes the drainage capacity of the lymphatic system [71, 72]. Usually ascites does not occur until the portal-systemic pressure gradient is greater than 12 mmHg and disappears if the gradient falls below 12 mmHg following shunting.

Serum-ascites albumin gradient (SAAG) is more useful than the total protein concentration of ascitic fluid in the classification of ascites into portal hypertensive and nonportal hypertensive aetiologies. This gradient is physiologically based on oncotic-hydrostatic balance and is related directly to portal pressure. The serum-ascites albumin gradient is calculated by subtracting the albumin concentration of ascitic fluid from the albumin concentration of serum obtained on the same day, and the result correlates directly with portal pressure [73]. Under normal circumstances the SAAG is ≤1.1 g/dL because serum oncotic pressure (pulling fluid back into circulation) is exactly compensated by the serum hydrostatic pressure (which pushes fluid out of the circulatory system). In presence of PH, there is an increase in the hydrostatic pressure causing more fluid and more albumin to move from the circulation into the peritoneal space with ascites formation; hence the SAAG increases (≥1.1 g/dL). Therefore, patients with SAAG of 1.1 g/dL or greater have portal hypertension, whereas patients with gradients less than 1.1 g/dL do not (Table 19.5) [73].

Different factors may influence the proper value of the SAAG such as the sampling of ascites and serum in different states of hydration or the impact of serum globulin concentration [74]. Ascites should also be analysed to diagnose an underlying spontaneous bacterial peritonitis (SBP), a bacterial infection in the peritoneum causing peritonitis, despite the absence of an obvious source for the infection. The diagnosis is made by ascitic fluid cell count: the absolute polymorphonuclear cell (PMN) count in the ascitic fluid is calculated by multiplying the total white blood cell count (or total 'nucleated cell' count) by the percentage of PMNs in the differential. SBP is diagnosed by an elevated ascitic fluid absolute PMN count (≥250 cells/mm^3), a positive ascitic fluid bacterial culture and absence of secondary causes of peritonitis [75].

Table 19.5 Causes of ascites based on serum-ascites albumin gradient (SAAG)

SAAG ≥ 1.1 g/dL = portal hypertension	SAAG ≤ 1.1 g/dL = other causes of ascites
Cirrhosis	Peritoneal lymphoma
Non-cirrhotic liver disease	Serositis
Fulminant hepatic failure	Chronic peritoneal infection
	Tuberculosis
	Other (bacteria, viruses, fungi)
Vascular/heart disease	Low serum colloid osmotic pressure
Portal vein thrombosis	Nephrotic syndrome
Veno-occlusive disease	Protein-losing gastroenteropathy
Budd-Chiari syndrome	Kwashiorkor
IVC obstruction/right heart failure	Hollow organ leak
Benign and malignant neoplasms	Lymphatic
Myxoedema	Other (pancreatic, biliary, intestinal)

IVC inferior vena cava, *TBC* tuberculosis

Patients with SBP should receive antibiotic therapy, such as intravenous third-generation cephalosporin, and be considered for liver transplantation. The duration of therapy, according to the guidelines in adults, should be a minimum of 5 days [76].

The first-line treatment of uncomplicated ascites is a moderate sodium-restricted diet combined with diuretic treatment. Spironolactone is the first-line diuretic of choice, as it is an aldosterone antagonist [77].

Large-volume paracentesis (LVP) for treatment of refractory ascites is fast and effective, but it may result in impaired circulatory function, named paracentesis-induced circulatory dysfunction (PICD), associated with a disruption in the renin-angiotensin axis and a hyperdynamic state [77, 78]. Albumin infusion may prevent this complication as demonstrated in a study on 32 children with severe ascites due to liver disease in whom the authors reported that LVP was safe in all age groups but best performed under albumin infusion to overcome the problems related to PICD and hyponatremia [79].

When ascites does not recede, a more aggressive treatment includes transjugular intrahepatic portosystemic shunt (TIPS), a radiological procedure which has been proved as effective also in children [70].

Liver transplantation is indicated when ascites is accompanied by impaired liver function or severe cholestasis. The presence of ascites along with hyponatremia in children with end-stage liver disease is considered a risk factor for severe complications and death as demonstrated in a study of 520 children with cirrhosis. The authors demonstrated the presence of ascites and serum sodium levels were associated with decreased patient survival while awaiting a liver graft [80].

Chylous ascites (CA) refers to the accumulation of lipid-rich lymph in the peritoneal cavity due to disruption of the lymphatic system secondary to traumatic injury or obstruction. Abdominal malignancy, cirrhosis and tuberculosis are the most common causes of CA in adults, the latter being most prevalent in developing countries, whereas congenital abnormalities of the lymphatic system and trauma are the most common causes in children. Chylous ascites can present also in patients with PH due to portal vein thrombosis or congenital portal venous malformation. In this setting, in spite of the absence of strong evidences, the management includes high-protein and low-fat diets supplemented with medium-chain triglycerides, therapeutic paracentesis if indicated, total parenteral nutrition and somatostatins [81].

19.4.4 Pulmonary Complications

Hepatopulmonary syndrome (HPS) and portopulmonary hypertension (PPH) are two distinct pulmonary vascular complications of hepatic and extrahepatic portal hypertension. The proposed theories suggest that these disorders result from a combination of portosystemic shunting, the hyperdynamic circulation, the increased cardiac output, the sheer injury to the pulmonary vascular walls and an imbalance of circulating vasoactive peptides. It is assumed that peptides such as EN-1, cytokines and neurohormones may reach the pulmonary vascular bed via portosystemic shunting and may alter the vessel tone leading to arteriovenous shunting in HPS and to increased pulmonary vascular resistance in PPH [82–84].

Hepatopulmonary syndrome (HPS). HPS is defined as dilated pulmonary capillaries and precapillary arteriovenous malformations resulting in intrapulmonary vascular shunting (IPVS), ventilation-perfusion mismatching and chronic hypoxemia in the setting of liver disease or portal hypertension [84].

The combined effect of reduced erythrocyte transit time associated with the hyperdynamic circulatory state typical of patients with liver disease and incomplete diffusion of oxygen to erythrocytes traversing through IPVS are thought to be important factors for the development of ventilation-perfusion mismatch and hypoxemia in patients with HPS. It is likely that vasoactive substances such as NO and EN-1 are involved in the development of HPS [85–87]. However, the current understanding of the pathophysiology of HPS remains incomplete and represents an active area of investigation.

HPS has been described not only in patients with liver disease but also in those with congenital portosystemic shunting (PSS) (i.e. the Abernethy malformation) suggesting a key role of the vascular shunts in the pathogenesis of the HPS, even in absence of PH. The main clinical symptoms are shortness of breath, exercise intolerance and digital clubbing. Since these symptoms are often mild at onset, the disease may be overlooked in the early stage and become overt only when advanced. Transcutaneous oxygen saturation is a simple and valuable tool to screen the patients for HPS; if it is <96%, further investigations are required to evaluate the real presence of IPVS.

The two main procedures to confirm the presence of IPVS and diagnose HPS are the echocardiography with agitated saline (bubble test) and the macroaggregated albumin scan. The former is simple and sensitive both in symptomatic and in asymptomatic children but it requires an expert operator. The latter may be used to quantify the degree of shunting, which can be useful in clinical decision-making and to test the progression of HPS over time [88–90]. Medical management of HPS is supportive, as there are no proven medical therapies. Liver transplantation is the only effective option for treating children with advanced HPS. Al-Hussaini et al. reported a study on 18 children with HPS over 14 years. Fourteen underwent LTX with resolution of HPS in 13, 6 patients developed vascular or biliary complications and 4 died (2 before transplantation) [91].

Portopulmonary hypertension (PPH). PPH is defined as pulmonary artery hypertension with an elevated mean pulmonary artery pressure and increased vascular resistance caused by an arteriopathy in the setting of portal hypertension and in the absence of underlying cardiopulmonary disease [90]. The prevalence in childhood liver disease can be estimated to be <1% both in children with end-stage liver disease awaiting liver transplantation and in the group of children with portal hypertension, corresponding to <5% and < 2% reported in adults, respectively [92, 93].

The pathophysiology of this disorder is still unclear although it seems to be related to a decreased hepatic clearance and portosystemic shunting of biochemical mediators in the setting of liver dysfunction and PH. The result is that of a progressive remodelling of the wall of the small pulmonary arteries with vasoconstriction and thickening of the arterial wall resulting in a histopathological pattern of plexogenic arteriopathy. Dyspnoea, fatigue, palpitations and syncope or chest pain are the most common symptoms at presentation. However, these symptoms are often subtle and therefore a high index of suspicion is required to diagnose PPH in asymptomatic patients before they develop severe and irreversible pulmonary hypertension [92, 93].

The physical examination in advanced PPH mimics other forms of pulmonary artery hypertension and can include an accentuated and split second heart sound, right ventricular heave, right-sided S3 gallop, jugular venous distention, ascites and declivous oedema.

The most useful screening modality in patients with suspected pulmonary hypertension is the echocardiography with Doppler flow analysis. Chest X-ray and ECG definitely lack sensitivity, while the high-resolution computed tomography of the chest and ventilation-perfusion lung scanning are helpful to exclude other pulmonary diseases [89]. The right heart catheter study is the goal standard for diagnosing and staging PPH as mild, moderate and severe if the mean pulmonary artery pressure is 25–35, 35–45 or ≥45 mmHg, respectively. PPH can be treated with LTX successfully if the diagnosis is made early and the pulmonary vasculopathy is reversible. Conversely, if PPH is advanced (with a mean pulmonary pressure >40 mmHg) and associated with right-sided heart failure, LT becomes very risky because of the functionally obstructed liver outflow that leads to graft failure and death in at least 50% of cases. Recent studies demonstrated that perioperative use of inhaled and intravenous pulmonary vasodilators (nitric oxide and epoprostenol) as well as oral drugs (sildenafil and bosentan) can remarkably reduce the pulmonary pressure to a safe level, allowing to perform LT [94]. However, if there is no response or the pressures remain very high, the only viable option is a combined lung-liver transplant.

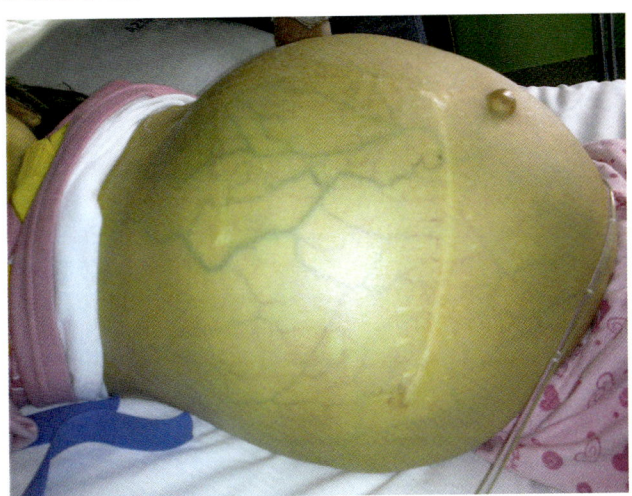

Fig. 19.4 Tense ascites and abdominal venous patterning in a child with biliary atresia, failed Kasai and end-stage liver disease

19.4.5 Other Major Complications of Portal Hypertension

Cutaneous vascular patterns. Prominent vascular markings on the abdomen are the result of porto-collateral shunting through subcutaneous vessels (Fig. 19.4). This is the result of the attempt at decompressing the portal venous system. Decompression through the umbilical vein results in prominent periumbilical collaterals, referred to as *caput medusae*. An audible venous hum (Cruveilhier-Baumgarten murmur) may occasionally be heard. Caput medusae is rare in children, partly because of the high prevalence of portal vein obstruction associated with umbilical vein obliteration. However, both umbilical venous shunts and rectal varices can be observed in children with long-standing PH, whereas in children with PH and an intestinal stoma (i.e. in short bowel syndrome associated with liver disease), stomal varices often occur and represent a site of low resistance and bleeding [95].

Hepatorenal syndrome (HRS). HRS is defined as a syndrome that occurs in patients with advanced liver disease, characterized by impaired renal function and marked abnormalities in the arterial circulation and overactivity of the endogenous vasoactive systems with associated vascular changes [96].

HRS results from a tentative to compensate the characteristic circulatory imbalance of advanced cirrhosis. Hence, in the kidney, there is marked renal vasoconstriction that results in a low GFR, while in the extrarenal circulation, there is a predominance of arterial vasodilation that results in the reduction of systemic vascular resistance and arterial hypotension. The small volume of the produced ultrafiltrate is then reabsorbed almost completely in the proximal tubule whereas no solutes (such as sodium) flow to the Henle's loop with nearly no hyperosmolar natriuresis, activation of adiuretin-vasopressin and reduced urine output. As a result, standard diuretic treatment may have little effect on diuresis [96].

The criteria for HRS proposed by American Association of the Study of the Liver (AASLD) include (1) cirrhosis with ascites, (2) serum creatinine greater than 1.5 mg/dL (132 mmol/L), (3) no improvement in serum creatinine after at least 2 days of diuretic withdrawal and volume expansion with albumin, (4) absence of shock, (5) no current or recent treatment with nephrotoxic drugs and (6) absence of parenchymal kidney disease [97]. The diagnostic criteria mentioned above are difficult to be applied in young children because of the lack of paediatric data. In fact, in children HRS is rare, probably due to the relatively short time that cirrhotic children spend on the transplantation waiting list.

HRS can be classified in type 1 and 2. Type 1 HRS is an acute and rapidly progressive form that often develops after a precipitating factor such as gastrointestinal bleeding or spontaneous bacterial peritonitis. Type 2 HRS is a slowly progressive form of renal failure that often occurs without a sudden trigger in the setting of chronic and refractory ascites.

HRS is a potentially reversible condition, but its natural prognosis is poor. Regarding the medical treatment, all diuretics should be stopped in patients on diagnosis, but furosemide may be used for maintaining urine output and treating volume overload. Various vasoconstrictors are useful in the treatment of HRS, and terlipressin is the first choice [98].

Hepatic encephalopathy (HE). HE refers to a variety of serious but often reversible neurologic abnormalities that arise when the liver cannot detoxify the portal venous blood in patients with cirrhosis and PH associated with anatomical and functional portosystemic shunting [99, 100].

In children, HE can be subtle and the condition seems to appear at a later stage of liver disease and be difficult to diagnose, especially in ill infants [101]. Various neurotoxins (especially ammonia) and inflammatory mediators have significant roles in its pathogenesis, inducing low-grade brain oedema, and producing a wide range of neuropsychiatric manifestations including disturbed consciousness (including coma), personality changes, intellectual deterioration and speech and motor dysfunction are common in older children with HE. The sudden onset and rapid reversibility of encephalopathy in liver disease suggest that it has a metabolic origin [99]. The most effective options for treating HE include protein diet restriction, cleansing enemas, oral antibiotic and lactulose [100, 102].

19.4.6 Non-cirrhotic Portal Hypertension

NCPH is a heterogeneous group of liver disorders of probable vascular origin, leading to PH in absence of cirrhosis [103]. Unlike cirrhotic PH, in the NCPH, HVPG is normal or only mildly elevated [104]. It can be classified as prehepatic, hepatic and posthepatic. Hepatic causes are further subdivided into presinusoidal, sinusoidal and postsinusoidal. The most common causes of NCPH are presinusoidal disorders such as non-cirrhotic portal fibrosis (NCPF) and extrahepatic portal vein obstruction (EHPVO).

Both entities present with clinically significant PH but with preserved liver functions [104]. Different theories have been proposed to explain the pathogenesis of this disorder. Recently, the so-called unifying hypothesis proposes infection/inflammation as a precipitating event in an individual with a prothrombotic status, in both EHPVO and NCPF. It is postulated that a major thrombotic event, occurring at young age, involves the main portal vein and causes EHPVO, while repeated microthrombotic events during adolescence involving medium and small branches of portal vein lead to NCPF [105]. In this session, we will focus on such two disorders.

19.4.7 Non-cirrhotic Portal Fibrosis (NCPF)

Non-cirrhotic portal fibrosis (NCPF) is a disorder of presinusoidal portal hypertension clinically characterized by features of PH, variously described in literature as idiopathic portal hypertension (IPH), hepatoportal sclerosis or obliterative venopathy [106, 107].

The term NCPF was used first by Basu et al. in 1967 and subsequently was endorsed by the Indian Council of Medical Research [108]. The disease has been reported from all parts of the world, more so from the developing countries. Differences in socioeconomic status, living conditions, average lifespan and ethnic background may be responsible for the higher occurrence in lower socioeconomic classes, though this is probably related to poor sanitation and hygiene and poor access to healthcare. NCPF is considered a very rare disorder in young children while it has been described mainly in young adults or middle-aged women. However, since the awareness among paediatric specialists is still low, this condition is probably underdiagnosed, especially in the western countries.

The precise etiopathogenesis of NCPF is an area of ongoing research and different theories have been postulated. The infection theory assumes that an intra-abdominal infection and infections affecting any of the portal vein-drained organs may result in septic embolization to the liver, portal pyaemia or pylephlebitis causing perivenular sclerosis or thrombosis, resulting in relative obstruction of small- and medium-sized portal venous radicles. Rarity of the disease in the west, a declining trend with improved standards of living and hygienic conditions, supports the role of infections of imprecise nature at an early age in the disease pathogenesis [109]. The role of prothrombotic disorders in the pathogenesis is supported by autopsy studies showing high prevalence of PV thrombosis (PVT) and studies from the west indicating association with prothrombotic states. There is also an immunological theory which is based on numerous immunological abnormalities seen in patients with NCPF including an increased incidence of upregulation of vascular cell adhesion molecule-1 (VCAM-1); an increased concentration of ET-1 in periportal hepatocytes, portal venules and hepatic sinusoids of patients with IPH; and increased connective tissue growth factor (CTGF) promoting fibrosis and phlebosclerosis.

Chronic exposure to inorganic arsenic, vinyl chloride polymers or to copper sulphate in vineyard sprayers have been widely investigated and thought as probable factors inducing the development of NCPF. Moreover, endotoxin-mediated liver injury and xenobiotic exposure, with or without induced autoimmunity, represent further etiopathogenetic factors involved in the development of NCPF [110].

The clinical pattern of presentation of NCPF is that of PH in the absence of an evident cause, such as liver fibrosis/cirrhosis or vascular obstruction. The most common presentations include episodes of variceal bleed, long-standing splenomegaly and anaemia.

On clinical examination, the liver may be normal, enlarged or slightly shrunken. Splenomegaly is common while peripheral stigmata of chronic liver disease are absent [111]. Liver biopsy features include phlebosclerosis, fibroelastosis, periportal and perisinusoidal fibrosis, aberrant vessels in portal tract (portal angiomatosis) with preserved lobular architecture and differential atrophy. The main portal vein branch is dilated, with thick sclerosed walls, along with thrombosis in the medium and small PV branches, giving a picture of 'obliterative portal venopathy' [106, 112]. However in children these features are often subtle and the condition may be overlooked [108].

Management in both NCPF/IPH is primarily focused on prevention and treatment of an acute episode of variceal bleeding. The prognosis of NCPF in paediatric age group is favourable as well as in adult population. Management primarily involves prevention (primary or secondary) and acute treatment of variceal bleeding [113, 114].

Poddar published the experience on 388 Indian children with PH (median age 11 years). Eleven of them (3%) were diagnosed with NCPF. Variceal bleeding, splenomegaly and a lump in the left upper abdomen were the most common symptoms at onset [115]. In a recent Indian study, the author described 19 patients diagnosed with NCPF with median age at onset of symptoms and diagnosis of 10 years and 13.8 years, respectively. Majority presented with left upper quadrant discomfort or mass. Laboratory parameters showed hypersplenism in majority with preserved liver synthetic functions. During follow-up, majority of the patients did not show disease progression. The authors concluded that NCPF was not an uncommon entity in paediatric population with age of onset in early second decade suggesting any patient presenting with evidence of portal hypertension with preserved hepatic functions, irrespective of the age, should be evaluated for possible NCPF [107, 116].

19.4.8 Extrahepatic Portal Vein Obstruction (EHPVO)

Extrahepatic portal vein obstruction (EHPVO) is defined by the obstruction of the extrahepatic portal vein with or without the involvement of the intrahepatic portal veins and does not include isolated thrombosis of the splenic vein. It may include occlusion of the splenic, superior mesenteric and coronary veins but excludes the isolated thrombosis of the splenic vein. It is the most common cause of non-cirrhotic, presinusoidal and prehepatic PH in children [55]. Up to 70% of children with EHPVO initially present to medical services with upper gastrointestinal haemorrhage, which mostly occurs before 10 years of age [117].

The term EHPVO implies chronicity and refers primarily to a long-standing condition that usually does not progress to end-stage liver disease and has no indication for liver transplantation. As a consequence, the EHPVO comprises the group of paediatric patients in which there is the largest experience with long-term complications and care of PH [61, 118].

The precise aetiology of the development of EHPVO in the majority of these children is unknown, but various factors including umbilical vascular catheterization, sepsis and an underlying hypercoagulable states (or thrombophilia) play a key role in the pathogenesis of the thrombus formation. Therefore, a full hypercoagulability panel including genetic factors has to be performed whenever the diagnosis is made [27].

Neonatal disorders may play an important role in determining the development of EHPVO. In a multicentre Italian study on 187 children with EHPVO, the mean age at diagnosis was 4 years, and the most common symptoms at onset were splenomegaly (39.5%) and bleeding (36.6%). The authors demonstrated that the development of EHPVO was strictly associated with a neonatal disorder including history of prematurity, neonatal illness and umbilical venous catheter. Thus, they suggested to perform a liver Doppler ultrasound before discharge from the neonatal unit and at the follow-up to allow an early recognition of the disease and avoid bleeding from oesophageal varices that are present from the early stages (personal, unpublished data).

Pathogenetic mechanisms which lead to PH are mainly related to the increased vascular resistance in the portal venous system due to thrombus formation. Portal vein obstruction is usually well tolerated, and patients are often asymptomatic, but two important mechanisms can play an important role in portal venous obstruction: the arterial vasodilation or arterial rescue, which can preserve the liver function in acute settings, and the formation of the portal cavernoma, which represents a tentative to bypass thrombus and replace a physiological portal venous flow. This process of neovascularization or neoangiogenesis takes around 4–6 weeks; the cavernoma is usually located at the hilum of the liver and can extend for a variable length inside and outside the liver.

Studies on adults demonstrated an increase in the cardiac index and a decrease in the total peripheral resistance in patients with EHPVO compared to control patients; other studies also reported the presence of alterations in the systemic and pulmonary vascular systems [61, 119, 120]. The results from these studies showed that EHPVO patients had similar hyperdynamic circulation manifested by high cardiac index and low systemic and pulmonary vascular resistance indices compared to cirrhotic patients suggesting a predominant role of portal hypertension per se in the genesis of systemic and pulmonary haemodynamic alterations [118, 121–124]. There are no studies evaluating the presence of a hyperdynamic circulation in children with EHPVO because the radiological procedures to assess haemodynamic changes (i.e. HVPG) are considered too invasive and are not routinely performed in children except in selected cases [125]. However, from the clinical point of view, children with EHPVO usually do not manifest symptoms in keeping with the hyperdynamic circulation nor its major complications including high cardiac output, hepatorenal syndrome and spontaneous bacterial peritonitis.

The common presentations in infancy are variceal bleeding, ascites and growth failure. Later in childhood and early adult life, variceal bleeding, growth retardation and hypersplenism are the main presenting clinical problems. Ascites is quite rare, more common in adults than in children. On physical examination the liver is normal or shrunken. Liver function tests are usually normal, at least in the early phases, whereas thy can be deranged in the long term [126]. An increase in gamma-glutamyl transpeptidase, total bilirubin and bile salts levels should raise the suspicion of the development of portal hypertensive biliopathy [127–129]. The diagnosis is based on radiological investigations (Doppler ultrasound, CT scan or nuclear magnetic resonance) aiming to demonstrate portal vein obstruction or portal vein cavernoma [55, 130].

HVPG, when performed, shows wedged hepatic venous pressure within normal limits and intrasplenic pressure significantly elevated, indicating the presinusoidal nature of portal hypertension in EHPVO patients. There is no indication to perform liver biopsy except when an underlying chronic liver disease is suspected, but if performed, a picture similar to what described in NCPF can be found. Anticoagulation therapy is not indicated outside of the acute phase, unless a hypercoagulable state has been documented [3]. The management is mainly direct to prevent the episodes of GI bleeding from rupture of upper varices. The patients may be asymptomatic for many years and the mortality from bleeding appeared to be negligible in this group of patients [131, 132]. However morbidity is very high, including complications such as variceal bleeding, growth retardation, portal hypertensive biliopathy and hepatic encephalopathy.

Growth retardation. Stunting and wasting is present in 37–54% and 31–57% of children with EHPVO, respectively (Fig. 19.5). Growth depends on duration of PH and declines further on follow-up despite appropriate energy intake. The pathogenetic mechanism is not well understood, but many factors seem to play an important role in determining growth failure in this setting including the reduced portal blood supply to the liver and the consequent deprivation of hepatotropic factors, the poor substrate utilization associated with the malabsorption due to portal hypertensive enteropathy as well as growth hormone resistance. Restoration of portal blood flow to the liver that follows a successful meso-portal bypass results in improved growth in these patients [133–135].

Portal hypertensive biliopathy (PHB). PHB is a complication characterized by cholestasis and liver dysfunction with elevated serum bilirubin and aminotransferases which may

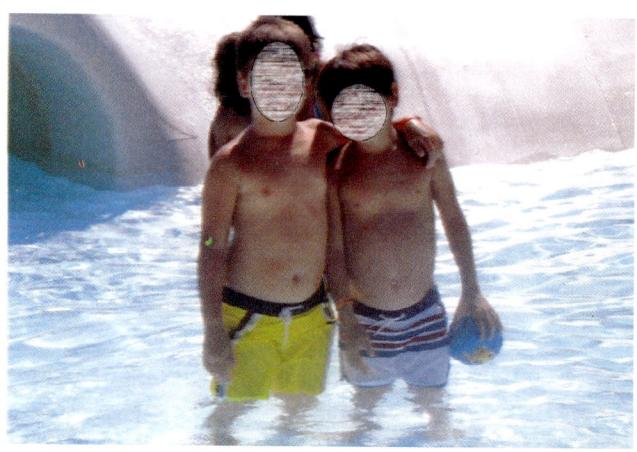

Fig. 19.5 Twins; one with portal vein thrombosis has growth retardation

occur in children with portal vein thrombosis as a result of external compression of bile ducts by cavernous transformation of the portal vein. The pathogenesis is mainly related to long-standing portal cavernoma in the biliary and peribiliary region, causing compressive and ischemic changes of the biliary tree, and more frequently in the left hepatic duct [128].

Major anatomical and functional abnormalities of the intrahepatic, extrahepatic and pancreatic ducts include intrahepatic biliary radicles dilation, indentations, calibre irregularities, displacements, angulations, ectasias, strictures, common bile duct stones, filling defects, compressions, gallbladder and pericholedochal varices or mass [127]. Patients with EHPVO occurring in infancy almost invariably develop radiological evidence of PHB as young adults; nevertheless only 20–30% develop clinical signs of cholestasis [136]. When symptomatic, PHB presents with jaundice, biliary colic, abdominal pain and recurrent cholangitis. Magnetic resonance cholangiopancreatography (MRCP) is the first choice tool to diagnose PHB in children [137]. ERCP is the diagnostic gold standard but, being invasive, is indicated in symptomatic cases requiring endotherapy. MRCP with portography has equal efficacy and is also helpful in differentiating choledochal varices from stones. Natural history of biliopathy is ill-defined and varies from asymptomatic state to development of various sequelae like choledocholithiasis, cholangitis and secondary biliary cirrhosis. The decision to treat biliary obstruction in these patients depends on the presence of symptoms. In asymptomatic patients, no intervention is recommended. In symptomatic children biliary stenting (by endoscopic retrograde cholangiopancreatography or percutaneous transhepatic cholangiography) may temporarily improve the symptoms restoring a normal bile flow. Nevertheless some patients may require shunt surgery to decompress the biliary varices and resolve the obstruction [136].

Minimal hepatic encephalopathy (MHE). MHE is a brain dysfunction caused by liver insufficiency and/or portosystemic shunting. The term 'minimal hepatic encephalopathy' has been used to describe a subset of patients with the mildest form of encephalopathy, not detected on clinical examination, but detected on psychometric testing or electrophysiological techniques [102]. It manifests as a wide spectrum of neurological/psychiatric abnormalities ranging from subclinical alterations to coma. In particular, MHE would compromise attention, processing speed and psychomotor performance, in some cases affecting the academic performance of the patients. It has been reported in about one-third of children with EHPVO and normal liver function [101, 138, 139]. The diagnosis is made by psychometric tests, critical flicker frequency and MR spectroscopy [140]. Hyperammonemia seems to play a key role in the pathogenesis of this complication [141]. The literature in this setting is limited, but this disorder is likely underestimated. MHE seems solved by restoring blood flow to the liver by the meso-portal bypass (MPB), while surgical portosystemic shunts may eventually worsen it [102, 138]. In a recent prospective study carried out on 30 patients with EHPVO, the prevalence of MHE among children with EHPVO was 20% (6/30). After randomization to treatment and no-treatment groups using lactulose, all tests were repeated after 3 months. Results showed an improvement on psychometric tests in 75% of the patients after treatment with lactulose [142]. Further studies need to best understand prevalence and characteristics of this disorder in children with EHVPO.

Management of EHPVO. It is primarily direct to treatment of PH complications. First-line treatment usually includes endoscopic procedures and NSBB. However, there are no prospective studies which provided evidences on efficacy of non-selective beta blockers (NSBBs), endoscopic varices obliteration (EVO) and different types of surgical operations in children [55]. Therefore, in absence of standardized guidelines, the management of EHPVO needs to be individualized case by case [143, 144].

The consensus opinion of the panel at the Baveno VI Pediatric Satellite reported that, in light of the morbidity associated with EHPVO and the physiologic responses to MPB, MPB should be considered as the primary approach in children with EHPVO who have evidence of a cavernoma, especially if there have been any clinical complications of EHPVO [145]. In a retrospective study we reviewed 65 children with EHPVO (median age at diagnosis 3.5 years) and proposed a stepwise approach to manage such a cohort of patients. After retrograde portogram, MPB resulted feasible only in 44% of cases. Patients in whom medical and endoscopic treatment failed in controlling large varices were treated by surgery including MPB in 13 (38.2%) patients, proximal splenorenal shunt in 13 (38.2%), meso-caval shunt in 3 (8.8%), distal splenorenal shunt in 2 (5.9%), and by transjugular intrahepatic portosystemic shunt (TIPS) in 2 (5.9%); LTX was performed in case 1 (3%) because of hepatopulmonary syndrome. Such a stepwise approach, comprising of medical, endoscopic and surgical options, provided excellent survival and bleeding control in more than 90% of patients [117]. A lively debate is still ongoing as to whether MPB should be considered as a pre-emptive technique or as a second line option after failure of medical and endoscopic management [146, 147]. However, it seems reasonable to consider MPB to restore the normal liver flow to in the early phase of the disease, whenever possible [60, 148].

19.5 Diagnosis

In patients with PH, all investigations should aim at identifying the liver disease responsible of PH and quantify the degree and severity of PH and its complications. Information on prematurity, neonatal jaundice, umbilical catheterization and organ malformations are helpful to give an explanation to signs or symptoms highly suspicious for PH (e.g. history of unexplained splenomegaly). Physical examination is directed to assess liver size and consistency, splenomegaly, abdominal venous pattering (site and direction of venous flow), ascites, skin signs of chronic liver disease (e.g. spider naevi, telangiectasias, palmar erythema), bruises and oedema. Laboratory tests provide information on liver function, blood cell and platelet count and clotting. Radiological and endoscopic procedures are mandatory to diagnose and quantify the degree of PH including abdominal Doppler ultrasound, upper gastrointestinal endoscopy, CT scan of the abdomen, invasive measurements of portal venous pressure and liver biopsy (Table 19.3).

19.5.1 Doppler Ultrasound

Ultrasound is the first-line imaging examination to be performed in patients with suspected portal hypertension, both adults and children. Ultrasound is safe, can be repeated easily, is not expensive and is highly sensitive. It provides information on liver size and texture, patency of portal and hepatic veins, hepatic artery patency and flow pattern (including the resistance index), portal-systemic shunting, ascites, splenomegaly and associated intra-abdominal abnormalities [149]. Colour Doppler and spectral waveform analysis allow haemodynamic assessment of the hepatic vessels and provide rapid information that may not be evident on more complex imaging techniques such as multi-detector (MD) CT or MRI, especially in young children.

On liver ultrasound the echogenicity of the parenchyma may be increased in cirrhosis and in some diseases in which steatosis is a histological feature (i.e. Wilson's disease and α1-antitripsin deficiency) [150]. The liver is usually normal in size in prehepatic PH, while in the other forms (hepatic and posthepatic), it appears enlarged as occurs in children with biliary atresia, ciliopathies, genetic cholestasis or in those with Budd-Chiari syndrome. Besides, liver scan may document the presence of major abnormalities involving the bile ducts and gallbladder (e.g. biliary dilation, the presence of gallstones), whereas small irregularities require more powerful imaging studies to be detected [150].

The colour Doppler technique provides information on blood flow in the portal venous system, the hepatic artery and the hepatic veins, where it is possible to calculate the flow velocity, although it is not possible to estimate pressures [151, 152]. It may show several features suggestive of PH including dilation of the portal venous system, lack of or reduced respiratory variations of splenic and superior mesenteric vein diameter and flow, reduced portal vein velocity, increased congestion index of the portal vein and an altered Doppler pattern in the liver veins. However, only two signs are highly specific of portal hypertension: portosystemic collaterals (e.g. paraumbilical vein, splenorenal collaterals, etc.) and reversal of flow in the portal venous system. The splenic size is easily measured and compared to normal values for age, since the presence of splenomegaly is a major complication related to PH [149]. The assessment of the renal parenchyma may be helpful to exclude the presence of cysts which may suggest an underlying ciliopathy [150]. Bi-dimensional ultrasonography can easily detect and confirm the presence of ascites suspected clinically. Hepatofugal flow towards the left gastric, paraduodenal or paraumbilical veins is a sign of a worsening of PH; also reversal of flow in the superior mesenteric vein or splenic vein may be suggestive of spontaneous mesentericocaval or splenorenal shunts, respectively [153]. The hepatic veins are straight, anechoic and tubular structures that converge towards the inferior vena cava approximately 1 cm below its confluence with the right atrium. The normal hepatic vein waveform is triphasic as result of transmitted cardiac activity [154]. Varices are formed in the lower oesophagus by portosystemic shunting via the left gastric vein through the lesser omentum. As a consequence, the lesser omentum gets thickened in PH [155–157].

Although the 'gold-standard' method for liver fibrosis assessment is liver biopsy, in the last years, non-invasive methods have increasingly been used in adult hepatology. Among ultrasound-elastography methods, transient elastography (TE) has been the first developed to assess liver stiffness. Given that liver fibrosis is the major component of hepatic resistance, and given that hepatic resistance is the major factor leading to portal hypertension in patients with compensated cirrhosis, liver stiffness has been tested as a surrogate of portal pressure in cirrhosis. Interestingly, it was observed that liver stiffness is able to identify clinically significant portal hypertension with a high accuracy (AUC of 0.93 on meta-analysis) [158, 159]. Data on its use in children are still scarce. In a study on 527 children (229 girls, ages 0.1–17.8 [median 6.0] years, including 400 healthy controls), the feasibility rate was 90%, but it decreased to 83% in children younger than 24 months even in ideal conditions and general anaesthesia significantly increased liver stiffness in healthy children [160].

19.5.2 Endoscopy

In children with PH, endoscopy plays an essential role in the management of upper varices which represent one of the major complications related to PH. A large multicentre study has demonstrated that there is good agreement among paediatric endoscopists evaluating and grading varices [161]. The primary aim of endoscopy is that of detecting the eventual presence of gastrointestinal signs suggestive for PH (e.g. upper varices or hypertensive gastropathy) [162]. The secondary aim will be that of treating the oesophageal and gastric varices, if indicated. In children upper GI endoscopies are routinely performed under general anaesthesia, and this represents a limitation because of the invasiveness of the procedure. Despite there is no recommendation to screen for the presence of varices in children, studies from Europe and North America demonstrated that many paediatric hepatologists prefer their patients to undergo endoscopic surveillance to best define and prevent the risk of bleeding from varix rupture [103, 143, 163]. Strategy and technique of endoscopic treatment are reported in the session on 'management of portal hypertension'.

19.5.3 Measurement of Hepatic Venous Pressure Gradient (HVPG)

Portal hypertension means elevated pressure within the portal system, including the portal vein and the tributary veins that drain into it. The pressure within the portal system is not routinely measured unless specific procedures are performed. Such an increased venous pressure may be detected by a direct measurement of the pressure into the portal vein or by the measurement of a portal pressure gradient (PPG) resulting from the difference, in pressure, between the portal vein and the inferior vena cava (IVC). Direct measurement of portal pressure through transhepatic or transvenous catheterization of the portal vein is invasive, inconvenient, associated with high risk of major intraperitoneal bleeding and therefore often clinically impractical. However it is the only effective way for measuring the portal pressure in cases in which the wedged pressure is unreliable, such as presinusoidal portal hypertension [164].

Currently, the most commonly used parameter is the hepatic venous pressure gradient (HVPG), which represents the gradient between pressures in the portal vein and the intra-abdominal portion of the IVC. In particular, HVPG measures the portal pressure gradient (PPG) as the difference between 'wedged' hepatic vein pressure (WHVP) and 'free' hepatic vein pressure (FHVP). The WHVP is measured by occluding the hepatic vein by inflating a balloon at the tip of the catheter; the injection of 5 mL of contrast dye into the vein with the balloon inflated can confirm an adequate occlusion of the hepatic vein. In this way, WHVP reflects the portal vein pressure basing on the concept that when blood flow in a hepatic vein is stopped by a wedged catheter, the proximal static column of blood transmits the pressure from the preceding communicated vascular territory (hepatic sinusoids) to the catheter. WHVP reflects hepatic sinusoidal pressure and not the portal pressure itself [40]. In the normal liver, due to pressure equilibration through interconnected sinusoids, the wedged pressure is slightly lower than the portal pressure, though this difference is clinically insignificant. Conversely, in liver cirrhosis, since the intersinusoidal communications are lost due to fibrosis, septa and nodule formation, the sinusoidal pressure equilibrates with portal pressure, and therefore WHVP gives an accurate estimation of portal pressure. The difference between WHPV and FHPV provides HVPG values (HVPG = WHVP − FHVP). Normal HVPG ranges from 1 to 5 mmHg in adults. Subclinical PH is defined when HVPG ranges from 6 to 9 mmHg, whereas complications of portal hypertension are expected when HVPG is greater than 10 mmHg. An HVPG greater than 20 mmHg correlates with variceal bleeding, rebleeding and increased mortality [165].

Classification of different forms of PH is based on HVPG values.

- Presinusoidal: normal or slightly increased HVPG values, normal or slightly increased wedged hepatic venous pressure (WHVP) and normal free hepatic venous pressure (FHVP).
- Sinusoidal: increase in WHVP with normal FHVP, resulting in high HVPG (cirrhosis is the most common cause).
- Postsinusoidal: HVPG is normal and both WHVP and FHVP are increased, such as in the Budd-Chiari syndrome (Table 19.2).

The HVPG is considered the diagnostic method of choice to measure portal venous pressure, and in adults it is also recognized as a surrogate marker for evaluating therapeutic efficacy and for predicting the outcome in portal hypertension [166–168].

Measurement of HVPG in paediatrics is uncommon. Thus, there are only few published date on HVPG measurements in the paediatric setting [169]. In a recent study, 49 children with liver disease (both acute and chronic) underwent 52 HVPG measurements. Results showed that the procedure was feasible in all patients, with no major complications [170].

19.5.4 Other Investigations

Findings of computed tomographic (CT) scanning with intravenous contrast and magnetic resonance (MR) angiography may support the diagnosis of PH in children. These procedures have the advantage of evaluating the surrounding anatomic structures, both above and below the diaphragm, as well as the liver and the entire portal circulation. Both procedures may provide information on liver parenchyma, presence of focal liver lesions, portal vein and hepatic veins patency, presence of collateral circulation and arteriovenous shunts, as well as presence of ascites and splenic malformation [171].

In the detection of oesophageal varices, CT scanning has a sensitivity of 85% compared to endoscopy. In a study performed in adult patients, magnetic resonance angiography proved more reliable than Doppler ultrasound for evaluating the portal venous system in patients with portal hypertension caused by cirrhosis [172].

19.6 Management

Key Definitions:

- Pre-primary prophylaxis: indicates the prevention of the formation of varices.
- Primary prophylaxis: indicates the prevention of the first bleeding episode.
- Secondary prophylaxis: indicates the prevention of the second bleeding episode.

The role of primary prophylaxis of variceal haemorrhage and the indications for meso-Rex bypass (MPB) in extrahepatic portal vein obstruction (EHPVO) are the two major unresolved issues in the management of PH in children [145, 173]. Despite the absence of data supporting the role of any type of prophylaxis to prevent variceal bleeding in children, many clinicians consider a cirrhotic child with large varices at risk of mortality or severe morbidity from the first bleed and therefore a definite candidate for primary prophylaxis [103]. On the other hand, consensus on indication to perform only secondary prophylaxis (prevention of rebleeding) in cirrhotic children appears to be wide [55].

19.6.1 Non-selective β-Blockers

Non-selective β-blockers (NSBBs) are widely used for managing PH complications in adult population. In this setting the optimal use of NSBBs may be restricted to a 'window' of optimal effectiveness with minimal harm. Propranolol is one of the most common NSBBs used in patients with PH.

These drugs work in two ways: (1) by blocking β1-receptors and reducing cardiac output and (2) by blocking β2-receptors, producing splanchnic vasoconstriction reducing portal flow and in turn reducing portal pressure [174].

Studies in adults have shown that a dose reducing the heart rate by 25% (or the HVPG by 20%) does decrease the bleeding rate in cirrhosis [167]. Conversely, in paediatrics, there are no randomized trials assessing the efficacy of propranolol as prophylaxis of variceal bleeding, and the paediatric experience is based on small case series reports which did not include the measurement of HVPG before and after treatment start. Studies demonstrated that in children the evaluation of heart rate at rest is problematic and the range of drug dosage required to reduce it by 25% is very wide, making achievement of adequate NSBBs dosage impractical and time-consuming [175–177]. Furthermore, paediatric patients with presinusoidal PH have no or very mild features of the hyperdynamic circulation; thus the real benefit from treatment with NSBBs has yet to be demonstrated [124].

Despite these findings, NSBBs are commonly used by paediatric hepatologist as confirmed by a survey on the management of PHT in children with BA, showing that propranolol appears to be safe in children, even at high doses [122, 176, 178].

A panel of experts, at last Baveno conference, confirmed that there are no enough evidences to support the routine use of NSBBs for the primary prophylaxis of oesophageal varices bleeding in infants, children or adolescents with PH. The physiologic impact of NSBBs on the hyperdynamic physiology of children with PHT with or without liver disease as well as on haemodynamic after a bleeding episode is still not known.

Conversely, in children unable or unwilling to be treated with endoscopy, the use of NSBBs may be considered, as secondary prophylaxis, although evidence for appropriate dosing is lacking [145].

Well-designed studies are required to determine the efficacy and safety of NSBBs in children with PHT. Unfortunately, a great difficulty in carrying out trials with NSBBs is that in Europe propranolol is not licensed for use in children.

19.6.2 Endoscopy

There are no standardized guidelines for the management of upper gastrointestinal bleeding in children due to different issues. First of all, in the paediatric population, there are few reports on the prevalence of varices in children with PH, and it is therefore difficult to predict how many children would benefit from endoscopic screening [162]. Secondly, how to grade varices in this setting? Recently, the old classification has been simplified, and the proposed description of small or large varices, with or without red marks, appears to be more practical [58]. Large varices, varices of any size but with red marks and gastric varices are likely at higher risk of bleeding in the short term, but again this has not been proven in children so far [179]. The scoring systems adopted in adults have not been validated in children, but such information is mandatory to determine the effectiveness of prophylaxis of variceal bleeding by either non-selective β-blockers (NSBBs) or endoscopic treatment. Encouraging results have been reported from studies on the interobserver agreement on paediatric varices grading in which the preliminary results suggested that accordance in the recognition of large varices is satisfactory [161]. Third, the usefulness of diagnostic endoscopy and primary prophylaxis of bleeding by endoscopic obliteration is still unproven [55].

Therefore, a panel of expert at last Baveno conference concluded that because of the lack of sufficient evidence, no consensus has been achieved related to surveillance endoscopy or primary prophylaxis of varices in children due to cirrhosis. They strengthened the concept that the indication for primary prophylaxis in children is unclear because mortality from the first bleed appears to be very low and the associated morbidity needs to be better defined, ideally in prospective longitudinal studies. Furthermore, the authors were concerned by the possible adverse neurodevelopmental consequences of repeated general anaesthesia in young children, as required for primary endoscopic prophylaxis.

Nevertheless, they concluded that some social factors have the potential to impact clinical decision-making related to primary prophylaxis including family circumstances, distance from the hospital and easy access to medical care in the event of an episode of bleeding [4].

Still, if in this setting mortality is not a relevant risk, morbidity is. For this reason several centres, including ours, have adopted the policy of performing surveillance endoscopies and primary prophylaxis by banding ligation [103]. In our centre this decision comes from the fact that special attention should be paid to patient and family quality of life, clearly hampered by the fear of a bleed, and to the cost of managing a child bleeding acutely that may be greater than the cost of elective endoscopies and treatments.

Conversely, secondary prophylaxis of oesophageal varices bleeding is recommended both in children with cirrhosis and in those with EHPVO.

Currently variceal band ligation (EVL) has become more popular and has been shown to be superior to sclerotherapy as far as efficacy, safety and degree of standardization are concerned, both in adults and in children [180–182]. However, in small children, in whom the banding devices available on the market cannot be used with small paediatric endoscopes, sclerotherapy remains the only feasible treatment option to manage large varices [182].

A real challenge in this setting is the presence of large gastric varices; evidence for the management of gastric variceal bleeding in children is limited to case reports and uncontrolled case series. Large gastric varices are a threat because they are difficult to obliterate prophylactically and even more so if actively bleeding; in this situation, balloon tamponade is often ineffective and the only option is to perform sclerotherapy with tissue glue (such as *N*-butyl-cyanoacrylate).

Failure to eradicate oesophageal or gastric varices should lead to consideration of an alternative approach such as TIPS, surgical portosystemic shunting and LT.

19.6.3 Management of Acute Variceal Bleeding

The diagnosis of acute variceal bleeding from varix rupture is suspected in presence of haematemesis or melena in a child with an underlying known liver disease and eventually confirmed by emergency endoscopy which shows one of the following signs: active variceal bleeding (blood spurting or oozing from a varix), a white nipple or clot adherent to a varix or the presence of blood in stomach and varices without other potential sources of bleeding.

The treatment goals for acute variceal bleeding aim to correct hypovolaemia, achieve rapid hemostasis and prevent early rebleeding as well as deterioration of liver function.

It is therefore mandatory to monitor vital signs, obtain venous access to perform blood tests (full blood count, international normalized ratio, liver function and electrolytes, C-reactive protein and a blood crossmatch) and start blood volume correction [183]. Stabilizing the patient is the initial focus of management of gastrointestinal haemorrhage. Packed red blood cells (PRC) should be provided with the aim to maintain the haemoglobin >7 g/dL, carefully avoiding a rebound overload of fluids that favour the increase of portal pressure and rebleeding [184]. In patients with coagulopathy from hepatic dysfunction and thrombocytopenia, the administration of vitamin K, fresh frozen plasma, cryoprecipitate and/or platelets can be required to stop the bleeding. Nasogastric tube placement is helpful to confirm the source and to monitor the persistence of active bleeding. Vasoactive drugs, such as octreotide, are effective in stopping bleeding from varices and should be started immediately to bridge the child to endoscopy and continued thereafter for a total of 4–5 days [185]. Proton-pump inhibitor helps to decrease the risk of bleeding from erosions or ulcerations. In adults, it has been proven that infectious complications commonly follow an episode of variceal bleeding in cirrhotic patients [186].

In adults one of the main complications associated with variceal haemorrhage is bacterial infection. Therefore, a short-term antibiotic prophylaxis not only decreases the rate infections but also decreases variceal rebleeding and increases survival. Although in children there is no such evidence so far, it is recommended to monitor them for any sign of infection and, if present, to start antibiotic treatment promptly, especially in cirrhotic children with advanced disease.

After the initial step, the child should be managed according to haemodynamic stability and the control of bleeding. If unstable, the patient should be sent to an intensive care unit, have a central venous catheter placed and monitored for circulating blood volume and preload (Fig. 19.6). Usually

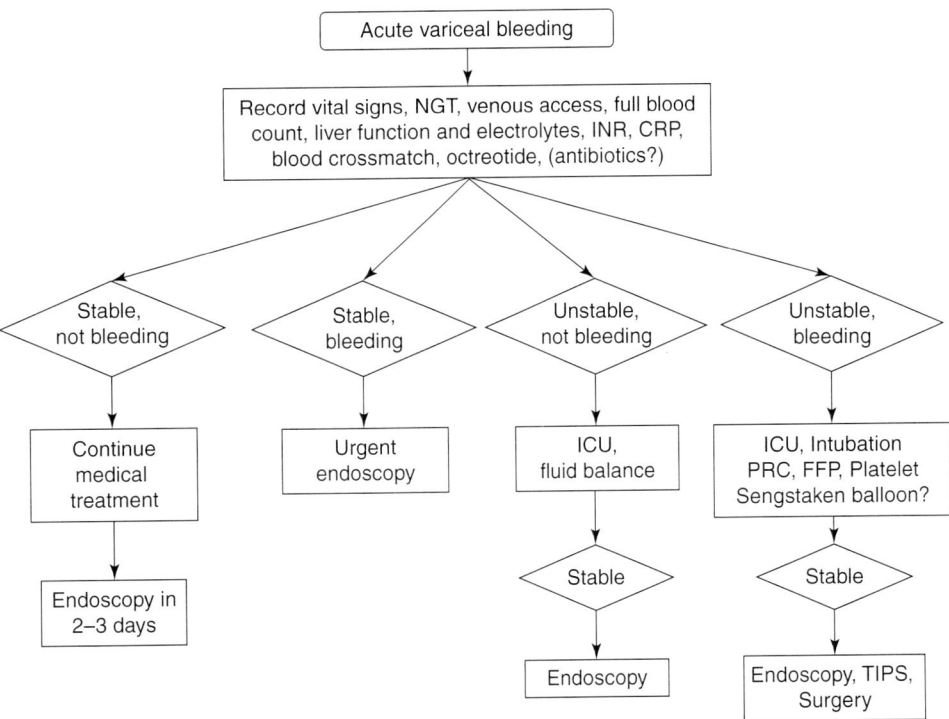

Fig. 19.6 Proposed algorithm for the management of acute variceal bleeding. *NGT* nasogastric tube, *INR* international normalized ratio, *CRP* C-reactive protein, *ICU* intensive care unit, *PRC* packed red cells, *FFP* fresh frozen plasma, *TIPS* transjugular intrahepatic portosystemic shunt

bleeding stops spontaneously after the ruptured varix empties. After cessation, it is usually acceptable to schedule an elective endoscopy in the following 24–72 h because rebleeding is uncommon during this time frame. Performing endoscopy too soon, when the bleeding is active, is disadvantageous, since endoscopic treatment is likely to be jeopardized by the difficult visualization of the bleeding source. However, if bleeding does not stop despite appropriate fluid load and correction of coagulopathy, the child may require urgent endoscopy and, rarely, the placement of a Sengstaken balloon as a bridge to TIPS or urgent shunt surgery (Fig. 19.6). Endoscopic sclerotherapy around the vessel may be the only option to treat an acutely bleeding varix that is underfilled and therefore difficult to be strangulated by a rubber band placed by endoscopic variceal ligation devices.

19.6.4 Surgical Procedures

When medical and endoscopic treatment of bleeding varices fails, an alternative option is to decompress the portal system by a shunt or a bypass [187]. Surgical strategy regarding the type of procedure depends on the underlying liver disease. In children with normal liver function, a surgical shunt or a bypass is advised to manage the complications of PH. In those with EHPVO, the first choice is represented by the meso-portal bypass (MPB) if the Rex recessus is patent [144, 148, 188] (Fig. 19.7).

If it is unfeasible, these patients can be treated by surgical portosystemic shunting or TIPS [189]. Surgical portosystemic shunts are classified as 'selective' or 'non-selective'. Selective shunts divert selectively a region of the abdomen, for example, the stomach and spleen, to decompress oesophagogastric varices. Blood is predominantly shunted into the low-pressure systemic venous circulation, and the varices then flow at a lower pressure with no residual risk of bleeding. Distal splenorenal shunt ('Warren' shunt) is an example of 'selective shunt'; in this procedure, the distal splenic vein is attached to the left renal vein (a part of the systemic venous system). Conversely, the non-selective shunts create a direct communication between the portal system and the systemic circulation, and depending on the flow, a full diversion can be achieved, with a consequent fall in the portal pressure. All these shunts have been associated with a significant risk of hepatic encephalopathy compared with selective shunts. Examples are the 'end-to-side portocaval shunt' or the 'proximal splenorenal shunt' [189, 190].

If the liver function is compromised, as in cirrhotic patients (e.g. children with biliary atresia, intrahepatic cholestasis and Alagille syndrome), surgical shunts are not indicated since the best treatment option is represented by liver transplantation [191]. However, as reported below, TIPS may play a role as a bridge to liver transplantation [70].

19.6.5 Transjugular Intrahepatic Portosystemic Shunt (TIPS)

TIPS is a radiological procedure which consists of placing an intrahepatic portosystemic shunt (between the portal vein and hepatic vein) to decompress the portal venous system (Fig. 19.8) [70].

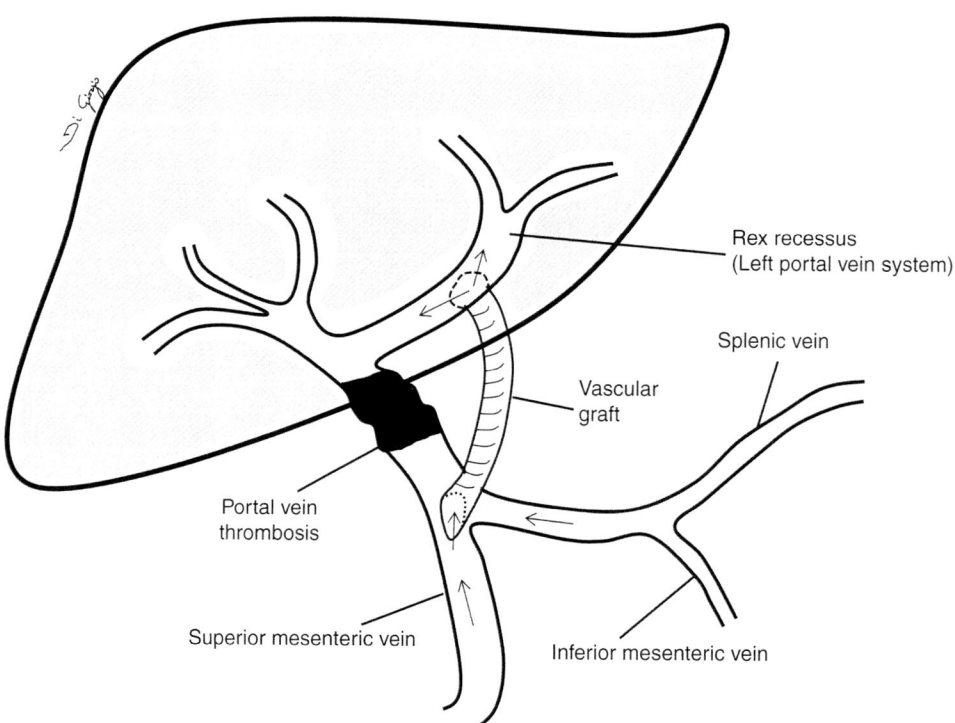

Fig. 19.7 Portal circulation after the operation of meso-portal bypass that re-establishes the hepatopetal flow to the liver

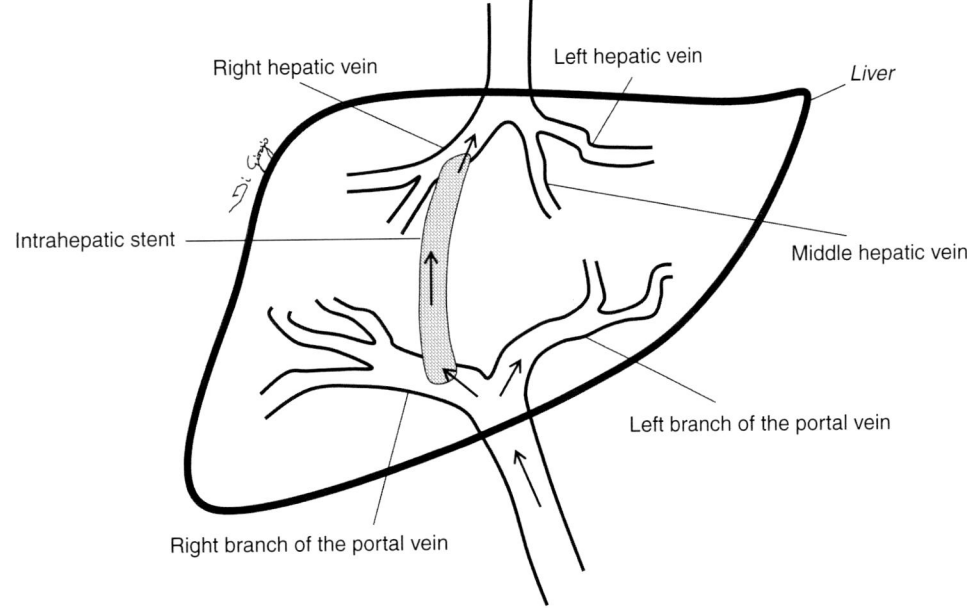

Fig. 19.8 Portal circulation after the placement of transjugular intrahepatic portosystemic shunt

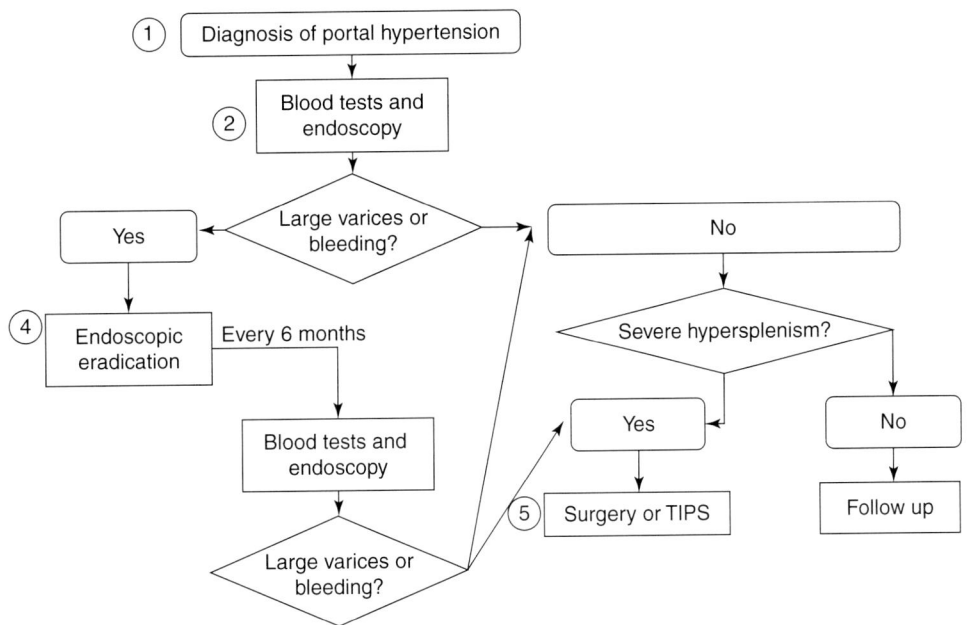

Fig. 19.9 Proposed algorithm for the approach to the child with portal hypertension. *TIPS* transjugular intrahepatic portosystemic shunt. Modified from [103]

TIPS is an extensively utilized procedure to treat PH complications in adults, while in children the experience is limited and the literature is poor. In our institution 24 children (median age 10.2 years [range 2.2–17.4 years], median weight 30.0 kg [11.5–96.0 kg]) affected by cirrhotic and non-cirrhotic PH (both transplanted and not, including 5 patients with EHPVO) unresponsive to NSBBs and endoscopic treatment, and in absence of coagulopathy and jaundice, were considered candidates for TIPS. Indications included persistent ascites in 7 patients and recurrent gastrointestinal bleeding in 16. TIPS was successfully placed in 22/23 (96%) patients. The median PPG before and after TIPS was 18 [12–35] and 8 mmHg [3–12], respectively ($p<0.01$). Complications of PH resolved completely in 18/22 (82%), partially in 3 (14%), persisted in 1 (4%). No patients developed overt encephalopathy. At last follow-up all patients (100%) had a patent TIPS, 9 (41%) had required LT after a median time from TIPS insertion of 0.8 years (range 0.1–4.9 years), 12 still have a patent shunt and 1 (with cystic fibrosis) died from respiratory tract infection. In our experience TIPS insertion was technically feasible in children with both native liver and split liver graft. TIPS was effective to normalize the PPG and control the severe complications of PH both in children with non-cirrhotic PH, as a permanent portosystemic shunt, and in those who may develop a cirrhotic PH, as a bridge to LT [192]. Figure 19.9 reports a possible protocol for the management of children with PH based on the development of oesophageal varices. In our centre NSBBs are not part of the standard management of these patients anymore and are used only when endoscopic treatment cannot solve the bleeding and transplantation is not indicated.

19.7 Implications for Liver Transplantation

The complications of portal hypertension can be managed temporarily by several therapeutic options such as drug therapy, interventional endoscopy, transjugular intrahepatic portosystemic shunt (TIPS) or surgical shunting procedures. Nevertheless there is nearly no patient with PH that can definitely be cured by these options, representing a sort of palliation. In fact, even non-cirrhotic portal hypertension and its complications tend to progress over time. This is particularly relevant if the condition started during the paediatric age.

There is no doubt that liver transplantation (LT) is the treatment of choice for PH in end-stage liver disease and should not be considered a specific treatment for portal hypertension in this setting. Strikingly enough, among children undergoing LT, three-quarters show evidence of PH and one-quarter have suffered a major gastrointestinal (GI) haemorrhage, usually due to rupture of oesophageal varices [69]. Therefore in cirrhotic patients PH plays an important role on timing of listing rather than on the obvious decision to perform LT.

More complex is the situation of children with non-cirrhotic PH, in whom there is no or trivial liver damage, normal synthetic and biliary functions and symptoms purely related to PH (upper intestinal varices, ascites and splenomegaly) [60]. These patients may be managed satisfactorily without LT for a relatively long period of time but may come to for consideration for LT in the very long-term, when extrahepatic complications of PH arise (i.e. hepatic encephalopathy, hepatopulmonary syndrome and portopulmonary syndrome, portal hypertensive biliopathy).

Indication and timing for LT have to be evaluated carefully, considering not only aetiology, severity and activity of underlying liver disease but also comorbidities and possible contraindications. Therefore, while treating the patient conservatively, the optimal time point for placing the patient on the waiting list should not be missed, in particular with regard to increasing waiting time and higher perioperative morbidity and mortality after liver transplantation in advanced liver failure.

Unfortunately, in some cases, LT cannot be performed because of complications of portal hypertension (e.g. severe portopulmonary hypertension) that contraindicate liver transplantation. Although these situations are becoming less and less frequent, prior to listing it is paramount to rule out complications of PH that can jeopardize liver transplantation [191].

References

1. Dooley JS, Lok A, Burroughs AK, Heathcote J. Sherlock's diseases of the liver and biliary system. 12th ed. Oxford: Wiley-Blackwell; 2011. 792 p.
2. Lautt WW. Hepatic circulation: physiology and pathophysiology. San Rafael: Morgan & Claypool; 2009.
3. Shneider B. Approaches to the management of pediatric portal hypertension: results of an informal survey. In: Groszmann RJ, Bosch J, editors. Portal hypertension in the 21st century. Montreal: Springer Netherlands; 2004.
4. Vorobioff J, Bredfeldt JE, Groszmann RJ. Hyperdynamic circulation in portal-hypertensive rat model: a primary factor for maintenance of chronic portal hypertension. Am J Physiol. 1983;244(1):G52–7. Epub 1983/01/01.
5. Orrego H, Blendis LM, Crossley IR, Medline A, Macdonald A, Ritchie S, et al. Correlation of intrahepatic pressure with collagen in the Disse space and hepatomegaly in humans and in the rat. Gastroenterology. 1981;80(3):546–56. Epub 1981/03/01.
6. Reddy SI, Grace ND. Liver imaging. A hepatologist's perspective. Clin Liver Dis. 2002;6(1):297–310, ix. Epub 2002/04/06.
7. Gupta TK, Chen L, Groszmann RJ. Pathophysiology of portal hypertension. Clin Liver Dis. 1997;1(1):1–12. Epub 1997/05/01.
8. Kowalski HJ, Abelmann WH. The cardiac output at rest in Laennec's cirrhosis. J Clin Invest. 1953;32(10):1025–33. Epub 1953/10/01.
9. Groszmann RJ, Vorobioff J, Riley E. Splanchnic hemodynamics in portal-hypertensive rats: measurement with gamma-labeled microspheres. Am J Physiol. 1982;242(2):G156–60. Epub 1982/02/01.
10. Iwakiri Y, Groszmann RJ. The hyperdynamic circulation of chronic liver diseases: from the patient to the molecule. Hepatology. 2006;43(2 Suppl 1):S121–31. Epub 2006/02/01.
11. Groszmann RJ. Hyperdynamic circulation of liver disease 40 years later: pathophysiology and clinical consequences. Hepatology. 1994;20(5):1359–63. Epub 1994/11/01.
12. Vorobioff J, Bredfeldt JE, Groszmann RJ. Increased blood flow through the portal system in cirrhotic rats. Gastroenterology. 1984;87(5):1120–6. Epub 1984/11/01.
13. Colombato LA, Albillos A, Groszmann RJ. Temporal relationship of peripheral vasodilatation, plasma volume expansion and the hyperdynamic circulatory state in portal-hypertensive rats. Hepatology. 1992;15(2):323–8. Epub 1992/02/01.
14. Hadengue A, Lee SS, Koshy A, Girod C, Lebrec D. Regional blood flows by the microsphere method: reproducibility in portal hypertensive rats and influence of a portal vein catheter. Proc Soc Exp Biol Med. 1988;187(4):461–8. Epub 1988/04/01.
15. Genecin P, Polio J, Groszmann RJ. Na restriction blunts expansion of plasma volume and ameliorates hyperdynamic circulation in portal hypertension. Am J Physiol. 1990;259(3 Pt 1):G498–503. Epub 1990/09/01.
16. Morgan JS, Groszmann RJ, Rojkind M, Enriquez R. Hemodynamic mechanisms of emerging portal hypertension caused by schistosomiasis in the hamster. Hepatology. 1990;11(1):98–104. Epub 1990/01/01.
17. Fallon MB. Mechanisms of pulmonary vascular complications of liver disease: hepatopulmonary syndrome. J Clin Gastroenterol. 2005;39(4 Suppl 2):S138–42. Epub 2005/03/11.
18. Katsuta Y, Honma H, Zhang XJ, Ohsuga M, Komeichi H, Shimizu S, et al. Pulmonary blood transit time and impaired arterial oxy-

genation in patients with chronic liver disease. J Gastroenterol. 2005;40(1):57–63. Epub 2005/02/05.
19. Agusti AG, Roca J, Bosch J, Garcia-Pagan JC, Wagner PD, Rodriguez-Roisin R. Effects of propranolol on arterial oxygenation and oxygen transport to tissues in patients with cirrhosis. Am Rev Respir Dis. 1990;142(2):306–10. Epub 1990/08/01.
20. Moller S, Henriksen JH, Bendtsen F. Central and noncentral blood volumes in cirrhosis: relationship to anthropometrics and gender. Am J Physiol Gastrointest Liver Physiol. 2003;284(6):G970–9. Epub 2003/02/28.
21. Shapiro MD, Nicholls KM, Groves BM, Kluge R, Chung HM, Bichet DG, et al. Interrelationship between cardiac output and vascular resistance as determinants of effective arterial blood volume in cirrhotic patients. Kidney Int. 1985;28(2):206–11. Epub 1985/08/01.
22. Schrier RW, Arroyo V, Bernardi M, Epstein M, Henriksen JH, Rodes J. Peripheral arterial vasodilation hypothesis: a proposal for the initiation of renal sodium and water retention in cirrhosis. Hepatology. 1988;8(5):1151–7. Epub 1988/09/01.
23. Moller S, Bendtsen F, Schifter S, Henriksen JH. Relation of calcitonin gene-related peptide to systemic vasodilatation and central hypovolaemia in cirrhosis. Scand J Gastroenterol. 1996;31(9):928–33. Epub 1996/09/01.
24. Chawla Y, Duseja A, Dhiman RK. Review article: the modern management of portal vein thrombosis. Aliment Pharmacol Ther. 2009;30(9):881–94. Epub 2009/08/15.
25. Giouleme O, Theocharidou E. Management of portal hypertension in children with portal vein thrombosis. J Pediatr Gastroenterol Nutr. 2013;57(4):419–25. Epub 2013/07/04.
26. DeLeve LD, Valla DC, Garcia-Tsao G. Vascular disorders of the liver. Hepatology. 2009;49(5):1729–64. Epub 2009/04/29.
27. Webb LJ, Sherlock S. The aetiology, presentation and natural history of extra-hepatic portal venous obstruction. Q J Med. 1979;48(192):627–39. Epub 1979/10/01.
28. de Ville de Goyet J, Alberti D, Clapuyt P, Falchetti D, Rigamonti V, Bax NM, et al. Direct bypassing of extrahepatic portal venous obstruction in children: a new technique for combined hepatic portal revascularization and treatment of extrahepatic portal hypertension. J Pediatr Surg. 1998;33(4):597–601. Epub 1998/05/09.
29. Bambini DA, Superina R, Almond PS, Whitington PF, Alonso E. Experience with the Rex shunt (mesenterico-left portal bypass) in children with extrahepatic portal hypertension. J Pediatr Surg. 2000;35(1):13–8; discussion 8–9. Epub 2000/01/26.
30. Camposilvan S, Milanesi O, Stellin G, Pettenazzo A, Zancan L, D'Antiga L. Liver and cardiac function in the long term after Fontan operation. Ann Thorac Surg. 2008;86(1):177–82. Epub 2008/06/25.
31. Rychik J, Veldtman G, Rand E, Russo P, Rome JJ, Krok K, et al. The precarious state of the liver after a Fontan operation: summary of a multidisciplinary symposium. Pediatr Cardiol. 2012;33(7):1001–12. Epub 2012/04/27.
32. Horton JD, San Miguel FL, Membreno F, Wright F, Paima J, Foster P, et al. Budd-Chiari syndrome: illustrated review of current management. Liver Int. 2008;28(4):455–66. Epub 2008/03/15.
33. Shrestha SM, Okuda K, Uchida T, Maharjan KG, Shrestha S, Joshi BL, et al. Endemicity and clinical picture of liver disease due to obstruction of the hepatic portion of the inferior vena cava in Nepal. J Gastroenterol Hepatol. 1996;11(2):170–9. Epub 1996/02/01.
34. Simson IW. Membranous obstruction of the inferior vena cava and hepatocellular carcinoma in South Africa. Gastroenterology. 1982;82(2):171–8. Epub 1982/02/01.
35. Cauchi JA, Oliff S, Baumann U, Mirza D, Kelly DA, Hewitson J, et al. The Budd-Chiari syndrome in children: the spectrum of management. J Pediatr Surg. 2006;41(11):1919–23. Epub 2006/11/15.
36. Doehring-Schwerdtfeger E, Abdel-Rahim IM, Kardorff R, Kaiser C, Franke D, Schlake J, et al. Ultrasonographical investigation of periportal fibrosis in children with Schistosoma mansoni infection: reversibility of morbidity twenty-three months after treatment with praziquantel. Am J Trop Med Hyg. 1992;46(4):409–15. Epub 1992/04/01.
37. Ross AG, Bartley PB, Sleigh AC, Olds GR, Li Y, Williams GM, et al. Schistosomiasis. N Engl J Med. 2002;346(16):1212–20. Epub 2002/04/19.
38. Ruiz-Guevara R, de Noya BA, Valero SK, Lecuna P, Garassini M, Noya O. Clinical and ultrasound findings before and after praziquantel treatment among Venezuelan schistosomiasis patients. Rev Soc Bras Med Trop. 2007;40(5):505–11. Epub 2007/11/10.
39. Thalheimer U, Leandro G, Samonakis DN, Triantos CK, Patch D, Burroughs AK. Assessment of the agreement between wedge hepatic vein pressure and portal vein pressure in cirrhotic patients. Dig Liver Dis. 2005;37(8):601–8. Epub 2005/05/24.
40. D'Amico G, Garcia-Pagan JC, Luca A, Bosch J. Hepatic vein pressure gradient reduction and prevention of variceal bleeding in cirrhosis: a systematic review. Gastroenterology. 2006;131(5):1611–24. Epub 2006/11/15.
41. Colman JC, Britton RS, Orrego H, Saldivia V, Medline A, Israel Y. Relation between osmotically induced hepatocyte enlargement and portal hypertension. Am J Physiol. 1983;245(3):G382–7. Epub 1983/09/01.
42. Dudenhoefer AA, Loureiro-Silva MR, Cadelina GW, Gupta T, Groszmann RJ. Bioactivation of nitroglycerin and vasomotor response to nitric oxide are impaired in cirrhotic rat livers. Hepatology. 2002;36(2):381–5. Epub 2002/07/27.
43. Zafra C, Abraldes JG, Turnes J, Berzigotti A, Fernandez M, Garca-Pagan JC, et al. Simvastatin enhances hepatic nitric oxide production and decreases the hepatic vascular tone in patients with cirrhosis. Gastroenterology. 2004;126(3):749–55. Epub 2004/02/28.
44. Moore K, Wendon J, Frazer M, Karani J, Williams R, Badr K. Plasma endothelin immunoreactivity in liver disease and the hepatorenal syndrome. N Engl J Med. 1992;327(25):1774–8. Epub 1992/12/17.
45. Martinet JP, Legault L, Cernacek P, Roy L, Dufresne MP, Spahr L, et al. Changes in plasma endothelin-1 and Big endothelin-1 induced by transjugular intrahepatic portosystemic shunts in patients with cirrhosis and refractory ascites. J Hepatol. 1996;25(5):700–6. Epub 1996/11/01.
46. Rockey D. The cellular pathogenesis of portal hypertension: stellate cell contractility, endothelin, and nitric oxide. Hepatology. 1997;25(1):2–5. Epub 1997/01/01.
47. Shulman HM, Fisher LB, Schoch HG, Henne KW, McDonald GB. Veno-occlusive disease of the liver after marrow transplantation: histological correlates of clinical signs and symptoms. Hepatology. 1994;19(5):1171–81. Epub 1994/05/01.
48. McDonald GB, Sharma P, Matthews DE, Shulman HM, Thomas ED. Venocclusive disease of the liver after bone marrow transplantation: diagnosis, incidence, and predisposing factors. Hepatology. 1984;4(1):116–22. Epub 1984/01/01.
49. Sperl W, Stuppner H, Gassner I, Judmaier W, Dietze O, Vogel W. Reversible hepatic veno-occlusive disease in an infant after consumption of pyrrolizidine-containing herbal tea. Eur J Pediatr. 1995;154(2):112–6. Epub 1995/02/01.
50. Corbacioglu S, Greil J, Peters C, Wulffraat N, Laws HJ, Dilloo D, et al. Defibrotide in the treatment of children with veno-occlusive disease (VOD): a retrospective multicentre study demonstrates therapeutic efficacy upon early intervention. Bone Marrow Transplant. 2004;33(2):189–95. Epub 2003/12/09.
51. D'Antiga L, Baker A, Pritchard J, Pryor D, Mieli-Vergani G. Veno-occlusive disease with multi-organ involvement following actinomycin-D. Eur J Cancer. 2001;37(9):1141–8. Epub 2001/05/30.

52. Reiss U, Cowan M, McMillan A, Horn B. Hepatic venoocclusive disease in blood and bone marrow transplantation in children and young adults: incidence, risk factors, and outcome in a cohort of 241 patients. J Pediatr Hematol Oncol. 2002;24(9):746–50. Epub 2002/12/07.
53. Arslan N, Buyukgebiz B, Ozturk Y, Hizli S, Bekem O, Sagol O, et al. Hepatoportal sclerosis in a child. Eur J Pediatr. 2004;163(11):683–4. Epub 2004/08/19.
54. Guzman EA, McCahill LE, Rogers FB. Arterioportal fistulas: introduction of a novel classification with therapeutic implications. J Gastrointest Surg. 2006;10(4):543–50. Epub 2006/04/22.
55. Shneider BL, Bosch J, de Franchis R, Emre SH, Groszmann RJ, Ling SC, et al. Portal hypertension in children: expert pediatric opinion on the report of the Baveno v Consensus Workshop on Methodology of Diagnosis and Therapy in Portal Hypertension. Pediatr Transplant. 2012;16(5):426–37. Epub 2012/03/14.
56. Gugig R, Rosenthal P. Management of portal hypertension in children. World J Gastroenterol. 2012;18(11):1176–84. Epub 2012/04/03.
57. Spence RA, Johnston GW, Odling-Smee GW, Rodgers HW. Bleeding oesophageal varices with long term follow up. Arch Dis Child. 1984;59(4):336–40. Epub 1984/04/01.
58. Garcia-Tsao G, Sanyal AJ, Grace ND, Carey WD. Prevention and management of gastroesophageal varices and variceal hemorrhage in cirrhosis. Am J Gastroenterol. 2007;102(9):2086–102. Epub 2007/08/31.
59. Sarin SK, Shahi HM, Jain M, Jain AK, Issar SK, Murthy NS. The natural history of portal hypertensive gastropathy: influence of variceal eradication. Am J Gastroenterol. 2000;95(10):2888–93. Epub 2000/10/29.
60. Alberti D, Colusso M, Cheli M, Ravelli P, Indriolo A, Signorelli S, et al. Results of a stepwise approach to extra-hepatic portal vein obstruction in children. J Pediatr Gastroenterol Nutr. 2013;57(5):619–26. Epub 2013/06/21.
61. Alvarez F, Bernard O, Brunelle F, Hadchouel P, Odievre M, Alagille D. Portal obstruction in children. I. Clinical investigation and hemorrhage risk. J Pediatr. 1983;103(5):696–702. Epub 1983/11/01.
62. Beppu K, Inokuchi K, Koyanagi N, Nakayama S, Sakata H, Kitano S, et al. Prediction of variceal hemorrhage by esophageal endoscopy. Gastrointest Endosc. 1981;27(4):213–8. Epub 1981/11/01.
63. van Heurn LW, Saing H, Tam PK. Portoenterostomy for biliary atresia: long-term survival and prognosis after esophageal variceal bleeding. J Pediatr Surg. 2004;39(1):6–9. Epub 2003/12/25.
64. Misra SP, Dwivedi M, Misra V. Prevalence and factors influencing hemorrhoids, anorectal varices, and colopathy in patients with portal hypertension. Endoscopy. 1996;28(4):340–5. Epub 1996/05/01.
65. Triger DR. Extra hepatic portal venous obstruction. Gut. 1987;28(10):1193–7. Epub 1987/10/01.
66. Bolognesi M, Merkel C, Sacerdoti D, Nava V, Gatta A. Role of spleen enlargement in cirrhosis with portal hypertension. Dig Liver Dis. 2002;34(2):144–50. Epub 2002/04/03.
67. Shah SH, Hayes PC, Allan PL, Nicoll J, Finlayson ND. Measurement of spleen size and its relation to hypersplenism and portal hemodynamics in portal hypertension due to hepatic cirrhosis. Am J Gastroenterol. 1996;91(12):2580–3. Epub 1996/12/01.
68. Gana JC, Turner D, Mieli-Vergani G, Davenport M, Miloh T, Avitzur Y, et al. A clinical prediction rule and platelet count predict esophageal varices in children. Gastroenterology. 2011;141(6):2009–16. Epub 2011/09/20.
69. Ling SC, Pfeiffer A, Avitzur Y, Fecteau A, Grant D, Ng VL. Long-term follow-up of portal hypertension after liver transplantation in children. Pediatr Transplant. 2009;13(2):206–9. Epub 2008/06/20.
70. Di Giorgio A, Agazzi R, Alberti D, Colledan M, D'Antiga L. Feasibility and efficacy of transjugular intrahepatic portosystemic shunt (TIPS) in children. J Pediatr Gastroenterol Nutr. 2012;54(5):594–600. Epub 2012/01/10.
71. Narahara Y, Kanazawa H, Fukuda T, Matsushita Y, Harimoto H, Kidokoro H, et al. Transjugular intrahepatic portosystemic shunt versus paracentesis plus albumin in patients with refractory ascites who have good hepatic and renal function: a prospective randomized trial. J Gastroenterol. 2011;46(1):78–85. Epub 2010/07/16.
72. Ginés P, Arroyo V, Rodés J, Schrier RW, editors. Ascites and renal dysfunction in liver disease: pathogenesis, diagnosis, and treatment. Oxford: Wiley-Blackwell; 2005. 464 p.
73. Khandwalla HE, Fasakin Y, El-Serag HB. The utility of evaluating low serum albumin gradient ascites in patients with cirrhosis. Am J Gastroenterol. 2009;104(6):1401–5. Epub 2009/06/06.
74. Annamalai A, Wisdom L, Herada M, Nourredin M, Ayoub W, Sundaram V, et al. Management of refractory ascites in cirrhosis: are we out of date? World journal of hepatology. 2016;8(28):1182–93. Epub 2016/10/13.
75. Such J, Runyon BA. Spontaneous bacterial peritonitis. Clin Infect Dis. 1998;27(4):669–74; quiz 75–6. Epub 1998/11/03.
76. Di Giorgio A, D'Antiga L. Diagnosing spontaneous bacterial peritonitis in children: tap-in for higher scores. J Pediatr Gastroenterol Nutr. 2017;64(2):171–2. Epub 2016/08/31.
77. Arikan C, Ozgenc F, Akman SA, Yagci RV, Tokat Y, Aydogdu S. Large-volume paracentesis and liver transplantation. J Pediatr Gastroenterol Nutr. 2003;37(2):207–8. Epub 2003/07/29.
78. Kramer RE, Sokol RJ, Yerushalmi B, Liu E, MacKenzie T, Hoffenberg EJ, et al. Large-volume paracentesis in the management of ascites in children. J Pediatr Gastroenterol Nutr. 2001;33(3):245–9. Epub 2001/10/11.
79. Sen Sarma M, Yachha SK, Bhatia V, Srivastava A, Poddar U. Safety, complications and outcome of large volume paracentesis with or without albumin therapy in children with severe ascites due to liver disease. J Hepatol. 2015;63(5):1126–32. Epub 2015/07/03.
80. Pugliese R, Fonseca EA, Porta G, Danesi V, Guimaraes T, Porta A, et al. Ascites and serum sodium are markers of increased waiting list mortality in children with chronic liver failure. Hepatology. 2014;59(5):1964–71. Epub 2013/10/15.
81. Leong RW, House AK, Jeffrey GP. Chylous ascites caused by portal vein thrombosis treated with octreotide. J Gastroenterol Hepatol. 2003;18(10):1211–3. Epub 2003/09/17.
82. Whitworth JR, Ivy DD, Gralla J, Narkewicz MR, Sokol RJ. Pulmonary vascular complications in asymptomatic children with portal hypertension. J Pediatr Gastroenterol Nutr. 2009;49(5):607–12. Epub 2009/10/13.
83. Barbe T, Losay J, Grimon G, Devictor D, Sardet A, Gauthier F, et al. Pulmonary arteriovenous shunting in children with liver disease. J Pediatr. 1995;126(4):571–9. Epub 1995/04/01.
84. Krowka MJ. Portopulmonary hypertension. Semin Respir Crit Care Med. 2012;33(1):17–25. Epub 2012/03/27.
85. Fallon MB, Abrams GA, Luo B, Hou Z, Dai J, Ku DD. The role of endothelial nitric oxide synthase in the pathogenesis of a rat model of hepatopulmonary syndrome. Gastroenterology. 1997;113(2):606–14. Epub 1997/08/01.
86. Zhang M, Luo B, Chen SJ, Abrams GA, Fallon MB. Endothelin-1 stimulation of endothelial nitric oxide synthase in the pathogenesis of hepatopulmonary syndrome. Am J Physiol. 1999;277(5 Pt 1):G944–52. Epub 1999/11/24.
87. Kinane TB, Westra SJ. Case records of the Massachusetts General Hospital. Weekly clinicopathological exercises. Case 31-2004. A four-year-old boy with hypoxemia. N Engl J Med. 2004;351(16):1667–75. Epub 2004/10/16.
88. Abrams GA, Jaffe CC, Hoffer PB, Binder HJ, Fallon MB. Diagnostic utility of contrast echocardiography and lung

perfusion scan in patients with hepatopulmonary syndrome. Gastroenterology. 1995;109(4):1283–8. Epub 1995/10/01.
89. Santamaria F, Sarnelli P, Celentano L, Farina V, Vegnente A, Mansi A, et al. Noninvasive investigation of hepatopulmonary syndrome in children and adolescents with chronic cholestasis. Pediatr Pulmonol. 2002;33(5):374–9. Epub 2002/04/12.
90. Hoeper MM, Krowka MJ, Strassburg CP. Portopulmonary hypertension and hepatopulmonary syndrome. Lancet. 2004;363(9419):1461–8. Epub 2004/05/04.
91. Al-Hussaini A, Taylor RM, Samyn M, Bansal S, Heaton N, Rela M, et al. Long-term outcome and management of hepatopulmonary syndrome in children. Pediatr Transplant. 2010;14(2):276–82. Epub 2009/08/19.
92. Ridaura-Sanz C, Mejia-Hernandez C, Lopez-Corella E. Portopulmonary hypertension in children. A study in pediatric autopsies. Arch Med Res. 2009;40(7):635–9. Epub 2010/01/20.
93. Ecochard-Dugelay E, Lambert V, Schleich JM, Duche M, Jacquemin E, Bernard O. Portopulmonary Hypertension in liver disease presenting in childhood. J Pediatr Gastroenterol Nutr. 2015;61(3):346–54. Epub 2015/04/18.
94. Condino AA, Ivy DD, O'Connor JA, Narkewicz MR, Mengshol S, Whitworth JR, et al. Portopulmonary hypertension in pediatric patients. J Pediatr. 2005;147(1):20–6. Epub 2005/07/20.
95. Iyer VB, McKiernan PJ, Foster K, Gupte GL. Stomal varices manifestation of portal hypertension in advanced intestinal failure-associated liver disease. J Pediatr Gastroenterol Nutr. 2011;52(5):630–1.
96. European Association for the Study of the Liver. EASL clinical practice guidelines on the management of ascites, spontaneous bacterial peritonitis, and hepatorenal syndrome in cirrhosis. J Hepatol. 2010;53(3):397–417. Epub 2010/07/17.
97. Pericleous M, Sarnowski A, Moore A, Fijten R, Zaman M. The clinical management of abdominal ascites, spontaneous bacterial peritonitis and hepatorenal syndrome: a review of current guidelines and recommendations. Eur J Gastroenterol Hepatol. 2016;28(3):e10–8. Epub 2015/12/17.
98. Lata J. Hepatorenal syndrome. World J Gastroenterol. 2012;18(36):4978–84. Epub 2012/10/11.
99. Amodio P. The liver, the brain and nitrogen metabolism. Metab Brain Dis. 2009;24(1):1–4. Epub 2008/12/25.
100. Amodio P, Bemeur C, Butterworth R, Cordoba J, Kato A, Montagnese S, et al. The nutritional management of hepatic encephalopathy in patients with cirrhosis: Ishen consensus. Hepatology. 2013;58(1):325–36. Epub 2013/03/09.
101. D'Antiga L, Dacchille P, Boniver C, Poledri S, Schiff S, Zancan L, et al. Clues for minimal hepatic encephalopathy in children with noncirrhotic portal hypertension. J Pediatr Gastroenterol Nutr. 2014;59(6):689–94. Epub 2014/08/21.
102. Ferenci P, Lockwood A, Mullen K, Tarter R, Weissenborn K, Blei AT. Hepatic encephalopathy—definition, nomenclature, diagnosis, and quantification: final report of the working party at the 11th World Congresses of Gastroenterology, Vienna, 1998. Hepatology. 2002;35(3):716–21. Epub 2002/03/01.
103. D'Antiga L. Medical management of esophageal varices and portal hypertension in children. Semin Pediatr Surg. 2012;21(3):211–8. Epub 2012/07/18.
104. Khanna R, Sarin SK. Non-cirrhotic portal hypertension—diagnosis and management. J Hepatol. 2014;60(2):421–41. Epub 2013/08/28.
105. Sarin SK. Non-cirrhotic portal fibrosis. J Gastroenterol Hepatol. 2002;17(Suppl 3):S214–23. Epub 2002/12/11.
106. Okudaira M, Ohbu M, Okuda K. Idiopathic portal hypertension and its pathology. Semin Liver Dis. 2002;22(1):59–72. Epub 2002/04/03.
107. Sood V, Lal BB, Khanna R, Rawat D, Bihari C, Alam S. Noncirrhotic portal fibrosis in pediatric population. J Pediatr Gastroenterol Nutr. 2017;64(5):748–53. Epub 2017/04/25.
108. Rajekar H, Vasishta RK, Chawla YK, Dhiman RK. Noncirrhotic portal hypertension. J Clin Exp Hepatol. 2011;1(2):94–108.
109. Sarin SK, Kumar A, Chawla YK, Baijal SS, Dhiman RK, Jafri W, et al. Noncirrhotic portal fibrosis/idiopathic portal hypertension: APASL recommendations for diagnosis and treatment. Hepatol Int. 2007;1(3):398–413. Epub 2007/09/01.
110. Schouten JN, Garcia-Pagan JC, Valla DC, Janssen HL. Idiopathic noncirrhotic portal hypertension. Hepatology. 2011;54(3):1071–81. Epub 2011/05/17.
111. Dhiman RK, Chawla Y, Vasishta RK, Kakkar N, Dilawari JB, Trehan MS, et al. Non-cirrhotic portal fibrosis (idiopathic portal hypertension): experience with 151 patients and a review of the literature. J Gastroenterol Hepatol. 2002;17(1):6–16. Epub 2002/03/16.
112. Nakanuma Y, Tsuneyama K, Ohbu M, Katayanagi K. Pathology and pathogenesis of idiopathic portal hypertension with an emphasis on the liver. Pathol Res Pract. 2001;197(2):65–76. Epub 2001/03/23.
113. Krasinskas AM, Eghtesad B, Kamath PS, Demetris AJ, Abraham SC. Liver transplantation for severe intrahepatic noncirrhotic portal hypertension. Liver Transplant. 2005;11(6):627–34; discussion 10–1. Epub 2005/05/26.
114. Sawada S, Sato Y, Aoyama H, Harada K, Nakanuma Y. Pathological study of idiopathic portal hypertension with an emphasis on cause of death based on records of Annuals of Pathological Autopsy Cases in Japan. J Gastroenterol Hepatol. 2007;22(2):204–9. Epub 2007/02/14.
115. Poddar U, Thapa BR, Puri P, Girish CS, Vaiphei K, Vasishta RK, et al. Non-cirrhotic portal fibrosis in children. Indian J Gastroenterol. 2000;19(1):12–3. Epub 2000/02/05.
116. Cantez MS, Gerenli N, Ertekin V, Gulluoglu M, Durmaz O. Hepatoportal sclerosis in childhood: descriptive analysis of 12 patients. J Korean Med Sci. 2013;28(10):1507–11. Epub 2013/10/18.
117. Alberti D, Colusso M, Cheli M, Ravelli P, Indriolo A, Signorelli S, et al. Results of a stepwise approach to extrahepatic portal vein obstruction in children. J Pediatr Gastroenterol Nutr. 2013;57(5):619–26. Epub 2013/06/21.
118. Sarin SK, Sollano JD, Chawla YK, Amarapurkar D, Hamid S, Hashizume M, et al. Consensus on extra-hepatic portal vein obstruction. Liver Int. 2006;26(5):512–9. Epub 2006/06/10.
119. Thompson EN, Williams R, Sherlock S. Liver function in extrahepatic portal hypertension. Lancet. 1964;2(7374):1352–6. Epub 1964/12/26.
120. Sarin SK, Agarwal SR. Extrahepatic portal vein obstruction. Semin Liver Dis. 2002;22(1):43–58. Epub 2002/04/03.
121. Bosch J, Mastai R, Kravetz D, Navasa M, Rodes J. Hemodynamic evaluation of the patient with portal hypertension. Semin Liver Dis. 1986;6(4):309–17. Epub 1986/11/01.
122. Lebrec D, Bataille C, Bercoff E, Valla D. Hemodynamic changes in patients with portal venous obstruction. Hepatology. 1983;3(4):550–3. Epub 1983/07/01.
123. Harada A, Nonami T, Kasai Y, Nakao A, Takagi H. Systemic hemodynamics in non-cirrhotic portal hypertension—a clinical study of 19 patients. Jpn J Surg. 1988;18(6):620–5. Epub 1988/11/01.
124. Braillon A, Moreau R, Hadengue A, Roulot D, Sayegh R, Lebrec D. Hyperkinetic circulatory syndrome in patients with presinusoidal portal hypertension. Effect of propranolol. J Hepatol. 1989;9(3):312–8. Epub 1989/11/01.
125. Sarin SK, Sethi KK, Nanda R. Measurement and correlation of wedged hepatic, intrahepatic, intrasplenic and intravariceal pressures in patients with cirrhosis of liver and non-cirrhotic portal fibrosis. Gut. 1987;28(3):260–6. Epub 1987/03/01.

126. Rangari M, Gupta R, Jain M, Malhotra V, Sarin SK. Hepatic dysfunction in patients with extrahepatic portal venous obstruction. Liver Int. 2003;23(6):434–9. Epub 2004/02/28.
127. Chandra R, Kapoor D, Tharakan A, Chaudhary A, Sarin SK. Portal biliopathy. J Gastroenterol Hepatol. 2001;16(10):1086–92. Epub 2001/11/01.
128. El-Matary W, Roberts EA, Kim P, Temple M, Cutz E, Ling SC. Portal hypertensive biliopathy: a rare cause of childhood cholestasis. Eur J Pediatr. 2008;167(11):1339–42. Epub 2008/02/14.
129. Suarez V, Puerta A, Santos LF, Perez JM, Varon A, Botero RC. Portal hypertensive biliopathy: a single center experience and literature review. World J Hepatol. 2013;5(3):137–44. Epub 2013/04/05.
130. Schettino GC, Fagundes ED, Roquete ML, Ferreira AR, Penna FJ. Portal vein thrombosis in children and adolescents. J Pediatr (Rio J). 2006;82(3):171–8. Epub 2006/06/15.
131. Orloff MJ, Orloff MS, Rambotti M. Treatment of bleeding esophagogastric varices due to extrahepatic portal hypertension: results of portal-systemic shunts during 35 years. J Pediatr Surg. 1994;29(2):142–51; discussion 51–4. Epub 1994/02/01.
132. Orloff MJ, Orloff MS, Girard B, Orloff SL. Bleeding esophagogastric varices from extrahepatic portal hypertension: 40 years' experience with portal-systemic shunt. J Am Coll Surg. 2002;194(6):717–28; discussion 28–30. Epub 2002/06/26.
133. Sarin SK, Bansal A, Sasan S, Nigam A. Portal-vein obstruction in children leads to growth retardation. Hepatology. 1992;15(2):229–33. Epub 1992/02/01.
134. Mehrotra RN, Bhatia V, Dabadghao P, Yachha SK. Extrahepatic portal vein obstruction in children: anthropometry, growth hormone, and insulin-like growth factor I. J Pediatr Gastroenterol Nutr. 1997;25(5):520–3. Epub 1997/11/14.
135. Superina R, Bambini DA, Lokar J, Rigsby C, Whitington PF. Correction of extrahepatic portal vein thrombosis by the mesenteric to left portal vein bypass. Ann Surg. 2006;243(4):515–21. Epub 2006/03/23.
136. Gauthier-Villars M, Franchi S, Gauthier F, Fabre M, Pariente D, Bernard O. Cholestasis in children with portal vein obstruction. J Pediatr. 2005;146(4):568–73. Epub 2005/04/07.
137. Superina R, Shneider B, Emre S, Sarin S, de Ville de Goyet J. Surgical guidelines for the management of extra-hepatic portal vein obstruction. Pediatr Transplant. 2006;10(8):908–13. Epub 2006/11/14.
138. Chiu B, Superina RA. Encephalopathy caused by a splenorenal shunt can be reversed by performing a mesenteric-to-left portal vein bypass. J Pediatr Surg. 2006;41(6):1177–9. Epub 2006/06/14/.
139. Mack CL, Zelko FA, Lokar J, Superina R, Alonso EM, Blei AT, et al. Surgically restoring portal blood flow to the liver in children with primary extrahepatic portal vein thrombosis improves fluid neurocognitive ability. Pediatrics. 2006;117(3):e405–12. Epub 2006/02/17.
140. Yadav SK, Srivastava A, Thomas MA, Agarwal J, Pandey CM, Lal R, et al. Encephalopathy assessment in children with extra-hepatic portal vein obstruction with MR, psychometry and critical flicker frequency. J Hepatol. 2010;52(3):348–54. Epub 2010/02/09.
141. Yadav SK, Saksena S, Srivastava A, Saraswat VA, Thomas MA, Rathore RK, et al. Brain MR imaging and 1H-MR spectroscopy changes in patients with extrahepatic portal vein obstruction from early childhood to adulthood. AJNR Am J Neuroradiol. 2010;31(7):1337–42. Epub 2010/03/13.
142. El-Karaksy HM, Afifi O, Bakry A, Kader AA, Saber N. A pilot study using lactulose in management of minimal hepatic encephalopathy in children with extrahepatic portal vein obstruction. World J Pediatr. 2017;13(1):70–5. Epub 2016/11/24.
143. Ling SC, Shneider BL. Portal hypertension in children: current practice and the need for evidence. Oxford: Wiley-Blackwell; 2011. p. 189–96.
144. Superina RA, de Ville de Goyet J. Pre-emptive Meso-Rex bypass for children with idiopathic pre-hepatic portal hypertension: trick or treat? J Pediatr Gastroenterol Nutr. 2014;58(4):e41. Epub 2013/12/24.
145. Shneider BL, de Ville de Goyet J, Leung DH, Srivastava A, Ling SC, Duche M, et al. Primary prophylaxis of variceal bleeding in children and the role of MesoRex Bypass: summary of the Baveno VI Pediatric Satellite Symposium. Hepatology. 2016;63(4):1368–80. Epub 2015/09/12.
146. Superina RA, de Ville de Goyet J. Preemptive meso-rex bypass for children with idiopathic prehepatic portal hypertension: trick or treat? J Pediatr Gastroenterol Nutr. 2014;58(4):e41. Epub 2013/12/24
147. Alberti D, D'Antiga L. Authors' response. J Pediatr Gastroenterol Nutr. 2014;58(4):e41. Epub 2013/12/24.
148. Sharif K, McKiernan P, de Ville de Goyet J. Mesoportal bypass for extrahepatic portal vein obstruction in children: close to a cure for most! J Pediatr Surg. 2010;45(1):272–6. Epub 2010/01/29.
149. Uno A, Ishida H, Konno K, Ohnami Y, Naganuma H, Niizawa M, et al. Portal hypertension in children and young adults: sonographic and color Doppler findings. Abdom Imaging. 1997;22(1):72–8. Epub 1997/01/01.
150. Gorka W, Kagalwalla A, McParland BJ, Kagalwalla Y, al Zaben A. Diagnostic value of Doppler ultrasound in the assessment of liver cirrhosis in children: histopathological correlation. J Clin Ultrasound. 1996;24(6):287–95. Epub 1996/07/01.
151. Martinez-Noguera A, Montserrat E, Torrubia S, Villalba J. Doppler in hepatic cirrhosis and chronic hepatitis. Semin Ultrasound CT MR. 2002;23(1):19–36. Epub 2002/02/28.
152. Goyal N, Jain N, Rachapalli V, Cochlin DL, Robinson M. Non-invasive evaluation of liver cirrhosis using ultrasound. Clin Radiol. 2009;64(11):1056–66. Epub 2009/10/14.
153. Gaiani S, Bolondi L, Li Bassi S, Zironi G, Siringo S, Barbara L. Prevalence of spontaneous hepatofugal portal flow in liver cirrhosis. Clinical and endoscopic correlation in 228 patients. Gastroenterology. 1991;100(1):160–7. Epub 1991/01/01.
154. Annet L, Materne R, Danse E, Jamart J, Horsmans Y, Van Beers BE. Hepatic flow parameters measured with MR imaging and Doppler US: correlations with degree of cirrhosis and portal hypertension. Radiology. 2003;229(2):409–14. Epub 2003/09/13.
155. Patriquin H, Lafortune M, Weber A, Blanchard H, Garel L, Roy C. Surgical portosystemic shunts in children: assessment with duplex Doppler US. Work in progress. Radiology. 1987;165(1):25–8. Epub 1987/10/01.
156. De Giacomo C, Tomasi G, Gatti C, Rosa G, Maggiore G. Ultrasonographic prediction of the presence and severity of esophageal varices in children. J Pediatr Gastroenterol Nutr. 1989;9(4):431–5. Epub 1989/11/01.
157. Patriquin H, Tessier G, Grignon A, Boisvert J. Lesser omental thickness in normal children: baseline for detection of portal hypertension. AJR Am J Roentgenol. 1985;145(4):693–6. Epub 1985/10/01.
158. Piscaglia F, Marinelli S, Bota S, Serra C, Venerandi L, Leoni S, et al. The role of ultrasound elastographic techniques in chronic liver disease: current status and future perspectives. Eur J Radiol. 2014;83(3):450–5. Epub 2013/07/31.
159. Sporea I, Gilja OH, Bota S, Sirli R, Popescu A. Liver elastography—an update. Med Ultrason. 2013;15(4):304–14. Epub 2013/11/29.
160. Goldschmidt I, Streckenbach C, Dingemann C, Pfister ED, di Nanni A, Zapf A, et al. Application and limitations of transient

liver elastography in children. J Pediatr Gastroenterol Nutr. 2013;57(1):109–13. Epub 2013/03/30.
161. D'Antiga L, Betalli P, De Angelis P, Davenport M, Di Giorgio A, McKiernan PJ, et al. Interobserver agreement on endoscopic classification of oesophageal varices in children. J Pediatr Gastroenterol Nutr. 2015;61(2):176–81. Epub 2015/04/18.
162. Yachha SK, Sharma BC, Kumar M, Khanduri A. Endoscopic sclerotherapy for esophageal varices in children with extrahepatic portal venous obstruction: a follow-up study. J Pediatr Gastroenterol Nutr. 1997;24(1):49–52. Epub 1997/01/01.
163. Ling SC, Walters T, McKiernan PJ, Schwarz KB, Garcia-Tsao G, Shneider BL. Primary prophylaxis of variceal hemorrhage in children with portal hypertension: a framework for future research. J Pediatr Gastroenterol Nutr. 2011;52(3):254–61. Epub 2011/02/22.
164. Berzigotti A, Seijo S, Reverter E, Bosch J. Assessing portal hypertension in liver diseases. Expert Rev Gastroenterol Hepatol. 2013;7(2):141–55. Epub 2013/02/01.
165. Bosch J, García-Pagán JC. Prevention of variceal rebleeding. Lancet. 2003;361(9361):952–4.
166. Ripoll C, Groszmann R, Garcia-Tsao G, Grace N, Burroughs A, Planas R, et al. Hepatic venous pressure gradient predicts clinical decompensation in patients with compensated cirrhosis. Gastroenterology. 2007;133(2):481–8. Epub 2007/08/08.
167. Turnes J, Garcia-Pagan JC, Abraldes JG, Hernandez-Guerra M, Dell'Era A, Bosch J. Pharmacological reduction of portal pressure and long-term risk of first variceal bleeding in patients with cirrhosis. Am J Gastroenterol. 2006;101(3):506–12. Epub 2006/03/18.
168. de Franchis R. Revising consensus in portal hypertension: report of the Baveno V consensus workshop on methodology of diagnosis and therapy in portal hypertension. J Hepatol. 2010;53(4):762–8. Epub 2010/07/20.
169. Miraglia R, Luca A, Maruzzelli L, Spada M, Riva S, Caruso S, et al. Measurement of hepatic vein pressure gradient in children with chronic liver diseases. J Hepatol. 2010;53(4):624–9. Epub 2010/07/10.
170. Woolfson J, John P, Kamath B, Ng VL, Ling SC. Measurement of hepatic venous pressure gradient is feasible and safe in children. J Pediatr Gastroenterol Nutr. 2013;57(5):634–7. Epub 2013/06/27.
171. Taylor CR. Computed tomography in the evaluation of the portal venous system. J Clin Gastroenterol. 1992;14(2):167–72. Epub 1992/03/01.
172. Finn JP, Kane RA, Edelman RR, Jenkins RL, Lewis WD, Muller M, et al. Imaging of the portal venous system in patients with cirrhosis: MR angiography vs duplex Doppler sonography. AJR Am J Roentgenol. 1993;161(5):989–94. Epub 1993/11/01.
173. de Franchis R, Baveno VIF. Expanding consensus in portal hypertension: report of the Baveno VI Consensus Workshop: stratifying risk and individualizing care for portal hypertension. J Hepatol. 2015;63(3):743–52. Epub 2015/06/07.
174. Lebrec D. Pharmacological treatment of portal hypertension: hemodynamic effects and prevention of bleeding. Pharmacol Ther. 1994;61(1-2):65–107. Epub 1994/01/01.
175. Shashidhar H, Langhans N, Grand RJ. Propranolol in prevention of portal hypertensive hemorrhage in children: a pilot study. J Pediatr Gastroenterol Nutr. 1999;29(1):12–7. Epub 1999/07/10.
176. Ozsoylu S, Kocak N, Demir H, Yuce A, Gurakan F, Ozen H. Propranolol for primary and secondary prophylaxis of variceal bleeding in children with cirrhosis. Turk J Pediatr. 2000;42(1):31–3. Epub 2000/03/25.
177. Ozsoylu S, Kocak N, Yuce A. Propranolol therapy for portal hypertension in children. J Pediatr. 1985;106(2):317–21. Epub 1985/02/01.
178. Ostman-Smith I, Wettrell G, Riesenfeld T. A cohort study of childhood hypertrophic cardiomyopathy: improved survival following high-dose beta-adrenoceptor antagonist treatment. J Am Coll Cardiol. 1999;34(6):1813–22. Epub 1999/11/30.
179. Duche M, Ducot B, Tournay E, Fabre M, Cohen J, Jacquemin E, et al. Prognostic value of endoscopy in children with biliary atresia at risk for early development of varices and bleeding. Gastroenterology. 2010;139(6):1952–60. Epub 2010/07/20.
180. Zargar SA, Javid G, Khan BA, Shah OJ, Yattoo GN, Shah AH, et al. Endoscopic ligation vs. sclerotherapy in adults with extrahepatic portal venous obstruction: a prospective randomized study. Gastrointest Endosc. 2005;61(1):58–66. Epub 2005/01/27.
181. Zargar SA, Javid G, Khan BA, Yattoo GN, Shah AH, Gulzar GM, et al. Endoscopic ligation compared with sclerotherapy for bleeding esophageal varices in children with extrahepatic portal venous obstruction. Hepatology. 2002;36(3):666–72. Epub 2002/08/29.
182. Zargar SA, Yattoo GN, Javid G, Khan BA, Shah AH, Shah NA, et al. Fifteen-year follow up of endoscopic injection sclerotherapy in children with extrahepatic portal venous obstruction. J Gastroenterol Hepatol. 2004;19(2):139–45. Epub 2004/01/21.
183. Lacroix J, Hebert PC, Hutchison JS, Hume HA, Tucci M, Ducruet T, et al. Transfusion strategies for patients in pediatric intensive care units. N Engl J Med. 2007;356(16):1609–19. Epub 2007/04/20.
184. Villanueva C, Colomo A, Bosch A, Concepcion M, Hernandez-Gea V, Aracil C, et al. Transfusion strategies for acute upper gastrointestinal bleeding. N Engl J Med. 2013;368(1):11–21. Epub 2013/01/04.
185. Eroglu Y, Emerick KM, Whitingon PF, Alonso EM. Octreotide therapy for control of acute gastrointestinal bleeding in children. J Pediatr Gastroenterol Nutr. 2004;38(1):41–7. Epub 2003/12/17.
186. Goulis J, Armonis A, Patch D, Sabin C, Greenslade L, Burroughs AK. Bacterial infection is independently associated with failure to control bleeding in cirrhotic patients with gastrointestinal hemorrhage. Hepatology. 1998;27(5):1207–12. Epub 1998/05/15.
187. Botha JF, Campos BD, Grant WJ, Horslen SP, Sudan DL, Shaw BW Jr, et al. Portosystemic shunts in children: a 15-year experience. J Am Coll Surg. 2004;199(2):179–85. Epub 2004/07/28.
188. Alberti D, D'Antiga L. Meso-portal bypass carried out pre-emptively or as second line treatment? Facts and opinions. J Pediatr Gastroenterol Nutr. 2013. Online letter
189. Evans S, Stovroff M, Heiss K, Ricketts R. Selective distal splenorenal shunts for intractable variceal bleeding in pediatric portal hypertension. J Pediatr Surg. 1995;30(8):1115–8. Epub 1995/08/01.
190. Lykavieris P, Gauthier F, Hadchouel P, Duche M, Bernard O. Risk of gastrointestinal bleeding during adolescence and early adulthood in children with portal vein obstruction. J Pediatr. 2000;136(6):805–8. Epub 2000/06/06.
191. Klupp J, Kohler S, Pascher A, Neuhaus P. Liver transplantation as ultimate tool to treat portal hypertension. Dig Dis. 2005;23(1):65–71. Epub 2005/05/28.
192. Di Giorgio AAR, Colusso M, Cheli M, Colledan M, D'Antiga L. Transjugular Intrahepatic Portosystemic Shunt (TIPS): a valuable treatment option for the management of portal hypertension in children. A single centre experience. J Pediatr Gastroenterol Nutr. 2017;64:592A.

Vascular Liver Disease

Simon C. Ling and Ines Loverdos

Key Points
- Management options for chronic portal vein thrombosis include meso-Rex bypass surgery to prevent variceal bleeding and restore portal venous flow to the liver.
- Sinusoidal obstruction syndrome is diagnosed by clinical criteria and may be managed with defibrotide.
- Prothrombotic abnormalities are commonly identified in children with Budd-Chiari syndrome and may require lifelong anticoagulation therapy.
- Idiopathic non-cirrhotic portal hypertension encompasses a variety of histological abnormalities and may be associated with infections, medications, toxins, malignancies, genetic abnormalities, or disorders of the immune system, circulation, or coagulation.
- Accurate diagnosis of congenital vascular malformations and their hemodynamic and other consequences determines most appropriate therapy with medications, image-guided interventions, or surgery.

Research Needed in the Field
- Multicenter registry research to characterize the natural history and improve understanding of therapeutic interventions in rare congenital vascular disorders
- Determining the role of endoluminal recanalization techniques for portal vein thrombosis and Budd-Chiari syndrome
- Identification of interventions to prevent and treat endothelial damage and small vessel disorders in the liver, including sinusoidal obstruction syndrome and idiopathic non-cirrhotic portal hypertension

20.1 Extrahepatic Portal Vein Obstruction

20.1.1 Definition

Extrahepatic portal vein obstruction (EHPVO) occurs when the extrahepatic portal vein is obstructed, most commonly by thrombosis. EHPVO may occur with or without associated obstruction of the intrahepatic portal veins, splenic veins, or mesenteric veins. Isolated occlusion of the splenic vein or superior mesenteric vein does not constitute EHPVO. EHPVO due to thrombosis may occur as a complication of liver cirrhosis or abdominal neoplasm. EHPVO is usually diagnosed as an established chronic disorder, although may be recognized in the acute phase when the management options differ [1–4].

20.1.2 Epidemiology

EHPVO is the second most common cause of portal hypertension in the world, after cirrhosis. It is responsible for up to 30% of all variceal bleeding in developing countries and is the most common cause of variceal bleeding in children [1, 3, 5].

S. C. Ling (✉)
Division of Gastroenterology, Hepatology and Nutrition, The Hospital for Sick Children, Toronto, ON, Canada

Department of Paediatrics, University of Toronto, Toronto, ON, Canada
e-mail: simon.ling@sickkids.ca

I. Loverdos
Unidad de Gastroenterología, Hepatología y Nutrición pediátrica, Corporació Sanitària Universitària Parc Taulí. Sabadell, Barcelona, Spain

20.1.3 Etiology

EHPVO in children is almost always due to thrombosis. Other rare causes include infiltration or compression by hepatic or intra-abdominal tumor, including hepatoblastoma and hepatocellular carcinoma. The cause of thrombosis causing EHPVO in children remains unclear in approximately 50% of patients, although several variables are relevant to understanding the cause in individual children.

Local factors: Thrombosis may occur following omphalitis, umbilical vein catheterization (UVC), episodes of dehydration, neonatal septicemia, or abdominal sepsis. The role of UVC as a risk factor for problematic EHPVO is well recognized, although the associated thrombi will often resolve spontaneously during infancy and may be limited to the left portal vein without important clinical sequelae. Published reports show the incidence of portal vein thrombosis following neonatal UVC ranges from 0 to 43% [6–9].

Prothrombotic state: It is unclear how often a hypercoagulable condition plays a role in pediatric EHPVO [1, 3, 10–12]. Case-control studies comparing children with EHPVO to controls report odds ratios for a thrombophilic state ranging from 1 to 11.9. The commonest reported abnormalities are factor V Leiden mutation and protein C and/or S deficiency [12–14]. Up to 12.5% of children with EHPVO have more than one thrombophilic disorder [15]. However, not all reports have found thrombophilic abnormalities [10] and measured levels of coagulation-inhibitor proteins may be misleading, because restoration of portal flow by performing mesenterico-left portal vein bypass surgery has been shown to improve previously depressed circulating levels of protein C, S, and prothrombin time in children with EHPVO [16]. Genetic testing for thrombophilic disorders is therefore preferred over functional testing. The occurrence of portal vein thrombosis in patients with cirrhosis may relate to increased gut permeability causing elevated concentration of bacterial lipopolysaccharide in the splanchnic venous blood, which in turn increases local endothelial production of factor VIII [17].

Congenital anomaly: EHPVO is sometimes found in association with congenital abnormalities of other systems, such as cardiovascular or urinary tract, suggesting the potential for a congenital anomaly of the portal vein as well [12, 18].

20.1.4 Pathophysiology

EHPVO in children is usually a chronic condition that is not associated with intrinsic liver disease. The symptoms of EHPVO can be classified into those derived from portal hypertension and those secondary to spontaneous portosystemic shunting.

The portal vein is responsible for approximately two thirds of the hepatic blood supply. When thrombosis in the portal system occurs, two mechanisms maintain hepatic blood flow. Firstly, arterial flow increases due to hepatic artery vasodilatation. Secondly, a portal cavernoma develops, consisting of a network of collaterals which enable portal blood to partially bypass the thrombosed portal vein. Cavernous transformation of the portal vein starts to develop within days of the onset of occlusive thrombosis. The collaterals are insufficient to carry all the portal blood flow, and thus presinusoidal and prehepatic portal hypertension occurs [19–21].

20.1.5 Diagnosis

Acute portal vein thrombosis should be suspected in patients presenting with abdominal pain, ascites, fever, or symptoms consistent with intestinal ischemia in the absence of portal cavernoma.

EHPVO in children is usually a chronic condition that presents coincidentally when splenomegaly is felt on physical examination or is noted on an abdominal ultrasound ordered for other reasons. Alternatively, acute variceal bleeding may be the first presenting symptom. In a cohort of 108 children with EHPVO, 79% of the patients had an episode of gastrointestinal bleeding and in 42% occurred before 4 years of age [1, 3, 12, 21]. Ascites is usually absent. Abnormally low platelet and white cell counts may be found, resulting from hypersplenism. Liver enzyme levels in blood are usually normal.

Children with EHPVO may have growth retardation and decreased growth velocity. The mechanism has not been clearly defined but may relate to reduced passage to the liver of hepatotrophic hormones generated in the splanchnic circulation. Whether resistance to growth hormone plays a role in the setting of EHPVO is unclear [22, 23]. Covert hepatic encephalopathy may impair neurocognitive function, due to portosystemic shunting. Rarely, portal biliopathy may cause clinical, biochemical, and/or imaging features of biliary obstruction or stricturing, which may arise due to extrinsic bile duct compression by the portal cavernoma, due to ischemic damage secondary to portal vein thrombosis, or due to the presence of varices within the bile duct wall [12, 21, 24–26]. Other associations include hepatopulmonary syndrome and portopulmonary hypertension that may be identified by reduced exercise tolerance and low oxygen saturation levels.

EHPVO is best diagnosed by Doppler ultrasound, which will show portal vein obstruction, intraluminal material, or portal cavernoma (Table 20.1). Computerized tomography (CT), magnetic resonance imaging (MRI), and invasive venography are used to demonstrate the extent of thrombosis

Table 20.1 Important components to consider in the evaluation of EHPVO

Medical history	Umbilical vein catheterization, omphalitis, pancreatitis, appendicitis, abdominal surgery, inflammatory bowel disease, liver abscess, family history of thrombosis
Physical exam	Growth parameters, splenomegaly, spider naevi, palmar erythema, abdominal wall veins
Imaging studies	Doppler ultrasound Second-line studies: MRI, CT
Initial laboratory investigations	CBC, INR, liver enzymes, bilirubins, albumin
Thrombophilia panel	Protein C, protein S, antithrombin III, factor VIII level, factor V Leiden, prothrombin gene mutation, homocysteine, antiphospholipid antibody, anticardiolipin antibody, dysfibrinogenemia screen, JAK2 mutation, paroxysmal nocturnal hemoglobinuria screen
Contrast-enhanced echocardiography	Hepatopulmonary syndrome, portopulmonary hypertension
Neuropsychologist assessment	Neurocognitive testing for minimal hepatic encephalopathy

and in planning for therapeutic intervention. The patency of intrahepatic portal veins can be demonstrated by transjugular retrograde or transhepatic portal venography. Assessment of underlying thrombophilic disorders should be undertaken, relying where possible on genetic rather than functional testing. Liver biopsy is indicated when there is suspicion of intrinsic liver disease. In children with exercise intolerance or hypoxemia, echocardiography with intravenous contrast enhancement is utilized to identify associated congenital heart disease, hepatopulmonary syndrome, or portopulmonary hypertension [1, 3, 21, 27].

20.1.6 Treatment

20.1.6.1 Acute Portal Vein Thrombosis

Systemic anticoagulation for 3–6 months is usually recommended to treat acute portal vein thrombosis due to the low likelihood of spontaneous recanalization, although there is a lack of evidence to guide therapeutic choices for these children. Limited experience with other therapeutic approaches such as thrombectomy, thrombolysis, or transjugular intrahepatic portosystemic shunt (TIPS) has been reported. While appropriate clinical indications and contraindications have not yet been defined, their use must currently be based upon careful case-by-case consideration and availability of local expertise [4, 28].

20.1.6.2 Chronic Portal Vein Thrombosis

There is no role for anticoagulation therapy in the management of chronic portal vein thrombosis, unless a prothrombotic disorder has been identified [3]. The approach to management is focused on the alleviation of portal hypertension and/or the reduction of portosystemic shunting. There is widespread agreement that therapeutic interventions are indicated when significant morbidity occurs, for example, due to variceal hemorrhage. Expert consensus now also recommends a role for surgical therapy to prevent complications [16, 29–32].

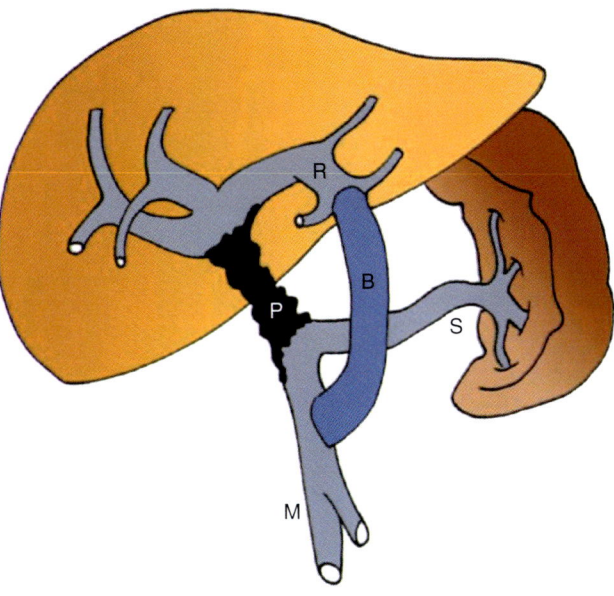

Fig. 20.1 Anatomy of the meso-left portal vein bypass. *B* bypass, *M* superior mesenteric vein, *P* portal vein thrombosis, *S* splenic vein, *R* Rex recessus (From reference 32, with permission)

The preferred surgical procedure for chronic EHPVO due to thrombosis is the meso-Rex bypass (mesenteric to left portal vein bypass). When feasible, this procedure results in restoration of portal blood flow to the liver, without resulting in portosystemic shunting (Fig. 20.1). An autologous internal jugular vein graft is used as the conduit from the superior mesenteric vein to the intrahepatic left portal vein where it is located in the Rex recessus. Before surgery is undertaken, efforts must be made to ascertain the patency of the left portal vein by Doppler ultrasound, CT or MR venography, and invasive hepatic venography. When successful, the meso-Rex bypass provides a corrective treatment for EHPVO that resolves symptoms related to portal hypertension and portosystemic shunting, including variceal bleeding, hypersplenism, hepatopulmonary syndrome, and encephalopathy. Mack et al. studied eight children with EHPVO who underwent meso-Rex bypass surgery and demonstrated improvement of fluid cognitive ability indices [29]. Meso-Rex bypass surgery should be performed early in life if possible, when the intrahepatic portal venous system is more able to adapt to accommodate the high portal venous blood flow that is re-established postoperatively.

Expert consensus now recommends the use of meso-Rex bypass to prevent the onset of complications such as variceal hemorrhage, if surgery is undertaken for selected patients and in a center where a successful outcome is at least 90% likely [32]. The outcome of such primary prophylactic surgery is optimized by ensuring favorable patient characteristics, including patency of the intrahepatic portal venous system and mesenteric veins, absence of parenchymal liver disease, absence of or effective treatment for any underlying prothrombotic condition, normal echocardiography, and body weight above 8 kg. Furthermore, appropriate surgical and center expertise must be demonstrated.

If a meso-Rex bypass cannot be performed, then either a distal splenorenal shunt should be considered as an alternative or conservative management of the presenting complications such as ongoing management of varices with endoscopic variceal ligation. Children with complications due to spontaneous portosystemic shunting are usually not considered to be candidates for surgical portosystemic shunt procedures, which may worsen symptoms of encephalopathy, portopulmonary hypertension, or hepatopulmonary syndrome. Successful insertion of TIPS has been described in adults with portal vein thrombosis and may improve hepatopulmonary syndrome or portopulmonary hypertension, although it also creates a portosystemic shunt that may worsen encephalopathy. Liver transplantation is an alternative therapeutic option for these children, although it requires a careful case-by-case determination of risks and benefits.

Acute variceal bleeding in the setting of EHPVO is rarely fatal in the absence of intrinsic liver disease but is often associated with significant morbidity. There is little high-quality evidence to guide clinical decision making for the prevention and management of variceal bleeding in children with EHPVO [3, 21, 33].

20.2 Sinusoidal Obstruction Syndrome (Hepatic Veno-occlusive Disease)

20.2.1 Definition

Sinusoidal obstruction syndrome (SOS) is a non-thrombotic obstruction of the hepatic sinusoids that can extend to the adjacent central veins, but in the absence of an underlying disorder of the hepatic veins. The initial injury is to the hepatic sinusoids and involvement of the central vein can be absent. In fact, occlusion of the central vein was only seen in 55% of patients with mild to moderate SOS and in 75% of patients with severe SOS. Therefore the previous term of "hepatic veno-occlusive disease" is considered inaccurate [4, 28].

Table 20.2 Risk factors for development of SOS after bone marrow transplantation

Risk factors for SOS after bone marrow transplantation
Younger age
Preexisting liver disease
Chronic hepatitis B and C
Nonalcoholic steatohepatitis
Parenteral nutrition-associated liver disease
Cirrhosis
Cholestatic liver diseases
HLA-mismatched or HLA-unrelated donor transplant
Use of concomitant drugs
Itraconazole
Sirolimus
Norethisterone
Previous abdominal irradiation
High-dose conditioning regimens
High-risk primary diagnoses
Osteopetrosis
Neuroblastoma
Adrenoleukodystrophy
Primary hemophagocytic lymphohistiocytosis

20.2.2 Epidemiology

The overall incidence of SOS after myeloablative therapy for hematopoietic stem cell transplantation (HSCT) has reduced over recent decades to approximately 7%, largely owing to improvements in low-intensity conditioning regimens [34, 35]. SOS is also more rarely associated with other clinical settings, such as the use of azathioprine and several other medications detailed below, or exposure to dietary toxins found in Jamaican "bush tea" or other natural health products containing pyrrolizidine alkaloids.

20.2.3 Etiology

SOS occurs most commonly after hematopoietic stem cell transplantation (HSCT), when it is caused by toxicity from the conditioning therapy. The most hepatotoxic regimens are those that contain cyclophosphamide in combination with busulfan or total body irradiation. Several risk factors have been identified for development of SOS in HSCT recipients (Table 20.2). SOS also occurs in patients receiving radiotherapy and other drugs, including gemtuzumab ozogamicin, 6-thioguanine, cytosine arabinoside, urethane, 6-mercaptopurine, azathioprine, actinomycin D, dacarbazine, oxaliplatin, and tacrolimus.

SOS can be caused by the ingestion of plants including *Senecio, Crotalaria, Heliotropium,* and *Symphytum.*

Pyrrolizidine alkaloids contained in herbal teas, naturopathic remedies, or contaminated food may also cause SOS. The severity of the liver damage depends on the ingested dose and individual susceptibility [36].

20.2.4 Pathophysiology

SOS is primarily a vascular disorder that causes liver dysfunction as a secondary phenomenon. Initially, liver sinusoidal endothelial cells are damaged by drug effects and irradiation. The first morphological change of SOS to appear is ballooning of the endothelial cells of hepatic sinusoids, detected by electron microscopy. Inflammation and endothelial cell death ensue, with detachment of endothelial cells allowing penetration of red blood cells to the space of Disse. Endothelial dysfunction, altered vascular tone, and dissection of endothelial cells into the sinusoidal lumen contribute to an increased resistance to sinusoidal blood flow, and consequently portal hypertension ensues. These initial changes are followed by deposition of collagen in the sinusoids and central and sublobular veins.

20.2.5 Diagnosis

SOS is diagnosed using clinical criteria, because there is no specific laboratory or imaging marker that has adequate diagnostic or prognostic value. SOS should be suspected when a patient who has received a hepatotoxic myeloablative regimen develops tender hepatomegaly, abdominal pain localized to the right upper quadrant, and weight gain secondary to fluid retention and ascites. The patient may develop jaundice. There are two widely accepted diagnostic criteria for SOS; the Seattle criteria and the Baltimore criteria, each based on the clinical features of a large cohort of patients with SOS (Table 20.3). The Seattle criteria have chronologic consideration that can only be applied to cyclophosphamide-containing regimens because other drugs can induce SOS beyond 20 days post-HSCT. Therefore the concept of late SOS, presenting beyond 20 days after HSCT, and the coexistence of multiorgan failure (especially renal and pulmonary failure) have been introduced as features of the clinical spectrum of SOS [28, 37, 38]. The severity of SOS can be classified as mild (no requirement for treatment and self-resolving), moderate (need for treatment to manage fluid balance or pain but resolves completely), or severe (leading to death or failure to resolve after day 100 post initiation of therapy) [37]. Severe SOS is associated with a mortality rate of more than 84% [37, 39].

The poor sensitivity of the Baltimore and Seattle criteria must be remembered when trying to reach a diagnosis. Accurate diagnosis can be complicated by the presence of multiple comorbidities in this complex patient group. The differential diagnosis includes sepsis, graft-versus-host disease, hemolysis, total parenteral nutrition-induced cholestasis, congestive heart failure, and toxicity due to the concomitant use of other hepatotoxic drugs.

In SOS, imaging will usually show hepatomegaly, splenomegaly, and ascites. Edema of the gallbladder wall may be identified but is a non-specific finding. Doppler ultrasound may appear normal, or reveal reversal of portal venous flow, or reduced hepatic venous flow, or increased hepatic artery resistive index [28, 36]. Imaging studies are mainly useful to rule out other conditions such as biliary obstruction, portal vein thrombosis, or liver abscess.

When undertaken, liver biopsy may provide supportive evidence of SOS. However, there is a very high risk associated with this procedure early after HSCT when pancytopenia is present. Therefore, most practitioners are reluctant to consider liver biopsy even when clinical and radiological features do not provide enough information to make a confident diagnosis of SOS. The histological features of SOS include dilatation of sinusoids, extravasation of red cells through the space of Disse, and widening of the subendothelial zone in the central veins. As the disease progresses, hemorrhage in zones 2 and 3 of the liver acinus, dislodgement of hepatocytes into portal and hepatic venules, collagenization of sinusoids and vein walls, and cirrhosis may appear. If undertaken, the liver biopsy must be interpreted in the knowledge that involvement may be patchy and the histological features evolve with time [4, 36].

Measurement of the hepatic venous pressure gradient may improve diagnostic accuracy. A pressure gradient above 10 mmHg was highly specific for SOS in one study [40]. The transjugular, intrahepatic approach to this measurement allows performance of a liver biopsy at the same time in those children in whom the diagnosis is unclear.

20.2.6 Treatment

SOS resolves with time in the majority of patients. Treatment is focused on the management of fluid balance, reduced sodium intake, diuresis for ascites, and maintaining adequate

Table 20.3 Diagnostic criteria for SOS

Baltimore criteria [42]
Hyperbilirubinemia >2 mg/dL (34.2 μmol/L) and ≥2 of the following: • Hepatomegaly (usually painful) • ≥5% weight gain • Ascites
Seattle criteria [37]
Two of three findings within 20 days of HSCT: • Hepatomegaly or R upper quadrant pain • Sudden >2% weight gain (due to fluid retention) • Bilirubin >2 mg/dL (34.2 μmol/L)

renal blood flow. Studies have explored approaches to reduce endothelial cell injury and intravascular thrombosis while trying to avoid any increased risk of bleeding. Unfortunately, many therapies have shown either no benefit or an unacceptable risk profile, including tissue plasminogen activator, N-acetylcysteine, antithrombin III, prostaglandin E1, prednisone, or vitamin E with glutamine.

Defibrotide is a single-stranded polydeoxyribonucleotide with antithrombotic and profibrinolytic effects that has been studied as an anti-ischemic, endothelium-protective agent. Defibrotide has shown promise for the management of severe SOS [41, 42]. In a recent cohort of 102 patients including children with severe SOS and multiorgan failure, 38% survived to 100 days after HSCT compared to 25% of historical controls that did not receive defibrotide [43]. Using analysis adjusting for propensity score, the difference in survival between the treatment groups was 23%. Pediatric rates of survival are higher compared to adults [42]. Poor prognostic factors include multiorgan failure, high serum alanine aminotransferase levels, and high hepatic venous pressure gradient. Complications of multiorgan failure are the usual cause of death, rather than hepatic insufficiency itself [28, 44].

TIPS have been used to reduce portal hypertension with no improvement in outcome. Liver transplantation has been undertaken for selected children with HSCT for benign conditions [36, 45].

Prevention of SOS involves the use of less toxic myeloablative regimens and the identification of high-risk children that may benefit while not decreasing the chances of engraftment or increasing the relapse rate of the primary disease. Several groups have demonstrated good results by using this strategy and particularly by avoiding cyclophosphamide [46, 47]. There is no clear evidence that other treatments given to prevent SOS are effective. Prospective studies have not shown any benefit from the use of unfractionated or low molecular weight heparin, antithrombin III, pentoxifylline, or prostaglandin E1 [36]. However, ursodeoxycholic acid was shown to be effective in preventing SOS in a meta-analysis of three randomized trials [48].

In the first pediatric prospective, open-label, randomized trial to evaluate the prophylactic use of defibrotide in children at high risk for SOS, Corbacioglu et al. showed that defibrotide might offer benefit for SOS prophylaxis. The incidence of SOS was reduced in the defibrotide treatment group, as was the incidence of graft-versus-host disease and renal failure, without significant increase in adverse effects [28, 39]. Recommended prophylactic regimens therefore include the use of reduced intensity myeloablative regimens, ursodeoxycholic acid, and defibrotide.

20.3 Budd-Chiari Syndrome (Hepatic Venous Outflow Obstruction)

20.3.1 Definition

Budd-Chiari syndrome (BCS) is defined as the clinical syndrome associated with obstruction of the hepatic venous outflow, in the absence of right heart failure, constrictive pericarditis, and sinusoidal obstruction syndrome [49, 50]. Secondary BCS occurs when the obstruction is due to a compression or invasion of veins by tumor, abscess, or cyst or when obstruction is due to blunt abdominal trauma or following liver transplantation.

20.3.2 Epidemiology

The incidence of primary BCS in children is unknown. The estimated overall incidence in adults ranges from 0.2 to 0.8 per million per year, and it is likely to be more rare in children. The location of the venous obstruction varies according to geographical region, with obstruction of the inferior vena cava more common in Asia and involvement of the hepatic veins more common in Western countries [50, 51].

20.3.3 Etiology

Primary BCS is commonly associated with risk factors for thrombosis. At least one prothrombotic risk factor is identified in 84% of affected adults [52]. Myeloproliferative disorders (MPD) are found most frequently, accounting for 50% of adult BCS cases. Testing for MPD should always be undertaken, even when peripheral blood counts are unremarkable, because hypersplenism, hemodilution, and iron deficiency in BCS may mask the peripheral blood count abnormalities. Guidelines recommend genetic testing for the V617F mutation in the Janus tyrosine kinase 2 (JAK2) gene in granulocytes in all adult BCS patients. This mutation is found in 80% of adults with MPD and BCS. If the genetic testing is negative, a bone marrow biopsy should be considered to assess for MPD [21, 50, 53]. There is inadequate data to determine if this approach is also appropriate in children.

BCS is associated with paroxysmal nocturnal hemoglobinuria and Behçet's disease. [53] Antiphospholipid antibodies and hyperhomocysteinemia have also been associated with cases of BCS, but it remains unclear whether they are a cause or a consequence.

The major causes of inherited thrombophilia can be classified as gain-of-function mutations (factor V Leiden G1691A and prothrombin G20210A polymorphism) or loss of anticoagulant function (deficiencies of protein C, S, or antithrombin).

Factor V Leiden mutation is the commonest thrombophilia marker in the general population; the relative risk for venous thrombosis is 5–10-fold for heterozygotes and 50–100-fold for homozygotes. Factor V Leiden mutation has been found in 16–26% of adults with BCS and seems to be more common in patients presenting with inferior vena cava obstruction. However, this abnormality is commonly associated with other prothrombotic risk factors, and its individual role in promoting BCS is therefore unclear [53, 54]. Inherited deficiencies of protein C, S, and antithrombin have been implicated in BCS, but low levels of these proteins in serum should be carefully interpreted because impaired liver function or thrombosis may also reduce the circulating levels of these anticoagulant proteins.

In a series of 22 children with BCS, JAK2 mutations were negative in the 5 children who were tested, 2 patients had protein C deficiency, 1 had antiphospholipid antibodies, and 1 had antithrombin III deficiency [55]. In another series of 7 children presenting to one institution over 15 years, all 7 had identifiable prothrombotic risk factors including 2 with JAK2 mutations [56].

In some patients, venous obstruction is localized to a small area of the IVC or hepatic veins, appearing as a membrane or web. Although these webs have sometimes been considered as congenital malformations, they are now more commonly explained as sequelae of prior thrombus, resulting in fibrous thickened regions which may form a valve-like membrane or be several centimeters in length [50, 57, 58].

20.3.4 Pathophysiology

Hepatic venous obstruction causes congestion of the central veins and sinusoids of the liver, with secondary effects on portal venous and hepatic arterial flow. Regional variation of hepatic involvement arises due to the different levels of obstruction in the venous outflow tract (three hepatic veins and the IVC) and differences in available collateral venous drainage (e.g., the caudate lobe is usually spared due to its alternative venous drainage). Imaging therefore typically demonstrates a heterogeneous liver parenchyma.

Acute hepatocellular dysfunction may occur, with coagulopathy and jaundice, and sinusoidal hypertension exacerbates the development of ascites. Hepatic congestion contributes to hepatomegaly. Portal hypertension results in splenomegaly and the risk of development of esophageal varices.

Fibrosis due to BCS develops first in centrilobular regions and then spreads into diffuse fibrous septa. The difference in mechanisms driving hepatic fibrosis due to BCS, compared to other infectious or toxic liver diseases, is supported by different gene expression profiles in BCS livers [59]. Patients in whom the initial venous obstruction is symptomatically and functionally well tolerated may present later with established cirrhosis [28, 60].

20.3.5 Diagnosis

BCS should be considered in children presenting with abdominal pain, hepatosplenomegaly, and ascites with or without abdominal pain [61]. Prominent cutaneous abdominal veins may be seen. Liver enzymes, albumin, and INR may be normal or abnormal, and jaundice is uncommon. BCS should also be considered in patients presenting with idiopathic cirrhosis, portal hypertension, and hypersplenism or variceal bleeding. The duration of disease correlates poorly with the type of clinical presentation [28].

Doppler ultrasound is the most reliable imaging method with which to identify obstruction in the hepatic veins or suprahepatic IVC. The typical ultrasonographic features for BCS are an absent flow signal in the hepatic veins, reversed or turbulent flow, collateral veins connecting the hepatic veins or the diaphragmatic or intercostal veins, a weblike appearance near the hepatic vein ostia, or the replacement of a normal vein by a hyperechoic cord. Doppler ultrasound is more effective than MRI in the assessment of intrahepatic collaterals and does not provide information on blood flow direction. However, MRI may provide useful complimentary information, including the presence of webs, extraneous masses, or other abdominal and thoracic pathology. On CT scan the absence of visualization of the hepatic veins suggests obstruction, but indeterminate results are frequent. Multiphasic helical CT provides better results in BCS. Venography has a little role in the diagnostic phase but may have a therapeutic role [4, 21].

Two additional imaging features are highly supportive of a diagnosis of BCS: firstly, the presence of regenerative hypervascular nodules due to impaired hepatic perfusion and, secondly, hypertrophy of the caudate lobe, due to this lobe having separate venous drainage directly to the IVC [28].

Liver biopsy is not usually required when imaging studies clearly demonstrate venous obstruction, but it may be helpful when imaging is less clear-cut, such as when obstruction primarily involves the small intrahepatic veins. Liver biopsy must be interpreted with caution due to the histological features of BCS showing marked regional variation in severity, dependent upon the affected vessel(s). Two biopsies from different lobes are therefore preferred to improve sensitivity. Liver biopsy can be normal in the early stages of acute BCS. The initial features are dilatation of veins and sinusoids with a variable degree of necrosis. Following the acute phase, the sinusoids become collagenized and dilated, and the hepatic veins become incorporated into the fibrous septa and may disappear. These septa lead to venocentric cirrhosis with relative sparing of the portal triads [62].

Nagral et al. described 16 cases of BCS in children. Abdominal Doppler ultrasound led to the diagnosis in ten children. Liver biopsy was performed in the six children in whom ultrasound was not diagnostic; histology confirmed

BCS in four. A diagnosis of BCS was reached in the other two children following invasive hepatic venography. Collaterals between the hepatic veins and caudate lobe hypertrophy were found in half of the patients. Once the diagnosis was established, invasive venography was undertaken in 14 cases to enable image-guided therapy [55].

20.3.6 Treatment

In the absence of clinical trials for therapy of BCS, the preferred therapeutic approach is based upon expert opinion arising from the experience of adult hepatologists. The main aim of treatment is to decompress the liver and restore hepatic venous flow, and a stepwise approach is usually recommended. Anticoagulation should be commenced in all patients unless there is a major contraindication. Previous gastrointestinal bleeding due to portal hypertension is not considered to be a sufficient contraindication for anticoagulation. Patients with an underlying thrombophilia should receive lifelong anticoagulation treatment [4, 21]. For other patients, there is no consensus on the optimal duration of anticoagulation treatment. If a short-length stenosis of the IVC or hepatic vein is identified, then an attempt at recanalization by percutaneous angioplasty or stenting techniques should be undertaken. If this approach to therapy is unsuccessful, TIPS is the next treatment of choice in adults. Liver transplantation is considered in patients unresponsive to the above procedures and in those who present with acute liver failure [4, 21].

Literature regarding treatment in children with BCS is scarce and composed only of small case series and case reports. In a series of 16 children in India, 11 underwent radiological interventions that included angioplasty in four children, stenting in two children, and TIPS in six children (one child had both angioplasty and TIPS). The outcome seemed better with stenting and TIPS than with angioplasty [55]. In a pediatric case series from King's College Hospital, London, three of the seven patients received radiological interventions (two TIPS, one hepatic vein stent), two underwent liver transplantation, and one a surgical meso-caval shunt [56]. Thrombolytic therapy, pericardial patch atriocavoplasty, surgical repair, surgical portosystemic shunting, and liver transplant have also been described in case series of pediatric BCS [61, 63–66].

20.4 Idiopathic Non-cirrhotic Portal Hypertension

20.4.1 Definition

Idiopathic non-cirrhotic portal hypertension (INCPH) represents a group of conditions characterized by portal hypertension without cirrhosis. The conditions share many histological and clinical features in common and are likely to be caused by abnormalities of the small intrahepatic portal vein radicles [67–69]. Different terminology has been reported in the literature regarding INCPH, including non-cirrhotic intrahepatic portal hypertension, non-cirrhotic portal hypertension, idiopathic portal hypertension, non-cirrhotic portal fibrosis, nodular regenerative hyperplasia, obliterative portal venopathy, hepatoportal sclerosis, and incomplete septal cirrhosis.

20.4.2 Epidemiology

The prevalence of INCPH varies around the world, for reasons that have not been determined. The prevalence and incidence of INCPH in children are unknown, but overall in adults INCPH accounts for 3–5% of cases of portal hypertension in Europe and North America and is responsible for 15–30% in India [67, 70]. In a large study of 2500 adult autopsies, INCPH due to nodular regenerative hyperplasia (NRH) was found in 2.6%, mostly related to other systemic diseases [71].

20.4.3 Etiology

Although its exact etiology remains elusive, INCPH is associated with several factors that are likely to be important in its causation [67, 72–75]:

Immunological and autoimmune disorders. INCPH is associated with systemic immunological disorders such as systemic lupus erythematosus, systemic sclerosis, polyarteritis nodosa, celiac disease, and primary hypogammaglobulinemia.

Infections. Intestinal bacterial infections may give rise to septic embolization to the portal circulation causing small portal vein obliteration.

Medications and toxins. INCPH occurs in a subgroup of patients treated with azathioprine, 6-thioguanine, busulfan, doxorubicin, cyclophosphamide, and other drugs and following prolonged ingestion of arsenic.

Circulatory disorders. INCPH, and specifically nodular regenerative hyperplasia, has been described in congestive heart failure, other cardiac abnormalities, and portal vein agenesis.

Malignancy: INCPH has been described in patients with leukemia and lymphoma.

Genetic disorders. A genetic background to some cases of INCPH is suggested by occasional reports of familial recurrence and its association with congenital disorders such as Turner, Felty, and Adams-Oliver syndromes. There is a high frequency of HLA-DR3 in patients with INCPH.

Thrombophilia. Thrombophilic risk factors are often identified in patients with INCPH, suggesting a potential etiological role.

20.4.4 Pathophysiology

Wanless et al. studied autopsy liver tissue and liver biopsies and demonstrated a loss or obstruction of portal vein radicles, an obliterative portal venopathy, in patients with nodular regenerative hyperplasia [71, 76]. They showed that regenerative nodules are supplied by patent portal vein radicles, whereas neighboring atrophic areas are not. Due to the nature of the associated conditions and drug therapies, INCPH is suspected to arise due to primary thrombotic disorder or secondary to endothelial damage by toxins, infection, or inflammatory mediators. The presence of vasculitis in many of the associated conditions raises the possibility of portal venous radicle thrombosis occurring due to inflammation of the closely neighboring hepatic arterial radicles [77]. The pathology leads to portal hypertension, but does not otherwise impair liver function.

20.4.5 Diagnosis

INCPH should be considered in children who present with splenomegaly with or without other evidence of portal hypertension on imaging, in whom other more common causes of these manifestations have been ruled out. Complications from portal hypertension such as gastrointestinal bleeding and ascites may occur and for some patients may be the initial reason for seeking medical attention. Liver enzymes are frequently normal or only slightly elevated, and synthetic liver function is normal. Hypersplenism may cause cytopenias in the peripheral blood count. Hyperammonemia and hepatopulmonary syndrome have been reported in children with INCPH.

Imaging studies help to demonstrate findings of portal hypertension, to rule out other causes of portal hypertension, and to confirm that the portal vein is patent. Transient elastography of the liver may show that its stiffness is elevated in the intermediate range between normal and values found in cirrhosis [78].

Liver biopsy is required to confirm the diagnosis of INCPH. However, interpretation of the biopsy may be difficult because this is a rare disease in pediatrics with changes that are often subtle and patchy. The histological lesion includes obliteration of small intrahepatic portal veins [69]. Many portal tracts lack a normal-sized portal vein, and portal veins that are present have thickening of the media of the wall. Inflammation is absent or mild. Reduction of portal blood flow leads to atrophy of liver cell plates in the perivenular areas, resulting in portal tracts being abnormally close to each other. Compensatory hyperplasia of hepatocytes in the areas that remain well perfused results in regenerative small nodules from 1 to 3 mm (nodular regenerative hyperplasia). Fine fibrous septa may appear in the areas of parenchymal atrophy, but do not link to each other (incomplete septal cirrhosis). Biliary features may be present in the form of periductular fibrosis without loss of bile ducts [68, 74].

20.4.6 Treatment

Treatment of INCPH consists of the management of the complications of portal hypertension. It is currently unclear whether there is a role for anticoagulation therapy to address the possible etiological role of small vessel thrombosis [67, 79, 80].

20.5 Congenital Vascular Malformations

20.5.1 Definition

Pediatric vascular malformations can be classified as hemangiomas if the lesion exhibits cellular proliferation and hyperplasia or as vascular malformations if there is normal endothelial turnover. Liver hemangiomas may regress, but arteriovenous malformations do not regress and are associated with higher morbidity and mortality [81, 82].

Liver vascular malformations cause abnormal shunting of blood in the liver. These malformations are most often congenital but may be acquired after abdominal blunt trauma, liver biopsy, cholangiography, or surgery. Shunting can occur from the hepatic artery to the hepatic vein (arteriovenous or arteriohepatic), from the hepatic artery to the portal vein (arterioportal), or from the portal vein to the systemic circulation (portosystemic). In hereditary hemorrhagic telangiectasia, these three types of shunts may coexist.

20.5.1.1 Arteriovenous Malformation (AVM)
Isolated AVM is a rare malformation presenting in the perinatal period with the clinical triad of hepatomegaly, anemia, and cardiac congestive failure. Persistent pulmonary hypertension has also been reported. The literature is scarce, and in many publications, the term AVM is used to refer to infantile hepatic hemangioma. The mortality rate among reported cases is high, and it is therefore important to strive for early diagnosis before cardiopulmonary vascular complications become irreversible. The treatment options include embolization, surgical ligation, or liver transplantation [81, 83, 84].

20.5.1.2 Liver Involvement in Hereditary Hemorrhagic Telangiectasia

Epidemiology

Hereditary hemorrhagic telangiectasia (HHT), or Rendu-Osler-Weber disease, has an estimated prevalence of 1–2 cases per 10,000 population. Liver vascular malformations are present in 32–78% of the patients, but only about 8% are symptomatic [85–87].

20.5.2 Etiology

HHT is an autosomal dominant disease that can arise from mutations in one of three genes involved in the TGF-beta pathway, endoglin (*ENG*, in 39–59% of patients), activin A receptor type II-like 1 (*ACVRL1*, in 25–57%), and *SMAD4* (in 1–2% of patients, 10% of those testing negative for *ENG* and *ACVRL1* mutations). Juvenile polyposis may occur simultaneously in patients with *SMAD4* mutations [85, 86].

20.5.3 Pathophysiology

Hepatic vascular lesions in HHT range from small telangiectases to the coexistence of the three types of intrahepatic shunting (arteriovenous, arterioportal, and portosystemic). Usually one type of shunt is predominant, although the type of predominant shunt may change with time. Shunting of blood through these malformations may result in high-output cardiac failure, portal hypertension, and impaired arterial blood supply to neighboring areas or organs due to arterial steal. This steal syndrome may result in biliary ischemia and biliary strictures.

20.5.4 Diagnosis of HHT

HHT should be considered in patients with vascular malformation in the liver, especially those who also present with cutaneous and/or mucosal telangiectasias (e.g., epistaxis or GI bleeding) or visceral vascular malformations especially involving the lungs or brain. The diagnosis of liver involvement can occur at any age, from infancy onwards [88]. Clinical features at presentation may include hepatomegaly, a palpable thrill over the liver, features of portal hypertension, and jaundice [28, 85–87, 89, 90].

HHT is diagnosed by clinical criteria and genetic testing. The Curaçao criteria are based on four diagnostic clinical features: spontaneous and recurrent epistaxis; multiple telangiectasias located in the oral cavity and lips, fingers, or nose; the presence of visceral lesions such as gastrointestinal telangiectasias and pulmonary, hepatic cerebral, or spinal AVMs; and the presence of a first-degree relative with HHT. Patients who fulfill three or more criteria are considered to be definite HHT, two criteria indicate possible HHT, and the diagnosis is unlikely if only one or none of the criteria are present [91]. Genetic testing is used to identify a specific mutation in a family and enables diagnostic screening among relatives of affected individuals.

Diagnosis of hepatic vascular lesions begins with Doppler ultrasound evaluation, which may show a dilated hepatic artery with elevated hepatic artery flow and intrahepatic vascularity that is suggestive of vascular malformations. CT scan and/or MRI may enable further understanding of the vascular anatomy when planning for therapeutic interventions. Irregular blood flow to different areas of the liver may cause nodular regenerative hyperplasia and a nodular appearance on imaging. Liver biopsy is not usually required for diagnosis and is best avoided due to the high risk of bleeding [92, 93].

20.5.5 Treatment of Liver Manifestations of HHT

AVMs may be amenable to interventional radiology approaches to embolization, but the balance between risks and benefits of hepatic arterial embolization may not be favorable. Improvement in cardiac symptoms may only be temporary, and there are considerable risks for ischemic hepatobiliary complications. Liver transplantation should be considered in the setting of ischemic biliary necrosis, intractable heart failure, or intractable portal hypertension [85].

Bevacizumab, an anti-vascular endothelial growth factor antibody, may be a therapeutic option in the treatment of associated complications of liver vascular malformations in HHT. Initial studies suggest that it reduces cardiac output in patients with hepatic vascular malformations and potentially avoids the need for liver transplantation. Further studies are needed to more clearly determine its role [94–96].

20.6 Congenital Portosystemic Shunts

20.6.1 Definition

Congenital portosystemic shunts (CPSS) are rare venous malformations that allow intestinal blood to bypass the hepatic sinusoids.

20.6.2 Epidemiology

The incidence of CPSS is not known, although it is a rare pathology. It can be diagnosed at any age from infancy to late adulthood. Approximately 9% of reported cases have associated chromosomal abnormalities, and 22% have congenital heart disease.

20.6.3 Etiology

The precise causes of this developmental abnormality have not been elucidated.

20.6.4 Pathophysiology

Intrahepatic shunts can occur in one or in both lobes and consist of one or multiple connections between branches of the portal and hepatic veins [97]. Extrahepatic portosystemic shunts are also known as the "Abernethy malformation" and may be associated with apparent absence (Abernethy type 1) or preservation (Abernethy type 2) of portal venous flow to the liver [98]. A patent ductus venosus is sometimes included within the classification of intrahepatic CPSS, despite its course in the ligamentum venosum from the left portal vein to a hepatic vein.

Complications arise due to portosystemic shunting of intestinal blood (minimal hepatic encephalopathy, hepatopulmonary syndrome, portopulmonary hypertension) and associated abnormal hepatic blood flow (focal nodular hyperplasia, nodular regenerative hyperplasia). No mechanistic explanation has yet been found for the rare occurrence of hepatic adenoma, hepatocellular carcinoma, and hepatoblastoma in children with CPSS.

20.6.5 Diagnosis

CPSS may present in asymptomatic children or adults following abdominal imaging that was ordered for other reasons or may present with neurodevelopmental, hepatic, or cardiopulmonary manifestations. Portal hypertension is not a feature of CPSS, in which shunting of blood is not associated with increased resistance to flow. Associated laboratory abnormalities include elevated blood ammonia, galactose, conjugated bilirubin, bile acids, and aminotransferases.

CPSS may cause hepatic encephalopathy that can present with learning difficulties, behavioral issues, or developmental delay. Approximately a quarter of children with CPSS develop benign liver masses, most commonly associated with extrahepatic shunts [99]. Rare occurrence of malignant tumors has also been reported, necessitating careful imaging and possible biopsy when hepatic masses are identified [100, 101]. Both hepatopulmonary syndrome and portopulmonary hypertension have been reported in association with CPSS [102].

20.6.6 Treatment

Intrahepatic CPSS may close spontaneously within the first year of life, and interventions for this subtype are therefore best delayed until after the first birthday. Larger caliber extrahepatic shunts, including Abernethy type 1 malformations, are not expected to close spontaneously.

It is unclear whether all persistent CPSS will eventually cause problems and therefore the decision to provide an intervention to close a shunt in an asymptomatic child is addressed on a case-by-case basis and related to the availability of appropriate expertise and a calculation of the potential risks and benefits. Therapeutic intervention is indicated for lesions with deleterious associated clinical manifestations in a child in whom spontaneous closure is not expected. Current therapeutic options include interventional radiology embolization or closure devices, surgical ligation, or liver transplantation [103, 104]. Closure is likely to be successful even when the intrahepatic venous circulation is not apparent on Doppler ultrasound or other imaging techniques, although a two-stage surgical approach may be required to enable gradual adaptation of the atrophied intrahepatic portal veins to accommodate the newly increased blood flow [105].

20.7 Infantile Hepatic Hemangiomas (IHH)

20.7.1 Epidemiology

Infantile hemangiomas are the most common benign tumor in infancy, affecting 1–2% of newborns and around 10% of infants by 1 year of age [81]. The majority of the lesions involve the skin and subcutaneous tissue, but a subset of infants may also present with lesions elsewhere, including the liver. Infantile hepatic hemangioma (IHH) is the most common pediatric liver tumor and affects females more frequently than males. This tumor may also be called a hemangioendothelioma.

20.7.2 Etiology

The cause of this developmental vascular abnormality has not been clearly defined.

20.7.3 Pathophysiology

IHH are characterized by excess endothelial proliferation and hyperplasia. Endothelial cells demonstrate positive immunohistochemical staining for GLUT1 that distinguishes these lesions from other vascular malformations [106].

IHH can be divided into three groups, focal, multifocal, and diffuse [107]. Lesions follow a natural history of initial proliferation (from birth to 9–12 months), a variable period of stability, and then slow involution (2–10 years) [108].

In some infants, overproduction of type III iodothyronine deiodinase by the IHH promotes inactivation of thyroxine and results in hypothyroidism. Other rare clinical presentations include fulminant hepatic failure when the lesion replaces nearly all the liver parenchyma and intraperitoneal hemorrhage following rupture of hemangiomas located at the liver surface [83, 109, 110].

20.7.4 Diagnosis

Single focal IHH are usually asymptomatic, without associated skin lesions, and diagnosed incidentally when an ultrasound scan of the liver is performed for other reasons. In larger lesions containing high-flow arteriovenous shunts, high-output cardiac failure may occur [111, 112].

Diagnosis of single, focal IHH relies on characteristic findings on imaging studies [83], especially because liver biopsy of these vascular lesions carries a high risk of bleeding. When imaged by ultrasound scan, IHH appears as a well-defined hypo- or hyperechoic lesion with heterogeneous echotexture. Doppler findings vary depending on the presence and type of vascular shunt. MRI scan reveals a well-defined, hypointense lesion on T1-weighted images and hyperintense on T2-weighted scans, with centripetal enhancement after gadolinium contrast [81]. Areas of necrosis, thrombosis, or hemorrhage lead to a heterogeneous appearance on imaging studies. Calcifications are present in about 16% of cases.

Multifocal and diffuse IHH may also be asymptomatic and diagnosed only when visceral screening is undertaken in a child with more than five skin hemangiomas. Symptomatic presentation usually involves hepatomegaly and high-output congestive heart failure. Anemia and thrombocytopenia occur secondary to consumption, hemorrhage, or thrombosis within the hemangiomas. Hemolysis may give rise to jaundice. In rare cases, severe hepatomegaly may lead to respiratory compromise or abdominal compartment syndrome [83, 109, 111, 113]. Ultrasound imaging usually confirms the diagnosis in the clinical scenario of a child with multiple cutaneous lesions, showing small multifocal hepatic lesions that are homogenous and most commonly hypoechoic. The hepatic vessels may appear enlarged, and the scan may show feeding arteries and draining veins associated with the lesions.

Children with IHH should be tested for hypothyroidism. Cases of hepatic angiosarcoma have been reported in association with multiple cutaneous infantile hemangiomas. Children with an unclear imaging diagnosis and those who present after 1 year of age may require liver biopsy [114].

20.7.5 Treatment

Asymptomatic focal IHH lesions usually do not proliferate in the postnatal period and can be observed with serial imaging studies. Although the efficacy of medical treatment for larger single symptomatic lesions is unknown, a trial of medical therapy (see below) is recommended before considering embolization or surgical resection [109].

Asymptomatic infants with multinodular IHH without shunts or hypothyroidism can also be observed. In diffuse forms and symptomatic multinodular IHH with high-output cardiac failure or hypothyroidism, medical treatment is the first step of therapy [109, 111].

First-line therapy for IHH in infants requiring treatment is propranolol 1–3 mg/kg/day. Treatment with this nonselective β-blocker usually causes a few side effects. The mechanism of action is incompletely understood but may include vasoconstriction, decreased expression of angiogenic factors, increased apoptosis, and effects on the differentiation of mesenchymal stem cells. Treatment should continue until the end of the proliferation phase of IHH (usually 8–12 months of age). Second-line medical options include steroids, vincristine, and alfa-2a interferon, which are each troubled by more adverse effects than propranolol [115–118].

Surgical resection or embolization therapy is usually reserved for children in whom medical therapy has failed or those with life-threatening complications.

Embolization can result in improved cardiac function but IHH proliferation may continue. Early involvement of the liver transplant team is recommended in the presence of progressive cardiac failure or severe shunting [108, 111].

20.8 Vascular Malignancies

Hepatic angiosarcoma is a malignant neoplasm that is very rare in childhood. The clinical presentation is often as abdominal distension or hepatomegaly secondary to the presence of a hepatic mass. In some patients, associated multiple cutaneous hemangiomas lead to the misdiagnosis of multifocal IHH. The age of presentation is variable with a range from newborns to adolescence. Pulmonary metastases are common, and the overall prognosis is very poor with death often occurring within 6 months of diagnosis. Imaging characteristics are variable, often multifocal, and usually showing a heterogeneous enhancement pattern. Treatment options reported in the pediatric literature are vascular ablation, chemotherapy, and resection. Liver transplantation is controversial due to reported cases of posttransplant recurrence [114, 119, 120].

20.8.1 Hepatic Epithelioid Hemangioendothelioma

Hepatic epithelioid hemangioendothelioma is a low-grade malignant tumor mostly seen in adults but with occasional pediatric cases also reported. The appearance on ultrasound imaging is variable, including an individual nodule, multinodular changes, or a diffusely heterogeneous echotexture of the liver [83, 121]. It is commonly associated with bone and brain involvement. Surgery is the treatment of choice, because this tumor is not responsive to chemotherapy. Liver transplantation should be considered.

References

1. Sarin SK, Sollano JD, Chawla YK, Amarapurkar D, Hamid S, Hashizume M, et al. Consensus on extra-hepatic portal vein obstruction. Liver Int. 2006;26(5):512–9.
2. Senzolo M, Riggio O, Primignani M. Vascular disorders of the liver: recommendations from the Italian Association for the Study of the Liver (AISF) ad hoc committee. Dig Liver Dis. 2011;43(7):503–14.
3. Shneider BL, Bosch J, de Franchis R, Emre SH, Groszmann RJ, Ling SC, et al. Portal hypertension in children: expert pediatric opinion on the report of the Baveno V Consensus Workshop on Methodology of Diagnosis and Therapy in Portal Hypertension. Pediatr Transplant. 2012;16(5):426–37.
4. Plessier A, Rautou PE, Valla DC. Management of hepatic vascular diseases. J Hepatol. 2012;56(Suppl 1):S25–38. England: 2012 European Association for the Study of the Liver. Published by Elsevier B.V.
5. Garcia-Pagan JC, Hernandez-Guerra M, Bosch J. Extrahepatic portal vein thrombosis. Semin Liver Dis. 2008;28(3):282–92. PubMed PMID: 18814081. Epub 2008/09/25. eng.
6. Williams S, Chan AK. Neonatal portal vein thrombosis: diagnosis and management. Semin Fetal Neonatal Med. 2011;16(6):329–39.
7. Sakha SH, Rafeey M, Tarzamani MK. Portal venous thrombosis after umbilical vein catheterization. Indian J Gastroenterol. 2007;26(6):283–4. PubMed PMID: 18431012.
8. Morag I, Epelman M, Daneman A, Moineddin R, Parvez B, Shechter T, et al. Portal vein thrombosis in the neonate: risk factors, course, and outcome. J Pediatr. 2006;148(6):735–9. PubMed PMID: 16769378.
9. Morag I, Shah PS, Epelman M, Daneman A, Strauss T, Moore AM. Childhood outcomes of neonates diagnosed with portal vein thrombosis. J Paediatr Child Health. 2011;47(6):356–60. PubMed PMID: 21309882.
10. Seixas CA, Hessel G, Siqueira LH, Machado TF, Gallizoni AM, Annichino-Bizzacchi JM. Study of hemostasis in pediatric patients with portal vein thrombosis. Haematologica. 1998;83(10):955–6. PubMed PMID: 9830810.
11. Pinto RB, Silveira TR, Bandinelli E, Rohsig L. Portal vein thrombosis in children and adolescents: the low prevalence of hereditary thrombophilic disorders. J Pediatr Surg. 2004;39(9):1356–61. PubMed PMID: 15359390.
12. Abd El-Hamid N, Taylor RM, Marinello D, Mufti GJ, Patel R, Mieli-Vergani G, et al. Aetiology and management of extrahepatic portal vein obstruction in children: King's College Hospital experience. J Pediatr Gastroenterol Nutr. 2008;47(5):630–4. PubMed PMID: 18955865.
13. Pietrobattista A, Luciani M, Abraldes JG, Candusso M, Pancotti S, Soldati M, et al. Extrahepatic portal vein thrombosis in children and adolescents: influence of genetic thrombophilic disorders. World J Gastroenterol. 2010;16(48):6123–7. PubMed PMID: 21182228. Pubmed Central PMCID: 3012577.
14. Heller C, Schobess R, Kurnik K, Junker R, Gunther G, Kreuz W, et al. Abdominal venous thrombosis in neonates and infants: role of prothrombotic risk factors—a multicentre case-control study. For the Childhood Thrombophilia Study Group. Br J Haematol. 2000;111(2):534–9. PubMed PMID: 11122096.
15. El-Karaksy H, El-Koofy N, El-Hawary M, Mostafa A, Aziz M, El-Shabrawi M, et al. Prevalence of factor V Leiden mutation and other hereditary thrombophilic factors in Egyptian children with portal vein thrombosis: results of a single-center case-control study. Ann Hematol. 2004;83(11):712–5. PubMed PMID: 15309526.
16. Mack CL, Superina RA, Whitington PF. Surgical restoration of portal flow corrects procoagulant and anticoagulant deficiencies associated with extrahepatic portal vein thrombosis. J Pediatr. 2003;142(2):197–9. PubMed PMID: 12584545.
17. Carnevale R, Raparelli V, Nocella C, Bartimoccia S, Novo M, Severino A, et al. Gut-derived endotoxin stimulates factor VIII secretion from endothelial cells. Implications for hypercoagulability in cirrhosis. J Hepatol. 2017;67(5):950–6.
18. Odievre M, Pige G, Alagille D. Congenital abnormalities associated with extrahepatic portal hypertension. Arch Dis Child. 1977;52(5):383–5. PubMed PMID: 869567. Pubmed Central PMCID: PMC1544565. Epub 1977/05/01. eng.
19. Suchy FJ, Sokol RJ, Balistreri WF. Liver disease in children. 3rd ed. Cambridge: Cambridge University Press; 2007. xvii, 1030 p., 22 p. of plates p.
20. Valla DC, Condat B. Portal vein thrombosis in adults: pathophysiology, pathogenesis and management. J Hepatol. 2000;32(5):865–71. PubMed PMID: WOS:000086871500022.
21. Shneider B, Emre S, Groszmann R, Karani J, McKiernan P, Sarin S, et al. Expert pediatric opinion on the Report of the Baveno IV consensus workshop on methodology of diagnosis and therapy in portal hypertension. Pediatr Transplant. 2006;10(8):893–907. PubMed PMID: 17096755.
22. Sarin SK, Bansal A, Sasan S, Nigam A. Portal-vein obstruction in children leads to growth retardation. Hepatology. 1992;15(2):229–33. PubMed PMID: 1735525.
23. Mehrotra RN, Bhatia V, Dabadghao P, Yachha SK. Extrahepatic portal vein obstruction in children: anthropometry, growth hormone, and insulin-like growth factor I. J Pediatr Gastroenterol Nutr. 1997;25(5):520–3. PubMed PMID: 9360206.
24. Alvarez F, Bernard O, Brunelle F, Hadchouel P, Odievre M, Alagille D. Portal obstruction in children. I. Clinical investigation and hemorrhage risk. J Pediatr. 1983;103(5):696–702. PubMed PMID: 6605419.
25. Khuroo MS, Yattoo GN, Zargar SA, Javid G, Dar MY, Khan BA, et al. Biliary abnormalities associated with extrahepatic portal venous obstruction. Hepatology. 1993;17(5):807–13. PubMed PMID: 8491448.
26. Gauthier-Villars M, Franchi S, Gauthier F, Fabre M, Pariente D, Bernard O. Cholestasis in children with portal vein obstruction. J Pediatr. 2005;146(4):568–73. PubMed PMID: 15812469.
27. de Franchis R, Baveno VF. Revising consensus in portal hypertension: report of the Baveno V consensus workshop on methodology of diagnosis and therapy in portal hypertension. J Hepatol. 2010;53(4):762–8. PubMed PMID: 20638742.
28. DeLeve LD, Valla DC, Garcia-Tsao G. Vascular disorders of the liver. Hepatology. 2009;49(5):1729–64. PubMed PMID: 19399912. Epub 2009/04/29. eng
29. Mack CL, Zelko FA, Lokar J, Superina R, Alonso EM, Blei AT, et al. Surgically restoring portal blood flow to the liver in children

with primary extrahepatic portal vein thrombosis improves fluid neurocognitive ability. Pediatrics. 2006;117(3):e405–12.
30. Superina R, Bambini DA, Lokar J, Rigsby C, Whitington PF. Correction of extrahepatic portal vein thrombosis by the mesenteric to left portal vein bypass. Ann Surg. 2006;243(4):515–21. PubMed PMID: 16552203. Pubmed Central PMCID: 1448975.
31. Superina R, Shneider B, Emre S, Sarin S, de Ville de Goyet J. Surgical guidelines for the management of extra-hepatic portal vein obstruction. Pediatr Transplant. 2006;10(8):908–13. PubMed PMID: 17096756.
32. Shneider BL, de Ville de Goyet J, Leung DH, Srivastava A, Ling SC, Duché M, et al. Primary prophylaxis of variceal bleeding in children and the role of MesoRex Bypass: summary of the Baveno VI Pediatric Satellite Symposium. Hepatology. 2016;63(4):1368–80.
33. Ling SC, Walters T, McKiernan PJ, Schwarz KB, Garcia-Tsao G, Shneider BL. Primary prophylaxis of variceal hemorrhage in children with portal hypertension: a framework for future research. J Pediatr Gastroenterol Nutr. 2011;52(3):254–61. PubMed PMID: 21336158.
34. Coppell JA, Richardson PG, Soiffer R, Martin PL, Kernan NA, Chen A, et al. Hepatic veno-occlusive disease following stem cell transplantation: incidence, clinical course, and outcome. Biol Blood Marrow Transplant. 2010;16(2):157–68. PubMed PMID: 19766729. Pubmed Central PMCID: 3018714.
35. Carreras E, Diaz-Beya M, Rosinol L, Martinez C, Fernandez-Aviles F, Rovira M. The incidence of veno-occlusive disease following allogeneic hematopoietic stem cell transplantation has diminished and the outcome improved over the last decade. Biol Blood Marrow Transplant. 2011;17(11):1713–20.
36. McDonald GB. Hepatobiliary complications of hematopoietic cell transplantation, 40 years on. Hepatology. 2010;51(4):1450–60. PubMed PMID: 20373370. Pubmed Central PMCID: PMC2914093. Epub 2010/04/08. eng
37. McDonald GB, Hinds MS, Fisher LD, Schoch HG, Wolford JL, Banaji M, et al. Veno-occlusive disease of the liver and multiorgan failure after bone marrow transplantation: a cohort study of 355 patients. Ann Intern Med. 1993;118(4):255–67. PubMed PMID: 8420443.
38. Jones RJ, Lee KS, Beschorner WE, Vogel VG, Grochow LB, Braine HG, et al. Venoocclusive disease of the liver following bone marrow transplantation. Transplantation. 1987;44(6):778–83. PubMed PMID: 3321587.
39. Corbacioglu S, Cesaro S, Faraci M, Valteau-Couanet D, Gruhn B, Rovelli A, et al. Defibrotide for prophylaxis of hepatic veno-occlusive disease in paediatric haemopoietic stem-cell transplantation: an open-label, phase 3, randomised controlled trial. Lancet. 2012;379(9823):1301–9. PubMed PMID: 22364685. Epub 2012/03/01. eng.
40. Carreras E, Granena A, Navasa M, Bruguera M, Marco V, Sierra J, et al. On the reliability of clinical criteria for the diagnosis of hepatic veno-occlusive disease. Ann Hematol. 1993;66(2):77–80. PubMed PMID: 8448243. Epub 1993/02/01. eng.
41. Richardson PG, Murakami C, Jin Z, Warren D, Momtaz P, Hoppensteadt D, et al. Multi-institutional use of defibrotide in 88 patients after stem cell transplantation with severe veno-occlusive disease and multisystem organ failure: response without significant toxicity in a high-risk population and factors predictive of outcome. Blood. 2002;100(13):4337–43. PubMed PMID: 12393437.
42. Richardson PG, Soiffer RJ, Antin JH, Uno H, Jin Z, Kurtzberg J, et al. Defibrotide for the treatment of severe hepatic veno-occlusive disease and multiorgan failure after stem cell transplantation: a multicenter, randomized, dose-finding trial. Biol Blood Marrow Transplant. 2010;16(7):1005–17. PubMed PMID: 20167278. Pubmed Central PMCID: PMC2956581. Epub 2010/02/20. eng.
43. Richardson PG, Riches ML, Kernan NA, Brochstein JA, Mineishi S, Termuhlenet AM, et al. Phase 3 trial of defibrotide for the treatment of severe veno-occlusive disease and multi-organ failure. Blood. 2016;127(13):1656–65.
44. Reiss U, Cowan M, McMillan A, Horn B. Hepatic venoocclusive disease in blood and bone marrow transplantation in children and young adults: incidence, risk factors, and outcome in a cohort of 241 patients. J Pediatr Hematol Oncol. 2002;24(9):746–50. PubMed PMID: 12468917. Epub 2002/12/07. eng.
45. DeLeve LD. Vascular liver diseases. Curr Gastroenterol Rep. 2003;5(1):63–70. PubMed PMID: 12530950. Epub 2003/01/18. eng.
46. Puig N, de la Rubia J, Remigia MJ, Jarque I, Martin G, Cupelli L, et al. Morbidity and transplant-related mortality of CBV and BEAM preparative regimens for patients with lymphoid malignancies undergoing autologous stem-cell transplantation. Leuk Lymphoma. 2006;47(8):1488–94. PubMed PMID: 16966258. Epub 2006/09/13. eng.
47. de Lima M, Couriel D, Thall PF, Wang X, Madden T, Jones R, et al. Once-daily intravenous busulfan and fludarabine: clinical and pharmacokinetic results of a myeloablative, reduced-toxicity conditioning regimen for allogeneic stem cell transplantation in AML and MDS. Blood. 2004;104(3):857–64. PubMed PMID: 15073038. Epub 2004/04/10. eng.
48. Tay J, Tinmouth A, Fergusson D, Huebsch L, Allan DS. Systematic review of controlled clinical trials on the use of ursodeoxycholic acid for the prevention of hepatic veno-occlusive disease in hematopoietic stem cell transplantation. Biol Blood Marrow Transplant. 2007;13(2):206–17. PubMed PMID: 17241926. Epub 2007/01/24. eng.
49. Horton JD, San Miguel FL, Membreno F, Wright F, Paima J, Foster P, et al. Budd-Chiari syndrome: illustrated review of current management. Liver Int. 2008;28(4):455–66.
50. Valla DC. Primary Budd-Chiari syndrome. J Hepatol. 2009;50(1):195–203.
51. Valla D-C. Hepatic venous outflow tract obstruction etiopathogenesis: Asia versus the West. J Gastroenterol Hepatol. 2004;19:S204–S11.
52. Darwish Murad S, Plessier A, Hernandez-Guerra M, Fabris F, Eapen CE, Bahr MJ, et al. Etiology, management, and outcome of the Budd-Chiari syndrome. Ann Intern Med. 2009;151:167–75.
53. Shetty S, Ghosh K. Thrombophilic dimension of Budd chiari syndrome and portal venous thrombosis—a concise review. Thromb Res. 2011;127:505–12.
54. Deltenre P, Denninger MH, Hillaire S, Guillin MC, Casadevall N, Briere J, et al. Factor V Leiden related Budd-Chiari syndrome. Gut. 2001;48(2):264–8. PubMed PMID: 11156651. Pubmed Central PMCID: PMC1728208. Epub 2001/01/13. eng.
55. Nagral A, Hasija RP, Marar S, Nabi F. Budd-Chiari syndrome in children: experience with therapeutic radiological intervention. J Pediatr Gastroenterol Nutr. 2010;50(1):74–8. PubMed PMID: 19915494. Epub 2009/11/17. eng.
56. Nobre S, Khanna R, Bab N, Kyranam E, Height S, Karani J, et al. Primary Budd-Chiari Syndrome in Children: King's College Hospital Experience. J Pediatr Gastroenterol Nutr. 2017;65(1):93–6.
57. Vickers CR, West RJ, Hubscher SG, Elias E. Hepatic vein webs and resistant ascites. Diagnosis, management and implications. J Hepatol. 1989;8(3):287–93. PubMed PMID: 2732442. Epub 1989/05/01. eng.
58. Kage M, Arakawa M, Kojiro M, Okuda K. Histopathology of membranous obstruction of the inferior vena cava in the Budd-Chiari syndrome. Gastroenterology. 1992;102(6):2081–90. PubMed PMID: 1587428.
59. Paradis V, Bièche I, Dargère D, et al. Quantitative gene expression in Budd-Chiari syndrome: a molecular approach to the pathogenesis of the disease. Gut. 2005;54:1776–81.

60. Hadengue A, Poliquin M, Vilgrain V, Belghiti J, Degott C, Erlinger S, et al. The changing scene of hepatic vein thrombosis: recognition of asymptomatic cases. Gastroenterology. 1994;106(4):1042–7. PubMed PMID: 8143970. Epub 1994/04/01. eng.
61. Gentil-Kocher S, Bernard O, Brunelle F, Hadchouel M, Maillard JN, Valayer J, et al. Budd-Chiari syndrome in children: report of 22 cases. J Pediatr. 1988;113(1 Pt 1):30–8. PubMed PMID: 3290415. Epub 1988/07/01. eng.
62. MacSween RNM, Anthony PP, Scheuer PJ. Pathology of the liver. New York: Churchill Livingstone; 1979; distributed in U.S. by Longman. 458 p.
63. Cauchi JA, Oliff S, Baumann U, Mirza D, Kelly DA, Hewitson J, et al. The Budd-Chiari syndrome in children: the spectrum of management. J Pediatr Surg. 2006;41(11):1919–23. PubMed PMID: 17101371. Epub 2006/11/15. eng.
64. Gomes AC, Rubino G, Pinto C, Cipriano A, Furtado E, Goncalves I. Budd-Chiari syndrome in children and outcome after liver transplant. Pediatr Transplant. 2012;16(8):E338–41. PubMed PMID: 22452639.
65. Nezakatgoo N, Shokouh-Amiri MH, Gaber AO, Grewal HP, Vera SR, Chamsuddin AA, et al. Liver transplantation for acute Budd-Chiari syndrome in identical twin sisters with Factor V leiden mutation. Transplantation. 2003;76(1):195–8. PubMed PMID: 12865809. Epub 2003/07/17. eng.
66. Odell JA, Rode H, Millar AJ, Hoffman HD. Surgical repair in children with the Budd-Chiari syndrome. J Thorac Cardiovasc Surg. 1995;110(4 Pt 1):916–23. PubMed PMID: 7475157. Epub 1995/10/01. eng.
67. Schouten JN, Garcia-Pagan JC, Valla DC, Janssen HL. Idiopathic noncirrhotic portal hypertension. Hepatology. 2011;54(3):1071–81. PubMed PMID: 21574171. Epub 2011/05/17. eng.
68. Hübscher SG. Pathology of non-cirrhotic portal hypertension and incomplete septal cirrhosis. Diagnost Histopathol. 2011;17(12):530–8.
69. Nakanuma Y, Hoso M, Sasaki M, Terada T, Katayanagi K, Nonomura A, et al. Histopathology of the liver in non-cirrhotic portal hypertension of unknown aetiology. Histopathology. 1996;28(3):195–204. PubMed PMID: 8729037. Epub 1996/03/01. eng.
70. Dhiman RK, Chawla Y, Vasishta RK, Kakkar N, Dilawari JB, Trehan MS, et al. Non-cirrhotic portal fibrosis (idiopathic portal hypertension): experience with 151 patients and a review of the literature. J Gastroenterol Hepatol. 2002;17:6–16.
71. Wanless IR. Micronodular transformation (nodular regenerative hyperplasia) of the liver: a report of 64 cases among 2,500 autopsies and a new classification of benign hepatocellular nodules. Hepatology. 1990;11(5):787–97.
72. Hillaire S, Bonte E, Denninger MH, Casadevall N, Cadranel JF, Lebrec D, et al. Idiopathic non-cirrhotic intrahepatic portal hypertension in the West: a re-evaluation in 28 patients. Gut. 2002;51(2):275–80. PubMed PMID: 12117894. Pubmed Central PMCID: PMC1773310. Epub 2002/07/16. eng.
73. Sarin SK, Agarwal SR. Extrahepatic portal vein obstruction. Semin Liver Dis. 2002;22(1):43–58. PubMed PMID: 11928078.
74. Yilmaz G, Sari S, Egritas O, Dalgic B, Akyol G. Hepatoportal sclerosis in childhood: some presenting with cholestatic features (a re-evaluation of 12 children). Pediatr Dev Pathol. 2012;15(2):107–13. PubMed PMID: 22150463. Epub 2011/12/14. eng.
75. Eapen CE, Nightingale P, Hubscher SG, Lane PJ, Plant T, Velissaris D, et al. Non-cirrhotic intrahepatic portal hypertension: associated gut diseases and prognostic factors. Dig Dis Sci. 2011;56(1):227–35. PubMed PMID: 20499175. Epub 2010/05/26. eng.
76. Wanless IR, Godwin TA, Allen F, Feder A. Nodular regenerative hyperplasia of the liver in hematologic disorders: a possible response to obliterative portal venopathy. A morphometric study of nine cases with an hypothesis on the pathogenesis. Medicine (Baltimore). 1980;59(5):367–79.
77. Reynolds WJ, Wanless IR. Nodular regenerative hyperplasia of the liver in a patient with rheumatoid vasculitis: a morphometric study suggesting a role for hepatic arteritis in the pathogenesis. J Rheumatol. 1984;11(6):838–42.
78. Seijo S, Reverter E, Miquel R, Berzigotti A, Abraldes JG, Bosch J, García-Pagán JC. Role of hepatic vein catheterisation and transient elastography in the diagnosis of idiopathic portal hypertension. Dig Liver Dis. 2012;44(10):855–60. https://doi.org/10.1016/j.dld.2012.05.005. Epub 2012 Jun 19. PubMed PMID: 22721839.
79. Dabritz J, Worch J, Materna U, Koch B, Koehler G, Duck C, et al. Life-threatening hypersplenism due to idiopathic portal hypertension in early childhood: case report and review of the literature. BMC Gastroenterol. 2010;10:122. PubMed PMID: 20961440. Pubmed Central PMCID: PMC2988068. Epub 2010/10/22. eng.
80. Al-Mukhaizeem KA, Rosenberg A, Sherker AH. Nodular regenerative hyperplasia of the liver: an under-recognized cause of portal hypertension in hematological disorders. Am J Hematol. 2004;75(4):225–30. PubMed PMID: 15054815. Epub 2004/04/01. eng.
81. Boon LM, Burrows PE, Paltiel HJ, Lund DP, Ezekowitz RA, Folkman J, et al. Hepatic vascular anomalies in infancy: a twenty-seven-year experience. J Pediatr. 1996;129(3):346–54.
82. Mulliken JB, Glowacki J. Classification of pediatric vascular lesions. Plast Reconstr Surg. 1982;70(1):120–1.
83. Burrows PE, Dubois J, Kassarjian A. Pediatric hepatic vascular anomalies. Pediatr Radiol. 2001;31(8):533–45.
84. Alexander CP, Sood BG, Zilberman MV, Becker C, Bedard MP. Congenital hepatic arteriovenous malformation: an unusual cause of neonatal persistent pulmonary hypertension. J Perinatol. 2006;26(5):316–8.
85. Faughnan ME, Palda VA, Garcia-Tsao G, Geisthoff UW, McDonald J, Proctor DD, et al. International guidelines for the diagnosis and management of hereditary haemorrhagic telangiectasia. J Med Genet. 2011;48(2):73–87.
86. Garcia-Tsao G. Liver involvement in hereditary hemorrhagic telangiectasia (HHT). J Hepatol. 2007;46(3):499–507.
87. Buscarini E, Leandro G, Conte D, Danesino C, Daina E, Manfredi G, et al. Natural history and outcome of hepatic vascular malformations in a large cohort of patients with hereditary hemorrhagic teleangiectasia. Dig Dis Sci. 2011;56(7):2166–78.
88. Al-Saleh S, John PR, Letarte M, Faughnan ME, Belik J, Ratjen F. Symptomatic liver involvement in neonatal hereditary hemorrhagic telangiectasia. Pediatrics. 2011;127(6):e1615–20.
89. Brenard R, Chapaux X, Deltenre P, Henrion J, De Maeght S, Horsmans Y, et al. Large spectrum of liver vascular lesions including high prevalence of focal nodular hyperplasia in patients with hereditary haemorrhagic telangiectasia: the Belgian Registry based on 30 patients. Eur J Gastroenterol Hepatol. 2010;22(10):1253–9.
90. Garcia-Tsao G, Korzenik JR, Young L, Henderson KJ, Jain D, Byrd B, et al. Liver disease in patients with hereditary hemorrhagic telangiectasia. N Engl J Med. 2000;343(13):931–6.
91. Shovlin CL, Guttmacher AE, Buscarini E, Faughnan ME, Hyland RH, Westermann CJ, et al. Diagnostic criteria for hereditary hemorrhagic telangiectasia (Rendu-Osler-Weber syndrome). Am J Med Genet. 2000;91(1):66–7.
92. Memeo M, Stabile Ianora AA, Scardapane A, Suppressa P, Cirulli A, Sabba C, et al. Hereditary haemorrhagic telangiectasia: study of hepatic vascular alterations with multi-detector row helical CT and reconstruction programs. Radiol Med. 2005;109(1–2):125–38.
93. Buscarini E, Plauchu H, Garcia Tsao G, White RI Jr, Sabba C, Miller F, et al. Liver involvement in hereditary hemorrhagic telangiectasia: consensus recommendations. Liver Int. 2006;26(9):1040–6.

94. Dupuis-Girod S, Ginon I, Saurin JC, Marion D, Guillot E, Decullier E, et al. Bevacizumab in patients with hereditary hemorrhagic telangiectasia and severe hepatic vascular malformations and high cardiac output. JAMA. 2012;307(9):948–55.
95. Mitchell A, Adams LA, MacQuillan G, Tibballs J, vanden Driesen R, Delriviere L. Bevacizumab reverses need for liver transplantation in hereditary hemorrhagic telangiectasia. Liver Transplant. 2008;14(2):210–3.
96. Guilhem A, Fargeton AE, Simon AC, Duffau P, Harle JR, Lavigne C, et al. Intra-venous bevacizumab in hereditary hemorrhagic telangiectasia (HHT): a retrospective study of 46 patients. PLoS One. 2017;12(11):e0188943.
97. Park JH, Cha SH, Han JK, Han MC. Intrahepatic portosystemic venous shunt. AJR Am J Roentgenol. 1990;155(3):527–8.
98. Morgan G, Superina R. Congenital absence of the portal vein: two cases and a proposed classification system for portasystemic vascular anomalies. J Pediatr Surg. 1994;29(9):1239–41.
99. Kondo F. Benign nodular hepatocellular lesions caused by abnormal hepatic circulation: etiological analysis and introduction of a new concept. J Gastroenterol Hepatol. 2001;16(12):1319–28.
100. Barton JW 3rd, Keller MS. Liver transplantation for hepatoblastoma in a child with congenital absence of the portal vein. Pediatr Radiol. 1989;20(1–2):113–4.
101. Pichon N, Maisonnette F, Pichon-Lefievre F, Valleix D, Pillegand B. Hepatocarcinoma with congenital agenesis of the portal vein. Jpn J Clin Oncol. 2003;33(6):314–6.
102. Yagi H, Takada Y, Fujimoto Y, Ogura Y, Kozaki K, Ueda M, et al. Successful surgical ligation under intraoperative portal vein pressure monitoring of a large portosystemic shunt presenting as an intrapulmonary shunt: report of a case. Surg Today. 2004;34(12):1049–52.
103. Gillespie MJ, Golden A, Sivarajan VB, Rome JJ. Transcatheter closure of patent ductus venosus with the Amplatzer vascular plug in twin brothers. Pediatr Cardiol. 2006;27(1):142–5.
104. Ohnishi Y, Ueda M, Doi H, Kasahara M, Haga H, Kamei H, et al. Successful liver transplantation for congenital absence of the portal vein complicated by intrapulmonary shunt and brain abscess. J Pediatr Surg. 2005;40(5):e1–3.
105. Franchi-Abella S, Branchereau S, Lambert V, Fabre M, Steimberg C, Losay J, et al. Complications of congenital portosystemic shunts in children: therapeutic options and outcomes. J Pediatr Gastroenterol Nutr. 2010;51(3):322–30.
106. Mo JQ, Dimashkieh HH, Bove KE. GLUT1 endothelial reactivity distinguishes hepatic infantile hemangioma from congenital hepatic vascular malformation with associated capillary proliferation. Hum Pathol. 2004;35(2):200–9.
107. Frieden IJ, Haggstrom AN, Drolet BA, Mancini AJ, Friedlander SF, Boon L, et al. Infantile hemangiomas: current knowledge, future directions. Proceedings of a research workshop on infantile hemangiomas, April 7-9, 2005, Bethesda, Maryland, USA. Pediatr Dermatol. 2005;22(5):383–406.
108. Christison-Lagay ER, Burrows PE, Alomari A, Dubois J, Kozakewich HP, Lane TS, et al. Hepatic hemangiomas: subtype classification and development of a clinical practice algorithm and registry. J Pediatr Surg. 2007;42(1):62–7; discussion 7–8.
109. Kulungowski AM, Alomari AI, Chawla A, Christison-Lagay ER, Fishman SJ. Lessons from a liver hemangioma registry: subtype classification. J Pediatr Surg. 2012;47(1):165–70.
110. Huang SA, Tu HM, Harney JW, Venihaki M, Butte AJ, Kozakewich HP, et al. Severe hypothyroidism caused by type 3 iodothyronine deiodinase in infantile hemangiomas. N Engl J Med. 2000;343(3):185–9.
111. Dickie B, Dasgupta R, Nair R, Alonso MH, Ryckman FC, Tiao GM, et al. Spectrum of hepatic hemangiomas: management and outcome. J Pediatr Surg. 2009;44(1):125–33.
112. Hernandez F, Navarro M, Encinas JL, Lopez Gutierrez JC, Lopez Santamaria M, Leal N, et al. The role of GLUT1 immunostaining in the diagnosis and classification of liver vascular tumors in children. J Pediatr Surg. 2005;40(5):801–4.
113. Murphy AA, Herrmann E, Osinusi AO, Wu L, Sachau W, Lempicki RA, et al. Twice weekly PegIFN-Alfa 2a and ribavirin results in superior viral kinetics in HIV/HCV co-infected patients compared to standard therapy. AIDS. 2011;25(9):1179–87.
114. Nord KM, Kandel J, Lefkowitch JH, Lobritto SJ, Morel KD, North PE, et al. Multiple cutaneous infantile hemangiomas associated with hepatic angiosarcoma: case report and review of the literature. Pediatrics. 2006;118(3):e907–13.
115. Leaute-Labreze C, Dumas de la Roque E, Hubiche T, Boralevi F, Thambo JB, Taieb A Propranolol for severe hemangiomas of infancy. N Engl J Med. 2008;358(24):2649–51.
116. Mhanna A, Franklin WH, Mancini AJ. Hepatic infantile hemangiomas treated with oral propranolol—a case series. Pediatr Dermatol. 2011;28(1):39–45.
117. Sans V, de la Roque ED, Berge J, Grenier N, Boralevi F, Mazereeuw-Hautier J, et al. Propranolol for severe infantile hemangiomas: follow-up report. Pediatrics. 2009;124(3):e423–31.
118. Mazereeuw-Hautier J, Hoeger PH, Benlahrech S, Ammour A, Broue P, Vial J, et al. Efficacy of propranolol in hepatic infantile hemangiomas with diffuse neonatal hemangiomatosis. J Pediatr. 2010;157(2):340–2.
119. Geramizadeh B, Safari A, Bahador A, Nikeghbalian S, Salahi H, Kazemi K, et al. Hepatic angiosarcoma of childhood: a case report and review of literature. J Pediatr Surg. 2011;46(1):e9–11.
120. Awan S, Davenport M, Portmann B, Howard ER. Angiosarcoma of the liver in children. J Pediatr Surg. 1996;31(12):1729–32.
121. Chung EM, Lattin GE Jr, Cube R, Lewis RB, Marichal-Hernandez C, Shawhan R, et al. From the archives of the AFIP: pediatric liver masses: radiologic-pathologic correlation. Part 2. Malignant tumors. Radiographics. 2011;31(2):483–507.

Liver Tumours and Nodular Lesions

Chayarani Kelgeri, Khalid Sharif, and Ulrich Baumann

Key Points
- Widespread use of high-resolution imaging modalities has led to increased detection of hepatic lesions.
- Hepatic lesions need to be distinguished as benign or malignant to guide therapy.
- A good understanding of radioimaging physics helps increase diagnostic yield and plan surgical and medical treatment.
- Histology is required if the lesion is suspected to be malignant.
- Liver transplant is an accepted indication with excellent long-term prognosis for unresectable hepatoblastoma, while the transplant decision for other liver tumours including hepatocellular carcinoma should be individualised.

Research Needed in the Field
- Identify the most appropriate immunosuppression protocol in a patient requiring liver transplantation for malignancy.
- Identify genotype-phenotype correlations in benign and malignant liver tumours in children and its impact on outcome and therapeutic options.
- Identify specific radioimaging features in paediatric hepatic adenoma and HCC to prognosticate outcome and guide management.
- Define indications for liver transplantation in childhood HCC.

C. Kelgeri · K. Sharif
Liver Unit and Small Bowel Transplant, Birmingham Women's and Children's Hospital, Birmingham, UK
e-mail: khalid.sharif1@nhs.net

U. Baumann (✉)
Liver Unit and Small Bowel Transplant, Birmingham Women's and Children's Hospital, Birmingham, UK

Hannover Medical School, Hannover, Germany
e-mail: Baumann.U@mh-hannover.de

21.1 Introduction

21.1.1 Clinical Approach to a Newly Detected Liver Mass

A liver tumour may be detected in one of the following scenarios:

1. Routine antenatal imaging.
2. Incidental finding because of radioimaging done for unrelated conditions such as abdominal pain, cholestasis or abnormal liver function tests.
3. Medical surveillance of a recognised chronic liver disease or a cancer predisposing genetic condition.
4. Child presenting with abdominal distention and/or abdominal lump.

An early diagnosis following the detection of a mass usually incorporates a staged approach with detailed clinical history, physical examination, blood tests including tumour markers, imaging procedures and finally often liver histology. This stepwise approach is paramount to distinguish malignant lesions from benign ones and to facilitate swift appropriate treatment. Age and gender of the patient, the presenting complaint and any predisposing factors to develop liver masses, such as foreign travel and medication history, offer important clues especially if lesions have no clear diagnostic features on radioimaging.

21.1.2 Clinical History

Age and gender are important as the tumours to be considered in less than 3 years include haemangioma, mesenchymal hamartomas, simple hepatic cysts, hepatoblastoma and metastases from other malignancies most common being neuroblastoma and Wilms tumour [1] (Table 21.1). Children with metastatic malignancies are generally unwell with fever, anorexia, weight loss, irritability and

Table 21.1 Risk factors for liver tumours

Hepatoblastoma	Hepatocellular carcinoma	Adenoma	Focal nodular hyperplasia
Prematurity Low birth weight Beckwith-Weidman syndrome Simpson-Golabi-Behmel syndrome Li-Fraumeni syndrome Familial adenomatous polyposis Gardener syndrome Budd-Chiari syndrome Trisomy 18	Chronic hepatitis B infection Hepatitis C infection Tyrosinaemia 1 Familial cholestasis syndrome Fanconi anaemia Ataxia telangiectasia Biliary atresia Alpha-1 antitrypsin deficiency Alagille syndrome Glycogen storage disease Wilson's disease Congenital hepatic fibrosis Portosystemic shunt Drugs: methotrexate, oestrogens	Oestrogens Tyrosinaemia 1 GSD 1 and GSD 3	Vascular malformation Congenital portosystemic malformations

Table 21.2 Age distribution of Liver lesions

Age in years	Benign	Malignant	
		Primary	Metastatic
0–3	Haemangioma Mesenchymal hamartoma Teratoma	Hepatoblastoma Rhabdomyosarcoma Rhabdoid tumours Yolk sac tumour	Neuroblastoma Wilms tumour Leukaemia Pancreaticoblastoma
3–10	Focal nodular hyperplasia Adenoma	Rhabdomyosarcoma Undifferentiated embryonal sarcoma Hepatocellular carcinoma Angiosarcoma	
Adolescence	Adenoma Focal nodular hyperplasia	Hepatocellular carcinoma Angiosarcoma Undifferentiated embryonal sarcoma Epithelioid haemangioendothelioma Cholangiocarcinoma	Hodgkin's and non-Hodgkin's lymphoma Metastasis from extrahepatic malignancies
Any age	Hepatic cyst Hepatic abscess Nodular regenerative hyperplasia Hepatic foregut cyst Inflammatory fibroblastic tumour		

bony pains [2]. Adenomas are usually seen in adolescent females on oestrogen-based contraceptive pills or metabolic conditions such as glycogen storage disease. Hepatocellular carcinoma (HCC) is typically seen in school-aged children. It may be associated with metabolic disease (tyrosinaemia type I) but can also be sporadic. Enquiries should be made for genetic conditions like Beckwith-Wiedemann syndrome, Li-Fraumeni syndrome, Simpson-Golabi-Behmel syndrome and familial adenomatous polyposis as these conditions have a higher incidence of hepatoblastoma as compared to the general paediatric population (Table 21.2).

Liver lesions on a background of abnormal blood flow like Budd-Chiari or Abernethy malformation are usually focal nodular hyperplasia (FNH). Children treated in the past with chemotherapy or radiotherapy for solid tumours are also known to have a higher incidence of FNH.

21.1.3 Clinical Findings

Cutaneous haemangiomas or a swirl on auscultation of the fontanelle favours a diagnosis of infantile haemangioma [3]. One should look for signs of chronic liver disease, organomegaly and features suggestive of genetic syndromes in the clinical examination of the patient. "Blueberry" skin nodules seen with neuroblastoma and leukaemias metastasising to subcutaneous tissue are a diagnostic feature [4]. Complications of hepatic haemangiomas like congestive cardiac failure [3] or shock in tumour bleeds may be evident at presentation [5].

21.1.4 Blood Tests

Baseline liver function tests and viral markers are done to exclude chronic viral hepatitis. Thrombocytosis may be seen in hepatoblastomas as the tumours are known to secrete thrombopoietin [5].

21.1.5 Tumour Markers

Alpha-fetoprotein (AFP) is a glycoprotein that is produced by foetal liver cells and yolk sac tumours. In foetal life it precedes the emergence of albumin. The different glycosylation forms of AFP help to differentiate the origin of the AFP. AFP originating from the yolk sac has a different glycosylation pattern than AFP from malignant tumours and from benign hepatocytes. Standard tests usually measure all isoforms, but specific tests for the different isoforms are available. Neonates often have markedly elevated AFP levels that rapidly fall in the first 6 months of life and reach normal reference ranges by the age of 1 year. Nomograms are available to interpret AFP levels below 1 year of age. Certain cancers like teratomas and liver malignant lesions such as hepatoblastoma and hepatocellular carcinoma produce AFP which is used as an adjunct for diagnosis, prognostication, response to treatment and surveillance for recurrence. Hepatoblastomas with very high or low AFP at diagnosis and the ones that fail to respond to chemotherapy are suggestive of unfavourable histology and indicate poor prognosis. The biological half-life of AFP is approximately 5 days [6].

Levels of AFP above the reference range may be found in patients with viral hepatitis and chronic liver disease with regenerating hepatocytes. Not all hepatoblastomas and HCC have AFP above the reference range, and hence AFP alone cannot be used for diagnosis or screening. Additional biomarkers like des-γ-carboxy prothrombin, *Lens culinaris* AFP–L3 (fucosylated isoform of AFP) and Golgi protein 73 when used individually are not very useful but when combined may improve the diagnostic yield in HCC especially in the early stages [6, 7]. Vitamin B12-binding proteins such as transcobalamin 100 have been found to be elevated in fibrolamellar variant of HCC and can been used in monitoring response to treatment.

β-Human chorionic gonadotrophin (β-HCG) is produced by some hepatoblastomas causing precocious puberty. This too can be used for monitoring similar to AFP in these patients. Extremely high levels are seen in infantile choriocarcinoma of the liver [5, 7].

Urine catecholamines are helpful in suspected infiltrative neuroblastoma of the liver as they can mimic other liver tumours on radioimaging (Fig. 21.1).

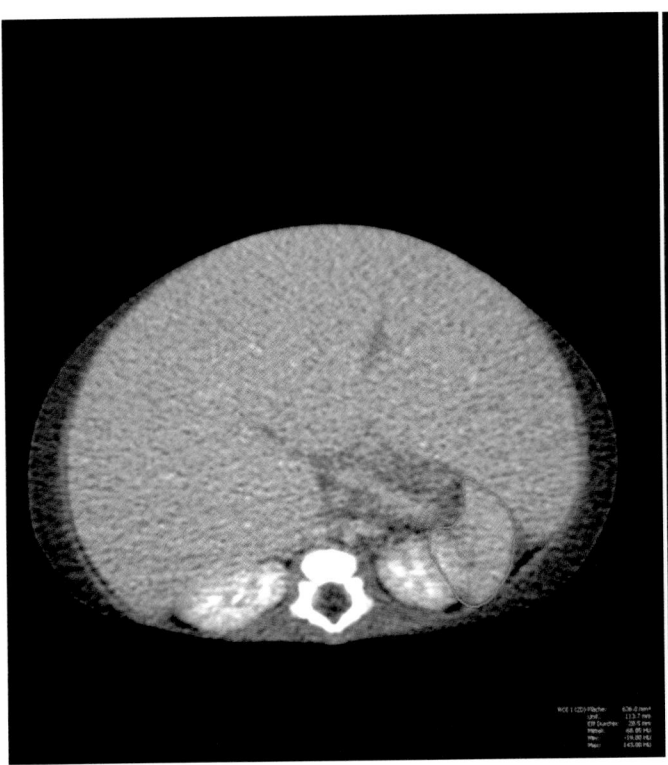
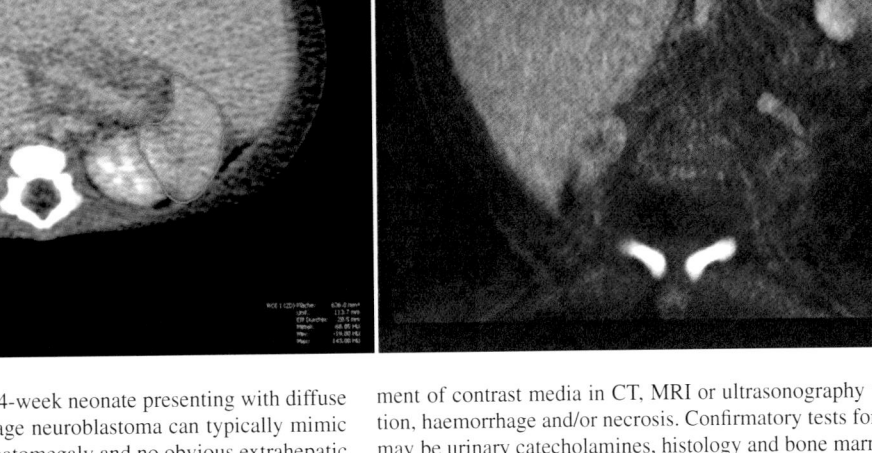

Fig. 21.1 Neuroblastoma of a 4-week neonate presenting with diffuse infiltration of the liver. At this age neuroblastoma can typically mimic metabolic liver disease with hepatomegaly and no obvious extrahepatic tumour mass. Diagnosis is may be suspected by heterogeneous enhancement of contrast media in CT, MRI or ultrasonography with calcification, haemorrhage and/or necrosis. Confirmatory tests for the diagnosis may be urinary catecholamines, histology and bone marrow aspirate

21.1.6 Choosing Appropriate Imaging Modality

Ultrasound (USS) is usually the first radioimaging modality to screen a liver lesion. It confirms the mass arising from the liver and can differentiate between cystic or solid lesions. Dopplers are helpful in determining vascularity of the lesions, and at times USS alone is sufficient in making a diagnosis. However, its sensitivity and specificity are limited in hepatic steatosis, diffuse liver disease and solid liver lesions less than 1 centimetre (cm) [8, 9]. USS if inconclusive can guide clinicians in choosing further imaging modality to characterise the lesion and stage and detect metastasis if malignant and delineate the vascular anatomy if surgical resection or liver transplantation is anticipated (Fig. 21.2).

Visibility of the liver lesion depends on the attenuation difference between the lesion and the background liver. Unenhanced CT scan is unhelpful if this attenuation difference is absent, and this is overcome by using an intravenous contrast. Due to the dual blood supply from the artery and portal vein, the liver has three distinct phases after injecting intravenous contrast. First is the arterial phase occurring 10–15 s after injecting the contrast followed by the portal venous phase, also called the hepatic phase, after 60–75 s. Finally in the equilibrium phase, also called the delayed venous phase, the contrast starts leaving the liver. Liver masses, if vascular, receive their blood supply from the hepatic artery. This vascular architecture results in different enhancement patterns during various phases of intravenous contrast circulation which is then exploited to characterise the lesion.

Hypervascular lesions such as focal nodular hyperplasia and hepatic adenoma will enhance in the late arterial phase as the liver parenchyma is comparatively hypodense and will fade out in the late portal phase as the liver brightens up

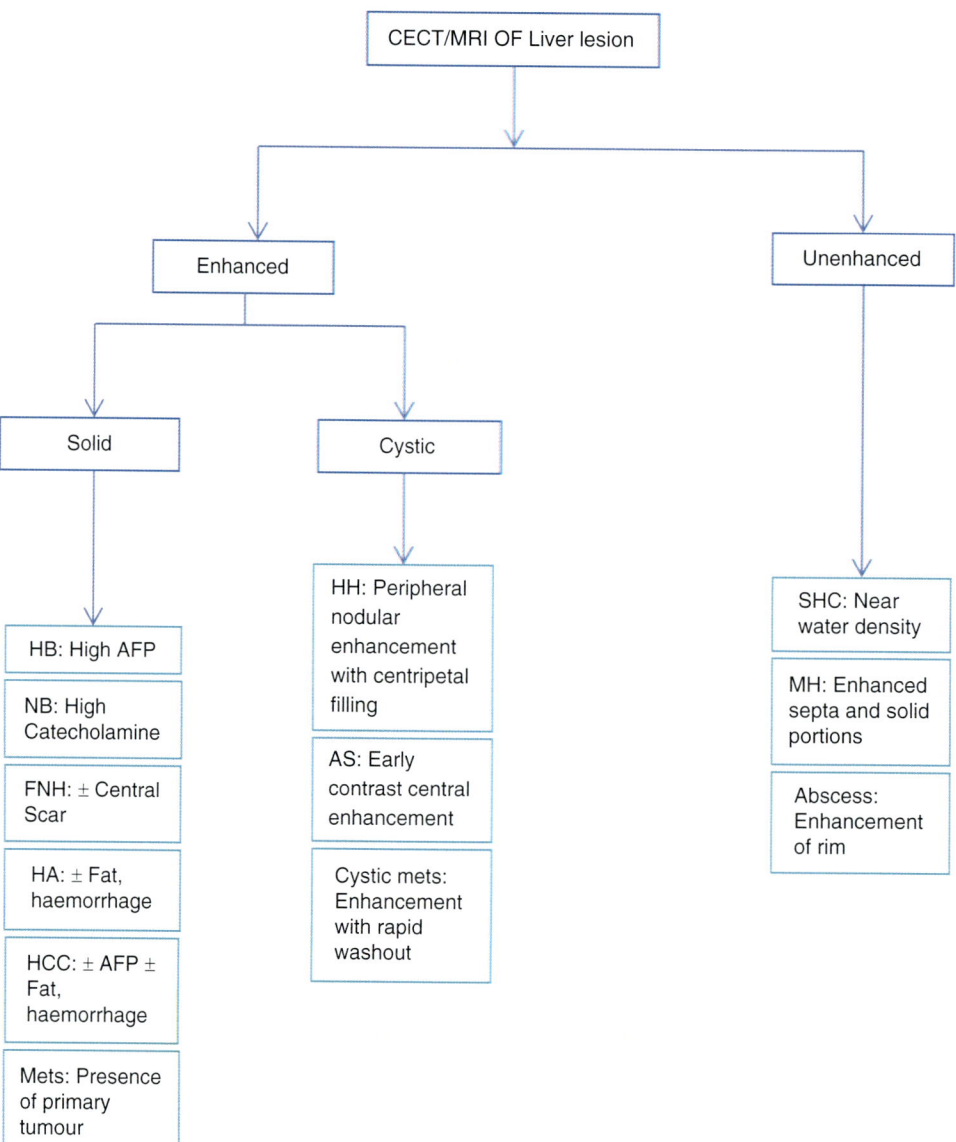

Fig. 21.2 Characterising a liver lesion on radioimaging. A flow chart approach incorporating radioimaging characteristics and biochemical tests helps in differentiating liver lesions. *HB* hepatoblastoma, *NB* neuroblastoma, *HH* hepatic haemangioma, *AS* angiosarcoma, *MH* mesenchymal hamartoma, *FNH* focal nodular hyperplasia, *HA* hepatic adenoma, *HCC* hepatocellular carcinoma, *SHC* simple hepatic cyst, *AFP* alpha fetoprotein, *Mets* metastasis

because of the portal venous supply. In contrast hypovascular lesions will be best seen in the portal venous phase. Liver lesions will be hypodense or hyperdense as compared to liver parenchyma in the equilibrium phase (scans taken 10 min after contrast) depending on the washout or retention of the contrast in the lesion [8].

Magnetic resonance imaging (MRI) with gadolinium contrast provides the best spatial resolution for liver lesions in the rapid dynamic T1-weighted images. It avoids ionising radiation making it the modality of choice. Better lesion characterisation is achieved by defining signal intensity characteristics of the lesion, vascularity, stromal component, presence of necrosis, fat and haemorrhages [8].

The characterisation and location of lesions are further enhanced by using mixed extracellular hepatobiliary gadolinium-based contrast agents such as gadoxetate disodium and gadobenate dimeglumine. Delayed hepatobiliary phase with delineation of biliary anatomy is possible as these contrast agents are partially excreted in bile after being taken up by hepatocytes, thus providing functional and morphologic information [10, 11].

This is particularly useful for differentiating adenomas and hepatocellular carcinomas from focal nodular hyperplasia. Magnetic resonance elastography and acoustic radiation force impulse imaging are currently under investigation and may potentially be useful techniques in the characterisation of liver masses [8]. In spite of these advantages, cost, long duration of procedure and need for sedation or anaesthesia limit its use in children [10, 11].

21.1.7 Histology

Liver histology often is the key to the diagnosis of a solid mass; however, liver biopsy is an invasive procedure and should be prepared following detailed radioimaging for a maximum result. Benign lesions seldom require biopsy unless the clinical picture and radioimaging have been inconclusive. Immunohistochemistry further adds to the diagnostic accuracy and is helpful in prognostication of a liver lesion. It is advisable to biopsy both the liver lesion and the back ground liver tissue in patients with sporadic adenomas or focal nodular hyperplasia to rule out underlying liver disease. Suspected malignant lesions almost always require histopathological diagnosis to guide therapy and prognosis.

21.2 Benign Lesions of Liver

21.2.1 Hepatic Haemangiomas (HH)

Paediatric hepatic haemangiomas are the most common benign liver tumours. Their nomenclature in the past has been confusing causing an irrational management approach. The Liver Haemangioma Registry from Boston in 2007 categorised hepatic haemangiomas into focal, multifocal and diffuse subtypes [3, 12]. The Boston group proposed a management algorithm of these subtypes based on their similarities in biological behaviour and natural history to the congenital and infantile cutaneous haemangiomas described in the International Society for the Study of Vascular Anomalies (ISSVA) classification [13]. HH are endothelial lined vascular mass in the liver with feeding and draining vessels and are distinct from the epithelioid haemangioendotheliomas, hepatic arteriovenous malformations and hepatic haemangiomas of adults.

Focal hepatic haemangiomas (FHH), also called congenital haemangiomas, account for one third of the HH. They are variable in size ranging from a few millimetres to more than 10 cm. Most are asymptomatic and are picked up incidentally on antenatal or postnatal scans. The large ones though can be symptomatic because of their size, location or haemodynamic effects caused by high-flow shunts. FHH begin to evolve in utero, are fully formed at birth and do not have a postnatal growth phase. They are rarely associated with cutaneous haemangiomas and have no sex predilection. These lesions begin to involute soon after birth, decreasing in size and regressing by 14–18 months of age [12]. FHH thus behave similar to the congenital cutaneous haemangiomas of rapid involuting type of the ISSVA classification.

Multifocal and diffuse hepatic haemangiomas are the true infantile hepatic haemangiomas (IHH) of the ISSVA classification [13]. They are similar to the cutaneous infantile haemangioma in their biologic behaviour and are associated with cutaneous haemangiomas at other sites. They are encountered more commonly in females and white population. Multifocal hepatic haemangiomas (MHH) appear after birth and are most commonly picked up on visceral screening for multiple cutaneous haemangiomas. About 90% are diagnosed in first 6 months of life with one third of them in the first month [2]. Some of them like the focal ones can be symptomatic with features of high-output cardiac failure, and these patients will need additional monitoring with echocardiogram and brain natriuretic peptide to guide and monitor treatment. Similar to cutaneous infantile haemangiomas, these lesions proliferate up to a year after birth, then stabilise and finally involute over several years [3, 12, 13].

The diffuse infantile haemangioma (DIH) is almost always symptomatic with abdominal distension because of hepatomegaly as majority of the liver parenchyma is replaced by the haemangioma. Hepatomegaly can be severe enough to cause abdominal compartment syndrome, inferior vena cava and renal vein compression causing poor venous return, impaired ventilation and multiorgan failure [3, 12].

Patients with IHH especially the diffuse type are likely to develop hypothyroidism. This is because the vascular endothelium of IHH produces type 3 iodothyronine deiodinase which inactivates the active form of thyroxine (T3) into an inactive form. Hypothyroidism may be severe enough to cause heart failure and mental growth retardation. These patients need large doses of thyroxine, sometimes intravenously, to get to euthyroid state. This complication has not been described in the focal or congenital hepatic haemangioma [3, 12].

Mild anaemia and thrombocytopenia have been reported with hepatic haemangiomas unlike the severe thrombocytopenia with consumption coagulopathy of Kasabach-Merritt syndrome associated with haemangioendotheliomas. Complications associated with HH resolve once they have involuted either spontaneously or medically [3, 12].

On USS, FHH are seen as a well-demarcated hypoechoic vascular mass with heterogeneous echotexture. Feeding and draining vessels have been described but may be difficult to visualise on ultrasound. Non-contrast CT of these lesions appears as low attenuation hypodense lesions with calcifications that are more frequently seen in the involution phase. Early peripheral nodular enhancement with progressive fill-in causing centripetal enhancement is seen on contrast-enhanced CT scan (CECT). Central areas may be anechoic because of haemorrhage, necrosis or fibrosis. Multifocal and diffuse lesions have multiple well-defined lesions on USS and CT scan. The MHH are homogenous in echotexture with normal intervening liver parenchyma and enhance uniformly with contrast. In the diffuse type, liver tissue is replaced by numerous lesions with no normal intervening liver parenchyma [3].

MRI has the highest sensitivity and specificity for diagnosing haemangiomas up to 95%. On MRI they appear as hypointense on T1-weighted images and hyperintense on T2. Enhancement pattern is similar to CT scan in the gadolinium-enhanced MRI [9]. Occasionally haemangiomas are atypical and mimic other liver lesions like metastatic neuroblastoma necessitating biopsy [9]. Other indications for biopsy include late presentation beyond 1 year of life and lack of response to treatment.

Tissue diagnosis is rarely necessary but when performed in cases of uncertainty shows the tumour to be composed of vascular channels lined by endothelial cells. The cellularity is replaced by loose fibro-fatty stroma as the tumour involutes. These lesions are differentiated from other vascular lesions based on immunostaining of the endothelial cells to erythrocyte-type glucose transporter protein 1 (GLUT 1). Focal haemangiomas (congenital) are negative, while the multifocal (infantile) ones are positive for GLUT1 staining. The GLUT1 staining status is not yet established in the diffuse subtype [3, 12].

21.2.2 Management

Asymptomatic FHH are best left alone as they are known to spontaneously involute. Large focal haemangiomas with symptomatic shunts causing heart failure are considered for embolisation or selective hepatic artery ligation. The multifocal or GLUT1-positive haemangiomas are amenable to medical therapy. Recently propranolol has found favour with many clinicians as it has shown significant efficacy in multiple case reports including those with hypothyroidism and heart failure. Exact mechanism of action is not known but is thought to possibly decrease renin which in turn decreases vascular endothelial growth factor and causes vasoconstriction. Other medications such as steroids, interferon and vincristine have been used in some cases. Medically resistant symptomatic tumours may need hepatic embolisation or resection. Diffuse types are the most difficult to manage. Decompressive laparotomy may be needed for abdominal compartment syndrome, and hypothyroidism needs to be treated aggressively. Liver transplant has been reported in patients with MIH and diffuse subtypes which are not amenable to medical or surgical resection [3, 12–14].

21.2.2.1 Mesenchymal Hamartoma (MH)

Mesenchymal hamartoma is a multicystic hepatic tumour with variable amounts of solid tissue. They are seen below the age of 2 years and have a slight male preponderance. MH usually presents as a painless abdominal distension caused by enlarging liver mass but can have an acute presentation because of rapid increase in size causing mass effect. Prenatal lesions have been reported, most often in the last trimester of pregnancy, and it may be a cause of hydrops [17, 18].

Findings on radioimaging are variable and range from multiseptated cystic mass to predominantly solid mass with cysts. The cysts appear as anechoic, while the solid tissue is echogenic. On contrast-enhanced CT, the solid component, septae and peripheral rim enhance. MH commonly involves the right hepatic lobe and is not typically associated with calcification or haemorrhage [17, 18].

On MRI, the cystic content gives variable signal intensity depending on the protein content of the cyst fluid. With contrast, enhancement is limited to the septa and solid components of the tumour. Biopsy is warranted if radiology is doubtful [17].

Histologically, MH is characterised by the presence of mesenchymal stroma, cysts and bile ducts interspersed with hepatocytes. Although benign, MH shares several common histopathologic, immunohistochemical and cytogenetic features of undifferentiated embryonic sarcoma (UES). There are suggestions that UES can develop in pre-existing MH. Calcifications, haemorrhage and necrosis are not frequently seen in these tumours. MH has been considered a focal tumour, but small satellite lesions at the tumour margin have been described which could explain tumour recurrence after apparent tumour resection [17].

21.2.3 Management

MH requires surgical resection as they can grow in size and have a potential for malignant transformation. Percutaneous aspiration and drainage may initially be required for large cystic lesions causing mass effects followed by surgical resection. Liver transplant has been considered for unresectable tumours [18].

21.2.3.1 Focal Nodular Hyperplasia (FNH)

FNH is uncommon in children and accounts for 2–4% of all paediatric liver tumours [1, 15]. A marked female preponderance has been noticed. FNH lesions are solitary in about 70–80% and less than 5 cm although larger lesions have been documented. Multiple lesions may be seen in patients with underlying vascular liver diseases like Budd-Chiari syndrome, portal vein agenesis and congenital disorders such as hereditary haemorrhagic telangiectasia [16, 17]. FNH is considered to be a proliferative or a hyperplastic cell response to increased blood flow by an aberrant vascular malformation. A higher incidence has been noted in patients with a history of previously treated malignancy as compared to general paediatric population and is possibly related to treatment-related vascular injury. The mean time to develop FNH after treatment is estimated to be between 4 and 12 years (range 2–27 years). It has also been reported in congenital portosystemic shunts and may be because of impaired portal flow with compensatory arterialisation of the liver parenchyma (Table 21.2). Compared to other liver lesions, the size of FNH remains stable over time. They are rarely symptomatic and are picked up incidentally on radioimaging although few patients may be symptomatic with abdominal pain and distension. Tumour rupture and haemorrhage are extremely rare.

The echogenicity of both FNH and its scar is variable and may not be picked up on ultrasound if they are isoechoic with the surrounding liver parenchyma. Some may be visible because of a pseudocapsule formed by compression of surrounding liver parenchyma. The diagnostic feature is the presence of a central scar which may be hyperechoic to the rest of the lesion. The central scar on Doppler examination is fed by an artery and extends to the periphery in a spoke wheel pattern. On unenhanced CT scan, FNH appears as a well-circumscribed, homogeneous hypoattenuating mass. After contrast, FNH enhances homogeneously relative to the background liver in the late arterial phase. In the portal and subsequent phases, the lesion becomes isoattenuated except for the central scar which is hyperintense as compared to the rest of the liver because of accumulation of the contrast. A typical scar may not be seen in as many as 20% of cases [16, 17].

MRI is comparatively more sensitive and specific to USS and CT scan in diagnosis of FNH. These lesions are seen as homogeneous, slightly hypointense on T1-weighted images and hyper- or isointense on T2 images with a bright central scar in about 80% of patients. The use of hepatobiliary MR contrast agents demonstrates features similar to contrast-enhanced CT scan.

Regenerative nodules may have similar features to FNH, and pre-contrast features may be useful to make the differentiation. Atypical features of FNH, like the presence of steatosis, strong hyperintensity on T2-weighted images, pseudocapsule mimicking true capsule and washout in the equilibrium phase, cause difficulties in characterisation of the lesion and need a biopsy for definitive diagnosis [11, 17].

Histologically, FNH is composed of hyperplastic hepatocytes arranged in nodules separated by fibrous septa that originate from the central scar. Ductular proliferation, blood vessels and inflammatory cells seen in the fibrous septa are highly suggestive of FNH. Immunohistochemical staining for glutamine synthase is specific to FNH and is used for diagnostic accuracy [17].

21.2.4 Management

A conservative approach is recommended in asymptomatic FNH given the rarity of complications [16]. However it can be difficult to distinguish from hepatocellular carcinoma (fibrolamellar) and may require surgical resection. Resection has also been considered if the FNH is pedunculated, expanding or exophytic for the theoretical risk of rupture secondary to trauma. In the past this has been a reason to consider surgical resection of this benign tumour.

21.2.4.1 Hepatic Adenoma (HA)

Hepatic adenoma is a rare benign neoplasm of the liver commonly seen in adolescent girls using oestrogen-based oral contraceptives. Conditions associated with adenomas without a sex predilection include glycogen storage disease types 1 and 3, maturity-onset diabetes mellitus, androgens (either endogenous production or exogenous therapy), congenital or portosystemic shunts, germline mutation of hepatic nuclear factor-1α (HNF-1α) gene and familial adenomatous polyposis [16–18] (Table 21.2).

HA is usually a solitary tumour, asymptomatic and discovered incidentally. Some adenomas come to medical attention because of abdominal pain, palpable mass or haemodynamic instability because of tumour rupture with bleeds. Multiple adenomas may be noticed on a background of glycogen storage disease or androgen therapy. "Adenomatosis" is a term used when there are more than ten adenomas, seen in adults without an underlying background liver disease and unrelated to oestrogen or androgen therapy. They are invariably symptomatic and need medical intervention [19].

Hepatic adenomas on USS or CT scan appear hypodense but are heterogeneous in echotexture because of necrosis, fat and haemorrhage. Doppler examination demonstrates internal vascularity. On contrast-enhanced CT scan, they show a variable pattern of enhancement in the late arterial phase and become isodense to the liver in delayed images [16, 17].

MRI is the best imaging modality for hepatic adenomas as it is sensitive in detecting fat and haemorrhage. They are seen as heterogeneous lesions on both T1- and T2-weighted images, and the imaging features reflect the tumour subtype. Enhancement patterns with gadolinium are similar to contrast-enhanced CT, but chemical shift and fat suppression techniques facilitate identification of lesions with fat. Some HCC lesions contain fat and may make the differentiation from HA difficult warranting histopathological investigations [16].

On histological examination, HA is seen as well-demarcated tumour composed of sheets of liver cells without a fibrous capsule or portal tract elements. Very few Kupffer cells can be seen with no bile ducts, a feature that distinguishes it from FNH. Areas of necrosis and haemorrhage can be seen within the tumour [17].

Adult hepatic adenomas have been classified into four subtypes based on immunohistochemical markers: HA inactivated for HNF-1α (H-HA) characteristically associated with steatosis, inflammatory HA (I-HA) associated with mutations activating the JAK/STAT pathway, β-catenin-activated HA (β-HA) and the unclassified HA (U-HA) which do not have any specific mutation or morphology. Among these the β-HA subgroup has the highest risk for malignancy. In addition telangiectatic FNH has now been classified as I-HA based on molecular studies. This classification is helpful in prognosticating HA, thereby guiding management strategies [20, 21]. There are no reported studies on molecular subtyping exclusive to paediatric population to our knowledge.

21.2.5 Management

Good metabolic control in glycogen storage disease, androgen withdrawal, stopping oral contraceptives, weight loss and closure of congenital portosystemic shunts regress HA when associated with these conditions. Close follow-up is advised in all cases to document regression or detect any malignant change [16].

A study published by the Bordeaux group reported half of HA to be the inflammatory subtype but a significant 28% to have the β-catenin mutation explaining the higher incidence of malignant change in HA associated with glycogen storage disease [22].

Lesions more than 5 cm, growing lesions, male sex irrespective of tumour size and β-catenin-expressing adenomas are considered high risk for bleeds and malignant transformation in adults and hence surgically resected. These risk factors should be taken into consideration in paediatric HA as well. Embolisation can be performed in case of haemorrhage followed by resection for residual viable lesion. Management strategies should be discussed in a multidisciplinary team to plan the best possible surgical option [18].

21.2.5.1 Nodular Regenerative Hyperplasia (NRH)

NRH previously thought to be rare is now increasingly being reported as a cause of noncirrhotic portal hypertension. It can occur at any age and is characterised by hepatic parenchyma architecture changing into regenerative nodules surrounded by atrophic liver with no perisinusoidal or periportal fibrosis. The nodules are of variable size and small ones can coalesce to form bigger ones.

The pathogenesis of NRH is unclear but is probably a hepatocytic hyperplastic response related to altered small vessel blood flows. It has been reported in patients with Abernethy malformations and portal vein thrombosis. Other causes implicated are drugs like steroids, azathioprine, immunosuppressive drugs, autoimmune conditions, collagen vascular disease, neoplastic and myeloproliferative diseases and congenital thrombophilia.

About half of the patients with NRH will present with portal hypertension, while the others may be picked up incidentally.

It is difficult to make a definitive diagnosis of NRH on radioimaging alone as the nodules may be too small to be picked up. Nodules, even if the nodules are large, are difficult to differentiate from normal liver parenchyma. Findings related to portal hypertension may be seen. The lesions are hypoattenuated on non-contrast CT scan and do not enhance in the arterial phase of contrast-enhanced CT scan. On MR imaging, the nodules are homogeneous, slightly hyperintense to the surrounding liver parenchyma on T1-weighted images and variable on T2-weighted images. Liver biopsy is the gold standard in diagnosing NRH [17, 19].

21.2.6 Management

Managing portal hypertension is the mainstay of treatment, and the aetiological factor should be eliminated if possible. Other causes of portal hypertension should be excluded before making a diagnosis of NRH. Outcome and prognosis depend on underlying aetiological factor and severity of portal hypertension [17].

21.2.6.1 Inflammatory Myofibroblastic Tumours (IMT)

They are benign, also called as inflammatory pseudotumours. They can arise from any organ system. Histologically, they are masses of inflammatory infiltrate with collagen stroma. IMT may be difficult to differentiate from malignant lesions. Symptoms because of local effects need resection including liver transplant for unresectable hilar tumours, while asymptomatic ones are treated conservatively [23].

21.2.6.2 Hepatic Cyst

It is a benign congenital lesion resulting from abnormal exclusion of the intrahepatic biliary ducts. These lesions do not communicate with the biliary tree. They occur in approximately 2.5% of the general population, are usually asymptomatic and are discovered incidentally, but large big cysts may present with abdominal pain and distension or complications including infection and bleeding [24].

Simple hepatic cysts are thin-walled anechoic masses without septae or vascularity on USS. On CT and MRI, they appear as non-enhancing masses with attenuation and signal intensity of water.

Atypical cysts with fenestrations, septations, multiple cysts, calcifications and daughter cysts warrant further investigations to exclude cystic metastasis, hydatid or parasitic cysts. Multiple hepatic cysts (more than ten) should raise the possibility of polycystic liver disease, often referred to as ciliopathy.

Histologically simple hepatic cysts are composed of an outer layer of fibrous tissue and are lined by cuboidal, columnar epithelium that produces cystic fluid.

Asymptomatic cysts do not require treatment or follow-up. Large symptomatic cysts or cysts with complications need surgical intervention.

Ciliated hepatic foregut cyst (CHFC) is very rare in children with only a handful of cases being reported in literature. They originate from the embryological foregut. They are usually seen in segment 4 although a few have been described in the anterior segments of the liver. CHFC have similar appearances to hepatic cyst radiologically but may be iso- or hyperdense in a few because of soft tissue density. The presence of ciliated epithelium on histology differentiates them from hepatic cyst. Surgical approach is recommended given the risk for malignant transformation and biliary communication [24].

21.3 Malignant Hepatic Tumours

Malignant tumours can be classified as the most common liver tumours accounting for two thirds of all liver tumours in the paediatric population, 80% of these being hepatoblastoma (HB) [5, 25]. Hepatocellular carcinoma, mesenchymal stromal tumours, epithelioid haemangioendothelioma (which are rarely described in childhood), cholangiocarcinoma and nested tumours account for the remainder [5, 26]. The incidence of HB is rising, while the remainder have more or less remained static. This could be because of increased survival of premature babies which is a risk factor for HB. The incidence of HCC is expected to decline with universal hepatitis B vaccination, as worldwide, a large proportion of HCC in children is seen with chronic hepatitis B carriers. Surgery with or without chemo- and radiotherapy is the essence of treatment, and hence these children should be referred early to a multidisciplinary team with expertise in hepatobiliary surgery and liver transplant.

21.3.1 Hepatoblastoma

Hepatoblastomas usually present in children less than 3 years of age, and about 4% are present at the time of birth. Maternal smoking, parental occupation and genetic susceptibility have been associated with HB, and an increased risk has been reported in low-birth-weight infants with supplemental oxygen therapy, phototherapy, drugs and use of parental nutrition. Hepatoblastomas are also picked up during surveillance programmes for certain conditions like Beckwith-Weidman syndrome and familial polyposis coli (Table 21.2) [5].

Clinically, HBs are often picked up by carer or clinician as an abdominal lump. Atypical presentations include precocious puberty because of β-HCG being secreted by some tumours, osteoporotic fractures or an acute abdomen because of rupture causing intraperitoneal bleed [14]. Hepatoblastoma is often associated with underlying associated syndromes or prematurity (Table 21.1).

Blood investigations may show thrombocytosis because of thrombopoietin and interleukin 6 secreted by these tumours which stimulate the megakaryotic cell line. AFP is an important marker for diagnosis, follow-up and prognosis. It is raised in 90% of the tumours, and a falling AFP to chemotherapy indicates a good prognosis. A rise again after initial fall may mean relapse. Similarly, AFP should fall to normal ranges after surgery, and a rising AFP during postoperative follow-up should prompt the physician to look for recurrence. A tumour with low AFP or AFP that fails to fall with chemotherapy is regarded as biologically aggressive with poor prognosis [5, 14].

β-HCG can be monitored similar to AFP in tumours secreting this marker. Molecular markers like glypican 3, nuclear β-catenin and membranous EpCAM currently have limited clinical application. Research is ongoing to find molecular-genetic markers which can not only help in diagnosis but will have therapeutic and prognostic implications [27].

The first radioimaging done is usually USS. This confirms the origin of the mass to be hepatic. Further imaging with CT scan is required to characterise the lesions, stage them, investigate for pulmonary metastasis and determine if they are amenable to resection. On CT scan, HB appears as heterogeneous, low attenuation mass enhancing on arterial phase and hypoattenuates in the portal phase. Calcifications are frequently seen. MRI is becoming more popular as it avoids radiation. It shows HB as hypointense in comparison to normal liver in T1-weighted sequences and hyperintense in T2-weighted sequences, while post gadolinium, it enhances in a heterogeneous fashion with rapid washout.

Rarely angiography may be required if more clarity on vascular structures is required to aid resection [11].

Biopsy is required before start of chemotherapy in SIOPEL (Childhood Liver Tumor Strategy Group of the Societe Internationale d'Oncologie Pediatrique) protocol although the COG (Children's Oncology Group) from the United States proceeds to resection without biopsy or adjuvant chemotherapy if the presentation and evaluation are suggestive of pure foetal histology subtype. The histology is confirmed on the resected specimen [14].

HB are heterogeneous with varying combination of cell types. The international paediatric liver tumour consensus classifies HB into various subtypes that correlate well with clinical outcome [27]. The well-differentiated foetal cell type has a favourable outcome, whereas the undifferentiated small-cell subtype often has a poor outcome. Consensus has been achieved regarding a general need for pretreatment tumour histology.

21.4 Staging and Stratification of Hepatoblastoma

Children's Hepatic Tumours International Collaboration (CHIC) in an attempt to unify the approach to tumour staging and risk stratification across various tumour groups has recently proposed the new Children's Hepatic Tumours International Collaboration-Hepatoblastoma Stratification (CHIC-HS) [28]. It is based on 5-year event-free survival (EFS) and incorporates PRETreatment EXTent of disease (PRETEXT) staging, age, AFP level and the PRETEXT annotation factors, namely, metastatic disease (M), macrovascular involvement of all hepatic veins (V) or portal bifurcation (P), contiguous extrahepatic tumour (E), multifocal tumour (F) and spontaneous rupture (R) which have been identified as statistically important prognostic factors.

This risk stratification divides all hepatoblastoma cases into low risk (EFS >90%), intermediate risk (EFS 70–90%), high risk (EFS 50–70%) and very high risk (EFS <50%).

CHIC-HS will be further refined in coming years to include CHIC histology subtype review. This stratification will allow comparison of various treatment strategies and in conjunction with biological and molecular markers will pave a path for individualised approach for hepatoblastoma.

21.4.1 Management

The cornerstone of management of HB is to achieve a tumour-free resection state. Chemotherapy is able to downstage about 60% of HB that are unresectable at diagnosis. It is important to identify risk factors for unresectability at presentation so that discussions are initiated early on with a hepatobiliary centre with multidisciplinary expertise in managing these children [29–31].

Risk stratification helps guide treatment of HB, and the mainstay of treatment is cisplatin-based chemotherapy and surgery. SIOPEL treats PRETEXT 1, 2 and 3 hepatoblastomas with a combination of chemotherapy and surgery [28]. The tumours shrink because of fibrosis with chemotherapy and provide easy resectability. Usually four cycles of chemotherapy are given, and surgery is planned around this time followed by two more cycles of chemotherapy.

Multifocal as compared to focal disease, even with similar histology, is associated with poor EFS and overall survival and should have intensive chemotherapy [32]. The COG approach is to offer primary resection at diagnosis if feasible followed by chemotherapy, exception being the tumour with pure foetal cell-type histology which does not receive chemotherapy after resection. Unresectable tumours are treated with neoadjuvant chemotherapy in an attempt to shrink the tumour to facilitate resection. This is a strategy to limit the use of chemotherapy [31, 33].

Liver transplant is considered in unresectable hepatoblastomas in carefully selected patients and is discussed in the later section.

The outcomes of HB have changed significantly in the last few years, and the initiation of Paediatric Hepatic International Tumour Trial will add more to our understanding and hopefully provide solutions for tumours that are currently high risk with increased recurrence rates.

21.4.1.1 Hepatocellular Carcinoma (HCC)

HCC is uncommon in children and its incidence increases with age. They are picked up on surveillance programmes in children with a background of liver disease that predisposes them to develop HCC (Table 21.2) (Fig. 21.3). On rare occasions,

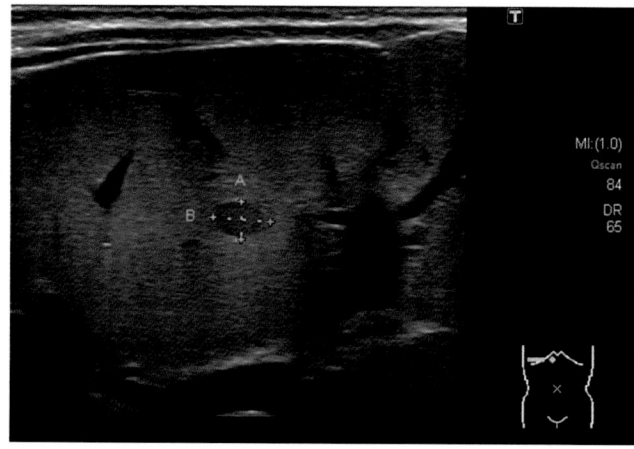

Fig. 21.3 HCC in a 1-year-old girl with TJP2 deficiency, waiting for liver transplantation for end-stage liver disease. Total AFP was 40 ng/mL, and L3 AFP was detectable at low levels of 7 ng/mL. Histology post-liver transplantation confirmed the suspicion of HCC

they are identified because of abdominal pain, a lump or jaundice because of biliary tree compression or invasion without a pre-existing liver disease where the prognosis is not so good.

AFP is used as a tumour marker for diagnosis, monitoring response to therapy and for recurrence of tumour. Some HCC may not produce AFP. Transcobalamin I 100 (vitamin B12-binding protein) is a useful monitoring marker in the fibrolamellar variant of HCC which occurs on a background of noncirrhotic liver [5, 14]. CECT and MRI are imaging modalities of choice for evaluation of HCC. The characteristic imaging appearance of HCC is early arterial enhancement followed by washout during delayed imaging. Fibrolamellar type, a variant of HCC, can have a central hypodense, hypervascular area mimicking a central scar of FNH. MRI is useful in distinguishing these two conditions [11].

Special stains (reticulin stains) can sometimes be helpful because the reticulin framework is completely lost in well-differentiated HCC. Positive immunostaining with markers such as glypican-3 and heat shock protein 70 is highly specific but not sensitive in differentiating HCC from HA [21].

21.4.2 Management

Management of paediatric HCC is challenging. Complete surgical resection is required for cure. Resectable HCC without metastasis have a 5-year EFS of 80–90%, but only 20% of HCC have been reported to be amenable to resection at the time of diagnosis. Results for unresectable HCC or HCC with metastasis are poor. Neoadjuvant chemotherapy for HCC is derived from experiences with paediatric hepatoblastoma. In contrast to adults, about 40% of tumours are chemosensitive which however does not translate to resectability. Resectability is achieved in approximately 36% even with intensification of chemotherapy. Sorafenib, gemcitabine and oxaliplatin have improved resectability in adults and need to be investigated in children. Transarterial chemoembolisation (TACE) chemotherapy has been reported in a few paediatric cases to achieve resectability. Studies are ongoing in adults with new drugs like bevacizumab, c-met inhibitors and immune checkpoint blockade agents like nivolumab [33].

Experience with liver transplantation in HCC is limited. The outcome of HCC after liver transplantation in childhood is greater than in adult patients (see below).

The radioimaging features of various liver tumours and nodular lesions is summarised in Table 21.3.

21.4.2.1 Biliary Tract Rhabdomyosarcoma (BRS)

BRS is rare and accounts for 0.8% of all rhabdomyosarcomas. It arises in the biliary system and can extend into the liver parenchyma or down into the biliary system and typically presents with symptoms and biochemical features of obstructive jaundice. It is seen in the younger age group with a median age of 3 years. After the initial radioimaging, biopsy is required to confirm the diagnosis. The pathology of the intraductal lesions is similar to that of rhabdomyosarcoma at other sites. The intraductal tumour is usually either the botryoid or embryonal subtype, unless the lesion involves predominantly the hepatic parenchyma, in which case the alveolar subtype predominates. MRCP is particularly useful in diagnosis as it delineates the biliary system. These tumours are chemosensitive and are managed with a combination of chemotherapy followed by resection [18].

21.4.2.2 Undifferentiated Embryonal Sarcoma (UES)

It is an aggressive mesenchymal tumour seen more frequently in older children. Abdominal pain, poor appetite and weight loss are typical presenting features. Malignant transformation from mesenchymal hamartomas is reported. They appear as solid on USS while cystic without solid components on CT and MRI. This discrepancy is highly suggestive of UES. Diagnosis is by histology showing spindle-shaped tumour cells in a myxoid matrix with positive immunostaining (positive expression of SMA, a-ACT, desmin, vimentin). Multimodal approach with chemotherapy, radiation and surgery has improved the outcome in recent years. Liver transplant experience in unresectable UES is limited to a few case reports [5, 18].

21.4.2.3 Angiosarcoma

This is a malignant spindle cell tumour of the liver derived from endothelial cells. Prognosis is poor with early metastasis often to the lungs. Cases treated with chemotherapy followed by hepatectomy and liver transplant have been reported [18].

21.4.2.4 Malignant Rhabdoid Tumour (MRT)

MRT shares some clinical features and may be difficult to distinguish from HB in some cases. Immunohistochemistry for INI1 is necessary for accurate diagnosis. It is treated with chemotherapy with aims of complete resection. However, outcomes are very poor [18].

21.4.2.5 Epithelioid Haemangioendothelioma

This is a very aggressive tumour with extrahepatic spread and may be difficult to resect even after chemotherapy and TACE (Fig. 21.4). Diagnosis is usually made because of symptoms related to tumour growth like pain, portal hypertension or liver failure. Newer chemotherapeutic agents have shown promising results in tumour shrinkage and may help in achieving resection. Response to chemotherapy may also help in selecting patients for liver transplant if they are unresectable [5].

Table 21.3 Radioimaging features of Liver lesions

Liver lesion	USS findings	Contrast CT scan		MRI		Other tests
		Arterial phase	Delayed portal phase	T1 weighted	T2 weighted	
HH	Heterogeneous Hypoechoic ± calcifications	Peripheral nodular enhancement	Centripetal fill-in	Hypointense	Hyperintense	Thyroid function tests, Glut1 immunohistochemistry
HB	Heterogeneous, septa Hypoechoic ± calcifications	Enhancement seen	Hypoattenuates	Hypointense	Hyperintense	High AFP ± vascular invasion
MH	Hypoechoic, echogenic septa	Unenhanced	Enhancement of septa and solid portions	Hypointense	Variable intensity Enhanced septa	
FNH	Variable echogenicity Central scar	Homogeneous enhancement, hypodense scar	Isoattenuated lesion, bright scar	Iso- to hypointense	Hyper- to isointense Scar mildly hyperintense	
HA	Variable echogenicity Heterogeneous	Enhance actively	Hypodense	Variable intensity	Hyperintense, fat, haemorrhage	MRI with chemical shift or fat suppression useful in high lipid content
HCC	Heterogeneous, Hyperechoic	Enhance actively	Hypodense, rapid washout	Variable intensity	Hyperintense ± fat ± haemorrhage	Scar may be seen in fibrolamellar variant ± vascular invasion ± high AFP
HC	Anechoic Homogeneous	No enhancement, near-water density		Hypointense, homogeneous, no enhancement	Hyperintense	
Abscess	Anechoic	Enhancement of rim		Hypointense	Hyperintense	
NB	Similar to haemangioma					Urine catecholamines, additional sites of metastasis, presence of primary tumour

HB hepatoblastoma, *HH* hepatic haemangioma, *MH* mesenchymal hamartoma, *FNH* focal nodular hyperplasia, *HA* hepatic adenoma, *HCC* hepatocellular carcinoma, *HC* hepatic cyst, *NB* neuroblastoma

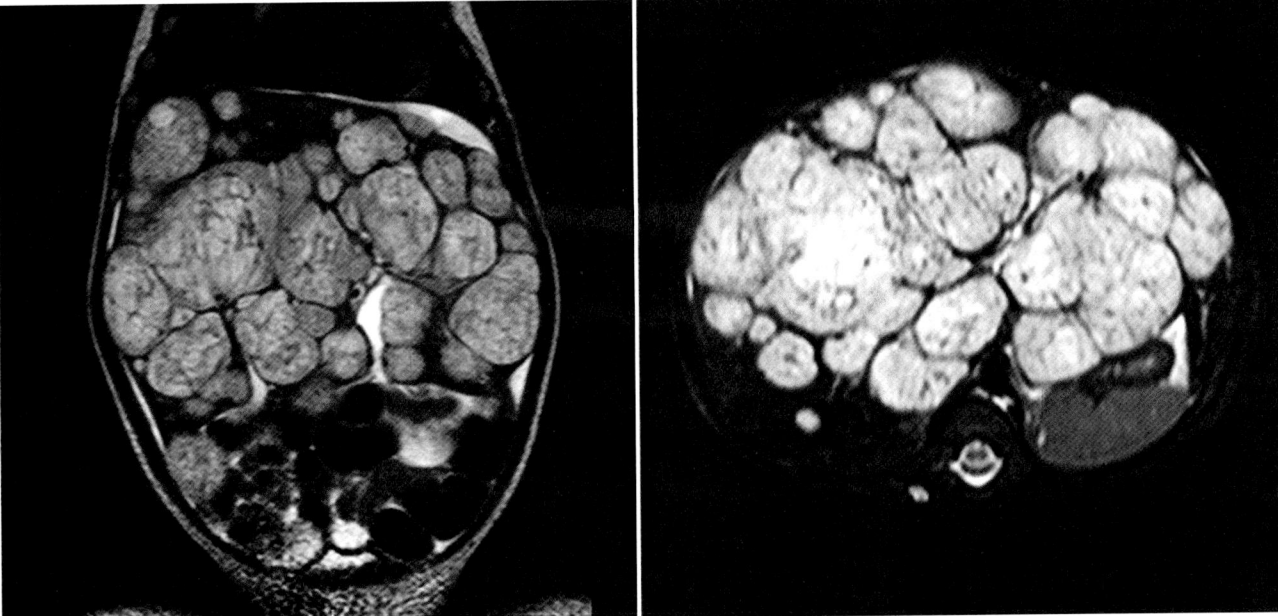

Fig. 21.4 Hepatic haemangioendothelioma in a 3-month-old child

21.5 Indications of Liver Transplant in Liver Tumours

The 5-year survival in unresectable and metastatic HB has improved following liver transplant in a select group of children, and indeed liver transplant is now an acceptable indication for this condition. Audacious attempts at resection are discouraged as outcome after primary liver transplants has proved to be far superior to ones done after recurrence following resection [25, 30, 31]. It is hence important that these tumours are staged accurately so as to plan the best surgical option.

Liver transplant is considered for unresectable HB without extrahepatic disease, exception being pulmonary metastasis provided they have been treated medically with chemotherapy or resected surgically before transplant. Recurrence of disease after resection, involvement of the hilar structures or the main portal vein and its branches and involvement of all hepatic veins which is unlikely to be amenable to resection should also be considered for liver transplant. Each patient should be individualised and discussed within the multidisciplinary team to ensure best possible outcome.

The timing to schedule liver transplant after chemotherapy is narrow, and this is overcome by prioritising them on the waiting list. Living related liver transplant options are also considered to circumvent this problem [30, 31].

The role of post-transplant chemotherapy is not very clear, and the recommendations vary from centre to centre. Some have reported it to be beneficial and some not [34].

In contrast to HB, experience with liver transplantation that is offered to unresectable HCC without extrahepatic spread or macroscopic vascular invasion is limited. Results are improving due to appropriate patient selection and advances made in surgical techniques and chemotherapy. It is currently under debate if the adult Milan criteria should be applied in children as biology of tumours is different and each patient needs to be individualised [35]. Successful liver transplants have been reported in children even when transplanted beyond the more liberal University of California, San Francisco, criteria (single tumour ≤6.5 cm or maximum of three tumours ≤4.5 cm and cumulative tumour size ≤8 cm) or the up-to-seven criteria (absence of angioinvasion, number of nodules plus the maximum size of the largest nodule ≤7 cm) and the United Kingdom criteria (single tumour ≤5 cm or maximum of three tumours ≤3 cm or tumour >5 cm and ≤ 7 cm without tumour progression, extrahepatic spread and no new lesions over a 6-month period) [36–38]. Outcome for liver transplantation for primary HCC is generally better in children than in adult patients. It is not clear if this statistic is solely due to less cirrhotic liver disease in the background of tumourigenesis, superior grafts in younger patients or different tumour biology. Favourable outcomes of liver transplants have been reported if HCC is found incidentally on explant livers as compared to children transplanted for HCC [39]. A recent analysis of the European Liver Transplant Registry data for patient and graft survival in children and adults transplanted for HCC found superior long-term survival in paediatric HCC on a background of inherited liver disease when compared to paediatric HCC without underlying inherited liver disease and adult HCC patients with or without inherited liver disease. They suggest factoring in this advantage when considering liver transplantation in this subgroup of children [40].

Other rare tumours that may be amenable to liver transplant are epithelial haemangioendothelioma, embryonal cell sarcomas and metastatic neuroendocrine liver tumours after removal of the primary tumour. Although good outcomes have been reported with the exception of angiosarcomas [30, 34, 39], the role of liver transplant is uncertain as very few patients are transplanted because of these tumours and the long-term data is awaited.

Among the benign tumours, liver transplants in symptomatic mesenchymal hamartomas, hepatic haemangiomas and inflammatory myofibroblastic tumours have been reported to have failed medical therapy and are not amenable to resection [41].

Paediatric liver unresectable tumour observatory (PLUTO) is a multicentre, multi-institutional registry that provides database of children transplanted for an unresectable malignant liver tumour. As malignant liver tumours are so rare, results from this registry may provide some answers in the future [42].

References

1. Adeyiga AO, Lee EY, Eisenberg RL. Focal hepatic masses in pediatric patients. Am J Roentgenol. 2012;199(4):422–40.
2. Fernandez-Pineda I, Sandoval JA, Davidoff AM. Hepatic metastatic disease in pediatric and adolescent solid tumors. World Hepatol. 2015;7(14):1807–17.
3. Christison-Lagay ER, Burrows PE, Alomari A, Dubois J, Kozakewich HP, Lane TS, et al. Hepatic hemangiomas: subtype classification and development of a clinical practice algorithm and registry. J Pediatr Surg. 2007;42(1):62–8.
4. Latham WD. Blueberry muffin baby: neonatal neuroblastoma with subcutaneous metastases. Plast Reconstr Surg. 1971;47(1):98.
5. Chunbao G, Zhang M. Liver tumors in infancy and children, hepatic surgery. 2013. https://www.intechopen.com/books/hepatic-surgery/liver-tumors-in-infancy-and-children. Accessed 4 March 2018.
6. Lai Q, Melandro F, Pinheiro RS, Donfrancesco A, Fadel BA, Levi Sandri GB, et al. Alpha-fetoprotein and novel tumor biomarkers as predictors of hepatocellular carcinoma recurrence after surgery: a brilliant star raises again. Int J Hepatol. 2012;2012:893103.
7. Singal AK, Agarwala S. Tumour markers in pediatric solid tumours. J Indian Assoc Pediatr Surg. 2005;10(3):183–90.
8. Thyagarajan MS, Sharif K. Space occupying lesions in the liver. Indian J Pediatr. 2016;83(11):1291–302.
9. Sahani DV, Kalva SP. Imaging the liver. Oncologist. 2004;9(4):385–97.
10. Neri E, Bali MA, Ba-Ssalamah A, Boraschi P, Brancatelli G, Alves FC, et al. ESGAR consensus statement on liver MR imaging and clinical use of liver-specific contrast agents. Eur Radiol. 2016;26(4):921–31.
11. Shelmerdine SC, Roebuck DJ, Towbin AJ, McHugh K. MR of paediatric liver tumours: how we review and report. Cancer Imaging. 2016;16(1):21.
12. Kulungowski AM, Alomari AI, Chawla A, Christison-Lagay ER, Fishman SJ. Lessons from a liver hemangioma registry: subtype classification. J Pediatr Surg. 2012;47(1):165–70.
13. Wassef M, Blei F, Adams D, Alomari A, Baselga E, Berenstein A, et al. Vascular anomalies classification: recommendations from the International Society for the Study of Vascular Anomalies. Pediatrics. 2015;136(1):e203–15.
14. Morland B, Sharif K. Primary hepatic tumors. In: Kelly DA, editor. Diseases of the liver and biliary system in children. 4th ed. West Sussex: Wiley; 2017. p. 459–78.
15. Maillette de Buy Wenniger L, Terpstra V, Beuers U. Focal nodular hyperplasia and hepatic adenoma: epidemiology and pathology. Dig Surg. 2010;27(1):24–3.
16. Franchi-Abella S, Branchereau S. Benign hepatocellular tumors in children: focal nodular hyperplasia and hepatocellular adenoma. Int J Hepatol. 2013;2013:1–11.
17. Chung EM, Cube R, Lewis RB, Conran RM. Pediatric liver masses: radiologic-pathologic correlation. Part 1. Benign tumors. Radiographics. 2010;30(3):801–26.
18. Fernandez-Pineda I, Cabello-Laureano R. Differential diagnosis and management of liver tumors in infants. World J Hepatol. 2014;6(7):486–95.
19. Bahirwani R, Reddy KR. Review article: the evaluation of solitary liver masses. Aliment Pharmacol Ther. 2008;28(8):953–65.
20. European Association for the Study of the Liver (EASL). EASL Clinical Practice Guidelines on the management of benign liver tumours. J Hepatol. 2016;65(2):386–98.
21. Dhingra S, Fiel MI. Update on the new classification of hepatic adenomas. Arch Pathol Lab Med. 2014;138:1090–7.
22. Calderaro J, Labrune P, Morcrette G, Rebouissou S, Franco D, Prevot S, et al. Molecular characterization of hepatocellular adenomas developed in patients with glycogen storage disease type I. J Hepatol. 2013;58(2):350–7.
23. Nagarajan S, Jayabose S, McBride W, Prasadh I, Tanjavur V, Marvin MR, Rodriguez-Davalos MI. Inflammatory myofibroblastic tumor of the liver in children. J Pediatr Gastroenterol Nutr. 2013;57(3):277–80.
24. Marrero JA, Ahn J, Reddy KR. ACG clinical guideline: the diagnosis and management of focal liver lesions. Am J Gastroenterol. 2014;109(9):1328–47.
25. Otte JB, Pritchard J, Aronson DC, Brown J, Czauderna P, Maibach R, Maibach R, et al. Liver transplantation for hepatoblastoma: results from the International Society of Paediatric Oncology (SIOP) study SIOPEL-1 and review of the world experience. Pediatr Blood Cancer. 2004;42(1):74–83.
26. Newsome JR, Venkatramani R, Heczey A, Danysh HE, Fishman DS, Miloh T. Cholangiocarcinoma among children and adolescents: a review of the literature and surveillance, epidemiology, and end results program database analysis. J Pediatr Gastroenterol Nutr. 2018;66(1):e12–8.
27. López-Terrada D, Alaggio R, de Dávila MT, Czauderna P, Hiyama E, Katzenstein H, et al. Towards an international pediatric liver tumor consensus classification: proceedings of the Los Angeles COG liver tumors symposium. Mod Pathol. 2014;27(3):472–91.
28. Meyers RL, Maibach R, Hiyama E, Haberle B, Krailo M, Rangaswami A, et al. Risk-stratified staging in paediatric hepatoblastoma: a unified analysis from the Children's Hepatic Tumors International Collaboration. Lancet Oncol. 2017;18(1):122–31.
29. D'Antiga L, Vallortigara F, Cillo U, Talenti E, Rugge M, Zancan L, et al. Features predicting unresectability in hepatoblastoma. Cancer. 2007;110(5):1050–8.
30. McDiarmid SV. Liver transplantation for malignancies in children. Liver Transpl. 2010;16(S2):S13–21.
31. Meyers RL, Tiao G, de Ville de Goyet J, Superina R, Aronson DC. Hepatoblastoma state of the art: pre-treatment extent of

31. disease, surgical resection guidelines and the role of liver transplantation. Curr Opin Pediatr. 2014;26(1):29–36.
32. Saettini F, Conter V, Provenzi M, Rota M, Giraldi E, Foglia C, et al. Is multifocality a prognostic factor in childhood hepatoblastoma? Pediatr Blood Cancer. 2014;61(9):1593–7.
33. Schmid I, von Schweinitz D. Pediatric hepatocellular carcinoma: challenges and solutions. J Hepatocell Carcinoma. 2017;4:15–21.
34. Khan AS, Brecklin B, Vachharajani N, Subramanian V, Nadler M, Stoll J, et al. Liver transplantation for malignant primary pediatric hepatic tumors. J Am Coll Surg. 2017;225(1):103.
35. Squires RH, Ng V, Romero R, Ekong U, Hardikar W, Emres S, et al. Evaluation of the pediatric patient for liver transplantation: 2014 practice guideline by the American Association for the Study of Liver Diseases, American Society of Transplantation and the North American Society for Pediatric Gastroenterology, Hepatology and Nutrition. Hepatology. 2014;60(1):362–98.
36. Romano F, Stroppa P, Bravi M, Casotti V, Lucianetti A, Guizzetti M, et al. Favorable outcome of primary liver transplantation in children with cirrhosis and hepatocellular carcinoma. Pediatr Transplant. 2011;15(6):573–9.
37. Yu SB, Kim HY, Eo H, Won JK, Jung SE, Park KW, et al. Clinical characteristics and prognosis of pediatric hepatocellular carcinoma. World J Surg. 2006;30(1):43–50.
38. Ismail H, Broniszczak D, Kalicinski P, Markiewicz-Kijewska M, Teisseyre J, Stefanowicz M, et al. Liver transplantation in children with hepatocellular carcinoma. Do Milan criteria apply to pediatric patients? Pediatr Transplant. 2009;13:682–92.
39. Vinayak R, Cruz RJ, Ranganathan S, Mohanka R, Mazariegos G, Soltys K, et al. Pediatric liver transplantation for hepatocellular cancer and rare liver malignancies: US multicenter and single-center experience (1981-2015). Liver Transpl. 2017;23(12):1577–88.
40. Baumann U, Adam R, Duvoux C, Mikolajczyk R, Karam V, D'Antiga L, et al. Survival of children after liver transplantation for hepatocellular carcinoma. Liver Transpl. 2018;24(2):246–55.
41. Stringer MD. The role of liver transplantation in the management of paediatric liver tumours. Ann Royal Coll Surg Engl. 2007;89(1):12–21.
42. Otte JB, Meyers R. PLUTO first report. Pediatr Transplant. 2010;14(7):830–5.

The Liver in Systemic Illness

Melanie Schranz, Maria Grazia Lucà, Lorenzo D'Antiga, and Stefano Fagiuoli

Key Points

- The liver can be frequently involved in systemic diseases; consciousness about this fact is essential to avoid an even worse issue than the underlying disease.
- Due to various development stadiums of the liver with different availabilities of enzymes that are responsible for metabolic processes or detoxification, liver involvement in children sometimes expresses in different ways compared to adults.
- Systemic diseases can injure the liver in a chronic manner finally leading to cirrhosis; acute severe liver involvement may result in liver failure.
- Treatment of the systemic illness is most of the times sufficient to treat the liver disease, but sometimes specific interventions may be necessary.
- Primary liver damage may be of vascular, hepatocellular, or cholestatic nature.

Research Needed in the Field

- Large studies on the liver involvement during the course of a systemic disease dedicated to the paediatric population are often missing, rendering impossible to answer epidemiologic questions.
- Pathophysiologic mechanisms responsible for liver involvement are widely unrevealed; thus drawing conclusions on the effect of an immature liver in children is delicate.
- Diagnostic non-invasive methods (e.g. contrast-enhanced ultrasound) to assess liver involvement need to be improved and especially evaluated in children to avoid liver biopsies.

22.1 Endocrine Disorders

22.1.1 Thyroid Disease

Thyroid disorders in childhood affect growth and maturation of thyroid-dependent tissues. The interaction between the thyroid and the liver is critical for maintaining homeostasis in both organs. The liver is responsible for glucuronidation and sulfation of thyroid hormones prior to secretion into the bile. In addition, these hormones play an important role in bilirubin metabolism by interacting with the enzymatic activity of glucuronyltransferase and by regulating the level of ligandin, a major organic anion-binding protein [1]. The main causes of hypothyroidism and hyperthyroidism in childhood are autoimmune thyroid diseases (AITD), chronic lymphocytic thyroiditis, and Graves' disease, respectively [2].

22.1.1.1 Hyperthyroidism
Introduction
Hyperthyroidism rarely occurs in childhood, most frequently as a consequence of Graves' disease (GD) resulting from thyrotropin (TSH) receptor stimulation by autoantibodies. GD is more frequent in female than in male patients and increases in frequency with age, from about 0.1 per 100,000 person-years in young children to 3 per 100,000 person-years in adolescents [3]. The major symptoms of Graves'

disease are the clinical manifestations of hyperthyroidism, as anxiety or attention-deficit, exercise-induced asthma, or primary cardiac arrhythmia [4]. Neonatal Graves' disease develops in 1.5–2.5% of infants, whose mother is affected by this disorder. Well-known signs and symptoms include goitre causing tracheal compression, hyperthermia, tachycardia, irritability, heart failure, hydrops, hypertension, diarrhoea, and craniosynostosis [5]. Autoimmune neonatal hyperthyroidism is commonly triggered by maternal antibodies, which pass the placenta and stimulate the thyrotropin (TSH) receptor (TRAb), leading to thyroid hormone hypersecretion in the foetal thyrocytes [6].

Liver Involvement

Cholestatic jaundice with hepatosplenomegaly and hepatitis are unusual complications of neonatal Graves' disease [7]. The aetiology of neonatal hyperthyroidism-associated cholestasis and liver failure is unknown. One possible explanation is enlargement of the reticuloendothelial system seen in neonatal Graves' disease, which might disrupt hepatic architecture and thus cause cholestasis [8]. Treatment is conducted by administering antithyroid drugs (ATD) to mothers of affected foetus. ATDs encompass carbimazole and its active metabolites, methimazole (MMI) and propylthiouracil (PTU). Treatment with ATDs is also the first choice in childhood and adolescence; other treatment options include subtotal or near-total thyroidectomy and radioactive iodine (RAI)—I131. Since hepatotoxicity has been increasingly seen with the use of PTU, including the risk of drug-induced fulminant hepatic necrosis, MMI is currently recommended [4].

22.1.1.2 Hypothyroidism

Introduction

Congenital hypothyroidism (CH) is diagnosed in 1 in 1500 to 3000 new-borns [3]. Early treatment of thyroid hormone deficiency allows normal development and cognition. The most common cause is thyroid dysgenesis, which is responsible for up to 85% of all cases, followed by defects in thyroid hormone biosynthesis or secretion known as thyroid dyshormonogenesis [9]. Central hypothyroidism, which is often linked to additional pituitary hormone deficiencies, occurs less frequently.

Liver Involvement

Isolated hypothyroidism causes neonatal unconjugated hyperbilirubinemia, which is prolonged due to immaturity of hepatic glucuronyl transferase, and usually lasts for more than 3 weeks [9]. Infants with multiple pituitary hormone deficiencies often present with cholestatic hepatitis, in addition to hypoglycaemia, microphallus, and ocular abnormalities, which are the clinical hallmarks of septo-optic dysplasia [10]. Cholestasis and hepatosplenomegaly seem to resolve within several weeks after replacement of glucocorticoid and thyroid hormones, while transaminase levels remain high [4, 11].

22.1.1.3 Thyroid Dysfunction and Non-alcoholic Fatty Liver Disease

The liver is the major site for cholesterol and triglyceride metabolism. Thyroid hormones play an integral part in hepatic lipid homeostasis. Thyroid hormones cause increased expression of low-density lipoprotein (LDL) receptors on hepatocytes, thus incrementing activity of lipid-lowering liver enzymes, which results in a reduction of LDL levels [12]. In adult patients with clinically manifested hypothyroidism, increased levels of total cholesterol and low-density lipoprotein cholesterol have been observed [13]. Reduced beta-oxidation of fatty acids and increased peroxidation of lipids lead to oxidative stress that causes liver tissue injury and increased insulin resistance. These pathologic mechanisms occur in both non-alcoholic fatty liver disease/non-alcoholic steatohepatitis (NAFLD/NASH) and in hypothyroidism [14]. In addition, hypothyroidism seems to increase the levels of leptin, which may contribute to hepatic insulin resistance and hepatic collagen synthesis [15]. There is growing evidence that increased TSH is an independent risk factor for the development of hepatic steatosis as demonstrated by ultrasound imaging in severely obese children and adolescents [16]. Already discreet elevations of TSH could thus be initial indicators for NAFLD and negatively contribute to the metabolic risk of children and adolescents [17].

22.1.2 Cushing Syndrome

Introduction

Cushing syndrome (CS) affects multiple organ systems due to excessive exposure of glucocorticoids. Truncal obesity, hypertension, growth deceleration, and hirsutism are the main clinical signs of this disorder. Exogenous administration of glucocorticoids causing CS is seen frequently, while endogenous hypercortisolism is rare in children. The annual incidence per million children is approximately 0.35 [18]. Pituitary adenomas are the most common endogenous cause of adrenocorticotropic hormone (ACTH) overproduction [19].

Liver Involvement

Apart from the well-known clinical signs of CS, insulin resistance may increase due to direct interaction of cortisol with the insulin receptor on the one hand and stimulation of lipolysis and proteolysis causing increase of free fatty acids and amino acid release on the other hand. In addition, accelerated gluconeogenesis causes elevated levels of plasma glucose and thus contributes to enhanced insulin resistance [20]. The prevalence of hepatic steatosis in adult patients with CS is approximately 20% [21]. No epidemiologic data are available for children. Several studies indicate that increase enzymatic conversion from cortisone to active cortisol and decreased enzymatic clearance of cortisol may have an impact on NAFLD development in CS [22]. Moreover, increased expression of glucocorticoid receptor and decreased enzymatic activity to reduce active cortisol leads to hepatic lipid accumulation in progressed NAFLD [23].

22.1.3 Adrenal Insufficiency

Introduction
Adrenal insufficiency is a potentially life-threatening condition characterized by decreased production or action of glucocorticoids and/or mineralocorticoids and adrenal androgens. This disorder is classified according to the affected location; primary, secondary, or tertiary insufficiency results from involvement of the adrenal cortex, the anterior pituitary gland, or the hypothalamus, respectively. The clinical manifestations of adrenal insufficiency include anorexia, abdominal pain, weakness, weight loss, fatigue, hypotension, salt craving, and hyperpigmentation of the skin in case of primary adrenal insufficiency. Diagnosis is based on low cortisol levels. Prompt replacement of glucocorticoid and/or mineralocorticoid is the treatment of choice [24].

Liver Involvement
The liver is rarely affected by adrenal insufficiency; however, since hypocortisolism is a well-known cause of neonatal cholestasis, its investigation should be part of the diagnostic workup of jaundiced infants. Only few cases in adults have been described so far [25]. Mildly elevated levels of aspartate transaminase (AST) and alanine transaminase (ALT) were found in association with adrenal insufficiency without signs of liver function impairment. Histological evaluation shows portal lymphocyte infiltration. Short-course steroid therapy for the treatment of Addison's disease led to normalization of liver enzymes in all cases [25]. However, in one case adrenal insufficiency, which was induced by suspension of long-term treatment with dexamethasone, caused severe elevation of liver enzymes and liver failure requiring admission to an intensive care unit. Coagulopathy and hypertransaminasemia completely resolved under prednisolone treatment [26].

22.2 Connective Tissue Disorders and Vasculitides

22.2.1 Lupus Erythematosus

22.2.1.1 Systemic Lupus Erythematosus

Introduction
Systemic lupus erythematosus (SLE) is an autoimmune disorder of the connective tissue that affects multiple organ systems and manifests with a vast number of clinical symptoms.

In about 20% of the cases, diagnosis is made in childhood, usually between 12 and 14 years of age, rarely before the age of 5 [27]. The female to male ratio in paediatric SLE increases with age, from 4:3 during the first decade of life to 4:1 during the second decade [28].

For classification of SLE, the American College of Rheumatology (ACR) criteria were applied, which have been lastly updated in 1997. The Systemic Lupus International Collaborating Clinics (SLICC) developed the SLICC classification criteria in 2012. The SLICC criteria have also been validated in children and show higher sensitivity than the former ACR criteria [29].

Liver Involvement
Since the liver is less frequently involved in SLE, liver function tests usually do not make part of the diagnostic workup, even though mild transient liver enzyme abnormalities are reported in up to 25% of paediatric patients [30]. A significantly higher prevalence of autoimmune liver diseases (AILD) in juvenile lupus patients compared with adult patients has been reported. Moreover, it seems that the liver disease precedes the diagnosis of SLE in the juvenile patients [30].

SLE predisposes for thromboembolic disorders, and occasionally circulating antiphospholipid antibodies can impair hepatic circulation, inducing portal thrombosis and Budd-Chiari syndrome [31]. Focal disturbances of vascularization linked to SLE may also facilitate the development of benign hepatic lesions, such as focal nodular hyperplasia (FNH) or haemangioma, which have been identified to a higher degree in patients with SLE compared to healthy controls [32, 33].

Lupus hepatitis manifests with fluctuations in the levels of ALT that correlate with the activity of SLE [34]. Presentation in most cases is subclinical and shows a low rate of progression to end-stage liver disease. Serum anti-ribosomal P antibody can be detected to a high extent [31]. There may be a link between disease progression and appearance of high antibody levels in the serum of SLE patients [31]. Histological analysis reveals lobular and occasionally periportal inflammation with a paucity of lymphoid infiltrates typical for this entity [35]. Liver enzyme elevation responds well to steroid treatment [33].

Juvenile SLE and autoimmune hepatitis (AIH) rarely appear contemporarily in children [36]. It is assumed that AIH develops in genetically predisposed individuals after their exposure to triggering factors like microbes, viruses, and xenobiotics. Subsequently, the autoimmune attack is induced by molecular mimicry mechanisms and promoted by the reduced control of regulatory T cells [37]. AIH is characterized by increased liver enzymes, hypergammaglobulinemia, the appearance of autoantibodies and typical histological changes [36] such as periportal piecemeal necrosis and lobular activity, rosettes formation of hepatocytes, and lymphocytic infiltrates [33, 35]. AIH sometimes progresses to fulminant hepatic failure or cirrhosis [38]. In adults, discrimination between AIH/SLE overlap and lupus hepatitis plays an important role in patients with SLE [39]. Anti-ribosomal P antibodies are not specific for lupus hepatitis, because patients with overlapping AIH/SLE or AIH alone also result positive [39], and anti-double-stranded DNA antibodies can also be detected in ANA-positive AIH [40]. As in AIH, immunosuppressive therapy is indicated [33].

22.2.1.2 Neonatal Lupus Erythematosus
Introduction
Neonatal lupus erythematosus (NLE) is an acquired autoimmune disease of the developing foetus and neonate resulting from anti-SSA/Ro autoantibodies (anti-Sjögren's syndrome-related antigen A) that cross the placenta. A considerable proportion of mothers of affected infants are asymptomatic (40–60%), while the remaining women have clear evidence of SLE, Sjögren's syndrome, or of some undifferentiated connective tissue disease [33, 41]. The clinical manifestations of NLE include congenital heart block (CHB), cutaneous lesions, thrombocytopenia, pulmonary and neurologic disease, and hepatitis.

Liver Involvement

Liver involvement can be detected in about 10–24% of NLE cases [41] and manifests as cholestatic syndrome. Histology may show bile duct obstruction, portal fibrosis, and inflammation. In general, cholestasis resolves spontaneously, but severe liver failure has also been reported [42]. For the diagnosis of NLE liver disease, conjugated hyperbilirubinemia and increased liver enzyme levels are required, along with detection of antibodies to SSA/Ro and/or SSB/La.

22.2.1.3 Discoid Lupus Erythematosus
Discoid lupus erythematosus (DLE) is rare in children, but studies indicate a higher rate of progression from DLE to SLE compared with adults roughly 20% [43]. However, systemic disease seems to manifest with a milder phenotype. A female predominance of 2:1 is found. On average, progression to SLE occurs at 11 years of age, and the risk is highest during the first year after the diagnosis of DLE. Diagnostic criteria include mucocutaneous lesions in the form of discus and oral or nasal ulcerations, positive antibodies, and/or cytopenia without developing end-organ damage [44]. Disseminated lesions are much more frequent in patients with criteria for systemic lupus erythematosus [45]. Liver involvement is a sign for systemic disease evolution and it has been discussed above.

22.2.2 Systemic Juvenile Idiopathic Arthritis (sJIA) (Formerly Reported as Still's Disease)

Introduction
The prevalence of sJIA is 3.5 per 100,000 [46]. The most common age at presentation is 2 years [47]. sJIA is a multifactorial disease caused by uncontrolled inflammation due to dysregulation of cytokines, innate immune abnormalities resembling auto-inflammatory diseases, and/or certain genetic variants. Most patients present with altered inflammatory parameters including erythrocyte sedimentation rate (ESR), CRP, and leucocytosis. Diagnostic criteria in children under 16 years of age include arthritis of one or more joints with or preceded by documented fever since at least 2 weeks and is accompanied by one or more of the following symptoms: (1) evanescent erythematosus rash, (2) generalized lymph node enlargement, (3) hepatomegaly and/or splenomegaly, and (4) serositis [48, 49].

Liver Involvement

Besides anaemia of inflammation, increase of D-dimers, ferritin, and aldolase and elevated liver enzymes are frequent laboratory findings [47]. The most common symptom at presentation is fever, followed by arthritis and rash. Hepatosplenomegaly, lymphadenopathy, and pericarditis occur less frequently [47]. Splenomegaly occurs in about 50% of patients; hepatomegaly instead seems to correlate with the disease activity [50]. Liver biopsy reveals periportal infiltrates of inflammatory cells [51]. Progression of hepatosplenomegaly may be a manifestation of amyloidosis and requires particular attention since it may result in renal failure [50].

Treatment of sJIA is based on NSAIDs, steroids, and IL-1 blockers, whose administration depends on the type and severity of symptoms at presentation [49].

22.2.2.1 Macrophage Activation Syndrome
Another life-threatening complication of sJIA is the macrophage activation syndrome (MAS) [52], which is caused by uninhibited production and activation of both macrophages and T lymphocytes resulting in fever, liver dysfunction, coagulopathy, pancytopenia, lymphadenopathy, and neurological impairment [53]. The incidence of MAS ranges from 6.7 to 13% with a mortality rate of 8–22% [49, 54]. Females are affected more frequently (6:4), and a recent large retrospective study identified a median time interval between the onset of sJIA and MAS of 4 months [54]. The cause of MAS cannot always be determined; its onset has been associated with the activity of the underlying disease, infections, or the administration of certain medications [54]. Bone marrow examination sometimes reveals the presence of macrophages with hemophagocytic activity, which can also infiltrate other

organs such as the lymph nodes, liver, and spleen; MAS can thus be classified as secondary or acquired form of hemophagocytic lymphohistiocytosis (HLH) syndromes [55]. Fever is the major symptom of this disorder and is recorded in almost all patients. Hepato- and/or splenomegaly are described in up to 70% of cases and CNS dysfunction in more than one third of patients. Frequent laboratory abnormalities include decreased platelet count, elevation of aspartate and alanine aminotransferases, and increase of ferritin, lactate dehydrogenase, triglycerides, and D-dimer. However, serum ferritin levels show major changes over time, and the ratio of ferritin to ESR seems to be a good identifier of MAS with high sensitivity and specificity [54, 56]. This ratio reflects two pathologic mechanisms occurring during MAS: on the one hand, the rise of an acute phase protein and, on the other hand, the decrease of ESR due to low fibrinogen levels as a result of hepatic dysfunction and elevated consumption [54]. The new PRINTO criteria have recently been developed based on these clinical and biochemical findings, which consider fever and elevated ferritin levels >684 ng/mL the main criteria in addition to two of the following laboratory abnormalities: platelet count ≤181 × 109/L, aspartate aminotransferase >48 U/L, triglycerides >156 mg/dL, and/or fibrinogen ≤360 mg/dL [57]. Once the diagnosis of MAS is confirmed, treatment should be started. High-dose corticosteroid therapy is recommended as first-line treatment [58].

22.2.3 Juvenile Dermatomyositis

Introduction
Juvenile dermatomyositis (JDM) is an autoimmune disease in children and adolescents that affects blood vessels of muscles and skin. The mean age of onset is 7 years, and girls have a slight predominance. Manifestations include erythematosus rash and proximal muscle weakness potentially leading to debilitation [59, 60].

Liver Involvement
Hepatomegaly has been reported in patients with juvenile DM. However, plasma AST, ALT, and LDH levels may be elevated due the myositis independently of the presence of hepatitis. Few case reports exist, describing the occurrence of cholestasis, especially in the beginning of the underlying disease, without histological signs of sclerosing cholangitis or primary biliary cholangitis, which have been reported in association with DM in adults. In this series patients presented with hyperbilirubinemia, hepatomegaly, acholic stools, and elevated liver enzymes with histologic signs of noninflammatory cytoplasmic and ductal cholestasis with intact architecture. Liver function was not usually impaired and liver enzyme elevation reverted with steroids [61]. The authors hypothesized that cholestasis is due to cytokines that disappear after treatment with steroids. Indeed, certain proinflammatory cytokines, such as tumour necrosis factor (TNF) and interleukin-1 (IL-1), IL-6, and IL-8, may induce intrahepatic cholestasis by interfering with hepatocellular mechanisms that are responsible for biliary excretion of bile salts and bilirubin [61]. Indeed, these cytokines are elevated in patients with polymyositis [62]. Similar changes during the acute phase of juvenile DM may be responsible for cholestasis [61].

22.2.4 Childhood Scleroderma

Introduction
Scleroderma is a rare disease with an estimated prevalence of 276–300 cases per million. Females are more commonly affected (4.6 to 1) [63]. Scleroderma is an autoimmune rheumatic disorder characterized by fibrosis of the skin and certain internal organs. It is rare in children, and peak age of onset is between 45 and 60 years [64].

Liver Involvement
PBC is the most common liver disorder in patients with scleroderma with a prevalence of about 2% [65]. Vice versa, the prevalence of scleroderma in patients with PBC is estimated to be around 8% [66]. PBC has been rarely described in children; therefore this association has never been identified so far.

22.2.5 Mixed Connective Tissue Disease

Introduction
Mixed connective tissue disease (MCTD) is one of the least common paediatric rheumatology disorders occurring with a frequency varying from 0.1 to 0.5%. Girls are six times more often affected than boys, and median disease onset is 11 years of age [67]. MCTD is a systemic disorder, which shows clinical features of systemic lupus erythematosus (SLE), scleroderma, polymyositis/dermatomyositis, and rheumatoid arthritis (RA). Association with human leukocyte antigen (HLA)-DR4 and HLA-B8 and the presence of high titters of anti-U1 ribonucleoprotein antibodies (anti-U1 RNP) support the diagnosis of MCTD. Both the innate and adaptive immune systems are involved in the development of MCTD [68]. The most common manifestations include polyarthritis, Raynaud's phenomenon, swollen fingers or hands, myositis, oesophageal dysfunction, and nonspecific symptoms such as fever, fatigue, arthralgia, or myalgia [69].

Liver Involvement
Two paediatric cases, a 16-year-old girl and an 11-year-old boy, have been reported in literature, where MCTD occurred in association with autoimmune hepatitis (AIH). Diagnosis was based either on the presence of specific autoantibodies (anti-nuclear antibody, anti-smooth muscle antibody,

liver-kidney microsomal antibody) in the absence of other aetiologies or on typical histological findings. Both cases were successfully treated with immunosuppressive agents [69].

22.2.6 Sjögren's Syndrome

Introduction

Sjögren's syndrome (SS) is a chronic autoimmune disease primarily affecting the lachrymal and salivary glands with varying degrees of systemic involvement. SS can occur (primary SS or pSS) alone or in association with other autoimmune diseases, such as rheumatoid arthritis, systemic lupus erythematosus, or scleroderma (secondary SS or sSS). Middle-aged women are commonly affected by pSS; its occurrence in childhood is rare, even though pSS may be overlooked, as there are no specific diagnostic criteria for children, and manifestations are sometimes different [70, 71]. Recurrent parotide swelling is a common feature observed in up to 100% of affected children, while sicca symptoms are rarely referred [71]. Other symptoms observed at disease onset include arthritis (10%), fever (10%), fatigue (7.5%), and submandibular swelling (5%) [71]. Even though a strong association with HLA-DR3 was found, pSS resembles more a complex, polygenic disorder with sharing common genetic determinants with autoimmune-related diseases, such as systemic lupus erythematosus (SLE) and rheumatoid arthritis (RA) [72].

Liver Involvement

Only few reports of adult patients describe liver involvement in pSS. There seems to be an association between primary biliary cholangitis, type 1 autoimmune hepatitis, and sclerosing cholangitis [73]. No such data exist from the paediatric population.

22.2.7 The Ehlers-Danlos Syndrome

The Ehlers-Danlos syndrome (EDS) belongs to a group of heritable connective tissue disorders, which are genetically heterogeneous and manifest with joint hypermobility, skin hyper extensibility, and tissue fragility [74]. *Liver involvement* in young adults with vascular type EDS has been reported in few severe cases of spontaneous rupture of both the liver and spleen [75].

22.2.8 Childhood Vasculitides

Introduction

Childhood vasculitides are multisystemic complex diseases. The annual incidence of primary vasculitis in the paediatric population up to 17 years of age is approximately 23 per 100,000 [76]. Vasculitis is an inflammation of the blood vessel wall, whose phenotype and severity is related to the location, the vessel size, the extent of affection, and the underlying pathology. Primary forms are distinguished from secondary forms, which are caused by infection, malignancies, drug exposure, and other rheumatic disorders such as SLE and juvenile DM [77]. Symptoms at presentation may be unspecific and include fever, discomfort, and diffuse pain, and blood tests may reveal increased acute phase proteins suggesting systemic inflammation. Disease progression leads to the occurrence of more specific clinical features such as a purpuric rash and signs of organ dysfunction. Subsequent detection of anti-neutrophil cytoplasmic antibodies (ANCA) is highly indicative for the diagnosis of vasculitis [77].

22.2.8.1 Henoch-Schönlein Purpura

Henoch-Schönlein purpura (HSP) is a leukocytoclastic vasculitis that predominantly affects the small blood vessels. HSP is the vasculitis with the highest annual incidence of approximately 20 per 100,000 children, and it usually manifests between 4 and 6 years of age [76]. Unlike most vasculitides, boys are more commonly affected than girls (2:1). HSP occurs with a higher frequency during winter and spring, which indicates that infections may play a role in triggering this disease [78]. Typical symptoms include abdominal pain, arthritis, purpura on lower-extremity, and renal disease [77].

Liver Involvement

Hepatobiliary involvement is rarely reported. One study including 225 patients with HSP found elevated serum alanine transaminase (ALT) or gamma-glutamyl transpeptidase (GGT) or the presence of hepatomegaly in 9% of the children [79]. A recent prospective study revealed that 10% of patients at presentation had mildly elevated liver parameters, which self-remitted within 4 weeks, but liver alterations with ultrasound imaging, on the contrary, were not detectable [80].

22.2.8.2 Kawasaki Disease

Kawasaki disease (KD) primarily affects medium-sized blood vessels. The annual incidence is around 2 per 100,000, and together with HSP it constitutes 99.5% of childhood vasculitides among children below 10 years of age. Both are associated with a seasonal onset pattern paralleling infections. As described for HSP, KD also primarily affects boys [76]. Pathogenesis has not been clarified, but it seems that bacterial and viral infections, genetic predisposition, and autoimmunity play a role in the development of the disease [77].

Liver involvement: Gastrointestinal (GI) involvement is not a common finding; however, abdominal pain, liver function impairment, or gall bladder abnormalities are reported in some patients [81]. Hepatic manifestations may range from asymptomatic increase of liver enzymes to severe cholestatic hepatitis. At least one abnormal liver function test including bilirubin, aspartate aminotransferase, alanine aminotransferase, or GGT has been found in up to 45% of patients diagnosed with KD [82]. A multifactorial mechanism involving generalized inflammation, vasculitis, congestive heart failure secondary to myocarditis, and non-steroidal anti-inflammatory antipyretics may be responsible for the liver injury. In almost all cases, the resolution of hepatic manifestations is observed when the underlying disease is dissolved [83]. Gall bladder (GB) abnormalities are reported in up to 15% of KD patients during the first 2 weeks after disease onset [84]. Acute acalculous cholecystitis (AAC) is an inflammatory disease that is characterized by distension and wall thickening of the GB, sludge, and pericholecystic fluid. Symptoms usually last 1 month, and surgical treatment should be reserved for the appearance of complications. Laboratory deviations that could be indicative for the diagnosis together with typical ultrasound findings are neutrophil count, total bilirubin levels, and C-reactive protein. The aetiology of this disease has yet not been clarified, but it seems that the underlying vasculitis eventually affecting the gastrointestinal tract, the liver, and the biliary tract including the GB plays a pivotal role in the development of AAC. It has recently been shown that the occurrence of AAC is significantly associated with an increased risk for coronary artery abnormalities, which ultimately determine the outcome of KD [85].

22.2.8.3 Polyarteritis Nodosa

Polyarteritis nodosa (PAN) is predominantly a medium-sized vasculitis, and its annual incidence per 100,000 has recently been estimated to be 0.07 [76]. Disease onset is usually around 9 years of age. There is evidence that PAN is related to familial Mediterranean fever. Instead, the strong link with hepatitis B, seen in adults, is less common in the paediatric population. In general, any organ can be affected by the impaired vascular supply, but it is most commonly seen in muscles, skin, kidneys, and GI tract [77].

Liver involvement: Liver involvement occurs to a variable degree (16–56%) in adult patients, but clinical manifestations due to hepatic dysfunction are rare, even if necrotizing arteritis of hepatic vessels has been found in most patients with polyarteritis [86, 87]. Few case reports describe hepatobiliary complications due to PAN in children ranging from acalculous cholecystitis to cholestatic hepatitis and multiple visceral haematomas. Interestingly, association with familial Mediterranean fever is evident in most of these cases [88–90].

22.2.8.4 Takayasu's Arteritis

Takayasu's arteritis (TA) is a granulomatous vasculitis that predominantly affects the aorta and its major branches. The annual incidence rate in childhood is 0.04 per 100,000 [76]. TA is usually diagnosed during adolescence as reflected by its mean age of presentation of 13 years [91]. Girls are about three times more often affected than boys. In children, apart from the aorta, also subclavian and carotid arteries as well as renal arteries are commonly involved. The most frequent symptoms include headache, dizziness, abdominal pain, claudication of the extremities, fever, and weight loss. Roughly 90% of children initially present with hypertension [91]. Specific symptoms appear accordingly to the site of vessels, which are affected.

Liver involvement: Few cases of liver involvement are described in literature. One boy had alterations of liver enzymes and signs of portal hypertension as evidenced by Doppler ultrasonography [92]. Two young women, 18 and 20 years of age, presented with hepatomegaly and unexplained cholestasis, which arose during steroid treatment and was interpreted as a cause-and-effect relationship. The subsequent liver biopsy led to the diagnosis of hepatic sinusoidal dilatation (HSD). HSD can cause blood flow impairment manifesting as portal hypertension. The authors hypothesized that HSD might reflect endothelial cell damage observed in TA [93]. In a 17-year-old boy, hepatomegaly and elevated serum GGT and alkaline phosphatase (ALP) in association with lymph node swelling preceded typical pulseless stage of TA. Liver histology showed signs of non-specific reactive hepatitis [94]. Treatment in these cases included steroids and immunosuppressive agents, such as azathioprine and cyclophosphamide, but therapy of TA is challenging, and tapering of steroids is often associated with disease relapse [77].

22.2.8.5 Behçet's Disease

Behçet's disease (BD) occurs less frequently in children before the age of 16 years, roughly in 4–26% of paediatric cases. Peak age of onset is in young adulthood (25–30 years) [95]. BD is a systemic inflammatory disease involving primarily the oral and genital mucosa, skin, and eyes. Vasculitis can affect all sizes of vessels but prominently the veins [96]. As observed in auto-inflammatory diseases, BD attacks are recurrent and self-limited. Large vessel vasculitis is the leading cause of death, typically by multiple thrombosis or pulmonary arteritis. The aetiology of BD seems to rely on a strong genetic background and infectious triggers, which induce a detrimental mechanism implying the innate immune system [97].

Liver involvement: Budd-Chiari syndrome (BCS) is the most common manifestation of the liver in patients with BD. BCS may manifest as a serious condition, associated with a high mortality rate. Endothelial dysfunction from vasculitis with secondary venous thrombosis has been proposed as a possible mechanism. Studies in adult patients have reported prevalence rates between 1.3 and 3.2% [98]. Males are more likely to develop BCS than females. No data regarding the frequency of BCS in paediatrics exist; however, vascular involvement has been found in 5–20% of children with BD [97]. Presenting signs and symptoms of BCS include right upper quadrant abdominal pain, hepatosplenomegaly, and ascites [99]. Disease manifestation can be acute, subacute, or chronic. Acute BCS seems to carry a poor prognosis [100]. Thrombosis may occur in hepatic veins (HV), inferior vena cava (IVC), or portal vein (PV) [98].

22.2.8.6 ANCA-Associated Vasculitides
Introduction
ANCA-associated vasculitides (AAVs) are a group of necrotizing vasculitides that predominantly affect small blood vessels and are characterized by the presence of anti-neutrophil cytoplasmic antibodies (ANCA). Microscopic polyangiitis (MPA), granulomatosis with polyangiitis (GPA), and eosinophilic granulomatosis with polyangiitis (EGPA) belong to this disease entity. Data on AAVs in paediatrics are scarce, but recent cohort studies including GPA and MPA patients greatly impact on today's knowledge and contribute to determine the clinical phenotype of paediatric AAV [101, 102]. GPA and MPA are the most common forms of AAVs with an annual incidence rate of 0.14 per 100,000 [76]. Childhood AAVs affect primarily females in the early second decade of life. The formation of ANCAs seems to play an integral role in the pathogenesis of the disease [103], even if they are not necessarily detectable in children. Steroids and cyclophosphamide are considered the gold standard of treatment in children [102].

The hallmark of *granulomatosis with polyangiitis* (GPA, Wegener's granulomatosis) is the granulomatous inflammation of the arterial walls and perivascular areas usually occurring in the upper airways and manifesting as recurrent epistaxis or nasal septum perforation, while lower airways involvement presents with nodules, cavities, or fixed infiltrates detectable with X-ray or CT scan. Proteinuria and haematuria are typical findings of kidney involvement. Median age of onset is 14 years [101, 102]. Hepatic involvement in children has not been reported so far.

Microscopic polyangiitis (MPA) generally affects children with a median age of 12 years [101]. Unlike the other forms of AAVs, MPA does not manifest with granulomatous formations. Renal disease occurs frequently at the onset and presents usually as rapidly progressive glomerulonephritis. In addition, musculoskeletal, cutaneous, lower airways, and gastrointestinal tract involvement can occur [104]. Liver manifestations have not been described in children.

Eosinophilic granulomatosis with polyangiitis (EGPA/Churg-Strauss syndrome) is defined as one of the anti-neutrophil cytoplasmic antibody-associated (ANCA) vasculitides, but the ANCA positivity is less reported in paediatric cases (about 40%). Childhood-onset EGPA is more frequent in females with a male/female ratio of 0.7, and the mean age at diagnosis is 12 years [105]. EGPA occurs rarely in childhood with an annual incidence rate of 0.04 per 100,000 [76]. Three clinical stages have been described: first is the prodromal phase, involving allergic rhinitis and asthma, the second phase is characterized by peripheral eosinophilia and eosinophilic tissue infiltration, and finally, the third phase is defined by the occurrence of systemic vasculitis. Pulmonary manifestations are a central feature of paediatric EGPA. Hepatomegaly occurs in 9% and abnormal liver tests in 6–7% of adult patients with EGPA [106]. No such data exist from paediatric populations.

22.3 Haematological Diseases and Coagulation Disorders

22.3.1 Lymphomas

22.3.1.1 Hodgkin Lymphoma
Introduction
Hodgkin lymphoma (HL) has the highest annual incidence in adolescents from 15 to 19 years of age with 2.9 cases per 100,000. In this age group there is a slight female predominance (m/f = 0.8), while in younger children under 5 years, boys are clearly more often affected (m/f = 5.3) [107]. Hodgkin lymphoma is characterized by giant cells with multiple nuclei (Reed-Sternberg cells) or large mononuclear variants (lymphocytic and histiocytic cells, termed Hodgkin's cells), which are associated with a variable number of inflammatory cells including lymphocytes, granulocytes, macrophages, plasma cells, and fibroblasts. Reed-Sternberg cells and Hodgkin's cells belong to the same clonal population and derive in almost all cases from peripheral B cells in lymph nodes and disseminate across the lymphatic system [108]. One possible cause for the development of HL is Epstein-Barr virus (EBV) infection. Accordingly, individuals with immunodeficiency are at higher risk to develop HL [109]. Symptoms of Hodgkin lymphoma depend on the effects of the nodal or extra-nodal disease manifestations. Cytokine release from Reed-Sternberg cells causes constitutional symptoms including weight loss, night sweats, and fever, which are known as B symptoms and appear to correlate with the prognosis.

Liver Involvement
In 5% of patients hepatic infiltration by malignant cells can be found [110]. Hepatomegaly seems to increase with the stage of the HL and is detected in up to 45% of patients with advanced tumour disease. Hepatic manifestations span from slight increase of aminotransferases and alkaline phosphatase to symptomatic cholestasis possibly due to tumour cell infiltration, extrahepatic biliary obstruction, viral hepatitis, vanishing bile duct syndrome, or drug-induced liver

injury [111]. Acute liver failure has also been reported and was ascribed to ischemic injury as a result of compression of the hepatic sinusoids and massive hepatocyte destruction by infiltrating lymphoma cells [112, 113].

22.3.1.2 Non-Hodgkin Lymphoma
Introduction
The 5-year survival rate for non-Hodgkin lymphoma (NHL) has increased by around 45% over the last 40 years in children and adolescents [114]. Depending on immunophenotype, molecular biology, and response to treatment, NHL can be divided in the following three main categories: mature B-cell NHL (Burkitt lymphoma, diffuse large B-cell lymphoma), anaplastic large cell lymphoma, and lymphoblastic lymphoma. NHL represents about 7% of cancers in children and adolescence. The annual incidence is approximately 1 case per 100,000. NHL has its peak onset in the second decade of life and affects predominantly males [115]. An association between EBV and NHL has been reported in the immune-deficient population. Both congenital and acquired (human immunodeficiency virus infection or immunosuppression after transplantation) immunodeficiency display a risk factor for the development of NHL [116]. Children tend to develop NHL in extra-nodal locations such as the abdomen, mediastinum, neck, head, and central nerve system [116].

Liver Involvement
Lymphoma cell in infiltration of the liver may result in hepatomegaly, but hepatic function is usually preserved [113]. However, acute hepatic failure caused by ischemic injury due to massive infiltration of the sinusoids by malignant cells and subsequent necrosis of the liver parenchyma has been described [117], as well as extrahepatic biliary obstruction by the tumour mass [118]. Also intrahepatic lesions are sometimes detectable especially in the highly aggressive subtypes. Nevertheless, data show a higher occurrence of benign lesions at disease onset compared to focal lesions due to NHL [119]. Ascites, in particular chylous ascites due to lymphatic obstruction, may be present [113, 120].

Primary hepatic NHL are rare in children and occur usually in middle-aged men [121]. Manifestations include hepatomegaly, abdominal pain, fever, and deviations of liver enzymes, in particular LDH and ALT elevations. Diffuse large B-cell lymphoma is the most frequently found histological subtype that may manifest with in the form of liver nodules or diffuse portal infiltration with sinusoidal spread [122]. Hepatitis C viral infection or autoimmune disease my play a causative role in the lymphoma-genesis of hepatic B cells [123]. Liver transplantation and subsequent chemotherapy is an option for the treatment of acute liver failure caused by primary hepatic lymphoma [124].

Hepatosplenic T-cell lymphoma is a very rare type of aggressive NHL in children [125]. Liver function tests, in particular AST, ALT, and ALP, are frequently elevated. Antitumour necrosis factor-alpha therapy and purine analogues may play a role in the pathogenesis of this type of lymphoma [126].

22.3.2 Acute Leukaemias

Introduction
Acute leukaemias are one of the most frequent occurring haematologic malignancies in children. About 80% are classified as acute lymphoblastic leukaemia (ALL) and 15–20% as acute myeloid leukaemia (AML) [127]. Presenting symptoms are induced by superseding growth of leukaemic blasts and include bleedings due to thrombocytopenia, pallor and fatigue from anaemia, and infection caused by neutropenia.

22.3.2.1 Acute Lymphoblastic Leukaemia
Acute lymphoblastic leukaemia (ALL) is the most common cancer among children and the most frequent cause of death from cancer before 20 years of age [128]. Leukaemic infiltration of the liver, spleen, lymph nodes, and mediastinum can be seen frequently at diagnosis. The incidence of ALL is about 30 cases per million persons under 20 years of age, with a peak between 3 and 5 years [129]. It occurs more frequently in boys than in girls (male/female ratio, 55%:45%). Genetic mutations influence key cellular processes, including the transcriptional regulation of lymphoid development and differentiation or cell cycle regulation [130]. ALL may be of B-cell precursor or T-cell lineage.

Liver Involvement
Hepatic involvement in acute leukaemia is frequent at presentation and usually manifests as transaminase elevation due to hepatic injury from leukaemic infiltrates. Conjugated hyperbilirubinemia is seen less often in about 3% of ALL cases in children but may require a short course of steroids prior to initiation of induction chemotherapy in order to provide full dosing of induction chemotherapy [131]. Acute hepatitis with or without jaundice as early manifestation of ALL has been described as well as fulminant liver failure [132]. One case is reported in literature describing successful liver transplantation for acute liver failure as a consequence of ALL in an adolescent [133]. Liver biopsy specimens of patients with severe liver injury show infiltration with blast cells and ischemic necrosis, while less impaired liver disease was histologically characterized by a few blast cells in the portal tracts and eventually a hemophagocytic pattern [132]. Regression of liver disease was observed along with leukaemia treatment [132].

22.3.2.2 Acute Myeloid Leukaemia
The incidence of *AML* in infants is 1.5 per 100,000 individuals per year and increases with age. The clinical outcome has

improved significantly over the past few decades, with current long-term survival rates of about 70% [134]. The cause of AML is still unknown. It generally occurs de novo in childhood. The generation of chimeric fusion genes in a permissive haematopoietic stem/progenitor cell is considered to be the critical initiating step in the pathogenesis of a significant proportion of AML arising in children and younger adults [134].

Liver involvement: Diffuse hepatomegaly is a common sign at presentation of paediatric leukaemia, but there are only few case reports describing acute hepatitis with or without liver failure in children due to AML. Also ascites may occur in this context likely due to occlusion of the venous flow [135]. As for ALL ischemic damage caused by blast infiltration is the proposed mechanism of tissue injury as suggested by liver histology and imaging [135]. Initiation of chemotherapy should be aimed, since significant improvement in liver biochemical results have subsequently been seen [132].

22.3.3 Myeloproliferative Neoplasms

Introduction
Myeloproliferative neoplasms (MPN) are characterized by malignant proliferation of one or more myeloid lineages that often lead to the appearance of increased immature cells in the peripheral blood. The BCR-ABL-negative MPNs are polycythaemia vera (PV), essential thrombocythemia (ET), and primary myelofibrosis (PMF), whereas chronic myeloid leukaemia (CML) is BCR-ABL-positive [136]. These classical forms typically occur in older adults and are very rare in children. Mutations in the tyrosine kinase (JAK2), the thrombopoietin receptor (MPL), or the calreticulin (CALR) have been identified to play a causative role in the pathogenesis of these neoplasms. While the majority of adult patients present with mutations in JAK2, children seem to be affected less frequently by this alteration [136].

Liver Involvement
MPNs can sometimes induce the development of portal vein thrombosis [137]. The prevalence of JAK2 mutations in paediatric patients with PVT has not been defined yet [138]. One 17-year-old girl has been reported with splenic and portal vein thrombosis linked to a JAK2 mutation [139]. In up to 60 % of adult patients with Budd-Chiari syndrome, JAK2 mutations have been identified with or without apparent findings of MPNs [113, 140]. However, in the paediatric population only few cases of Budd-Chiari syndrome due to JAK2 mutations have been described [139, 141, 142].

22.3.3.1 Polycythemia Vera
Polycythemia vera (PV) is characterized by an increased red cell mass after other potentially disease-causing conditions such as hypoxia or erythropoietin overproduction have been excluded. Bone marrow biopsy reveals significant increase of erythropoiesis and a simultaneous rise of platelets and granulocytes in the peripheral blood. Experience in the paediatric population is based on few case reports. The annual incidence is estimated to be around two cases per ten million individuals less than 20 years of age. Main symptoms include, pruritus, headache, and fatigue, but only about half of the affected children are symptomatic at disease onset [143]. Thrombotic or bleeding complications have in comparison to adult PV patients not yet been reported in paediatrics [143].

Liver involvement: Hepatomegaly is a common finding in adults but seems less common in children. Splenomegaly occurs in about one third of affected children [136].

22.3.3.2 Essential Thrombocythemia
Essential thrombocythemia (ET) is defined by increased megakaryopoiesis leading to thrombocytosis, which is associated with an elevated risk of thrombi formation on the one hand and bleeding complications on the other hand. Moreover, since ET originates from haematopoietic stem cells as member of the group of the myeloproliferative neoplasms, a risk of leukaemia exists. The annual incidence in children is approximately one case in ten million children under 14 years of age [144]. Usually thrombocytosis in children is an incidental finding without any clinical sign (65–75%). If symptoms appear, they are mainly due to impaired vasomotor functions caused by abnormal platelet-endothelial interactions. Headaches occur most commonly in children [143].

Liver involvement: In 19% of paediatric patients splenomegaly has been reported, while hepatomegaly can be found only in few cases [136].

22.3.3.3 Myelofibrosis
Myelofibrosis (MF) occurs alone (primary MF) or as a result of marrow fibrosis after PV or ET (secondary MF). MF can also be triggered by CML. Primary MF (PMF) is characterized by reticulin and/or collagen fibrosis in the bone marrow (BM) leading to ineffective haematopoiesis, which causes cytopenia, proliferation of dysfunctional megakaryocytes, and leukoerythroblastosis. Moreover, extramedullary haematopoiesis (EMH) is induced that leads to organomegaly [136, 145]. Among the myeloproliferative neoplasms, MF has the worst prognosis. PMF in children is very rare; roughly 46 cases have been reported so far. It usually occurs in children below 3 years of age with female predominance (ratio 2:1) [145]. The disease expression in children is variable and ranges from mild presentations with spontaneous resolution to aggressive disease manifestations with rapid progression and potentially fatal outcome, which is curable only by HSCT. Increased BM fibrosis is due to elevated lev-

els of cytokines and growth factors released by haematopoietic stem cell clones which induce proliferation of fibroblasts and mesenchymal cells [136]. The main JAK2 and most frequent MPL mutations seem to be less detectable in children, whereas CALR mutations are identified in roughly 50% [146]. Symptoms at presentation in paediatric patients are mostly related to cytopenia and organomegaly as a result of EMH [136].

Liver involvement: Hepatic manifestations consist of hepatomegaly [145]. PMF can only be cured by HSCT; to avoid complications related to disease progression such as infections or repeated transfusions, children should rapidly be directed versus HSCT [136].

22.3.3.4 Chronic Myeloid Leukaemia

Chronic myeloid leukaemia (CML) is rare in paediatrics (2–3% of leukaemias) with an incidence of 0.6–1.2 per million children per year. Its incidence increases with age. CML is a Philadelphia chromosome-positive MPN with the characteristic reciprocal translocation t (9;22)(q34;q11), which leads to the formation of the BCR-ABL fusion gene and protein. The only definite etiological factor in CML is ionizing radiation. Imatinib (tyrosine kinase inhibitor) treatment has significantly decreased the rate of transformation to blast crisis [147]. Different trials evidence that 96% of children on imatinib achieved complete haematological response [148]. At disease onset 20–50% of patients do not bear any symptoms. Manifestations may be unspecific such as malaise or fatigue, but also B symptoms can occur. Space-occupying abdominal symptoms such as pain or satiety due to an enlarged spleen may be present. In addition, splenomegaly can lead to splenic infarction. No specific data on hepatic manifestations concerning the paediatric population exist so far.

22.3.3.5 Juvenile Myelomonocytic Leukaemia

Juvenile myelomonocytic leukaemia (JMML) is an aggressive myeloid neoplasm of the childhood, which is clinically characterized by overproduction of monocytic cells that may infiltrate different organs, including the spleen, the liver, the gastrointestinal tract, and the lungs. JMML is categorized by the World Health Organization as an overlap disease between myeloproliferative neoplasm and myelodysplastic syndrome [149]. The incidence rate is 1.2 per million children per year. The median age at diagnosis is 20 months. Symptoms such as lymphadenopathy, hepatosplenomegaly, and skin lesions are provoked by organ infiltration by malignant cells, as well as by replacement of the production of other blood components, which causes cytopenia resulting in pallor, fever, and bleeding complications. Impairment of signal transduction on the MAPK/ERK pathway, which induces increased sensitivity of the malignant cells to granulocyte-macrophage colony-stimulating factor (GM-CSF), is supposed to be responsible for the pathogenesis. Disease expression ranges from rapid progression in one third of the cases to relatively mild course [150].

Liver Involvement

Hepatosplenomegaly can be found in over 90% of patients and thus makes up part of the diagnostic criteria for JMML. Its persistence after treatment indicates poor prognosis [151]. Allogeneic HSCT is until now the only curative therapy; without transplantation the median survival time is 10–12 months [150].

22.3.4 Histiocytic Disorders

22.3.4.1 Langerhans Cell Histiocytosis

Introduction

The hallmarks of Langerhans cell histiocytosis (LCH) are lesions including pathologic CD207+ dendritic cells (DCs) that resemble epidermal Langerhans cells. These pathognomonic cells are associated with an accumulation of inflammatory cells including variable numbers of lymphocytes, eosinophilic granulocytes, and macrophages [152]. The presence of the somatic mutation BRAF-V600E in haematopoietic precursor cells underlines the neoplastic origin, while the inflammatory nature of LCH lesions, cytokine abnormalities, and a myeloid cell maturation defect in the LCH cell indicates dysfunctional immune responses [153]. Single skin or bone lesions may be the only manifestations of LCH, but dissemination can result in life-threatening multiple organ failure. The annual incidence of LCH is about 0.5 cases per 100,000 children under 15 years of age with a median disease onset of 30 months. Girls and boys are equally affected [154]. Almost any organ system can be involved: clinical high-risk LCH is defined by infiltration of the liver, spleen, and/or bone marrow, while LCH of clinical low-risk is defined by lesions anywhere else [152]. The 5-year overall survival in patients with high-risk LCH is more than 85% with adequate treatment, while low-risk LCH patients have a long-term survival of nearly 100% [153].

Liver Involvement

Among children with LCH, liver involvement occurs frequently between 10 and 45%. Moreover, misdiagnosis does not occur rarely, especially in localized disease [155]. Positive immunohistochemistry staining of CD1a and S100 protein in lesion tissue is required for the diagnosis [156]. Frequent hepatic manifestations and clinical signs include hepatomegaly, abnormal liver enzymes, and cholestasis with additional increase of associated biochemical markers (ALP, GGT, conjugated bilirubin). Langerhans cells directly infiltrate the periportal regions of the liver showing remarkable selectivity for the bile ducts, which may lead to sclerosing cholangitis that can rapidly progress to cirrhosis. The incidence of sclerosing cholangitis in multisystem LCH ranges from 10 to 18% [157]. Bile duct infiltration by

Langerhans cells is histologically not always demonstrable [157, 158]. GGT represents a sensitive marker for liver infiltration in children. Indirect effects on the liver without direct involvement may arise from macrophage activation that seems to be responsible for hepatomegaly and hypoalbuminemia [159]. Ribbon-like or nodular areas of relative hypo-attenuation in computed tomography (CT) imaging may reflect infiltration and periportal proliferative or formation of granulomatous lesions, respectively. Hepatic nodules may also present hypodense with ring enhancement [155]. Actual standard of care for children is basically 1 year of vinblastine, and prednisone is recommended as management of multisystem disease [152]. Also liver transplantation has rarely been reported as an option for patients with advanced liver disease [156].

22.3.4.2 Hemophagocytic Lymphohistiocytosis
Introduction
Hemophagocytic lymphohistiocytosis (HLH) is characterized by pathologically activated T cells and macrophages that engulf erythrocytes and to a lesser extent also leukocytes, which finally results in organ damage. Primary HLH is caused by germline mutations that play a role in the cytotoxic function of NK cells and lymphocytes [160], while secondary HLH is a pathologic inflammation occurring in malignancy or autoimmune disease. HLH manifestations include fever and splenomegaly; laboratory abnormalities show cytopenia, hyperferritinemia, and increased levels of soluble IL2 receptor, and hemophagocytosis can be detected on bone marrow biopsies [161]. Symptoms are mainly caused by circulating cytokines released from activated natural killer cells and cytotoxic T cells [162].

Liver Involvement

Liver manifestations play a central role in HLH and range from hepatomegaly occurring in half of the cases, cholestasis and transaminase elevation, to decreased hepatic function and fulminant hepatic failure [163]. Cholestasis among others determines the prognosis of HLH [164]. Hepatotoxicity is induced by hemophagocytosis in the hepatic sinusoids and the cytokine impact with focal hepatocellular necrosis [113, 163]. Liver histology may show large portal infiltrates of lymphocytes, immunoblasts, and histiocytes [165]. Prognosis is fatal if HLH remains unrecognized and untreated. Treatment is immunosuppression or, in cases of irreversible immune injury or persistent inflammation, haematopoietic stem cell transplantation [162].

22.3.5 Multiple Myeloma

Introduction
Multiple myeloma (MM) arises from plasma cell clones that are derived from post-germinal-centre B cells. Myeloma is thought to originate from monoclonal gammopathy of undetermined clinical significance (MGUS) that progresses to smouldering myeloma and finally to symptomatic myeloma [166]. It occurs increasingly with age. Experience in children is scarce and relies on few case reports [167]. Malignant plasma cells reside mainly in the bone marrow, but they can also be found in the peripheral blood and other organs. In most patients, MM is characterized by the secretion of a monoclonal immunoglobulin or monoclonal free light chains, which are produced by the abnormal plasma cells. Liver involvement in children has not been reported.

22.3.6 Sinusoidal Obstruction Syndrome/Veno-Occlusive Disease

Sinusoidal obstruction syndrome (SOS), formerly referred to as hepatic veno-occlusive disease (VOD), is primarily an issue in patients undergoing haematopoietic cell transplantation (HCT) [168]. SOS is caused by toxic injury of the sinusoidal endothelium, from where cells detach from the sinusoidal wall are transported downstream and finally block the sinusoidal blood flow. Furthermore dissection of red blood cells and leukocytes into the space of Disse leads to accumulation of cell components in the terminal hepatic vein, which triggers proliferation of perisinusoidal stellate cells and fibroblasts and thus induces formation of extracellular matrix [169]. Subsequent lumen constriction increases the resistance to blood flow and augments post-sinusoidal portal hypertension that worsens liver dysfunction and ascites and may finally result in multi-organ failure (MOF) [170]. Sinusoidal endothelial cells can be injured by chemotherapy or radiotherapy used for conditioning therapy and cytokine release due to inflammation and engraftment, endotoxins, alloreactivity, and calcineurin inhibitors [168]. Another rare cause of SOS is liver transplantation [171]. In children the incidence of SOS ranges from 20 to 60%, which exceeds two- to threefold the incidence reported for adults [172]. A number of diseases typically manifesting in childhood carry a higher risk for the development of SOS, for example, infantile osteopetrosis [173]; also certain congenital diseases such as congenital macrophage activation syndromes, familial hemophagocytic lymphohistiocytosis, Griscelli syndrome, and X-linked lymphoproliferative disease are frequently linked to the occurrence of SOS [168]. In addition, hepatic iron overload due to thalassemia or sickle cell disease is related with an increased risk of SOS development [174]. Taken together, the paediatric population represents probably the largest group at risk of SOS, which may be due to the immaturity of the liver in this age group [168]. In children SOS seems to occur later in the course of the posttransplant period, in one fifth of the cases after 30 days. Clinical manifestations include hepatomegaly, ascites, and weight gain. Progression to MOF has been documented for 30–60% of the affected children [175].

Significant differences of disease manifestations between adult and paediatric patients, in particular concerning time of onset and occurrence of hyperbilirubinemia, have been identified. The recently proposed diagnostic and severity criteria for SOS in paediatric patients on behalf of the European Society for Blood and Marrow Transplantation (EBMT) consider these diagnostic deviations from existing guidelines adjusted for adults. The diagnostic EBMT criteria for SOS in paediatric patients are summarized in Table 22.1 (adapted from Corbacioglu et al. 2018 [168]). Defibrotide is approved for the treatment of post-HCT severe hepatic SOS in the European Union [176]. Preclinical studies indicate that defibrotide induces endothelial cell protection, reduces activation, and enhances plasmin enzymatic activity [177]. Its early use was associated, particularly in children, with a better outcome and overall survival [178]. In addition, supportive care aiming to control extracellular fluid accumulation without exacerbating renal damage should be provided [179]. Patients at very high risk to be affected by this life-threatening disease, for example, children with osteopetrosis, hemophagocytic lymphohistiocytosis, or other macrophage activation syndromes, benefit from the prophylactic use of defibrotide [180].

22.3.7 Graft Versus Host Disease (GVHD)

Allogeneic haematopoietic stem cell transplant (HSCT) allows to treat many malignant and non-malignant disorders achieving survival rates over 90% and cure for some disease due to significant improvements in human leukocyte antigen (HLA)-typing techniques, less toxic conditioning regimens, and better supportive care [181]. Previous subdivision between acute GVHD (aGVHD) and chronic GVHD (cGVHD), which were exclusively based on the time of presentation, before or after day 100, respectively, gives nowadays more and more way to a classification depending on the clinico-pathological constellation. The combination of inflammatory dermatitis, enteritis, and hepatitis that is caused by cytotoxic lymphocytes and inflammatory cytokines due to T-cell activation characterizes aGVHD, while signs of cGHVD include manifestations, which resemble autoimmune diseases [182]. Even though grading of liver involvement is accomplished according to the degree of the hyperbilirubinemia, it is often preceded or accompanied by elevations of serum transaminases, in particular ALT, and later on by elevations of serum alkaline phosphatase. The liver is rarely the sole organ affected by aGVHD, and usually it occurs with co-involvement of the gut, which requires additional systemic treatment. Systemic glucocorticoids are used as first-line therapy in this case [182].

Chronic GVHD is characterized by variable clinical features resembling autoimmune or other immunologic disorders such as scleroderma, Sjögren's syndrome, primary biliary cirrhosis, wasting syndrome, bronchiolitis obliterans, immune cytopenia, and chronic immunodeficiency [183]. The rates of cGVHD in children (20–50%) are lower than in adults (60–70%), but the incidence seems to increase due to the more frequent implementation of peripheral blood stem cells and unrelated donors. cGVHD usually occurs approximately 6 months after allo-HSCT and can affect almost any organ [184]. The pathophysiology of cGVHD may include inflammation, cell-mediated immunity, humoral immunity, and fibrosis [183]. The 2014 NIH Chronic GVHD Diagnosis and Staging Consensus Recommendations discuss in detail diagnostic criteria and organ-specific severity scores [183]. There are no hepatic manifestations that are pathognomonic for cGVHD, moreover liver injury may be due to a variable number of other causes such as infection, drug toxicity, iron overload, focal nodular hyperplasia, etc. that need to be investigated [184]. Hepatic cGVHD can present as cholestatic or hepatitic form. Portal fibrosis and bile duct reduction causing obstructive jaundice characterized by increased alkaline phosphatase, gamma-glutamyl transferase (GGT), and serum bilirubin is a typical disease expression, while hepatitis-like isolated elevation of serum alanine aminotransferase (ALT) and aspartate aminotransferase (AST) with epithelial bile duct damage, significant portal/periportal inflammation, and lobular necro-inflammation is rarely seen. The hepatitic form usually requires prompt immunosuppressive intervention with glucocorticoids. Ursodeoxycholic acid may be useful in the case of hyperbilirubinemia [184, 185].

Table 22.1 EBMT diagnostic criteria for hepatic SOS in children

EBMT diagnostic criteria for hepatic SOS in children [168]
• No limitation for time of onset of SOS
The presence of two or more of the following:[a]
• Unexplained consumptive and transfusion-refractory thrombocytopenia[b]
• Otherwise unexplained weight gain on three consecutive days despite the use of diuretics or a weight gain
• ≥5% above baseline value
• Hepatomegaly (best if confirmed by imaging) above baseline value[c]
• Ascites (best if confirmed by imaging) above baseline value[c]
• Rising bilirubin from a baseline value on three consecutive days or bilirubin ≥2 mg/dL within 72 h

CT computed tomography; *HCT* haematopoietic cell transplantation; *MRI* magnetic resonance imaging; *SOS/VOD* sinusoidal obstruction syndrome/veno-occlusive disease; *US* ultrasonography
[a]With the exclusion of other potential differential diagnoses
[b]≥1 weight-adjusted platelet substitution/day to maintain institutional transfusion guidelines
[c]Suggested: imaging (US, CT, or MRI) immediately before HCT to determine baseline value for both hepatomegaly and ascites

22.3.8 Anaemias

22.3.8.1 Thalassemia

Introduction

The thalassemias belong to a group of inherited disorders, which are characterized by haemolytic anaemia due to decreased or absent synthesis of a globin chain [186]. Both sexes are affected equally and the annual incidence is about 44 per 100,000. Alpha thalassemia is mainly seen in Africa and Southeast Asia, while beta thalassemia also occurs commonly in Mediterranean countries [187].

Alpha thalassemia is caused by deficient or absent synthesis of alpha globin chains, which induces production of excess beta globin chains. Disease expression correlates with quantity of gene deletions and related substitution of haemoglobin A (HbA) by haemoglobin H (HbH) that consists of four beta chains manifesting as alpha thalassemia intermediate and resulting in microcytic anaemia, haemolysis, and splenomegaly. Deletion of all four alpha genes induces increased production of haemoglobin Bart's (Hb Bart's), which is assembled by four gamma chains and has a causes course resulting in hydrops fetalis [187, 188].

Beta thalassemia is characterized by deficient or absent synthesis of beta globin chains, which causes overproduction of alpha genes. The amount of beta globin chains inversely correlates with the quantity of alpha globins and thus with the degree of disease manifestation. Beta thalassemia trait (minor) means that one gene is defect and leads to mild disease expression with microcytosis and benign anaemia. If both genes are absent or severely affected, the disease expresses as beta thalassemia major also called Cooley anaemia. The phenotypic expression of beta thalassemia intermedia is less severe with minor reduction of beta chains [187]. Beta thalassemia major manifests during infancy usually after 6 months of life with pallor, jaundice, growth retardation, and hepatosplenomegaly. After this period HbF is almost entirely substituted by defective Hb. The only curative therapy for this form of thalassemia is HSCT. Beta thalassemia intermedia causes symptoms due to microcytic anaemia later in life. Complications that may develop due to beta thalassemia major or intermedia are caused by increased stimulation of the BM, defective erythropoiesis, and iron overload resulting from repeated blood transfusions.

Increased iron storage is seen mainly in the liver, the heart, and in endocrine glands. Cardiac complications due to iron overload are the main cause of mortality in these cases [189]. Endocrinopathies due to iron overload include hypogonadism and diabetes mellitus. Splenomegaly develops in symptomatic thalassemias and can furthermore deteriorate the cytopenia. Thromboembolic events may occur, especially after splenectomy. In general, management of patients with thalassemias is supportive with on-demand blood transfusions and iron chelation if required, while HSCT is reserved for major disease expression. Excellent outcome has been reported for low-risk patients with no hepatomegaly, no portal fibrosis on liver biopsy, and regular chelation therapy [190].

Liver Involvement

The liver is the initial site of iron deposition, which results in fibrosis and cirrhosis. In blood supply-dependent thalassemias, the degree of liver injury directly depends on the patient's age, number of blood units transfused, and liver iron concentration. Liver fibrosis can worsen after HSCT without adequate iron depletion, whereas regression of cirrhosis has been shown after phlebotomy or the use of iron chelators such as deferoxamine after HSCT [191].

22.3.8.2 Sickle Cell Disease

Introduction

Sickle cell disease (SCD) is a highly prevalent monogenic disorder. Initially SCD was seen in areas with malarial disease (Africa, the Mediterranean, Southern Asia), whereas in Europe, it was present only in Greece and Southern Italy, but due to migration nowadays its prevalence all over the continent is increasing. In general, around 300,000 children with sickle cell syndromes are born every year [192]. SCD follows an autosomal recessive inheritance of the haemoglobin S (Hb S) variant. Its most frequent genotype (sickle cell anaemia or homozygous SS disease) is caused by a single amino acid substitution at the sixth residue of the beta globin chain (p.Glu6Val), which results in the production of the characteristic sickle Hb that may result in haemolytic anaemia, vaso-occlusion, and vasculopathy, which are the hallmarks of SCD. Clinical manifestations range from a virtually asymptomatic to repeated acute events and chronic organ damage.

Liver Involvement

Liver involvement is mainly based on vascular diseases. Moreover, repeated transfusions for the treatment of anaemia may lead to iron overload, elevated risk of viral hepatitis, and gallstone formation, all of which can contribute to the development of a liver disease termed sickle cell hepatopathy, which is characterized by marked hyperbilirubinemia and impaired hepatic function [193]. However, aberrations of putative cholestasis parameters such as indirect bilirubin, LDH, ALP, and AST are frequently observed in patients with SCD without evidence of liver disease, since they are rather related to haemolysis and ineffective erythropoiesis [194], whereas acute increase in serum aminotransferases can be an indicator for hepatic ischemia in vaso-occlusive crisis [113]. There seem to be an association between autoimmune liver disease (AILD) and SCD. It is noteworthy that 17% of SCD patients in a cohort of 77 children showed serologic and/or histologic signs of AILD affecting mainly female patients and responding well to immunosuppression [195].

22.3.8.3 Haemolytic Anaemia

Introduction

Sever damage of red blood cells leads to preterm destruction or removal of red blood cells from the circulation. Minor haemolysis can occur lifelong without causing any symptoms, but usually erythrocytosis cannot keep pace with red cell destruction, which leads to manifestation of anaemia. Typical clinical manifestations of haemolytic anaemia (HA) include jaundice, cholelithiasis, and splenomegaly [196]. Intravascular haemolysis occurs as a consequence of red blood cell destruction due to a mechanical trauma caused by endothelium injury, complement binding and activation, and infectious agents. The more common extravascular haemolysis results from removal of erythrocyte by macrophages within the reticuloendothelial system due to membrane alterations [196]. Most intrinsic causes are hereditary such as glucose-6-phosphate dehydrogenase deficiency, spherocytosis, thalassemia, and sickle cell anaemia with the exception of paroxysmal nocturnal haemoglobinuria (PNH). Extrinsic HA is induced by immune or non-immune mechanisms that include systemic diseases, for example, infections, hepatic, or renal diseases [113]. Liver involvement in specific disease entities is discussed in detail in the subsequent sections.

Autoimmune haemolytic anaemia (AIHA) is a rare condition in children. The annual incidence is estimated to range from 0.2 to 4 per million individuals under 20 years of age [197]. Most children affected are less than 5 years old and of female gender [198]. The hallmark of this disease is lysis of erythrocytes triggered by binding of autoantibodies to the cell surface. In children AIHA is the main cause of acquired extrinsic haemolysis [197]. In more than half of the cases, AIHA develops in the background of an underlying disease such as infections, immune, or lymphoproliferative disorder (secondary AIHA). When this condition is missing, AIHA is termed idiopathic or primary [198].

Liver Involvement

An unusual association with Coombs-positive haemolytic anaemia is giant cell hepatitis (GCH), which is characterized by the appearance of large multinucleated hepatocytes, so-called giant cells, and progressive liver function impairment. GCH-AIHA occurs early in childhood and has a severe disease course potentially leading to liver failure. In general outcome is poor with a mortality rate of 39% of the reported cases. Treatment response to standard immunosuppression is poor in most cases, and high recurrence rates have been seen after liver transplantation [199]. A humoral immune mechanism has been proposed as probable cause for GCH-AIHA. Authors argue that Coombs-positivity results from activation of complement cascade on the red cell surface as a consequence of immunoglobulin G (IgG) binding. Since hepatocyte injury also seems to be induced by complement binding and portal inflammatory infiltrates include mainly macrophages and neutrophils, B-cell-mediated autoimmunity seems the mechanism, which is responsible for disease development [200]. Furthermore, others have shown association with different autoimmune conditions such as type 1 diabetes, thyroiditis, and psoriasis [199]. Another hypothesis suspects a non-controlled release of cytokines by activated T lymphocytes and Kupffer cells to play a role in the disease development [201]. Several immune-modulatory drugs have been applied for the treatment of GCH-AIHA including corticoids, azathioprine, cyclosporine, tacrolimus, mycophenolate mofetil, intravenous immunoglobulins, and anti-CD20 (rituximab) [202].

22.3.8.4 Paroxysmal Nocturnal Haemoglobinuria

Introduction

Paroxysmal nocturnal haemoglobinuria (PNH) is a rare disease characterized by dark urine (haemoglobinuria), usually in the morning, intravascular haemolysis, thrombotic events, bone marrow failure, and serious infections. In children, PNH is even rarer and predominantly affects teenagers [203]. Somatic mutations of the X-linked PIG-A gene in haematopoietic stem cells that expresses a protein involved in the synthesis of glycosylphosphatidylinositol (GPI) are responsible for the development of classic PNH. GPI anchors various proteins on the cell surface of blood cells. Mutations at this site lead to the loss of inhibitors of the complement system, thereby inducing increased susceptibility of the affected cells to complement-mediated lysis [204]. Classic PNH is distinguished from PNH/BMD, where bone marrow disorder (BMD) like aplastic anaemia (AA) or myelodysplastic syndrome (MDS) predominates and PNH develops as secondary condition. In comparison to adult patients classic PNH is seen less frequently in children than PNH/BMD.

Liver Involvement

Serious complications associated with PNH include development of a hypercoagulable state and formation of thrombi. A significantly higher thrombosis risk has been found for adult patients with more than 50% of PNH GPI-anchor deficient granulocytes [205]. In a retrospective study, including 26 children, 31% experienced venous thrombotic events including Budd-Chiari syndrome [203]. In adults PNH can cause also de novo portal vein thrombosis, which has not yet been described in the paediatric population [206].

22.3.9 Disseminated Intravascular Coagulation

Introduction

Disseminated intravascular coagulation (DIC) is characterized by systemic activation of coagulation that results in intravascular thrombin and fibrin generation. Thromboembolism can lead to organ dysfunction on the one hand and due to increased consumption to severe bleeding complications on the other hand. In older infants and children, the major causes of DIC include sepsis, trauma, and malignancies. In the neonate, DIC is caused primarily by sepsis and perinatal complications (i.e. birth asphyxia) [207]. The underlying aetiology essentially determines the treatment of DIC. Clinical manifestations vary in relation to the severity of DIC and range from mild bleeding venipuncture sites to severe life-threating haemorrhage and thrombosis with end-organ damage especially of kidneys, liver, lungs, central nervous system, and extremities. The diagnosis of overt DIC is based upon clinical findings of haemorrhage and microthrombi in patients with predisposing medical conditions and abnormal coagulation studies. Developed scoring systems essentially imply the medical condition known to be associated with DIC and readily available coagulation tests. The major treatment approach should include the therapy of the underlying disease, for example, administering antibiotics, placing surgical drainages, or introducing anticancer drugs. However, additional adjustments of coagulation abnormalities are sometimes required [208].

Liver Involvement

Hepatic manifestations include jaundice, which may apart from liver impairment also be due to increased bilirubin production secondary to haemolysis. Sepsis and hypotension, as well as thromboembolism, can cause ischemic hepatocellular injury. Thrombosis with end-organ dysfunction was found in up to 35% of patients [209]. Since the liver itself plays a pivotal role in the synthesis, not only of coagulation factors but also of inhibitors, hepatic injury significantly impacts on the deterioration of DIC. Moreover, thrombocytopenia may also aggravate by hypersplenism due to portal hypertension [113].

22.3.10 Thrombophilia

Introduction

Thrombophilias are hereditary or acquired conditions which can increase the risk of venous or arterial thrombosis. Since the aetiology of thrombosis is multifactorial, other elements in addition to the thrombophilic defect are usually required to determine the risk. Hereditary thrombophilia is due to a genetic mutation that affects the amount or function of a protein in the coagulation system. The most frequent mutations and their function are summarized in Table 22.2 [210]. The antiphospholipid syndrome (APS) is an example of acquired thrombophilia, even though familial mutations have been described. However, transient elevations of antiphospholipid antibodies (APAs) frequently occur in otherwise healthy children after an infection without pathogenic significance. Diagnosis of APS thus requires persistently positive APAs [211]. The majority of young children who develop thrombosis have several coexisting risk factors. There are divergent data concerning the risk of inherited thrombophilia for thrombotic events in children. Accordingly, the reported prevalence of thrombophilia in children with venous and arterial thrombotic events varies greatly, from as low as 13% to as high as 79%.

Liver Involvement

Thrombophilia impacts on liver function on a microscopic and macroscopic level and is among many other one possible cause for the development of liver fibrosis. Hepatic vein thrombosis in Budd-Chiari syndrome, for example, may induce hepatic fibrosis [212]. In addition, data suggest accelerated fibrogenesis in the presence of hypercoagulability. In patients with chronic viral hepatitis and NAFLD, advanced fibrosis is significantly more often associated with thrombophilia than earlier stadium of liver disease. Patients with factor V Leiden (FVL) mutation and hepatitis C have an increased risk of fibrosis progression. Similar observations of higher fibrosis grades are reported for patients with protein C deficiency, increased FVIII expression and hyperhomocysteinaemia [213]. Intrahepatic micro-infarcts in hepatic and portal veins may cause ischemia and finally fibrosis. Moreover, hepatic stellate cell activation induced by liver injury stimulates myofibroblasts with pro-inflammatory and pro-fibrogenic abilities. Moreover, interaction with thrombin causes secretion of extracellular matrix proteins and stimulation of fibrogenesis [214]. Taken together, these findings suggest that hypercoagulability may play a role in fibrogenesis through stellate cell activation [213]. Also Budd-Chiari syndrome and portal vein thrombosis are frequently linked to prothrombotic disorders. Moreover, thrombophilia seems to be involved in the development of idiopathic non-cirrhotic portal hypertension (INCPH), since an association has been found in up to 50% of the cases [215].

Table 22.2 Most common hereditary thrombophilias

Thrombophilia	Mutation type
Factor V Leiden mutation	Gain of function
Prothrombin 20210 mutation	Gain of function
Protein S deficiency	Loss of function
Protein C deficiency	Loss of function
Antithrombin deficiency	Loss of function
Elevated lipoprotein(a)	Gain of function
Elevated factor VIII	Gain of function
Hyperhomocysteinaemia	Loss of function

22.4 Chronic Inflammatory Diseases

22.4.1 Celiac Disease

Introduction

Celiac disease (CD) develops as chronic inflammatory intestinal disorder in genetically predisposed persons when exposure to dietary gluten occurs. CD is a highly prevalent systemic disease that affects around 1% of individuals of any age in Europe and North America [216]. In first-degree relatives prevalence is as high as 15% [217]. Certain HLA-haplotypes are significantly associated with CD, especially DQ2 and DQ8 are expressed in 90% or 5% of the cases, respectively [216]. Dietary gliadin peptides are deamidated by small intestinal tissue transglutaminase, become immunogenic, and cause activation of pro-inflammatory CD4+ T cells. Mainly dendritic cells that carry HLA-DQ2 and DQ8 molecules present these immunogenic peptides. Activation of T cells subsequently manifests in cytokine production, clonal T-cell expansion, and B-cell recruitment, which leads to the production of anti-gliadin (AGA) and anti-transglutaminase antibodies (tTGA) [218]. Chronic diarrhoea, weight loss, and abdominal pain occur in almost half of CD patients. Other symptoms include iron deficiency, aphthous stomatitis, growth retardation, and chronic fatigue. To avoid clinical manifestations and especially complications such as osteoporosis, neurologic impairment, ulcerative jejuno-ileitis, and cancer, which may appear when the disease remains untreated, gluten-free diet has to be introduced [216]. Diagnosis is based on the combination of serologic findings and biopsy of the small intestine. Tissue transglutaminase antibodies (tTGA) and anti-endomysial antibodies (EMA) of the immunoglobulin A (IgA) class show high sensitivity (98%) and a specificity between 90 and 99%. IgG-deamidated gliadin peptide antibodies (DGP) can be used in patents with IgA deficiency and in children under 2 years of age. Recommendations for children and adolescence do not necessarily imply a small bowel biopsy, when symptoms are present and tTGA titter is high (>10× ULN), in the background of EMA and HLA-DQ2/-DQ8 positivity [219].

Liver Involvement

Mild to moderate hypertransaminasemia has been reported in approximately 60% of symptomatic Italian children with CD [220]. Frequent histological changes include Kupffer cell hyperplasia, mononuclear cell infiltration, and steatosis [221]. In children with increased transaminase levels, biopsies show reactive hepatitis as well as moderately active chronic hepatitis. The reported children did not have any symptoms, but jejunal histology revealed the presence of CD. Transaminases returned to normal levels in all patients on gluten-free diet (GFD), and resolution of histologic changes could be shown in some cases [222]. In a large prospective study involving children and adolescents with isolated hypertransaminasemia for more than 6 months, 1.8% were diagnosed with CD. It is therefore advisable to test for CD in children with otherwise unexplained hypertransaminasemia [223]. Autoimmune liver disorders (AILD), namely, autoimmune hepatitis (AIH), autoimmune cholangitis (AIC), and overlap syndrome, are frequently associated with CD in up to 16% of children, and in about one fifth of the cases, the AILD precedes the CD. Liver histology revealed typical signs of auto-inflammatory injury and variable degrees of fibrosis including cirrhosis in all patients. After strict GFD and immunosuppression, remission could be observed in all subjects [224]. Another study showed normalization of hypertransaminasemia after introduction of GFD, while children with associated AIH required additional immunosuppressive treatment [225]. Moreover, AILD has been reported more frequently among adolescents and young adults with CD than in an age-matched control group without the disease [226]. Within the paediatric population, a linkage between CD and PSC has less frequently been observed [224, 227]. There is growing evidence that CD is associated with NAFLD as shown by a large study from Sweden including more than 26,000 CD patients (about 40% ≤19 years of age). It seems that the risk to develop NAFLD is highest during the first year after diagnosis of CD, but as discussed by the authors, one cannot exclude a surveillance bias due to intensified medical evaluation in this period. However, even after 15 years significantly more CD patients were diagnosed with NAFLD. The pathogenesis is unclear, but it is hypothesized that small intestinal bacterial overgrowth and increased intestinal permeability are involved as well as cellular stress. TNF-α may play a role, since it induces tissue injury in CD on the one hand and potentially promotes progression to NASH in NAFLD on the other hand [228]. In general, liver involvement in CD is not well understood. As discussed for NAFLD, it may be due to the combination of increased permeability of the gut and bacterial overgrowth at the same time. In addition, more than 70% of the blood supply derives from the intestine and thus delivers also its toxic products [229]. In conclusion, liver involvement in CD should be routinely tested, and vice versa association with CD should be excluded in children with hepatic disease [223].

22.4.2 Hepatic Amyloidosis

Introduction

Amyloidosis is an extremely rare finding in children and has been mentioned mainly in association with sJIA as described elsewhere in this chapter. Amyloid is characterized by fibril deposits composed of different low molecular weight subunits of serum proteins [230].

Liver Involvement

Within the liver amyloid deposits are found in hepatic stellate cells and induce a pro-fibrogenic state that resembles other fibrotic liver disorders. Clinical manifestations include hepatomegaly and increased ALP levels. Progressed liver injury with portal hypertension and hepatic malfunction is rarely observed. The gold standard to diagnose amyloidosis is liver biopsy, but it should only be encouraged after exclusion of other easier accessible disease locations, since increased bleeding risk has been reported in some cases. The primary aim is to treat the underlying disease such as malignancy, auto-inflammatory disorder, or infection, and other therapeutic interventions are solely supportive [230, 231].

22.4.3 Hepatic Granulomas

Introduction

Hepatic granulomas are unspecific features, which may indicate a systemic disease. Granulomas themselves do generally not cause liver injury, but their histologic characterization and intrahepatic localization together with the clinical manifestations can be suggestive for the underlying disorder. A selection of possible disease aetiologies of hepatic granulomas and their histological features are summarized in Table 22.3.

Granulomas are circumscribed structures caused by inflammatory reactions of various origins. A rim of lymphocytes and fibroblasts surrounds central macrophages, which have been stimulated by cytokines. Thereby activated macrophages, also called epithelioid cells, from sarcoidosis patients, for example, are able to release different proteins, e.g. the well-known and diagnostically important angiotensin-converting enzyme (ACE). However, one has to keep in mind that ACE levels vary according to the age; healthy children have up to 50% higher values than adults [232]. The presence of eosinophil's suggested a drug-induced injury or a parasitic infection. Other histologic characteristics that may lead to the diagnosis of the provoking disease include caseating and noncaseating conditions, which describe the presence or absence of central necrosis, as seen in tuberculosis or sarcoidosis, respectively. When epithelioid cells build a circle around a vacuole often with a fibrin ring, the differential diagnoses rather point to Hodgkin lymphoma, cytomegalovirus (CMV), or allopurinol drug toxicity. Lipogranulomas containing a central lipid vacuole occur in association with fatty liver disease (Table 22.3). Intrahepatic localization of the granulomas can be another indicator for the pathogenesis; portal or periportal lesions, for example, are usually observed in sarcoidosis or PBC [233]. In general granulomas emerge, when foreign material

Table 22.3 Disease Aetiologies of Hepatic Granulomas

Selected causes of hepatic granulomas		Histopathologic features
Autoimmune disease	Sarcoidosis	Noncaseating epithelioid cell granuloma [239]
	PBC	Noncaseating often adjacent to portal tracts [240]
Bacteria	Mycobacterium tuberculosis	Caseating [236]
	Bartonella henselae (cat scratch disease)	Fibrin-rim and characteristic stellate abscesses [241]
	Listeriosis	Micro-abscesses with small granulomas [242]
Viral	Cytomegalovirus	Fibrin-ring granuloma [243]
	Epstein-Barr virus	Fibrin-ring granuloma [244]
	Hepatitis C	Epithelioid granulomas [245]
Fungal	Histoplasmosis	Foamy macrophage aggregates [237]
Parasitic	Schistosomiasis	Granuloma surrounding schistosomal egg often accompanied by portal fibrosis [246]
Drugs	Amoxicillin/clavulanate	Epithelioid granulomas [247]
	Bacillus Calmette-Guérin	Epithelioid granulomas [248]
Inherited	Chronic granulomatous disease	Epithelioid granulomas, sometimes pigmented macrophages in sinusoids [249]
Metabolic	Fatty liver disease	Lipogranulomas [250]

is inefficiently clearable by the immune system, which thus aims to isolate and neutralize difficult-to-eradicate pathogenic substrates [234].

Clinical manifestations are multifactorial and depend on the pathophysiologic mechanism. Patients often present with fever, particularly in the case of a systemic infection, and also night sweats and weight loss can occur. Hepatosplenomegaly has been observed primarily in association with schistosomiasis [235]. Increased levels of alkaline phosphatase are noticed frequently, while jaundice occurs mainly in the case of bile duct injury. In addition, advanced liver disease with portal hypertension has been observed, especially in sarcoidosis, PBC, and schistosomiasis [233].

The most frequent causes of hepatic granulomas accounting for approximately three quarters of cases in the Western world are sarcoidosis, drugs, mycobacterial infections, malignancies, and PBC. Data from children are scarce. A single centre study from Southern Iran involving patients from 10 days to 75 years of age found mainly infectious causes as trigger for hepatic granuloma formation, above all mycobacterial infections that accounted for more than 50% of the cases [236]. Another small study from North America revealed that the aetiology of two third of children, who underwent a liver biopsy, which evidenced granulomas, was histoplasma infection, followed by sarcoidosis and schistosomiasis [237]. The pathogenesis therefore seems to vary slightly between children and adults and markedly depends on the geographic area. However, the aetiology cannot be clarified in up to 36% of cases despite profound workup [233].

The primary aim is to treat the underlying disease. If no specific disorder can be identified, clinical symptoms, granulomas, and liver function should regularly be monitored. Immunosuppressive treatment with corticoids can be taken into consideration in the case of idiopathic granulomatous hepatitis after exclusion of mycobacterial tuberculosis infection. If the response is unsatisfying, one should consider neoplastic disease or atypical infections [238].

22.4.4 Primary Antiphospholipid Syndrome and Budd-Chiari Syndrome

Introduction
Antiphospholipid syndrome (APS) is an autoimmune disease leading to arterial and venous thrombosis and is generally defined by the persistence of antiphospholipid antibodies (aPL) and pregnancy morbidity [251]. In children primary APS is not well characterized but implies the presence of aPL associated with thrombosis [252]. Other autoimmune disorders may be linked to APS, especially childhood-onset systemic lupus erythematosus (SLE). Paediatric primary APS is rare, data from a large European cohort including 1000 patients (mean age 42 years) evidenced disease onset under 15 years of age in only 2.8% of the cases [253]. Out of 121 children with APS in Europe, 50% were primary disease and 41% associated with SLE [254].

While vascular thrombosis is a valid criterion for the diagnosis of APS in children, pregnancy morbidity is less relevant. In comparison to adults, the paediatric population is more frequently affected by non-thrombotic manifestations of haematological or neurological nature. Screening for APS should include all three types of aPL, namely, lupus anticoagulant (LA), anticardiolipin antibodies (aCL), and anti-β2 glycoprotein-I antibodies (anti-β2GPI). aPL can be detected in 11–87% of patients with SLE; it is therefore recommended to determine the titer in all SLE patients at the disease onset. However, without the occurrence of a thrombotic event, APS cannot be diagnosed, even if aPL are detectable [255].

In case of an associated disease, the underlying disorder needs to be treated adequately. Preventive treatment of APS in children with SLE and positivity for aPL should include an antiplatelet agent such as aspirin in addition to hydroxychloroquine. After manifestation of a thrombosis, long-term anticoagulation is recommended, only if the thrombotic event was related to persisting aPL. In the case of arterial thrombotic events and aPL positivity, a combination of anticoagulation and antiaggregation should be taken into consideration [255].

Liver Involvement
The lower limbs are the most frequent location of thrombotic events in children, while thrombosis of the vena cava, hepatic (Budd-Chiari syndrome, BCS), or portal veins occurs rarely [256]. Primary BCS is characterized by hepatic outflow obstruction regardless of the precise location or the entity of the obstruction [257]. Obstruction can affect the entire venous tract from the small hepatic veins to the right atrium. BCS typically manifests within 6 months with abdominal pain, ascites, hepatosplenomegaly, and to a lower degree with gastrointestinal varices. Also a fulminant presentation with disease manifestations within a few days has been described leading to severe liver dysfunction with increased aminotransferases, hyperbilirubinemia, hepatic encephalopathy, and hepatorenal syndrome [258]. Symptoms correlate with the number of vessels involved, the grade of occlusion, and the velocity of appearance that determines the possibility of compensation. However, one has to keep in mind that BCS due to APS in children is rarely reported and experience relies on some case reports [259–261].

22.4.5 IgG4-Related Disease

Introduction
IgG4-related disease (IgG4-RD) is characterized by the presence of IgG4 positive plasma cells that may form tumorous lesions in variable parts of the body leading to local inflammation and fibrosis. Only recently this disorder has been described, and, especially in the paediatric population, knowledge is based mainly on case reports. Awareness of this disease is important, since, if left untreated, progressive fibrosis causes persistent tissue injury. Data from a recent literature review involving 25 children from 22 months to 17 years of age (median, 13 years) show a female predominance (two thirds), while in adults, male patients seem to be affected more frequently [262]. Organ manifestations determine the symptomatic presentation of the disease. It seems that the disease locations in children are comparable to those in adults; orbital disease is also in the paediatric population on top of the list affecting almost half of the patients. IgG4-related pancreatitis was observed in 12% of children, followed by IgG4-related cholangitis and pulmonary disease occurring in 8% of cases each, other organs involved include the thyroid and the salivary glands, the mesenterium, lymph nodes, and the liver. Renal manifestations were reported in association with other

disease locations. In approximately 40% of the cases, two or more organs were affected [262]. IgG4-RD requires a histologic evidence; hence diagnosis is based on typical histological features including lymphoplasmacytic infiltrate, obliterative phlebitis, and storiform-type fibrosis; the ratio and absolute IgG4 counts in various tissues contribute to the final evaluation and are defined by the Boston Consensus [263]. Increased serum IgG4 levels were found in a similar proportion of children compared to adults (70%). Even if the positive predictive value of serum IgG4 is low, it may be useful to assess treatment response [263]. The pathogenesis of IgG4-RD has not been clarified yet, but it is supposed that T-helper cells and regulatory T cells, triggered by an antigen, activate B cells by cytokine stimulation, which in turn express IgG4 and induce generation of fibrosis [264]. Glucocorticoids are the first treatment choice [265]. In more than 80% of children, prednisone was effective, but in only half of the cases, remission was achieved by a monotherapy, and addition of an immunosuppressive maintenance treatment using MMF, azathioprine, or methotrexate was required [262].

Liver Involvement

IgG4-associated cholangitis (IAC) or IgG4-related sclerosing cholangitis (IgG4-RSC) is characterized by marked lymphocytic infiltration of the bile duct wall that is mainly composed of IgG4-positive plasma cells. Clinical manifestations usually consist of jaundice, abdominal pain, and weight loss. Pancreatic contribution (autoimmune pancreatitis) may occur leading to diabetes mellitus or symptoms of exocrine dysfunction. Radiological features include the detection of hepatic masses or sclerosing lesions rendering the distinction, between IAC from pancreatic biliary malignancies or sclerosing cholangiopathies, challenging [266]. Laboratory abnormalities may, apart from increased cholestatic parameters such as bilirubin, ALP, and gamma-GT, also consist of elevated IgG4 serum levels and heightened tumour marker CA19-9. But neither IgG4 levels, if less than fourfold increased [267], nor CA19-9 is specific for IAC. Typical histological features have already been described, and the organ-specific threshold for IgG4 positive plasma cells per high-power field has been set >10 in the case of IAC [263]. However, its sensitivity and specificity are low, applying this cut off level [268]. Thus, in the absence of specific diagnostic tools, several criteria for adults have been developed during the past few years, for example, the HISORt criteria [269] or the international consensus diagnostic criteria (ICDC) [270], which take in consideration clinical, radiological, histological, and serological features, involvement of other organs, and treatment response. Few paediatric case reports of IAC have been published until now. Children presented with asymptomatic liver enzyme abnormalities, apparent jaundice, or recurrent fever, while radiologic imaging varied, showing bile duct strictures, diffuse thickening of intrahepatic ducts, or a hepatic mass, respectively. Serum IgG4 levels were suggestive and histologic features clearly indicated IgG4-RD. In addition, the children responded well to immunosuppressive treatment [271–274].

22.5 The Liver in Cardiac Diseases

22.5.1 The Pathogenesis of Liver Involvement in Cardiac Diseases

The main two causes of hepatic dysfunction due to heart failure (HF) are passive congestion as a result of increased filling pressures in chronic heart failure, backward failure, or impaired perfusion secondary to low cardiac output, forward failure. The congestion-related perisinusoidal oedema can interfere with the transport of oxygen and nutrients to the hepatocytes, causing zone 3 sinusoidal dilation and haemorrhagic necrosis [275]. Augmented lymph formation may lead to ascites when the draining capacity of the lymphatic system is exhausted. Moreover, the occurrence of microthrombi is favoured by stagnant flow conditions. These mechanisms taken together can contribute to centrilobular fibrosis and ultimately cirrhosis ("cardiac cirrhosis") [276, 277]. Zonal enhancement on computed tomography scans has been found in correlation with inferior hepatic congestion and thus lower risk of cardiac cirrhosis, while reticular enhancement seems to be linked to extensive hepatic fibrosis. Isolated gamma-GT elevation is often the first sign of hepatic passive venous congestion, followed by moderate increase of AST and ALT levels as well as ALP and LDH elevation and rise of conjugated and nonconjugated bilirubin [278]. ALT deviations have been shown to correlate well with the right atrial pressure, the free hepatic venous pressure, and the wedge hepatic venous pressure, but not with the hepatic venous pressure gradient (HVPG). Elevated prothrombin time has been detected in association with congestive liver injury, while hypoalbuminemia is only described in decompensated cirrhosis [279]. Also ischemic hepatitis can appear in patients with right heart failure, since it results in reduced portal flow due to augmented hepatic sinusoidal pressure, and as a consequence increased sensitivity to alterations of the artery flow may occur [279]. Ascites is usually not a sign of decompensated liver disease but rather triggered by worsening right heart failure. Measuring serum-ascites albumin gradient and total protein may help in distinguishing between the two origins [280], but an HVPG measurement and/or a transjugular liver biopsy is often required to determine the underlying cause. The general management of complications of portal hypertension is in accordance with the standard guidelines, but some aspects need to be specified:

- Transjugular intrahepatic portosystemic shunt (TIPS) implantation is not recommended in the presence of high right-sided pressures, due to the risk of shunt dysfunction as well as potentially severe elevation of preload.

- Gastric variceal bleeding is more difficult to treat, because variceal obliteration with tissue adhesive glues is linked to a higher risk of systemic emboli due to right-to-left intracardiac shunts.
- Higher-grade varices should be excluded or treated before starting an anticoagulation treatment.

Forward heart failure with impaired hepatic perfusion leads to ischemic tissue injury. The liver can protect itself from hypoxia-related damages by improved hepatocyte extraction of oxygen up to 95% [279]. When this protective mechanism is exhausted, an acute ischemic injury can occur. Low cardiac output can cause a variable degree of hepatic perfusion damage, which may range from clinically not evident to acute hypoxic hepatitis due to severe systemic hypotension in cardiopulmonary failure [279]. Also forward heart failure leading to ischemic liver injury is characterized by centrilobular necrosis, but without any sign of histological inflammation as seen in viral hepatitis [281]. Acute cardiac dysfunction usually causes both low cardiac output liver disease and passive hepatic congestion. Distinguishing this entity from primary liver disorders may be difficultly, but the ALT/LDH ratio of less than 1.5 can be a hint for ischemic injury [282]. Moreover, rapid significant elevation of AST and ALT levels in association with acute decrease in cardiac output and systemic hypotension also indicates ischemic liver injury. Acute cardiac failure is rather linked to jaundice with significantly increased bilirubin and encephalopathy in comparison to chronic or acute on chronic cardiac dysfunction [279]. AST is usually the primary marker of ischemic liver injury, reaching levels of more than ten times ULN, and also important increase in LDH and high ALP serum levels as well as prolonged prothrombin time are frequently noticed. In general, these changes reach highest values after 1 to 3 days and return to normal within 4–10 days once the underlying cardiac disorder has been resolved [278].

22.5.1.1 Altered Pharmacokinetics in Liver Dysfunction

Liver dysfunction can interfere with the pharmacokinetic of cardiovascular drugs, which may cause altered harmful blood concentrations of the agents. Awareness of these circumstances is necessary to adjust the doses. For instance, losartan or propranolol is primarily metabolized in the liver; thus liver dysfunction may lead to a bioavailability of these drugs almost twice as high as normal, while ACE inhibitors, which are prod rugs, and need to be activated in the liver, often do not reach the expected levels of the activated agent. Response to warfarin is usually potentiated in patients with liver dysfunction, since its inactivation by hepatic cytochrome P-450 is reduced. Statins have to be used carefully in patients with liver dysfunction due to their potential hepatotoxicity and should be avoided in the case of acute liver failure. Digoxin does not undergo hepatic metabolism, but due to the lower distribution volume, lower drug dosage may be required. Normal dosage can usually be kept for diuretic treatment [278].

22.5.2 Congenital Heart Defects

Liver involvement occurs frequently in patients with congenital heart defects (CHD), since the primary cardiac defect itself as well as the palliative surgical procedure can cause hepatic injury. Moreover, repeated transfusions and drug-related hepatotoxicity may contribute to the liver damage. Congenital heart disease (CHD) affects approximately 1.35 million new-borns globally every year and thus represent the most frequent congenital anomaly [283]. The prevalence of CHD is 8 per 1000 live births [284], and in 10–40% of the cases, CHD leads to HF in infancy [285, 286].

22.5.2.1 Left-to-Right Shunt

Shunting may cause right atrial and ventricular enlargement and tricuspid regurgitation due to dilatation of the tricuspid annulus. Ventricular septal defects, atrial septal defects, complete atrioventricular canal defects, patent ductus arteriosus, and aortopulmonary windows may induce this pathophysiologic mechanism [287]. Pulmonary hypertension can sometimes be a consequence of the volume overload, which reverses the shunt from right to left and thus causes cyanosis (Eisenmenger's syndrome). Pulmonary hypertension is more frequently seen in patients with a VSD. Passive congestion with central venous hypertension is the pathophysiologic mechanism responsible for the liver injury in these cases [279]. After repair of complete atrioventricular septal defects, left ventricular outflow tract obstruction can occur in approximately 3.5% of cases, which may result in hypoxic liver injury [288].

22.5.2.2 Tetralogy of Fallot (TOF)

This combination of lesions occurs in about 30 of every 100,000 live births and accounts for 7–10% of all congenital cardiac malformations [289]. The main features consist of a ventricular septal defect, pulmonary stenosis, overriding aorta, and right ventricular hypertrophy [290]. Surgical repair of the pulmonary stenosis may lead to pulmonary regurgitation, which in turn can cause right ventricular dilatation and consequently tricuspid regurgitation that finally results in right ventricular dysfunction. Communication between the ventricles may also impair the left ventricle. As a consequence, besides passive congestion with central venous hypertension, here also hepatic ischemia can occur due to the low-flow state [279].

22.5.2.3 Ebstein's Anomaly

Ebstein's anomaly (EA) is a rare disease; it is described in less than 1% of cases with CHD [291]. The mean annual incidence is 11.4 per 100,000 live births [284]. Even though it is a congenital anomaly, it can clinically manifest at any age. EA is a special form of tricuspid valve dysplasia due to failed delamination from the right ventricular endothelium [292]. Associations with different cardiac congenital disorders have been identified such as mitral valve prolapse and left ventricular non-compaction (LVNC) [293]. Regurgitation across the defective tricuspid valve may cause dilatation and dysfunction of the right ventricle, which can in part remain, even after surgical repair of the tricuspid valve, and lead to liver injury by passive congestion [279].

22.5.2.4 D-Transposition of the Great Arteries (D-TGA)

The prevalence of D-TGA is 3 per 100,000 live births [284]. Male sex is predominantly affected [294]. D-TGA is characterized by the transposition of the aorta, which originates from the right ventricle, and the pulmonary artery that arises from the left ventricle. The arterial switch operation is nowadays applied to manage this disorder, which has led to a 20-year survival of almost 90% [295]. The formerly used atrial switch procedure according to Mustard and Senning resulted in ventricular failure and tricuspid regurgitation, because the morphology of the right ventricle did not resist to systemic pressures. Passive congestion of the liver occurred, which can now be avoided by the arterial switch procedure [279].

22.5.2.5 Coronary Insufficiency

Cardiomyopathies due to ischemic injury can result from congenital anomalies such as an anomalous left coronary artery from the pulmonary artery and an anomalous aortic origin of a coronary artery. Also surgical procedures may cause ischemic cardiomyopathies as, for example, the Ross procedure, a pulmonary autograft replacement for the aortic valve, or the arterial switch operation for the D-TGA. Ischemic cardiac injury may lead to forward failure and thus to hypoxic liver impairment.

22.5.2.6 Outflow Tract Obstruction

Supravalvular aortic stenosis and pulmonary stenosis are examples of cardiac pressure overload disorders that may induce different types of hepatic pathophysiologic mechanisms. Supravalvular aortic stenosis (SAS) includes variable degrees of obstructive anomalies that range from an unimpressive membrane to tunnel-like obstruction. It is a relatively common CHD with a prevalence of 6.5% [296]. In more than 70% of the cases, SAS can lead to aortic regurgitation, which has been shown to be a significant predictor for surgical intervention. Even after surgery recurrence of the obstruction has been observed [297]. Forward cardiac failure is the main mechanism that causes liver disease in these patients, since it leads to low-flow state and thus hypoxic injury. Instead, pulmonary stenosis, which occurs with an annual incidence of about 73 per 100,000 live births [284], leads to increase of right ventricular and right atrial pressure and thus causes congestive liver injury [298].

22.5.2.7 Single-Ventricle Physiology and Fontan Operation

The Fontan procedure, previously reported in patients with tricuspid atresia, is commonly performed in patients with single-ventricle physiology. A similar condition results from the univentricular correction of the hypoplastic left heart syndrome following the Norwood procedure [299]. A single-ventricle causes intracardiac mixing of low and highly oxygenized blood and thus leads to arterial hypoxemia and exorbitant volume load on a single ventricle. The Fontan operation bypasses the hypoplastic right ventricle by creating a caval-pulmonary anastomosis using either an intra-atrial tunnel or an extra-cardiac conduit, which is interposed between the vena cava and the pulmonary arteries [279]. Even though the Fontan operation is considered a definite solution, as time passes it may get out of balance [300]. Indeed, liver disease can develop as a result of inevitable rise in central venous pressure [301]. However, variable factors contribute to significant hepatic injury after a Fontan procedure. Increased pulmonary vascular resistance due to thrombi, scarring in the Fontan pathway, or failure of the systemic ventricle resulting in increased pressure in the pulmonary conduit may lead to Fontan circuit failure. Moreover, atrial arrhythmias and formation of pulmonary veno-venous collaterals can have an impact on the hypoxia. Low cardiac output with hypoxic liver injury and more commonly marked congestive liver injury expanding from zone 3 towards the periportal zone lead to significant structural and functional hepatic impairment after a Fontan correction. Occurrence of liver complications derived from a failed Fontan operation correlate with the duration of the follow-up. Progression to cirrhosis can already be observed 10 years after the initial Fontan surgery [279]. The differential diagnosis between hepatic congestion and fibrosis by non-invasive methods is still challenging. Since liver stiffness progressively increases over time after a Fontan procedure, monitoring with transient elastography may be of use particularly in patients without significant liver congestion [302]. However, since the diagnostic gold standard of fibrosis remains liver histology, a transjugular liver biopsy should be considered during follow-up cardiac catheter studies. In order to reduce the venous congestion of the Fontan circulation, therapies aimed at lowering pulmonary vascular resistance have been administered immediately after total cavopulmonary connection (TCPC) [300]. Another option might be to perform combined heart-liver transplant in patients with overt cirrhosis or consider cardiac transplant before cirrhosis occurs [300]. Another possible option includes the creation of a conduit to left atrium fenestration, thus accepting a moderate degree of right-to-left shunting, which may contribute to limit venous congestion [300].

Besides focal nodular hyperplasia (FNH), which is frequently found in patients with high Fontan venous pressure, also HCC is increasingly observed in cardiac cirrhosis after Fontan procedure. Since the risk to develop cirrhosis correlates with the duration of the Fontan circulation, it has been suggested to start HCC surveillance at least 10 years after Fontan correction [279].

22.5.3 Cardiomyopathies

Cardiomyopathies (CMP) occur rarely in childhood with an annual incidence of approximately 1.3 per 100,000. Dilated and hypertrophic CMP are more frequently diagnosed, while restrictive, non-compaction, and mixed CMP are less common, and arrhythmogenic right ventricular CMP is rare. Their pathogenesis includes coronary artery abnormalities, infection, toxins, and to an increasing extent they are ascribed to genetic mutations [303]. Growth retardation, tachypnea, and hepatomegaly with abdominal pain are possible symptoms associated with CMP [304], but the wide range of manifestations are reflected in the eventual absence of symptoms on the one hand and acute cardiac failure or sudden death due to arrhythmias on the other hand [305]. The hepatic injury depends on the mechanism and type of cardiac failure and includes congestion due to increased filling pressure in right-sided heart failure or hypoxic injury due to left-sided heart failure with low cardiac output.

22.5.4 Rheumatic Fever

Cardiac manifestations of rheumatic fever (RF) may cause a persistent heart injury in 14 to 99% of patients. This wide range of prevalence results from diagnostic issues in the recognition of the disease that often presents with only mild symptoms, in addition echocardiography was previously not available to identify subclinical carditis [306, 307]. Apart from carditis, RF causes arthritis and can affect the CNS and subcutaneous tissue after a pharyngeal infection by a group A beta-haemolytic streptococci (*Streptococcus pyogenes*). RF usually manifests in children between 5 and 15 years of age [308]. Pathogenesis is still not completely clarified, but it is suggested that a streptococcal protein binds to collagen type IV, and thus antibody response is induced resulting in an inflammatory reaction of the matrix presumably without causing molecular mimicry and an autoimmune reaction [309]. The mitral valve is primarily affected, most commonly presenting regurgitation (MR), while mitral stenosis (MS) in this context is pathognomonic for rheumatic heart disease. When MR persists the left atrium and left ventricle may dilate. In patients with MS, the left atrium is enlarged, and regurgitation with right-sided heart failure may occur, especially when marked pulmonary hypertension is present. Aortic valve involvement is often seen in combination with MR or MS [308]. Liver injury is mainly caused by excessive filling pressure and congestion.

22.5.5 Liver Diseases in Children with Cardiac Malformations

22.5.5.1 Biliary Atresia

Biliary atresia (BA) is characterized by obstructed or absent bile ducts due to inflammatory sclerosis [7]. The estimated annual incidence is 0.06 to 0.13 in 1000 live births. BA is the most frequent cause for paediatric liver transplantation [310]. It leads to cholestatic liver disease in infancy, and 20% of the patients show other anatomic anomalies including defects in situ determination and laterality that causes heterotaxy and complex heart defects. Cardiovascular malformations are reported in up to 50% of cases with associated anomalies [311]. When patients are treated first with Kasai operation and subsequently, if indicated, directed to liver transplantation, survival rates almost reach 90%. Since the outcome of the Kasai operation depends on the early diagnosis of this disease, awareness and prompt intervention are essential [312].

22.5.5.2 Polysplenia Syndrome

The polysplenia syndrome (PS) is characterized by the presence of multiple spleens commonly between two and six. The annual incidence is 2.5 per 100,000 live births. However, less than 5% of patients survive longer than 5 years as a consequence of severe congenital malformations that occur in association with PS and may affect solid organs and the gastrointestinal tract, the heart, and the great vessels [313]. In 10% of BA cases with linked anomalies, PS is present [314].

22.6 Systemic Infections and Sepsis

Besides the typical hepatotropic viruses, hepatitis A to E, also systemic infections can involve the liver and lead to hepatic injury. In general the liver can either be damaged by direct interaction with the pathogen or through toxins and cytokines that institute pro- inflammatory triggers.

22.6.1 Bacterial Infections

22.6.1.1 Pneumonia

The gram-positive *Streptococcus pneumoniae* usually affects children, elderly, and immune-compromised individuals. Pneumococcal infection is still a worldwide health issue and the main cause of bacterial pneumonia in children [315]. Pneumococcal pneumonia is sometimes associated with elevated concentrations of serum aminotransferases and bilirubin. Occurrence of jaundice could be an indicator for severe tissue damage with necrotic hepatocellular injury [316].

Mycoplasma pneumoniae infection is a common infection of the lower respiratory tract in children and adolescents, and up to 40% of community-acquired pneumonia can be ascribed to this pathogen [317]. Several pathomechanisms for the liver injury have been discussed including autoimmune cross-reactions and direct damage of epithelial cells. In a large Korean study including children, mainly from 0 to 6 years of age, antibiotic treatment resulted in prompt response with rapid restoration of the liver function. The incidence of *M. pneumoniae* hepatitis was 7.7% and presented with abnormal serum aminotransferase levels, while increased bilirubin concentrations were less common [318]. Liver biopsies show hepatocellular injury with inflammatory infiltration [319].

22.6.1.2 Food-Borne Disease

Microbial food-borne disease is common and usually manifests with gastrointestinal symptoms, but complications including hepatitis, renal failure, or neurogenic symptoms may occur.

Typhoid fever is still frequently seen in the developing countries, sometimes accompanied by hepatomegaly and moderately increased serum aminotransferase levels [320], but severe hepatitis is a rare event during the course of the infection. Its presentation can mimic acute viral hepatitis [321, 322], which is distinguishable from the typhoid-associated form by the ALT/LDH ratio [323]. Jaundice usually appears within the first 2 weeks after onset of the typhoid fever [324]. Since hepatic involvement can occur by haematogenous seeding, liver biopsies may show in focal areas typhoid nodules with ballooning degeneration and mononuclear cell infiltration [325]. Administration of the appropriate antibiotics generally results in resolution of the infection and the liver disease. Even though typhoid hepatitis is not frequently reported among children, it remains an important differential diagnosis in tropical areas [321].

22.6.1.3 Tuberculosis

Hepatobiliary tuberculosis is a rare presentation of a common infection by *Mycobacterium tuberculosis*. In most of the cases the generalized disease, miliary TB, involves the liver by clustered miliary tubercles. Focal involvement by the tuberculosis primary complex through affection of hilar lymph nodes, or in a continuous manner by confluence of miliary foci, occurs to a lesser extent [326]. Males are twice as much affected by this manifestation, and the age peak is between 11 and 50 years [327]. Prenatally and perinatal infections of the liver occur through the umbilical vein or the amniotic fluid. Postnatal hepatic involvement is due to haematogenous or lymphatic dissemination. Immune response causes hepatobiliary granulomas, which can be asymptomatic, or causes in most cases unspecific upper abdominal pain [328]. Liver enzyme abnormalities especially ALP and aminotransferase elevations occur frequently in patients with hepatic tuberculosis [329]. Jaundice is less common, but suggests biliary involvement and may reflect biliary obstruction that is either caused by hilar lymph nodes, or by direct affection of the biliary epithelium, or by ruptured granulomas into the bile ducts [330]. Treatment still relies on the conventional antituberculosis therapy including at least four drugs. However, drug-induced liver injury, especially due to isoniazid, occurs. Cumulative mortality rates for hepatobiliary TB range from 15 to 42% [326].

22.6.2 Fungal Infections

Invasive fungal diseases are life-threatening infections that affect different organs. Especially immune-compromised children, premature neonates, and children, who reside in zones where mycoses like histoplasmosis, blastomycosis, and coccidioidomycosis are endemic, are at risk for an infection [331].

22.6.2.1 Candidiasis

Hepatosplenic candidiasis is caused by candidaemia. The portal of entry can be the gut, when the barrier of the gastrointestinal mucosa is damaged. Disseminated disease often affects patients with haematologic malignancies and significant prolonged neutropenia. Clinical manifestations may include fever with spikes, abdominal pain, and nausea. Laboratory abnormalities rather resemble cholestasis with elevated concentrations of ALP and GGT, possibly reflecting the presence of small liver abscesses or granulomas [332]. Frequently microbiologic assessment from blood cultures results negative, probably due to major dissemination through the portal vein system. MRI and CT are validated imaging tools to diagnose hepatosplenic candidiasis. Recently also contrast-enhanced ultrasound (CEUS) becomes more important, especially in children. Treatment differs regionally and includes amphotericin B, fluconazole, micafungin, flucytosine, echinocandin, and caspofungin [333]. However, mortality due to paediatric candidiasis is still approximately 10% [334].

22.6.3 Parasitic Infections

Liver involvement occurs frequently during parasitic infections; the two most common infections worldwide are schistosomiasis and malaria.

22.6.3.1 Schistosomiasis

Schistosomiasis is caused by dissemination of trematode worms through the blood stream that infect different organs. Globally, there are over 200 million people with schistosomiasis, more than half of the patients are symptomatic, and approximately 10% have severe disease [335]. Endemic areas spread across tropical and subtropical regions of Africa, Asia, and South America [325]. Excreted eggs of the parasite contaminate water, especially in zones without functioning sanitation. After reproduction in susceptible snails, cercariae penetrate through the human skin and enter the blood flow and lymph as schistosomula. During the initial infections, worms reside in different organs and deposit eggs, which induces an immune response that results in tissue injury, especially in granuloma formation [336]. Hepatic granulomas are typically found in children. After several years of infection, fibrosis can appear as a result of the chronic inflammation. Most of the time liver function parameters are within the normal range. Nonetheless, ongoing fibrosis can cause portal hypertension with its well-known complications [325]. Praziquantel is still the first treatment of choice for schistosomiasis [337].

22.6.3.2 Malaria

The WHO estimated approximately 214 million cases of malaria worldwide in 2015. Almost 100,000 deaths were reported, but this number does not represent the true mortality rate, since most deaths occur outside the health system. The disease is transmitted by the bite of an infected anopheles mosquito mostly in underdeveloped tropical countries. Sporozoites are then released into the bloodstream and infect hepatocytes of the liver. Mature sporozoites, termed schizonts, produce merozoites that reach the blood after rupture of the hepatocyte and invade erythrocytes, where they further replicate. The cycle restarts when erythrocytes rupture and release the merozoites. Some malaria strains are able to produce dormant hypnozoites after hepatocyte infection, which are responsible for disease relapse. Symptomatic infection may thus occur months after the first infection [325]. In comparison to adults, children report less chills, headaches, or arthralgia/myalgia, but rather unspecific symptoms such as fever, lethargy, malaise, nausea, and abdominal pain. Hepatomegaly and splenomegaly in children occur in half of the cases, twice as much as in adults. Jaundice and elevated concentrations of liver enzymes are also seen more frequently in children (50% vs. 30%) [338, 339]. Jaundice in the course of a malaria infection may indicate different pathologies including liver dysfunction, haemolysis due to ruptured erythrocytes, septicaemic hepatitis, and DIC-associated haemolysis [340]. Liver histology may show necrosis, portal inflammation, pigmented Kupffer cell hyperplasia caused by engulfed erythrocytes, and cholestasis [341]. The type of anti-malaria drug is chosen according to the plasmodium species, the knowledge about the local resistance situation, the patient's comorbidities, and the disease severity. In general drug combinations are preferred to monotherapy. Artemisinin and its derivatives combined with either mefloquine or amodiaquine or lumefantrine or piperaquine are the treatment of choice in children. Severe malaria infections, characterized by cerebral malaria with altered consciousness, signs of organ failure, shock, or intractable vomiting with dehydration, are an emergency and should be treated accordingly [339].

22.6.4 Sepsis

Introduction

Sepsis is still one of the main causes worldwide for death in childhood and adolescence [342]. In 2013, a global multi-centre study on the burden of paediatric severe sepsis in the developed and the developing world including 26 countries was performed (SPROUT study). A prevalence of severe sepsis of 8.2% among children in ICU was shown with a related mortality rate of 25%, but no difference in age or developing status [343]. Data from Italy reveal an overall incidence of sepsis, severe sepsis, and septic shock of 7.9, 1.6, and 2.1%, respectively, and a mean mortality rate of severe sepsis and septic shock takes together of 34% [344]. The main reasons for almost half of the cases are infections of the respiratory tract, followed by bacteraemia that accounts for about 20% of the cases [343]. The milestones for the management of sepsis are early administration of antibiotics and stabilization of circulation by resuscitation of fluids and vasopressor support. Similar to data from Kumar et al. among adults demonstrating a higher survival rate for septic shock patients after early administration of appropriate antibiotics, Weiss et al. reported in children with severe sepsis or septic shock that a delay of more than 3 h was related to a significant increase in ICU mortality. However, unlike in adults, this does not concern delays of appropriate antibiotic administration within these 3 h [345, 346].

Liver Involvement

Inflammatory stimuli and hypoxia can result in liver injury followed by liver failure. Liver dysfunction may occur early in sepsis and represents an independent risk factor for poor outcome [347]. As demonstrated by the large international study including almost 7000 children (SPROUT study), hepatic dysfunction was present at screening in 25% of the cases ranking on place four after respiratory, cardiovascular, and haematologic dysfunction [343]. It has been shown for adults that liver dysfunction was related to severe complications in sepsis and that mortality rates were higher among patients with liver failure than with respiratory failure [348]. It seems that liver involvement in sepsis is a common finding. Needle biopsies taken from adult patients immediately after death from sepsis without known underlying liver disease revealed that 60% of patients had the hepatitic pattern with portal or lobular inflammation and centrilobular often haemorrhagic necrosis, while the reminiscent 40% showed a mixed histological pattern composed of variable biliary lesions including hyperplasia, cholangitis, and cholestasis, portal or lobular inflammation, and centrilobular necrosis. Steatosis was observed in about 70% of patients. Laboratory alterations mainly affected gamma-GT, ALP, and bilirubin, whereas AST and ALT elevations were only mild [349]. A rise in aminotransferase levels has been reported later in the course of sepsis after a prolonged period of hypotension [348]. Liver dysfunction usually occurs early as shown in a rat model by Muftuoglu et al., where first signs of impaired liver function appeared already 1.5 h after induction of sepsis and concern mainly glucose metabolism and drug detoxification, while alterations on the transcriptional level occurred around 6 h after induction. Fifteen hours post initiation of sepsis in the animals, conjugation of bilirubin was severely disturbed, and a steep rise of unconjugated bilirubin could be noticed [350].

The liver is markedly involved in removal of bacteria and toxins during sepsis. Even lipopolysaccharides (LPS), which are important stimuli for the inflammatory reaction in bacterial infection, are to the major extent degraded by the liver [351]. When hepatic function is impaired, the risk of bacteraemia increases due to disturbed bacteria removal; accordingly, cirrhosis has been associated with an increased risk of bacterial infection. Moreover, the function of the reticuloendothelial system, neutrophil phagocytosis, complement production, and antigen presentation via monocyte HLA-DR expression is impaired, which contributes to the reduced bacterial clearance [352]. Kupffer cells, stellate cells, and liver sinusoidal endothelial cells (LSECs) play a pivotal role in the protection from bacterial spread and inflammatory activation through chemotaxins [351, 353]. Endotoxin exposure leads to mainly hepatic release of cytokines and NO [354]. Hepatic natural killer T (NKT) cells additionally stimulate the pro-inflammatory response. One has to keep in mind that exorbitant inflammatory stimulation may result in necrosis and finally in liver injury. Therefore, hepatic response to sepsis also includes simultaneous induction of anti-inflammatory mediators [355]. LPS-induced tolerance in the liver is a key mechanism to prevent excessive inflammation, but this effect also contributes significantly to immunosuppression with potentially fatal outcome [356]. In addition, myeloid-derived suppressor cells (MDSCs) populate the liver during sepsis to trigger immunosuppression. In the mouse model, MDSCs markedly suppress CD4+ and CD8+ T-cell proliferation after sepsis induction. Moreover, MDSCs act on dendritic cell development and block NK-cell cytotoxicity [357]. In conclusion, sepsis induced liver injury aliments and worsens the inflammation; therefore interference with pro- and anti-inflammatory factors seems an important aim to improve the outcome of this disease.

22.7 Drug-Induced Liver Injury

Drug-induced liver injury (DILI) seems to be primarily of idiosyncratic nature, which describes an adverse reaction characterized by (1) occurrence in a small proportion of patients taking the drug, (2) the missing relation to the pharmacological effect, (3) no dose dependency, and (4) the delay between the drug exposure and the onset of symptoms, which can be triggered and accelerated by re-challenge [358]. Ten percent of the adverse drug reactions (ADRs) can be ascribed to DILI [359]. Its annual incidence is 0.1 per 100,000 patients. The host factors attributing to DILI include genetic and nutritional factors, interactions with other medications, comorbidities, and age, which seems of particular importance [360]. Less than 10% of all DILI cases affect children (cDILI), and in approximately 20% it results in acute liver failure (ALF) [361, 362]. Fatal outcome of cDILI differs between 4 and 31% in different studies [362, 363]. Idiosyncratic DILI (IDILI) is characterized by an individual response to a drug due to genetic and acquired factors. To understand and to eventually prevent IDILI by identifying susceptibility to adverse reactions due to certain genetic features is an important research issue. Certain HLA subtypes have been linked to higher risk of IDILI in children because of their frequent identification in sick children. Also IL-10, which is a potent anti-inflammatory molecule that stimulates release of Th2 cytokines, seems to be involved in paediatric hepatotoxic reactions [364]. The time between drug exposure and disease onset is usually 1–3 months, but IDILI may have a delay of even more than 1 year [365], while, for example, fluoroquinolone-induced liver injury can appear within a few days [366]. DILI can lead to hepatocellular, cholestatic, or mixed liver injury as indicated by hypertransaminasemia, or ALP, bilirubin, and gamma-GT elevations, respectively. In cDILI the hepatocellular pattern seems more common, and a lower fibrosis stadium is often associated, while advanced fibrosis, which is frequently found in adults, has not been observed in children [360]. The occurrence of hyperbilirubinemia, after exclusion of mechanic cholestasis or other comorbidities, in addition to mild DILI indicates that a drug is more likely to induce liver failure, as described by the Hy's law established in adults, which might simplify the identification of drugs causing liver failure [358, 367].

22 The Liver in Systemic Illness

Drug metabolism is characterized by three different phases: the first mainly involves hepatic cytochrome P450 (CYP450) enzymes that modify the medication to obtain a better water solubility. During organ development the quality and quantity of CYP enzymes vary as reflected by the predominant expression of CYP3A7 in the neonatal liver, while in adults drugs are mainly metabolized by CYP3A4 that is increasingly expressed with age [368]. These differences in the expression patterns are transferable also to other CYP enzymes and may cause differences in drug sensitivity in various development stages. As a result of phase 1 metabolism, reactive toxic intermediate products may emerge that need to be modified to enable their elimination by the kidneys or the liver. This conjugation step including glucuronidation, sulfation, acetylation, methylation, and glutathione conjugation describes phase 2 of the drug metabolism [360]. An age-dependent variability of the involved cofactors has been described, which plays a role for the metabolic pathway to which a certain drug is destined [369]. The third and last step of drug metabolism, even if the drug is not further altered in its chemical structure, involves drug transporters that excrete the conjugated metabolites across membranes of the renal tubular cells or hepatocytes for elimination. The multidrug resistance protein (P-glycoprotein) is a well-known member of this group of molecules. Inhibition of drug transporters can cause accumulation of the drug reaching toxic levels. Just few data exist on the ontogeny of these transporters, but age-dependent variations may exist that lead to differential drug elimination and DILI [370, 371]. Other contributing factors include intestinal drug absorption that in general increases with age, and its subsequent metabolism seems to be diminished during the first year of life [372]. The drug clearance is fastest between 2 and 10 years of age and decreases afterwards. The proportion of body water and ratio of surface area to mass index are higher in children, while body fat and binding capacity of plasma proteins for drugs are lower. Pharmacokinetics may therefore be significantly influenced by these factors [373]. Pharmacodynamics addresses the molecular mode of interaction between a drug and its target. Even though age differences in receptor ligand binding and subsequent intracellular signal transduction seem probable, little is known concerning the developmental changes [360].

Clinical features may be absent and DILI may evidence solely with laboratory abnormalities (Table 22.4). Possible manifestations include nausea, vomiting, and weight loss and in case of cholestasis also pruritus and jaundice. When endothelial cells are involved, vaso-occlusion can occur causing ascites [247]. The R-value has been introduced to discriminate between hepatocellular and cholestatic liver injury ((ALT * ULN ALP)/(ALP * ULN ALT)). A value of 5 or more indicates a hepatocellular damage, while R of 2 or less cholestatic DILI values in between suggest a mixed injury [374].

Table 22.4 Selection of drugs causing cDILI in children [360]

Drugs	Characteristics
Acetaminophen	Leading cause of cDILI in the Western world, second most frequent reason for ALF; hypertransaminasemia within 12–36 h; centrilobular necrosis
Halothane	Severe hepatitis: 1 in 6000–30,000 adults, children seem less susceptible
Propylthiouracil	Third most common cause of drug-induced ALF in children, who seem more sensitive for DILI than adults
Valproic acid	Hepatotoxicity more frequently in children than in adults, DILI risk up to 1/600 in children < 2 years of age; spectrum of liver injury ranges from transient increase of transaminases to hepatic dysfunction/failure
Isoniazid	Hypertransaminasemia most frequent abnormality, in 7% to 14% of children receiving INH, more severe cDILI less frequently, incidence of liver failure estimated 3.2 per 100,000 patients
Rifampicin + isoniazid	The incidence of cDILI is 3.3%, earlier manifestation than with either medication alone
Ketoconazole	Incidence of hepatotoxicity in general estimated 134 per 100,000; hypertransaminasemia in 2% to 17% starting after weeks of therapy; mainly hepatocellular injury; cases of ALF reported in children
Sulfonamides	Induces idiosyncratic DILI; ALF is rare in children; onset of symptoms after days to 1 month; mainly centrilobular cholestasis with portal infiltration

However, the R-value has yet not been validated for children.

Liver histology greatly differs depending on the drug and especially on the provoked reaction. Liver injury may be observed more in the centrilobular region, the location of the highest concentration of cytochrome P450 enzymes, but also diffuse patterns can be found. IDILI often causes development of antidrug or autoantibodies, but their detection is still an issue due to the missing availability of the specific reagents [358].

The key task in the treatment of DILI is to stop the triggering agent and supportive care. Few drugs such as acetaminophen and valproate have antidotes. For the use of corticosteroid in children, no controlled trials have yet been carried out. In the case of acute liver failure (ALF), children should be referred to a transplant centre as soon as possible. Different prognostic scores have been applied in children, and according to a recent single centre study involving 128 patients, it seems that the MELD score and ALFSG prognostic models have a good predictive value for ALF due to DILI [375]. In general, follow-up of DILI has to proceed until clinical symptoms and laboratory abnormalities have normalized.

References

1. Khemichian S, Fong TL. Hepatic dysfunction in hyperthyroidism. Gastroenterol Hepatol. 2011;7(5):337–9.
2. Segni M. Disorders of the thyroid gland in infancy, childhood and adolescence. In: De Groot LJ, Chrousos G, Dungan K, et al., editors. Endotext. South Dartmouth, MA: MDText.com, Inc; 2000.
3. Wassner AJ, Brown RS. Congenital hypothyroidism: recent advances. Curr Opin Endocrinol Diabetes Obes. 2015;22(5):407–12.
4. Hanley P, Lord K, Bauer AJ. Thyroid disorders in children and adolescents: a review. JAMA Pediatr. 2016;170(10):1008–19.
5. Akangire G, Cuna A, Lachica C, Fischer R, Raman S, Sampath V. Neonatal Graves' disease with maternal hypothyroidism. AJP Rep. 2017;7(3):e181–4.
6. Leger J, Carel JC. Hyperthyroidism in childhood: causes, when and how to treat. J Clin Res Pediatr Endocrinol. 2013;5(Suppl 1):50–6.
7. Hasosah M, Alsaleem K, Qurashi M, Alzaben A. Neonatal hyperthyroidism with fulminant liver failure: a case report. J Clin Diagn Res. 2017;11(4):SD01–2.
8. Foley TP Jr. Maternally transferred thyroid disease in the infant: recognition and treatment. Adv Exp Med Biol. 1991;299:209–26.
9. Rastogi MV, Lafranchi SH. Congenital hypothyroidism. Orphanet J Rare Dis. 2010;5:17.
10. Nebesio TD, Mckenna MP, Nabhan ZM, Eugster EA. Newborn screening results in children with central hypothyroidism. J Pediatr. 2010;156(6):990–3.
11. Karnsakul W, Sawathiparnich P, Nimkarn S, Likitmaskul S, Santiprabhob J, Aanpreung P. Anterior pituitary hormone effects on hepatic functions in infants with congenital hypopituitarism. Ann Hepatol. 2007;6(2):97–103.
12. Malik R, Hodgson H. The relationship between the thyroid gland and the liver. QJM. 2002;95(9):559–69.
13. Cappola AR, Ladenson PW. Hypothyroidism and atherosclerosis. J Clin Endocrinol Metab. 2003;88(6):2438–44.
14. Bakker SJ, Ter Maaten JC, Popp-Snijders C, Slaets JP, Heine RJ, Gans RO. The relationship between thyrotropin and low density lipoprotein cholesterol is modified by insulin sensitivity in healthy euthyroid subjects. J Clin Endocrinol Metab. 2001;86(3):1206–11.
15. Saxena NK, Ikeda K, Rockey DC, Friedman SL, Anania FA. Leptin in hepatic fibrosis: evidence for increased collagen production in stellate cells and lean littermates of ob/ob mice. Hepatology. 2002;35(4):762–71.
16. Kaltenbach TE, Graeter T, Oezturk S, et al. Thyroid dysfunction and hepatic steatosis in overweight children and adolescents. Pediatr Obes. 2017;12(1):67–74.
17. Denzer C, Karges B, Nake A, et al. Subclinical hypothyroidism and dyslipidemia in children and adolescents with type 1 diabetes mellitus. Eur J Endocrinol. 2013;168(4):601–8.
18. Lodish M. Cushing's syndrome in childhood: update on genetics, treatment, and outcomes. Curr Opin Endocrinol Diabetes Obes. 2015;22(1):48–54.
19. More J, Young J, Reznik Y, et al. Ectopic ACTH syndrome in children and adolescents. J Clin Endocrinol Metab. 2011;96(5):1213–22.
20. Pivonello R, De Leo M, Vitale P, et al. Pathophysiology of diabetes mellitus in Cushing's syndrome. Neuroendocrinology. 2010;92(Suppl 1):77–81.
21. Tarantino G, Finelli C. Pathogenesis of hepatic steatosis: the link between hypercortisolism and non-alcoholic fatty liver disease. World J Gastroenterol. 2013;19(40):6735–43.
22. Dowman JK, Hopkins LJ, Reynolds GM, et al. Loss of 5alpha-reductase type 1 accelerates the development of hepatic steatosis but protects against hepatocellular carcinoma in male mice. Endocrinology. 2013;154(12):4536–47.
23. Marino L, Jornayvaz FR. Endocrine causes of nonalcoholic fatty liver disease. World J Gastroenterol. 2015;21(39):11053–76.
24. Charmandari E, Nicolaides NC, Chrousos GP. Adrenal insufficiency. Lancet. 2014;383(9935):2152–67.
25. Boulton R, Hamilton MI, Dhillon AP, Kinloch JD, Burroughs AK. Subclinical Addison's disease: a cause of persistent abnormalities in transaminase values. Gastroenterology. 1995;109(4):1324–7.
26. Vafaeimanesh J, Bagherzadeh M, Parham M. Adrenal insufficiency as a cause of acute liver failure: a case report. Case Rep Endocrinol. 2013;2013:487189.
27. Font J, Cervera R, Espinosa G, et al. Systemic lupus erythematosus (SLE) in childhood: analysis of clinical and immunological findings in 34 patients and comparison with SLE characteristics in adults. Ann Rheum Dis. 1998;57(8):456–9.
28. Mina R, Brunner HI. Pediatric lupus—are there differences in presentation, genetics, response to therapy, and damage accrual compared with adult lupus? Rheum Dis Clin North Am. 2010;36(1):53–80., vii-viii.
29. Thakral A, Klein-Gitelman MS. An update on treatment and management of pediatric systemic lupus erythematosus. Rheumatol Ther. 2016;3(2):209–19.
30. Irving KS, Sen D, Tahir H, Pilkington C, Isenberg DA. A comparison of autoimmune liver disease in juvenile and adult populations with systemic lupus erythematosus—a retrospective review of cases. Rheumatology (Oxford). 2007;46(7):1171–3.
31. Bessone F, Poles N, Roma MG. Challenge of liver disease in systemic lupus erythematosus: clues for diagnosis and hints for pathogenesis. World J Hepatol. 2014;6(6):394–409.
32. Berzigotti A, Frigato M, Manfredini E, et al. Liver hemangioma and vascular liver diseases in patients with systemic lupus erythematosus. World J Gastroenterol. 2011;17(40):4503–8.
33. Shizuma T. Clinical characteristics of concomitant systemic lupus erythematosus and primary biliary cirrhosis: a literature review. J Immunol Res. 2015;2015:713728.
34. Piga M, Vacca A, Porru G, Cauli A, Mathieu A. Liver involvement in systemic lupus erythematosus: incidence, clinical course and outcome of lupus hepatitis. Clin Exp Rheumatol. 2010;28(4):504–10.
35. Koshy JM, John M. Autoimmune hepatitis—SLE overlap syndrome. J Assoc Physicians India. 2012;60:59–60.
36. Deen ME, Porta G, Fiorot FJ, Campos LM, Sallum AM, Silva CA. Autoimmune hepatitis and juvenile systemic lupus erythematosus. Lupus. 2009;18(8):747–51.
37. Gatselis NK, Zachou K, Koukoulis GK, Dalekos GN. Autoimmune hepatitis, one disease with many faces: etiopathogenetic, clinico-laboratory and histological characteristics. World J Gastroenterol. 2015;21(1):60–83.
38. Di Giorgio A, Bravi M, Bonanomi E, et al. Fulminant hepatic failure of autoimmune aetiology in children. J Pediatr Gastroenterol Nutr. 2015;60(2):159–64.
39. Takahashi A, Abe K, Saito R, et al. Liver dysfunction in patients with systemic lupus erythematosus. Intern Med. 2013;52(13):1461–5.
40. Czaja AJ, Morshed SA, Parveen S, Nishioka M. Antibodies to single-stranded and double-stranded DNA in antinuclear antibody-positive type 1-autoimmune hepatitis. Hepatology. 1997;26(3):567–72.
41. Shahian M, Khosravi A, Anbardar MH. Early cholestasis in neonatal lupus erythematosus. Ann Saudi Med. 2011;31(1):80–2.
42. Lin SC, Shyur SD, Huang LH, Wu JY, Chuo HT, Lee HC. Neonatal lupus erythematosus with cholestatic hepatitis. J Microbiol Immunol Infect. 2004;37(2):131–4.

43. Timpane S, Brandling-Bennett H, Kristjansson AK. Autoimmune collagen vascular diseases: Kids are not just little people. Clin Dermatol. 2016;34(6):678–89.
44. Arkin LM, Ansell L, Rademaker A, et al. The natural history of pediatric-onset discoid lupus erythematosus. J Am Acad Dermatol. 2015;72(4):628–33.
45. Sampaio MC, De Oliveira ZN, Machado MC, Dos Reis VM, Vilela MA. Discoid lupus erythematosus in children—a retrospective study of 34 patients. Pediatr Dermatol. 2008;25(2):163–7.
46. Modesto C, Anton J, Rodriguez B, et al. Incidence and prevalence of juvenile idiopathic arthritis in Catalonia (Spain). Scand J Rheumatol. 2010;39(6):472–9.
47. Behrens EM, Beukelman T, Gallo L, et al. Evaluation of the presentation of systemic onset juvenile rheumatoid arthritis: data from the Pennsylvania Systemic Onset Juvenile Arthritis Registry (PASOJAR). J Rheumatol. 2008;35(2):343–8.
48. Petty RE, Southwood TR, Manners P, et al. International League of Associations for Rheumatology classification of juvenile idiopathic arthritis: second revision, Edmonton, 2001. J Rheumatol. 2004;31(2):390–2.
49. Gurion R, Lehman TJ, Moorthy LN. Systemic arthritis in children: a review of clinical presentation and treatment. Int J Inflam. 2012;2012:271569.
50. Schneider R, Laxer RM. Systemic onset juvenile rheumatoid arthritis. Baillieres Clin Rhesumatol. 1998;12(2):245–71.
51. Schaller J, Beckwith B, Wedgwood RJ. Hepatic involvement in juvenile rheumatoid arthritis. J Pediatr. 1970;77(2):203–10.
52. Stephan JL, Zeller J, Hubert P, Herbelin C, Dayer JM, Prieur AM. Macrophage activation syndrome and rheumatic disease in childhood: a report of four new cases. Clin Exp Rheumatol. 1993;11(4):451–6.
53. Grom AA, Passo M. Macrophage activation syndrome in systemic juvenile rheumatoid arthritis. J Pediatr. 1996;129(5):630–2.
54. Minoia F, Davi S, Horne A, et al. Clinical features, treatment, and outcome of macrophage activation syndrome complicating systemic juvenile idiopathic arthritis: a multinational, multicenter study of 362 patients. Arthritis Rheumatol. 2014;66(11):3160–9.
55. Ramanan AV, Schneider R. Macrophage activation syndrome—what's in a name! J Rheumatol. 2003;30(12):2513–6.
56. Gorelik M, Fall N, Altaye M, et al. Follistatin-like protein 1 and the ferritin/erythrocyte sedimentation rate ratio are potential biomarkers for dysregulated gene expression and macrophage activation syndrome in systemic juvenile idiopathic arthritis. J Rheumatol. 2013;40(7):1191–9.
57. Ravelli A, Minoia F, Davi S, et al. 2016 Classification criteria for macrophage activation syndrome complicating systemic juvenile idiopathic arthritis: a European League Against Rheumatism/American College of Rheumatology/Paediatric Rheumatology International Trials Organisation Collaborative Initiative. Arthritis Rheumatol. 2016;68(3):566–76.
58. Boom V, Anton J, Lahdenne P, et al. Evidence-based diagnosis and treatment of macrophage activation syndrome in systemic juvenile idiopathic arthritis. Pediatr Rheumatol Online J. 2015;13:55.
59. Patwardhan A, Rennebohm R, Dvorchik I, Spencer CH. Is juvenile dermatomyositis a different disease in children up to three years of age at onset than in children above three years at onset? A retrospective review of 23 years of a single center's experience. Pediatr Rheumatol Online J. 2012;10(1):34.
60. Cojocaru M, Cojocaru IM, Silosi I, Vrabie CD. Liver involvement in patients with systemic autoimmune diseases. Maedica (Buchar). 2013;8(4):394–7.
61. Russo RA, Katsicas MM, Davila M, Ciocca M, Zelazko M. Cholestasis in juvenile dermatomyositis: report of three cases. Arthritis Rheum. 2001;44(5):1139–42.
62. Chwalinska-Sadowska H, Maldykowa H. Polymyositis-dermatomyositis: 25 years of follow-up of 50 patients disease course, treatment, prognostic factors. Mater Med Pol. 1990;22(3):213–8.
63. Mayes MD, Lacey JV Jr, Beebe-Dimmer J, et al. Prevalence, incidence, survival, and disease characteristics of systemic sclerosis in a large US population. Arthritis Rheum. 2003;48(8):2246–55.
64. Shah AA, Wigley FM. My approach to the treatment of scleroderma. Mayo Clin Proc. 2013;88(4):377–93.
65. Assassi S, Fritzler MJ, Arnett FC, et al. Primary biliary cirrhosis (PBC), PBC autoantibodies, and hepatic parameter abnormalities in a large population of systemic sclerosis patients. J Rheumatol. 2009;36(10):2250–6.
66. Rigamonti C, Shand LM, Feudjo M, et al. Clinical features and prognosis of primary biliary cirrhosis associated with systemic sclerosis. Gut. 2006;55(3):388–94.
67. Swart JF, Wulffraat NM. Diagnostic workup for mixed connective tissue disease in childhood. Isr Med Assoc J. 2008;10(8-9):650–2.
68. Berard RA, Laxer RM. Pediatric mixed connective tissue disease. Curr Rheumatol Rep. 2016;18(5):28.
69. Sedej K, Toplak N, Praprotnik M, Luzar B, Brecelj J, Avcin T. Autoimmune hepatitis as a presenting manifestation of mixed connective tissue disease in a child. Case report and review of the literature. Pediatr Rheumatol Online J. 2015;13(1):47.
70. Civilibal M, Canpolat N, Yurt A, et al. A child with primary Sjogren syndrome and a review of the literature. Clin Pediatr (Phila). 2007;46(8):738–42.
71. Cimaz R, Casadei A, Rose C, et al. Primary Sjogren syndrome in the paediatric age: a multicentre survey. Eur J Pediatr. 2003;162(10):661–5.
72. Longhi BS, Appenzeller S, Centeville M, Gusmao RJ, Marini R. Primary Sjogren's syndrome in children: is a family approach indicated? Clinics (Sao Paulo). 2011;66(11):1991–3.
73. Zeron PB, Retamozo S, Bove A, Kostov BA, Siso A, Ramos-Casals M. Diagnosis of liver involvement in primary Sjogren syndrome. J Clin Transl Hepatol. 2013;1(2):94–102.
74. Malfait F, Francomano C, Byers P, et al. The 2017 international classification of the Ehlers-Danlos syndromes. Am J Med Genet C Semin Med Genet. 2017;175(1):8–26.
75. Fikree A, Chelimsky G, Collins H, Kovacic K, Aziz Q. Gastrointestinal involvement in the Ehlers-Danlos syndromes. Am J Med Genet C Semin Med Genet. 2017;175(1):181–7.
76. Mossberg M, Segelmark M, Kahn R, Englund M, Mohammad AJ. Epidemiology of primary systemic vasculitis in children: a population-based study from southern Sweden. Scand J Rheumatol. 2018;47(4):295–302. https://doi.org/10.1080/03009742.2017.1412497.
77. Weiss PF. Pediatric vasculitis. Pediatr Clin North Am. 2012;59(2):407–23.
78. Weiss PF, Klink AJ, Luan X, Feudtner C. Temporal association of Streptococcus, Staphylococcus, and parainfluenza pediatric hospitalizations and hospitalized cases of Henoch-Schonlein purpura. J Rheumatol. 2010;37(12):2587–94.
79. Chao HC, Kong MS, Lin SJ. Hepatobiliary involvement of Henoch-Schonlein purpura in children. Acta Paediatr Taiwan. 2000;41(2):63–8.
80. Rosti G, Milani GP, Laicini EA, Fossali EF, Bianchetti MG. Liver chemistry in new-onset Henoch-Schonlein syndrome. Ital J Pediatr. 2017;43(1):85.
81. O'Connor N, Dargan PI, Jones AL. Hepatocellular damage from non-steroidal anti-inflammatory drugs. QJM. 2003;96(11):787–91.
82. Eladawy M, Dominguez SR, Anderson MS, Glode MP. Abnormal liver panel in acute Kawasaki disease. Pediatr Infect Dis J. 2011;30(2):141–4.
83. Pawlowska J, Naorniakowska M, Liber A. Liver involvement in children with collagen vascular diseases. Clin Exp Hepatol. 2015;1(3):117–9.

84. Newburger JW, Takahashi M, Gerber MA, et al. Diagnosis, treatment, and long-term management of Kawasaki disease: a statement for health professionals from the Committee on Rheumatic Fever, Endocarditis and Kawasaki Disease, Council on Cardiovascular Disease in the Young, American Heart Association. Circulation. 2004;110(17):2747–71.
85. Yi DY, Kim JY, Choi EY, Choi JY, Yang HR. Hepatobiliary risk factors for clinical outcome of Kawasaki disease in children. BMC Pediatr. 2014;14:51.
86. Matsumoto T, Kobayashi S, Shimizu H, et al. The liver in collagen diseases: pathologic study of 160 cases with particular reference to hepatic arteritis, primary biliary cirrhosis, autoimmune hepatitis and nodular regenerative hyperplasia of the liver. Liver. 2000;20(5):366–73.
87. Selmi C, De Santis M, Gershwin ME. Liver involvement in subjects with rheumatic disease. Arthritis Res Ther. 2011;13(3):226.
88. Oguzkurt P, Akcoren Z, Kale G, Tanyel FC. Polyarteritis nodosa involving the hepatobiliary system in an eight-year-old girl with a previous diagnosis of familial Mediterranean fever. Eur J Pediatr Surg. 2000;10(2):145–7.
89. Park HJ, Choi YJ, Kim JE, Ye YM, Park HS, Suh CH. Successful treatment of pediatric systemic polyarteritis nodosa with cholestatic hepatitis. Clin Rheumatol. 2007;26(1):122–4.
90. Baysun S, Demircin G, Erdodan O, Bulbul M, Yildiz YT, Oner A. Multiple visceral hematomas in a child with familial Mediterranean fever: polyarteritis nodosa. Pediatr Nephrol. 2008;23(8):1233., 1235-1237.
91. Cakar N, Yalcinkaya F, Duzova A, et al. Takayasu arteritis in children. J Rheumatol. 2008;35(5):913–9.
92. Herrera CN, Tomala-Haz JE. Portal hypertension: an uncommon clinical manifestation of Takayasu arteritis in a 9-year-old child. Open Access Rheumatol. 2016;8:115–8.
93. Durant C, Martin J, Hervier B, Gournay J, Hamidou M. Takayasu arteritis associated with hepatic sinusoidal dilatation. Ann Hepatol. 2011;10(4):559–61.
94. Yotsuyanagi H, Chikatsu N, Kaneko Y, Kurokawa K. Takayasu's arteritis in prepulseless stage manifesting lymph node swelling and hepatosplenomegaly. Intern Med. 1995;34(5):455–9.
95. Karincaoglu Y, Borlu M, Toker SC, et al. Demographic and clinical properties of juvenile-onset Behcet's disease: a controlled multicenter study. J Am Acad Dermatol. 2008;58(4):579–84.
96. Jennette JC, Falk RJ, Bacon PA, et al. 2012 revised International Chapel Hill Consensus Conference Nomenclature of Vasculitides. Arthritis Rheum. 2013;65(1):1–11.
97. Kone-Paut I. Behcet's disease in children, an overview. Pediatr Rheumatol Online J. 2016;14(1):10.
98. Skef W, Hamilton MJ, Arayssi T. Gastrointestinal Behcet's disease: a review. World J Gastroenterol. 2015;21(13):3801–12.
99. Calamia KT, Schirmer M, Melikoglu M. Major vessel involvement in Behcet's disease: an update. Curr Opin Rheumatol. 2011;23(1):24–31.
100. Orloff LA, Orloff MJ. Budd-Chiari syndrome caused by Behcet's disease: treatment by side-to-side portacaval shunt. J Am Coll Surg. 1999;188(4):396–407.
101. Cabral DA, Canter DL, Muscal E, et al. Comparing presenting clinical features in 48 children with microscopic polyangiitis to 183 children who have granulomatosis with polyangiitis (Wegener's): an ARChiVe cohort study. Arthritis Rheumatol. 2016;68(10):2514–26.
102. Calatroni M, Oliva E, Gianfreda D, et al. ANCA-associated vasculitis in childhood: recent advances. Ital J Pediatr. 2017;43(1):46.
103. Alberici F, Martorana D, Vaglio A. Genetic aspects of antineutrophil cytoplasmic antibody-associated vasculitis. Nephrol Dial Transplant. 2015;30(Suppl 1):i37–45.
104. Iudici M, Quartier P, Terrier B, Mouthon L, Guillevin L, Puechal X. Childhood-onset granulomatosis with polyangiitis and microscopic polyangiitis: systematic review and meta-analysis. Orphanet J Rare Dis. 2016;11(1):141.
105. Zwerina J, Eger G, Englbrecht M, Manger B, Schett G. Churg-Strauss syndrome in childhood: a systematic literature review and clinical comparison with adult patients. Semin Arthritis Rheum. 2009;39(2):108–15.
106. Singh R, Singh D, Abdou N. Churg-Strauss syndrome presenting as acute abdomen: are gastrointestinal manifestations an indicator of poor prognosis? Int J Rheum Dis. 2009;12(2):161–5.
107. Childhood Hodgkin Lymphoma Treatment (PDQ(R)). Health Professional Version. In PDQ Cancer Information Summaries, Bethesda, MD; 2002.
108. Pileri SA, Ascani S, Leoncini L, et al. Hodgkin's lymphoma: the pathologist's viewpoint. J Clin Pathol. 2002;55(3):162–76.
109. Kennedy-Nasser AA, Hanley P, Bollard CM. Hodgkin disease and the role of the immune system. Pediatr Hematol Oncol. 2011;28(3):176–86.
110. Pourtsidis A, Doganis D, Baka M, et al. Differences between younger and older patients with childhood Hodgkin lymphoma. Pediatr Hematol Oncol. 2013;30(6):532–6.
111. Yusuf MA, Elias E, Hubscher SG. Jaundice caused by the vanishing bile duct syndrome in a child with Hodgkin lymphoma. J Pediatr Hematol Oncol. 2000;22(2):154–7.
112. Vardareli E, Dundar E, Aslan V, Gulbas Z. Acute liver failure due to Hodgkin's lymphoma. Med Princ Pract. 2004;13(6):372–4.
113. Murakami J, Shimizu Y. Hepatic manifestations in hematological disorders. Int J Hepatol. 2013;2013:484903.
114. Smith MA, Altekruse SF, Adamson PC, Reaman GH, Seibel NL. Declining childhood and adolescent cancer mortality. Cancer. 2014;120(16):2497–506.
115. Childhood Non-Hodgkin Lymphoma Treatment (PDQ(R)). Health Professional Version. In PDQ Cancer Information Summaries, Bethesda, MD; 2002.
116. Sandlund JT, Downing JR, Crist WM. Non-Hodgkin's lymphoma in childhood. N Engl J Med. 1996;334(19):1238–48.
117. Hong FS, Smith CL, Angus PW, Crowley P, Ho WK. Hodgkin lymphoma and fulminant hepatic failure. Leuk Lymphoma. 2010;51(5):947–51.
118. Ghosh I, Bakhshi S. Jaundice as a presenting manifestation of pediatric non-Hodgkin lymphoma: etiology, management, and outcome. J Pediatr Hematol Oncol. 2010;32(4):e131–5.
119. Civardi G, Vallisa D, Berte R, Lazzaro A, Moroni CF, Cavanna L. Focal liver lesions in non-Hodgkin's lymphoma: investigation of their prevalence, clinical significance and the role of Hepatitis C virus infection. Eur J Cancer. 2002;38(18):2382–7.
120. Karaosmanoglu D, Karcaaltincaba M, Oguz B, Akata D, Ozmen M, Akhan O. CT findings of lymphoma with peritoneal, omental and mesenteric involvement: peritoneal lymphomatosis. Eur J Radiol. 2009;71(2):313–7.
121. Miller ST, Wollner N, Meyers PA, Exelby P, Jereb B, Miller DR. Primary hepatic or hepatosplenic non-Hodgkin's lymphoma in children. Cancer. 1983;52(12):2285–8.
122. Masood A, Kairouz S, Hudhud KH, Hegazi AZ, Banu A, Gupta NC. Primary non-Hodgkin lymphoma of liver. Curr Oncol. 2009;16(4):74–7.
123. Kikuma K, Watanabe J, Oshiro Y, et al. Etiological factors in primary hepatic B-cell lymphoma. Virchows Arch. 2012;460(4):379–87.
124. Cameron AM, Truty J, Truell J, et al. Fulminant hepatic failure from primary hepatic lymphoma: successful treatment with orthotopic liver transplantation and chemotherapy. Transplantation. 2005;80(7):993–6.

125. Guo X, Li Q, Zhu YP. Childhood hepatosplenic T-cell lymphoma with skin involvement. Indian Pediatr. 2015;52(5):427–8.
126. Beigel F, Jurgens M, Tillack C, et al. Hepatosplenic T-cell lymphoma in a patient with Crohn's disease. Nat Rev Gastroenterol Hepatol. 2009;6(7):433–6.
127. De Rooij JD, Zwaan CM, Van Den Heuvel-Eibrink M. Pediatric AML: from biology to clinical management. J Clin Forensic Med. 2015;4(1):127–49.
128. Smith MA, Seibel NL, Altekruse SF, et al. Outcomes for children and adolescents with cancer: challenges for the twenty-first century. J Clin Oncol. 2010;28(15):2625–34.
129. Linabery AM, Ross JA. Trends in childhood cancer incidence in the U.S. (1992-2004). Cancer. 2008;112(2):416–32.
130. Hunger SP, Mullighan CG. Acute lymphoblastic leukemia in children. N Engl J Med. 2015;373(16):1541–52.
131. Segal I, Rassekh SR, Bond MC, Senger C, Schreiber RA. Abnormal liver transaminases and conjugated hyperbilirubinemia at presentation of acute lymphoblastic leukemia. Pediatr Blood Cancer. 2010;55(3):434–9.
132. Rivet C, Leverger G, Jacquemin E, Bernard O. Acute leukemia presenting as acute hepatitis without liver failure. J Pediatr Gastroenterol Nutr. 2014;59(5):640–1.
133. Reddi DM, Barbas AS, Castleberry AW, et al. Liver transplantation in an adolescent with acute liver failure from acute lymphoblastic leukemia. Pediatr Transplant. 2014;18(2):E57–63.
134. Grimwade D, Ivey A, Huntly BJ. Molecular landscape of acute myeloid leukemia in younger adults and its clinical relevance. Blood. 2016;127(1):29–41.
135. Nakano Y, Yamasaki K, Otsuka Y, et al. Acute myeloid leukemia with RBM15-MKL1 presenting as severe hepatic failure. Glob Pediatr Health. 2017;4:2333794X16689011.
136. Hofmann I. Myeloproliferative neoplasms in children. J Hematop. 2015;8(3):143–57.
137. Hoekstra J, Bresser EL, Smalberg JH, Spaander MC, Leebeek FW, Janssen HL. Long-term follow-up of patients with portal vein thrombosis and myeloproliferative neoplasms. J Thromb Haemost. 2011;9(11):2208–14.
138. Ferri PM, Rodrigues Ferreira A, Fagundes ED, et al. Evaluation of the presence of hereditary and acquired thrombophilias in Brazilian children and adolescents with diagnoses of portal vein thrombosis. J Pediatr Gastroenterol Nutr. 2012;55(5):599–604.
139. Bertrand A, Heissat S, Caron N, et al. Deep vein thrombosis revealing myeloproliferative syndrome in two adolescents. Arch Pediatr. 2014;21(5):497–500.
140. Valla D, Casadevall N, Lacombe C, et al. Primary myeloproliferative disorder and hepatic vein thrombosis. A prospective study of erythroid colony formation in vitro in 20 patients with Budd-Chiari syndrome. Ann Intern Med. 1985;103(3):329–34.
141. Coskun ME, Height S, Dhawan A, Hadzic N. Ruxolitinib treatment in an infant with JAK2+ polycythaemia vera-associated Budd-Chiari syndrome. BMJ Case Rep. 2017;2017.
142. Randi ML, Putti MC, Scapin M, et al. Pediatric patients with essential thrombocythemia are mostly polyclonal and V617FJAK2 negative. Blood. 2006;108(10):3600–2.
143. Giona F, Teofili L, Moleti ML, et al. Thrombocythemia and polycythemia in patients younger than 20 years at diagnosis: clinical and biologic features, treatment, and long-term outcome. Blood. 2012;119(10):2219–27.
144. Hasle H. Incidence of essential thrombocythaemia in children. Br J Haematol. 2000;110(3):751.
145. Saksena A, Arora P, Khurana N, Sethi GR, Singh T. Paediatric idiopathic myelofibrosis. Indian J Hematol Blood Transfus. 2014;30(Suppl 1):363–5.
146. An W, Wan Y, Guo Y, et al. CALR mutation screening in pediatric primary myelofibrosis. Pediatr Blood Cancer. 2014;61(12):2256–62.
147. Druker BJ, Guilhot F, O'brien SG, et al. Five-year follow-up of patients receiving imatinib for chronic myeloid leukemia. N Engl J Med. 2006;355(23):2408–17.
148. De La Fuente J, Baruchel A, Biondi A, et al. Managing children with chronic myeloid leukaemia (CML): recommendations for the management of CML in children and young people up to the age of 18 years. Br J Haematol. 2014;167(1):33–47.
149. Loh ML. Recent advances in the pathogenesis and treatment of juvenile myelomonocytic leukaemia. Br J Haematol. 2011;152(6):677–87.
150. Sakashita K, Matsuda K, Koike K. Diagnosis and treatment of juvenile myelomonocytic leukemia. Pediatr Int. 2016;58(8):681–90.
151. Emanuel PD. Juvenile myelomonocytic leukemia and chronic myelomonocytic leukemia. Leukemia. 2008;22(7):1335–42.
152. Allen CE, Kelly KM, Bollard CM. Pediatric lymphomas and histiocytic disorders of childhood. Pediatr Clin North Am. 2015;62(1):139–65.
153. Gadner H, Minkov M, Grois N, et al. Therapy prolongation improves outcome in multisystem Langerhans cell histiocytosis. Blood. 2013;121(25):5006–14.
154. Stalemark H, Laurencikas E, Karis J, Gavhed D, Fadeel B, Henter JI. Incidence of Langerhans cell histiocytosis in children: a population-based study. Pediatr Blood Cancer. 2008;51(1):76–81.
155. Yi X, Han T, Zai H, Long X, Wang X, Li W. Liver involvement of Langerhans' cell histiocytosis in children. Int J Clin Exp Med. 2015;8(5):7098–106.
156. Tang Y, Zhang Z, Chen M, et al. Severe sclerosing cholangitis after Langerhans cell histiocytosis treated by liver transplantation: An adult case report. Medicine (Baltimore). 2017;96(9):e5994.
157. Braier J, Ciocca M, Latella A, De Davila MG, Drajer M, Inventarza O. Cholestasis, sclerosing cholangitis, and liver transplantation in Langerhans cell Histiocytosis. Med Pediatr Oncol. 2002;38(3):178–82.
158. Kaplan KJ, Goodman ZD, Ishak KG. Liver involvement in Langerhans' cell histiocytosis: a study of nine cases. Mod Pathol. 1999;12(4):370–8.
159. Jaffe R. Liver involvement in the histiocytic disorders of childhood. Pediatr Dev Pathol. 2004;7(3):214–25.
160. Meeths M, Chiang SC, Lofstedt A, et al. Pathophysiology and spectrum of diseases caused by defects in lymphocyte cytotoxicity. Exp Cell Res. 2014;325(1):10–7.
161. Creput C, Galicier L, Buyse S, Azoulay E. Understanding organ dysfunction in hemophagocytic lymphohistiocytosis. Intensive Care Med. 2008;34(7):1177–87.
162. Ishii E. Hemophagocytic lymphohistiocytosis in children: pathogenesis and treatment. Front Pediatr. 2016;4:47.
163. Amin N, Shah I, Bhatnagar S. Hemophagocytic lymphohistiocytosis (HLH) in children presenting as liver disease. J Clin Exp Hepatol. 2014;4(2):175–7.
164. Larroche C, Ziol M, Zidi S, Dhote R, Roulot D. Liver involvement in hemophagocytic syndrome. Gastroenterol Clin Biol. 2007;31(11):959–66.
165. Favara BE. Histopathology of the liver in histiocytosis syndromes. Pediatr Pathol Lab Med. 1996;16(3):413–33.
166. Palumbo A, Anderson K. Multiple myeloma. N Engl J Med. 2011;364(11):1046–60.
167. Pilbeam KL, Lund TC. Pediatric multiple myeloma. Blood. 2017;129(3):395.
168. Corbacioglu S, Carreras E, Ansari M, et al. Diagnosis and severity criteria for sinusoidal obstruction syndrome/veno-occlusive dis-

ease in pediatric patients: a new classification from the European society for blood and marrow transplantation. Bone Marrow Transplant. 2018;53(2):138–45.
169. Fan CQ, Crawford JM. Sinusoidal obstruction syndrome (hepatic veno-occlusive disease). J Clin Exp Hepatol. 2014;4(4):332–46.
170. Deleve LD, Shulman HM, Mcdonald GB. Toxic injury to hepatic sinusoids: sinusoidal obstruction syndrome (veno-occlusive disease). Semin Liver Dis. 2002;22(1):27–42.
171. Sakamoto S, Nakazawa A, Shigeta T, et al. Devastating outflow obstruction after pediatric split liver transplantation. Pediatr Transplant. 2013;17(1):E25–8.
172. Cesaro S, Pillon M, Talenti E, et al. A prospective survey on incidence, risk factors and therapy of hepatic veno-occlusive disease in children after hematopoietic stem cell transplantation. Haematologica. 2005;90(10):1396–404.
173. Schulz AS, Classen CF, Mihatsch WA, et al. HLA-haploidentical blood progenitor cell transplantation in osteopetrosis. Blood. 2002;99(9):3458–60.
174. Cheuk DK, Wang P, Lee TL, et al. Risk factors and mortality predictors of hepatic veno-occlusive disease after pediatric hematopoietic stem cell transplantation. Bone Marrow Transplant. 2007;40(10):935–44.
175. Coppell JA, Richardson PG, Soiffer R, et al. Hepatic veno-occlusive disease following stem cell transplantation: incidence, clinical course, and outcome. Biol Blood Marrow Transplant. 2010;16(2):157–68.
176. Mohty M, Malard F, Abecassis M, et al. Sinusoidal obstruction syndrome/veno-occlusive disease: current situation and perspectives-a position statement from the European Society for Blood and Marrow Transplantation (EBMT). Bone Marrow Transplant. 2015;50(6):781–9.
177. Palomo M, Mir E, Rovira M, Escolar G, Carreras E, Diaz-Ricart M. What is going on between defibrotide and endothelial cells? Snapshots reveal the hot spots of their romance. Blood. 2016;127(13):1719–27.
178. Corbacioglu S, Greil J, Peters C, et al. Defibrotide in the treatment of children with veno-occlusive disease (VOD): a retrospective multicentre study demonstrates therapeutic efficacy upon early intervention. Bone Marrow Transplant. 2004;33(2):189–95.
179. Dalle JH, Giralt SA. Hepatic veno-occlusive disease after hematopoietic stem cell transplantation: risk factors and stratification, prophylaxis, and treatment. Biol Blood Marrow Transplant. 2016;22(3):400–9.
180. Corbacioglu S, Richardson PG. Defibrotide for children and adults with hepatic veno-occlusive disease post hematopoietic cell transplantation. Expert Rev Gastroenterol Hepatol. 2017;11(10):885–98.
181. Flinn AM, Gennery AR. Treatment of pediatric acute graft-versus-host disease-lessons from primary immunodeficiency? Front Immunol. 2017;8:328.
182. Carpenter PA, Macmillan ML. Management of acute graft-versus-host disease in children. Pediatr Clin North Am. 2010;57(1):273–95.
183. Jagasia MH, Greinix HT, Arora M, et al. National Institutes of Health Consensus Development Project on criteria for clinical trials in chronic graft-versus-host disease: I. The 2014 Diagnosis and Staging Working Group report. Biol Blood Marrow Transplant. 2015;21(3):389–401 e381.
184. Baird K, Cooke K, Schultz KR. Chronic graft-versus-host disease (GVHD) in children. Pediatr Clin North Am. 2010;57(1):297–322.
185. Melin-Aldana H, Thormann K, Duerst R, Kletzel M, Jacobsohn DA. Hepatitic pattern of graft versus host disease in children. Pediatr Blood Cancer. 2007;49(5):727–30.
186. Rund D, Rachmilewitz E. Beta-thalassemia. N Engl J Med. 2005;353(11):1135–46.
187. Muncie HL Jr, Campbell J. Alpha and beta thalassemia. Am Fam Physician. 2009;80(4):339–44.
188. Galanello R, Cao A. Gene test review. Alpha-thalassemia. Genet Med. 2011;13(2):83–8.
189. Modell B, Khan M, Darlison M. Survival in beta-thalassaemia major in the UK: data from the UK Thalassaemia Register. Lancet. 2000;355(9220):2051–2.
190. Lucarelli G, Andreani M, Angelucci E. The cure of thalassemia by bone marrow transplantation. Blood Rev. 2002;16(2):81–5.
191. Ghavamzadeh A, Mirzania M, Kamalian N, Sedighi N, Azimi P. Hepatic iron overload and fibrosis in patients with beta-thalassemia major after hematopoietic stem cell transplantation: a pilot study. Int J Hematol Oncol Stem Cell Res. 2015;9(2):55–9.
192. Aguilar Martinez P, Angastiniotis M, Eleftheriou A, et al. Haemoglobinopathies in Europe: health & migration policy perspectives. Orphanet J Rare Dis. 2014;9:97.
193. Ahn H, Li CS, Wang W. Sickle cell hepatopathy: clinical presentation, treatment, and outcome in pediatric and adult patients. Pediatr Blood Cancer. 2005;45(2):184–90.
194. Johnson CS, Omata M, Tong MJ, Simmons JF Jr, Weiner J, Tatter D. Liver involvement in sickle cell disease. Medicine (Baltimore). 1985;64(5):349–56.
195. Jitraruch S, Fitzpatrick E, Deheragoda M, et al. Autoimmune liver disease in children with Sickle cell disease. J Pediatr. 2017;189:79–85.e2.
196. Dhaliwal G, Cornett PA, Tierney LM Jr. Hemolytic anemia. Am Fam Physician. 2004;69(11):2599–606.
197. Aladjidi N, Leverger G, Leblanc T, et al. New insights into childhood autoimmune hemolytic anemia: a French national observational study of 265 children. Haematologica. 2011;96(5):655–63.
198. Hill QA, Stamps R, Massey E, et al. The diagnosis and management of primary autoimmune haemolytic anaemia. Br J Haematol. 2017;176(3):395–411.
199. Maggiore G, Sciveres M, Fabre M, et al. Giant cell hepatitis with autoimmune hemolytic anemia in early childhood: long-term outcome in 16 children. J Pediatr. 2011;159(1):127–132.e121.
200. Paganelli M, Patey N, Bass LM, Alvarez F. Anti-CD20 treatment of giant cell hepatitis with autoimmune hemolytic anemia. Pediatrics. 2014;134(4):e1206–10.
201. Rovelli A, Corti P, Beretta C, Bovo G, Conter V, Mieli-Vergani G. Alemtuzumab for giant cell hepatitis with autoimmune hemolytic anemia. J Pediatr Gastroenterol Nutr. 2007;45(5):596–9.
202. Bouguila J, Mabrouk S, Tilouche S, et al. Giant cell hepatitis with autoimmune hemolytic anemia in a nine month old infant. World J Hepatol. 2013;5(4):226–9.
203. Ware RE, Hall SE, Rosse WF. Paroxysmal nocturnal hemoglobinuria with onset in childhood and adolescence. N Engl J Med. 1991;325(14):991–6.
204. Mercuri A, Farruggia P, Timeus F, et al. A retrospective study of paroxysmal nocturnal hemoglobinuria in pediatric and adolescent patients. Blood Cells Mol Dis. 2017;64:45–50.
205. Hall C, Richards S, Hillmen P. Primary prophylaxis with warfarin prevents thrombosis in paroxysmal nocturnal hemoglobinuria (PNH). Blood. 2003;102(10):3587–91.
206. Van Den Heuvel-Eibrink MM, Bredius RG, Te Winkel ML, et al. Childhood paroxysmal nocturnal haemoglobinuria (PNH), a report of 11 cases in the Netherlands. Br J Haematol. 2005;128(4):571–7.
207. Rajagopal R, Thachil J, Monagle P. Disseminated intravascular coagulation in paediatrics. Arch Dis Child. 2017;102(2):187–93.
208. Wada H, Matsumoto T, Yamashita Y. Diagnosis and treatment of disseminated intravascular coagulation (DIC) according to four DIC guidelines. J Intensive Care. 2014;2(1):15.
209. Bakhshi S, Arya LS. Diagnosis and treatment of disseminated intravascular coagulation. Indian Pediatr. 2003;40(8):721–30.

210. Stevens SM, Woller SC, Bauer KA, et al. Guidance for the evaluation and treatment of hereditary and acquired thrombophilia. J Thromb Thrombolysis. 2016;41(1):154–64.
211. Raffini L, Thornburg C. Testing children for inherited thrombophilia: more questions than answers. Br J Haematol. 2009;147(3):277–88.
212. Tanaka M, Wanless IR. Pathology of the liver in Budd-Chiari syndrome: portal vein thrombosis and the histogenesis of venocentric cirrhosis, veno-portal cirrhosis, and large regenerative nodules. Hepatology. 1998;27(2):488–96.
213. Tripodi A, Anstee QM, Sogaard KK, Primignani M, Valla DC. Hypercoagulability in cirrhosis: causes and consequences. J Thromb Haemost. 2011;9(9):1713–23.
214. Mann DA, Marra F. Fibrogenic signalling in hepatic stellate cells. J Hepatol. 2010;52(6):949–50.
215. Schouten JN, Verheij J, Seijo S. Idiopathic non-cirrhotic portal hypertension: a review. Orphanet J Rare Dis. 2015;10:67.
216. Fasano A, Catassi C. Clinical practice. Celiac disease. N Engl J Med. 2012;367(25):2419–26.
217. Tack GJ, Verbeek WH, Schreurs MW, Mulder CJ. The spectrum of celiac disease: epidemiology, clinical aspects and treatment. Nat Rev Gastroenterol Hepatol. 2010;7(4):204–13.
218. Newton KP, Singer SA. Celiac disease in children and adolescents: special considerations. Semin Immunopathol. 2012;34(4):479–96.
219. Husby S, Koletzko S, Korponay-Szabo IR, et al. European Society for Pediatric Gastroenterology, Hepatology, and Nutrition guidelines for the diagnosis of coeliac disease. J Pediatr Gastroenterol Nutr. 2012;54(1):136–60.
220. Bonamico M, Pitzalis G, Culasso F, et al. Hepatic damage in celiac disease in children. Minerva Pediatr. 1986;38(21):959–62.
221. Volta U, De Franceschi L, Lari F, Molinaro N, Zoli M, Bianchi FB. Coeliac disease hidden by cryptogenic hypertransaminasaemia. Lancet. 1998;352(9121):26–9.
222. Vajro P, Fontanella A, Mayer M, et al. Elevated serum aminotransferase activity as an early manifestation of gluten-sensitive enteropathy. J Pediatr. 1993;122(3):416–9.
223. Anania C, De Luca E, De Castro G, Chiesa C, Pacifico L. Liver involvement in pediatric celiac disease. World J Gastroenterol. 2015;21(19):5813–22.
224. Caprai S, Vajro P, Ventura A, Sciveres M, Maggiore G. Disease SSGFaLDIC. Autoimmune liver disease associated with celiac disease in childhood: a multicenter study. Clin Gastroenterol Hepatol. 2008;6(7):803–6.
225. Di Biase AR, Colecchia A, Scaioli E, et al. Autoimmune liver diseases in a paediatric population with coeliac disease—a 10-year single-centre experience. Aliment Pharmacol Ther. 2010;31(2):253–60.
226. Ventura A, Magazzu G, Greco L. Duration of exposure to gluten and risk for autoimmune disorders in patients with celiac disease. SIGEP Study Group for autoimmune disorders in celiac disease. Gastroenterology. 1999;117(2):297–303.
227. Lacaille F, Canioni D, Bernard O, Fabre M, Brousse N, Schmitz J. Celiac disease, inflammatory colitis, and primary sclerosing cholangitis in a girl with Turner's syndrome. J Pediatr Gastroenterol Nutr. 1995;21(4):463–7.
228. Reilly NR, Lebwohl B, Hultcrantz R, Green PH, Ludvigsson JF. Increased risk of non-alcoholic fatty liver disease after diagnosis of celiac disease. J Hepatol. 2015;62(6):1405–11.
229. Miele L, Marrone G, Lauritano C, et al. Gut-liver axis and microbiota in NAFLD: insight pathophysiology for novel therapeutic target. Curr Pharm Des. 2013;19(29):5314–24.
230. Rowe K, Pankow J, Nehme F, Salyers W. Gastrointestinal amyloidosis: review of the literature. Cureus. 2017;9(5):e1228.
231. Cowan AJ, Skinner M, Seldin DC, et al. Amyloidosis of the gastrointestinal tract: a 13-year, single-center, referral experience. Haematologica. 2013;98(1):141–6.
232. Beneteau-Burnat B, Baudin B, Morgant G, Baumann FC, Giboudeau J. Serum angiotensin-converting enzyme in healthy and sarcoidotic children: comparison with the reference interval for adults. Clin Chem. 1990;36(2):344–6.
233. Coash M, Forouhar F, Wu CH, Wu GY. Granulomatous liver diseases: a review. J Formos Med Assoc. 2012;111(1):3–13.
234. Wahl SM. Hepatic granuloma as a model of inflammation and repair: an overview. Methods Enzymol. 1988;163:605–22.
235. Hams E, Aviello G, Fallon PG. The schistosoma granuloma: friend or foe? Front Immunol. 2013;4:89.
236. Geramizadeh B, Jahangiri R, Moradi E. Causes of hepatic granuloma: a 12-year single center experience from southern Iran. Arch Iran Med. 2011;14(4):288–9.
237. Collins MH, Jiang B, Croffie JM, Chong SK, Lee CH. Hepatic granulomas in children. A clinicopathologic analysis of 23 cases including polymerase chain reaction for histoplasma. Am J Surg Pathol. 1996;20(3):332–8.
238. Lagana SM, Moreira RK, Lefkowitch JH. Hepatic granulomas: pathogenesis and differential diagnosis. Clin Liver Dis. 2010;14(4):605–17.
239. Shetty AK, Gedalia A. Childhood sarcoidosis: a rare but fascinating disorder. Pediatr Rheumatol Online J. 2008;6:16.
240. Dahlan Y, Smith L, Simmonds D, et al. Pediatric-onset primary biliary cirrhosis. Gastroenterology. 2003;125(5):1476–9.
241. Murano I, Yoshii H, Kurashige H, Sugio Y, Tsukahara M. Giant hepatic granuloma caused by Bartonella henselae. Pediatr Infect Dis J. 2001;20(3):319–20.
242. Teixeira AB, Lana AM, Lamounier JA, Pereira Da Silva O, Eloi-Santos SM. Neonatal listeriosis: the importance of placenta histological examination-a case report. AJP Rep. 2011;1(1):3–6.
243. Ozkan TB, Mistik R, Dikici B, Nazlioglu HO. Antiviral therapy in neonatal cholestatic cytomegalovirus hepatitis. BMC Gastroenterol. 2007;7:9.
244. Bolis V, Karadedos C, Chiotis I, Chaliasos N, Tsabouri S. Atypical manifestations of Epstein-Barr virus in children: a diagnostic challenge. J Pediatr (Rio J). 2016;92(2):113–21.
245. Egritas O, Sari S, Dalgic B, Vural C, Akyol G. Granulomatous hepatitis, perihepatic lymphadenopathies, and autoantibody positivity: an unusual association in a child with hepatitis C. Eur J Pediatr. 2009;168(3):275–9.
246. Elbaz T, Esmat G. Hepatic and intestinal schistosomiasis: review. J Adv Res. 2013;4(5):445–52.
247. Amin MD, Harpavat S, Leung DH. Drug-induced liver injury in children. Curr Opin Pediatr. 2015;27(5):625–33.
248. Tajima Y, Takagi R, Nakajima T, Kominato Y. An infant with asymptomatic hepatic granuloma probably caused by bacillus Calmette-Guerin (BCG) vaccination found incidentally at autopsy: a case report. Cases J. 2008;1(1):337.
249. Levine S, Smith VV, Malone M, Sebire NJ. Histopathological features of chronic granulomatous disease (CGD) in childhood. Histopathology. 2005;47(5):508–16.
250. Schwimmer JB, Behling C, Newbury R, et al. Histopathology of pediatric nonalcoholic fatty liver disease. Hepatology. 2005;42(3):641–9.
251. Shoenfeld Y. Systemic antiphospholipid syndrome. Lupus. 2003;12(7):497–8.
252. Avcin T, Cimaz R, Rozman B, Ped-APS Registry Collaborative Group. The Ped-APS Registry: the antiphospholipid syndrome in childhood. Lupus. 2009;18(10):894–9.
253. Cervera R, Piette JC, Font J, et al. Antiphospholipid syndrome: clinical and immunologic manifestations and patterns of disease expression in a cohort of 1,000 patients. Arthritis Rheum. 2002;46(4):1019–27.

254. Avcin T, Cimaz R, Silverman ED, et al. Pediatric antiphospholipid syndrome: clinical and immunologic features of 121 patients in an international registry. Pediatrics. 2008;122(5):e1100–7.
255. Groot N, De Graeff N, Avcin T, et al. European evidence-based recommendations for diagnosis and treatment of paediatric antiphospholipid syndrome: the SHARE initiative. Ann Rheum Dis. 2017;76(10):1637–41.
256. Berkun Y, Padeh S, Barash J, et al. Antiphospholipid syndrome and recurrent thrombosis in children. Arthritis Rheum. 2006;55(6):850–5.
257. Deleve LD, Valla DC, Garcia-Tsao G. American Association for the Study Liver D. Vascular disorders of the liver. Hepatology. 2009;49(5):1729–64.
258. Boudhina T, Ghram N, Ben Becher S, et al. Budd-Chiari syndrome in children. Apropos of 7 cases. Arch Fr Pediatr. 1991;48(4):243–8.
259. Khubchandani RP, D'souza S. Antiphospholipid antibody syndrome as a cause of Budd-Chiari syndrome. Indian Pediatr. 2003;40(9):907–8.
260. Ravelli A, Martini A. Antiphospholipid syndrome. Pediatr Clin North Am. 2005;52(2):469–91., vi.
261. Saca LF, Szer IS, Henar E, Nanjundiah P, Haddad ZH, Quismorio FP Jr. Budd-Chiari syndrome associated with antiphospholipid antibodies in a child: report of a case and review of the literature. J Rheumatol. 1994;21(3):545–8.
262. Karim F, Loeffen J, Bramer W, et al. IgG4-related disease: a systematic review of this unrecognized disease in pediatrics. Pediatr Rheumatol Online J. 2016;14(1):18.
263. Deshpande V, Zen Y, Chan JK, et al. Consensus statement on the pathology of IgG4-related disease. Mod Pathol. 2012;25(9):1181–92.
264. Kamisawa T, Zen Y, Pillai S, Stone JH. IgG4-related disease. Lancet. 2015;385(9976):1460–71.
265. Khosroshahi A, Wallace ZS, Crowe JL, et al. International Consensus Guidance Statement on the management and treatment of IgG4-related disease. Arthritis Rheumatol. 2015;67(7):1688–99.
266. Hubers LM, Maillette De Buy Wenniger LJ, Doorenspleet ME, et al. IgG4-associated cholangitis: a comprehensive review. Clin Rev Allergy Immunol. 2015;48(2-3):198–206.
267. Nakazawa T, Naitoh I, Hayashi K, Miyabe K, Simizu S, Joh T. Diagnosis of IgG4-related sclerosing cholangitis. World J Gastroenterol. 2013;19(43):7661–70.
268. Kawakami H, Zen Y, Kuwatani M, et al. IgG4-related sclerosing cholangitis and autoimmune pancreatitis: histological assessment of biopsies from Vater's ampulla and the bile duct. J Gastroenterol Hepatol. 2010;25(10):1648–55.
269. Chari ST, Smyrk TC, Levy MJ, et al. Diagnosis of autoimmune pancreatitis: the Mayo Clinic experience. Clin Gastroenterol Hepatol. 2006;4(8):1010–6.; quiz 1934.
270. Shimosegawa T, Chari ST, Frulloni L, et al. International consensus diagnostic criteria for autoimmune pancreatitis: guidelines of the International Association of Pancreatology. Pancreas. 2011;40(3):352–8.
271. Rosen D, Thung S, Sheflin-Findling S, et al. IgG4-sclerosing cholangitis in a pediatric patient. Semin Liver Dis. 2015;35(1):89–94.
272. Ibrahim SH, Zhang L, Freese DK. A 3-year-old with immunoglobulin G4-associated cholangitis. J Pediatr Gastroenterol Nutr. 2011;53(1):109–11.
273. Nada R, Gupta A, Kang M, et al. Hepatic mass and coagulopathy in a ten-year-old boy with fever. Arthritis Rheumatol. 2015;67(7):1977.
274. Zen Y. The pathology of IgG4-related disease in the bile duct and pancreas. Semin Liver Dis. 2016;36(3):242–56.
275. Safran AP, Schaffner F. Chronic passive congestion of the liver in man. Electron microscopic study of cell atrophy and intralobular fibrosis. Am J Pathol. 1967;50(3):447–63.
276. Moller S, Bernardi M. Interactions of the heart and the liver. Eur Heart J. 2013;34(36):2804–11.
277. Wanless IR, Liu JJ, Butany J. Role of thrombosis in the pathogenesis of congestive hepatic fibrosis (cardiac cirrhosis). Hepatology. 1995;21(5):1232–7.
278. Alvarez AM, Mukherjee D. Liver abnormalities in cardiac diseases and heart failure. Int J Angiol. 2011;20(3):135–42.
279. Asrani SK, Asrani NS, Freese DK, et al. Congenital heart disease and the liver. Hepatology. 2012;56(3):1160–9.
280. Runyon BA, Committee APG. Management of adult patients with ascites due to cirrhosis: an update. Hepatology. 2009;49(6):2087–107.
281. Birgens HS, Henriksen J, Matzen P, Poulsen H. The shock liver. Clinical and biochemical findings in patients with centrilobular liver necrosis following cardiogenic shock. Acta Med Scand. 1978;204(5):417–21.
282. Cassidy WM, Reynolds TB. Serum lactic dehydrogenase in the differential diagnosis of acute hepatocellular injury. J Clin Gastroenterol. 1994;19(2):118–21.
283. Van Der Linde D, Konings EE, Slager MA, et al. Birth prevalence of congenital heart disease worldwide: a systematic review and meta-analysis. J Am Coll Cardiol. 2011;58(21):2241–7.
284. Hoffman JI, Kaplan S. The incidence of congenital heart disease. J Am Coll Cardiol. 2002;39(12):1890–900.
285. Massin MM, Astadicko I, Dessy H. Epidemiology of heart failure in a tertiary pediatric center. Clin Cardiol. 2008;31(8):388–91.
286. Sommers C, Nagel BH, Neudorf U, Schmaltz AA. Congestive heart failure in childhood. An epidemiologic study. Herz. 2005;30(7):652–62.
287. Masarone D, Valente F, Rubino M, et al. Pediatric heart failure: a practical guide to diagnosis and management. Pediatr Neonatol. 2017;58(4):303–12.
288. Ginde S, Lam J, Hill GD, et al. Long-term outcomes after surgical repair of complete atrioventricular septal defect. J Thorac Cardiovasc Surg. 2015;150(2):369–74.
289. O'laughlin MP, Slack MC, Grifka RG, Perry SB, Lock JE, Mullins CE. Implantation and intermediate-term follow-up of stents in congenital heart disease. Circulation. 1993;88(2):605–14.
290. Becker AE, Connor M, Anderson RH. Tetralogy of Fallot: a morphometric and geometric study. Am J Cardiol. 1975;35(3):402–12.
291. Dearani JA, Danielson GK. Surgical management of Ebstein's anomaly in the adult. Semin Thorac Cardiovasc Surg. 2005;17(2):148–54.
292. Nihoyannopoulos P, Mckenna WJ, Smith G, Foale R. Echocardiographic assessment of the right ventricle in Ebstein's anomaly: relation to clinical outcome. J Am Coll Cardiol. 1986;8(3):627–35.
293. Yuan SM. Ebstein's Anomaly: Genetics, Clinical Manifestations, and Management. Pediatr Neonatol. 2017;58(3):211–5.
294. Samanek M. Congenital heart malformations: prevalence, severity, survival, and quality of life. Cardiol Young. 2000;10(3):179–85.
295. Jatene AD, Fontes VF, Paulista PP, et al. Anatomic correction of transposition of the great vessels. J Thorac Cardiovasc Surg. 1976;72(3):364–70.
296. Devabhaktuni SR, Chakfeh E, Malik AO, Pengson JA, Rana J, Ahsan CH. Subvalvular aortic stenosis: a review of current literature. Clin Cardiol. 2018;41(1):131–6.
297. Etnel JR, Takkenberg JJ, Spaans LG, Bogers AJ, Helbing WA. Paediatric subvalvular aortic stenosis: a systematic review and meta-analysis of natural history and surgical outcome. Eur J Cardiothorac Surg. 2015;48(2):212–20.
298. Kim DH, Park SJ, Jung JW, Kim NK, Choi JY. The comparison between the echocardiographic data to the cardiac catheterization data on the diagnosis, treatment, and follow-up in patients

298. diagnosed as pulmonary valve stenosis. J Cardiovasc Ultrasound. 2013;21(1):18–22.
299. Norwood WI, Lang P, Hansen DD. Physiologic repair of aortic atresia-hypoplastic left heart syndrome. N Engl J Med. 1983;308(1):23–6.
300. Agnoletti G, Ferraro G, Bordese R, et al. Fontan circulation causes early, severe liver damage. Should we offer patients a tailored strategy? Int J Cardiol. 2016;209:60–5.
301. Camposilvan S, Milanesi O, Stellin G, Pettenazzo A, Zancan L, D'antiga L. Liver and cardiac function in the long term after Fontan operation. Ann Thorac Surg. 2008;86(1):177–82.
302. Fidai A, Dallaire F, Alvarez N, et al. Non-invasive investigations for the diagnosis of Fontan-associated liver disease in pediatric and adult Fontan patients. Front Cardiovasc Med. 2017;4:15.
303. Lee TM, Hsu DT, Kantor P, et al. Pediatric cardiomyopathies. Circ Res. 2017;121(7):855–73.
304. Hollander SA, Addonizio LJ, Chin C, et al. Abdominal complaints as a common first presentation of heart failure in adolescents with dilated cardiomyopathy. Am J Emerg Med. 2013;31(4):684–6.
305. Rossano JW, Shaddy RE. Heart failure in children: etiology and treatment. J Pediatr. 2014;165(2):228–33.
306. Juneja R, Tandon R. Rheumatic carditis: a reappraisal. Indian Heart J. 2004;56(3):252–5.
307. De Rosa G, Pardeo M, Stabile A, Rigante D. Rheumatic heart disease in children: from clinical assessment to therapeutic management. Eur Rev Med Pharmacol Sci. 2006;10(3):107–10.
308. Zuhlke LJ, Beaton A, Engel ME, et al. Group A Streptococcus, acute rheumatic fever and rheumatic heart disease: epidemiology and clinical considerations. Curr Treat Options Cardiovasc Med. 2017;19(2):15.
309. Tandon R, Sharma M, Chandrashekhar Y, Kotb M, Yacoub MH, Narula J. Revisiting the pathogenesis of rheumatic fever and carditis. Nat Rev Cardiol. 2013;10(3):171–7.
310. Perlmutter DH, Shepherd RW. Extrahepatic biliary atresia: a disease or a phenotype? Hepatology. 2002;35(6):1297–304.
311. Silveira TR, Salzano FM, Howard ER, Mowat AP. Congenital structural abnormalities in biliary atresia: evidence for etiopathogenic heterogeneity and therapeutic implications. Acta Paediatr Scand. 1991;80(12):1192–9.
312. Nizery L, Chardot C, Sissaoui S, et al. Biliary atresia: clinical advances and perspectives. Clin Res Hepatol Gastroenterol. 2016;40(3):281–7.
313. De La Villeon B, Le Goudeveze S, Goudard Y, Fondin M, Vauchaussade De Chaumont A, Duverger V. Polysplenia syndrome. J Visc Surg. 2011;148(5):e395–6.
314. Davenport M, Tizzard SA, Underhill J, Mieli-Vergani G, Portmann B, Hadzic N. The biliary atresia splenic malformation syndrome: a 28-year single-center retrospective study. J Pediatr. 2006;149(3):393–400.
315. Bridy-Pappas AE, Margolis MB, Center KJ, Isaacman DJ. Streptococcus pneumoniae: description of the pathogen, disease epidemiology, treatment, and prevention. Pharmacotherapy. 2005;25(9):1193–212.
316. Minemura M, Tajiri K, Shimizu Y. Liver involvement in systemic infection. World J Hepatol. 2014;6(9):632–42.
317. Defilippi A, Silvestri M, Tacchella A, et al. Epidemiology and clinical features of mycoplasma pneumoniae infection in children. Respir Med. 2008;102(12):1762–8.
318. Kim KW, Sung JJ, Tchah H, et al. Hepatitis associated with mycoplasma pneumoniae infection in Korean children: a prospective study. Korean J Pediatr. 2015;58(6):211–7.
319. Suzuyama Y, Iwasaki H, Izumikawa K, Hara K. Clinical complications of mycoplasma pneumoniae disease—other organs. Yale J Biol Med. 1983;56(5-6):487–91.
320. Morgenstern R, Hayes PC. The liver in typhoid fever: always affected, not just a complication. Am J Gastroenterol. 1991;86(9):1235–9.
321. Karoli R, Fatima J, Chandra A, Singh G. Salmonella hepatitis: an uncommon complication of a common disease. J Family Med Prim Care. 2012;1(2):160–2.
322. El-Newihi HM, Alamy ME, Reynolds TB. Salmonella hepatitis: analysis of 27 cases and comparison with acute viral hepatitis. Hepatology. 1996;24(3):516–9.
323. Balasubramanian S, Kaarthigeyan K, Srinivas S, Rajeswari R. Serum ALT: LDH ratio in typhoid fever and acute viral hepatitis. Indian Pediatr. 2010;47(4):339–41.
324. Maher D, Harries A. Pitfalls in the diagnosis and management of the jaundiced patient in the tropics. Trop Doct. 1994;24(3):128–30.
325. Talwani R, Gilliam BL, Howell C. Infectious diseases and the liver. Clin Liver Dis. 2011;15(1):111–30.
326. Chaudhary P. Hepatobiliary tuberculosis. Ann Gastroenterol. 2014;27(3):207–11.
327. Oliva A, Duarte B, Jonasson O, Nadimpalli V. The nodular form of local hepatic tuberculosis. A review. J Clin Gastroenterol. 1990;12(2):166–73.
328. Essop AR, Posen JA, Savitch I, Levin J, Kew MC. Radiocolloid liver imaging in tuberculous hepatitis. Clin Nucl Med. 1984;9(2):81–4.
329. Maartens G, Willcox PA, Benatar SR. Miliary tuberculosis: rapid diagnosis, hematologic abnormalities, and outcome in 109 treated adults. Am J Med. 1990;89(3):291–6.
330. Kok KY, Yapp SK. Tuberculosis of the bile duct: a rare cause of obstructive jaundice. J Clin Gastroenterol. 1999;29(2):161–4.
331. Chu JH, Feudtner C, Heydon K, Walsh TJ, Zaoutis TE. Hospitalizations for endemic mycoses: a population-based national study. Clin Infect Dis. 2006;42(6):822–5.
332. Lewis JH, Patel HR, Zimmerman HJ. The spectrum of hepatic candidiasis. Hepatology. 1982;2(4):479–87.
333. Steinbach WJ. Pediatric invasive candidiasis: epidemiology and diagnosis in children. J Fungi (Basel). 2016;2(1).
334. Zaoutis TE, Argon J, Chu J, Berlin JA, Walsh TJ, Feudtner C. The epidemiology and attributable outcomes of candidemia in adults and children hospitalized in the United States: a propensity analysis. Clin Infect Dis. 2005;41(9):1232–9.
335. Chitsulo L, Loverde P, Engels D. Schistosomiasis. Nat Rev Microbiol. 2004;2(1):12–3.
336. Gryseels B, Polman K, Clerinx J, Kestens L. Human schistosomiasis. Lancet. 2006;368(9541):1106–18.
337. Osakunor DNM, Woolhouse MEJ, Mutapi F. Paediatric schistosomiasis: what we know and what we need to know. PLoS Negl Trop Dis. 2018;12(2):e0006144.
338. Ladhani S, Aibara RJ, Riordan FA, Shingadia D. Imported malaria in children: a review of clinical studies. Lancet Infect Dis. 2007;7(5):349–57.
339. Schumacher RF, Spinelli E. Malaria in children. Mediterr J Hematol Infect Dis. 2012;4(1):e2012073.
340. Anand AC, Puri P. Jaundice in malaria. J Gastroenterol Hepatol. 2005;20(9):1322–32.
341. Rupani AB, Amarapurkar AD. Hepatic changes in fatal malaria: an emerging problem. Ann Trop Med Parasitol. 2009;103(2):119–27.
342. Kawasaki T. Update on pediatric sepsis: a review. J Intensive Care. 2017;5:47.
343. Weiss SL, Fitzgerald JC, Pappachan J, et al. Global epidemiology of pediatric severe sepsis: the sepsis prevalence, outcomes, and therapies study. Am J Respir Crit Care Med. 2015;191(10):1147–57.
344. Wolfler A, Silvani P, Musicco M, Antonelli M, Salvo I, Italian Pediatric Sepsis Study Group. Incidence of and mortality due to sepsis, severe sepsis and septic shock in Italian Pediatric Intensive Care Units: a prospective national survey. Intensive Care Med. 2008;34(9):1690–7.

345. Kumar A, Roberts D, Wood KE, et al. Duration of hypotension before initiation of effective antimicrobial therapy is the critical determinant of survival in human septic shock. Crit Care Med. 2006;34(6):1589–96.
346. Weiss SL, Fitzgerald JC, Balamuth F, et al. Delayed antimicrobial therapy increases mortality and organ dysfunction duration in pediatric sepsis. Crit Care Med. 2014;42(11):2409–17.
347. Kramer L, Jordan B, Druml W, Bauer P, Metnitz PG. Austrian Epidemiologic Study on Intensive Care ASG. Incidence and prognosis of early hepatic dysfunction in critically ill patients—a prospective multicenter study. Crit Care Med. 2007;35(4):1099–104.
348. Yan J, Li S, Li S. The role of the liver in sepsis. Int Rev Immunol. 2014;33(6):498–510.
349. Koskinas J, Gomatos IP, Tiniakos DG, et al. Liver histology in ICU patients dying from sepsis: a clinico-pathological study. World J Gastroenterol. 2008;14(9):1389–93.
350. Muftuoglu MA, Aktekin A, Ozdemir NC, Saglam A. Liver injury in sepsis and abdominal compartment syndrome in rats. Surg Today. 2006;36(6):519–24.
351. Deng M, Scott MJ, Loughran P, et al. Lipopolysaccharide clearance, bacterial clearance, and systemic inflammatory responses are regulated by cell type-specific functions of TLR4 during sepsis. J Immunol. 2013;190(10):5152–60.
352. Wasmuth HE, Kunz D, Yagmur E, et al. Patients with acute on chronic liver failure display "sepsis-like" immune paralysis. J Hepatol. 2005;42(2):195–201.
353. Dhainaut JF, Marin N, Mignon A, Vinsonneau C. Hepatic response to sepsis: interaction between coagulation and inflammatory processes. Crit Care Med. 2001;29(7 Suppl):S42–7.
354. Siore AM, Parker RE, Stecenko AA, et al. Endotoxin-induced acute lung injury requires interaction with the liver. Am J Physiol Lung Cell Mol Physiol. 2005;289(5):L769–76.
355. Gustot T, Durand F, Lebrec D, Vincent JL, Moreau R. Severe sepsis in cirrhosis. Hepatology. 2009;50(6):2022–33.
356. Li F, Tian Z. The liver works as a school to educate regulatory immune cells. Cell Mol Immunol. 2013;10(4):292–302.
357. Ren D, Bi Q, Li L, et al. Myeloid-derived suppressor cells accumulate in the liver site after sepsis to induce immunosuppression. Cell Immunol. 2012;279(1):12–20.
358. Uetrecht J, Naisbitt DJ. Idiosyncratic adverse drug reactions: current concepts. Pharmacol Rev. 2013;65(2):779–808.
359. Aithal GP, Rawlins MD, Day CP. Clinical diagnostic scale: a useful tool in the evaluation of suspected hepatotoxic adverse drug reactions. J Hepatol. 2000;33(6):949–52.
360. Shi Q, Yang X, Greenhaw JJ, Salminen AT, Russotti GM, Salminen WF. Drug-induced liver injury in children: clinical observations, animal models, and regulatory status. Int J Toxicol. 2017;36(5):365–79.
361. Chalasani N, Fontana RJ, Bonkovsky HL, et al. Causes, clinical features, and outcomes from a prospective study of drug-induced liver injury in the United States. Gastroenterology. 2008;135(6):1924–34.
362. Molleston JP, Fontana RJ, Lopez MJ, et al. Characteristics of idiosyncratic drug-induced liver injury in children: results from the DILIN prospective study. J Pediatr Gastroenterol Nutr. 2011;53(2):182–9.
363. Devarbhavi H, Karanth D, Prasanna KS, Adarsh CK, Patil M. Drug-induced liver injury with hypersensitivity features has a better outcome: a single-center experience of 39 children and adolescents. Hepatology. 2011;54(4):1344–50.
364. Ocete-Hita E, Salmeron-Fernandez M, Urrutia-Maldonado E, et al. Analysis of immunogenetic factors in idiosyncratic drug-induced liver injury in the pediatric population. J Pediatr Gastroenterol Nutr. 2017;64(5):742–7.
365. Bjornsson E, Talwalkar J, Treeprasertsuk S, et al. Drug-induced autoimmune hepatitis: clinical characteristics and prognosis. Hepatology. 2010;51(6):2040–8.
366. Orman ES, Conjeevaram HS, Vuppalanchi R, et al. Clinical and histopathologic features of fluoroquinolone-induced liver injury. Clin Gastroenterol Hepatol. 2011;9(6):517–523.e513.
367. Temple R. Hy's law: predicting serious hepatotoxicity. Pharmacoepidemiol Drug Saf. 2006;15(4):241–3.
368. Chen YT, Trzoss L, Yang D, Yan B. Ontogenic expression of human carboxylesterase-2 and cytochrome P450 3A4 in liver and duodenum: postnatal surge and organ-dependent regulation. Toxicology. 2015;330:55–61.
369. Allegaert K, Van Den Anker JN, Naulaers G, De Hoon J. Determinants of drug metabolism in early neonatal life. Curr Clin Pharmacol. 2007;2(1):23–9.
370. Kearns GL, Abdel-Rahman SM, Alander SW, Blowey DL, Leeder JS, Kauffman RE. Developmental pharmacology—drug disposition, action, and therapy in infants and children. N Engl J Med. 2003;349(12):1157–67.
371. Brouwer KL, Aleksunes LM, Brandys B, et al. Human ontogeny of drug transporters: review and recommendations of the Pediatric Transporter Working Group. Clin Pharmacol Ther. 2015;98(3):266–87.
372. Bartelink IH, Rademaker CM, Schobben AF, Van Den Anker JN. Guidelines on paediatric dosing on the basis of developmental physiology and pharmacokinetic considerations. Clin Pharmacokinet. 2006;45(11):1077–97.
373. Mahmood I. Prediction of drug clearance in children: a review of different methodologies. Expert Opin Drug Metab Toxicol. 2015;11(4):573–87.
374. Benichou C. Criteria of drug-induced liver disorders. Report of an international consensus meeting. J Hepatol. 1990;11(2):272–6.
375. Devarbhavi H, Patil M, Reddy VV, Singh R, Joseph T, Ganga D. Drug-induced acute liver failure in children and adults: results of a single-centre study of 128 patients. Liver Int. 2018;38(7):1322–9. https://doi.org/10.1111/liv.13662.

Nutrition and Liver Disease

Florence Lacaille

Key Points

- Protein-energy malnutrition is highly prevalent in children with chronic liver diseases.
- Sarcopenia or muscle wasting is a central element in the evolution, poorly responsive to nutritional therapy.
- Fat malabsorption is an important factor in cholestatic disorders.
- Exercise should be maintained.
- Intestinal failure-associated liver disease (IFALD) is the most prevalent complication in children on long-term parenteral nutrition.
- The etiology of IFALD is multifactorial, with toxic, anatomical, infectious risk factors, many of them preventable.
- The maintenance of enterohepatic circulation and control of infections are major factors.
- Lipid emulsions play a significant role in the pathogenesis of IFALD, and the less toxic are probably those containing fish oil.

Research Needed in the Field

- Longitudinal and bedside evaluation of nutritional status with easily available methods, such as bioimpedance analysis, and validation of scores
- Mechanisms of sarcopenia in children with chronic liver disease
- Evaluation of sarcopenia and its relationship with prognosis
- The role of branched-chain amino acids in the treatment of children with chronic liver disease
- The understanding of the role of microbiota and its modifications in children with IFALD
- The real advantage provided by fish oil-containing lipid emulsions on the liver of children on long-term PN

23.1 Nutrition in Chronic Liver Disease

23.1.1 Epidemiology

Protein-energy malnutrition is one of the most frequent complications of chronic liver diseases (CLD) and is associated with an increased risk of morbidity and mortality [1–5]. As the nutritional status is a modifiable condition, it has to be assessed regularly so that therapy can be rapidly instituted. Prevention and treatment of malnutrition in children with CLD should be a daily concern [6, 7].

Children normally rely on fat to meet their high energy needs. However, the most frequent and severe CLD in childhood are cholestatic disorders, which impact early on nutrition due to their consequences on fat absorption [8]. A majority of children with CLD have therefore nutritional deficiencies. These are due to impaired absorption but also insufficient intakes and disorders in hepatic homeostasis and regulation of energy and carbohydrate and fat metabolism.

The depletion of muscle mass ("sarcopenia") has emerged as central in the evolution of "frailty" in chronic diseases. It has been correlated to prognosis in CLD and after liver transplantation [9–11], with the new paradox of "sarcopenic obesity" in adults with nonalcoholic steatohepatitis (NASH) and end-stage liver disease. Muscle wasting is however not consistently

F. Lacaille (✉)
Pediatric Gastroenterology-Hepatology-Nutrition Unit, Hôpital Universitaire Necker-Enfants Malades, University Paris Cité Sorbonne Paris Descartes Medical School, Paris, France
e-mail: florence.lacaille@aphp.fr

responsive to nutritional supplementation. The muscle plays a key role in mobility, heart and respiratory function, regulation of glucose and lipid metabolism, and immune function. It stores amino acids and proteins, which can be mobilized in catabolic conditions. Insufficient food intakes, hypermetabolism, decreased activity, endotoxemia, and disturbed energy metabolism may all contribute to sarcopenia. Hyperammonemia has recently been recognized as a key mediator in the metabolic dysfunctions leading to sarcopenia [9]. The evaluation of sarcopenia is therefore becoming increasingly important in the nutritional assessment and management of cirrhosis.

23.1.2 Etiology and Pathophysiology

23.1.2.1 Insufficient Intakes
A child with CLD has increased energy requirements but is often anorectic. This can be related to several factors:

- Mechanical disturbances caused by the enlarged liver or spleen or ascites.
- Delayed gastric emptying.
- Impaired gut motility.
- Abdominal pain secondary to the diarrhea of malabsorption.
- Frequent vomiting, especially on enteral nutrition.
- Altered taste sensation, especially with zinc deficiency.
- Chronic inflammation, frequent infections.
- General wasting.
- Iatrogenic, with the prescription of inhospital fasting, or unpalatable diets or unnecessary restrictions.

23.1.2.2 Malabsorption
Fat malabsorption is one of the main complications of chronic cholestasis. It is due to the lack of bile salts in the intestinal lumen and the defective solubilization of long-chain triglycerides (the main fat component of a normal diet) in micelles (lipids in the center, surrounded by bile salts), necessary for their uptake by enterocytes. The nonabsorbed fat induces diarrhea (steatorrhea), with fermentation, bloating, and secondary malabsorption of other nutrients. The absorption of fat-soluble vitamins (A, D, E, K) is also impaired.

In addition, severe portal hypertension may induce mucosal lesions and protein-losing enteropathy.

The changes in the intestinal microbiota secondary to liver disease have variable consequences on a range of functions, including the intraluminal digestion of nutrients [12]. In children with concomitant intestinal diseases, or in some patients with Roux-en-Y loop and blind loop syndrome, bacterial overgrowth and its consequences on intraluminal digestion (such as de-conjugation of bile acids, impairing the formation of micelles) may be contributing factors to malabsorption.

Some patients may also have a pancreatic disease, further impairing the intraluminal digestion of nutrients.

23.1.2.3 Hypermetabolism and Inflammation
A significant proportion of adult cirrhotic patients (15–35%) have an increased metabolic activity, due at least in part to an increase in beta-adrenergic activity and measured by an increased resting energy expenditure [13]. The increased energy requirements may also be due to the disordered use of substrates. In children, the energy expenditure is increased for height, but not for age [14]. Most patients with severe CLD have a hyperdynamic circulation, with a high heart rate and cardiac output, reflecting the high sympathetic tonus. In addition, in small children, the polypnea induced by ascites or organomegaly further increases the energy requirements.

Patients with stable cirrhosis may have a mild-to-moderate chronic inflammation, reflected by hypergammaglobulinemia. An acute event such as infection increases the level of inflammation and the subsequent catabolism.

23.1.2.4 Impaired Hormonal Function
The liver produces the major part of plasma IGF and IGF-binding proteins in response to growth hormone. The normal response of IGF-1 and IGF-BP decreases with the progression of liver disease and malnutrition [15]. Growth hormone is an important mediator of the liver-muscle axis. Its decreased concentration, or the impaired response in the muscle, are likely contributors to sarcopenia [9].

23.1.2.5 Altered Nutrient Metabolism

Carbohydrate and Lipid Metabolism
Ingested carbohydrates are normally taken up by the liver and stored as glycogen. In the fasting state, glucose is produced in the liver via glycogenolysis and gluconeogenesis. Patients with CLD have reduced glycogen stores and gluconeogenesis capacity and enter into a starvation state far earlier (overnight in adults) than healthy subjects. In this situation, the energy metabolism shifts from carbohydrate to lipid oxidation, increasing the free fatty acid level [16]. In advanced CLD, insulin resistance develops and disturbs the normal delivery of glucose to tissue, switching the energy metabolism toward an increased use of free fatty acids [4, 7, 8]. Younger children with CLD have a risk of hypoglycemia, as well as hyperinsulinemia and peripheral insulin resistance. Fat and proteins are used as alternative energy sources. In chronic cholestasis however, the fat absorption is impaired by the defective micelle formation.

Essential fatty acids are decreased in correlation with nutritional status and severity of liver disease [4, 17]. This can be worsened by a deficient diet in young children.

Essential fatty acids are however necessary for the growth and development of brain and retina and as precursors of polyunsaturated fatty acids and important biological mediators such as eicosanoids [8].

Proteins

The negative nitrogen balance in CLD is the resultant of several factors. Albumin synthesis is decreased, and its serum level inversely correlates with the degree of liver failure. The protein breakdown from skeletal muscle is an important mechanism of sarcopenia [11]. The protein catabolism is accelerated to provide amino acids, mainly branched-chain amino acids (BCAA), for protein synthesis and energy supply. Amino acids are used for gluconeogenesis far earlier than in healthy subjects (12 h as compared to 3 days), further worsening the protein deficiency [18].

The metabolism of BCAA (leucine, isoleucine, valine) is profoundly disturbed. They are consumed as energy substrates but also as a source of glutamate, which detoxifies ammonia by glutamine synthesis in the skeletal muscle. An imbalance between BCAA and aromatic amino acids is thought to play a central role in hepatic encephalopathy [19].

In addition, proteins may be lost by bleeding through the digestive tract.

Vitamins

Fat-soluble vitamins (A, D, E, and K) are normally absorbed together with triglycerides in micelles and are therefore deficient in patients with cholestasis. Their storage capacity is limited, and deficiencies can have devastating consequences, such as bleeding (K), ocular lesions (A), neurological symptoms (E), and rickets (D) [2, 4, 8]. The vitamin D status may also be low due to a lack of sun exposure. However the hydroxylation of 25-OH-vitamin D in the liver is conserved very late. Water-soluble vitamins also are decreased, because of alterations of the intermediary metabolism in the liver [2, 5, 8].

Oligo-elements

Calcium may form soaps with the malabsorbed lipids in the intestinal lumen, especially in chronic cholestatic conditions. This, together with vitamin D deficiency, participates in the bone disease. Iron deficiency is frequent and multifactorial: insufficient intake, chronic bleeding from portal hypertension, and frequent blood tests. Zinc status is difficult to assess but may be deficient [2, 4], especially on diuretic treatment. On the contrary, copper and manganese are usually high, due to their defective excretion in bile. It may be useful to check for magnesium on diuretics.

23.1.2.6 Hyperammonemia

Ammonia appears as an important mediator of sarcopenia. Ammonia disposal by ureagenesis in the liver is critical, but the metabolism is impaired by the hepatocellular dysfunction and portosystemic shunting. Ammonia is generated by amino acid metabolism, purine metabolism, enterocyte glutaminase activity, and urealysis in the gut. In liver disease, the muscle acts as a metabolic sink for ammonia. Ammonia activates in the muscle metabolic responses, such as reduced ATP synthesis, impaired mitochondrial function, and increased autophagy, all contributing to sarcopenia [9].

23.1.3 Diagnosis: Assessment of Nutritional Status

23.1.3.1 Clinical Data

The usual anthropometric data, body mass index, and growth curve should be collected. The measure of weight can be misleading, due to hepatosplenomegaly, edema, or ascites. The height curve may be a good reflection of the chronicity of the disease. However the growth may be normal for a long time in non-cholestatic disorders. The ratio of arm to head circumference is easy to measure and reliable up to 4 years of age. It is normally more than 0.35, and malnutrition is significant under 0.3. Isolated mid-arm circumference is also a reliable measure, to be compared to the reference values for the patient's age, ethnical background, and gender [20]. Triceps skinfold thickness is easy to use and reliable, when the device and tables are available [4, 5].

23.1.3.2 Dietary Assessment

It should be performed at each visit in at-risk patients. It is easiest in young children, drinking recorded amounts of milk. In older patients, a 3-day diary is at best completed, including all food, fluids and supplements, and instructions (size of servings, etc.).

23.1.3.3 Biological Parameters

Albumin is not a very reliable marker of malnutrition. It is synthesized by the liver, with a half-life of 3 weeks, and the synthesis is decreased in CLD together with coagulation factors. It can be lost through protein-losing enteropathy, nephrotic syndrome, and extensive dermatitis. It may also be decreased because of malnutrition and chronic inflammation.

Prealbumin has a short half-life and is highly affected by liver disease, which make it unreliable as a screening tool for malnutrition [4]. Cholesterol level is increased in most cholestatic disorders and decreased in malnutrition: it should thus be individually interpreted.

Fat-soluble vitamins should be regularly checked to adapt the supplementation (Table 23.1). Vitamins A, D, and E are directly measured in the plasma. The vitamin A to RBP and vitamin E to total lipids ratio are adequate to evaluate the stores. Vitamin K is indirectly controlled with the prothrombin time [8]. Alkaline phosphatases as a marker of bone remodeling are both a marker of growth and vitamin D supply.

Table 23.1 Children with chronic liver disease: requirements in vitamins [8]

	Requirements	Comments, controls
Vitamin A	<10 kg: 5000 IU/day >10 kg: 10000 IU/day IM: 50000 IU/month or 2 months	Oral if bilirubin <100 μM Serum retinol/RBP ≥ 0.8
Vitamin D	25-OH vitamin D: 2–5 μg/kg/day IM: 30–50,000 IU/month or 3 months	Oral if bilirubin <100 μM IM dose: Depends on availability and clinical situation Alkaline phosphatases (liver + bone) as indirect control
Vitamin E	25 IU/kg	Water-soluble solution (tocofersolan) Vitamin E/total lipids ≥0.6 mg/g Control knee reflexes
Vitamin K	2–10 mg/week IM: 5–10 mg/2 weeks	Micellar solution Oral if bilirubin <120–150 μM Usually IM needed if higher bilirubin Prothrombin time (factors II, VII, X vitamin K-dependent)
Water-soluble vitamins	Twice recommended amount	

23.1.3.4 Measure of Body Composition

- Indirect calorimetry measures the oxygen consumption and carbon dioxide production per minute, thus calculating energy expenditure and nonprotein respiratory quotient. This latter is a good marker for protein-energy malnutrition. In CLD, it is decreased due to the shift of energy metabolism from carbohydrate to lipid oxidation and has been correlated to survival. The technique is however difficult to implement in daily clinical practice, due to practicability and cost [4, 7, 21].
- Bioimpedance analysis is based on the measurement of tissue conductivity. The skeletal muscle is a major body component with low resistance and is therefore a dominant conductor. The bioimpedance analysis is a reliable bedside tool to evaluate the body cell mass, separating lean (water and bone) and fat (storage of energy) mass, although ascites and edema are confounding factors. The values obtained for the skeletal mass are not significantly different than with magnetic resonance imaging (MRI) or dual-energy X-ray absorptiometry, making it a convenient and cheapest alternative, if the device is available [22].
- Dual-energy X-ray absorptiometry (DEXA) is easy, reproducible, available in many pediatric centers, and causing minimal irradiation, although fluid retention can be confounding. It can measure the fat, lean tissue, and bone mass and therefore evaluate the sarcopenia and osteopenia [5, 7].

23.1.3.5 Assessment of Muscle Wasting or Sarcopenia

The diagnosis of muscle mass depletion requires analysis of the body composition using one of the available techniques, as well as normal values for age and gender [9]. CT scan has been the most used in adults: the measures of the psoas or the total abdominal muscle areas at the level of the third or fourth lumbar vertebra are accurate, objective, and reproducible and have been validated after normalization for stature (cm^2/m^2) [9, 23]. Less data are available with MRI in cirrhotic patients. The irradiation is significant with CT scan, but imaging performed for clinical reasons (exploration of a liver nodule, etc.) can readily be used. Ultrasonography is under study for this purpose, with measurement of the muscle mass in the thigh or on four sites. DEXA has the same accuracy as CT scan or MRI, although fluid retention may modify the results. Very few data are available in children, even less so in children with CLD.

The functional assessment may be more sensitive in the early stages, but no scales for age are available in children. Tests such as handgrip or 6-min walk have been correlated to clinical decompensation in adult cirrhotic patients [7, 9].

23.1.3.6 Scores

Global assessment tools have been developed in adults, to be used as screening and follow-up tools. They include the BMI, weight loss, food intake, gastrointestinal symptoms, some markers of severity (days in hospital, acute illness, etc.), mobility, neuropsychological problems, or scores such as APACHE (Acute Physiology and Chronic Health Evaluation) [3]. No such scores are available in children with CLD. The "Pediatric Hepatology Dependency Score" is a global score for the severity of CLD and includes one only nutritional item [24]. Pediatricians should rely on the growth curve and its changes, taking into account ascites or edema, the mid-arm circumference, the dietary assessment, and the clinical situation, chronic or acute decompensation with catabolism or inflammation.

23.1.4 Treatment

23.1.4.1 Oral

Oral nutritional treatment is the first step and should be implemented from the diagnosis, especially in young cholestatic children (Table 23.2). The choice of the milk formula depends on the degree of cholestasis, availability, and cost. Protein hydrolysates are enriched in medium-chain triglycerides (MCT), which are absorbed without needing micelles. They should be preferred in case of cholestasis but are poorly palatable and expensive. If the child is breast-fed, the breast-feeding may be continued, with increased number of feeds or addition of glucose polymers (maltodextrin) to drawn milk.

Table 23.2 Nutritional requirements for children with chronic liver disease [8]

	Daily requirements	Comments
Lipids	30–50% of energy, 30–50% of which medium-chain triglycerides	Depends on degree of malabsorption
Proteins	2–4 g/kg	Depends on age and clinical situation. Treatment of hyperammonemia without decreasing protein intake
Carbohydrates	50–70% of nonprotein energy	Glucose polymers, starch
Energy	Normal for age or 120–150% of recommended for weight	Depends on severity of growth, failure, and ascites (weight)
Sodium	1 mM/kg	Water-sodium retention in cirrhosis. Regular control of natremia on diuretics
Potassium	2–3 mM/kg	Regular control on diuretics

If the child receives a formula, it can be concentrated, and glucose polymers or MCT oil added, up to 1–1.5 kcal per mL. The enrichment should be careful and progressive, to avoid the lactose-induced or hyperosmotic diarrhea. In older children, food is selected from its caloric content (potatoes better than green beans, etc.) and enriched with glucose polymers or MCT oil or alternatively starch, sugar, oil, butter, etc. The limitation may be the diarrhea induced by nonabsorbed long-chain triglycerides, but it is usually moderate. Caloric supplements may be used and should be given at the end or between meals. The caloric amount should be 130–150% of recommended for weight or 100% of recommended for age, depending on the severity of growth failure. The content of proteins should be 2–3 g/kg. Lipids should be 30–50% of the nonprotein calories, 30–50% of them MCT. Depending on the formula used, extra essential fatty acids may have to be given (vegetable oil, egg yolk).

A low protein diet is not recommended in children with CLD, except if the liver failure is severe, as the requirements for growth are high. If ammonia increases, lactulose or sodium benzoate should be prescribed, without decreasing the protein intake [8].

Sodium restriction of 1 mM/kg/day is appropriate. Fluid restriction is usually not necessary, and fluid overload should be controlled with diuretics.

The timing of food intake can influence energy metabolism. Because cirrhotic patients enter a starvation state after a short fasting period, a large number of small meals ("nibbling" pattern) is preferable to a small number of large meals ("gorging" pattern) to maintain optimal energy metabolism [25].

23.1.4.2 Enteral

Enteral nutrition is indicated when the oral caloric intake is insufficient to maintain growth [26]. A silicone or polyurethane nasogastric tube is usually well tolerated, even with esophageal varices. Gastrostomy is contraindicated if portal hypertension is significant, due to the risk of peristomial varices. The formula used should be enriched in MCT that means in young children a protein hydrolysate, concentrated as needed, and a commercial MCT-containing formula in older children. If possible, half of the total amount is given with enteral nutrition and half orally. Preserving a normal daytime pattern of feeding is important to avoid the development of oral aversion. The enteral feeding is preferentially administered at night, in order to preserve the feeding behavior and motor activity [8]. It has also been shown in adult cirrhotic patients that late nocturnal energy supplementation shifted the energy metabolism from preferred lipid oxidation back to preferred carbohydrate metabolism. It may also better support protein accretion than daytime supplementation [27].

23.1.4.3 Parenteral

The indications for parenteral nutrition are rare, limited to the failure or intolerance to enteral nutrition, and usually as a bridge to liver transplantation. A large amount of calories can be brought in a limited volume of fluid, decreasing the risk of ascites. Even with severe cholestasis or liver insufficiency, amino acids and fat can be brought without restrictions [28].

23.1.4.4 Other Supplementations

- Fat-soluble vitamins A, D, E, and K should be supplied as needed with blood controls (Table 23.1). When cholestasis is absent or mild (bilirubin less than 100–120 μM), they can be administered in large oral doses. When the cholestasis worsens, micellar oral solutions are available only for vitamin K and E [29]. Vitamins A and D have to be administered by (painful) intramuscular injections, monthly, bi-, or tri-monthly depending on the available formulations.
- Zinc, magnesium, and iron may have to be supplemented, following controls.
- Water-soluble vitamins should be given at twice the recommended dose [8], due to altered hepatic metabolism.
- The supplementation in BCAA has been advocated, as a nutritional but also pharmacological therapy. They have a positive effect on albumin synthesis, insulin resistance, and development of encephalopathy. A large adult trial has demonstrated an improved prognosis and quality of life, and a small pediatric study an improvement in mid-arm circumference and skinfold thickness, with oral supplementation [30, 31]. But meta-analysis has shown a positive effect on encephalopathy only [4].

23.1.4.5 Exercise

Children with CLD and protein-energy malnutrition have decreased physical activity, which leads to muscle weakness and sarcopenia. In adults, the maximal oxygen consumption is reduced and correlated to the severity of the liver disease [32]. The preservation of physical activity, both resistance and endurance, in children with CLD, is crucial to prevent sarcopenia and also to improve the quality of life, with the maintenance of exercise capacity and interactions with peers [7, 9].

However a moderate exercise can increase the portal pressure, with a theoretical increased risk of variceal bleeding. An insufficient caloric intake can promote protein catabolism and thereby sarcopenia. There is however no risk of wounds of the enlarged fibrotic liver and spleen in normal conditions of exercise. The benefits of exercise performed with caloric supplementation and adapted to the clinical situation far outweigh the theoretical risks [7, 9]. Care should be taken about iatrogenic limitations of motor activity and excessive protection from the caregivers.

23.1.5 Implications for Liver Transplantation

It has been demonstrated that the prognosis of liver transplantation depends on the patient's nutritional status. It has also become clear that sarcopenia is the most important risk factor. The careful maintenance or correction of the nutritional status and muscle mass is therefore key to the success of transplantation.

Children with disorders of protein metabolism, especially organic acidurias, are severely sarcopenic and should be considered high-risk patients when they are listed for liver transplantation.

23.2 Intestinal Failure-Associated Liver Disease

23.2.1 Epidemiology

Intestinal failure-associated liver disease (IFALD) is the most prevalent complication in children with intestinal failure (IF) receiving long-term parenteral nutrition (PN) [33–35]. Liver disease is the consequence of different types of aggression, toxic effects of the PN solution, physiological and anatomical abnormalities associated with the underlying cause of IF, and infections from the central line. In children, the majority of diseases responsible for IF begin at birth, when the liver is extremely sensitive to aggression, even more when the child is premature. Many functions are immature, such as detoxification and bile formation. This explains the prevalence and frequent severity and rapid evolution of liver disease in this age group.

IFALD is defined as "hepatobiliary dysfunction as a consequence of medical and surgical management strategies for intestinal failure, which can variably progress to end-stage liver disease, or can be stabilized or reversed with promotion of intestinal adaptation" [36]. The diagnosis depends on the criteria, whether clinical, biological, or histological. It is usually made on clinical grounds in children with IF, long-term PN dependency, and cholestasis. With the new fish oil-containing lipid emulsions, it has also become clear that IFALD can develop without cholestasis. IFALD may present at early reversible stages or become evident as an end-stage liver disease. Many of the factors contributing to its development are preventable, and this should be a daily concern in the care of children on long-term PN. The shared care with an experienced IF center is key to prevention and treatment of IFALD and also timely referral for transplantation in the small proportion of children with irreversible and severe liver disease.

The prevalence of IFALD depends on the criteria used. In series from large experienced centers, about 20–25% of children on long-term PN develop IFALD, with end-stage liver failure leading to death or transplantation in 2–4% [37, 38]. However, even severe fibrosis or cirrhosis can remain clinically silent on the long term, if risk factors can be controlled [39].

23.2.2 Etiology and Pathophysiology
(Table 23.3)

23.2.2.1 Patient-Dependent Risk Factors

Prematurity

The mechanisms of bile secretion are immature in the newborn's liver. The bile salt pool is reduced, and important detoxification pathways such as sulfation are insufficient. The premature liver is also more sensitive to lipid peroxidation. The PN is administered in continuous rather than cyclical infusion to avoid hypoglycemia and provides high

Table 23.3 Risk factors for intestinal failure-associated liver disease (IFALD)

– Age: premature, newborn child
– Disruption of the enterohepatic circulation: bowel resection, stoma, intestinal stasis
– Lack of oral or enteral feeding
– Early infections (all sites)
– Mode of administration of parenteral nutrition: continuous versus cyclical
– Type of fat emulsion: fish oil-based emulsions seem protective
– Excessive dose of lipids
– Excessive dose of amino acids
– Excessive dose of glucose: promotes steatosis
– Changes in microbiota

amounts of fat and glucose to meet the energy needs, thus promoting steatosis. Frequent complications such as necrotizing enterocolitis and its gastrointestinal consequences (short bowel, disruption of the enterohepatic cycle, stasis), surgery, infections, lack of enteral nutrition further contribute to cholestasis [40].

Anatomy

The disruption of the enterohepatic circulation, due to bowel resection, presence of a stoma, or intestinal obstruction and stasis, is a major contributor to cholestasis. Bile acids, the major organic component of bile, are physiologically secreted from hepatocytes into bile, are reabsorbed in the ileum, and return to the liver through the portal flow and the liver sinusoids, where they are very efficiently taken up into hepatocytes. A small amount spills over to the systemic circulation, where other tissues get exposed (adipose tissues, muscle, kidney, etc.). Bile acids and gut microbiota interact at many levels during this journey. In addition to their detergent function for lipid absorption, bile acids have important signaling properties in the gut and liver, mediated by the nuclear farnesoid X receptor (FXR) and the membrane-bound TGR5. They are particularly involved in lipid and glucose metabolism, liver inflammation and fibrosis, and intestinal integrity and permeability. Enterokines such as FGF19 in the ileum and GLP-1 in the small intestine and colon are induced through FXR [41]. The consequences of interruption of the enterohepatic circulation and gut-liver enterokine axis are likely important and depend on the postsurgical anatomy.

Lack of Oral or Enteral Feeding

The absence of food in the mouth prevents the release of epidermal growth factor from salivary glands and the normal secretion by the gastrointestinal tract of trophic factors, which should stimulate villus hyperplasia. Normal intestinal motility should also be promoted by the ingestion of food and the alternation of fasting and feeding [42].

Infections

All infections, whether catheter-related or gastrointestinal, may induce cholestasis. Several studies emphasized the role of early infections on the development of fibrosis in children on PN [43]. Bacteria should be neutralized by acid in the stomach, but H$_2$ blockers or proton pump inhibitors allow them to successfully enter the small bowel. They should then be eliminated by the normal anterograde peristalsis and mucosal immune factors, which are both often deficient, promoting small bowel bacterial overgrowth, which in turn cause endotoxemia and portal inflammation. The presence of large dilated dysmotile loops increases the risk [42]. The prescription of large-spectrum antibiotics should be restricted, to limit the emergence of multiresistant bacteria.

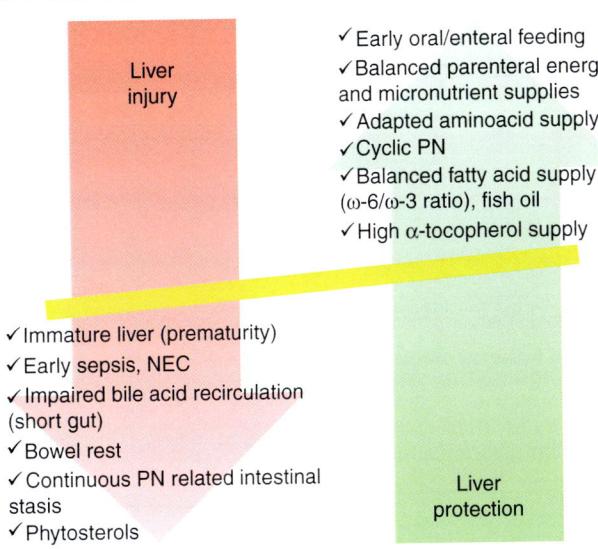

Fig. 23.1 Factors affecting intestinal failure-associated liver disease. *PN* parenteral nutrition, *NEC* necrotizing enterocololitis

Microbiota

The microbiota is strongly impacted by the medical situation and treatments, such as H$_2$ blockers, antibiotics, and surgery. The real effect however of its changes, spontaneous or with probiotics, is still unclear [34, 42]. Figure 23.1 shows the factors that have been implicated in causing or protecting against IFALD.

23.2.2.2 PN-Dependent Risk Factors

Lipids

Intravenous lipid emulsions based on soybean, safflower, or olive oil are implicated in IFALD, due to their content in pro-inflammatory omega-6 polyunsaturated fatty acids and plant sterols. The composition of fish oil-based lipid emulsions has several potential advantages, including omega-3 polyunsaturated fatty acids, a high amount of alpha-tocopherol, their content in the anti-inflammatory eicosapentaenoic acid, and the absence of phytosterols [44] (Table 23.4). They have been showed to reverse cholestasis in premature or postsurgical infants and children on long-term parenteral nutrition. Pure fish oil-based lipid emulsions (Omegaven®) do not contain the recommended amount of essential fatty acids and may not provide enough calories for growth. In Europe, the preferred lipid emulsions are nowadays a mixture of fish, olive, coconut, and soybean oil (SMOFlipid®) [45]. Fibrosis may however develop or worsen, despite a normal bilirubin level, as was seen in small series of children on long-term PN, some of them ultimately needing transplantation [46, 47].

The dose of lipids is clearly an important factor, at least with non-fish oil-based emulsions. Severe cholestasis has been linked to high doses (more than 2 g/kg/day) and

Table 23.4 Composition of fat emulsions for parenteral nutrition

	Intralipid®	Medialipid®	ClinOleic®	SMOFlipid®	Omegaven®
Soybean oil %	100	50	20	30	0
MCT %	0	50	0	30	0
Olive oil %	0	0	80	25	0
Fish oil %	0	0	0	15	100
Phytosterols mg/L	350	200	330	48	0
α-tocopherol mg/L	38	<30	200	200	150–300
ω-3 fatty acids	+	±	+	++	+++
ω-6 fatty acids	+++	++	+	++	+

MCT medium-chain triglycerides

reversed with temporary suspension of fat administration [48]. However, increasing glucose intake to maintain an adequate energy supply induces steatosis. PN should provide 15–30% of nonprotein calories as fat, with a minimum of 0.5 g/kg/day of a lipid emulsion containing essential fatty acids.

Proteins
An excess in amino acid supply has been associated with cholestasis, especially in infants. Only solutions adapted to children should be used and the dose adapted to age.

Carbohydrates and Energy
Carbohydrates (usually 8–18 g/kg/day of glucose, according to age and disease state) are, together with fat, the source of energy. Carbohydrates and fat delivered in excess promote steatosis, through hyperinsulinemia, and the delivery of lipids to the liver in liposomes instead of chylomicrons. A balanced PN formulation provides 75% of nonprotein calories as carbohydrate and 25% as fat.

Mode of Infusion of PN
Cyclic infusion of PN over less than 24 h results in more lipid oxidation, less hyperinsulinemia, and less fat deposition in the liver, than continuous PN. Liver enzymes and bilirubin are also less elevated [49]. Figure 23.2 provides a suggested prescription of PN in children older than 6 months.

23.2.3 Diagnosis and Evaluation of Severity of IFALD

The limitations of "usual" liver tests for the prediction of severity in any liver disease is well known. Historically, the degree of IFALD was evaluated on the level of bilirubin. This has been challenged: some studies showed complete reversion of severe cholestasis with changes in fat intake; and progression of IFALD without overt cholestasis has been observed with fish oil-based lipid emulsions. Noninvasive markers of fibrosis, such as Fibroscan®, have not been validated in IFALD but can be used to follow an individual patient

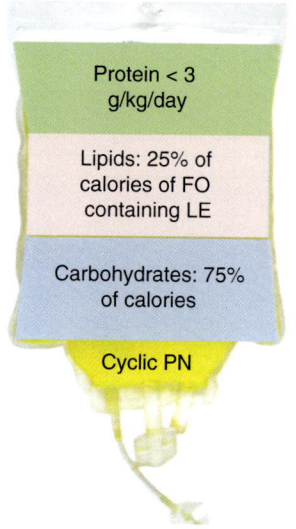

Fig. 23.2 Recommended nutrients doses for long-term parenteral nutrition preparation in children above 6 months of age. *FO* fish oil, *LE* lipid emulsion, *PN* parenteral nutrition

[50]. The presence of splenomegaly, also reflected in the level of platelets (outside of an episode of sepsis or macrophage activation), can be due to portal hypertension. In children after abdominal surgery, esophageal varices usually are not found, as collaterals develop along intraperitoneal scars.

The evaluation of IFALD is a combination of clinical findings (size and consistency of the liver, splenomegaly, collaterals), blood tests such as bilirubin, coagulation (although factors can be decreased due to consumption in an enlarged spleen), albumin (which can also decrease with protein-losing enteropathy, malnutrition, or inflammation), ultrasonography, upper gastrointestinal endoscopy, and ultimately liver biopsy.

23.2.4 Prevention and Treatment

All risk factors need to be addressed together and early on, from the diagnosis of intestinal failure, in the surgical or intensive care unit.

23.2.4.1 Medical Treatment

The prevention of infections includes continuous training of the hospital staff, nutritional care teams, early discharge on home PN with regular outpatient controls, and ethanol or taurolidine locks.

Oral or enteral nutrition should be introduced as soon as possible, to promote mucosal hyperplasia and hypertrophy, gastrointestinal hormone secretion, gut motility, and enterohepatic circulation. Oral nutrition is always preferred, because of the maintenance of the normal suckling and oral activity, the physiological stimulation of hormonal secretion and gut motility, and the self-limitation of overfeeding in case of dysmotility, reducing the risk of bacterial overgrowth [42, 51].

The close adaptation of the PN supply follows growth and significant events, such as surgery or the development of cholestasis. If bilirubin increases, manipulations in the type and delivery of lipid emulsions, including a transient suspension, may be enough to reverse cholestasis.

Trophic factors such as growth hormone, insulin, short-chain fatty acids and recently GLP-2 have been used in short bowel syndrome, to promote villous growth and thus decrease the need for PN and its side effects. Studies with GLP-2 have shown promising effects in adults and begin in children [52, 53].

23.2.4.2 Non-transplant Surgery

A primary anastomosis after resection, the early closure of a stoma when the anastomosis was not feasible, and restoring bowel continuity with unused segments of small or large bowel are important to improve the absorptive capacities and enterohepatic circulation. In children with short bowel syndrome, dilatation of one or several bowel loops is frequent, promoting dysmotility, bacterial overgrowth, and sepsis. A lengthening procedure, such as serial transverse enteroplasty (STEP) or longitudinal intestinal lengthening and tailoring (LILT), should be discussed in a multidisciplinary setting, taking into account the child's age, the remaining small bowel length, its potential of growth and adaptation, the enteral feed tolerance, and the degree of IFALD [54]. Both procedures should be very cautiously performed in children with advanced IFALD, due to portal hypertension, and risk of bleeding and surgical failure.

23.2.4.3 Intestinal Transplantation

Liver and small bowel transplantation is the ultimate treatment of severe IFALD (Table 23.5). It must be emphasized though that in 2017 the mortality is far higher after intestinal transplantation than on long-term PN and that the long-term survival after transplantation is unsatisfactory. The Intestinal Transplant Registry reported in 2015 on 1730 children, less than 1000 alive at last report, 1060 with a liver-containing graft, with a 1- and 5-year patient survival rates of, respectively, 80% and 70%, and a 10-year graft survival of 55% [55]. The 10-year survival in large pediatric IF units is close to 100% in children with primary digestive diseases on long-term PN [37, 56, 57].

The technique of transplantation depends on the degree of IFALD and the child's disease. Isolated small bowel transplantation can be performed only if IFALD is mild or moderate. In other cases, the liver-containing graft can be a combined liver and small bowel or a multivisceral graft including the stomach and duodenum, if the child has an extensive motility disorder or a severe portal hypertension. The right colon is usually included if the indication is a congenital enteropathy or a motility disorder [58, 59].

Isolated liver transplantation can be discussed as a lifesaving procedure in a patient with end-stage IFALD and reasonable expectations for intestinal autonomy after the resolution of portal hypertension. It is a difficult procedure, which should be discussed and performed only in units experienced both in transplantation and IF [60].

Table 23.5 Indications for intestinal transplantation in children [57, 58]

– Severe irreversible intestinal failure-associated liver disease: see text for prevention and treatment
– Loss of venous access: loss of 3 or more central venous catheter sites
– Repeated life-threatening infections: if all preventive measures (caregiver training, hygiene, ethanol or taurolidine locks) are ineffective
– Severe hydro-electrolytic disorders: for example, microvillous inclusion disease with very high stool volume
– Growth failure: despite adapted parenteral nutrition
– Impossibility to carry on home parenteral nutrition
– Psychological intolerance to long-term parenteral nutrition: debatable and difficult indication

References

1. Merli M, Riggio O, Dally L. Does malnutrition affect survival in cirrhosis ? PINC (Policentrica Italiana Nutrizione Cirrosi). Hepatology. 1996;23:1341–6.
2. Chin SE, Shepherd RW, Thomas BJ, Cleghorn GJ, Patrick MK, Wilcox JA, et al. The nature of malnutrition in children with end-stage liver disease awaiting orthotopic liver transplantation. Am J Clin Nutr. 1992;56:164–8.
3. Tandon P, Raman M, Mourtzakis M, Merli M. A practical approach to nutritional screening and assessment in cirrhosis. Hepatology. 2017;65:1044–57.
4. Plauth M, Merli M, Kondrup J, Weimann A, Ferenci P, Müller MJ. ESPEN guidelines for nutrition in liver disease and transplantation. Clin Nutr. 1997;16:43–55.
5. Ramaccioni V, Soriano HE, Arumugam R, Klish WJ. Nutritional aspects of chronic liver disease and liver transplantation in children. J Pediatr Gastroenterol Nutr. 2000;30:361–7.
6. O'Brien A, Williams R. Nutrition in end-stage liver disease: principles and practice. Gastroenterology. 2008;134:1729–40.

7. Toshikuni N, Arisawa T, Tsutsumi M. Nutrition and exercise in the management of liver cirrhosis. World J Gastroenterol. 2014;20:7286–97.
8. Baker A, Stevenson R, Dhawan A, Goncalves I, Socha P, Sokal E. Guidelines for nutritional care for infants with cholestatic liver disease before liver transplantation. Pediatr Transplant. 2007;11:825–34.
9. Dasarathy S, Merli M. Sarcopenia from mechanism to diagnosis and treatment in liver disease. J Hepatol. 2016;65:1232–44.
10. Englesbe MJ, Patel SP, He K, Lynch RJ, Schaubel DE, Harbaugh C, et al. Sarcopenia and mortality after liver transplantation. J Am Coll Surg. 2010;211:271–8.
11. Kim HY, Jang JW. Sarcopenia in the prognosis of cirrhosis: going beyond the MELD score. World J Gastroenterol. 2015;21:7637–47.
12. Giannelli V, Di Gregorio V, Iebba V, Giusto M, Schippa S, Merli M, Thalheimer U. Microbiota and the gut-liver axis: bacterial translocation, inflammation and infection in cirrhosis. World J Gastroenterol. 2014;20:16795–810.
13. Müller MJ, Lautz HU, Plogmann B, Bürger M, Körber J, Schmidt FW. Energy expenditure and substrate oxidation in patients with cirrhosis: the impact of cause, clinical staging and nutritional state. Hepatology. 1992;15:782–94.
14. Greer R, Lehnert M, Lewindon P, Cleghorn GJ, Shepherd RW. Body composition and components of energy expenditure in children with end-stage liver disease. J Pediatr Gastroenterol Nutr. 2003;36:358–63.
15. Holt RI, Baker AJ, Jones JS, Miell JP. The insulin-like growth factor and binding protein axis in children with end-stage liver disease before and after liver transplantation. Pediatr Transplant. 1998;2:76–84.
16. Changani KK, Jalan R, Cox IJ, Ala-Korpela M, Bhakoo K, Taylor-Robinson SD, et al. Evidence for altered hepatic gluconeogenesis in patients with cirrhosis using in vivo 32-phosphorus magnetic resonance spectroscopy. Gut. 2001;49:557–64.
17. Socha P, Koletzko B, Pawlowska J, Socha J. Essential fatty acid status in children with cholestasis, in relation to serum bilirubin concentration. J Pediatr. 1997;131:700–6.
18. Tessari P. Protein metabolism in liver cirrhosis: from albumin to muscle myofibrils. Curr Opin Clin Nutr Metab Care. 2003;6:79–85.
19. Kawaguchi T, Izumi N, Charlton MR, Sata M. Branched-chain amino acids as pharmacological nutrients in chronic liver disease. Hepatology. 2011;54:1063–70.
20. World Health Organization, UNICEF. WHO child growth standards and the identification of severe acute malnutrition in infants and children. Geneva: World Health Organization; 2009.
21. Tajika M, Kato M, Mohri H, Miwa Y, Kato T, Ohnishi H, et al. Prognostic value of energy metabolism in patients with viral liver cirrhosis. Nutrition. 2002;18:229–34.
22. Pirlich M, Schütz T, Spachos T, Ertl S, Weiss ML, Lochs H, et al. Bioelectric impedance analysis is a useful bedside technique to asssess malnutrition in cirrhotic patients with and without ascites. Hepatology. 2000;32:1208–15.
23. Durand F, Buyse S, Francoz C, Laouénan C, Bruno O, Belghiti J, et al. Prognostic value of muscle atrophy in cirrhosis using psoas muscle thickness on computed tomography. J Hepatol. 2014;60:1151–7.
24. Cowley AD, Cummins C, Beath SV, Lloyd C, van Mourik ID, McKiernan PJ, Kelly DA. Paediatric hepatology dependency score (PHD score): an audit tool. J Pediatr Gastroenterol Nutr. 2007;44:108–15.
25. Verboeket-van de Venne WP, Westerterp KR, van Hoek B, Swart GR. Energy expenditure and substrate metabolism in patients with cirrhosis of the liver: effects of the pattern of food intake. Gut. 1995;36:110–6.
26. Plauth M, Cabré E, Riggio O, Assis-Camilo M, Pirlich M, Kondrup J, et al. ESPEN guidelines on enteral nutrition: liver disease. Clin Nutr. 2006;25:285–94.
27. Planck LD, Gane EJ, Peng S, Muthu C, Mathur S, Gillanders L, et al. Nocturnal nutritional supplementation improves total body protein status of patients with liver cirrhosis: a randomized 12-month trial. Hepatology. 2008;48:557–66.
28. Grimber D, Michaud L, Ategbo S, Turck D, Gottrand F. Experience of parenteral nutrition for nutritional rescue in children with severe liver disease following failure of enteral nutrition. Pediatr Transplant. 1999;3:139–45.
29. Thébault A, Nemeth A, Le Mouhaër J, Scheenstra R, Baumann U, Koot B, et al. Oral tocofersolan corrects or prevents vitamin E deficiency in children with chronic cholestasis. J Pediatr Gastroenterol Nutr. 2016;63:610–5.
30. Marchesini G, Bianchi G, Merli M, Amodio P, Panella C, Loguercio C, et al. Nutritional supplementation with branched-chain amino acids in cirrhosis: a randomized double blind trial. Gastroenterology. 2003;124:1792–801.
31. Chin SE, Shepherd RW, Thomas BJ, Cleghorn GJ, Patrick MK, Wilcox JA, et al. Nutritional support in children with end-stage liver disease: a randomized crossover trial of a branched-chain amino acid supplement. Am J Clin Nutr. 1992;56:158–63.
32. Lemize D, Dharancy S, Wallaert B. Response to exercise in patients with liver cirrhosis: implications for liver transplantation. Dig Liver Dis. 2013;45:362–6.
33. Lacaille F, Gupte G, Colomb V, D'Antiga L, Hartman C, Hojsak I, et al. Intestinal failure—associated liver disease. A position paper by the ESPGHAN Working Group of Intestinal failure and intestinal transplantation. J Pediatr Gastroenterol Nutr. 2015;60:272–83.
34. D'Antiga L, Goulet O. Intestinal failure in children. The European view. J Pediatr Gastroenterol Nutr. 2012;56:118–26.
35. Koletzko B, Goulet O, Hunt J, Krohn K, Shamir R, Parenteral Nutrition Guidelines Working Group; European Society for Clinical Nutrition and Metabolism; European Society of Paediatric Gastroenterology, Hepatology and Nutrition (ESPGHAN); European Society of Paediatric Research (ESPR). Guidelines on Paediatric Parenteral Nutrition of the European Society of Paediatric Gastroenterology, Hepatology and Nutrition (ESPGHAN) and the European Society for Clinical Nutrition and Metabolism (ESPEN), Supported by the European Society of Paediatric Research (ESPR). J Pediatr Gastroenterol Nutr. 2005;41:S1–87.
36. Kocoshis SA. Medical management of intestinal failure. Semin Pediatr Surg. 2010;19:20–6.
37. Colomb V, Dabbas-Tyan M, Taupin P, Talbotec C, Révillon Y, Jan D, et al. Long term outcome of children receiving home parenteral nutrition: a 20 year single center experience in 302 patients. J Pediatr Gastroenterol Nutr. 2007;44:347–53.
38. Pichler J, Horn V, Macdonald S, Hill S. Intestinal failure-associated liver disease in hospitalised children. Arch Dis Child. 2012;97:211–4.
39. Ganousse-Mazeron S, Lacaille F, Colomb-Jung V, Talbotec C, Ruemmele F, Sauvat F, Chardot C, Canioni D, Jan D, Revillon Y, Goulet O. Assessment and outcome of children with intestinal failure referred for intestinal transplantation. Clin Nutr. 2015;34:428–35.
40. Black DD, Suttle A, Whitington PF, Whitington GL, Korones SD. The effect of short-term parenteral nutrition on hepatic function in human neonate: a prospective randomized study demonstrating alteration of hepatic canalicular function. J Pediatr. 1981;99:445–9.
41. Trauner M, Fuchs CD, Halibasic E, Paumgartner G. New therapeutic concepts in bile acid transport and signaling for management of cholestasis. Hepatology. 2017;65:1393–404.
42. Goulet O, Olieman J, Ksiazyk J, Spolidoro J, Tibboe D, Köhler H, et al. Neonatal short bowel syndrome as a model of intestinal failure: physiological background for enteral feeding. Clin Nutr. 2013;32:162–71.
43. Hermans D, Talbotec C, Lacaille F, Goulet O, Ricour C, Colomb V. Early central catheter infections may contribute to hepatic fibro-

sis in children receiving long-term parenteral nutrition. J Pediatr Gastroenterol Nutr. 2007;44:459–63.
44. Goulet O, Lambe C. Intravenous lipid emulsions in pediatric patients with intestinal failure. Curr Opin Organ Transplant. 2017;22:142–8.
45. Seida JC, Mager DR, Hartling L, Vandermeer B, Turner JM. Parenteral ω-3 fatty acid lipid emulsions for children with intestinal failure and other conditions: a systematic review. J Parenter Enter Nutr. 2013;37:44–55.
46. Mercer DF, Hobson BD, Fischer RT, Talmon GA, Perry DA, Gerhardt BK, et al. Hepatic fibrosis persists and progresses despite biochemical improvement in children treated with intravenous fish oil emulsion. J Pediatr Gastroenterol Nutr. 2013;56:354–9.
47. Belza C, Thompson R, Somers GR, de Silva N, Fitzgerald K, Steinberg K, et al. Persistence of hepatic fibrosis in pediatric intestinal failure patients treated with intravenous fish oil lipid emulsion. J Pediatr Surg. 2017;52:795–801.
48. Colomb V, Jobert-Giraud A, Lacaille F, Goulet O, Fournet JC, Ricour C. Role of lipid emulsions in cholestasis associated with long-term parenteral nutrition in children. J Parenter Enter Nutr. 2000;24:345–50.
49. Stout SM, Cober MP. Metabolic effects of cyclic parenteral nutrition infusion in adults and children. Nutr Clin Pract. 2010;25:277–81.
50. Van Gossum A, Pironi L, Messing B, Moreno C, Colecchia A, D'Errico A, et al. Transient elastography (Fibroscan) is not correlated with fibrosis but to cholestasis in patients with long term home parenteral nutrition. J Parenter Enteral Nutr. 2015;39:719–24.
51. Braegger C, Decsi T, Dias JA, Hartman C, Kolacek S, Koletzko B, et al. Practical approach to paediatric enteral nutrition: a comment by the ESPGHAN committee on nutrition. J Pediatr Gastroenterol Nutr. 2010;51:110–22.
52. Jeppesen PB, Gilroy R, Pertkiewicz M, et al. Randomised placebo-controlled trial of teduglutide in reducing parenteral nutrition and/or intravenous fluid requirements in patients with short bowel syndrome. Gut. 2011;60:902–14.
53. Carter BA, Cohran VC, Cole CR, Corkins MR, Dimmitt RA, Duggan C, et al. Outcomes from a 12-week, open-label, multicenter clinical trial of teduglutide in pediatric short bowel syndrome. J Pediatr. 2017;181:102–11.
54. Frongia G, Kessler M, Weih S, Nickkholgh A, Mehrabi A, Holland-Cunz S. Comparison of LILT and STEP procedures in children with short bowel syndrome—a systematic review of the literature. J Pediatr Surg. 2013;48:1794–805.
55. Intestinal Transplant Registry. http://www.intransplant/org.
56. Abi Nader E, Lambe C, Talbotec C, Pigneur B, Lacaille F, Garnier-Lengliné H, et al. Outcome of home parenteral nutrition in 251 children over a 14-y period: report of a single center. Am J Clin Nutr. 2016;103:1327–36.
57. Burghardt KM, Wales PW, de Silva N, Stephens D, Yap J, Grant D, Avitzur Y. Pediatric intestinal transplant listing criteria. A call for a change in the new era of intestinal failure outcomes. Am J Transplant. 2015;15:1674–81.
58. Grant D, Abu-Elmagd K, Mazariegos G, Vianna R, Langnas A, Mangus R, et al. Intestinal transplant association. Intestinal transplant registry report: global activity and trends. Am J Transplant. 2015;15:210–9.
59. Lacaille F, Irtan S, Dupic L, Talbotec C, Lesage F, Colomb V, et al. Twenty-eight years of intestinal transplantation in Paris: experience of the oldest European center. Transpl Int. 2017;30:178–86.
60. Taha AMI, Sharif K, Johnson T, Clarke S, Murphy MS, Gupte GL. Long-term outcomes of isolated liver transplantation for short bowel syndrome and intestinal failure-associated liver disease. J Pediatr Gastroenterol Nutr. 2012;54:547–51.

Intensive Care Management of Children with Liver Disease

Isabella Pellicioli, Angelo Di Giorgio, and Lorenzo D'Antiga

Key Points

- Children with liver disease may require intensive care/general anesthesia in case of complications of portal hypertension, acute liver failure, and perioperative period after transplant.
- The intensivist should be able to maintain hemodynamic stability; control acid/base balance, electrolyte, and glucose; and monitor and correct coagulopathy.
- Pediatric acute liver failure is a complex and rapidly progressive condition requiring supportive care provided in a pediatric intensive care unit of a transplantation center.
- Acute liver failure is characterized by coagulopathy, encephalopathy, hypoglycemia, and severe jaundice and has a high mortality risk.
- Careful monitoring is required after pediatric liver transplantation, to detect promptly acute rejection and vascular and biliary complications.
- A tight liaison between the pediatric hepatologist and the pediatric intensivist offers the highest standards of care to children with liver disease and need for intensive care management.

Research Needed in the Field

- Investigate the features of coagulopathy in acute and chronic liver disease, as well as in the perioperative transplant period, and the possible treatments affecting the outcome.
- Define better the etiology of ALF patients currently classified as having indeterminate cause.
- Develop liver support systems able to stabilize the patients with acute liver failure, allowing longer time for spontaneous recovery or graft procurement.

24.1 Introduction

Many children suffering from liver disease experience at least one admission to pediatric intensive care unit (PICU) during their life. The most common causes are (1) an episode of acute liver failure presenting with severe coagulopathy and encephalopathy, (2) an acute decompensation in a patient with a known chronic liver disease, (3) complications of cirrhosis and portal hypertension, and (4) an admission following surgical operations such as hepatic resection or liver transplantation (LT) [1, 2].

Since hepatic dysfunction may affect many other organ functions, intensive care management should be holistic, including medical interventions and invasive procedures. Cardiovascular, respiratory, neurological, renal, infectious, metabolic, hematological, and nutritional dysfunctions may need to be addressed. Due to the complexity of these patients, a multidisciplinary approach is of paramount importance to offer these children the best opportunity to recover quickly and without sequelae. After an initial evaluation of the patient condition, the intensive care support should focus on patient monitoring, choosing an age-appropriate diagnostic approach, supporting organ functions, and treating complications [3].

I. Pellicioli (✉)
Paediatric Intensive Care Unit, Hospital Papa Giovanni XXIII, Bergamo, Italy
e-mail: ipellicioli@asst-pg23.it

A. Di Giorgio · L. D'Antiga
Paediatric Hepatology, Gastroenterology and Transplantation, Hospital Papa Giovanni XXIII, Bergamo, Italy
e-mail: adigiorgio@asst-pg23.it; ldantiga@asst-pg23.it

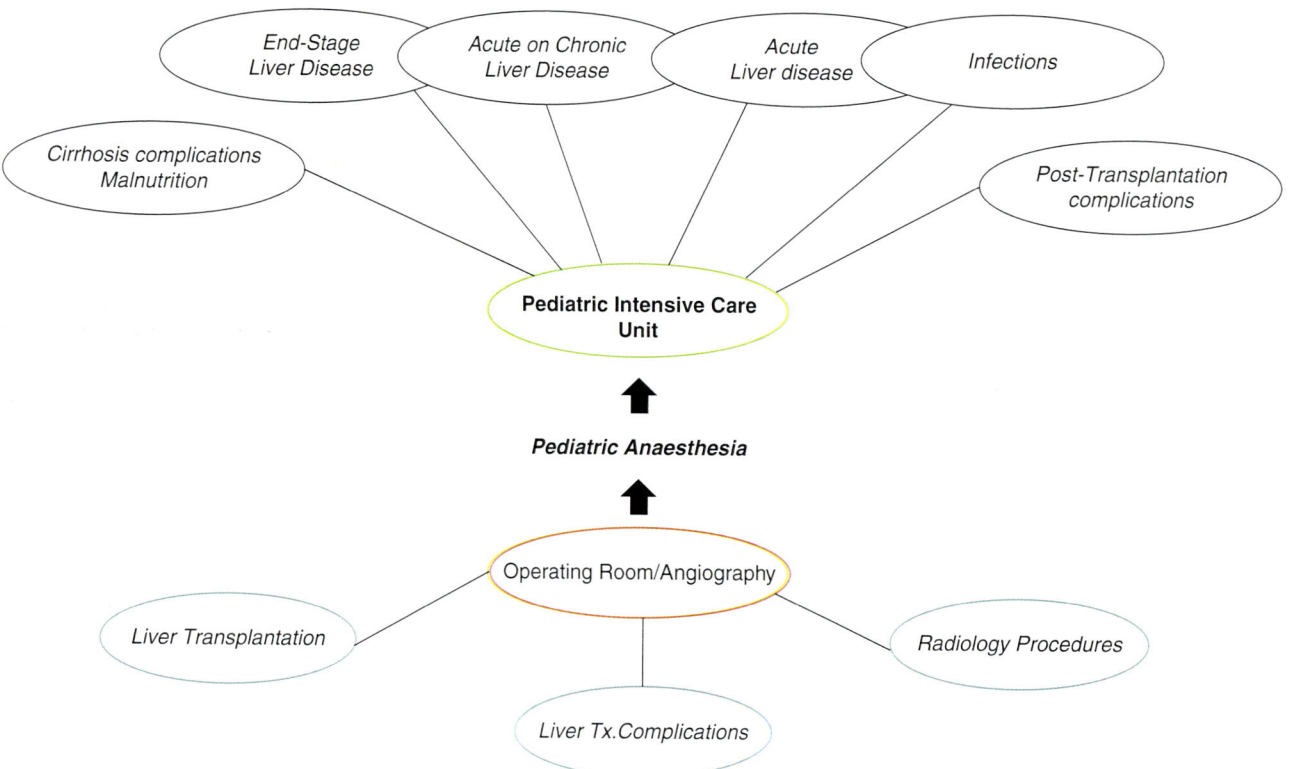

Fig. 24.1 Reasons for referral to PICU in the management of children with liver disease

Many different reasons indicate the referral to PICU in these patients, as shown in Fig. 24.1.

24.2 General Principles of Anesthesia for Children with Liver Disease

Radiological and endoscopic investigations, as well as liver biopsy and surgical procedures, need general anesthesia to temporarily obliterate consciousness and control pain. Anesthetic agents and techniques may have potential side effects on organ system function, so that sick children may be exposed to further organ injury [4]. Therefore, a careful clinical evaluation is of vital importance to estimate the risk/benefit ratio of the procedure and predict potential complications.

24.2.1 Cardiovascular System

High-output, low-resistance state is the typical cardiovascular condition in both acute and chronic liver disease. In these patients the volume loss is poorly tolerated due to inability to compensate the intravascular depletion through vasoconstriction, so that the organ perfusion is only supported by elevated heart rate. Thus, hypovolemia, dehydration, or diuretic therapy should be managed prudently [5]. Coexistent congenital cardiac defects, mainly those characterized by an outflow tract obstruction (such as severe pulmonary stenosis/hypoplasia in Alagille syndrome), make the management of these patients challenging and at higher risk of complications. Congenital heart defects with intracardiac defects may lose the balance in presence of changes of volume load or inotropic support, potentially switching a left-to-right shunt into a right-to-left one, with consequent hypoxemia [6]. During liver transplantation, at the time of graft reperfusion via the portal vein, important hemodynamic changes occur: myocardial depression, arterial hypotension due to a fall in systemic vascular resistance, and increase in pulmonary vascular resistance are frequently observed. If there is insufficient increase in cardiac output by inotrope support and judicious administration of intravenous fluid, the graft may remain poorly perfused, and its function may be compromised. For this reason it is important to verify if the patient has sufficient cardiac reserve to support the surgical stress and cardiovascular changes that might take place during the planned intervention. Preoperative cardiac assessment and therapy optimization are necessary; a stress test with inotropic agents may add more information, but it is complex and sometimes has high risks of complications [4]. Figure 24.2 summarizes the effects of anesthesia on different organ systems.

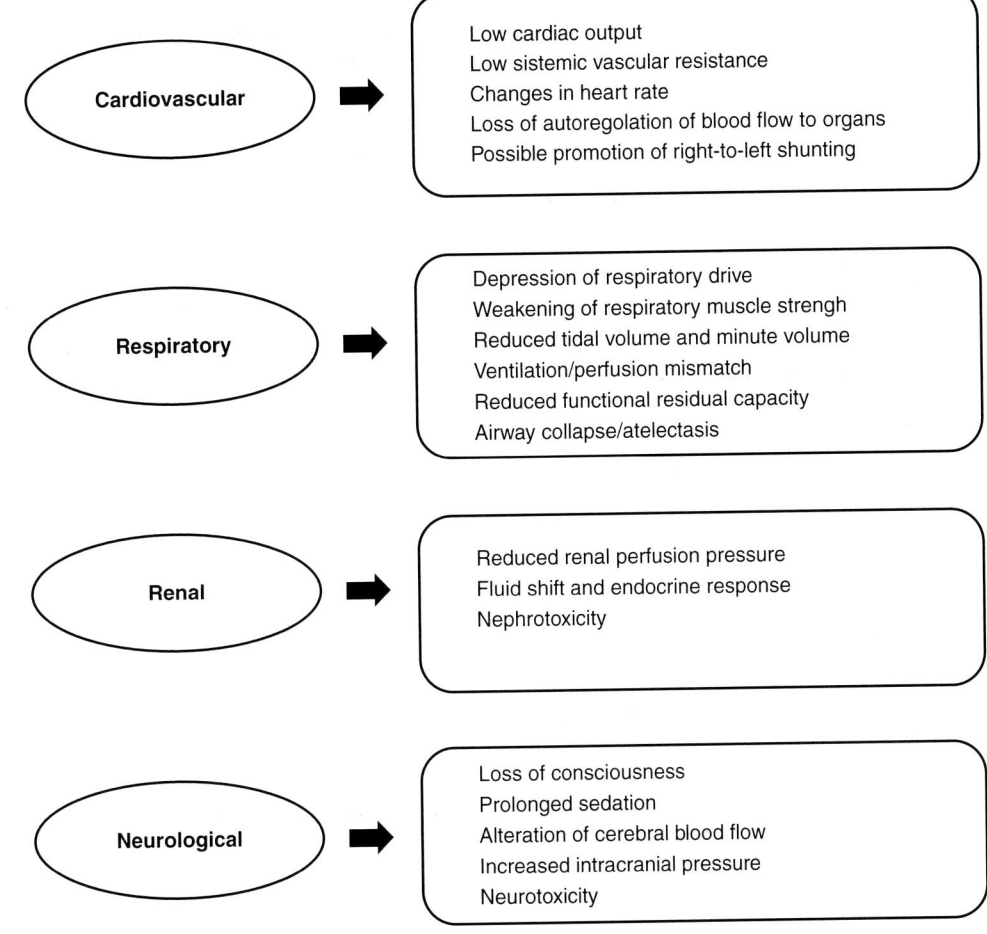

Fig. 24.2 Effects of anesthesia on different organ systems

24.2.2 Respiratory System

In patients with liver disease, respiratory problems may depend on diaphragmatic splinting caused by ascites and organomegaly. This condition can lead to decrease of functional residual capacity, exclusion of small airways, and increased work of breathing, so that patients quickly become hypoxemic during the perioperative period. Poor nutritional status affects growth and development of muscle tone and may worsen respiratory impairment [7]. Pleural effusion and hepatopulmonary syndrome may aggravate the situation. Hepatopulmonary syndrome causes hypoxemia due to redistribution of pulmonary blood flow with ventilation/perfusion mismatch and formation of new blood vessels causing a true right-to-left shunt. The degree of hypoxemia is not proportional to the severity of liver disease. Hypoxemia may progress over time and the only effective treatment is liver transplantation. Its resolution may take several months after surgery. Therefore, it is important to know not only the magnitude of true shunt but also the response of hypoxemia to inspired oxygen fraction and nitric oxide inhalation (iNO), to avoid intraoperative hypoxic injury to the graft and the patients' organ systems. Weaning from mechanical ventilation in this situation may not be straightforward, and sometimes prolonged intubation and iNO inhalation may be required [8].

24.2.3 Renal

Usually renal impairment in children with liver disease does not correspond to hepatorenal syndrome, a complication of cirrhosis seen commonly in adults with end-stage liver disease and caused by intense renal vasoconstriction. More frequently, children with liver disease have a genetic disorder involving also the kidney function (such as Alagille syndrome, Wilson disease, alpha-1 antitrypsin deficiency, fibrocystic liver disease, etc.) [9]. However an acute renal impairment may be caused by acute intravascular depletion and reduction in total body water. Achieving a hemodynamic balance is crucial, and the key anesthetic management consists of adequate preoperative hydration, optimal volume loading, good cardiac output, adequate perfusion pressure, good oxygen delivery, and maintenance of a normal acid/

base balance. When renal failure occurs and diuretic therapy is insufficient, renal replacement therapy is the only option. Continuous veno-venous hemofiltration (CVVH) or diafiltration (CVVHDF) with high fluid turnover may be used to optimize fluid balance and promote clearance of ammonia and other unmeasured toxins. Continuous hemofiltration rather than intermittent hemodialysis is better tolerated from the hemodynamic point of view [10, 11].

Correcting the abnormalities of serum electrolytes is of utmost importance in this setting. Serum potassium, which has the potential to cause dysrhythmias under anesthesia, is the most common alteration to be corrected. Both hyper- and hyponatremia are frequent, and their slow correction is mandatory to avoid central pontine myelinolysis [12]. Besides, fluctuation in serum sodium is detrimental for the central nervous system, especially in presence of raised intracranial pressure, due to the potential to cause rapid fluid shifts between compartments. Neuronal instability with paresthesias, muscle spasms, tetany, and seizures may be caused by hypocalcemia. Hypocalcemia may also contribute to heart failure, hypotension, insensitivity to inotropic agents, and a prolonged QT interval. Hypomagnesemia may determine membrane instability with prolonged PR and QT intervals and ventricular arrhythmias and is relatively common after liver transplantation, under immunosuppressive treatment. Hypophosphatemia may determine respiratory muscle weakness and respiratory failure, encephalopathy, seizures, and paresthesias [13, 14].

24.2.4 Coagulopathy

In liver patients coagulopathy is a typical problem, usually not causing spontaneous bleeding, especially in acute liver failure. However when invasive or surgical procedures are planned, the risk increases remarkably; therefore clotting should be supported perioperatively [4]. Noteworthy, infusion of large volumes of clotting factors might cause many problems, including thrombotic complications. During acute bleeding the administration of large amounts of plasma is associated with persistent, repeated bleedings because of fluid overload [15]. A prothrombin time twice the normal value is usually adequate to accomplish surgical hemostasis, if the number of platelets is $>50 \times 10^9/L$.

24.2.5 Encephalopathy

Encephalopathy is a serious complications of both acute and end-stage liver disease, and its severity is related to the combination of hyperammonemia, raised intracranial pressure, and neuronal inflammation. Although under anesthesia cerebral perfusion may fall due to the decrease of mean arterial pressure, severe encephalopathy leading to cerebral edema should be treated by deep neuroprotective sedation, following the rules of the management of raised intracranial pressure due to head traumas. Respiratory depression may increase PCO_2 causing intense vasoconstriction in the cerebral vessels thereby decreasing cerebral perfusion. Maintaining normocarbia, avoiding hyperventilation, is recommendable [16, 17].

With regard to anesthetic drugs, more or less all agents may interfere with liver function and consequently with central nervous system function. Inhaled agents such as isoflurane and sevoflurane are both acceptable; desflurane has the advantage of having only partial liver metabolism and consequently a lower toxicity [18, 19]. For muscle paralysis atracurium is safe, but cisatracurium offers the advantage of lower levels of metabolites and a lower risk of neurotoxicity from its accumulation [7].

24.2.6 Liver Transplantation (LT)

LT represents the only effective treatment of end-stage liver disease. Technically the procedure has three different phases. The "dissection phase" which is characterized by skeletonization of the native liver and preparation of the liver vessels. Here, the main problem is the high risk of bleeding. The "anhepatic phase" starts when the portal vein and hepatic artery are clamped and divided. During this phase the main problems include serious derangements of acid/base balance with an increase in lactate and decrease in ionized calcium and glucose. The last is the "reperfusion phase" which is characterized by hemodynamic instability from the effects of reperfusion of an ischemic organ (releasing inflammatory molecules), transient depression of myocardial systolic function, wide fluctuations in circulating volume due to blood losses from the cut surface, and vascular anastomoses together with filling of the new liver [20].

From the anesthesiology point of view, this surgical procedure requires some special considerations. A central venous catheter is essential, because it allows central venous pressure monitoring, the rapid infusion of fluids and blood products, and the infusion of inotropes and other drugs. Usually a non-tunneled catheter is put in place, since long-lasting Silastic® catheters are unsuitable for intraoperative use. Catheter insertion, in the internal jugular or subclavian veins, is associated with potential complications including bleeding, accidental carotid artery puncture, pneumothorax, hemothorax, and pericardial tamponade [21]. The use of real-time ultrasound guidance has dramatically decreased the incidence of these complications [22].

Core temperature should be monitored continuously, because of the risks of hypothermia that during liver transplant may cause cardiac arrhythmias, impaired coagulation, and poor platelet function. Increasing the ambient temperature, using warm intravenous fluids and blood products, and heating the patient with air blanket and warm mattresses are essential precautions.

A close hemodynamic observation is also necessary, with continuous electrocardiogram, oxygen saturation, central venous pressure, and invasive arterial pressure monitoring. In infants and small children, cardiac output monitoring is difficult and risky. The most commonly used methods include thermodilution through a pulmonary artery catheter (Swan-Ganz), lithium dilution cardiac output (LiDCO), and pulse contour analysis using pulse contour cardiac output (PiCCO) [23]. Monitoring and assessment of coagulation, which changes rapidly during the surgical procedure, is important, and currently several handy assays have become popular in the operatory room. The thromboelastograph (TEG®) has different patterns indicating a range of clotting abnormalities such as dilution coagulopathy, thrombocytopenia, disseminated intravascular coagulation (DIC), or hyperfibrinolysis. The addition in the blood sample of heparinase provides information about the influence of heparin-like substances released during graft reperfusion [24]. Thromboelastometry (ROTEM®) and the platelet function analyzer (PFA-100®) perform similar tests with additional information that may offer some advantages. These tests are considered useful for the monitoring of whole blood coagulation and have been shown to reduce blood components transfusion during liver transplantation [25].

24.3 Pediatric Acute Liver Failure (PALF)

The term pediatric acute liver failure refers to a rare but dramatic, complex, and rapidly progressive syndrome caused by acute hepatocellular injury or death. It is characterized by an acute abnormality of liver blood tests revealing hepatocyte necrosis, coagulopathy, and altered level of consciousness due to hepatic encephalopathy (HE) that occurs in a previously healthy patient [26]. Although acute HE remains a hallmark of PALF as well, usually it is difficult to detect it in infants and small children and may not be clinically evident until the final stages of the disease [27]. Furthermore, some specific and important pediatric disorders (such as inborn errors of metabolism) cause a syndrome similar to PALF where the encephalopathy is due to direct metabolic damage to the brain, rather than being secondary to liver failure (the so-called Reye-like syndrome). Finally, in seriously ill children, other clinical conditions like sepsis or metabolic failure might cause mental status alterations independently of hepatic dysfunction. Consequently a consensus of the members of the Pediatric Acute Liver Failure study group, a multicenter and multinational consortium, proposed the PALF criteria, shown in Table 24.1 [26].

Table 24.1 Pediatric acute liver failure study group entry criteria

• Child with no known evidence of chronic liver disease
• Biochemical and/or clinical evidence of severe liver dysfunction
• Hepatic-based coagulopathy with a prothrombin time (PT) ≥2.0 or international normalized ratio (INR) ≥2.0 that is not corrected by parenteral vitamin K
• And/or hepatic encephalopathy (must be present if the PT is 15–19.9 s or INR 1.5–1.9, but not if PT ≥20 s or INR ≥2.0)

Despite the PALF criteria had the merit to provide an attempt to classify and compare groups of patients presenting with an acute, severe liver disease, the patients fulfilling them are likely to be very heterogeneous. For instance, these criteria deliberately include patients with Rye-like syndrome (having usually hepatic encephalopathy despite an INR <2) and those having a chronic liver disease presenting as acute liver failure (such as autoimmune hepatitis or Wilson disease) [28]. Besides the PALF criteria are very wide, including patients with a mild and benign disease as well as those with a rapidly fulminant course.

PALF is the indication of about 10–15% of all pediatric liver transplants (LT), and the outcome in this group is known to be worse compared to more common, elective indications [29].

24.3.1 Etiology

The etiology of PALF is variable, depending on age and geographical areas (Fig. 24.3). The most common causes are infectious, immunologic, or metabolic disorders and toxins or drug-related events. In about 30–50% of cases, the cause remains unknown, and the PALF is defined indeterminate [1, 26, 30].

24.3.1.1 Infectious Disease

Viral hepatitis is the most frequent cause of PALF in children of all ages [31].

Herpes simplex virus (HSV) represents the most common virus causing liver failure in newborns, with an incidence of 27% in infants <28 days of age [32]. Among hepatotropic viruses that cause PALF, hepatitis B virus (HBV) is the commonest one worldwide with a worse prognosis compared to other etiologies, since spontaneous recovery occurs in fewer than 20% of cases. Hepatitis A virus (HAV) is prevalent in developing countries, while hepatitis E virus (HEV) has rarely been associated with PALF although hepatitis E infection is common in developing countries. Other viruses such as varicella zoster, cytomegalovirus, and Epstein-Barr virus have been reported to cause PALF, especially in immunocompromised patients, with EBV most frequently implicated.

Infectious agents other than viruses rarely lead to PALF [33, 34].

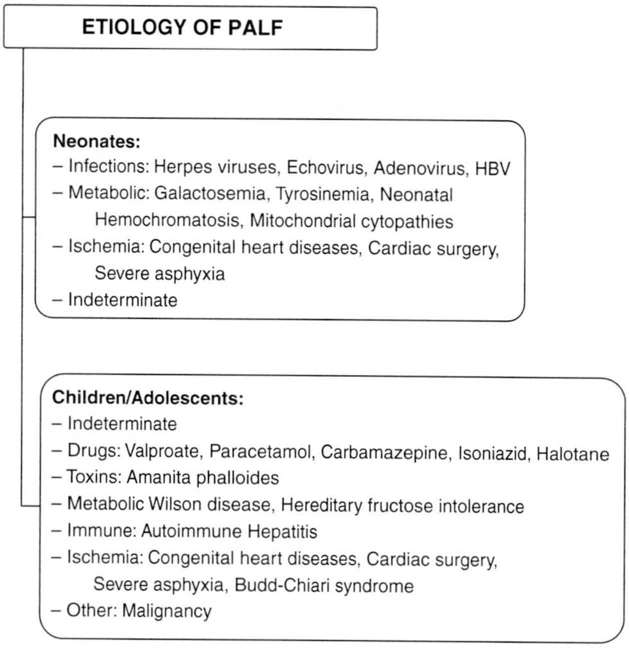

ETIOLOGY OF PALF

Neonates:
- Infections: Herpes viruses, Echovirus, Adenovirus, HBV
- Metabolic: Galactosemia, Tyrosinemia, Neonatal Hemochromatosis, Mitochondrial cytopathies
- Ischemia: Congenital heart diseases, Cardiac surgery, Severe asphyxia
- Indeterminate

Children/Adolescents:
- Indeterminate
- Drugs: Valproate, Paracetamol, Carbamazepine, Isoniazid, Halotane
- Toxins: Amanita phalloides
- Metabolic Wilson disease, Hereditary fructose intolerance
- Immune: Autoimmune Hepatitis
- Ischemia: Congenital heart diseases, Cardiac surgery, Severe asphyxia, Budd-Chiari syndrome
- Other: Malignancy

Fig. 24.3 Etiology of PALF according to age

Table 24.2 Comparison of clinical features, laboratory investigations at presentation, and outcome in children with fulminant hepatic failure of autoimmune and indeterminate etiology

Clinical features/laboratory investigations	Autoimmune ($n = 10$)	Indeterminate ($n = 20$)	P value
Age at onset	7.6 (4.8)	3.5 (3.9)	0.017
ALT (IU/L)	1140 (459)	3086 (2637)	0.029
Total bilirubin (mg/dL)	19 (10.8)	23.0 (2.0–46.1)	0.637
INR	3.6 (0.8)	4.7 (1.66)	0.130
Ammonia (μmol/L)	191 (85)	179 (84)	0.716
IgG (mg/dL)	2070 (114)	948 (388)	<0.001
IgM (mg/dL)	166 (91)	126 (52)	0.141
IgG/ULN	1.6 (0.8)	1.01 (0.58)	0.004
IgG/IgM ratio	13.7 (6.6)	8.2 (4.2)	0.011
Female prevalence	40%	55%	0.349
Prevalence of autoantibodies	100%	15%	<0.001
LT	50%	70%	0.250
Overall survival	90%	90%	0.748

ALT alanine aminotransferase, *INR* international normalized ratio, *LT* liver transplantation, *IgG/ULN* IgG corrected by the upper level of normal for age. Age and laboratory values are expressed as a mean (standard deviation) (see [35])

24.3.1.2 Autoimmune Hepatitis

Autoimmune hepatitis (AIH) is a chronic and progressive liver disease affecting all age groups with a higher incidence among females. The hallmarks of AIH are the presence of autoantibodies, elevated serum immunoglobulin G (IgG), and histological features of interface hepatitis. Up to 30–40% of children with AIH can have an acute presentation, but a minority of them have a fulminant course characterized by encephalopathy and need for transplantation. The cause of ALF in children can be determined in approximately half of patients, whereas in the other half it remains indeterminate. In particular the autoimmune etiology may be underestimated [35].

AIH represents a potentially reversible cause of acute liver failure (ALF), and in adults its early identification and treatment with steroids have been shown to avoid liver transplantation (LT) in about one third of patients [36–38].

ALF represents a life-threatening event in which coagulopathy often contraindicates liver biopsy, the mainstay of the diagnosis of AIH. The picture is made further complicated by the fact that autoantibodies may be negative at presentation, and antinuclear autoantibodies (ANA) as well as smooth muscle autoantibodies (SMA) can be positive even in patients with liver diseases of different etiologies [39–41].

In our experience AIH is a much more common cause of ALF than previously suggested and confirmed in 22% of our series of 46 patients. A complete autoantibody testing including LKM-type is essential in this setting, since autoantibodies are uncommon in the so-called "indeterminate" ALF. We found histology is not helpful to distinguish the different ALF etiologies, but, when serology is suggestive of AIH, a cautious steroids trial avoided transplantation in half cases [35] (Table 24.2).

24.3.1.3 Neonatal Hemochromatosis (NH) and Gestational Alloimmune Liver Disease (GALD)

Neonatal hemochromatosis (NH) is the most common cause of neonatal liver failure and is characterized by a hepatopathy starting in the prenatal life and coming to the medical attention acutely at birth despite being a chronic, end-stage liver disease [42]. NH is characterized by neonatal liver failure with hepatic and extrahepatic iron accumulation in parenchymal cells (liver, pancreas, kidney, brain, thyroid, salivary glands) rather than in reticuloendothelial cells (as seen in hemosiderosis) [43]. GALD represents a condition that is part of the wider group of diseases presenting with NH, resulting from an intrauterine alloimmune liver injury. Maternal immunoglobulin G appears to activate fetal complement that leads to the formation of membrane attack complex, causing liver cell injury [44]. Hypoglycemia, severe coagulopathy, hypoalbuminemia, elevated serum ferritin (>1000 ng/mL), normal or near-normal serum aminotransferase, and ascites are common clinical features of neonatal NH, including GALD. Iron deposition can be easily demonstrated in a buccal biopsy sampling the minor salivary glands (Fig. 24.4). A large proportion of patients with GALD respond to plasmapheresis and the administration of high-dose immunoglobulins [45]. Nonresponders to this treatment

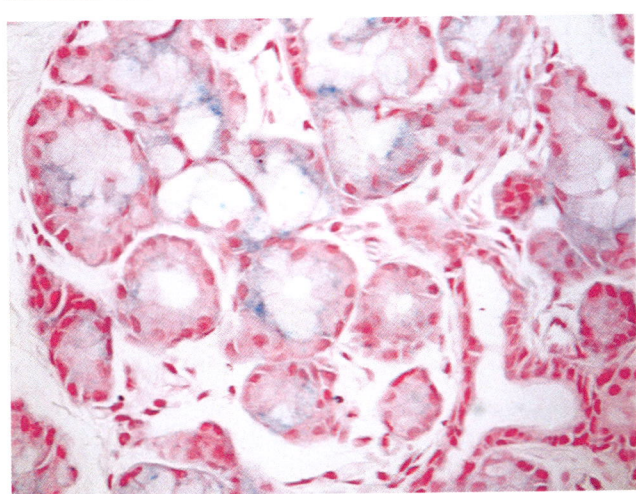

Fig. 24.4 Microphotograph of buccal biopsy histology showing accumulation of iron in the acinar cells of the salivary glands (blue spots) from a patient with neonatal hemochromatosis (Perl stain)

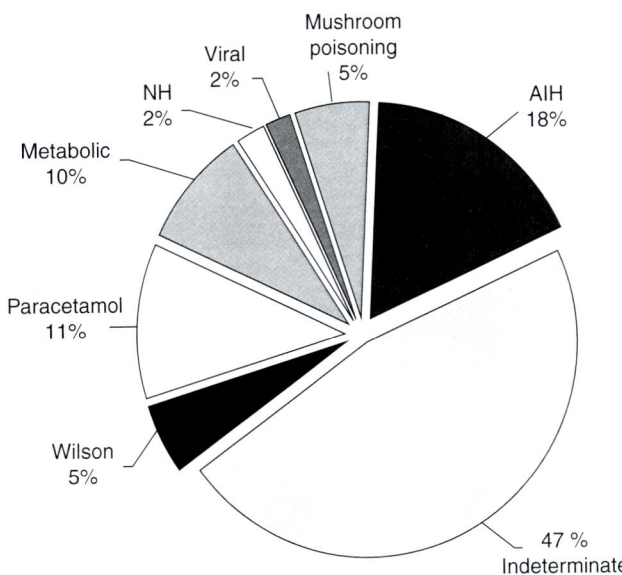

Fig. 24.5 Etiology distribution of a cohort of 55 Italian children presenting with acute liver failure. *AIH* autoimmune hepatitis, *NH* neonatal hemochromatosis

become candidate to a technically demanding liver transplant, having therefore worse patient and graft outcomes compared to LT performed at older ages.

24.3.1.4 Inherited and Metabolic Diseases

Metabolic diseases account for at least 10% cases of PALF (Fig. 24.5). While some conditions, such as mitochondrial cytopathies, may present at any age, most metabolic disorders presenting as liver failure segregate within particular age groups.

In infants metabolic disorders causing PALF are galactosemia, tyrosinemia, Niemann-Pick type C, urea cycle defects, and mitochondrial cytopathies. In older infants and young children up to 5 years of age, hereditary fructose intolerance, tyrosinemia, urea cycle defects, and mitochondrial cytopathies represent the most common etiologies. Finally, in older children and adolescents, Wilson disease should be suspected, as it is the most common inheritable disorder causing PALF at this age [46].

24.3.1.5 Toxic and Drug-Related PALF

Drugs and toxin represent the second cause of PALF in the pediatric population. The mechanism of toxicity may be directly related to the agent (paracetamol, amanitin, salicylate, etc.) or due to idiosyncratic reaction (isoniazid, propylthiouracil, halothane, etc.) [47–50].

24.3.1.6 Indeterminate PALF

In about 40–50% of pediatric ALF patients, it is not possible to recognize a specific etiology, and, after proper workup ruling out known causes of PALF, these cases are classified as indeterminate. Indeterminate PALF is likely to be due to viral infections, although a significant number of patients may have an undiagnosed autoimmune hepatitis [35, 51]. The etiology distribution in our country is shown in Fig. 24.5.

24.3.2 Pathophysiology of PALF

Main factors involved in the pathogenesis of liver injury in ALF are innate immunity and cytokines storm, mechanisms of apoptosis, signal transduction pathways, sterile inflammation, and liver regeneration.

24.3.2.1 Innate Immunity and Cytokines Storm

This pathogenic mechanism depends on the relationship between the molecular sensors that trigger the innate immune response and the effector cells of this response. There are two molecular patterns involved in the pathogenesis of liver injury in patients with ALF. The first one is the pathogen-associated molecular patterns (PAMPs), more important in ALF caused by hepatotropic viruses, and the second one is the damage-associated molecular patterns (DAMPs), more relevant in toxic etiologies [52]. Many cells participate in the innate immune response (e.g., monocytes, macrophages, dendritic cells, leukocytes, natural killer cells) by expressing receptors that can recognize both PAMPs and DAMPs of injury. Cells like monocytes, macrophages, and leukocytes regulate the inflammatory response by producing reactive oxygen radicals and pro- and anti-inflammatory cytokines, while the dendritic cells present antigens and induce T cells through expression of co-stimulatory molecules. These processes eventually lead to activation of adaptive immunity targeting viral- or drug-specific antigens. Of the various receptors of recognition, Toll-like receptors (TLRs), RNA helicase receptors, and Nod-like receptors/inflammasomes sense endogenous and exogenous danger signals and induce pro-inflammatory cytokines and type I interferons. At this stage, the clinical characteristics and outcome of the ALF syndrome will be influenced by the specificity of ligands, pattern recognition receptors, intracellular adaptor molecules, and signal transduction pathways. Moreover, the relative concentration of each innate immune cell type will determine the pattern of cytokines released locally within the liver and ultimately in the systemic circulation [53].

Thus, ALF is a clinical syndrome which results from pro- and anti-inflammatory cytokines spilling into the systemic circulation from the liver. Consistent with this, the two main causes of death, such as cerebral edema and multiorgan system failure, are a consequence of systemic inflammatory response syndrome (SIRS) which is mediated by release of pro-inflammatory cytokines including tumor necrosis factor (TNF), interleukin (IL)-1β, and IL-6. These SIRS mediators contribute to cerebral edema by decreasing cerebrovascular tone causing cerebral hyperperfusion.

Although a compensatory anti-inflammatory response syndrome mediated by anti-inflammatory cytokines (IL-4, IL-10, transforming growth factor-β) mounts concomitantly in patients with ALF to contrast SIRS, a persistent inflammatory state can certainly lead to multiorgan failure and late mortality [54].

24.3.2.2 Apoptosis in ALF

ALF occurs when hepatocyte death is so acute and massive that exceeds the liver regeneration. In ALF the hepatocyte death follows one of two patterns, apoptosis or necrosis. Apoptosis represents the execution of an adenosine triphosphate-dependent death program, leading to orderly resorption of cell nuclei and cytoplasm, minimizing the inflammatory response. Conversely, the necrosis involves depletion of adenosine triphosphate leading to cell lysis and secondary inflammation from lytic by-products. Current understanding supports the idea that a massive apoptosis constitutes the major path of hepatocyte death in ALF, particularly if due to viral and toxic etiologies.

In a study from ALF study group aiming to determine whether circulating apoptotic markers were altered in ALF, the authors demonstrated that the activity of the apoptosis-associated proteins TNF-α, HGF, IL-6, and M-30 antigen was significantly higher in ALF patients than in either chronic HCV or healthy controls, confirming the dramatic activation of apoptotic mechanisms in the cell death attending ALF. Also, they showed that high levels of soluble Fas and HGF supported the diagnosis of drug-induced liver injury or acetaminophen-related ALF, while higher levels of M-30 antigen were associated with poor clinical outcomes.

These results suggested a scientific rationale for future treatment trials with agents such as caspase inhibitors that block apoptotic pathways [55].

24.3.2.3 Signal Transduction Pathways

In humans or experimental models of hepatocyte injury by paracetamol or galactosamine, the cell stress results in the activation of pro-death and pro-survival pathways. In this area an important role is played by c-Jun N-terminal kinases (JNKs) which are a family of serine/threonine kinases belonging to the MAPK family. In most cells, including hepatocytes, two JNK isoforms, JNK1 and JNK2, are expressed. Studies showed JNK plays an important role in stress response and once activated, JNK regulates many metabolic and survival pathways but also mediates cell death.

In particular, the ability of JNK to mediate both cell survival and cell death pathways is often determined by the duration of JNK activation [56]. In fact, a prolonged JNK activation has been shown to mediate liver injury caused by paracetamol, and an important role seems to be played by a mitochondrial Sab protein which is required to sustained JNK activation leading to hepatocyte death. These data indicate specific pathways traversed by specific etiologic agents of ALF like paracetamol and suggest rational targets for modulating hepatocyte injury [57, 58].

24.3.2.4 Role of Sterile Inflammation

Two phenomena can be distinguished: septic inflammation and sterile inflammation. The former indicates an inflammatory response triggered by damage mediated by infectious sources, therefore called "septic inflammation." In the setting of ALF, inflammation and necrosis predispose patients to infections due to complement deficiency and/or impaired polymorphonuclear or Kupffer cell function. As a consequence, the patients are at risk of developing bacterial and fungal infections [59].

Conversely, "sterile inflammation" (SI) indicates a systemic response triggered by damage mediated by noninfectious sources. In the liver, SI is particularly important because it is a major component of the pathophysiology of a wide range of diseases, such as alcoholic steatohepatitis (ASH), nonalcoholic steatohepatitis (NASH), drug-induced liver injury, and ischemia/reperfusion (I/R).

The issue of SI has recently undergone advances in the understanding of how tissue injury results in inflammation. It has been demonstrated that the intracellular molecules released during pathological cell death (necrosis or apoptosis) are responsible for the sterile inflammation that occurs not only locally but also in distant organs and it is driven by DAMP pathway. Activation of pattern recognition receptors by DAMPs results in a wide range of immune responses, including production of pro-inflammatory cytokines and localization of immune cells to the site of injury. In the liver,

DAMPs can stimulate local intravascular sentinel cells (Kupffer cells) to produce IL-1, which induces upregulation of ICAM-1 on sinusoidal endothelial cells. Neutrophils are then recruited via integrin (Mac-1)-dependent adhesion to endothelial ICAM-1, to sustain the inflammatory process. As a result, the activation of these inflammatory mechanisms promotes further cell damage rather than repair, both in the liver and in other organs.

24.3.2.5 Liver Regeneration

In ALF patients, spontaneous survival has improved over the years. Nevertheless around 50% still require liver transplantation. The key point is liver regeneration. This is a complex phenomenon which aims at maintaining a constant liver mass in the event of injury resulting in loss of hepatic parenchyma. Pathogenetic mechanisms of liver regeneration associated with ALF are less well established compared to those associated to partial hepatectomy, in which it has been demonstrated that a series of events involving multiple signaling pathways controlled by mitogenic growth factors (HGF, EGF) and their receptors (MET and EGFR) may be activated.

During liver regeneration, whether following surgical resection or parenchymal injury and loss, all cell types of the liver can proliferate to replace their own cell population. When unable to do so, however, there are internal or external (e.g., hematopoietic) sources of progenitor cells that are able to differentiate into the various cells of the liver to restore cell compartments.

In presence of an acute liver injury, the outcome of a patient with ALF depends on the capacity of the liver of regenerating and restoring a normal liver synthetic function. If liver regeneration exceeds liver necrosis and apoptosis, the survival will occur; diversely, there will not be survival without LT. A relevant issue is also the time required to regenerate that can be much longer than the time a patient can survive with a failing liver. This supported the rationale for the use of auxiliary partial liver transplantation in ALF [60].

Certain etiologies of ALF (e.g., paracetamol overdose or ischemic liver injury) carry a much better prognosis than most other etiologies (e.g., mushroom poisoning or viral) suggesting that liver regeneration is influenced by different etiopathogenic mechanisms.

Initial clinical studies focused on alpha-fetoprotein as a marker of liver regeneration. Further studies showed that an early activation of the b-catenin signaling system contributes to liver regeneration in animal models and in patients with paracetamol-induced ALF and thus it may also serve as a marker of liver regeneration. Studies showed prostaglandin E2 (PGE2) increases liver size and hepatocyte number in zebrafish, while in paracetamol toxicity PGE2 injections reduced mortality and prolonged the therapeutic window for the effects of n-acetylcysteine, suggesting a possible therapeutic role for PGE2 in the treatment of patients with ALF.

These results suggest that liver regenerative pathways may be manipulated and offer hope for advances and future therapies in patients with this condition [61].

24.3.3 Diagnosis of PALF

Severe PALF, invariably leading to a multiorgan failure, represents a medical emergency that requires a multidisciplinary support (hepatologist, intensivist, liver transplant surgeon) and management in pediatric intensive care unit (PICU).

Liver dysfunction, hypoglycemia, coagulopathy, and jaundice are typical signs of PALF. Renal and neurological dysfunctions (with encephalopathy and cerebral edema), cardiovascular and respiratory dysfunctions, and a particular sensitivity to infections are also common. On admission, a careful clinical assessment of the patient and his/her history is of utmost importance. Specific questions to seek the etiology and possible comorbidities may be collected from the relatives. The age and the clinical history are helpful to guide the diagnostic process. All the patients should have a complete physical exam paying particular attention to the signs of a possible underlying chronic liver disease and to the neurological competence. To define nature and severity of liver injury, complete biochemical evaluation should include liver tests with synthetic function, arterial blood gas, lactate, and ammonia. An age-related metabolic workup including Wilson disease, the complete blood count, renal function (low urea is a marker of severe liver dysfunction, while creatinine may be difficult to assay in the context of elevated bilirubin), age-appropriate testing for infectious causes (serological screen for virus infection), and autoimmune markers (including ANA, SMA, and LKM autoantibodies) is mandatory. Chest radiography, baseline echocardiography, and liver ultrasound (with particular attention to the patency and direction of flow, liver texture, and size, splenic size) should be carried out to complete the diagnosis [62]. Liver biopsy is contraindicated in patients with ALF, because of the high risk of bleeding, and, when done, was shown to be unhelpful to determine the underlying etiology. In a minor proportion of patients who can benefit from a liver biopsy, the transjugular approach offers a reasonable risk/benefit ratio [35].

24.3.3.1 Serum Biochemistry

Typical serological signs of PALF are very high levels of INR and aminotransferases (ALT, AST) with an increasing bilirubin. The transaminase drop may be an ominous sign, in keeping with burnt out liver parenchyma (reflecting severe necrosis and collapse of hepatic cells); persistence of coagulopathy unresponsive to vitamin K, persistence of jaundice, hyperammonemia, and hypoglycemia difficult to correct are also signs of end-stage liver failure. According to the classical

King's criteria, mortality without transplantation in non-paracetamol overdose patients is best predicted by elevated INR and bilirubin, etiology, and timing of appearance of encephalopathy (Table 24.3) [63].

24.3.3.2 Hepatic Encephalopathy and Cerebral Edema

Hepatic encephalopathy (HE) is a neuropsychiatric disturbance in a patient with liver insufficiency, having no history of preexisting neurological disease. The diagnosis is clinical and at electroencephalogram (EEG).

Figure 24.6 shows the classical classification of HE in children and adolescents. However this scale has less value for neonates and infants especially in the early phases of encephalopathy, since at this age HE is more difficult to evaluate and infants are more resistant to the neurological effects of a failing liver.

The Pediatric Acute Liver Failure study group database, consisting of 348 patients, reported that 55% of children developed HE. The majority (75%) of patients had grade 1–2 encephalopathy. Grade 3 and 4 encephalopathy was seen in 17% and 7% of patients, respectively [64].

HE is characterized by a wide range of manifestations from confusion, disorientation or irritability, and inactivity to frank coma. In many occasions early clinical symptoms are subtle and difficult to assess. For neonates and infants, a better defined classification of HE has been proposed, and it is reported in Table 24.4 [3].

The real pathogenesis of HE remains incompletely understood. In general it is considered the consequence of a complex interaction between cerebral blood flow, systemic and cerebral inflammation, and metabolic disturbances including hyperammonemia, which plays a crucial role. Ammonia is a by-product of nitrogen metabolism, generated by the enzyme glutaminase in the enterocytes of the small intestine and the colon. Ammonia enters the urea cycle and is transformed in urea and excreted by the kidneys. The part of ammonia which bypasses this way is usually metabolized to glutamine in hepatocytes, skeletal myocytes, and astrocytes. Astrocytes are abundant cerebral cells, particularly sensitive to the increase of ammonia. When ammonia blood level increases, astrocytes metabolize it to glutamine which passes into the cerebral cells increasing their osmolarity. This generates an osmotic stress leading to an influx of water into astrocytes determining cellular swelling and in turn cerebral edema (CE). Plasma level of ammonia not always correlates with the gravity of HE. Probably also systemic circulation of pro-inflammatory mediators as interleukins (IL)-1 and IL-6 and tumor necrosis factor-alpha (TNF-α) may play a crucial role in the development of HE and CE. These molecules alter cerebral endothelial permeability to neurotoxins and modify intracranial vascular resistance. Cerebral edema and consequent intracranial hypertension are related to the severity of HE and typically occur at the later stages (grade 3 or 4) of HE [65].

Both generalized or focal and convulsive or nonconvulsive (electrographic) seizures may occur during PALF.

Table 24.3 King's College Hospital criteria for predicting mortality in non-paracetamol overdose acute liver failure

Prothrombin time > 100 s (INR > 6.5)
Or
Any three of the following (irrespective of grade of encephalopathy):
• Age < 10 or > 40 years
• Etiology: indeterminate, drug-induced (not paracetamol)
• Duration of jaundice to hepatic encephalopathy >7 days
• Prothrombin time > 50 (INR > 3.5)
• Serum bilirubin >300 μmol/L

Fig. 24.6 Classical classification of hepatic encephalopathy in children older than 3 years of age

Grade	Clinical findings	Reflexes
Grade 0	normal	normal
Grade 1	confused, mood changes, crying	normal or hyperreflexic
Grade 2	drowsy, inappropriate behavior, crying	normal or hyperreflexic
Grade 3	stupor, somnolence, may obey to simple commands	normal or hyperreflexic
Grade 4	comatose, arousable with painful stimoli or no responses	absent

Table 24.4 Assessment of encephalopathy for children from birth to age 3 years

Grade	Clinical	Asterixis/reflexes	Neurologic signs
Early (I and II)	Inconsolable crying, sleep reversal, inattention to task	Unreliable/normal or hyperreflexic	Untestable
Mid (III)	Somnolence, stupor, combativeness	Unreliable/hyperreflexic	Most likely untestable
Late (IV)	Comatose, arouses with painful stimuli (IVa) or no response (IVb)	Absent	Decerebrate or decorticate

In most cases the treatment of choice is intravenous phenytoin, but, till now, there is no definitive consensus on the best option. When the crisis is refractory to phenytoin, other therapeutic options may be midazolam infusion, phenobarbital, levetiracetam, or topiramate. The choice will depend on the patient's mental status, physiologic stability, and the possibility of continuous EEG monitoring to titrate drug infusion [66].

The neurologic scenario, with its spectrum of signs and symptoms, together with different bedside diagnostic tools like transcranial Doppler, cerebral near-infrared spectrophotometry, and continuous EEG monitoring may help to make an early and precise diagnosis of HE [67, 68]. Further studies are needed to improve early detection of neurological impairment since neurologic morbidity represents the major determinant of PALF outcome.

24.3.4 Treatment of PALF

PALF is a medical emergency because of its multiorgan system involvement and rapid neurological deterioration. Medical management should focus on careful monitoring of organ function to provide specific support in case of failure, prevention and prompt treatment of infections, and careful evaluation and monitoring of cardiovascular, respiratory, renal, and nutritional status, to buy time for hepatic regeneration as well as optimize clinical conditions to prepare the patient to liver transplantation.

24.3.4.1 General

As in all patients with prolonged INR, vitamin K should always be administered to see the real extent of hepatic failure; H2 antagonists or proton pump inhibitors should be administered prophylactically to prevent gastrointestinal hemorrhage from stress erosions. The use of N-acetylcysteine (NAC) in non-paracetamol toxicity has been abandoned after a multicenter randomized placebo-controlled study supported by the National Institutes of Health could not demonstrate its efficacy. In this study of 184 children with PALF, those receiving NAC were not more likely to survive compared to the ones receiving placebo [69]. Nonetheless, NAC may be considered at the onset of PALF, at least for the time needed to carefully rule out paracetamol overdose.

24.3.4.2 Neurological Dysfunction

Encephalopathy is a serious manifestation of PALF and may be exacerbated by sepsis, gastrointestinal bleeding, electrolyte disturbances, or sedation, especially benzodiazepine administration. Its early recognition and appropriate management in PICU are of paramount importance to reduce associated mortality and morbidity [70, 71]. The patient should be kept in a quiet environment with minimal stimuli. Neurological evaluations should be routinely performed (2–4 h) to estimate the grade of HE. The earliest neurological manifestations include personality changes with regression, irritability, apathy, and occasionally euphoria; sleep disturbances such as insomnia or sleep inversion; and apraxia due to disturbed spatial recognition. With the progression of HE, drowsiness and lethargy followed by deep somnolence and stupor are common manifestations. Seizures may develop. At stage 4 of HE, coma appears, and the patient responds only to intense painful stimuli and usually presents a decerebrate posture. Since ammonia plays a crucial role in the pathogenesis of HE, treatment aimed at reducing its production and accumulation is indicated [72].

The components of therapy should be:

- *Control of hyperammonemia:* Reduction of dietary protein to an intake of 1–2 g/kg/d, administered enterally or parenterally, and minimization of the formation of nitrogenous substances in the intestine are recommended. The use of a cathartic product such as nonabsorbable disaccharides (lactulose) is indicated and may be administered orally or via a nasogastric tube. The nonabsorbable antibiotics rifaximin or neomycin may also be used to reduce ammonia production [73]. A recent preliminary report of the adult ALF study group suggests L-ornithine phenylacetate may be considered as adjunctive therapy to reduce ammonia level in ALF [74].
- *Control of blood glucose:* An additional factor that may worsen the neurological pattern is hypoglycemia, resulting from failure of hepatic glucose synthesis and release, increased glucose utilization, and hyperinsulinemia due to failure of hepatic degradation. The infusion of a 10–33% glucose solution is indicated, although avoiding hyperglycemia that may worsen cerebral edema.
- *Airway protection:* Once neurological conditions deteriorate and grade 3 HE appears, intubation and mechanical ventilation should be carried out to prevent aspiration,

provide safer respiratory care avoiding hyper- and hypocapnia and hypoxemia, and avoid any sensory neural trigger. The main complication of HE is cerebral edema (CE) which causes intracranial hypertension.

- *Prevent and treat cerebral edema:* Factors affecting CE are fluid overload, failure to maintain normal glucose concentration in the blood, and hemodynamic instability with failure to maintain systemic blood pressure causing the reduction of cerebral perfusion pressure (CPP), which in turn ends up to cerebral ischemia. Monitoring of CE and intracranial hypertension is problematic with noninvasive tests. Head CT scan remains the best tool to evaluate CE. The surgical placement of an intracranial pressure (ICP) catheter to monitor the pressure is very useful to assess the response to treatment of cerebral hypertension, but severe coagulopathy, hallmark of ALF, puts the patient at high risk of intracranial bleeding. A small retrospective study showed that intracranial pressure monitoring allowed targeted interventions to manage elevated ICP, without improvement in survival [75]. At the moment there are insufficient data to recommend the routine use of ICP monitoring in patients with PALF. An alternative might be transcranial Doppler ultrasonography that evaluates middle cerebral artery flow and resistance, but, till now, no studies have been carried out in the pediatric setting. The standard management of CE involves adequate sedation, head elevation at 20°–30° with neutral head position, fluid restriction (80% of maintenance), and close monitoring of blood glucose (glucose infusion rate of 10–15 mg/kg/min avoiding hyperglycemia).

The management of acute intracranial hypertensive crisis comprises:

- *Osmotic therapy.* 3% saline and mannitol represent the fundamental therapy to reduce ICP. 3% saline decreases brain water content, improves cerebral blood flow, and stabilizes cerebral endothelial cell volume. Serum sodium should be monitored during this therapy and should be maintained between 145 and 150 mmol/L [14]. Mannitol increases serum osmolarity and therefore oncotic pressure, causing outward movement of water from brain parenchyma and decreasing blood viscosity and cerebral blood volume. Usually the dose of 0.5–1 g/kg/dose is recommended to treat an acute rise in ICP; no prophylactic therapy is recommended. Serum osmolarity should be maintained between 300 and 320 mOsm, keeping in mind that it should be measured with an osmometer, not calculated. Guidelines on treatment of traumatic brain injury in children and infants suggest to prefer the use of 3% saline over mannitol in the management of intracranial hypertension, due to insufficient evidence to support the use of mannitol [76].

- *Body temperature control.* A gradual increase of body temperature, having detrimental effects on the brain, typically accompanies the development of intracranial hypertension. The control of hyperthermia is essential to avoid further cerebral damage. Measures to induce hypothermia may protect the brain reducing its metabolism and neuronal inflammation. However hypothermia causes side effects such as cardiac arrhythmias, increased risk of bleeding and infection, and electrolyte imbalance. Till now, after several studies have been carried out especially in the setting of adult ALF, there is no clear consensus regarding the use of hypothermia in ALF. Active normothermia (36°–37°), though, is highly recommended [77].

- *Sedation and pain control.* Historically thiopentone has been used in severe HE and coma, due to its deep neuroprotective effects. However it can easily accumulate, leading to a long period before consciousness is regained upon suspension; this eliminates the possibility to monitor any clinical sign of brain dysfunction, apart from pupil reaction to light. Besides thiopentone affects the cardiovascular stability through depression of cardiac contractility and reduction of the cardiac output, leading to arterial hypotension. Short-acting agents may be a better choice in this condition. The use of propofol is safe and may offer some neurological protection through decreased cerebral blood flow and consequently ICP [78]. Benzodiazepines may worsen neurological pattern by increasing gamma-aminobutyric acid neurotransmission in addition to protracted sedative effect due to hepatic impairment. Short-acting opioids such as fentanyl and remifentanil are good options, and their concomitant use with sedatives may allow a dose reduction. If neuromuscular blockade is necessary, the best choice is cisatracurium, due to the fact that its elimination is not affected by liver function [7].

- *Hemodynamic control.* Adequate cerebral perfusion pressure (CPP = mean arterial pressure − intracranial pressure) is of paramount importance to protect the brain. The use of inotropes, such as norepinephrine, permits to maintain arterial pressure, reduces the amount of volume load needed to treat systemic hypotension, and consequently maintains CPP reducing CE [79].

Table 24.5 reports the general PICU measures for the management of hepatic encephalopathy in children with ALF.

24.3.4.3 Cardiovascular Dysfunction

In children with PALF, the use of a central venous catheter and an arterial line is necessary to drive both hemodynamic evaluation and treatment. Echocardiography provides information on systolic and diastolic function and often will show increased cardiac output and reduced vascular resistance

Table 24.5 Neuroprotection in acute liver failure and hepatic encephalopathy

General measures:
- Elevate head at 15–30 °C
- Maintain the neck in neutral position
- Maintain normoglycemia
- Mannitol bolus only if impending herniation and measured serum osmolality <320 mOsm/L
- Phenytoin if seizures (clinical or EEG)

Fluids:
- 70% of maintenance
- 3% hypertonic saline infusion (aim for serum sodium between 145 and 150 mEq/L)

Hyperammonemia:
- Oral/rectal lactulose
- Rifaximin or neomycin
- Consider CVVH if no response to medical treatment

Body temperature:
- Ensure normothermia with drugs and other cooling systems
- If resistant raised ICP (>20 mmHg): therapeutic hypothermia at 33–34 °C (with paralysis)

Blood pressure:
- Maintain BP > 50th percentile for age
- Maintain CPP > 50 mmHg (use inotropes if required)

Sedation (if evidence of raised ICP):
- Propofol ± opioids ± paralysis
- Fentanyl or propofol boluses before any procedure (airways suction, movements) to avoid ICP spikes
- If resistant raised ICP (>20 mmHg): thiopentone infusion with continuous EEG monitoring

Mechanical ventilation:
- Aim for normocarbia
- Avoid hyperventilation, except when there is impending herniation (apply temporarily)

with hyperdynamic status. Vasodilation may be due to elevated levels of circulating cytokines, gut-derived endotoxins, and substances released from the necrotic liver. Maintaining adequate intravascular volume should be the first step to avoid organ hypoperfusion and hyperlactacidemia. After appropriate volume load, ongoing hyperlactacidemia is likely to reflect the inability of the failing liver to metabolize the increased lactate production seen in response to sympathetic drive, with accelerated aerobic glycolysis. Till now there are no clear indications concerning the type of fluid to be preferred in PALF patients. In general, the literature on critical care medicine supports the use of crystalloids over colloids, but the choice should be done considering the biochemical parameters and the clinical status of the patient. Ringer lactate or balanced solutions (buffered with either bicarbonate or acetate) may be an alternative to normal saline, while the use of albumin in this specific situation has not been investigated. Once hemodynamic stability is achieved, fluid maintenance may run around 70–80% of the normal maintenance and consist of 10% dextrose in 0.45% or NaCl solution. If, after adequate volume, hypotension persists, a vasopressor agent may be used. Given the high-output and low-resistance status, the vasopressor recommended is norepinephrine [80]. Additional low-dose vasopressin has not shown any benefit and could be detrimental with regard to cerebral complication of PALF. In the presence of persistent hypotension, it is unclear whether hydrocortisone may have any benefit, possibly decreasing vasopressors requirement [81]. A rather large proportion of PALF patients may have evidence of adrenal dysfunction, requiring glucocorticoid supplements.

24.3.4.4 Respiratory Dysfunction

Patients with grade 2 and 3 encephalopathy tend to hyperventilate shifting acid/base balance toward respiratory alkalosis. In stage 4, profound neurological impairment causes hypoventilation, hypoxia, and hypercapnia. Elective airway protection with endotracheal intubation is recommended when grade 3 encephalopathy develops, when patients with grade 1 or 2 require sedation, and in case of respiratory dysfunction secondary to infection, pulmonary hemorrhage, or pediatric respiratory distress syndrome (PARDS) [1]. Noninvasive ventilation in patients with neurological impairment should be avoided because of high risk of aspiration. For intubation, the induction of anesthesia may be carried out with a short-acting opiate and propofol that decreases cerebral oxygen consumption and has anticonvulsant properties. With conventional ventilation the strategy should be lung-protective, with low tidal volume and appropriate level of positive end expiratory pressure (PEEP) to minimize ventilator-induced lung injury and warrant normocarbia and normoxia. Hyperventilation should be used to manage increased intracranial pressure crisis just for some instances, while sustained hyperventilation should be avoided. The recommendations of the Pediatric Acute Lung Injury Consensus Conference, in case of preserved respiratory system compliance, support ventilation with tidal volume of 5–8 mL/kg predicted body weight, low levels of PEEP (5 cmH$_2$O), and inspiratory plateau pressure limit of 28 cmH$_2$O [82]. In case of PARDS, characterized by poor respiratory system compliance, these guidelines suggest ventilation with tidal volume of 3–6 mL/kg predicted body weight, moderately elevated levels of PEEP (10–15 cmH$_2$O) titrated to maintain an open lung and normal oxygenation, and slightly higher plateau pressure of 29–32 cmH$_2$O. In addition, careful recruitment maneuvers in the attempt to improve severe oxygenation failure by slow incremental and decremental PEEP steps are suggested.

The role of nursing is crucial and includes patient mobilization (except prone position due to neurological impairment and possible development of intracranial hypertension), airway suction, and periodic control of endotracheal tube cuff, keeping in mind that any maneuver can trigger a crisis of intracranial hypertension.

24.3.4.5 Renal Dysfunction

The exact incidence of acute kidney injury (AKI) in PALF is unknown, but in an analysis of 583 pediatric patients with PALF, AKI was noted in 17.5% of subjects and was associated to increased mortality [26, 83]. The causes may be prerenal uremia, acute tubular necrosis, and functional renal failure. Prerenal uremia is the consequence of dehydration or absorption of a big amount of nitrogenous substances derived from gastrointestinal bleeding. Acute tubular necrosis is the consequence of hemodynamic instability due to hypovolemia or dehydration related to diuretic therapy. Typical signs of this condition are oliguria (urine output <0.5 mL/kg/h), decreased creatinine clearance, and urinary sodium concentration >20 mmol/L [84]. Functional renal failure, usually named hepatorenal syndrome, resulting from intrarenal vasoconstriction leading to decreased perfusion, has multifactorial etiology, including hypovolemia, cytokine storm, sepsis, and electrolyte disturbances. Typical signs are urinary sodium concentration < 20 mmol/L and oliguria with urinary output <1 mL/kg/h. While functional renal failure recovers well with liver transplantation, acute tubular necrosis may sustain renal impairment for a long period of time. Renal-protective measures to be applied are the minimization of the use of intravenous contrast or nephrotoxic drugs, the avoidance of excessive diuretic therapy, and the maintenance of adequate renal perfusion pressure. The reasons to start continuous renal replacement therapy (CRRT) are uremia, fluid overload, serious metabolic acidosis, sodium imbalance, and sepsis. CRRT should be considered also in presence of markedly elevated ammonia or progression of encephalopathy. Continuous veno-venous modes of renal replacement treatment are better than intermittent ones, due to better hemodynamic stability. Anticoagulation therapy during CRRT is controversial. The options are either no anticoagulation or prostacyclins, while regional citrate is usually discouraged since the liver is unable to metabolize it [11, 85, 86].

24.3.4.6 Hematological Dysfunction

Coagulopathy is the hallmark of PALF, and prolongation of prothrombin time (PT/INR) assesses both the severity of liver impairment and the risk of bleeding. Coagulopathy is due to balanced reduction in procoagulant (factors V, VII, and X and fibrinogen) and anticoagulant (antithrombin, protein C, and protein S) proteins, and this explains why episodes of bleeding are relatively infrequent in the absence of a provocative trigger such as invasive procedures, infections, or portal hypertension. Clinically significant hemorrhage is seen in <5% of patients with PALF, and < 1% have spontaneous intracranial bleeding [87]. PT prolongation reflects only a reduction of some of the liver-based coagulation proteins, and not the real risk of bleeding. In PALF a more detailed study of coagulation is mandatory to evaluate the risk of bleeding and consequently the need of transfusions of blood products. Measurement of factor VII, which has a shorter half-life and decreases more quickly than other factors, appears to be more sensitive to detect liver dysfunction. The level of fibrinogen is usually normal till disseminated intravascular coagulation (DIC) takes place. In this circumstance the measurement of factor VIII may help distinguishing between DIC and PALF, as this factor is synthesized by the vascular endothelium and therefore in PALF is normal or increased. There may be a reduction in platelet count, although in the pediatric population is less frequent than in adults. Severe thrombocytopenia suggests hypersplenism, DIC, or development of aplastic anemia. Transfusion strategy should take advantage of plasma or cryoprecipitates before invasive procedures, in the setting of active bleeding, or when INR is steadily above 4. Recombinant factor VII, although very potent, should be used very sparingly due to the high risk of systemic venous thrombosis [88]. Platelet transfusion is indicated if the platelet count is <10,000, or in presence of bleeding with platelet count <50,000. A condition associated with indeterminate PALF is bone marrow failure. A spectrum of features ranging from mild pancytopenia to aplastic anemia may occur in these patients. In most cases this condition presents overtly just after liver transplantation. Different treatments include hematopoietic stem cell transplantation or, if no matched donor is available, the use of powerful immunosuppressive agents [89].

24.3.4.7 Nutrition, Fluids, and Electrolytes

Patients with liver disease have increased resting energy expenditure as other critically ill patients. Their resting status is catabolic; therefore a correct amount of calories should be guaranteed. Early introduction of enteral feeding, if possible, should be encouraged because it minimizes loss of muscle mass and reduces the risk of gastrointestinal bleeding. The aims of nutritional support include adequate calorie intake to decrease catabolism, maintain normal blood glucose, and provide a correct amount of protein without favoring hyperammonemia. The advantage of using branched-chain amino acid compared to standard solutions is insufficiently supported. LCT/MCT emulsions are those most commonly utilized. The use of parenteral nutrition depends on nutritional status of the patient, ability to tolerate enteral feeds, and duration of low-calorie intake. Meticulous and frequent monitoring of serum electrolyte concentration and prompt correction of abnormalities are essential. Hypokalemia may occur because of dilution and volume overload, ascites, or renal loss. Hyponatremia is relatively frequent and should be avoided because of detrimental effects on central nervous system. Alterations in serum phosphate, magnesium, and ionized calcium are commonly observed and should be monitored and corrected. Hypophosphatemia has been reported as a positive prognostic sign of liver regeneration [90].

24.3.4.8 Infections

Children with liver failure are particularly susceptible to infections due to impairment of cellular and humoral immune system. About 50% of children will develop significant infections, sepsis, or septic shock. The increased need of invasive organ supports and monitoring may contribute in these critically ill patients, who commonly experience colonization with multidrug-resistant bacteria and the development of severe infections. The most common infection sites are the lung (especially in intubated patients), urinary tract infections, intravenous catheter-related bloodstream bacteremia, and spontaneous bacteremia. Gram-negative enteric bacilli and Gram-positive cocci are the most frequently isolated. There are no retrospective nor prospective data delineating infection-related complications in PALF. Constant attention to handwashing, strict asepsis during invasive procedures, and manipulation of intravascular lines, in addition to appropriate bronchial toilet, are essential in the care of these patients. Careful clinical evaluation, blood examinations including biomarkers of sepsis (RCP and PCT), and strict microbiologic surveillance with blood, urine, and other biological sample for cultures should be performed if suspicion of infection is high. Although there are no clear guidelines that recommend the routine use of antibiotics or antifungals drugs in patients presenting with ALF, prophylaxis with a cephalosporin is widely used in transplantation centers to decrease mortality of these subjects [71]. Empirical broad-spectrum antibiotics is particularly indicated in patients who have signs of SIRS, refractory hypotension, or progression of HE. Empiric antibiotic therapy should be recommended also for patients listed for super urgent liver transplantation, since the development of infection may force prompt delisting [91].

24.3.4.9 Liver Support Systems

Extracorporeal liver support (ELS) systems are used as bridge to liver transplantation or to assist the liver during recovery. They replace the failing liver securing metabolic and excretory functions, replacing liver-derived proteins and peptides and mitigating the innate immune activation following acute hepatocyte injury [11]. In addition to ammonia and urea (removed also from hemodialysis), ELS remove large albumin-bound molecules such as bilirubin, bile acid, metabolites of aromatic amino acids, medium-chain fatty acids, and cytokine [92].

They consist of two different systems: the bioartificial (BALS) and artificial (ALS) liver supports (Fig. 24.7) [93]. BALS combines plasma separation with perfusion of biocells containing either human hepatoblastoma cells or porcine hepatocytes. The main advantage of this method over the noncell-mediated artificial systems is the replication of metabolic and biosynthetic function in addition to detoxication. Up to now, few studies have been carried out, and their evidence for efficacy and safety on BALS is not convincing, especially in the pediatric population [94–96].

The two commercially available ALS are albumin dialysis devices based on filtration and adsorption. MARS (molecular absorbent and recirculating system) consists of a first circuit in which the patient's blood passes through a specialized hemofilter with a size selection threshold (<60 kDa) and a second circuit, containing albumin-enriched dialysate, passing the filter in a counter directional flow. A hemofiltration pump is required simultaneously to control the blood and dialysate circuit. For the MARS device, two different filters are available on the market: the adult filter (2.1 m^2, filling volume 152 mL) is recommended for patients of >25 kg of body weight, whereas the MARSmini filter (0.6 m^2, filling volume 57 mL) is used below 25 kg of body weight [97–99]. A second device, the Prometheus, consists of a first circuit in which the patient's blood passes through an albumin-permeable membrane, enabling the patient's albumin fraction to pass into a second circuit in which albumin-bound toxins are removed via two adsorbing columns. The cleansed dialysate can then reenter the first circuit. This device can be

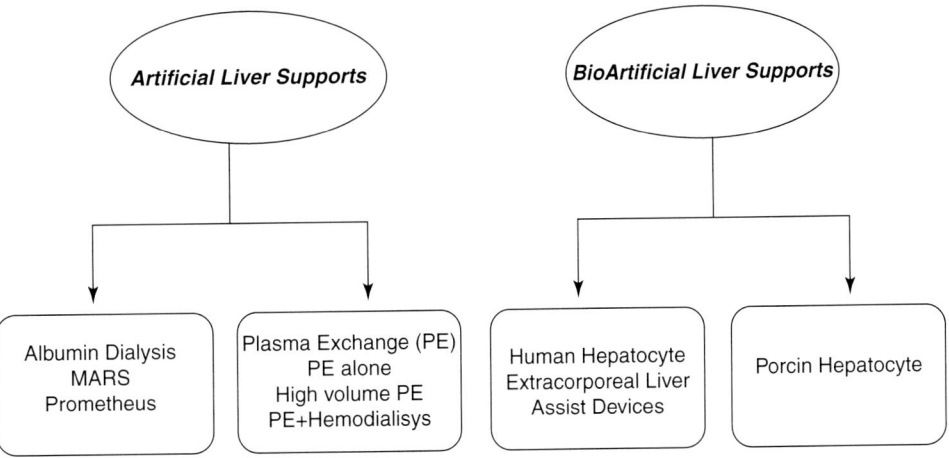

Fig. 24.7 Different types of extracorporeal liver supports (ELS). *BALS* bioartificial liver supports, *ALS* artificial liver supports

utilized only in adult-sized patients [100]. Despite albumin dialysis has shown the ability to provide a marked improvement in biochemical parameters (including serum ammonia, bilirubin, bile acid), there is no evidence of its benefit on patient survival. In the pediatric population, there are only case reports and case series that show results similar to those of adults. Given the scarcity of evidence of survival advantage, there is currently no indication to use MARS routinely in PALF, although some centers use it as a supportive critical care treatment in selected patients [101, 102]. Plasma exchange (PE) alone or with high volume exchange (defined as exchange of 15% of ideal body weight) represents another therapeutic ELS, in which the patient's plasma is removed by blood filtration and replaced by fresh-frozen plasma or albumin. PE methods allow improvement in serum biochemical parameters, neurological impairment, and coagulation profile and are used more commonly in pediatric liver ICUs, since PE devices are widely available [103–106]. PE combined with hemodialysis (HD) may offer a better tool to improve toxin removal. Some case reports and reports of small case series of PALF have suggested the superiority of this strategy to MARS [107]. Controlled trials are needed to better understand the real role of these tools. Whatever the choice of ELS, it should always be kept in mind that all these devices need the placement of large catheters and the availability of appropriate size circuits; this frequently represents a major limitation of their use, especially in newborns and infants.

24.3.4.10 Liver Transplantation

Liver transplantation is the only definitive treatment of PALF and represents 5–10% of all transplants performed at pediatric age. Spontaneous recovery has been reported in about one third of patients [90]. The outcome of LT for PALF is poorer when compared to other indications. Nevertheless survival is improving, approaching that of children transplanted for chronic liver disease [30]. In the SPLIT database, 1-year patient survival was 76% in the PALF group compared to 89% for other groups. The factors predicting poor outcome included age <1 year, grade 4 HE, and the need for dialysis before transplantation [108].

24.4 Intensive Care Management Following Liver Transplantation

The recent history of pediatric liver transplantation has been very successful because of the progressive improvement in preoperative management of end-stage liver disease, innovative surgical techniques, immunosuppression therapy, and intensive care management of posttransplant complications. Nowadays liver transplantation is considered the standard treatment of acute and chronic liver failure [109].

Timing for listing for LT is crucial and should be guided by good knowledge of the underlying disease, the organs' availability and waiting time on the list, and the allocation rules of the local organ-sharing network [110]. There are several different clinical situations indicating listing for transplantation. Usually, the persistent alteration of some biochemical parameters, such as persistent rise in total bilirubin, prolongation of prothrombin ratio and international normalized ratio (INR), and a fall in serum albumin in the contest of severe liver disease, represents the condition to list the patient. These parameters have been utilized to develop the pediatric end-stage liver disease (PELD) score to predict death and have confirmed their accuracy in predicting need for transplantation [111] (Fig. 24.8).

Most pediatric liver transplantations are performed following graft splitting procedure, to prepare a size-matched segmental graft, while the other segments are used for an adult patient. There are four main types of segmental liver grafts: the left lateral (segments II–III), the left lobe (segments I–IV), the right lobe (segments V–VIII), and the right extended lobe (segments I + IV–VIII) [112]. Although technically demanding, a monosegmental graft (segment II) or a reduced thickness graft can also be used for very small infants (neonates) [113]. Liver matching is based on blood group typing and not on human leukocyte antigen (HLA) matching, because the liver is less susceptible to HLA-mediated rejection. An alternative option, especially in neonates and infants <1 year of age, in whom the level of isohemagglutinins is very low, is the use of ABO blood-mismatched grafts, with good results. In patients older than 1 year, removal of anti-A/B antibodies is necessary and achieved with plasmapheresis and, if needed, the administration of rituximab [114].

Factors that strongly impact the posttransplantation course include the underlying disease and complications, the type of liver graft used, and the tolerance to the graft on immunosuppression therapy. In PICU, after transplantation,

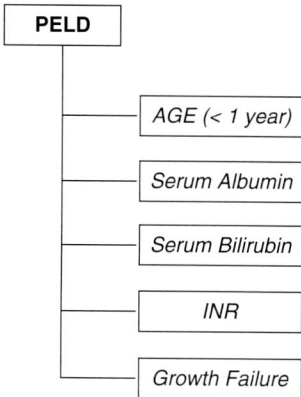

Fig. 24.8 Pediatric end-stage liver disease (PELD) score

the patient is maintained sedated with the infusion of sedatives and analgesic medications until liver function is regained; there is good hepatic artery and portal vein flow on Doppler ultrasound; no bleed from surgical site is seen; abdominal drainage produces only a small amount of fluid (less than 10 mL/kg/day); serum glucose, electrolytes, acid-base balance, albumin, and lactate are in range; and all organ functions are stable and normal. The interruption of anesthetic drugs allows assessment of level of consciousness, which is an accurate parameter for the function of the newly transplanted liver. Neurological complications such as seizures are uncommon in our experience, but they have been described in up to 30% of patients. High serum levels of immunosuppressive drugs, hypoglycemia, and electrolyte alterations represent the main causes of seizures [5].

If the patient is stable, mechanical ventilation weaning can start, and successful extubation can be achieved when sufficient respiratory autonomy is established, usually within 24 h from surgery. Noninvasive ventilatory support (with helmet CPAP or facial mask) has become widely available and has shown to be very helpful in reducing the respiratory work and the intubation period in patients arrived to transplant with malnutrition and poor muscle mass. Longer respiratory support may be required in case of pulmonary edema, pleural effusion (typically on the right side due to passage of ascitic fluid through the right diaphragm), atelectasis, neurological dysfunction, or chest infections [115].

From the hemodynamic point of view, it is useful to continuously monitor arterial and venous blood pressure and the arterial hemoglobin saturation of oxygen. Adequate fluid resuscitation with crystalloids rather than colloids is essential for organ perfusion in patients that are often vasoconstricted and relatively hypovolemic [116]. The target is normal pressure and central venous pressure of 8–10 mmHg [117]. Over 70% of patients have hypertension, which in some occasions requires pharmacological treatment. The reasons of hypertension include volume overload, elevated renin levels, and the use of steroid and calcineurin inhibitors [118].

Renal impairment with oliguria should be managed with inotrope support and diuretic therapy. Anuria with a rising urea, creatinine, and potassium should be treated with renal replacement treatments (CVVH, CVVHDF). Hemoglobin should be kept between 8 and 10 g/L because higher values may increase the risk of hepatic artery thrombosis thorough increase of blood viscosity. Early administration of antiplatelet therapy (such as aspirin at 5 mg/kg/day) is used by many centers if there is no major risk of bleeding. Blood products should be used sparingly, to limit the potential risk of thrombosis at the level of vascular anastomosis [119]. The infusion of low-dose sodium heparin (10 IU/kg/h) is also used in most centers to decrease the risk of vascular thrombosis in the immediate postoperative period, although the evidence on its efficacy is scarce.

Strict body temperature monitoring and control are fundamental to limit coagulation disorders.

In the presence of worsening liver function or lack of improvement, it is mandatory to perform a thorough evaluation to exclude vascular complications, primary nonfunction, rejection, infections, or biliary complications. In these circumstances, abdominal ultrasound represents the best first-line tool, because it's widely available and noninvasive and has good sensitivity in expert hands. However angio-CT scan may often be required. All patients need an adequate immunosuppressive therapy to protect the graft against rejection. Immunosuppression should be titrated to balance control of rejection and over-immunosuppression side effects. Remarkably, many medications interact with the main immunosuppressant tacrolimus, through cytochrome p-450 or p-glycoprotein efflux pump, affecting its serum levels, either reducing or increasing its activity and side effects (Table 24.6).

The use of segmental grafts has reduced waiting list time and mortality but increased postoperative complications. However, long-term patient and graft survival is similar to that seen with whole liver transplantation [120].

PICU length of stay is extremely variable, since it is influenced by preexisting conditions of the recipient (malnutrition, renal dysfunction), the quality of the graft (primary nonfunction, coagulopathy), adverse intraoperative events (intra-abdominal hemorrhage, vascular thrombosis, venous outflow obstruction), or postoperative complications (acute rejection, persistent wound drainage or large amounts of ascites, sepsis, biliary leak, arterial or portal stenosis/thrombosis). Using a temporal criterion, postoperative complications may be separated in early and late (Figs. 24.9 and 24.10). Late complications are extensively discussed elsewhere in this book.

24.4.1 Early Complications

24.4.1.1 Primary Nonfunction

Primary nonfunction (PNF) is a severe condition occurring in the first 48 h after transplantation and requiring urgent retransplantation. Although rare, probably occurring in less than 2% of cases, it accounts for about 25% of severe graft dysfunction in the first days posttransplantation.

The suspicion of this condition is based on worsening coagulopathy, acidosis, rising liver enzymes and cholestasis, and development of organ dysfunctions (hepatic encephalopathy, vasoplegic shock, renal failure) [121, 122].

24.4.1.2 Vascular Thrombosis

Hepatic artery thrombosis (HAT) and portal vein thrombosis (PVT) occur in 1–5% of recipients and account for some 40% of graft loss in the first days after transplant [121]. Hepatic artery thrombosis occurs three to four times more

Table 24.6 Drugs interacting with tacrolimus metabolism through cytochrome p-450 CYP3A and P-glycoprotein efflux pump

Inhibitors (increase levels)		Substrates (increase levels)	Inducers (reduce levels)	
Interaction with tacrolimus through CYP3A				
Bromocriptine	Macrolides	Alprazolam	Lidocaine	Aluminum hydroxide
Verapamil	Methylprednisolone	Alfentanil	Lovastatin	Dexamethasone
Voriconazole	Metoclopramide	Amiodarone	Loratadine	Ethosuximide
Glibenclamide	Metronidazole	Amlodipine	Nevirapine	Isoniazid
Grapefruit	Midazolam	Atorvastatin	Nicardipine	Carbamazepine
Dalfopristin	Midecamycin	Warfarin	Nifedipine	Magnesium oxide
Danazol	Miconazole	Venlafaxine	Omeprazole	Methylprednisolone
Delavirdine	Nelfinavir	Vinblastine	Paclitaxel	Nevirapine
Diltiazem	Nefazodone	Dabigatran	Progesterone	Orlistat
Erythromycin	Nicardipine	Dantrolene	Propafenone	Prednisone
Etinilestradiol	Prednisolone	Dapsone	Sertraline	Rifabutin
Zafirlukast	Prednisone	Diazepam	Simvastatin	Rifampicin
Indinavir	Progesterone	Disopyramide	Tamoxifen	Sirolimus
Itraconazole	Ritonavir	Enalapril	Testosterone	Sodium bicarbonate
Quinupristin	Saquinavir	Estradiol	Triazolam	Sulfapyridine
Ketoconazole	Troleandomycin	Estrogen	Felodipine	Phenylbutazone
Clarithromycin	Fluvoxamine	Etoposide	Flutamide	Phenytoin
Clotrimazole	Fluconazole	Zolpidem	Chlorpromazine	Phenobarbital
Cortisol	Fluoxetine	Quinidine	Cyclophosphamide	
Lansoprazole	Chloramphenicol	Clonazepam	Cilostazol	
Levofloxacin	Cyclosporine	Cocaine	Cisapride	
Lopinavir	Cimetidine	Cortisol		
Inhibitors (increase levels)		Substrates (increase levels)	Inducers (reduce levels)	
Interaction with tacrolimus through P-glycoprotein efflux pump				
Azithromycin		Azithromycin	Avasimibe	
Amiodarone		Actinomycin	Ambrisentan	
Conivaptan		Vinblastine	Dabigatran	
Verapamil		Vincristine	Everolimus	
Diltiazem		Dexamethasone	Imatinib	
Dronedarone		Digoxin	Carbamazepine	
Erythromycin		Doxorubicin	Ranolazine	
Indinavir		Etoposide	Ritonavir	
Itraconazole		Colchicine	Rifampin	
Captopril		Cortisol	Rifampicin	
Carvedilol		Lovastatin	Sirolimus	
Quinidine		Paclitaxel	Talinolol	
Ketoconazole		Terfenadine	Tipranavir	
Clarithromycin		Fexofenadine	Topotecan	
Conivaptan		Phenytoin	Phenytoin	
Lopinavir				
Ranolazine				
Ritonavir				
Felodipine				
Cyclosporine				

frequently in children than in adult transplants, and its presentation is abrupt and dramatic, characterized by acute liver failure due to sudden hepatic necrosis [123, 124].

Diagnosis is based on Doppler ultrasound at bedside and confirmed by computed tomography and angiography [125]. The two therapeutic options are endovascular catheter-directed thrombolysis or surgical revision of arterial anastomosis. Retransplantation is indicated if extensive parenchymal necrosis occurs. Biliary leaks or strictures and hepatic abscesses represent the late complications of hepatic artery thrombosis.

Portal vein thrombosis (PVT) is more common in children transplanted for biliary atresia, due to preexisting portal vein hypoplasia, which needs a complex surgical anastomosis [126]. The consequences of portal vein thrombosis are ascites, intestinal congestion with possible bacterial translocation and infection, and portal hypertension with gastrointestinal bleeding [127].

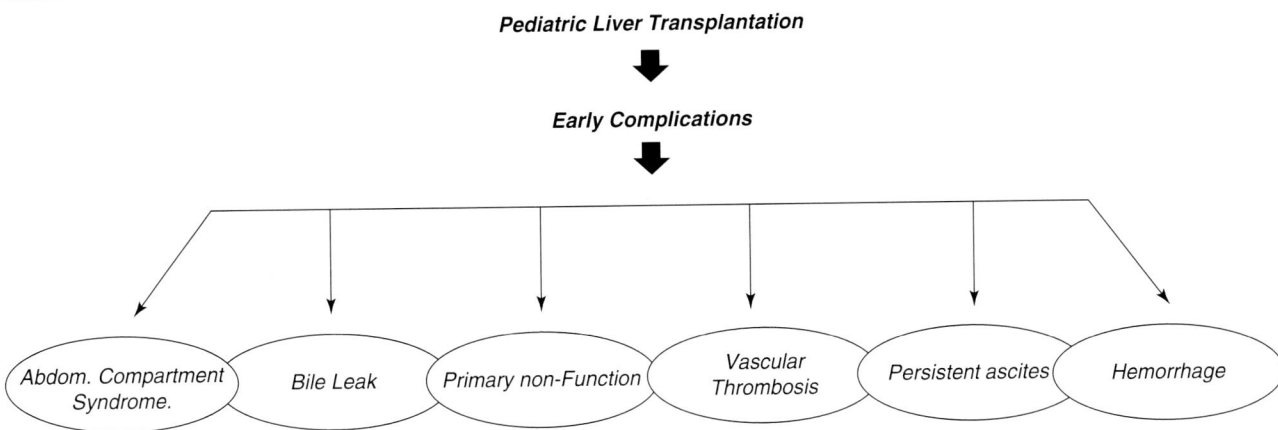

Fig. 24.9 Early complications after pediatric liver transplantation

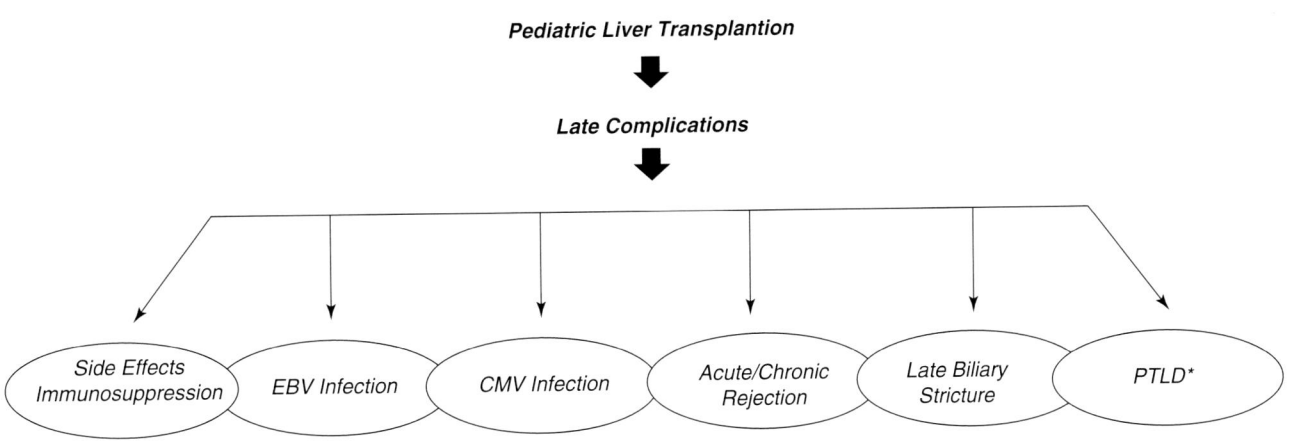

❖ Post Transplant Lynphoproliferative Disease

Fig. 24.10 Late complications after pediatric liver transplantation

The therapeutic options are urgent surgical thrombectomy, which may be effective and lead to successful revascularization and graft salvage, or local thrombolysis using a catheter inserted in the portal vein by the surgeon in operating room.

24.4.1.3 Hemorrhage

Coagulopathy and bleeding due to altered hemostatic profile are critical issues typical of patients with liver disease and represent a real problem in the immediate posttransplant period too. After transplantation, hemorrhage, though transitionally, remains a risk due to increased capillary fragility, dilutional hemostatic coagulopathy, and lacking of full graft ability to synthesize all coagulation factors. Remarkably, data available in literature report both a tendency to bleed and a prothrombotic status after transplantation, with a subsequent and gradual recovery of balanced coagulation activity in 2–3 weeks [128, 129]. Early intravenous infusion of low dose of sodium heparin (10 UI/kg/h) and antiplatelet aggregation therapy are useful but expose the patients to bleeding. Noteworthy, the standard coagulation tests such as prothrombin time (PT) and activated partial prothrombin time (APTT) are unable to give a complete and clear picture of the real coagulation status, because of their insensibility to plasma levels of anticoagulant proteins (protein C pathway, antithrombin, and tissue factor pathway inhibitor) and their inability to show the role of endothelium and cells in the hemostatic process [130, 131].

An aid to approach this issue and facilitate intensive care management and decision-making in transfusional policy and point-of-care (POC) devices, providing visual, rapid, and reliable results at bedside, has been developed. TEG® and ROTEM® represent two of these devices. They provide a real-time assessment of viscoelastic clot strength using a little amount of whole blood [25].

The official recommendations suggest the following thresholds to react and transfuse in the presence of perioperative bleeding: hemoglobin of 8 mg/dL, PLT count

<50.000/μL, transfusion of fibrinogen concentrate (30–50 mg/kg), or cryoprecipitate (5 mL/kg) to increase plasma fibrinogen concentrations above trigger values of 1.5–2.0 g/L [132].

24.4.1.4 Abdominal Compartment Syndrome

Normally, the intra-abdominal pressure (IAP) is 5–7 mmHg. Higher pressure values may cause dysfunction of intra-abdominal organs with the development of abdominal compartment syndrome (ACS). ACS may be defined as IAP >20 mmHg and abdominal perfusion pressure (the difference between mean systemic pressure and intra-abdominal pressure) <60 mmHg with consequent organ hypoperfusion. The main cause of the syndrome after transplant is the use of a large-for-size graft, which renders difficult the abdomen wall closure. It is important to monitor the IAP at least every 4–6 h in case of implantation of a large-for-size graft. The measurement is easily accomplished via a transurethral intravesical pressure catheter and the intermittent filling of the bladder with saline solution [133].

The medical management considers:

- Improvement of abdominal wall compliance (sedation, analgesia, neuromuscular blockade, no head of bed >30°)
- Emptying intraluminal contents (nasogastric decompression, rectal decompression, prokinetic agents)
- Careful control of fluid balance
- Hemodynamic stability: use vasopressors aiming for a mean arterial pressure > 60 mmHg
- Emptying abdominal fluid collection (paracentesis or percutaneous drainage)

If intra-abdominal hypertension and compartment syndrome persist, decompressive laparotomy is mandatory, with the placement of a Silastic® abdominal wall patch and a vacuum occlusive dressing [134].

24.4.1.5 Acute Rejection

Early postoperative period is the time of highest risk for immunologic reactions between host and graft. In this phase, aggressive immune therapy with its various combinations is required. Nevertheless, acute cellular rejection remains common after transplantation. About 40–70% of pediatric liver transplant recipients experience rejection, most of them in the first 2 weeks after surgery. Clinical manifestation of very early, severe rejection may consists in fever and abdominal pain/discomfort, while laboratory tests reveal rising or lack of decrease of serum bilirubin, aspartate and alanine transaminases, and γ-glutamyl transpeptidase. Confirmation of liver rejection always requires a liver biopsy. Clinical and histological features of cellular rejection as well as its management are discussed extensively elsewhere in this book.

24.4.1.6 Bile Leak

Biliary tree complications, such as anastomosis stricture, biliary leak, and anastomosis dehiscence, are very frequent and occur in approximately 15% of patients after transplantation.

Biliary strictures may be the consequence of an anastomotic stenosis, edema of the bile ducts, or hepatic artery ischemia. Biliary leaks from the cut surface of a partial graft are more common after transplant. Minor biliary leaks settle spontaneously, while larger ones, causing large collections and biliary peritonitis or biliary abscesses, may require the percutaneous biliary drainage through the placement of an external biliary catheter to reduce the flow through the fistula.

24.4.1.7 Persistent Ascites

Prolonged presence of ascites may depend on preoperative ascites, acute rejection, hepatic vein obstruction, and bacterial or fungal peritonitis. The loss of big amount of fluid, abundant of protein like coagulation factors, and electrolytes, may compromise patient stability. The medical approach includes diuretic and careful fluid balance with volume restriction.

In a recent study, we found that large drain losses after transplant are associated with early graft dysfunction. Graft dysfunction was predicted by >20 mL/kg/d of ascites at age 0–2 years and > 10 mL/kg/d above 2 years. The measurement of drain losses after pediatric LT could be used as a noninvasive marker of graft dysfunction and prompt the decision to perform a liver biopsy [135]. In case of suspected hepatic vein obstruction, interventional radiology may diagnose and treat the problem [136].

24.5 Conclusion

In conclusion children with liver disease almost invariably require intensive care unit skills in case of complications of cirrhosis, acute decompensation of chronic liver disease, and acute and acute on chronic liver failure, after liver transplantation. Every transplantation center should have a pediatric intensive care unit with knowledge and experience on liver disease in childhood, since these patients are fragile during anesthesia and the pathophysiology of their condition is peculiar.

In this setting acute liver failure represents the main challenge, because of the rapid progression and high mortality and because of lack of evidence on predictors of survival, prevention, and management of its complications. The decision to use invasive tools such as mechanical ventilation and extracorporeal supports and to list the patient for transplantation is still mainly based on local center experience and organ availability. A tight liaison between the pediatric hepatologist and the pediatric intensivist offers the highest standards of care to children with liver disease and need for intensive care management.

References

1. Dhawan A. Acute liver failure in children and adolescents. Clin Res Hepatol Gastroenterol. 2012;36(3):278–83. Epub 2012/04/24.
2. Devictor D, Tissieres P, Afanetti M, Debray D. Acute liver failure in children. Clin Res Hepatol Gastroenterol. 2011;35(6–7):430–7. Epub 2011/05/03.
3. Lutfi R, Abulebda K, Nitu ME, Molleston JP, Bozic MA, Subbarao G. Intensive care management of pediatric acute liver failure. J Pediatr Gastroenterol Nutr. 2017;64(5):660–70.
4. Bennett J, Bromley P. Perioperative issues in pediatric liver transplantation. Int Anesthesiol Clin. 2006;44(3):125–47. Epub 2006/07/13.
5. Bromley P, Bennett J. Anaesthesia for children with liver disease. Contin Educ Anaesth Crit Care Pain. 2014;14(5):207–12.
6. Bonavia A, Pachuski J, Bezinover D. Perioperative anesthetic management of patients having liver transplantation for uncommon conditions. Semin Cardiothorac Vasc Anesth. 2018;22(2):197–210.
7. Djurberg H, Pothmann Facharzt W, Joseph D, Tjan D, Zuleika M, Ferns S, et al. Anesthesia care for living-related liver transplantation for infants and children with end-stage liver disease: report of our initial experience. J Clin Anesth. 2002;14(8):564–70. Epub 2003/02/05.
8. Schiller O, Avitzur Y, Kadmon G, Nahum E, Steinberg RM, Nachmias V, et al. Nitric oxide for post-liver-transplantation hypoxemia in pediatric hepatopulmonary syndrome: case report and review. Pediatr Transplant. 2011;15(7):E130–4. Epub 2010/04/23.
9. Deep A, Saxena R, Jose B. Acute kidney injury in children with chronic liver disease. Pediatr Nephrol. 2018.
10. Ringe H, Varnholt V, Zimmering M, Luck W, Gratopp A, Konig K, et al. Continuous veno-venous single-pass albumin hemodiafiltration in children with acute liver failure. Pediatr Crit Care Med. 2011;12(3):257–64. Epub 2010/10/06.
11. Aron J, Agarwal B, Davenport A. Extracorporeal support for patients with acute and acute on chronic liver failure. Expert Rev Med Devices. 2016;13(4):367–80.
12. Ranger AM, Chaudhary N, Avery M, Fraser D. Central pontine and extrapontine myelinolysis in children: a review of 76 patients. J Child Neurol. 2012;27(8):1027–37.
13. Rehman M, Taneja P, Gurnaney H. New-onset prolonged QTc leading to torsade de pointes in a child with acute liver disease. Paediatr Anaesth. 2012;22(6):593–5. Epub 2012/05/19.
14. Singh RK, Poddar B, Singhal S, Azim A. Continuous hypertonic saline for acute liver failure. Indian J Gastroenterol. 2011;30(4):178–80. Epub 2011/06/23.
15. Odutayo A, Desborough MJ, Trivella M, Stanley AJ, Doree C, Collins GS, et al. Restrictive versus liberal blood transfusion for gastrointestinal bleeding: a systematic review and meta-analysis of randomised controlled trials. Lancet Gastroenterol Hepatol. 2017;2(5):354–60.
16. Choquette M. 50 years ago in The Journal of Pediatrics: hepatic coma in childhood. J Pediatr. 2013;163(5):1360. Epub 2013/10/29.
17. Kelly DA. Managing liver failure. Postgrad Med J. 2002;78(925):660–7. Epub 2002/12/24.
18. Green DW, Ashley EM. The choice of inhalation anaesthetic for major abdominal surgery in children with liver disease. Paediatr Anaesth. 2002;12(8):665–73. Epub 2002/12/11.
19. Starczewska MH, Mon W, Shirley P. Anaesthesia in patients with liver disease. Curr Opin Anaesthesiol. 2017;30(3):392–8.
20. Camkiran A, Araz C, Seyhan Balli S, Torgay A, Moray G, Pirat A, et al. Anesthetic management in pediatric orthotopic liver transplant for fulminant hepatic failure and end-stage liver disease. Exp Clin Transplant. 2014;12(Suppl 1):106–9.
21. Frykholm P, Pikwer A, Hammarskjold F, Larsson AT, Lindgren S, Lindwall R, et al. Clinical guidelines on central venous catheterisation. Swedish Society of Anaesthesiology and Intensive Care Medicine. Acta Anaesthesiol Scand. 2014;58(5):508–24.
22. Denys BG, Uretsky BF, Reddy PS. Ultrasound-assisted cannulation of the internal jugular vein. A prospective comparison to the external landmark-guided technique. Circulation. 1993;87(5):1557–62.
23. Torgay A, Pirat A, Akpek E, Zeyneloglu P, Arslan G, Haberal M. Pulse contour cardiac output system use in pediatric orthotopic liver transplantation: preliminary report of nine patients. Transplant Proc. 2005;37(7):3168–70.
24. Pivalizza EG, Abramson DC, King FS Jr. Thromboelastography with heparinase in orthotopic liver transplantation. J Cardiothorac Vasc Anesth. 1998;12(3):305–8.
25. Smart L, Mumtaz K, Scharpf D, Gray NO, Traetow D, Black S, et al. Rotational thromboelastometry or conventional coagulation tests in liver transplantation: comparing blood loss, transfusions, and cost. Ann Hepatol. 2017;16(6):916–23.
26. Squires RH Jr, Shneider BL, Bucuvalas J, Alonso E, Sokol RJ, Narkewicz MR, et al. Acute liver failure in children: the first 348 patients in the pediatric acute liver failure study group. J Pediatr. 2006;148(5):652–8. Epub 2006/06/02.
27. Rivera-Penera T, Moreno J, Skaff C, McDiarmid S, Vargas J, Ament ME. Delayed encephalopathy in fulminant hepatic failure in the pediatric population and the role of liver transplantation. J Pediatr Gastroenterol Nutr. 1997;24(2):128–34. Epub 1997/02/01.
28. Di Giorgio A, Nicastro E, Dalla Rosa D, Nebbia G, Sonzogni A, D'Antiga L. Transplant-free survival in chronic liver disease presenting as acute liver failure in childhood. Transplantation. 2018; Epub ahead of printing.
29. Dhawan A, Cheeseman P, Mieli-Vergani G. Approaches to acute liver failure in children. Pediatr Transplant. 2004;8(6):584–8. Epub 2004/12/16.
30. Di Giorgio A, Sonzogni A, Picciche A, Alessio G, Bonanomi E, Colledan M, et al. Successful management of acute liver failure in Italian children: A 16-year experience at a referral centre for paediatric liver transplantation. Dig Liver Dis. 2017;49(10):1139–45. Epub 2017/07/01.
31. Schwarz KB, Dell Olio D, Lobritto SJ, Lopez MJ, Rodriguez-Baez N, Yazigi NA, et al. Analysis of viral testing in nonacetaminophen pediatric acute liver failure. J Pediatr Gastroenterol Nutr. 2014;59(5):616–23.
32. Devictor D, Tissieres P, Durand P, Chevret L, Debray D. Acute liver failure in neonates, infants and children. Expert Rev Gastroenterol Hepatol. 2011;5(6):717–29. Epub 2011/10/25.
33. Silverio CE, Smithen-Romany CY, Hondal NI, Diaz HO, Castellanos MI, Sosa O. Acute liver failure in Cuban children. MEDICC Rev. 2015;17(1):48–54. Epub 2015/03/03.
34. Uribe M, Alba A, Hunter B, Valverde C, Godoy J, Ferrario M, et al. Chilean experience in liver transplantation for acute liver failure in children. Transplant Proc. 2010;42(1):293–5. Epub 2010/02/23.
35. Di Giorgio A, Bravi M, Bonanomi E, Alessio G, Sonzogni A, Zen Y, et al. Fulminant hepatic failure of autoimmune aetiology in children. J Pediatr Gastroenterol Nutr. 2015;60(2):159–64. Epub 2014/10/12.
36. Potts JR, Verma S. Optimizing management in autoimmune hepatitis with liver failure at initial presentation. World J Gastroenterol. 2011;17(16):2070–5. Epub 2011/05/07.

37. Fujiwara K, Yasui S, Yokosuka O. Efforts at making the diagnosis of acute-onset autoimmune hepatitis. Hepatology. 2011;54(1):371–2. author reply 3. Epub 2011/04/01.
38. Duclos-Vallee JC, Ichai P, Samuel D. Autoimmune acute liver failure. Hepatology. 2011;54(1):372–3. author reply 3. Epub 2011/04/06.
39. Santos RG, Alissa F, Reyes J, Teot L, Ameen N. Fulminant hepatic failure: Wilson's disease or autoimmune hepatitis? Implications for transplantation. Pediatr Transplant. 2005;9(1):112–6. Epub 2005/01/26.
40. Stravitz RT, Lefkowitch JH, Fontana RJ, Gershwin ME, Leung PS, Sterling RK, et al. Autoimmune acute liver failure: proposed clinical and histological criteria. Hepatology. 2011;53(2):517–26. Epub 2011/01/29.
41. Hofer H, Oesterreicher C, Wrba F, Ferenci P, Penner E. Centrilobular necrosis in autoimmune hepatitis: a histological feature associated with acute clinical presentation. J Clin Pathol. 2006;59(3):246–9. Epub 2006/03/01.
42. Taylor SA, Whitington PF. Neonatal acute liver failure. Liver Transpl. 2016;22(5):677–85.
43. Rodrigues F, Kallas M, Nash R, Cheeseman P, D'Antiga L, Rela M, et al. Neonatal hemochromatosis--medical treatment vs. transplantation: the King's experience. Liver Transpl. 2005;11(11):1417–24.
44. Whitington PF. Gestational alloimmune liver disease and neonatal hemochromatosis. Semin Liver Dis. 2012;32(4):325–32.
45. Whitington PF, Hibbard JU. High-dose immunoglobulin during pregnancy for recurrent neonatal haemochromatosis. Lancet. 2004;364(9446):1690–8. Epub 2004/11/09.
46. Hegarty R, Hadzic N, Gissen P, Dhawan A. Inherited metabolic disorders presenting as acute liver failure in newborns and young children: King's College Hospital experience. Eur J Pediatr. 2015;174(10):1387–92. Epub 2015/04/24.
47. Reuben A, Koch DG, Lee WM, Acute Liver Failure Study Group. Drug-induced acute liver failure: results of a U.S. multicenter, prospective study. Hepatology. 2010;52(6):2065–76. Epub 2010/10/16.
48. Rajanayagam J, Bishop JR, Lewindon PJ, Evans HM. Paracetamol-associated acute liver failure in Australian and New Zealand children: high rate of medication errors. Arch Dis Child. 2015;100(1):77–80. Epub 2014/09/18.
49. Grabhorn E, Nielsen D, Hillebrand G, Brinkert F, Herden U, Fischer L, et al. Successful outcome of severe Amanita phalloides poisoning in children. Pediatr Transplant. 2013;17(6):550–5. Epub 2013/06/01.
50. Cillo U, Bassanello M, Vitale A, D'Antiga L, Zanus G, Brolese A, et al. Isoniazid-related fulminant hepatic failure in a child: assessment of the native liver's early regeneration after auxiliary partial orthotopic liver transplantation. Transpl Int. 2005;17(11):713–6. Epub 2005/02/18.
51. Alonso EM, Horslen SP, Behrens EM, Doo E. Pediatric acute liver failure of undetermined cause: a research workshop. Hepatology. 2017;65(3):1026–37. Epub 2016/11/20.
52. Chung RT, Stravitz RT, Fontana RJ, Schiodt FV, Mehal WZ, Reddy KR, et al. Pathogenesis of liver injury in acute liver failure. Gastroenterology. 2012;143(3):e1–7. Epub 2012/07/17.
53. Szabo G, Mandrekar P, Dolganiuc A. Innate immune response and hepatic inflammation. Semin Liver Dis. 2007;27(4):339–50.
54. Shubin NJ, Monaghan SF, Ayala A. Anti-inflammatory mechanisms of sepsis. Contrib Microbiol. 2011;17:108–24.
55. Rutherford AE, Hynan LS, Borges CB, Forcione DG, Blackard JT, Lin W, et al. Serum apoptosis markers in acute liver failure: a pilot study. Clin Gastroenterol Hepatol. 2007;5(12):1477–83.
56. Banerjee A, Gerondakis S. Coordinating TLR-activated signaling pathways in cells of the immune system. Immunol Cell Biol. 2007;85(6):420–4.
57. Win S, Than TA, Han D, Petrovic LM, Kaplowitz N. c-Jun N-terminal kinase (JNK)-dependent acute liver injury from acetaminophen or tumor necrosis factor (TNF) requires mitochondrial Sab protein expression in mice. J Biol Chem. 2011;286(40):35071–8.
58. Hanawa N, Shinohara M, Saberi B, Gaarde WA, Han D, Kaplowitz N. Role of JNK translocation to mitochondria leading to inhibition of mitochondria bioenergetics in acetaminophen-induced liver injury. J Biol Chem. 2008;283(20):13565–77.
59. Kubes P, Mehal WZ. Sterile inflammation in the liver. Gastroenterology. 2012;143(5):1158–72.
60. Quaglia A, Portmann BC, Knisely AS, Srinivasan P, Muiesan P, Wendon J, et al. Auxiliary transplantation for acute liver failure: Histopathological study of native liver regeneration. Liver Transpl. 2008;14(10):1437–48. Epub 2008/10/01.
61. Kang LI, Mars WM, Michalopoulos GK. Signals and cells involved in regulating liver regeneration. Cell. 2012;1(4):1261–92.
62. Squires RH Jr. Acute liver failure in children. Semin Liver Dis. 2008;28(2):153–66. Epub 2008/05/03.
63. O'Grady JG, Alexander GJM, Hayllar KM, Williams R. Early indicators of prognosis in fulminant hepatic failure. Gastroenterology. 1989;97(2):439–45.
64. Ng VL, Li R, Loomes KM, Leonis MA, Rudnick DA, Belle SH, et al. Outcomes of children with and without hepatic encephalopathy from the Pediatric Acute Liver Failure Study Group. J Pediatr Gastroenterol Nutr. 2016;63(3):357–64. Epub 2016/07/02.
65. Azhar N, Ziraldo C, Barclay D, Rudnick DA, Squires RH, Vodovotz Y. Analysis of serum inflammatory mediators identifies unique dynamic networks associated with death and spontaneous survival in pediatric acute liver failure. PLoS One. 2013;8(11):e78202.
66. Hussain E, Grimason M, Goldstein J, Smith CM, Alonso E, Whitington PF, et al. EEG abnormalities are associated with increased risk of transplant or poor outcome in children with acute liver failure. J Pediatr Gastroenterol Nutr. 2014;58(4):449–56.
67. Sijens PE, Alkefaji H, Lunsing RJ, van Spronsen FJ, Meiners LC, Oudkerk M, et al. Quantitative multivoxel 1H MR spectroscopy of the brain in children with acute liver failure. Eur Radiol. 2008;18(11):2601–9. Epub 2008/05/22.
68. Srivastava A, Yadav SK, Borkar VV, Yadav A, Yachha SK, Thomas MA, et al. Serial evaluation of children with ALF with advanced MRI, serum proinflammatory cytokines, thiamine, and cognition assessment. J Pediatr Gastroenterol Nutr. 2012;55(5):580–6. Epub 2012/05/23.
69. Squires RH, Dhawan A, Alonso E, Narkewicz MR, Shneider BL, Rodriguez-Baez N, et al. Intravenous N-acetylcysteine in pediatric patients with nonacetaminophen acute liver failure: a placebo-controlled clinical trial. Hepatology. 2013;57(4):1542–9. Epub 2012/08/14.
70. Wendon J, Lee W. Encephalopathy and cerebral edema in the setting of acute liver failure: pathogenesis and management. Neurocrit Care. 2008;9(1):97–102.
71. Stravitz RT, Kramer AH, Davern T, Shaikh AO, Caldwell SH, Mehta RL, et al. Intensive care of patients with acute liver failure: recommendations of the U.S. Acute Liver Failure Study Group. Crit Care Med. 2007;35(11):2498–508.
72. Ozanne B, Nelson J, Cousineau J, Lambert M, Phan V, Mitchell G, et al. Threshold for toxicity from hyperammonemia in critically ill children. J Hepatol. 2012;56(1):123–8.
73. Debray D, Yousef N, Durand P. New management options for end-stage chronic liver disease and acute liver failure: potential for pediatric patients. Paediatr Drugs. 2006;8(1):1–13.
74. Stravitz RT, Gottfried M, Durkalski V, Fontana RJ, Hanje AJ, Koch D, et al. Safety, tolerability, and pharmacokinetics of l-ornithine phenylacetate in patients with acute liver injury/failure and hyperammonemia. Hepatology. 2018;67(3):1003–13.

75. Kamat P, Kunde S, Vos M, Vats A, Gupta N, Heffron T, et al. Invasive intracranial pressure monitoring is a useful adjunct in the management of severe hepatic encephalopathy associated with pediatric acute liver failure. Pediatr Crit Care Med. 2012;13(1):e33–8. Epub 2011/01/26.
76. Kochanek PM, Carney N, Adelson PD, Ashwal S, Bell MJ, Bratton S, et al. Guidelines for the acute medical management of severe traumatic brain injury in infants, children, and adolescents—second edition. Pediatr Crit Care Med. 2012;13(Suppl 1):S1–82.
77. Bernal W, Murphy N, Brown S, Whitehouse T, Bjerring PN, Hauerberg J, et al. A multicentre randomized controlled trial of moderate hypothermia to prevent intracranial hypertension in acute liver failure. J Hepatol. 2016;65(2):273–9.
78. Mpabanzi L, Jalan R. Neurological complications of acute liver failure: pathophysiological basis of current management and emerging therapies. Neurochem Int. 2012;60(7):736–42.
79. Shawcross DL, Wendon JA. The neurological manifestations of acute liver failure. Neurochem Int. 2012;60(7):662–71.
80. Polson J, Lee WM. AASLD position paper: the management of acute liver failure. Hepatology. 2005;41(5):1179–97.
81. Wendon J, Cordoba J, Dhawan A, Larsen FS, Manns M, Samuel D, et al. EASL Clinical Practical Guidelines on the management of acute (fulminant) liver failure. J Hepatol. 2017;66(5):1047–81.
82. Khemani RG, Smith LS, Zimmerman JJ, Erickson S. Pediatric acute respiratory distress syndrome: definition, incidence, and epidemiology: proceedings from the Pediatric Acute Lung Injury Consensus Conference. Pediatr Crit Care Med. 2015;16(5 Suppl 1):S23–40.
83. Kulkarni S, Perez C, Pichardo C, Castillo L, Gagnon M, Beck-Sague C, et al. Use of Pediatric Health Information System database to study the trends in the incidence, management, etiology, and outcomes due to pediatric acute liver failure in the United States from 2008 to 2013. Pediatr Transplant. 2015;19(8):888–95.
84. Fortenberry JD, Paden ML, Goldstein SL. Acute kidney injury in children: an update on diagnosis and treatment. Pediatr Clin North Am. 2013;60(3):669–88.
85. Rodriguez K, Srivaths PR, Tal L, Watson MN, Riley AA, Himes RW, et al. Regional citrate anticoagulation for continuous renal replacement therapy in pediatric patients with liver failure. PLoS One. 2017;12(8):e0182134. Epub 2017/08/10.
86. Agarwal B, Gatt A, Riddell A, Wright G, Chowdary P, Jalan R, et al. Hemostasis in patients with acute kidney injury secondary to acute liver failure. Kidney Int. 2013;84(1):158–63.
87. Stravitz RT, Ellerbe C, Durkalski V, Schilsky M, Fontana RJ, Peterseim C, et al. Bleeding complications in acute liver failure. Hepatology. 2018;67(5):1931–42.
88. Levi M, Levy JH, Andersen HF, Truloff D. Safety of recombinant activated factor VII in randomized clinical trials. N Engl J Med. 2010;363(19):1791–800.
89. Hadzic N, Height S, Ball S, Rela M, Heaton ND, Veys P, et al. Evolution in the management of acute liver failure-associated aplastic anaemia in children: a single centre experience. J Hepatol. 2008;48(1):68–73.
90. Bernal W, Wendon J. Acute liver failure. N Engl J Med. 2013;369(26):2525–34.
91. Godbole G, Shanmugam N, Dhawan A, Verma A. Infectious complications in pediatric acute liver failure. J Pediatr Gastroenterol Nutr. 2011;53(3):320–5. Epub 2011/05/11.
92. Struecker B, Raschzok N, Sauer IM. Liver support strategies: cutting-edge technologies. Nat Rev Gastroenterol Hepatol. 2014;11(3):166–76.
93. Jain V, Dhawan A. Extracorporeal liver support systems in paediatric liver failure. J Pediatr Gastroenterol Nutr. 2017;64(6):855–63.
94. Chen SC, Hewitt WR, Watanabe FD, Eguchi S, Kahaku E, Middleton Y, et al. Clinical experience with a porcine hepatocyte-based liver support system. Int J Artif Organs. 1996;19(11):664–9. Epub 1996/11/01.
95. Horslen SP, Hammel JM, Fristoe LW, Kangas JA, Collier DS, Sudan DL, et al. Extracorporeal liver perfusion using human and pig livers for acute liver failure. Transplantation. 2000;70(10):1472–8. Epub 2000/12/16.
96. Rozga J, Podesta L, LePage E, Morsiani E, Moscioni AD, Hoffman A, et al. A bioartificial liver to treat severe acute liver failure. Ann Surg. 1994;219(5):538–44. discussion 44-6. Epub 1994/05/01.
97. Prokurat S, Grenda R, Lipowski D, Kalicinski P, Migdal M. MARS procedure as a bridge to combined liver-kidney transplantation in severe chromium-copper acute intoxication: a paediatric case report. Liver. 2002;22(Suppl 2):76–7. Epub 2002/09/11.
98. Schaefer B, Schaefer F, Engelmann G, Meyburg J, Heckert KH, Zorn M, et al. Comparison of Molecular Adsorbents Recirculating System (MARS) dialysis with combined plasma exchange and haemodialysis in children with acute liver failure. Nephrol Dial Transplant. 2011;26(11):3633–9. Epub 2011/03/23.
99. Tissieres P, Sasbon JS, Devictor D. Liver support for fulminant hepatic failure: is it time to use the molecular adsorbents recycling system in children? Pediatr Crit Care Med. 2005;6(5):585–91. Epub 2005/09/09.
100. Rodrigues J, Castro SG, Moya B, Fortuna P, Martins A, Pereira JP, et al. Liver depurative techniques: a single liver transplantation center experience. Transplant Proc. 2015;47(4):996–1000.
101. Novelli G, Rossi M, Morabito V, Pugliese F, Ruberto F, Perrella SM, et al. Pediatric acute liver failure with molecular adsorbent recirculating system treatment. Transplant Proc. 2008;40(6):1921–4.
102. Rustom N, Bost M, Cour-Andlauer F, Lachaux A, Brunet AS, Boillot O, et al. Effect of molecular adsorbents recirculating system treatment in children with acute liver failure caused by Wilson disease. J Pediatr Gastroenterol Nutr. 2014;58(2):160–4.
103. Akdogan M, Camci C, Gurakar A, Gilcher R, Alamian S, Wright H, et al. The effect of total plasma exchange on fulminant hepatic failure. J Clin Apher. 2006;21(2):96–9. Epub 2005/09/06.
104. De Palo T, Giordano M, Bellantuono R, Colella V, Troise D, Palumbo F, et al. Therapeutic apheresis in children: experience in a pediatric dialysis center. Int J Artif Organs. 2000;23(12):834–9. Epub 2001/02/24.
105. Sadahiro T, Hirasawa H, Oda S, Shiga H, Nakanishi K, Kitamura N, et al. Usefulness of plasma exchange plus continuous hemodiafiltration to reduce adverse effects associated with plasma exchange in patients with acute liver failure. Crit Care Med. 2001;29(7):1386–92. Epub 2001/07/11.
106. Morgan SM, Zantek ND. Therapeutic plasma exchange for fulminant hepatic failure secondary to Wilson's disease. J Clin Apher. 2012;27(5):282–6. Epub 2012/06/22.
107. Ide K, Muguruma T, Shinohara M, Toida C, Enomoto Y, Matsumoto S, et al. Continuous veno-venous hemodiafiltration and plasma exchange in infantile acute liver failure. Pediatr Crit Care Med. 2015;16(8):e268–74.
108. Baliga P, Alvarez S, Lindblad A, Zeng L, Studies of Pediatric Liver Transplantation Research Group. Posttransplant survival in pediatric fulminant hepatic failure: the SPLIT experience. Liver Transpl. 2004;10(11):1364–71. Epub 2004/10/22.
109. Kasahara M, Umeshita K, Sakamoto S, Fukuda A, Furukawa H, Uemoto S. Liver transplantation for biliary atresia: a systematic review. Pediatr Surg Int. 2017;33(12):1289–95.
110. Jimenez-Rivera C, Nightingale S, Benchimol EI, Mazariegos GV, Ng VL. Outcomes in infants listed for liver transplantation: a retrospective cohort study using the United Network for Organ Sharing database. Pediatr Transplant. 2016;20(7):904–11.
111. Freeman RB Jr, Wiesner RH, Roberts JP, McDiarmid S, Dykstra DM, Merion RM. Improving liver allocation: MELD and PELD. Am J Transplant. 2004;9:114–31.

112. Spada M, Cescon M, Aluffi A, Zambelli M, Guizzetti M, Lucianetti A, et al. Use of extended right grafts from in situ split livers in adult liver transplantation: a comparison with whole-liver transplants. Transplant Proc. 2005;37(2):1164–6.
113. Kasahara M, Sakamoto S, Shigeta T, Uchida H, Hamano I, Kanazawa H, et al. Reducing the thickness of left lateral segment grafts in neonatal living donor liver transplantation. Liver Transpl. 2013;19(2):226–8.
114. Kim JM, Kwon CH, Joh JW, Kang ES, Park JB, Lee JH, et al. ABO-incompatible living donor liver transplantation is suitable in patients without ABO-matched donor. J Hepatol. 2013;59(6):1215–22.
115. Murase K, Chihara Y, Takahashi K, Okamoto S, Segawa H, Fukuda K, et al. Use of noninvasive ventilation for pediatric patients after liver transplantation: decrease in the need for reintubation. Liver Transpl. 2012;18(10):1217–25.
116. Bunn F, Trivedi D. Colloid solutions for fluid resuscitation. Cochrane Database Syst Rev. 2012;13(6).
117. Englesbe MJ, Kelly B, Goss J, Fecteau A, Mitchell J, Andrews W, et al. Reducing pediatric liver transplant complications: a potential roadmap for transplant quality improvement initiatives within North America. Am J Transplant. 2012;12(9):2301–6.
118. Ganschow R, Nolkemper D, Helmke K, Harps E, Commentz JC, Broering DC, et al. Intensive care management after pediatric liver transplantation: a single-center experience. Pediatr Transplant. 2000;4(4):273–9.
119. Nacoti M, Corbella D, Fazzi F, Rapido F, Bonanomi E. Coagulopathy and transfusion therapy in pediatric liver transplantation. World J Gastroenterol. 2016;22(6):2005–23.
120. Colledan M, Andorno E, Valente U, Gridelli B. A new splitting technique for liver grafts. Lancet. 1999;353(9166):1763. https://doi.org/10.1016/S0140-6736(99)00661-3.
121. Razonable RR, Findlay JY, O'Riordan A, Burroughs SG, Ghobrial RM, Agarwal B, et al. Critical care issues in patients after liver transplantation. Liver Transpl. 2011;17(5):511–27.
122. Bolondi G, Mocchegiani F, Montalti R, Nicolini D, Vivarelli M, De Pietri L. Predictive factors of short term outcome after liver transplantation: a review. World J Gastroenterol. 2016;22(26):5936–49.
123. Agopian VG, Petrowsky H, Kaldas FM, Zarrinpar A, Farmer DG, Yersiz H, et al. The evolution of liver transplantation during 3 decades: analysis of 5347 consecutive liver transplants at a single center. Ann Surg. 2013;258(3):409–21.
124. Hardikar W, Poddar U, Chamberlain J, Teo S, Bhat R, Jones B, et al. Evaluation of a post-operative thrombin inhibitor replacement protocol to reduce haemorrhagic and thrombotic complications after paediatric liver transplantation. Thromb Res. 2010;126(3):191–4.
125. Stewart ZA, Locke JE, Segev DL, Dagher NN, Singer AL, Montgomery RA, et al. Increased risk of graft loss from hepatic artery thrombosis after liver transplantation with older donors. Liver Transpl. 2009;15(12):1688–95.
126. Cheng YF, Chen CL, Huang TL, Chen TY, Chen YS, Takatsuki M, et al. Risk factors for intraoperative portal vein thrombosis in pediatric living donor liver transplantation. Clin Transpl. 2004;18(4):390–4.
127. Spada M, Riva S, Maggiore G, Cintorino D, Gridelli B. Pediatric liver transplantation. World J Gastroenterol. 2009;15(6):648–74.
128. Lisman T, Platto M, Meijers JC, Haagsma EB, Colledan M, Porte RJ. The hemostatic status of pediatric recipients of adult liver grafts suggests that plasma levels of hemostatic proteins are not regulated by the liver. Blood. 2011;117(6):2070–2.
129. Mimuro J, Mizuta K, Kawano Y, Hishikawa S, Hamano A, Kashiwakura Y, et al. Impact of acute cellular rejection on coagulation and fibrinolysis biomarkers within the immediate post-operative period in pediatric liver transplantation. Pediatr Transplant. 2010;14(3):369–76.
130. Monagle P, Ignjatovic V, Savoia H. Hemostasis in neonates and children: pitfalls and dilemmas. Blood Rev. 2010;24(2):63–8.
131. Caldwell SH, Hoffman M, Lisman T, Macik BG, Northup PG, Reddy KR, et al. Coagulation disorders and hemostasis in liver disease: pathophysiology and critical assessment of current management. Hepatology. 2006;44(4):1039–46. https://doi.org/10.1002/hep.21303.
132. Kozek-Langenecker SA, Afshari A, Albaladejo P, Santullano CA, De Robertis E, Filipescu DC, et al. Management of severe perioperative bleeding: guidelines from the European Society of Anaesthesiology. Eur J Anaesthesiol. 2013;30(6):270–382.
133. Handschin AE, Weber M, Renner E, Clavien PA. Abdominal compartment syndrome after liver transplantation. Liver Transpl. 2005;11(1):98–100.
134. Sheth J, Sharif K, Lloyd C, Gupte G, Kelly D, de Ville de Goyet J, et al. Staged abdominal closure after small bowel or multivisceral transplantation. Pediatr Transplant. 2012;16(1):36–40.
135. Marseglia A, Ginammi M, Bosisio M, Stroppa P, Colledan M, D'Antiga L. Determinants of large drain losses early after pediatric liver transplantation. Pediatr Transplant. 2017;21(5):17.
136. Tannuri U, Mello ES, Carnevale FC, Santos MM, Gibelli NE, Ayoub AA, et al. Hepatic venous reconstruction in pediatric living-related donor liver transplantation—experience of a single center. Pediatr Transplant. 2005;9(3):293–8.

Part II

Paediatric Liver Transplantation

"For God's sake, save children!"

(Thomas Starzl, 1926–2017)

Precision Medicine in Liver Transplantation

Alastair Baker

Key Points

- Liver transplantation is established as a highly effective treatment for liver diseases and liver-based metabolic diseases.
- The long-term prognosis is improving but still uncertain in the context of a child's lifetime.
- Quality of life over all is better than for chronic liver disease or cancer, similar to other organ transplants but worse than diabetes type 1.
- Quality of life is a professionalised concept that would benefit from patient definition.
- Education and employment achievements are impaired compared with peers.
- Adaptation toward normality is better at home but less good at school and with peer groups.
- Long-term immunosuppression itself may compromise long-term survival.
- Transition and retransplantation carry additional morbidity and mortality.

Research Needed in the Field

- An international registry of metabolic transplants of rare and diverse conditions with information of outcomes including neurodevelopmental status would allow better counselling of families at transplant assessment.
- Current immunosuppression carries risk of severe morbidity and mortality. Long-term tolerance seems a vain expectation. Radically different immunosuppression with lesser risk of organ damage and metabolic syndrome must be sought.
- Understanding chronic graft damage and loss is already being undertaken. Given the risks of retransplantation, we need to understand late graft dysfunction and manage it more effectively.
- Quality of life research based more on patient and family defined outcomes and achievements rather than on deficits would help in clarifying what transplantation can achieve, particularly among adults who underwent transplantation as children.
- Impaired peer socialisation appears to be a barrier to educational achievement, employment and problems with treatment adherence. Research into optimising socialisation from before transplantation may improve long-term outcomes.

25.1 Introduction

The story has been told often, including by the great Tom Starzl himself, how the technical and immunological impediments were overcome by persevering application of scientific endeavour, to take liver transplantation (OLT) from experimentation to its present status: a routine if complex therapy for diverse liver conditions and their complications [1]. It is acknowledged, often from personal experience because the progress has been so rapid, how liver transplantation has steadily improved in outcomes and how various problems such as organ-recipient size relationship and organ availability have been addressed, relative risks have been recognised and accommodated, new indications have been accepted and immunosuppression has been improved. Progress continues, but it is salutary, briefly, to review the present situation for OLT for paediatric patients,

A. Baker (✉)
Paediatric Liver Centre, King's College Hospital, London, UK
e-mail: alastair.baker@nhs.net

for whom the benefits for long-term survival, development, complications and quality of life may be argued to matter most, with the most life in front of them. We can then proceed to consider the peculiar indications, requirements and outcomes of what are now many and diverse indications for OLT, including some without clinical liver disease. We will reflect on what we know of the risks and benefits for the children who receive OLT for these less frequent but important, and sometimes new, indications and consider some challenges.

Transplantation must be recognised as carrying its own chronic morbidity, and it is for children in particular where OLT must be considered a long-term undertaking [2]. It is self-evident that with the complications of transplantation and long-term immunosuppression, patients exchange the natural history and prognosis of their primary condition, usually at the end stages, for the natural history and prognosis of transplantation but at an early stage. The very long-term prognosis of transplantation is not yet clear as will be illustrated later and may change as a result of improvements during children's lives. Comparison of what is known of the natural histories of both the existing disease and the specific application of OLT allows risk-benefit analysis in clinical decisions for OLT. While this process is undertaken more or less explicitly during the discussion process of transplant assessment and listing, it is important that clinicians with knowledge of rare or poorly predictable conditions suffered by patients being considered for transplantation, particularly those not seen frequently by paediatric hepatologists, contribute intimately to the decisions for transplantation. This is especially the case when transplantation incompletely corrects the primary condition or secondary morbidity has accrued that will not be corrected by transplantation. The risk-benefit analysis is further complicated when the benefit is anticipated primarily in terms of quality of life, while the risk could be realised primarily in terms of mortality.

OLT only became genuinely successful in 1981 and has been undertaken in significant numbers of children since the mid-1980s giving just over 30 years total follow-up experience [3]. Paediatric patients account for about 12.5% of liver transplant recipients and have different indications, management requirements and outcomes to adults. Early belief from the 1980s was that the condition of the recipient scarcely impacted on the short-term outcome so that patients were often referred in poor condition, a misconception that was gradually corrected, so improving results. Technical aspects of transplantation, quality of immunosuppression and organ sourcing and availability have improved steadily over the years. Indications have broadened meanwhile. There have never been sufficient numbers of ideal organs, due to increasing referrals and new indications more than keeping place with investment in necessary resources. Paediatric transplant programmes have tended to be small. In addition, different OLT services have developed with particular referral arrangements and some differences in clinical practices. Children develop, progress through education, undergo adolescence and seek employment as adults, changes that occur over up to 25 years, and themselves have a complex reciprocal effect on outcomes. Large international data sets have been collected prospectively for liver transplantation but lack the granularity to drill down on personal influences on prognosis [4]. These conditions of evolution of services and outcomes, diverse pathologies and practice, small cohort numbers, rapid changes in the treatment and the development of the individuals receiving it limit the quality of our current data for predicting long-term prognosis. However, with those constraints in mind, we should consider what liver transplantation currently offers children who need it.

25.1.1 The Profile of Diagnoses Referred to Transplant Units

Units tend to have their own profile of referral diagnoses based on their referral geography and clinical relationships and the reputations and expertise that have developed. The diagnoses of patients listed for transplantation in a typical paediatric OLT unit are represented in Fig. 25.1. Biliary atresia is the commonest indication for transplantation in all paediatric programmes, as it is the commonest reason for chronic liver failure in children, but it is represented relatively less at KCH than shown here because of increased representation of other indications. Acute liver failure has been traditionally strongly represented at KCH, as have metabolic diseases particularly organic acidaemias for which we have had good outcomes justifying willingness to accept them. Metabolic conditions without chronic liver disease such as Crigler-Najjar type 1, coagulation factor 7 deficiency and some urea cycle disorders may be managed well by auxiliary transplant leading to increased referrals to our centre. The availability of intestinal transplantation may lead to patients with marginal gut receiving liver transplantation alone. Larger programmes may be able to accommodate a proportion of patients of higher or unknown risk, more readily allowing innovation. Older programmes may see more patients coming to retransplant due to graft loss over time. An active co-located renal transplant programme may mean more patients referred for combined transplantation. Figures 25.1 and 25.2 show the most common indications and ages in paediatric liver transplantation.

25 Precision Medicine in Liver Transplantation

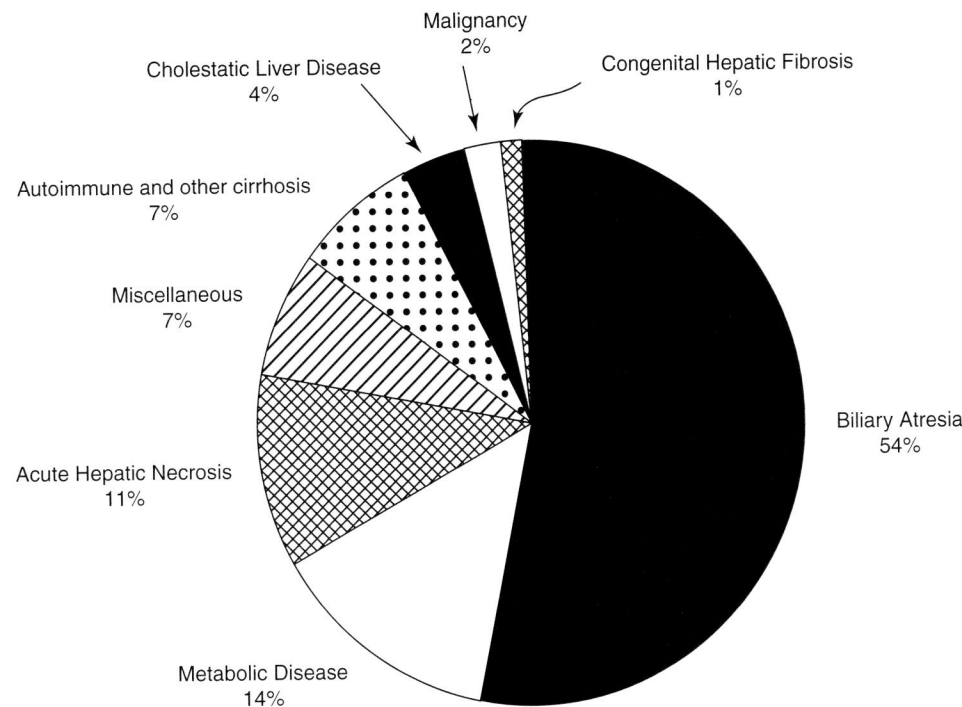

Fig. 25.1 A generic profile of diagnoses of patients receiving liver transplantation at a paediatric transplant unit. Biliary atresia is generally the commonest single diagnosis in most such units at 40% or more. Acute hepatic necrosis represents all forms of acute and acute on chronic liver failure

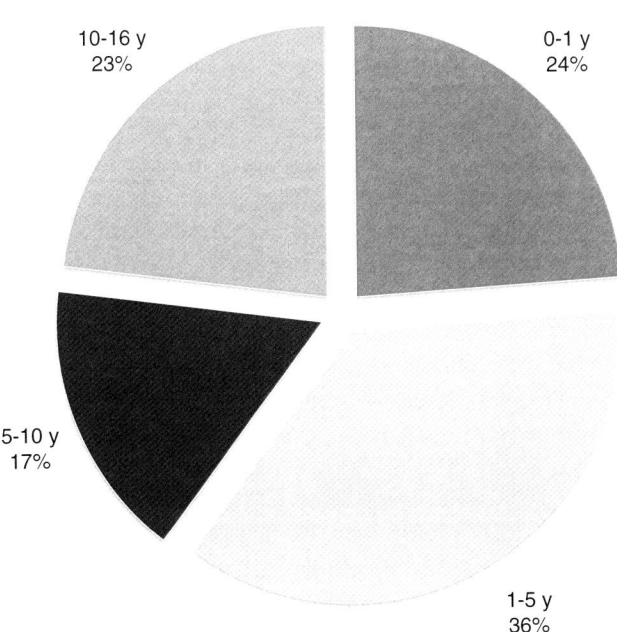

Fig. 25.2 The proportions of patients receiving liver transplantation by age in a paediatric transplant unit. Mean age at operation was 4 years (5 days–16 years). The majority will receive reduced or split organs from an adult donor

25.2 Current Survival After OLT

In considering the risk-benefit balance of OLT, the long-term outcomes bear consideration. For example, overall patient and graft survival rates reported in 2018 for 806 US children at 5, 10 and 20 years with a typical spectrum of indications were 81%, 78%, and 69% and 67%, 63% and 53%, respectively, while among 128 consecutive children who underwent cadaveric transplantation in France from 1988 to 1993 patient survival rates recorded at 5, 10 and 20 years were 84%, 82% and 79%, and graft survival rates were 73%, 72% and 65% [5, 6]. Transplant nephropathy stage 2 or more was present in one third of the French patients, pointing to significant morbidity for the even longer term. We will consider transition later, but data from Birmingham UK showed 12 deaths among 137 patients (8.8%) and 5 retransplants while under transition to adult services, believed to be related mostly to non-adherence with medication. After transition was complete, 10-year patient and graft survival for the ensuing period was 89.9% and 86.2%, respectively [7]. National adult data from the UK showed adult 5-year survival is 80%, evidence that adults and children suffer similar medium-term post-transplant attenuation [4]. Outcomes are improving so that 20-year survival will undoubtedly be better in 10 years, but the side effects of current immunosuppressives with nephropathy and features similar to metabolic syndrome imply that a normal population life expectancy is unlikely to be achievable for the majority with current therapeutic strategies.

25.2.1 Graft Prognosis

As illustrated above, graft survival is consistently 10–15% below patient survival with the difference increasing gradually during the follow-up period, representing retransplantation from continuous low-level graft loss. Immunological processes and imperfections of bile and blood flow probably contribute to graft attrition. While hepatocytes appear resistant to ageing, they are affected by replicative senescence and stress-related senescence, both probably exacerbated by OLT [8]. Even when children appear clinically well with normal graft function, histological abnormalities are commonly seen in late post-transplant protocol biopsies that may progress and lead to graft loss. A high frequency of unexplained chronic hepatitis in late post-transplant biopsies from children is associated with the development of graft fibrosis and cirrhosis [9]. This phenomenon is replacing the characteristic chronic or ductopenic rejection that historically accounted for later graft loss. Adolescents in particular may be more prone to developing late rejection possibly related to immunosuppression non-adherence or perhaps the developmental strength of their immune system. Children's liver diseases recur infrequently in their grafts compared with adults'. De novo auto-immune hepatitis occurs in up to 10% of children probably also representing a hepatitic form of late rejection and responding to treatment with increased immunosuppression. The relationship of late hepatitic graft dysfunction to antibody-mediated rejection is currently a matter for debate as is the question of graft senescence.

25.2.2 Quality of Life (QoL) After OLT

Raw patient and graft survival might be seen as the picture frame within which we can hope to appreciate the individual portrait and collective landscape of patients' experienced outcomes of transplantation. The paediatric patients and ultimately the adults with liver transplants into whom they develop have the most to gain from OLT in the quality of their daily life, which has become an increasing clinical emphasis since OLT began to anticipate good medium-term survival. However, quality of life is by its nature an extremely difficult concept to define and is even harder still to make comparisons between two individuals or between the outcome for a single individual and the opportunity costs of the choice of a line of irreversible management. It varies with perception, with external influences and circumstances and with individual constitutional tendencies as well as habituation and expectations. Qualitative information inherently defies being converted to numbers or classifications. Group assessments of QoL outcomes, in order to predict the outcome on embarking on treatment for an individual, have value, but understanding of the predictive variables is weak and their interactions highly complex. Our insights into QoL gained from clinical interactions and biased by our own incomplete knowledge of patients and families can be misleading for individuals and for many reasons simply asking about QoL in consultations only helps a little, although of course it is mandatory.

Two longitudinal and 23 cross-sectional studies were reviewed reporting various measures. The most common indication for OLT was biliary atresia. Median age was 8 or above in all except one study illustrating the added difficulty of assessing small children for QoL. Domain scores were lowest in school functioning and physical functioning scores and most consistently normal in family functioning. Admissions, operations, short stature, medicine adherence, family function and sleep disturbance, particularly associated with fatigue, have been variously associated with effects on QoL. Height growth typically matters more to boys, and it has more effect on their life opportunities. In 101 survivors of 128 paediatric OLT followed for over 20 years, final height was below the target height in 37 patients, but final height was within the normal range for most patients. There were some consistent differences between questionnaire methodologies: The general health perception domain was the lowest of all domain scores when included. Disease-specific questionnaires have the advantage of offering greater sensitivity and specificity with lower total scores on the disease-specific tool when employed simultaneously with general health tools. Children with a genetic-metabolic disease performed worse than the other diagnoses. The strongest relationship was shown between height at OLT and verbal comprehension, perceptual reasoning, working memory and total IQ. The results suggest a consequence of primary diagnosis and nutritional impairment on children's long-term cognitive performance [6, 10].

Health-related QoL in paediatric OLT recipients is lower than healthy controls, but there were no significant differences noted in PedsQL scores between OLT recipients and renal or cardiac transplant recipients. Compared with type 1 diabetes patients, two studies reported significantly lower domain scores in paediatric OLT patients but higher than patients with childhood cancer. QoL was significantly better in 20-year survivors than in patients with chronic liver disease, congestive heart failure or diabetes.

A longitudinal study found infant QoL scores increased steadily 1 year after OLT in sub-scales except global mental health. Liver transplant recipients showed twice more "serious delays" (IQ < 70) compared to a control group (9.4% vs. 4.7%). HRQoL is also known to be poorer in patients transplanted at an older age and at the other end of the age scale, and lower physical function and physical component summary scores were seen in over-10-year OLT survivors, while among 20-year survivors, one study showed very good self-reported QoL, while another described lower role physical, general health, social functioning, mental health and summary scores [11].

More young liver transplantation recipients than expected are at increased risk for lasting cognitive and academic deficits with implications for educational attainment. One hundred and forty-four patients tested 2 years after OLT occurring at age 5–6 years were retested at age 7–9 years. More participants than expected had below-average IQ, verbal comprehension, working memory and mental arithmetic skills, as well as deficits on teacher Behaviour Rating Inventory of Executive Function. At 7–9 years, 42% of children had received some sort of special education. Fourteen percent had a previous diagnosis of attention-deficit/hyperactivity disorder, while 5% required hearing aids. Pre-transplant markers of nutritional status and operative complications predicted outcome. Among OLT survivors with below-average functioning, deficits tend to remain mostly static after the initial recovery period, in contrast to patterns of early recovery in head injury or deterioration of late cancer effects. In summary long-term liver transplant survivors exhibit fixed difficulties in executive function and are more likely to have attention-deficit/hyperactivity disorder despite stable and relatively maintained intellect and cognition [11–13].

In-depth interviews with 27 of the now-adult survivors of the pioneer cohort of children receiving liver transplants in Britain in the early 1980s and 1990s explored how childhood identities were shaped at home by parents, with survival the current goal. Their body and therapies applied to it were interpreted mechanistically, while the children were simultaneously trying to be normal despite a serious illness. In hospital they felt normal in being the same as other children, yet at school the differences between their own interpretation of normal and that of others caused most tension which was represented in their narratives and sense of identity. These interviews revealed a helpful frame through which to consider the relationship between healthcare and society and the consequences for the social development of patients with chronic illnesses [14].

The extent of economic independence and employment attainment of this pioneering OLT cohort remain to be determined as much as their long-term survival. After OLT, 34% of paediatric recipients married, and 79% remained married at 20 years follow-up. Meanwhile, functional outcomes are extremely important in transplant recipients. Many families care about school performance for their children after OLT as much as graft function, and of course both need to be achieved. Thus, the picture of the prognosis has yet to develop full detail and depth of focus, but as patients' specific needs become clearer, the necessary social and educational support required to develop their future are more evident. Having invested in their survival, we should be making every effort to provide the necessary resources [15].

25.2.3 The Effect of Indications on Survival/Complications

Acute liver failure (ALF) is dealt with elsewhere. However certain aspects pertaining to the decision for transplantation bear comparison to other diagnoses leading to OLT, in particular the risk-benefit analysis related to the prognosis.

Most causes of ALF are potentially recoverable if liver regeneration were to occur before the patient died of complications of liver failure. Good intensive care can reduce the risk of mortality related to complications, with the risk of mortality being dependent on primary diagnosis. The decision for transplantation is justified when the expected outcome of transplantation is better than the expected outcome of conservative management of ALF. The implications of this comparison are that firstly intensive care must be as good as possible, also to prolong the time to make a transplant organ available, and secondly that all efforts should be made to get a correct diagnosis for ALF since it may change the prognosis both for spontaneous recovery (e.g. Mitochondrial disorders, Walcott-Rallinson syndrome, LARS) and disease progression despite transplantation (also mitochondrial disorders, X-Linked lymphoproliferative disease, giant cell hepatitis, malignancies) [16–24]. Thirdly, a prognostic scoring system should take account of the current risk to the patient of the clinical condition of the ALF and the diagnosis. Various scoring systems are in use including for NonA-NonE ALF, paracetamol hepatotoxicity and Wilson disease [25]. They are discussed elsewhere in this book. None are perfectly sensitive and specific predictors of mortality.

In considering the risk-benefit balance of OLT versus acute management, a specific diagnosis and implied prognosis may not be available at the time of decision-making. For currently cryptogenic liver failure, the timescale of the natural history of the condition described for adults as subacute, acute and hyperacute helps in predicting the outcome. Acute liver failure equates most nearly to fulminant hepatic failure (FHF) described by Trey and Davidson, although children manifest encephalopathy less readily than adults. The paediatric prognostic markers currently used for ALF at KCH are shown elsewhere, but INR > 4 is taken as the major predictor. Hyperacute liver failure manifests over a shorter timescale typified by shock hepatopathy, acute paracetamol toxicity and Amanita poisoning and is only rarely cryptogenic. Subacute hepatic failure (SHF) is typified by the course of Wilson disease and auto-immune hepatitis with liver failure evident more than 8 weeks after onset of symptoms. Coagulopathy may be indolent, but encephalopathy is ominous in SHF.

Neonatal acute liver failure (ALF) is recognised to have a worse prognosis than ALF for older children, partly because various metabolic conditions presenting with ALF have a poor prognosis, because of poorer availability of smaller organs and because of the demanding technical requirements of OLT in small infants. Neonatal haemochromatosis is the most common identifiable cause of ALF in neonates. Among 38 patients who received OLT, 1- and 5-year patient survival were 84.2% and 81.6% and graft survival were 71.1% and

68.4%, respectively. There is no specific prognostic system for determining OLT in the first weeks of life, but it is essential to exclude conditions with an overall poor outcome, such as lysosomal storage disorders, and haemophagocytic lymphohistiocytosis. Infants appear resistant to the features of encephalopathy yet may still suffer long-term consequences. We have used the prognostic score developed for older children with knowledge that prognosis tends to be worse in newborns and infants [19, 20].

25.3 Practical Aspects Before and After OLT

25.3.1 Transplant Assessment

Assessment for OLT has two simultaneous roles: Firstly, to evaluate the risk-benefit balance of providing transplantation as implied above and secondly to agree to proceed to OLT with benefit exceeding risk, while providing the patient and caregivers with sufficient information that they can make an informed decision to proceed to OLT when an organ becomes available. Clearly the former requires an understanding of the circumstances of the patient beyond those of a generic patient with life-threatening liver disease. If there is significant delay while on the transplant list, repeat and considered re-evaluation must be undertaken to anticipate possible deterioration, recognising increasing morbidity that may occur with prolonged list waiting times. Some of the aspects that require attention at OLT assessment are considered beneath.

25.3.2 Exclusion of Severe Systemic and Potentially Recurrent Diseases

The correct primary diagnosis is extremely important, yet patients may present with severe liver disease requiring transplantation when a definite diagnosis is not possible. Reasons include severity of illness precluding investigations, limited time available before deterioration, liver disease obscuring features of metabolic disease or metabolic diseases being asymptomatic between crises. After OLT, patients may then develop unforeseen complications of the primary illness such as severe neurological features, e.g. in lysosomal storage disorders such as Niemann-Pick C disease (but not B disease), or severe recurrent disease such as Giant Cell hepatitis with Coombs positive haemolytic anaemia. With the advent of precision medicine, many of these situations may be avoided when results can be reported in a timely manner for clinical decision-making. Meanwhile, very occasionally patients receive OLT which might appear, with the benefit of hindsight, to have been an error [23, 24].

25.3.3 Planning OLT and Anticipating Complications

Pre-existing complications of liver disease are recognised to be associated with specific peri-transplant problems. Anticipating their occurrence usually reduces their consequences.

Rapid electrolyte changes resulting in central pontine myelinolysis or osmotic demyelination syndrome are associated with entering OLT with severe hyponatraemia and overly rapid plasma level correction. The hyponatraemia is often in part due to sodium restriction to control oedema in severely decompensated liver disease. Fatality is possible, but considerable recovery from the CNS injury of lesser episodes is also possible in children. Electrolyte management becomes progressively more critical as liver disease becomes more severe [26].

Relative polycythaemia with packed cell volume (PCV) above 0.35 has an association with hepatic artery thrombosis with small donor and recipient arteries. The problem may be alleviated by dilution venesections. Patients with massive hypersplenism may 'autotransfuse' themselves as their portal pressure normalises early after OLT when several sequential venesections may be necessary to control PCV [27].

Patients with prolonged metabolic bone disease, related to liver disease typically of cholestatic aetiology and with refractory or overlooked rickets, can suffer respiratory complications from a highly compliant thoracic cage. Some are driven to metabolic correction in the first days after OLT as the liver causes hypoparathyroidism with hypophosphataemia and hypocalcaemia known as 'hungry bone syndrome' [28].

The commonest indication for transplantation in children is biliary atresia. Patients have end-stage liver disease with cholestasis and portal hypertension having had extensive abdominal surgery at Kasai operation. Portal collaterals form through peritoneal adhesions requiring meticulous division at OLT that inevitably leaves surfaces without mucous membrane cover and with divided lymphatics. Portal hypertension may not settle rapidly from preservation effects on the liver or a small-for-size graft so that high exudative drain losses can be a problem needing high-volume plasma replacement. Interpretation of liver and renal function may be compromised by dilution from such losses. When the lymphatics are interrupted, chylous ascites may follow introduction of lipid-containing feeds. Medium-chain triglyceride-based feeds, e.g. Monogen (Nutricia), given for 2 weeks with a very low fat diet reliably solve this problem.

The procedure of dissecting adhesions during hepatectomy at OLT following previous abdominal surgery, particularly in patients with poor nutritional state, risks early GI perforation which may be difficult to detect in patients receiving steroids. CMV infection can be associated with perforation. A high index of suspicion for early laparotomy is appropriate.

Toxic liver syndrome and auxiliary OLT for ALF. Auxiliary OLT for acute liver failure is associated with a persistent SIRS-like phenomenon related to inflammation continuing in the remaining failing liver lobe. Patients continue to have fevers, raised inflammatory markers and other general features of infection. Broad spectrum antibiotics and antifungals are given although evidence of specific organisms is often not forthcoming. The episode settles eventually when recovery of the native liver occurs so long as the correct decision for auxiliary OLT has been made.

25.3.4 Planning Tailored Immunosuppression

The concept of 'tailored immunosuppression' whereby a combination of immunosuppressive medications and their doses and levels are selected in anticipation of their benefits and side effects including in the long term is a helpful one.

Patients with renal glomerulopathy or tubulopathy should be allocated a renal-sparing regime. The one we currently use requires Basiliximab at day 1 and 4, introduction of mycophenolate mofetil (MMF) as soon as feeding is possible and low levels of tacrolimus from 3 months or before. Occasionally, tacrolimus is replaced with Sirolimus after 3 months for worsening renal dysfunction.

A low- or nonsteroid regimen may be indicated by diabetes mellitus, poor height growth, severe metabolic bone disease or hypertension. Azathioprine or MMF are introduced with the introduction of feeding and prednisolone tapered and stopped. Patients with auto-immune liver disease generally maintain a higher prednisolone regimen also with azathioprine or MMF but lower tacrolimus levels from 3 months or before.

Immunological imbalance is seen from immunosuppression, generally more often from tacrolimus including de novo autoimmune hepatitis, eosinophilic GI disease, eczema and even Guillain-Barre syndrome. Tacrolimus must be reduced or even withdrawn, and a course of increased steroids may be beneficial and immunosuppression rebalanced based on azathioprine or MMF.

Cytopaenia is seen following chemotherapy, in severe hypersplenism and as a side effect of azathioprine or MMF but also occasionally tacrolimus. Such patients may benefit from cyclosporin A in preference.

The side effects of the various immunosuppression agents for OLT, hypertension, glucose intolerance, hyperlipidaemia, nephropathy, fatty liver and weight gain have a common resemblance to metabolic syndrome. These features are associated with reduced telomere length in peripheral lymphocytes suggesting senescence. An important future challenge, especially for OLT patients genetically at risk of the consequences of metabolic syndrome will be the choice of a combination of medicines that avoid the life-shortening consequences of the current first-line treatments [29].

25.4 Specific Liver Conditions

25.4.1 Cholangiopathies and Cholestatic Disorders

As the commonest indication for OLT in children, Biliary Atresia represents the archetype against which peculiarities are considered. Nevertheless syndromic associations are seen in up to 20% of patients. Of particular relevance are hepato-pulmonary syndrome, which is considered below, and congenital cardiac anomalies. Minor cardiac anomalies are compatible with uncomplicated OLT, but major defects with atrial, ventricular or outflow tract shunts have the possibility of major right to left shunting or cardiac failure during reperfusion at OLT. Open heart surgery on bypass is poorly tolerated by patients with cirrhosis, so that late cardiac repair is contraindicated. We have required full cardiac repair *before* Kasai porto-enterostomy so that if the patient proceeds to OLT cardiac function is effectively normal. However, OLT in patients with a single ventricle has been achieved successfully [30].

Alagille syndrome (ALGS). Indications for OLT in ALGS are more frequently quality of life related such as pruritus, poor growth and metabolic bone disease than the complications of cirrhosis. Meanwhile, the risks of repercussion at OLT to the graft and patient are increased with increased right-sided heart pressures seen with peripheral pulmonary artery stenosis. The risk-benefit equation must therefore be assessed in detail for each patient. We have used a MRI catheter under dobutamine challenge to mimic transplant repercussion and assess the possible effects on the new graft, since when we have not incurred perioperative deaths but have declined a small number of patients. Cardiac index must be able to increase by 40% under 20 mg/kg/min dobutamine without increasing right ventricular pressure to more than 50% of left ventricular/aortic pressure [31].

About 30% of ALGS patients will have renal abnormalities. The commonest and most insidious form is renal tubular acidosis. Patients are at increased risk of immunosuppressive nephropathy and particularly electrolyte and pH imbalances. We have employed an early renal-sparing immunosuppressive regime as tailored immunosuppression for all ALGS patients.

Some ALGS patients have been shown to have a pro-inflammatory immune dysregulation. However this appears not to be a clinical problem in the ALGS cohorts after OLT, who have good survival outcomes comparable to biliary atresia [32].

Caroli disease is the extreme manifestation of the ductal plate malformation of congenital hepatic fibrosis (CHF). It predisposes to impaired bile flow with secondary biliary damage compared with CHF. Patients tend to come to liver transplantation in combination with renal transplantation for autosomal recessive polycystic kidney disease. However adult Caroli disease has a better OLT outcome than other adult biliary diseases such as PBC, PSC and secondary biliary cirrhosis with patient and allograft survivals at 10 years of 77.8% and 67.9%, respectively [33, 34].

25.4.1.1 PFIC Variants

PFIC1 is a whole-body condition resulting in defects in transmembrane transporters in many tissues including the GI tract, pancreas and kidney. OLT is often considered for poor quality of life especially related to pruritus and poor growth. Graft dysfunction with persistent steatosis occurs soon after transplantation often with diarrhoea, presumably due to an existing imbalance in bile acid trafficking at intestinal level being exposed by hepatic bile flow. Patients still do not grow well. Quality of life may not be alleviated greatly by OLT.

BSEP deficiency. The bile salt export pump is found on the basolateral hepatocyte membrane where it is normally exposed to surveillance by the immune system. Patients who have never expressed immunologically recognisable protein in the anatomically correct position are at risk of developing alloantibodies after transplantation that block BSEP function leading to a clinical phenotype similar to the original disease with low plasma gGT and pruritus. Increased immunosuppression reduces the alloantibodies. We have preferentially used B cell-targeted treatment based on antibodies, rituximab, MMF and, if necessary, Sirolimus to a good effect.

25.4.2 Cystic Fibrosis

While cystic fibrosis (CF) is a common condition in developed countries, and evidence of liver disease is relatively common among its sufferers, progression to end-stage liver disease is uncommon, and liver transplantation is precluded by other CF complications among some of those who could otherwise benefit. The characteristic features of CF LD and its natural history are illustrated in Fig. 25.3 with portal hypertension (PHT) associated with varices and hypersplenism as the commonest liver-related complications.

Indications for OLT focus predominantly poor synthetic function (albumin <30 g/L, jaundice), liver decompensation with ascites or encephalopathy, spontaneous bacterial peritonitis, intractable malnutrition and hepato-pulmonary syndrome, but not other complications of PHT. Contraindications are particularly focused on impaired respiratory function when intensive treatment should be able to achieve results of at least 50% of predicted for height and age and infection or colonisation with highly resistant organisms such as *Mycobacterium abscessus*, *Aspergillus* and *Pseudomonas* Sp. Renal function in CF is often impaired more than recognised so that a measured GFR is required of over 50 mL/min/1.73 m². Impaired glucose tolerance is not a contraindi-

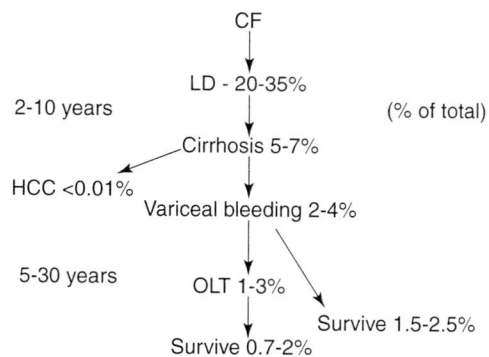

Fig. 25.3 The characteristic features of CF LD and its natural history. Portal hypertension (PHT) associated with varices and hypersplenism are the commonest liver-related complications

cation by itself as it may improve after OLT with improved nutrition, and a pancreas may be transplanted simultaneously with the liver if glucose intolerance is more severe. Respiratory function has been shown to improve after OLT probably due to improved muscle function from better nutrition.

While the co-morbidities of CF tend to increase the short term complications so increasing duration of the hospital stay, medium term results are good with 5 year survival 70–100%, and no difference if a pancreas is also transplanted. Patients who received a liver but not a pancreas were at risk of developing diabetes mellitus, while those receiving a pancreas also did not develop diabetes and complications were low. A low threshold for transplanting a pancreas with a liver seems appropriate (Table 25.1). Results of multi-organ transplantation for CF however are poor (with one series exception) giving perhaps 30% survival approximated from the various small series. Cystic fibrosis is not a common indication for liver transplantation, and the decision to proceed is often complex because of comorbidities. Nevertheless careful patient selection and judicious timing of transplantation can yield good medium-term results [35–44].

25.4.3 Tumours

The key to long-term survival in hepatocellular malignancies is recognised to be removal of the complete primary tumour, particularly for hepatoblastoma but also rhabdomyosarcoma and rare chemosensitive pancreaticoblastomas. Following OLT typically two cycles of chemotherapy are retained for eradication of residual or chance micro-dissemination at the time of surgery. Unfortunately, some tumours either do not

Table 25.1 Citations for transplantation in adults and children with cystic fibrosis (CF) showing survival rates and duration

Ref	Number	Duration FU	Survival %	Notes
Noble-Jamieson [35]	11	5.5 years	75	2 adults
Mieles [36]	9	Up to 4 years	78	5 adults
Lamireau [37]	5	8 years	60	2 adults
Milkiewicz [39]	7	1 years	100	20% survival for 3 organs
Fridell [40]	12	5	75	
Nash [41]	12	5 years	37.5	Triple
Nash [41]	19	4 years	85	Liver
Mekeel [43]	9	5 years	100	3 liver and pancreas
Mendizabal [44]	148	5 years	85.8	UNOS data children
Mendizabal [44]	55	5 years	72.7	UNOS data adults

While the comorbidities of CF tend to increase the short-term complications increasing duration of the hospital stay, medium-term results are good with 5-year survival 70–100% and no difference if a pancreas is also transplanted. Transplantation of the lungs in particular worsens prognosis considerably

retract anatomically completely under chemotherapy or retract such that simple complete resection is not possible. For these patients OLT offers the probability of cure. Results show 90% + 5-year survival. Live-related transplantation works well for such patients because the timescale window between cycles of chemotherapy is limited and further cycles are likely to increase toxicity. The bone marrow and renal effects of the various chemotherapy regimes require early tailoring of the immunosuppressive regimes. Management of neutropenia after OLT with GCSF can increase the risk of rejection [45, 46].

25.4.3.1 Non-Malignant Tumours of the Liver

Non-malignant tumours are rarely an indication for OLT, but there are important exceptions when either local effects, mass effects or haemodynamic effects may be inaccessible or refractory to other medical and surgical management. Examples are:

Haemangioendothelioma. Such tumours are usually seen in early infancy when they may present with rapid growth in the first weeks after birth. At that time they may exhibit a shunt effect with arteriovenous connections allowing arteriovenous high-output cardiac failure. An alternative form of presentation is with a sump-like trapping of cellular blood components known as Kasabach-Merritt syndrome. This effect may lead to rapid growth in size of the liver and abdominal compartment syndrome. The lesions tend to involute spontaneously in 1–4 years but with risk of mortality meanwhile in the worst cases. Recent conventional treatment consists sequentially of propranolol, arterial embolisation, hepatic artery ligation and partial hepatectomy. Liver transplantation can remove the space-occupying and haemodynamic effects in severely life-threatening circumstances.

Langerhans cell histiocytosis is a low-grade invasive malignant condition with a predilection for the skin, flat bones, brain, lung, liver and biliary system and with a tendency to 'burn itself out'. Treatment is based on low-toxicity chemotherapy and immunotherapy, being orientated to controlling active disease rather than rapid elimination. The biliary disease tends to leave a cholangiopathy on attaining remission leading to secondary biliary cirrhosis with profound cholestasis and associated complications. If the primary disease is not in complete remission, it may recur in the transplanted organ. Patients are at increased risk of post-transplant lymphoproliferative disease probably due to the total effect of immunosuppression they have been given for the primary disease and the transplant.

Budd-Chiari syndrome (BCS) is a rare indication for OLT as a last resort rescue treatment. Paediatric patients can benefit despite the complexity of management leading to OLT. In adults, the aetiology of the procoagulant condition leading to hepatic venous thrombosis seems not to affect the prognosis. JAK2 mutations are a frequent cause of BCS in children. Ruxolitinib, a novel-JAK-2 inhibitor, may improve outlook and reduce the need for OLT in BCS [47–49].

25.4.4 Metabolic Diseases

Liver-related inborn errors of metabolism are conventionally divided into those that primarily cause cirrhosis, those that do not cause liver disease but where the defective gene product is entirely or effectively entirely confined to the liver and those where the gene product is distributed throughout the body but with a significant proportion in the liver. The significance for OLT is that for the first group the decision for OLT is based on the development of cirrhosis and its complications, and these patients have historically been the majority with metabolic diseases requiring OLT. In the second group, the decision is based on the risk of extrahepatic complications with the expectation of effective cure of the primary disease. In the third group of diseases, full cure cannot be expected, but the enzyme capacity of the liver acts as a 'buffer' against accumulation of toxic metabolites and the effects of metabolic crises. Those without liver disease may be suitable for domino liver donation. In the latter two groups, the question of anticipated quality of life colours the decision for OLT, and these patients are increasingly being considered as candidates. The risk-benefit calculation including taking into consideration long-term survival versus short-term quality of life is often very complicated and would be helped if we knew more about long-term prognosis.

Five- and 20-year survival rates for 74 paediatric patients for diverse metabolic diseases were 89 and 77%, with paediatric results superior to adults and similar to other indications for paediatric OLT. However, the long-term prognosis for neurodevelopment after OLT of some of the conditions described is unknown and likely to be inferior to transplantation for conditions such as the benchmark, biliary atresia. It is therefore possible that in benefitting from OLT, a cohort of patients with significant ongoing long-term social care needs will require special provision during transition and as adults [50, 51].

Alpha-1 antitrypsin deficiency (α1ATD) is the commonest metabolic disease complicated by cirrhosis, requiring OLT in childhood. The factors for more rapid deterioration in a minority are unclear, but those that remain jaundiced after neonatal hepatitis progress almost as rapidly as a failed Kasai for biliary atresia to biliary cirrhosis and soon need OLT. Those who clear the jaundice but continue to suffer chronic hepatitis with fluctuating transaminases and particularly with biliary features on liver biopsy tend to develop cirrhosis and portal hypertension. While these patients may remain remarkably well and stable for years, onset of jaundice, ascites or spontaneous bacterial peritonitis heralds rapid deterioration mandating OLT [52, 53].

Patients with PIZ A-1-ATD are known to be at risk of IgA nephropathy associated with hypertension and increased risk of immunosuppression-related nephropathy after OLT. Renal assessment at OLT assessment and a tailored renal-sparing immunosuppressive regimen if indicated are required. We recorded a heterozygous (PiMZ) alpha 1 antitrypsin (α1AT) living-related donor liver in a homozygous (PiZ) child that was complicated by massive ascites early after transplant and died [54].

Recommendations for paediatric transplantation for Wilson disease (WD) have yet to achieve evidence-based guidelines, although consensus is forming for overall management. Transplantation may be indicated for acute liver failure, subacute liver failure, decompensated liver disease and possibly neurological WD. Medical therapy is effective for most patients, and OLT can rescue those with acute liver failure or with advanced liver disease refractory to medical therapy. However, the response Ito penicillamine in subacute liver failure and chronic liver disease may be gradual making the decision prolonged and difficult. The decision for OLT can be supported by the revised WD scoring system (Table 25.2) with hepatic encephalopathy a strong additional

Table 25.2 The revised Wilson disease (WD) scoring system for children based on serum bilirubin, international normalised ratio, aspartate aminotransferase (AST) and white cell count (WCC) at presentation identified a cutoff score of 11 for death and proved to be 93% sensitive and 98% specific, with a positive predictive value of 88%

Prognostic score	Bilirubin (μmol/L)	INR	AST (IU/L)	WCC (109/L)
0	0–100	0–1.29	0–100	0–6.7
1	101–150	1.3–1.6	101–150	6.8–8.3
2	151–200	1.7–1.9	151–300	8.4–10.3
3	201–300	2.0–2.4	301–400	10.4–15.3
4	>301	>2.5	>401	>15.4

adverse predictor. The revised WD scoring system for children based on serum bilirubin, international normalised ratio, aspartate aminotransferase (AST) and white cell count (WCC) at presentation identified a cutoff score of 11 for death and proved to be 93% sensitive and 98% specific, with a positive predictive value of 88% [25, 55].

Two adult patients transplanted due to progressive neurological impairment only despite optimal WD treatment had pre-OLT Modified Rankin Debility Score (MRDS) of 4 compared to 3 and 2, respectively, post OLT. (Grade 0 MRDS is no handicap; grade 1 is minor symptoms that do not interfere with lifestyle extending to grade 5, severe handicap, totally dependent, requiring constant attention day and night). WD neurological disease neurological status is refractory to optimal conservative management [56].

Glycogen storage disease type IV is very rare and unlike other GSDs associated with rapid hepatic cirrhosis. Skeletal and cardiomyopathy with uncertain prognosis make the decision for transplantation very difficult. Our own experience of poor tolerance of complications and neurodevelopment dysfunction advises caution in future. GSD111 is less prone to hepatic fibrosis than GSD IV with OLT possible in the second decade or later.

25.4.4.1 Non-Cirrhotic Conditions: Prevention of Crises/Other Complications

The role of OLT is developing as a prophylactic therapy for metabolic conditions where there is no significant primary liver disease either to prevent end-stage organ failure elsewhere in the body or to prevent neurological injury either progressively from continuous toxicity or from crises. Organ damage may be renal as in methylmalonic acidaemia, vascular as in primary oxaluria, cardiac as in hypercholesterolaemia or haemorrhagic as in coagulation factor disorders such as Factor VII deficiency. Neurological injury may come about by hyperammonaemia, hypoglycaemia or other toxins or events.

Glycogen storage disease type 1 (GSD 1) is complicated by nephropathy, poor growth, hyperlipidaemia, hyperuricaemia, metabolic bone disease and hepatic adenomas but not cirrhosis. Early hypoglycaemia may lead to developmental delay that is typically mild. In combination, these features tend more compromise quality of life than risk mortality, but renal failure may supervene in the second decade. OLT should be considered for patients with multifocal, growing adenomatous lesions that do not regress with improved dietary regimens and who do not have evidence of distant metastatic disease. Poor control with resulting complications, or poor quality of life from the efforts to achieve dietary control but still suffering complications are also relative indications. More than 100 children and adults with GSD Ia have undergone liver transplantation in North America with 1-, 5- and 10-year survival rate of 82%, 76% and 64%, respectively. Survival rates after OLT have improved over the past 20 years, but complications in the postoperative course remain. Chronic renal failure is a well-documented complication of liver transplantation in GSD Ia sometimes within a few years of OLT, warranting renal-sparing immunosuppression [57, 58].

25.4.4.2 Urea Cycle Disorders (UCDs)

The urea cycle takes place in the hepatocyte where ammonia and bicarbonate are consumed in its production. The inborn errors of ureagenesis that are more frequently encountered are illustrated in Fig. 25.4 that shows the enzymes of the cycle and the names of the associated clinical conditions. Crises with ammonia levels above 400 μmol/L have been shown to predict major neurological consequences and are more likely in those with severe defects presenting in infancy. Patients with unstable disease or likely to suffer neurological injury would be better to be offered OLT to be timed when stable. UCDs may differ in liver involvement according to the enzymatic deficiency. Hepatocellular carcinomas are frequent in some UCDs, such as in citrin deficiency, and can sometimes occur in non-cirrhotic patients. Ornithine transcarbamylase deficiency may be associated more with acute liver failure and argininosuccinic aciduria with chronic liver failure and cirrhosis [59].

All urea cycle defects are inherited in autosomal recessive fashion with the exception of ornithine transcarbamylase deficiency (OTC), which is X-linked. OTC deficiency in Lyonised female patients may be asymptomatic or manifest as neuropsychiatric features or even as severe crises precipitated by a protein load. Long-term neurological outcomes can be guarded with significant impairment justifying OLT in rare circumstances [60].

There has been a debate about management of early neonatal urea cycle disorders because survival rates are lower and intact neurological survival lower still, with a traditional argument applied that the inevitably poor neurological outcome does not warrant OLT. Hepatocyte transplantation has been used as an early bridge to liver transplantation with a good neurological outcome in our unit [61, 62].

In addition there are carrier defects where the role of OLT is less clear. They are mitochondrial ornithine carrier defect (hyperornithinaemia, hyperammonaemia, homocitrullinuria or HHH syndrome), mitochondrial aspartate/glutamate carrier deficiency (citrullinaemia type 2 or citrin deficiency) and dibasic amino acid carrier defect (hyperdibasic aminoaciduria or lysinuric protein intolerance). OLT has shown good

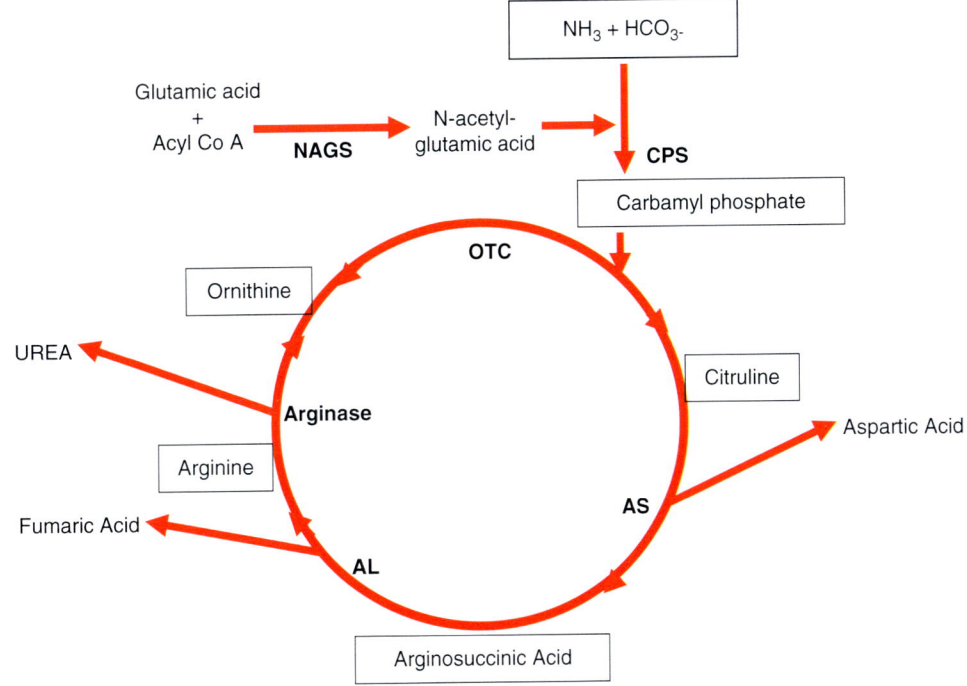

Fig. 25.4 The components and metabolites of the urea cycle. *OTC* ornithine transcarbamylase deficiency; *CPS* carbamoyl phosphate synthetase deficiency; *NAGS* N-acetylglutamate synthetase deficiency; Arginase, arginase deficiency; *AL* argininosuccinate lyase deficiency (Argininosuccinic aciduria); *AS* argininosuccinic acid synthetase 1 (citrullinaemia). Of these only citrullinaemia is recognised to develop progressive fibrotic liver disease

results in HHH and citrin deficiency but not Lysinuric protein intolerance. Its role versus conservative management is yet to be clarified [63].

Tyrosinemia type 1 is associated with progressive liver disease and development of early hepatocellular carcinomas. Nitisinone therapy inhibiting the enzyme 4-hydroxyphenylpyruvate dioxygenase and preventing accumulation of succinyl acetone is started in the newborn period and prevents HCC, liver disease, kidney dysfunction, rickets and neurological crises so that OLT is now only required for late diagnosis or non-adherence to treatment [64].

25.4.4.3 Diseases Not 'Cured' by OLT

Methylmalonic Acidaemia

About half of both mut0 and mut- phenotype patients will have developed renal failure with hyperkalaemia by 5–10 years of age. Suboptimal growth and muscle wasting are associated with dietary restriction. Risk of neurological injury attends recurrent crises and strokes. Quality of life for families tends to be poor in attempting to prevent crises and managing those that occur. Following OLT those transplanted with normal GFR retained kidney function. Neurodevelopmental stabilisation was typically achieved. An increase in natural protein intake has been possible, to average up to 2.1 g/kg/day. Combined renal transplant when necessary has comparable outcomes, but earlier transplantation is indicated in more severe disease and before nephropathy has developed.

Medium-term survival (3–5 years) after OLT in small series combined is 72–80%. The key to better results seems to be the condition of the patient at transplantation. Those with muscle wasting and poor nutrition may be at increased risk of sepsis. Those with marginal renal function may deteriorate to need renal support, while those transplanted in incipient metabolic crisis may deteriorate during the process and suffer neurological injury deterring some units from pursuing this indication for OLT [65].

Propionic Acidaemia

Indications for OLT are based on control of hyperammonaemic crises and controlling their risk and complications, normalising diet and improving nutrition and better quality of life. As with other metabolic disorders, patients with developmental delay may still benefit from OLT although the limitations of treatment must be clear to the family. After OLT patients continue to have a degree of immune deficiency so that they are at increased risk of severe and opportunist infections as well as post-transplant lymphoproliferative disease. There may also be increased risk of pancreatitis. Patients are managed during OLT for risk of early metabolic crisis with a form of emergency regime to try to avoid catabolism [66].

Mitochondrial diseases with MtD and somatic mutations: The debate concerning a role for OLT. A group of younger children and newborns present with acute liver failure and genetic markers of primary mitochondrial dysfunction such as POLG, DGUOK, TRMU and MPV17 mutations. Experience with OLT for MtD has been disappointing in terms of extrahepatic complications, perhaps predictably given the whole-body distribution of mitochondria, yet a proportion of patients benefit from life-saving OLT. Among 9 patients of whom 5 had pre OLT evidence of MtD, 7 survived (77.8%) but 2 with mitochondrial depletion syndrome developed pulmonary hypertension after OLT, so that only 2 had long term healthy survival [67].

A new and somewhat similar group of syndromes, aminoacyl-tRNA synthetase (ARS) disorders, has been shown to be an infrequent cause of liver disease usually in infants and younger children, who may present with ALF also with neurological features similar to MtD and with mechanism possibly through Mt. dysfunction, attributable to the LARS gene. The liver failure typically settles spontaneously but may recur under metabolic stress. The role of OLT in preventing liver crises or modifying other features, particularly neurological, remains to be clarified [68].

Walcott-Rallinson syndrome is the phenotype of defects in the gene encoding eukaryotic translation initiation factor 2α kinase 3 (EIF2AK3), also known as PKR-like endoplasmic reticulum kinase (PERK). Patients suffer from early-onset diabetes, recurrent ALF, renal dysfunction, exocrine pancreas insufficiency, intellectual deficit, hypothyroidism, neutropenia and recurrent infections. OLT has been undertaken for sporadic cases including with the pancreas and also kidney. In our experience neurologic crises continue to occur after OLT potentially with a poor prognosis. Decision for OLT should be taken with caution [21].

25.4.4.4 Liver Inborn Errors Without (Significant) Liver Disease

Crigler-Najjar type1 (CN-1) is characterised by absent or nearly absent Bilirubin UGT1A1 enzyme activity. Unconjugated hyperbilirubinaemia presents shortly after birth with serum bilirubin levels greater than 350 μmol/L. The risk for kernicterus persists into adult life, but the level and conditions at which risk becomes critical are unknown. Liver transplantation remains the only definitive treatment for this disease, but hepatocyte transplantation and gene therapy both show promise. Auxiliary OLT has been undertaken successfully for CN-1 retaining the native liver for future gene therapy in expectation of avoiding life-long immunosuppression [69, 70].

Maple syrup urine disease (MSUD) is an inherited disorder of branched chain keto acid (BCKA) oxidation with chronic brain disease and metabolic crises. OLT provides 9–13% whole-body BCKA oxidation capacity and stabilises

MSUD removing or reducing crises but does not represent a cure. Domino donated liver segments from MSUD patients effectively maintain steady-state BCAA and BCKA homeostasis on an unrestricted diet in their recipients but might have lesser effects than grafts from unrelated deceased donors.

Eight MSUD patients underwent OLT for poor quality of life related to poor control and were followed up 5–21 years with 87.5% survival. Patients achieved a normal diet and crises were almost prevented. Amino acid abnormalities reduced by more than 50% and neurological abnormalities stabilised, representing a considerable improvement for the families [71, 72].

Congenital factor VII (FVII) deficiency is a rare, autosomal recessive condition with phenotype that may be as severe as life-threatening intracranial haemorrhage. OLT has been undertaken with good results including from non-heart beating donors. Rarely, patients with congenital FVII deficiency develop inhibitor to therapeutic FVII when liver transplant is considered to be the definitive treatment.

Primary hyperoxaluria Oxalate production is obligate but with additional source from diet and removal is by the liver with variable removal also by gut commensal bacteria (e.g. *Oxalobacter* Sp.) with oxalate-degrading activity. Primary hyperoxaluria type 1 derives from a deficiency of the liver enzyme alanine-glyoxylate aminotransferase (AGT) that results in hyperoxaluria and oxalate kidney stones leading to progressive loss of glomerular function rate (GFR). As GFR falls, oxalate clearance falls even faster leading to renal failure. Oxalate deposition then occurs in other tissues particularly bones and arterial vessel walls leading to loss of compliance and hypertension. Dialysis cannot achieve oxalate clearance approaching obligate production. Pre-emptive liver transplantation before the GFR falls to 50 mL/min/m^2 allows renal stabilisation before end-stage renal disease develops. Once GFR has fallen below 40 mL/min/m^2, liver and kidney transplantation is required. Acceptable vascular compliance allows combined liver and kidney transplantation, while worsening arteriopathy requires stabilisation of oxalate balance by OLT followed by renal transplant. A high oxalate load considerably increases the risk of the procedure including rarely through bone marrow deposition of oxalate crystals [73–75].

Primary hyperoxaluria type 2 (PH2) is caused by deficiency of the enzyme glyoxylate reductase/hydroxypyruvate reductase (GR/HPR), which is expressed in the liver but also more generally in the body including in leucocytes. The phenotype is similar with end-stage renal disease occurring in childhood or early adulthood. Combined liver and renal transplantation have been used successfully [76, 77].

OLT is considered an alternative to complex pharmacotherapy in severe familial hypercholesterolaemia, which replaces the missing LDL receptors and normalises cholesterol. However, vascular calcifications and valve disease have been reported after liver transplant in the setting of rejection. Calcific aortic stenosis has also been seen to continue to progress by 20 months after OLT despite normalisation of lipid levels and the absence of rejection. It is possible that the rate of progression of aortic valve disease may not be able to be slowed once vascular disease has been established or that there are a subgroup still prone to progressive calcific valve disease. The role of OLT in preventing calcific valve disease therefore needs to be reconsidered [78–80].

25.4.5 Diseases at Risk of Recurrence After OLT

Primary Sclerosing Cholangitis (SC), Auto-immune Sclerosing Cholangitis and Auto-Immune Hepatitis. Features of recurrence of these conditions are often difficult to distinguish from other technical and immunological causes of graft dysfunction after OLT, and while recurrence is well recognised, with the differences in definitions and natural history between adults and children, it is difficult to know exactly what parallels can be drawn. For adults with PSC disease, recurrence ranges between 17 and 37% at 14–55 months with 8.4% graft loss and for AIH 17–33% at 14–55 months with 6.2% graft loss. Graft survival rate for PSC was 56.3% at 5 years and 21.9% at 10 years after the recurrence. The complexity of immune dysregulation in auto-immunity and immunosuppression may mean that active colitis, SC and rejection contribute adversely to each other [81–83].

The role of colectomy in preventing recurrence of SC among adults with ulcerative colitis is becoming clearer. Colitis tends to worsen in about 30% of adults after OLT, although some improve, and there is a threefold increased risk of colon cancer. Colectomy before liver transplantation is associated with decreased risk of recurrence of SC. Activity of IBD before OLT is not predictive of recurrence, but tacrolimus immunosuppression is an independent risk factor for SC recurrence. The optimal rationale for colectomy and immunosuppression is not yet clear [84, 85].

It is extremely rare for paediatric patients with hepatitis B (HBV) infection to progress to need OLT either for cirrhosis or the development of hepatocellular carcinoma. Patients are occasionally found to be HBV positive when being evaluated for other conditions, for example, in the UK as the cause of ALF. Eradication of all evidence of HBV infection and risk of viral replication under immunosuppression cannot yet be achieved. Long-term suppression of HBV replication after OLT comes from adult studies. The combination of long-term lamivudine plus HB immunoglobulin (HBIG) has been used for many years, but HBIG is costly, and lamivudine induces viral resistance. Entecavir- or tenofovir-based treatment with HBIG withdrawn after 1 year or longer have been shown to maintain viral remission of over 95% provided there is good adherence to treatment [86]. HBV vaccination is not effective.

The hepatitis C (HCV) epidemic once appeared to be a looming catastrophe with need for OLT in adults for cirrhosis and hepatocellular carcinoma and retransplantation due to aggressive recurrence of disease threatening to overwhelm available sources of organs. Paediatric HCV has very rarely been an indication for OLT. With highly effective combination oral antivirals effective even in cirrhosis, HCV is set to become a vanishingly rare indication for OLT [87]. Recognition and cure of HCV represents one of the great achievements of hepatology of the last 30 years.

However, a new epidemic has arisen as HCV has been overcome: Non-alcoholic fatty liver disease (NAFLD). It is highly unlikely to progress to cirrhosis in the paediatric period unless associated with a second hepatotoxic factor [88]. However the persistence of the previous lifestyle and predisposition towards metabolic syndrome from the side effects of immunosuppressive medications make this a condition at high risk of recurrence [89].

The prognosis of intestinal transplantation continues to improve but remains poorer in terms of survival and quality of life than liver transplant alone. Patients with intestinal failure-associated liver disease (IFALD) develop worsening intestinal function due to portal hypertension and cholestasis. Some patients, particularly those referred late, deteriorate before a suitable length of gut is available. Another subgroup can be recognised to have theoretically functional gut length, mucosa and motility that were not rehabilitated before the onset of liver disease. For the first group of patients, OLT can be a bridge to intestinal transplantation, and for the second group, OLT is a second opportunity for gut rehabilitation [90].

25.4.6 Transplantation of Liver and Kidney

Simultaneously transplanted livers and kidneys were less likely to develop rejection than sequentially transplanted livers with the kidneys. The liver can protect the kidney from hyperacute rejection and may also decrease acute cellular rejection rates. In a comparison of combined liver and kidney transplants (LKT) with renal alone (RT) to consider chronic graft loss in high-risk situations for renal rejection, among patients with similar levels of donor-specific antibodies (DSAs), acute antibody-mediated rejection was higher in RT: 46.4% against 7.1%, as was chronic transplant glomerulopathy at 53.6% against 0%. Cumulative incidence of T cell-mediated rejection was 30.6% against 7.4%. Over 5 years renal allograft loss or greater than 50% decline in GFR was 20.4% against 7.4%. Overall long-term outcome in LKT in terms of graft survival is good and not different from isolated liver or kidney transplantation; however, patient survival is inferior due to complexity of this procedure. Quality of life after LKD, either due to ARPKD or primary oxaluria, is similar in childhood to liver or kidney transplant alone [91–94].

25.4.7 Extrahepatic Liver Complications

25.4.7.1 Hepato-Pulmonary Syndrome (HPS)

HPS is a complication of porto-systemic shunting usually associated with chronic liver disease. It is seen in up to 10% of cirrhosis and about 20% of biliary atresia splenic malformation patients where presentation of portal effluent to the pulmonary circulation results in vasodilatation and then new vessel formation as illustrated in Fig. 25.5. Nitric oxide is thought to be the final common pathway. When ventilation-perfusion mismatch comes about either through diffusion limitation or fixed shunts, patients experience exertional dyspnoea, then dyspnoea at rest and finally cyanosis. Orthodeoxia is present with greater cyanosis erect than supine because V/Q mismatch deteriorates with posture. The shunting develops progressively but at a variable rate. While various treatments have been proposed such as garlic, somatostatin analogues, cyclooxygenase inhibitors and immunosuppressants such as glucocorticoids and cyclophosphamide all have showed disappointing results. Methylene blue has showed variable improvements in gas exchange. Liver transplantation is the only established curative treatment. However after OLT V/Q, mismatch may be exacerbated by surgical and PICU complications such as pleural effusion or lobar collapse that can be managed by ventilatory techniques or by paradoxically NO. Graft dysfunction may cause the HPS to recur or worsen. Patients may remain cyanosed for weeks but usually tolerate it very well. We have used nebulised N(G)-nitro-L-arginine methyl ester (L-NAME), an inhibitor of NO synthesis, to improve V/Q with some success while the fixed shunts resolve, occasionally taking months [95–98].

25.4.8 Portopulmonary Hypertension

Portopulmonary hypertension (PPH) is characterised by an elevated pulmonary vascular resistance as a consequence of obstruction to pulmonary arterial blood flow. Patients are not cyanosed or typically even symptomatic even though shunts may also be present, but right heart failure and death may occur regardless of the severity of portal hypertension or liver disease. Pulmonary pressures may be found at transplant assessment to represent increased transplant risk even to prohibitive levels. Bosentan, ambrisentan, sildenafil and tadalafil can achieve hemodynamic conditions allowing adult PPH patients access to liver transplantation. Similarly

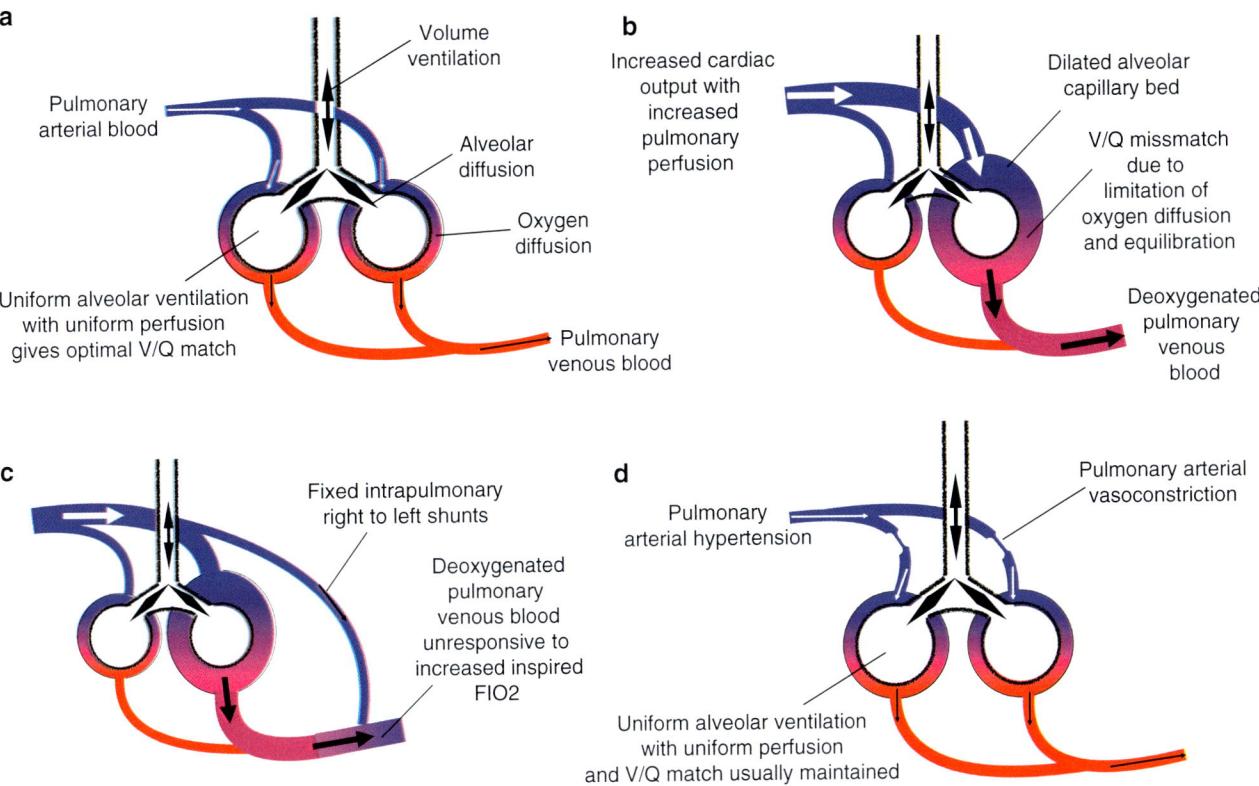

Fig. 25.5 (**a**–**d**) Hepato-pulmonary syndrome is a complication of porto-systemic shunting associated with chronic liver disease with pulmonary vasodilatation resulting in a progressive oxygen perfusion defect and then new vessel formation of intrapulmonary shunts. Both of these reactions result in V/Q mismatch but typically normal pulmonary pressures. Vasoconstriction due to portopulmonary hypertension is associated increased pulmonary pressures but not typical V/Q mismatches

epoprostenol can bridge PPH patients to OLT, which resolves PPH and currently represents the only curative treatment. Interestingly HPS may be improved or masked by an accidental overlap with pulmonary hypertension in the terminal stage of liver disease, which makes vigilance of HPS on the transplant list important because their already increased risk may paradoxically worsen as their cardinal feature, cyanosis, improves [99–102].

25.4.9 Chronic Hepatic Encephalopathy

Chronic hepatic encephalopathy is well recognised in adults with subtle neurological features found in many patients with cirrhosis. In children, encephalopathy may be present subclinically as 50% of children with chronic liver disease develop minimal hepatic encephalopathy (MHE) with impaired neuropsychological testing. It is believed that chronic encephalopathy compromises neurodevelopment outcomes for children with anecdotal experience that prolonged chronic encephalopathy has an irreversible element. Having accepted that encephalopathy is an indication for OLT, it is unclear what tests show the presence of encephalopathy to justify OLT on this basis. There may be a role for screening as children have raised blood ammonia, inflammatory cytokines and mild cerebral oedema on diffusion tensor imaging as compared to children without MHE. Neurocognitive assessments, EEG and magnetic resonance spectroscopy (HMRS) may be required for confirmation [103–105].

25.5 Challenges

25.5.1 The Challenge of Transition

Transition is covered comprehensively elsewhere in this book. However, it is appropriate to consider its effects as a 'peculiarity' of OLT. The emergence is seen of a new balance between relationships at home, in the hospital and at school. The latter is the major arena for interaction with peer groups that tends to lead during adolescence to social pressures away from health-related behaviour such as adherence with medicines and towards independent and risk-taking behaviours including alcohol and recreational drugs. Such behaviours, which are recognised as representing aspects of development of emotional independence, are reasonably believed to predispose to increased rejection rate, risk of graft loss and risk of mortality. An answer could be to offer an alternative peer group that recognises the special health requirements of young adults after transplantation, which is similar to the solution that some third sector organisations have created with great success [7, 14].

25.5.2 The Challenge of Retransplantation

Hepatic retransplantation (re-OLT) has been recognised as surgically and medically challenging since the beginning of liver transplant. Patient survival with re-OLT continues to be significantly worse than that of primary transplant, and 9–29% of paediatric liver transplant recipients have required re-OLT accounting for 5–10% of OLT, of which late re-OLT are now the biggest group. Unlike in adults, recurrent disease is rarely the reason for re-OLT in children. Perioperative events are now seldom the cause of re-OLT mortality, but waiting list mortality and complications of long-term immunosuppression, particularly from efforts to save the graft, remain problematic. Among adults, of whom 33% were retransplanted from ICU, 56% had significant comorbidities by the time of re-OLT, particularly renal dysfunction in 44%. The presence of any comorbidity was associated with greater than five times the risk of death on the waiting list. Patients who received three or more grafts had 40% 5-year survival, compared to 64% in patients who received two previous grafts and 72% in those who received only one graft. Re-OLT could be optimally restricted to centres familiar with the increased risks and should be expedited in anticipation of developing comorbidities. More than three grafts may not represent appropriate use of donated organs [106–108].

25.6 Conclusions

Liver transplantation although still radical and expensive has become the major modality of treatment of chronic liver disease, applicable to many liver-based conditions, not only those resulting in liver failure. It is highly successful for at least the first 20 years and probably also for decades beyond with low early mortality for most indications. In that sense we might consider that the second, non-experimental era of liver transplantation is upon us. For most patients it achieves the quality of life of a chronic condition and quite close to that of patients' peers. Nevertheless OLT has its own natural history and prognosis. Its complications are largely determined by graft-related and immunological–/immunosuppression-related events. For children surviving beyond 20 years, graft loss leading to need for re-OLT appears likely to be the major association with patient mortality with a greater risk than primary transplantation, especially the third graft or more. Therefore, the first transplant will usually have the best outcome and warrants appropriate investment in the first attempt.

Transition to adult services which accompanies progress to independent life as an adult is also associated with a period of increased risk, probably associated with the burden of patients taking responsibility for their own care. However, the mechanisms of late graft loss are currently unclear in many cases. Services including for long-term psychosocial support are often found inadequate to allow paediatric transplant patients to benefit fully from their transplant investment in the long term. Maximising transplant benefits and return requires further investment in medical and social services for young people after OLT. We anticipate that these efforts can lead to the third era of liver transplantation in children represented by the expectation of normal life and survival.

References

1. Starzl TE. The Puzzle People: memoirs of a transplant surgeon. University of Pittsburgh Press; Reprint edition; 2003.
2. Kohli R, Cortes M, Heaton ND, Dhawan A. Liver transplantation in children: state of the art and future perspectives. Arch Dis Child. 2018;103(2):192–8.
3. Venick RS, Farmer DG, Soto JR, Vargas J, Yersiz H, Kaldas FM, Agopian VG, Hiatt JR, SV MD, Busuttil RW. One thousand pediatric liver transplants during thirty years: lessons learned. J Am Coll Surg. 2018;226(4):355–66.
4. Neuberger J. Liver transplantation in the United Kingdom. Liver Transpl. 2016;22:1129–35.
5. Duffy JP, Kao K, Ko CY, Farmer DG, McDiarmid SV, Hong JC, Venick RS, Feist S, Goldstein L, Saab S, Hiatt JR, Busuttil RW. Long-term patient outcome and quality of life after liver transplantation: analysis of 20-year survivors. Ann Surg. 2010;252(4):652–61.
6. Martinelli J, Habes D, Majed L, Guettier C, Gonzalès E, Linglart A, Larue C, Furlan V, Pariente D, Baujard C, Branchereau S, Gauthier F, Jacquemin E, Bernard O. Long-term outcome of liver transplantation in childhood: a study of 20-year survivors. Am J Transplant. 2018;18(7):1680–9.
7. Sagar N, Leithead JA, Lloyd C, Smith M, Gunson BK, Adams DH, Kelly D, Ferguson JW. Pediatric liver transplant recipients who undergo transfer to the adult healthcare service have good long-term outcomes. Am J Transplant. 2015;15(7):1864–73.
8. Hodgson R, Christophi C. What determines ageing of the transplanted liver? HPB (Oxford). 2015;17(3):222–5. Epub 2014 Sep 28.
9. Kelly D, Verkade HJ, Rajanayagam J, McKiernan P, Mazariegos G, Hübscher S. Late graft hepatitis and fibrosis in pediatric liver allograft recipients: current concepts and future developments. Liver Transpl. 2016;22(11):1593–602.
10. Parmar A, Vandriel SM, Ng VL. Health-related quality of life after pediatric liver transplantation: a systematic review. Liver Transpl. 2017;23(3):361–74.
11. Ee LC, Lloyd O, Beale K, Fawcett J, Cleghorn GJ. Academic potential and cognitive functioning of long-term survivors after childhood liver transplantation. Pediatr Transplant. 2014;18(3):272–9.
12. Kaller T, Langguth N, Petermann F, Ganschow R, Nashan B, Schulz KH. Cognitive performance in pediatric liver transplant

recipients. Am J Transplant. 2013;13(11):2956–65. Epub 2013 Sep 18.
13. Sorensen LG, Neighbors K, Martz K, Zelko F, Bucuvalas JC, Alonso EM, Studies of Pediatric Liver Transplantation (SPLIT) Research Group and the Functional Outcomes Group (FOG). Longitudinal study of cognitive and academic outcomes after pediatric liver transplantation. J Pediatr. 2014l;165(1):65–72.
14. Lowton K, Hiley C, Higgs P. Constructing embodied identity in a 'new' ageing population: a qualitative study of the pioneer cohort of childhood liver transplant recipients in the UK. Soc Sci Med. 2017;172:1–9.
15. Shemesh E. Beyond graft survival and into the classroom: should school performance become a new post-transplant outcome measure? Liver Transpl. 2010;16(9):1013–5.
16. Rivera E, Gupta S, Chavers B, Quinones L, Berger MR, Schwarzenberg SJ, Pruett T, Verghese P, Chinnakotla S. En bloc multiorgan transplant (liver, pancreas, and kidney) for acute liver and renal failure in a patient with Wolcott-Rallison syndrome. Liver Transpl. 2016;22(3):371–4.
17. Hegarty R, Hadzic N, Gissen P, Dhawan A. Inherited metabolic disorders presenting as acute liver failure in newborns and young children: King's College Hospital experience. Eur J Pediatr. 2015;174(10):1387–92.
18. Casey JP, McGettigan P, Lynam-Lennon N, McDermott M, Regan R, Conroy J, Bourke B, O'Sullivan J, Crushell E, Lynch S, Ennis S. Identification of a mutation in LARS as a novel cause of infantile hepatopathy. Mol Genet Metab. 2012;106(3):351–8.
19. Jimenez-Rivera C, Nightingale S, Benchimol E, Mazariegos G, Ng V. Outcomes in infants listed for liver transplantation: a retrospective cohort study using the United Network for Organ Sharing database. Pediatr Transplant. 2016;20(7):904–11.
20. Sheflin-Findling S, Annunziato RA, Chu J, Arvelakis A, Mahon D, Arnon R. Liver transplantation for neonatal hemochromatosis: analysis of the UNOS database. Pediatr Transplant. 2015;19(2):164–9.
21. Engelmann G, Meyburg J, Shahbek N, Al-Ali M, Hairetis MH, Baker AJ, Rodenburg RJ, Wenning D, Flechtenmacher C, Ellard S, Smeitink JA, Hoffmann GF, Buchanan CR. Recurrent acute liver failure and mitochondriopathy in a case of Wolcott-Rallison syndrome. J Inherit Metab Dis. 2008;31(4):540–6.
22. Coelho GR, Praciano AM, Rodrigues JP, Viana CF, Brandão KP, Valenca JT Jr, Garcia JH. Liver transplantation in patients with Niemann-Pick Disease—Single-Center Experience. Transplant Proc. 2015;47(10):2929–31.
23. Melendez HV1, Rela M, Baker AJ, Ball C, Portmann B, Mieli-Vergani G, Heaton ND. Liver transplant for giant cell hepatitis with autoimmune haemolytic anaemia. Arch Dis Child. 1997;77(3):249–51.
24. Akyildiz M, Karasu Z, Arikan C, Nart D, Kilic M. Successful liver transplantation for giant cell hepatitis and Coombs-positive hemolytic anemia: a case report. Pediatr Transplant. 2005;9(5):630–3.
25. Dhawan A, Taylor RM, Cheeseman P, De Silva P, Katsiyiannakis L, Mieli-Vergani G. Wilson's disease in children: 37-year experience and revised King's score for liver transplantation. Liver Transpl. 2005;11(4):441–8.
26. Wu SY, Chen TW, Feng AC, Fan HL, Hsieh CB, Chung KP. Comprehensive risk assessment for early neurologic complications after liver transplantation. World J Gastroenterol. 2016;22(24):5548–57.
27. Buckels JA, Tisone G, Gunson BK, McMaster P. Low haematocrit reduces hepatic artery thrombosis after liver transplantation. Transplant Proc. 1989;21(1 Pt 2):2460–1.
28. Jain N, Reilly RF. Hungry bone syndrome. Curr Opin Nephrol Hypertens. 2017;26(4):250–5.
29. Uziel O, Laish I, Bulcheniko M, Harif Y, Kochavi-Shalem N, Aharoni M, Braunstein R, Lahav M, Ben-Ari Z. Telomere shortening in liver transplant recipients is not influenced by underlying disease or metabolic derangements. Ann Transplant. 2013;18:567–75.
30. Yamada Y, Hoshino K, Oyanagi T, Gatayama R, Maeda J, Katori N, Fuchimoto Y, Hibi T, Shinoda M, Matsubara K, Obara H, Aeba R, Kitagawa Y, Yamagishi H, Kuroda T. Successful management of living donor liver transplantation for biliary atresia with single ventricle physiology-from peri-transplant through total cavopulmonary connection: a case report. Pediatr Transplant. 2018.
31. Kamath BM, Schwarz KB, Hadžić N. Alagille syndrome and liver transplantation. J Pediatr Gastroenterol Nutr. 2010;50(1):11–5.
32. Tilib Shamoun S, Le Friec G, Spinner N, Kemper C, Baker AJ. Immune dysregulation in Alagille syndrome: a new feature of the evolving phenotype. Clin Res Hepatol Gastroenterol. 2015;39(5):566–9.
33. Rawat D, Kelly DA, Milford DV, Sharif K, Lloyd C, McKiernan PJ. Phenotypic variation and long-term outcome in children with congenital hepatic fibrosis. J Pediatr Gastroenterol Nutr. 2013;57(2):161–6.
34. Harring TR, Nguyen NT, Liu H, Goss JA, O'Mahony CA. Caroli disease patients have excellent survival after liver transplant. J Surg Res. 2012;177(2):365–72.
35. Noble-Jamieson G, Barnes N, Jamieson N, Friend P, Calne R. Liver transplantation for hepatic cirrhosis in cystic fibrosis. J R Soc Med. 1996;89(Suppl 27):31–7.
36. Mieles LA, Orenstein DM, Toussaint RM, Selby R, Gordon RD, Starzl TE. Outcome after liver transplantation for cystic fibrosis. Pediatr Pulmonol Suppl. 1991;11(S1):130–1.
37. Lamireau T, Martin S, Lallier M, Marcotte JE, Alvarez F. Liver transplantation for cirrhosis in cystic fibrosis. Can J Gastroenterol. 2006;20(7):475–8.
38. Couetil JP, Soubrane O, Houssin DP, Dousset BE, Chevalier PG, Guinvarch A, Loulmet D, Achkar A, Carpentier AF. Combined heart-lung-liver, double lung-liver, and isolated liver transplantation for cystic fibrosis in children. Transpl Int. 1997;10(1):33–9.
39. Milkiewicz P, Skiba G, Kelly D, Weller P, Bonser R, Gur U, Mirza D, Buckels J, Stableforth D, Elias E. Transplantation for cystic fibrosis: outcome following early liver transplantation. J Gastroenterol Hepatol. 2002;17(2):208–13.
40. Fridell JA, Bond GJ, Mazariegos GV, Orenstein DM, Jain A, Sindhi R, Finder JD, Molmenti E, Reyes J. Liver transplantation in children with cystic fibrosis: a long-term longitudinal review of a single center's experience. J Pediatr Surg. 2003;38(8):1152–6.
41. Nash KL, Collier JD, French J, McKeon D, Gimson AE, Jamieson NV, Wallwork J, Bilton D, Alexander GJ. Cystic fibrosis liver disease: to transplant or not to transplant? Am J Transplant. 2008;8(1):162–9.
42. Dowman JK, Watson D, Loganathan S, Gunson BK, Hodson J, Mirza DF, Clarke J, Lloyd C, Honeybourne D, Whitehouse JL, Nash EF, Kelly D, van Mourik I, Newsome PN. Long-term impact of liver transplantation on respiratory function and nutritional status in children and adults with cystic fibrosis. Am J Transplant. 2012;12(4):954–64.
43. Mekeel KL, Langham MR Jr, Gonzalez-Perralta R, Reed A, Hemming AW. Combined en bloc liver pancreas transplantation for children with CF. Liver Transpl. 2007;13(3):406–9.
44. Mendizabal M, Reddy KR, Cassuto J, Olthoff KM, Faust TW, Makar GA, Rand EB, Shaked A, Abt PL. Liver transplantation in patients with cystic fibrosis: analysis of United Network for Organ Sharing data. Liver Transpl. 2011;17(3):243–50.
45. Aronson DC, Meyers RL. Malignant tumors of the liver in children. Semin Pediatr Surg. 2016;25(5):265–75.
46. Tajiri T, Kimura O, Fumino S, Furukawa T, Iehara T, Souzaki R, Kinoshita Y, Koga Y, Suminoe A, Hara T, Kohashi K, Oda Y, Hishiki T, Hosoi H, Hiyama E, Taguchi T. Surgical strategies for unresectable hepatoblastomas. J Pediatr Surg. 2012;47(12):2194–8.

47. Nobre S, Khanna R, Bab N, Kyrana E, Height S, Karani J, Kane P, Heaton N, Dhawan A. Primary Budd-Chiari syndrome in children: King's College Hospital Experience. J Pediatr Gastroenterol Nutr. 2017;65(1):93–6.
48. Potthoff A, Attia D, Pischke S, Mederacke I, Beutel G, Rifai K, Deterding K, Heiringhoff K, Klempnauer J, Strassburg CP, Manns MP, Bahr MJ. Long-term outcome of liver transplant patients with Budd-Chiari syndrome secondary to myeloproliferative neoplasms. Liver Int. 2015;35(8):2042–9.
49. Coskun ME, Height S, Dhawan A, Hadzic N. Ruxolitinib treatment in an infant with JAK2+ polycythaemia vera-associated Budd-Chiari syndrome. BMJ Case Rep. 2017;2017.
50. Petrowsky H, Brunicardi FC, Leow VM, Venick RS, Agopian V, Kaldas FM, Zarrinpar A, Markovic D, McDiarmid SV, Hong JC, Farmer DG, Hiatt JR, Busuttil RW. Liver transplantation for lethal genetic syndromes: a novel model of personalized genomic medicine. J Am Coll Surg. 2013;216(4):534–43.
51. Fagiuoli S, Daina E, D'Antiga L, Colledan M, Remuzzi G. Monogenic diseases that can be cured by liver transplantation. J Hepatol. 2013;59(3):595–612.
52. Prachalias AA, Kalife M, Francavilla R, Muiesan P, Dhawan A, Baker AJ, Hadzic N, Mieli-Vergani G, Rela M, Heaton N. Liver transplantation for alpha-1-antitrypsin deficiency in children. Transpl Int. 2000;13(3):207–10.
53. Carey EJ, Iyer VN, Nelson DR, Nguyen JH, Krowka MJ. Outcomes for recipients of liver transplantation for alpha-1-antitrypsin deficiency–related cirrhosis. Liver Transpl. 2013;19(12):1370–6.
54. Khorsandi SE, Thompson R, Vilca-Melendez H, Dhawan A, Heaton N. Massive ascites and the heterozygous alpha 1 antitrypsin (α1 AT) living related donor liver in the homozygous child. Pediatr Transplant. 2018;22(1).
55. Socha P, Janczyk W, Dhawan A, Baumann U, D'Antiga L, Tanner S, Iorio R, Vajro P, Houwen R, Fischler B, Dezsofi A, Hadzic N, Hierro L, Jahnel J, McLin V, Nobili V, Smets F, Verkade HJ, Debray D. Wilson's disease in children: a Position Paper by the Hepatology Committee of the European Society for Paediatric Gastroenterology, Hepatology and Nutrition. J Pediatr Gastroenterol Nutr. 2018;66(2):334–44.
56. Laurencin C, Brunet AS, Dumortier J, Lion-Francois L, Thobois S, Mabrut JY, Dubois R, Woimant F, Poujois A, Guillaud O, Lachaux A, Broussolle E. Liver transplantation in Wilson's disease with neurological impairment: evaluation in 4 patients. Eur Neurol. 2017;77(1-2):5–15.
57. Kishnani PS, Austin SL, Abdenur JE, Arn P, Bali DS, Boney A, Chung WK, Dagli AI, Dale D, Koeberl D, Somers MJ, Wechsler SB, Weinstein DA, Wolfsdorf JI, Watson MS, American College of Medical Genetics and Genomics. Diagnosis and management of glycogen storage disease type I: a practice guideline of the American College of Medical Genetics and Genomics. Genet Med. 2014;16(11):e1.
58. Maheshwari A, Rankin R, Segev DL, Thuluvath PJ. Outcomes of liver transplantation for glycogen storage disease: a matched-control study and a review of literature. Clin Transplant. 2012;26:432–6.
59. Bigot A, Tchan MC, Thoreau B, Blasco H, Maillot F. Liver involvement in urea cycle disorders: a review of the literature. J Inherit Metab Dis. 2017;40(6):757–69.
60. Pridmore CL, Clarke JT, Blaser S. Ornithine transcarbamylase deficiency in females: an often overlooked cause of treatable encephalopathy. J Child Neurol. 1995;10(5):369–74.
61. Saudubray JM, Touati G, Delonlay P, Jouvet P, Narcy C, Laurent J, Rabier D, Kamoun P, Jan D, Revillon Y. Liver transplantation in urea cycle disorders. Eur J Pediatr. 1999;158(Suppl 2):S55–9.
62. Puppi J, Tan N, Mitry RR, Hughes RD, Lehec S, Mieli-Vergani G, Karani J, Champion MP, Heaton N, Mohamed R, Dhawan A. Hepatocyte transplantation followed by auxiliary liver transplantation-a novel treatment for ornithine transcarbamylase deficiency. Am J Transplant. 2008;8(2):452–7.
63. Fecarotta S, Parenti G, Vajro P, Zuppaldi A, Della Casa R, Carbone MT, Correra A, Torre G, Riva S, Dionisi-Vici C, Santorelli FM, Andria G. HHH syndrome (hyperornithinaemia, hyperammonaemia, homocitrullinuria), with fulminant hepatitis-like presentation. J Inherit Metab Dis. 2006;29(1):186–9.
64. Das AM. Clinical utility of nitisinone for the treatment of hereditary tyrosinemia type-1 (HT-1). Appl Clin Genet. 2017;10:43–8.
65. Niemi AK, Kim IK, Krueger CE, Cowan TM, Baugh N, Farrell R, Bonham CA, Concepcion W, Esquivel CO, Enns GM. Treatment of methylmalonic acidemia by liver or combined liver-kidney transplantation. J Pediatr. 2015;166(6):1455–61.
66. Vara R, Turner C, Mundy H, Heaton ND, Rela M, Mieli-Vergani G, Champion M, Hadzic N. Liver transplantation for propionic acidemia in children. Liver Transpl. 2011;17(6):661–7.
67. Meyer-Schuman R, Antonellis A. Emerging mechanisms of aminoacyl-tRNA synthetase mutations in recessive and dominant human disease. Hum Mol Genet. 2017;26(R2):R114–27.
68. Memon N, Weinberger BI, Hegyi T, Aleksunes LM. Inherited disorders of bilirubin clearance. Pediatr Res. 2016;79(3):378–86.
69. Rela M, Muiesan P, Vilca-Melendez H, Dhawan A, Baker AJ, Mieli-Vergani G, Heaton ND. Auxiliary partial orthotopic liver transplantation for Crigler-Najjar syndrome type I. Ann Surg. 1999;229(4):565–9.
70. Díaz VM, Camarena C, de la Vega Á, Martínez-Pardo M, Díaz C, López M, Hernández F, Andrés A, Jara P. Liver transplantation for classical maple syrup urine disease: long-term follow-up. J Pediatr Gastroenterol Nutr. 2014;59(5):636–9.
71. Feier F, Schwartz IV, Benkert AR, Seda Neto J, Miura I, Chapchap P, da Fonseca EA, Vieira S, Zanotelli ML, Pinto e Vairo F, Camelo JS Jr, Margutti AV, Mazariegos GV, Puffenberger EG, Strauss KA. Living related versus deceased donor liver transplantation for maple syrup urine disease. Mol Genet Metab. 2016;117(3):336–43.
72. Hatch M. Gut microbiota and oxalate homeostasis. Ann Transl Med. 2017;5(2):36.
73. Mykytiv V, Campoy Garcia F. Anemia in patient with primary hyperoxaluria and bone marrow involvement by oxalate crystals. Hematol Oncol Stem Cell Ther. 2018;11(2):118–21.
74. Khorsandi SE, Samyn M, Hassan A, Vilca-Melendez H, Waller S, Shroff R, Koffman G, Van't Hoff W, Baker A, Dhawan A, Heaton N. An institutional experience of pre-emptive liver transplantation for pediatric primary hyperoxaluria type 1. Pediatr Transplant. 2016;20(4):523–9.
75. Dhondup T, Lorenz EC, Milliner DS, Lieske JC. Combined liver-kidney transplantation for primary Hyperoxaluria type 2: a case report. Am J Transplant. 2018;18(1):253–7.
76. Rumsby G, Hulton SA. Primary Hyperoxaluria Type 2. In: Adam MP, Ardinger HH, Pagon RA, Wallace SE, LJH B, Stephens K, Amemiya A, editors. GeneReviews® [Internet]. Seattle, WA: University of Washington; 2008. [updated 2017 Dec 21].
77. France M. Homozygous familial hypercholesterolaemia: update on management. Paediatr Int Child Health. 2016;36(4):243–7.
78. Martinez M, Brodlie S, Griesemer A, Kato T, Harren P, Gordon B, Parker T, Levine D, Tyberg T, Starc T, Cho I, Min J, Elmore K, Lobritto S, Hudgins LC. Effects of liver transplantation on lipids and cardiovascular disease in children with homozygous familial hypercholesterolemia. Am J Cardiol. 2016;118(4):504–10.
79. Greco M, Robinson JD, Eltayeb O, Benuck I. Progressive aortic stenosis in homozygous familial hypercholesterolemia after liver transplant. Pediatrics. 2016;138(5).
80. Maggiore G, Riva S, Sciveres M. Autoimmune diseases of the liver and biliary tract and overlap syndromes in childhood. Minerva Gastroenterol Dietol. 2009;55(1):53–70.

81. Tillmann HL, Jäckel E, Manns MP. Liver transplantation in autoimmune liver disease--selection of patients. Hepatogastroenterology. 1999;46(30):3053–9.
82. Carbone M, Neuberger JM. Autoimmune liver disease, autoimmunity and liver transplantation. J Hepatol. 2014;60(1):210–23.
83. Lindström L, Jørgensen KK Boberg KM, Castedal M, Rasmussen A, Rostved AA, Isoniemi H, Bottai M, Bergquist A. Risk factors and prognosis for recurrent primary sclerosing cholangitis after liver transplantation: a Nordic multicentre study. Scand J Gastroenterol. 2018;53(3):297–304.
84. Ueda Y, Kaido T, Okajima H, Hata K, Anazawa T, Yoshizawa A, Yagi S, Taura K, Masui T, Yamashiki N, Haga H, Nagao M, Marusawa H, Seno H, Uemoto S. Long-term prognosis and recurrence of primary sclerosing cholangitis after liver transplantation: a single-center experience. Transplant Direct. 2017;3(12):e334.
85. Sasaki K, Sakamoto S, Uchida H, Narumoto S, Shigeta T, Fukuda A, Ito R, Irie R, Yoshioka T, Murayama K, Kasahara M. Liver transplantation for mitochondrial respiratory chain disorder: a single-center experience and excellent marker of differential diagnosis. Transplant Proc. 2017;49(5):1097–102.
86. Wong SN, Chu CJ, Wai CT, Howell T, Moore C, Fontana RJ, Lok AS. Low risk of hepatitis B virus recurrence after withdrawal of long-term hepatitis B immunoglobulin in patients receiving maintenance nucleos(t)ide analogue therapy. Liver Transpl. 2007;13(3):374–81.
87. Gupta M, Bahirwani R, Levine MH, Malik S, Goldberg D, Reddy KR, Shaked A. Outcomes in pediatric hepatitis C transplant recipients: analysis of the UNOS database. Pediatr Transplant. 2015;19(2):153–63.
88. Fujio A, Kawagishi N, Echizenya T, Tokodai K, Nakanishi C, Miyagi S, Sato K, Fujimori K, Ohuchi N. Long-term survival with growth hormone replacement after liver transplantation of pediatric non alcoholic steatohepatitis complicating acquired hypopituitarism. Tohoku J Exp Med. 2015;235(1):61–7.
89. Perito ER, Vase T, Ramachandran R, Phelps A, Jen KY, Lustig RH, Feldstein VA, Rosenthal P. Hepatic steatosis after pediatric liver transplant. Liver Transpl. 2017;23(7):957–67.
90. Muiesan P, Dhawan A, Novelli M, Mieli-Vergani G, Rela M, Heaton ND. Isolated liver transplant and sequential small bowel transplantation for intestinal failure and related liver disease in children. Transplantation. 2000;69(11):2323–6.
91. Grenda R, Kaliciński P. Combined and sequential liver-kidney transplantation in children. Pediatr Nephrol. 2018. https://doi.org/10.1007/s00467-017-3880-4.
92. Rogers J, Bueno J, Shapiro R, Scantlebury V, Mazariegos G, Fung J, Reyes J. Results of simultaneous and sequential pediatric liver and kidney transplantation. Transplantation. 2001;72(10):1666–70.
93. Taner T, Heimbach JK, Rosen CB, Nyberg SL, Park WD, Stegall MD. Decreased chronic cellular and antibody-mediated injury in the kidney following simultaneous liver-kidney transplantation. Kidney Int. 2016;89(4):909–17.
94. Schmaeschke K, Lezius S, Grabhorn E, Kemper MJ, Brinkert F. Health-related quality of life after combined liver and kidney transplantation in children. Pediatr Transplant. 2017;21(4).
95. Krowka MJ, Fallon MB, Kawut SM, Fuhrmann V, Heimbach JK, Ramsay MA, Sitbon O, Sokol RJ. International Liver Transplant Society Practice Guidelines: diagnosis and management of hepatopulmonary syndrome and portopulmonary hypertension. Transplantation. 2016;100(7):1440–52.
96. Alexander J, Greenough A, Baker AJ, Rela M, Heaton N, Potter D. Nitric oxide treatment of severe hypoxemia after liver transplantation in hepatopulmonary syndrome: case report. Liver Transpl Surg. 1997;3(1):54–5.
97. Brussino L, Bucca C, Morello M, Scappaticci E, Mauro M, Rolla G. Effect on dyspnoea and hypoxaemia of inhaled N(G)-nitro-L-arginine methyl ester in hepatopulmonary syndrome. Lancet. 2003;362(9377):43–4.
98. Iqbal CW, Krowka MJ, Pham TH, Freese DK, El Youssef M, Ishitani MB. Liver transplantation for pulmonary vascular complications of pediatric end-stage liver disease. J Pediatr Surg. 2008;43(10):1813–20.
99. Golbin JM, Krowka MJ. Portopulmonary hypertension. Clin Chest Med. 2007;28(1):203–18. ix.
100. Fussner LA, Iyer VN, Cartin-Ceba R, Lin G, Watt KD, Krowka MJ. Intrapulmonary vascular dilatations are common in portopulmonary hypertension and may be associated with decreased survival. Liver Transpl. 2015;21(11):1355–64.
101. Legros L, Chabanne C, Camus C, Fournet M, Houssel-Debry P, Latournerie M, Jezequel C, Rayar M, Boudjema K, Guyader D, Bardou-Jacquet E. Oral pulmonary vasoactive drugs achieve hemodynamic eligibility for liver transplantation in portopulmonary hypertension. Dig Liver Dis. 2017;49(3):301–7.
102. Umeda A, Tagawa M, Kohsaka T, Miyakawa T, Kawasaki K, Kitamura M, Nakano M. Hepatopulmonary syndrome can show spontaneous resolution: possible mechanism of portopulmonary hypertension overlap? Respirology. 2006;11(1):120–3.
103. Esmat S, Garem NE, Raslan H, Elfekki M, Sleem GA. Critical flicker frequency is diagnostic of minimal hepatic encephalopathy. J Invest Med. 2017;65(8):1131–5.
104. Wakamoto H, Manabe K, Kobayashi H, Hayashi M. Subclinical portal-systemic encephalopathy in a child with congenital absence of the portal vein. Brain Dev. 1999;21(6):425–8.
105. Srivastava A, Chaturvedi S, Gupta RK, Malik R, Mathias A, Jagannathan NR, Jain S, Pandey CM, Yachha SK, Rathore RKS. Minimal hepatic encephalopathy in children with chronic liver disease: prevalence, pathogenesis and magnetic resonance-based diagnosis. J Hepatol. 2017;66(3):528–36.
106. Dreyzin A, Lunz J, Venkat V, Martin L, Bond GJ, Soltys KA, Sindhi R, Mazariegos GV. Long-term outcomes and predictors in pediatric liver retransplantation. Pediatr Transplant. 2015 Dec;19(8):866–74.
107. Kitchens WH, Yeh H, Markmann JF. Hepatic retransplant: what have we learned? Clin Liver Dis. 2014;18(3):731–51.
108. Al-Freah MAB, Moran C, Foxton MR, Agarwal K, Wendon JA, Heaton ND, Heneghan MA. Impact of comorbidity on waiting list and post-transplant outcomes in patients undergoing liver retransplantation. World J Hepatol. 2017;9(20):884–95.

Liver Allograft Donor Selection and Allocation

26

James E. Squires and George V. Mazariegos

Key Points
- Globally, children have varying access to transplantation. Improvements have been made in waitlist mortality in the United States. Selected centers in Europe or Asia have further improved waitlist results by adopting strict intentional technical innovations such as liver splitting or living related transplantation as well as by advocating for policy change that supports pediatric prioritization.
- Results for living related and split liver technical variant transplantation are now equivalent to outcomes of whole organ transplantation. Technical variant use in the United States lags behind the use of such grafts in other parts of the world.

Research Needed in the Field
- Further research in optimizing utilization of all suitable allografts is important to the field. Decision support methods for graft selection based on multiple factors may be able to be achieved using large data and newer analytics.

26.1 Pediatric Liver Disease Prioritization and Allocation

Pediatric liver disease prioritization varies globally but frequently is based on the pediatric end-stage liver disease (PELD) and model for end-stage liver disease (MELD) allocation scores. These United States (US) disease scores have been extensively reviewed in detail [1] and are listed in Table 26.1.

Beginning in 2002, MELD and PELD scoring systems were incorporated into pediatric allocation based on their ability to predict mortality in adults waiting for liver transplantation. The MELD score is calculated using total bilirubin, INR, and creatinine and has a maximum score of 40. The PELD score, which has no maximum, was generated from the database of Studies of Pediatric Transplantation (SPLIT) to predict death, transplantation, or transfer to the intensive care unit and adds albumin, growth failure, and age <1 year to the MELD criteria without the creatinine. However, there were often discrepancies felt to exist between the calculated score and the perceived urgent need for liver transplant resulting in the introduction of exception point requests. Briefly, these appeals to increase the patients calculated score are made by the transplant care team to Regional Review Boards (RRB) and may be granted or denied on a case-by-case basis. Further recognition of the inherent weakness of PELD in addressing mortality risk in children with specific, rare conditions, where intrinsic liver dysfunction was not present, led to the creation of standardized exceptions for these conditions which do not require RRB approval (Table 26.2). Additional PELD and allocation modifications have been significant over time and are summarized in Fig. 26.1 [2].

Table 26.1 MELD/PELD calculator documentation

Formula[a]	
PELD score	= 0.480 × $\log_e$ (bilirubin mg/dL)
	+ 1.857 × $\log_e$ (INR)
	− 0.687 × $\log_e$ (albumin g/dL)
	+ 0.436 if the patient is less than 1 year old
	+ 0.667 if the patient has growth failure
MELD score	= 0.957 × $\log_e$ (creatinine mg/dL)
	+ 0.378 × $\log_e$ (bilirubin mg/dL)
	+ 1.120 × $\log_e$ (INR)
	+ 0.643

[a]Multiply the score by 10 and round to the nearest whole number

J. E. Squires · G. V. Mazariegos (✉)
UPMC Children's Hospital of Pittsburgh, Pittsburgh, PA, USA
e-mail: james.squires2@chp.edu; george.mazariegos@chp.edu

The utilization of exception scores has led to concern over inequity in application [2, 3] while recognizing the multifactorial contributions of waitlist management and other complex behaviors that may be center, region, or disease specific [1, 4–6]. Recent reports have highlighted some of the shortcomings of the current system including disparity in the use of exception points [2] and variability in organ acceptance rates for those who have been granted exception points [7]. As such, a current modification of this system has led to the creation of a National Review Board with a pediatric arm that will use guidelines to help in the standardization of criteria for granting of exceptions (https://optn.transplant.hrsa.gov/resources/guidance/liver-review-board-guidance).

Table 26.2 Standardized MELD/PELD exceptions not needing RRB approval

Cholangiocarcinoma
Cystic fibrosis
Familial amyloid polyneuropathy
Hepatic artery thrombosis
Hepatocellular carcinoma
Hepatopulmonary syndrome
Metabolic disease (urea cycle disorder or organic acidemia)
Portopulmonary hypertension
Primary hyperoxaluria

Globally, pediatric liver allocation models are heterogeneous. In the United States, allocation is complex and based on local/regional prioritization before national allocation (Fig. 26.2). Age is a consideration with pediatric age donors less than 11 being allocated more widely to children than pediatric donors aged 12–18 or adult livers. Yet recent data has shown that 6% of adult liver transplant recipients received livers from pediatric donors, highlighting an opportunity for improvement in the current system [5]. Notably, universal pediatric prioritization is lacking, and the use of split liver grafts (discussed below) is not incorporated into the current US allocation system. In contrast, other countries have successfully prioritized pediatric liver allocation in a definitive manner without detriment to adult liver access. Table 26.3 demonstrates pediatric prioritization and utilization of split liver policies in selected European countries.

26.2 Pediatric Liver Allograft Type

The surgical techniques utilized in contemporary pediatric liver transplantation will be summarized expertly in the subsequent chapters. Pertinent decision-making elements and outcomes that are relevant to best recipient outcomes are summarized herein.

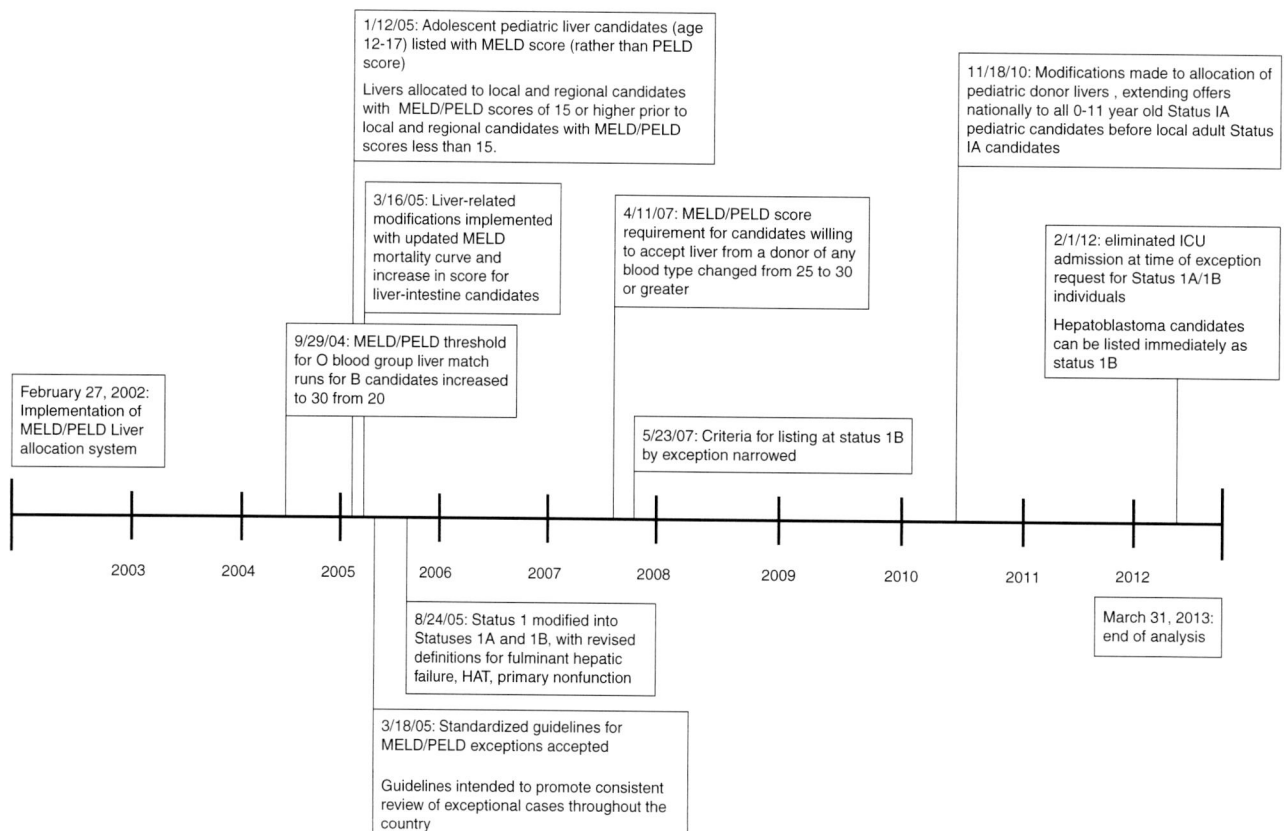

Fig. 26.1 Pediatric liver allocation policy modifications made since the implementation of the MELD/PELD scoring system in 2002. (Adapted from Hsu et al., 2015 [2])

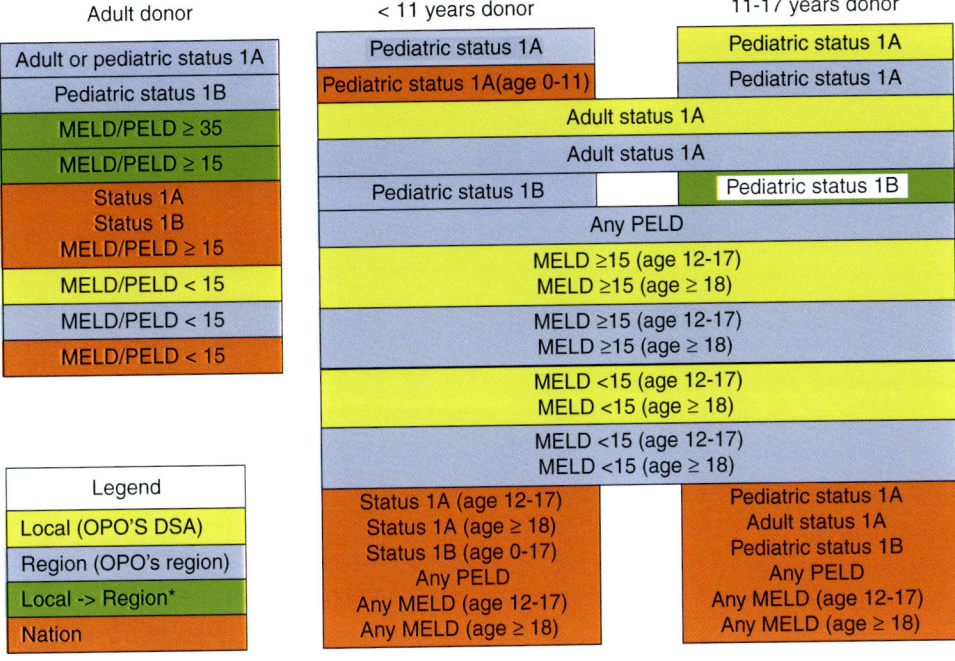

Fig. 26.2 US allocation algorithm by donor age (from Hsu et al., 2017 [5]). *Allocation will occur at the OPO's DSA followed by OPO's region. For MELD/PELD scores, allocation will occur at each given score prior to proceeding to next lower score

Pediatric allograft selection must be made in the context of optimizing or eliminating waitlist morbidity and mortality as well as achieving long-term survival. In the United States, pediatric liver waitlist morbidity and mortality remain significant considerations for the youngest patients [8]. Waitlist morbidity often accrues with time while awaiting transplant. Therefore, it is notable that approximately 45% of children spend over a year on the waitlist, often with detrimental effects during a critical time of growth and development [9]. Furthermore, mortality in children awaiting transplant remains unacceptably high. In 2016, 34/577 (5.9%) of candidates died while waiting for transplant, and an additional 23 (4%) were removed after they were considered too sick to transplant [9]. The greatest mortality is in listed children under the age of 2 where more than 10% die awaiting transplant. Consequently, there is a critical need to increase organ availability to children awaiting this lifesaving intervention.

Graft types available to children include deceased donor grafts (with whole organs or technical variant split grafts) or living donor grafts (live donor segmental or domino organ) [10, 11]. *Reduced Liver Grafts*: Technical variant grafts (Fig. 26.3) initially were conceived by the development of "reduced" liver grafts [12] which entail decreasing the size of large, deceased donor grafts for use in a small child where the size of the abdomen or vessels may prohibit the use of a whole organ. While this advancement successfully extended organ availability to the very young, it did not expand the donor pool as the remainder of the allograft following reduction was discarded.

Split Liver Grafts: In contrast, split liver transplantation, whereby the donor liver is divided into usable grafts for two recipients, was initially developed by German and US teams [13, 14] and has been used successfully to increase organ availability to those awaiting transplant [15]. In situ splitting was developed as a proposed advantage to ex situ splitting [16, 17], although modern preservation and surgical techniques have lessened the importance of the splitting technique. Regrettably, despite data suggesting that split liver transplantation may provide opportunities to reduce pediatric waitlist mortality while maintaining current accessibility to adults [18], the practice had not been widely utilized in the United States [1].

Living Donor Grafts: A natural progression of split liver transplantation is the concept of living donor liver transplant (LDLT) whereby part of the liver from a healthy donor is used to treat a sick recipient. Living donor grafts were first applied to a child with biliary atresia from a maternal donor successfully in 1989 [19] (Fig. 26.4). Subsequent shortages of acceptable donor organs have led to the development of unique technical, physiological, and logistical innovations in LDLT [20]. As a result, LDLT has been used in a variety of disorders including metabolic liver disease, acute liver failure, liver tumors, and autoimmune liver disease [20]. Despite these advancements, LDLT is only performed in the minority of pediatric liver transplants with most recent US data indicating its use in only 193/1683 (11.5%) of cases [9]. A particularly extraordinary subset of LDLT includes the apt-termed "domino" liver transplant where the explanted liver

Table 26.3 Pediatric prioritization and split liver policy in selected European countries (Adapted from Hsu, Mazariegos, 2017 [1])

	France	United Kingdom	Spain	Italy	ET	Switzerland
Prioritization of pediatric patients	Children have access to emergency status (wait time 0–6 months for AHN, emergent retransplantation, hepatoblastoma, acute/chronic decompensation, or metabolic disease after external expert review)	Children are prioritized for all donors under age 16 years immediately after super-urgent local and national patients, hepatoblastoma, and IFALD patients	Children (under age 16 years) listed for emergent retransplantation	Donor livers under age 18 years offered to children first. Single national waiting list with specific allocation rules for pediatric recipients	Children aged 16 years and under receive allocation equivalent to 35% 3-month mortality with automatic 15% monthly increase	Donor organ <18 years offered to patients age <18 years by priority score and following sequence: 1. Patient <12 years 2. Patient 12–18 years 3. >18 years of age
Split policy	Donors under age 30 years are first proposed to pediatric liver teams	Donor age <40 years, >50 kg, and <5 days in PICU	Donors less than age 16 years are offered to children first	Donors aged 18–50 years not allocated to super-urgent or the MELD >30 list are offered to pediatric centers to decide split feasibility	Donors under age 50 years and >50 kg are considered splittable livers	Liver can be split if the patient with the highest priority consents to the split
Liver disease severity score used	PELD not used	Liver is allocated to center for patient selection	Liver is allocated to center for patient selection	Grafts are allocated among pediatric recipients according to PELD (MELD in adolescents) + exceptions	Liver is allocated to center for patient selection	
Additional notes	No prioritization for multivisceral candidates	Approximately 20% donors used are split	<2% livers used are split	Right lobe returned to normal allocation	Right lobe returned to normal allocation	MELD-based system with exception point accrual for children
Additional reference	Agence de la Biomédecine www.agence-biomedecine.fr	Organ Donation and Transplantation. Liver Advisory Group Papers http://www.odt.nhs.uk/transplantation/liver/	Organización Nacional de Trasplantes www.ont.es		Eurotransplant. Eurotransplant Manual https://www.eurotransplant.org/cms/index.php?page=et_manual	Schweizerische Eidgenossenschaft Confédération Suisse. Ordonnance du DFI sur l'attribution d'organes destinés à une transplantation https://www.admin.ch/opc/fr/classified-compilation/20062074/index.html

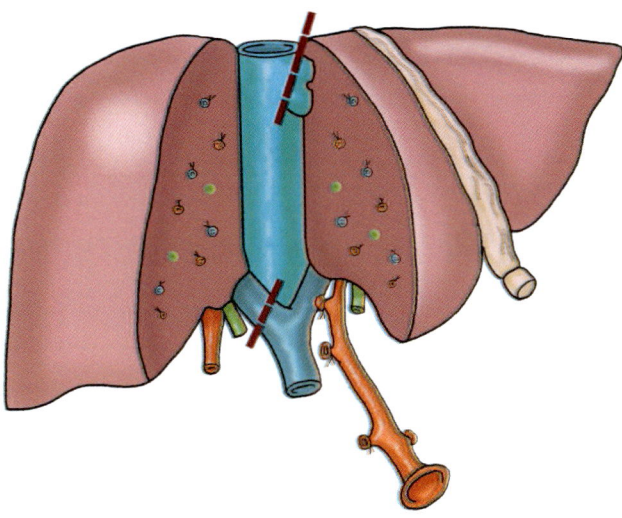

Fig. 26.3 Deceased donor recovery along with utilization of graft vessels may allow for anatomic requirements of the recipient

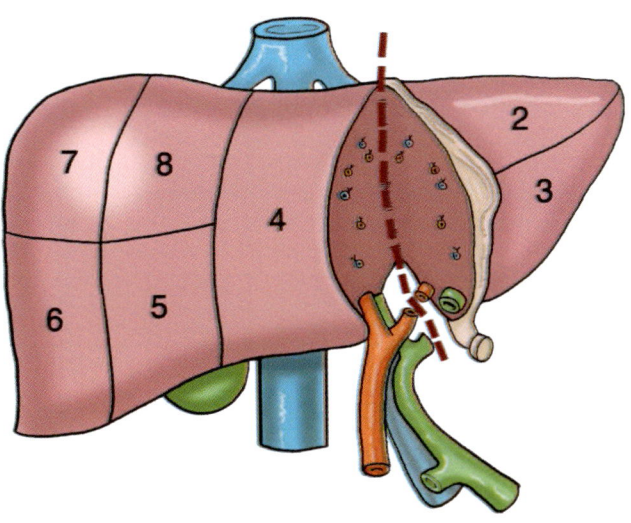

Fig. 26.4 Live donor split segment anatomical considerations

26.3 Determinants Affecting Graft Selection

Pediatric liver allograft selection must be made in the context of optimizing or eliminating waitlist mortality while improving long-term survival [10]. Multiple factors can affect and complicate the decision process.

Organ Accessibility: In the United States, the Department of Health and Human Services (HHS) stipulates that organ allocation be based on medical criteria, and not "accidents of geography" [25]. Still, regional variation in access to liver transplantation persists [26]. Donor access itself varies across countries. For example, deceased donor organs which may be routinely available in the United States are often in short supply in East Asian countries, driving the development of LDLT [27]. Some variation in accessibility can be traced to differences in regional trauma patterns or disease prevalence which can affect utility and availability of organs [28]. Additional accessibility may be in part related to disparities in public safety laws, healthcare infrastructure, and public funding which may influence the regional risk of death and subsequent availability of a deceased donor. In other words, some of the variation in liver availability may not be reflective of geography but rather a by-product of societal disadvantage [29]. Among-center variability in liver offer acceptance rates, not explained by donor or recipient factors, can also impact organ availability and waitlist mortality [7]. Half of pediatric patients who die awaiting liver transplant had been offered an organ that was eventually transplanted into another pediatric patient [5]. Ultimately, the final determinants of liver allograft availability are complex and interrelated, based on geographical and center expertise, and dependent on local organ donor availability.

Recipient Determinants: Physiologic criteria involved in graft selection for children [10] include determining optimal graft volume for the degree of portal hypertension [30], anatomic constraints, and degree of metabolic enzyme required for phenotypic cure of metabolic disease [31]. A schematic of these considerations is shown in Fig. 26.5.

Donor Determinants: Donor criteria for pediatric liver allografts have not been well studied but typically are considered to be hemodynamically feasible for donors >age 3–6 months or for adult livers are based around clinical criteria for the graft that may be considered "split-able" such as proposed by Battula et al. [15] (Table 26.4).

Graft Determinants: Graft type as a determinant of outcomes has been extensively reviewed, and results have demonstrated an evolution of experience. Initial data from the Studies in Pediatric Liver Transplantation (SPLIT) database showed that whole liver grafts enjoyed superior outcomes over technical variant grafts [32]. Although single-center experiences later reported similar outcomes among the various graft types, it has not been until recently that data suggests the "learning curve" has been reached nationwide [33]

of one patient is used to transplant into a recipient with the expectation that the disease will not be expressed [21]. The classical scenario is a patient with maple syrup urine disease (MSUD) who is the recipient of a liver transplant and who then donates their liver to another individual without MSUD where the extrahepatic enzyme mass can compensate for the absence in the liver and prevent the MSUD phenotype in the domino recipient [22]. Outcomes of domino liver transplant have shown to be comparable with traditional deceased donor transplant [23], and successful splitting of the domino graft has been reported [24]. While the technical expertise and team coordination required to perform successful domino transplantation cannot be underestimated, its potential represents additional opportunity to meet the increasing demands or organ shortage.

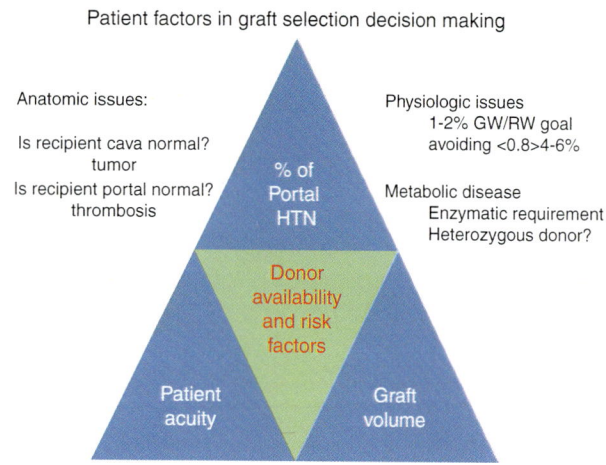

Fig. 26.5 Recipient considerations in liver graft type for children (from Mazariegos, 2017 [10])

Table 26.4 Deceased donor liver criteria for "split-able" liver (Adapted from Battula et al., 2017 [15])

Donation after brain death donor criteria to accept liver for split procedure
Age < 40 years
Weight > 50 kg < 90 kg
Liver function tests up to two to three times normal
Intensive care stay <5 days
No sepsis
Low-dose vasopressors
Satisfactory macroscopic appearance of the graft

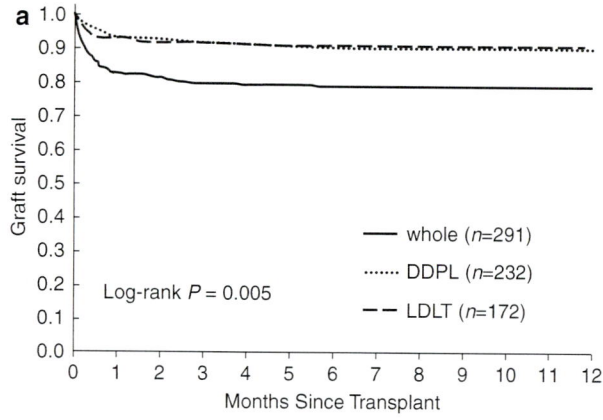
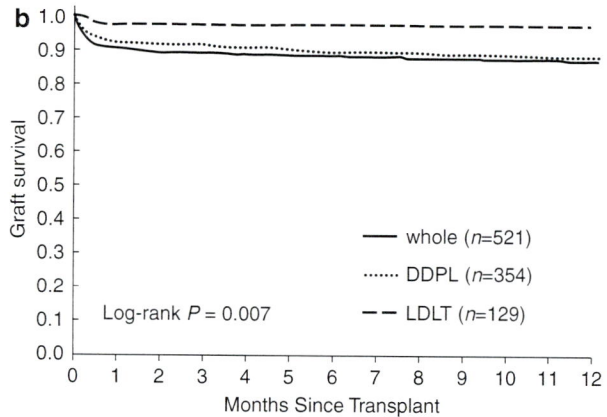

Fig. 26.6 Overall graft survival for pediatric recipients weighing (**a**) ≤ 7 kg, (**b**) 7–14 kg

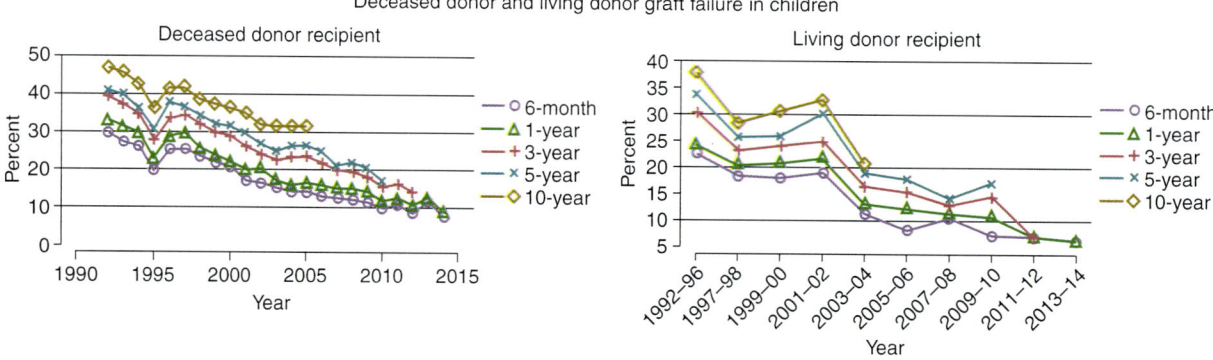

Fig. 26.7 Living donor outcomes over time compared to deceased donors in children receiving liver allografts (from Kim et al., 2017 [8])

and that outcomes are similar between whole livers and technical variant grafts [18, 34, 35]. More recent data suggests that technical variant grafts should no longer be considered inferior to whole grafts for children, particularly for those under the age of 2 years who are the most at risk for waitlist mortality. In fact, technical variant grafts, including LDLT, may be the preferred graft [34]. In a recent analysis of 2123 children in the United Network for Organ Sharing (UNOS) database undergoing transplant for biliary atresia, patient and graft survival advantages were demonstrated for technical variant grafts in children under 7 kg in weight [36]. Vascular thrombosis and retransplantation rates were higher in the youngest cohort when whole organs were utilized. Live donor grafts for these children were also shown to have improved graft survival over whole liver recipients for children <7 kg as well as those weighing 7–14 kg [36] (Fig. 26.6). Long-term data from the Scientific Registry of Transplant Recipients (SRTR) database supports these reports, finding a survival advantage for recipients of live donor allografts at 10 years [8] (Fig. 26.7).

26.4 Extended Criteria Grafts

In children, there is a limited but growing experience utilizing extended criteria grafts to expand the donor pool to address the growing disparity between those awaiting organ transplant and the availability of acceptable organs (Table 26.5).

Donation After Cardiac Death: The utilization of organs from donors with circulatory death has been limited by concern for organ hypoperfusion with resultant ischemic organ injury in the allograft [37]. Yet liver grafts from donation after cardiac death (DCD) are endorsed by the World Health Organization (WHO), practiced worldwide, and increasingly accepted as an extension of the organ pool for liver transplantation [38]. DCD has been increasing in the pediatric population [39–41]. Excellent long-term outcomes have been reported in DCD recipients with absent ischemic cholangiopathy and vascular complications and comparable biliary anastomotic stricture development compared to children who underwent more traditional donation after brain death (DBD) [41]. Furthermore, transplantation of livers from pediatric DCD donors has shown good long-term outcomes with patient and graft survival similar to pediatric DBD donor livers [38].

ABO Incompatibility: Despite the risk of antibody-mediated acute rejection, ABO incompatible (ABOi) grafts, often combined with B-cell desensitization protocols, have been used in Asia and other selected patient populations as a mechanism to compensate for donor shortage. In very small transplant recipients (<5 kg) where mortality awaiting transplant is high, ABOi transplants have been shown to have comparable outcomes, even with standard immunosuppression [42]. Long-term outcomes of pediatric ABOi LDLT demonstrated lower, though not significant, graft survival at 1, 3, and 5 years following transplant. Notably, desensitization did not completely prevent the development of antibody-mediated rejection, highlighting opportunities for improvement [43]. A recent review of US data supports equivalent outcomes in ABOi grafts for recipients under the age of 2 years, although the study volume remains limited [44]. Still, additional complications such as acute kidney injury [45] and biliary stricture development [46] have been reported to have an increased incidence in ABOi transplantation in adult populations.

Hypernatremic Donors: The use of livers from donors with hypernatremia has been associated with graft dysfunction and poor outcomes in adult recipients [47]. However, there is a growing body of evidence that use of grafts from donors with hypernatremia may be acceptable in children awaiting transplant. In a single-center experience from Switzerland, pediatric recipients from hypernatremic donors experienced no significant increases in rates of mortality, rejection, early biliary complications, or infection. While there was an increased relative risk of thrombotic complications, it did not reach significance [47]. In a separate registry study of over 2300 pediatric liver transplant recipients, 722 (31%) of participants received a graft from a donor with a serum sodium level ≥ 150 mmol/L, 155 of whom received a liver from a donor with levels ≥ 160 mmol/L. In the analysis, no negative effects on mortality or graft failure were seen 30 days following transplant [48].

Donors with Increased Body Mass Index: In adult liver transplant recipients, the donor body mass index (dBMI) is associated with posttransplant obesity, but not increased graft loss [49]. In an effort to clarify whether similar results recapitulate in the pediatric population, data on 3788 transplants from UNOS were analyzed. The authors report that while overweight and obese donors are commonly used, the use of donors with BMI of $25 < 35$ kg/m^2 was not associated with decreased graft or patient survival. However, severely obese donors (BMI ≥ 35 kg/m^2) did increase the risk of graft loss and mortality. Posttransplant obesity was not associated with dBMI [50].

Donors of Increased Age: Older donor age has universally been recognized as a significant risk factor that may negatively affect transplant outcomes due to increases in graft failure, perioperative complications, and mortality [51, 52]. While recent reports in adults suggest that grafts from older donors grant equivalent perioperative courses to ideal young donors (aged 18–39), data on their use in children is sparse [51]. While there is a paucity of data in pediatrics, children receiving livers from older donors are at increased risk for the development of intrahepatic biliary strictures [53].

Drowned Donors: Liver donation from drowned donors has often been considered high risk given concerns for infection and graft dysfunction [54]. However, recent studies have shown an increasing trend in the use of grafts from drowned donors [28]. Thus, it is notable that a recent single-center experience suggests that select drowned donor organs can be utilized at no greater risk to transplant patients than that of organs from a matched cohort of head trauma victims [54].

In adults, the utilization of other expanded criteria grafts such as those with extended cold ischemia time; from donors with infectious diseases such as hepatitis B, C, and HIV; from donors with a history of malignancy; and grafts with substantial macrovesicular steatosis is being used in select

Table 26.5 Expanded criteria grafts

Grafts associated with increased risk of dysfunction	Older donor age ABO incompatibility Donation after cardiac death Steatosis Increased cold ischemia time Increased donor body mass index
Grafts associated with increased risk of disease transmission	Hepatitis B core antibody positive Hepatitis B surface antigen positive Hepatitis C infection Human immunodeficiency virus infection History of malignancy

circumstances in order to address the challenge of organ shortage. However, with each use of a high-risk graft, there is a theoretical trade-off between waitlist and posttransplant morbidity and mortality [55]. Ultimately, in pediatrics, these decisions are made that much more complex given the life-years expected following transplantation and the desire to provide the greatest opportunity for optimized quantity and quality of life.

26.5 Decision Support Models

The acceptance of an organ for transplantation is a high-risk medical decision with often little certainty of whether a more suitable graft will become available before death. Thus, various models and decision support indices have been developed to aid in the decision-making process with the goal to better evaluate liver quality and predict perioperative complications [56, 57]. In pediatrics, donor selection is a particularly complex analysis that may benefit from algorithms based in large data analytics. While modeling of decision support systems aimed at pediatric data will be of significant utility in the field [57], to date the field of decision modeling exists mainly as an adjunct to clinical judgment when organ offers are being considered.

26.6 Summary

Allocation of pediatric liver allografts varies widely across the world. Living related liver transplantation has dominated experience in Asia but has been an underutilized technique in the United States. Deceased donor allocation that has coupled pediatric prioritization with split liver technical variant usage has resulted in reduction of pediatric waitlist mortality while minimizing detriments to adult liver transplant outcomes or volumes.

Current data suggests that optimal outcomes can be achieved by developing expertise in all appropriate allograft types and utilizing them in a timely fashion to minimize morbidity on the waitlist and optimize long-term outcomes.

References

1. Hsu EK, Mazariegos GV. Global lessons in graft type and pediatric liver allocation: a path toward improving outcomes and eliminating wait-list mortality. Liver Transpl. 2017;23(1):86–95.
2. Hsu EK, et al. Heterogeneity and disparities in the use of exception scores in pediatric liver allocation. Am J Transplant. 2015;15(2):436–44.
3. Perito ER, et al. Justifying nonstandard exception requests for pediatric liver transplant candidates: an analysis of narratives submitted to the United Network for Organ Sharing, 2009-2014. Am J Transplant. 2017;17(8):2144–54.
4. Ebel NH, et al. Disparities in waitlist and posttransplantation outcomes in liver transplant registrants and recipients aged 18 to 24 years: analysis of the UNOS database. Transplantation. 2017;101(7):1616–27.
5. Hsu EK, et al. Analysis of liver offers to pediatric candidates on the transplant wait list. Gastroenterology. 2017;153(4):988–95.
6. Rana A, et al. Geographic inequity results in disparate mortality: a multivariate intent-to-treat analysis of liver transplant data. Clin Transplant. 2015;29(6):484–91.
7. Mitchell E, et al. Variability in acceptance of organ offers by pediatric transplant centers and its impact on wait-list mortality. Liver Transpl. 2018;24(6):803–9.
8. Kim WR, et al. OPTN/SRTR 2015 annual data report: liver. Am J Transplant. 2017;17(Suppl 1):174–251.
9. Kim WR, et al. OPTN/SRTR 2016 annual data report: liver. Am J Transplant. 2018;18(Suppl 1):172–253.
10. Mazariegos GV. Critical elements in pediatric allograft selection. Liver Transpl. 2017;23(S1):S56–8.
11. Kelly D, et al. Late graft hepatitis and fibrosis in pediatric liver allograft recipients: current concepts and future developments. Liver Transpl. 2016;22(11):1593–602.
12. Bismuth H, Houssin D. Reduced-sized orthotopic liver graft in hepatic transplantation in children. Surgery. 1984;95(3):367–70.
13. Emond JC, et al. Transplantation of two patients with one liver. Analysis of a preliminary experience with 'split-liver' grafting. Ann Surg. 1990;212(1):14–22.
14. Pichlmayr R, et al. [Transplantation of a donor liver to 2 recipients (splitting transplantation)—a new method in the further development of segmental liver transplantation]. Langenbecks Arch Chir. 1988;373(2):127–30.
15. Battula NR, et al. Intention to split policy: a successful strategy in a combined pediatric and adult liver transplant center. Ann Surg. 2017;265(5):1009–15.
16. Rogiers X, et al. In situ splitting of cadaveric livers. The ultimate expansion of a limited donor pool. Ann Surg. 1996;224(3):331–9; discussion 339–41.
17. Rogiers X, et al. In situ splitting of the liver in the heart-beating cadaveric organ donor for transplantation in two recipients. Transplantation. 1995;59(8):1081–3.
18. Perito ER, et al. Split liver transplantation and pediatric waitlist mortality in the United States: potential for improvement. Transplantation. 2018. [Epub ahead of print] PMID: 29684000
19. Strong RW, et al. Successful liver transplantation from a living donor to her son. N Engl J Med. 1990;322(21):1505–7.
20. Kasahara M, Sakamoto S, Fukuda A. Pediatric living-donor liver transplantation. Semin Pediatr Surg. 2017;26(4):224–32.
21. Mc Kiernan PJ. Recent advances in liver transplantation for metabolic disease. J Inherit Metab Dis. 2017;40(4):491–5.
22. Matsunami M, et al. Living donor domino liver transplantation using a maple syrup urine disease donor: a case series of three children—the first report from Japan. Pediatr Transplant. 2016;20(5):633–9.
23. Geyer ED, et al. Outcomes of domino liver transplantation compared to deceased donor liver transplantation: a propensity-matching approach. Transpl Int. 2018;31(11):1200–6.
24. Herden U, et al. The first case of domino-split-liver transplantation in maple syrup urine disease. Pediatr Transplant. 2017;21(6).
25. Organ Procurement and Transplantation Network—HRSA. Final rule with comment period. Fed Regist. 1998;63(63):16296–338.
26. Axelrod DA, Vagefi PA, Roberts JP. The evolution of organ allocation for liver transplantation: tackling geographic disparity through broader sharing. Ann Surg. 2015;262(2):224–7.
27. Shukla A, et al. Liver transplantation: east versus west. J Clin Exp Hepatol. 2013;3(3):243–53.
28. Yoeli D, et al. Trends in pediatric liver transplant donors and deceased donor circumstance of death in the United States, 2002-2015. Pediatr Transplant. 2018;22(3):e13156.

29. Ladin K, Zhang G, Hanto DW. Geographic disparities in liver availability: accidents of geography, or consequences of poor social policy? Am J Transplant. 2017;17(9):2277–84.
30. Squires RH, et al. Evaluation of the pediatric patient for liver transplantation: 2014 practice guideline by the American Association for the Study of Liver Diseases, American Society of Transplantation and the North American Society for Pediatric Gastroenterology, Hepatology and Nutrition. Hepatology. 2014;60(1):362–98.
31. Mazariegos G, et al. Liver transplantation for pediatric metabolic disease. Mol Genet Metab. 2014;111(4):418–27.
32. Diamond IR, et al. Impact of graft type on outcome in pediatric liver transplantation: a report From Studies of Pediatric Liver Transplantation (SPLIT). Ann Surg. 2007;246(2):301–10.
33. Cauley RP, et al. Deceased donor liver transplantation in infants and small children: are partial grafts riskier than whole organs? Liver Transpl. 2013;19(7):721–9.
34. Mogul DB, et al. Fifteen-year trends in pediatric liver transplants: split, whole deceased, and living donor grafts. J Pediatr. 2018;196:148–53.e2.
35. Rodriguez-Davalos MI, et al. Segmental grafts in adult and pediatric liver transplantation: improving outcomes by minimizing vascular complications. JAMA Surg. 2014;149(1):63–70.
36. Alexopoulos SP, et al. Effects of recipient size and allograft type on pediatric liver transplantation for biliary atresia. Liver Transpl. 2017;23(2):221–33.
37. Morrissey PE, Monaco AP. Donation after circulatory death: current practices, ongoing challenges, and potential improvements. Transplantation. 2014;97(3):258–64.
38. van Rijn R, et al. Long-term results after transplantation of pediatric liver grafts from donation after circulatory death donors. PLoS One. 2017;12(4):e0175097.
39. Harring TR, et al. Liver transplantation with donation after cardiac death donors: a comprehensive update. J Surg Res. 2012;178(1):502–11.
40. Bartlett A, et al. A single center experience of donation after cardiac death liver transplantation in pediatric recipients. Pediatr Transplant. 2010;14(3):388–92.
41. Hong JC, et al. Liver transplantation in children using organ donation after circulatory death: a case-control outcomes analysis of a 20-year experience in a single center. JAMA Surg. 2014;149(1):77–82.
42. Gelas T, et al. ABO-incompatible pediatric liver transplantation in very small recipients: Birmingham's experience. Pediatr Transplant. 2011;15(7):706–11.
43. Honda M, et al. Long-term outcomes of ABO-incompatible pediatric living donor liver transplantation. Transplantation. 2018;102(10):1702–9.
44. Rana A, et al. Pediatric liver transplantation across the ABO blood group barrier: is it an obstacle in the modern era? J Am Coll Surg. 2016;222(4):681–9.
45. Jun IG, et al. Comparison of acute kidney injury between ABO-compatible and ABO-incompatible living donor liver transplantation: a propensity matching analysis. Liver Transpl. 2016;22(12):1656–65.
46. Song GW, et al. Biliary stricture is the only concern in ABO-incompatible adult living donor liver transplantation in the rituximab era. J Hepatol. 2014;61(3):575–82.
47. Kaseje N, et al. Donor hypernatremia influences outcomes following pediatric liver transplantation. Eur J Pediatr Surg. 2013;23(1):8–13.
48. Kaseje N, et al. Donor hypernatremia before procurement and early outcomes following pediatric liver transplantation. Liver Transpl. 2015;21(8):1076–81.
49. Everhart JE, et al. Weight change and obesity after liver transplantation: incidence and risk factors. Liver Transpl Surg. 1998;4(4):285–96.
50. Perito ER, et al. Impact of the donor body mass index on the survival of pediatric liver transplant recipients and post-transplant obesity. Liver Transpl. 2012;18(8):930–9.
51. Biancofiore G, et al. Octogenarian donors in liver transplantation grant an equivalent perioperative course to ideal young donors. Dig Liver Dis. 2017;49(6):676–82.
52. Pirenne J, et al. Liver transplantation using livers from septuagenarian and octogenarian donors: an underused strategy to reduce mortality on the waiting list. Transplant Proc. 2005;37(2):1180–1.
53. Luthold SC, et al. Risk factors for early and late biliary complications in pediatric liver transplantation. Pediatr Transplant. 2014;18(8):822–30.
54. Kumm KR, et al. Are drowned donors marginal donors? A single pediatric center experience. Pediatr Transplant. 2017;21(6).
55. Feng S, Lai JC. Expanded criteria donors. Clin Liver Dis. 2014;18(3):633–49.
56. Mataya L, et al. Decision making in liver transplantation—limited application of the liver donor risk index. Liver Transpl. 2014;20(7):831–7.
57. Volk ML, et al. Decision support for organ offers in liver transplantation. Liver Transpl. 2015;21(6):784–91.

Surgical Techniques

Michele Colledan and Stefania Camagni

Key Points

- Different types of technical variant grafts and full-size grafts have been used in paediatric LT. Nowadays, transplantation of LLSs from split liver and living donation appears the most effective strategy to transplant small children.
- Organ availability and donor-to-recipient size matching guide the choice of a specific graft type on a case-by-case basis.
- The best results overall may be achieved at high-volume centres with extensive experience with all graft types and age groups, which may allow transplantation according to each recipient's special needs. A liberal split policy and an active LDLT program should be complementary resources in Western countries for the purpose of eliminating paediatric wait-list mortality.
- For a safe and effective implantation of a LLS, it is important to keep in mind some recipient-related and graft-related peculiarities:
  - Small children easily tolerate cross-clamping of the infrahepatic and the suprahepatic vena cava, so total clamping is preferred to side clamping even in case of caval preservation since it allows a large opening over the orifices of the hepatic veins for outflow reconstruction.
  - A hypoplastic portal vein is a common feature in patients with biliary atresia, so the need for a specific technical solution is not that unusual.
  - The arterial anastomosis site depends on both the recipient's arterial axis and the graft arterial pedicle.
  - Biliary reconstruction consists of a single or double end-to-side hepaticojejunostomy, depending on the presence of the left bile duct or of two separate segmental ducts.
  - An optimal graft orientation is fundamental to avoid portal vein kinking and outflow obstruction.
- Further reduction of LLSs, the use of LLSs from small deceased paediatric donors and delayed abdominal closure may be useful strategies to transplant infants less than 5–6 kg in weight.
- In experienced hands, APOLT is being increasingly accepted as a valid alternative to standard LT in selected cases of ALF, allowing over two-thirds of these patients the chance of an immunosuppression-free life. Even though its acceptance is controversial, APOLT may be a safe alternative to standard LT also in the setting of NCMLD, preserving the option of later gene therapy without lifelong immunosuppression.

Research Needed in the Field

- **Size Matching**

  Size matching is crucial for the outcome of paediatric LT but any of the current approaches to this issue may be questionable since no evidence-based guidelines exist and the safe size matching range is unknown [1]. So, research on this issue may help improve both graft and patient survival.

M. Colledan (✉) · S. Camagni
Department of Organ Failure and Transplantation,
Hospital Papa Giovanni XXIII, Bergamo, Italy
e-mail: mcolledan@asst-pg23.it; scamagni@asst-pg23.it

- **Graft Inflow Modulation**

  When transplanting a cirrhotic child with portal hypertension, graft inflow modulation may allow optimal portal and arterial flow. The most appropriate haemodynamic parameters to guide the application of graft inflow modulation and the best graft inflow modulation strategies are still a topic of debate [2, 3]. So, prospective multicentre trials should be encouraged to further explore this issue.

- **Prevention of Biliary Complications**

  Biliary complications are a major source of morbidity after paediatric SLT and LDLT. No gold standard for their prophylaxis has been established so far [4, 5]. Thus, the need for further investigation into this issue is undeniable. Provided a high index of clinical suspicion and an attitude to early aggressive diagnosis are shared, prospective multicentre trials would be advisable.

- **APOLT**

  The best candidates to APOLT have not been clearly identified yet. Besides, in the setting of NCMLD, the required auxiliary graft volume to replace the deficient enzymatic activity is unknown and the ideal strategy to manage portal steal has not been defined yet [6, 7]. So, APOLT appears as another field needing further research.

27.1 Graft Types for Paediatric Liver Transplantation

27.1.1 From Full-Size to Reduced-Sized Grafts

Since 1967, when Starzl accomplished the first successful case [8], for almost two decades, all paediatric liver transplantations (LT) have been performed using size-matched whole organs from deceased donors. Unfortunately, such grafts were hardly available. In 1984, Bismuth firstly reported a paediatric LT with a segmental graft obtained by reducing the size of an adult liver [9]. Actually, a similar case had been previously performed by Starzl in 1975 but was reported only in 1990 [10]. The reduced-sized technique appeared to be the solution to the shortage of appropriate-sized donors for small children and soon became the procedure of choice for this population with good results [11–13]. Anyway, as the reduction of an adult liver generated only one transplantable graft, the problem of organ shortage was merely shifted from the paediatric to the adult population. So, two strategies were developed to supply the paediatric demand for small-sized grafts without detriment to the adult waiting list: split LT (SLT), resulting from the division of a deceased donor liver into two transplantable parts, and living donor LT (LDLT). The first ex situ split (see paragraph "Ex situ versus in situ split liver") was described by Pichlmayr in 1988 [14], while the first successful LDLT was reported by Strong in 1989 [15]. Initially, SLT had a limited diffusion because the outcomes reported by the early series were worse than those obtained by full-size LT and LDLT [16–18]. In 1995, a retrospective analysis of the European Split Registry showed improved survival for the first time, raising new interest in SLT [19]. In the same year, Rogiers described the first in situ split [20] (see paragraph "Ex situ versus in situ split liver"). The introduction of the in situ technique offered another big contribution to the progressively increasing diffusion of SLT [21–28].

Nowadays, transplantation of left lateral segment grafts (LLSs), from split liver or living donation, is the most common strategy to transplant small children, who represent the largest portion of paediatric candidates to LT.

Figures 27.1 and 27.2 present the evolution over time of graft types for paediatric LT in Europe according to ELRT/ELITA data [29].

This chapter will focus on deceased donor paediatric LT, particularly on SLT, LDLT being the object of another specific chapter of this textbook.

The use of a specific graft type from a deceased donor depends on donor-to-recipient size matching.

27.2 Split Liver

Split liver, namely the division of a deceased donor liver into two transplantable parts, is based on the fundamental principle that a partial liver graft with a suitable arterial and portal inflow together with the corresponding venous and biliary drainage and sufficient hepatocyte mass can fulfil the role of a whole organ [30, 31]. Along with LDLT, SLT evolved from the advancements of hepatobiliary surgery and an improved understanding of liver segmental anatomy (Fig. 27.3).

27.2.1 Ex Situ Versus In Situ Split Liver

Split liver can be performed ex situ or in situ. The former technique consists of dividing the whole liver on the back-table after standard procurement. The latter, derived from the experience of living donor liver procurement, consists of dividing the whole liver in the heart-beating deceased donor. The in situ technique offers the advantage of shortening the ischaemia time, which allows for long-distance sharing between transplant centres as well. Theoretically, it may also improve the control of bleeding from the cut parenchymal surface of the grafts [22]. On the other hand, it significantly increases the donor operation time and general complexity, which must be

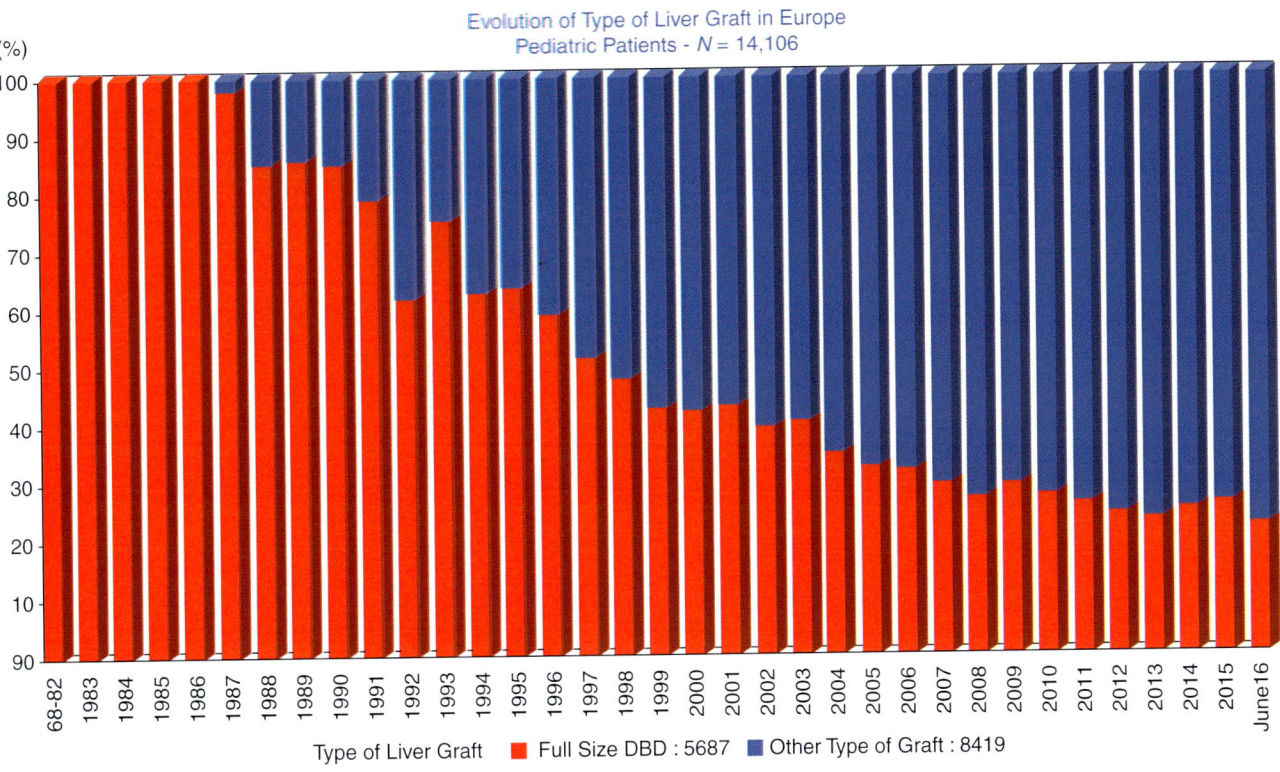

Fig. 27.1 Evolution over time of graft types for paediatric LT in Europe (ELTR/ELITA data, kindly provided by Dr. Vincent Karam)

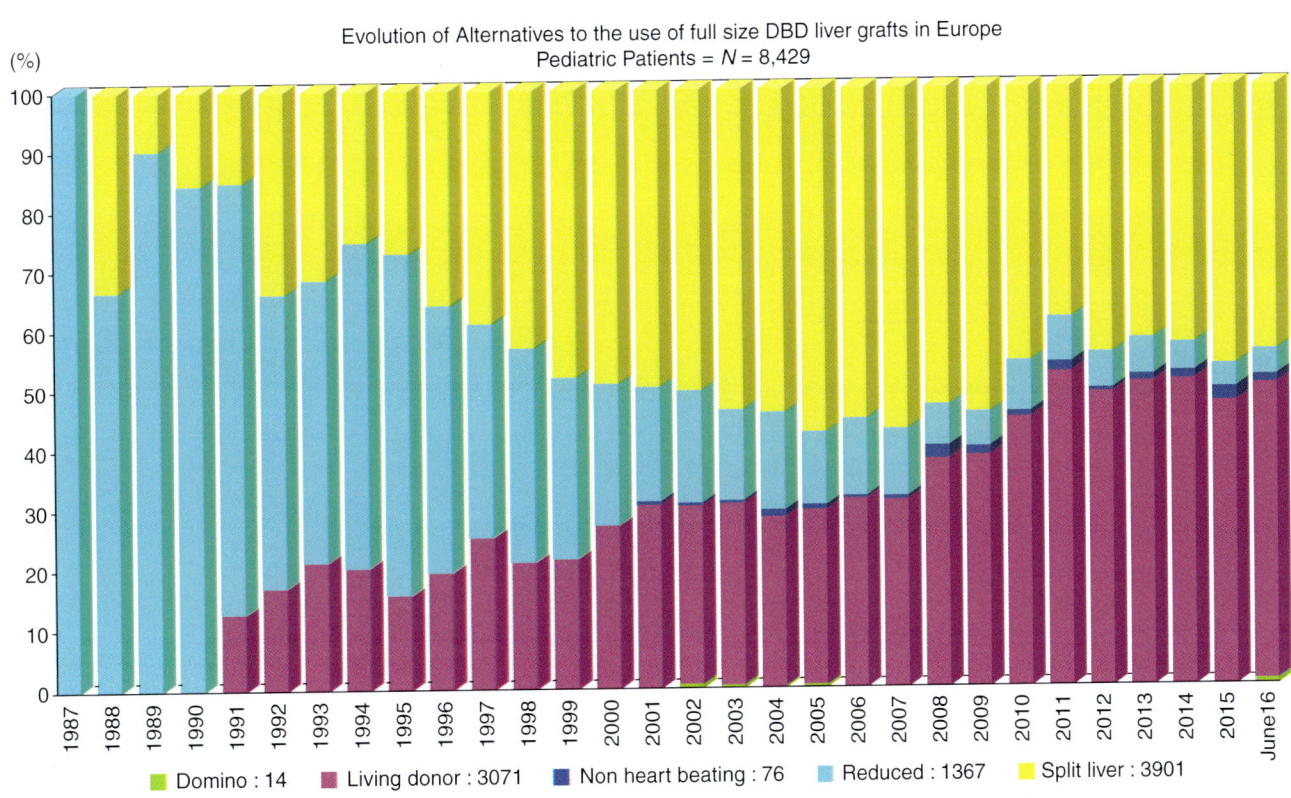

Fig. 27.2 Evolution over time of the alternatives to full-size grafts from donors after neurological determination of death (DBD) for paediatric LT in Europe (ELTR/ELITA data, kindly provided by Dr. Vincent Karam)

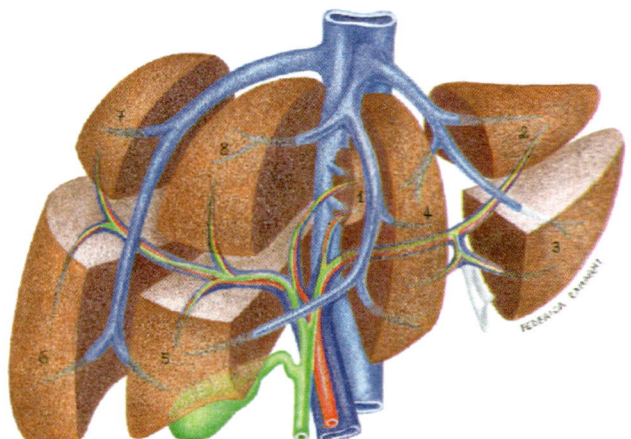

Fig. 27.3 Liver segmental anatomy

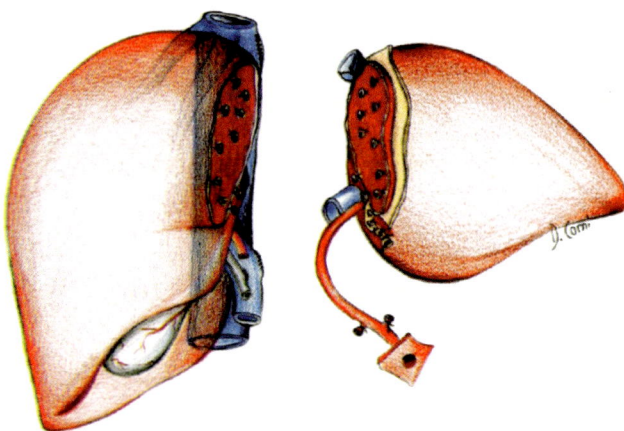

Fig. 27.4 ACSL (this figure, published in "Transplant Rev 2005;19:221–231", has been reproduced with permission from Elsevier)

considered for organisational aims. No prospective studies comparing the two techniques are available but the reported series of ex situ and in situ split liver show similar outcomes [32, 33]. The in situ technique is the preferred and substantially exclusive choice for split liver at our centre.

27.2.2 Types of Split Liver

The concept of split liver involves two different entities.

The adult/child split liver (ACSL) generates an extended right graft (ERG), including the Couinaud segments I and IV to VIII [34], and a LLS, including segments II and III (Fig. 27.4). The former is suitable for transplantation into an adult (or an adult-sized child), while the latter is appropriate for transplantation into a small child usually not exceeding 30 kg in weight [33]. Despite controversies on the quality of this kind of grafts still exist and the debate on the outcomes of SLT is still open [35], the ACSL represents a well-established procedure at the main paediatric transplant centres in Western countries.

The adult/adult split liver (AASL) generates two similar-sized grafts, usually a full-right one (FRG), including segments V to VIII, and a full-left one (FLG), including segments I to IV (Fig. 27.5). These grafts are suitable for transplantation into two small adults or large children exceeding 25–30 kg in weight [33]. The first attempt of dividing an adult whole liver into two grafts to be transplanted into two adult-sized recipients was made in 1989 by Bismuth, who used this strategy for emergency grafting of two patients with fulminant hepatic failure [36]. Unfortunately, both of them died of causes not specifically related to the surgical technique. In 1999, our group first reported the long-term successful application of an original technique of AASL, derived from the experience of living donor right lobe procurement [37]. Subsequently, case reports and larger series

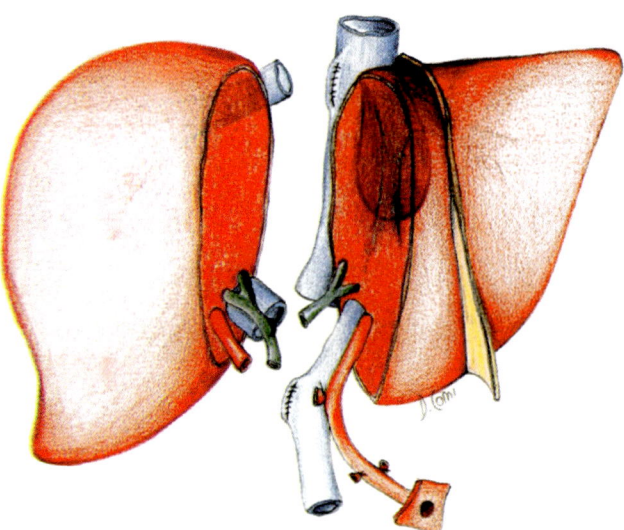

Fig. 27.5 AASL (this figure, published in "Transplant Rev 2005;19:221–231", has been reproduced with permission from Elsevier)

of AASL from Western transplant centres were published with encouraging results [38–45]. Anyway, this very complex procedure is still less standardized than ACSL and its diffusion remains limited.

27.3 Adult/Child Split Liver

27.3.1 Donor Selection

Although specific selection criteria vary among centres [30, 33, 46–49], it is agreed that the ideal donor for ACSL should be young and not obese, should not have a history of liver disease, should have a short intensive care unit stay, should be haemodynamically stable and should have normal or near normal liver function tests [50]. The North Italian Transplant program, the referral organization to which our centre belongs, identified the following donor eligibility criteria: age <60 years, intensive care unit stay <5 days, low inotropic support and normal or near normal liver function tests [49]. At our centre, the split liver technique is used aggressively for size adapting in any donor whose liver is deemed suitable for transplanting a child on the waiting list, with no specific criteria for the split procedure itself [33, 51]. The only exception is haemodynamic instability, which represents a reasonable technical contraindication to the in situ technique [33].

27.3.2 Size Matching

Size matching is crucial for the outcome of paediatric LT. A too small graft may be unable to meet the functional demands of the recipient, leading to small-for-size syndrome. Conversely, a too large graft may be damaged by vascular thrombosis or necrosis due to inadequate perfusion and may result in the impossibility to close the abdomen, with increased mortality [33, 52–54]. Unlike LDLT, generally SLT cannot rely on a precise preoperative assessment of the volume of the donor LLS. In theory, the LLS accounts for the 25–30% of the total liver volume. Anyway, the LLS volume is highly variable and cannot be predicted by simple anthropometric variables [53]. No evidence-based guidelines concerning size matching are available, and the safe size matching range remains unknown [1]. At our centre, when the recipient is a small child, the rule about size matching provides for transplanting the liver as a whole (Fig. 27.6) or ERG for a donor-to-recipient weight ratio (DRWR) between 0.5 and 2 and for transplanting a LLS for a DRWR between 2 and 12 [33], which usually translates into a graft-to-recipient weight ratio (GRWR) between 1.5% and 6% or somewhat more. In case of ERGs, it has to be kept in mind that they are expected to represent about 70–75% of the total liver volume.

27.3.3 Attribution of the Vascular and Biliary Supply and Choice of the Transection Plane

No consensus exists on the allocation of the whole arterial axis, including the celiac, common and proper hepatic artery [33, 55]. One of the grafts has necessarily to rely only on its named branch. The policy of most paediatric transplant centres provides for retaining the celiac axis with the LLS [26, 27, 33, 56, 57]. In fact, the size of the right hepatic artery is usually larger than that of the left hepatic artery and appropriate for a safe anastomosis. Devascularisation of segment IV, which happens when its arterial supply arises from the proper of left hepatic artery, is generally only an occasional cause of minor morbidity in the recipient of the ERG. Anyway, the allocation of the whole arterial axis should be discussed time after time with the ERG team, taking into consideration the specific arterial anatomy and reciprocal needs. Figure 27.7 shows two different LLS, one retaining the whole arterial axis (a) while the other retaining only the left hepatic artery (b).

Conversely, the allocation of the portal, biliary and hepatocaval pedicles is unanimously agreed upon: the LLS retains the left branch of the portal vein, the left hepatic duct and the left hepatic vein, while the ERG retains the portal vein, the common bile duct and the inferior vena cava (Fig. 27.4).

Two techniques have been employed for ACLS, the trans-umbilical and the trans-hilar [14, 16, 17, 36, 58]. One of the distinctive characteristics of the two approaches is the line for liver division. The trans-umbilical technique sets the cut surface through the umbilical fissure, thus producing a pure LLS, including only segments II and III. Instead, the trans-hilar technique sets the transection line somewhat on the right of the umbilical fissure, thus including a variable portion of segment IV along with the LLS. Recently, de Ville de Goyet retrospectively compared the outcomes of the two approaches, which appeared to be equally safe and effective [55]. At our centre, almost all ACSL have been performed following the trans-umbilical technique, which will be described in the next paragraph.

27.3.4 Surgical Technique

This paragraph describes the technique for in situ ACLS adopted at our centre [33].

The donor operation begins with the evaluation of the LLS. The definitive judgement on size matching depends on the estimation of its volume. The feasibility of the splitting procedure is assessed by excluding technical contraindications such

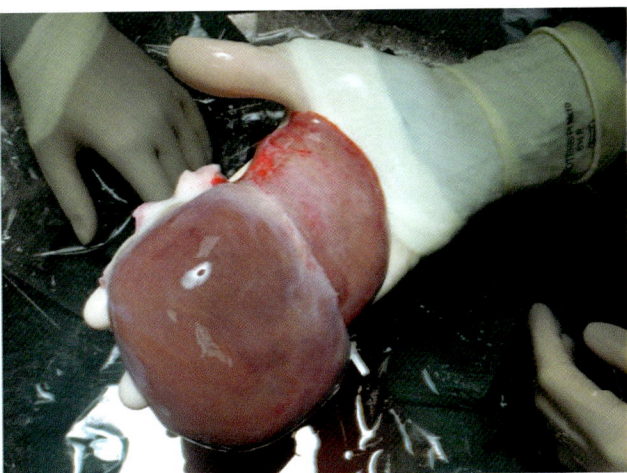

Fig. 27.6 Full-size liver graft from a paediatric donor

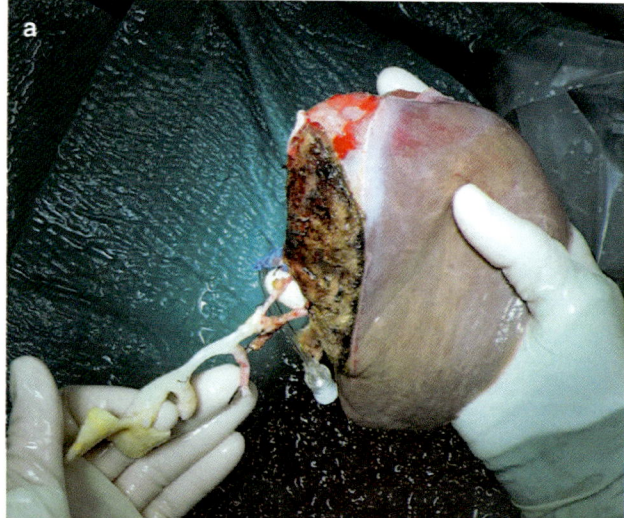

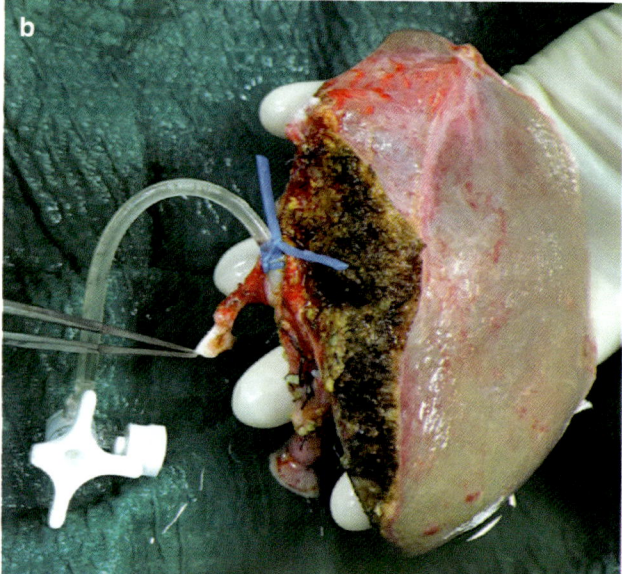

Fig. 27.7 (a) The LLS retains the whole arterial axis. (b) The LLS retains only its named branch (indicated by the forceps), which, anyway, appears to be large enough to allow for a safe anastomosis in a primary transplant recipient

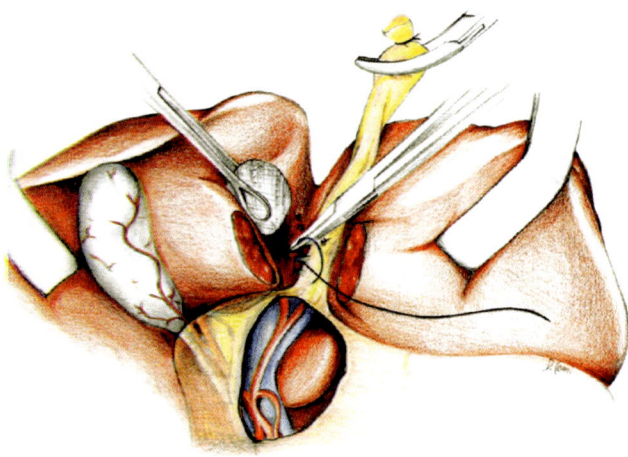

Fig. 27.8 ACSL: dissection of the umbilical fissure (this figure, published in "Transplant Rev 2005;19:221–231", has been reproduced with permission from Elsevier)

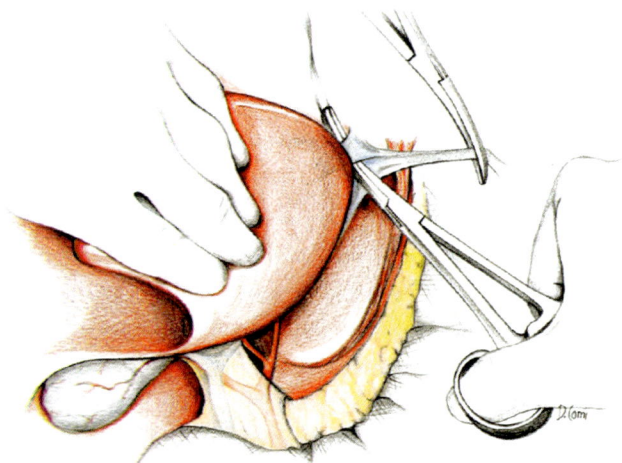

Fig. 27.9 ACLS: isolation of the left hepatic vein (this figure, published in "Transplant Rev 2005;19:221–231", has been reproduced with permission from Elsevier)

as an undivided portal vein at the hilum [59, 60] and a left-sided gallbladder, which may be associated with portal and biliary anomalies [61]. Finally, a biopsy may occasionally help assess the liver quality at the surgeon's discretion: at our centre, macrovescicular steatosis >10% is considered a relative contraindication to split liver, depending on the recipient's conditions.

After standard manoeuvres for aortic control, the division of the liver is started.

The origin of the right hepatic artery is identified and the left hepatic artery is isolated. Then, the umbilical fissure is dissected with suture ligation and section of the portal branches connecting the round ligament and the Rex recessus with segment IV (Fig. 27.8). The left branch of the portal vein is encircled. So, the left aspect of the hilar plate is exposed. After sectioning the hepatogastric, left triangular and coronary ligaments and dissecting the Arantius' ligament, the left hepatic vein is encircled at its confluence into the inferior vena cava (Fig. 27.9). Returning to the hepatic pedicle, the left portion of the hilar plate is encircled and sectioned sharply with the knife at the level of the planned parenchymal transection. Then, an umbilical tape is passed around the left hepatic vein, along the sulcus of Arantius and between the left hepatic pedicle and the parenchyma to emerge in the umbilical fissure. Traction on its edges helps the subsequent parenchymal transection [62], which is carried along the falciform ligament. After parenchymal transection, the liver is divided into two still perfused grafts, connected only by their vascular pedicles (Fig. 27.10).

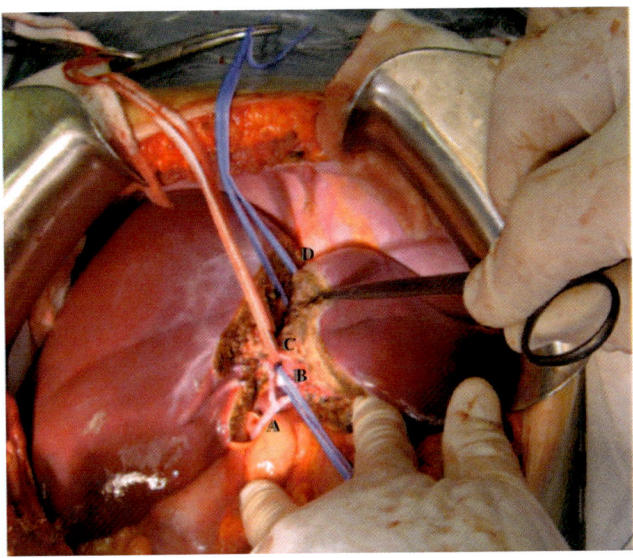

Fig. 27.10 LLS and ERG from in situ split connected only by their vascular pedicles and by the hilar plate. (A) Left hepatic artery. (B) Left branch of the portal vein. (C) Left portion of the hilar plate (the hilar plate can be sectioned either before or after aortic cross-clamping and cold flushing). (D) Left hepatic vein

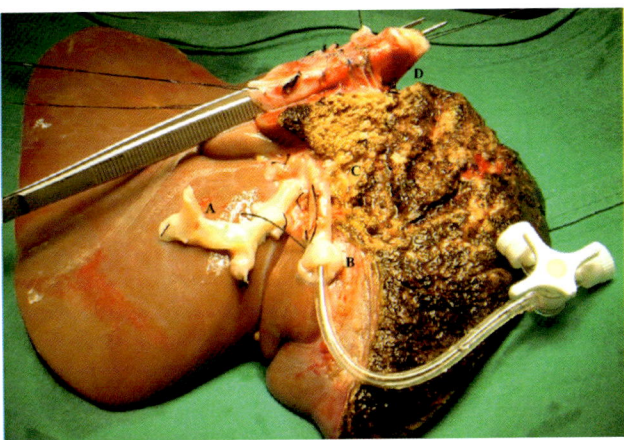

Fig. 27.11 FLG retaining the whole arterial axis (A), the portal trunk (B), the left hepatic duct (C) and the inferior vena cava (D)

The multiorgan procurement is then carried on in the standard fashion. After aortic cross-clamping and cold flushing, the two liver grafts are retrieved separately.

In the ex situ technique, the procedure for liver division on the back-table is the same as in the in situ technique.

27.4 Adult/Adult Split Liver

27.4.1 Donor Selection and Size Matching

Even if precise parameters have not been identified, consensus exists on limiting the AASL procedure to optimal donors; thus selection criteria are more restrictive than for ACSL [45, 50, 63–65].

Size matching is a delicate issue, too. As for ACSL, an accurate preoperative measurement of FLG and FRG volume is generally not feasible. So, size matching is based on the estimation of FLG and FRG volume as about the 40 and 60% of the donor total liver volume respectively, FLG volume being particularly unpredictable, and on a desired GRWR of at least 1% [33, 45, 65]. When the grafts from AASL are shared between a child and an adult, the FLG is usually assigned to the former.

27.4.2 Attribution of the Vascular and Biliary Supply

It is agreed that the whole arterial axis and the portal trunk should be left with the FLG to ensure optimal blood supply to segments I and IV, FRG blood supply relying on the right arterial and portal branches. The common bile duct is preferentially kept with the FRG, whereas the left hepatic duct, normally longer than the right, is left with the FLG [31]. The retrohepatic vena cava is generally attributed to the FLG, the FRG retaining the right hepatic vein [66, 67], or divided into two patches, one for each graft [68]. Optimal outflow may be obtained by dividing also the middle hepatic vein longitudinally into two halves to be shared between the two grafts [69].

Figure 27.5 illustrates the most common allocation of the vascular and biliary supply in AASL. Figure 27.11 shows a FLG retaining the whole arterial axis, the portal trunk, the left hepatic duct and the retrohepatic inferior vena cava, as more commonly performed at our centre.

27.5 Recipient Operation

The following paragraphs will describe the surgical techniques adopted at our centre [33].

27.5.1 Total Hepatectomy

A bilateral subcostal incision is performed (Fig. 27.12). The round ligament is ligated and divided and the falciform ligament is sectioned. Being biliary atresia the most common indication to paediatric LT, adhesions from a previous Kasai procedure are a frequent finding and have to be carefully dissected. In the presence of a Roux-en-Y loop from a previous Kasai procedure, it is divided at the porta hepatis and preserved for reuse. Otherwise, in the presence of the biliary tree, both the cystic duct and the common hepatic duct or the common bile duct are ligated and sectioned (Fig. 27.13). The left and right hepatic arteries are isolated, ligated and dissected as close to the liver as possible to keep any options for

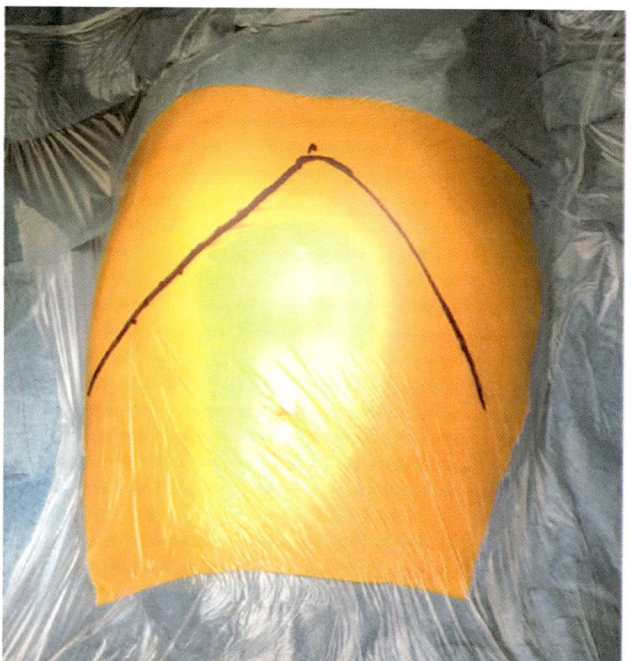

Fig. 27.12 Planned bilateral subcostal incision

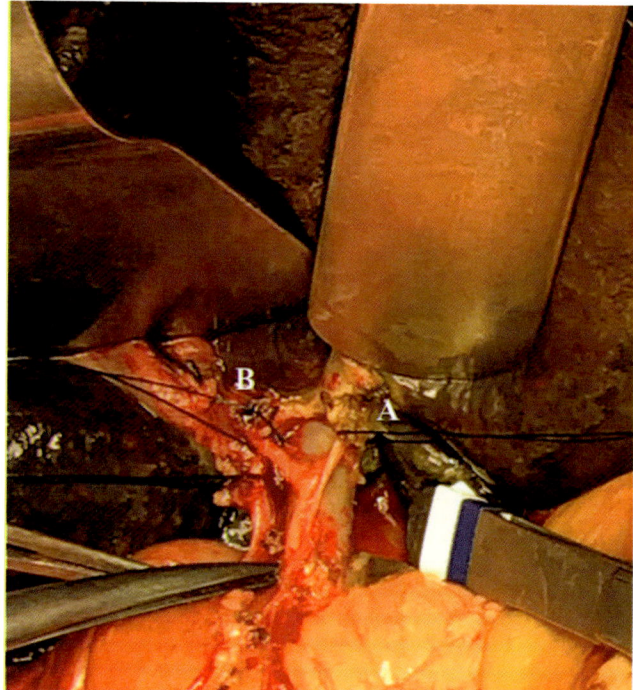

Fig. 27.14 Suture ligation and dissection of the left (A) and right (B) hepatic arteries as close to the liver as possible

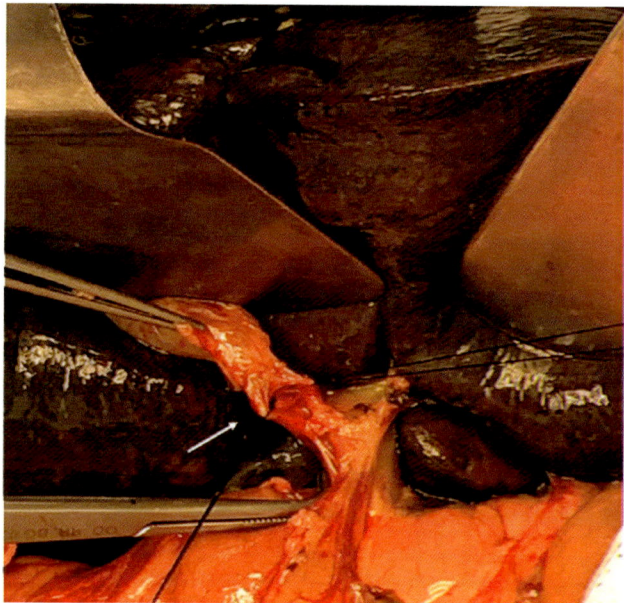

Fig. 27.13 Suture ligation of the cystic duct (indicated by the arrow)

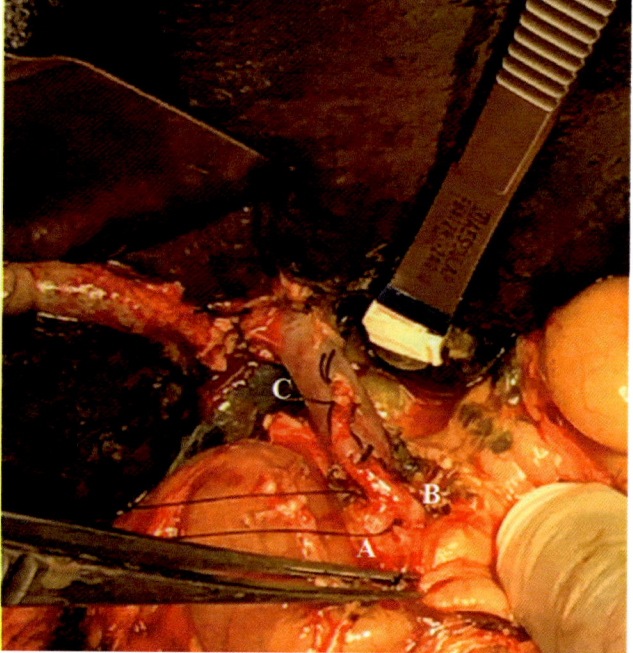

Fig. 27.15 Mobilisation of the arterial axis from the proper hepatic artery to the gastroduodenal artery (A) and the common hepatic artery (B). Isolation of the portal vein (C) from its bifurcation to the spleno-mesenteric confluence

the subsequent graft implantation (Fig. 27.14). For the same purpose, it may be useful to mobilise the arterial axis from the proper hepatic artery to the gastroduodenal artery or even further. The portal vein is then skeletonized from its bifurcation to a level depending on its calibre (Fig. 27.15). After hilar dissection, the left and right liver lobes are mobilised. On the left, the hepatogastric, triangular and coronary ligaments are divided (Fig. 27.16). On the right, the triangular and coronary ligaments are sectioned, and the right lobe is freed from its retroperitoneal attachments (Fig. 27.17). Depending on the graft type or on the specific condition or on the preferred technique for hepatic venous outflow recon-

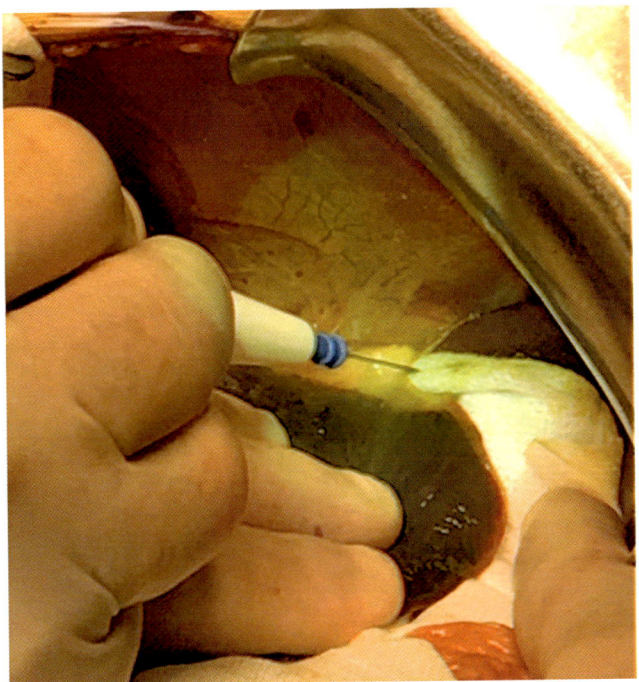

Fig. 27.16 Division of the left triangular and coronary ligament

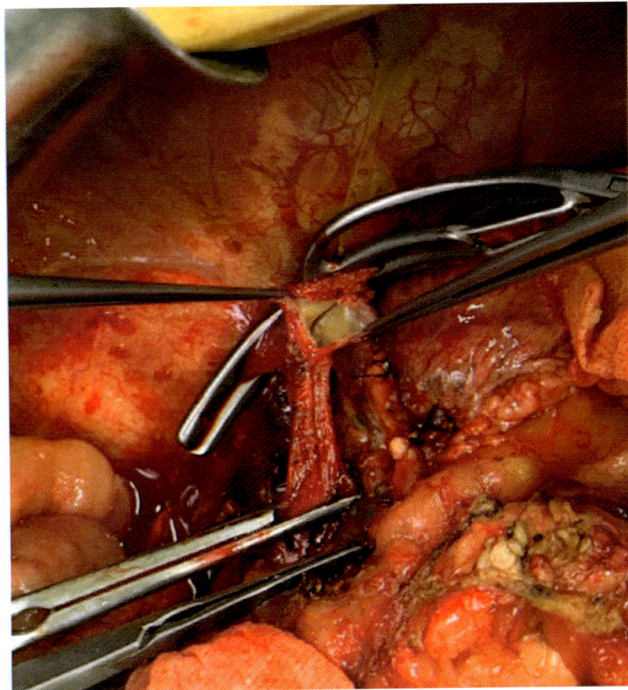

Fig. 27.18 Preserved native vena cava after total hepatectomy. Double cross-clamping of the infrahepatic and the suprahepatic vena cava allows a large opening over the orifices of the hepatic veins

27.5.2 Implantation of the Left Lateral Segment

Being transplantation of LLSs from split liver or living donors the most common strategy for LT in small children, the implantation of this kind of graft will be discussed extensively while the implantation of other types of graft will be just briefly mentioned.

Although relatively well tolerated in small children, it is important to limit the cross-clamp time in order to avoid prolonged stasis in both systemic and portal circulation. Moreover, once the graft is put into the operative field, any effort should be made to keep the implantation rewarming time as short as possible.

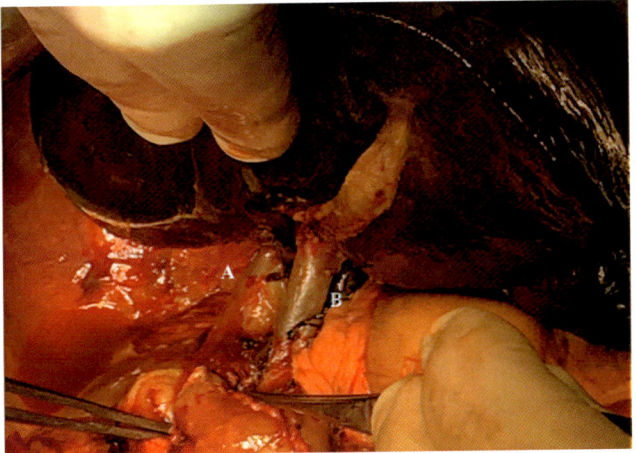

Fig. 27.17 Mobilisation of the right lobe (A, inferior vena cava; B, portal vein)

struction, the retrohepatic vena cava can be preserved or removed with the native liver. In small children, cross-clamping of the infrahepatic and the suprahepatic vena cava is easily tolerated, so it is preferred to side clamping even in case of caval preservation since it allows for a large opening over the orifices of the hepatic veins for outflow reconstruction (Fig. 27.18). After cross-clamping of the portal vein and of the infrahepatic and the suprahepatic vena cava, the native liver is excised.

If the native vena cava has been preserved, as it usually happens, a triangular end-to-side anastomosis is performed between the graft hepatic vein and an opening including one, two or all the orifices of the native right, middle and left hepatic veins using non-absorbable polypropylene sutures (Fig. 27.19). This technique, first proposed by Broelsch and Emond [70, 71], enables a large anastomosis for outflow optimization. Other techniques have been described with a similar rate of outflow complications [72–76]. If the retrohepatic vena cava has been removed with the native liver to achieve a radical resection in case of liver malignancies or for anatomical or technical reasons, it may be replaced by a donor venous graft. At our centre, first the venous graft is implanted on the LLS hepatic vein at the back-table, and then a double caval end-to-end anastomosis is performed (Fig. 27.20). The back-table preparation of the neo-cava allows to limit the cross-clamp time. Literature on caval replacement in paediatric LT with LLSs is scanty. We have recently presented the results of a monocentric retrospective cohort study comparing caval preservation and caval replacement in paediatric recipients of primary LT with deceased donor LLSs. Since no statistical difference in the incidence of hepatic venous outflow complications has been verified, we deem caval replacement safe and effective and consider it a useful option in case of liver malignancies, Budd-Chiari syndrome or severe hypoplasia of the retrohepatic vena cava [77]. Occasionally, in case of congenital interruption or absence of the inferior vena cava with azygous or hemiazygos continuation, a third approach is needed: an end-to-end anastomosis may be performed between the graft hepatic vein and the cloaca of the recipient's hepatic veins, directly draining into the right atrium [78]. Whatever the technique, during the outflow reconstruction the liver graft is flushed with Ringer's lactate solution.

Then comes the end-to-end anastomosis between the graft left portal branch and the recipient's portal vein. In the presence of a hypoplastic portal vein, which is a common feature in patients with biliary atresia, a donor venous graft may be interposed between the spleno-mesenteric confluence and the LLS portal branch [79]. Portoplasty may be an alternative option: after dissection of the portal vein down to the spleno-mesenteric confluence, a longitudinal venotomy is performed, and a donor patch venous graft is sutured to the recipient's portal vein; then, an end-to-end anastomosis between this reconstructed vessel and the graft portal stump is done [80, 81]. In the event of haemodynamically significant portosystemic shunts, their ligature should be attempted in order to avoid portal flow diversion from the liver and subsequent portal vein thrombosis. A singular condition is represented by Abernethy malformation type 1, which is characterized by the congenital absence of the portal vein and by an extrahepatic end-to-side portocaval shunt (Fig. 27.21) [82]. In this case, the portocaval shunt is discontinued, and a standard end-to-end portal anastomosis is performed with the interrupted vessel. Whatever the technique, the orientation of the liver graft is crucial to prevent portal vein kinking and subsequent thrombosis. We are used to place it in a rather central position, rotated about 30–45° to the right on an axial plane and clockwise on a coronal plane [33].

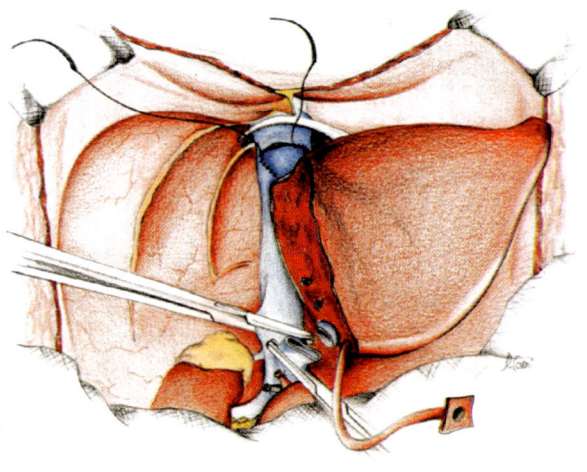

Fig. 27.19 Caval preservation: triangular end-to-side anastomosis between the graft hepatic vein and the orifices of the native hepatic veins (this figure, published in "Transplant Rev 2005;19:221–231", has been reproduced with permission from Elsevier)

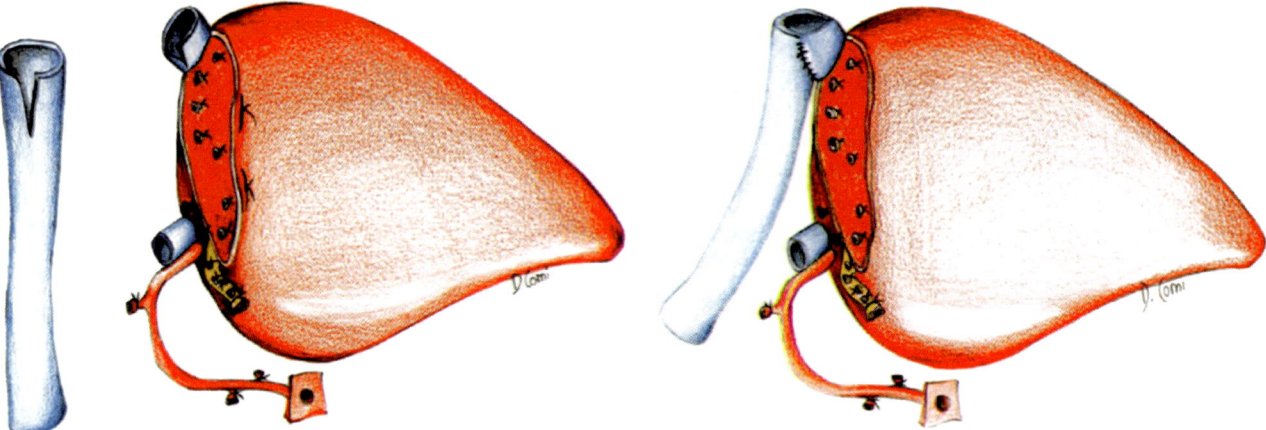

Fig. 27.20 Caval replacement by back-table implantation of a venous graft on the LLS hepatic vein

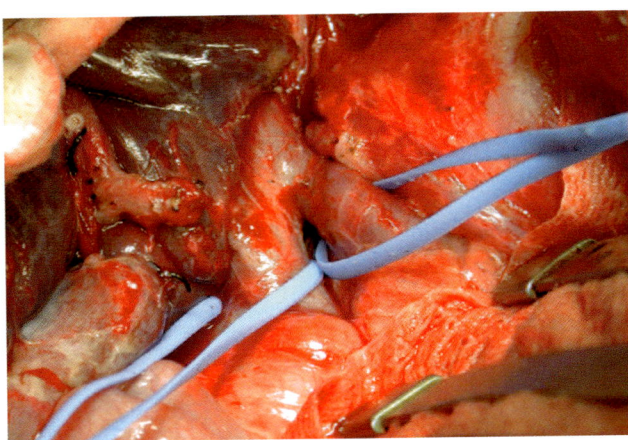

Fig. 27.21 Abernethy malformation type 1

Once the portal anastomosis has been completed, the removal of portal and caval clamps allows graft reperfusion by portal flow and ends the warm ischaemic time.

The next step consists of restoration of hepatic arterial flow. The choice of the arterial anastomosis site depends on the graft arterial pedicle and on the recipient's arterial axis. The graft and the recipient's arterial branches to be anastomosed should be congruent in calibre, and the resulting vessel should not kink or twist. Children affected by biliary atresia often have a large arterial axis, so the anastomosis can be safely performed on their common or proper hepatic artery most of the times. On the contrary, Alagille syndrome is characterized by a hypoplastic arterial axis, so the supraceliac or infrarenal aorta could be an option for the anastomosis, with or without an interposition graft. Microvascular techniques using both intraoperative microscopy and high-power loupe magnification have been described, with the most recent series showing similar results with any of these strategies [83–87].

At our centre, it is common practice to use absorbable polydioxanone sutures for portal anastomosis in order to prevent stricture formation by allowing these small calibre vascular anastomoses to grow over time.

Finally, biliary reconstruction is accomplished by end-to-side hepaticojejunostomy, using the same loop of the previous Kasai operation, if present, or preparing a new Roux-en-Y loop. Even in the presence of a normal native bile duct, a direct duct-to-duct anastomosis is generally avoided. A single or double anastomosis may be necessary, depending on the presence of the left bile duct or of two separate segmental ducts (Fig. 27.22). As few interrupted stitches as possible of absorbable polydioxanone suture are used for the hepaticojejunostomy, with careful mucosa-to-mucosa apposition. At our centre, a transanastomotic stent is usually placed with the purpose of preventing biliary complications.

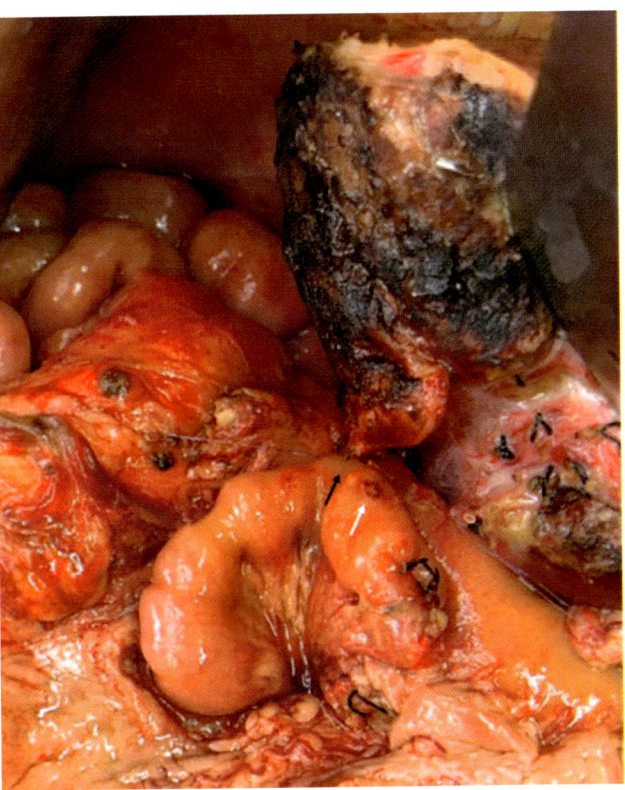

Fig. 27.22 Double hepaticojejunostomy: the black arrow indicates the first anastomosis, the white arrow indicates the enterotomy for the second one

27.5.3 Implantation of the Extended Right Graft and of the Full-Size Graft

Since the ERG retains the inferior vena cava, the portal vein and the common bile duct, its implantation and that of a full-size graft are almost identical.

If the native vena cava has been removed, a double caval anastomosis is performed. If, instead, the native vena cava has been preserved, the piggyback technique is adopted, so an end-to-side anastomosis is performed between the graft suprahepatic vena cava and a common cuff at the confluence of the native hepatic veins. In this case, side clamping may be an option in large children with a native vena cava of adequate calibre.

As described in the previous paragraph, the next steps are portal and arterial anastomosis and biliary reconstruction.

In the particular above-mentioned case of Abernethy malformation type 1, if a caval side clamping is feasible, arterial prior to portal reperfusion may be an option, leaving the congenital portocaval shunt intact until arterial reperfusion (Fig. 27.23).

For biliary reconstruction, the choice between an end-to-end duct-to-duct anastomosis and an end-to-side hepaticojejunostomy is guided by both anatomical and technical considerations.

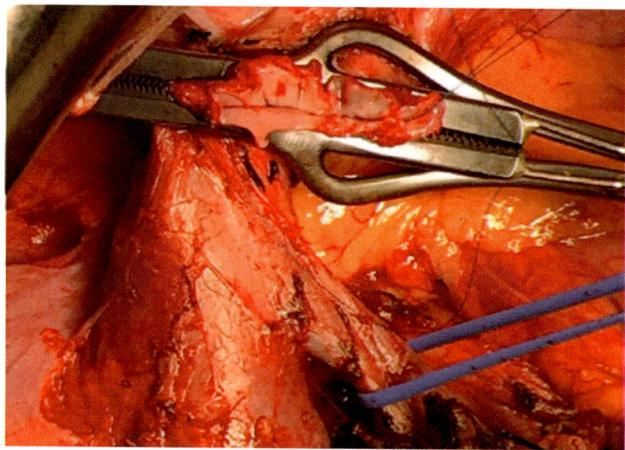

Fig. 27.23 Preservation of the congenital portocaval shunt during side clamping of the native vena cava

In the presence of an ERG, a careful check for biliary leaks from the sutured orifice of the left hepatic duct or from the small caudate lobe ducts is mandatory.

27.5.4 Implantation of the Full-Left Graft and of the Full-Right Graft

Size-matching is the main reason why the most commonly used graft from AASL for paediatric LT is the FLG, whose volume is smaller than that of the FRG.

Since the FLG retains the inferior vena cava, the portal vein and the whole arterial axis, its implantation is very similar to that of a full-size graft. The implantation of the FRG, instead, is very similar to that of a right lobe from a living donor.

In case of split cava technique, the caval patch of any graft is anastomosed to the recipient's side clamped inferior vena cava in a side-to-side fashion.

Whatever the biliary pedicle of any graft, biliary reconstruction may be performed by both an end-to-end duct-to-duct anastomosis and an end-to-side hepaticojejunostomy.

27.5.5 Retransplantation

Basically, surgical technique of paediatric liver retransplantation is the same as just described for primary LT. Anyway, enhanced complexity due to the previous transplant itself is almost the rule. Sometimes, retransplantation is really a surgical challenge. Explantation of the previous graft may be highly demanding due to adhesions, whose dissection may be particularly laborious, and to peculiar anatomical conditions. Available vascular pedicles for the new anastomoses are the result of both the ability of dissecting them free and the complications of the previous transplant. For instance, the isolation of the retrohepatic vena cava may occasionally be so troublesome that it may not be preserved. Chronic portal vein thrombosis not timely treated by Meso-Rex bypass [88] may entail the need for an alternative vessel for the new anastomosis: a jump graft between the recipient's splenomesenteric confluence and the graft portal stump may be an option; a varix or, in the presence of a splenorenal shunt, the left renal vein may be considered in adults but are hardly ever a viable option in children. It is worthwhile to underline that chronic portal vein thrombosis is an important risk factor for early mortality after retransplantation (personal unpublished data), hence the need for a timely and aggressive management of this complication [88]. Occasionally, neither the hepatic artery nor its branches are available for the arterial anastomosis, which therefore has to be performed with the supraceliac or the infrarenal aorta, with or without an interposition graft. Finally, if hepaticojejunostomy is the choice for biliary reconstruction, the same loop of the previous transplant is usually reused.

27.6 Results of Paediatric LT by Graft Type

The impact of graft type on the outcome of paediatric LT has been a matter of lively debate for more than two decades. Anyway, it still remains unclear. Several studies using data from different transplant systems, both registry and single centre data, have reported conflicting results. Actually, these studies are heterogeneous in that they analyse different geographical realities with different organ supply and allocation policy. Besides, they share limitations due to their common retrospective nature: on the one hand, centres with a wide range of experience contribute to registry data to different extents; on the other hand, even the biggest single centre series does not have the statistical power of registry-based studies. We are going to elucidate what just stated by describing some important studies published in the last 15 years.

First, we are going to focus on North America. In 2004, Roberts presented an analysis of the Scientific Registry of Transplant Recipients database. Among the 2277 children aged less than 2 years who had received their first transplant between 1989 and 2000, those transplanted with living donor grafts had a significantly lower risk of graft failure during the first post-transplant year than those transplanted with both full-size and split or reduced grafts from deceased donors. They had a significantly lower mortality risk than those transplanted with split or reduced grafts from deceased donors, too. The benefits of LDLT seemed to be lost for older children [89]. In 2007, two different studies using data from the Studies of Pediatric Liver Transplantation registry reported discrepant results. Soltys, who investigated late events among children who had received their first transplant between 1995 and 2004, demonstrated similar rates of graft loss after the first post-transplant year for technical variant grafts from both deceased and living donors and full-size grafts [90]. Instead, Diamond showed increased morbidity and mortality for children who had received their first transplant between 1995 and 2006 with technical variant grafts from both deceased and living donors compared to those transplanted with full-size grafts. 30-day and 2-year morbidity was significantly increased for any type of technical variant compared to full-size grafts. Moreover, split and reduced grafts from deceased donors represented an independent predictor of retransplantation or death [91]. Moving to the United Network for Organ Sharing (UNOS) database, different studies reported conflicting results once again. In 2004, Abt presented the outcomes of 3125 children who had received their first transplant between 1991 and 2001. For those aged less than 3 years, 3-year graft survival was significantly higher after LDLT compared to transplantation with both full-size and split or reduced grafts from deceased donors. Conversely, for those aged between 3 and 12 years, it was transplantation with full-size grafts to offer a significant 3-year graft survival advantage over any type of technical variant grafts [92]. In 2008, Becker reported an analysis of 1260 LT performed between 2002 and 2004 in children aged less than 12 years. 30-day patient survival was significantly higher after transplantation with full-size compared to any type of technical variant grafts, including living donor ones. However, adjusted 1-year graft and patient survival was comparable among all graft types and age groups [93]. In 2013, Cauley published a study on 2683 children aged less than 2 years who had received their first transplant with both full-size and split or reduced grafts from deceased donors between 1995 and 2010. Graft and patient survival turned out to be similar among graft types for patients transplanted after 2000 [94]. In 2017, Alexopoulos showed that, among children who had received their first transplant for biliary atresia between 2002 and 2014, those less than 7 kg in body weight had significantly better graft survival after transplantation with technical variant grafts from both deceased and living donors compared to those transplanted with full-size grafts [95]. We are going to complete this picture of paediatric LT in North America with a monocentric study published by Hong in 2009. He focused on the Dumont UCLA Transplant Center experience. Among the 442 paediatric LT performed between 1993 and 2006, he found no significant difference in long-term graft and patient survival by graft type (full-size grafts and LLSs from both split liver and living donation). Anyway, LLSs from split liver showed a significantly higher rate of primary non-function, while LLSs from living donation had a significantly higher rate of portal vein thrombosis [96].

Now, let us move to Europe. In 2004, Broering presented the first ever reported series with more than 100 paediatric LT recipients with an actual 6-month patient survival of 100%. He analysed 132 consecutive LT performed at the University Hospital Hamburg-Eppendorf between 2001 and 2003. Actual graft survival and the rate of biliary complications appeared to be similar among LDLT and split and full-size LT [97]. In 2003, Gridelli described Bergamo experience with 124 paediatric patients transplanted for end-stage cholestatic liver disease between 1997 and 2002. He demonstrated comparable 4-year graft and patient survival after split and full-size LT [98]. In 2007, Bourdeaux reported on 235 consecutive paediatric primary LT performed at Saint-Luc University Clinics between 1993 and 2002. Of them, 100 were LDLT, while 135 were deceased donor LT with both full-size and split and reduced grafts. Actuarial 1- and 5-year graft survival was significantly higher after LDLT compared to deceased donor LT. Moreover, actuarial 1- and 5-year graft and patient survival was significantly higher after LDLT compared to deceased donor LT for children aged less than 2 years. At multivariate analysis, deceased donor grafts appeared to be significantly correlated with hepatic artery thrombosis, while living donor grafts turned out to be significantly correlated with acute rejection [99]. ELTR analysis revealed comparable early up to 10-year graft survival after SLT and whole LT for 14,022 children transplanted between 1988 and 2016; instead, longer-term graft survival resulted to be significantly better for children transplanted with full-size graft [29]. Finally, in 2017, Battula showed the very good results of the intention to split policy adopted at Birmingham transplant centre. Of the 724 paediatric LT performed between 1992 and 2014, 516 were split LT. 1-, 5- and 10-year graft and patient survival was excellent after split LT, and paediatric wait-list mortality was eliminated during the last 4 years of the study period [100].

In conclusion, as paediatric waiting lists everywhere include mostly small children but size-matched whole organs from deceased donors are a scarce resource, there is no alternative to the use of LLSs from split liver and living donors for this population. Actually, not being whole organs as timely disposable as LLSs, it might be worthless to compare the outcomes of LT by this kind of grafts. Technical variant grafts from both split liver and living donation have greatly contributed to virtually eliminate paediatric wait-list mortality in some European countries [98, 100, 101]. Technical variant grafts have become significantly safer over time. This is likely the effect of a learning curve regarding surgical experience, donor and recipient selection and matching and short- and long-term post-transplant patient management. The contradictory reported results of paediatric LT with LLSs from split liver and living donation should be interpreted critically in light of both data sources and centre-specific variables [32, 102]. LDLT with LLSs offers the indisputable advantage of scheduling transplantation at a recipient-controlled time, before the development of life-threatening complications or severe malnutrition, with very low donor mortality and morbidity [32, 89, 99, 103]. Anyway, the adoption of a liberal split policy timely provides grafts of excellent quality to transplant most paediatric patients when they are still clinically stable [98].

We think that the best results overall may be achieved at high-volume centres with extensive experience with all graft types and age groups, which may allow transplantation according to each recipient's special needs. We agree with Mazariegos that the ability to use the appropriate graft type in a timely fashion implies a clear understanding of each recipient's specific condition, including the degree of portal hypertension, anatomical variations and risk factors [104]. We firmly believe that deceased donor SLT and LDLT should be complementary resources in Western countries, with regular access to both of them. If, on the one hand, LLSs from split liver and living donation represent an adequate pool to fulfil the needs of small children, on the other hand, the supply of size-matched grafts for large children is actually a problem. Whole organs or ERGs from paediatric donors and LLSs of sufficient volume are a scarce resource, so a possible solution lies in enhancing the program of AASL and providing size-matched FLGs.

27.7 Liver Transplantation in Very Small Infants

LT in newborns and infants weighting less than 5–6 kg has always represented a surgical challenge because of both the difficulty of a safe size matching and technical issues. The related literature reports conflicting results. Cauley's analysis of the UNOS database showed a significantly higher risk of graft failure and mortality for recipients weighting less than 6 kg [94]. In the few small series looking exclusively at children under 5 kg in weight, graft and patient survival ranges between 50% and 77% and between 55% and 86%, respectively [105–110]. Mekeel described comparable overall graft and patient survival for recipients weighting less than 5 kg and for those weighting more than 5 kg [110]. Broering observed no disadvantage concerning mortality in children under 5 kg in weight [97]. Our group reported satisfactory long-term graft and patient survival and a low rate of surgical complications after LT in children less than 6 kg [111]. For sure, the best results of LT in very small infants are the effect of a learning curve for both surgical aspects and perioperative care.

Whole organs from matched paediatric donors are rarely available. Besides, neonatal livers are mostly considered not suitable for transplantation due to their immature function [112–114]. The outcomes of full-size grafts from donors weighting less than 6 kg, regardless of donor age, are controversial. Concerns are about the functional maturity of newborn donor livers and the risk of vascular thrombosis. Mekeel reported comparable overall graft survival for children transplanted with full-size grafts from donors weighting less than 6 kg and for those transplanted with full-size grafts from donors weighting more than 6 kg [110]; others, instead, have described high rates of graft failure due to vascular complications and primary non-function with the same kind of grafts [95, 107, 112].

LLSs from adult or adult-sized donors are often too big for recipients less than 5–6 kg in weight. A GRWR more than 6% may occasionally result in insufficient blood supply to the graft, in the risk of compartment syndrome in case of abdominal closure and in a higher rate of early episodes of acute rejection [33, 52–54, 115, 116]. So, two approaches have been developed to transplant very small infants without the deleterious effects of large-for-size grafts: further reduction of LLSs from both deceased and living adult donors, in order to tailor them to the recipient size, and transplantation of LLSs from deceased paediatric donors less than 10 years old or 40 kg in weight. A third strategy to address this problem is represented by delayed abdominal closure, which will be discussed in a specific paragraph, since it may be useful not only in the presence of large-for-size grafts. However, it is worthwhile to underline that, even in case of GRWR more than 6%, LT has been safely performed without any need for neither further graft reduction nor delayed abdominal closure [98].

Further reduction of a LLS may be both anatomical, leading to a monosegment, and nonanatomical, providing a hyper-reduced graft that is larger than a monosegment but smaller than a LLS. Both these techniques were first adopted in deceased donor LT and subsequently borrowed by LDLT. Experience with transplantation of monosegments and hyper-reduced grafts is limited, and no data directly comparing the outcomes of these two techniques are available. They both seem to be satisfactory options for very small infants, but it is still unknown which of these grafts represents the best choice [117]. Regarding monosegmental LT, reduction of a LLS to segment II appears technically more demanding than creating a segment III graft, since it involves a hazardous dissection at the base of the umbilical fissure [118]. Besides, segment II is usually smaller than segment III. So, monosegmental LT seems safer and easier with segment III rather than with segment II [115]. Hyper-reduced grafts were proposed as a versatile alternative to monosegments. The supporters of this approach advocate that it allows to tailor the graft size to any specific needs on a case-by-case basis much more than monosegmental LT and that it oversteps some technical pitfalls of monosegmental LT. The basic principle is to reduce the size of a LLS without compromising its vascular inflow and outflow. So, parenchymal planes of resection are usually a sagittal plane resecting the graft left lateral edge and a transverse plane resecting the graft inferior edge. No dissection at the base of the umbilical

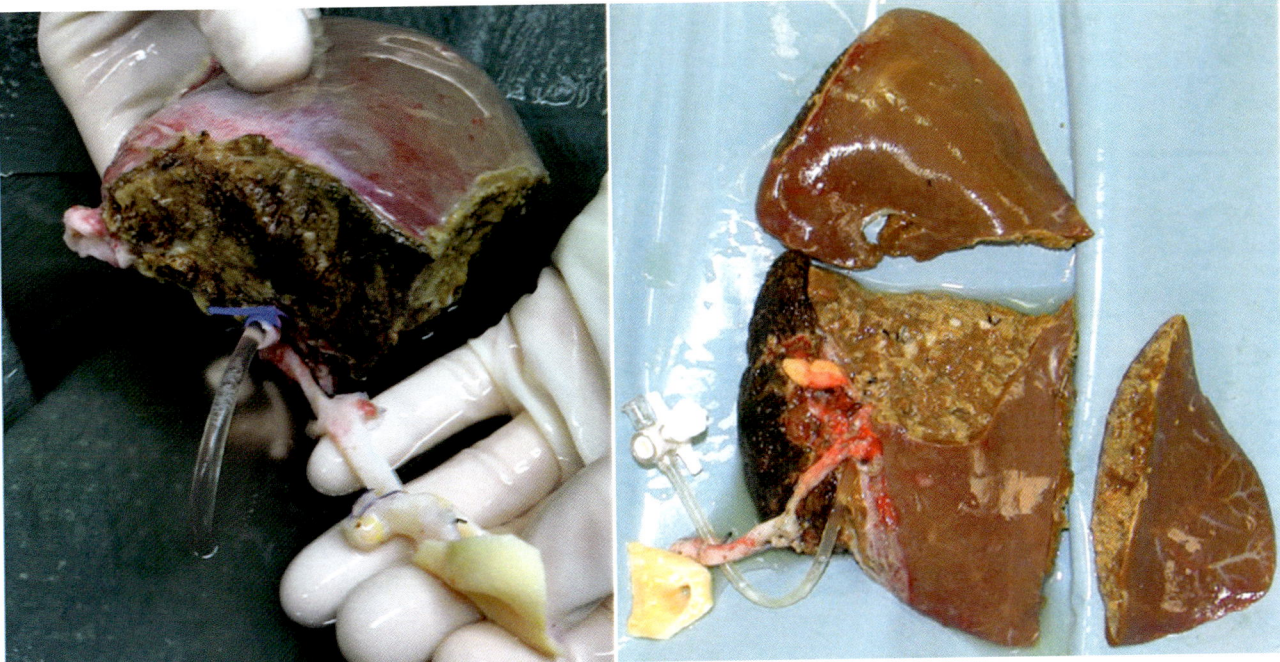

Fig. 27.24 Two different types of hyper-reduced LLSs. Both LLSs were derived from in situ split of a deceased donor liver and further reduced ex situ

fissure is needed. The implantation of a hyper-reduced graft is similar to that of a LLS, being their vascular pedicles exactly the same [119, 120] (Fig. 27.24).

Split LT from paediatric donors less than 10 years old or under 40 kg in weight was proved to be an effective strategy to increase organ availability by a prospective Italian multicentre study. Survival and complication rates were not significantly different between recipients of grafts from paediatric donors aged less than 10 years or weighting less than 40 kg and recipients of grafts from older or larger paediatric donors. Difficulties in vascular and biliary reconstructions appeared to be balanced by optimal graft quality [121, 122] (Fig. 27.25).

27.8 Delayed Abdominal Closure

Delayed abdominal closure after paediatric LT may be a useful option in some particular conditions. It may avoid abdominal compartment syndrome not only in the presence of a large-for-size graft, as previously mentioned, but also in case of massive intestinal oedema due to prolonged stasis in portal circulation [123]. Moreover, it may allow the ideal orientation of the graft, which is fundamental for an optimal inflow and outflow, in case of an unfavourable relationship between the graft anteroposterior diameter and anteroposterior abdominal depth [120, 123]. So, it gives time either for graft or abdominal wall remodelling or for resolution of portal hypertension.

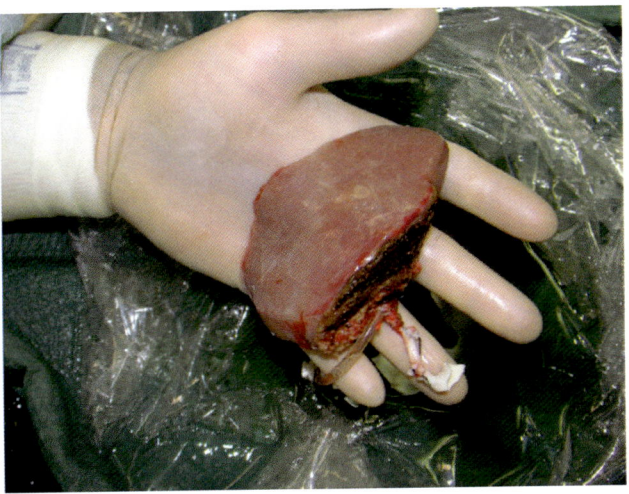

Fig. 27.25 LLS from in situ split of the liver of a paediatric deceased donor of 20 kg in weight

Many strategies for delayed abdominal closure have been described, each with pros and contra, and different materials have been used as well.

Available meshes are both non-absorbable and absorbable synthetic ones, such as polypropylene, polytetrafluoroethylene, Gore-tex and polyglactin meshes and extracellular matrix-derived biological ones [123].

One approach consists of temporarily abdominal dressing with subsequent staged reduction in size until definitive closure with or without a prosthesis. Some

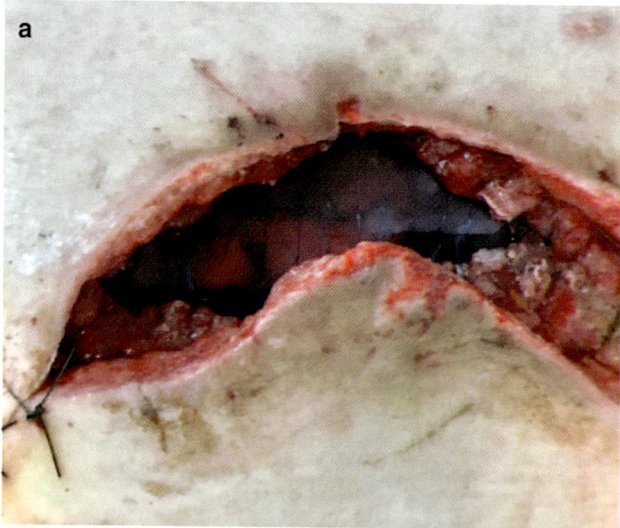

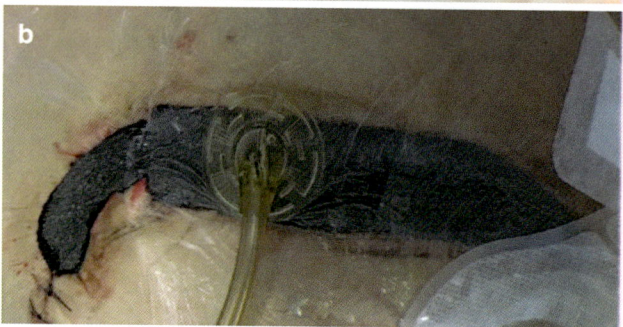

Fig. 27.26 (a) Downsized silastic mesh secured to the muscle fascia. (b) Sealed wound dressing connected to a vacuum pump over the silastic mesh

Finally, abdominal closure with a non-vascularized allotransplantation of the same donor abdominal rectus fascia has been reported [127].

Delayed abdominal closure and graft size reduction are not mutually exclusive; they may rather be complementary options in the presence of a large-for-size graft. They may be further combined with the use of prosthetic materials supporting the graft in order to avoid outflow obstruction due to caval compression [120, 128].

27.9 Auxiliary Partial Orthotopic Liver Transplantation

Auxiliary partial orthotopic liver transplantation (APOLT) is a special technique of LT where a portion of the native liver is resected and replaced by a size-matched partial graft, which is implanted in an orthotopic position. In small children, a LLS from split liver or living donation is generally an adequate auxiliary graft. Although technically easier, a left lobectomy of the native liver does not create enough space for an adult LLS to be implanted, so a left hepatectomy appears to be the best option.

The main indications for APOLT are ALF and NCMLD. APOLT has also been reported for Abernethy malformation type 1 complicated by hyperammonaemia and hepatopulmonary syndrome with complete resolution of symptoms [129].

groups, including ours, have adopted the following two- or multistep technique: a silastic mesh, which is a reinforced silicone sheet, is secured to the muscle fascia and subsequently downsized until definitive mass muscle closure or definitive closure with interposition of an absorbable synthetic mesh to fill in the fascial defect; the skin may be closed over the silastic mesh; otherwise a sealed wound dressing connected to a vacuum pump may be employed [123, 124] (Fig. 27.26). Others have used a similar approach, with a synthetic mesh for temporarily abdominal dressing and a biological one for an early definitive closure [125].

Very early primary abdominal wall augmentation by means of a biological mesh represents an alternative strategy. The rationale for this technique is both to limit any possible risk of infection associated with an open abdomen and to avoid any possible complication associated with the use of synthetic meshes [126]. Biological meshes seem to integrate into the abdominal wall as a result of a process of incorporation [125, 126].

27.9.1 Auxiliary Partial Orthotopic Liver Transplantation in Acute Liver Failure

In the setting of ALF, APOLT can act as a bridge to native liver regeneration, so that patients can be spared lifelong immunosuppression [103, 117, 130]. Children with a high potential for native liver regeneration and with a favourable clinical status are the best candidates for APOLT. Conditions with an excellent regenerative potential are represented by acetaminophen overdose, hepatitis A and E and mushroom poisoning. Patient's clinical status is fundamental since APOLT is more technically demanding and consequently more time consuming than standard LT, so patients with haemodynamic instability, severe systemic inflammatory response syndrome or intracranial hypertension may not tolerate this prolonged procedure [6]. In experienced hands and in carefully selected recipients, APOLT has provided excellent results in terms of both graft and patient survival and complication rate, allowing over two-thirds of these patients the chance of an immunosuppression-free life [131, 132]. Thus, it is being increasingly accepted as a valid treatment option for children with ALF [6].

27.9.2 Auxiliary Partial Orthotopic Liver Transplantation in Non-cirrhotic Metabolic Liver Diseases

The rationale for APOLT in the setting of NCMLD is to provide sufficient liver mass to produce the missing enzyme and correct the metabolic abnormality. It would be reasonable to think that APOLT may be limited to NCMLD with the liver as the main site of the defective gene expression [133]. As a matter of fact, among NCMLD, Crigler-Najjar syndrome type 1 (CNS1) and urea cycle disorders are the main indications to APOLT [7]. In particular, CNS1 represents the archetypal NCMLD suitable for it since it has been shown to be corrected by the replacement of less than 12% of total hepatocyte volume and less than 5% of hepatic enzymatic activity. Anyway, APOLT has been reported in case of propionic acidaemia, characterized by the liver as a part of a multisystem disorder, with adequate metabolic control and stabilization of the disease [7, 133]. APOLT has some advantages over standard LT: first, in case of failure of the auxiliary graft, the native remnant can support general liver function without any risks for the patient's life; second, if gene therapy becomes clinically available, the native remnant can be treated and lifelong immunosuppression can be avoided [103, 117, 130]. Anyway, there is some scepticism in accepting APOLT for NCMLD. In fact, concerns for technical difficulties and for the risk of long-term graft atrophy due to the functional competition with a structurally normal native remnant exist. Slow progress in gene therapy research does not help, too. However, most of the above-mentioned issues have been recently addressed, and APOLT for NCMLS has been proved to be feasible with good results in experienced hands [133].

In the setting of NCMLD, domino APOLT represents an original strategy aiming at expanding the organ pool. A donor partial graft is used for APOLT in a NCMLD recipient, whose resected partial graft is transplanted into a child affected by a different NCMLD as an auxiliary graft. A further evolution of domino APOLT for the purpose of "donorless" transplantation may be cross-domino APOLT, where LLSs may be swapped between children with different NCMLD with no need for a donor [7, 133].

27.9.3 Surgical Technique

In small children, the preferred practice is to perform a left hepatectomy of the native liver and to replace it with a LLS.

The implantation of this auxiliary graft is similar to that of a LLS in standard LT. Outflow reconstruction is accomplished by means of an end-to-side anastomosis between the graft left hepatic vein and the stump of the native left and middle hepatic veins. For portal anastomosis, either the orifice of the left portal branch or a fresh venotomy on the main portal trunk may be used. In case of NCMLD, portal vein modulation is necessary to avoid portal steal and achieve preferential portal flow to the graft. On the contrary, portal vein modulation is usually unneeded in the setting of ALF since portal flow is preferentially directed to the graft due to the stiffness of the collapsed native remnant. Arterial anastomosis often represents a technical challenge because discrepancy between the left hepatic artery of the graft, from an adult donor, and the left hepatic artery of the paediatric recipient is common. Finally, hepaticojejunostomy is performed for biliary reconstruction [6, 133].

27.10 Conclusions

A wide range of technical options, in terms of both graft type and surgical strategies, are available for paediatric LT. Extensive experience with any graft type and any age group may timely allow for the appropriate solution. A clear understanding of each recipient's specific condition and awareness of graft-related peculiarities are the keys for the success of paediatric LT.

References

1. Herden U, Wischhusen F, Heinemann A, Ganschow R, Grabhorn E, Vettorazzi E, Nashan B, Fischer L. A formula to calculate the standard liver volume in children and its application in pediatric liver transplantation. Transpl Int. 2013;26:1217–24.
2. Feng AC, Fan HL, Chen TW, Hsieh CB. Hepatic hemodynamic changes during liver transplantation: a review. World J Gastroenterol. 2014;20:11131–41.
3. De Magnee C, Veyckemans F, Pirotte T, Menten R, Dumitriu D, Clapuyt P, Carbonez K, Barrea C, Sluysmans T, Sempoux C, Leclercq I, Zech F, Stephenne X, Reding R. Liver and systemic hemodynamics in children with cirrhosis: impact on the surgical management in pediatric living donor liver transplantation. Liver Transpl. 2017;23:1440–50.
4. Seehofer D, Eurich D, Veltzke-Schlieker W, Neuhaus P. Biliary complications after liver transplantation: old problems and new challenges. Am J Transplant. 2013;13:253–65.
5. Anderson CD, Turmelle YP, Darcy M, Shepherd RW, Weymann A, Nadler M, Guelker S, Chapman WC, Lowell JA. Biliary strictures in pediatric liver transplant recipients—early diagnosis and treatment results in excellent graft outcomes. Pediatr Transplant. 2010;14:358–63.
6. Rela M, Kaliamoorthy I, Reddy MS. Current status of auxiliary partial orthotopic liver transplantation for acute liver failure. Liver Transpl. 2016;22:1265–74.
7. Reddy MS, Rajalingam R, Rela M. Revisiting APOLT for metabolic liver disease: a new look at an old idea. Transplantation. 2017;101:260–6.
8. Starzl TE, Koep LJ, Schroter GP, Halgrimson CG, Porter KA, Weil R 3rd. Liver replacement for pediatric patients. Pediatrics. 1979;63:825–9.
9. Bismuth H, Houssin D. Reduced-sized orthotopic liver graft in hepatic transplantation in children. Surgery. 1984;95:367–70.

10. Starzl TE, Demetris AJ. Liver transplantation. Chicago, IL: Year Book Medical Publisher, Inc.; 1990.
11. Broelsch CE, Emond JC, Thistlethwaite JR, Rouch DA, Whitington PF, Lichtor JL. Liver transplantation with reduced-size donor organs. Transplantation. 1988;45:519–24.
12. Emond JC, Whitington PF, Thistlethwaite JR, Alonso EM, Broelsch CE. Reduced-size orthotopic liver transplantation: use in the management of children with chronic liver disease. Hepatology. 1989;10:867–72.
13. Houssin D, Soubrane O, Boillot O, Dousset B, Ozier Y, Devictor D, Bernard O, Chapuis Y. Orthotopic liver transplantation with a reduced-size graft: an ideal compromise in pediatrics? Surgery. 1992;111:532–42.
14. Pichlmayr R, Ringe B, Gubernatis G, Hauss J, Bunzendahl H. Transplantation of a donor liver to 2 recipients (splitting transplantation). A new method in the further development of segmental liver transplantation. Langenbecks Arch Chir. 1988;373:127–30.
15. Strong R, Lynch S, Ong T, Matsunami H, Koido Y, Balderson G. Successful liver transplantation from a living donor to her son. N Engl J Med. 1990;322:1505–7.
16. Otte JB, de Ville de Goyet J, Alberti D, Balladur P, de Hemptinne B. The concept and technique of the split liver in clinical transplantation. Surgery. 1990;107:605–12.
17. Emond JC, Whitington PF, Thistlethwaite JR, Cherqui D, Alonso EA, Woodle IS, Vogelbach P, Busse-Henry SM, Zucker AR, Broelsch CE. Transplantation of two patients with one liver. Analysis of a preliminary experience with "split-liver" grafting. Ann Surg. 1990;212:14–22.
18. Emond J, Heffron T, Thistlethwaite JR. Innovative approaches to donor scarcity. A critical comparison between split liver and living related liver transplantation. Hepatology. 1991;14:92A.
19. De Ville de Goyet J. Split liver transplantation in Europe: 1988 to 1993. Transplantation. 1995;59:1371–6.
20. Rogiers X, Malagó M, Habib N, Knoefel WT, Pothmann W, Burdelski M, Meyer-Moldenhauer WH, Broelsch CE. In situ splitting of the liver in the heart-beating cadaveric organ donor for transplantation in two recipients. Transplantation. 1995;59:1081–3.
21. Rogiers X, Malagó M, Gawad K, Kuhlencordt R, Fröschle G, Sturm E, Sterneck M, Pothmann W, Schulte am Esch J, Burdelski M, Broelsch C. One year experience with extended application and modified techniques of split liver transplantation. Transplantation. 1996;61:1059–61.
22. Rogiers X, Malagó M, Gawad K, Jauch KW, Olausson M, Knoefel WT, Gundlach M, Bassas A, Fischer L, Sterneck M, Burdelski M, Broelsch CE. In situ splitting of cadaveric livers. The ultimate expansion of a limited donor pool. Ann Surg. 1996;224:331–9.
23. Azoulay DF, Astarcioglu I, Bismuth H, Castaing D, Majno P, Adam R, Johann M. Split-liver transplantation, The Paul Brousse policy. Ann Surg. 1996;224:737–46.
24. Goss JA, Jersiz H, Shackleton CR, Seu P, Smith CV, Markowitz JS, Farmer DG, Gobrial RM, Markmann JF, Arnaout WS, Imagawa DK, Colquhoun SD, Fraiman MH, McDiarmid SV, Busuttil RW. In situ splitting of the cadaveric liver for transplantation. Transplantation. 1997;64:871–7.
25. Olausson M, Backman L, Friman S, Mjornstedt L, Krantz M, Broelsch CE, Rogiers X. In situ split liver procedures in cadaver and living related donors. Transplant Proc. 1997;29:3094–5.
26. Mirza DF, Achilleos O, Pirenne J, Buckels JA, McMaster P, Mayer AD. Encouraging results of split-liver transplantation. Br J Surg. 1998;85:494–7.
27. Rela M, Vougas V, Muiesan P, Vilca-Melendez H, Smyrniotis V, Gibbs P, Karani J, Williams R, Heaton N. Split liver transplantation: King's College Hospital experience. Ann Surg. 1998;227:282–8.
28. Colledan M, Segalin A, Spada M, Lucianetti A, Corno V, Gridelli B. Liberal policy of split liver for pediatric liver transplantation. A single centre experience. Transpl Int. 2000;13:S131–3.
29. ELTR/ELITA data, Data Analysis Booklet Pediatric patients (kindly provided by Dr. Vincent Karam).
30. Busuttil RW, Goss JA. Split liver transplantation. Ann Surg. 1999;229:313–21.
31. Ghobrial RM, Farmer DG, Amersi F, Busuttil RW. Advances in pediatric liver and intestinal transplantation. Am J Surg. 2000;180:328–34.
32. Spada M, Riva S, Maggiore G, Cintorino D, Gridelli B. Pediatric liver transplantation. World J Gastroenterol. 2009;15:648–74.
33. Colledan M. Split liver transplantation: technique and results. Transplant Rev. 2005;19:221–31.
34. Bismuth H. Surgical anatomy and anatomical surgery of the liver. World J Surg. 1982;6:3–9.
35. Moussaoui D, Toso C, Nowacka A, McLin VA, Bednarkiewicz M, Andres A, Berney T, Majno P, Wildhaber BE. Early complications after liver transplantation in children and adults: are split grafts equal to each other and equal to whole livers? Pediatr Transplant. 2017;21:e12908.
36. Bismuth H, Morino M, Castaing D, Gillon MC, Descorps Declere A, Saliba F, Samuel D. Emergency orthotopic liver transplantation in two patients using one donor liver. Br J Surg. 1989;76:722–4.
37. Colledan M, Andorno E, Valente U, Gridelli B. A new splitting technique for liver grafts. Lancet. 1999;353:1763.
38. Azoulay D, Castaing D, Adam R, Savier E, Delvart V, Karam V, Ming BY, Dannaoui M, Krissat J, Bismuth H. Split-liver transplantation for two adult recipients: feasibility and long-term outcomes. Ann Surg. 2001;233:565–74.
39. Sommacale D, Farges O, Ettorre GM, Lebigot P, Sauvanet A, Marty J, Durand F, Belghiti J. In situ split liver transplantation for two adult recipients. Transplantation. 2000;15:1005–7.
40. Humar A, Ramcharan T, Sielaff TD, Kandaswamy R, Gruessner RW, Lake JR, Payne WD. Split liver transplantation for two adult recipients: an initial experience. Am J Transplant. 2001;1:366–72.
41. Zamir G, Olthoff KM, Desai N, Markmann JF, Shaked A. Toward further expansion of the organ pool for adult liver recipients: splitting the cadaveric liver into right and left lobes. Transplantation. 2002;74:1757–61.
42. Hwang S, Lee SG, Park KM, Kim KH, Ahn CS, Moon DB, Ha TY. A case report of split liver transplantation for two adult recipients in Korea. Transplant Proc. 2004;36:2736–40.
43. Colledan M, Segalin A, Andorno E, Corno V, Lucianetti A, Spada M, Gridelli B. Modified splitting technique for liver transplantation in adult-sized recipients. Technique and preliminary results. Acta Chir Belg. 2000;100:289–91.
44. Giacomoni A, Lauterio A, Donadon M, De Gasperi A, Belli L, Slim A, Dorobantu B, Mangoni I, De Carlis L. Should we still offer split-liver transplantation for two adult recipients? A retrospective study of our experience. Liver Transpl. 2008;14:999–1006.
45. Zambelli M, Andorno E, De Carlis L, Rossi G, Cillo U, De Feo T, Carobbio A, Giacomoni A, Bottino G, Colledan M. Full-right-full-left split liver transplantation: the retrospective analysis of an early multicenter experience including graft sharing. Am J Transplant. 2012;12:2198–210.
46. Emond JC, Freeman RB, Renz JF, Yersiz H, Rogiers X, Busuttil RW. Optimizing the use of donated cadaver livers: analysis and policy development to increase the application of spit liver transplantation. Liver Transpl. 2002;8:863–72.
47. Schlitt HJ. Which liver is splittable? In: Rogiers X, Bismuth H, Busuttil RW, Broering DC, Azoulay D, editors. Split liver transplantation. Theoretical and practical aspects. Darmstadt: Steinkopff Verlag; 2002. p. 63.

48. Toso C, Ris F, Mentha G, Oberholzer J, Morel P, Majno P. Potential impact of in situ liver splitting on the number of available grafts. Transplantation. 2002;74:222–6.
49. Cardillo M, De Fazio N, Pedotti P, De Feo T, Fassati LR, Mazzaferro V, Colledan M, Gridelli B, Caccamo L, De Carlis L, Valente U, Andorno E, Cossolini M, Martini C, Antonucci A, Cillo U, Zanus G, Baccarani U, Scalamogna M, NITp Liver Transplantation Working Group. Split and whole liver transplantation outcomes: a comparative cohort study. Liver Transpl. 2006;12:402–10.
50. Lauterio A, Di Sandro S, Concone G, De Carlis R, Giacomoni A, De Carlis L. Current status and perspectives in split liver transplantation. World J Gastroenterol. 2015;21:11003–15.
51. Petz W, Spada M, Sonzogni A, Colledan M, Segalin A, Lucianetti A, Bertani A, Guizzetti M, Peloni G, Gridelli B. Pediatric split liver transplantation using elderly donors. Transplant Proc. 2001;33:1361–3.
52. Fukazawa K, Nishida S, Volsky A, Tzakis AG, Pretto EA. Body surface area index predicts outcome in orthotopic liver transplantation. J Hepatobiliary Pancreat Sci. 2011;18:216–25.
53. Gelas T, Mirza DF, Boillot O, Muiesan P, Sharif K. Can donor liver left lateral sector weight be predicted from anthropometric variables? Pediatr Transplant. 2012;16:239–43.
54. Fukazawa K, Yamada Y, Nishida S, Hibi T, Arheart KL, Pretto EA. Determination of the safe range of graft size mismatch using body surface area index in deceased liver transplantation. Transpl Int. 2013;26:724–33.
55. De Ville de Goyet J, di Francesco F, Sottani V, Grimaldi C, Tozzi AE, Monti L, Muiesan P. Splitting livers: trans-hilar or trans-umbilical division? Technical aspects and comparative outcomes. Pediatr Transplant. 2015;19:517–26.
56. Kilic M, Seu P, Goss JA. Maintenance of the celiac trunk with the left-sided liver allograft for in-situ split liver transplantation. Transplantation. 2002;73:1252–7.
57. Maggi U, De Feo TM, Andorno E, Cillo U, De Carlis L, Colledan M, Burra P, De Fazio N, Rossi G, Liver Transplantation and Intestine North Italy Transplant Study Group. Fifteen years and 382 extended right grafts from in situ split livers in a multicenter study: are these still extended criteria liver grafts? Liver Transpl. 2015;21:500–11.
58. Broelsch CE, Whitington PF, Emond JC, Heffron TG, Thistlethwaite JR, Stevens L, Piper J, Whitington SH, Lichtor JL. Liver transplantation in children from living related donors. Surgical technique and results. Ann Surg. 1991;214:428–37.
59. Deshpande RR, Heaton ND, Rela M. Surgical anatomy of segmental liver transplantation. Br J Surg. 2002;89:1078–88.
60. Chaib E, Bertevello P, Saad WA, Pinotti HW, Gama-Rodrigues J. The main hepatic anatomic variations for the purpose of split-liver transplantation. Hepato-Gastroenterology. 2007;75:688–92.
61. Hsu SL, Chen TY, Huang TL, Sun CK, Concejero AM, Tsang LL, Cheng YF. Left-sided gallbladder: its clinical significance and imaging presentations. World J Gastroenterol. 2007;13:6404–9.
62. Broering DC, Rogiers X, Malagò M, Bassas A, Broelsch CE. Vessel loop-guided technique for parenchymal transection in living donor or in situ split-liver procurement. Liver Transpl Surg. 1998;4:241.
63. Strasberg SM, Lowell JA, Howard TK. Reducing the shortage of donor livers: what would it take to reliably split livers for transplantation into two adult recipients? Liver Transpl Surg. 1999;5:437–50.
64. Rogiers X, Broering DC, Topp S, Gundlach M. Technical and physiological limits of split liver transplantation into two adults. Acta Chir Belg. 2000;100:272–5.
65. Azoulay D, Castaing D, Adam R, Savier E, Delvart V, Karam V, Ming BY, Dannaoui M, Krissat J, Bismuth H. Split-liver transplantation for two adult recipients: feasibility and long-term outcomes. Ann Surg. 2001;233:565–74.
66. Renz JF, Yersiz H, Reichert PR, Hisatake GM, Farmer DG, Emond JC, Busuttil RW. Split-liver transplantation: a review. Am J Transplant. 2003;3:1323–35.
67. Humar A, Khwaja K, Sielaff TD, Lake JR, Payne WD. Technique of split liver transplant for two adult recipients. Liver Transpl. 2002;8:725–9.
68. Gundlach M, Broering D, Topp S, Sterneck M, Rogiers X. Split-cava technique: liver splitting for two adult recipients. Liver Transpl. 2000;6:703–6.
69. Broering DC, Bok P, Mueller L, Wilms C, Rogiers X. Splitting of the middle hepatic vein in full right-full left splitting of the liver. Liver Transpl. 2005;11:350–2.
70. Broelsch CE, Whitington PF, Emond JC, Heffron TG, Thistlethwaite JR, Stevens L, Piper J, Whitington SH, Lichtor JL. Liver transplantation in children from living related donors. Surgical techniques and results. Ann Surg. 1991;214:428–37.
71. Emond JC, Heffron TG, Whitington PF, Broelsch CE. Reconstruction of the hepatic vein in reduced size hepatic transplantation. Surg Gynecol Obstet. 1993;176:11–7.
72. Kilic M, Aydinli B, Aydin U, Alper M, Zeytunlu M. A new surgical technique for hepatic vein reconstruction in pediatric live donor liver transplantation. Pediatr Transplant. 2008;12:677–81.
73. Sommovilla J, Doyle MM, Vachharajani N, Saad N, Nadler M, Turmelle YP, Weymann A, Chapman WC, Lowell JA. Hepatic venous outflow obstruction in pediatric liver transplantation: technical considerations in prevention, diagnosis, and management. Pediatr Transplant. 2014;18:497–502.
74. Tannuri U, Tannuri ACA, Santos MM, Miyatani HT. Technique advance to avoid hepatic venous outflow obstruction in pediatric living-donor liver transplantation. Pediatr Transplant. 2015;19:261–6.
75. Sakamoto S, Egawa H, Kanazawa H, Shibata T, Miyagawa-Hayashino A, Haga H, Ogura Y, Kasahara M, Tanaka K, Uemoto S. Hepatic venous outflow obstruction in pediatric living donor liver transplantation using left-sided lobe grafts: Kyoto University experience. Liver Transpl. 2010;16:1207–14.
76. Tannuri U, Santos MM, Tannuri ACA, Gibelli NE, Moreira A, Carnevale FC, Ayoub AA, Maksoud-Filho JC, Andrade WC, Velhote MC, Silva MM, Pinho-Apezzato ML, Miyatani HT, Guimaraes RR. Which is the best technique for hepatic venous reconstruction in pediatric living-donor liver transplantation? Experience from a single center. J Pediatr Surg. 2011;46:1379–84.
77. Camagni S, Lucianetti A, Pinelli D, D'Antiga L, Colledan M. Replacement versus preservation of the native vena cava in pediatric liver transplantation with left lateral segment grafts. Abstracts of the 18th Congress of the European Society for Organ Transplantation, 24-27 September 2017, Barcelona. Transpl Int. 2017;30:331.
78. Varela-Fascinetto G, Castaldo P, Fox IJ, Sudan D, Heffron TG, Shaw BW, Langnas AN. Biliary atresia-polysplenia syndrome. Surgical and clinical relevance in liver transplantation. Ann Surg. 1998;227:583–9.
79. Mitchell A, John PR, Mayer DA, Mirza DF, Buckels JA, de Ville de Goyet J. Improved technique of portal vein reconstruction in pediatric liver transplant recipient with portal vein hypoplasia. Transplantation. 2002;73:1244–7.
80. Marwan IK, Fawzy AT, Egawa H, Inomata Y, Uemoto S, Asonuma K, Kiuchi T, Hayashi M, Fujita S, Ogura Y, Tanaka K. Innovative techniques for and results of portal vein reconstruction in living-related liver transplantation. Surgery. 1999;125:265–70.
81. De Magnee C, Bourdeaux C, De Dobbeleer F, Janssen M, Menten R, Clapuyt P, Reding R. Impact of pre-transplant liver hemodynamics and portal reconstruction techniques on post-transplant portal vein complications in pediatric liver transplantation—a retrospective analysis in 197 recipients. Ann Surg. 2011;254:55–61.

82. Howard ER, Davenport M. Congenital extrahepatic portocaval shunts: the Abernethy malformation. J Pediatr Surg. 1997;32:494–7.
83. Guarrera JV, Sinha P, Lobritto SJ, Brown RS Jr, Kinkhabwala M, Emond JC. Microvascular hepatic artery anastomosis in pediatric segmental liver transplantation: microscope vs loupe. Transpl Int. 2004;17:585–8.
84. Heffron TG, Welch D, Pillen T, Fasola C, Redd D, Smallwood GA, Martinez E, Atkinson G, Guy M, Nam C, Henry S, Romero R. Low incidence of hepatic artery thrombosis after pediatric liver transplantation without the use of intraoperative microscope or parenteral anticoagulation. Pediatr Transplant. 2005;9:486–90.
85. Darwish AA, Bourdeaux C, Kader HA, Janssen M, Sokal E, Lerut J, Ciccarelli O, Veyckemans F, Otte JB, de Ville de Goyet J, Reding R. Pediatric liver transplantation using left hepatic segments from living related donors: surgical experience in 100 recipients at Saint-Luc University Clinics. Pediatr Transplant. 2006;10:345–53.
86. Enne M, Pacheco-Moreira L, Balbi E, Cerqueira A, Alves J, Valladares MA, Santalucia G, Martinho JM. Hepatic artery reconstruction in pediatric living donor liver transplantation under 10 Kg, without microscope use. Pediatr Transplant. 2010;14:48–51.
87. Tannuri AC, Monteiro RF, Santos MM, Miyatani HT, Tannuri U. A new simplified technique of arterial reconstruction in pediatric living-donor liver transplantation: a comparison with the classical technique. J Pediatr Surg. 2014;49:1518–21.
88. De Ville de Goyet J, Lo Zupone C, Grimaldi C, D'Ambrosio G, Candusso M, Monti L. Meso-Rex bypass as an alternative technique for portal vein reconstruction at or after liver transplantation in children: review and perspectives. Pediatr Transplant. 2013;17:19–26.
89. Roberts JP, Hulbert-Shearon TE, Merion RM, Wolfe RA, Port FK. Influence of graft type on outcomes after pediatric liver transplantation. Am J Transplant. 2004;4:373–7.
90. Soltys KA, Mazariegos GV, Squires RH, Sindhi RK, Anand R, the SPLIT Research Group. Late graft loss or death in pediatric liver transplantation: an analysis of the SPLIT database. Am J Transplant. 2007;7:2165–71.
91. Diamond IR, Fecteau A, Millis JM, Losanoff JE, Ng V, Anand R, Song C, the SPLIT Research Group. Impact of graft type on outcome in pediatric liver transplantation. A report from Studies of Pediatric Liver Transplantation (SPLIT). Ann Surg. 2007;246:301–10.
92. Abt PL, Rapaport-Kelz R, Desai NM, Frank A, Sonnad S, Rand E, Markmann JF, Shaked A, Olthoff KM. Survival among pediatric liver transplant recipients: impact of segmental grafts. Liver Transpl. 2004;10:1287–93.
93. Becker NS, Barshes NR, Aloia TA, Nguyen T, Rojo J, Rodriguez JA, O'Mahony CA, Karpen SJ, Goss JA. Analysis of recent pediatric orthotopic liver transplantation outcomes indicates that allograft type is no longer a predictor of survivals. Liver Transpl. 2008;14:1125–32.
94. Cauley RP, Vakili K, Potanos K, Fullington N, Graham DA, Finkelstein JA, Kim HB. Deceased donor liver transplantation in infants and small children: are partial grafts riskier than whole organs? Liver Transpl. 2013;19:721–9.
95. Alexopoulos SP, Nekrasov V, Cao S, Groshen S, Kaur N, Genyk YS, Matsuoka L. Effect of recipient size and allograft type on pediatric liver transplantation for biliary atresia. Liver Transpl. 2017;23:221–33.
96. Hong JC, Yersiz H, Farmer DG, Duffy JP, Ghobrial RM, Nonthasoot B, Collins TE, Hiatt JR, Busuttil RW. Longterm outcomes for whole and segmental liver grafts in adult and pediatric liver transplant recipients: 1 10-year comparative analysis of 2988 cases. J Am Coll Surg. 2009;208:682–91.
97. Broering DC, Kim JS, Mueller T, Fischer L, Ganschow R, Bicak T, Mueller L, Hillert C, Wilms C, Hinrichs B, Helmke K, Pothmann W, Burdelski M, Rogiers X. One hundred thirty-two consecutive pediatric liver transplants without hospital mortality. Lessons learned and outlook for the future. Ann Surg. 2004;240:1002–12.
98. Gridelli B, Spada M, Petz W, Bertani A, Lucianetti A, Colledan M, Altobelli M, Alberti D, Guizzetti M, Riva S, Melzi ML, Stroppa P, Torre G. Split-liver transplantation eliminates the need for living-donor liver transplantation in children with end-stage cholestatic liver disease. Transplantation. 2003;75:1197–203.
99. Bourdeaux C, Darwish A, Jamart J, Tri TT, Janssen M, Lerut J, Otte JB, Sokal E, de Ville de Goyet J, Reding R. Living-related versus deceased donor pediatric liver transplantation: a multivariate analysis of technical and immunological complications in 235 recipients. Am J Transplant. 2007;7:440–7.
100. Battula NR, Platto M, Anbarasan R, Perera MT, Ong E, Roll GR, Ferraz Neto BH, Mergental H, Isaac J, Muiesan P, Sharif K, Mirza DF. Intention to split policy. A successful strategy in a combined pediatric and adult liver transplant center. Ann Surg. 2017;265:1009–15.
101. Spada M, Gridelli B, Colledan M, Segalin A, Lucianetti A, Petz W, Riva S, Torre G. Extensive use of split liver for pediatric liver transplantation: a single-center experience. Liver Transpl. 2000;6:415–28.
102. Hsu EK, Mazariegos GV. Global lessons in graft type and pediatric liver allocation: a path toward improving outcomes and eliminating wait-list mortality. Liver Transpl. 2017;23:86–95.
103. Hackl C, Schlitt HJ, Melter M, Knoppke B, Loss M. Current developments in pediatric liver transplantation. World J Hepatol. 2015;7:1509–20.
104. Mazariegos GV. Critical elements in pediatric allograft selection. Liver Transpl. 2017;23:S56–8.
105. Lund DP, Lillehei CW, Kevy S, Perez-Atayde A, Maller E, Treacy S, Vacanti JP. Liver transplantation in newborn liver failure: treatment for neonatal hemochromatosis. Transplant Proc. 1993;25:1068–71.
106. Bonatti H, Muiesan P, Connelly S, Baker A, Mieli-Vergani G, Gibbs P, Heaton N, Rela M. Hepatic transplantation in children under 3 months of age: a single centre's experience. J Pediatr Surg. 1997;32:486–8.
107. Cacciarelli TV, Esquivel CO, Moore DH, Cox KL, Berquist WE, Concepcion W, Hammer GB, So SK. Factors affecting survival after orthotopic liver transplantation in infants. Transplantation. 1997;64:242–8.
108. Woodle ES, Millis JM, So SK, McDiarmid SV, Busuttil RW, Esquivel CO, Whitington PF, Thistlethwaite JR. Liver transplantation in the first three months of life. Transplantation. 1998;66:606–9.
109. Noujaim HM, Mayer DA, Buckles JA, Beath SV, Kelly DA, McKiernan PJ, Mirza DF, de Ville de Goyet J. Techniques for and outcome of liver transplantation in neonates and infants weighting up to 5 kilograms. J Pediatr Surg. 2002;37:159–64.
110. Mekeel KL, Langham MR, Gonzalez-Peralta RP, Hemming AW. Liver transplantation in very small infants. Pediatr Transplant. 2007;11:66–72.
111. Lucianetti A, Guizzetti M, Bertani A, Corno V, Maldini G, Pinelli D, Aluffi A, Codazzi D, Spotti A, Spada M, Gridelli B, Torre G, Colledan M. Liver transplantation in children weighting less than 6 Kg: the Bergamo experience. Transplant Proc. 2005;37:1143–5.
112. Sundaram SS, Alonso EM, Whitington PF. Liver transplantation in neonates. Liver Transpl. 2003;9:783–8.
113. Tolosa L, Pareja-Ibars E, Donato MT, Cortes M, Lopez S, Jimenez N, Mir J, Castell JV, Gomez-Lechon MJ. Neonatal livers: a source for the isolation of good-performing hepatocytes for cell transplantation. Cell Transplant. 2014;23:1229–42.

114. Pareja-Ibars E, Cortes M, Tolosa L, Gomez-Lechon MJ, Lopez S, Castell JV, Mir J. Hepatocyte transplantation program: lessons learned and future strategies. World J Gastroenterol. 2016;22:874–86.
115. Enne M, Pacheco-Moreira L, Balbi E, Cerqueira A, Santalucia G, Martinho JM. Liver transplantation with monosegments. Technical aspects and outcome: a meta-analysis. Liver Transpl. 2005;11:564–9.
116. Kiuchi T, Kasahara M, Uryuhara K, Inomata Y, Uemoto S, Asonuma K, Egawa H, Fujita S, Hayashi M, Tanaka K. Impact of graft size mismatching on graft prognosis in liver transplantation from living donors. Transplantation. 1999;67:321–7.
117. Azouz SM, Diamond IR, Fecteau A. Graft type in pediatric liver transplantation. Curr Opin Organ Transplant. 2011;16:494–8.
118. Srinivasan P, Vilca-Melendez H, Muiesan P, Prachalias A, Heaton ND, Rela M. Liver transplantation with monosegments. Surgery. 1999;126:10–2.
119. Attia MS, Stringer MD, McClean P, Prasad KR. The reduced left lateral segment in pediatric liver transplantation: an alternative to the monosegment graft. Pediatr Transplant. 2008;12:696–700.
120. Thomas N, Thomas G, Verran D, Stormon M, O'Loughlin E, Shun A. Liver transplantation in children with hyper-reduced grafts. A single-center experience. Pediatr Transplant. 2010;14:426–30.
121. Cescon M, Spada M, Colledan M, Andorno E, Valente U, Rossi G, Reggiani P, Grazi GL, Tisone G, Majno P, Rogiers X, Santamaria ML, Baccarani U, Ettorre GM, Cillo U, Rossi M, Scalamogna M, Gridelli B. Split-liver transplantation with pediatric donors: a multicenter experience. Transplantation. 2005;79:1148–53.
122. Cescon M, Spada M, Colledan M, Torre G, Andorno E, Valente U, Rossi G, Reggiani P, Cillo U, Baccarani U, Grazi GL, Tisone G, Filipponi F, Rossi M, Ettorre GM, Salizzoni M, Cuomo O, De Feo T, Gridelli B. Feasibility and limits of split liver transplantation from pediatric donors. An Italian multicenter experience. Ann Surg. 2006;244:805–14.
123. Khorsandi SE, Day AW, Cortes M, Deep A, Dhawan A, Vilca-Melendez H, Heaton N. Is size the only determinant of delayed abdominal closure in pediatric liver transplant? Liver Transpl. 2017;23:352–60.
124. De Ville de Goyet J, Struye de Swielande Y, Reding R, Sokal EM, Otte JB. Delayed primary closure of the abdominal wall after cadaveric and living related donor liver graft transplantation in children: a safe and useful technique. Transpl Int. 1998;11:117–22.
125. Caso Maestro O, Abradelo de Usera M, Justo Alonso I, Calvo Pulido J, Manrique Municio A, Cambra Molero F, Garcia Sesma A, Loinaz Segurola C, Moreno Gonzalez E, Jimenez Romero C. Porcine acellular dermal matrix for delayed abdominal wall closure after pediatric liver transplantation. Pediatr Transplant. 2014;18:594–8.
126. Karpelowsky JS, Thomas G, Shun A. Definitive abdominal wall closure using a porcine intestinal submucosa biodegradable membrane in pediatric transplantation. Pediatr Transplant. 2009;13:285–9.
127. Gondolesi G, Selvaggi G, Tzakis A, Rodriguez-Laiz G, Gonzalez-Campana A, Fauda M, Angelis M, Levi D, Nishida S, Iyer K, Sauter B, Podesta L, Kato T. Use of the abdominal rectus fascia as a nonvascularized allograft for abdominal wall closure after liver, intestinal, and multivisceral transplantation. Transplantation. 2009;87:1884–8.
128. Jones VS, Thomas G, Stormon M, Shun A. The ping-pong ball as a surgical aid in liver transplantation. J Pediatr Surg. 2008;43:1745–8.
129. Matsuura T, Soejima Y, Taguchi T. Auxiliary partial orthotopic living donor liver transplantation with a small-for-size graft for congenital absence of the portal vein. Liver Transpl. 2010;16:1437–9.
130. Bartlett A, Rela M. Progress in surgical techniques in pediatric liver transplantation. Pediatr Transplant. 2010;14:33–40.
131. Faraj W, Dar F, Bartlett A, Vilca-Melendez H, Marangoni G, Mukherji D, Mieli-Vergani G, Dhawan A, Heaton N, Rela M. Auxiliary liver transplantation for acute liver failure in children. Ann Surg. 2010;251:351–6.
132. Weiner J, Griesemer A, Island E, Lobritto S, Martinez M, Selvaggi G, Lefkowitch J, Velasco M, Tryphonopoulos P, Emond J, Tzakis A, Kato T. Longterm outcomes of auxiliary partial orthotopic liver transplantation in preadolescent children with fulminant hepatic failure. Liver Transpl. 2016;22:485–94.
133. D'Antiga L, Colledan M. Surgical gene therapy by domino auxiliary liver transplantation. Liver Transpl. 2015;21:1338–9.

Pediatric Living Donor Liver Transplantation

Mureo Kasahara, Seisuke Sakamoto, and Akinari Fukuda

Key Points
- The advantages of obtaining a liver graft from living donors include the preoperative control of graft steatosis by diet and exercise, as well as short ischemic time.
- The outcome of ABO-incompatible living donor liver transplantation is largely dependent on patient age.
- Potential LDLT donors for Alagille syndrome recipients must be cautiously evaluated to rule out unsuspected bile duct paucity by magnetic resonance cholangiopancreatography.
- The modified-reduced left lateral segment grafts, including hyper-reduced grafts and monosegmental grafts, have the potential to allow these children to undergo transplantation safely without the associated complications of large-for-size grafts.
- In recipient operation, the collateral vessels must be carefully devascularized to obtain sufficient portal venous front flow.
- If the native portal vein is sclerotic with insufficient front flow, portal venous anastomosis by using interpositional vein graft is indicated.

Research Needed in the Field
- Long-term outcomes of living donors, especially "quality of life" after donor operation
- Long-term outcomes of recipients undergoing living donor liver transplants, especially growth and development
- Long-term outcomes of the recipients receiving technical variant grafts, especially modified-reduced left lateral segments grafts
- Long-term patency of portal venous anastomosis by using interpositional vein graft
- Immunological benefits of living donors, such as haplo-identical HLA matching
- Significance of preformed or de novo donor-specific antibody and the treatment of antibody-mediated rejection
- Possibility of withdrawal of immunosuppressants related to immunological tolerance

28.1 Introduction

The concept of living donor liver transplantation (LDLT), using a part of the liver from a healthy individual to treat another sick individual, is likely as far back as the mid-twentieth century. When deceased whole liver transplantation became a universal standard procedure in the 1980s, transplantation medicine in turn began to face the inevitable issue of organ shortage so far. Deceased organ shortage in the pediatric population soon led to the technical innovations of reduced-size and split-liver transplantation [1, 2]. The emergence of LDLT as a special extension to the concept of split-liver transplantation, i.e., the sharing of a liver between a donor and a recipient, seemed to be a natural consequence of these changes. Difference of these two procedures is that no mortality/morbidity is allowed in living donors. There are also many anatomical, physiological, and surgical similarities between split-liver transplantation and LDLT.

M. Kasahara (✉) · S. Sakamoto · A. Fukuda
Organ Transplantation Center, National Center for Child Health and Development, Tokyo, Japan
e-mail: kasahara-m@ncchd.go.jp; sakamoto-si@ncchd.go.jp; fukuda-a@ncchd.go.jp

When the first cases of LDLT in children were tried and successful in 1988, no one imagined that this treatment modality would be passed onto the adult patients and spread all over the world. Graft selection has been extended from left lateral segment to the left lobe, right lobe, and some modification of the left lateral segment to save infants. The process has always been accompanied by caseless controversies about the donor safety. Today the role of the LDLT is increasing rapidly even in countries where deceased donor transplantation program is working nicely, especially pediatric liver transplantation program.

Living donor liver transplantation (LDLT) was introduced in Japan in 1989 as a lifesaving procedure for a patient with biliary atresia due to the absolute scarcity of organs available for deceased donor transplantation [3]. The shortage of deceased organ donors led to the development of unique technical, physiological, and logistical innovations in LDLT [4, 5]. Experience with technical improvements in living donor surgery has led to the generalization of pediatric LDLT, and even adult LDLT, with excellent patient and graft survival outcomes [6]. These techniques have expanded the potential donor pool and decreased waiting list mortality in the setting of pediatric liver transplantation (LT) [7]. Living donor candidates are strictly limited to relatives up to the third civil degree or spouses of the recipient who show a strong voluntary will to donate.

The number of LDLTs performed in Japan showed an initial increase to a maximum of 562 in 2005 followed by a decrease and return to the status quo of approximately 400–450 annually (Fig. 28.1). During these 25 years (November 1989 to December 2015), 7862 LDLTs were performed in Japan; 2897 were children less than 18 years of age (36.8%). The annual number of pediatric LDLT cases has been 120–140 over the past 5 years. During the same study period, 45 deceased LTs, including 20 split-liver transplantations in pediatric patients, were performed [8].

There have been technical and immunological refinements in the Japanese pediatric LDLT program, such as resolving graft size matching and overcoming blood type mismatches. The Kyoto group reported that the use of small-for-size grafts, defined as grafts with a graft-to-recipient body weight ratio (GRWR) less than 0.8%, is associated with small-for-size syndrome, the development of massive ascites, renal insufficiency, persistent cholestasis, coagulopathy, and infectious complications in patients with lower grafts and reduced patient survival, especially in adolescents, most likely due to enhanced parenchymal cell injury and reduced metabolic and synthetic graft capacity [9]. Meanwhile, large-for-size grafts are used in neonatal and infantile LDLT. The main problems associated with large-for-size grafts include the small size of the recipient's abdominal cavity, size discrepancies between vascular calibers, and insufficient blood supply to the graft. Further reducing the left lateral segment (LLS) increases the possibility of supplying an adequate graft size, while reduced or hyper-reduced LLS has been introduced to mitigate the problems of large-for-size grafts

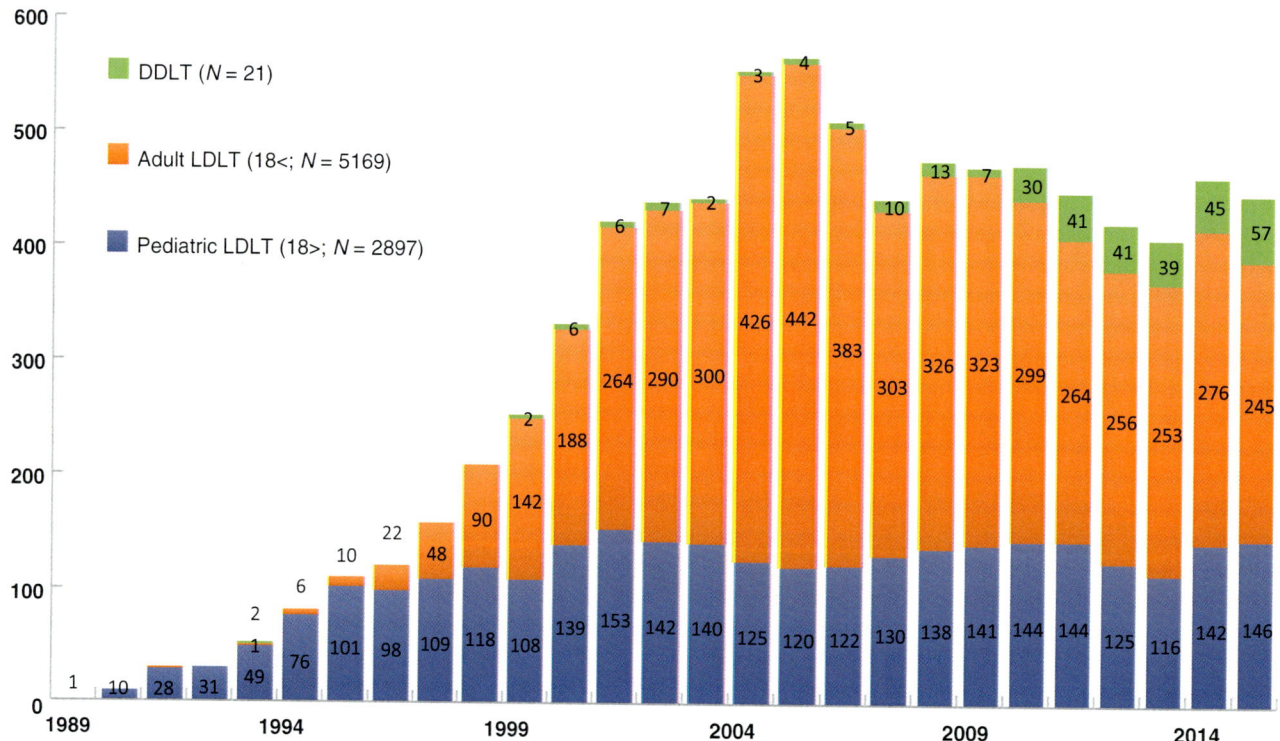

Fig. 28.1 Liver transplantation in Japan (1989~2015; $n = 7862$)

with GRWRs estimated to be over 4.0% especially in the neonatal acute liver failure patients [10].

28.1.1 Blood Type Combination in LDLT

ABO-incompatible LDLT was introduced in Japan to overcome the potential donor shortage. ABO-incompatible grafts were used in nearly 13% of the recipients included in the Japanese LDLT series. It has been reported that, despite the application of preoperative plasma exchange, splenectomy, and enhanced immunosuppression, the 5-year graft survival rate is less than 70% in the pediatric population. A Japanese LDLT series reported that ABO-incompatible liver transplantations were performed with relative safety in infants less than 2 years of age, although the long-term results were not satisfactory in children over 2 years of age [11, 12] (Fig. 28.2). Patients over 10 years of age remain at considerable risk for early fatal outcomes due to complications such as hepatic necrosis and late ischemic cholangitis. New strategies to prevent antibody-mediated rejection are required. New strategies for preventing antibody-mediated rejection using rituximab prophylaxis have been routinely applied since 2005 to overcome the ABO-blood barrier. The current immunosuppression protocol for ABO-incompatible LDLT in NCCHD consists of rituximab infusion (375 mg/m^2) 4 weeks prior to planned LDLT, pre-LDLT plasma exchange (targeted at recipient isoagglutinin titer $\leq 1:8$), and mycophenolate mofetil as an additional immunosuppressant (Fig. 28.3). Significant improvements in the graft survival, however, were obtained in more recent transplants within 5 years with a 5-year graft survival rate of 88.9% (Fig. 28.4).

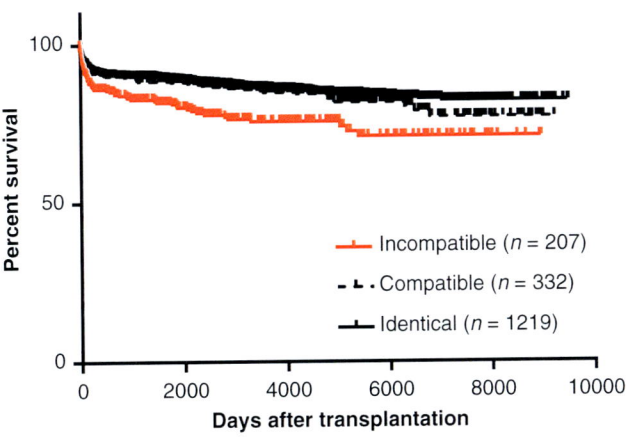

Fig. 28.2 Graft survival after pediatric living donor live transplantation in Japan

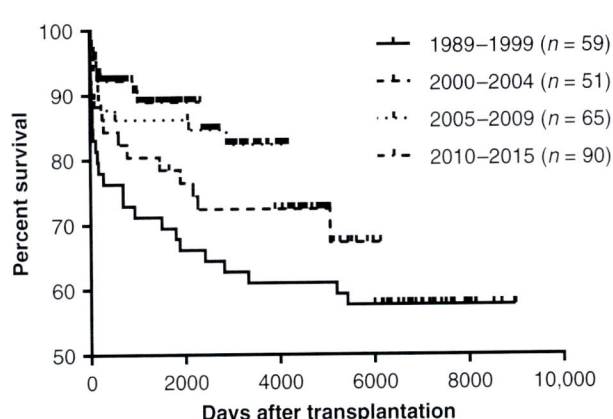

Fig. 28.4 Graft survival in ABO-I LDLT according to LDLT era

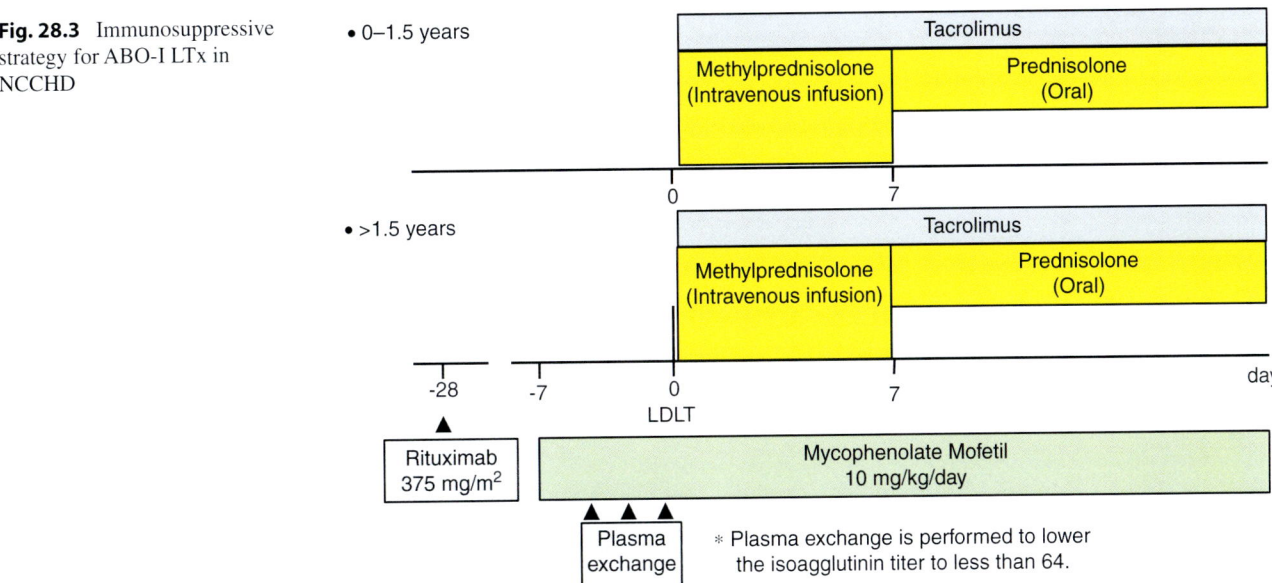

Fig. 28.3 Immunosuppressive strategy for ABO-I LTx in NCCHD

28.1.2 Indication of LDLT

The indications for LT include cholestatic liver disease, metabolic liver disease, acute liver failure, neoplastic disease, vascular disease, graft failure, and other indications. Specific diseases and preoperative patient conditions might be associated with transplantation outcomes [13, 14]. During the past two decades, medical and surgical innovations have established pediatric LDLT to be the optimal therapy for patients suffering from acute and chronic liver disease. This has allowed expansion of the indications for LT to assess patient severity and body weight in association with various diseases. The profiles of current pediatric LT recipients differ significantly from those of earlier eras [15] (Fig. 28.5). If we reviewed the outcomes of 270 pediatric LDLT recipients with metabolic disorders, the 1-, 5-, 10-, and 15-year patient and graft survival rates of the patients with metabolic disorders undergoing LDLT were 91.2%, 87.9%, 87.0%, and 79.3% and 91.2%, 87.9%, 86.1%, and 74.4%, respectively (Fig. 28.6). There are increasing incidence of urea cycle disorders and decreasing in Wilson's disease in JLTS series (Fig. 28.7).

28.1.3 Intraoperative Findings of Specific Liver Disease

There are many textbooks illustrating the indication of various liver diseases in children; however, few have been reported regarding actual intraoperative findings of specific

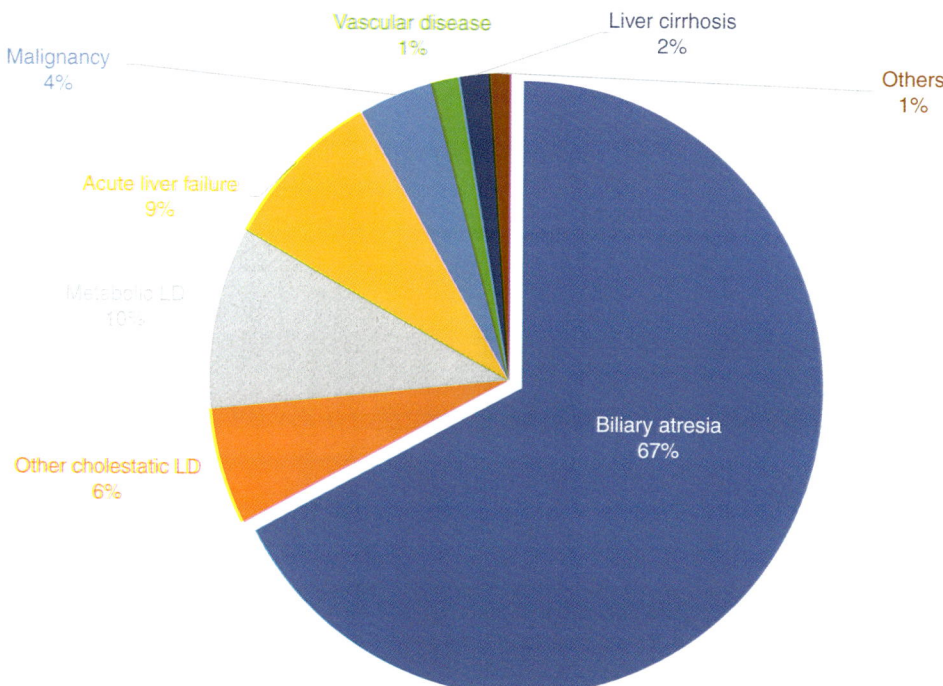

Fig. 28.5 Indication of pediatric living donor liver transplantation in Japan (1989~2015: $n = 2897$)

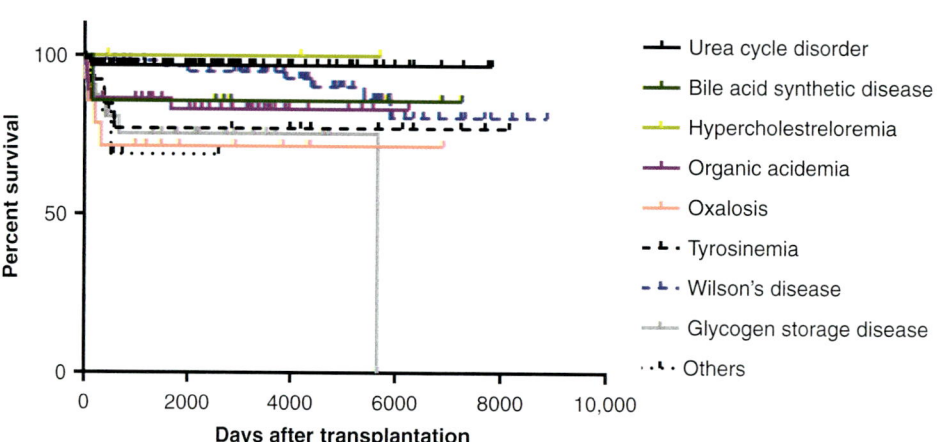

Fig. 28.6 Graft survival in metabolic LD in Japan

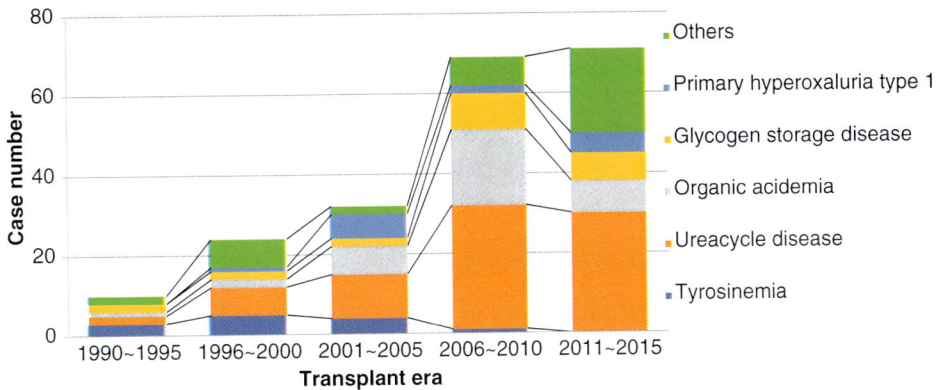

Fig. 28.7 Metabolic disorders according to transplant era ($N = 270$)

liver diseases. The following figure shows intraoperative findings of specific liver disease indicating living donor liver transplantation in the National Center for Child Health and Development, Tokyo, Japan.

(a) Biliary atresia	(b) Biliary atresia with situs inversus, absence of inferior vena cava, preduodenal portal vein, and poly splenia. The stomach in the right side
(c) Alagille syndrome	(d) Budd-Chiari syndrome

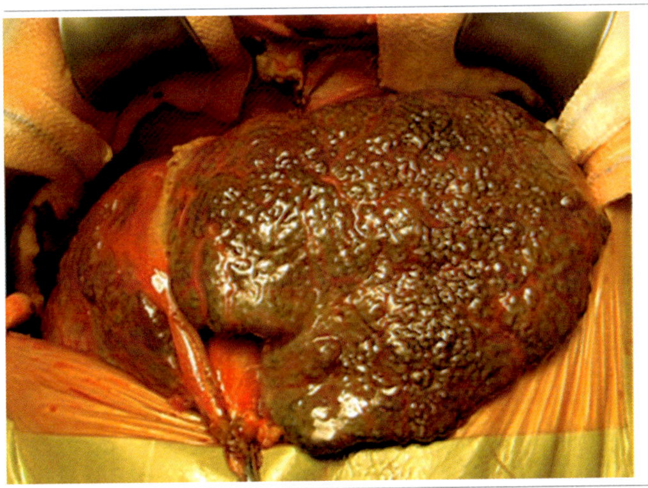

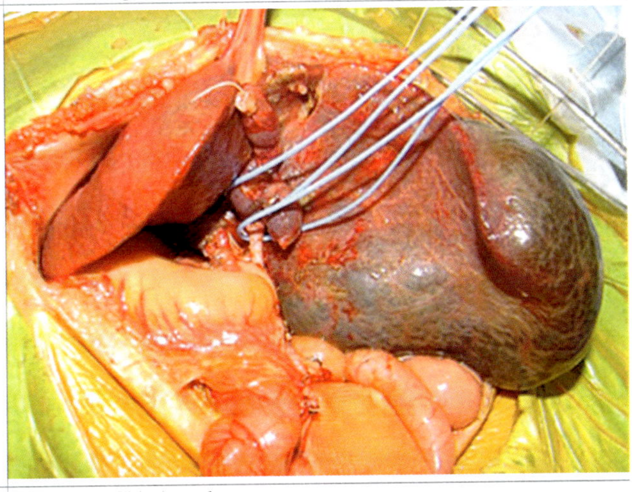

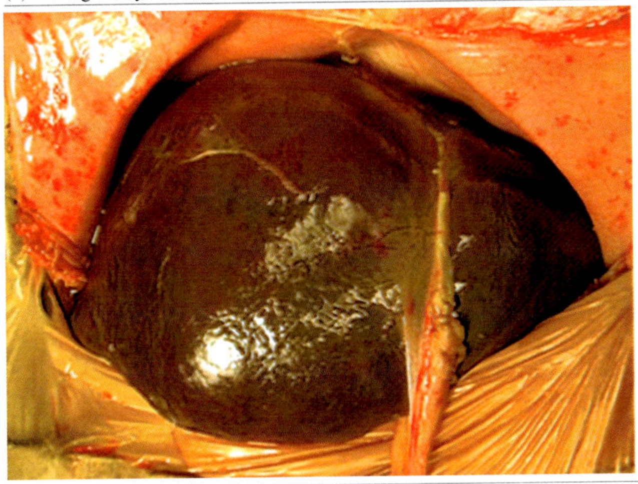

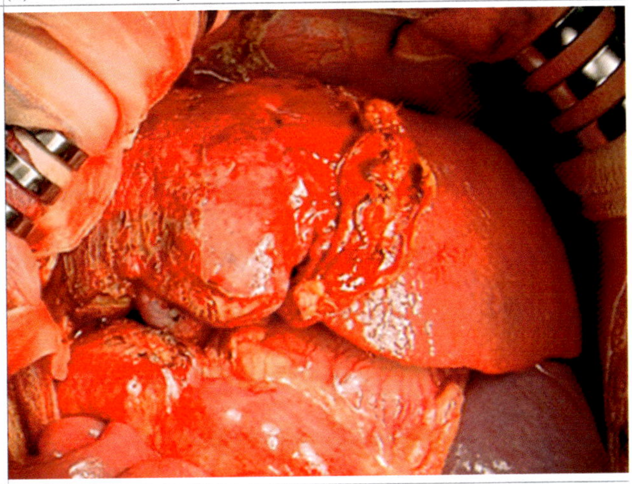

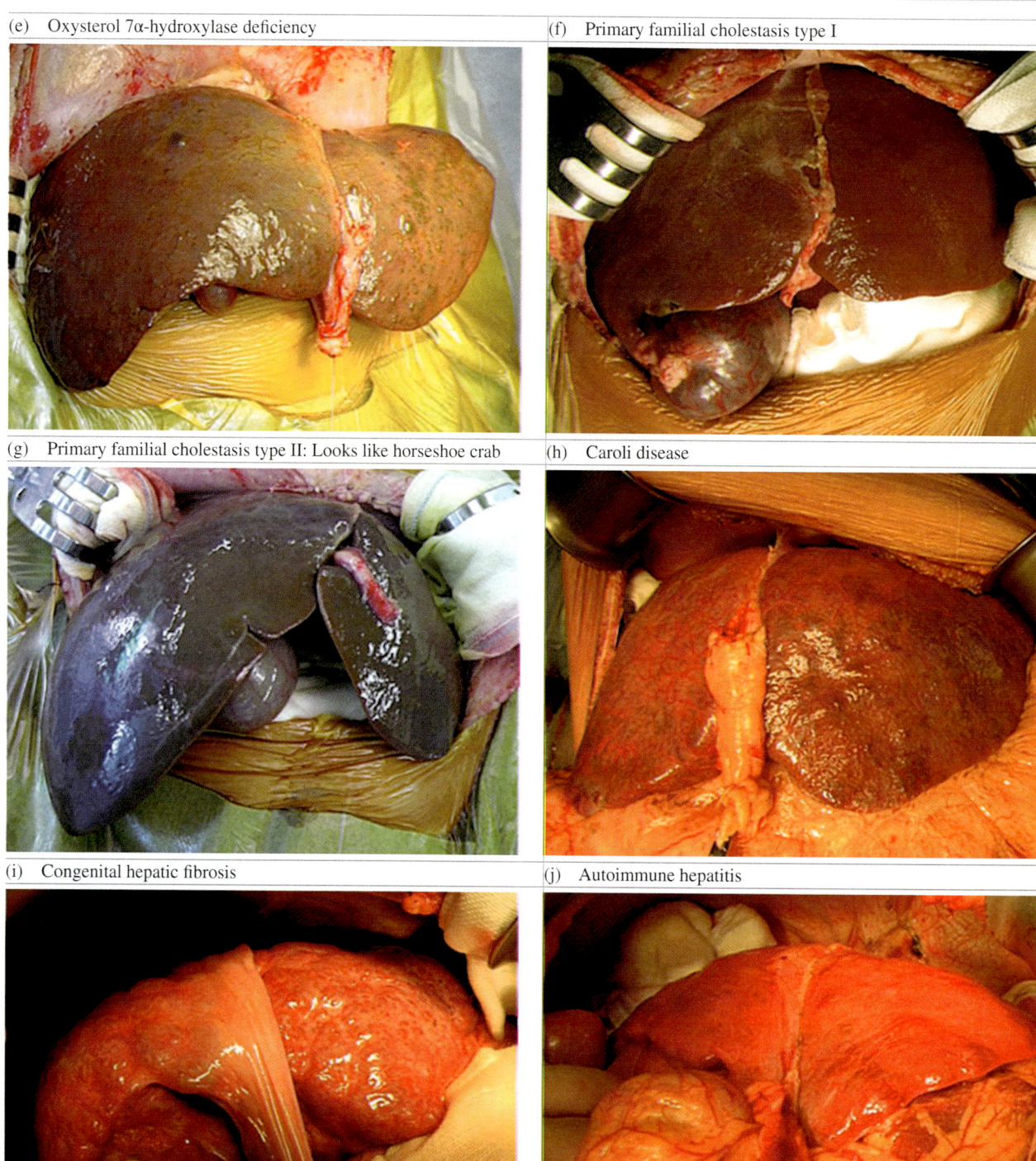

(k) Primary sclerosing cholangitis

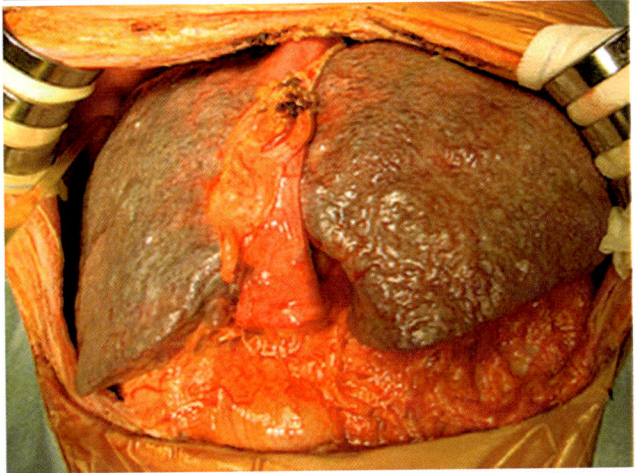

(l) Neonatal intrahepatic cholestasis caused by citrulline deficiency

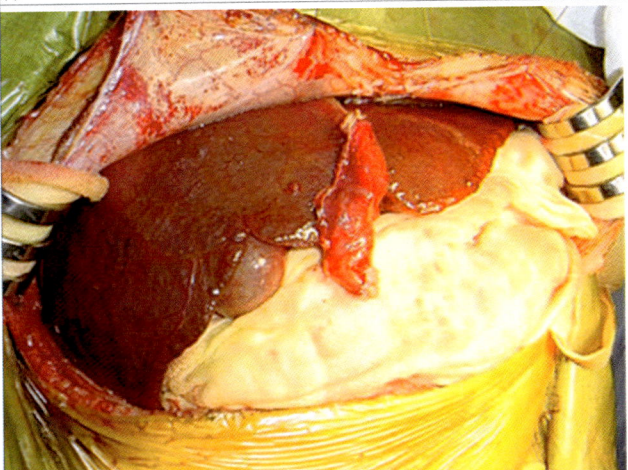

(m) Ornithine transcarbamylase deficiency: steatosis due to protein restriction

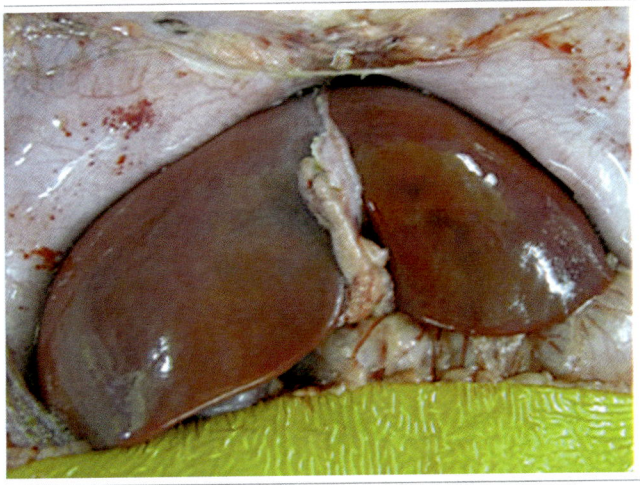

(n) Carbamoyl phosphate synthetase 1 deficiency

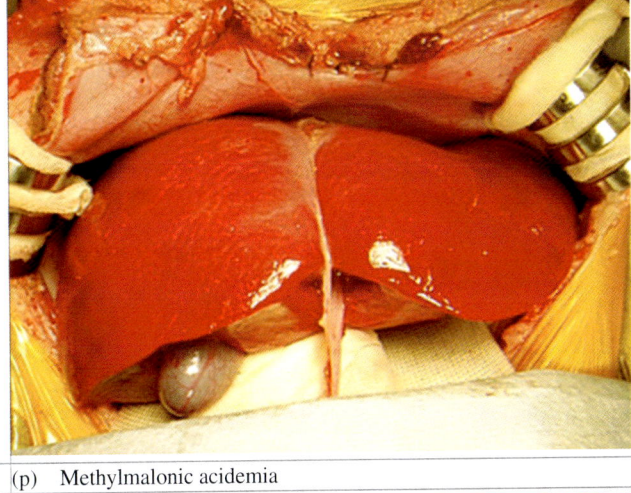

(o) Citrullinemia type I

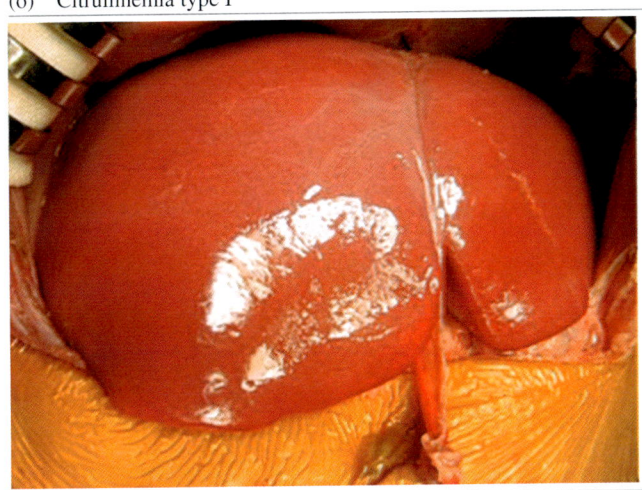

(p) Methylmalonic acidemia

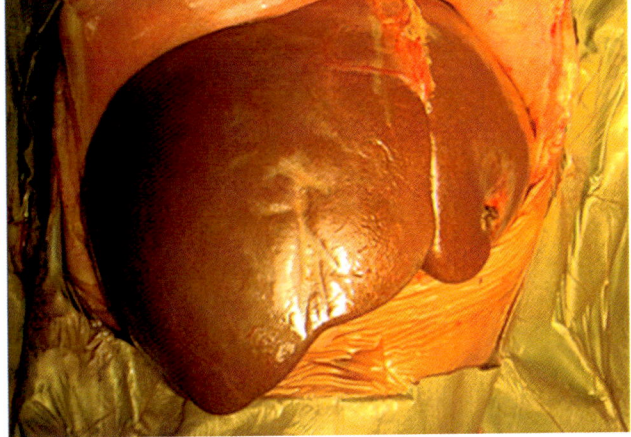

(q) Propionic acidemia

(r) Primary hyperoxaluria type I: slimy abdominal cavity

(s) Glycogen storage type Ib: hepatomegaly with steatosis

(t) Glycogen storage type IIIb

(u) Wilson's disease

(v) Acute liver failure: fluorescent red color

(w) Hemangioma: multiple pulsating tumor

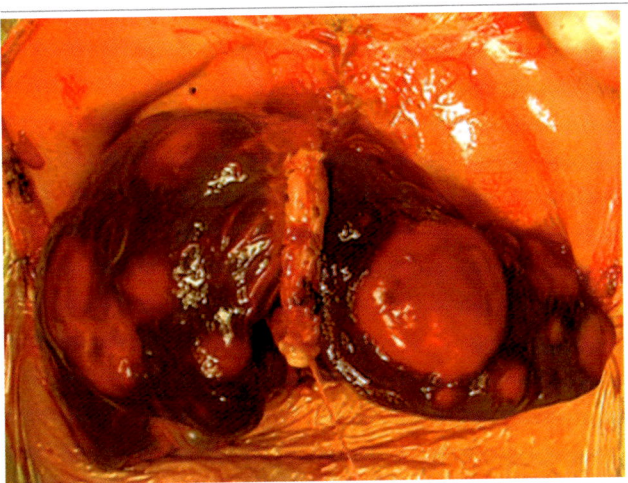

(x) Congenital absence of portal vein: symmetric liver with left-sided gall bladder

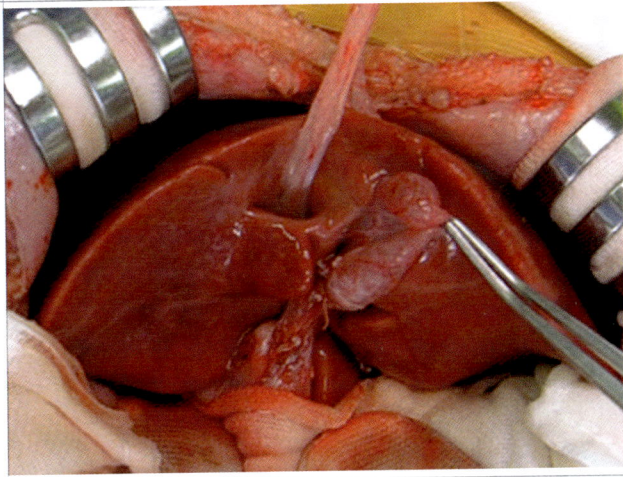

(y) Gestational alloimmune liver disease: already cirrhotic at 13 days after birth

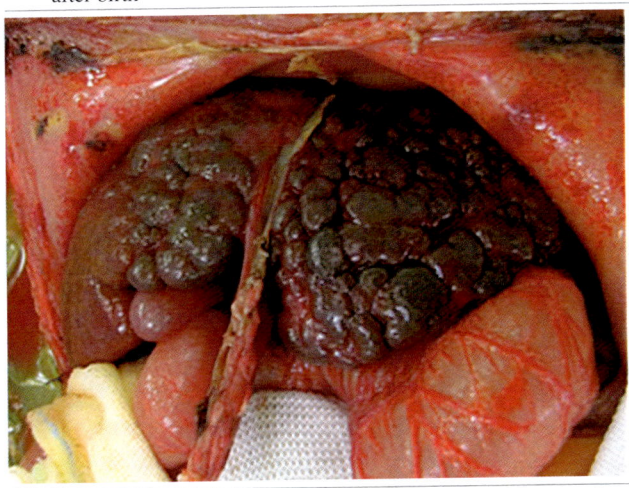

(z) Mitochondrial depletion syndrome: small cobble stonelike appearance

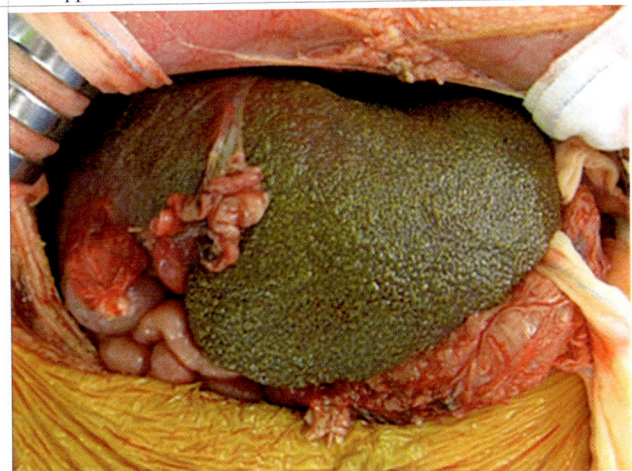

(aa) Hepatoblastoma: centrally located, unresectable without total hepatectomy

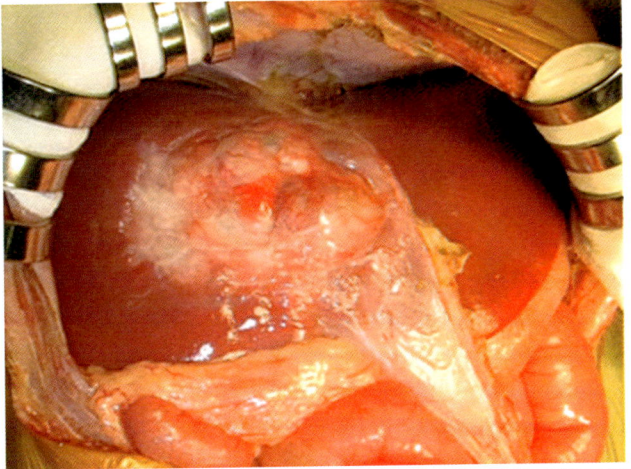

The Organ Transplantation Center of National Center for Child Health and Development (NCCHD), Tokyo, Japan, has been established in 2005, and based on these 10-year experiences in pediatric LDLT and liver surgery, we have demonstrated our innovative surgical procedure, including standard technique and complicated case presentations with beautiful surgical videos, to standardize and continue to improve the quality of surgery for end-stage pediatric liver disease (Pediatric Liver Surgery and Transplantation E-learning: Surgical Technique:

- http://www.ncchd.go.jp/recruitment/movie/organ_index.html
- ID: seiiku-guest
- Password: otLEZYjC).

This LDLT chapter is useful in maintaining high-quality surgery in all pediatric patients and in avoiding unrecognized changes in surgical strategy for all involved in this field. We are also grateful for our patients from whom we have learned so much indeed.

28.2 Living Donor

28.2.1 Preoperative Evaluation and Management

In living donor liver transplantation (LDLT), the concept of "choosing voluntarily to donate an organ" is incredibly important. Once a family realizes that their child needs a liver transplant, they start thinking of who will be the donor. This is an extremely important decision, because two members of the family will undergo surgery at the same time in a LDLT.

The main examinations involve the blood type, general biochemistry, infectious diseases, tumor markers, occult blood test, urinalysis, the respiratory functions, electrocardiography (including an examination by the cardiovascular department if abnormalities are found), a chest/abdominal radiography, and contrast computed tomography (for fatty liver and lesions and to estimate the vessel paths and the size of the liver).

The donor candidate has been fully informed of the donation process and its risks and has chosen to participate; they must undergo a series of evaluations [16]. A list of the tests necessary for donor evaluation is shown in Table 28.1.

If the child receiving the transplant has any of the following diseases, additional tests are performed. When the donor candidate is a blood relative of a recipient whose transplant indication is autoimmune liver disease, such as primary biliary cirrhosis or autoimmune hepatitis, screening for autoimmune antibodies, e.g., antinuclear antibody or antimitochondrial antibody, should be conducted. When the donor candidate is a blood relative of a patient with primary sclerosing cholangitis, Caroli disease, polycystic liver disease, or congenital hepatic fibrosis, these diseases should be excluded using imaging studies [17, 18].

The advantages of obtaining a liver graft from living donors compared with deceased donors include the preoperative control of graft steatosis by diet and exercise, as well as short ischemic time during transplantation. However, thorough evaluation of potential donors is necessary to exclude serious conditions such as nonalcoholic steatohepatitis (NASH). This is possible as there is ample time for evaluation in LDLT [18, 19]. Detailed medical history and family history of donor candidates are necessary to start the evaluation for steatosis. In cases where the body mass index (BMI) is greater than 25, suggesting obesity, every effort is taken to reduce body weight to reduce the risk of perioperative complications, such as deep vein thrombosis, as well as to control graft steatosis. Ultrasound and CT are useful measures to aid the understanding of the vasculature of the graft, as well as to evaluate steatosis of the graft. Ultrasound is a noninvasive method for donor screening. However, for the quantitative evaluation, the liver/spleen ratio can also be used, i.e., the ratio of CT values of the liver divided by that of the spleen, measured using plain CT. If the ratio is greater than 1.2, the percent of macrovesicular steatosis is less than 30% in most cases based on zero-biopsy findings [19]. We do not perform liver biopsy unless there is a need to exclude NASH because liver biopsy carries a small risk of bleeding and damaging the graft. The important underlying factor in NASH is believed to be insulin tolerance. Diabetes mellitus, hypertension, hyperlipidemia, obesity, and hyperuricemia are risk factors for insulin intolerance. Family history of liver cirrhosis of unknown etiology is a warning factor as NASH can progress to cirrhosis without any other virological background. We use the homeostasis model assessment for insulin resistance [HOMA-IR; fasting blood glucose (mg/dL) × fasting insulin (μU/mL)/405] as an indicator for insulin intolerance [20]. If HOMA-IR is greater than 1.64, insulin intolerance is suspected.

The upper age limit permitted for donor candidates varies in each institute [21, 22]. In view of donor safety, as a general rule, 64 years is the maximum age permitted for living donors at our center. With regard to graft quality, despite the belief of many transplant surgeons that grafts from aged donors are somewhat worse than grafts from younger donors, no conclusive data to support this belief have been found in LDLT [21].

In liver transplantation, there are only a few reports in the literature indicating the importance of human leukocyte antigen (HLA) matching in reducing the incidence of rejection [23]. In deceased donor liver transplantation, HLA matching is of less importance for donor selection. In terms of the role of HLA matching in rejection, it may also be the case in LDLT. However, in order to mitigate the risk of graft-versus-host disease (GVHD), HLA typing is essential in the donor evaluation process when a living donor is a person who potentially shares one haplotype with a recipient [24]. Since a parent and a child share one haplotype, one-way matching is established when the donor has homozygous HLA [25]. Liver transplant from an HLA-homozygous individual to a haplo-identical HLA-heterozygous individual in loci A, B, and DR is contraindicated because GVHD is a devastating and fatal complication.

Since it is widely known that ABO-incompatible liver transplantation has a very poor outcome, it is usually a contraindication or is performed only in exceptional situations [23, 24]. However, in Japan ABO-incompatible transplants are sometimes inevitable because a cadaveric transplant program has not yet been well established [26, 27]. It is not rare for all available living donor candidates to be ABO-incompatible. The outcome of ABO-incompatible liver transplantation is largely dependent on patient age [12, 28]. ABO-incompatible LDLT for patients aged less than 1 year and 6 months old is not necessarily contraindicated because the outcome is comparable to that of a compatible combination. We made original protocol for ABO-incompatible according to the age of the recipients. The patients younger than 1.5 years old have the standard immunosuppressive therapy consisting of tacrolimus and steroids. The patients 1.5 years old or older have additional immunosuppression using rituximab (375 mg/m^2) and mycophenolate mofetil. Plasma exchange is indicated when the recipient has the titer of blood type antibody of more than 64. ABO-incompatible LDLT is no longer considered an absolute contraindication, but an ABO-incompatible transplant should be avoided when other compatible donor candidates are available.

In order to avoid transmission of infection from donor to recipient, a thorough investigation must be performed to ensure that the donor candidate is free from infectious diseases. Human T-lymphotropic virus type I (HTLV-I) is the virus causing adult T-cell leukemia and HTLV-I-associated myelopathy. Hepatitis B virus (HBV) can often be transmitted from donor to recipient through liver transplantation if the donor has antibodies to hepatitis B core antigen [29]. When the only donor candidate is HBc positive, recipients should undergo prophylactic passive immunization with hyperimmune hepatitis B immunoglobulin (HB-IgG). Hepatitis C virus antibody-positive individuals should be excluded from the donor pool. A case of hepatic graft tuberculosis was reported, which was most likely transmitted by the graft from the living related donor [30]. This emphasizes the importance of tuberculosis screening for the donor. The tuberculin skin test (TST) was often indicated for the diagnosis of tuberculosis. However, an interferon-gamma release assay, commonly known as an IGRA or QuantiFERON-TB Gold, is a modern alternative to the tuberculin skin test (TST). Unlike the TST, QFT is a controlled laboratory test that requires only one patient visit and is unaffected by previous vaccination with bacille Calmette-Guérin (BCG) [31, 32]. Screening for syphilis is carried out using a combination of the *Treponema pallidum* hemagglutination (TPHA) test and serological tests for syphilis (STS). STS have a biological false-positive reaction.

Alagille syndrome is an autosomal dominant genetic disorder characterized by chronic cholestasis, congenital heart disease, peculiar facies, butterfly-like vertebrae, and posterior embryotoxon. Liver dysfunction is the common presentation of Alagille syndrome, and liver transplantation may be indicated. Donor selection must be carried out carefully in LDLT for patients with Alagille syndrome, because this disease can be inherited by multiple family members. One of the cases died after an operation in which a graft with unsuspected bile duct paucity was received, which resulted in persistent hyperbilirubinemia and graft dysfunction [33]. When the donor is a blood relative of the recipient, preoperative magnetic resonance cholangiopancreatography or endoscopic retrograde cholangiopancreatography should be a routine component of the pretransplant evaluation.

An inherited defect of the urea cycle enzyme often manifests soon after birth as a severe and fatal syndrome marked by hyperammonemia, coma, and devastating central nervous system impairment [34]. Ornithine transcarbamylase (OTC) deficiency is an X-linked dominant disease. Most patients who show a variety of symptoms in the neonatal period are male, and the severe cases die at a few days of life due to apnea, convulsion, and hyperammonemia-induced coma. In female patients, symptoms appear later [35]. Liver transplantation represents the best presently available therapeutic approach to cure this metabolic defect. In LDLT, many recipients with OTC deficiency may receive a liver graft from a blood relative who is a heterozygous carrier of the disease. Therefore, donors need to be assessed with regard to disease potential by urinary orotic acid excretion using the allopurinol loading test. Furthermore, it can often be confirmed by gene assays [36]. LDLT was performed in six cases of OTC deficiency: the donors were four fathers who were not considered carriers by allopurinol loading test and two mothers who were heterozygous carriers with subclinical abnormalities in the allopurinol loading test. Nonetheless, neither the donors nor the recipients who received heterozygous livers have experienced any episodes suggestive of hyperammonemia [37]. We experienced two OTCD patients who were performed LDLT from asymptomatic OTCD heterozygous donors and just after their LDLT transiently required continuous veno-venous hemodialysis [38]. They are currently doing well without intensive medical treatment. The use of asymptomatic OTCD heterozygous donors in LDLT has been accepted with careful examination. However, an OTCD heterozygous carrier donor should be avoided if there is another donor candidate, due to the potentially fatal condition of hyperammonemia following LDLT.

Gilbert's syndrome is defined as benign, familial, mild, unconjugated hyperbilirubinemia (serum bilirubin 1–5 mg/dL) not due to hemolysis and with normal routine tests of liver function and hepatic histology. Its incidence appears to be approximately 3–7% of the population. The diagnosis of Gilbert's syndrome is based on the finding that serum bilirubin increases with fasting and nicotinic acid administration and falls on phenobarbitone administration. In liver transplantation, Gilbert's syndrome is not a donor contraindication. Recipients of transplanted grafts which had been diagnosed as Gilbert's syndrome have only a slightly elevated serum bilirubin level, and this does not affect the graft function [39, 40].

Hypertension, diabetes mellitus, hypercholesterolemia, other hyperlipidemia, and high BMI are risk factors for atherosclerosis and other cardiovascular diseases. Hypertension itself may not be a contraindication for donation if it is well controlled, but close evaluation for cardiovascular diseases is necessary, including ECG and stress testing. Arrhythmia can be a reason to preclude donor candidacy if it is ventricular and potentially associated with the risk of serious tachycardia. For an individual with bronchial asthma, complete control of attacks is the absolute requirement before becoming a living donor, and full surveillance by a respiratory specialist is needed. Usually a candidate with a significant history of asthma attack and medication is excluded from candidacy. Chronic obstructive pulmonary disease revealed by spirogram also precludes donor candidacy. The screening tests for renal disease are also very important. For example, if a candidate has immunoglobulin A nephritis, a careful assessment by a specialist is necessary even when it is asymptomatic.

Lack of organ donors is one of the most pressing problems in transplantation. Therefore, people with a history of malignancy can also be eligible to be organ donor candidates, although donation is often contraindicated in those in the active phase of malignancy. There are no apparent exclusion criteria for organ donor candidates with a history of malignancy. Of 17,639 donors, 202 (1.1%) had a history of cancer, including 61 donors with cancers classed as having an unacceptable/high risk of transmission from the transplanted and cancer registry in the United Kingdom. No cancer transmission was noted in 133 recipients of organs from these 61 donors [41]. To prevent donor transmission of malignancy, donor selection should be assessed carefully. The lung, colon, breast, and prostate also demonstrate higher rates of transmission [42]. It has been recommended that donors with a history of any of these cancers be avoided because of the transmission risks. Regarding the safe period between curative treatment and organ donation, no consensus has been obtained to date. In LDLT, more careful donor evaluations can be carried out than in deceased donor liver transplantation. Moreover if possible, other candidates who have no history of malignancy should be assessed. If there are no candidates except those with a history of malignancy, donor selection should be based on not only confirming no disease recurrence with laboratory data, radiography, endoscopy, and radioscintigraphy but also bearing in mind the biological propensity of tumor recurrence. Some types of tumor, such as the breast and lung, are known to recur in the long term after the initial diagnosis and treatment.

28.2.2 Technical Aspects of the Donor Surgery for Pediatric LDLT

28.2.2.1 Standard Left Lateral Segment Graft

The operative procedure has been previously described [43]. After 10 cm midline incision, left triangular ligament was dissected, and left lateral segment was freed from diaphragm attachment. Lesser omentum, which sometimes includes left hepatic artery from left gastric artery, was carefully opened, and sizable left gastric vein was ligated. After isolation of the donor left hepatic artery, hepatic duct, and portal branch, cholecystectomy and cholangiogram were applied. Sugita clip was placed on 3 mm left side of biliary bifurcation to make sure exact cutting line by cholangiogram. After taking liver biopsy, hepatic parenchyma of the medial segment was transected 5 mm to the right side of the falciform ligament without blood inflow occlusion or graft manipulation. Left bile duct was encircled and dissected with sharp knife. Hepatic artery, portal vein, and hepatic vein were gently clumped and dissected, and the graft was preserved in cold preservation solution. The graft liver volume, size of vessels, and bile duct were measured and were prepared for implantation on the bench surgery [44].

28.2.2.2 Reduced and Hyper-reduced Left Lateral Segment Graft (Nonanatomical Volume Reduction)

There have been technical refinements in the Japanese pediatric LDLT program, such as resolving graft size matching. The main problems associated with large-for-size grafts include the small size of the recipient's abdominal cavity, size discrepancies between vascular calibers, and insufficient blood supply to the graft, particularly in neonatal and infantile LDLT. Liver volume is one of the key determinant factors for graft liver function for recipients as well as for remnant liver function for donors. Routine use of CT volumetry is indispensable both for donor safety and for recipient survival. For the evaluation of graft volume in relation to recipient body weight, graft-to-recipient weight ratio (GRWR), which is calculated as graft weight divided by recipient body weight, is useful. The risk of vascular complications such as portal vein thrombosis and/or acute rejection is reported to be high [45]. One-year graft survival is 82% with large-for-size graft (3% GRWR <5%) and 71% with extra-large-for-size graft (GRWR ≥5%), respectively. The lack of size-matched pediatric liver grafts has led to the development of reduced, split, and living donor liver transplantation. These techniques have expanded the potential donor pool and have decreased waiting-list mortality for children [46]. Transplantation in children who weigh less than 5 kg remains a problem because the left lateral segment (LLS) from an adult may be too large when the graft-to-recipient weight ratio is greater than 4.0% and thus may result in a large-for-size graft and its associated morbidity [45]. Further reduced LLS grafts that can be transplanted safely without compromise to patient survival have been introduced for these children to mitigate the problem of large-for-size grafts [47]. In very small children (neonates) who have no portal hypertension, hepatomegaly, or ascites, the abdominal cavity may be small, and the anteroposterior thickness of the graft remains a problem [48, 49]. The disadvantages of using large-for-size grafts include graft compression, the use of silastic mesh to close the abdomen and associated infections, splinting of the diaphragm, and delayed extubation, all of which contribute to poor outcomes [50]. These complications are amplified by the small recipient size and often associated malnutrition in a patient population that already presents a technical challenge and postoperative complexity [51]. To relieve the problem of large-for-size grafts in small babies, reduced LLS grafts have been introduced [45, 47, 48, 52]. After isolation of the left lateral segment graft, the LLSs of the donors were reduced in situ as previously reported [48, 53]. The transection line was dependent on the anatomical variation of the hepatic rather than the portal venous system. The caudal part and lateral part of LLS were resected in situ while preserving the medial branch of the left hepatic vein (Fig. 28.8). Intraoperative Doppler ultrasonography was used to avoid vessel injury. We defined "reduced LLS graft" as reduced lateral part of the LLS graft and "hyper-reduced LLS graft" as reduced both lateral and caudate part of LLS graft. The resected liver volume was weighted and was prepared for "hepatocyte transplantation program," if the informed consent is available. This procedure is useful for the small baby; however, there still remained an issue that the thickness of the graft could not be reduced.

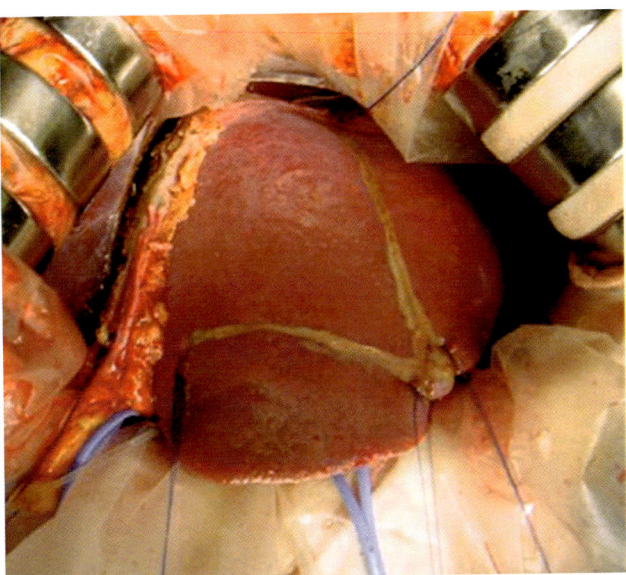

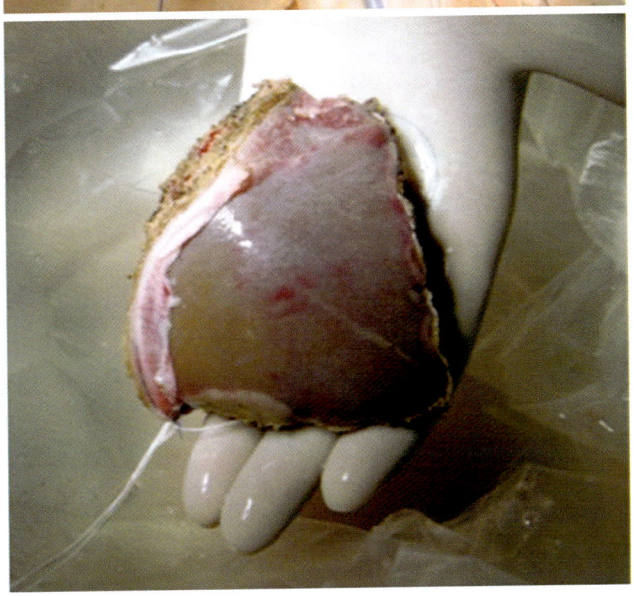

Fig. 28.8 After isolation of the left lateral segment graft, additional resection was made of reduction of caudal and lateral part of left lateral segment. It actually worked well, but there still remained an issue that the thickness of the graft could not be reduced in this procedure

28.2.2.3 Reduced-Thickness LLS Graft

Segment II Graft (Anatomical Reduction)

In addition, the size and shape of the LLS of the donor should be taken into consideration. Some LLSs are short and thick, whereas others are thin and long (Fig. 28.9). We have developed a modified LLS reduction by which the thickness of the graft is addressed and transplantation is allowed in very small infants. In the donor operation, after the isolation of the LLS graft, segment II graft can be available with meticulous technique. Following the falciform ligament toward the hepatic parenchyma and then each PV branch feeding to segment III was separately exposed (Fig. 28.10a). According to the preoperative assessment of the anatomical patterns of the PV, the relevant PV branches feeding to the reduction part of segment III were occluded to make demarcation lines on the surface between segments II and III (Fig. 28.10b). At that point, the intraoperative Doppler ultrasonography (US) could visualize the portal venous flow feeding to the graft, which planned to be preserved inside the liver. The further transection of hepatic parenchyma was horizontally performed, following those demarcation lines. If required the further reduction from the perspective of the graft volume, the removal of the lateral part of segment III was added [54, 55].

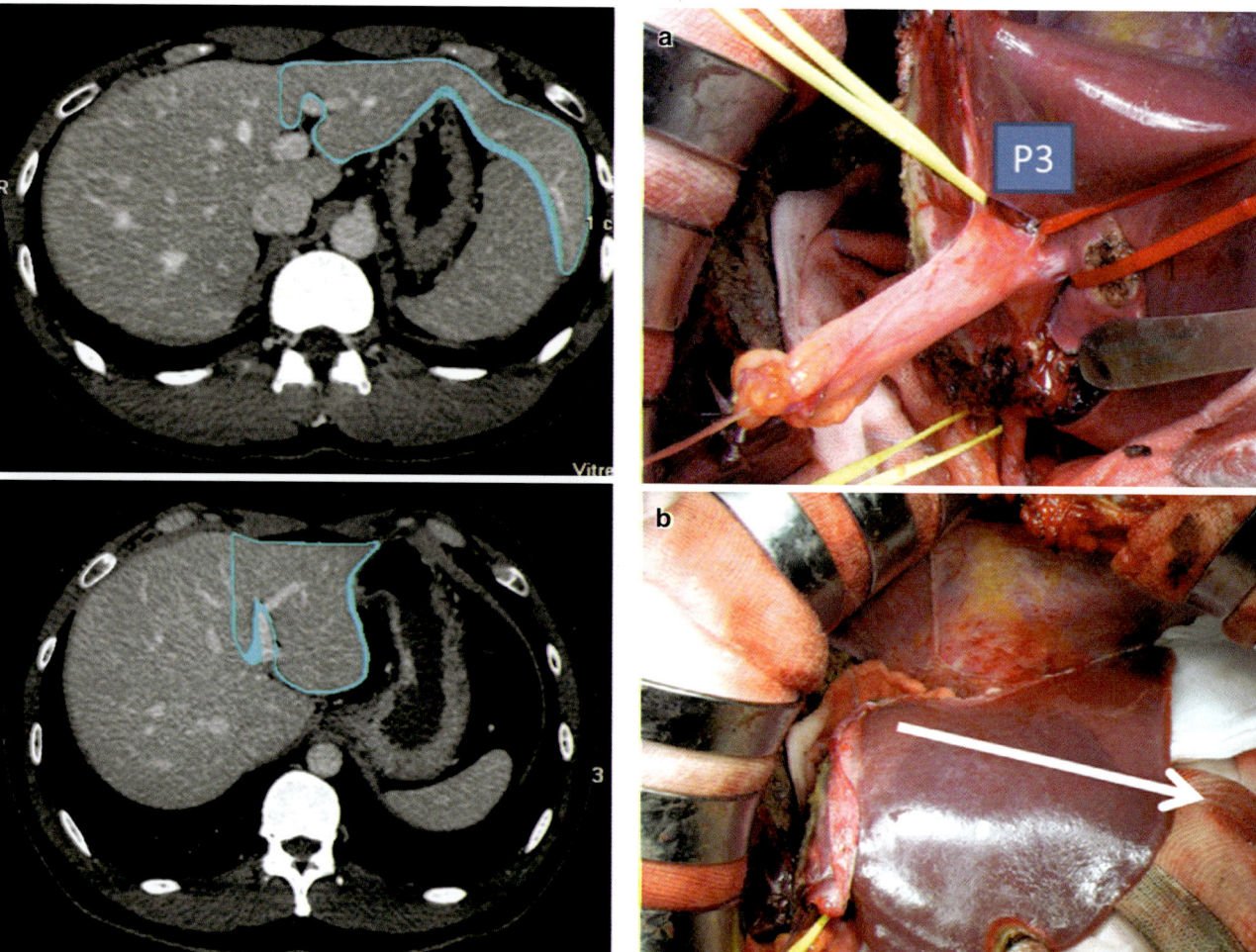

Fig. 28.9 If the LLS graft shape is flat fish-shaped type, modification as HRLLS graft is suitable. If the LLS graft shape is puffy fish-shaped type, S2 monosegment graft should be considered

Fig. 28.10 Segment III Glissonian sheath was encircled, and parenchymal dissection has been made according to the demarcation lines between segments II and III

We have faced anatomical limitation for reducing the graft especially segment II graft. In this particular case, segments II and III hepatic arteries are raised from left hepatic artery separately; at the time of reduction, we may not know which artery should be reconstructed without proper imaging study. In this case we have sufficient imaging study and made hepatic arterial anastomosis without misunderstanding A2 and A3 (Fig. 28.11). There was another anatomical problem which had left portal vein branched to P2 and P3 inside of the left lateral segment parenchyma. This kind of anatomical variant is not suitable for taking the segment II graft (Fig. 28.12). And the crucial point of this procedure is underlying the risk of the drainage vein of the graft, because main left hepatic vein is running between P2 and P3 branch (Fig. 28.13). During that procedure, we have to paid attention to preserve the drainage veins of the graft.

Modified (P3 Preserving) Segment II Graft (Modified Anatomical Reduction)

We have developed "the modified (p-3 preserving) segment II graft" to overcome the disadvantage of segment II graft. After the left lateral segment graft is transected in the donor, segment III Glissonian sheath was encircled, and parenchymal dissection has been made according to the demarcation lines between segments II and III. During transection, we keep the cutting plain just above the main P3; the transection line for this was located horizontally on the level of the segment III branch of the PV (oblique line). Normally, main LHV is running between P2 and P3 branch. As far as one preserves P3 main branch, it never compromises outflow of the graft. This transection line could preserve the drainage vein of the graft, which drained into the inferior vena cava between the segment II and III branches of the PV (Fig. 28.10).

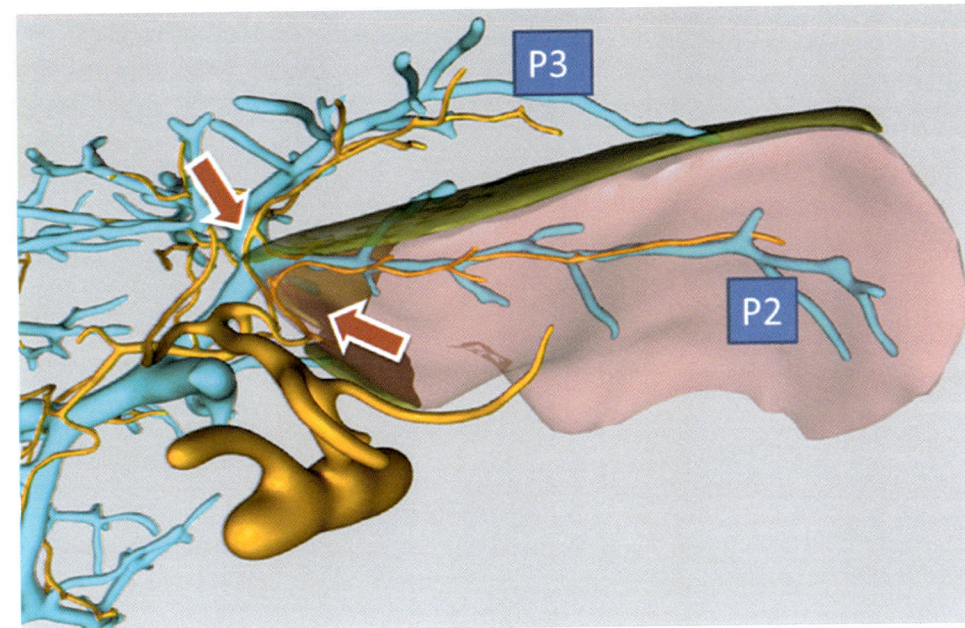

Fig. 28.11 We have anatomical limitation for reducing the graft especially segment II graft. In this particular case, segments II and III hepatic arteries arise from left hepatic artery separately; at the time of reduction, we may not know which artery should be reconstructed without proper imaging study. In this case we have sufficient imaging study and made hepatic arterial anastomosis without misunderstanding A2 and A3

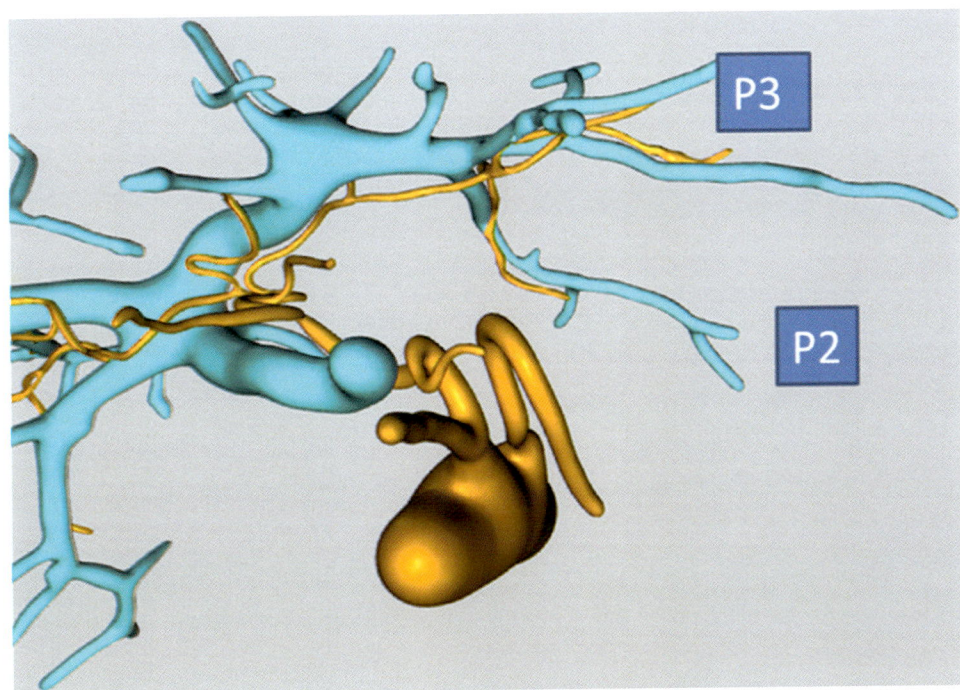

Fig. 28.12 The P2 and P3 divided inside the parenchyma; it would be tricky and better to be done by experienced surgeon with intraoperative ultrasonography

Tailoring the graft size and especially reducing the thickness of the graft might be important for small infants with end-stage liver disease. Although steps 2 and 3 of the procedure presented in this article could be done ex situ to protect the donor from the risk of bleeding and possible air embolisms, prolonged cold ischemia times and rewarming of the graft during back-table surgery have been found to be associated with increased susceptibility to ischemic/reperfusion injury in ex situ split-liver transplantation, and it might be postulated that these factors contribute to a higher incidence of graft dysfunction [56]. The procedure is associated with a much higher rate of biliary fistulas, and meticulous surgical technique and pre-/intraoperative anatomical evaluations with cholangiography/echography are recommended to prevent compromises to donor and recipient safety. By limiting adhesions in unexpected re-laparotomy during follow-up, the use of hemostatic fleeces to protect the cutting edges might be effective (Fig. 28.14).

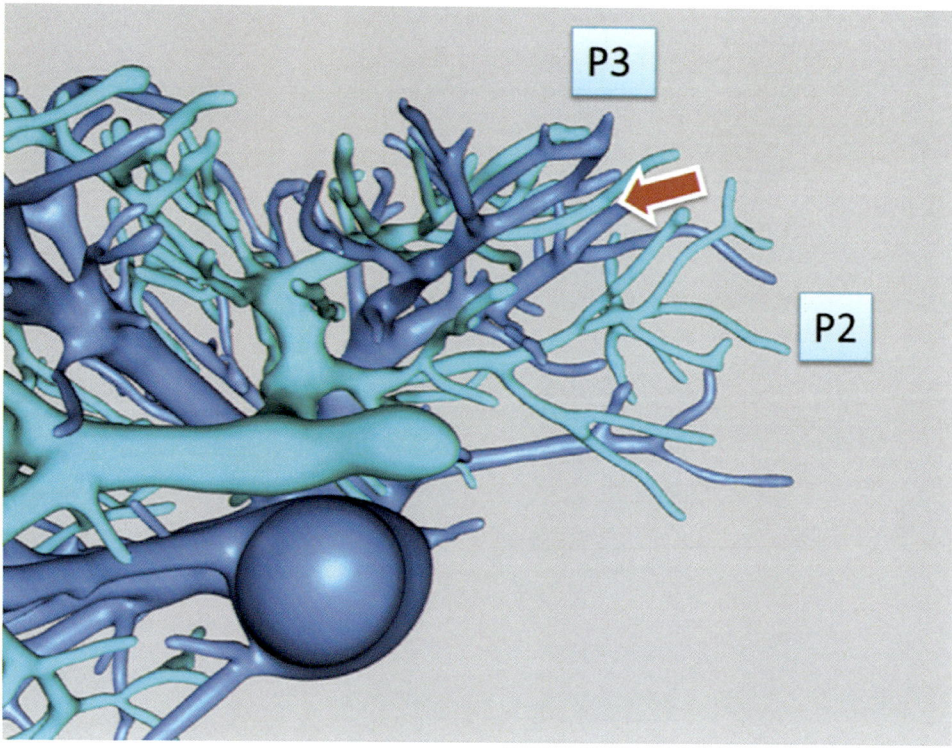

Fig. 28.13 Main LHV is always running between P2 and P3. As far as one preserves P3 branch, it never compromises the outflow of the graft

28.2.2.4 The Algorithm of Graft-Type Selection in LDLT for Smaller Children

Our series proposes the algorithm that can be used to select the graft type in LDLT for smaller children, which is simply framed in terms of the GRWR and the ratio of the thickness of the LLS to the AP diameter in the recipient's abdominal cavity. Furthermore, performing a preoperative analysis using a 3D, computer-generated model of the donor's liver can provide valuable information for the decision-making process in regard to graft-type selection.

As shown in Fig. 28.15a, b, if the maximum thickness of the donor's LLS is smaller than the AP diameter in the recipient's abdominal cavity (ratio of thickness <1.0), then segment II grafts may not be necessary for the majority of recipients. However, if a recipient is associated with a profoundly ill status before the operation, and shows severe subcutaneous edema of the abdominal wall or edematous intestines, then nonanatomically reduced LLS is unlikely to fit into the small abdominal cavity of the child. Therefore, the algorithm proposed in our experience should be refined through the further accumulation of experience, especially considering various preoperative conditions of the recipients as reference indices for graft-type selection [57].

The modified-reduced LLSs have the potential to allow these children to undergo transplantation safely without the associated complications of large-for-size grafts. Although long-term observation should be necessary to establish this technical modification, we hope that increasing experience with the technique and refinements will lead to improved outcomes in liver transplantation for small babies.

28.2.3 Postoperative Management and Outcome of the Living Donor

Between November 2005 and December 2016, 406 children underwent LDLT in the National Center for Child Health and Development (NCCHD). There were 168 male donors (41.4%) and 238 female donors (58.6%) with a median age of 35 years (range, 1–62 years) and a median body weight of 56.7 kg (range, 8.5–85.0 kg). The donors were parents in 96.3% cases, including fathers and mothers in 56.9% and 39.4% of cases, respectively, followed by domino donor (Maple syrup urinary disease) in 1.0% of cases. The blood type combination was identical in 59.6% and compatible in 22.9%, while 17.5% recipients received ABO-incompatible grafts. The graft types included modified left lateral segment in 23.6%, left lateral segment (LLS) in 64.8, left lobe in 9.9%, right lobe grafts in 1.0%, and domino whole graft in 0.7%. There are 15 donor complications (3.7%) including wound hernia in 3, wound infection in 3, duodenal ulcer in 3, paralytic ileus in 2, deep vein thrombosis in 1, biliary leakage in 1, radial nerve palsy in 1, and meningitis related to epidural tube in 1. There were no donor mortalities in our series.

28.3.1.1 Cholestatic Liver Diseases

Biliary atresia (BA) was the most common cholestatic liver diseases indicated for LDLT. Most of the patients received Kasai operation; some of them underwent redo surgeries, which might induce tight adhesions in the abdominal cavity; however, LDLT tended to be indicated earlier once the first Kasai operation was failed and anti-adhesive materials were used at the time of the operation for most of the recent cases. When the BA patients were considered to indicate LDLT, there were several important clinical features specific to BA as follows: comorbid congenital anomalies, hepatopulmonary syndrome, incidental malignancy, and portal vein hypoplasia with collateral development. Determining the surgical priority in the BA recipients with congenital heart diseases is a challenge due to the hemodynamic alterations that increase surgical risks. In order to prioritize the choice of surgery, it is essential to analyze the advantages and disadvantages of performing each procedure first. Giving priority to cardiac surgery as the first procedure would stabilize the vascular system dynamics during the subsequent LDLT, but the patient would face the risk of a coagulation disorder during cardiac surgery, as well as the risk of hepatic dysfunction after the cardiac intervention. Alternatively, if LDLT were carried out first, the patient would have good hepatic function during the cardiac intervention but would have the risk of an air embolism during the liver replacement, as well as the risk of infectious endocarditis after liver transplantation. Definitive criteria do not exist for prioritizing heart and liver operations in cases with coexistent end-stage liver disease and congenital cardiac malformations that require surgical correction. Therefore, one needs to evaluate the patient's specific situation with respect to heart disease and liver failure and carefully analyze the available data to determine the order of surgery [58].

Situs inversus (SI) occurs in association with the polysplenia syndrome with midgut malrotation, preduodenal PV, aberrant hepatic arterial supply, and absence of inferior vena cava (IVC) (Fig. 28.16). Consideration has to be given to additional vascular reconstruction at LT for BA with SI. Native liver appears asymmetric, and hepatic arteries often arise at the celiac trunk more cranially; therefore, it might be sometimes difficult to orientate hepatic arteries' anatomy, and hepatic arterial anastomosis is exposed to be with the tension. The evaluation of intrapulmonary shunting (IPS) of portal hypertensive pulmonary hypertension is important when the patients are indicated for LDLT. If those pulmonary complications have already become severe, LT should be carefully indicated. The case with IPS is often susceptible to surgical morbidities, such as biliary complications and vascular thrombosis [59]. BA cases have a risk of development of malignant tumors, such as hepatoblastoma or hepatocellular carcinoma.

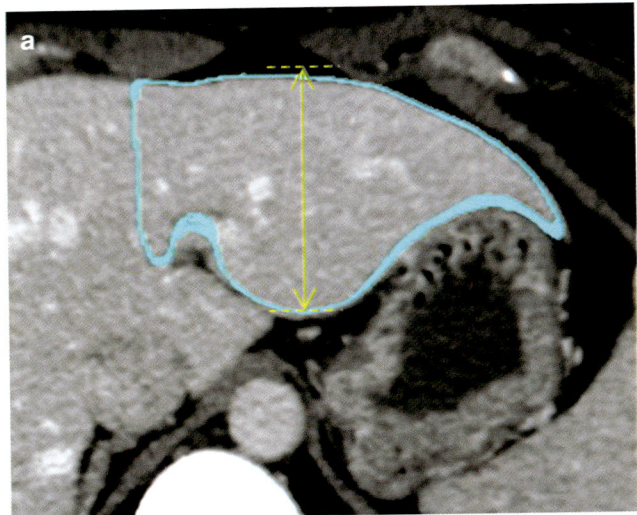

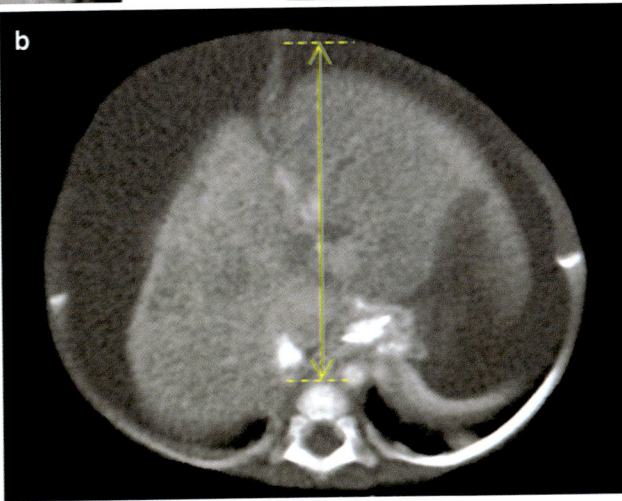

Fig. 28.14 (a) The maximum thickness of the donor left lateral segment graft. (b) The anteroposterior (A-P) diameter in the recipient abdominal cavity. From the perspective of the graft shape, if the LLS of the donor was bulky, and its maximum thickness was larger than the anteroposterior (AP) diameter in the recipient's abdominal cavity, which was identified as the length from the inside abdominal wall to the front of the vertebra on axial computed tomography images, a segment II graft was considered (when the ratio of thickness [= graft thickness/recipient A] more than 1.0)

28.3 Recipient

28.3.1 Characteristics of Recipients with Each Liver Disease Undergoing Living Donor Liver Transplantation

The indications of living donor liver transplantation (LDLT) for pediatric liver disease are mostly similar to those of deceased donor liver transplantation (DDLT). In this chapter, some of the difference in the characteristics of the recipients with each liver disease is separately described below.

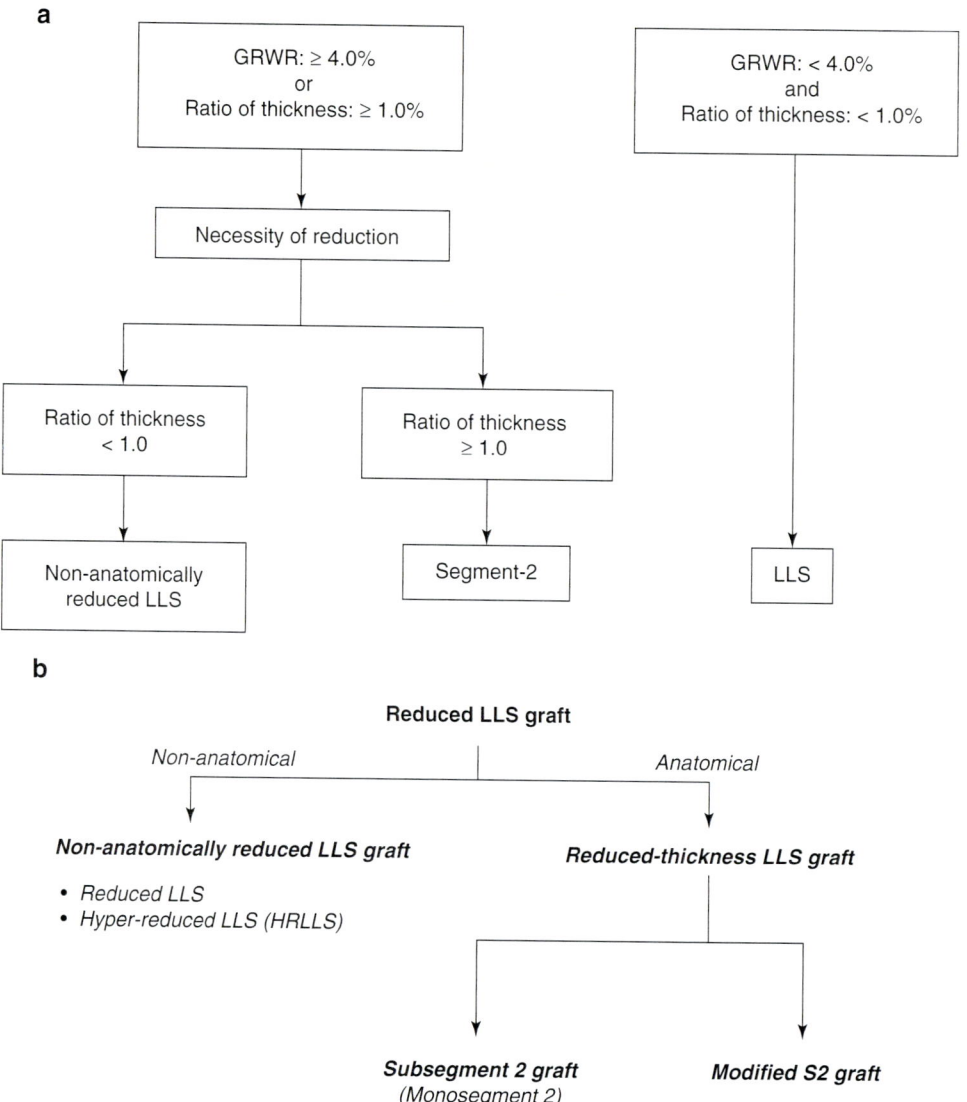

Fig. 28.15 The algorithm of graft-type selection in LDLT for smaller children: algorithm used for the preoperative assessment for graft-type selection. *GRWR* graft-to-recipient weight ratio, *LLS* left lateral segment, *ratio of thickness* the ratio of the maximum thickness of the LLS to the anteroposterior diameter in the recipient's abdominal cavity

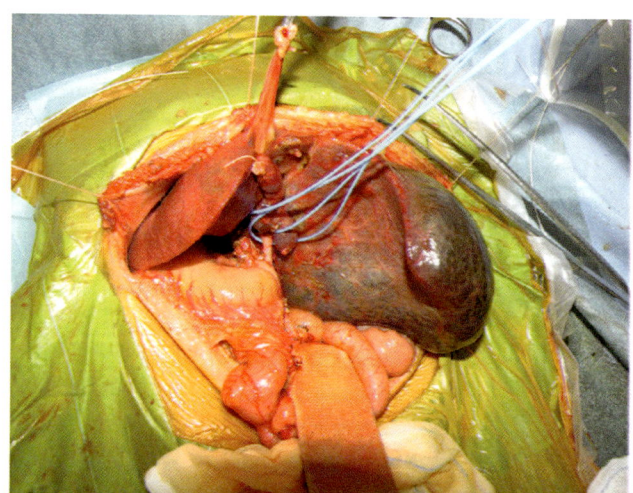

Fig. 28.16 Intraoperative findings of biliary atresia with situs inversus

Alagille syndrome (AGS) is an autosomal dominant genetic disorder, and therefore, potential LDLT donors, commonly recipients' parents, may have intrahepatic bile duct paucity or anatomical anomalies of hepatic vasculatures [60]. LDLT donors must be cautiously evaluated to rule out unsuspected bile duct paucity (Fig. 28.17). Progressive familial intrahepatic cholestasis (PFIC), including type 1 and type 2, is also indicated for LDLT. PFIC type 1, which is caused by mutations in ATP8B1 gene on hepatocytes, cholangiocytes, and enterocytes leading to cholestatic jaundice, diarrhea, and growth retardation, is often complicated by postoperative diarrhea and recurrent graft steatosis, and therefore, LT might be cautiously indicated for this type of PFIC [61].

28.3.1.2 Metabolic Liver Diseases

Urea cycle disorders (UCD), consisting of ornithine transcarbamylase deficiency (OTCD) and carbamoyl phosphate synthetase 1 deficiency (CPS1D), are the most common metabolic

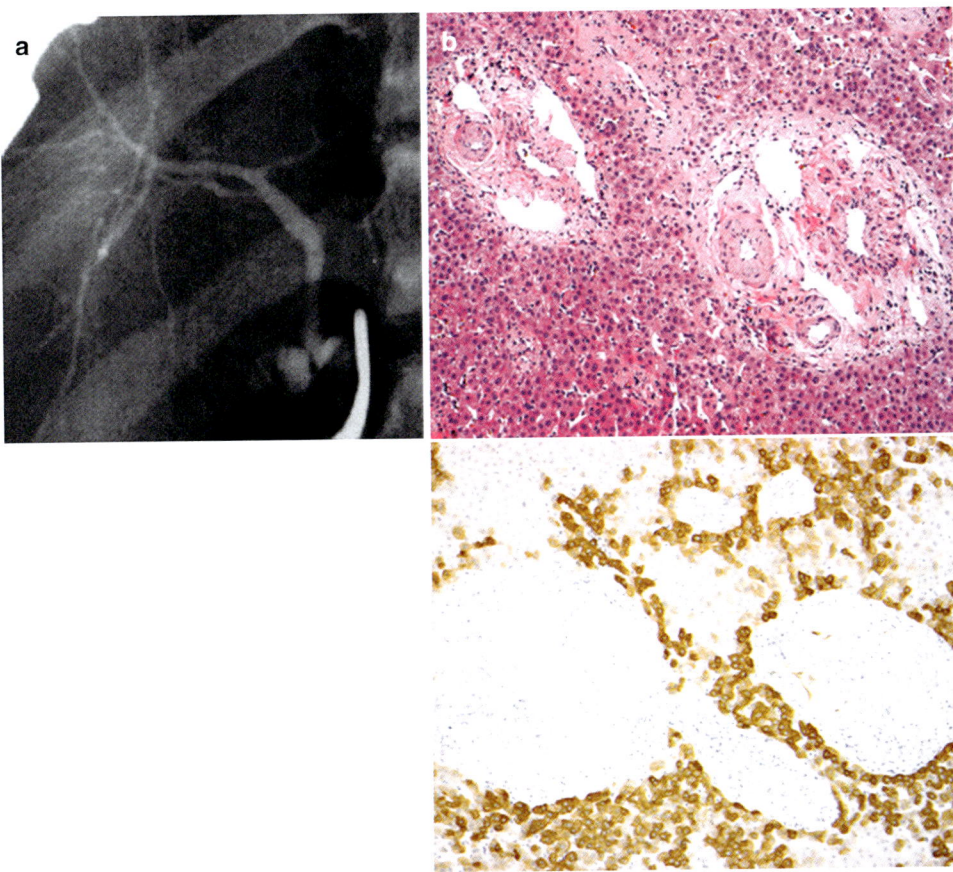

Fig. 28.17 Living donor for the recipient with Alagille syndrome. (**a**) Intraoperative cholangiogram showed scrimpy biliary trees. (**b**) Liver biopsy revealed unsuspected bile duct paucity

liver diseases indicated for LDLT [62]. If the patients with UCD are diagnosed by prenatal diagnosis, hepatocyte transplantation can be considered as a therapeutic option to bridge LDLT once their body weight reached 6.0 kg. The source of hepatocytes is derived from remnant liver tissue, which is voluntarily donated from unrelated living donors receiving in situ reduction procedure at the time of left lateral segmentectomy for their recipients [63]. Although OTCD is an X-linked inheritance, the use of asymptomatic heterozygous donors has been accepted with careful examinations in LDLT. However, few cases with OTCD, receiving grafts from their mothers, may experience severe hyperammonemia following LDLT, and therefore, an OTCD heterozygous carrier donor should be avoided if there is another donor candidate [38].

Organic acidemias, consisting of methylmalonic academia and propionic academia, are also indicated for LDLT. Although implanted liver grafts produce deficient enzymes, LDLT only partially corrects the biochemical defects. However, the benefits of an improved quality of life associated with the elimination of episodes of decompensation and improved protein tolerance must be weighed against the potential for renal and neurological injury [64].

Glycogen storage disease (GSD) 1b shows the added features of neutropenia and neutrophil dysfunction, which require the regular administration of recombinant human granulocyte colony stimulating factor (G-CSF). GSD1b recipients are susceptible to infection, especially catheter-related blood stream infection, and therefore, unnecessary catheter placement has to be avoided. Neutropenia may not be able to be cured by LDLT, and it thus remains an open question whether LT improves neutropenia in patients with GSD1b [65].

In the patients with primary hyperoxaluria type 1 (PH1), overproduction and urinary excretion of oxalate lead to urolithiasis, and nephrocalcinosis may consequently result in renal failure. Transplantation strategies for PH1 have been proposed based on concomitant renal insufficiency. If renal insufficiency becomes chronic kidney disease (CKD) stage 5 under dialysis at the time of LDLT, concomitant or sequential liver-kidney transplantation have to be considered. Preemptive LDLT for PH1 patient with mild renal insufficiency, below CKD stage 3, may be a reasonable therapeutic option to avoid further renal replacement therapy, including kidney transplantation [66].

28.3.1.3 Acute Liver Failure

All of the patients suspected of ALF are admitted to the pediatric intensive care unit, and multidisciplinary management is commenced. Consultation with a pediatrician who specialized in neurology, electroencephalogram, and brain computed tomography imaging findings is considered to evaluate the neurological impairment. Artificial liver support therapy in combination with continuous veno-venous hemodiafiltration (CVVHDF) and plasma exchange (PE) is initially performed for all patients under mechanical ventilation, while the precipitating cause of ALF is searched as much as possible; once the cause of ALF is determined, specific therapy is initiated [67]. If the liver function does not sufficiently recover despite conservative treatment, while preparing for LT, then the indications for LT are discussed based on the clinical course and liver pathology. LT is mainly considered when there is at least one of the following symptoms: exacerbation of hepatic encephalopathy by analysis of electroencephalogram and/or progression of liver atrophy on ultrasound (US) and/or prolonged international normalized ratio of prothrombin time (PT-INR) [68]. While the patients are put on the waiting list for DDLT, the living donor candidates are also evaluated in parallel. The rejection rate appears to be higher than the other liver diseases, and moreover the majority of them suffer from repeated episodes of rejection. The pathological findings of liver biopsies at the time of severe liver dysfunction commonly reveal centrilobular injuries, consisting of central venulitis, hemorrhage, and necrosis, which are considered as pathological features refractory to steroid bolus therapy [69]. Anti-thymocyte globulin can be effective to rejection presenting centrilobular injuries.

28.3.1.4 Congenital Hepatic Fibrosis/Caroli Disease

Congenital hepatic fibrosis (CHF) and Caroli disease are often associated with autosomal recessive polycystic kidney disease (ARPKD). The concomitant renal insufficiency may lead to a poor prognosis for the patients undergoing LDLT. Recent remarkable advances in LDLT have yielded survival for pediatric recipients. Therefore, LDLT should be performed before renal insufficiency becomes far advanced to avoid missing the proper timing [70]. Even though sequential KT has to be considered when there is progression of renal insufficiency after LDLT, the recovery of liver function provides advantages for the successful outcome of this procedure.

28.3.1.5 Liver Tumors

Hepatoblastoma (HBL) is the most common pediatric liver tumor indicated for LDLT. Therapeutic strategy for advanced HBL, classified into pretreatment extent of disease (PRETEXT) III and IV, consists of neoadjuvant chemotherapy and surgical interventions. Neoadjuvant chemotherapy (NAC) includes the Société Internationale d'Oncologie Pédiatrique-Epithelial Liver Tumor Study Group (SIOPEL), the Children's Oncology Group (COG), or the Japanese Study Group for Pediatric Liver Tumor (JPLT) guidelines. After 2–4 cycles of NAC, the possibility of surgical interventions including LDLT is assessed [71]. If lung metastases still exist, however, the number of metastases becomes countable after NAC, lung resection is performed, and then surgical intervention to primary liver tumors is scheduled 2 weeks later. LDLT is considered to be a better option than DDLT, because LDLT can be timely scheduled LT. A final judgment of surgical resectability is made during the operation by macroscopic findings and intraoperative US, and therefore, LDLT donors have been already prepared for a backup option of LDLT at the same time. Adjuvant chemotherapy depends on the patients' general conditions, especially liver and renal functions; however, there are no promising guidelines for adjuvant chemotherapy after LT. In contrast to the total hepatectomy for the other liver diseases, the procedures including limited mobilization of the native liver and inflow occlusion at the hepatic hilum are always introduced to prevent tumor spread during the operation. Furthermore, if portal vein thrombosis is not suspected, temporary portocaval shunt is made in the beginning of the operation to reduce intraoperative blood loss and maintain hemodynamic stability (Fig. 28.18) [72]. LDLT provides a valuable alternative treatment, given the appropriate timing for scheduled LT, with excellent results in children with HBL [73].

28.3.1.6 Retransplants

Retransplants using grafts from living donors (Re-LDLT) are challenging. At the time of re-LDLT, surgical procedures are always complicated, especially vascular reconstructions. The length of vasculatures, such as portal vein and hepatic artery, at the recipient side often becomes short, and therefore, interpositional vein graft is needed. DDLT may cope with the complexity of vascular reconstructions in re-LT because of the necessity of vascular grafts.

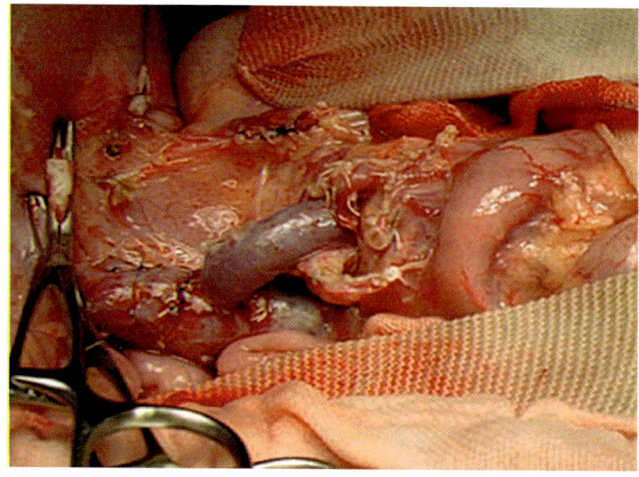

Fig. 28.18 Temporary portocaval shunt during total hepatectomy of hepatoblastoma

28.3.1.7 ABO-Incompatible Donors

Previous reports related to ABO-incompatible liver transplantation (ABO-I LT), including Kyoto University experience [74], showed that ABO-I LT was safely performed for pediatric cases, especially under 1 year. However, elderly patients might have considerable risk of antibody-mediated rejection (AMR) similarly as adult patients. Various preconditioning regimens for B-cell desensitization, including rituximab, have been applied for pediatric ABO-I living donor LT (LDLT), although the regimens appropriate to pediatric candidates still remain controversial. Preconditioning regimens for B-cell desensitization have been changed reflecting emerging trends. Until rituximab was indicated for ABO-I LDLT in the early 2000s, several sessions of plasmapheresis were performed to decrease anti-donor AB antibodies immediately before LDLT, and local infusion therapy through portal vein or hepatic artery, including steroids, was indicated for the elder children [75]. Recent standard preconditioning regimens for B-cell desensitization consist of rituximab administration 1 month before a scheduled LDLT, and mycophenolate mofetil is added to the conventional immunosuppressive regimens with calcineurin inhibitor and low-dose steroids. Additional splenectomy is controversial in the setting of pediatric ABO-I LDLT, and it is contraindicated for the recipients younger than 2 years.

28.3.2 Surgical Challenges in Recipient Operation in Living Donor Liver Transplantation

28.3.2.1 Standard Recipient Operation

The standard recipient operation for post-Kasai BA patient is demonstrated. After reverse T incision, left and right triangular ligament is dissected. Then the liver is mobilized from the right side until it reaches to the left lesser omental cavity. Roux-en-Y (RY) limb for Kasai operation is identified just above the duodenum. Hepatic arteries (HA) and portal veins (PV) are dissected as distally as possible. If preoperative US shows retrograde PV flow, one can cut PV completely because the patient has collaterals. And if the PV diameter is less than 4 mm and looks attenuated, it is better to use interpositional vein graft for reconstruction [76]. Otherwise, left PV is preserved to prevent intestinal congestion. Potential collaterals are devascularlized to get sufficient PV front flow. After a total hepatectomy, the top vena cava is freed from its diaphragmatic attachments, by dividing the phrenic veins, and is skeletonized to allow adequate spacing for the hepatic vein anastomosis. During anhepatic period, a portosystemic shunt is made between the right portal branch and the inferior vena cava (IVC) to prevent portal hypertension in the patients without collaterals. The orifice of the left, middle, and right hepatic veins are enlarged with a transverse incision, making a natural triangular orifice to obtain sufficient outflow. Anastomosis of the hepatic veins (HV) is accomplished in an end-to-end fashion with interrupted sutures for anterior wall and a continuous suture for posterior wall (*5-0 Prolene*). Portal vein reconstruction is made with interrupted sutures for anterior wall and a continuous suture for posterior wall (*6-0 PDS*) using native PV branch patch technique. Arterial reconstruction is carried out using *9-0 Prolene* with surgical microscope. Biliary reconstruction is carried out with RY hepaticojejunostomy with *four Fr* biliary stent tubes.

28.3.2.2 HA Reconstruction with Surgical Microscope

HA anastomosis might be one of the key factors for successful pediatric liver transplantation, and the use of operative microscope has dramatically reduced the incidence of HA thrombosis in pediatric segmental LT. Peripheral branch of native HA is used for HA reconstruction with *9-0 Prolene* interrupted suture. Because of the short stump of graft left HA and size discrepancy between native HA and graft left HA, nonanatomical HA reconstruction could be applied in some cases using gastroduodenal artery, right gastroepiploic artery, sigmoid artery interposition, mesentery artery of Roux-en-Y limb, and donor/recipient radial artery (Fig. 28.19). If gastroduodenal artery is dissected, elongation of PV would be easier.

Although several hepatic arteries may supply the segmental graft in LDLT, it is not necessary to reconstruct all of them as far as backflow of remnant looks sufficient.

28.3.2.3 How to Get Sufficient Portal Front Flow? Cruise Technique

It has been reported that the vascular complication rate in pediatric LDLT is higher than that of adult LDLT, because of the size discrepancy between the graft and native vasculature. Obtaining sufficient PV front flow may contribute to prevent PV complications in children. The collateral vessels, including left gastric vein, splenorenal shunts, and retroperitoneal shunts, must be carefully devascularized. Splenorenal shunt ligation from anterior approach would be effective to get sufficient front flow (Fig. 28.20) [77]. The measurement of PV pressure might be a feasible index of PV front flow; if PV pressure after the devascularization of collateral vessels shows more than 30 mmH$_2$O, PV front flow may be sufficient enough.

28.3.2.4 Interpositional Vein Graft for PV Reconstruction

If the native PV is sclerotic with insufficient front flow, especially small caliber of the native PV (less than 4 mm), PV anastomosis by using interpositional vein graft is

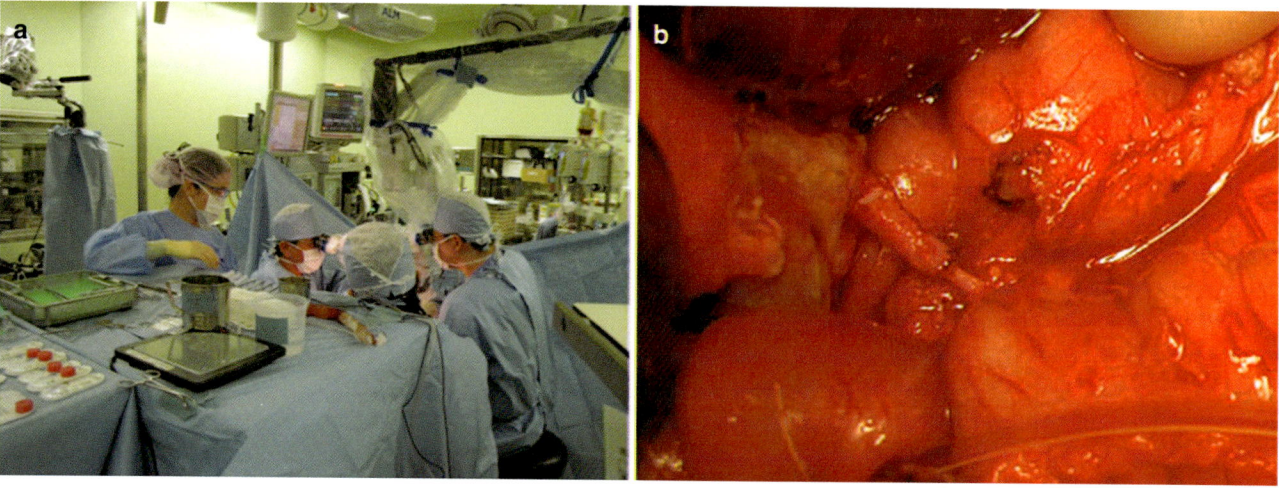

Fig. 28.19 Hepatic artery reconstruction. (**a**) Operative microscope. (**b**) Nonanatomical reconstruction with native right gastroepiploic artery and graft left hepatic artery

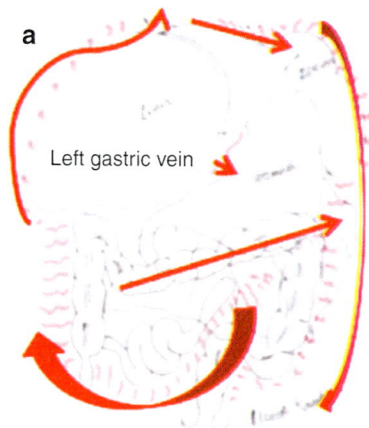
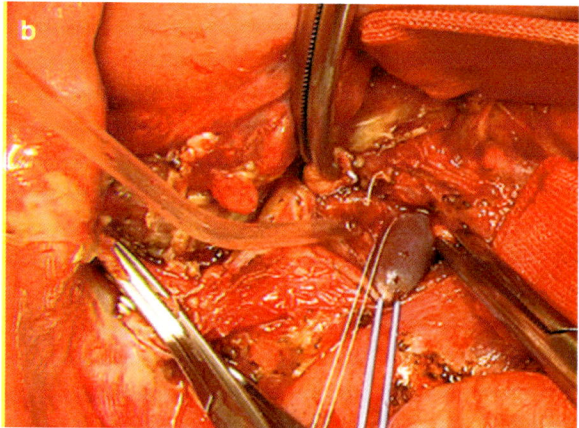

Fig. 28.20 The devascularization of collateral vessels. (**a**) Cruise technique. (**b**) Splenorenal shunt ligation with anterior approach. Left renal vein (blue sling) and splenorenal shunt (white sling)

indicated [76]. Donor ovarian vein or inferior mesenteric vein is usually used for interpositional vein graft. An interposition vein graft is first anastomosed to the confluence of the superior mesenteric vein and the splenic vein after cutting the narrowing and sclerotic native PV trunk (Fig. 28.21). Branch patch between the stump of left gastric vein and main PV trunk can be used for anastomosis. Perioperative anticoagulant therapy is not routinely performed. The use of the interposition vein graft appears to be a feasible option, with better graft survival and fewer PV complications than conventional methods.

28.3.2.5 Pediatric Living Donor Domino Transplantation from Maple Syrup Urinary Disease

Due to the organ shortage in liver transplantation, domino liver transplantation has been increasingly applied using the explanted liver from maple syrup urinary disease (MSUD) without compromising *second* recipient long-term survival [78]. Because the recipients of liver grafts from MSUD donors are not likely to develop protein intolerance, 60% of branched-chain ketoacid dehydrogenase activity occurs in the muscle. In the setting of living donor domino liver transplantation, livers obtained from patients with MSUD, who had undergone LDLT, inherently lack the retro-hepatic IVC and have multiple vessel and bile duct orifices. It is important to evaluate the transection site of the vessels based on the findings of *3D*-CT of the first donor and recipient before the operations. The first recipient's intraoperative findings are sent to second recipient operators to make sure cutting line of each vessel. Vascular plasty of the HVs is needed to be conducted on the back table (Fig. 28.22). The right HV, middle HV, left HV, and left superficial vein are sutured together to create one orifice. The unified graft HVs are anastomosed with the orifice of the united recipient HVs. PV, HA, and biliary reconstructions are performed in the standard manner as described above.

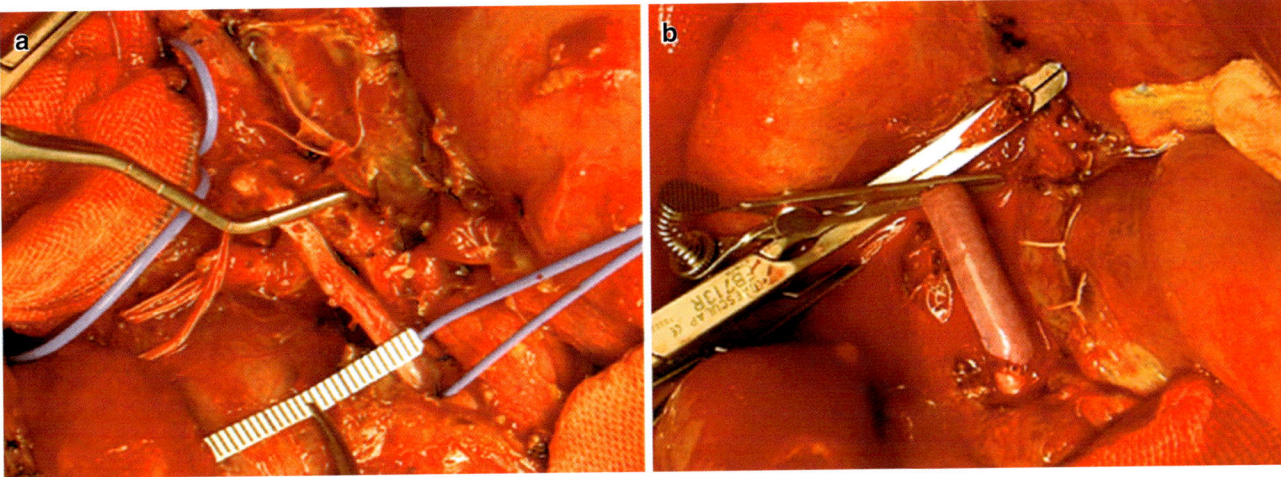

Fig. 28.21 Interpositional vein graft for portal vein reconstruction. (**a**) The native portal vein appears narrowing, and its diameter is smaller than 4 mm. (**b**) Vein graft with ovarian vein graft is obtained from the maternal donor

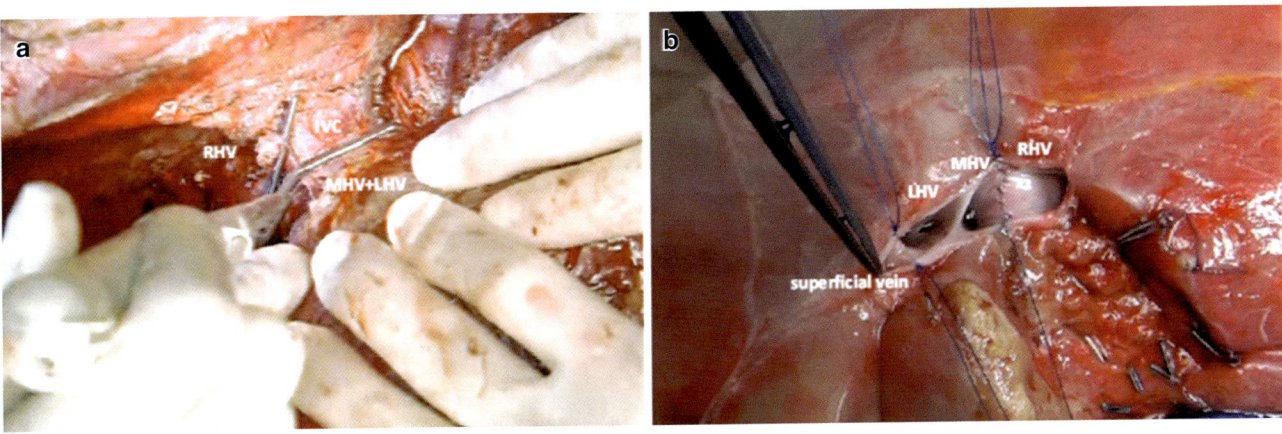

Fig. 28.22 Pediatric living donor domino transplantation. (**a**) The HVs were exteriorized as far as possible in the native liver parenchyma. (**b**) The RHV, MHV, LHV, and superficial vein were sutured together by venoplasty at the back table

28.3.3 The Outcomes of Living Donor Liver Transplantation

In a multicenter Organ Procurement and Transplant Network (OPTN) analysis, LDLT has been associated with improved outcomes particularly in the youngest recipients under the age of 2 years [79]. Unmatched overall living donor outcomes at 5 and 10 years are incrementally better as compared with deceased donor outcomes in the Scientific Registry of Transplant Recipient database between 1991 and 2013 [80]. A recent study from the Registry of the Japanese Liver Transplantation Society analyzed the results of the largest world cohort of 2224 LDLT pediatric recipients; the 1-year, 5-year, and 10-year patient survival rates were 88.3%, 85.4%, and 82.8%, respectively [81]. In that study, etiology of liver disease, recipient age, ABO incompatibility, and the transplant era were found to be significant predictors of overall survival. Patients with cholestatic liver disease showed a significantly better patient survival rate than those with metabolic disease, neoplastic disease, or acute liver failure (Fig. 28.23). Retransplantation with living donors, accounted for 3.3% of cases, showed a significant worse patient survival rate compared with the patients receiving single grafts (48.1% and 84.0% at 10 years, respectively). Liver graft size matching is one of the major factors determining a successful outcome in pediatric LDLT. Relative to the older pediatric recipients, infants had worse overall patient survival rates. The disadvantage of using large-for-size grafts in infants is that insufficient tissue oxygenation and graft compression are observed in association with a relatively high incidence of vascular complications that result in poor outcomes. Reduction procedures for adult left lateral segments (LLSs) have been developed to eliminate size mismatch in living donor LT for small children [82, 83]. Reduced LLS grafts have been changed reflecting emerging trends, from nonanatomically reduced LLS grafts to reduced-thickness LLS grafts. In our recent series accumulating 96 infants receiving

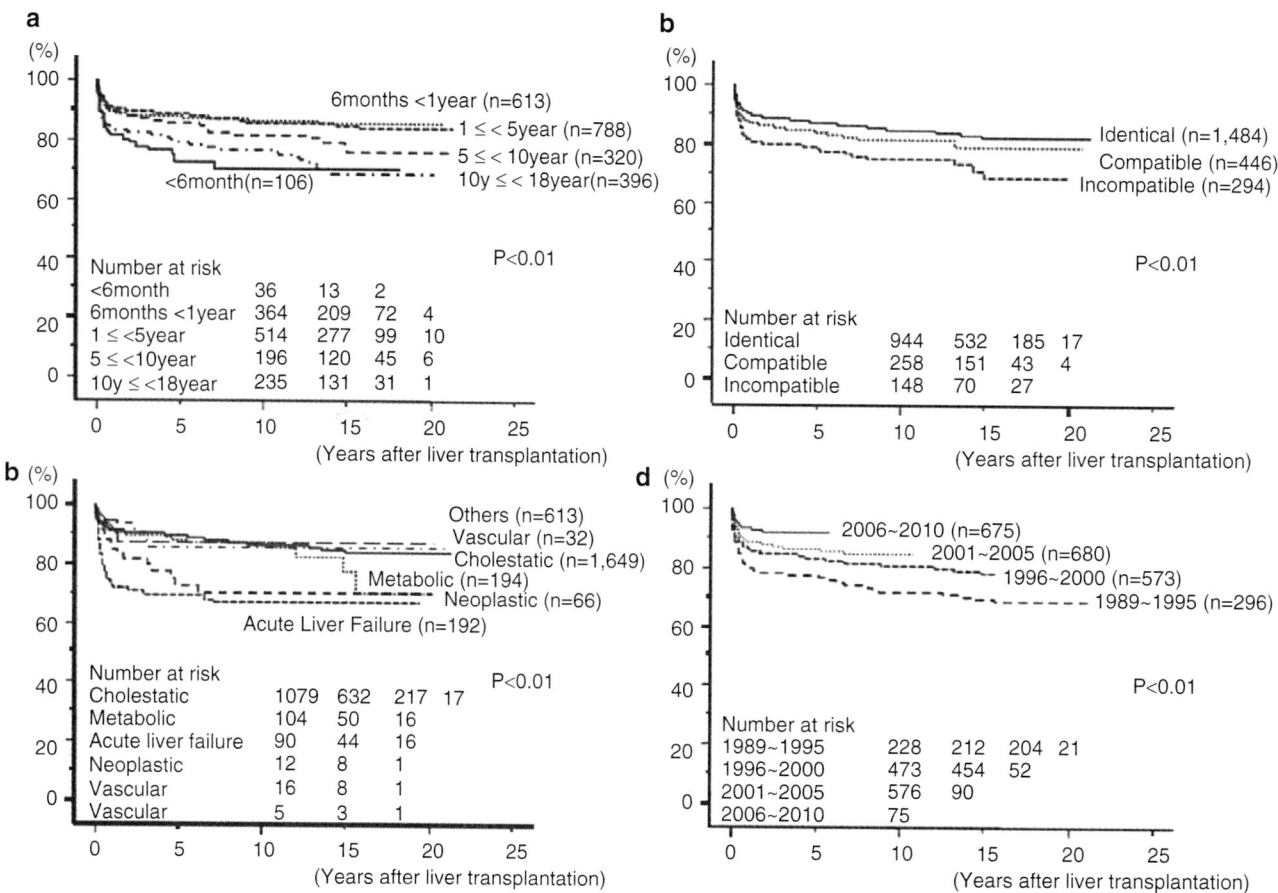

Fig. 28.23 Recipient survival in pediatric living donor liver transplantation from the Registry of the Japanese Liver Transplantation Society [81]. (**a**) Recipient age, (**b**) ABO compatibility, (**c**) original liver disease, (**d**) transplant era

Table 28.1 Surgical complications in living donor liver transplantation at National Center for Child Health and Development

Surgical complications		Number	Incidence
Portal vein	Thrombosis	4	0.9%
	Stricture	19	4.3%
Hepatic vein	Stricture	5	1.1%
Hepatic artery	Thrombosis	0	0.0%
Bile duct	Leakage	7	1.6%
	Stricture	25	5.7%
	Accidental ligation of B2	5	1.1%

reduced LLS grafts, reduced-thickness LLS grafts showed a significantly better patient survival rate compared with the patients receiving nonanatomically reduced LLS grafts (94.8% and 80.8% at 3 years, respectively, unpublished data). LDLT for smaller children is technically more challenging due to the smaller vascular structures and size discrepancies with the grafts. Various surgical innovations have overcome the technical issues in LDLT for smaller children, as described in the "surgical procedures" above. According to recent published studies, the incidence of hepatic artery, portal vein, and hepatic venous outflow complications were decreasing, below 3% [84], 10% [85], and 5% [86], respectively. Portal vein complications are reported as the most frequent vascular complications in pediatric LDLT. Biliary atresia, the most common disease indicated for pediatric LDLT, is often associated with PV hypoplasia, which is caused by rapidly progressing sclerosis and fibrosis, previous Kasai procedure, and repeated attacks of cholangitis that could lead to PV inflammation [85]. Although various techniques to enlarge the diameter of hypoplastic PV, including the use of interpositional vein graft, have been applied to PV reconstruction, obtaining sufficient PV front flow, which can be provided by careful devascularization of collateral vessels, may contribute to prevent PV complications.

In terms of vascular and biliary complications in our series of 440 LDLT cases until the end of 2016, there were PV complications in 23 cases (5.2%); 3 cases required stent placement for PV stricture, and 4 cases underwent reanastomosis of PV and HV complications in five cases (1.1%); 2 cases required stent placement for HV stricture, and 1 case underwent reanastomosis of HV and biliary complications in 32 cases (7.3%), including biliary leakage in 7 cases and biliary stricture in 25 cases. Fortunately, we have not yet encountered any HA thrombosis. All of the patients with biliary stricture were successfully treated by percutaneous biliary balloon dilatation; however, two cases of them finally received biliary reanastomosis after repeated episodes of restricture. Biliary duct of segment 2 (B2) was accidentally ligated during the donor operation, and biliary reconstruction of B2 had to be performed in five cases (Table 28.1).

References

1. Broelsch CE, Emond JC, Whichington PF, Thistlethwaite JR, Baker AL, Lichter JL. Application of reduced-sized liver transplants as split grafts, auxiliary orthotopic grafts, and living related segmental transplants. Ann Surg. 1990;212:368–77.
2. Raia S, Navy JR, Miles S. Liver transplantation from live donors. Lancet. 1989;8661:497.
3. Nagasue N, Kohno H, Matsuo S, et al. Segmental (partial) liver transplantation from a living donor. Transplant Proc. 1992;24:1958–9.
4. Tanaka K, Uemoto S, Tokunaga Y, et al. Surgical techniques and innovations in living related liver transplantation. Ann Surg. 1993;217:82–91.
5. Makuuchi M, Kawasaki S, Noguchi T, et al. Donor hepatectomy for living related partial liver transplantation. Surgery. 1993;113:395–402.
6. Egawa H, Tanabe K, Fukushima N, et al. Current status of organ transplantation in Japan. Am J Transplant. 2012;12:523–30.
7. Goyet JD, Hausleithner V, Reding R, et al. Impact of innovative techniques on the waiting list and result in pediatric liver transplantation. Transplantation. 1993;56:1130–6.
8. Kasahara M, Umeshita K, Inomata Y, et al. Long-term outcomes of pediatric living donor liver transplantation in Japan: an analysis of more than 2200 cases listed in the registry of the Japanese Liver Transplantation Society. Am J Transplant. 2013;13(7):1830–9.
9. Kiuchi T, Kasahara M, Uryuhara K, et al. Impact of graft-size mismatching on graft prognosis in liver transplantation from living donors. Transplantation. 1999;67:321–7.
10. Kasahara M, Fukuda A, Yokoyama S, et al. Living donor liver transplantation with hyper-reduced left lateral segments. J Pediatr Surg. 2008;43:1575–8.
11. Egawa H, Oike F, Buhler L, et al. Impact of recipient age on outcome of ABO-incompatible living-donor liver transplantation. Transplantation. 2004;77:403–11.
12. Egawa H, Teramukai S, Haga H, et al. Present status of ABO-incompatible living donor liver transplantation in Japan. Hepatology. 2008;47:143–52.
13. Farmer DG, Venick RS, McDiarmid SV, et al. Predictors of outcomes after pediatric liver transplantation: an analysis of more than 800 cases performed at single institution. J Am Coll Surg. 2007;204:904–16.
14. McDiarmid SV, Anand R, Martz K, et al. A multivariate analysis of pre-, peri-, and post-transplant factors affecting outcome after pediatric liver transplantation. Ann Surg. 2011;254:145–54.
15. Feng S, Si M, Taranto S, et al. Trends over a decade of pediatric liver transplantation in the United States. Liver Transpl. 2006;12:578–84.
16. Barr ML, Belghiti J, Villamil FG, Pomfret EA, Sutherland DS, Gruessner RW, Langnas AN, et al. A report of the Vancouver Forum on the care of the live organ donor: lung, liver, pancreas, and intestine data and medical guidelines. Transplantation. 2006;81:1373–85.
17. Sakamoto S, Nosaka S, Shigeta T, Uchida H, Hamano I, Karaki C, Kanazawa H, et al. Living donor liver transplantation using grafts with hepatic cysts. Liver Transpl. 2012;18:1415–20.
18. Yamamoto K, Takada Y, Fujimoto Y, Haga H, Oike F, Kobayashi N, Tanaka K. Nonalcoholic steatohepatitis in donors for living donor liver transplantation. Transplantation. 2007;83:257–62.
19. Iwasaki M, Takada Y, Hayashi M, Minamiguchi S, Haga H, Maetani Y, Fujii K, et al. Noninvasive evaluation of graft steatosis in living donor liver transplantation. Transplantation. 2004;78:1501–5.
20. Chu CJ, Hung TH, Hwang SJ, Wang YJ, Yang CF, Lin HC, Lee FY, et al. Association of insulin resistance with hepatic steatosis and progression of fibrosis in Chinese patients with chronic hepatitis C. Hepato-Gastroenterology. 2008;55:2157–61.
21. Yoshizumi T, Taketomi A, Soejima Y, Uchiyama H, Ikegami T, Harada N, Kayashima H, et al. Impact of donor age and recipient status on left-lobe graft for living donor adult liver transplantation. Transpl Int. 2008;21:81–8.
22. Akamatsu N, Kokudo N. Living Liver Donor Selection and Resection at the University of Tokyo Hospital. Transplant Proc. 2016;48:998–1002.
23. Kasahara M, Kiuchi T, Uryuhara K, Uemoto S, Fujimoto Y, Ogura Y, Oike F, et al. Role of HLA compatibility in pediatric living-related liver transplantation. Transplantation. 2002;74:1175–80.
24. Kamei H, Oike F, Fujimoto Y, Yamamoto H, Tanaka K, Kiuchi T. Fatal graft-versus-host disease after living donor liver transplantation: differential impact of donor-dominant one-way HLA matching. Liver Transpl. 2006;12:140–5.
25. Kiuchi T, Harada H, Matsukawa H, Kasahara M, Inomata Y, Uemoto S, Asonuma K, et al. One-way donor-recipient HLA-matching as a risk factor for graft-versus-host disease in living-related liver transplantation. Transpl Int. 1998;11(Suppl 1):S383–4.
26. Gugenheim J, Samuel D, Reynes M, Bismuth H. Liver transplantation across ABO blood group barriers. Lancet. 1990;336:519–23.
27. Farges O, Nocci Kalil A, Samuel D, Arulnaden JL, Bismuth A, Castaing D, Bismuth H. Long-term results of ABO-incompatible liver transplantation. Transplant Proc. 1995;27:1701–2.
28. Egawa H, Oike F, Buhler L, Shapiro AM, Minamiguchi S, Haga H, Uryuhara K, et al. Impact of recipient age on outcome of ABO-incompatible living-donor liver transplantation. Transplantation. 2004;77:403–11.
29. Uemoto S, Sugiyama K, Marusawa H, Inomata Y, Asonuma K, Egawa H, Kiuchi T, et al. Transmission of hepatitis B virus from hepatitis B core antibody-positive donors in living related liver transplants. Transplantation. 1998;65:494–9.
30. Kiuchi T, Inomata Y, Uemoto S, Satomura K, Egawa H, Okajima H, Yamaoka Y, et al. A hepatic graft tuberculosis transmitted from a living-related donor. Transplantation. 1997;63:905–7.
31. Huaman MA, Deepe GS Jr, Fichtenbaum CJ. Elevated Circulating Concentrations of Interferon-Gamma in Latent Tuberculosis Infection. Pathog Immun. 2016;1:291–303.
32. Kowada A. Cost effectiveness of interferon-gamma release assay for tuberculosis screening using three months of rifapentine and isoniazid among long-term expatriates from low to high incidence countries. Travel Med Infect Dis. 2016;14:489–98.
33. Kasahara M, Kiuchi T, Inomata Y, Uryuhara K, Sakamoto S, Ito T, Fujimoto Y, et al. Living-related liver transplantation for Alagille syndrome. Transplantation. 2003;75:2147–50.
34. Whitington PF, Alonso EM, Boyle JT, Molleston JP, Rosenthal P, Emond JC, Millis JM. Liver transplantation for the treatment of urea cycle disorders. J Inherit Metab Dis. 1998;21(Suppl 1):112–8.
35. Maestri NE, Brusilow SW, Clissold DB, Bassett SS. Long-term treatment of girls with ornithine transcarbamylase deficiency. N Engl J Med. 1996;335:855–9.
36. Nagasaka H, Yorifuji T, Egawa H, Kikuta H, Tanaka K, Kobayashi K. Successful living-donor liver transplantation from an asymptomatic carrier mother in ornithine transcarbamylase deficiency. J Pediatr. 2001;138:432–4.
37. Morioka D, Takada Y, Kasahara M, Ito T, Uryuhara K, Ogawa K, Egawa H, et al. Living donor liver transplantation for noncirrhotic inheritable metabolic liver diseases: impact of the use of heterozygous donors. Transplantation. 2005;80:623–8.

38. Rahayatri TH, Uchida H, Sasaki K, Shigeta T, Hirata Y, Kanazawa H, Mali V, et al. Hyperammonemia in ornithine transcarbamylase-deficient recipients following living donor liver transplantation from heterozygous carrier donors. Pediatr Transplant. 2017;21(1).
39. Te HS, Schiano TD, Das S, Kuan SF, DasGupta K, Conjeevaram HS, Baker AL. Donor liver uridine diphosphate (UDP)-glucuronosyltransferase-1A1 deficiency causing Gilbert's syndrome in liver transplant recipients. Transplantation. 2000;69:1882–6.
40. Lachaux A, Aboufadel A, Chambon M, Boillot O, Le Gall C, Gille D, Hermier M. Gilbert's syndrome: a possible cause of hyperbilirubinemia after orthotopic liver transplantation. Transplant Proc. 1996;28:2846.
41. Desai R, Collett D, Watson CJ, Johnson P, Evans T, Neuberger J. Estimated risk of cancer transmission from organ donor to graft recipient in a national transplantation registry. Br J Surg. 2014;101:768–74.
42. Feng S, Buell JF, Cherikh WS, Deng MC, Hanto DW, Kauffman HM, Leichtman AB, et al. Organ donors with positive viral serology or malignancy: risk of disease transmission by transplantation. Transplantation. 2002;74:1657–63.
43. Tanaka K, Uemoto S, Tokunaga Y, Fujita S, Sano K, Nishizawa T, Sawada H, et al. Surgical techniques and innovations in living related liver transplantation. Ann Surg. 1993;217:82–91.
44. Sakamoto S, Shigeta T, Hamano I, Fukuda A, Kakiuchi T, Matsuno N, Tanaka H, et al. Graft outflow venoplasty on reduced left lateral segments in living donor liver transplantation for small babies. Transplantation. 2011;91:e38–40.
45. Kasahara M, Kaihara S, Oike F, Ito T, Fujimoto Y, Ogura Y, Ogawa K, et al. Living-donor liver transplantation with monosegments. Transplantation. 2003;76:694–6.
46. Diamond IR, Fecteau A, Millis JM, Losanoff JE, Ng V, Anand R, Song C, et al. Impact of graft type on outcome in pediatric liver transplantation: a report From Studies of Pediatric Liver Transplantation (SPLIT). Ann Surg. 2007;246:301–10.
47. Srinivasan P, Vilca-Melendez H, Muiesan P, Prachalias A, Heaton ND, Rela M. Liver transplantation with monosegments. Surgery. 1999;126:10–2.
48. Kasahara M, Fukuda A, Yokoyama S, Sato S, Tanaka H, Kuroda T, Honna T. Living donor liver transplantation with hyperreduced left lateral segments. J Pediatr Surg. 2008;43:1575–8.
49. McDiarmid SV, Anand R, Martz K, Millis MJ, Mazariegos G. A multivariate analysis of pre-, peri-, and post-transplant factors affecting outcome after pediatric liver transplantation. Ann Surg. 2011;254:145–54.
50. Kiuchi T, Kasahara M, Uryuhara K, Inomata Y, Uemoto S, Asonuma K, Egawa H, et al. Impact of graft size mismatching on graft prognosis in liver transplantation from living donors. Transplantation. 1999;67:321–7.
51. McDiarmid SV. Management of the pediatric liver transplant patient. Liver Transpl. 2001;7:S77–86.
52. Enne M, Pacheco-Moreira L, Balbi E, Cerqueira A, Santalucia G, Martinho JM. Liver transplantation with monosegments. Technical aspects and outcome: a meta-analysis. Liver Transpl. 2005;11:564–9.
53. Kanazawa H, Sakamoto S, Fukuda A, Uchida H, Hamano I, Shigeta T, Kobayashi M, et al. Living-donor liver transplantation with hyperreduced left lateral segment grafts: a single-center experience. Transplantation. 2013;95:750–4.
54. Kasahara M, Sakamoto S, Shigeta T, Uchida H, Hamano I, Kanazawa H, Kobayashi M, et al. Reducing the thickness of left lateral segment grafts in neonatal living donor liver transplantation. Liver Transpl. 2013;19:226–8.
55. Sakamoto S, Kanazawa H, Shigeta T, Uchida H, Sasaki K, Hamano I, Fukuda A, et al. Technical considerations of living donor hepatectomy of segment 2 grafts for infants. Surgery. 2014;156:1232–7.
56. Busuttil RW, Goss JA. Split liver transplantation. Ann Surg. 1999;229:313–21.
57. Kasahara M, de Ville de Goyet J. Reducing left liver lobe grafts, more or less? Don't throw out the baby with the bath water. Pediatr Transplant. 2015;19:815–7.
58. Garbanzo JP, Kasahara M, Egawa H, Ikeda T, Doi H, Sakamoto S, Morioka D, Castro E, Takada Y, Tanaka K. Results of living donor liver transplantation in five children with congenital cardiac malformations requiring cardiac surgery. Pediatr Transplant. 2006;10:923–7.
59. Egawa H, Kasahara M, Inomata Y, Uemoto S, Asonuma K, Fujita S, Kiuchi T, Hayashi M, Yonemura T, Yoshibayashi M, Adachi Y, Shapiro JA, Tanaka K. Long-term outcome of living related liver transplantation for patients with intrapulmonary shunting and strategy for complications. Transplantation. 1999;67:712–7.
60. Kasahara M, Kiuchi T, Inomata Y, Uryuhara K, Sakamoto S, Ito T, Fujimoto Y, Ogura Y, Oike F, Tanaka K. Living-related liver transplantation for Alagille syndrome. Transplantation. 2003;75:2147–50.
61. Miyagawa-Hayashino A, Egawa H, Yorifuji T, Hasegawa M, Haga H, Tsuruyama T, Wen MC, Sumazaki R, Manabe T, Uemoto S. Allograft steatohepatitis in progressive familial intrahepatic cholestasis type 1 after living donor liver transplantation. Liver Transpl. 2009;15:610–8.
62. Kasahara M, Sakamoto S, Horikawa R, Koji U, Mizuta K, Shinkai M, Takahito Y, Taguchi T, Inomata Y, Uemoto S, Tatsuo K, Kato S. Living donor liver transplantation for pediatric patients with metabolic disorders: the Japanese multicenter registry. Pediatr Transplant. 2014;18:6–15.
63. Enosawa S, Horikawa R, Yamamoto A, Sakamoto S, Shigeta T, Nosaka S, Fujimoto J, Nakazawa A, Tanoue A, Nakamura K, Umezawa A, Matsubara Y, Matsui A, Kasahara M. Hepatocyte transplantation using a living donor reduced graft in a baby with ornithine transcarbamylase deficiency: a novel source of hepatocytes. Liver Transpl. 2014;20:391–3.
64. Kasahara M, Sakamoto S, Kanazawa H, Karaki C, Kakiuchi T, Shigeta T, Fukuda A, Kosaki R, Nakazawa A, Ishige M, Nagao M, Shigematsu Y, Yorifuji T, Naiki Y, Horikawa R. Living-donor liver transplantation for propionic acidemia. Pediatr Transplant. 2012;16:230–4.
65. Kasahara M, Horikawa R, Sakamoto S, Shigeta T, Tanaka H, Fukuda A, Abe K, Yoshii K, Naiki Y, Kosaki R, Nakagawa A. Living donor liver transplantation for glycogen storage disease type Ib. Liver Transpl. 2009;15:1867–71.
66. Sasaki K, Sakamoto S, Uchida H, Shigeta T, Matsunami M, Kanazawa H, Fukuda A, Nakazawa A, Sato M, Ito S, Horikawa R, Yokoi T, Azuma N, Kasahara M. Two-step transplantation for primary hyperoxaluria: a winning strategy to prevent progression of systemic oxalosis in early onset renal insufficiency cases. Pediatr Transplant. 2015;19:E1–6.
67. Ide K, Muguruma T, Shinohara M, Toida C, Enomoto Y, Matsumoto S, Aoki K, Fukuda A, Sakamoto S, Kasahara M. Continuous venovenous hemodiafiltration and plasma exchange in infantile acute liver failure. Pediatr Crit Care Med. 2015;16:e268–74.
68. Uchida H, Sakamoto S, Fukuda A, Sasaki K, Shigeta T, Nosaka S, Kubota M, Nakazawa A, Nakagawa S, Kasahara M. Sequential analysis of variable markers for predicting outcomes in pediatric patients with acute liver failure. Hepatol Res. 2017;47(12):1241–51.
69. Sakamoto S, Haga H, Egawa H, Kasahara M, Ogawa K, Takada Y, Uemoto S. Living donor liver transplantation for acute liver failure in infants: the impact of unknown etiology. Pediatr Transplant. 2008;12:167–73.
70. Sakamoto S, Kasahara M, Fukuda A, Tanaka H, Kakiuchi T, Karaki C, Kanazawa H, Kamei K, Ito S, Nakazawa A. Pediatric liver-kidney transplantation for hepatorenal fibrocystic disease from a living donor. Pediatr Transplant. 2012;16:99–102.

71. Sakamoto S, Kasahara M, Mizuta K, Kuroda T, Yagi T, Taguchi T, Inomata Y, Umeshita K, Uemoto S. Japanese Liver Transplantation Society. Nationwide survey of the outcomes of living donor liver transplantation for hepatoblastoma in Japan. Liver Transpl. 2014;20:333–46.
72. Uchida H, Fukuda A, Sasaki K, Hirata Y, Shigeta T, Kanazawa H, Nakazawa A, Miyazaki O, Nosaka S, Mali VP, Sakamoto S, Kasahara M. Benefit of early inflow exclusion during living donor liver transplantation for unresectable hepatoblastoma. J Pediatr Surg. 2016;51:1807–11.
73. Kasahara M, Ueda M, Haga H, Hiramatsu H, Kobayashi M, Adachi S, Sakamoto S, Oike F, Egawa H, Takada Y, Tanaka K. Living-donor liver transplantation for hepatoblastoma. Am J Transplant. 2005;5:2229–35.
74. Egawa H, Oike F, Buhler L, Shapiro AM, Minamiguchi S, Haga H, Uryuhara K, Kiuchi T, Kaihara S, Tanaka K. Impact of recipient age on outcome of ABO-incompatible living-donor liver transplantation. Transplantation. 2004;77:403–11.
75. Egawa H, Teramukai S, Haga H, Tanabe M, Fukushima M, Shimazu M. Present status of ABO-incompatible living donor liver transplantation in Japan. Hepatology. 2008;47:143–52.
76. Kanazawa H, Sakamoto S, Fukuda A, Shigeta T, Loh DL, Kakiuchi T, Karaki C, Miyazaki O, Nosaka S, Nakazawa A, Kasahara M. Portal vein reconstruction in pediatric living donor liver transplantation for patients younger than 1 year with biliary atresia. J Pediatr Surg. 2012;47:523–7.
77. Uchida H, Fukuda A, Masatoshi M, Sasaki K, Shigeta T, Kanazawa H, Nakazawa A, Miyazaki O, Nosaka S, Sakamoto S, Kasahara M. A central approach to splenorenal shunt in pediatric living donor liver transplantation. Pediatr Transplant. 2015;19:E142–5.
78. Matsunami M, Ishiguro A, Fukuda A, Sasaki K, Uchida H, Shigeta T, Kanazawa H, Sakamoto S, Ohta M, Nakadate H, Horikawa R, Nakazawa A, Ishige M, Mizuta K, Kasahara M. Successful living domino liver transplantation in a child with protein C deficiency. Pediatr Transplant. 2015;19:E70–4.
79. Roberts JP, Hulbert-Shearon TE, Merion RM, Wolfe RA, Port FK. Influence of graft type on outcomes after pediatric liver transplantation. Am J Transplant. 2004;4:373–7.
80. Kim WR, Lake JR, Smith JM, Skeans MA, Schladt DP, Edwards EB, Harper AM, Wainright JL, Snyder JJ, Israni AK, Kasiske BL. OPTN/SRTR 2013 Annual Data Report: liver. Am J Transplant. 2015;15(Suppl 2):1–28.
81. Kasahara M, Umeshita K, Inomata Y, Uemoto S, Japanese Liver Transplantation Society. Long-term outcomes of pediatric living donor liver transplantation in Japan: an analysis of more than 2200 cases listed in the registry of the Japanese Liver Transplantation Society. Am J Transplant. 2013;13:1830–9.
82. Sakamoto S, Kanazawa H, Shigeta T, Uchida H, Sasaki K, Hamano I, Fukuda A, Nosaka S, Egawa H, Kasahara M. Technical considerations of living donor hepatectomy of segment 2 grafts for infants. Surgery. 2014;156:1232–7.
83. Kasahara M, Sakamoto S, Sasaki K, Uchida H, Kitajima T, Shigeta T, Narumoto S, Hirata Y, Fukuda A. Living donor liver transplantation during the first 3 months of life. Liver Transpl. 2017;23:1051–7.
84. Seda-Neto J, Antunes da Fonseca E, Pugliese R, Candido HL, Benavides MR, Carballo Afonso R, Neiva R, Porta G, Miura IK, Teng HW, Iwase FC, Rodrigues ML, Carneiro de Albuquerque LA, Kondo M, Chapchap P. Twenty years of experience in pediatric living donor liver transplantation: focus on hepatic artery reconstruction, complications, and outcomes. Transplantation. 2016;100:1066–72.
85. Gurevich M, Guy-Viterbo V, Janssen M, Stephenne X, Smets F, Sokal E, Lefebvre C, Balligand JL, Pirotte T, Veyckemans F, Clapuyt P, Menten R, Dumitriu D, Danse E, Annet L, Clety SC, Detaille T, Latinne D, Sempoux C, Laterre PF, de Magnée C, Lerut J, Reding R. Living donor liver transplantation in children: surgical and immunological results in 250 recipients at Université Catholique de Louvain. Ann Surg. 2015;262:1141–9.
86. Sakamoto S, Egawa H, Kanazawa H, Shibata T, Miyagawa-Hayashino A, Haga H, Ogura Y, Kasahara M, Tanaka K, Uemoto S. Hepatic venous outflow obstruction in pediatric living donor liver transplantation using left-sided lobe grafts: Kyoto University experience. Liver Transpl. 2010;16:1207–14.

29. Listing for Transplantation; Postoperative Management and Long-Term Follow-Up

Nathalie Marie Rock and Valérie Anne McLin

Key Points

- Standardization of protocols in each center adapted to local resources is the foundation of successful management of pretransplant, transplant, and posttransplant period.
- The aims of the pretransplantation evaluation are (1) evaluation of the indication, (2) recognition of any contraindications, (3) social and psychological evaluation, and (4) early family education. A system-based approach is recommended.
- The most common early and late complications following pediatric liver transplantation are infection and rejection.
- The long-term outcome of the patients after liver transplantation is affected by kidney disease, hypertension, cardiovascular risk, metabolic syndrome, and secondary malignancies.
- Long-term complications can be subclinical. A regular and standardized follow-up of pediatric liver transplant recipients allows for preventative or early care.

Research Needed in the Field

- **In the pretransplant assessment**: establish the indications for CNS imaging, the role of frailty tool, and the role of psychological assessment in the prevention of psychosocial complications posttransplant.
- **In the early postoperative management**: establish the indications and timing of viral prophylaxis; study how to prevent vascular thrombosis as far as monitoring of coagulation and use of medications.
- **Long-term follow-up**: establish the role of protocol biopsies, the use of attenuated vaccines, and the management of renal impairment and high blood pressure.

Abbreviations

AIH	Autoimmune hepatitis
AILD	Autoimmune liver disease
BA	Biliary atresia
CNI	Calcineurin inhibitor
DSA	Donor-specific antibodies
FFP	Fresh frozen plasma
HB	Hepatoblastoma
HCC	Hepatocarcinoma
HPS	Hepatopulmonary syndrome
IS	Immunosuppressive drugs
LT	Liver transplantation
PH	Portal hypertension
POPH	Portopulmonary hypertension
PPI	Proton-pump inhibitor
UCDA	Ursodeoxycholic acid

29.1 Listing for Transplantation

29.1.1 Introduction

The first step to listing a patient for transplantation is to perform a pretransplant evaluation, *the aims of which are to evaluate the risk and benefits of transplantation, identify*

N. M. Rock (✉) · V. A. McLin (✉)
Pediatric Gastroenterology, Hepatology and Nutrition Unit, Department of Pediatrics, Swiss Pediatric Liver Center, University Hospitals of Geneva, Geneva, Switzerland
e-mail: Nathalie.Rock@hcuge.ch; Valerie.McLin@hcuge.ch

contraindications to transplant, and anticipate postoperative care based on individual patient needs. Other goals of the pretransplant evaluation include assessment of the current medical condition, early patient and family education, and social and psychological assessment. It is also an opportunity to reassess initial diagnosis when appropriate and to discuss living-related donor transplantation. A holistic approach using a thorough head-to-toe approach is essential to mitigate risk and optimize outcomes. Indications for LT, morbidity, and mortality are explained in previous chapters.

A multidisciplinary review board formalizes the listing for transplantation. The patient is placed on a waiting list according to highly regulated, country-specific allocation rules and regulations. In case of acute liver failure, the pretransplant evaluation is often time sensitive but must nonetheless be performed focusing specifically on any signs pointing to an underlying cause and to extrahepatic disease that may compromise patient outcome following LT.

29.1.2 Timing of Referral

The patient should be referred to a transplant center of reference for evaluation when the child begins to present signs of decompensation of chronic liver disease or when it is clear that liver transplantation may be a therapeutic option. In addition, early referral affords the opportunity for the development of a strong working relationship between caregivers and family. Finally, timing of referral will differ according to countries depending on their respective resources and allocation policies.

Timing of referral differs according to underlying diagnosis. For patients with biliary atresia, referral to a transplant center should be initiated in the face of persistent cholestasis, progressive portal hypertension, nutritional impairment, or life-threatening cholangitis. In patients with cirrhosis, evidence of portal hypertension and some of its complications are an indication for referral. Patients with acute liver failure should be stabilized at the referring hospital and transferred shortly thereafter. In case of liver-based inborn errors of metabolism, patients are referred either when conventional therapy fails or when extrahepatic complications are progressive and may be stabilized or partially corrected by liver replacement. Rarely, an acute metabolic crisis may be an indication for urgent LT [1].

LT is the treatment of choice for unresectable hepatoblastoma (HB) after three courses of chemotherapy (SIOPEL protocol). Early referral by the oncology team is essential to assess resectability prior to chemotherapy (PRETEXT stage) (http://www.siopel.org). Both multifocal HB and HB in which R0 resection is uncertain should benefit from total hepatectomy and LT. Metastatic HB is not a contraindication to LT [2]. Hepatocellular carcinoma (HCC) is rarer in children. When HCC is present, it is often an incidental finding within a cirrhotic liver or, more frequently, suspected in patients with tyrosinemia type I. Either way, prompt referral for transplant affords pediatric recipients an excellent prognosis [3].

29.1.3 Pretransplant Evaluation

The pretransplant evaluation is an important step to ensure favorable outcomes. It is sometimes the first contact between the family and transplant center. It is often practical to conduct the head-to-toe, multidisciplinary assessment during a short, elective hospitalization. Table 29.1 summarizes suggested medical, surgical, and social components of a standard pretransplant evaluation. Although the pretransplant evaluation should be rigorously standardized so as to leave no stone unturned, it should of course be individualized to each patient with the aim to anticipate preoperative, intraoperative, and postoperative course and complications. The pretransplant evaluation is the opportunity to reassess the patient's underlying diagnosis if need be, keeping in mind that there may be therapeutic alternatives to transplantation. Importantly, this is also the time for the transplant team to anticipate extrahepatic disease-specific requirements after transplantation, in those cases in which LT is not entirely curative. Indications for pediatric LT are evolving; as clinicians are confronted with novel indications, an anticipatory, systemic approach will help ensure that disease-specific needs are met either pre- or post-LT.

A significant part of the pretransplant evaluation is centered around psychosocial and financial assessment. Psychologists will take time to evaluate the family and the patient to assess if psychological support will be necessary either before or following liver transplantation. A non-exhaustive list of some of the issues to consider is outlined below:

- Who will be the primary caregiver after liver transplant? Who will be the backup of the primary caregiver?
- What are family needs and plans regarding daycare/kindergarten/school after LT?
- Do parents have financial resources to cover the hidden costs of transplantation (accommodation, food, travel)?
- Is insurance coverage adequate? Are there any restrictions or caps?
- Family organization at time of transplant: who will take care of the siblings? Does the family have support?
- Accommodation before and at time of transplantation.
- Parent employment: are parents at risk of losing their job in case of a prolonged absence?

In addition to medical and psychosocial assessment, the pre-LT evaluation is an opportunity for the main caregivers (surgery, hepatology, anesthesia, specialized nurse, transplant coordinator) to take time to "sit, listen, and talk" with the family and child if age-appropriate. Giving them the opportunity to hear the practical and technical details of transplant, the expected short-term and long-term outcomes, and the pos-

Table 29.1 Pretransplant assessment by system [88–98]

	Exam	Purpose
Medical		
Hepatology	Esogastroduodenoscopy Liver panel test Liver biopsy, genetic exam, metabolic workup Diagnostic workup	Varices and hypertensive gastritis in case of portal hypertension Systematic screening is not recommended Pretransplant liver status Any abnormalities if the diagnosis is uncertain
Gastroenterology	Colonoscopy	In case of unexplained blood loss. IBD in case of AILD
Infectiology	CMV, EBV	CMV and EBV status before transplantation
	HIV, toxoplasmosis HAV, HBV, HEV, HCV, HSV, VZV, HHV6 Parvovirus B19, measles, rubeola, mumps Multidrug-resistant bacteria, parasitology in stool TB spot or tuberculin purified protein derivative	Any other active infection or colonization
	Sputum culture in CF patient	Bacterial carrier status before LT
Immunology	IgG, IgM, IgA Vaccinology dosage	Seroprotection Delay of vaccination (see Table 29.2)
Nutrition	Weight, height, BMI, growth curves Nutrition scores and status (mid-arm circumference and tricipital skinfold) Vitamins dosage	Nutritional status; risk of sarcopenia *Weight alone is an insufficient measure owing to ascites*
Endocrinology	Bone age Blood sugar, Hb1Ac AM cortisol level, IGF1, IGF-BP3, TSH, T3, T4	Pretransplant endocrine comorbidities/abnormalities
Cardiology	EKG 12lead Echocardiogram with saline contrast injection	Pretransplant ventricular dysfunction (cardiomyopathy in BA); underlying heart disease (BA, Alagille); HPS and POPH
Pneumology	Thorax X-ray Pulse oximetry in upright position	HPS, isomerism, hydrothorax
	Pulmonary scintigraphy	HPS
	Pulmonary functions tests	Pulmonary function of cystic fibrosis patient
Neurology	Cerebral MRI Electroencephalogram (EEG) NH4 Neurocognitive exam and/or developmental exam	Signs if chronic hepatic encephalopathy (globus pallidus, T1 on MRI) Acute hepatic encephalopathy Complications from chronic liver disease
Hematology	CBC, complete coagulation tests	Pretransplant correctible abnormalities
Oncology	CT scan, PET scanner, alpha-fetoprotein	Pretext staging
Nephrology	Urea, creatinine, cystatin-C GFR (Schwartz formula, EDTA clearance, inulin clearance) Electrolytes (N, K, Alb, Prot, Ca, PO$_4$) Urinary cells and electrolytes Renal ultrasonography	Preexisting renal dysfunction and hepatorenal syndrome, ciliopathy
	Vit D, PTH Bone mineral density	Hepatic osteodystrophy
Allergology	IgE total; IgE specific if necessary Prick tests if pertinent history	Pretransplant allergic disease
Dermatology	Clinical exam	Premalignant lesions, previous scars
Ophthalmology	Eye examination including fundoscopy	Pretransplant eye condition including papilledema, embryotoxon, or other condition. Assessment of intraocular hypertension prior to steroid treatment
Dental	Dental exam	Caries or treatable conditions
Overall general condition	Frailty tool	Measure of physiologic decline, risk management
Surgical assessment		
	Liver ultrasonography and Doppler Abdominal angio-CT	Vascular anatomy, biliary anatomy, any intra-abdominal abnormalities
	Doppler assessment of jugular veins	Vascular anatomy and patency for CVC placement
	Anesthesiologist consultation	Pretransplant discussion
Social assessment		
	Social and financial assessment (fundraising) Psychological evaluation of patient and family Education of patient and family School and community resource assessment Meeting with transplantation coordination team	

BA biliary atresia, *PH* portal hypertension, *HPS* hepatopulmonary syndrome, *POPH* portopulmonary hypertension, *AILD* autoimmune liver disease

sible complications including the risk of death is crucial. When appropriate, the help of a translator affords families the opportunity to use their native language. The collaborative nature of pre- and post-LT care between family and caregivers is emphasized. Typically, this is an appropriate time to obtain consent and to outline practical details prior to transplant: frequency of pretransplant follow-up visits, contact persons to call in case of illness/need, when to call, and collaboration with local pediatricians and specialists.

During the pre-LT evaluation, the patient and family will meet with transplant coordinators to go over the logistics of the day of transplant including transportation or special dietary needs at the time transfer. This is also a good time to show patients the operating room, the intensive care unit, and the emergency department, if they are not familiar with the premises. The use of additional learning materials is encouraged to help families make sense of the huge body of information. For example, several hospitals have family-oriented websites. Storybooks and dolls are available to help children comprehend basic principles of their health condition.

29.1.4 Patient Listing

After the patient and the families have undergone pretransplant evaluation, the patient is customarily presented to the "institutional review board," the institutional body habilitated to place a patient on the national/regional waiting list. Generally, patients are presented in a systematic protocoled fashion. A suggested minimal summary is outlined in Table 29.2. Families are informed of the final decision according to local customs (phone call or letter from physician, coordinator, specialized nurse).

29.1.5 Pretransplant Follow-Up

The goal of management during the wait period is to bring the patient to transplant in the most stable condition and to mitigate known risk factors for complications. Frequency of follow-up visits will depend on age, diagnosis, and severity of liver disease or of any complications warranting management prior to LT. MELD/PELD renewal is generally managed by the coordinators according to score. Figure 29.1 summarizes the main aims of pre-LT follow-up, and Table 29.3 summarizes the management of complications of chronic liver disease. Much of pre-LT care focuses on nutritional management, especially in the small, cholestatic infants (recommendations are outlined elsewhere) [4]. For patients with liver-based inborn errors of metabolism, close collaboration with metabolicians for nutrition is essential. Careful cardiopulmonary follow-up is important because of the risk of developing hepatopulmonary syndrome and portopulmonary hypertension in older children.

The diagnosis and care of encephalopathy is of importance to optimize long-term outcomes. Chronic encephalopathy is insidious in children and may only transpire as school difficulties ascribed to school absenteeism secondary to medical visits. It may also manifest as fatigue which should prompt workup for other causes including anemia, infectious disease, and vitamin deficiencies [4]. Special attention to neurocognitive development is paramount to offer appropriate guidance and avoid long-term deficits [5].

29.1.6 Transplant Day

The coordinator informs the medical and surgical teams when an offer is accepted and organizes patient transport. A multidisciplinary team welcomes the patient and family in an orchestrated fashion that is outlined in the individualized preoperative protocol. For patients with inborn errors of metabolism, this is a critical window in which the risks of fasting have to be mitigated with appropriate IV nutrition and tight monitoring.

29.1.7 Living Donor Transplantation

In certain conditions, LDLT may be the only life-saving solution for the child. Although living donor liver transplantation (LDLT) is explained in detail in a previous chapter, a few points are worth mentioning in the setting of pretransplant assessment.

The living donor may or may not be related to the recipient. It is important to consider that in recessive, inherited conditions, a parental donor is an obligate heterozygote. Depending on the underlying gene defect, this may or may not impact the risk for the donor or the recipient. Inborn errors of carbohydrate or amino-acid metabolism may have no histological repercussions in the donor, while bile acid transporter defects may harbor significant histological changes. Although the data are sparse, structural and architectural changes associated with such inherited conditions may theoretically increase the risks

Table 29.2 Patient presentation at review board

Patient characteristics	Age, weight, height Diagnosis Brief history of the patient
Pretransplant evaluation	Anatomic evaluation and surgical assessment (including vessel measurement) Medical assessment of comorbidities Last laboratory values MELD/PELD
Type of graft	Living related donor or deceased donor Split or whole organ Recipient CMV/EBV status
Disease-specific requirements	Pretransplant management of metabolic disease

Fig. 29.1 Follow-up of patient on waiting list (Modified from [4])

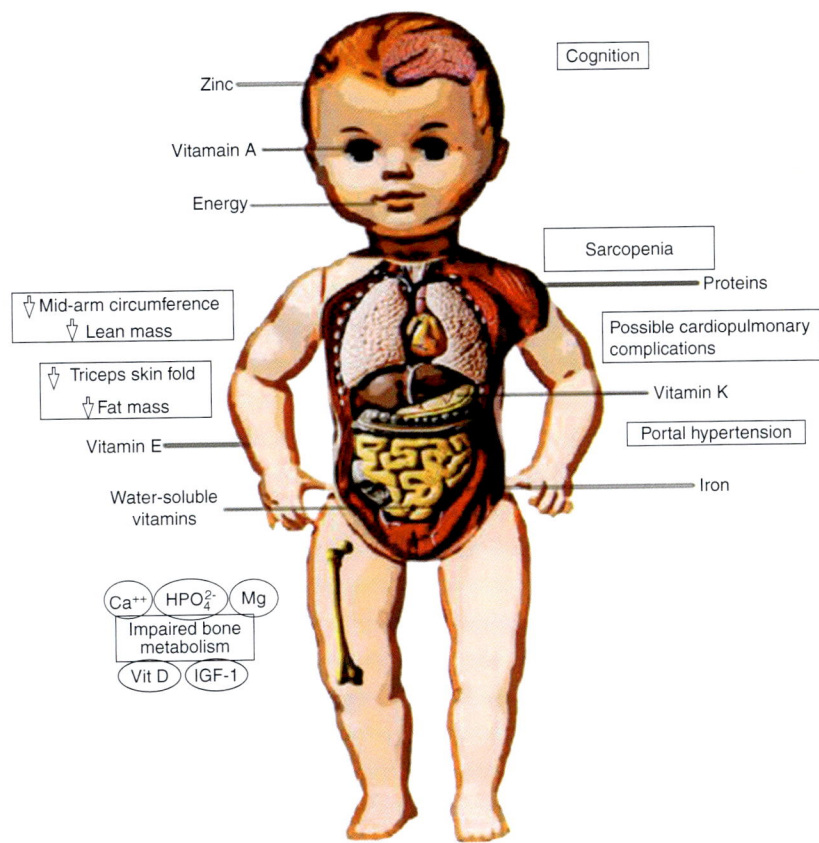

Table 29.3 Pretransplant medical follow-up and management while on transplant list

	Complication	Management
Medical		

Gastroenterology/hepatology	Portal hypertension
	– Ascites
	– Varices
	Cholestasis
	   Pruritus
	   Cholangitis
		Low sodium diet, spironolactone, IV albumin
		Variceal ligation in cases of bleeding, discuss propranolol
		Rifampicin
		Extended treatment with broad-range antibodies

Infectious disease	Infectious disease susceptibility due to chronic disease and impaired reticuloendothelial system	Treat according to the cause Discuss temporary inactivation on the list
Immunology	Vaccination delay	Accelerated vaccine schedule for patients likely to require early LT Catch-up of immunization according to the antibody titer according to the accelerated protocol Live virus vaccine with temporary inactivation on the list (4 weeks), including varicella vaccination Yearly influenza immunization Family immunization status up to date
Nutrition	Vitamin deficiency Energy deficit and growth failure	ADEK supplementation, parenteral supplementation if bilirubinemia >60 µM/L trace element and soluble vitamins Fortified milk with medium chain triglycerides Nasogastric tube feeding or parenteral nutrition
Cardiology, pneumology	HPS, POPH	Diuretics, specific cardiologic follow-up and treatment, O2 therapy as required
Neurology—psychology	Neurocognitive and neurodevelopment delay	Early intervention with physical therapy, occupational therapy, and nutritional management
Nephrology	Renal failure—hepatorenal syndrome Glomerular hyperfiltration Abnormal bone metabolism and hepatic osteodystrophy	Discuss renal replacement therapy Close follow-up Vitamin D supplementation, calcium and phosphate supplementation
Hematology	Thrombocytopenia Anemia	Transfusion in case of surgical intervention or cerebral traumatism Iron supplementation

HPS hepatopulmonary syndrome, *POPH* portopulmonary hypertension

of hepatectomy in the donor and of short- and long-term graft dysfunction in the recipient.

Donor assessment should be completely separate from recipient assessment. The donor, regardless of his/her relationship to the child, should benefit from full confidentiality and an opportunity to ask questions and evaluate risks and benefits free of family or spousal pressure. Generally, the transplant coordinator acts as the interface between the donor and recipient medical teams. A date for LT is set when both evaluations are complete. Pretransplant recipient management is the same as for deceased donor LT.

29.2 Early Postoperative Management (<30 Days)

29.2.1 Introduction

Medical management during the early period posttransplantation (<30 days) should follow a standardized diagnostic and therapeutic protocol. The routine use of standardized protocols helps detect and may prevent early complications. A short description of common complications is outlined below, together with a systematic approach to postoperative management. The major early complications in children include infectious, biliary, and vascular disease. Table 29.4 summarizes a proposed routine approach to the early posttransplant period, while Table 29.5 summarizes posttransplant management. It must be emphasized that there is no standardized management. In fact, it is recommended that the perioperative and postoperative protocol be personalized to the needs of each pediatric liver transplant recipient.

29.2.2 Hepatology

Close follow-up of liver function and liver enzymes is performed to monitor graft function. Primary non-function is the major early cause of retransplantation but is increasingly rare. Elevated aminotransferase levels in blood and insufficient synthetic function within 7 days after LT (coagulation factors, glucose, ammonia) are suggestive signs [6]. Primary non-function may be associated with multiple organ failure. Delayed graft function is generally defined by persistently elevated INR, AST/ALT, and bilirubin 1 week after liver transplantation.

Liver function is monitored by factor V/VII or INR and typically normalizes within 1 or 2 days after LT. Ammonium is cleared rapidly, but levels >1 × ULN may persist for a few days. These are insignificant if the patient is awake, extubated, and otherwise well.

Liver enzymes (ASAT, ALAT) generally are high (10e3) immediately following LT and decrease within 2–4 days. Normal values are reached 2–3 weeks after LT [7]. Initially, these are followed daily and then on an every other day basis, to ensure that they continue to normalize. Rising LFTs or a plateau suggests any of the following: vascular complications, primary non-function/delayed graft function, and rejection (covered in later chapters). Some centers use prostaglandin infusion to minimize ischemia-reperfusion injury [8]. Other causes of abnormal LFTs include infection, sepsis, cardiac dysfunction, drug toxicity, and rejection.

Bilirubin and gGT tend to take longer to normalize. Cholestasis is concerning for biliary leak, vascular complications, infections, drug-induced liver injury, and rejection [9]. Treatment with UDCA is commonly accepted to favor bile drainage and is used in many centers.

Table 29.4 Proposed standard follow-up in early transplant period

Exam	D0	D1	D2	D3	D4	D5	D6	D7	D8	D9	D10	D11–D14	D15–D30
Blood													
Blood gas	2×	2×	2×	2×	2×	2×	2×	2×	1×	1×	1×	1×/2 days	Weekly
CBC, reticulocytes	2×	2×	2×	1×	1×	1×	1×	1×	1×	1×	1×	1×/2 days	Weekly
ACT, anti-Xa, antithrombin III	As needed to insure correct anticoagulation												
INR, PT, PTT, fibrinogen	1×	1×	1×	1×	1×	1×	1×	1×	–	–	–	–	Weekly
Factor V and factors VII–X	1×	1×	1×	1×	–	–	–	–	–	–	–	–	–
Electrolytes (glucose, Na, K, Cl, CO$_2$, Mg, Ph, Alb, Ca)	2×	2×	2×	1×	1×	1×	1×	1×	1×	1×	1×	1×/2 days	Weekly
Renal function (BUN, creatinine)	2×	2×	2×	1×	1×	1×	1×	1×	1×	1×	1×	1×/2 days	Weekly
Liver function tests (ASAT, ALAT, Bili tot and conj, γGT)	2×	2×	2×	1×	1×	1×	1×	1×	1×	1×	1×	1×	Weekly
Tacrolimus trough level	1×	1×	1×	1×	1×	1×	1×	1×	1×	1×	1×	1×/2 days	Weekly
Ammonium	1×	–	–	–	–	–	–	–	–	–	–	–	–
Lipid profile	1×	Weekly											
EBV and CMV PCR Serum protein electrophoresis	1×	Weekly											
Radiology													
Abdominal liver Doppler and US	2×	2×	2×	2×	2×	2×	2×	2×	1×	1×	1×	1×/day	1×/2 days

Table 29.5 Proposed early postoperative treatment by system

	Treatment	Posology	Timing	Remark
Medical management				
Hepatology	Ursodeoxycholic acid	10 mg/kg Q8–Q12	D[b]–M6	Increased according to tolerance
	Prostacyclin	0.2 µg/kg/h–0.6 µg/kg/h	D0–D5	
Gastroenterology	Proton-pump inhibitor	2 mg/kg Q24	D0–M3	Until end of steroids
	Ranitidine	2 mg/kg Q8		
Infectiology	**Antibiotic prophylaxis**[a]	50 mg/kg Q8h	D0–D5	First dose before LT
	Cefuroxime	25 mg/kg Q8h	D0–D5	First doses before LT
	or cefazolin	2.25 mg/kg Q8h	D[b]–M12	According to D/R status
	Digestive decontamination	15 mg/kg Q8h	D0–D10	In case of low risk of CMV infection, immediate use of valganciclovir or preemptive strategy
	Polymyxin	6 mg/kg TMP–3 day/week	D11–M6	
	Neomycin	300 mg/month	D0–D5	
	PCP prophylaxis	5 mg/kg Q12–24		First doses before LT
	Sulfamethoxazole/trimethoprim	15–18 mg/kg/j Q24		Some team pursue antifungal therapy until M3
	or inhale/IV pentamidine	10 mg/kg Q24		
	Viral prophylaxis	200,000–500,000 U Q24		
	Ganciclovir IV			
	Valganciclovir PO			
	Antifungal prophylaxis			
	Amphotericin			
	Or nystatin			
Immunology	Tacrolimus	0.3 mg/kg	D0	First dose 6 h after closing of abdominal wall
	Basiliximab	0.3 mg/kg Q12h	D1–D2	Target 12–15 µg/mL[b]
	Steroids (prednisone or methylprednisolone)	0.1 mg/kg Q12h	D3–D30	Target 10–12 µg/mL
		10 mg if <35 kg	M1–M3	Target 8–10 µg/mL
		20 mg if >35 kg	M3–M6	Target 6–8 µg/mL
		1 mg/kg Q24h	M > 6	Steroid-sparing protocols are often used, while some centers never discontinue low-dose steroids
		0.5 mg/kg Q24h	D0 + D4	
		0.25 mg/kg Q24h	D0–D30	
			D30–D60	
			D60–D90	
Cardiology	Fluid maintenance	80–100%		
	Albumin	1 g/kg per 24 h		
	Diuretics	as needed		
Pneumology	Intubation—noninvasive ventilation	Positive pressure or controlled volume		Begin respiratory physiotherapy as soon as possible
	Oxygenotherapy			
Hematology	Platelets transfusion	According to weight	J0–J5	If active bleeding
	Blood transfusion	To reach 10 g/dL		
	Vitamin K	<10 kg–2 mg Q24		
		>10 kg–5 mg Q24		
Nephrology	**Antihypertensive therapy**	Continuous IV 0.5–4 µg/kg/h	If needed, every 20 min	If TA > 95 percentile for age
	Sodium nitroprusside (rare)	0–5 kg:1 mg		If persistent high blood pressure
	Nifedipine	5–10 kg:2.5 mg		Increased according to tolerance (diarrhea)
	Chronic antihypertensive therapy	10–20 kg:5 mg		If bicarbonates <22 mmol/L
	Nifedipine sustained release	>20 kg:10 mg		
	Enalapril	0.25–3 mg/kg Q24		
	Amlodipine	0.05 mg/kg Q12		
	Magnesium	0.05 mg/kg Q24		
	Sodium bicarbonate	0.3–1 mmol/kg/jr		
		0.25 mmol/kg/jr Q6–Q12		
Surgical treatment				
	Thrombosis prophylaxis	10 UI/kg/H	D0	When platelets >20 G/L
	Heparin	5 mg/kg Q24	D1–D90	When platelets >50 G/L
	Acetylsalicylic acid	1–2 mg/kg Q8	D0–D5	
	Dipyridamole	1/2 or 1/3 of losses		
	Drainage compensation			
	Colloid solution or			
	Fresh frozen plasma			
Others				
	Social follow-up (financial, accommodation; feeding; school, etc.)			
	Education of patients, families, schools, primary care: treatment, food, hygiene measures, infection prevention			
	Psychological follow-up of patient and families			

D day, *M* month, *H* hours, *TID* three times daily

This table gives a wide description of treatment use in the following transplantation. Management varies according to center

[a]Or according to the patient (previous cholangitis, bacterial carrier status)

[b]When oral feeding initiated

29.2.3 Surgical Management

Technical complications are the major cause of retransplantation and/or death after LT [10]. Surgical complications are described in detail in a later chapter. Early follow-up includes regular ultrasonography and Doppler. Monitoring of abdominal drainage helps to define type of fluid (bile, ass, bleeding, fecal, etc.) and consequent replacement. In case of massive abdominal drainage, chylous ascites, infectious ascites, and a posthepatic venous outflow obstruction should be excluded and targeted therapy initiated. Hepatic artery thrombosis (HAT) should be suspected in case of a drop in platelet count, rise of aminotransferases, fever, ascites, liver dysfunction, or sepsis [11]. Portal vein thrombosis should be suspected in case of portal hypertension after LT, splenomegaly, and ascites. Early biliary complications include leaks (cut surface or anastomotic), hemobilia, and acute bile duct dilation [12, 13]. Bowel perforation should be suspected as soon as there is a change of drainage color, but is frequently discovered when the child begins to present signs of peritonitis or sepsis, often after feeding has resumed. Many pediatric recipients will have a fresh Roux-en-Y anastomosis and thus delayed feeding. Intra-abdominal clots should be suspected in case an acute drop in Hb, especially in centers where posttransplant anticoagulation is prescribed.

29.2.4 Gastroenterology

Akin to any ICU patient, pediatric LT recipients are at risk of developing ulcers or gastritis after LT due to stress and corticosteroid therapy. A proton-pump inhibitor is typically prescribed until p.o. feeding is resumed or until steroid taper is complete. Diarrhea is often observed during the first week after LT. This may be due to any number of reasons including drugs, viruses, and bile acid pool recirculation; it is usually self-limited and benign and uncommonly leads to electrolyte imbalance.

29.2.5 Infectious Disease

Early infection is common after LT because of high levels of immunosuppression, ascites, and invasive equipment [14]. Most centers use prophylactic antibiotic and antiviral treatments, and some add an antifungal. Close monitoring for fever and other clinical signs of infection should allow for prompt workup and treatment. Two points are important to consider: first, signs may be subtle owing to the use of steroids or broad-spectrum antibiotics, and second, commonly used inflammatory markers such as CRP and PCT may be of limited use in the early course posttransplant [15].

During the first month, the most common infectious agents are bacteria (30%) and *Candida* sp. (8%) [16]. Pneumonia is common during first week and may delay extubation. Pneumococcal infection is frequent, emphasizing the importance of immunization before transplant. Gram-positive bacteremia is associated with central venous access and Gram-negative bacteremia with biliary leak or bowel perforation [16]. In case of persistent fever and an elevated white count despite broad-spectrum antibiotics, an invasive fungal infection should be suspected and empirically treated [17].

Beyond the first month, viral infections are the most common infectious disease [18, 19]. Viral load quantification of EBV and CMV is performed regularly during the first month. While CMV prophylaxis is common according to donor-recipient risk, some teams use a preemptive strategy for CMV [20, 21]. In those teams who choose to use prophylaxis, ganciclovir is the IV drug of choice, while oral valganciclovir is the drug of choice when patients are taking p.o. medications. Historically, CMV has been watched carefully owing to its association with rejection.

29.2.6 Immunology

Immunosuppression is discussed in detail in the next chapter. Induction of immunosuppression treatment will begin during the intraoperative or postoperative phase. Currently, immunosuppression typically combines a calcineurin inhibitor (CNI) and interleukin-2 receptor monoclonal antibodies (basiliximab) [22], although the latter is not used in all centers. Tacrolimus is generally preferred to cyclosporine if available because of its side effect profile and efficacy. Early management of immunosuppression is characterized by fluctuating levels owing to multiple variables including fluid balance, drug interactions, fasting, and the use of nasogastric tubes. As soon as patients stabilize, families should be instructed on the purpose of the drugs and their administration. This is the best way to make sure that all caregivers get the same information about current medications. Signs of tacrolimus toxicity include headache, myalgia, hypertension, low magnesium, renal insufficiency, and neurological manifestations (see below), all of which should prompt families to get a trough level drawn quickly and communicate with the transplant center.

Symptoms of acute rejection are non-specific and include fever, fatigue, pain, and new rise of AST/ALT. Treatment is discussed in the following chapters. Most often, however, rejection is asymptomatic and detected via serial blood tests.

29.2.7 Nutrition

During the acute phase after liver transplantation, energy needs are usually met by a glucose and electrolyte infusion, and parental nutrition is not required. Overnutrition should be avoided because of the risk of CO_2 overload and hyperglycemia which may delay extubation [23, 24]. Parenteral nutrition is not necessary during the acute phase (when the patient requires intensive support), but there is some evidence that it is of benefit during the recovery phase (e.g., after weaning of intensive support such as ventilation).

Nutrition during recovery phase is a key part of management and is associated with better outcomes [24, 25]. Enteral nutrition should begin as soon as possible and will usually require nasogastric feeding at least transiently. When the patient feeds on his own, many centers recommend avoiding raw meat and seafood during the 3 first months, although this varies according to local ecology and customs. There is a general agreement that all drinks should be pasteurized. Grapefruit is forbidden for life owing to its interactions with CNIs.

29.2.8 Endocrinology

Abnormalities in glucose metabolism are the most common endocrine/metabolic finding early after LT. Hyperglycemia is most common and has several etiologies: liver graft dysfunction, side effect of corticosteroids, and other medications including CNIs. Occasionally, patients require may require insulin. Hypoglycemia is rarer and is a sign of liver dysfunction or sepsis.

29.2.9 Cardiology

Fluid management is the cornerstone of early postoperative management to ensure adequate graft perfusion. Third-spacing is a common occurrence owing to a combination of capillary leak, fluid losses, and postoperative ileus. The mainstay of ICU management (covered elsewhere in this book) consists in maintaining intravascular volume while avoiding total body fluid overload. Intravascular volume repletion is preferred to avoid vascular thromboses, as is the avoidance of large fluid shifts. Therefore, diuretics should be used with caution. It has been recommended that central venous pressure be maintained around 10 mmHg [26]. Rarely, patients with ventricular dysfunction will need vasoactive and or inotropic support. Left ventricular hypertrophy is frequently observed following LT owing to increased afterload and side effects of steroids and CNIs. Arrhythmias are another drug-induced side effect [19, 27].

29.2.10 Pulmonary

Early extubation is the goal of ICU respiratory management. It is accepted to reduce morbidity and length of stay. Common obstacles to early ET tube removal include atelectasis, pulmonary infection, increased intra-abdominal pressure, diaphragmatic paresis, and fluid overload. After extubation, noninvasive support or oxygen supplementation are frequently needed during the first week after transplantation. Right hydrothorax is commonly associated to abdominal third-spacing. Chest tube insertion may be warranted in case of respiratory distress. Chylothorax typically presents when the child begins to feed; it is diagnosed based on fluid composition and cell count. It typically responds to an MCT-rich formula or total parenteral nutrition. Octreotide can be used safely beyond 1 month post-LT. Young children with an upper respiratory infection before LT can develop viral pneumonitis or reactive airway disease [19].

29.2.11 Neurology

Postoperative neurologic evaluation is often difficult owing to sedation. The effect of sedatives can be potentiated by drug interactions and delayed hepatic or renal clearance. Awakening the patient immediately postoperatively is essential to assess organ function. Neurological issues that can arise in the early postoperative period include seizures either due to metabolic abnormalities or preexisting disease, intracranial bleeding, or high serum levels of immunosuppressants [19]. Other manifestations of elevated CNI trough levels include migraine and tremors [28, 29]. Other neurologic complications include encephalopathy with symptoms of decrease of consciousness, lethargy, and coma and may be due to one of the following: liver failure, CNS infections, hypertension, or hypoxemia. Posterior reversible encephalopathy syndrome (PRES) occurs in 0.8–1% of LT patients and is due to toxicity of tacrolimus or cyclosporine and hypertension. Typical MR imaging reveals lesions of the posterior cerebral hemisphere and may be associated with symptoms such as stupor, blindness, and seizures [29].

29.2.12 Hematology

The typical hematological problems in the early postoperative period include cytopenias and coagulation problems (hyper- or hypocoagulable states). An acute drop in hemoglobin and/or platelets indicates the need to rule out bleeding. A slower, more insidious onset suggests medication adverse effects, infections, new-onset portal hypertension, or immune-mediated problems. Early hemolytic anemia can be drug-induced or due to lymphocyte passenger syndrome (LPS). In this case, indirect Coombs test will be positive, and elution shows positive alloantibodies from the donor [30]. Lymphopenia after liver transplantation is common and due to side effects of medication and infection or can be observed in case of chylous losses.

Transfusion should be avoided as long as the patient remains hemodynamically stable. A level of hemoglobin around 10 g/dL during perioperative period is generally the accepted target. Levels in excess of this are typically considered to be associated with hyperviscosity and therefore worrisome for risk of vascular thrombosis. In case of active bleeding, transfusion should be carefully given under surgical advice [26]. Of note, many patients receive pRBCs intraoperatively, supplying them with a large iron load. Therefore, in spite of ongoing losses owing to repetitive blood draws, few patients require Fe supplementation in the early posttransplant period.

Coagulopathy is common, and vitamin K supplementation is typically administered during the first few postoperative days. Prevention of vascular thrombosis is a subject of much interest and debate, yet there is no universal protocol. It is accepted that the synthesis of liver-derived pro- and anti-coagulants reaches physiological levels at different rates as liver function recovers, thereby putting patients at risk both of bleeding and thrombosis. For example, ATIII, required for heparin efficacy, reaches normal plasma levels within 1 week postoperatively [31]. There is some consensus about the use of continuous heparin followed by aspirin, but this is practice-based. The systematic use of FFP for ATIII substitution has been reported but is controversial because it leads to fluid overload among several downsides [32, 33]. Some teams use dipyridamole and prostaglandin, but evidence is limited [8, 34, 35].

Among centers using prophylactic anticoagulation, there is still controversy about how to monitor for over- and under-anticoagulation. At the present time, all we can recommend is for each center to decide which test is most reliable in their hands.

29.2.13 Nephrology

Renal function is often impaired during early period as patient will receive nephrotoxic drugs and is confronted to volume variation. In case of preexisting renal impairment, a renal-sparing immunosuppressive regimen may be tailor-made for the child. Ensuring adequate intravascular volume and managing hypertension are two ways to protect renal function. In case of severe renal dysfunction, acute tubular necrosis caused by drug toxicity should be ruled out. The need for hemofiltration is rare and occurs generally when there is a preexisting renal impairment either owing to underlying disease or to CNI toxicity (retransplantation).

High blood pressure is common after LT and should be treated as soon as detected to avoid cardiac and renal complications. Causes are multiple: renal impairment and side effect of medication including tacrolimus and vascular overload. Unless BP is excessively high, it is common practice to wait until the patient is stable on the conventional ward before starting calcium channel blockers. CCBs are the drugs of choice owing to the effect of CNIs on the vascular afferent tubule. Amlodipine is favored over nifedipine for its interaction profile. Nifedipine has the advantage of being fast acting, but it is also metabolized via CYP3A4 and may contribute to the variations in IS trough levels early during the posttransplant course. Further, it is impractical for home and induces gingival hyperplasia. If a second drug is required, it will typically be an ACEi [36–39].

Most common electrolytes abnormalities are hyponatremia due to dilution or excessive diuretic use and hyperkaliemia due to cell lysis or transfusion. Close follow-up affords the opportunity to adjust electrolyte supplementation as needed. Hypomagnesemia and hyperchloremic acidemia, both due to tubular losses, are common and easily correctable [19].

29.2.14 Transition from PICU to Home

Decision to transfer the patient from the ICU to the ward is made by the multidisciplinary team and based on local resources. The child is typically transferred when all systems are stable and major complications managed.

The transition between time of stability in hospital and going home should offer families the opportunity to ask questions and feel comfortable with the treatment plan. If the child is at an age to understand, he must be involved in his daily care. Written guidelines with practical tips should be provided because of the amount of new informations to remember given during a short and stressful time. These guidelines are typically offered online and should include the following: (1) whom to call and when (pediatrician, gastroenterologist, nurse, transplant center) and (2) signs and symptoms indicating a call to a caregiver.

In addition, patients benefit hugely from a personalized summary of their medications, and many enjoy peer-to-peer mentoring programs, and play tools should be provided to the child and family. The typical schedule for early, outpatient, posttransplant care is the following:

- First month: 1×/week
- Second to third months: 2×/week
- >third month: 1×/month if patient is stable

Close communication between community hospitals and the transplant center is essential during this early phase. It is also recommended that during the first months at least, immunosuppression management should be provided by the transplant center owing to the many variables that can influence trough levels. Return to school or kindergarten is a function of different factors including patient age and degree of immunosuppression. For young infants this can be delayed to 3 months during the winter. Sports are generally accepted after 6–12 weeks but vary according to center.

29.3 Long-Term Follow-Up Protocol and Complications Surveillance

29.3.1 Introduction

As currently the survival of patients having received a liver transplant as a child is in excess of 90% at 1 year and 75% at 15–20 years, the new challenge faced by physicians in managing these patients is to ensure longevity while minimizing long-term complications [39]. Management of complications following pediatric LT is best summarized as anticipatory, because complications can remain silent or with minimal symptoms for a long time. Among the key complications to watch for are rejection, infection renal disease, metabolic syndrome, and secondary malignancies. The use of a systematic follow-up protocol affords clinicians following these patients to leave no stone unturned, thereby increasing the likelihood of detecting potential problems early [39].

Table 29.6 provides a proposed follow-up schedule including complementary testing and treatment schedule. Table 29.7 provides an overview of the main complications observed late after LT including pointers for diagnosis and treatment. Our purpose here is to offer a practical approach to the diagnosis and management of these late complications.

29.3.2 Hepatology

Late graft complications such as rejection, chronic hepatitis, fibrosis, and autoimmune hepatitis are discussed in the following chapters. The follow-up for patients with biliary or vascular complications is also summarized elsewhere.

Abnormalities of liver function tests are most often related to rejection, viral disease, vascular problems, drug-induced toxicity, and rarely recurrence of disease. Follow-up will depend on clinical suspicion and severity of LFT abnormality. Cholestasis or rising GGT without significant hepatitis is most often seen in biliary abnormalities, hepatic artery problems, and drug toxicity. Any unexplained, persistent LFT abnormality should be discussed with the transplant center who will evaluate the need for biopsy.

Development of **progressive fibrosis** and hepatitis leading to graft loss is one of the major concerns about long-term outcome [40–43]. Chronic antibody-mediated rejection (AMR) and donor-specific antibodies are likely contributive [40, 44]. Identification of chronic fibrosis is more difficult as it occurs in patients with normal liver biology. Noninvasive measures of fibrosis are increasingly used clinically [43, 45]. The role of protocol biopsy to diagnose chronic fibrosis and rejection is still debated. Performing a protocol liver biopsy after 1 year and after 5 years to assess the graft seems reasonable [39, 46]. In case of positive findings, the immunosuppression may be modified. In addition, it is recommended that patients having undergone transplant for sclerosing cholangitis, autoimmune hepatitis, and PFIC2 be monitored closely for recurrence of disease. Likewise, patients having undergone LT for unresectable hepatoblastoma should be closely followed-up for recurrence.

29.3.3 Gastroenterology

Children following LT often present with abdominal complaints which may be overlooked. The transplant team should consider these symptoms seriously as they are sometimes the only physicians seeing the child on a regular basis and will consider the differential diagnosis in the setting of LT. Chronic diarrhea is a frequent symptom after liver transplantation and could be due to various causes and should be investigated if growth or quality of life is affected. One of the first causes is persistent viral infection secondary to immune suppression. Positive stools PCR may suffice for diagnosis, but on occasion colonoscopy is required to identify the pathogen and rule out other causes of mucosal inflammation. Portal hypertension or posthepatic venous obstruction should be suspected in case of protein losing enteropathy. Medication can also be a culprit of bothersome diarrhea (mycophenolate mofetil, tacrolimus, cyclosporine). The other causes of post-transplant diarrhea include eosinophilic GI disease or new-onset IBD [47–49]. Diarrhea and failure to thrive can also be the presenting symptoms of PTLD (25–30% of the cases). Abdominal pain, heartburn, and vomiting are also frequent symptoms after liver transplantation. Side effects of medication and viral disease should be also suspected. Intracranial hypertension is a rare but with severe consequence cause of recurrent vomiting after LT. Surgical obstruction should also always be considered [50].

29.3.4 Infectious Diseases

Infection post-LT causes more deaths than rejection [16]. Any fever in an immunocompromised patient should be carefully investigated, and the patient should be examined with necessary lab tests to understand the source of the fever. Viral PCRs should be performed in case of fever or LFT abnormalities. In the latter case, the absence of normalization after the viral disease is cleared warrants a workup for rejection. During the first 6 months post-LT, patients are at high risk of opportunistic infection like CMV or *Pneumocystis jirovecii* infection. Prophylaxis for *Pneumocystis jirovecii* is typically continued until 12 months. CMV and EBV infections cause severe complications and should be sought regularly. They are discussed in the following chapter. In addition, HBV, HCV, HEV, and HHV6 are rare but possible culprits of abnormal liver

Table 29.6 Long-term follow-up schedule

	Assessment		Treatment	
	Test	Schedule	To be continued	Stop
>1 month	Tacrolimus trough level Renal function, CBC, liver panel Electrolytes (Mg) CMV-EBV PCR Clinical evaluation Doppler and liver US + Fibroscan	1×/2 weeks 1×/month 1×/2 weeks 1×/month	Tacrolimus Prednisone Valganciclovir TMP-SMZ or pentacarinat Ursodeoxycholic acid	Magnesium according to level Antihypertensive drugs according to blood pressure
>3 months	Tacrolimus trough level Renal function, CBC, liver panel Electrolytes (Mg) CMV-EBV PCR Clinical evaluation Doppler and liver US + Fibroscan Eye examination with measure of intraocular pressure if steroid treatment	1×/2 weeks 1×/month 1×/month 1×/month 1×	Tacrolimus Valganciclovir TMP-SMZ or pentacarinat Ursodeoxycholic acid	Prednisone PPI
>6 months	Tacrolimus trough level Renal function, CBC, liver panel Electrolytes (Mg) CMV-EBV PCR AIH panel Vaccination control test DSA test Clinical evaluation Doppler and liver US + Fibroscan	1/month 1×/2 month 1× at 6-month visit 1×/month 1× at 6-month visit	Tacrolimus TMP-SMZ or pentamidine	Ursodeoxycholic acid Valganciclovir
>12 months	Tacrolimus trough level Renal function, CBC, liver panel Electrolytes (Mg), uric acid CMV-EBV PCR HEV AIH panel Control of immunization DSA test Clinical evaluation Doppler and liver US + Fibroscan Liver biopsy Mineralometry >5 years Evaluation of GFR by creatinine clearance or inulin clearance Eye examination with fundoscopy	1×/2 months 1×/2–3 months 1× at 12-month visit 1× at 12-month visit 1×/2–3 months 1× at 12-month visit 1× at 12-month visit 1× at 12-month visit 1× at 12-month visit	Tacrolimus Vaccination catch-up	TMP-SMZ or pentamidine
>24 months	Tacrolimus level Renal function, CBC, liver panel Electrolytes (Mg), uric acid CMV-EBV PCR HEV AIH panel Control of immunization DSA test Clinical evaluation Doppler and liver US + Fibroscan Liver biopsy Mineralometry >5 years Evaluation of GFR by creatinine clearance or inulin clearance 24 h blood pressure control Cardiac ultrasonography	1×/3–6 months 1×/6–12 months 1×/year 1×/year 1×/3–6 months 1×/year 1×/5 year According to previous result 1×/1–2 years If BP elevated If BP elevated	Tacrolimus Influenza immunization 1×/year	

Treatment according to protocol of the patient. *AIH* autoimmune hepatitis panel (including FAN)

Table 29.7 Medical follow-up and treatment of posttransplant complication

	Complication	Diagnosis	Management
Medical			
Hepatology Gastroenterology	Acute rejection	Abnormal LFTs, Doppler or Fibroscan, DSA, liver biopsy	See next chapter
	Chronic rejection	Endoscopy	Budesonide
	Antibody-mediated rejection	Colonoscopy	Food eviction
	Eosinophilic gastritis or enteropathy	IgE-specific positive and positive history	
	IBD new onset		
	Food allergic disease		
Infectious disease	CMV-HHV6	Positive PCR	Ganciclovir for 3 weeks
	Adenovirus		Cidofovir
	HSV 1–II; HZV		Acyclovir for 5 days, 4 for HSV/HZV
	EBV		Decrease immunosuppression
Immunology	Immunization	Antibody titers	Vaccination with recombinant
	Autoimmune hepatitis	Positive antibodies during schedule F/u and biopsy if perturbations of liver panel test	HPV in young adolescent
	Autoimmune cytopenias	Control for presence of antibodies against erythrocytes (Coombs test with elution) antineutrophil or antiplatelet	Add steroids or azathioprine
			Immunoglobulins for immune thrombocytopenia
			Steroids and rituximab for hemolytic anemia
Endocrinology	Diabetes mellitus	Screening by oral glucose tolerance 1×/year in at-risk patient	Insulin as required, diet
	– Due to steroids and tacrolimus	ACTH stimulation test	Hydrocortisone, steroid stress doses
	Adrenal insufficiency	High blood pressure, hypertriglyceridemia. Obesity	Diet, physical activity
	– Due to steroids		
	Risk of metabolic syndrome		
Cardiology	Ventricular hypertrophy, cardiac dysfunction	Echocardiogram	Address to cardiologist
ORL/pneumology	Allergic rhinitis, asthma	Clinical diagnosis, pulmonary function	Local steroids or steroid inhaled/montelukast
Neurology	Neurocognitive and neurodevelopment delay	Neuropsychological assessment	Intensive physiotherapy and occupational therapy support
	Migraine and tremor	Low magnesemia	Decrease tacrolimus level
	Leg cramps		
Hematology/ Oncology	Anemia, thrombopenia, leucopenia	CBC	Treat according to the cause
	Iron deficit	Low ferritin and low transferrin saturation	Iron supplementation
	PTLD	Persistent adenopathy, positive EBV PCR, oligoclonal high IgG in electrophoresis	Decreased IS, chemotherapy
	Other malignancies	According to physical exam and history	Treat according to the cause

(continued)

Table 29.7 Continued

	Complication	Diagnosis	Management
Medical			
Nephrology	Glomerular hyperfiltration, renal insufficiency or dysfunction Hypertension Abnormal bone metabolism and hepatic osteodystrophy	Creatinine clearance, renal function test 24 h blood pressure measurement DEXA scan Low vitamin D, high PTH	Discuss substitution to mycophenolate or mTOR inhibitor Decrease other nephrotoxic drugs Antihypertensive drugs Vitamin D supplementation, calcium supplementation
Allergology	Transplant-related food allergy Respiratory allergy Eczema	IgE specific Prick tests	Food eviction and specific treatment
Dermatology	Skin malignancy Eczema	Regular dermatologic screening Skin biopsy if uncertain diagnosis	Prevention by sunscreen Removal of any suspicious nevi Local treatment
Ophthalmology	Glaucoma Cataract Intracranial hypertension	Increase intracranial pressure Lens examination Papilledema	Tapering steroids, topical treatment Tapering steroids, cataract surgery Acetazolamide
Dental hygiene	Caries, gingivitis, greenish coloration, bleeding	Routine but close follow-up	Consider antibiotic prophylaxis
Surgical			
	Biliary complication Vascular complication	Liver ultrasonography, liver panel and biopsy	Surgery or interventional radiology
Social			
	Quality of life School difficulties Financial difficulties Loss of compliance Psychiatric problem Transition issue	Use Pediatric Liver transplant Quality of Life (HRQOL) [99] Thorough history taking by MD or specialized nurse	Address to social services, psychiatry if necessary

biology posttransplant. Patients in contact with varicella who are nonimmune should receive immunoglobulins within 72 h of exposure [18]. Viral respiratory disease are common, but their course may be more protracted in transplant recipients who may in addition have some degree of reactive airway disease [16, 18, 39]. Community-acquired bacterial diseases such as *Haemophilus influenzae* and pneumococcus are also frequent.

29.3.5 Immunology

After liver transplantation, antibody titers should be monitored 6 and 12 months [51, 52]. Immunization schedule should resume, including catch-up when immunosuppression permits. There is no known cutoff trough level. For live attenuated vaccines, monotherapy and trough levels <8 µg/mL have been recommended to ensure response [53]. Indeed, recent evidence convincingly suggests that live attenuated vaccines after transplantation are safe and effective starting 1 year posttransplant [51]. MMR is currently under study. Annual influenza vaccine is recommended as is HPV in adolescents [54, 55].

Development of autoimmune disease is quite frequent after LT. Many patients will develop autoantibodies of unknown clinical significance. De novo autoimmune hepatitis should be suspected in case of abnormal liver enzymes, with rising of total IgG levels, and the presence of autoantibodies known to be associated with AIH. A biopsy is needed to confirm diagnosis and guide treatment. Other immune complications are autoimmune cytopenias and new-onset IBD [30, 47, 56].

29.3.6 Nutrition-Growth: Puberty

Generally, patients requiring liver transplantation for chronic liver disease will experience growth and weight delay owing to many factors including feeding intolerance, increased protein/calorie needs, and liver endocrine dysfunction. Liver transplantation improves digestion and feeding, thereby leading to appropriate intake. It also restores IGF-1, GH, and sex hormone metabolism [57, 58]. Catch-up generally will occur during the 2 first years after LT, but 25% of patients will keep a growth delay. The use of steroids posttransplant may be a modifiable factor, and some centers have chosen a steroid-free approach to avoid growth delay [36, 59]. Pubertal delay is also frequent posttransplant and may require specialist referral. Pretransplant growth impairment may be a modifiable risk factor of delayed puberty, something increasingly addressed with pretransplant feeding regimens, especially in cholestatic infants [60].

29.3.7 Endocrinology

In addition to the impact on growth, the use of steroids may induce adrenal insufficiency. A slow steroid taper and the hydrocortisone supplementation may help reduce the risk. It is generally recommended that in the first year posttransplant, patients having received steroids receive a stress dose in case of acute illness or surgery. An ACTH stimulation test or a cortisol measurement can help guide the need for supplementation.

Posttransplantation diabetes mellitus (PTDM) is another frequent complication of steroid use which can require insulin, but usually resolves as steroid dose is tapered. In some patients, however, DM may persist, a known side effect of CNIs. Certain patients seem at increased risk of developing DM: patients with elevated BMI or family history of MS, patients with cystic fibrosis, patients with primary sclerosing cholangitis patients, and those having presented with acute liver failure [18, 39, 61]. A rare complication of steroid treatment is avascular necrosis of the hip and should be suspected in case of hip pain.

Metabolic syndrome (MS) should be suspected in any overweight patient, following plasma triglyceride levels. Hypertriglyceridemia should be sought in all patients on a routine basis to identify CNI-induced metabolic abnormalities even in patients with a normal BMI, the rationale being that MS is associated with NASH which will compromise allograft longevity [43, 57].

29.3.8 Bone Health

Patients with a history of liver disease or liver transplantation can present with several skeletal or bone health issues. Hepatic osteodystrophy is caused by liver disease and cholestasis and is improved by LT. Nonetheless, fracture risk remains high, especially asymptomatic vertebral fractures in patients with persistently lower bone mineral density [62]. This may be in part due to incomplete recovery of sarcopenia, at least in adults, something not yet confirmed in children [57]. Next, the risk of developing scoliosis during puberty may also be increased in LT patients [63]. In general, it is recommended that patients undergo regular DEXA measurements through puberty and benefit from routine serum vitamin D and PTH monitoring [57, 64]. Adequate calcium and vitamin D intake should be maintained. Of note, vitamin D sufficiency is in contradiction with another posttransplant recommendation: avoidance of excessive sun exposure!

29.3.9 Cardiology

Compared to normal population, patients having undergone SOT have an increased risk of developing cardiac disease in their adult life as they are subject to metabolic syndrome, dyslipidemia, and hypertension. Cardiovascular death is the most common cause of death in adult LT recipients, and it is known that hypertensive children become hypertensive adults. Therefore, close follow-up of these complications and early treatment are recommended [65, 66]. Follow-up of cardiac function using cardiac ultrasound is recommended in case of hypertension and of preexisting cardiac abnormalities. Increasing evidence points to the measure of intima media thickness and share wave elastography to assess the complication of high blood pressure [67, 68].

29.3.10 Nephrology

Decreased renal function is one of the major long-term concerns that plagues pediatric liver transplant recipients, mostly owing to CNI toxicity, together with other insults such as antibiotics and acute renal failure in the pre- or posttransplant period. Among those patients with an unremarkable early posttransplant course, it is not clear who will develop renal disease. Yet, as many as 30 percent (30%) of patients may present with stage III renal failure 15 years after transplant [36, 39, 69]. Early recognition is important to try to halt progression, yet there is no consensus on management, either preemptive or when renal failure is present. Recommendations are to decrease CNI target trough levels and add a less nephrotoxic drug such as mycophenolate if GFR is less than 90 mL/min/1.73 m^2. Currently mTOR inhibitors are an interesting alternative but may be associated with proteinuria [39, 65, 70–72].

More than 50% of pediatric liver-transplanted patient will present with elevated blood pressure during a routine follow-up visit 5–10 years post-LT. The concern is that hypertensive children become hypertensive adults. Further, hypertension likely acts as a second hit on kidneys injured by CNIs. Therefore, current recommendations suggest that 24 h ambulatory blood pressure monitoring be performed to detect subclinical evidence of elevated BP [65]. There is some controversy about when to start treating BP abnormalities in SOT recipients. The most recent AAP updated guidelines suggested >90 percentile, while in practice, it is probably cautious to begin sooner [73].

There is no consensus on the treatment of hypertension in children post-LT. Commonly, in the early posttransplant period, amlodipine is the preferred and first-line agent, because it has minimal interaction with CNI, is administered daily, and acts on the afferent arteriole, the known site of vasoconstriction in animal models. ACEi are used as a second-line drug, in later cases of hypertension, and in case of associated proteinuria. Close follow-up of renal impairment due to hypertensive disease is also recommended as a measure of end-organ damage. Each center will use the method that works in their hands, but the preferred methods are Cr EDTA or inulin clearance.

In addition, a less well-known complication of CNI nephrotoxicity is hyperuricemia. Patients should benefit from annual serum uric acid levels, as these may be increased in chronic renal disease owing to increased tubular absorption. Rarely, gout has been described in adolescents [74, 75].

29.3.11 Hematology

Anemia is a very common complication after liver transplantation. Iron deficiency is the first cause and should be ruled out first with adequate treatment. Other causes of anemia are renal insufficiency, chronic bleeding, side effects of medication, and immune-mediated hemolytic anemia.

Leucopenia and thrombocytopenia are also relatively frequent in a child after LT. Drug toxicity is one of the most frequent etiologies. Typical agents with bone marrow toxicity include trimethoprim-sulfamethoxazole, valganciclovir, azathioprine, and mycophenolate. Drug discontinuation may be necessary if the cell counts lead to clinical complications. The differential diagnosis includes acute or chronic viral infection which should be sought in peripheral blood using PCR. Persistent hypersplenism due to persistence of splenomegaly after LT even in absence of portal hypertension can occur, and rarely, partial splenectomy may be indicated. Both thrombocytopenia and neutropenia may be immune in origin; the presence of peripheral antibodies does not necessarily imply causality. Post-liver transplantation aplasia is a rare severe complication and could be due to side effect of medication or infection. There is a described association between acute liver failure and bone marrow failure which could persist even if the child was transplanted [76, 77].

29.3.12 Oncology

Posttransplant lymphoproliferative disease is a dreaded posttransplant complication. PTLD should be suspected in case of persistent diarrhea, unexplained fever, failure to thrive, or any unexplained symptoms. Clinical examination can reveal tonsil hypertrophy or persisting adenopathy. PTLD and its management are explained in the next chapter.

Secondary malignancies are very rare during pediatric age after liver transplantation, although there are no reliable epidemiological data, but should be ruled out in case of clinical signs [78]. In adult population, the most frequent is skin cancer (see dermatology). Particular attention should be paid to the prevention of other risk factor of malignancies with appropriate counseling during adolescence (tobacco, alcohol, sunscreen, etc.).

29.3.13 Allergy

Transplant-acquired food allergies (TAFA) often arise during first year posttransplantation but are often misdiagnosed [79]. This condition appears to be more frequent after liver transplantation than following other SOT. There are two ways to acquire TAFA. The first and most common is thought to arise secondary to CNI-induced Th2 response. It can present clinically as angioedema or urticaria. It can also present with acute or chronic GI symptoms such as diarrhea or growth failure with or without peripheral eosinophilia or atopy. Diagnosis and management are similar to that in patients without CNI treatment [47, 48, 80]. The course can be self-limited, but more typically patients remain allergic even if CNI treatment is tapered. Rarely, CNI will be discontinued or combination therapy initiated with another class of immunosuppressant. The other mode of TAFA presentation is via passive transmission through the graft, from a patient without or without known allergic disease. Most often, the passive transfer of IgE is short-lived. Once patients are off steroids, they undergo an oral food challenge, and serial IgE titers help in documenting the disappearance of sensitization. Exceptionally, memory B cells persist and the allergy remains [80, 81].

New onset of asthma or allergic rhinitis is rarer than TAFA. Again, diagnosis and management are conventional. Posttransplant drug allergy and eczema are described below [80, 82].

29.3.14 Dermatology

Atopic disease is frequent posttransplant. Much like in the non-transplanted population, a cause is rarely identified, and management is the same. Calcineurin inhibitors favor a Th2 response and as such have been incriminated in post-SOT atopic disease. Some centers have reported decreasing CNI trough levels to abate symptoms with some success [83]. In general, the differential diagnosis of skin lesions in SOT recipients includes drug reaction, infections, or graft-versus-host disease. Skin biopsy may be useful for diagnosis. Finally, long-term immunosuppressive treatment has been associated with a higher risk of skin malignancies in adults [84]. An annual dermatology consult is recommended, but may not be necessary in the first decade following transplant or as long as parents are very closely involved in the skin care/hygiene of the child. Sun protective clothing or mineral barriers are recommended in case of sun exposure. Abnormal nevi should be removed as indicated by a dermatologist. Some centers now have a specialized consultation for immunosuppressed patients—including this in annual follow-up visits may be more appropriate than referring patients to their local dermatologist.

29.3.15 Ophthalmology

Ophthalmological complications after liver transplantation include (1) infection (CMV retinitis; bacterial cellulitis); (2) cataract due to long-term steroid use or labile blood glucose; (3) glaucoma, a short-term complication of steroids; and (4) rarely ocular PTLD.

Patients with Alagille syndrome are known for pretransplant ocular abnormalities including embryotoxon and drusen. It is recommended that patients undergo an ophthalmological exam after 3 months of steroid use and 1 year after LT for complete fundoscopy.

29.3.16 Dental Care

Poor dental status is frequent before and after liver transplantation [85, 86]. The most commonly observed problem is greenish tooth discoloration due to cholestasis prior to LT during early windows of dental development. This is a cosmetic problem that can be managed in late adolescence. Gingivitis is also more frequent in transplant recipients and associated with the presence of plaque and immunosuppressive level. Gingival hyperplasia is associated with the use of calcium channel blockers and cyclosporine. A close follow-up of caries is crucial as they can lead to severe dental infection, bacteremia, and systemic infection [86, 87]. Oral hygiene is also paramount and should be reinforced during annual control. Antibiotic prophylaxis is rarely recommended for dental care, except in cases of very profound immunosuppression.

References

1. Squires RH, Ng V, Romero R, et al. AASLD practice guideline evaluation of the pediatric patient for liver transplantation: 2014 practice guideline by the American Association for the Study of Liver Diseases, American Society of Transplantation and the North American Society for Pediatric. Hepatology. 2014;60(1):362–98.
2. D'Antiga L, Vallortigara F, Cillo U, et al. Features predicting unresectability in hepatoblastoma. Cancer. 2007;110(5):1050–8.
3. Baumann U, Adam R, Duvoux C, et al. Survival of children after liver transplantation for hepatocellular carcinoma. Liver Transpl. 2018;24(2):246–55.

4. Tsouka A, McLin VA. Complications of chronic liver disease. Clin Res Hepatol Gastroenterol. 2012;36(3):262–7.
5. Caudle SE, Katzenstein JM, Karpen S, McLin V. Developmental assessment of infants with biliary atresia: differences between boys and girls. J Pediatr Gastroenterol Nutr. 2012;55:384–9.
6. Ploeg RJ, D'Alessandro AM, Knechtle SJ, Stegall MD, Pirsch JD, Hoffmann RM, et al. Risk factors for primary dysfunction after liver transplantation—a multivariate analysis. Transplantation. 1993;55:807–13.
7. Maddrey WC, Schiff ER, Sorrell MF, editors. Transplant of the liver. Philadelphia: Lippincott Williams & Wilkins; 2001.
8. Lironi C, McLin VA, Wildhaber BE. The effect and safety of prostaglandin administration in pediatric liver transplantation. Transplant Direct. 2017;3(6):e163.
9. Angelico R, Gerlach UA, Gunson BK, et al. Severe unresolved cholestasis due to unknown aetiology leading to early allograft failure within the fir. Transplantation. 2018;102(8):1307–15.
10. Kuang AA, Rosenthal P, Roberts JP, et al. Decreased mortality from technical failure improves results in pediatric liver transplantation. Arch Surg. 1996;131:887–92.
11. Hashikura Y, Kawasaki S, Okumura N, et al. Prevention of hepatic artery thrombosis in pediatric liver transplantation. Transplantation. 1995;60(10):1109–12.
12. Lüthold SC, Kaseje N, Jannot A-S, et al. Risk factors for early and late biliary complications in pediatric liver transplantation. Pediatr Transplant. 2014;18(8):822–30.
13. Kamran Hejazi Kenari S, Mirzakhani H, Eslami M, Saidi RF. Current state of the art in management of vascular complications after pediatric liver transplantation. Pediatr Transplant. 2015;19(1):18–26.
14. Cousin VL, Wildhaber BE, Verolet CM, Belli DC, Posfay-Barbe KM, McLin VA. Complications of indwelling central venous catheters in pediatric liver transplant recipients. Pediatr Transplant. 2016;20(6):798–806.
15. Cousin VL, Lambert K, Trabelsi S, et al. Procalcitonin for infections in the first week after pediatric liver transplantation. BMC Infect Dis. 2017;17(1):1–7.
16. Shepherd RW, Turmelle Y, Nadler M, et al. Risk factors for rejection and infection in pediatric liver transplantation. Am J Transplant. 2008;8(2):396–403.
17. Vilca-Melendez H, Heaton ND. Paediatric liver transplantation: the surgical view. Postgrad Med J. 2004;80(948):571–6.
18. Miloh T. Medical management of children after liver transplantation. Curr Opin Organ Transplant. 2014;19(5):474–9.
19. Tannuri AC, Gibelli NE, Ricardi LR, Santos MM, Maksoud-Filho JG, Pinho-Apezzato ML, et al. Living related donor liver transplantation in children. Transplant Proc. 2011;43:161–4.
20. Danziger-Isakov L, Bucavalas J. Current prevention strategies against cytomegalovirus in the studies in pediatric liver transplantation (SPLIT) centers. Am J Transplant. 2014;14(8):1908–11.
21. Nicastro E, Giovannozzi S, Stroppa P, et al. Effectiveness of preemptive therapy for cytomegalovirus disease in pediatric liver transplantation. Transplantation. 2017;101(4):804–10.
22. McDiarmid SV. Management of the pediatric liver transplant patient. Liver Transpl. 2001;7(11 Suppl 1):77–86.
23. Fivez T, Kerklaan D, Mesotten D, et al. Early versus late parenteral nutrition in critically ill children. N Engl J Med. 2016;374(12):1111–22.
24. Joosten KF, Kerklaan D, Verbruggen SC. Nutritional support and the role of the stress response in critically ill children. Curr Opin Clin Nutr Metab Care. 2016;19(3):226–33.
25. Joffe A, Anton N, Lequier L, et al. Nutritional support for critically ill children (review). Cochrane Database Syst Rev. 2016;(5):1–31.
26. Englesbe M, Kelly B, Goss J, et al. Reducing pediatric liver transplant complications: a potential roadmap for transplant quality improvement initiatives within North America. Am J Transplant. 2012;12(9):2301–6.
27. Feltracco P, Barbieri S, Galligioni H, Michieletto E, Carollo C, Ori C. Intensive care management of liver transplanted patients. World J Hepatol. 2011;3(3):61–71.
28. Ghosh PS, Hupertz V, Ghosh D. Neurological complications following pediatric liver transplant. J Pediatr Gastroenterol Nutr. 2012;54(4):540–6.
29. Gungor S, Kilic B, Arslan M, Selimoglu MA, Karabiber H, Yilmaz S. Early and late neurological complications of liver transplantation in pediatric patients. Pediatr Transplant. 2017;21(3):1–6.
30. Rock N, Ansari M, Villard J, Ferrari-Lacraz S, Waldvogel S, McLin VA. Factors associated with immune hemolytic anemia after pediatric liver transplantation. Pediatr Transplant. 2018;22(5):e13230.
31. Stahl RL, Duncan A, Hooks MA, Henderson JM, Millikan WJ, Warren WD. A hypercoagulable state follows orthotopic liver transplantation. Hepatology. 1990;12(3 Pt 1):553–8.
32. McLin VA, Rimensberger P, Belli DC, Wildhaber BE. Anticoagulation following pediatric liver transplantation reduces early thrombotic events. Pediatr Transplant. 2011;15(1):117–8.
33. Arni D, Wildhaber BE, McLin VA, Rimensberger PC, et al. Effects of plasma transfusion on antithrombin levels after pediatric liver transplantation. Vox Sang. 2018;113:569–76.
34. Quintero J, Ortega J, Miserachs M, Bueno J, Bilbao I, Charco R. Low plasma levels of antithrombin III in the early postoperative period following pediatric liver transplantation: should they be replaced? A single-center pilot study. Pediatr Transplant. 2014;18(2):185–9.
35. Taniguchi M, Magata S, Suzuki T, Shimamura T, Jin MB, Iida J, Furukawa H, Todo S. Dipyridamole protects the liver against warm ischemia and reperfusion injury. J Am Coll Surg. 2004;198(5):758–69.
36. McLin VA, Allen U, Boyer O, et al. Early and late factors impacting patient and graft outcome in pediatric liver transplantation: summary of an ESPGHAN monothematic conference. J Pediatr Gastroenterol Nutr. 2017;65(3):e53–9.
37. Campbell K, Ng V, Martin S, et al. Glomerular filtration rate following pediatric liver transplantation—the SPLIT experience. Liver Transpl. 2010;10(3):1593–602.
38. Galioto A, Semplicini A, Zanus G, et al. Nifedipine versus carvedilol in the treatment of de novo arterial hypertension after liver transplantation: results of a controlled clinical Trial. Liver Transpl. 2008;14:1020–8.
39. Kelly DA, Bucuvalas JC, et al. Long-term medical management of the pediatric patient after liver transplantation: 2013 practice guideline by the American Association for the Study of Liver Diseases and the American Society of Transplantation. Liver Transpl. 2013;19(8):798–825.
40. Evans HM, Kelly DA, McKiernan PJ, et al. Progressive histological damage in liver allografts following pediatric liver transplantation. Hepatology. 2006;43(5):1109–17. 25.
41. Scheenstra R, Gerver WJ, Odink RJ, et al. Growth and final height after liver transplantation during childhood. J Pediatr Gastroenterol Nutr. 2008;47:165–71.
42. Ekong UD, Melin-Aldana H, Seshadri R, Lokar J, Harris D, Whitington PF, Alonso EM. Graft histology characteristics in long-term survivors of pediatric liver transplantation. Liver Transpl. 2008;14:1582–7.
43. Kelly D, Verkade HJ, Rajanayagam J, McKiernan P, Mazariegos G, Hübscher S. Late graft hepatitis and fibrosis in pediatric liver allograft recipients: current concepts and future developments. Liver Transpl. 2016;22(11):1593–602.
44. Varma S, Ambroise J, Komuta M, et al. Progressive fibrosis is driven by genetic predisposition, allo-immunity, and inflammation in pediatric liver transplant recipients. EBioMedicine. 2016;9:346–55.
45. Hanquinet S, Rougemont AL, Courvoisier D, Rubbia-Brandt L, McLin V, Tempia M, Anooshiravani M. Acoustic radiation force

impulse (ARFI) elastography for the noninvasive diagnosis of liver fibrosis in children. Pediatr Radiol. 2013;43:545–51.
46. Kelly D, Verkade HJ, Rajanayagam J, McKiernan P, et al. Late graft hepatitis and fibrosis in pediatric liver allograft recipients: current concepts and future developments. Liver Transpl. 2016;22(11):1593–602.
47. Hampton DD, Poleski MH, Onken JE. Inflammatory bowel disease following solid organ transplantation. Clin Immunol. 2008;128(3):287–93.
48. Wisniewski J, Lieberman J, Nowak-Weogonekgrzyn A, et al. De novo food sensitization and eosinophilic gastrointestinal disease in children post-liver transplantation. Clin Transplant. 2012;26(4):365–71.
49. Lee JH, Park HY, Choe YH, Lee SK, Lee SI. The development of eosinophilic colitis after liver transplantation in children. Pediatr Transplant. 2007;11(5):518–23.
50. Eberhardt C, Merlini L, McLin V, Wildhaber B. Cholestasis as the leading sign of a transmesenteric hernia in a split-liver transplanted child—a case report and review of literature. Pediatr Transplant. 2012;16(5):E172–6.
51. Pittet L, Posfay-Barbe K. Immunization in transplantation: review of the recent literature. Curr Opin Organ Transplant. 2013;18(5):543–8.
52. L'Huillier AG, Wildhaber BE, Belli DC, et al. Successful serology-based intervention to increase protection against vaccine-preventable diseases in liver-transplanted children: a 19-yr review of the Swiss national reference center. Pediatr Transplant. 2012;16(1):50–7.
53. Posfay-Barbe KM, Pittet LF, Sottas C. Varicella-zoster immunization in pediatric liver transplant recipients: safe and immunogenic. Am J Transplant. 2012;12(11):2974–85.
54. Feldman AG, Kempe A, Beaty BL, Sundaram SS. Immunization practices among pediatric transplant hepatologists. Studies of Pediatric Liver Transplantation (SPLIT) Research Group. Pediatr Transplant. 2016;20(8):1038–44.
55. Barshes NR, Chang IF, Karpen SJ, et al. Successful serology-based intervention to increase protection against vaccine-preventable diseases in liver-transplanted children: a 19-yr review of the Swiss national reference center. J Pediatr Gastroenterol Nutr. 2017;39(3):362–98.
56. Liberal R, Vergani D, Mieli-vergani G. Recurrence of autoimmune liver disease and inflammatory bowel disease after pediatric liver transplantation. Liver Transpl. 2016;22(9):1275–83.
57. Hogler W, Baumann U, Kelly D. Endocrine and bone metabolic complications in chronic liver disease and after liver transplantation in children. J Pediatr Gastroenterol Nutr. 2012;54(3):313–21.
58. Maes M, Sokal E, Otte JB. Growth factors in children with end-stage liver disease before and after liver transplantation: a review. Pediatr Transplant. 1997;1:171–5.
59. Reding R, Gras J, Sokal E, Otte J, Davies H. Steroid-free liver transplantation in children. Lancet. 2003;362:2068–70.
60. Mohammad S, Grimberg A, Rand E, Anand R, Yin W, Alonso EM. Long-term linear growth and puberty in pediatric liver transplant recipients. J Pediatr. 2013;163(5):1354–60.
61. Kuo HT, Sampaio MS, Ye X, Reddy P, Martin P, Bunnapradist S. Risk factors for new-onset diabetes mellitus in adult liver transplant recipients, an analysis of the organ procurement and transplant network/united network for organ sharing database. Transplantation. 2010;89(9):1134–40.
62. Guichelaar MM, Schmoll J, Malinchoc M, et al. Fractures and avascular necrosis before and after orthotopic liver transplantation: long-term follow-up and predictive factors. Hepatology. 2007;46:1198–207.
63. Helenius I, Jalanko H, Remes V, et al. Scoliosis after solid organ transplantation in children and adolescents. Am J Transplant. 2006;6:324–30.
64. Gordon CM, Bachrach LK, Carpenter TO, et al. Dual energy x-ray absorptiometry interpretation and reporting in children and adolescents: the 2007 ISCD Pediatric official positions. J Clin Densitom. 2008;11:43–58.
65. McLin VA, Anand R, Daniels SR, Yin W, Alonso EM. Blood pressure elevation in long-term survivors of pediatric liver transplantation. Am J Transplant. 2012;12(1):183–90.
66. Lauer RM, Clarke WR. Childhood risk factors for high adult blood pressure: the Muscatine study. Pediatrics. 1989;84:633–41.
67. Yang JW, Cho KI, Kim JH, Kim SY, Kim CS, You GI, Lee JY, Choi SY, Lee SW, Kim HS, Heo JH, Cha TJ, Lee JW. Wall shear stress in hypertensive patients is associated with carotid vascular deformation assessed by speckle tracking strain imaging. Clin Hypertens. 2014;20:10.
68. Memaran N, Blöte R, Kirchner M, Bauer R, Beier R, et al. Ambulatory blood pressure monitoring detects high prevalence of hypertension in recipients of non-renal transplants. Paper presented at the 9th Congress of the International Pediatric Transplant Association, Barcelona, Spain, May 27, 2017.
69. Basso MS, Subramaniam P, et al. Sirolimus as renal and immunological rescue agent in pediatric liver transplant recipients. Pediatr Transplant. 2011;15:722–7.
70. Campbell MS, Kotlyar DS, Brensinger CM, et al. Renal function after orthotopic liver transplantation is predicted by duration of pretransplantation creatinine elevation. Liver Transpl. 2005;11(9):1048–55.
71. Campbell K, Ng V, Martin S, et al. Glomerular filtration rate following pediatric liver transplantation—the SPLIT experience. Am J Transplant. 2010;10(12):2673–82.
72. Kivela JM, Raisanen-Sokolowski A, et al. Long-term renal function in children after liver transplantation. Transplantation. 2011;91:115–20.
73. Flynn J, Kaelber D, Baker-Smith C, Al E. Clinical practice guideline for screening and management of high blood pressure in children and adolescents. Pediatrics. 2017;140(3).
74. Tumgor G, Arikan C, Kilic M, Frequency AS. Frequency of hyperuricemia and effect of calcineurin inhibitors on serum uric acid levels in liver transplanted children. Pediatr Transplant. 2006;10:665–8.
75. Sullivan PM, William A, Tichy EM. Hyperuricemia and gout in solid-organ transplant: update in pharmacological management. Prog Transplant. 2015;25(3):263–70.
76. Tung J, Hadzic N, Layton M, et al. Bone marrow failure in children with acute liver failure. J Pediatr Gastroenterol Nutr. 2000;31(5):557–61.
77. Itterbeek P, Demuynck H, Roskams T. Aplastic anemia after transplantation for non-A, non-B, non-C fulminant hepatic failure: case report and review of the literature. Transpl Int. 2002;15(2–3):117–23.
78. Debray D, Baudouin V, Lacaille F, Charbit M, Rivet C, et al. Pediatric Transplantation Working Group of the French Speaking Society of Transplantation. De novo malignancy after solid organ transplantation in children. Transplant Proc. 2009;41(2):674–5.
79. Lebel MJ, Chapdelaine H, Paradis L, Des Roches A, Alvarez F. Increase in de novo food allergies after pediatric liver transplantation: tacrolimus vs. cyclosporine immunosuppression. Pediatr Transplant. 2014;18(7):733–9.
80. Noble C, Peake J, Lewindon PJ. Increase in de novo allergies after paediatric liver transplantation: the Brisbane experience. Pediatr Transplant. 2011;15(5):451–4.
81. Legendre C, Caillat-Zucman S, Samuel D, et al. Transfer of symptomatic peanut allergy to the recipient of a combined liver-and-kidney transplant. N Engl J Med. 1997;337:822–4. 26.
82. Lee Y, Lee YM, Kim MJ, Lee SK, Choe YH. Long-term follow-up of de novo allergy in pediatric liver transplantation—10 yr experience of a single center. Pediatr Transplant. 2013;17(3):251–5.

83. Shroff P, Mehta RS, Chinen J, Karpen SJ, Davis CM. Presentation of atopic disease in a large cohort of pediatric liver transplant recipients. Pediatr Transplant. 2012;16(4):379–84.
84. Ducroux E, Boillot O, Ocampo MA, et al. Skin cancers after liver transplantation: retrospective single-center study on 371 recipients. Transplantation. 2014;98(3):335–40.
85. Wondimu B, Nemeth A, Modeer T. Oral health in liver transplant children administered cyclosporin A or tacrolimus. Int J Paediatr Dent. 2001;11:424–9.
86. Funakoshi Y, Ohshita C, Moritani Y, Hieda T. Dental findings of patients who underwent liver transplantation. J Clin Pediatr Dent. 1992;16:259–62.
87. Sandoval MJ, Zekeridou A, Spyropoulou V, et al. Oral health of pediatric liver transplant recipients. Pediatr Transplant. 2017;21(7):1–7. https://doi.org/10.1111/petr.13019.
88. Sundaram SS, Alonso EM, Anand R. Outcomes after liver transplantation in young infants. J Pediatr Gastroenterol Nutr. 2008;47(5):486–92.
89. Högler W, Baumann U, Kelly D. Endocrine and bone metabolic complications in chronic liver disease and after liver transplantation in children. J Pediatr Gastroenterol Nutr. 2012;54(3):313–21.
90. Yudkowitz FS, Chietero M. Anesthetic issues in pediatric liver transplantation. Pediatr Transplant. 2005;9(5):666–72.
91. Barshes NR, Chang IF, Karpen SJ, Carter BA, Goss JA. Impact of pretransplant growth retardation in pediatric liver transplantation. J Pediatr Gastroenterol Nutr. 2006;43(1):89–94.
92. Desai M, Zainuer S, Kennedy C, Kearney D, Goss J, Karpen S. Cardiac structural and functional alterations in infants and children with biliary atresia, listed for liver transplantation. Gastroenterology. 2011;141:1264–72.
93. Madan N, Arnon R. Evaluation of cardiac manifestations in pediatric liver transplant candidates. Pediatr Transplant. 2012;16:318–28.
94. Anastaze Stelle K, Belli DC, Parvex P, et al. Glomerular and tubular function following orthotopic liver transplantation in children treated with tacrolimus. Pediatr Transplant. 2012;16(3):250–6.
95. Lurz E, Quammie C, Englesbe M, Alonso EM, et al. Frailty in children with liver disease: a prospective multicenter study. J Pediatr. 2018;194:109–15.
96. Dehghani S, Aleyasin S, Honar N, et al. Pulmonary evaluation in pediatric liver transplant candidates. Indian J Pediatr. 2011;78:171–5.
97. Sahani D, Mehta A, Blake M, Prasad S, Harris G, Saini S. Preoperative hepatic vascular evaluation with CT and MR angiography: implications for surgery. Radiographics. 2004;24(5):1367–80.
98. Wasson N, Deer J, Suresh S. Anesthetic management of pediatric liver and kidney transplantation. Anesthesiol Clin. 2017;35(3):421–38.
99. Ng V, Nicholas D, Dhawan A, et al. Development and validation of the pediatric liver transplantation quality of life: a disease-specific quality of life measure for pediatric liver transplant recipients. J Pediatr. 2014;165(3):547–55.

Surgical Complications Following Transplantation

Michele Colledan, Domenico Pinelli, and Laura Fontanella

Key Points
- Surgical complications after pediatric liver transplantation are common. Occasionally, they are extremely serious and may lead to graft loss or patient death.
- Typically, life-threatening surgical complications are primary non-function, arterial and portal vein thrombosis, and acute outflow obstruction.
- Biliary complications are relatively frequent, but their management is more often successful.
- Multidisciplinary technical expertise is critical to early success of pediatric liver transplantation.

Research Needed in the Field
- To define homogeneous criteria identifying any surgical complications for a better data sharing among centers.
- To provide prospective trials on etiopathogenesis, treatment, and outcome of any complications, particularly biliary ones.
- To implement the use of "failure to rescue" as a tool improving quality assessment.

30.1 Introduction

Although liver transplantation currently achieves excellent patient and graft survival, the procedure is indeed affected by a relevant morbidity, both in the short and in the long term. This is not surprising if one considers its extreme technical and biological complexity.

M. Colledan (✉) · D. Pinelli · L. Fontanella
Department of Organ Failure and Transplantation,
Hospital Papa Giovanni XXIII, Bergamo, Italy
e-mail: mcolledan@asst-pg23.it; dpinelli@asst-pg23.it; laura.fontanella02@universitadipavia.it

Complications are commonly classified as "surgical" and "medical." However the distinction between these two different entities is not always evident. Surgical complications are generally considered as those directly related to the surgical operation or requiring a surgical treatment. In fact, often, neither of these criteria allows an absolute distinction. The etiology of complications is in most cases multifactorial, a vascular thrombosis, for example, being the possible consequence of an anastomotic defect, but also of an abnormal hypercoagulable state or of immunological phenomena on a perfect anastomosis. Similarly, a bowel perforation may be the consequence of a viral infection. On the other hand, the treatment of a single complication may require, according to its severity, a medical or a surgical management. For example, chronic rejection, which is typically an immunological event, may require a pharmacological approach or a retransplantation.

This chapter will focus on non-immunological impairments of the early function of the liver allograft, on vascular and biliary complication, on bowel perforations, and on hemorrhagic complications.

In general, the available epidemiological data on morbidity after liver transplantation are often controversial, mainly due to the lack of uniform diagnostic criteria for each complication. Also, classification of severity of the events is somewhat confusing. The Clavien-Dindo classification, mostly grading the complications on the intensity of the required management and, for example, on the need for general anesthesia, although very useful to grade surgical morbidity in adults, is of limited help in the specific setting of pediatric LT for at least two reasons. The first is that important differences exist among centers in terms of diagnostic or therapeutic aggressiveness, the same complication being managed conservatively in some centers and with aggressive procedures in others. The second is that most diagnostic and interventional procedures in small children require sedation or general anesthesia [1, 2].

Obviously, complications impact the final outcome of LT. The Studies of Pediatric Liver Transplantation (SPLIT), multicenter database including data on children undergoing liver transplantation in the USA and Canada, was analyzed for a comprehensive range of factors that may influence the outcome from the time of listing through the peri- and postoperative period. In the final model, post-transplant complications had the highest relative risk of death or graft loss; reoperation for any cause increased the risk for both patient and graft loss by 11-fold whereas reoperation exclusive of specific complications by four-fold. Vascular thrombosis, bowel perforation, septicemia, and retransplantation, each independently increased the risk of patient and graft loss by three- to fourfold [3].

Outcomes after transplantation vary between centers. Centers' capacities to quickly recognize and appropriately manage postoperative complications may be an important reason for this variation.

Reducing mortality requires addressing both the rate of complications themselves and the ability to rescue patients and grafts once complications occur. This includes both recognizing and effectively managing them.

In this sense, the concept of "failure to rescue" (FTR) is expressed by the rate of mortality in those patients who suffered a major complication:

$$FTR = \frac{\text{Patients who had a complication and died}}{\text{Patients who had a complication}}$$

FTR may help to better characterize the inter-center variability, and it may represent a useful quality improvement tool in the field of transplantation [4].

30.2 Inadequate Graft Function Recovery

Typically, the progressive recover of graft function is very rapid after LT. The earliest predictor of graft function is probably the appearance and consistency of the liver after reperfusion in the operative room. Bile production is commonly observed during the operation. Hemodynamic stability with adequate urine production, good acid-base balance, and signs of neurological recovery are all indicators too.

Elevated aminotransferase levels are common in the early hours and days and usually are not—per se—a major matter of concern as long as they remain below ×50/×80 the normal values [5]. This is particularly true for segmental grafts, which may show some degree of tissue necrosis on the cut parenchymal edge. Similarly, serum bilirubin levels are not very useful in the early assessment of organ function. Abnormalities in coagulation are common too in the first 24–48 h after transplantation but usually show a progressive improvement. It is not recommended to routinely correct coagulation abnormalities in the absence of bleeding. Lactate is mainly metabolized by the liver, and a damaged liver can itself be a source of this metabolite. Therefore, serum lactate level and more so early clearance over the first 36 h are reliable markers of early graft function [6]. Serum ammonium has been reported too as a reliable marker [5].

30.2.1 Primary Non-function (PNF)

The term "primary non-function" (PNF) is best defined as graft failure soon after graft reperfusion with no discernible cause leading to either retransplantation or death of the patient in the early postoperative phase. When the severe dysfunction appears soon but after a short initial apparently good functional recovery, the term "delayed PNF" is preferred. Although the best is currently available, these definitions are still relatively unsatisfactory for several reasons. First of all, the fact that treatment (retransplantation) is included in the definition is somewhat potentially misleading, since an aggressive retransplantation policy may preclude a spontaneous recovery of the graft function. Furthermore, the lack of a discernible cause is still questionable. In fact, graft failure due to any clearly identifiable technical problems such as hepatic artery, portal vein, or hepatic venous outflow abnormalities is excluded from the definition of PNF. Nevertheless, even in the absence of these causes, some causal factor, generally related to technical difficulties emerged during the operation and leading, for example, to an excessively long total or implantation "warm" ischemia time, or to a severe hemodynamic impairment with very low cardiac output at the time of reperfusion, can usually be identified. However, not all the patients with these factors developed a PNF. The incidence of PNF is reported between 0.9 and 7.2% [7].

Typically, its features are severe neurological impairment, with uncorrectable coagulopathy, very high transaminases, and persistently high serum lactate and ammonia, together with hypoglycemia, metabolic acidosis, and oliguria. The situation is substantially similar to acute liver failure in that spontaneous recovery of the graft is theoretically possible, if the patients survive long enough. The choice between adding the risk of a retransplantation and that of waiting for a spontaneous recovery, which may not be rapid enough, requires a high level of clinical judgment and is related to the specific national or local availability of donors.

In the SPLIT database, PNF was the indication in 44% of the pediatric recipients who were retransplanted within the first 30 postoperative days [8].

By definition, the outcome is death or graft loss.

30.2.2 Initial Poor Function (IPF) or Early Graft Dysfunction (EGD)

All other conditions of early graft dysfunction, which do not result in retransplantation or death, represent a borderline, reversible syndrome and are defined as initial poor function (IPF) or early graft dysfunction (EGD), with an incidence ranging between 5.2 and 36.3%.

Most studies assess IPF based on time intervals during the first postoperative days or weeks and use liver-related laboratory parameters.

Olthoff, for example, proposed that IPF is present when one or more of the following variables are observed: bilirubin ≥ 10 mg/dL and international normalized ratio (INR) ≥ 1.6 on postoperative day 7, with a peak of transaminases >2000 IU/L in the first week [9].

30.2.3 Graft/Recipient Size Mismatch

A graft excessively small for the recipient size or, more frequent in children, too large to fit in the abdominal cavity may be a relevant cause of failure of the graft itself or, more in general, of morbidity. Small-for-size syndrome (SFSS) is a well-known entity in adult patients, particularly in those receiving a segmental graft. When the liver graft is excessively small, an imbalance between the excessive portal flow and the arterial one generates SFSS, which typically appears after the fourth/fifth postoperative day and is characterized by coagulopathy ascites and progressive cholestasis. The evolution is toward sepsis and multiple organ failure and ultimately death in up to 50% of cases [10]. In fact, since most pediatric candidates to LT are very small, the problem of an excessively small liver, although possible, is very uncommon. On the other hand, the opposite is more easily the case, when the liver graft is excessively large to fit the space available in the recipient's abdominal cavity. In this situation, the blood inflow may be insufficient to supply the needs of the graft itself. Furthermore, the closure of the abdominal cavity under tension may worsen perfusion of the graft [11] and more in general of the abdominal viscera, generating an abdominal compartment syndrome with graft and even multiple organ failure [12, 13]. Few studies have targeted the problem of size matching in pediatric LT, and no strict consensus is available on how to deal with it. The relevant parameter, well studied in adults, is graft-to-recipient weight ratio (GRWR). The normal ratio between the native liver and the body weight in healthy adults is generally about 2%, and the minimal safe GRWR is currently considered to be 0.8/1%. The minimal safe GRWR for pediatric LT has never been precisely defined but, considering that the ratio between the native liver and body weight, varies with age, ranging from 4% in infants and small children to 3% in younger adolescents; it has been suggested to be above 1.9/2% [14, 15].

On the other hand, the safe upper limit of GRWR is considered to range between 4 and 6 or even above [14–17].

Prevention of relevant size mismatch relies, obviously, on proper donor selection. However, this is not always possible: in deceased donors, prediction of a segmental graft volume based on anthropometric data is not completely reliable, and a CT scan, which would allow for adequate volume measurement, is not always available. On the other hand, when liver donation is considered, in countries with limited or no deceased donor availability, there is often little donor choice. When the risk of a SFSS is expected, portal flow modulation may help preventing the complication. This may be achieved by splenic artery ligation or embolization or, very uncommonly in children, by surgical or radiological partial portal flow diversion. On the other hand, the options for prevention of a "large-for-size syndrome" (LFSS) range from the use of mono-segmental or hyper-reduced grafts to delayed closure of the abdomen or the use of prosthesis to enlarge the abdominal wall. These are described in the chapter on surgical techniques. A very aggressive attitude in preventing relevant size mismatching and managing its manifestations is strongly recommended since, once SFSS or LFSS are established, retransplantation may be the only alternative to patient's death.

30.3 Vascular Complications

Vascular complications after pediatric liver transplantation are rare but potentially devastating. These may involve the reconstruction of the hepatic artery, the portal vein, or the graft venous outflow and may range from complete thrombosis, representing the most serious form, to strictures, flow abnormalities, or other alterations.

30.3.1 Arterial Complications

Arterial problems after pediatric LT include hepatic artery thrombosis (HAT), hepatic artery strictures (including twisting or kinking), and hepatic artery aneurisms (HAA) (Table 30.1).

30.3.1.1 Hepatic Artery Thrombosis (HAT)
HAT is the most common form of vascular complication and the main cause of graft loss in pediatric LT.

HAT is classified into two categories: early (<4 weeks) HAT (e-HAT) and late (>4 weeks) HAT (l-HAT).

In a systematic literature review, Bekker et al. reported an overall incidence of 8.3% in children for e-HAT with 34.3% mortality [18].

30.3.1.2 HAT Risk Factors

A number of predisposing factors were described. Besides obvious technical causes (such as narrow anastomosis, kinking, twisting, small and mismatched vessel size, and complex anatomy), hypercoagulable state, rejection, prolonged ischemia, and cytomegalovirus infection are also reported (Table 30.1).

It is a general belief that technical variant grafts (reduced SL, SLT, and LDLT) may be associated with a lower incidence of HAT than WL grafts. The underlying thought is that segmental liver grafts mostly come from adult donors with potentially larger vessel diameter; however, this is not true for grafts with living donors that only rely on segmental arteries and in split grafts when the choice is made to leave the main arterial axis with the other graft. Publications dealing with these issues showed contradictory results, and a recent meta-analysis comparing pediatric whole liver transplantation and technical variant liver transplantation showed a comparable incidence between the two groups [19]. Also, Bekker found no significant difference and reported an incidence of 3.1% and 4.6% in living donor LT and deceased donor LT, respectively [18]. An accurate microsurgical technique with the use of magnification is considered relevant in preventing HAT; however, again, no difference was reported in incidence among centers using the operation microscope for the arterial anastomosis (3.1%) versus centers using loupe magnification (2.1%) [20]. Anticoagulation/antiplatelet agents have also been advocated as effective prevention means.

Table 30.1 Arterial complications

Incidence	*Risk factors*
Overall Arterial Complications Incidence 3–9%	**Donor factors**
Classification	Hypercoagulable state
Hepatic artery thrombosis (HAT)	CMV D/R mismatch
Hepatic artery stenosis (HAS)	Complex donor arterial anatomy
Aneurism	**Recipient factors**
Onset	Complex arterial anatomy
Early HAT : <30 days 8.3% [18]	Immunological or genetic factors
Late HAT : >30 days <5% [33]	Infection
	Celiac stenosis or compression by arcuate ligament
	Multiple rejections
	Operative factors
	Difficult anastomosis
	Complex back-table arterial reconstruction
	HAS and kinking
	Ischemia time
	Number of FFP and/or blood transfusions
	Aortic conduit for arterial reconstruction
	Roux-en-Y biliary reconstruction
	Postoperative factors
	Ischemia-reperfusion injury
	Bile leak
	Cholangitis
	Re-laparotomy
Manifestation	*Treatment approaches*
Early HAT (<30 days)	**Early HAT**
Mild elevation in transaminases and bilirubin	• *Endovascular Intervention (EI)*
Ischemia/necrosis of bile duct	Intra-arterial thrombolysis
Sepsis	Percutaneous transarterial angioplasty (PTA)
Fulminant liver necrosis (48 h)	Stent placement
Acidosis	• *Surgical revision*
Transaminase values rise abruptly	Thrombectomy and reanastomosis
Coagulopathy/encephalopathy/oliguria	• *Urgent retransplantation*
Late HAT (>30 days)	• *Observation*
Asymptomatic (radiological investigations)	**Late HAT**
Insidious course: cholangitis, relapsing fever, bacteremia	• *Biliary stent placement*
Symptomatic: from biliary complications to liver failure	• *Endovascular treatment*
Diagnosis	• Retransplantation
Doppler US protocol surveillance	**HAS**
HAS diagnosis: peak systolic velocity < 20 cm/s	• *Medical treatment*: anticoagulation and observation
and/or resistive index <0.6	• *Interventional PTA ± stent*
Angiogram indications despite normal serum liver tests:	• *Surgical redo*
peak systolic velocity < 10 cm/s	• *Retransplantation*
and/or resistive index <0.5	
CT Angiogram - Angiography	

The reported median time to detection of HAT was 6.9 days in e-HAT (range 1–17.5 days postoperative) and 6 months in l-HAT (range 1.8–79 months) [18].

The early form is mostly considered as caused by technical factors, whereas l-HAT, on which a more limited number of reports are available, is often thought to be the consequence of immunological events. The reported incidence rates are generally higher for e-HAT than for l-HAT but, since the latter may remain clinically indolent, with nonspecific symptoms like back pain, shoulder pain, or fatigue, or even completely silent, this may only reflect a lack of appropriate diagnosis.

Retransplantation is an important risk factor for e-HAT. Oh et al. reported that primary transplantations were associated with an e-HAT incidence of 1.6%, increasing to 4.8% and 12.5% in second and third retransplantation, respectively [21].

30.3.1.3 HAT Manifestations/Diagnosis

The natural history of acute HAT is characterized by ischemic necrosis of the bile ducts, whose vascularization solely relies on arterial blood supply, which is usually followed by uncontrollable sepsis, occasionally gangrene of the liver, and ultimately by patient's death (Table 30.1).

In fact, however, the time and rapidity of onset of the thrombosis and the possibility of development of collaterals have a strong influence on its clinical manifestations to a spectrum that ranges from the catastrophic pattern described above to completely asymptomatic situations. Collaterals may develop, particularly in children, from the superior mesenteric (mostly via the vessels of the Roux-en-Y loop of the biliary reconstruction) and/or from the splenic and phrenic arteries. As a result, three main patterns of clinical manifestation were identified by Tzakis et al. [22]:

1. Massive hepatic necrosis. It is more typical of e-HAT and generally represents a dramatic clinical emergency, requiring urgent retransplantation for survival.
2. Delayed biliary leak.
3. Intermittent episodes of sepsis without an immediately evident source but generally related to intrahepatic biliary injury.

Early diagnosis is of fundamental relevance, allowing to immediately take the appropriate measures, in order to improve the success rate, and reducing mortality.

All liver transplant centers apply a screening protocol for preemptive detection of vascular complication post-LT, based on Doppler ultrasonography (DUS), which is a proven noninvasive investigation for the assessment of hepatic artery patency [23, 24].

The protocols differ for frequency, interval, and duration of screening. Generally DUS is performed at least daily, or more frequently, for a period of at least 1 week after transplantation and less frequently later on. After discharge of the patient, it is repeated at any follow-up control and whenever clinical manifestations suggest the possibility of HAT.

The most common findings on Doppler US are the absence of arterial signals (sensitivity 92%). Resistance index (RI) is a useful parameter that reflects vascular resistance and compliance. Kaneko and associates observed that sensitivity and specificity of RI for HAT detection were 83% and 85% when the threshold was set at 0.6 (normal range 0.6–0.8). Other experiences confirmed that RI of <0.6 is the most sensitive and specific single parameter for predicting HAT [25, 26].

The diagnosis is then confirmed by multi-detector computed tomographic angiography (MDCTA), which has emerged as an accurate, fast, and noninvasive imaging technique, alternative to the more invasive catheter angiography, for the diagnosis of vascular complications following LT [27].

MDCTA can precisely delineate the patency of the hepatic artery and anatomical defects such as stenosis or kinks with a sensitivity of 100%, a specificity of 89%, and an accuracy of 95% [28].

Conventional catheter angiography is usually reserved as a next step, when an interventional treatment is contemplated.

30.3.1.4 HAT: Treatment

Because HAT, particularly in the early form, has a high mortality, an aggressive management is required.

Retransplantation is typically the treatment of choice, which may be required urgently, mostly in the early forms, or electively or semi-electively, mostly in the late forms. However, in e-HAT, since the clinical evolution may be extremely rapid, some revascularization procedure is generally attempted while waiting for retransplantation, in order to gain time and possibly salvage the graft (Table 30.1).

There are two major options for revascularization: endovascular procedures and open surgery. The former includes intra-arterial thrombolysis, percutaneous transluminal angioplasty (PTA), and stent placement. The latter includes thrombectomy and reanastomosis. The most effective treatment approach remains controversial.

Endovascular intervention (EI) is performed by abdominal angiography and carried out under general anesthesia. If a decrease or disappearance of blood flow through the anastomosed site is confirmed, the first treatment may be the intra-arterial thrombolysis [20].

There is no consensus on the dosage nor on the optimal technique for catheter-directed delivery of any thrombolytic agent as they have been successfully used as continuous infusion or bolus push. Vasodilators may be associated.

Selective intra-arterial thrombolysis via hepatic artery has several advantages versus a systemic one, such as small thrombolytic dose, high local concentration, and little influence on systemic hemostasis.

Most of the studies recommended the association of heparin with thrombolytic therapy to maintain the partial thromboplastin time between 1.5 and 2.5 times the control value.

Careful monitoring of coagulation profile and clinical symptoms are mandatory.

Hemorrhage was the most common complication seen in about 20% of the patients as bloody abdominal fluid drainage or leakage of contrast medium during the procedure [20].

Dilation of the obstructed artery with a PTA balloon catheter is an alternative or may be associated to thrombolysis, with stenting in case of recurrent stricture.

The revascularization is defined as successful when the peak systolic velocity is >20.0 cm/s and/or the resistive index is 0.6 [20, 29].

On the other hand, arterial revascularization may be performed surgically by laparotomy. The arterial anastomosis is exposed and carefully observed: when a hematoma, abscess, and/or kinking of the anastomotic site is thought to be the cause of the obstruction, it is removed. Generally the anastomosis is explored and thrombectomy is performed. When an improvement in blood flow is not obtained a new anastomosis is performed either directly or by an interposition graft. Although the principal aim of these procedures is to gain time while waiting for retransplantation, occasionally, when they are performed very early, usually at a pre-symptomatic stage, their effectiveness may go beyond. The patient's clinical condition dictates management, and if the liver function remains stable, retransplantation may cautiously be postponed or possibly avoided [30].

In fact in some series, children with hepatic artery thrombosis survived without retransplantation.

Ackermann et al. reported Hospital Bicetre experience in 45 pediatric liver transplants complicated by early HAT (<15 pod) adopting an aggressive surgical revascularization strategy. Over a period of 20 years, four main results emerged: (1) early detection of e-HAT by DUS is of paramount importance; (2) successful surgical revascularization was associated with significantly higher survival than failed or unattempted revascularization; (3) unsuccessful revascularization was not detrimental compared to unattempted revascularization; and (4) the aggressive combination of urgent surgical HA revascularization, biliary interventional radiology, and/or surgery and retransplantation led to long-term patient survival of 80%, identical to that of children who did not experience HAT [31].

Regardless the revascularization strategy adopted (surgical or radiological intervention), when timely availability of grafts for retransplantation is lacking, mortality of HAT will be higher [30, 32].

Approximately, one half of the patients presenting with "late" HAT are asymptomatic, and the thrombosis is detected during routine ultrasonographic evaluation of the hepatic vasculature. Survival of patients who are symptomatic at the time of diagnosis is lower than for asymptomatic ones (40% vs. 82%, respectively). Most patients with l-HAT may initially be managed conservatively, but 25–30% will develop graft failure or biliary strictures in spite of the possibility to initially treat them with biliary stents or with surgical reconstructions, virtually all of these patients will, in the long term, require retransplantation. Importantly, the window of opportunity in which these patients can be retransplanted is narrow, as biliary sepsis is common and contributes significantly up to 50% mortality rate observed with retransplantation [33].

30.3.1.5 Other Arterial Complications

Arterial strictures may be the consequence of a defective technique (twisting, kinking, stenosis, intimal flap) or of intimal proliferation or extrinsic compression. They may be completely asymptomatic or present with different patterns, most commonly related to ischemia of the bile ducts. They are generally suspected when an intrahepatic Doppler US waveform shows a prolonged systolic acceleration time and a low RI (<0.5) with a "tardus parvus" pattern [34]. In this case a focal peak velocity greater than 2 m/s along the course of the main hepatic artery is diagnostic (if not detected the differential diagnosis must include HAT with development of collateral vessels). The diagnosis is then confirmed by MDCTA. Since they may predispose to subsequent HAT, an aggressive management may be recommended. This is usually achieved by PTA with or without stenting.

Another arterial cause of graft arterial impairment is so-called splenic artery steal syndrome. This is represented by an abnormally low flow in the hepatic artery in the presence of an enlarged splenic artery which is so common in children with portal hypertension. In fact, the name is inappropriate since the arterial flow reduction is not caused by a steal phenomenon but rather by a hepatic artery buffer response to the excess of flow in the portal vein from an extremely enlarged spleen. The more appropriated name "splenic artery syndrome" has therefore been suggested. This condition may be a cause of functional impairment of the liver graft or cholangiopathy and may predispose to HAT. When identified, it may be effectively managed by ligation or embolization of the splenic artery, achieving a reduction in the portal flow [35].

Extrahepatic and intrahepatic arterial aneurysms and pseudoaneurysms represent an uncommon but serious complication of pediatric liver transplantation. Management is variable according to the circumstances, but an aggressive approach is generally recommended. A peculiar, rare, but severe entity is represented by mycotic aneurysms. In spite of the name, these may be caused by both bacterial and fungal infections. Early symptoms and diagnosis are extremely rare. Actually, they most often present acutely, with dissection or rupture, which explains the high related mortality [36, 37]. Treatment consists of both bleeding control, in an emergency setting, and eradication of the infection. Despite the risk of graft loss and need for retransplantation, ligation of the hepatic artery seems to better cope with this goal rather than immediate revascularization in an infected field [38].

30.3.2 Portal Vein Complications

Portal vein complications (PVCs) are another significant cause of postoperative morbidity and occasionally of graft failure, occurring in 3–19% of pediatric LT [39].

They are also generally classified as "early" (which may include intraoperative forms) or "late," according to the date of presentation, with a cutoff at the third postoperative month [40], the former being generally deemed as caused by technical problems and the latter by fibrous hyperplasia of the new intima followed by fibrous and organic thrombus [40, 41].

The spectrum ranges from portal vein thrombosis (PVT) to portal vein stenosis and to flow abnormalities [42] (Table 30.2).

30.3.2.1 Portal Vein Thrombosis (PVT)

PVT causes a partial or complete obstruction of the vessel; it's a rare (2–7%) but serious event that may lead to occasionally serious graft impairment [43].

30.3.2.2 PVT: Risk Factors

The low incidence makes it difficult to estimate the variables associated with early and late PVT, but, clearly, the development of PVT is multifactorial (Table 30.2).

Risk factors for early PVT include graft-, recipient-, and technique-related issues.

Table 30.2 Portal vein complications

Incidence		Risk factors
Portal vein complications (PVC)	0–33%	**Early PVT**
Classification		Recipient-related issues (young age, body weight < 6 kg, BA)
Portal vein thrombosis (PVT)	1–4%	Recipient portal hypoplasia
Portal vein stenosis (PVS)	3%	Preexistent portosystemic shunt
– Anastomotic		Prior splenectomy
– Non-anastomotic		Segmental graft (reduced size, split, living related)
Portal flow anomalies		Other technical-related issues
Onset		Large-for-size graft (GBWR >4%)
Early PVC: <30/90 POD		D/R vessel size mismatch
Late PVC: >30/90 POD		Anastomotic stricture or HVOO
		Anastomotic twisting/kinking
		Interposition vein grafts (cryopreserved)
		Long cold ischemia time (>12 h) retransplantation
		Late PVT
		Younger and smaller recipients
		Other vascular or biliary complications
		Chronic graft rejection
		Chronic cholangitis
Manifestation/diagnosis		*Treatment approaches*
PVT: Early onset		**PVT**
Graft dysfunction: from mild to acute graft failure		**Early onset**[a]
Late onset		• *Open surgery*: anastomotic revision and thrombectomy
Mild liver impairment		• *Radiological interventional approach*
Portal hypertension manifestations*		Transhepatic
Symptomatic portal biliopathy		Transplenic
Growth delay, neurocognitive impairment		Transjugular
PVS: Portal hypertension manifestations		Transmesenteric
Portal hypertension manifestations *:Ascites		• *Early retransplantation*
Splenomegaly		**Late onset**[a]
GI (variceal) bleeding		• *Systemic anticoagulation only*
Hypersplenism		• *Interventional management (including TIPPS)*
Abnormal liver function tests		• *Meso-REX shunt*
Portosystemic shunt-related hyper-IgA		• *Surgical portosystemic shunt*
Screening : Doppler; TAC		• *Retransplantation*
Diagnosis: angiography/venogram (gold standard)		**PVS**
		Early/late onset[a]
		• Percutaneous transhepatic angioplasty (PTA) ± stenting

[a]Starting systemic anticoagulant therapy

1. *Graft-Related Issues*

    In general terms, PVT is more frequent with segmental grafts (necessarily and by far more frequently used in children) than with whole size ones [44]. Graft to recipient size matching is also relevant, a higher incidence of PVT being reported for GRWR >4% [45].

2. *Recipient-Related Issues*

    Any condition in the recipient that may lead to a reduced flow in the portal vein may represent a risk factor for PVT. The most common condition is the presence of large collaterals with spontaneous portosystemic shunts causing a "steal syndrome" [42]. Such shunts, when evident, should be ligated.

    In BA, the rapid evolution of fibrosis and portal hypertension, besides the development of large collaterals, may lead to hypoplasia of the portal vein with thickening of its wall [46]. These conditions predispose to the development of PVT; a small portal vein diameter was reported as a highly significant risk factor with cutoffs at 3.5 or 5 mm [47, 48].

    The size of the recipient matters too, with smaller children being more exposed: in the series from Kyoto, a body weight < 6 kg was the only significant risk factor for PVT at multivariate analysis [49]. Less common conditions in children may be a preexistent thrombosis or a previous splenectomy [50].

3. *Technical Issues*

In general, size or length discrepancy between the donor and recipient vascular stumps, leading to anastomotic excessive tension, or kinking, or twisting, may predispose to PVT. Little consensus exists on the best technical option to face the caliber or length mismatch when performing the portal anastomosis. In Kyoto experience there were no significant differences in PVT rates among five types of reconstruction: standard end-to-end method, branch-patch or bifurcation method, spleno-mesenteric confluence method, patch graft method, and interposition graft [49].

In the Saint Luc University Hospital experience, portoplasty (patch graft method) seemed to provide the best results when an end-to-end anastomosis was not feasible because of PV hypoplasia [51]. The use of interposition grafts doesn't seem to be a significant risk factor [49] at least with increasing experience [52] and except when cryopreserved grafts are used [53].

Long ischemia time, compartment syndrome due to LFSS, outflow disturbances, and a high intra- and postoperative hematocrit may increase the incidence of thrombosis. A low portal flow (<7 cm/s) after reperfusion of the liver graft is a relevant predictor [49, 50].

30.3.2.3 PVT: Manifestations/Diagnosis

Early PVT presentation may range from a completely silent situation to acute graft necrosis and failure. This latter is an uncommon manifestation, generally limited to cases with very early occurrence, usually in the first 24 postoperative hours. The more typical pattern is that of a mild to moderate graft functional impairment (Table 30.2).

In late-onset PVT (or in the chronic evolution of the early form), the function of the graft shows generally little or no impairment. The picture is initially silent and thereafter progressively dominated by the portal hypertension, with ascites, splenomegaly, hypersplenism, and gastrointestinal bleeding. This latter is more often chronic than acute and usually comes from the bowel, since classical gastroesophageal varices seldom develop. The same pattern is observed in the chronic evolution of the untreated early forms.

In the long term, the further evolution may include portal cavernoma, symptomatic portal biliopathy, growth retardation, neurocognitive impairment, hepatopulmonary or portopulmonary syndrome, and in general severe limitations of the quality of life.

Doppler US is the first-level exam for detecting PVT and more in general abnormalities in the portal vein. As previously mentioned, in the Arterial Complications section, most centers perform this exam systematically, at least daily in the first postoperative days, and in any case of clinical suspicion. It is sensitive and specific in detecting complete and partial PVT even when asymptomatic. In case of doubt, CT scan precisely confirms the diagnosis and allows for prompt treatment.

30.3.2.4 PVT: Treatment

Aggressive early management of PVT is strongly advisable in order to prevent early and long-term consequences; the earlier it is, the more likely it is to be effective (Table 30.2).

Systemic anticoagulation is usually employed but never sufficient. Except for rare cases showing acute liver failure and prompting for urgent retransplantation, generally the early forms are managed by surgical thrombectomy. This may be achieved through the recessus of Rex or, more commonly and effectively, by disunion of the anastomosis. This allows a careful removal of the thrombus both on the proximal and distal side, and a new anastomosis is then performed. Any possible cause of reduced flow that might have been overlooked at the transplant operation, such as significant portal collaterals causing a "steal" phenomenon or mispositioning of the liver graft resulting in kinking, should then be looked for and removed. However, the reoperation may be very complex due to the need for a cross-clamping of both the proximal and the distal stump, this latter typically very short in segmental grafts, as well as to the presence of the biliary anastomosis that may easily be partially or totally disrupted during the maneuvers. For this reason an interventional approach by a percutaneous [54], surgical, or hybrid access is increasingly being proposed allowing a "no-touch hilum" procedure [55]. This requires a catheter access to the portal system that may be achieved either percutaneously, via transjugular, transhepatic [56], or even trans-splenic route [57, 58], or surgically, by cannulation of the branches of the recessus of Rex (that were ligated during the splitting or the living donor procedure) [59] or of the ileocolic vein at the jejunal mesenterium [55, 60].

This latter allows anterograde control of all the portal system. After cannulation, pharmacological or mechanical direct thrombolysis may be performed. Significant diverting collaterals may also be identified and embolized [61–63] (Fig. 30.1).

The same aggressiveness is warranted in late PVT, be it primary or recurrent after failure of the management of an early form. In these cases, surgical exploration and redo anastomosis are not an advisable option and, in fact, seldom performed. Interventional radiological management is more commonly used, through the accesses listed above, and includes recanalization of the thrombosed vessel, with controversy on the use of stents, due to the concern of growth and to the possible future need for retransplantation. When increased intraparenchymal resistance, such as in chronic rejection, is considered to be a cause of the thrombosis, a transjugular intrahepatic portosystemic shunt (TIPS) may also be placed. This resolves the portal hypertension but in the long term may lead to the consequences of hyperdynamic splanchnic flow, such as pulmonary hypertension and development of splanchnic aneurisms.

Failure of these interventional maneuvers may worsen the situation, causing extension of the thrombosis to both the mesenteric and the intrahepatic branches, thus precluding any further management. An elegant and very effective surgical alternative, when allowed by the anatomical condition, is therefore represented by the meso-Rex shunt. This option effectively restores a physiological situation achieving an optimal and persistent result and represents probably the most appropriate management [40, 64]. However it has to be performed early after the diagnosis since the required dissection when a chronic TVP with portal cavernoma is established is always absolutely troublesome.

Patients with established PVT, who failed interventional treatment and/or are not suitable to meso-Rex procedure,

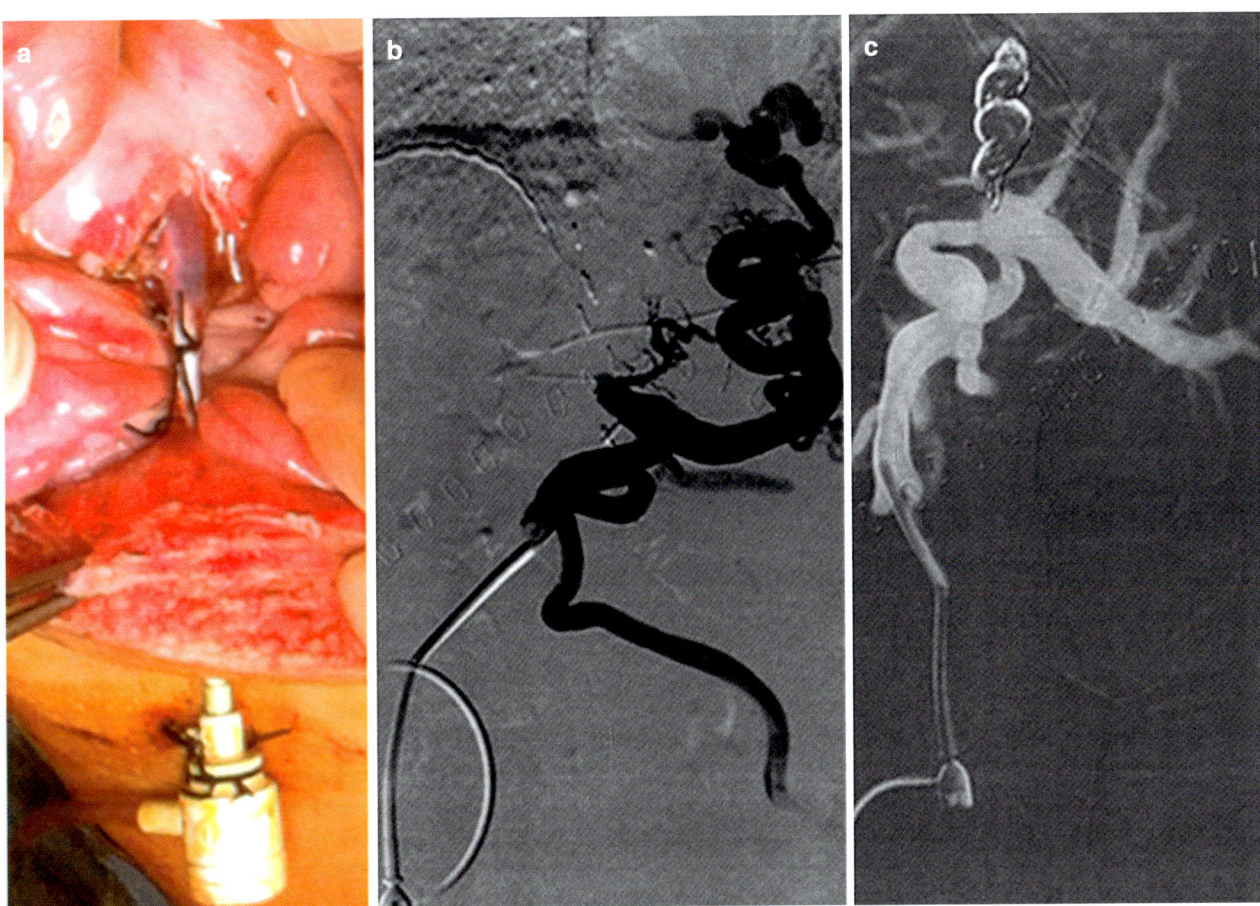

Fig. 30.1 Intraoperative portal vein thrombosis: successful combined surgical and radiological approach. (**a**) Transabdominal angiographic sheath inserted through a collateral of the mesenteric vein. (**b**) Anterograde portal venography showing portal vein thrombosis (white arrow) and large portosystemic shunts. (**c**) Resolution of portal vein thrombosis after fibrinolysis and shunts embolization

may temporarily benefit from a palliative portosystemic shunt. However, in the long run, they will all inevitably need a retransplantation that is usually very challenging. In fact, dissection of the liver in these cases, when portal cavernoma is fully developed, is really troublesome and extraordinarily hemorrhagic; mortality is therefore very high. Furthermore, in some instances, the thrombosis may completely extend in the roots of the portal vein. Finally, the hyperdynamic splanchnic flow may cause the formation of diffuse multiple splanchnic aneurysms, to extents that may preclude the possibility of retransplantation itself.

30.3.2.5 Other Portal Vein Complications

Portal vein stenosis or other flow disturbances, such as turbulence or flow inversion, usually present with little signs and symptoms if any and are detected by systematic DUS. The diagnosis of stenosis may be confirmed by CT scan. Careful evaluation of these conditions is to be encouraged, including assessment of the liver graft condition. In general, an aggressive approach is probably advisable, particularly when they exceed 50% of the lumen, since these may evolve in PVT. With the exception of some very early case that is considered caused by a technical defect and may be managed by redo surgery [65], stenoses are usually best treated by interventional radiology dilatation and in case of recoil or recurrence by stent placement [66]. If so, placement of the stent should always be performed in agreement with the surgeon, keeping in mind the possible future need for a retransplantation.

30.3.3 Hepatic Vein Outflow Obstruction (HVOO)

HVOO is a general term reflecting any impairment of the HV outflow by any cause. Its incidence after pediatric LT varies from 0 to 28% (Table 30.3).

Complete occlusion, with an acute Budd-Chiari syndrome, is a very uncommon event, usually requiring urgent retransplantation, whereas mild to moderate obstruction is more often the case (Table 30.3A).

30.3.3.1 HVOO: Risk Factors

Outflow reconstruction is one of the crucial factors in the recipient operation, and the creation of a wide anastomosis is a keypoint for preventing HVOO. This is particularly true when segmental grafts are used and the outflow reconstruction is by an anastomosis, typically end-to-side, between the graft hepatic vein(s) and the preserved recipient's vena cava, which is by far most commonly the case in pediatric LT. On the other hand, HVOO are very rare in the less common situations where the liver graft includes the donor's vena cava and a cavo-caval anastomosis of any kind is performed.

Typically, the most common anastomosis [67] is preferably single and has a triangular shape to ensure an adequate width, and it is short to avoid kinking (by using the margin of the graft vein at its entry point in the parenchyma) [68]. Several variants have however been reported, mostly in retrospective studies, with controversial results, and no advantage can objectively be advocated to any alternative option [69, 70].

Table 30.3 Caval/hepatic vein complications

Incidence		Risk factors
Hepatic vein outflow obstruction (HVOO)	0–28%	**Segmental livers in pediatric patients (DDSLT/LDLT)**
Classification		Small anastomotic orifice
Mechanical outflow obstruction		Venoplasty of the graft hepatic veins
Technical problems		Preservation of the retro-hepatic vena cava?
Compression and twisting caused by graft regeneration		Graft dislocation
Intimal hyperplasia and fibrosis at the anastomotic sites		Stenotic anastomosis
Sinusoidal obstruction syndrome (SOS)		**Late causes**
		Growth/dislocation of the graft
		Retransplantation
Manifestation/diagnosis		*Treatment approaches*
Early onset		• *Balloon angioplasty* = gold standard
Insidious presentation may make diagnosis challenging		If early or multiple recurrences:
Classical presentation (acute Budd-Chiari syndrome)		*Expandable metallic stent (EMS)*
Ascites (delayed resolution)		(consider child growth; difficulty in retransplantation)
Right-sided pleural effusion. Pericardial effusion		• *Reoperation* (rarely employed)
Low serum levels of albumin and high levels of bilirubin		• *Retransplantation* in case of severe organ dysfunction
Center lobular necrosis (CLN) at liver biopsy		
Less commonly coagulopathy or even fulminant graft failure		
Late onset		
Ascites		
Splenomegaly		
Abnormal liver function tests		
Screening study: Doppler US		
Diagnosis: Venogram		
Hepatic vein-cava P. gradient >3–5 mmHg		

The presence of multiple suprahepatic veins in the graft requiring a venoplasty or multiple anastomoses is however an important risk factor. In Kyoto experience, the cases with presence of multiple graft veins treated by venoplasty showed a significantly high incidence of HVOO ($p = 0.030$) [69].

In the same series at the univariate analysis, a low recipient-to-donor body weight ratio (i.e., a high donor-to-recipient weight ratio) and a hyper-reduced graft were significant risk factors for HVOO, while recipient's age (<1 vs. >1 year) did not affect the incidence of obstructive complications, unlike other authors stated [71].

Anteroposterior compression of the graft at closure of the abdomen has deemed as the causal element. And an alternative hyper-reduction technique to modify the anteroposterior diameter of the graft was proposed.

All these surgical factors contribute to early outflow obstruction (Table 30.3).

Late-onset HVOO are rather correlated with parenchymal regeneration and graft growth after LT causing twisting, stretching, or compression of the vessels.

30.3.3.2 HVOO: Manifestations/Diagnosis

Patients with HVOO most commonly present with ascites and/or right-sided pleural effusion, often in the setting of otherwise normal graft function. The presenting sign may only be a marked delay in resolution of ascites following transplant. Less commonly, patients have been reported to present with altered liver function or even severe graft failure [69] (Table 30.3).

As for other vascular complications, DUS is the first-level imaging technique, followed by CT scan. However these investigations are seldom very helpful since the alterations may be subtle, even in the presence of relevant clinical manifestations. Histology may show centrilobular necrosis that may possibly be mistaken for acute cellular rejection [72]. In most cases, the diagnosis may be confirmed only by venogram with measurement of hepatic vein-vena cava pressure gradient which is considered the gold standard, and a measurement of a trans-anastomotic pressure gradient >3–5 mmHg may be diagnostic.

30.3.3.3 HVOO: Treatment

The most common treatment for HVOO is pneumatic anastomosis dilation performed during the diagnostic angiography (Table 30.3).

At the end of the procedure, the morphology and the reduction of the pressure gradient define the success of the procedure itself.

A relapse is possible in about 50% of cases and may be treated successfully with the same technique.

In early or repeated recurrences, the placement of a self-expandable metallic stent may be considered, yet keeping in mind the possibility of displacement with growth and the problems that may arise in case of retransplantation.

Exceptional options are represented by surgical stricturoplasty with venous patch and veno-atrial anastomosis; however the difficult anatomic position and the risks related with re-intervention limit these indications [73].

In cases presenting with acute graft failure or those with failure of percutaneous radiological interventions and concomitant worsening of graft function, retransplantation may be the only surgical option.

30.4 Biliary Complications (BCs)

BCs represent a relevant cause of morbidity in pediatric LT. Their incidence is reported with a high variability, ranging between 10% and 35% which is probably related to the lack of homogeneous diagnostic criteria.

In general the incidence is higher in recipients of segmental grafts [74–78].

They are classified as early or late with a cutoff ranging, according to the different authors, between 1 and 3 months, early ones being generally considered more as the consequence of technical issues.

Different types of complications may be recognized (Table 30.4):

1. Biliary leak (BL), typically early and occurring either at the anastomosis or at the cut surface of segmental grafts, with an incidence ranging from 2 to 15% [79, 80]. When BL is small and self-limited, it may result in bilomas.
2. Anastomotic stricture (AS), representing a focal narrowing of the anastomosis, with an incidence ranging between 2 and 35% [75, 81].
3. Non-anastomotic stricture (NAS), including strictures located other than at the anastomosis site, generally in the graft intrahepatic biliary system or in extrahepatic one, when present [82].
4. Missing or excluded duct is a segmental bile duct not in continuity with the main biliary tree of a partial allograft that remains unrecognized, and therefore ligated, during the donor procedure. Its incidence may reach 40% after LDLT.

30.4.1 BCs: Risk Factors

Ischemia is a crucial element. As previously mentioned, the blood supply to the wall of the biliary ducts relies solely on the hepatic arterial flow and is provided by thin periductal arterial plexuses. Furthermore, the plexus for the left hepatic duct, which is the anastomotic site for left segmental grafts, most commonly used in children, arises generally from the

Table 30.4 Biliary complications (BCs)

Incidence	*Risk factors*
Overall Biliary Complications (BCs) Incidence 15–40%	**BL-BS**
Classification	**Contradictory data about**
Bile leakage (BL)	Type of anastomosis: bilioenteric/duct to duct
Anastomotic leak/disruption	Graft type: segmental grafts
Non-anastomotic leak (graft's cut surface)	Multiple ducts
Biliary stricture (BS)	Technical factors:
Anastomotic strictures (AS)	Ductoplasty
Non-anastomotic strictures (NAS)	Microsurgery
Missing or excluded segmental duct	Sutures (running/interrupted)
Ligated duct: segmental bile duct excluded (40% in LDLT)	Stenting
	NAS
	Ischemic (arterial or other)
	Microangiopathic injury (donor factors):
	Preservation injury, prolonged ischemia times, DCD
	Immunogenetic injury:
	ABO incompatibility, rejection, autoimmune dis., CMV
Manifestation/diagnosis	*Treatment approaches*
BL	**BL - Anastomotic leak, cut surface leak**
Observation of the contents of abdominal drain	• *Conservative* (low output)
Comparison of bilirubin levels from abdominal drainage	• *Radiological interventional/surgical* (high output)
BS High degree of clinical suspicion	**BS**
Clinical findings	• *Rad. interventional*: percutaneous dilatation and temporary stent
Fever, jaundice, acholic stools, pruritus often totally absent	(permanent stent only as bridge to retransplantation)
Laboratory results	• *Surgical approach*
Gamma-glutamyl transferase (GGT) always increased	• *Retransplantation* in repeated failures with secondary cirrhosis
Aminotransferases of the normal	**Missing Duct**
Bilirubin often normal	• *Conservative*
US findings	• *New anastomosis*
Intrahepatic bile duct dilatation often absent	**NAS**
Liver biopsy (LB)	• *Rad. interventional for focal dominant strictures*/palliation
Ductular-type interface activity	• *Retransplantation*
Portal and periportal edema	
Periductal edema-ductular proliferation-cholestasis	
Diagnosis	
MRCP magnetic resonance cholangiopancreatography	
Percutaneous transhepatic cholangiography (gold standard)	
Endoscopic retrograde cholangiography (uncommon)	
Missing duct or excluded segmental duct	
Segmental bile duct dilation without a leak	

right branch of the hepatic artery which is typically not included with the graft itself but left with the right liver. Vascularization is therefore anyway precarious.

Any added arterial abnormality such as stenosis or thrombosis has always a further detrimental effect on the integrity of the biliary tree and represents a significant risk factor as well as CMV infection and chronic rejection [75, 83–85] (Table 30.4).

A second relevant element is the aggressive effect of bile salts on the biliary epithelium, which is enhanced by ischemia. The biliary tree is therefore more exposed to the ischemic damage than liver parenchyma during the phases of organ procurement, preservation, and implantation, and both total and warm ischemia time are significant risk factors. Extremely important is also thorough rinsing of bile from the biliary lumen during these phases.

Generally, segmental grafts are reported as more likely to develop any type of complication within 30 days than are whole organ recipients [76], although this correlation is not confirmed in some series [75] and reported to disappear with increasing experience [84].

Other technical issues are probably relevant too, although supporting data are controversially reported in the literature. As for the type of biliary anastomosis, for several reasons, in children, this is more commonly bilioenteric than duct to duct. However, a choice between the techniques is sometimes possible. In these cases, the preference more frequently goes to the former, although contradictory results are reported favoring either option [86, 87].

The presence of multiple bile ducts was found to be an independent risk factor for the development of BC after pediatric liver transplantation and has a higher incidence of BL compared with single duct (21% vs. 9%, respectively) [75], particularly when a ductoplasty with single anastomosis, rather than two distinct anastomoses, is performed [83].

The use of wide-interval interrupted sutures has been reported to decrease the incidence of BCs [79], whereas the use and the effect of biliary stents are also controversial.

Finally, the use of magnification, be it with operative microscope or with loupes, and microsurgical techniques may be helpful in preventing complications [88].

Non-anastomotic strictures, also called "ischemic-type biliary lesions," may also be related with immunologic injury such as in ABO incompatibility, rejection episodes, or autoimmunity.

30.4.2 BCs: Manifestations/Diagnosis
(Table 30.4)

1. Biliary Leaks

    Usually, leaks (or fistulas) appear during the first weeks after LT and in most cases are self-evident as the appearance of bile in the drain(s) placed either at surgery or secondarily to evacuate a collection [84, 85].

    Biliary leaks can occur at the anastomosis site or cut surface of partial liver grafts. The daily output is relevant for the prognosis, low output situations being more likely to heal spontaneously.

    Infection may frequently be associated; major leaks due to partial or total anastomotic disruption may present as massive choleperitoneum and peritonitis.

2. Anastomotic Strictures

    Strictures of anastomosis (AS) have a more indolent evolution and present somewhat later after LT.

    The presentation pattern may be extremely variable. Classical features of biliary obstruction such as jaundice, acholic stools, and itching may frequently be only mild or even completely absent in a significant proportion of cases. Bilirubin levels are normal in nearly half of those patients with a high gamma-glutamyl transferase (GGT) being the only biochemical feature [89, 90]. Less than 50% of the patients present with cholangitis.

    The ability of US to make the diagnosis varies widely in literature and ranges from 25 to 95% of patients suspected of having BSs [89, 91]. Particularly, bile duct dilation can be persistently absent, in up to 60% of patients, even in the presence of a severe BS. For all these reasons, a high level of suspicion should always be kept in mind and (Fig. 30.2).

    Liver biopsy, performed for elevated cholestasis in asymptomatic patients, can provide the diagnosis or at least its suspicion in 69–83% of patients [89] showing the typical pattern of periportal fibrosis and proliferation of biliary neoductules. Cholangio-magnetic resonance may significantly help confirming the diagnosis. However, since it requires anyway a general anesthesia, some groups (including ourselves) prefer to skip it and perform a direct cholangiography, representing the diagnostic gold standard. This is more commonly achieved by the percutaneous than the retrograde endoscopic approach because the latter is particularly awkward in small children and most anastomoses are bilioenteric rather than bilio-biliary. A very experienced interventional radiologist virtually always succeeds in the procedure, even in the absence of bile duct dilation.

3. Non-anastomotic Strictures (NAS)

    NAS, also called ischemic-type biliary lesions, are to be expected in patients recovering from early HAT, in those with late HAT [81], or whenever the graft has undergone a particularly relevant ischemic damage [82]. The manifestations are similar to those of AS, although they may more easily present with cholangitis [92, 93].

4. Missing Duct

    A missing duct may be suspected when a patient presents biochemical signs of cholestasis and histology fails to show alterations. This happens when the biopsy sampling falls on a segment or sub-segment of the graft different from that drained by the missing duct itself.

30.4.3 BCs: Treatment

Treatment of BC plays a fundamental role in medium-long-term prognosis after LT (Table 30.4).

Untreated or improperly treated BC can lead to secondary biliary cirrhosis and graft loss or even to sepsis and patient's death.

An analysis of the American SPLIT database showed that non-HAT-related biliary strictures contribute to approximately 8.6% of all late graft losses in pediatric transplantation [94].

On the other hand, treatment is very effective; an aggressive approach is therefore strongly advisable. As previously alluded to, differently from the adult population, interventional endoscopy is generally of little help in pediatric LT. Management rather includes a combination of surgical and interventional radiology and procedures, these latter mostly based on percutaneous transhepatic cholangiography (PTC) techniques. An experienced interventional radiology team is paramount: the small liver volume, the frequent absence of intrahepatic biliary dilatation, and the possibility of multiple biliary anastomoses render pediatric biliary interventional procedures challenging with the occasional need for long fluoroscopy times [95].

As for bile leaks, generally, only minor, low-output ones may be effectively managed conservatively by simply assuring optimal drainage until resolution. Conversely, higher

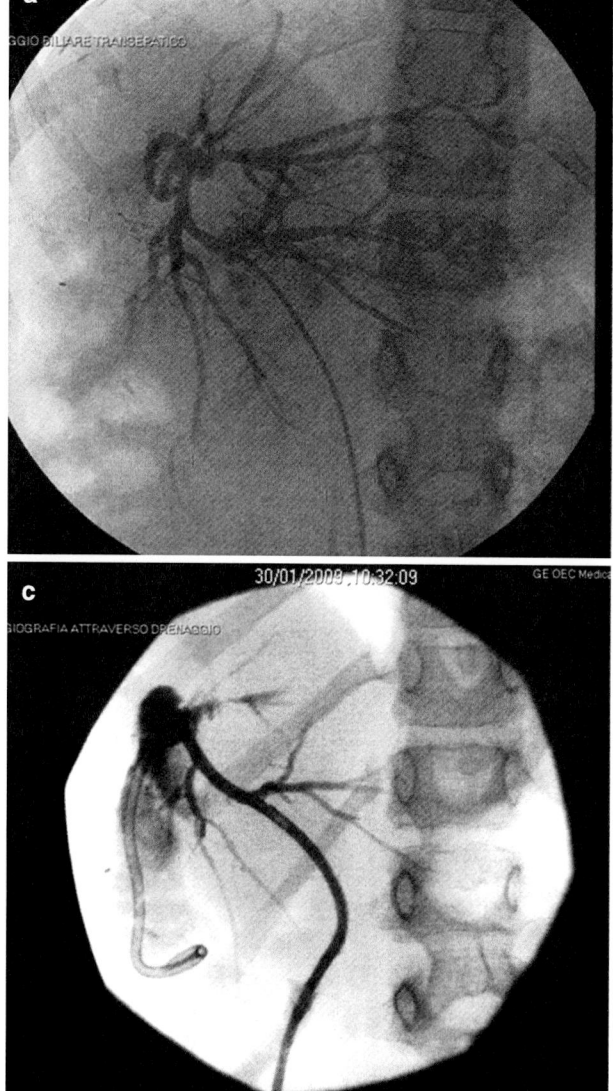

Fig. 30.2 Complete obstruction of bilioenteric anastomosis in an asymptomatic transplanted child: US minimal dilatation of biliary tree, no jaundice, no itching, and bilirubin <1.5 mg/dL; (**a**, **b**) percutaneous transhepatic cholangiography (PTC) showing the impossibility to negotiate the stricture and an extra-luminal effusion of contrast medium; (**c**) cholangiography after surgical redo of bilioenteric anastomosis and placement of a percutaneous transhepatic biliary drainage

output leaks may be treated either by percutaneous decompressive drainage of the biliary tree, allowing a significant reduction of the leak output until its closure, or by reoperation and surgical closure of the leak itself that may require complete redo of the biliary anastomosis. The choice of the approach may depend on the clinical situation but is also very variable among the different institutions, and very little evidence supports the preference of either option. A combination of the percutaneous and surgical procedures may also be used. Whatever the management, since a previous leak appears to be an independent factor for the development of a BS, with a 2.25-fold increase, patients with a previous BL should be followed closely to detect a possible BS in the future [83].

Similarly, AS may also be treated by primary surgical redo of the anastomosis or by percutaneous balloon dilatation and temporary stenting. Again, controversial results are supporting the preference for either approach [96].

Regardless of the adopted approach, the treatment success rates are satisfactory, ranging between 75 and 100%.

The main advantages claimed for surgical treatment include the fact of being a single-stage procedure allowing for a better quality of life, since no temporary anterograde stent is in place, and the high success rate.

Its main disadvantages are the related morbidity and mortality [84].

The advantage attributed to the percutaneous treatment is its low morbidity. However, Lorenz observed a major complication rate of 1.7% and a minor complication rate of 10.8%. The associated 30-day mortality rate was 2.5% (3/120) [97]. The main disadvantage negatively influencing the quality of life is the necessity of temporary internal-external stenting for 3–6 months (for at least 3–6 months) and the need for repeated treatment sessions under general anesthesia.

The recurrence rate of percutaneous treatments for anastomotic BCs in single-center reports varied from 0 to 66% [84].

Recurrences after two or more attempts are generally an indication for surgery. Permanent stenting is generally avoided due to concern for the patient's growth and for the long-term patency. It is reserved for palliation of those cases that are deemed unavoidably destined to retransplantation.

NAS may be managed by interventional radiology in terms of drainage of biliary intrahepatic abscesses and dilatation of isolated or dominant strictures. This management is however to be considered as palliative, and most cases ultimately require retransplantation.

30.5 Other Surgical Complications

30.5.1 Hemorrhage: Transfusions

Technical complexity including the necessity of adhesiolysis, portal hypertension, and coagulopathy all contribute to the risk of intra- and early postoperative hemorrhage. Management of intraperitoneal bleeding is not substantially different from that commonly used in other types of surgery.

Moreover gastrointestinal bleeding has been observed in 2.4–25% of recipients and, in the early postoperative period (within 30 days), is mostly related to variceal bleeding or peptic ulcer bleeding. Persistence of esophageal varices after LT is usually due to small graft ("small-for-size") or persistent portal hypertension possibly related to portal vein thrombosis.

Bleeding from Roux-en-Y anastomosis is also a possible early postoperative complication, usually self-limiting.

Several studies have shown a negative impact of transfusion therapy on patient and graft survival in adult and pediatric populations [98, 99].

On the other hand, studies have demonstrated that pediatric patients may tolerate lower hemoglobin levels without significant morbidity if meticulous monitoring of normovolemia is performed [100].

Both attentions to surgical technique in order to decrease perioperative blood loss and transfusion algorithms to avoid unnecessary and inappropriate transfusions as well as overtransfusion should be implemented. Blood conservation strategies include acute normovolemic hemodilution, hypervolemic hemodilution, deliberate hypotension, antifibrinolytics, intraoperative blood salvage, and preoperative autologous donations [101].

Intraoperative cell salvage systems, commonly used as a blood conservation technique in adults, are available for children too; however there is very little evidence supporting its use in children.

30.5.2 Bowel Perforation

Bowel perforation after LT has been reported to occur at a frequency of 6.4–20% and may carry a poor prognosis, with a mortality rate up to 30–50% [102].

Risk factors for bowel perforation include previous laparotomy (especially portoenterostomy for biliary atresia, BA), a long duration of surgery, subsequent laparotomies, early PVT, treatment with high-dose steroids, and cytomegalovirus infection.

Two other possible risk factors are thermal injury to the adherent bowel wall during the hepatectomy and prolonged portal clamping that may cause bowel congestion [103].

Only a minimum degree of gentle detachment should be performed for intra-abdominal adhesions at transplant, in order to avoid any thermal injury caused by electrocautery.

Clinical manifestations may be scanty in the early phases, and clear signs of peritonitis, as commonly seen in adults, are seldom present. Generally the child presents with pain and irritability, possibly associated with abdominal distension. Signs of infection as fever and leukocytosis are almost always present. Positivity of cultures for enterobacteria is not typical of the early phase but may be an important sign.

Examination of the abdominal fluid for count of neutrophils or research for amylase may be helpful, whereas plain x-ray of the abdomen seldom adds relevant information. In doubtful situations exploratory laparotomy may be the only way to confirm or exclude the diagnosis, and a systematic exploration on postoperative day 5 has been proposed.

Immediate surgical treatment is mandatory.

During surgery to repair bowel perforation, in addition to simple closure, bowl resection and/or enterostomy may also be necessary.

Careful attention should be paid to the possibility that multiple perforations may be present. In case of diffuse purulent peritonitis, open treatment with second look at 24/48 h may be appropriate. Perforation may recur, even repeatedly in some rare cases, requiring prolonged open treatment and multiple surgical revisions.

30.5.3 Ascites

Ascites after LT is quite common. Herzog reports an overall incidence of ascites after pediatric liver transplantation of 31.2% [104].

Besides being a manifestation of impaired venous outflow (see above) [105], or other postoperative complications, thrombosis, infections, biliary leakage, and relevant ascites may be associated with other conditions such as of graft dysfunction, low patient and graft weight, greater native organ-to-recipient weight ratio (NRWR), greater native liver-to-graft weight difference (NGWD), and microvascular changes during acute rejection. A specific entity is chylous ascites, whose diagnosis requires the detection of high chilomicrones dosage in the fluid [104, 106] and which may require prolonged total parenteral nutrition.

30.6 Retransplantation Policies

The natural evolution of most complications, or the failure of their management, may eventually lead to graft failure and need for retransplantation.

The need may be urgent or elective, more commonly in the early and in the late forms, respectively [8, 107].

Particularly, as long-term survival of transplanted patients progressively improves, it is easy to expect that the need for late retransplantation will progressively increase generating a competition for grafts in all other patients listed for primary transplantation [108].

The attitude with respect to retransplantation may be subject to significant variations among different institutions, based on the interaction of several local factors, such as (1) experience and expertise, (2) availability of the appropriate multidisciplinary skills (e.g., pediatric interventional radiologist), and (3) organ availability.

This latter is particularly relevant; profound differences exist among countries from this standpoint. For example, in most eastern countries, cultural, religious, and legal issues represent a huge limit to postmortem donation, and transplantation relies mainly on living donation. In case of need for retransplantation, a second living donor may not exist, and a deceased donor may not be timely available, making in fact the procedure nearly impossible [109].

On the other hand, in countries where deceased donors are more available, allocation policies based on utility (or even on benefit) or alternatively on urgency may limit or favor the access or the prioritization for retransplantation.

The final result is that the indication and actual use of retransplantation may be significantly different among institutions with attitudes alternatively more aggressive "procedure-wise" and conservative "graft-wise" or vice versa.

Acknowledgments We thank Dr. Roberto Agazzi for kindly providing the pictures of Figs. 30.1 and 30.2.

References

1. Dindo D, Demartines N, Clavien P-A. Classification of surgical complication. A new proposal with evaluation in a cohort of 6336 Patients and results of a Survey. Ann Surg. 2004;240:205–2013.
2. Clavien P-A, Camargo CA, Croxford R, Langer B, Levy GA, Greig PD. Definition and classification of negative outcomes in solid organ transplantation. Ann Surg. 1994;220(2):109–20.
3. McDiarmid SV, Anand R, Martz K, Millis MJ, Mazariegos GV. A multivariate analysis of pre-,peri-, and post-transplant factors affecting outcome after pediatric liver transplantation. Ann Surg. 2011;254:145–54.
4. Cramm SL, Waits SA, Englesbe MJ, Bucuvalas JC, Horslen SP, Mazariegos GV, Soltys K, Anand R, Magee JC. Failure to rescue as a quality improvement approach in transplantation: a first effort to evaluate this tool in pediatric liver transplantation. Transplantation. 2016;4:801–7.
5. Nacoti M, Barlera S, Codazzi D, Bonanomi E, Passoni M, Vedovati S, Rota sperti L, Colledan M, Fumagalli R. Early detection of the graft failure after pediatric liver transplantation: a Bergamo experience. Acta Anaesthesiol Scand. 2011;55:842–50.
6. Wu J-F, Wu R-Y, Chen J, Ou-Yang B, Chen M-Y, Guan X-D. Early lactate clearance as a reliable predictor of initial poor graft function after orthotopic liver transplantation. Hepatobiliary Pancreat Dis Int. 2011;10(6):587–92.
7. Chen X-B, Xu M-Q. Primary graft dysfunction after liver transplantation. Hepatobiliary Pancreat Dis Int. 2014;13:125–37.
8. Ng V, Anand R, Martz K, Fetau A. Liver retransplantation in children: a SPLIT database analysis of outcome and predictive factors for survival. Am J Transplant. 2008;8:386–95.
9. Olthoff K, Kulik L, Samstein B, Kaminski M, Abecassis M, Emond J. Validation of a current definition of early allograft dysfunction in liver transplant recipients and analysis of risk factors. Hepatobiliary Pancreat Dis Int. 2014;13:125–37.
10. Neaton N. Small-for-size liver syndrome after auxiliary and split liver transplantation: donor selection. Liver Transpl. 2003;9(9):S26–8.
11. Rangel Moreira Dde A, Aoun Tannuri AC, Belon AR, Mendonça Coelho MC, et al. Large-for-size liver transplantation: a flowmetry study in pigs. J Surg Res. 2014;189:313–20.
12. Kiuchi T, Kasahara M, uryuhara K, Inomata Y, Uemoto S, Asonuma K, Egawa H, Fujita S, Hayashi M, Tanaka K. Impact of graft size mismatching on graft prognosis in liver transplantation from living donors. Transplantation. 1999;67(2):321–7.
13. Dahm F, Georgiev P, Clavien P-A. Small-for-size syndrome after partial liver transplantation: definition, mechanisms of disease and clinical implications. Am J Transplant. 2005;5:2605–10.
14. Li J-J, Zu C-H, Li S-p, Gao W, Shen Z-Y, Cai J-Z. Effect of graft size matching on pediatric living-donor liver transplantation at single center. Clin Transpl. 2018;32:e13160.
15. Yamada N, Sanada Y, Hirata Y, Okada N, Ihara Y, Sasanuma H, Urahashi t, Sukuma Y, Yasuda Y, Mizuta K. The outcomes of pediatric living donor liver transplantation using small-for-size grafts: experience of a single institute. Pediatr Surg Int. 2016;32:363–8.
16. Colledan A, Segalin M, Spada L, Lucianetti V, Corno BG. Liberal policy of split liver for pediatric liver transplantation. A single centre experience. Transpl Int. 2000;13(suppl 1):131–3.
17. Gridelli B, Spada M, Petz W, Bertani A, Lucianetti A, Colledan M, Altobelli M, Alberto D, Guizzetti M, Riva S. Split-liver transplantation eliminates the need for living-donor liver transplantation in

children with end-stage cholestatic liver disease. Transplantation. 2003;75(8):1197–203.
18. Bekker J, Ploem S, Jong K. Early hepatic artery thrombosis after liver transplantation: a systematic review of the incidence, outcome and risk factors. Am J Transplant. 2009;9:746–57.
19. Ye H, Zhao Q, Wang Y, Zheng Z, Schroder P, et al. Outcomes of technical variant liver transplantation versus whole liver transplantation for pediatric patients: a meta-analysis. PLoS One. 2015;10(9):e0138202.
20. Singhal A, Stokes K, Sebastian A, Wright HI, Kohli V. Endovascular treatment of hepatic artery thrombosis following liver transplantation. Transpl Int. 2010;23:245–56.
21. Oh C, Pelletier S, Sawyer R, et al. Uni- and multi-variate analysis of risk factors for early and late hepatic artery thrombosis after liver transplantation. Transplantation. 2001;71:767–72.
22. Tzakis AG, Gordon RD, Shaw BW, Iwatsuki S, Starzl T. Clinical presentation of hepatic artery thrombosis after liver transplantation in the cyclosporine era. Transplantation. 1985;40(6):667–71.
23. Nishida S, Kato T, Levi D, Naveen M, Berney T, Vianna R, Selvaggi G, Buitorago E, Al-Niami A, Nakamura N, Vaidya J, Tzakis A. Effect of protocol Doppler ultrasonography and urgent revascularization on early hepatic artery thrombosis after pediatric liver transplantation. Arch Surg. 2002;137:1279–83.
24. Vignali C, Bargellini I, Cioni R. Diagnosis and treatment of hepatic artery stenosis after orthotopic liver transplantation. Transplant Proc. 2004;36:2771–8.
25. Gu L, Fang H, Li F, Li P, Zhu C, Zhu J, Zhang S. Prediction of early hepatic artery thrombosis by intraoperative color Doppler ultrasound in pediatric segmental liver transplantation. Clin Transpl. 2012;26:571–6.
26. Ahmad T, Chavhan GB, Avitzur Y, Moineddin R, Oudjhane K. Doppler parameters of the hepatic artery as predictors of graft status in pediatric liver transplantation. AJR Am J Roentgenol. 2017;209:671–5.
27. Saba L, Mallarini G. Multidetector row CT angiography in the evaluation of the hepatic artery and its anatomical variants. Clin Radiol. 2008;63:312–9.
28. Brancatelli G, Katyal S, Federle M, Fontes P. Three dimensional multislice helical computed tomography with the volume rendering technique in the detection of vascular complications after liver transplantation. Transplantation. 2002;73:237–43.
29. Uller W, Knoppke B, Schreyer A, Heiss A. Interventional radiological treatment of perihepatic vascular stenosis or occlusion in pediatric patients after liver transplantation. Cardiovasc Intervent Radiol. 2013;36:1562–71.
30. Uchida Y, Sakamoto S, Egawa K, Ogura Y, Taira K, Kasahara M, Uryuhara K, Takada Y, Uemoto S. The impact of meticulous management for hepatic artery thrombosis on long-term outcome after pediatric living donor liver transplantation. Clin Transpl. 2009;23:392–299.
31. Ackermann O, Branchereau S, Franchi-Abella S, Pariente D, Chevret L, Debray D, Jacquemin E, Gauthier F, Hill C, Bernard O. The long-term outcome of hepatic artery thrombosis after liver transplantation in children: role of urgent revascularization. Am J Transplant. 2012;12:1496–503.
32. Seda-Neto J, Antunes de Fonseca E, Pugliese R, Candido EL, Benavides MR, Afonso RC, Neiva R, Porta G, et al. Twenty years of experience in pediatric living donor liver transplantation: focus on hepatic artery reconstruction, complications, and outcomes. Transplantation. 2016;100(5):1066–72.
33. Porrett PM, Hsu J, Saked A. Late surgical complications following liver transplantation. Liver Transpl. 2009;15:s12–8.
34. Stafford WL, Stevens SD, Krohmer S, DiSantis D. "Tardus-Parvus" waveform. Abdom Radiol. 2016;41:344–6.
35. Quintini C, Hirose K, Hashimoto K, Diago t, Aucejo F, Eghtesad B, Vogt d, Pierce G, Baker M, Kelly D, Miller CM. "Splenic artery Steal Syndrome" is a misnomer: the cause is portal hyperperfusion, not arterial siphon. Liver Transpl. 2008;14:374–9.
36. Jones V, Chennapragada M, Lord D, Stormon M, Shun A. Post liver transplantation mycotic aneurysm of the hepatic artery. J Pediatr Surg. 2008;43(3):555–8.
37. Volpin E, Pessaux P, Sauvanet A, Sibert A, Kianmanesh R, Durand A. Preservation of arterial vascularization after hepatic artery pseudoaneurysm following orthotopic liver transplantation: long term results. Ann Transplant. 2014;19:346–52.
38. Camagni S, Stroppa P, Tebaldi A, Lucianetti A, Pinelli D, Colledan M. Mycotic aneurysm of the hepatic artery in pediatric liver transplantation: a case series and literature review. Transpl Infect Dis. 2018;20(3):e12861.
39. Kenari K, Mirzakhani H, Eslami M, Saidi R. Current state of the art in management of vascular complications after pediatric liver r transplantation. Pediatr Transplant. 2015;19:18–26.
40. Cho Y-P, Kim K-M, Ha T-Y, Ko G-Y, Hwang J-Y, Park H, Chung YS, Yoon T, Hwang S, Jun H, Kwan T-W, Lee S-G. Management of late-onset portal vein complications in pediatric living-donor liver transplantation. Pediatr Transplant. 2014;18:64–71.
41. Moon J, Jung GO, Choi G-S, Kim JM, Shin E, Kim E, Kwon C, Kim S-J, Joh J-W, Lee S-K. Risk factors for portal vein complications after pediatric living donor liver transplantation with left-sided grafts. Transplant Proc. 2010;42:871–5.
42. Alvarez F. Portal vein complications after pediatric liver transplantation. Curr Gastroenterol Rep. 2012;14:270–4.
43. Duffy JP, Hong JC, Farmer DG, Ghobrial R, Yerziz H, Hiatt J, Busuttil RW. Vascular complications of orthotopic liver transplantation: experience in more than 4,200 patients. J Am Coll Surg. 2009;208:896–903.
44. Mazariegos GV. Critical elements in pediatric allograft selection. Liver Transpl. 2017;23(S1):S56–8.
45. Ueda M, Egawa H, Ogawa K, Uryuhara K, Fujimoto Y, Kasahara M, Ogura Y, Kozaki K, Takada Y, Tanaka K. Portal vein complications in the long-term course after pediatric living donor liver transplantation. Transplant Proc. 2005;37:1138–40.
46. de Magnée C, Veyckemans F, Pirotte T, Menten R, Dumitru D, Clapuyt P, Carbonez K, et al. Liver and systemic hemodynamics in children with cirrhosis: impact on the surgical management in pediatric living donor liver transplantation. Liver Transpl. 2017;23:1440–50.
47. Suzuki L, de oliveira IR, Widman A, Gibeli NEM, Carnevale F, Maksound J, Hubbard A, Cerri G. Real-time and Doppler US after pediatric segmental liver transplantation. Pediatr Radiol. 2008;38:403–8.
48. Gu L-H, Fang H, Li F-H, Zhang S-J, Han L-Z, Li Q-G. Preoperative hepatic hemodynamics in the prediction of early portal vein thrombosis after liver transplantation in pediatric patients with biliary atresia. Hepatobiliary Pancreat Dis Int. 2015;4:380–5.
49. Ueda M, Oike F, Kasahara M, Ogura Y, Ogawa K, Haga H, Takada Y, Egawa H, Tanaka K, Uemoto S. Portal vein complications in pediatric living donor liver transplantation using left-side grafts. Am J Transplant. 2008;8:2097–105.
50. Kishi Y, Sugawara Y, Matsui Y, Akamatsu N, Makuuchi M. Late onset portal vein thrombosis and its risk factors. Hepato-Gastroenterology. 2008;55(84):1008–9.
51. de Magnée C, Bourdeaux C, De Dobbeleer F, Janssen M, Menten R, Clapuyt P, Reding R. Impact of pre-transplant liver hemodynamics and portal reconstruction techniques on post-transplant portal vein complications in pediatric liver transplantation. Ann Surg. 2011;254(1):55–61.
52. Seda-Neto J, Fonseca EA, Feier FH, Pugliese R, Candido HL, Benavides M, Porta G, Miura IK, Danesi VB, Guimaraes T, Porta A, Borges C, Godoy A, Kondo M, Chapchap P. Analysis factor associated with portal vein thrombosis in pediatric living donor liver transplant recipients. Liver Transpl. 2014;20:1157–67.

53. Buell J, Funaki B, Cronin DC, Yoshida A, Perlman MK, Lorenz J, Kelłly S, Brady L, Leef JA, Mills J. Long-term venous complications after full-size and segmental pediatric liver transplantation. Ann Surg. 2002;236(5):658–66.
54. Cheng Y, Ou H-Y, Yu C-Y, Tsang LL-C, Huang T-L, Chen T-YA. Section 8. Management of portal venous complications in pediatric living donor liver transplantation. Transplantation. 2014;97(8s):s32–4.
55. Bueno J, Perez-Lafuente M, Venturi C, Segarra A, Barber I, Molino J, Romero A, Ortega J, Bilbao I, Martinez-Ibanez VR. No-touch hepatic hilum technique to treat early portal vein thrombosis after pediatric liver transplantation. Am J Transplant. 2010;10:2148–53.
56. Ko G-Y, Sung K-B, Yoon H-K, Lee S. Early posttransplantation portal vein stenosis: following living donor liver transplantation: percutaneous transhepatic primary stent placement. Liver Transpl. 2007;13:530–6.
57. Chick JFB, Jo A, Dasika N, Saad W, Sirinivasa R. Transsplenic endovascular recanalization and stenting of a completely occluded portal vein jejunal variceal embolization in a pediatric liver transplant recipient. Pediatr Radiol. 2017;47:1212–015.
58. Bertram H, Pfister E-D, Becker T, Schoof S. Transsplenic endovascular therapy of portal vein stenosis and subsequent complete portal vein thrombosis in a 2.year-old child. J Vasc Interv Radiol. 2010;21:1760–4.
59. Chen C-L, Conceiero AM, Ou H-Y, Chen Y-F, Yu C-Y, Huang T-L. Intraoperative portal vein stent placement in pediatric living donor liver transplantation. J Vasc Interv Radiol. 2012;23(5):725–6.
60. Kensinger CD, Sexton KW, Baron CM, Lipnik AJ, Meranze SG, Gorden DL. Management of portal vein thrombosis after liver transplantation with a combined open and endovascular approach. Liver Transpl. 2015;21:132–4.
61. Carnevale F, Santos A, Seda-Neto J, Zurstrassen C, Moreira A, Carone E, Marcelino A, Porta G, Pugliese R, Miura I, Baggio V, Guimaraes T, Cerri G, Chapchap P. Portal vein obstruction after liver transplantation in children treated by simultaneous minilaparotomy and transhepatic approaches: initial experience. Pediatr Transplant. 2011;15:47–52.
62. Miura K, Sato Y, Nakatsuka H, Yamamoto S, Oya H, Hara Y, kokai H, Hatakeyama K. Catheter-directed continuous thrombolysis following aspiration thrombectomy via ileocolic route for acute portal venous thrombosis: report of two cases. Surg Today. 2013;43:1310–5.
63. Nosaka YI, Kasahara M, Miyazaki O, Sakamoto S, Uchida H, Shigeta T, Masaki H. Recanalization of post-transplant late-onset long segmental portal vein thrombosis with bidirectional transhepatic and transmesenteric approach. Pediatr Transplant. 2013;17:e71–5.
64. de Ville de Goyet J, Lo Zupone C, Grimaldi CA. Meso-Rex bypass as an alternative technique for portal vein reconstruction at or after liver transplantation in children: review and perspectives. Pediatr Transplant. 2013;17:19–26.
65. Shibasaki S, Taniguchi M, Shimamura T, Suzuki T, Yamashita K, et al. Risk factors for portal vein complications in pediatric living donor liver transplantation. Clin Transpl. 2010;24:550–6.
66. Woo D, LaBerge JM, Gordon RL, Wilson MW, Kerlan RK. Management of portal venous complications after liver transplantation. Tech Vasc Interv Radiol. 2007;10:233–9.
67. Emond J, Heffron T, Whitington A. Reconstruction of the hepatic vein in reduced size hepatic transplantation. Surg Gynecol Obstet. 1993;176:11–7.
68. Heffron T, Pillen T, Smallwood G, Henry S, Sekar S, Casper K, Solis D, Tang W, Fasola C, Romero R. Incidence, impact, and treatment of portal and hepatic venous complications following pediatric liver transplantation: a single-center 12 years experience. Pediatr Transplant. 2010;14:722–9.
69. Sakamoto S, Egawa H, Kanazawa H, Shibata A. Hepatic venous outflow obstruction in pediatric living donor liver transplantation using left-sided lobe grafts: Kyoto University experience. Liver Transpl. 2010;16:1207–14.
70. Tannuri U, Tannuri A, Santos M, Miyatani H. Technique advance to avoid hepatic venous outflow obstruction in pediatric living-donor liver transplantation. Pediatr Transplant. 2015;19:261–6.
71. Buell JF, Funaki B, Cronin D, Yoshida A, Perlman A. Long-term venous complications after full-size and segmental pediatric liver transplantation. Ann Surg. 2002;236(5):658–66.
72. Gibelli N, Tannuri A, Andrade W, Ricardi L, Tannuri U. Centrilobular necrosis as a manifestation of venous outflow block in pediatric malnourished liver transplant recipients - case reports. Pediatr Transplant. 2012;16:E383–7.
73. Akamatsu N, Sugawara Y, Kaneko J, Kishi Y, Niiya T, Kokudo N, Makuuchi M. Surgical repair for late-onset hepatic venous outflow block after living-donor liver transplantation. Transplantation. 2004;77(11):1768–70.
74. Yersiz H, Renz J, Farmer D, Hisatake G, McDiarmid S, Busuttil RW. One hundred in situ split-liver transplantations. A single-center experience. Ann Surg. 2003;238:496–507.
75. Salvalaggio R, Whitington PF, Alonso EM, Superina RA. Presence of multiple bile ducts in the liver graft increases the incidence of biliary complications in pediatric liver transplantation. Liver Transpl. 2005;11(2):161–6.
76. Diamond IR, Fecteau A, Millis JM, Lasanoff JE, Vicky N, Anand R, Song C. Impact of graft type on outcome in pediatric liver transplantation. A report from studies of pediatric liver transplantation (SPLIT). Ann Surg. 2007;246:301–10.
77. Becker NS, Barshes NR, Aloja T, Nguyen T, Rojo J, Rodriguez J, O'Mahony CA, Karpen SJ, Goss JA. Analysis of recent pediatric orthotopic liver transplantation outcomes indicates that allograft type is no longer a predictor of survivals. Liver Transpl. 2008;14:1125–32.
78. Anderson CD, Turmelle YP, Darcy M, Shepherd RW, Weymann A, Nadler M, Guelker S, Chapman WC, Lowell JA. Biliary strictures in pediatric liver transplant recipients – early diagnosis and treatment results in excellent graft outcomes. Pediatr Transplant. 2010;14:358–63.
79. Ando H, Kaneko K, Ono Y, Tainaka T, Kawai Y. Biliary reconstruction with wide-interval interrupted suture to prevent biliary complications in pediatric living-donor liver transplantation. J Hepatobiliary Pancreat Sci. 2011;18:26–31.
80. Liu C, Loong C-C, Hsia C-Y, Peng C-H, Tsai H-L, Tsou M-Y, Wei C. Duct-to-duct biliary reconstruction in selected cases in pediatric living-donor left-lobe liver transplantation. Pediatr Transplant. 2009;13:693–6.
81. Seehofer D, Eurich D, Veltzke-Schlieker W, Neuhaus P. Biliary complications after liver transplantation: old problems and new challenges. Am J Transplant. 2013;13:263–6.
82. Cursio R, Gugenheim J. Ischemia-reperfusion injury and ischemic-type biliary lesions following liver transplantation. J Transp Secur. 2012:164329.
83. Feier FH, Seda-Neto J, da fonseca EA, Candido HLL, Pugliese RS, Neiva R, Benavides MR, Chapchap P. Analysis of factors associated with biliary complications in children after liver transplantation. Transplantation. 2016;100(9):1944–54.
84. Darius T, Rivera J, Fusaro F, Lai Q, de Magnée C, Bourdeaux C, Janssen M, Clapuyt P, Reding R. Risk factors and surgical management of anastomotic biliary complications after pediatric liver transplantation. Liver Transpl. 2014;20:893–903.
85. Chok KSH, Chan SC, Chan KL, Sharr WW, Tam PK, Fan ST, Lo CM. Bile duct anastomotic stricture after pediatric living donor liver transplantation. J Pediatr Surg. 2012;47:1399–403.

86. Tanaka H, Fukuda A, Shigeta T, Kuroda T, Kimura T, Sakamoto S, Kasahara M. Biliary reconstruction in pediatric live donor liver transplantation: duct-to-duct or Roux-en-Y hepaticojejunostomy. J Pediatr Surg. 2010;45(8):1668–75.
87. Feier FH, da Fonseca E, Seda-Neto J, Chapchap P. Biliary complications after pediatric liver transplantation: risk factors, diagnosis and management. World J Hepatol. 2015;7(18):2162–70.
88. Lin T-S, Chen C-L, Concejero AM, Yap AQ, Lin Y-H, Liu C-Y, Chiang Y-C, Wang S-H, Lin C-C, Yong C-C, Chang Y-F. Early and long-term results of routine microsurgical biliary reconstruction in living donor liver transplantation. Liver Transpl. 2013;19:207–14.
89. Miraglia R, Maruzzelli L, Caruso S, Riva S, Spada S, Luca A, Gridelli B. Percutaneous management of biliary strictures after pediatric liver transplantation. Cardiovasc Intervent Radiol. 2008;31:993–8.
90. Seda-Neto J, Pugliese R, Fonseca EA, Vincenzi R, Pugliese V, Candido H, Stein A, Benavides M, Ketzer B, Teng H, Porta G, Miura IK, Baggio V, Guimaraes T, Porta A, Rodrigues CA, Carnevale FC, Carone E, Kondo M, Chapchap P. Four hundred thirty consecutive pediatric living donor liver transplants: variables associated with posttransplant patient and graft survival. Liver Transpl. 2012;18:577–84.
91. Feier FH, Chapchap P, Pugliese R, da Fonseca EA, Carnevale FC, Moreira AM, Zurstrassen C, Santos AC, Miura IK, Baggio V, Porta A, Guimaraes T, Candido H, Benavides M, Godoy A, Leite KMR, Porta G, Kondo M, Seda-neto J. Diagnosis and management of biliary complications in pediatric living donor liver transplant recipients. Liver Transpl. 2014;20:882–92.
92. Buis C, Verdonk R, Van der Jagt E, Van der Hilst C, Sloof M, Haagsma E, Porte R. Nonanastomotic biliary strictures after liver transplantation, part 1: radiological features and risk factors for early vs. late presentation. Liver Transpl. 2007;13:708–18.
93. Verdonk R, Buis C, Van der Jagt E, Gouw A, Limburg A, Sloof M, Kleibeuker J, Porte R, Haagsma E. Nonanastomotic biliary strictures after liver transplantation, part 2: management, outcome, and risk factors for disease progression. Liver Transpl. 2007;13:725.732.
94. Soltys KA, Mazariegos GV, Squires RH, Sindhi RK, Anand R, The SPLIT Research Group. Late graft loss or death in pediatric liver transplantation: an analysis of the SPLIT database. Am J Transplant. 2007;7:2165–71.
95. Miraglia R, Maruzzelli L, Tuzzolino F, Indovina P, Luca A. Radiation exposure in biliary procedures performed to manage anastomotic strictures in pediatric liver transplant recipients: comparison between radiation exposure levels using an image intensifier and a flat-panel detector-based system. Cardiovasc Intervent Radiol. 2013;36:1670–6.
96. Colledan M, D'Antiga L. Biliary complications after pediatric liver transplantation: the endless heel. Pediatr Transplant. 2014;18:786–7.
97. Lorenz JM, Funaki B, Leef JA, Rosenblum JD, Van Ha T. Percutaneous transhepatic cholangiography and biliary drainage in pediatric liver transplant patients. AJR. 2001;176:761–5.
98. Nacoti M, Cazzaniga S, Lorusso F, Naldi L, Brambillasca P, Benigni A, Corno V, Colledan M, Bonanomi EV, Buoro S, Falanga A, Lussana F, Barbui TS. The impact of perioperative transfusion of blood products on survival after pediatric liver transplantation. Pediatr Transplant. 2012;16(4):357–66.
99. De Boer M, Christensen M, Asmussen A. The impact of intraoperative transfusion of platelets and red blood cells on survival after liver transplantation. Anesth Analg. 2008;16:32–4.
100. Bhananker S, Ramamoorthy C, Geiduschek JA. Anesthesia-related cardiac arrest in children. Update from the pediatric Perioperative Cardiac Arrest registry. Anesth Analg. 2007;105:344–50.
101. Lavoie J. Blood transfusion risks and alternative strategies in pediatric patients. Pediatr Anesth. 2011;21:14–24.
102. Sanada Y, Mizuta K, Wakiya T, Umehara M, Egami S, Urahashi T, Hishikawa S, Fujiwara T, Sakuma Y, Hyodo M, Yasuda Y, Kawarasaki H. Bowel perforation after pediatric living donor liver transplantation. Pediatr Surg Int. 2011;27:23–7.
103. Dehghani SM, Nikeghbalian S, Kazemi K, Dehghani M, Gholami S, Bahador A, Salahi H, Malek-Hosseini SA. Outcome of bowel perforation after pediatric liver transplantation. Pediatr Transplant. 2008;12:146–9.
104. Herzog D, Martin S, Lallier M, Alvarez F. Ascites after orthotopic liver transplantation in children. Pediatr Transplant. 2005;9:74–9.
105. Krishna Kumar G, Sharif K, Mayer D, Mirza D, Foster K, Kelly D, Millar AJW. Hepatic venous out- flow obstruction in paediatric liver transplantation. Pediatr Surg Int. 2010;26:423–5.
106. Marseglia A, Ginammi M, Bosisio M, Stroppa P, Colledan M, D'Antiga L. Determinants of large drain losses early after pediatric liver transplantation. Pediatr Transplant. 2017;21:e12932.
107. Bourdeaux C, Brunati A, Janssen M, de Magnée C, Otte JB, Sokal E, Reding R. Liver retransplantation in children. A 21-year single-center experience. Transpl Int. 2009;22:416–22.
108. Dreyzin A, Lunz J, Venkat v, Martin L, Bond GJ, Soltys KA, Sindhi R, Mazariegos GV. Long-term outcomes and predictors in pediatric liver retransplantation. Pediatr Transplant. 2015;19:866–74.
109. Miura K, Sakamoto S, Shimata K, Honda M, Kobayashi T, Wakai T, Sugawara Y, Inomata Y. The outcomes of pediatric liver retransplantation from a living donor: a 17-year single-center experience. Surg Today. 2017;47:1405–14.

Immunosuppression in Pediatric Liver Transplant

Patrick McKiernan and Ellen Mitchell

Key Points
- Tacrolimus is the default immunosuppressive agent following pediatric liver transplantation.
- The use of induction agents is increasing internationally.
- Chronic rejection is now a rare cause for graft failure or retransplantation.
- Most immunosuppressive regimens are center specific with relatively little standardization.

Research Needed in the Field
- There is a need for randomized controlled trials to compare modern induction regimens.
- There is a need for randomized controlled trials to determine the appropriate treatment of antibody-mediated rejection.
- The impact of donor-specific antibodies on routine clinical practice should be tested in prospective clinical trials.
- There is a need for trials of individualized immunosuppression regimens based on pharmacogenetic factors and individual risks of rejection.

Immunosuppression in liver transplant is a constantly evolving field. The primary goal is to utilize the minimal level of therapy that prevents graft rejection while minimizing toxicity and promoting tolerance. The agents and dosing regimens used vary widely and evolve as new medications and data become available. Unfortunately, evidence-based data is often limited, and practice may be inferred from studies in adults or other transplant organs. This lack of evidence-based guidelines contributes to a wide variation in practice between centers.

31.1 Induction Agents

Induction is the use of intensive immunosuppression in the perioperative period as prophylaxis against acute rejection. The use of induction protocols has been shown to result in significantly improved graft and patient survival for up to 5-year posttransplant [1]. Initial induction protocols were largely corticosteroid based, while more recently steroid-sparing/steroid-avoiding protocols have become commoner. Most current induction protocols incorporate some modification of calcineurin inhibitor dosing with a view to nephroprotection. These agents are also used in the treatment of acute cellular rejection [ACR].

31.2 Anti-IL-2 Receptor Antibodies (Anti-CD25 Antibodies)

These can be used as an alternative to steroids for induction, with improvement in rates of both acute and chronic rejection and decreased infections.

Daclizumab is a humanized monoclonal antibody that blocks the CD25 component of interleukin-2 (IL-2) receptors on T cells. IL-2 receptors are found on activated T cells, so blocking these results in a more targeted blockage of T-cell clonal expansion, a key step in allograph organ rejection [2–4]. In adults, daclizumab has a half-life of just over 4 days and significantly reduces CD25+ cells for 28 days after liver transplantation [5].

Initially used in patients with renal insufficiency, daclizumab facilitated delaying the introduction of nephrotoxic calcineurin inhibitors without increasing the risk of rejection [6]. In an unselected transplant population, its use resulted in delaying the first episode of ACR and in decreasing the overall incidence of ACR without any increase in adverse events, including infection, compared to placebo [7]. While the literature in the adult population supported a two-dose regime, some initial pediatric studies only used a single dose. Despite this, patients given daclizumab for induction developed fewer episodes of ACR in the first 30 days (14.8% vs. 50% $P = 0.003$) and had fewer episodes of ACR at any time (39.3% vs. 75%, $P = 0.01$) compared to patients given tacrolimus immediately after transplant [8].

Basiliximab blocks the same receptor as daclizumab but has a tenfold higher binding affinity [5]. When basiliximab was added to a regimen of cyclosporine and prednisone, it significantly decreased the risk of ACR, although graft survival, patient survival, chronic rejection, posttransplant lymphoproliferative disorder [PTLD], and steroid-resistant rejection rates were similar for up to 4 years after transplant. When basiliximab was used in place of steroids, it did not affect overall patient or graft survival but resulted in less ACR, less overall rejection, and significantly fewer infections by 1 year [9]. In another study basiliximab showed a significantly improved rejection-free graft survival, in addition to improved patient and graft survival, just short of statistical significance, compared to historical controls given steroids. In addition there was a significant reduction in viral infection when patients were given basiliximab instead of steroids [10].

These drugs are generally very well tolerated, but potential side effects include hypersensitivity reaction, abdominal pain, vomiting, insomnia, edema, hypertension, anemia, dysuria, cough, dyspnea, and fever. If given as a bolus instead of an infusion, patients may experience nausea, vomiting, and local pain at injection site [11].

31.2.1 Thymoglobulin

Thymoglobulin is produced by immunizing animals with human T cells and thymocytes. The subsequent antisera are then purified to reduce the likelihood of serum sickness. Thymoglobulin is usually produced by horses or rabbits, and there may be significant variability in potency and antigen specificity between patches [12]. In addition to nonspecific T-cell depletion, thymoglobulin also causes decreased cell-to-cell interactions and inhibits leukocyte migration across capillary endothelial surfaces [13, 14].

An initial retrospective study showed less ACR, less steroid-resistant rejection, and prolonged rejection-free periods when thymoglobulin was added to cyclosporine, azathioprine, and steroids [15]. The subsequent prospective studies that followed were less convincing. When thymoglobulin was added to a tacrolimus [TAC] and steroid-based regimen and compared to these agents used alone, there was improvement in clinical signs of ischemia/reperfusion injury but no change in ACR incidence [16]. When thymoglobulin was added to TAC, mycophenolate mofetil [MMF], and steroids, there was again no change in the rate of ACR, and, unfortunately, there was an increase in leukopenia [17].

However, when Eason et al. replaced steroids with thymoglobulin combined with a maintenance regimen of TAC and MMF, patients treated with thymoglobulin had the same number of episodes of ACR, but these were less severe, and subjects experienced significantly less steroid exposure overall. Thymoglobulin induction was also associated with decreased recurrence of HCV, posttransplant diabetes mellitus, and CMV infection [18].

In other promising studies, thymoglobulin with delayed TAC reduction demonstrated improved 1-year graft survival and decreased ACR [19] despite less overall tacrolimus exposure [20].

While thymoglobulin is a useful replacement for steroids or to facilitate delayed early TAC use, it does require premedication to prevent significant systemic reactions including serum sickness, leukopenia, thrombocytopenia, and anemia.

31.2.2 Alemtuzumab

Alemtuzumab (Campath) is a recombinant anti-CD52 humanized rat monoclonal antibody. By targeting antigen CD52, a cell surface glycoprotein, it binds to lymphocytes, thymocytes, monocytes, and macrophages while sparing other cell lines. Receptor blockage triggers cell death and long-lasting lymphopenia [21]. While B lymphocyte counts return to normal levels within 3–12 months, CD4 and CD8 lymphocyte counts remain significantly depressed for as long as 3 years [22]. This profound lymphopenia is thought to create an environment for gradual engagement of the host immune system facilitating long-term low-dose immune suppression and even eventual immunosuppression withdrawal [23].

Much of the evidence based for alemtuzumab comes from the renal transplant population. In a randomized control trial in renal transplantation, alemtuzumab as monotherapy showed similar patient survival, graft survival, and ACR incidence compared to traditional triple therapy (cyclosporine, azathioprine, and prednisone) [24]. Another trial confirmed equivalent outcomes with alemtuzumab combined with TAC and MMF as opposed to thymoglobulin or daclizumab. However, alemtuzumab was superior to the other induction agents because patients required less steroids overall [25].

In a retrospective review of liver transplant patients, alemtuzumab was used instead of steroids with tacrolimus. There was no change in graft survival or the incidence of ACR when compared to steroids, but importantly, there was significantly less renal toxicity in those treated with alemtuzumab [26]. These results were subsequently confirmed in a prospective trial which showed a decrease in ACR in those treated with alemtuzumab [27].

Data is limited in the pediatric population to a small study from the University of Miami looking at ten patients transplanted for autoimmune hepatitis who were given alemtuzumab in addition to tacrolimus. There was a significantly longer period of rejection-free survival in those treated with alemtuzumab despite lower maintenance immunosuppression when compared to steroids [28].

Since alemtuzumab causes profound and long-lasting leukopenia, there are concerns about its effect on the immune system. Lymphoid depletion may increase the risk of infection; however, this has not been reported in patients treated with alemtuzumab [29–31]. Alemtuzumab is not recommended for patients with hepatitis C since lymphoid depletion may increase the risk of HCV recurrence [32]. There is also concern that this medication could alter the balance of immune regulatory cells and increase the risk of autoimmune disease. The development of autoimmune disease has only been reported in one study of transplant recipients, but the increased risk of autoimmune disease was well established when alemtuzumab was used in the treatment of multiple sclerosis [24, 33].

31.2.3 Corticosteroids

Corticosteroids have been the mainstay therapy for induction immunosuppression. High doses are typically given in the early postoperative period which are then tapered after the first few weeks to relative low doses which are continued for at least 3–6 months [34]. Steroids must be weaned carefully due to risk of adrenal insufficiency and rebound rejection.

Unfortunately, steroids have many well-established severe side effects including growth impairment [35] diabetes, hyperlipidemia, and hypertension [11]. Steroids also interfere with hepatocyte regeneration [36]. Children and adolescents are particularly sensitive to the cosmetic effects including cushingoid facies, striae, and weight gain. Steroids can also cause mood swings. Thankfully, many of these adverse effects resolve when steroids are weaned, and children often experience subsequent catch-up growth [37]. Concern for adverse effects from steroids has led to the development of steroid-free transplant protocols.

31.3 Maintenance Treatment

31.3.1 Calcineurin Inhibitors

There are two major calcineurin inhibitors [CNI], tacrolimus and cyclosporine. Tacrolimus binds to cyclophilin and cyclosporine binds to FKBP-12, which are both intracellular immunophilins. When bound, these molecules both inhibit the phosphatase action of calcineurin. This blocks transcription of interleukin-2 genes in T cells and greatly decreases the cytokine response, in addition to interfering with transcription of IL-3, IL-4, granulocyte-macrophage colony-stimulating factor, interferon gamma, and TNF-alpha [38].

There have been several studies comparing the two CNI drugs. The first trial comparing tacrolimus and cyclosporine found no overall difference in patient and graft survival but greater rejection-free survival with tacrolimus which was later confirmed in a large multicenter study [39, 40]. A later study with longer follow-up showed greater patient and graft survival with tacrolimus in addition to less steroid-resistant rejection [41].

All CNIs share the side effects of nephrotoxicity, neurotoxicity, glucose intolerance, increased susceptibility to infection, and malignancy. CNIs are metabolized by cytochrome P450 (CYP) 3A system, and so drug interactions are common. Absorption and metabolism can be impacted by grapefruit, star fruit, pomegranate, and Seville oranges.

Renal dysfunction related to CNI therapy can improve when CNIs are withdrawn. Discontinuing CNI also resulted in improved blood pressure and serum uric acid levels; however, hyperlipidemia may not completely resolve [42].

31.3.2 Tacrolimus

Tacrolimus is currently the most common maintenance therapy according to the Studies of Pediatric Liver Transplantation (SPLIT) registry [43]. Typical dose is 0.1–0.15 mg/kg/day divided into twice-daily dosing with initial goal levels of 10–15 ng/mL for the first month with subsequent target relaxation to levels of 8–10 ng/mL by 6 months, in the absence of rejection.

Compared to cyclosporine, there is a less rejection, hypertension, hyperlipidemia, and cosmetic side effects with tacrolimus [44] but higher rate of new-onset diabetes after transplant [45]. There is also an increased risk of PTLD in patients treated with tacrolimus especially if high levels are used [46]. Nephrotoxicity is the most common complication, being reported in 24–70% of patients [47]. It is important to note that nephrotoxicity may be subtle in pediatric patients as creatinine levels may overestimate true renal function and it may be difficult to accurately measure blood pressure.

There is also an increased risk for hypomagnesemia due to renal magnesium wasting [11]. More recently it has been recognized that there is a significant risk of developing food allergies and eosinophilic gastroenteritis in children treated with tacrolimus, which appears to be commoner in those transplanted at an earlier age [48].

Since nonadherence was the third leading cause of death in pediatric transplant recipients and the leading cause of late mortality in adolescents, there is the potential to significantly improve compliance with extended-release, once-a-day dosing (Astagraf XL, Advagraf) [49]. When compared to standard dosing, the extended-release preparation is more convenient and has been shown to have similar safety and efficacy in both adults and children [50, 51].

31.3.3 Cyclosporine

It was the introduction of cyclosporine that resulted in much improved results so that liver transplantation became viable [52]. It was later reformulated as a microemulsion with improved consistency in absorption [53]. Typical doses are 5–10 mg/kg/day divided into twice-daily dosing. Initial trough goals are 250–350 ng/mL during the first month, decreased to 150–250 ng/mL during the first 6 months, 150–200 ng/mL until 1 year, and subsequently 100–150. Cyclosporine has to be administered from a glass container, not plastic or Styrofoam. However, tacrolimus has been shown to be safer and more effective with lower mortality and graft loss, reduced ACR and less steroid-resistant rejection [54].

In addition to the class side effects of all CNIs, cyclosporine has an increased risk of hypertension [45], hirsutism, and gingival hyperplasia [55] compared to tacrolimus. Cyclosporine is currently much less commonly used compared to tacrolimus, but many patients transplanted some time ago remain stable on cyclosporine.

31.4 Antimetabolites

31.4.1 Azathioprine

Azathioprine is converted to 6-mercaptopurine (6-MP). An amino group can also be added to 6-MP to make 6-thioguanine. Subsequently 6-MP and 6-thioguanine are phosphorylated to form the nucleotides thioinosinic acid and thioguanylic acid, respectively. These are then incorporated into DNA and halt replication of lymphocytes [56].

Much of the data for the use of azathioprine is in renal transplant patients where it has been shown to improve renal function, reduce hypertension, lower uric acid concentration, and lower the risk of cardiovascular death when compared to cyclosporine [57]. Liver transplant patients also showed an initial improvement in renal function when compared to cyclosporine. However, long-term follow-up demonstrated that the improvement was not sustained [58] and patients switched from a cyclosporine to azathioprine had an increased incidence of ACR [59].

Azathioprine is typically used in combination with CNI as part of maintenance immunosuppression. However, its use has declined since the introduction of mycophenolate. A significant advantage of azathioprine is its lack of embryotoxicity, meaning it will continue to have useful role in the management of teenagers and young adults. It may have an increasing role in the management of chronic hepatitis of the allograft.

Side effects include neutropenia, pancreatitis, and hepatotoxicity. Its use can be optimized by monitoring the therapeutic metabolite 6-thioguanine [60].

31.4.2 Mycophenolate

Mycophenolate mofetil [MMF] is a prodrug hydrolyzed to mycophenolic acid which then binds to, and inhibits, inosine monophosphate dehydrogenase so preventing purine synthesis. Since lymphocytes rely on this pathway for DNA synthesis, mycophenolate inhibits the proliferative response of both T and B lymphocytes [61]. It is used more often than azathioprine because it is considered more potent [62].

As with any antimetabolite, the most common side effect of mycophenolate is gastrointestinal symptoms [42], but these are rarely severe enough to warrant discontinuation [63]. More life-threatening side effects include anemia [64], neutropenia, and sepsis [62, 63, 65]. With increased immunosuppression, there was concern that there would also be increased risk of PTLD, but this has not been confirmed [66]. There were initial reports of increased invasive CMV infections, but this was not confirmed with later studies [62, 67, 68].

Similar to azathioprine, mycophenolate has mostly been used either to minimize or replace CNIs for nephroprotection or as a step-up medication in the treatment of established rejection. In adult liver transplant patients with kidney disease, there was an increase in rejection episodes following withdrawal of CNI when MMF was used alone, but not when it was used with steroids. All patients who developed rejection responded to steroids and restarting CNI treatment [42].

In pediatrics, mycophenolate has been used as an adjunct therapy or for rescue in case of rejection, with a response rate of 62% [68]. For adjunct therapy, mycophenolate has been added to tacrolimus [66] or a combination of cyclosporine and prednisone [63]. Adding mycophenolate can facilitate significant reduction in steroid dose in those who are steroid dependent [68]. De novo autoimmune hepatitis is a recently recognized phenomenon in posttransplant patients which often responds well to MMF when combined with tacrolimus and steroids [69].

In children with renal dysfunction, mycophenolate can be used to prevent deterioration and even to improve kidney function during CNI withdrawal. This can rarely be used as monotherapy, usually requiring combination with low-dose corticosteroids or the reintroduction of low-dose CNI [70].

31.5 mTOR Inhibitors

Sirolimus and everolimus are mammalian target of rapamycin (mTOR) inhibitors. They reversibly bind and activate cytoplasmic FKBP12, which then binds to mTOR. When mTOR is inhibited, the cell cycle arrests in the G1 phase, therefore triggering apoptosis. Production of IL-6 and IL-10 halts in addition to preventing T-cell proliferation [71].

31.5.1 Sirolimus (Rapamycin)

Sirolimus is most commonly used in place of CNIs in the setting of renal impairment or less commonly neurotoxicity but can also be used as a step-up treatment in chronic rejection [72]. It can be used in combination with steroids, MMF, and CNIs or as monotherapy.

There is limited published data in pediatrics, but a retrospective review of 38 children who had sirolimus added to a tacrolimus-based regimen showed fewer episodes of rejection, and they were able to tolerate lower tacrolimus levels. The addition of sirolimus also significantly improved renal function in patients with established renal impairment [73].

Leg edema, dermatitis, oral ulcers [72], hyperlipidemia, and bone marrow suppression are the most common side effects of sirolimus and are dose related. More rare side effects include lymphedema, oral aphthae, proteinuria, and wound dehiscence [74]. The use of sirolimus soon after transplant was associated with hepatic artery thrombosis, and hence these drugs are avoided in the early postoperative period [75].

31.5.2 Everolimus

Everolimus is a derivative of sirolimus but with greater stability and solubility [76]. When combined with a CNI treatment, it resulted in reduced minimum effective doses of both drugs [77].

When everolimus was added to tacrolimus 30 days after transplant, there was a reduction in tacrolimus closure and improved renal function without increased risk of rejection [78]. Thirty days was chosen as a compromise, soon enough to prevent renal damage but also late enough to avoid the early complications of everolimus, including hepatic artery thrombosis and impaired wound healing. However, even with delayed introduction of everolimus, there were wound-related complications. There was also a trend toward hyperlipidemia and invasive infections, but these did not reach statistical significance. It is important to note that renal transplant centers have seen tubular damage and proteinuria with mTOR inhibitors [79] but that was not seen in liver transplant patients [78].

In a multicenter trial of everolimus in combination with reduced CNI following pediatric liver transplantation, it resulted in improved renal function without increased rejection. However the overall side effect profile was dose-limiting, and the combination appeared to be too potent for routine clinical use [80].

31.6 Anti-B-Cell Treatments

31.6.1 Rituximab

This is a monoclonal antibody against CD20, which is expressed on almost all B cells but not on plasma cells. It induces both antibody-dependent and complement-dependent natural killer cell cytotoxicities and promotes B-cell apoptosis. B-cell numbers are depleted rapidly for approximately 6 months with subsequent recovery by 1 year. IgG levels follow a similar trajectory, although levels may remain within the normal range.

Most liver transplant experience with rituximab has been in the treatment of PTLD. It is also a key component of induction regimens following ABO incompatible transplantation where it is often used in combination with plasmapheresis and immunoglobulin treatment. Its use as an antirejection agent is in the treatment of antibody-mediated rejection (AMR) which is off label, albeit it has been extensively used following renal transplantation [34].

31.6.2 Bortezomib

This is the first proteasome inhibitor to be used clinically. Proteasome inhibition prevents the breakdown of pro-apoptotic factors, promoting apoptosis in a range of cell types but particularly plasma cells [35]. Initial experience was in the treatment of antibody-mediated rejection [AMR] following renal transplantation. Subsequently it has been shown in small case series to be effective in the treatment of hepatic AMR [36, 37]. It appears to be systemically well tolerated but is associated with nausea, fatigue and malaise.

31.6.3 Pediatric Considerations

Many medications come in pill form; it can be difficult to find compounding pharmacies and preparations can vary between pharmacies. Dosing is usually weight based and hence needs frequent updating, especially in small children.

Trough levels may vary when different preparations are used. Suspensions are usually more expensive and require special care such as refrigeration and shaking before administration to assure consistent concentration.

Medications are often unpalatable, and children can require nasogastric tubes or even gastrostomy to administer. Children are also not typically in charge of their medications which can leave them more at risk if there are inconsistent caregivers.

Children also have a longer expected period of exposure to immunosuppression, which can impact growth, risk of infection (bacterial, viral, and fungal), carcinogenesis, and likelihood of nonadherence.

With these unique considerations, pediatric patients are likely to benefit from a multidisciplinary team including a child life specialist, social worker, financial counselor and transplant pharmacist to help navigate these potential barriers to optimal care.

31.6.4 Immunosuppression Regimens

Immunosuppression regimens have not been standardized and tend to be center specific. They may include an induction regimen and usually consist of a CNI in combination with either steroids or an antimetabolite. Higher levels of immunosuppression are usually used in the first 3 months with subsequent relaxation of targets until 1 year after transplant in the absence of rejection. An example regimen used at Children's Hospital of Pittsburgh is attached [Table 31.1].

Table 31.1 Routine immunosuppression for liver transplantation at Children's Hospital of Pittsburgh

1. Tacrolimus. Starting dose 0.1 mg/kg orally twice daily, subsequently adjusted to achive target levels			
Time posttransplant	Target trough level [Ng/mL]		
Month 1	12–15		
2–3 months	10–12		
>3 months	8–10		
This is combined with either thymoglobulin or corticosteroids			
(a) Thymoglobulin			
Preoperative 5 mg/kg infusion over 6–12 h with premedication			
(b) Corticosteroids			
Perioperative 10 mg/kg methylprednisolone [maximum dose 1 g]			
Postoperative day	Dose [mg/Kg]	Frequency	Maximum single dose (mg)
1	1.25	4 times daily	50
2	1.0	4 times daily	40
3	1.0	3 times daily	30
4	1.0	2 times daily	20

Subsequently move to oral prednisolone 2 mg/kg per day [maximum 40 mg]. Gradually wean toward discontinuation after 3 months [except autoimmune disease]

The use of induction therapy is gradually increasing and in 2015 was used in approximately one third of pediatric recipients in the USA [81]; these were IL-2 receptor antagonists in 23% and lymphocyte-depleting agents in 12%. These were commonly used as part of a steroid-free or minimization regimen. Tacrolimus continues to be the commonest maintenance agent, used in greater than 95% of cases in the USA. This was combined with corticosteroids in 80% and mycophenolate in 33%. By 1 year after transplant, corticosteroid use had decreased to 60%.

mTOR inhibitors are rarely used in the immediate perioperative period and may be introduced to maintenance therapy in selected cases for nephroprotection or where the primary diagnosis was hepatic malignancy. By 1 year after transplant, these were used less than 10% of cases in the USA in 2015 [81].

31.6.5 Acute Rejection

The incidence of acute rejection following pediatric transplantation remains approximately 40–60% in the first year, mostly occurring in the first 3 months [82]. Occasionally the presentation is with clinical features such as abdominal pain or fever but most commonly is marked by worsening laboratory function tests and should be confirmed histologically.

First-line treatment is with corticosteroids, usually given as an intravenous pulse for 1–5 days. Doses vary per institutional protocol but are usually in the range of 5–15 mg/kg methylprednisolone [with a maximum dose range of 500 mg to 1 g). Subsequently there is a steroid taper toward maintenance dose. Specific titration of therapy will depend on institutional practice, histological and biochemical severity, biochemical response, and therapy side effects. Corticosteroids alone are effective in more than 80% of cases [40, 83].

A single episode of acute rejection which responds quickly to therapy does not impact on long-term prognosis and may even promote subsequent tolerance [84, 85]. As a result, there is no absolute need to subsequently increase maintenance immunosuppression so long as close and careful monitoring is feasible. In this situation, specific monitoring of the immune response such as Pleximmune may help individualize subsequent management [86].

31.6.6 Steroid-Resistant Rejection

This is defined as no improvement in biochemical or histological features following pulsed steroids in the presence of adequate background immunosuppressive levels. The incidence is approximately 5% overall or 10% of those with acute rejection [40, 83]. First-line treatment is usually with either anti-IL-2 or lymphocyte-depleting antibodies. An antimetabolite should be added, if this is not already part of the regimen. Given its greater potency, mycophenolate is generally preferred to azathioprine in this situation [87]. Target levels of tacrolimus should be raised and maintained at a higher level for at least for the next 3 months.

If there is incomplete response, or intolerance of increased tacrolimus exposure, mTOR inhibitors may be used. These should initially be additional to tacrolimus, at least until therapeutic levels are achieved. After complete response is achieved, tacrolimus can be gradually withdrawn.

31.6.7 Chronic Rejection

With the evolution of immunosuppression, and particularly since the introduction of tacrolimus as the default maintenance agent, chronic rejection has become rare. Recent long-term studies found histologically confirmed chronic rejection in <10% after 10 years with repeat transplantation being required in <5% of cases [88].

Clinically chronic rejection presents with progressive cholestasis commonly, but not invariably, following previous and recurrent episodes of acute rejection. Histologically it is characterized by ductopenia, centrilobular inflammation, and a foam cell arteriopathy. It has classically been divided into early and late chronic rejection, with late rejection characterized by >50% bile duct loss and >25% arteriolar loss with bridging fibrosis [89]. Recently the frequency of de novo donor-specific antibodies [DSA] in the presence of chronic rejection has been appreciated, although there is still uncertainty as to whether these are pathogenic or epiphenomenon [84, 90].

The histological classifications are not absolutely guides as to whether the rejection is reversible. Even where there appears to be complete duct loss, reversal can occur [91]. Treatment consists of increasing immunosuppression and addressing any nonadherence issues. Where nonadherence was not an issue, mTOR inhibitors and/or mycophenolate should be added and are effective in greater than 50% of cases. In the absence of response, retransplantation is the only option, with excellent results so long as adherence can be assured.

31.6.8 Antibody-Mediated Rejection (AMR)

This is a rarely recognized entity which presents with fever, acute liver dysfunction, and thrombocytopenia, usually in the first 2 posttransplant weeks. It appears to be commoner in children, presumably because the smaller graft size limits the capacity of the liver to clear preformed DSA. Histology shows hepatocellular necrosis and ischemic injury which may progress to interstitial hemorrhage. Complement 4d (C4d) staining of the portal venous and capillary network is usually positive, but this is not specific for AMR [92]. Both class 1 and 2 DSA drive the process, and these may be preformed or, even in early cases, may be formed de novo [92, 93]. Diagnosis requires the combination of liver injury, C4d staining, and DSA.

Treatment is poorly standardized. Initial management includes bolus corticosteroids as this is difficult to distinguish from ACR and indeed these conditions may coexist. Subsequent options include immunoglobulin infusion, with or without plasmapheresis, anti-B-cell agents including rituximab and bortezomib, mycophenolate, and most recently the use of eculizumab [92]. The timing of an AMR episode impacts treatment choices with rituximab preferred for early acute AMR because it targets B cells and using bortezomib to target longer-living plasma cells in late acute AMR.

Historically the outlook was very poor with a high mortality, but recent experience has been more positive with 70% survival, albeit with a subsequent risk of malignancy because of increased immunosuppression exposure [92].

A very specific form of AMR is the recurrent cholestasis following transplantation for progressive familial intrahepatic cholestasis type 2. This seems to be caused by de novo anti-BSEP antibodies in those who had no BSEP expression in their native liver. These antibodies block the allograft BSEP receptor and reproduce the pretransplant phenotype [94]. Recently this has been shown to respond to conventional treatment for AMR with plasmapheresis, immunoglobulin, and rituximab [95].

References

1. Cai J, Terasaki PI. Induction immunosuppression improves long-term graft and patient outcome in organ transplantation: an analysis of United Network for Organ Sharing registry data. Transplantation. 2010;90:1511–5.
2. Queen C, Schneider WP, Selick HE, et al. A humanized antibody that binds to the interleukin 2 receptor. Proc Natl Acad Sci U S A. 1989;86:10029–33.
3. Smith KA. Interleukin-2: inception, impact, and implications. Science. 1988;240:1169–76.
4. Minami Y, Kono T, Miyazaki T, Taniguchi T. The IL-2 receptor complex: its structure, function, and target genes. Annu Rev Immunol. 1993;11:245–68.
5. Koch M, Niemeyer G, Patel I, Light S, Nashan B. Pharmacokinetics, pharmacodynamics, and immunodynamics of daclizumab in a two-dose regimen in liver transplantation. Transplantation. 2002;73:1640–6.
6. Eckhoff DE, McGuire B, Sellers M, et al. The safety and efficacy of a two-dose daclizumab (zenapax) induction therapy in liver transplant recipients. Transplantation. 2000;69:1867–72.
7. Vincenti F, Kirkman R, Light S, et al. Interleukin-2-receptor blockade with daclizumab to prevent acute rejection in renal transplantation. Daclizumab Triple Therapy Study Group. N Engl J Med. 1998;338:161–5.

8. Heffron TG, Pillen T, Smallwood GA, Welch D, Oakley B, Romero R. Pediatric liver transplantation with daclizumab induction. Transplantation. 2003;75:2040–3.
9. Spada M, Petz W, Bertani A, et al. Randomized trial of basiliximab induction versus steroid therapy in pediatric liver allograft recipients under tacrolimus immunosuppression. Am J Transplant. 2006;6:1913–21.
10. Gras JM, Gerkens S, Beguin C, et al. Steroid-free, tacrolimus-basiliximab immunosuppression in pediatric liver transplantation: clinical and pharmacoeconomic study in 50 children. Liver Transpl. 2008;14:469–77.
11. Miloh T, Barton A, Wheeler J, et al. Immunosuppression in pediatric liver transplant recipients: unique aspects. Liver Transpl. 2017;23:244–56.
12. Fung J, Kelly D, Kadry Z, Patel-Tom K, Eghtesad B. Immunosuppression in liver transplantation: beyond calcineurin inhibitors. Liver Transpl. 2005;11:267–80.
13. Beiras-Fernandez A, Thein E, Chappel D, et al. Polyclonal antithymocyte globulins influence apoptosis in reperfused tissues after ischaemia in a non-human primate model. Transpl Int. 2004;17:453–7.
14. Chappell D, Beiras-Fernandez A, Hammer C, Thein E. In vivo visualization of the effect of polyclonal antithymocyte globulins on the microcirculation after ischemia/reperfusion in a primate model. Transplantation. 2006;81:552–8.
15. Tchervenkov J, Flemming C, Guttmann RD, des Gachons G. Use of thymoglobulin induction therapy in the prevention of acute graft rejection episodes following liver transplantation. Transplant Proc. 1997;29:13S–5S.
16. Bogetti D, Sankary HN, Jarzembowski TM, et al. Thymoglobulin induction protects liver allografts from ischemia/reperfusion injury. Clin Transpl. 2005;19:507–11.
17. Boillot O, Seket B, Dumortier J, et al. Thymoglobulin induction in liver transplant recipients with a tacrolimus, mycophenolate mofetil, and steroid immunosuppressive regimen: a five-year randomized prospective study. Liver Transpl. 2009;15:1426–34.
18. Eason JD, Blazek J, Mason A, Nair S, Loss GE. Steroid-free immunosuppression through thymoglobulin induction in liver transplantation. Transplant Proc. 2001;33:1470–1.
19. Tector AJ, Fridell JA, Mangus RS, et al. Promising early results with immunosuppression using rabbit anti-thymocyte globulin and steroids with delayed introduction of tacrolimus in adult liver transplant recipients. Liver Transpl. 2004;10:404–7.
20. Starzl TE, Murase N, Abu-Elmagd K, et al. Tolerogenic immunosuppression for organ transplantation. Lancet. 2003;361:1502–10.
21. Frampton JE, Wagstaff AJ. Alemtuzumab. Drugs. 2003;63:1229–43. discussion 45–6
22. Bloom DD, Hu H, Fechner JH, Knechtle SJ. T-lymphocyte alloresponses of Campath-1H-treated kidney transplant patients. Transplantation. 2006;81:81–7.
23. Calne R, Friend P, Moffatt S, et al. Prope tolerance, perioperative campath 1H, and low-dose cyclosporin monotherapy in renal allograft recipients. Lancet. 1998;351:1701–2.
24. Watson CJ, Bradley JA, Friend PJ, et al. Alemtuzumab (CAMPATH 1H) induction therapy in cadaveric kidney transplantation--efficacy and safety at five years. Am J Transplant. 2005;5:1347–53.
25. Ciancio G, Burke GW, Gaynor JJ, et al. A randomized trial of three renal transplant induction antibodies: early comparison of tacrolimus, mycophenolate mofetil, and steroid dosing, and newer immune-monitoring. Transplantation. 2005;80:457–65.
26. Tzakis AG, Tryphonopoulos P, Kato T, et al. Preliminary experience with alemtuzumab (Campath-1H) and low-dose tacrolimus immunosuppression in adult liver transplantation. Transplantation. 2004;77:1209–14.
27. Tryphonopoulos P, Madariaga JR, Kato T, et al. The impact of Campath 1H induction in adult liver allotransplantation. Transplant Proc. 2005;37:1203–4.
28. Kato T, Selvaggi G, Panagiotis T, et al. Pediatric liver transplant with Campath 1H induction--preliminary report. Transplant Proc. 2006;38:3609–11.
29. Vathsala A, Ona ET, Tan SY, et al. Randomized trial of Alemtuzumab for prevention of graft rejection and preservation of renal function after kidney transplantation. Transplantation. 2005;80:765–74.
30. Silveira FP, Marcos A, Kwak EJ, et al. Bloodstream infections in organ transplant recipients receiving alemtuzumab: no evidence of occurrence of organisms typically associated with profound T cell depletion. J Infect. 2006;53:241–7.
31. Alcaide ML, Abbo L, Pano JR, et al. Herpes zoster infection after liver transplantation in patients receiving induction therapy with alemtuzumab. Clin Transpl. 2008;22:502–7.
32. Marcos A, Eghtesad B, Fung JJ, et al. Use of alemtuzumab and tacrolimus monotherapy for cadaveric liver transplantation: with particular reference to hepatitis C virus. Transplantation. 2004;78:966–71.
33. Coles AJ, Wing M, Smith S, et al. Pulsed monoclonal antibody treatment and autoimmune thyroid disease in multiple sclerosis. Lancet. 1999;354:1691–5.
34. Moini M, Schilsky ML, Tichy EM. Review on immunosuppression in liver transplantation. World J Hepatol. 2015;7:1355–68.
35. Viner RM, Forton JT, Cole TJ, Clark IH, Noble-Jamieson G, Barnes ND. Growth of long-term survivors of liver transplantation. Arch Dis Child. 1999;80:235–40.
36. Vintermyr OK, Doskeland SO. Characterization of the inhibitory effect of glucocorticoids on the DNA replication of adult rat hepatocytes growing at various cell densities. J Cell Physiol. 1989;138:29–37.
37. Diem HV, Sokal EM, Janssen M, Otte JB, Reding R. Steroid withdrawal after pediatric liver transplantation: a long-term follow-up study in 109 recipients. Transplantation. 2003;75:1664–70.
38. Kahan BD, Ghobrial R. Immunosuppressive agents. Surg Clin North Am. 1994;74:1029–54.
39. McDiarmid SV, Busuttil RW, Ascher NL, et al. FK506 (tacrolimus) compared with cyclosporine for primary immunosuppression after pediatric liver transplantation. Results from the U.S. Multicenter Trial. Transplantation. 1995;59:530–6.
40. Kelly D, Jara P, Rodeck B, et al. Tacrolimus and steroids versus ciclosporin microemulsion, steroids, and azathioprine in children undergoing liver transplantation: randomised European multicentre trial. Lancet. 2004;364:1054–61.
41. Jain A, Mazariegos G, Kashyap R, et al. Comparative long-term evaluation of tacrolimus and cyclosporine in pediatric liver transplantation. Transplantation. 2000;70:617–25.
42. Schlitt HJ, Barkmann A, Boker KH, et al. Replacement of calcineurin inhibitors with mycophenolate mofetil in liver-transplant patients with renal dysfunction: a randomised controlled study. Lancet. 2001;357:587–91.
43. Ng VL, Fecteau A, Shepherd R, et al. Outcomes of 5-year survivors of pediatric liver transplantation: report on 461 children from a North American multicenter registry. Pediatrics. 2008;122:e1128–35.
44. Kelly D. Safety and efficacy of tacrolimus in pediatric liver recipients. Pediatr Transplant. 2011;15:19–24.
45. Muduma G, Saunders R, Odeyemi I, Pollock RF. Systematic review and meta-analysis of tacrolimus versus ciclosporin as primary immunosuppression after liver transplant. PLoS One. 2016;11:e0160421.
46. Sokal EM, Antunes H, Beguin C, et al. Early signs and risk factors for the increased incidence of Epstein-Barr virus-related posttransplant lymphoproliferative diseases in pediatric liver transplant recipients treated with tacrolimus. Transplantation. 1997;64:1438–42.
47. Kelly DA, Bucuvalas JC, Alonso EM, et al. Long-term medical management of the pediatric patient after liver transplantation: 2013 practice guideline by the American Association for the Study

of Liver Diseases and the American Society of Transplantation. Liver Transpl. 2013;19:798–825.
48. Wisniewski J, Lieberman J, Nowak-Wegrzyn A, et al. De novo food sensitization and eosinophilic gastrointestinal disease in children post-liver transplantation. Clin Transpl. 2012;26:E365–71.
49. Sudan DL, Shaw BW Jr, Langnas AN. Causes of late mortality in pediatric liver transplant recipients. Ann Surg. 1998;227:289–95.
50. Coilly A, Calmus Y, Chermak F, et al. Once-daily prolonged release tacrolimus in liver transplantation: experts' literature review and recommendations. Liver Transpl. 2015;21:1312–21.
51. Heffron TG, Pescovitz MD, Florman S, et al. Once-daily tacrolimus extended-release formulation: 1-year post-conversion in stable pediatric liver transplant recipients. Am J Transplant. 2007;7:1609–15.
52. Starzl TE, Iwatsuki S, Shaw BW Jr, Gordon RD, Esquivel CO. Immunosuppression and other nonsurgical factors in the improved results of liver transplantation. Semin Liver Dis. 1985;5:334–43.
53. Otto MG, Mayer AD, Clavien PA, Cavallari A, Gunawardena KA, Mueller EA. Randomized trial of cyclosporine microemulsion (neoral) versus conventional cyclosporine in liver transplantation: MILTON study. Multicentre International Study in Liver Transplantation of Neoral. Transplantation. 1998;66:1632–40.
54. McAlister VC, Haddad E, Renouf E, Malthaner RA, Kjaer MS, Gluud LL. Cyclosporin versus tacrolimus as primary immunosuppressant after liver transplantation: a meta-analysis. Am J Transplant. 2006;6:1578–85.
55. Peters TG, Spinola KN, West JC, et al. Differences in patient and transplant professional perceptions of immunosuppression-induced cosmetic side effects. Transplantation. 2004;78:537–43.
56. Evans WE. Pharmacogenetics of thiopurine S-methyltransferase and thiopurine therapy. Ther Drug Monit. 2004;26:186–91.
57. Hollander AA, van Saase JL, Kootte AM, et al. Beneficial effects of conversion from cyclosporin to azathioprine after kidney transplantation. Lancet. 1995;345:610–4.
58. Eid A, Perkins JD, Rakela J, Krom RA. Conversion from standard cyclosporine to low-dose cyclosporine in liver transplant recipients: effect on nephrotoxicity and hypertension beyond one year. Transplant Proc. 1989;21:2238–9.
59. Sandborn WJ, Hay JE, Porayko MK, et al. Cyclosporine withdrawal for nephrotoxicity in liver transplant recipients does not result in sustained improvement in kidney function and causes cellular and ductopenic rejection. Hepatology. 1994;19:925–32.
60. Rumbo C, Shneider BL, Emre SH. Utility of azathioprine metabolite measurements in post-transplant recurrent autoimmune and immune-mediated hepatitis. Pediatr Transplant. 2004;8:571–5.
61. Allison AC, Eugui EM. Purine metabolism and immunosuppressive effects of mycophenolate mofetil (MMF). Clin Transpl. 1996;10:77–84.
62. Sollinger HW. Mycophenolate mofetil for the prevention of acute rejection in primary cadaveric renal allograft recipients. U.S. Renal Transplant Mycophenolate Mofetil Study Group. Transplantation. 1995;60:225–32.
63. Renz JF, Lightdale J, Mudge C, et al. Mycophenolate mofetil, microemulsion cyclosporine, and prednisone as primary immunosuppression for pediatric liver transplant recipients. Liver Transpl Surg. 1999;5:136–43.
64. Herrero JI, Quiroga J, Sangro B, et al. Conversion of liver transplant recipients on cyclosporine with renal impairment to mycophenolate mofetil. Liver Transpl Surg. 1999;5:414–20.
65. Wiesner R, Rabkin J, Klintmalm G, et al. A randomized double-blind comparative study of mycophenolate mofetil and azathioprine in combination with cyclosporine and corticosteroids in primary liver transplant recipients. Liver Transpl. 2001;7:442–50.
66. Colombani PM, Lau H, Prabhakaran K, et al. Cumulative experience with pediatric living related liver transplantation. J Pediatr Surg. 2000;35:9–12.
67. Sarmiento JM, Munn SR, Paya CV, Velosa JA, Nguyen JH. Is cytomegalovirus infection related to mycophenolate mofetil after kidney transplantation? A case-control study. Clin Transpl. 1998;12:371–4.
68. Chardot C, Nicoluzzi JE, Janssen M, et al. Use of mycophenolate mofetil as rescue therapy after pediatric liver transplantation. Transplantation. 2001;71:224–9.
69. Gibelli NE, Tannuri U, Mello ES, et al. Successful treatment of de novo autoimmune hepatitis and cirrhosis after pediatric liver transplantation. Pediatr Transplant. 2006;10:371–6.
70. Evans HM, McKiernan PJ, Kelly DA. Mycophenolate mofetil for renal dysfunction after pediatric liver transplantation. Transplantation. 2005;79:1575–80.
71. Dunn C, Croom KF. Everolimus: a review of its use in renal and cardiac transplantation. Drugs. 2006;66:547–70.
72. Montalbano M, Neff GW, Yamashiki N, et al. A retrospective review of liver transplant patients treated with sirolimus from a single center: an analysis of sirolimus-related complications. Transplantation. 2004;78:264–8.
73. Casas-Melley AT, Falkenstein KP, Flynn LM, Ziegler VL, Dunn SP. Improvement in renal function and rejection control in pediatric liver transplant recipients with the introduction of sirolimus. Pediatr Transplant. 2004;8:362–6.
74. Dean PG, Lund WJ, Larson TS, et al. Wound-healing complications after kidney transplantation: a prospective, randomized comparison of sirolimus and tacrolimus. Transplantation. 2004;77:1555–61.
75. Sindhi R, Ganjoo J, McGhee W, Mazariegos G, Reyes J. Preliminary immunosuppression withdrawal strategies with sirolimus in children with liver transplants. Transplant Proc. 2002;34:1972–3.
76. Kirchner GI, Meier-Wiedenbach I, Manns MP. Clinical pharmacokinetics of everolimus. Clin Pharmacokinet. 2004;43:83–95.
77. Schuurman HJ, Cottens S, Fuchs S, et al. SDZ RAD, a new rapamycin derivative: synergism with cyclosporine. Transplantation. 1997;64:32–5.
78. De Simone P, Nevens F, De Carlis L, et al. Everolimus with reduced tacrolimus improves renal function in de novo liver transplant recipients: a randomized controlled trial. Am J Transplant. 2012;12:3008–20.
79. Franz S, Regeniter A, Hopfer H, Mihatsch M, Dickenmann M. Tubular toxicity in sirolimus- and cyclosporine-based transplant immunosuppression strategies: an ancillary study from a randomized controlled trial. Am J Kidney Dis. 2010;55:335–43.
80. Ganschow R, Ericzon BG, Dhawan A, et al. Everolimus and reduced calcineurin inhibitor therapy in pediatric liver transplant recipients: results from a multicenter, prospective study. Pediatr Transplant. 2017;21(7).
81. Kim WR, Lake JR, Smith JM, et al. OPTN/SRTR 2015 annual data report: liver. Am J Transplant. 2017;17(Suppl 1):174–251.
82. Ng VL, Fecteau A, Shepherd R, et al. Outcomes of 5-year survivors of pediatric liver transplantation: report on 461 children from a North American Multicenter Registry. Pediatrics. 2008;122:e1128–e35.
83. Martin SR, Atkison P, Anand R, Lindblad AS, Group SR. Studies of Pediatric Liver Transplantation 2002: patient and graft survival and rejection in pediatric recipients of a first liver transplant in the United States and Canada. Pediatr Transplant. 2004;8:273–83.
84. Adams DH, Sanchez-Fueyo A, Samuel D. From immunosuppression to tolerance. J Hepatol. 2015;62:S170–85.
85. Wiesner RH, Demetris AJ, Belle SH, et al. Acute hepatic allograft rejection: incidence, risk factors, and impact on outcome. Hepatology. 1998;28:638–45.
86. Sindhi R, Ashokkumar C, Higgs BW, et al. Profile of the Pleximmune blood test for transplant rejection risk prediction. Expert Rev Mol Diagn. 2016;16:387–93.
87. Aw MM, Verma A, Rela M, Heaton N, Mieli-Vergani G, Dhawan A. Long-term outcome of mycophenolate mofetil rescue therapy

for resistant acute allograft rejection in pediatric liver transplant recipients. Liver Transpl. 2008;14:1303–8.
88. Ng VL, Alonso EM, Bucuvalas JC, et al. Health status of children alive 10 years after pediatric liver transplantation performed in the US and Canada: report of the studies of pediatric liver transplantation experience. J Pediatr. 2012;160:820–6.
89. Demetris AJ, Bellamy C, Hubscher SG, et al. 2016 Comprehensive Update of the Banff Working Group on Liver Allograft Pathology: introduction of antibody-mediated rejection. Am J Transplant. 2016;16:2816–35.
90. Grabhorn E, Binder TM, Obrecht D, et al. Long-term clinical relevance of de novo donor-specific antibodies after pediatric liver transplantation. Transplantation. 2015;99(9):1876–81.
91. Neff GW, Montalbano M, Slapak-Green G, et al. A retrospective review of sirolimus (Rapamune) therapy in orthotopic liver transplant recipients diagnosed with chronic rejection. Liver Transpl. 2003;9:477–83.
92. Wozniak LJ, Naini BV, Hickey MJ, et al. Acute antibody-mediated rejection in ABO-compatible pediatric liver transplant recipients: case series and review of the literature. Pediatr Transplant. 2017;21(1).
93. Yamada Y, Hoshino K, Mori T, et al. Successful living donor liver retransplantation for graft failure within 7 days due to acute de novo donor-specific anti-human leukocyte antigen antibody-mediated rejection. Hepatol Res. 2018;48:E360–E6.
94. Siebold L, Dick AA, Thompson R, et al. Recurrent low gamma-glutamyl transpeptidase cholestasis following liver transplantation for bile salt export pump (BSEP) disease (posttransplant recurrent BSEP disease). Liver Transpl. 2010;16:856–63.
95. Patel KR, Harpavat S, Finegold M, et al. Post-transplant recurrent bile salt export pump disease: a form of antibody-mediated graft dysfunction and utilization of C4d. J Pediatr Gastroenterol Nutr. 2017;65:364–9.

32. Pathology of Allograft Liver Dysfunction

Aurelio Sonzogni, Lisa Licini, and Lorenzo D'Antiga

32.1 Introduction

Long-term dysfunction and graft rejection have been a major concern since the beginning of liver transplantation (LT) era in the early 60s of the last century. Given the great improvements in post-transplant immunosuppression, the incidence of acute and chronic rejection has decreased significantly over the last few years. This has led to abnormalities in clinical and in histopathological presentation of rejection with more patients suffering from late acute rejection, which commonly has different histological appearances compared with the early posttransplant period; the term of atypical rejection has sometimes been applied to this conditions. Histological evaluation of biopsies is an integral part of the management of liver transplanted patients. From the time of donor hepatectomy onward, the allograft is susceptible to multiple insults, such as warm and cold ischemia, complications related to biliary and vascular anastomoses, rejection, and recurrence of native liver disease. It is often fairly challenging to distinguish these various entities by their clinical presentation alone.

The liver biopsy still remains a cornerstone in the diagnostic work-up of immunological and non-immunological complication of LT; due to incomplete maturation of immune system in pediatric patients, biological and histological dysfunction are usually polymorphic from many point of view, including morphological aspects in biopsy sample.

Liver biopsies can be performed by various technical support finalized to avoid complications, including a percutaneous approach (with marking liver by percussion/palpation, marking by ultrasounds under real-time US or computed tomography guidance), a trans-jugular approach, or a surgical/laparoscopic approach.

Despite its utility, liver biopsy carries anyway a small risk of potential complications in LT recipients. One study found a 1.8% rate of significant complications after each biopsy in this setting, including an increased rate of sepsis [1] that should be regarded as one of the most frequent and dangerous situation. In another report, infectious complications of liver biopsy were associated with the presence of biliary strictures and biliary anastomosis by choledochojejunostomy [2].

Due to relatively easy control of acute episodes of rejection, there is actually a shift in interest to the long-term outcome of liver allografts, mainly in pediatric groups, also regarding the possible rule of liver biopsy in weaning immunosuppression. Points of interest and discussion are the histological abnormalities commonly present in late posttransplant protocol and may be observed in recipients who are clinically well and with good graft function. The long-term immunosuppression leads to complex and atypical features on biopsy specimens and requires to achieve a strict clinical-pathological correlation. Even when standard liver tests are normal, ongoing inflammation in the graft could be present and, if immunosuppression is not modified, will lead to progressive fibrosis and cirrhosis. Conversely, normal liver histology may allow for reduction in the immunosuppression and so lower the risk of the complications associated with immunosuppression in long-term survivals. Most pediatric liver diseases are potentially curable with LT, and it is important to establish whether children who have undergone successful transplantation can expect a normal life or whether there will be a gradual decline in liver function and eventual graft loss.

A recent published paper by Banff group [3], an international panel of experts of LT histopathology, has proposed a systematic review of the previous terminology used in routinely diagnostic activity (Table 32.1) concerning immunological graft dysfunction that every center is encouraged to

A. Sonzogni (✉) · L. Licini
Department of Pathology, Papa Giovanni XXIII Hospital, Bergamo, Italy
e-mail: asonzogni@asst-pg23.it; unknown_user_453216@meteor.springer.com

L. D'Antiga
Paediatric Hepatology, Gastroenterology and Transplantation, Hospital Papa Giovanni XXIII, Bergamo, Italy
e-mail: ldantiga@asst-pg23.it

Table 32.1 Comparison between old and new proposed terminology for histological follow-up of LT

Old terms	New terms
Humoral or hyperacute rejection	Antibody-mediated rejection (AMR)
De novo autoimmune hepatitis	Plasma cell-rich rejection ("plasma cell hepatitis")
(Acute) cellular rejection	T cell-mediated rejection (TCMR)

follow in categorizing the various patterns of rejection. This classification could be useful to standardize and simplify terminology, avoiding confusing definitions and making histological diagnosis more comparable.

Liver biopsy is usually performed in two main settings: alterations of liver function tests with or without clinical signs and symptoms or scheduled procedure within a protocol.

This chapter will deal with the morphological features of more frequent adverse events in LT follow-up focusing about the main histological pictures that should be known by transplantation surgeons and pediatric hepatologists involved in transplantation activities. The detailed pathophysiology and histological features are beyond the scope of this chapter; only basic concepts will be provided tailored on daily practice, and for further information about these items, specific textbooks should be consulted.

32.2 Basic Requirements of Liver Biopsy

Liver biopsy is usually obtained on ultrasound-guided procedure basis, using a gauge needle. The tissue sample should include a satisfactory number of portal fields; small samples are at high risk of incorrect diagnosis, missing or underscoring fundamental microscopic lesions; definite diagnosis by pathologist in such cases has to be discouraged and liver sampling should be repeated.

According to guidelines for liver biopsy, adequacy as defined by AASLD/Banff Working Group includes two passes with a 16-gauge needle for adequate assessment of fibrosis. Smaller needle biopsies (<20 mm in length) are subject to sampling errors and possible underestimation of fibrosis. Needle liver samples containing <11 portal tracts might not be representative, mainly regarding biliary lesions that may be limited to few portal tracts in early phases up to 4–6 weeks from surgery.

Liver tissue will be usually processed routinely as any other bioptical sample; stained sections should be available for histological evaluation on next working day and for each liver biopsy should be routinely provided, besides standard hematoxylin-eosin staining, additional special histochemical stainings for collagen and iron. Other indispensable tools to be performed on demand are immunohistochemical stains to detect abnormal cell phenotype (i.e., liver cell biliary metaplasia demonstrated by staining with cytokeratin 7), degree of bile ducts proliferation, immunophenotyping of lymphocytic cell infiltrate, and demonstration of opportunistic viral infections (cytomegalovirus, herpes viruses, etc.).

In situ hybridization (ISH) is a technique that allows sharp localization of a specific segment of nucleic acid within a histologic section. The underlying basis of ISH is that nucleic acids, if preserved adequately within a histologic specimen, can be detected through the application of a complementary strand of nucleic acid to which a reporter molecule is attached. In LT follow-up setting, ISH is usually performed in paraffin-embedded tissue in order to detect the presence of Epstein-Barr virus or other opportunistic pathogens.

In case of urgent clinical background, a rapid processing method of biopsy specimens should be available in each transplantation center in order to get histological slides available for rush diagnosis in 2–3 h, and a liver-committed pathologist should be in charge to evaluate histopathological abnormalities.

32.3 T-Cell-Mediated Rejection (TCMR) (Synonym: Acute Rejection)

32.3.1 General Considerations

TMCR is an acute inflammation of allograft due to antigenic difference between donor and recipient commonly seen in every solid organ transplant; the main anatomic targets of this process in the liver are bile duct epithelium and vascular endothelium of portal vein branches, central veins and sometimes arteries, all of them expressing HLA class II antigens; involvement of arterial branches endothelium is possible, but is anyway rare and should be regarded as a sign of severity of rejection. The liver has peculiar immune characteristics (Kupffer cells, vascular and sinusoidal endothelial cells, large number of portal dendritic and inflammatory cells) that should promote graft rejection. In contrast there is minimal expression of class II HLA antigens on hepatocytes, which favors decreased antigenicity. It is also thought that donor Kupffer cells may be replaced with host macrophages, which would promote graft acceptance.

Lymphocyte trafficking through the allograft has been hypothesized to contribute to the development of a degree of immunological tolerance. On the other hand, approximately only 5–10% of liver transplantation recipients who develop acute cellular rejection progress to chronic rejection despite aggressive antirejection therapy.

The diagnosis of TCMR is suspected by elevations in serum aminotransferase and alkaline phosphatase levels, which typically precede clinical symptoms. However, biochemical parameters are not sensitive or specific for detecting acute cellular rejection and do not correlate with its severity [4]. Thus, the diagnosis should be always confirmed by liver biopsy before starting any treatment for rejection; previous medical treatment by steroids of clinically suspected TCMR may modified the degree of characteristic histological lesions and underscore the severity of the process.

Clinical signs and symptoms may include tachycardia, fever, malaise, right upper quadrant and right flank tenderness or pain, hepatomegaly, and increased ascites accumulation. The patient's mental status may also change, and disorientation may be noted in severe cases. The absence of abovementioned signs and symptoms does not anyway exclude the possibility of TCMR. The clinical-histological appearances of lesions are anyway very variable. At one end of the spectrum, graft function may remain stable in many patients found to have focal or mild histologic features of rejection on a protocol liver biopsy, even when no treatment is provided [5].

Most cases of TMCR occur within 30–40 days after liver transplantation, possibly related to massive migration of donor cells in lymphoid structures of the recipient. Early episodes may be seen in patients who undergone suboptimal baseline immunosuppression, but steroid boluses and increased immunosuppressive regimens usually are able to resolve TCMR. Early and late TCMR are anyway not strictly time-delineated, and considerable overlap exists so strict separation between the two patterns may be difficult. Poor compliance to immunosuppressive schedule or spontaneous withdrawn of drugs may be responsible of onset of TMCR also after many months or years from LT.

32.3.2 Histopathological Findings

TCMR manifests histologically as liver allograft infiltration by admixture of different inflammatory cells, mainly T lymphocytes accompanied by variable numbers of B lymphocytes, macrophages, plasma cells, eosinophils, and neutrophils granulocytes.

TCMR rejection severity grading is based on: (1) intensity and distribution of inflammation and tissue damage and (2) direct or indirect signs of vascular injury, such as lymphocytic arteritis, confluent liver cell necrosis, and non-procedural-related interstitial hemorrhage.

The three main histological lesions for the diagnosis of TCMR are (1) mixed portal inflammatory infiltrate represented by activated lymphocytes, neutrophils, plasma cells, and eosinophils (in most severe cases, inflammatory infiltrate extends around central veins), (2) subendothelial inflammation of portal and central vein (endothelitis) and (3) bile duct damage with acute inflammation (Fig. 32.1).

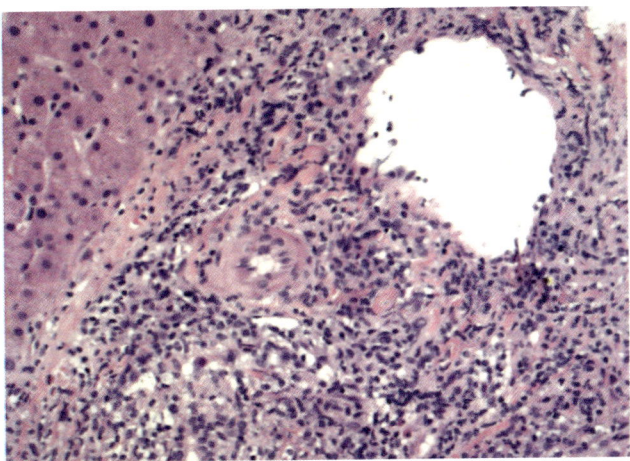

Fig. 32.1 Classical histological features allowing a diagnosis of severe TCMR, characterized by massive mixed portal field inflammatory infiltrate (lymphocytes, plasma cells, and eosinophils), portal vein branch circumferential endothelitis, and severe bile duct damage obscured by inflammatory cells; some degree of arteritis is also evident (H&E, 40×)

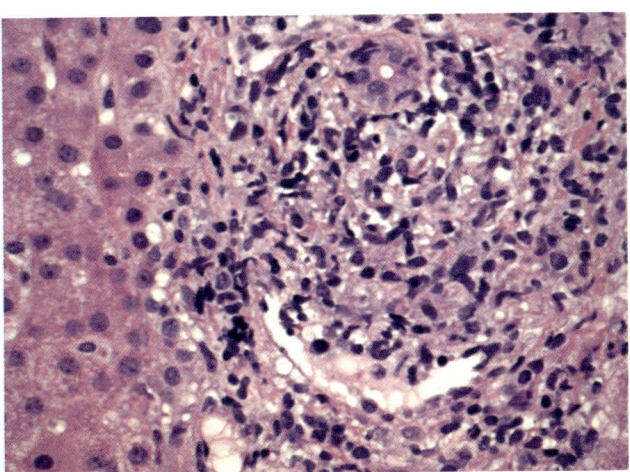

Fig. 32.2 Histological details of a portal field harboring classic lesions of severe TCMR; note inflammatory aggression of interlobular bile duct (top) and massive endothelitis with almost complete obliteration of portal branch vein lumen by a huge aggregate of lymphocytes and eosinophils under the endothelium (bottom) (H&E, 100×)

Endothelitis is the most representative histological alteration (Fig. 32.2), characterized by the attachment of lymphocytes and other inflammatory cells to the luminal surface of the vascular endothelium. Inflammatory infiltrate is mostly represented by T lymphocytes (mainly CD8-positive cells), while CD20-positive B lymphocytes usually represent a minor component of inflammatory infiltrate. The inflammatory process may be present only on a small segment of the vessel, and additional histological sections may be advisable to avoid this sampling pitfall. Lymphocytes also aggregate under the damaged endothelium, which is then lifted from the basement membrane with partial or complete obliteration of the lumen. In severe cases, there may be endothelitis and fibrinoid necrosis of the hepatic arteries branches. Severe forms of TCMR may also be associated with diffuse inflammatory infiltrates of T cells in sinusoids of variable entity, parenchymal bilirubinostasis, and liver cells apoptosis.

Bile inflammatory damage affects small bile ducts (less than 30 μm in diameter); lymphocytes are attached to basal membrane and dislocated within epithelium. Bile duct epithelium may show various degrees of degeneration and regression.

In severe TCMR, inflammatory infiltrate may expand to the liver cell plates in periportal areas showing interface activity and features similar to chronic hepatitis; infiltrate may also extend to sinusoids and central areas causing perivenular inflammation, centrilobular congestion and hemorrhages, liver cell necrosis, and dropout with reticulin frame denudation and collapse.

The International Banff Working group proposed in 1994 a semiquantitative grading method of acute rejection [5] applicable to TCMR (so-called RAI score), based of evaluation of three main parameters: portal inflammation, bile duct damage, and venous endothelial inflammation, each one scored from 0 (absent) to 3 (maximal degree) (Table 32.2). RAI score may be useful in transmitting intuitive information between pathologists and clinicians concerning the grade of TCMR severity in every single biopsy and is immediately informative about evolution of histological damage in follow-up biopsies.

Although there is no plenary consensus among different LT teams, pediatric patients with a RAI of ≥4 should undergo increased immunosuppressive regimen. While the Banff schema provides an indicator of the presence and severity of acute cellular rejection, a large retrospective analysis found that the RAI score did not correlate with response to corticosteroids or graft survival [6].

As RAI index does not mention pericentral lesions, description of these alterations are to be incorporated in final report as signs suggesting process severity.

Early (<6 months after surgery) TCMR shows more prevalent inflammatory bile duct damage, a mixed inflammation composition (lymphocytes, macrophages, eosinophils, neutrophils, and plasma cells), and minor degree of necroinflammatory-type interface activity compared to "late" TCMR. Hepatocytes are not involved until rejection is moderately advanced or in case of severe disease. The diagnosis in the early postoperative period is often clouded by bile duct damage, due to ischemic injury or caused by preservation solutions. For this reason, an intraoperative biopsy should be available for comparison.

Late TCMR shows less inflammatory bile duct damage, more homogeneous inflammatory infiltrate composition (lymphocytes, macrophages, plasma cells), and a greater tendency for low-grade interface and perivenular necro-inflammatory-type activity similar to active hepatitis; moreover it can present exclusively or predominately with perivenular necrotic and inflammatory modifications that are at high risk of progression to chronic rejection.

The consequences of TCMR are variable. While it can theoretically predispose to corticoid-resistant rejection and graft loss, most episodes do not have long-term adverse effects and are successfully treated. Furthermore, TCMR identified by protocol liver biopsy in the absence of biochemical dysfunction often resolves spontaneously without increasing immunosuppression [7]. There is even a suggestion that such subclinical immune activation might be beneficial in inducing a degree of tolerance [8]. The timing of rejection might affect outcomes; early TCMR was associated with better graft survival, and late acute rejection was associated with reduced graft survival, when compared with graft survival rates in patients without an episode of rejection [8]. Patients who developed late TCMR had an about 30% rate of chronic rejection and a 5% risk of final graft failure.

Table 32.2 Rejection activity index established by the Banff Working group

Rejection activity index (RAI score)		
Pathological alterations	Histological evaluation	Score
Portal field inflammation	Mixed inflammation involving, but not significantly expanding, a minority of the triads	1
	Expansion of most or all of the portal tracts by a mixed infiltrate containing lymphocytes, neutrophils, plasma cells, and eosinophils	2
	Marked expansion of most of the portal fields by a mixed inflammatory infiltrate containing numerous blasts and eosinophils with spillover into the periportal parenchyma	3
Bile duct inflammatory lesions	A minority of the ducts are cuffed and infiltrated by inflammatory cells; mild reactive alterations of the epithelial cells	1
	Majority of the bile ducts infiltrated by inflammatory cells. Few ducts affected by degenerative changes of the epithelium	2
	As for 2 score with most or all of the ducts showing degenerative changes	3
Venous endothelial inflammation	Subendothelial inflammatory infiltration of a minority of the portal/hepatic venules	1
	Subendothelial inflammatory infiltrate of most or all the portal/hepatic venules	2
	As 2 score with moderate or severe central perivenular inflammation extended into the perivenular parenchyma associated with perivenular hepatocyte necrosis	3
Total RAI score = 0–9/9		

A score greater than 4 is commonly considered the threshold to indicate treatment with pulsed steroid boluses

More recent novel approaches to the non-histological diagnosis of TCMR have been proposed in order to avoid biopsy for liver tissue sampling; they include measurement of alanine aminopeptidase N in bile [9], specific transcriptome patterns [10], and pattern of serum proteomic profile where complement component 4 (C4) and ALT were highly predictive of acute cellular rejection [11]. In addition, hepatocyte-derived microRNAs (HDmiRs, mir-122, miR-148a) have been evaluated as markers of acute cellular rejection. HDmiRs were elevated up to 20-fold during an episode of acute cellular rejection compared with levels 6 months after resolution of the episode. Further, miR-122 levels rose earlier than aminotransferases during the event of rejection, suggesting a role for such biomarkers in the earlier diagnosis of rejection [12].

However, it must be emphasized that these markers are investigational, are not widely available, and are not completely specific, so liver histology still remains mandatory to establish the diagnosis and subsequent management of TCMR.

32.3.3 Differential Diagnosis

The differential diagnosis of TCMR and other liver dysfunctions depends in part upon the time at which they occur. Within the first few days after transplantation, abnormal liver tests may reflect technical or functional problems, such as hepatic artery thrombosis, preservation injury, biliary anastomosis leakage or stenosis, primary graft nonfunction, or even consequences of shock and septicemia. Although many of these problems may be evident clinically or on imaging such as Doppler ultrasonography, the biopsy findings may sometimes be the first sign of a problem. Anyway an overt picture of moderate/severe TCMR is seldom evident in the first postoperative week.

Lesions related to preservation/reperfusion injury usually include mild microvesicular steatosis and some degree of hepatocyte damage and dropout in portal and periportal areas associated with some bile thrombi, perivenular necrosis, and neutrophilic inflammatory infiltrate in cases of severe necrosis (Fig. 32.3). Confluent necrosis may develop with reticulin frame collapse. Biliary tree is particularly exposed to ischemic or perfusion injury. Biliary sludge syndrome is the clinical result causing poor bile production and sludge of biliary material within bile ducts. Recovery needs usually 2 or 3 months and is characterized by liver cell mitosis and pluristratification of liver cell plates.

A rare and unpredictable complication after liver transplantation is acute graft necrosis and failure in the absence of vascular obstruction. Histologic features include widespread hemorrhage and infarction. This syndrome has been described as massive hemorrhagic necrosis.

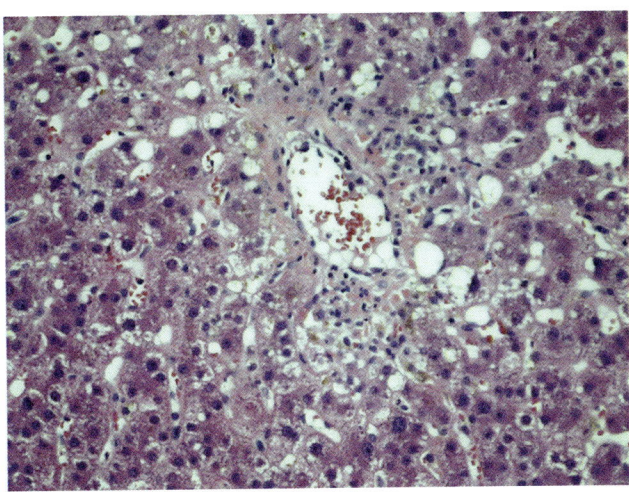

Fig. 32.3 Example of marked preservation injury in central area characterized by mild microvesicular steatosis, hepatocyte hydropic degeneration and dropout associated with some bile thrombi and neutrophilic inflammatory infiltrate (H&E, 40×)

Functional cholestasis is a unique entity that typically occurs in the early posttransplantation period. This form of cholestasis is independent of rejection, parenteral nutrition, or the use of specific drugs. Subcellular organelle damage produced by cold ischemia may play a central etiologic role, leading to bile flow dysfunction. Liver histology shows cholestasis in lobular and pericentral areas and may be associated with ballooning of hepatocytes cytoplasm in these areas [13].

Mechanical cholestasis due to anastomotic structures, bile linkage, cholangitis, and fistulas, occurs in 15–20% of patients, and, besides the type of biliary reconstruction during surgery, they are linked to ischemic damage to biliary tree during procedure. Liver biopsy shows portal edema and mixed inflammation, inflammatory lesions of bile ducts due to intraepithelial neutrophils, proliferation of bile ducts, and presence of bile in centrilobular areas. Liver histology abnormalities in case of mechanical obstruction of bile tree may be overt only 4–6 weeks after onset; morphological lesions are usually focal and minimal in the first phase and should be carefully searched for in the liver specimen.

Cholangitis, either septic or related to bile tree obstruction, is another frequent complication to mention in differential diagnosis of TCMR. The main histological picture, besides bile ducts proliferation, is prevalent neutrophilic infiltrate within portal tract with aggression of biliary epithelium. Sepsis is associated with a characteristic histological picture known as *cholangitis lenta*, which consists of bilirubinostasis and with bile plugs inside the lumen at the periphery of portal tracts.

32.4 Plasma Cell-Rich Rejection

32.4.1 General Considerations

Plasma cell-rich rejection (PCR) or plasma cell hepatitis (PCH), also previously known as de novo autoimmune hepatitis (DNAIH), is a poorly understood and uncommon (3–5% of recipients) cause of usually late (often >1 year) graft dysfunction, resembling clinically and histologically to native liver autoimmune hepatitis (AIH). It was described for the first time as a pure immunological graft dysfunction due to alloimmunity [14], but it became progressively clear that it represents a peculiar pattern of injury that should be regarded as an unusual manifestation of immunological dysfunction.

Transplantation of organs between individuals that are not genetically identical can cause a T-cell-mediated immune response that leads to rejection and graft destruction. The level of the alloimmune response is determined by the disparity of polymorphic antigens between individuals. Evidence supporting a contribution of autoimmunity include detection a variety of classical and other autoantibodies [15].

In the two past decades, several reports have appeared in the literature dealing with concerns about the development of a complex set of clinical, laboratory, and histological characteristics of a liver graft dysfunction that is compatible with autoimmune hepatitis. The *de novo* prefix was added to distinguish this entity from a pretransplant primary autoimmune hepatitis, but the globally accepted criteria for the diagnosis of autoimmune hepatitis have been adopted in the diagnostic algorithm. Indeed, DNAIH is characterized by the typical liver inflammation that is rich in plasma cells, the presence of interface hepatitis and the consequent laboratory findings of elevations in liver enzymes, increases in serum gamma globulin, and the appearance of non-organ-specific autoantibodies. Autoantibodies are frequently present without signs of graft dysfunction, particularly in the pediatric population, and liver biopsy is therefore required to determine the nature and the severity of any damage present.

There are many overlapping areas between DNAIH and rejection, including autoantibodies being present, sometimes transiently, in otherwise typical episodes of rejection (acute and chronic) [16, 17], previous episodes of rejection being a risk factor for the development of DNAIH and DNAIH occurring in the setting of under immunosuppression [18–20].

The presence of portal C4d deposits in cases of DNAIH, compared with absent C4d staining in chronic rejection, supports the suggestion that there may be also a component of mediated rejection in some cases.

Several mechanisms have been implicated in this loss of self-tolerance including impaired thymic regulation, reduced activity of T regulatory cells, molecular mimicry, calcineurin inhibitors, glutathione-s transferase, and genetic polymorphisms. In the pediatric transplant population, administering immunosuppressive therapy in the regimen used to treat autoimmune hepatitis has stabilized graft function in de novo autoimmune hepatitis.

Features supporting a contribution of alloimmunity in the disease are more prevalent and severe bile duct damage, plasma cell-rich central perivenulitis more aggressive than seen in typical AIH, IgG4+ plasma cells (not present in typical AIH) and DSA production.

Patients who received LT for non-autoimmune liver diseases can develop autoantibodies. Antinuclear antibodies are most frequently reported, followed by anti-smooth muscle antibodies. An atypical and peculiar form of the liver kidney microsomal antibody type 1 (LKM-1) has also been detected in these patients; this antibody has been reported to react with an unidentified cytosolic antigen instead of the microsomal liver fraction that contains cytochrome P4502D6, the target of LKM-1 in classic AIH type 2 [21]. Because we cannot yet determine with certainty the allo-specificity or auto-specificity of a liver-based immune response, diagnosis rely on surrogate markers, such as morphological evidence of significant necro-inflammatory interface activity, plasma cell prominence, hypergammaglobulinemia, autoantibodies and steroid dependence.

Long-term outcome is associated with continued allograft dysfunction and may lead to bile duct injury, CR, chronic graft histological changes of progressive fibrosis-cirrhosis, and portal hypertension necessitating liver re-transplantation in small number of patients [22].

32.4.2 Histopathological Findings

PCR is characterized by the typical liver necro-inflammation process that is rich in plasma cells, the presence of interface hepatitis, the gamma globulin high levels, and the appearance of non-organ-specific autoantibodies.

Morphological and clinical criteria suggestive for the diagnosis of PCR are (1) portal plasma cell-rich (estimated >30%) inflammatory infiltrates with periportal interface activity, often associated with perivenular necro-inflammatory lesions usually involving a majority of portal tracts and/or central veins (Figs. 32.4, 32.5, and 32.6). Varying degrees of lobular inflammation are frequently also present in more severe cases including areas of confluent or bridging necrosis (Fig. 32.7) and liver cell apoptosis; few patients will present with a predominant central venulitis with extensive perivenular liver cell dropout and reticulin frame collapse, (2) lymphocytic cholangitis and (3) native liver disease other than autoimmune hepatitis.

Immunostaining for CD79 antigen, even if not mandatory, may be useful to better identify and underline the marked presence of plasma cells within inflammatory infiltrate in portal and lobular areas (Fig. 32.8).

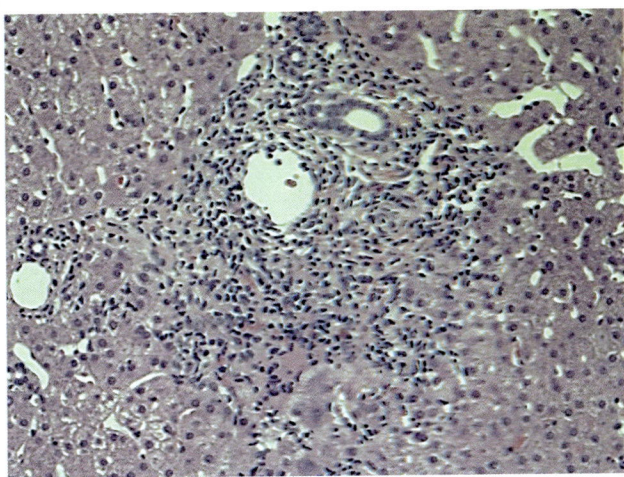

Fig. 32.4 Typical histological picture of PCR; portal area is expanded by mixed inflammatory infiltrate with lymphocytes, plasma cells, and eosinophils; marked interface activity and minimal degree of endothelitis of portal branch. Note also lobular inflammatory activity with spotty necrosis (H&E, 40×)

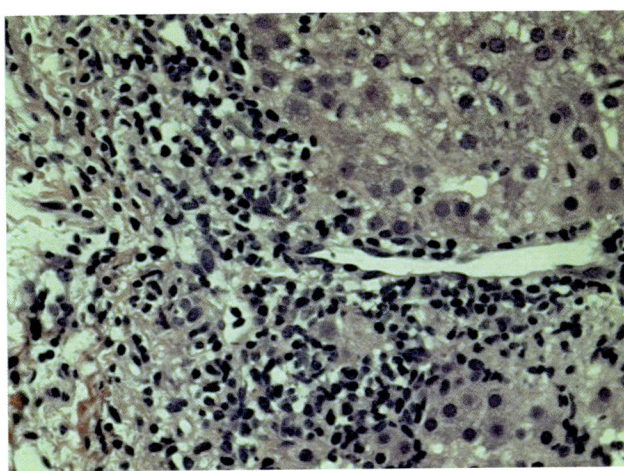

Fig. 32.6 Details of the previous microphotograph that highlight severe inflammatory infiltration of portal endothelium with evident plasma cells component, diffuse interface hepatitis and plurifocal lobular involvement with spotty and confluent necrosis, integrating the composite histological picture of TCMR associated with chronic hepatitis (H&E, 100×)

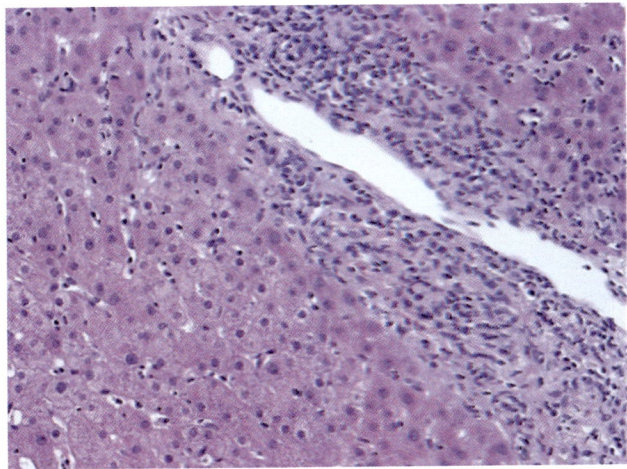

Fig. 32.5 Another typical case of PCR: massive inflammatory infiltrate in a portal tract represented by lymphocytes, eosinophils, and many plasma cells; note the aggression of vascular endothelium by inflammatory cells (endothelitis); fewer features of inflammatory activity at interface between portal tract and parenchyma (interface hepatitis) compared to the previous picture; some scattered foci of parenchymal necrosis (H&E, 40×)

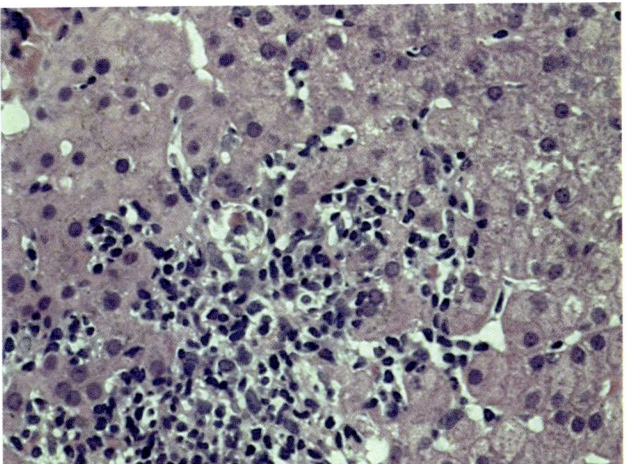

Fig. 32.7 Extensive lobular mixed inflammatory infiltrate mimicking lobular hepatitis, characterized by a focus of liver cells confluent necrosis and marked activation of Kupffer cells with expanded cytoplasm (H&E, 100×)

32.4.3 Differential Diagnosis

The main histological differential diagnosis is between TCMR and PCR, as both pathologies are characterized by inflammatory features in portal and parenchymal structures.

The use of strict morphological criteria for diagnosis of TCMR usually allows a confident diagnosis of this condition; besides inflammatory lesions present in both conditions, prevalent interface hepatitis and plasma cells-rich infiltrate are features in favor of PCR, while consistent bile duct damage and evidence of endothelitis address diagnosis to TCMR. To summarize histological distinction between PCH and TCMR rejection is mainly based on the presence of ≥30% plasma cells in the infiltrates and the prevalence of bile duct damage. If liver sample shows histologically severe necro-inflammatory pericentral lesions, the differential diagnosis with TCMR may be difficult; as previously mentioned, the presence of significant number of plasma cells, interface activity, absence of portal features of endothelitis, and bile duct aggression is more suggestive for diagnosis of PCR.

It should be mentioned that relapse of native AIH in LT transplanted patients is quite common and liver histology

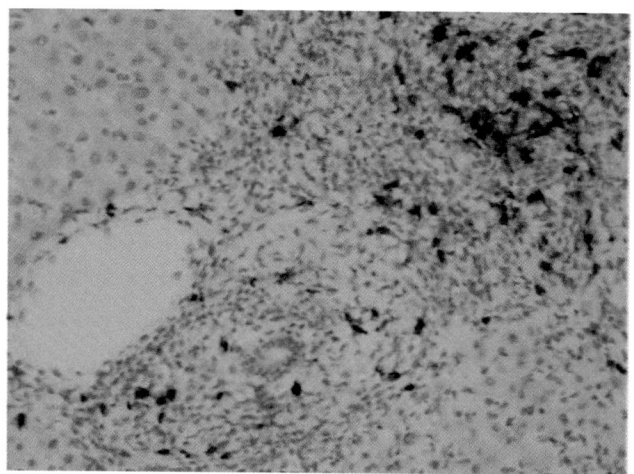

Fig. 32.8 Results of immunostaining by CD 79a decorating plasma cells in brown in a case of PCR; note the large proportion of these cells within inflammatory infiltrate (more than 30%), few of them infiltrating endothelium of portal vein branch. Scattered plasma cells are present in interface hepatitis areas (40×)

picture completely overlaps the histological aspects of DNAIH. In cases of relapse of native AIH, lobular inflammatory changes and liver cells necrosis tend to be more prominent and occur more frequently as a presenting feature before typical portal inflammatory changes are seen; on the other hand, mononuclear perivenular inflammation involving ≥50% of the terminal hepatic venules, associated with hepatocyte necrosis, usually with parenchymal dropout, is a frequent feature of PCH.

32.5 Chronic Rejection

32.5.1 General Considerations

Compared with other vascularized organ grafts, chronic liver rejection (CR) is uncommon chiefly in pediatric population [23], most likely due to the unique immunologic properties of the liver allograft, regenerative capacity of the liver, and improved recognition and treatment of TCMR. The liver seems to be quite insensitive to ongoing immunological damage, and only a short number of patients develop clinical features of chronic rejection 5 years after surgery. The incidence is approximately 1–5%. Indeed, there is clear evidence that the incidence of CR is actually declining over the past few years. This represents a dramatic decrease since first initial era of LT when incidence of chronic rejection was 5–20% at 5 years. The reason for this apparent decline is not completely clear, but it could be related to better immunosuppression management and detection of early histological lesions suggestive for graft dysfunction.

The term "chronic" implies a temporally prolonged course, and generally CR more indolently compromises graft organ function, in contrast to acute rejection that can cause clinically overt allograft dysfunction and severe alteration of liver biochemical parameters. However, many cases of CR possibly evolve from severe or inadequately controlled TCMR episodes and in patients not compliant with chronic maintenance immunosuppression. In such patients, ongoing immunologic injury leads to a progressive decline in organ function over a period of weeks to months. There is, however, a significant number of patients who do not fit these profiles and slowly develop graft failure over a period of years. This more indolent presentation may be attributable to "clinically silent" rejection episodes that go undetected.

To summarize, three main settings of clinical onset may present: persistent acute rejection unresponsive to increase or re-modulation of immunosuppressive therapy, end-stage result of multiple episode of acute rejection, or presentation without previous episodes of acute rejection.

32.5.2 Histopathological Findings

CR primary induces obliteration of large arteries at *ilum hepatis*, due to appearance of muscular layer hypertrophy, foamy cells arteritis and progressive narrowing of the lumen with consequential ischemia of the graft; biliary tree is the most sensible part of the liver to ischemic damage as supplied almost completely by arterial vascular system; histological lesions affect in liver biopsies portal fields and pericentral areas. The obliterative phase may be preceded by florid inflammatory lesions; the preferential localization of leukocytes in the adventitia and intima suggests that these are the most important antigenic targets or sites of damage.

Unfortunately the diagnosis of CR is easy to establish in failed explanted liver graft, evaluating the large arterial vessels at the hilum and finding obliterative arteriopathy with accumulation of foamy histiocytes within intimal layer (Fig. 32.9), triggering myofibroblastic activity and severe lumen narrowing. The thickened intimal layer may sometimes contain inflammatory cells, like T and B lymphocytes, macrophages, and occasionally dendritic cells that signal the presence of an ongoing immune reaction.

When rejection is mild, the inflammation is usually limited to the adventitia; if it is unusually severe, mononuclear and neutrophilic endothelitis, respectively, are usually also present. In many cases the intimal inflammation is quickly followed by fibrointimal hyperplasia, which marks the beginning of irreversible obliterative arteriopathy.

Based on Banff Consensus Paper [24], morphological damages are summarized and divided in two main catego-

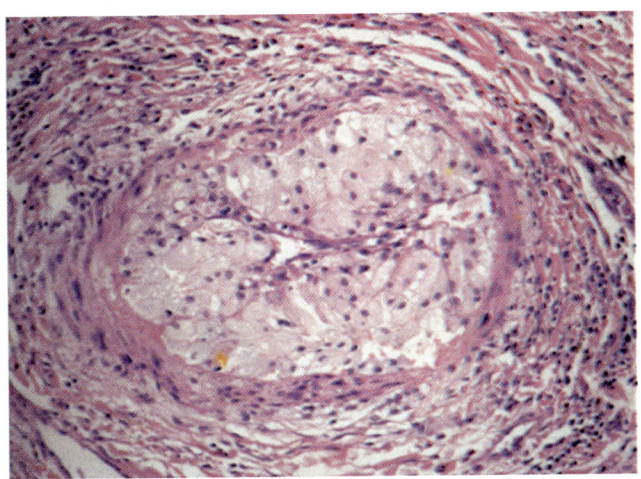

Fig. 32.9 Histological sample from a failed liver graft due to CR, demonstrating a large artery a *tilum hepatis* characterized by marked foamy cells accumulation in intimal layer, completely occluding the lumen (H&E, 40×)

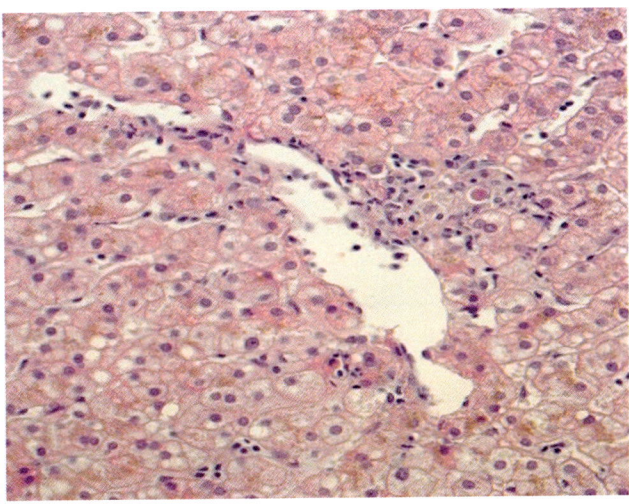

Fig. 32.10 Early CR. Central area typical lesions: lymphocytic inflammatory infiltrate with central vein endothelitis and pericentral liver cell dropout and apoptosis (H&E, 40×)

Table 32.3 Classification of chronic rejection according to the Banff Consensus Conference [24]

Anatomical targets	Early CR	Late CR
Small bile ducts (<60 μm)	Degenerative changes involving a majority of ducts (eosinophilia of the cytoplasm; increased N/C ratio; nuclear hyperchromasia; ulcerations of epithelium) Bile duct loss <50% of portal tracts	Degenerative changes in remaining bile ducts Loss in ≥50% of portal tracts
Terminal hepatic venules and central zone hepatocytes	Intimal layer inflammation Central zone liver cells necrosis and inflammation Mild central perivenular fibrosis	Focal obliteration Variable inflammation Severe (bridging) fibrosis
Portal tract hepatic arterioles branches	Loss involving <25% of portal tracts	Loss involving >25% of portal tracts
Large perihilar hepatic artery branches	Intimal layer inflammatory aggression, focal foam cell deposition, patent lumen	Lumen narrowing or obliteration by foam cells Fibrointimal proliferation
Large hilar bile ducts	Inflammation damage and focal foam cell degeneration	Foamy cells infiltration of intimal and medial layer, obliteration of the lumen

ries: early and late chronic rejection. Classification is summarized in Table 32.3.

Early CR is characterized mainly by inflammatory features such as central vein endothelitis, perivenular lymphocytic infiltration, and centrilobular hepatocytes dropout (Fig. 32.10); moreover some hepatitis-like pictures are often seen in liver biopsy. The early and potentially reversible stage of chronic rejection is identified primarily by degenerative changes of the biliary epithelium, even before overt duct loss is detected.

Main late CR lesion is loss of more than 50% of bile ducts in a graft with preserved lobular architecture (Fig. 32.11); liver cells usually show a diffuse biliary phenotype characterized by abnormal cytoplasmatic expression of CK7. Perivenular changes are characterized by severe perivenular fibrosis (Figs. 32.11 and 32.12) with development of central to central fibrotic bridging. A very mild accompanying inflammatory infiltrate, including infiltration of the epithelium by lymphoid cells, may be present, but the degree of inflammation is considerably lesser than is seen in TCMR. Bile ductular rejection is usually unremarkable or very weak. Arterial loss is also related to bile duct disappearance; the percentage of significance of these losses should be similar. Cirrhosis is really uncommon and, when present, is a feature of very late stages. Arteries with pathognomonic changes are seldom present in needle biopsies and in most cases are represented by obliteration of the lumen and myointimal hyperplasia of tunica media (Fig. 32.13).

Recognition of biliary senescence is the critical point of diagnosis of CR in initial stages; this diagnosis is based on identification of degenerative changes in biliary epithelium (eosinophilic degeneration of cytoplasm, nuclear enlargement, and hyperchromasia simulating atypia; biliary cells show positivity to staining for p21, a marker upregulated in cases of severe cellular stress suggesting senescence).

As diagnosis of late or ductopenic CR impacts severely the prognosis of the patient, it has to be based on a significant

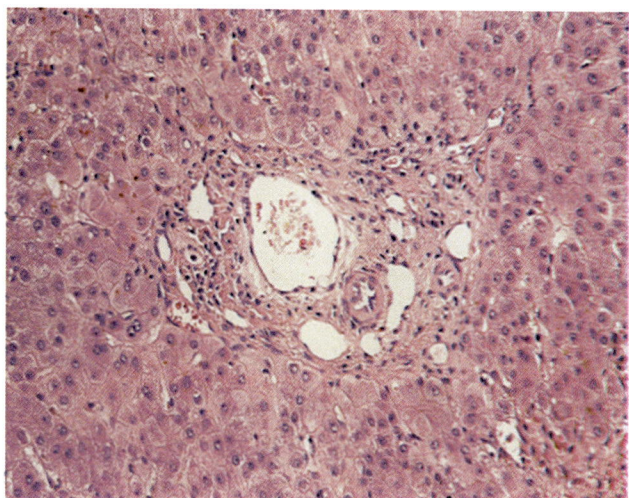

Fig. 32.11 Liver with normal lobular architecture, mild portal enlargement and minimal inflammatory infiltrate in portal field; complete absence of interlobular bile duct and some degree of obliterative arteriopathy with narrowing of the lumen (H&E, 40×)

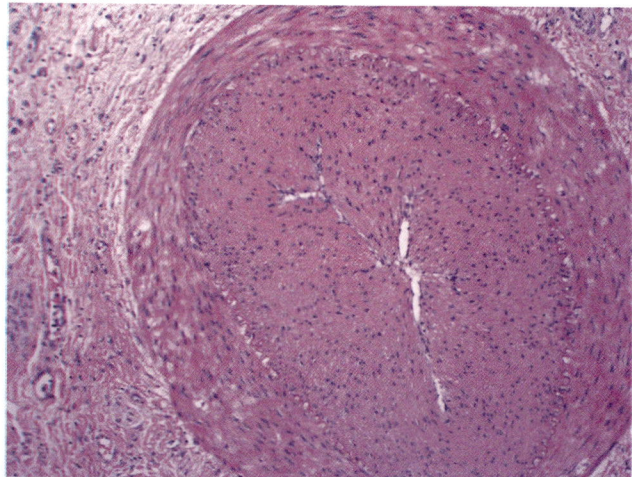

Fig. 32.13 Example of medium layer marked fibromuscular hypertrophy involving a large artery at *ilum hepatis*; sample obtained from a failed liver graft (H&E, 40×)

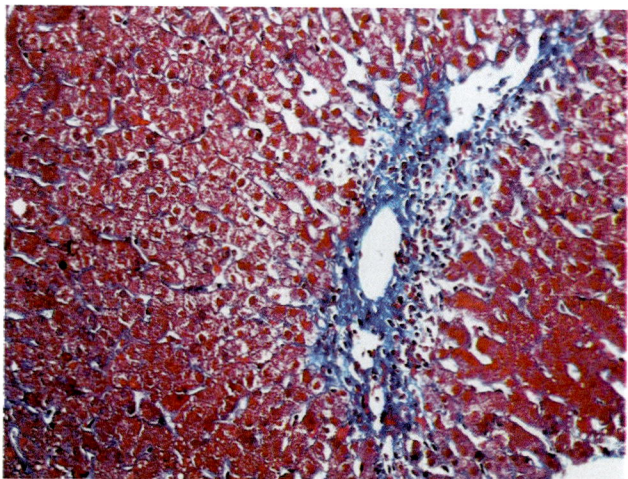

Fig. 32.12 Centrilobular damage with marked collagen deposition within central vein wall and in pericentral parenchymal area (trichrome stain, 40×)

needle liver sample containing at least 20 portal fields, in consideration of the issue that ratio in normal liver between portal tracts and interlobular bile duct is 10:9. CR is a more challenging diagnosis for the histopathologist than TMCR. On needle biopsy specimens, the arteriopathic changes are often not detected, although the downstream effects may be identified. In addition liver biopsy may not be completely diagnostic since small arteries are involved in only 10% of cases and bile duct loss may not be extensive.

Ductopenia involving less than 50% of bile ducts can be found in specimens without any significant alteration of liver function tests or clinical signs; it could represent an early phase of ductopenic CR. These findings are really questionable and are usually evident in protocol studies biopsies performed at scheduled time without any clinical concern.

32.5.3 Differential Diagnosis

Differential diagnoses of CR include many conditions such as ischemic cholangiopathy, obstructive cholestasis, and recurrent biliary disease (especially PSC). The most helpful diagnostic feature in distinguishing CR from these entities is a pattern consisting of cholestasis in combination with the absence of ductular proliferation or significant portal-periportal fibrosis.

The main differential diagnosis in long-term survivors is anyway obstructive cholestasis. Biliary complications are very common after LT and occur as biliary strictures, bile leaks, and bile duct stones, accounting for the majority of the complications. Risk factors include the type of biliary reconstruction, acute hepatic artery thrombosis, hepatic artery stenosis, prolonged warm or cold ischemia, cytomegalovirus infection, ABO blood group mismatch, donation after cardiac death, and primary sclerosing cholangitis as native liver disease. Histologic features of bile duct obstruction can sometimes be misleading and confused with rejection. Thus, correlation of histologic findings with results of imaging tests is important.

Unfortunately, abdominal US may not be sufficiently sensitive to detect biliary obstruction. Thus, in patients in whom there is clinical suspicion of biliary tract complications, the absence of bile duct dilation on US should not preclude further evaluation with other techniques and liver biopsy.

In liver biopsies biliary obstruction is diagnosed in presence of bile ducts proliferation, portal edema and mixed inflammation with granulocytes, variable degree of fibrosis from mild portal fibrosis to portal-portal bridging fibrosis and finally biliary type cirrhosis, opposite to CR presenting as progressive disappearance of bile ducts without significant inflammation and fibrosis in combination with atrophic changes of the biliary epithelium; moreover marked bile duct proliferation is not a feature of CR. In contrast to chronic rejection, the alterations typically involve larger ducts.

32.6 Antibody-Mediated Rejection (AMR) (Synonym: Humoral Rejection)

32.6.1 General Considerations

Antibody-mediated rejection (AMR) in liver transplants is a relatively new field compared with its allograft groups of the kidney and lung. AMR in liver transplantation was firstly described in cases of ABO-incompatible transplantation in which precipitous liver graft failure may occur few hours after LT; therefore it may manifest years later, and it is strictly associated with donor-specific antibodies (DSA). Susceptibility to AMR for any vascularized allograft is dependent on antibody class, titer, specificity, and timing, as well as density and distribution of target antigen expression, and AMR has been recognized in clinical liver transplantation practice for nearly three decades: first with ABO-incompatible allografts and later with lymphocytotoxic antibodies or DSA.

This pattern of rejection is anyway uncommon in LT setting [25], as liver seems to be less sensitive than other solid allografts to AMR. Different mechanisms have been postulated to explain this resistance: huge amount of Kupffer cells with high clearance activity of activated complement [26], reduced class II HLA antigen expression on microvascular endothelium [27], large size of the organ favoring dilution of antigens on endothelial cells surface [28], and marked liver regeneration capacity with small amount of fibrous tissue [29].

Diagnosis of liver AMR is anyway complex and requires concurrence of clinical, laboratory, and histologic data; exclusion of other causes is mandatory. Histologic features of AMR may overlap with those of biliary obstruction, preservation or reperfusion injury, and graft ischemia. Tissue examination for complement degradation product 4d (C4d) has been proved to support this diagnosis as in other allografts.

Criteria for establishing a definite diagnosis of AMR requires DSA testing, preferably obtained at the time of biopsy. AMR usually occurs in highly sensitized patients DSA. Complete donor and recipient HLA typing and pre-transplant crossmatch with DSA testing are needed; DSA testing should be repeated with a preference, if possible, to determine the IgG subtype and functional activity (C1q assay, etc.). IgM and IgG isoagglutinins are naturally encountered when blood group barriers are crossed and antibody titer and complement-fixing ability influence pathogenicity. Liver allograft injury is more often encountered when recipients harbor dilutions >1:64 usually manifest significant damage, but reduction to titers <1:16 by plasmapheresis has been suggested to largely avoid AMR. Only a minority of pre-LT positive crossmatch patients (about 20%) maintained positive crossmatch during the follow-up period and developed early severe AMR; most recipients spontaneously converted their positive crossmatch into negative and maintained good long-term liver function on routine immunosuppression. Pre-LT DSA with potential clinical relevance has been tentatively defined as mean fluorescence intensity (MFI) >5000. Most of class I DSA < 10,000 MFI recipients do not have significant clinical consequences.

Besides acute presentation within few days after surgery, AMR could manifest at any time during follow-up, and histological features may be absolutely variable and challenging.

Inclusion of ABO-incompatible AMR in the Banff schema is going to be considered, but inclusion of ABO-compatible AMR has been delayed because of widespread recognition that human liver allografts were less sensitive than kidney allografts to acute adverse consequences of pre-formed DSA and could possibly protect subsequent kidney and heart allografts from the same donor from AMR.

The main problem about the diagnosis of chronic AMR in liver allografts is the lack of specific or typical clinical or biochemical features. Instead, many of the histopathological features that have been postulated to occur as consequence of chronic AMR have been observed in protocol biopsies from liver allograft recipients (mostly pediatric) who appear to be clinically well with good graft function.

32.7 Acute AMR

Hyperacute liver allograft rejection DSA related manifests in the early postoperative hours as a fulminant hepatic failure. Although it may develop in the first few hours or days after transplantation, later presentations up to the end of the second week may occasionally occur. This cause of graft loss was previously seen more commonly in the early days of transplantation, when the procedure was done without avoiding ABO-incompatible matches. However, much has been learned from animal studies and from xenotransplantation.

With the increasing use of living donors, there has been a serious increase of ABO-incompatible transplants, and much interest has focused on the prevention of hyperacute rejection. A number of approaches have been adopted to download the effects of complement activation and damage to the vascular endothelium, such as plasmapheresis, intravenous infusion of immunoglobulin, anti-CD20 monoclonal antibody (rituximab), or even more invasive approaches like splenectomy.

These approaches may be helpful, but there is an associated morbidity, and because about 20% of recipients of ABO-incompatible livers develop significant problems, controlled studies are really needed to demonstrate an effective benefit.

The clinical picture of hyperacute AMR is a quickly onset of the signs and symptoms of acute liver failure, usually seen within hours of implantation of the graft. The serum transaminases become rapidly elevated, often reaching levels of 100 times the upper limit of normal. The clotting becomes profoundly deranged; lactic acidosis and hypoglycemia are seen. A thrombocytopenia is also seen.

The first changes occur after around 4 h with a deposition of microthrombi in the small intrahepatic blood vessels and sinusoids. This subsequently leads to congestion and coagulative liver cell necrosis, which is generally manifest by 48 h after transplantation.

The histological features of hyperacute AMR are usually identified in the removed liver at autopsy or after re-transplantation, since the severe coagulopathy usually precludes liver biopsy. The histological features are sinusoidal infiltrates of neutrophils, fibrin, and erythrocytes, progressing to hemorrhagic infarction. There is focal IgM, fibrin, C1q, and C4d deposition [30].

AMR may also present in acute form, not so rapidly catastrophic as hyperacute rejection. In this setting the main histological features are represented by microvascular endothelial cell hypertrophy, focal neutrophil sludging, capillary dilatation and rarefaction, and the so-called capillaritis or microvasculitis; in most severe cases in which isoagglutinins are usually present at high title, hemorrhages in portal fields, acidophilic liver cell necrosis and thrombi in portal and central veins may be present.

The morphological criteria to be satisfied for a confident diagnosis of AMR are actually considered (1) DSA in serum, (2) diffuse microvascular C4d positivity, (3) exclusion of other causes of a similar type of injury, and (4) histopathological evidence of diffuse microvascular injury.

C4d is an inactive component of complement activation cascade; endothelial localization of C4d deposits is considered one of the most specific signs for AMR in conjunction with other data. C4d staining should anyway be carefully evaluated; linear or granular sinusoidal pattern in non-necrotic areas correlates with presence of DSA and therefore considered specific for AMR. Immunofluorescence staining of frozen tissue for C4d is generally considered to be more sensitive than immunoperoxidase staining of formalin-fixed, paraffin-embedded tissue after antigen retrieval. Fresh frozen tissue samples have improved sensitivity to detect C4d deposits but have many practical limitations and require a time- and money-consuming organization of the laboratory. A possible alterative procedure could be based on a 3 mm fragment kept fresh frozen in OCT compound, and the remaining part of the core used routine formalin-fixed and paraffin- embedded processing. In most and largest transplantation centers, routine follow-up biopsy includes preparation of formalin-fixed, paraffin-embedded sections.

Liver biopsies are usually negative for endothelial cell C4d staining, but background and nonspecific C4d labeling can be seen in arterial elastic lamina, portal and perivenular elastic fibers, necrotic and steatotic hepatocytes, and areas of sinusoidal fibrosis; this not specific labeling should not be considered as diagnostic feature of AMR.

Intense Cd4 deposition is almost always associated with moderate to severe mixed inflammatory infiltrate within portal fields. Anyway C4d can also be activated via an alternative antibody-independent process. Thus C4d may be potentially deposited due to alternative pathway of activation of complement cascade, without previous antibody binding and in absence of DSA.

Portal microvascular (portal veins and capillaries) and sinusoidal endothelial cell C4d staining appears to be most specific for acute AMR, whereas portal C4d "stromal" staining seems to be more strongly associated with ABO-incompatible acute AMR.

Some histopathological changes resemble preservation/reperfusion injury and obstructive cholangiopathy, but microvascular dilatation, microvascular endothelial cell hypertrophy with thickening of the walls and narrowing of the lumen, and cytoplasmic eosinophilia and "microvasculitis," especially when involving central veins, distinguish acute AMR from these other complications. The presence of mixed inflammatory infiltrate represented by blastic lymphocytes and eosinophils, in addition to C4d positivity, should favor the diagnosis of AMR; additional clinical information, such as pre-sensitization state and laboratory profile, are helpful in differential diagnosis.

Microvasculitis or capillaritis (Fig. 32.14) is considered as most highly suggestive lesion of AMR and is recognized as intraluminal pooling and/or margination of various leukocytes and polymorphonucleated cells (monocytes, macrophages, lymphocytes, neutrophils, eosinophils) in dilated and irregularly shaped capillaries.

C4d staining is usually positive in endothelium of small caliber blood vessels affected by capillaritis (Fig. 32.15).

32.8 Chronic AMR

32.8.1 General Considerations

Chronic AMR is till now a partially known and controversial entity; the most supported hypothesis is that usually develops from severe persistent and therapy-resistant acute AMR; histological features may show patterns of usual liver

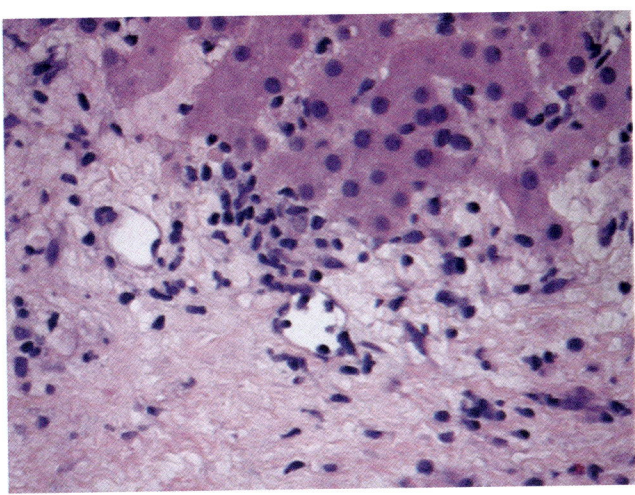

Fig. 32.14 Portal space widened by severe inflammatory infiltrate in a LT patient with high titers of DSA; note the presence of small blood vessels with adhesion of leucocytes to endothelium (so-called capillaritis) (H&E, 100×)

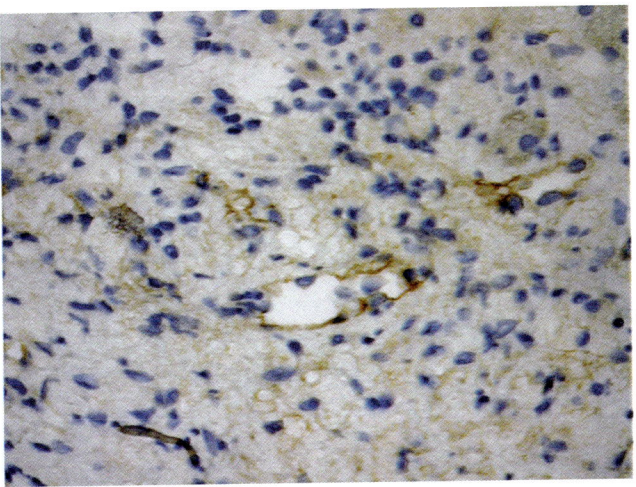

Fig. 32.15 C4d immunohistochemical staining decorating vascular venous vessels and some capillaries within portal field in a case of AMR; vessels in the center of the picture show infiltration of endothelium by lymphocytes (100×)

CR. Moreover candidate histopathological lesions suggestive for chronic liver allograft AMR are emerging primarily from long-term follow-up of pediatric liver allograft recipients, suboptimally immunosuppressed recipients, immunosuppression weaning studies, and transplantation centers that conduct protocol simultaneous serum and biopsy samplings.

Tissue injuries in a pattern consistent with chronic AMR are actually considered (1) perivenular and/or sub-sinusoidal fibrosis, (2) stellate cell activation, (3) portal inflammatory and portal vein damage, (4) diffuse microvascular C4d positivity in portal field vessels, and (5) reasonable exclusion of other causes of a similar pattern of injury.

32.9 Obstructive Cholestasis

32.9.1 General Considerations

Biliary tract complications are the most common adverse events after LT. These complications are encountered more commonly as a result of increased number of transplantation procedures and prolonged survival of transplant patients. The two most common forms of biliary reconstruction are choledochocholedochostomy (duct-to-duct anastomosis) and choledochojejunostomy (connection of the bile duct to a portion of jejunum); in pediatric patients, the latter type of biliary anastomosis is most commonly performed. The clinical presentation is very polymorphous from asymptomatic patient with moderate liver enzyme elevations to a septic patient with fever and hypotension due to ascending cholangitis.

Biliary strictures are usually classified as anastomotic or non-anastomotic. The incidence of biliary stricture ranges from 5 to 15% after deceased donor liver transplantation and 28–32% after living donor liver transplantation [31]. Strictures are due to fibrotic processes and are commonly seen as late complications, occurring many months after LT.

The two most frequent early complications include leaks from the anastomosis or cystic duct stump (of the donor or native duct) and obstruction at the surgical anastomosis. Not surgical management is often successful in early complications.

Late complications presenting with leaks and obstruction are often more difficult to treat conservatively as reactive fibrosis is usually present; frequently require surgical treatment or re-transplantation, though both endoscopic and percutaneous methods can be useful in the management of these complications or as a bridge to reparative surgical therapy.

32.9.2 Histopathological Findings

Pathological patterns of obstructive cholestasis complicating LT are absolutely comparable to histological alterations due to any other causes of biliary tree obstruction such as intraluminal stone or sclerosing cholangitis.

Complete secretory bile block causes bilirubinostasis (i.e., presence of bile plugs) in hepatocytes, in canaliculi and Kupffer cells, and in centrilobular areas; ductular proliferation in portal and periportal areas is another milestone in diagnosis. This latter lesion is an increase in a number of ductular bile structures, due to multiplication of preexisting ductules (Fig. 32.16), biliary metaplasia of periportal hepatocytes (Fig. 32.17), and activation of bile structures progenitors; it is usually associated with neutrophil infiltration.

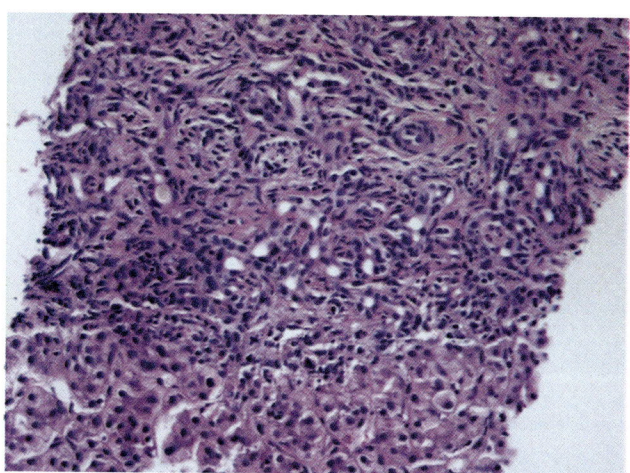

Fig. 32.16 Massive widening of a portal field characterized by diffuse bile duct proliferation and mixed inflammatory infiltrate with prevalent granulocytic component; histological features of severe obstructive cholestasis (H&E, 40×)

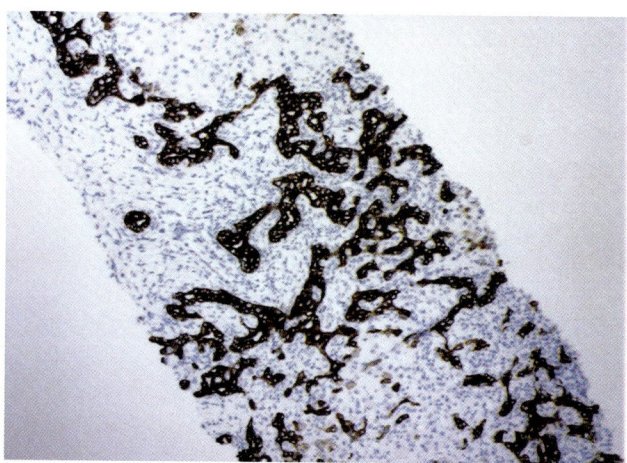

Fig. 32.17 Immunostaining by keratin 7 of the microscopic field shown in Fig. 32.14 highlights massive bile duct proliferation in a huge expanded portal tract extended in periportal areas; marked degree of periportal hepatocyte biliary metaplasia suggestive for long-standing cholestasis (40×)

Noteworthy, a mild ductular proliferation on histology may be the only clue revealing the presence of a subclinical biliary stricture.

Long-lasting cholestasis induces further histological lesions in liver samples: feathery degeneration of hepatocytes due to retention of detergent bile acids, liver cell rosettes representing a shift from hepatocellular to biliary differentiation, xanthomatous cells due to hyperlipidemia, cholatostasis in periportal hepatocytes due to overload of toxic bile acids and inducing foamy features of cytoplasm, bile infarcts, and progressive ductular reaction, always associated with portal and periductal fibrosis.

Bile ductular proliferation activates for increasing collagen matrix deposition, resulting in progressive biliary fibrosis ending to biliary cirrhosis. The most reliable markers of chronic cholestasis are cholatostasis, cholestatic liver cell rosettes, and bile ductular reaction. Bilirubinostasis is a late finding and often an ominous sign.

In most cases cholestatic features are accompanied by bile duct inflammatory injury of different degree; a confident diagnosis of cholangitis should be reserved to the cases characterized by extensive damage to biliary epithelium and presence of clusters of neutrophils in the epithelium and lumen of bile ducts. Evidence of neutrophilic sustained damage of bile ducts is not automatically associated with clinical manifestation of acute cholangitis.

32.9.3 Differential Diagnosis

Diagnosis of biliary tree obstruction may be challenging, and in pediatric population, causes include many different conditions as ischemia reperfusion injury, ABO blood group incompatibility, hepatic arterial thrombosis, cytomegalovirus infection, recurrent primary sclerosing cholangitis, and chronic rejection.

Strict adherence to diagnostic morphological criteria (i.e., portal edema and fibrosis, bile ductular proliferation, bilirubinostasis) and correlation with imaging technique findings allow a correct diagnosis in the large majority of cases. The most common differential diagnosis is CR; details are already discussed in the related section.

Preservation injury caused by hypothermic and hypoxic graft storage (cold ischemia) sustained ischemia during graft implantation and restoration of blood and oxygenation to the graft (reperfusion injury occurs at the level of the bile duct cells inducing a cholestatic syndrome). Histologically, the diagnosis of preservation-reperfusion injury is based on the presence of steatosis, diffuse bilirubinostasis and ballooning degeneration of hepatocytes in early posttransplantation biopsies [32]. After transplantation, transaminases normalize rapidly, while a prolonged cholestatic phase usually follows. Restoration of normal bilirubin concentration can take several months.

Primary graft nonfunction is poor function of the graft during the first week after transplantation. Hyperbilirubinemia is one of the findings, but the patient in most cases rapidly develops a syndrome of multiorgan failure. Risk factors include the use of marginal cadaveric donors: older donor age, presence of steatosis, and prolonged cold ischemia. Early histological are very similar to those related to preservation injury although liver cell ballooning and dropout may be more prominent and diffuse.

Hepatic artery thrombosis occurs in approximately 10–40% of pediatric recipients of primary liver grafts. The clinical presentation varies from a minimal alteration of biochemical tests to fulminant hepatic necrosis. Early thrombosis, associated with a high rate of allograft loss and patient mortality, results in massive injury to hepatocytes and ischemic bile duct injury that may lead to dehiscence of the biliary anastomosis, secondary bile duct strictures, intrahepatic bilomas, or abscesses. Late-onset thrombosis has a more benign course, often asymptomatic because of adequate portal vein flow or collateral circulation; thrombosis is suspected because of worsening biochemistry, episodes of cholangitis, or biliary complications such as anastomotic biliary strictures, intrahepatic abscesses, and bile leaks. In segmental liver allografts, a high incidence may be expected because of the smaller diameter of the arteries. The final diagnosis is confirmed by arteriography.

The recurrence rate for primary sclerosing cholangitis (PSC) after LT is quite common. Clinically, it may present as an increase in liver enzymes or fever and cholangitis. The diagnosis is based on cholangiographic findings of intrahepatic associated with extrahepatic biliary structuring, beading, and irregularity; histologic diagnostic findings are fibrous cholangitis and fibro-obliterative lesions with or without ductopenia, biliary fibrosis evolving rapidly in biliary cirrhosis. In pediatric population, fibro-obliterating lesions are often combined with intense inflammatory infiltrate, possibly due to the suggested autoimmune basis of this disease. Cholangiography, histology, and clinical correlation are necessary, owing to the histologic similarity of

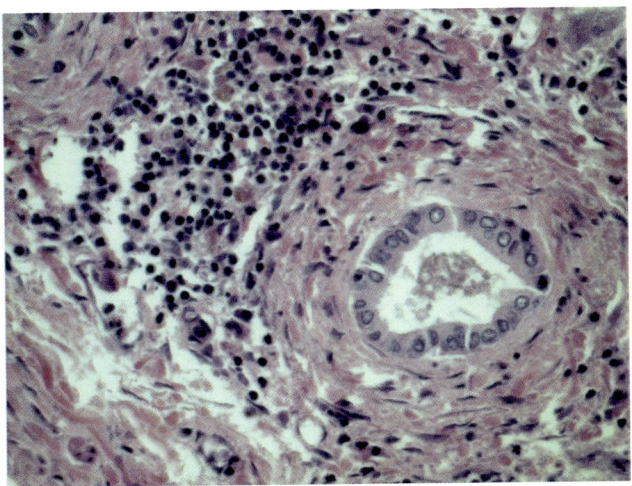

Fig. 32.19 High power view of liver biopsy in a case of PSC relapse after LT; note the typical periductal onion-skin fibrosis (H&E, 100×)

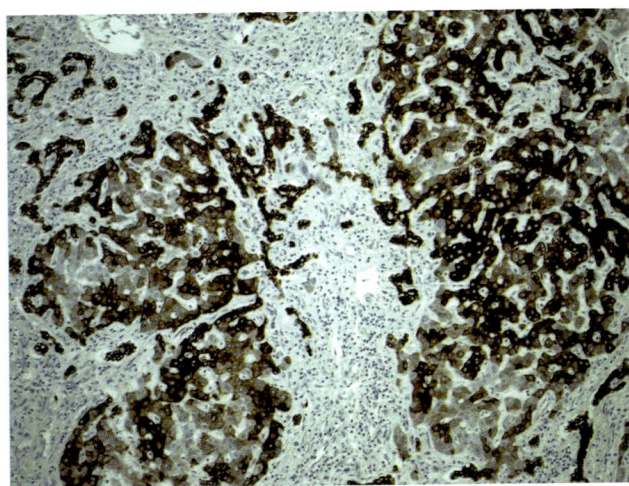

Fig. 32.20 Relapse of PSC; immunostaining for CK7 shows marked biliary metaplasia (brown coloration) of liver cells due to chronic cholestasis (40×)

recurrent PSC and chronic rejection (Figs. 32.18, 32.19, 32.20, and 32.21).

Advances in immunosuppressive therapy have played an important role in the evolution and success of LT. There may be difficulties in diagnosing drug toxicity related to immunosuppressive agents in liver allograft because of the multifactorial possibilities of liver damage in this setting. However, several other hepatotoxic medications (antibiotics, antifungal, antiviral) may also be prescribed for prophylaxis against opportunistic infections, manifested clinically as an asymptomatic increase in liver enzymes. Careful consideration of the characteristic features of drug-induced cholestasis after liver transplantation is crucial to improving patient management. Liver histology demonstrates diffuse eosinophilic inflammatory infiltrate with various degree of parenchymal necrosis; granulomas may be present within the lobule.

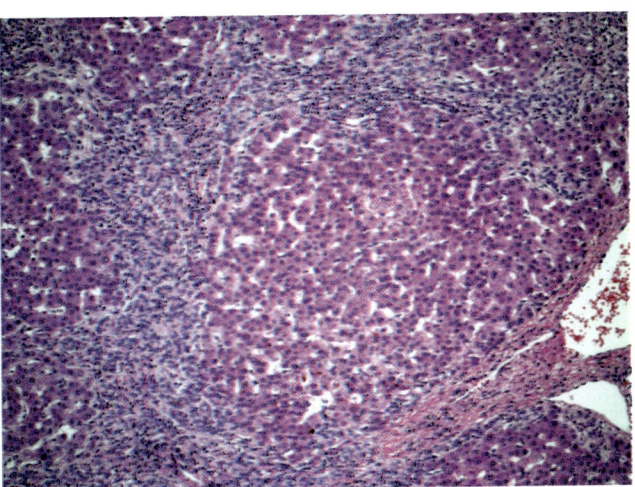

Fig. 32.18 Follow-up liver biopsy at 8 months form surgery of a patient transplanted for PSC; disease relapse with complete diffuse cirrhotic alteration and signs of ongoing bile ducts inflammatory damage (H&E, 40)

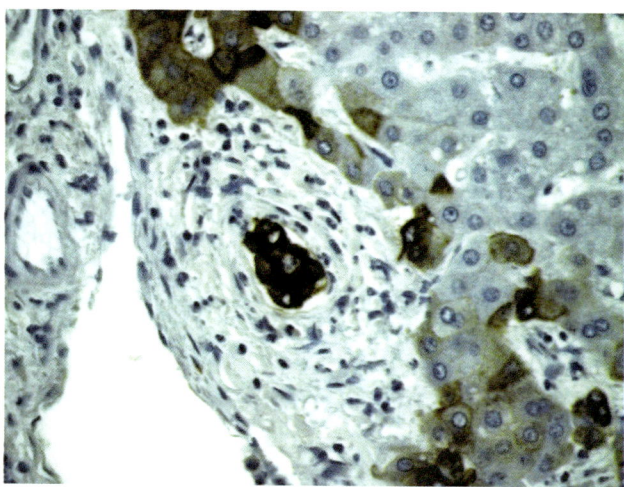

Fig. 32.21 Detail of CK7 staining in relapsing PSC; severely atrophic bile duct with degenerative changes of epithelium, periductal fibrosis, and narrowing of the lumen; periportal liver cells characterized by biliary metaplasia (100×)

32.10 Infections

32.10.1 General Considerations

Infections remain the main cause of death after LT [33]. Risk factors are the amount of intraoperative and perioperative blood products transfused, the length of stay on intensive care unit, renal dysfunction, immunosuppression and comorbid conditions (e.g., diabetes, lymphopenia, or neutropenia), and the presence of other infections [34, 35]. The occurrence of infections is conventionally described in time frames because it usually separates causative agents: first month, between the first and sixth month after liver transplantation, and after 6 months [36]. Most severe infections occur within the first 2 months and are mainly related to surgical and nosocomial risk factors. In the later period (after 6 months), infections are uncommon and are related to chronic rejection or are caused by opportunistic infections related to long-standing and overloaded immunosuppression. Most serious infectious opportunistic (*Mycobacterium tuberculosis*, *Pneumocystis*, *Listeria*, *Cryptococcus*, *Toxoplasma*, *Rhodococcus*, *Nocardia*, *Legionella*, etc.) complications usually occur in the first 8–10 weeks after surgery due to tissue damage and high levels of immunosuppressive drugs. Clinical presentation may be intriguing, and many signs and symptoms such as fever, unexplained abdominal pain, and late vascular thrombosis should address to the diagnosis of infectious concerns. Both the reactivation of previous infections and the exposition to new infectious agents are possible.

The liver is a regulatory organ in the host defense system, acting as a firewall against systemic diffusion of bacteria and pathogens; during infections, several pro-inflammatory cytokines (tumor necrosis factor alpha, interleukin [IL]-1, IL-6, and IL-8) are released, altering bile acid transport at the sinusoidal and canalicular membrane domains [37]. Cholestasis may precede the development of infectious life-threatening septic complications with high fever, cholestasis, and positive blood cultures.

Cytomegalovirus (CMV) infection is one of the most common viral complications of the early-intermediate post-LT period, involving about 30–50% of LT recipients, although a delayed onset can also be observed [38]. It is characterized by virus replication in the blood, defined as "CMV disease," in the presence of fever >38 °C for at least 2 days, neutropenia or thrombocytopenia, and signs of organ dysfunction of the lung, liver, kidney, and central nervous system. CMV infection can be primary (donor positive/recipient negative) or over-infection in a positive recipient. In the case of primary infection, in the absence of prophylaxis, over 90% of the recipients develop CMV infection compared to about 25% of the recipients in the case of superinfection; in the case of reactivation of previous infection (donor positive/recipient negative), only 15% of the recipients become clinically ill. Although CMV infection may increase alloantigen expression, making bile ducts more vulnerable to immunologic damage [39], large studies have failed to demonstrate any significant association between CMV infection and the graft cholangiopathy [40].

Epstein-Barr virus (EBV) infections are involved in the development of PTLD (post-transplant proliferative disease) EBV related. Three distinctive variants of PTLD have been recognized: reactive plasmacytic hyperplasia, polymorphic PTLD and monomorphic PTLD. During the early (polyclonal) stages of PTLD, the disease is frequently reversible, if immunosuppression is reduced. Measurement of EBV load by quantitative polymerase chain reaction assays is an important aid in the surveillance. Risk factors for PTLD include EBV seronegativity of the recipient, young age, intensity of immunosuppression, and the first year posttransplant.

Bacterial and fungal infections may be favored by high and prolonged levels of immunosuppressive drugs or by the presence of postsurgery necrotic tissues. Surgical complication such as dehiscence of biliary or intestinal anastomosis and vascular thrombosis puts the patient at high risk of infections sustained by these pathogens.

32.10.2 Histopathological Findings

Infections, independently from the type of pathogens, may induce polymorphic lesions in the liver, most of them not specific and unfortunately overlapping many other clinical-pathological conditions. Any infectious agents are able to determine intrahepatic cholestasis by release of toxic substances

[41, 42], manifested morphologically by diffuse bilirubinostasis and focal-mixed portal and lobular inflammatory infiltrate.

Viruses usually are responsible of a hepatitis-like picture characterized by diffuse reactive inflammatory infiltrate in portal field and lobule, spotty lobular necrosis, and Kupffer cell activation. Demonstration of pathogens in liver tissue may be useful in confirming the diagnosis, but, as germs are not always detected in tissue, identification of infectious agents and their components should relay mainly on microbiological tests on blood samples.

CMV usually induces typical intranuclear inclusions in hepatocytes and in other infected cells that may be very inconspicuous and scattered within the lobule (Fig. 32.22); some patients develop microabscesses around infected cells made by neutrophils [43] or in other instances aggregates of macrophages and lymphocytes form microgranuloma inside the lobule. Immunohistochemical staining confirms the diagnosis and is helpful in detecting smaller nuclear inclusions (Fig. 32.24) that could be missed in routine stained sections. Anyway failure in demonstrating inclusions does not exclude the diagnosis of CMV hepatitis. In most cases inflammatory damage of bile ducts may be detected that can resemble bile damage in rejection.

Herpes viruses may be responsible of a histological picture comparable to CMV hepatitis (Fig. 32.22); pathogens may be demonstrated by immunochemistry in nuclei of infected cells (Fig. 32.23). The infection may sometimes presents as a severe hepatitis leading to progressive liver failure and death; in these cases the liver biopsy may show extensive coagulative confluent hepatocytes necrosis.

EBV-related hepatitis causes in the liver a mild /moderate portal and sinusoidal lymphocytic infiltrate; some degree of liver cells necrosis may be present, sometimes confluent. The most severe effect of EBV infection is anyway the develop-

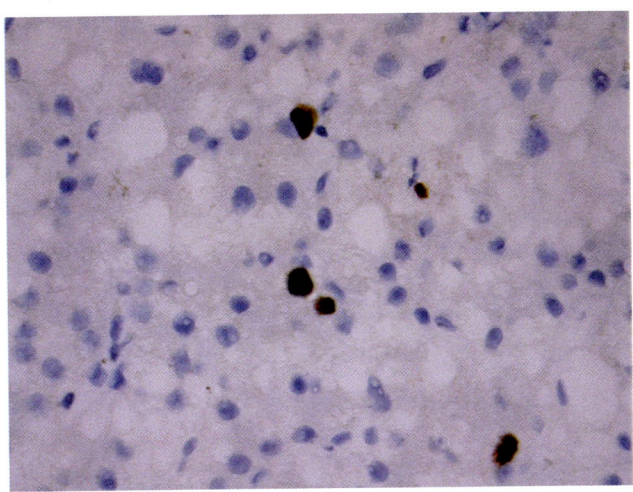

Fig. 32.23 Immunohistochemical staining of the microscopic field shown in Fig. 32.22 decorates few nuclei and confirms the diagnosis of CMV infection; note that stained nuclei are much more than suspected in H&E stain by owl eye alteration (100×)

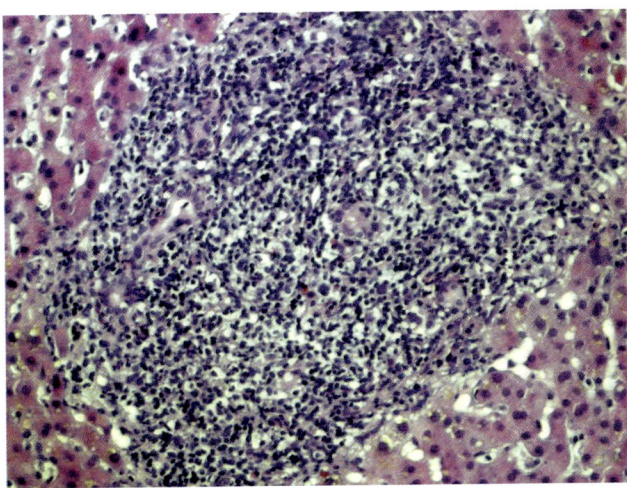

Fig. 32.24 Case of PTLD with liver involvement; portal area is severely expanded by monomorphic proliferation of large and activated lymphocytes; note diffuse aggression of biliary epithelium (H&E, 40×)

ment in some patients of unrestrained proliferation of lymphoid cells known as PTLD. PTLD in standard staining is suspected in case of diffuse lymphoid infiltrate of the graft (Fig. 32.24) or in other organs, mainly enlarged nodes; immunophenotyping and analysis of clonality of lymphoid infiltrate (Fig. 32.25) are mandatory in confirming the diagnosis of neoplastic or reactive nature of the process and in subclassifying the disease in order to treat patients with appropriated therapeutic strategy. EBV may be identified in lymphocyte nuclei by immunohistochemistry for the LMP1 antigen or by ISH technique (Fig. 32.26).

Bacterial and fungal infections arising in graft, mainly in biliary tree, or in other organs of transplant recipients usually are responsible for the histological picture known as "chol-

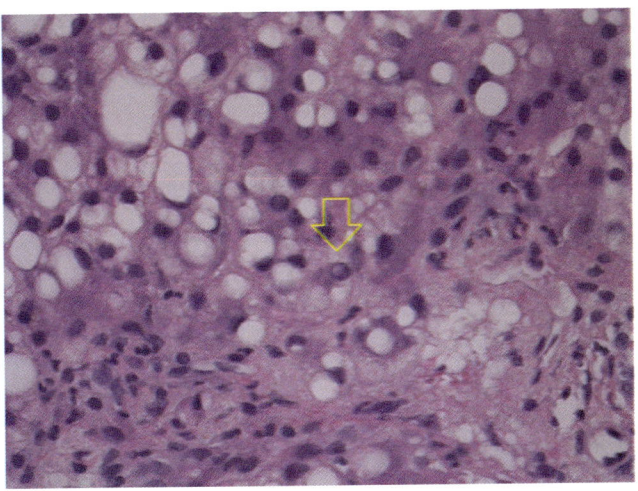

Fig. 32.22 Histological detail of a case of CMV post-LT hepatitis; typical owl eye aspect of an hepatocyte nucleus in periportal area (yellow arrow) (H&E, 100×)

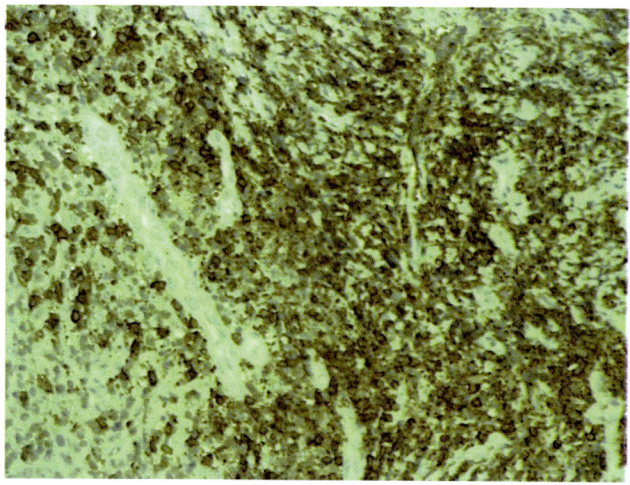

Fig. 32.25 Immunophenotyping of infiltrate seen in previous picture demonstrated a predominant component of large CD20 positive lymphocytes allowing histological diagnosis of B-cell monomorphic PTLD (100×)

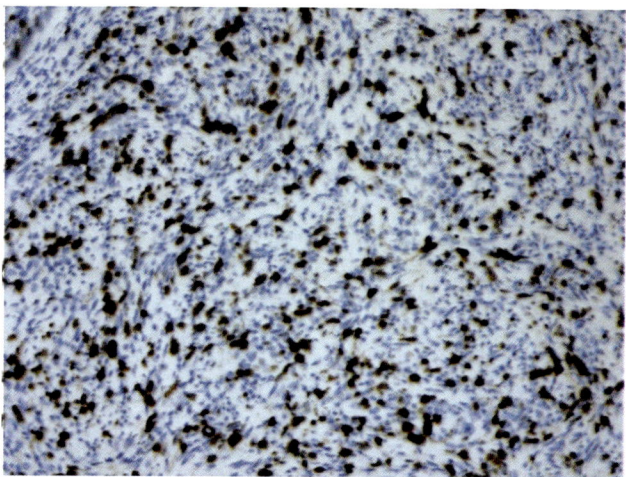

Fig. 32.26 Intense and diffuse positivity of ISH reaction for EBV in proliferating lymphoid cells nuclei (brown dots) (100×)

angitis lenta" due to toxic substances, characterized by neutrophilic infiltration of portal and lobular structures and inspissated bile plugs within dilated and proliferated portal and periportal bile ductules [44]. Fungi may be sometimes identified by special histochemical stains in liver specimens and in damaged tissues.

References

1. Bubak ME, Porayko MK, Krom RA, Wiesner RH. Complications of liver biopsy in liver transplant patients: increased sepsis associated with choledochojejunostomy. Hepatology. 1991;14:1063.
2. Larson AM, Chan GC, Wartelle CF, et al. Infection complicating percutaneous liver biopsy in liver transplant recipients. Hepatology. 1997;26:1406.
3. Anomynous. Comprehensive update of the Banff Working Group on Liver Allograft Pathology: introduction of antibody-mediated rejection. Am J Transplant. 2016;16(10):2816–35. https://doi.org/10.1111/ajt.13909. Epub 2016 Jul 14.
4. Abraham SC, Furth EE. Receiver operating characteristic analysis of serum chemical parameters as tests of liver transplant rejection and correlation with histology. Transplantation. 1995;59:740.
5. Anonymous. Banff schema for grading liver allograft rejection: an international consensus document. Hepatology. 1997;25(3):658–63.
6. McVicar JP, Kowdley KV, Bacchi CE, et al. The natural history of untreated focal allograft rejection in liver transplant recipients. Liver Transpl Surg. 1996;2:154.
7. Bartlett AS, Ramadas R, Furness S, et al. The natural history of acute histologic rejection without biochemical graft dysfunction in orthotopic liver transplantation: a systematic review. Liver Transpl. 2002;8:1147.
8. Thurairajah PH, Carbone M, Bridgestock H, et al. Late acute liver allograft rejection; a study of its natural history and graft survival in the current era. Transplantation. 2013;95:955.
9. Kim C, Aono S, Marubashi S, et al. Significance of alanine aminopeptidase N (APN) in bile in the diagnosis of acute cellular rejection after liver transplantation. J Surg Res. 2012;175:138.
10. Asaoka T, Kato T, Marubashi S, et al. Differential transcriptome patterns for acute cellular rejection in recipients with recurrent hepatitis C after liver transplantation. Liver Transpl. 2009;15:1738.
11. Massoud O, Heimbach J, Viker K, et al. Noninvasive diagnosis of acute cellular rejection in liver transplant recipients: a proteomic signature validated by enzyme-linked immunosorbent assay. Liver Transpl. 2011;17:723.
12. Shaked A, Chang BL, Barnes MR, et al. An ectopically expressed serum miRNA signature is prognostic, diagnostic, and biologically related to liver allograft rejection. Hepatology. 2017;65:269.
13. Goldstein NS, Hart J, Lewin KJ. Diffuse hepatocyte ballooning in liver biopsies from orthotopic liver transplant patients. Histopathology. 1991;18:331.
14. Kerkar N, Hadzic N, Davies ET, Portmann B, Donaldson PT, Rela M, Heaton ND, Vergani D, Mieli-Vergani G. De-novo autoimmune hepatitis after liver transplantation. Lancet. 1998;351(9100):409–13.
15. Fiel MI, Schiano TD. Plasma cell hepatitis (de-novo autoimmune hepatitis) developing post liver transplantation. Curr Opin Organ Transplant. 2012;17(3):287–92.
16. Avitzur B, Ngan M, Lao A, Fecteau VL. Prospective evaluation of the prevalence and clinical significance of positive autoantibodies after pediatric liver transplantation. J Pediatr Gastroenterol Nutr. 2007;45:222–7.
17. Duclos-Vallee JC, Johanet C, Bach JF, Yamamoto AM. Autoantibodies associated with acute rejection after liver transplantation for type-2 autoimmune hepatitis. J Hepatol. 2000;33:163–6.
18. D'Antiga L, Dhawan A, Portmann B, Francavilla R, Rela M, Heaton N, et al. Late cellular rejection in paediatric liver transplantation: aetiology and outcome. Transplantation. 2002;73:80–4.
19. Miyagawa-Hayashino HH, Egawa H, Hayashino Y, Sakurai T, Minamiguchi S, et al. Outcome and risk factors of de novo autoimmune hepatitis in living-donor liver transplantation Transplantation, vol. 78; 2004. p. 128–35.
20. Hubscer SG. Pathology of liver transplantation. Semin Liver Dis. 2009;29:74–90.
21. Ekong UD, McKiernan P, Martinez M, et al. Long-term outcomes of de novo autoimmune hepatitis in pediatric liver transplant recipients. Pediatr Transplant. 2017;21:e12945.
22. Porter KA. Pathology of liver transplantation. Transplant Rev. 1969;2:129–70.
23. Cuenca AG, Kim HB, Vakili K. Pediatric liver transplantation. Semin Pediatr Surg. 2017;26(4):217–23. https://doi.org/10.1053/j.sempedsurg.2017.07.014. Epub 2017 Jul 26.

24. Anonymous. Liver biopsy interpretation for causes of late liver allograft dysfunction. Hepatology. 2006;44:489–501. https://doi.org/10.1002/hep.21280.
25. Hubscher SG. Antibody-mediated rejection in the liver allograft. Curr Opin Organ Transplant. 2012;17:280–286.74.
26. Nakamura K, Murase N, Becich MJ, et al. Liver allograft rejection in sensitized recipients. Observations in a clinically relevant small animal model. Am J Pathol. 1993;142:1383–91.
27. Page C, Rose M, Yacoub M, Pigott R. Antigenic heterogeneity of vascular endothelium. Am J Pathol. 1992;141:673–83.
28. Astarcioglu I, Cursio R, Reynes M, Gugenheim J. Increased risk of antibody-mediated rejection of reduced-size liver allografts. J Surg Res. 1999;87:258–62.
29. Liu X, Xu J, Brenner DA, Kisseleva T. Reversibility of liver fibrosis and inactivation of fibrogenic myofibroblasts. Curr Pathobiol Rep. 2013;1:209–14.
30. Haga H, Egawa H, Fujimoto Y, et al. Acute humoral rejection and C4d immunostaining in ABO-blood type-incompatible liver transplantation. Liver Transpl. 2006;12:457–64.
31. Sharma S, Gurakar A, Jabbour N. Biliary strictures following liver transplantation: past, present and preventive strategies. Liver Transpl. 2008;14:759–69.
32. Neil DAH, Hubscher SG. Are parenchymal changes in early post-transplant biopsies related to preservation-reperfusion injury or rejection? Transplantation. 2001;71:1566–1572.5.
33. Romero FA, Razonable RR. Infections in liver transplant recipients. World J Hepatol. 2011;3:83–92.
34. Sun HY, Cacciarelli TV, Singh N. Identifying a targeted population at high risk for infections after liver transplantation in the MELD era. Clin Transpl. 2011;25:420–5.
35. van Hoek B, de Rooij BJ, Verspaget HW. Risk factors for infection after liver transplantation. Best Pract Res Clin Gastroenterol. 2012;26:61–72.
36. Fishman JA, Issa NC. Infection in organ transplantation: risk factors and evolving patterns of infection. Infect Dis Clin N Am. 2010;24:273–83.
37. Balmer ML, Slack E, de Gottardi A, Lawson MA, Hapfelmeier S, Miele L, Grieco A, Van Vlierberghe H, Fahrner R, Patuto N, Bernsmeier C, Ronchi F, Wyss M, Stroka D, Dickgreber N, Heim MH, McCoy KD, Macpherson AJ. The liver may act as a firewall mediating mutualism between the host and its gut commensal microbiota. Sci Transl Med. 2014;6:237ra66.
38. Fagiuoli S, Colli A, Bruno R, Craxi A, Gaeta GB, Grossi P, Mondelli MU, Puoti M, Sagnelli E, Stefani S, Toniutto P, Burra P, Group AST. Management of infections pre- and post-liver transplantation: report of an AISF consensus conference. J Hepatol. 2014;60:1075–89.
39. Waldman WJ, Knight DA, Adams PW, Orosz CG, Sedmak DD. In vitro induction of endothelial HLA class II antigen expression by cytomegalovirus-activated CD4+ T cells. Transplantation. 1993;56:1504–12.
40. Arnold JC, Portmann BC, O'Grady JG, Naoumov NV, Alexander GJ, Williams R. Cytomegalovirus infection persists in the liver graft in the vanishing bile duct syndrome. Hepatology. 1992;16:285–92.
41. Moseley RH, Wang W, Takeda H, Lown K, Shick L, Ananthanarayanan M, Suchy FJ. Effect of endotoxin. Post-liver transplant intrahepatic cholestasis: etiology, clinical presentation, therapy. Am J Phys. 1996;271(1 Pt 1):G137–46.
42. Bolder U, Ton-Nu HT, Schteingart CD, Frick E, Hofmann AF. Hepatocyte transport of bile acids and organic anions in endotoxemic rats: impaired uptake and secretion. Gastroenterology. 1997;112:214–25.
43. Lamps LW, Pinson CW, Raiford DS, Shyr Y, Scott MA, Washington MK. The significance of microabscesses in liver transplant biopsies: a clinicopathological study. Hepatology. 1998;28:1532–7.
44. Lefkowitch JH. Bile ductular cholestasis: an ominous histopathologic sign related to sepsis and "cholangitis lenta". Hum Pathol. 1982;13:19–24.

Chronic Rejection and Late Allograft Hepatitis

33

Deirdre Kelly

Key Points

- Liver transplantation (OLT) in children is highly successful (>80% 20-year survival).
- Most paediatric liver diseases are potentially curable with OLT.
- Long-term (>10 years) histological outcome of liver allografts is evolving.
- Chronic rejection may occur at any time posttransplant but is common in adolescence and post-transition to adult services because of nonadherence.
- Idiopathic posttransplant hepatitis (IPTH) and graft fibrosis in biopsies obtained >12 months post-LT in children with good graft function and normal liver biochemistry have been reported from many international centres.
- The cause of IPTH and graft fibrosis is unknown but progression to cirrhosis has been demonstrated and leads to graft loss.

Research Needed in the Field

Future research will focus on (1) potential immunological mechanisms such as DSA, allo- and autoantibodies; (2) mechanisms of graft fibrosis; (3) identification of non-invasive methods to detect graft fibrosis/hepatitis including longitudinal evaluation of multi-parametric MRI, miRNA's.

D. Kelly (✉)
The Liver Unit, Birmingham Womens and Childrens Hospital and University of Birmingham, Birmingham, UK
e-mail: deirdrekelly@nhs.net

33.1 Introduction

Liver transplantation (LTx) in children is highly successful with >80% having 20-year survival [1]. Most paediatric liver diseases are potentially curable with LTx, and so the long-term outcome of the graft is of particular concern [2]. This chapter will explore the incidence, aetiology, and pathophysiology of chronic rejection and late allograft hepatitis.

33.2 Chronic Rejection

33.2.1 Incidence and Risk Factors

The incidence of both acute (AR) and chronic rejection (CR) has been significantly reduced [3–5] by the development of effective immunosuppression with tacrolimus, sirolimus, mycophenolate mofetil [6–9], and/or interleukin-2 receptor blocking antibodies [10–12]. The majority of acute rejection episodes occur during the first month following transplantation, but chronic rejection may occur at any time posttransplant.

The incidence of chronic rejection is approximately 2–30% in recent series and needs early recognition because it may cause long-term graft dysfunction and fibrosis and be an indication for re-transplantation. The SPLIT consortium identified late graft loss in 35 of 872 children followed >1 year after transplantation [13]. Thirteen (37%) lost grafts due to CR and 4 (11%) to AR. Steroid-resistant AR was strongly associated with late graft loss, with a hazard ratio of 3.46 (1.81–6.44 95% CI). Having >1 AR episode was also associated with a twofold increased risk of late graft loss. Similar data was reported from a European study [14].

The choice of immunosuppressant is also a factor in the development of chronic rejection as other reports suggest that tacrolimus reduced CR compared with cyclosporine regimens [15, 16]. A longer-term prospective European trial comparing cyclosporine to tacrolimus indicated both reduced AR and CR with tacrolimus [6, 7].

Chronic rejection is a particular problem in adolescence and following transition to adult services because of the high incidence of nonadherence [17].

33.2.2 Clinical Presentation and Diagnosis

The clinical presentation is with jaundice, pruritus, and pale stools. The onset may be gradual and presentation may be late into the process. It is important to check compliance with medication in adolescents or young parents [17].

The differential diagnosis is with biliary obstruction, cholangitis, or recurrent sclerosing cholangitis, if relevant. Investigations include:

- Routine biochemical liver function tests which demonstrate an elevated conjugated bilirubin, AST, ALT, alkaline phosphatase, and GGT.
- An abdominal ultrasound of the liver is usually normal and excludes intra- or extrahepatic biliary obstruction.
- Additional imaging with MRCP is rarely required unless biliary obstruction or recurrent sclerosing cholangitis is suspected [17].
- Immunosuppression drug levels, particularly the standard deviation of trough levels, may indicate nonadherence [17].
- Liver histology is essential to make the diagnosis.

33.2.3 Histology

The Banff group defined the minimal histological features of CR as biliary epithelial changes affecting a majority of bile ducts with or without duct loss, foam cell obliterative arteriopathy (Fig. 33.1), or bile duct paucity or loss affecting >50% of portal tracts [18]. Biliary fibrosis or cirrhosis develops subsequently (Table 33.1).

33.2.4 Therapy

Treatment of chronic rejection depends on the severity of the rejection (Table 33.2). First-line therapy is to increase baseline immunosuppression, add pulse corticosteroids, and/or add an additional agent, such as mycophenolate mofetil (MMF) or conversion to tacrolimus or sirolimus [16–20].

33.2.5 Outcome

The prognosis is poor and most cases of severe rejection will lead to graft loss and the need for re-transplantation [13] although some will recover graft function on conversion to sirolimus.

A recent study from South America reported that chronic rejection occurred in 29/537 patients (5.4%). In 10 patients (10/29, 34.5%), chronic rejection resolved with immunosuppression, but in 19 patients (19/29, 65.5%), rejection was not controlled and led to re-transplantation (7 patients, 24.1%) or death (12 patients, 41.4%). The presence of ductopenia was associated with worse outcomes (risk ratio = 2.08, $p = 0.01$) [21].

In a long-term follow-up of 143 patients in Birmingham, who survived 15 years posttransplant, 20% required liver re-transplant after 1 year (28/143). The mean time re-transplant was 4.10 years (range 0–22.06 years) and leading indication was chronic rejection (75%) which did not respond to immunosuppression [22].

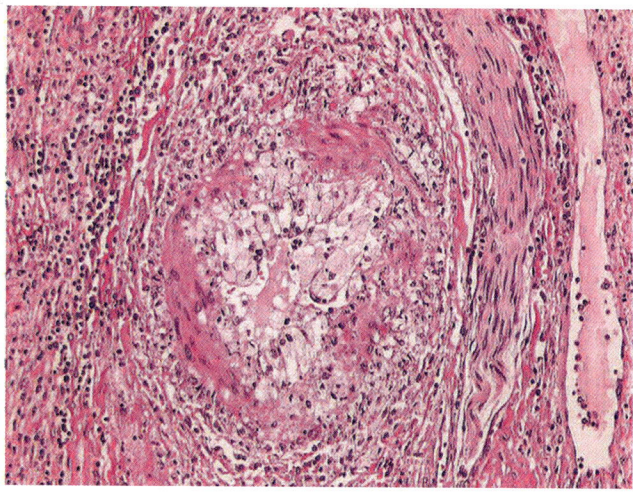

Fig. 33.1 Foam cell arteriopathy in chronic rejection. This biopsy demonstrates a large hepatic artery in an allograft liver. The lumen of the vessel is replaced by foamy macrophages typical of chronic rejection

Table 33.1 Evaluation of chronic rejection post-liver transplantation [18]

Structure	Early chronic rejection (at least two findings)	Late chronic rejection (at least two findings)
Small bile ducts (<60 μm)	Bile duct loss <50% of portal tracts	Loss ≥50% of portal tracts
Portal tract hepatic arterioles	Loss <25% of portal tracts	Loss >25% of portal tracts
Terminal hepatic venules and zone 3 hepatocytes	Perivenular mononuclear inflammation; lytic zone 3 necrosis and inflammation; mild perivenular fibrosis	Variable inflammation; moderate-to-severe bridging fibrosis
Large perihilar hepatic artery branches	Intimal inflammation, focal foam cell deposition without luminal compromise	Luminal narrowing by intimal foam cells; fibrointimal hyperplasia
Large perihilar bile ducts	Inflammation; focal foam cell deposition	Mural fibrosis

33.3 Late Graft Hepatitis

Table 33.2 Immunosuppressive drugs for chronic rejection

Drug	Class	Indications	Dose
Methyl prednisolone prednisone or prednisolone	Corticosteroid	Induction therapy Treatment of acute or chronic rejection maintenance immunosuppression	Pulse therapy IV (20 mg/kg/day) for 3 days (maximum 500 mg) or 1–2 mg/kg oral prednisone
Tacrolimus	CNI	Induction therapy Increased doses for chronic rejection Maintenance immunosuppression	0.1–0.15 mg/kg × 2/day Adjust dose to planned trough level
Cyclosporine	CNI	Not useful for chronic rejection Maintenance immunosuppression	10–15 mg/kg × 2/day Adjust dose to planned trough level
Mycophenolate mofetil	Anti-metabolite	Useful as additional therapy for chronic rejection Maintenance immunosuppression	15–20 mg/kg/dose (maximum 1 g) ×2
Azathioprine	Anti-metabolite	Not useful for chronic rejection Maintenance immunosuppression	0.5–2.0 mg/kg/day
Sirolimus	mTORI	Most effective for chronic rejection Maintenance immunosuppression	1–3 mg/M^2 Adjust dose to planned trough level

CNI calcineurin inhibitor, *mTORI* mammalian target of rapamycin inhibitor, *IV* intravenous

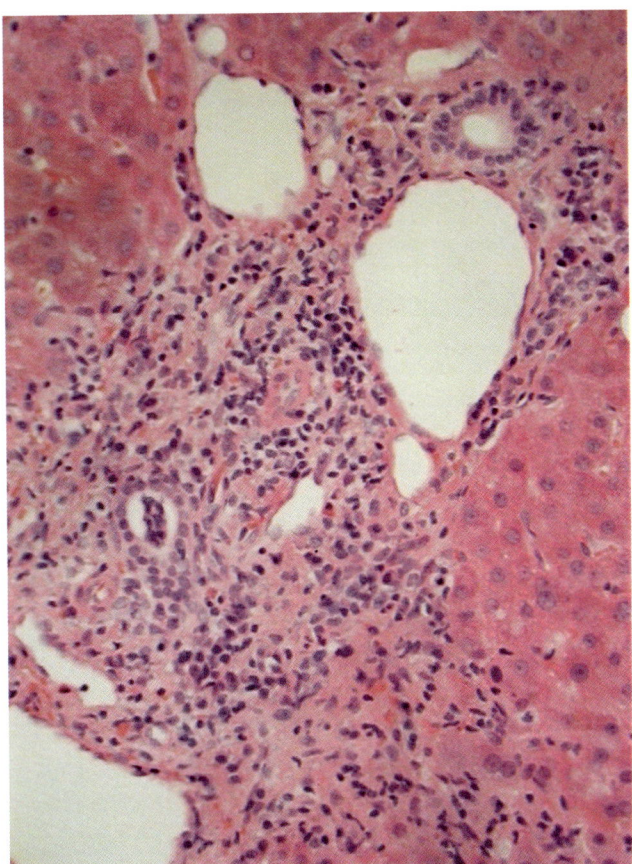

Fig. 33.2 De novo autoimmune hepatitis. This biopsy is similar to pre-transplant autoimmune hepatitis with a plasma cell portal inflammatory infiltrate with varying interface hepatitis and central perivenulitis

33.3 Late Graft Hepatitis

Late graft dysfunction is multifactorial and includes infection, rejection, recurrent disease, and technical complications such as late portal vein thrombosis, late hepatic artery thrombosis, and biliary strictures, all of which are covered elsewhere in this book. This chapter will focus on de novo autoimmune hepatitis ("plasma cell hepatitis", "immune-mediated graft hepatitis") and idiopathic graft hepatitis and fibrosis.

33.4 De Novo Autoimmune Hepatitis (Fig. 33.2)

33.4.1 Incidence and Risk Factors

"De novo autoimmune hepatitis" (DNAIH) describes the development of typical histological, biochemical, and immunological features of autoimmune hepatitis in patients transplanted for other diseases [23]. It is more common in paediatric patients (2.3–5.2%) perhaps because immunosuppression interferes with normal T-cell maturation in an immature immune system. It has been described in both cadaveric and live related LTx [23]. In studies in children, rejection and steroid dependence were identified as risk factors [24, 25].

The aetiology of DNAIH is unknown, but it may represent a form of late rejection as it often arises in a setting of under-immunosuppression or stimulation of host's immune system [25] and is associated with donor-specific antibodies, e.g. antibodies to the glutathione S-transferase T1 (GSTT1) enzyme in GSTT1-negative recipients of GSTT1-positive graft [26], and with features of acute or chronic rejection in 18–24% cases of DNAIH. Other postulated factors include molecular mimicry secondary to viruses with similar amino acid sequences to autoantigens, leading to cross-reactive immunity or polyclonal stimulation or interference with immunoregulatory cells [25]. Alternatively, calcineurin inhibitors may interfere with the maturation of T lymphocytes or the function of regulatory T cells, leading to the emergence and activation of auto-reactive T-cell clones [24, 25].

33.4.2 Clinical Presentation and Diagnosis

Clinical presentation is usually asymptomatic, and DNAIH is only suspected when biochemical liver function tests become abnormal in association with elevated immunoglobulins (IgG > 16 g/L) and the development of non-specific autoantibodies (ANA, SMA, and anti-LKM-1) [25].

Investigations include:
- Routine biochemical liver function tests which demonstrate raised transaminases
- Elevated immunoglobulins (IgG > 16 g/L)
- Raised titres of non-specific autoantibodies (ANA, SMA, and anti-LKM-1)
- Liver histology

33.4.3 Histology

Histological features include a plasma cell-rich portal inflammatory infiltrate with varying interface hepatitis and central perivenulitis [27], as seen with AIH in the native liver. Lobular inflammatory changes are more prominent in DNAIH in children often without interface necroinflammatory activity or prominent plasma cell infiltrates [28] (Fig. 33.2).

33.4.4 Therapy

Treatment with prednisolone (0.5–2 mg/kg/day) and azathioprine (0.5–2 mg/kg/day) is usually effective. It is essential to continue maintenance steroids of 5–10 mg/day to prevent relapse. Second-line therapy includes replacing azathioprine with mycophenolate mofetil or sirolimus as second-line therapy for those who do not respond. Awareness that treatment with prednisolone alone or in combination with azathioprine is successful in de novo AIH has led to excellent graft and patient survival [29].

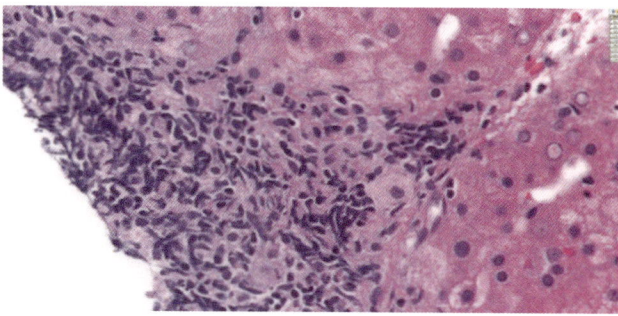

Fig. 33.3 Idiopathic graft hepatitis. This biopsy shows a portal-based inflammatory infiltrate with mononuclear inflammatory cells. Inflammation of bile ducts and portal vessels is minimal

33.4.5 Outcome

The long-term outcome is good with resolution of graft dysfunction. Progressive disease is rare, and re-transplantation is only required in those who do not respond or develop fibrosis and cirrhosis [30].

33.5 Graft Hepatitis and Fibrosis

The long-term outcome of liver grafts in children following transplantation is unknown, and hence a number of centres initialled routine protocol biopsies to determine graft histology.

33.5.1 Incidence and Risk Factors

Studies of 1-, 5-, and 10-year protocol biopsies obtained from children with normal liver biochemistry detected graft hepatitis and fibrosis in an increasing number of grafts, especially at 5- and 10-year posttransplant (Table 33.3) [27, 31–34]. In one study of 158 asymptomatic children on cyclosporine monotherapy, protocol liver biopsies at 1, 5, and 10 years after LTx demonstrated that although histology was normal at 1 year in most children,

Table 33.3 Histological findings in protocol biopsies in children with normal liver biochemistry

Centre	Time post-LTx	Abnormal histology	Main diagnoses
Birmingham (Evans 2006) [27]	1, 5, 10 years	32% at 1 year 55% at 5 years 69% at 10 years	Chronic hepatitis ± fibrosis (64%), biliary fibrosis (2%), recurrent PSC (2%), others (2%) at 10 years
Chicago (Ekong 2008) [31]	>3 years	97%	Fibrosis (97%), inflammation (70%)
Groningen (Scheenstra 2009) [32]	1, 3, 5, 10 years	34% at 1 year 48% at 3 years 65% at 5 years 69% at 10 years	Fibrosis (69%) at 10 years
Kyoto (Miyagawa-Hayashino 2012) [33]	>5 years	≥84%	Fibrosis (84%), inflammation (58%)
Brussels (Venturi 2012) [34]	7 years	94%	Fibrosis (94%), inflammation (74%), ductal proliferation (26%), steatosis (26%)

chronic hepatitis was present in 22%, 43%, and 64% of biopsies at 1, 5, and 10 years, respectively [27]. The prevalence and severity of fibrosis also increased with time, and by 10 years 50% had progressed to bridging fibrosis or cirrhosis.

No definite cause for chronic hepatitis was identified. In particular there was no evidence of chronic viral hepatitis or relationship with technical factors such as donor characteristics or cold/warm ischaemia times [35]. The only predictive risk factor [27] on multivariate analysis was the presence of non-specific autoantibody positivity with ANA and SMA.

More recently, an international consortium reviewed the incidence of graft hepatitis in 467 children [36]. Graft hepatitis was found in 43% biopsies at 5 years and 53% of biopsies at 10 years. Fifty-three percent of the children were positive for non-specific autoantibodies, which were higher in those children on cyclosporine and those on monotherapy without steroids. Factors such as age; gender; deceased- or living-related donor; and graft type (split, reduced, and whole grafts) were not associated with the presence of autoantibodies or hepatitis.

These histological studies also recorded an increase in posttransplant graft fibrosis (Table 33.3). An increase in graft fibrosis with time posttransplant was first reported by the group from Groningen who noted that the prevalence of fibrosis increased from 31 to 65% ($n = 66$) from 1 year to 5 years after LTx [32, 37]. There was no significant increase in the prevalence of fibrosis at 10 years (69%, $n = 55$), but the percentage of patients with severe fibrosis had increased from 10% (at 5 years) to 29%.

Fibrosis was not related to rejection, chronic hepatitis, or the immunosuppressive therapy used [27, 32, 37]. Risk factors for fibrosis included ischaemic biliary complications including prolonged cold ischaemia, the use of reduced-size allografts, and a high donor/recipient age ratio [37]. It was not possible to predict the severity of fibrosis based on liver biochemistry, and liver biopsy was required to detect this graft injury.

Donor-specific HLA antibodies (DSA) are found in 50–60% of children in the long-term following liver transplantation [33, 38]. These are largely class II DSA, mostly DQ. DSA are associated with graft fibrosis, chronic rejection, and de novo autoimmune hepatitis, and the higher the titre of DSA, the more likely there is associated graft injury.

It is possible that as the presence of hepatitis is associated with lower levels of immunosuppression and donor-specific antibodies, "idiopathic posttransplant chronic hepatitis" represents a form of late rejection particularly as graft inflammation, and/or fibrosis may improve or be prevented with increased immunosuppression [33, 39].

33.5.2 Clinical Presentation and Diagnosis

There are no clinical features associated with the development of either graft hepatitis or fibrosis, and the diagnosis is only made by protocol biopsy.

In children with advanced fibrosis, portal hypertension may develop with splenomegaly, thrombocytopenia, and oesophageal varices.

In those with cirrhosis, end-stage liver failure with malnutrition and decompensated liver disease may develop.

Investigations include:
- Protocol liver biopsies: Most centres who undertake protocol biopsies do so at 1, 5, and 10 years. The disadvantages are that liver biopsy is both invasive and expensive, and although complications are relatively rare in experienced hands, approximately 5% of children develop infection or haemorrhage post-biopsy, with a reported mortality of 0.6% [40]. Thus it is important to balance the risks and benefits and ensure the results of biopsies change management or outcome.
- Non-organ specific autoantibodies (SMA, ANA)
- Doppler ultrasonography/CT angiography is useful to detect vascular flow and biliary obstruction but is not useful for detecting graft hepatitis or fibrosis. It may identify splenomegaly or varices in those with advanced fibrosis.
- Transient elastography (TE) is useful in detecting cirrhosis in adults [41] although less accurate with mild fibrosis. A small paediatric study confirmed that TE correlates with histology posttransplant, but it is technically more difficult in split or live donor grafts [42].
- Liver biopsy is essential for making the diagnosis.

33.5.3 Histology

Most children with unexplained late graft hepatitis have a portal-based inflammatory infiltrate with mononuclear inflammatory cells. Inflammation of bile ducts and portal vessels is minimal or absent. Interface hepatitis is usually mild. Lobular inflammatory changes involving centrilobular regions with central perivenulitis are present [43, 44]. Scoring systems used to grade chronic hepatitis in the native liver (e.g. METAVIR, Ishak) are used to grade portal and periportal inflammatory changes, whereas the severity of central perivenulitis is scored according to the Banff Working Party proposal [45] (Fig. 33.4).

Graft fibrosis may be periportal, perisinusoidal, or perivenular [34] (9). It is possible that the periportal fibrosis is a result of portal inflammation and interface hepatitis [27, 31]. Centrilobular fibrosis may be secondary to the central perivenulitis or as a consequence of chronic rejection [44].

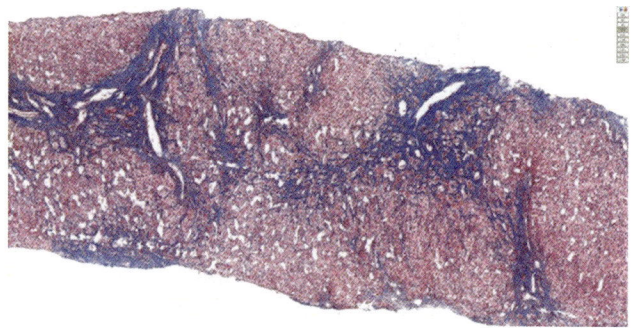

Fig. 33.4 Idiopathic graft fibrosis. This biopsy is typical of late graft fibrosis with periportal, perisinusoidal, and perivenular fibrosis. Note the sinusoidal dilation which is also seen

A semi-quantitative scoring system is useful to assess the severity of fibrosis around portal tracts (0–3), in sinusoids (0–3), and around centrilobular veins (0–3) and produces a liver allograft fibrosis (LAF) score (0–9) [34]. The LAF score correlates more effectively with morphometric fibrosis quantitation than METAVIR or Ishak fibrosis scores and may be useful for assessing the dynamics of fibrosis progression [46].

33.5.4 Outcome

Data on outcome of graft hepatitis and fibrosis are in evolution. An international consortium reviewed long-term outcomes of 289 asymptomatic (ALT < 50 IU/L) children who underwent 10-year (± 2 years) protocol biopsies. The histological findings were correlated with re-transplantation and survival over a 17-year follow-up after LTx [47].

Normal or near normal histology was reported in 68 (24%) and periportal or central fibrosis without bridging in 135 (47%); 59 (20%) had bridging fibrosis, and 27 (9%) had cirrhosis. A Kaplan-Meier analysis did not demonstrate reduced allograft survival in patients with periportal/central fibrosis and bridging fibrosis compared to patients without fibrosis at 10-year biopsy. In contrast, patients with cirrhosis at 10 years had a significantly ($p = 0.028$) higher risk of death (2 out of 27 patients) or re-transplantation (3 out of 27 patients) by the end of the second decade after LT, demonstrating the need to follow these patients long term into adult life.

33.6 Summary

The development of chronic rejection, de novo autoimmune hepatitis, idiopathic graft hepatitis, and fibrosis in paediatric liver grafts is well recognised, although the underlying mechanisms remain incompletely understood. The long-term outcome of graft hepatitis and fibrosis is evolving, but evidence of progression and graft loss confirms the necessity for life-long monitoring [48].

Evaluation of late graft outcomes should include pertinent clinical details and selected laboratory parameters (ALT, GGT, platelet count, serum autoantibodies) and imaging of graft vascular and biliary status (US, MRI, MRCP).

Transient elastography may prove to be a useful indicator of graft fibrosis and might eventually replace the need for liver biopsy, but in the meantime, protocol liver biopsies remain an important investigation in determining the long-term outcome of liver allografts.

33.7 Future Research

The underlying mechanisms for de novo autoimmune hepatitis, idiopathic graft hepatitis, and fibrosis in paediatric liver grafts are unknown, and future research is required to understand the aetiology and identify targets for therapy.

The Graft Injury Group Observing Long-Term Outcome (GIGOLO) is an international consortium which consists of clinicians, pathologists, and immunologists which was formed to determine the causes of long-term allograft injury in paediatric liver transplant recipients.

The group plans to perform long-term clinical outcome studies on patients with and without graft hepatitis/fibrosis, retrospective studies on stored tissue, and standardise histological reporting, procedures, and tissue samples for protocol biopsies in order to undertake prospective evaluation into aetiological mechanisms.

Initial focus will be on potential immunological mechanisms such as DSA and allo- and autoantibodies, while future projects will evaluate mechanisms of graft fibrosis and identification of non-invasive methods to study graft fibrosis/hepatitis including longitudinal evaluation of multi-parametric magnetic resonance imaging to standardise their applicability into standard operating procedures.

References

1. Duffy JP, Kao K, Ko CY, Farmer DG, McDiarmid SV, Hong JC, et al. Long-term patient outcome and quality of life after liver transplantation: analysis of 20-year survivors. Ann Surg. 2010;252(4):652–61.
2. Hubscher SG. What is the long-term outcome of the liver allograft? J Hepatol. 2011;55(3):702–17.
3. Dattani N, Baker A, Quaglia A, Melendez HV, Rela M, Heaton N. Clinical and histological outcomes following living-related liver transplantation in children. Clin Res Hepatol Gastroenterol. 2014;38(2):164–71.
4. Martin SR, Atkison P, Anand R, Lindblad AS. Studies of pediatric liver transplantation 2002: patient and graft survival and rejection

in pediatric recipients of a first liver transplant in the United States and Canada. Pediatr Transplant. 2004;8(3):273–83.
5. Oh SH, Kim KM, Kim DY, Lee YJ, Rhee KW, Jang JY, Chang SH, Lee SY, Kim JS, Choi BH, Park SJ, Yoon CH, Ko GY, Sung KB, Hwang GS, Choi KT, Yu E, Song GW, Ha TY, Moon DB, Ahn CS, Kim KH, Hwang S, Park KM, Lee YJ, Lee SG. Long-term outcomes of pediatric living donor liver transplantation at a single institution. Pediatr Transplant. 2010;14(7):870–8.
6. Kelly D, Jara P, Rodeck B, Lykavieris P, Burdelski M, Becker M, et al. Tacrolimus and steroids versus ciclosporin microemulsion, steroids, and azathioprine in children undergoing liver transplantation: randomised European multicentre trial. Lancet. 2004;364(9439):1054–61.
7. Kelly D. Safety and efficacy of tacrolimus in pediatric liver recipients. Pediatr Transplant. 2011;15(1):19–24.
8. Jimenez-Rivera C, Avitzur Y, Fecteau AH, Jones N, Grant D, Ng VL. Sirolimus for pediatric liver transplant recipients with post-transplant lymphoproliferative disease and hepatoblastoma. Pediatr Transplant. 2004;8(3):243–8.
9. Barau C, Furlan V, Debray D, Taburet AM, Barrail-Tran A. Population pharmacokinetics of mycophenolic acid and dose optimization with limited sampling strategy in liver transplant children. Br J Clin Pharmacol. 2012;74(3):515–24.
10. Spada M, Petz W, Bertani A, Riva S, Sonzogni A, Giovannelli M, et al. Randomized trial of basiliximab induction versus steroid therapy in pediatric liver allograft recipients under tacrolimus immunosuppression. Am J Transplant. 2006;6(8):1913–21.
11. Arora N, McKiernan PJ, Beath SV, deVille de Goyet J, Kelly DA. Concomitant basiliximab with low-dose calcineurin inhibitors in children post-liver transplantation. Pediatr Transplant. 2002;6(3):214–8.
12. Kerkar N, Morotti RA, Iyer K, Arnon R, Miloh T, Sturdevant M, et al. Anti-lymphocyte therapy successfully controls late "cholestatic" rejection in pediatric liver transplant recipients. Clin Transplant. 2011;25(6):E584–91.
13. Soltys K, Mazariegos G, Squires R, Sindhi R, Anand R. Late graft loss or death in pediatric liver transplantation: an analysis of the SPLIT database. Am J Transplant. 2007;7(9):2165–71.
14. Wallot MA, Mathot M, Janssen M, et al. Long-term survival and late graft loss in pediatric liver transplant recipients—a 15-year single-center experience. Liver Transpl. 2002;8(7):615–22.
15. Jain A, Mazariegos G, Pokharna R, et al. Almost total absence of chronic rejection in primary pediatric liver transplantation under tacrolimus. Transplant Proc. 2002;34(5):1968–9.
16. Jain A, Reyes J, Kashyap R, et al. Long-term survival after liver transplantation in 4,000 consecutive patients at a single center. Ann Surg. 2000;232(4):490–500.
17. Kelly DA, Bucuvalas JC, Alonso EM, Karpen SJ, Allen U, Green M, et al. Long-term medical management of the pediatric patient after liver transplantation: 2013 practice guideline by the American Association for the Study of Liver Diseases and the American Society of Transplantation. Liver Transpl. 2013;19(8):798–825.
18. Demetris A, Adams D, Bellamy C, Blakolmer K, Clouston A, Dhillon AP, et al. Update of the International Banff Schema for Liver Allograft Rejection: working recommendations for the histopathologic staging and reporting of chronic rejection. An International Panel. Hepatology. 2000;31(3):792–9.
19. Casas-Melley AT, Falkenstein KP, Flynn LM, Ziegler VL, Dunn SP. Improvement in renal function and rejection control in pediatric liver transplant recipients with the introduction of sirolimus. Pediatr Transplant. 2004;8(4):362–6.
20. Ganschow R, Pape L, Sturm E, Bauer J, Melter M, Gerner P, Höcker B, Ahlenstiel T, Kemper M, Brinkert F, Sachse MM, Tönshoff B. Growing experience with mTOR inhibitors in pediatric solid organ transplantation. Pediatr Transplant. 2013;17(7):694–706.
21. Tannuri AC, Lima F, Mello ES, Tanigawa RY, Tannuri U. Prognostic factors for the evolution and reversibility of chronic rejection in pediatric liver transplantation. Clinics (Sao Paulo). 2016;71(4):216–20.
22. Ruth ND, Legarda M, Smith M, Lewis PJ, Lloyd C, Paris S, Kelly DA. Long term outcome after liver transplant—a 15 year retrospective review. Hepatology. 2013;58(S1):146A.
23. Miyagawa-Hayashino A, Haga H, Egawa H, Hayashino Y, Sakurai T, Minamiguchi S, et al. Outcome and risk factors of de novo autoimmune hepatitis in living-donor liver transplantation. Transplantation. 2004;78(1):128–35.
24. Liberal R, Zen Y, Mieli-Vergani G, Vergani D. Liver transplantation and autoimmune liver diseases. Liver Transpl. 2013;19(10):1065–77.
25. Kerkar N, Yanni G. 'De novo' and 'recurrent' autoimmune hepatitis after liver transplantation: a comprehensive review. J Autoimmun. 2016;66:17–24.
26. Rodriguez-Mahou M, Salcedo M, Fernandez-Cruz E, et al. Antibodies against glutathione S-transferase T1 (GSTT1) in patients with GSTT1 null genotype as prognostic marker: long-term follow-up after liver transplantation. Transplantation. 2007;83(8):1126–9.
27. Evans HM, Kelly DA, McKiernan PJ, Hubscher S. Progressive histological damage in liver allografts following pediatric liver transplantation. Hepatology (Baltimore, Md.). 2006;43(5):1109–17.
28. Pongpaibul A, Venick RS, McDiarmid SV, Lassman CR. Histopathology of de novo autoimmune hepatitis. Liver Transpl. 2012;18(7):811–8.
29. Salcedo M, Vaquero J, Banares R, Rodriguez-Mahou M, Alvarez E, Vicario JL, et al. Response to steroids in de novo autoimmune hepatitis after liver transplantation. Hepatology. 2002;35(2):349–56.
30. Ekong UD, McKiernan P, Martinez M, Lobritto S, Kelly D, Ng VL, Alonso EM, Avitzur Y. Long-term outcomes of de novo autoimmune hepatitis in pediatric liver transplant recipients. Pediatr Transplant. 2017;21(6). Epub 2017 May 29.
31. Ekong UD, Melin-Aldana H, Seshadri R, et al. Graft histology characteristics in long-term survivors of pediatric liver transplantation. Liver Transpl. 2008;14(11):1582–7.
32. Scheenstra R, Peeters PM, Verkade HJ, Gouw AS. Graft fibrosis after pediatric liver transplantation: ten years of follow-up. Hepatology (Baltimore, Md.). 2009;49(3):880–6.
33. Miyagawa-Hayashino A, Yoshizawa A, Uchida Y, et al. Progressive graft fibrosis and donor-specific human leukocyte antigen antibodies in pediatric late liver allografts. Liver Transpl. 2012;18(11):1333–42.
34. Venturi C, Sempoux C, Bueno J, et al. Novel histologic scoring system for long-term allograft fibrosis after liver transplantation in children. Am J Transplant. 2012;12(11):2986–96.
35. Davison SM, Skidmore SJ, Collingham KE, Irving WL, Hubscher SG, Kelly DA. Chronic hepatitis in children after liver transplantation: role of hepatitis C virus and hepatitis G virus infections. J Hepatol. 1998;28(5):764–70.
36. Rajanayagam J. Haller W, Debray D, Verkade H, McLin V, Evans H, Sokal E, Sturm E, Scheenstra R, Gou A, Cousin V, Varma S, Hartleiff S, Hodson J, Kelly D. Serum autoantibodies are associated with chronic hepatitis and graft fibrosis after pediatric liver transplantation. Hepatology (Baltimore, Md.). 2015;62(Suppl 1).
37. Peeters PM, Sieders E, vd Heuvel M, et al. Predictive factors for portal fibrosis in pediatric liver transplant recipients. Transplantation. 2000;70(11):1581–7.
38. Wozniak LJ, Hickey MJ, Venick RS, Vargas JH, Farmer DG, Busuttil RW, et al. Donor-specific HLA antibodies are associated with late allograft dysfunction after pediatric liver transplantation. Transplantation. 2015;99(7):1416–22.
39. Haller W, Lloyd C, Hubscher SG, Brown RM, McKiernan PJ, Kelly DA. Is there a role of corticosteroids in preventing graft hepatitis

and fibrosis in liver allografts following paediatric liver transplantation? Hepatology. 2009;50(4):754a-a.
40. Azzam RK, Alonso EM, Emerick KM, Whitington PF. Safety of percutaneous liver biopsy in infants less than three months old. J Pediatr Gastroenterol Nutr. 2005;41(5):639–43.
41. Lutz HH, Schroeter B, Kroy DC, Neumann U, Trautwein C, Tischendorf JJ. Doppler ultrasound and transient elastography in liver transplant patients for noninvasive evaluation of liver fibrosis in comparison with histology: a prospective observational study. Dig Dis Sci. 2015;60(9):2825–31.
42. Goldschmidt I, Stieghorst H, Munteanu M, et al. The use of transient elastography and non-invasive serum markers of fibrosis in pediatric liver transplant recipients. Pediatr Transplant. 2013;17(6):525–34.
43. Hubscher S. What does the long-term liver allograft look like for the pediatric recipient? Liver Transpl. 2009;15(Suppl 2):S19–24.
44. Hubscher SG. Central perivenulitis: a common and potentially important finding in late posttransplant liver biopsies. Liver Transpl. 2008;14(5):596–600.
45. Demetris AJ, Adeyi O, Bellamy CO, Clouston A, Charlotte F, Czaja A, et al. Liver biopsy interpretation for causes of late liver allograft dysfunction. Hepatology. 2006;44(2):489–501.
46. Venturi C, Sempoux C, Quinones JA, et al. Dynamics of allograft fibrosis in pediatric liver transplantation. Am J Transplant. 2014;14(7):1648–56.
47. Hartleif S, Rajanayagam J, Cousin V, Debray D, Demetris J, Evans H, Fischler B, Gonzales E, Gouw A, Haller H, Hodson J, Hubscher S, Lacaille F, Malenicka S, Mazariegos G, McLin V, Squires J, Sturm E, Verkade H, Kelly D. Graft fibrosis and long-term outcome after paediatric liver transplantation. JPGN. 2017;62(Suppl 1).
48. Kelly D, Verkade HJ, Rajanayagam J, McKiernan P, Mazariegos G, Hübscher S. Late graft hepatitis and fibrosis in pediatric liver allograft recipients: Current concepts and future developments. Liver Transpl. 2016;22(11):1593–602. Review. Erratum in: Liver Transpl. 2017 Feb;23 (2):270).

Cytomegalovirus and Epstein-Barr Virus Infection and Disease

Emanuele Nicastro and Lorenzo D'Antiga

Key Points
- PTLD is a potentially fatal but preventable complication in paediatric liver transplant recipients, often related to EBV.
- In PTLD, stratifying the risk according to clinical and histological features and to response to immunosuppression withdrawal helps identifying the subset of patients who should benefit from rituximab and the few patients needing chemotherapy.
- CMV disease after liver transplantation can be effectively prevented by preemptive therapy, with reduced costs and antiviral exposure.
- CMV resistance should be suspected in patients not responding to 2 weeks of ganciclovir treatment and assessed through genotypic resistance testing.

Research Needed in the Field
- To find tools allowing to better understand the degree of immune competence of each patient during standard immunosuppressive treatment and tailor it to prevent severe viral infections
- To find strategies boosting the immune system and promoting the clearance of EBV infection, when occurred
- To identify prognostic factors defining patients with PTLD without satisfactory response to rituximab that benefit from the addition of cytoreductive chemotherapy
- To improve the monitoring of CMV infection and find new antiviral treatments efficacious on mutants resistant to ganciclovir

34.1 Introduction

Currently, the greatest rate of mortality following paediatric liver transplantation (LT) is related to infections, certainly related to excessive immunosuppression [1]. The impact of viral disease on LT outcome depends mainly on two factors: firstly, the time post-LT, thus the degree of immunosuppression, and secondly the serological status of the recipient. Most of the infectious complications following LT are caused by herpes viruses and are acquired with the donor organ [2]. Indeed, children are often seronegative recipients receiving livers from adult donors latently infected by cytomegalovirus (CMV), Epstein-Barr virus (EBV, and, less frequently, herpes simplex virus (HSV1-2) and human herpes virus 6 and 8 (HHV6, HHV8). Under maximum immunosuppression, this often leads to early infection/reactivation of the viruses, with different consequences.

In this chapter, the role of CMV and EBV, the main donor-associated viral pathogens, will be discussed.

34.2 EBV Infection and PTLD

34.2.1 Clinical Pictures and Epidemiology

EBV is responsible for a spectrum of clinical conditions that depend on the level of lymphoid tissue involvement and transformation, resulting from the interaction between the virus and the immune system. About 60–80% of seronegative children are expected to acquire EBV infection within 3 months of solid organ transplant, either from primary oropharyngeal EBV infection or via donor passenger lymphocytes in the transplanted organ from a seropositive donor.

Symptomatic EBV infection occurs in 8–22% of the cases and is not different from that of the immunocompetent host [3, 4]. It is commonly defined in the presence of IgM against the viral capsid (or positive viral load) along with either the

E. Nicastro (✉) · L. D'Antiga
Paediatric Hepatology, Gastroenterology and Transplantation, Hospital Papa Giovanni XXIII, Bergamo, Italy
e-mail: enicastro@asst-pg23.it; ldantiga@asst-pg23.it

histological evidence of an EBV infection or specific symptoms (fever, leukopenia, atypical lymphocytosis, exudative tonsillitis and/or lymphadenopathy, or hepatitis).

The most important and potentially fatal complication related to EBV is the post-transplant lymphoproliferative disorder (PTLD), which is defined on the basis of the histological criteria. PTLD represents a continuum of atypical lymphoid proliferations, ranging from lymphoid hyperplasia to malignant lymphomas, typically but not exclusively of B-cell origin.

The overall reported incidence of PTLD varies between 3 and 18%, with a mortality rate previously peaking at 60%, but nowadays ranging between 10 and 12% [3, 5–8].

In the North American centres of the SPLIT Consortium, comparing the periods 2002–2007 and 1995–2001, the incidence of symptomatic EBV infection and PTLD decreased from 11.3% to 5.9% and from 4.2% to 1.7%, respectively. This reduction seems to be related to an increased attention to immunosuppression, with most centres maintaining lower trough levels of both cyclosporine A and tacrolimus in the first months after LT [4].

Acknowledged risk factors for developing PTLD are the EBV seronegativity at LT, young recipient age, older donors, high levels of immunosuppression and the use of lymphocyte-depleting agents [3, 4, 9].

The majority of PTLDs in children occur within the first 2 years after LT (early PTLD), and this is related to EBV acquisition and intensive T-cell suppression [10, 11]. It can be said that 90% of childhood PTLDs are EBV-related and early-onset. Late-onset PTLD can occur in paediatric LT recipients as a consequence of lifelong immunosuppression and represents less than 10% of cases. Late forms present more frequently as disseminated, often monomorphic, disease, sometimes EBV-negative. Late PTLD tends to be less responsive to the sole immunosuppression reduction, displaying a worse clinical course. In a study carried out by our group, it has been shown that late PTLD seems to be related to sustained, long-term EBV detection in blood, although at low viral loads. The study concluded that long-term monitoring of EBV-PCR until negativisation is recommended to prevent or promptly diagnose late PTLD [12].

The current World Health Organization (WHO) classification recognises four types of PTLD:

- *Early lesions:* almost invariably represent the histologic picture of the early PTLD, with reactive infectious mononucleosis-like plasmacytic hyperplasia, always EBV-positive, occurring at the time of primary immunoconversion.
- *Polymorphic PTLD:* defined by the concomitant presence of monoclonal EBV-positive B lymphocytes and polyclonal T cells.

Table 34.1 Classification system for post-transplant lymphoproliferative disorder (PTLD)

Grading	Description
0	EBV lymphadenitis, hepatitis, not classified as PTLD
1	Early lesion, low-grade mononucleosis, plasma cell hyperplasia
2	Polymorphic, diffuse B-cell hyperplasia (PDBH) and polymorphic B-cell lymphoma (PBC)
3	Monomorphic or lymphomatous PTLD or lymphoma, immunoblastic lymphoma (IBL), diffuse large B-cell lymphoma (DLBCL) or diffuse small cell noncleaved (Burkitt-like)
4	Other Hodgkin's-like PTLD, plasma cell lesions, plasmacytoma, T-cell PTLD

Adapted from Harris NL et al.

- *Monomorphic PTLD:* this includes different subtypes. The vast majority are of B-cell origin and have large similarities with diffuse large B-cell lymphoma (DLBCL-like or PT-DLBCL). Burkitt and Burkitt-like lymphomas are less common, while the plasmablast/immunoblast lymphoma is exceptional.
- A fourth type encompasses Hodgkin's-like lymphoma, plasmacytoma-like PTLD and T-cell neoplasms.

The classification of PTLD lesions is summarised in Table 34.1. This classification has important implications for treatment, allowing a risk-adapted management of PTLD that—along with a high index of suspicion and surveillance—is the most effective strategy to reduce PTLD lethality.

Due to its importance in the EBV burden after solid organ transplantation, the following sections will discuss PTLD.

34.2.2 Pathophysiology of PTLD

Following EBV infection, the immunocompetent host develops a cytotoxic T-lymphocyte response to the viral proteins exposed on EBV-infected B lymphocytes [13]. After seroconversion, a lytic response leads to viral clearance, followed by a memory T-cell response. In the immunosuppressed patient failing to clear the infection, the EBV is capable of promoting the germinal centre T-cell-dependent pathway and starting different types of latency, resulting in a variable degree of resistance to apoptosis. This results in the proliferative stimulus to the activated B-blast (mainly mediated by LMP1 and EBNA2 expression) but also in the latent infection of the germinal centre blasts, in which EBV latency proteins lead to a failure in deleting low-affinity B-cell receptor clones that become immortalised. The resulting cells become differentiated mainly into memory B cells but also into plasma cells. The latter allow viral lytic replication, which is important for lymphomagenesis, especially for the early stages [14, 15].

Different EBV proteins are involved in the complex mechanism of PTLD, from B-cell hyperplasia to malignancy. LMP1 is analogous to CD40 and promotes cell transformation by inducing the NF-kB pathway, with consequent upregulation of BCL-2 and other genes involved in blocking apoptosis; nuclear EBNA1 and EBNA2 warrant viral episomal DNA replication and selective cellular and viral gene expression, respectively; LMP2 acts as a chronically active B-cell receptor and provides further survival signals [16].

The most common malignant PTLD subtype is the diffuse large B-cell lymphoma (PT-DLBCL), followed by Burkitt lymphoma (PT-BL) and plasmablastic lymphoma (PT-PBL). EBV-driven disruption of B-cell maturation is displayed in Fig. 34.1. However, around 10% of EBV-negative and a few T-cell origin post-transplant lymphomas have a different pathogenesis. Mechanisms that contribute to both EBV-positive and EBV-negative lymphomas are T-cell suppression, microsatellite instability, epigenetic alterations (such as hypermethylation and aberrant up- or downregulation of host microRNAs) and host polymorphisms in genes related to immune response.

34.2.3 Diagnosis

Since symptoms can be non-specific, the diagnosis of PTLD relies on a high index of suspicion. The lymphoid tissue involvement of diverse organs accounts for the heterogeneity of localisations and clinical signs, ranging from pharyngitis and/or Waldeyer ring enlargement to gastrointestinal symptoms.

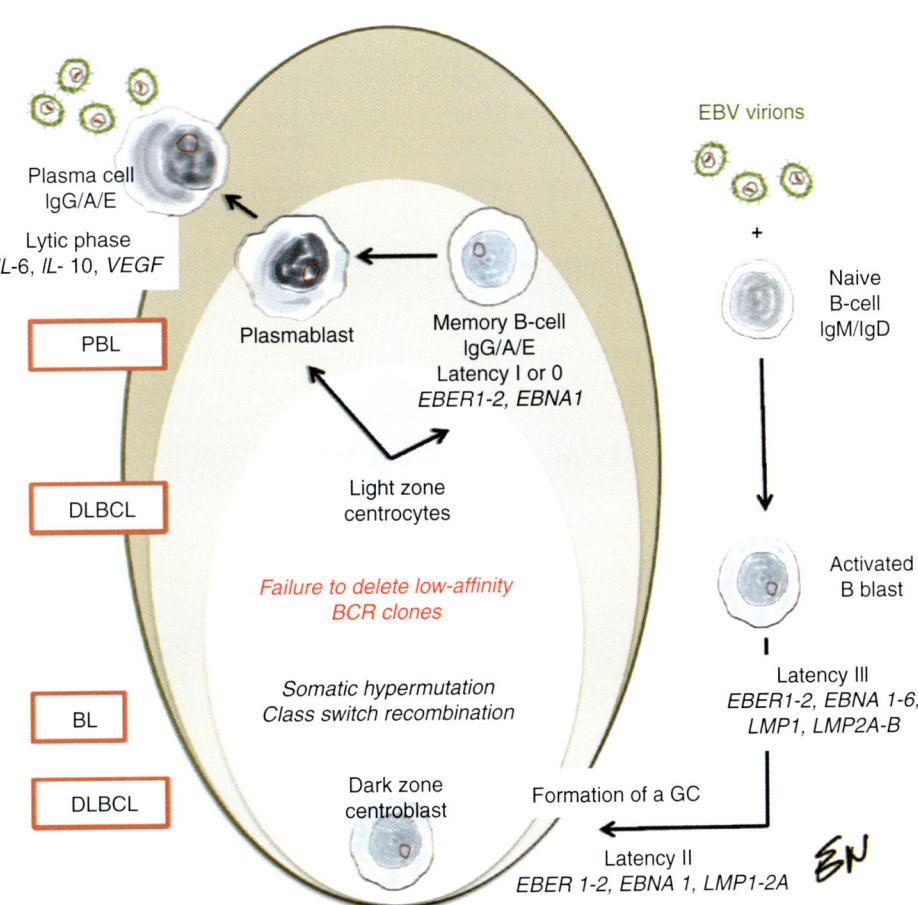

Fig. 34.1 Pathogenesis of the Epstein-Barr virus-mediated hyperplasia and malignancy in post-transplant lymphoproliferative disorder (PTLD). EBV exploits the normal B-cell activation pathway but succeeds to induce proliferation due to protein expression patterns. The activated EBV-infected blasts that enter the germinal centre (GC) express viral latency III pattern (LMP1+/EBNA2+), undergoing proliferation. Likewise, in the GC, latency II (LMP1+/EBNA2−) pattern is expressed by infected centroblasts undergoing somatic hypermutation and class switch recombination for antibody maturation. The selected B cells differentiate into plasma cells (that provide lytic phase that perpetuates the cycle) or memory cells (latency I, EBNA1+ or latency 0, no expression of viral proteins). The failure to control the EBV-associated proliferative stimulus by the immune system results in a spectrum of dysplastic and malignant B-cell subtypes that have features of their normal counterpart. *EBV* Epstein-Barr virus, *GC* germinal centre, *BCR* B-cell receptor, *DLBCL* diffuse large B-cell lymphoma, *BL* Burkitt lymphoma, *PBL* plasmablastic lymphoma. Adapted from [16]

Along with the clinical clues, the availability of viral nucleic acid monitoring has become a great tool to manage this complication. The viral load (measured in PBMC or in whole blood) is reliably correlated with the risk of developing symptomatic EBV infection and PTLD [17, 18]. However, EBV viral load, while useful to monitor EBV infection, is unable to reliably support the diagnosis of PTLD. Indeed, high viremia can be detected in the absence of PTLD, while, conversely, PTLD can be associated with low or even undetectable EBV viral loads, especially when it occurs in protected sites such as the graft itself or the gut. Furthermore, rather than the viremia per se, a more specific immune response conferring a substantial risk of developing PTLD is the high viral replication associated with a low number of anti-EBV cytotoxic T lymphocytes [19, 20].

The symptoms heralding PTLD are summarised in Table 34.2. The clinical presentation is often subtle and non-specific, with typically no or little involvement of peripheral lymph nodal stations. PTLD should be suspected in the case of otherwise unexplained fever, malaise or failure to thrive in a transplanted child, especially in the first year after LT or under augmented immunosuppression. Children with high or rapidly increasing EBV viral load, in the presence of physical signs or cytopenia, should also be considered at high risk of having PTLD. Clinical signs can be a mononucleosis-like syndrome, abdominal pain with or without diarrhoea or neurologic symptoms.

Imaging has a paramount role in confirming the suspicion of PTLD or staging a confirmed disease. Ultrasound has a limited role, while a neck, chest and/or abdominal CT or MR scan should be used as first-line tools as soon as the suspicion arises, since they can identify occult lesions amenable to tissue sampling.

In fact, histology is the pillar of the diagnosis of PTLD. Beyond the bulky lesions, histological evidence of the disease can be obtained from intestinal biopsies (early gastrointestinal endoscopy should be performed in case of even mild gastrointestinal symptoms or hypoalbuminemia due to protein-losing enteropathy) or from the graft, if evoked by specific clues. Histological analysis should always encompass in situ hybridisation to detect EBV-encoded small RNA (EBER), to confirm the disease is EBV-related, and CD3/CD20 stain for disease subtyping.

34.2.4 Treatment Algorithm

The basis of the treatment of PTLD are firstly restoring the cytotoxic T-lymphocyte immune response against the EBV and secondly targeting B-lymphocyte proliferation.

As for the first point, reduction or weaning of the immunosuppression is of great importance in controlling the lymphoproliferative modifications. This intervention is the gold standard for the early (usually polyclonal) PTLD, where it helps avoiding unnecessary medications, though exposing the patient to increased risk of rejection. The proportion of adult patients undergoing complete remission with this modulation alone shows a variation from 23 to 86% [21], reflecting the heterogeneity of the disease. Patients with monomorphic disease, or those having a poorer prognosis for disease extent or worse general conditions, are assigned to a more aggressive treatment.

Strategies to counteract B-cell proliferation are mainly based on the use of anti-CD20 antibodies and of cytoreductive chemotherapy regimens. Since the early 2000s, the availability of the humanised, chimeric anti-CD20 antibody *rituximab* has revolutionised the treatment of PTLD. Seventy percent of children who had an haematopoietic stem cell transplant (HSCT) and 64–84% of children undergoing a solid organ transplantation have prolonged disease-free survival after rituximab therapy, with better outcomes when this treatment is associated with immunosuppression reduction [22].

The association of rituximab with different low-dose chemotherapy regimens has been reported to warrant more robust results in children with PTLD, with an overall survival rate of between 83 and 86% and a 2-year event-free survival of 67–71% [11]. On the other hand, adding even a minimal cytoreductive regimen to rituximab leads to a non-negligible toxicity, essentially related to infections: chemotherapy-related mortality was 5–6% in two paediatric trials [11] and 11% in an adult trial [23], while it can be up to 50% for more intensive protocols [24, 25].

Thus it is important to identify prognostic factors defining patients not responding to rituximab that benefit from the addition of cytoreductive chemotherapy. Only few studies have translated this concern into a step-by-step approach to paediatric PTLD. In the non-randomised, response-adapted

Table 34.2 Clinical signs of post-transplant lymphoproliferative disorder (PTLD)

Systemic symptoms	Unexplained fever or night sweats
	Malaise
	Weight loss
	Sore throat
	Headache or focal neurologic symptoms
General and organ-specific signs	Pallor
	Lymphadenomegaly
	Tonsillar enlargement
	Focal neurologic signs
	Mass lesions
	Subcutaneous nodules
	Diarrhoea, abdominal pain, gastrointestinal bleeding
	Nausea and vomiting
	Hepatosplenomegaly
	Jaundice, graft dysfunction

German trial in CD20+ PTLDs after SOT, children with no response to rituximab were allocated to a moderate six-cycle chemotherapy regimen (mCOMP: vincristine, prednisone, cyclophosphamide and methotrexate). Fifteen out of 49 children in the trial required mCOMP. Complete remission was achieved in ten cases; further, more intensive chemotherapy was required in four cases, and only one child died from chemotherapy toxicity. Complete remission was achieved also in 81% of the children who were treated with rituximab alone, and the overall survival was 86% (PedPTLD).

Another study was conducted in Bergamo to prospectively evaluate a risk-adapted approach to PTLD after diverse paediatric SOT. In this study children with severe PTLDs (monomorphic or multiorgan disease, or not responding to immunosuppression withdrawal) were stratified according to the disease risk. Only high-risk patients (based on histology, staging, general functioning and LDH level) were treated with a reduced-intensity polychemotherapy, with overall satisfactory outcomes (overall and disease-free survival: 82% and 75%, respectively) and no mortality due to antineoplastic toxicity [8].

The proposed risk-adapted treatment algorithm for paediatric PTLD shown in Fig. 34.2 is designed to minimise patients' overtreatment, considering that:

- Rituximab treatment alone is relatively safe but is associated with a high rate of disease progression [23].
- Mortality from toxic effects of cytoreductive agents is substantial, also adopting sequential approaches with rituximab and low-dose chemotherapy [23].
- Rituximab effectiveness could be underestimated by some study endpoints, due to delayed effect.

In brief, patients with PTLD can be managed with weaning of immunosuppression in case of polymorphic, localised disease. On the contrary, patients with a monomorphic histology, involvement of more than one organ or bone marrow, with a poor performance status or failing to respond to previous tapering of immunosuppression are considered affected by a more aggressive form and treated with rituximab. Furthermore, those with a disseminated disease (stage III or IV) and those with higher LDH levels are considered at higher risk and treated with an additional reduced chemotherapy protocol.

Other treatments have a marginal role. Antivirals have an impact only on the lytic phase of the viral cycle, which has a limited role in lymphoid hyperplasia. In any case there is no evidence that antivirals can improve the outcome of PTLD when used as adjunctive treatment [26].

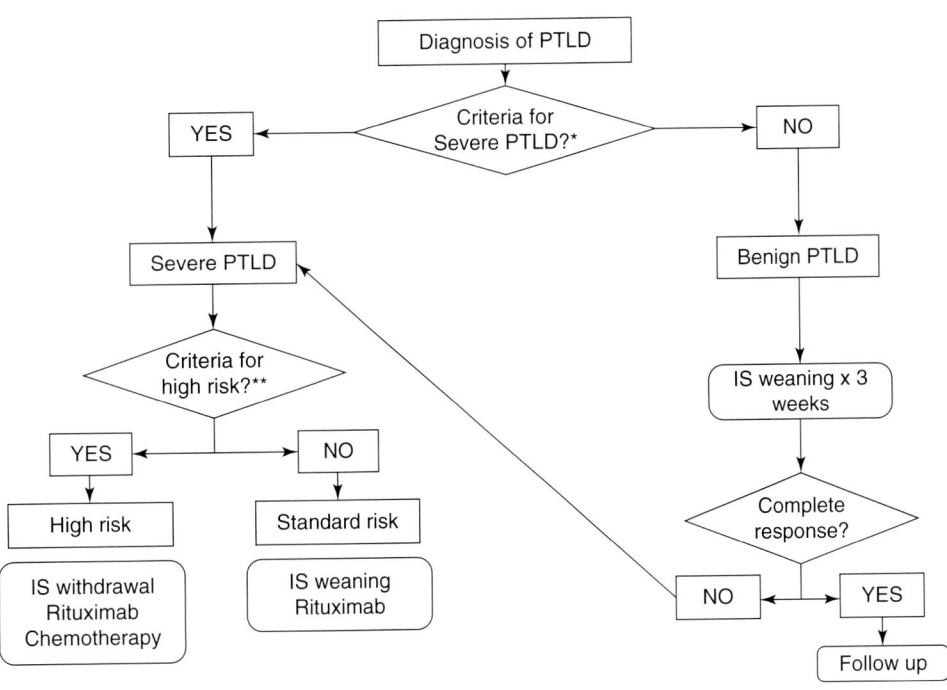

Fig. 34.2 Risk-adapted treatment algorithm for paediatric post-transplant lymphoproliferative disorder (PTLD) in solid organ transplantation. *Severe PTLD was diagnosed in the presence of at least one of the following criteria: (1) involvement of more than one organ, (2) involvement of the bone marrow, (3) organ dysfunction, (4) poor performance status, (5) monomorphic histology and (6) benign PTLD not responding to 3 weeks of immunosuppression withdrawal. **High-risk PTLD was diagnosed in the presence of at least two of the following criteria: (1) stage III or IV, (2) monomorphic histology, (3) poor performance status and (4) LDH ≥ 2 times the upper normal level for age (or ≥ 1000 IU/L). *IS* immunosuppression. In our centre, polychemotherapy includes blocks of fludarabine, cyclophosphamide, doxorubicin and rituximab (FCD-R) and reduced-intensity Berlin-Frankfurt-Münster (BFM) blocks for a maximum of six blocks

Since PTLD is a systemic disease, surgery and radiotherapy are useful only in selected cases, such as intestinal perforations (on intestinal localisations), or mass effect in central nervous system localisations.

Cell therapy strategies have been utilised to explore the competence of donor-derived and third-party EBV-specific T cells to restore the immunity against EBV, with promising but not definite results [27]. Another strategy is represented by the ex vivo production of EBV-specific T cells from autologous PBMC, obtained via the stimulation with lymphoblastoid cells as antigen-presenting cells [28]; however the limitation here is that these cells may not be rapidly available for a prompt clinical use.

34.3 CMV Infection and Disease

34.3.1 Clinical Pictures and Epidemiology

Cytomegalovirus (CMV) represents the most frequent opportunistic infection and a major threat in solid organ transplantation, especially in children. Because about 60% of adult donors have prior exposure to the virus, and most paediatric recipients receive an adult liver, the transplanted organ is often the source of infection.

In the absence of preventative measures (and similarly to EBV), the incidence of CMV infection (primary infection, reinfection or reactivation, defined as the detection of viral proteins or nucleic acid in any body fluid or tissue specimen), in this setting, depends mostly on the serological donor and recipient status. It is rare (1–2%) in case of both donor and recipient seronegativity; it occurs in 20–60% of the seropositive recipients as a reactivation, while almost all of the seronegative recipients receiving organs from seropositive donors get infected [29].

Another factor that has an impact on the risk of CMV infection and disease is the type of immunosuppression: the risk is greatest with lymphocyte-depleting agents and increased with the prolonged use of steroids and mycophenolic acid, when compared to standard tacrolimus monotherapy.

CMV infection in most cases has an asymptomatic course. However, about 20–30% of the infected patients develop a CMV disease, defined as the occurrence of consistent symptoms or tissue injury due to CMV [30, 31]. When overt, CMV disease most often causes a flu-like syndrome with fever, malaise, arthralgias and cytopenia. The virus can also cause direct injury to a wide range of target organs and tissues, due to its broad tropism. CMV is typically associated with colitis, retinitis, interstitial pneumonia and CNS disease with encephalitis, as well as other manifestations that are listed in Table 34.3. Importantly, CMV frequently causes graft hepatitis that resembles acute rejection. Beside these direct effects, it has been demonstrated that CMV replication is associated with "indirect" immunomodulatory effects ultimately leading to an increased risk of acute and chronic rejection, thrombotic events, opportunistic infections and PTLD [32, 33].

The combination of CMV infection and disease, in the absence of preventative measures, has been associated with a threefold higher risk of death or graft loss at 5 years post-LT [34–37].

34.3.2 Pathophysiology

CMV was historically perceived as a mild, slowly replicating virus capable of causing disease only in the presence of immune system impairment. However now it is regarded as a complex infection involving humoral and cellular, innate and adaptive immune responses.

CMV infection initially triggers innate immunity via the interaction of glycoprotein B- and Toll-like receptors and induces macrophage TLR4 and TLR5 ligand expression and TNF-alpha, IL-6 and IL-8 production. In parallel, NK cells stimulate the expression of IFN-gamma by effector

Table 34.3 Direct and indirect effects of cytomegalovirus in transplant recipients

Direct effects		Indirect effects	
CMV syndrome	Fever	Acute cellular rejection	
	Malaise	Chronic rejection	VBD syndrome
	Myelosuppression		Hepatitis
Tissue-invasive CMV disease	Colitis, enteritis		Fibrosis
	Hepatitis	Graft failure	
	Retinitis	Vascular thrombosis	
	Pneumonia/RDS	Opportunistic/secondary infections	Fungal
	Meningitis, encephalitis		Nocardia
	Carditis		Viruses (HHV6, EBV)
	MOF, death		PTLD

CMV cytomegalovirus, *RDS* respiratory distress syndrome, *MOF* multi-organ failure, *VBD* vanishing bile duct, *HHV6* human herpesvirus 6, *EBV* Epstein-Barr virus, *PTLD* post-transplant lymphoproliferative disorder. Modified from Marcelin JR et al.

cells and express Ig-like receptors which are relevant to viral control [38].

Turning to adaptive responses, the importance of humoral immunity is witnessed by the higher risk of developing CMV infection by seronegative recipients. However, pre-existing anti-CMV IgG may not protect from the strains introduced by the transplanted organ: among seropositive recipients, receiving a seropositive organ still increases the risk of CMV infection by threefold.

Finally, sustained control of CMV infection requires an adequate cellular response, as demonstrated by the crucial role of CMV-specific CD4 and CD8 cells in preventing CMV viremia and disease [39].

Data regarding the relationship between CMV infection and allograft tolerance are scarce and conflicting. Until recently, reports emphasised the correlation between CMV infection and disease and acute cellular rejection of the allograft, especially the liver [40], possibly as a consequence of the cross-reactivity of CMV-specific T-cell clones with allogeneic HLA molecules [41]. More recently, the link has been questioned, since most studies have not found an increased risk of acute rejection in CMV-infected patients [42–44] nor demonstrated a graft tolerogenic effect by the virus [45]. According to these latter findings, the hyporesponsiveness against the liver allograft would be accompanied and possibly caused by the relative shortage of donor-specific CD8 cells in liver allografts and by the higher Vdelta1/Vdelta2 γδ T-cell ratio, which is associated with operational tolerance [45].

34.3.3 Diagnosis

The diagnosis of CMV infection is based on the isolation of the virus or detection of viral proteins or nucleic acid in any body fluid or tissue specimen, regardless of symptoms. Nowadays, the best method is to use CMV-DNA detection via quantitative PCR. Both whole blood and plasma have proven suitable to determine and monitor the viral load and to provide prognostic information on the infection course [46]. However, decisional cut-off values in solid organ recipients have been better evaluated for whole blood samples [47–49]. Recently, the World Health Organization has released an international standard for CMV nucleic acid amplification technique (NIBSC 09/162) to homogenise the quantitative results worldwide.

Detection of the structural protein pp65 has lost importance, since it is technically more difficult and less precise than quantitative PCR and requires longer turnaround times. However, the equivalence between the two techniques is widely acknowledged.

CMV disease is defined as the evidence of infection in the presence of consistent symptoms, such as CMV syndrome (fever, malaise and myelosuppression) or proven CMV tissue-invasive disease (detection of CMV by immunohistochemical analysis and relevant histologic features on tissue biopsies, which are confirmed by in situ hybridisation or demonstration of CMV-DNA).

34.3.4 Treatment Algorithm

The goal of the anti-CMV management in the LT setting is to prevent overt disease and related complications. To achieve this result, two major strategies are currently employed: prophylaxis and preemptive therapy.

In the past, prophylaxis has been the most widely used approach and still remains the most used strategy by both the North American and the European paediatric transplant networks [50]. It consists of administering an antiviral agent (mainly ganciclovir or its orally absorbed prodrug valganciclovir) soon after LT to all, or only to high-risk, recipients regardless of the development of viremia, for a certain period of time. Undisputed advantages of this approach are that viral monitoring is not needed and infection does not develop soon after transplantation.

Preemptive therapy consists of administering the antiviral agents only in children with documented replication at an established viral load cut-off and continuing it till the obtainment of CMV-DNA clearance. The advantages of this approach are the reduced use of antiviral agents and the fact that a natural adaptive response is more rapidly achieved.

The pros and cons of each preventative strategy are showed in Table 34.4. However, any decision to choose either options should take into account the following issues:

– Overall outcomes do not differ between children who are managed with preemptive protocols and prophylaxis in terms of CMV disease incidence, graft-related

Table 34.4 Comparison between prophylaxis and preemptive therapy against cytomegalovirus

	Prophylaxis	Preemptive therapy
Early viremia/infection	Rare	Common
Late infection	Common	Rare
Prevention of CMV disease	Good efficacy	Good efficacy
Resistance	Uncommon	Uncommon (if weekly monitoring)
Feasibility	High	Needs CMV-DNA monitoring
Prevention of indirect effects	Unclear	Unclear
Costs	Drug costs	Monitoring costs
Drug exposure	High	Reduced
Graft survival	May improve	May improve

Modified from Kotton C, et al.

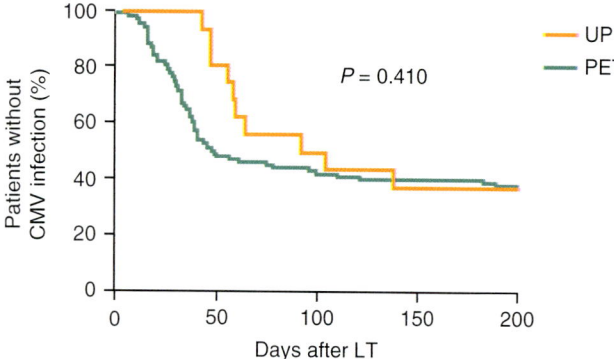

Fig. 34.3 Kaplan-Meier curve comparison showing the rate of cytomegalovirus (CMV) infection in patients managed with universal prophylaxis (UP) or preemptive therapy (PET) against cytomegalovirus. Although patients treated with UP get infected slightly later, by 100 days after transplantation, the rate of infection in the two groups is equal (see [44])

Table 34.5 Recommended preventative regimens against cytomegalovirus disease after LT in children

Serostatus	Risk level	Recommended	Alternative
D−/R−	Low	Monitoring of clinical symptoms	Preemptive therapy
D−/R+ D+/R+ D+/R−	Intermediate to high	2–4 weeks of GCV/VGCV with surveillance after prophylaxis[a]	3–4 months of VGCV Preemptive therapy

D donor, *R* recipient, *GCV* ganciclovir, *VGCV* valganciclovir
Modified from Kotton C, et al.
[a]Consider prolonged prophylaxis if T-cell-depleting agents

complications, graft loss and death, both in adults and children [44, 51, 52].
- Prophylaxis delays, but does not reduce, the overall infection rate by 200 days after LT (see Fig. 34.3, data of Bergamo Hospital) [44].
- Subclinical infection—which necessarily occurs with the preemptive approach—does not increase per se either the risk of acute cellular rejection nor that of other putative CMV indirect effects and has no effect on all causes of graft loss and death [44].
- Preemptive therapy is associated with less antiviral use, shorter length of hospitalisation and lower costs [44, 53].
- Virologic monitoring with acceptable turnaround time is a prerequisite for preemptive strategy.

Possible alternative preventative regimens recommended from the latest published guidelines are displayed in Table 34.5 [54]. In Bergamo, preemptive therapy is started at 100,000 CMV-DNA copies/mL (about 160,000 IU/mL) in whole blood samples (a cut-off established in a pilot study), regardless of the donor/recipient serostatus. This protocol has resulted in about 60% CMV infections and about 3% diseases, with no lethality associated to the virus. These results are similar to those recorded in other centres [31, 44, 52, 53]. Patients developing CMV disease are immediately treated with ganciclovir 5 mg/kg/dose every 12 h for at least 2 weeks and until resolution of symptoms and confirmed negative viremia. Other agents, such as foscarnet or cidofovir, are restricted to cases of suspected or confirmed resistance.

34.3.5 Management of CMV Antiviral Resistance

Drug resistance is defined as a viral genetic change that reduces the susceptibility of the virus to one or more antiviral drugs; it can present as a persistent or increasing viral load or the occurrence of symptoms despite adequate antiviral therapy [54]. The risk of harbouring resistance is present with both prophylaxis and preemptive protocols and is higher if the patient lacks pre-existing anti-CMV antibodies, in the case of highly immunosuppressed patients, or with inadequate antiviral drug delivery. Ganciclovir resistance has been reported to range from 5 to 12% in all solid organ transplant recipients [55–57], but it can be as high as 18 and 31% in lung and in intestinal transplant recipients, respectively [58–60]. The rate of viral resistance of other antiviral drugs is not well defined.

Patients who fail to achieve a substantial decrease in viral load after 2 weeks of treatment should be tested for resistance, especially if they have received a cumulative ganciclovir treatment longer than 6 weeks. Nowadays, the genotypic assay for viral resistance mutations in the UL97 kinase and UL54 DNA polymerase is the gold standard for the diagnosis. Interpretation of genetic testing should be conducted by an expert virologist. However, it is important to understand that the seven most common mutations in UL97 account for 80% of resistance pattern and that mutations in this gene do not confer cross-resistance to other drugs. On the other hand, mutations in UL54 occur in more conserved domains, and cross-resistance to foscarnet, cidofovir or both is likely.

For some low-grade resistance mutations (those that increase by two- to fivefold the drug concentration reducing viral growth by 50% [EC50]), doubling the ganciclovir dose may be sufficient and reduces the immunosuppression, if feasible. In other cases, a drug switch guided by the resistance test is recommended.

Alternative antiviral drugs are mainly foscarnet and cidofovir. Many other treatments are in development. Maribavir has succeeded as a salvage therapy in extensively resistant cases [54]. Letermovir is a potent UL56 terminase inhibitor and is being tested in prophylaxis regimens and as a rescue treatment in cases of resistant strains [61].

References

1. Shepherd RW, Turmelle Y, Nadler M, Lowell JA, Narkewicz MR, McDiarmid SV, et al. Risk factors for rejection and infection in pediatric liver transplantation. Am J Transplant. 2008;8:396–403. https://doi.org/10.1111/j.1600-6143.2007.02068.x.
2. Green M. Viral infections and pediatric liver transplantation. Pediatr Transplant. 2002;6:20–4.
3. Cox KL, Lawrence-Miyasaki LS, Garcia-Kennedy R, Lennette ET, Martinez OM, Krams SM, et al. An increased incidence of Epstein-Barr virus infection and lymphoproliferative disorder in young children on FK506 after liver transplantation. Transplantation. 1995;59:524–9.
4. Narkewicz MR, Green M, Dunn S, Millis M, McDiarmid S, Mazariegos G, et al. Decreasing incidence of symptomatic Epstein-Barr virus disease and posttransplant lymphoproliferative disorder in pediatric liver transplant recipients: report of the studies of pediatric liver transplantation experience. Liver Transpl. 2013;19:730–40. https://doi.org/10.1002/lt.23659.
5. Sokal EM, Antunes H, Beguin C, Bodeus M, Wallemacq P, de Ville de Goyet J, et al. Early signs and risk factors for the increased incidence of Epstein-Barr virus-related posttransplant lymphoproliferative diseases in pediatric liver transplant recipients treated with tacrolimus. Transplantation. 1997;64:1438–42.
6. Cacciarelli TV, Reyes J, Jaffe R, Mazariegos GV, Jain A, Fung JJ, et al. Primary tacrolimus (FK506) therapy and the long-term risk of post-transplant lymphoproliferative disease in pediatric liver transplant recipients. Pediatr Transplant. 2001;5:359–64.
7. Younes BS, McDiarmid SV, Martin MG, Vargas JH, Goss JA, Busuttil RW, et al. The effect of immunosuppression on posttransplant lymphoproliferative disease in pediatric liver transplant patients. Transplantation. 2000;70:94–9.
8. Giraldi E, Provenzi M, Conter V, Colledan M, Bolognini S, Foglia C, et al. Risk-adapted treatment for severe B-lineage posttransplant lymphoproliferative disease after solid organ transplantation in children. Transplantation. 2016;100:437–45. https://doi.org/10.1097/TP.0000000000000845.
9. Cao S, Cox KL, Berquist W, Hayashi M, Concepcion W, Hammes GB, et al. Long-term outcomes in pediatric liver recipients: comparison between cyclosporin A and tacrolimus. Pediatr Transplant. 1999;3:22–6.
10. Wistinghausen B, Gross TG, Bollard C. Post-transplant lymphoproliferative disease in pediatric solid organ transplant recipients. Pediatr Hematol Oncol. 2013;30:520–31. https://doi.org/10.3109/08880018.2013.798844.
11. Llaurador G, McLaughlin L, Wistinghausen B. Management of post-transplant lymphoproliferative disorders. Curr Opin Pediatr. 2017;29:34–40. https://doi.org/10.1097/MOP.0000000000000445.
12. D'Antiga L, Del Rizzo M, Mengoli C, Cillo U, Guariso G, Zancan L. Sustained Epstein-Barr virus detection in paediatric liver transplantation. Insights into the occurrence of late PTLD. Liver Transpl. 2007;13:343–8. https://doi.org/10.1002/lt.20958.
13. Münz C. Epstein Barr virus - a tumor virus that needs cytotoxic lymphocytes to persist asymptomatically. Curr Opin Virol. 2016;20:34–9. https://doi.org/10.1016/j.coviro.2016.08.010.
14. Miller G, El-Guindy A, Countryman J, Ye J, Gradoville L. Lytic cycle switches of oncogenic human gammaherpesviruses. Adv Cancer Res. 2007;97:81–109. https://doi.org/10.1016/S0065-230X(06)97004-3.
15. Whitehurst CB, Li G, Montgomery SA, Montgomery ND, Su L, Pagano JS. Knockout of Epstein-Barr virus BPLF1 retards B-cell transformation and lymphoma formation in humanized mice. MBio. 2015;6:e01574–15. https://doi.org/10.1128/mBio.01574-15.
16. Morscio J, Tousseyn T. Recent insights in the pathogenesis of posttransplantation lymphoproliferative disorders. World J Transplant. 2016;6:505–16. https://doi.org/10.5500/wjt.v6.i3.505.
17. Savoie A, Perpête C, Carpentier L, Joncas J, Alfieri C. Direct correlation between the load of Epstein-Barr virus-infected lymphocytes in the peripheral blood of pediatric transplant patients and risk of lymphoproliferative disease. Blood. 1994;83:2715–22.
18. Gridelli B, Spada M, Riva S, Colledan M, Segalin A, Lucianetti A, et al. Circulating Epstein-Barr virus DNA to monitor lymphoproliferative disease following pediatric liver transplantation. Transpl Int. 2000;13(Suppl 1):S399–401.
19. Macedo C, Zeevi A, Bentlejewski C, Popescu I, Green M, Rowe D, et al. The impact of EBV load on T-cell immunity in pediatric thoracic transplant recipients. Transplantation. 2009;88:123–8. https://doi.org/10.1097/TP.0b013e3181aacdd7.
20. Lee TC, Goss JA, Rooney CM, Heslop HE, Barshes NR, Caldwell YM, et al. Quantification of a low cellular immune response to aid in identification of pediatric liver transplant recipients at high-risk for EBV infection. Clin Transpl. 2006;20:689–94. https://doi.org/10.1111/j.1399-0012.2006.00537.x.
21. Reshef R, Vardhanabhuti S, Luskin MR, Heitjan DF, Hadjiliadis D, Goral S, et al. Reduction of immunosuppression as initial therapy for posttransplantation lymphoproliferative disorder(★). Am J Transplant. 2011;11:336–47. https://doi.org/10.1111/j.1600-6143.2010.03387.x.
22. Styczynski J, Gil L, Tridello G, Ljungman P, Donnelly JP, van der Velden W, et al. Response to rituximab-based therapy and risk factor analysis in Epstein Barr Virus-related lymphoproliferative disorder after hematopoietic stem cell transplant in children and adults: a study from the Infectious Diseases Working Party of the European Group for Blood and Marrow Transplantation. Clin Infect Dis. 2013;57:794–802. https://doi.org/10.1093/cid/cit391.
23. Trappe R, Oertel S, Leblond V, Mollee P, Sender M, Reinke P, et al. Sequential treatment with rituximab followed by CHOP chemotherapy in adult B-cell post-transplant lymphoproliferative disorder (PTLD): the prospective international multicentre phase 2 PTLD-1 trial. Lancet Oncol. 2012;13:196–206. https://doi.org/10.1016/S1470-2045(11)70300-X.
24. Dotti G, Fiocchi R, Motta T, Mammana C, Gotti E, Riva S, et al. Lymphomas occurring late after solid-organ transplantation: influence of treatment on the clinical outcome. Transplantation. 2002;74:1095–102. https://doi.org/10.1097/01.TP.0000030637.87507.3C.
25. Elstrom RL, Andreadis C, Aqui NA, Ahya VN, Bloom RD, Brozena SC, et al. Treatment of PTLD with rituximab or chemotherapy. Am J Transplant. 2006;6:569–76. https://doi.org/10.1111/j.1600-6143.2005.01211.x.
26. Østensen AB, Sanengen T, Holter E, Line P-D, Almaas R. No effect of treatment with intravenous ganciclovir on Epstein-Barr virus viremia demonstrated after pediatric liver transplantation. Pediatr Transplant. 2017;21:e13010. https://doi.org/10.1111/petr.13010.
27. Doubrovina E, Oflaz-Sozmen B, Prockop SE, Kernan NA, Abramson S, Teruya-Feldstein J, et al. Adoptive immunotherapy with unselected or EBV-specific T cells for biopsy-proven EBV+ lymphomas after allogeneic hematopoietic cell transplantation. Blood. 2012;119:2644–56. https://doi.org/10.1182/blood-2011-08-371971.
28. Gottschalk S, Rooney CM. Adoptive T-Cell Immunotherapy. Curr Top Microbiol Immunol. 2015;391:427–54. https://doi.org/10.1007/978-3-319-22834-1_15.
29. Razonable RR, Humar A. AST Infectious Diseases Community of Practice. Cytomegalovirus in solid organ transplantation. Am J Transplant. 2013;13(Suppl 4):93–106. https://doi.org/10.1111/ajt.12103.
30. Winston DJ, Emmanouilides C, Busuttil RW. Infections in liver transplant recipients. Clin Infect Dis. 1995;21:1077–89; quiz 1090–1.
31. Bruminhent J, Razonable RR. Management of cytomegalovirus infection and disease in liver transplant recipients. World J Hepatol. 2014;6:370–83. https://doi.org/10.4254/wjh.v6.i6.370.

32. Marcelin JR, Beam E, Razonable RR. Cytomegalovirus infection in liver transplant recipients: updates on clinical management. World J Gastroenterol. 2014;20:10658–67. https://doi.org/10.3748/wjg.v20.i31.10658.
33. Freeman HJ. Long-term natural history of Crohn's disease. World J Gastroenterol. 2009;15:1315–8.
34. Bosch W, Heckman MG, Diehl NN, Shalev JA, Pungpapong S, Hellinger WC. Association of cytomegalovirus infection and disease with death and graft loss after liver transplant in high-risk recipients. Am J Transplant. 2011;11:2181–9. https://doi.org/10.1111/j.1600-6143.2011.03618.x.
35. Razonable RR. Cytomegalovirus infection after liver transplantation: current concepts and challenges. World J Gastroenterol. 2008;14:4849–60. https://doi.org/10.3748/wjg.14.4849.
36. Stratta RJ, Shaefer MS, Markin RS, Wood RP, Kennedy EM, Langnas AN, et al. Clinical patterns of cytomegalovirus disease after liver transplantation. Arch Surg. 1989;124:1443–9; discussion 1449–50.
37. Burak KW, Kremers WK, Batts KP, Wiesner RH, Rosen CB, Razonable RR, et al. Impact of cytomegalovirus infection, year of transplantation, and donor age on outcomes after liver transplantation for hepatitis C. Liver Transpl. 2002;8:362–9. https://doi.org/10.1053/jlts.2002.32282.
38. Carbone J. The immunology of posttransplant CMV infection: potential effect of CMV immunoglobulins on distinct components of the immune response to CMV. Transplantation. 2016;100(Suppl 3):S11–8. https://doi.org/10.1097/TP.0000000000001095.
39. Manuel O, Husain S, Kumar D, Zayas C, Mawhorter S, Levi ME, et al. Assessment of cytomegalovirus-specific cell-mediated immunity for the prediction of cytomegalovirus disease in high-risk solid-organ transplant recipients: a multicenter cohort study. Clin Infect Dis. 2013;56:817–24. https://doi.org/10.1093/cid/cis993.
40. Gupta P, Hart J, Cronin D, Kelly S, Millis JM, Brady L. Risk factors for chronic rejection after pediatric liver transplantation. Transplantation. 2001;72:1098–102.
41. Amir AL, D'Orsogna LJA, Roelen DL, van Loenen MM, Hagedoorn RS, de Boer R, et al. Allo-HLA reactivity of virus-specific memory T cells is common. Blood. 2010;115:3146–57. https://doi.org/10.1182/blood-2009-07-234906.
42. Sun H-Y, Cacciarelli TV, Wagener MM, Singh N. Preemptive therapy for cytomegalovirus based on real-time measurement of viral load in liver transplant recipients. Transpl Immunol. 2010;23:166–9. https://doi.org/10.1016/j.trim.2010.06.013.
43. Indolfi G, Heaton N, Smith M, Mieli-Vergani G, Zuckerman M. Effect of early EBV and/or CMV viremia on graft function and acute cellular rejection in pediatric liver transplantation. Clin Transpl. 2012;26:E55–61. https://doi.org/10.1111/j.1399-0012.2011.01535.x.
44. Nicastro E, Giovannozzi S, Stroppa P, Casotti V, Callegaro AP, Tebaldi A, et al. Effectiveness of preemptive therapy for cytomegalovirus disease in pediatric liver transplantation. Transplantation. 2017;101:804–10. https://doi.org/10.1097/TP.0000000000001531.
45. Shi X-L, de Mare-Bredemeijer ELD, Tapirdamaz Ö, Hansen BE, van Gent R, van Campenhout MJH, et al. CMV primary infection is associated with donor-specific T cell hyporesponsiveness and fewer late acute rejections after liver transplantation. Am J Transplant. 2015;15:2431–42. https://doi.org/10.1111/ajt.13288.
46. Boaretti M, Sorrentino A, Zantedeschi C, Forni A, Boschiero L, Fontana R. Quantification of cytomegalovirus DNA by a fully automated real-time PCR for early diagnosis and monitoring of active viral infection in solid organ transplant recipients. J Clin Virol. 2013;56:124–8. https://doi.org/10.1016/j.jcv.2012.10.015.
47. Allice T, Cerutti F, Pittaluga F, Varetto S, Franchello A, Salizzoni M, et al. Evaluation of a novel real-time PCR system for cytomegalovirus DNA quantitation on whole blood and correlation with pp65-antigen test in guiding pre-emptive antiviral treatment. J Virol Methods. 2008;148:9–16. https://doi.org/10.1016/j.jviromet.2007.10.006.
48. Gerna G, Lilleri D, Furione M, Baldanti F. Management of human cytomegalovirus infection in transplantation: validation of virologic cut-offs for preemptive therapy and immunological cut-offs for protection. New Microbiol. 2011;34:229–54.
49. Lilleri D, Lazzarotto T, Ghisetti V, Ravanini P, Capobianchi MR, Baldanti F, et al. Multicenter quality control study for human cytomegalovirus DNAemia quantification. New Microbiol. 2009;32:245–53.
50. Danziger-Isakov L, Bucavalas J. Current prevention strategies against cytomegalovirus in the studies in pediatric liver transplantation (SPLIT) centers. Am J Transplant. 2014;14:1908–11. https://doi.org/10.1111/ajt.12755.
51. Mumtaz K, Faisal N, Husain S, Morillo A, Renner EL, Shah PS. Universal prophylaxis or preemptive strategy for cytomegalovirus disease after liver transplantation: a systematic review and meta-analysis. Am J Transplant. 2015;15:472–81. https://doi.org/10.1111/ajt.13044.
52. Saitoh A, Sakamoto S, Fukuda A, Shigeta T, Kakiuchi T, Kamiyama S, et al. A universal preemptive therapy for cytomegalovirus infections in children after live-donor liver transplantation. Transplantation. 2011;92:930–5. https://doi.org/10.1097/TP.0b013e31822d873d.
53. Gerna G, Lilleri D, Callegaro A, Goglio A, Cortese S, Stroppa P, et al. Prophylaxis followed by preemptive therapy versus preemptive therapy for prevention of human cytomegalovirus disease in pediatric patients undergoing liver transplantation. Transplantation. 2008;86:163–6. https://doi.org/10.1097/TP.0b013e31817889e4.
54. Kotton CN, Kumar D, Caliendo AM, Huprikar S, Chou S, Danziger-Isakov L, et al. The third international consensus guidelines on the management of cytomegalovirus in solid-organ transplantation. Transplantation. 2018;102:900–31. https://doi.org/10.1097/TP.0000000000002191.
55. Hantz S, Garnier-Geoffroy F, Mazeron M-C, Garrigue I, Merville P, Mengelle C, et al. Drug-resistant cytomegalovirus in transplant recipients: a French cohort study. J Antimicrob Chemother. 2010;65:2628–40. https://doi.org/10.1093/jac/dkq368.
56. Myhre H-A, Haug Dorenberg D, Kristiansen KI, Rollag H, Leivestad T, Asberg A, et al. Incidence and outcomes of ganciclovir-resistant cytomegalovirus infections in 1244 kidney transplant recipients. Transplantation. 2011;92:217–23. https://doi.org/10.1097/TP.0b013e31821fad25.
57. Young PG, Rubin R, Angarone M, Flaherty J, Penugonda S, Stosor V, et al. Ganciclovir-resistant cytomegalovirus infection in solid organ transplant recipients: a single-center retrospective cohort study. Transpl Infect Dis. 2016;18:390–5. https://doi.org/10.1111/tid.12537.
58. Boivin G, Goyette N, Rollag H, Jardine AG, Pescovitz MD, Asberg A, et al. Cytomegalovirus resistance in solid organ transplant recipients treated with intravenous ganciclovir or oral valganciclovir. Antivir Ther (Lond). 2009;14:697–704.
59. Lurain NS, Bhorade SM, Pursell KJ, Avery RK, Yeldandi VV, Isada CM, et al. Analysis and characterization of antiviral drug-resistant cytomegalovirus isolates from solid organ transplant recipients. J Infect Dis. 2002;186:760–8. https://doi.org/10.1086/342844.
60. Ambrose T, Sharkey LM, Louis-Auguste J, Rutter CS, Duncan S, English S, et al. Cytomegalovirus infection and rates of antiviral resistance following intestinal and multivisceral transplantation. Transplant Proc. 2016;48:492–6. https://doi.org/10.1016/j.transproceed.2015.09.070.
61. Chemaly RF, Ullmann AJ, Stoelben S, Richard MP, Bornhäuser M, Groth C, et al. Letermovir for cytomegalovirus prophylaxis in hematopoietic-cell transplantation. N Engl J Med. 2014;370:1781–9. https://doi.org/10.1056/NEJMoa1309533.

Liver Transplantation for Inherited Metabolic Disorders

Alberto Burlina and Lorenzo D'Antiga

Key Points
- Liver transplantation is an established treatment for inborn errors of metabolism.
- The success is mainly related to the severity of extrahepatic expression of the disease, providing only an improvement of the phenotype in defects that are not confined to the liver.
- Liver transplantation cures Crigler-Najjar syndrome, most urea cycle defects, maple syrup disease and primary hyperoxaluria type 1 and improves the phenotype of some organic acidurias.
- The overall outcome of liver transplantation in selected inborn errors defects of the liver is very good.

Research Needed in the Field
- Understand the factors affecting the success of LT in diseases expressed extrahepatically.
- Understand the impact of LT in large, multicentre series of rare inborn metabolic defects.
- Evaluate the success of LT in metabolic disorders when performed at early ages versus later in childhood.
- Improve perioperative management to reduce metabolic decompensations around the time of surgery.
- Explore the possibility of performing a successful LT in subgroups of patients with conditions so far regarded as contraindications to LT, such as mitochondrial disorders.

A. Burlina (✉)
Division of Inherited Metabolic Diseases, Reference Centre Expanded Newborn Screening, Department of Woman's and Child's Health, University of Padova, Padova, Italy
e-mail: alberto.burlina@unipd.it

L. D'Antiga
Paediatric Hepatology, Gastroenterology and Transplantation, Hospital Papa Giovanni XXIII, Bergamo, Italy
e-mail: ldantiga@asst-pg23.it

35.1 Introduction

Liver transplantation (LT) in paediatric age is usually carried out to restore hepatic synthetic function by replacing an organ with intrinsically defective structure (e.g. biliary atresia).

The use of LT for hereditary tyrosinemia type 1 (HT1) in 1976 [1] and ornithine transcarbamylase deficiency (OTCD) in 1989 [2] represented a new approach to replace a specific inherited enzymatic deficiency.

As the outcome for the procedure has progressively improved, the indications for LT have increased to encompass a growing number of inherited metabolic disorders (IMDs) (Fig. 35.1) [3]. Currently, IMDs represent approximately 15–25% of indications to LT in children [4].

Successful LT has been reported for a variety of metabolic conditions, including alpha-1-antitrypsin deficiency (A1At), urea cycle disorders (UCDs), hereditary tyrosinemia type 1 (HT1), maple syrup urine disease (MSUD), organic acidemias (OAs), glycogen storage disorders (GSD), familial cholestasis, primary hyperoxaluria type 1, Wilson's disease, mitochondrial disorders, porphyrias, inborn errors of lipid metabolism, acyl-CoA dehydrogenase deficiency and hemochromatosis [5–7].

While the list of potential IMDs amenable to treatment with LT has increased, the evaluation of the risk-benefit ratio has become more complicated. Advances in understanding of the pathogenesis of IMDs are essential for guiding patient selection [8].

When the primary cause of the disease resides within the liver cells, or is due to a structural liver disease (liver-specific metabolic disorders), there is the opportunity for LT to correct the underlying defect and provide a 'cure' for the disorder [7] (Table 35.1).

When the metabolic defect is also expressed in other tissues, LT is of potential use for metabolic disorders in which toxic intermediary metabolites from multiple organ systems

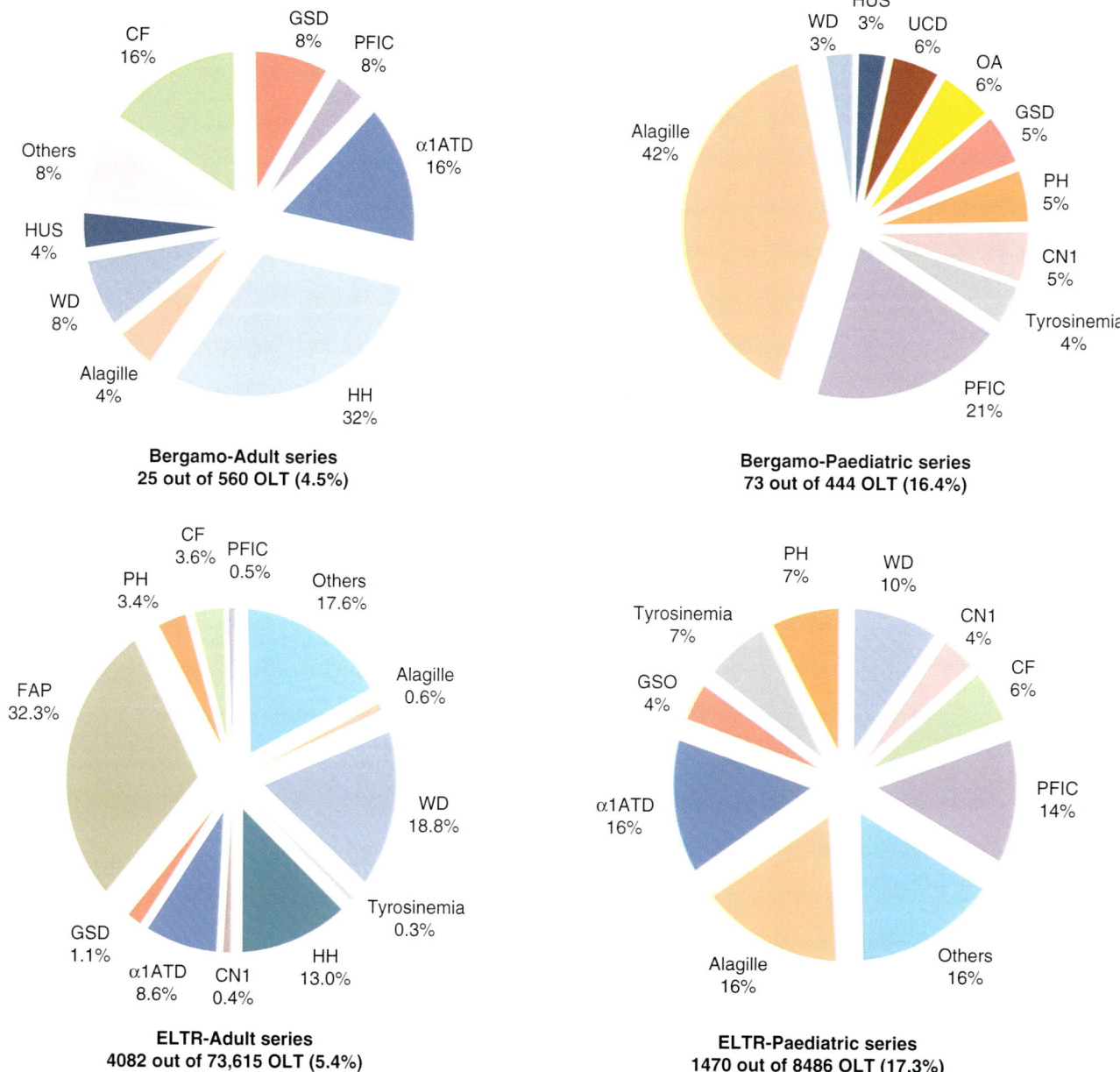

Fig. 35.1 ELTR and Bergamo experiences in adults and children transplanted for monogenic diseases: ELTR (1968–2010) and Bergamo (1998–2012). *α1ATD* alpha1 antitrypsin deficiency, *CF* cystic fibrosis, *CN1* Crigler-Najjar type 1, *FAP* familial amyloid polyneuropathy, *GSD* glycogen storage disease, *HH* hereditary haemochromatosis, *HUS* haemolytic uremic syndrome, *OA* organic acidurias, *PH* primary hyperoxaluria, *PFIC* progressive familial intrahepatic cholestasis, *UCD* urea cycle disorders, *WD* Wilson's disease (adapted from [3])

can freely interchange with other organs through the systemic circulation. In this setting, the residual abnormal metabolites generated by the rest of the body can be efficiently cleared by the donor liver [9]. Therefore, some IMDs that have significant extrahepatic expression may be effectively cured by LT. In these cases, the benefit of LT depends on the extent of extrahepatic manifestations, in particular neurological damage, at the time of LT (Fig. 35.2).

Even in the cases where LT cannot completely compensate the extrahepatic defects, it may provide substantial benefit by reducing the risk of acute metabolic crises, allowing a less stringent dietary restriction and reducing the progression of long-term organ dysfunctions, thereby significantly improving quality of life [10]. On the contrary, when a genetically normal liver is insufficient to compensates the extrahepatic defect, LT usually provides no or little benefit [11].

Over the last years, the implementation of expanded newborn screening (NBS) programmes in several countries has contributed to modify some IMD's natural history. The investment in an early neonatal screening can allow the early diagnosis and treatment in a pre-symptomatic period, avoiding severe clinical complications. LT may be a therapeutic option for several disorders detectable by NBS, such as UCDs, MSUD, OAs and tyrosinemia type 1, with the great advantage to offer a cure before the metabolic derangement has caused organs injury [12].

Table 35.1 Metabolic defects with expression mostly confined to the liver, amenable to correction by liver transplantation

Parenchymal injury	No significant parenchymal injury
α1 antitrypsin deficiency (PiZZ)	Crigler-Najjar
Tyrosinemia	Primary hyperoxaluria type 1
Wilson's disease	Urea cycle disorders
PFIC types 2 and 3	Familial hypercholesterolaemia
GSD type I (adenoma/HCC)	Haemophilia
Cholesteryl ester storage disease	Protein C and S deficiencies
	Factor H deficiency
	Acute intermittent porphyria
	Familial amyloid polyneuropathy

PFIC progressive familial intrahepatic cholestasis, *GSD* glycogen storage disease, *HCC* hepatocellular carcinoma

Therefore, IMDs that are candidates for LT can be broadly categorised into two groups depending on the extrahepatic expression and the outcome after LT:

1. Metabolic disease that can be cured by liver transplantation
2. Metabolic disease that can be treated by liver transplantation, improving the phenotype of the disease without providing a definitive cure

Table 35.2 provides an overview of the efficacy of LT in some metabolic disorders.

35.2 Liver Transplantation to Cure Inborn Errors of Metabolism

35.2.1 Urea Cycle Defects (UCDs)

The urea cycle is the metabolic pathway that allows the elimination of nitrogenous waste derived from protein catabolism through the production of urea. The degradation and synthesis of cellular proteins occurs continuously. Each day, humans turn over 1–2% of their total body protein, principally muscle proteins. Of the liberated amino acids, approximately 75% are reutilised. Since excess amino acids are not stored, those not immediately incorporated into new proteins are rapidly degraded to amphibolic intermediates such as ammonia. Endogenous ammonia, along with the portion coming from protein degradation in the colon, is converted into urea by the urea cycle, which is present almost exclusively in the liver. Any of the enzymes mediating the reactions converting ammonia into urea may be defective. In this situation, the block of the urea cycle results in life-threatening hyperammonemia with lethargy, poor feeding, vomiting, cerebral oedema, seizures, coma or death [13] (Fig. 35.3).

In patients with severe, early-onset UCD who survive the initial decompensation, irreversible brain damage and persistent neurocognitive impairment can occur [14]. Conversely, excellent post-transplant survival was seen in both children and adults who underwent LT for UCDs, and outcomes were similar across all ages. Patients with more severe defects (peak blood ammonia levels at disease onset >300 μmol/L) who underwent LT exhibit superior neurodevelopmental outcome than those who did not undergo LT [15]. Preventing neurological damage due to recurrent hyperammonemia and hepatic coma is critical, because some studies have demonstrated that LT can stop but doesn't reverse developmental delay [16–18].

The current consensus from the Urea Cycle Disorders Consortium on the management of patients with absent or very low enzyme function provides a strong indication to LT as a therapeutic approach in all UCDs (excluding NAGS and

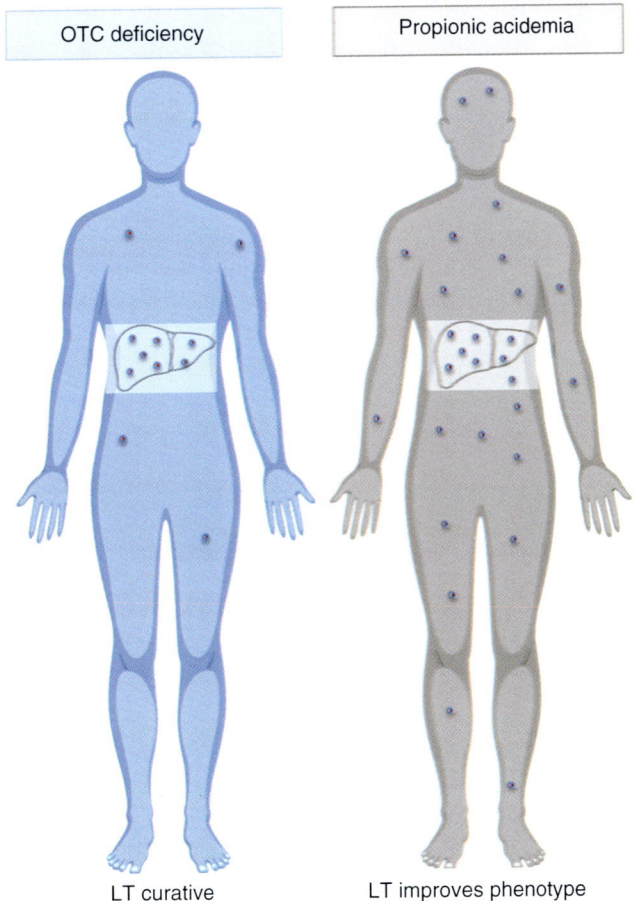

Fig. 35.2 Correction of the underlying metabolic condition by liver transplantation (LT) depends on extrahepatic expression of the defect. The diseases shown are given as examples. *OTC* ornithine transcarbamylase deficiency

Table 35.2 Examples of genetic/metabolic conditions that can be treated by liver transplantation

Disorder		Gene symbol	Inheritance	Mechanism of disease	Deficient enzyme	Tissue RNA expression[a]	Liver features	Clinical features	Correction by LT
Branched chain aminoacidopathies	MSUD	BCKDHA	AR	Elevated plasma-branched chain amino acids (leucine, isoleucine, valine)	Branched chain keto acid dehydrogenase E1, alpha polypeptide (MSUD 1a)	Liver 15% Others 85%	Normal liver architecture	Mental and physical retardation, feeding problems and a maple syrup odour to the urine	Good
	Propionic acidemia	PCC	AR	Excessive deamination of some amino acids in muscle, with consequent hyperammonemia and ketoacidosis	Propionyl-CoA carboxylase	Adrenals 25% Kidney 20% Liver 15% Others 40%		Vomiting, lethargy, hyperammonemia and ketosis, developmental retardation, intolerance to protein	Partial
	Methylmalonic acidemia	MUT	AR	Disorder of methylmalonate and cobalamin leading to methylmalonyl CoA accumulation in the body	Methylmalonyl CoA mutase	Liver 20% Kidney 10% Others 70%		Toxic encephalopathy, hyperammonemia, vomiting, failure to thrive, neutropenia, acidosis, ketosis	Poor
Ethylmalonic encephalopathy		ETHE1	AR	Mitochondrial malfunction. Ethylmalonic aciduria, increased plasma C4-/C5-acylcarnitines and lactate	Mitochondrial matrix protein oxidating a persulphide substrate to sulphite	Intestine 40% Liver 10% Others 50%	Normal liver architecture	Neurodevelopmental delay, pyramidal and extrapyramidal signs, recurrent petechiae, orthostatic acrocyanosis, chronic diarrhoea	Good? (single report)
Tyrosinemia	Type 1	FAH	AR	Lack of tyrosine degradation	Fumarylacetoacetate hydrolase (FAA)	Liver 40% Kidney 10% Others 50%	Hepatomegaly, acute liver failure, cirrhosis, hepatocellular carcinoma	Secondary renal tubular dysfunction (hypophosphatemic rickets), episodic weakness, self-mutilation, seizures	Optimal
Alpha-1 antitrypsin	PiZZ	SERPINA1	AR	Lack of inhibitory action against neutrophil elastase	Protease inhibitor-alpha 1 antitrypsin	Liver 90% Intestine 5% Others 5%	Cirrhosis Hepatocellular carcinoma	Emphysema, which becomes evident by the third to fourth decade	Optimal

Disorder		Gene symbol	Inheritance	Mechanism of disease	Deficient enzyme	Tissue RNA expression[a]	Liver features	Clinical features	Correction by LT
Urea cycle disorders	NAGS deficiency	NAGS	AR	Error of metabolism of the urea cycle with ammonia production	N-acetyl glutamate synthetase	Liver 60% Intestine 25% Others 15%	Near normal liver architecture at presentation Hepatomegaly, fibrosis, cirrhosis in late-onset cases	Somnolence, tachypnea, feeding difficulties, failure to thrive, hyperammonemia	Good
	CPS1 deficiency	CPS	AR		Carbamoyl phosphate synthetase	Liver 90% Intestine 10%		Protein intolerance, intermittent ataxia, seizures, lethargy and mental retardation	Optimal
	OTC deficiency	OTC	XL		Ornithine transcarbamylase	Liver 70% Intestine 30%		Neonatal hyperammonemic coma. Hyperammonemia and neurological delay	Optimal
	Argininosuccinic aciduria	ASL	AR		Argininosuccinate lyase	Liver 60% Intestine 20% Others 20%		Mental and physical retardation, skin lesions, dry and brittle hair, convulsions, unconsciousness	Good
	Argininemia	ARG 1	AR		Arginase	Liver 85% Skin 10% Spleen 5%		Developmental delay, seizures, ataxia, mental retardation, hypotonia, spastic quadriplegia	Good
	Citrullinemia	ASS1	AR		Argininosuccinate synthetase	Liver 60% Kidney 20% Others 20%		Lethargy, poor feeding, vomiting, seizures	Good
Primary hyperoxaluria	Type 1	AGXT	AR	Calcium oxalate accumulation in tissues	Alanine-glyoxylate-aminotransferase	Liver 100%	Normal liver architecture	Nephrolithiasis, renal failure	Optimal
Crigler–Najjar	Type 1	UGT1A1	AR	Impairment of bilirubin conjugation	Uridine diphosphate glucoronosyltransferase	Liver 90% Kidney 5% Intestine 5%	Normal liver architecture (some fibrosis in adulthood)	Unconjugated hyperbilirubinaemia, kernicterus	Optimal

OMIM Online Mendelian Inheritance in Man, *AR* autosomal recessive, *XL* X-linked recessive, *AD* autosomal dominant

[a]The human protein atlas https://www.proteinatlas.org/ (G-TEX dataset)

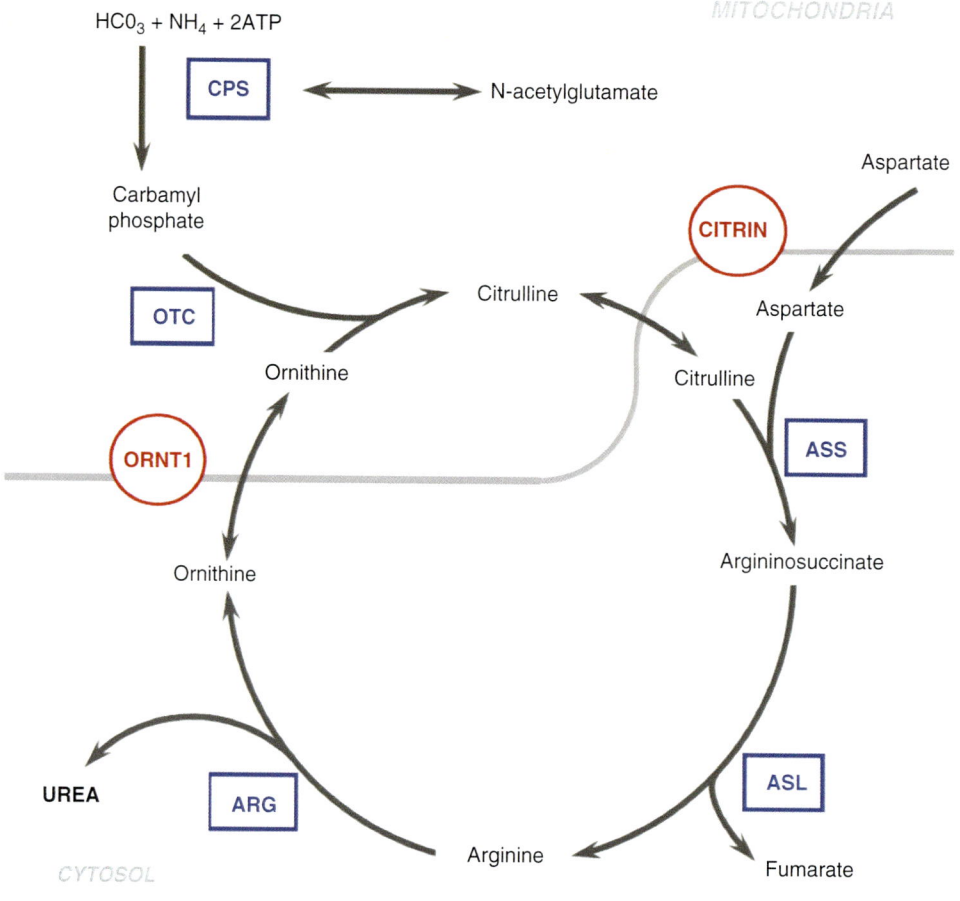

Fig. 35.3 The urea cycle. *CPS* carbamoyl phosphate synthetase, *ASS* argininosuccinate synthetase, *ASL* argininosuccinate lyase, *ARG* arginase, *OTC* ornithine transcarbamylase, *ORNT1* ornithine translocase-1 (ORNT1 and CITRIN are mitochondrial transporter)

arginase deficiency) [13, 19]. The European guidelines on the role of LT for citrullinemia (ASS) and ASL deficiencies are less definitive. Nonetheless LT has proven to be successful in all UCDs with a high survival rate and rapid normalisation of ammonia levels. Indeed, the transplanted liver corrects the deficiency and removes the risk of metabolic decompensation and the need for dietary protein restriction [20]. The first large series of LT in this setting was published by Morioka, who collected data from patients transplanted for UCDs either at the Kyoto University or elsewhere, as for the worldwide published literature, and described 51 patients (CPS1, n 4; OTCd, 22; citrullinemia, 4; citrin deficiency, 20; argininemia, 1) whose cumulative survival was 90% at 5 years after LT, with disappearance of hyperammonemic crises, interruption of drugs and restricted diet and therefore overall improvement of quality of life. Even in more recent reports, LT is confirmed as an effective treatment in UCDs, including when the organ comes from heterozygous donors (apart from OTC hemizygous parents) [15, 21, 22].

According to the SPLIT registry, among children who underwent LT for IMDs, UCDs were the most common indication, accounting for 25.6% of all cases [6, 23]. These include ornithine transcarbamylase deficiency (OTCd), N-acetyl glutamate synthetase deficiency (NAGSd), carbamoyl phosphate synthetase deficiency (CPS1d), argininosuccinic aciduria (ASL), argininemia (ARG1) and argininosuccinate synthetase deficiency (citrullinemia). Table 35.3 reports the results of liver transplantation in UCDs recorded in the UNOS database.

Ornithine transcarbamylase deficiency (OTCd) is the most prevalent urea cycle disorder in humans, with an estimated birth prevalence of approximately 1/50,000. Since OTC is a X-linked recessive genetic disease, hemizygous males with complete lack of enzymatic activity often present with a life-threatening hyperammonemia within few days after birth. Whereas patients with neonatal-onset OTCd are predominantly males, patients with late-onset OTCd are both hemizygous males and heterozygous females [24, 25].

OTCd is also the most common UCD in both adults and children who underwent liver transplantation [15]. The liver in patients with UCDs is commonly reported as histologically normal. Nevertheless during metabolic crisis, an acute hepatocyte necrosis occurs and can originate a picture of acute liver failure [26]. In this scenario, both the underlying defect and the hepatocellular injury contribute to the failure to metabolise urea, leading to devastating neurological consequences due to hyperammonemic coma. Despite a strict dietary protein restriction and the use of ammonia scavengers, metabolic decompensations can recur episodically.

Table 35.3 Characteristics of patients transplanted for urea cycle disorders versus all other transplants recorded in the UNOS database between 1988 and 2010

		UCDs ($n = 254$)	All others ($n = 12,198$)	P value
Age		2.6 ± 4.0	4.8 ± 5.6	<0.001
Female sex		33%	52%	<0.001
Albumin (g/L)		3.6 ± 0.80	3.1 ± 0.80	<0.001
Creatinine (mg/dL)		0.38 ± 0.45	0.60 ± 0.90	<0.001
Bilirubin (mg/dL)		1.28 ± 3.72	12.3 ± 12.0	<0.001
INR		1.29 ± 0.65	1.99 ± 2.54	<0.001
ALT (IU/l)		205 ± 670	357 ± 931	0.048
PELD or MELD		0.47 ± 8.0	15.9 ± 13.8	<0.001
Living donor (%)		6%	10.7%	0.015
Donor age (years)		9.9 ± 11.6	13.9 ± 14.7	<0.001
Diagnosis				
	OTCd	129 (51%)		
	Citrullinemia (ASS)	42 (16%)		
	CPS1d	26 (10%)		
	ASL	25 (10%)		
	Unspecified	32 (13%)		
Outcome				
	1 year survival	93%		
	5 year survival	89%		
Causes of death (27 pts, 10%)				
	Infections	12 (44%)		
	Multi organ failure	7 (26%)		
	Graft failure	4 (15%)		
	Others	4 (15%)		

UCDs urea cycle defects, *OTCd* ornithine transcarbamylase deficiency, *CPS1d* carbamoyl phosphate synthetase 1 deficiency, *ASL* argininosuccinic aciduria

These episodes can be fatal or cause permanent neurologic damage.

Table 35.4 reports the features of paediatric patients transplanted for OTCd published in the aforementioned studies.

A recent report showed that LT is effective also in patients with *citrullinemia (ASS)*. In this retrospective analysis, the authors described seven children who had a LT at a median age of 2.4 years (range, 1.3–6.5) because of frequent metabolic decompensations (4/7), ALF (1/7) or electively (2/7). Two patients received an auxiliary partial liver transplant (APOLT), whereas the others received a deceased donor left lateral segment or a whole liver. Graft and patient survivals were 86% and 100%, respectively. After a median follow-up of 3.1 years (range, 0.1–4.1), there have been no metabolic decompensations in six children, while one patient, a recipient of APOLT, developed asymptomatic hyperammonemia. All patients had a neurocognitive improvement after LT. Citrulline plasma levels decreased from a median of 2543 μmol/L (range, 1831–3460) to 586 μmol/L, (range, 282–1300), but in all it remained above the normal range (8–57 μmol/L) [27]. Table 35.5 summarises the features of the described patients.

Carbamoyl phosphate synthetase 1 deficiency (CPS1d) is a very rare UCD defect causing the lack of function of a mitochondrial matrix enzyme catalysing the first step of the urea cycle. Patients with CPS1 deficiency have severe hyperammonemia early after birth that results in serious neurologic sequelae and sometimes death. LT has been performed successfully in neonatal-onset CPS1 deficiency [5, 18, 28–31]. A study from Japan described five children with a diagnosis of CPS1 deficiency who underwent LDLT from heterozygous donors in Tokyo. All recipients achieved resolution of their metabolic derangement off medications and on unrestricted diet, although they remained with a nonreversible neurological impairment [32]. Table 35.6 shows a collection of published cases of CPS1 treated by LT reported in the current medical literature.

Argininosuccinic aciduria (ASL) is a rare disorder of urea cycle, with a prevalence of 5:100,000, characterised by either a severe, neonatal-onset form that manifests with hyperammonemia in the first few days of life or late-onset forms that manifest with stress or infection-induced episodic hyperammonemia. Very few reports are available on the efficacy of LT in ASL [33–37].

In the proceedings of a recent meeting, Ranucci and coworkers described pre- and post-LT features of five children transplanted for ASL. Mean arginine succinic acid levels decreased significantly after LT in plasma (from 445 ± 45 to 112 ± 7 μmol/L), along with other biochemical markers of the disease, but not in cerebrospinal fluid. The authors concluded that, despite good systemic metabolic control, LT has no impact on CNS disease and that this may contribute to the poor neurologic outcome in ASL patients after LT. Table 35.7 reports the published experience with LT in ASL.

It is well known that patients with proximal defects may present some residual biochemical derangement since the gut or other organs express the defect [27, 38].

In general, patients with UCDs are recommended to undergo LT in early childhood to prevent further metabolic decompensation episodes. Haberle et al. recommended LT between the ages of 3 and 12 months if the weight of the patients increases beyond 5 kg [13]. Recent data from Kido et al. suggest that, if the onset of UCD is during the neonatal period, LT may be indicated immediately to protect the brain [39].

35.2.2 Maple Syrup Urine Disease (MSUD)

Maple syrup urine disease (MSUD), also known as branched-chain ketoaciduria or leucinosis, is an aminoacidopathy due to an enzyme defect in the catabolic pathway of the branched-chain amino acids leucine, isoleucine and valine. The accu-

Table 35.4 Published series of paediatric patients transplanted for OTC deficiency

Disease	Gender	Age at LT (years)	Donor	Follow-up (months)	Outcome	Ref
OTCd	F	4	DDLT	42	Alive	Morioka
OTCd	M	1.1	APOLT	7	Dead	Morioka
OTCd		1.8	DDLT	60	Alive	Morioka
OTCd		5	DDLT	36	Alive	Morioka
OTCd		1.5	DDLT	0.5	Dead	Morioka
OTCd		2.2	DDLT	18	Alive	Morioka
OTCd	F	5	DDLT	24	Alive	Morioka
OTCd	M	0.2	DDLT	6	Alive	Morioka
OTCd	M	0.2	DDLT	63	Alive	Morioka
OTCd	M	0.5	DDLT	39	Alive	Morioka
OTCd	M	0.1	DDLT	9	Alive	Morioka
OTCd	M	0.9	DDLT	30	Alive	Morioka
OTCd	M	0.7	DDLT	30	Alive	Morioka
OTCd	F	2.9	DDLT	30	Alive	Morioka
OTCd	F	2.5	LDLT(m)	121	Alive	Morioka
OTCd	F	3	APOLT(f)	118	Alive	Morioka
OTCd	F	5.8	APOLT(f)	103	Alive	Morioka
OTCd	F	4.9	LDLT (m)	89	Alive	Morioka
OTCd	F	7.1	LDLT (f)	6	Dead	Morioka
OTCd	F	16.1	LDLT (f)	60	Alive	Morioka
OTCd	F	2.9	LDLT (f)	97	Alive	Wakiya
OTCd	M	1.8	LDLT (f)	61	Alive	Wakiya
OTCd	M	1.1	LDLT (f)	52	Alive	Wakiya
OTCd	F	8.1	LDLT (f)	3	Dead	Wakiya
OTCd	F	3.8	LDLT (m)	36	Alive	Wakiya
OTCd	M	3.3	LDLT (m)	24	Alive	Wakiya
OTCd	F	3.6	LDLT (m)	23	Alive	Wakiya
OTCd	F	11.6	LDLT (f)	23	Alive	Wakiya
OTCd	M	1.6	LDLT (f)	15	Alive	Wakiya
OTCd	F	3.5	LDLT (m)	10	Alive	Wakiya
OTCd	M	1.1	LDLT (f)	4	Alive	Wakiya
OTCd	M	0.7	LDLT (f)	3	Alive	Wakiya

OTCd ornithine transcarbamylase deficiency, *LT* liver transplant, *DDLT* deceased-donor liver transplant, *LDLT* living donor liver transplant, *APOLT* auxiliary partial liver transplant, *f* father, *m* mother. Modified from [15, 21]

Table 35.5 Published series of paediatric patients transplanted for citrullinemia

Disease	Age at LT (years)	Graft	Follow-up (months)	Outcome	Citrulline pre-LT (μmol/L)[a]	Citrulline post-LT (μmol/L)[a]	Ref
Citrullinemia	2.4	LLS	37.2	Alive	2400	500	Vara
Citrullinemia	1.3	LLS	32.4	Alive	1800	200	Vara
Citrullinemia	1.4	LLS	37.2	Alive	2400	400	Vara
Citrullinemia	3.3	LLS	49.2	Alive	3450	550	Vara
Citrullinemia	5.9	Left lobe	46.8	Alive	2550	450	Vara
Citrullinemia	1.8	APOLT	36	Alive	2300	1300	Vara
Citrullinemia	6.5	APOLT	1.2	Alive	2000	600	Vara

LT liver transplant, *LLS* left lateral segment, *APOLT* auxiliary partial liver transplantation. Modified from [27]
[a]Approximate values (plasma citrulline normal range 8–57 μmol/L)

mulation of these amino acids and their corresponding alpha-keto acids leads to progressive neurodegeneration in untreated infants.

Despite aggressive medical and nutritional management, patients with classical MSUD may suffer from bouts of metabolic decompensation during times of illness or stress, which may lead to a rapid and irreversible deterioration of neurologic function and even death [16].

In the recent years, LT has become a viable option for treatment of these patients, for which is considered potentially curative, offering protection from metabolic decompensations on a normal diet [40–45] (Table 35.8).

Table 35.6 Published series of paediatric patients transplanted for carbamoyl phosphate synthetase 1 deficiency (CPS1d)

Disease	Age at LT (months)	Graft	Follow-up (months)	Outcome	Neurological impairment	Glutamine post-LT (µmol/L)	Ref
CPS1d	4	LDLT (m)	24	Alive	Yes	697	Kasahara
CPS1d	6	LDLT (f)	30	Alive	Yes	773	Kasahara
CPS1d	8	LDLT (m)	20	Alive	No	779	Kasahara
CPS1d	10	LDLT (m)	12	Alive	Yes	602	Kasahara
CPS1d	31	LDLT (m)	48	Alive	Yes	523	Kasahara
CPS1d	20	DDLT	18	Dead	Yes		Tuchman
CPS1d	0.5	DDLT	37	Alive	Yes	650	Todo
CPS1d	5	DDLT	30	Alive	No		McBride
CPS1d	3.5	DDLT	30	Alive	Yes		McBride
CPS1d	10	LDLT	28	Alive	No	Normal	Ishida
CPS1d	14	DDLT	10	Alive	Yes	Normal	Huang
CPS1d	72	DDLT	24	Alive	Yes		Stevenson

LT liver transplant, *DDLT* deceased donor liver transplant, *LDLT* living donor liver transplant, *f* father, *m* mother. Modified from [32]

Table 35.7 Published series of paediatric patients transplanted for argininosuccinic aciduria (ASL)

Disease	Age at LT (months)	Graft	Country	N of pts	Follow-up (months)	Alive	Neurological impairment	Ref
ASL	18	DDLT	USA	1	48	Yes	Mild	Marble
ASL	5 adults	LDLT	Japan	7	NA	7/7	Moderate	Kido
ASL	19	LDLT (m)	Poland	1	32	Yes	Mild	Szymanska
ASL	13 years	DDLT	Poland	1	42	Yes	Mild	Szymanska
ASL	12	LDLT (m)	Poland	1	42	Yes	Moderate	Szymanska
ASL	18	LDLT (m)	Turkey	1	12	Yes	No	Ozkay
ASL	30		Turkey	1	60	Yes	Mild	Yankol
ASL		LDLT (m)	Turkey	1	54	Yes	Moderate	Yankol
ASL	40	WL	Belgium	1	24	Yes	Mild	Robberecht
ASL	24 years	DDLT	Australia	1	30	Yes	Moderate	Newnham

LT liver transplant, *DDLT* deceased donor liver transplant, *LDLT* living donor liver transplant, *m* mother

Although the percentage of hepatic expression of an enzymatic defect is considered important for the potential of LT to correct a disease, the experience with MSUD clearly proved that other aspects must be involved, such as the degree of toxicity of the disease by-products and the detoxifying potential of the new liver. Indeed, although branched-chain α-ketoacid dehydrogenase (BCKDH) activity in liver accounts for only about 10–15% of the whole-body BCKDH enzymatic pool, the experience with LT in MSUD has shown that restoring that function is sufficient to control branched-chain amino acids (BCAAs) metabolism on an unrestricted protein intake [46, 47]. In fact, immediately after LT, serum leucine returns within normal levels in the majority of cases, and BCAAs levels remain in the normal range in long term, without dietary protein restriction [44, 48]. In transplanted patients, leucine tolerance usually increases more than tenfold [41].

Moreover, neurological function stabilises, and the risk of strokes or death from cerebral oedema is greatly reduced or eliminated [16]. Nevertheless, LT does not reverse existing neurological damage because this may result from structural changes to the brain rather than reversible neurotransmitter deficiencies [41, 47]. Some authors assessed the cognitive and adaptive function of patients with MSUD treated by LT showing that the majority of patients evidenced no significant change in IQ and adaptive scores. Accordingly, the continuation of physical, occupational and speech therapies is highly recommended [44, 49]. Taken together, these findings suggest that, to improve neurological and cognitive outcomes, patients should receive LT early in life, before experiencing brain damage.

Despite the successful results, the protection afforded by LT in MSUD patients may have some limitations. For instance, the use of related heterozygous live donors has been associated to metabolic crises during major stresses. Heterozygous donors' livers may have a BCKDH deficiency that makes them unable to fully control BCAA metabolism during a metabolic stress [50]. This observation has an important clinical implication: clinicians should continue to monitor BCAAs in post-transplantation patients, particularly those who develop serious catabolic illness or unexplained encephalopathy.

Table 35.8 Published cases of paediatric patients transplanted for maple syrup urine disease (MSUD)

Disease	Age at LT (months)	Graft	Follow-up (months)	Outcome	Neurological impairment	Leucin post-LT (μmol/L)	Ref
MSUD	22	LDLT (d)	75	Alive	No	151	Mohan
MSUD	38	LDLT (d)	40	Alive	Mild	174	Mohan
MSUD	8.5	DDLT (w)	106	Alive	Yes	Normal	Strauss
MSUD	4.3	DDLT (w)	17.5	Alive	No	Normal	Strauss
MSUD	3.0	DDLT (w)	16.6	Alive	No	Normal	Strauss
MSUD	1.9	DDLT (w)	15.8	Alive	No	Normal	Strauss
MSUD	2.7	DDLT (w)	15.5	Alive	No	Normal	Strauss
MSUD	8.1	DDLT (w)	13.8	Alive	Yes	Normal	Strauss
MSUD	2.0	DDLT (w)	10.6	Alive	No	Normal	Strauss
MSUD	8.7	DDLT (w)	7.9	Alive	Yes	Normal	Strauss
MSUD	9.8	DDLT (w)	4.5	Alive	No	Normal	Strauss
MSUD	20.5	DDLT (w)	4	Alive	Yes	Normal	Strauss
MSUD	6.3	DDLT (w)		Alive	No	Normal	Strauss
MSUD	25	DDLT (w)	8	Alive	Yes	190	Khanna
MSUD	25	LDLT (m) (d)	37	Alive		Normal	Feier
MSUD	38	LDLT (m) (d)	16	Alive		Normal	Feier
MSUD	19	LDLT (m) (d)	13	Alive		Normal	Feier
MSUD	21	LDLT (m)	11	Alive		Normal	Feier

LT liver transplant, *DDLT* deceased donor liver transplant, *LDLT* living donor liver transplant, *m* mother, *d* used as domino, *w* whole organ. Leucine normal range: 80.9–154.3 μmol/L

Table 35.9 Published cases of patients transplanted with a domino maple syrup urine disease (MSUD) graft

Disease	Age at LT (months)	Graft	Follow-up (months)	Outcome	Metabolic derangement	Leucine post-LT (μmol/L)	Ref
Protein C def	23	MSUD	16	Alive	No	81	Matsunami
BA	28	MSUD	9	Alive	No	90	Matsunami
HHChol	34	MSUD	8	Alive	No	143	Matsunami
HCV	51 years	MSUD	8	Alive	No	190	Khanna

LT liver transplantation, *BA* biliary atresia, *HHChol* homozygous hypercholesterolemia, *HCV* hepatitis C. Leucine normal range, 80.9–154.3 μmol/L

Remarkably MSUD livers can be used for domino LT [51]. In the domino procedure, a donated liver is used for one recipient, and the recipient's liver is used for another patient [52]. The liver from an MSUD patient carries approximately 15% of the BCKDH activity of the body; therefore, its defective activity is well compensated by the large amount of extra-hepatic functional enzyme of a recipient with a different disease (Fig. 35.4). Normal BCAA metabolism has been documented in all domino recipients of MSUD livers thus far, with no sequelae of MSUD in any of them (Table 35.9) [53].

35.2.3 Other Aminoacidopathies

Prior to the availability of nitisinone (NTBC) in 1993, all children with hereditary *tyrosinemia type 1* (HT1) were referred for LT [1]. Due to the success of NTBC and the possibility to detect the disease at birth by expanded neonatal screening, the indication of LT for HT1 has been modified to patients who are resistant to NTBC treatment or who developed fulminant hepatic failure or hepatocellular carcinoma (HCC). Referral for transplantation has become the exception rather than the rule. Remarkably, patients who started nitisinone after the sixth month of age have a significant risk to develop HCC and require prompt listing for transplantation later in childhood [54]. Reflecting this trend, over the last decade, the rate of LT for children with HT1 has decreased, while the average age at the time of transplantation increased [6].

LT corrects the metabolic defect allowing an unrestricted diet in all cases. Persistent renal succinylacetone (SA) production is universal, but the functional significance of this is still not fully understood. At present, no correlation between post-transplant SA levels and any index of renal function has been found. In the NTBC era, patient survival reaches 100% [55].

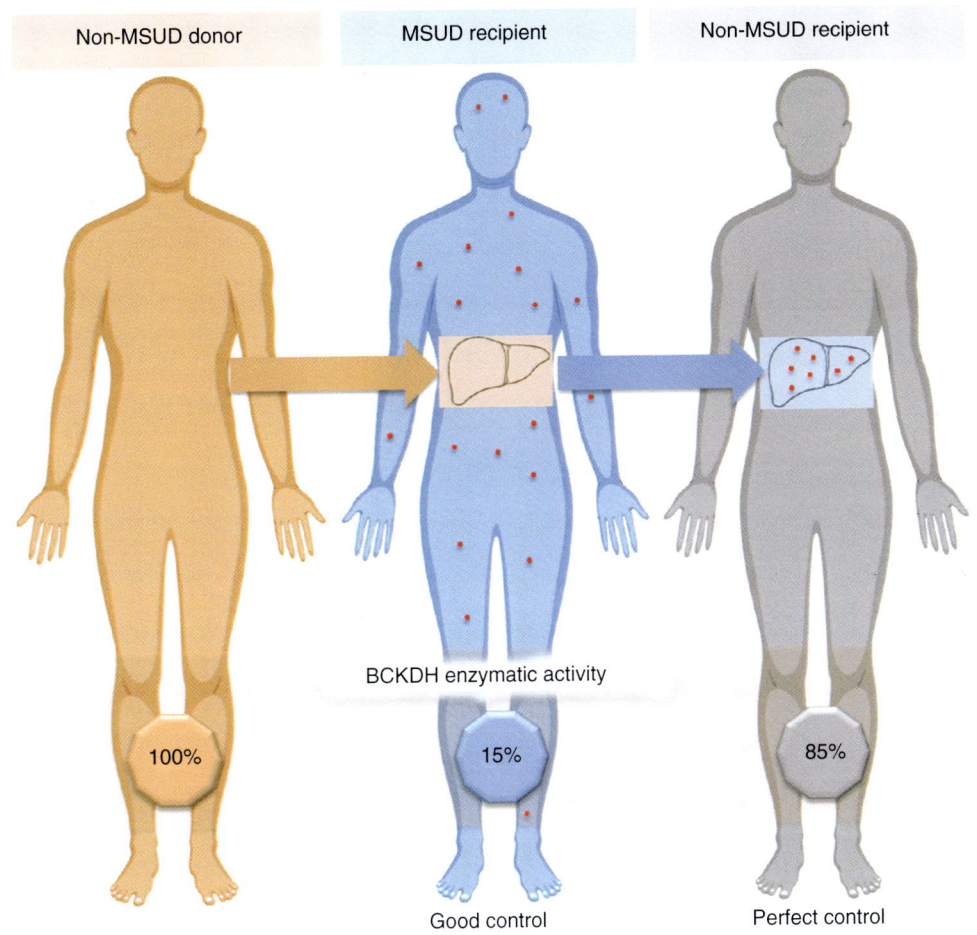

Fig. 35.4 MSUD livers can be used for domino liver transplantation. The MSUD recipient of a wild-type BCKDH liver gathers 15% of enzymatic activity, whereas the non-MSUD recipient of a MSUD liver reduces the BCKDH activity to 85%, with good and perfect metabolic control, respectively. *MSUD* maple syrup urine disease, *BCKDH* branched-chain α-ketoacid dehydrogenase

Other aminoacidopathies, such as *phenylketonuria*, could in theory be treated by LT, but effective dietary and medical therapy exists, making the risks of surgery exceeding potential benefits [56].

35.2.4 Crigler-Najjar Syndrome Type 1

Crigler-Najjar syndrome (CN) is a rare, autosomal recessive disorder of bilirubin metabolism that has been divided into two distinct forms based upon the severity of jaundice: Type I disease (CN1) is associated with severe jaundice and high risk of neurologic sequelae (kernicterus); Type II disease (CN2) is associated with a lower serum bilirubin concentration and no risk for kernicterus throughout the whole life [57].

Jaundice in CN is due to a variety of alterations in the coding sequences of the bilirubin-uridine diphosphate glucuronosyltransferase (UGT1A1) gene, which is responsible for bilirubin conjugation [58]. These mutations lead to the total loss or reduced levels of UGT1A1 activity respectively in CN1 and CN2. The hallmark of CN1 is unconjugated hyperbilirubinemia in the range of 20–25 mg/dL but can reach values as high as 50 mg/dL. Unlike CN1, CN2 has no indication to liver transplantation since it is characterised by bilirubin levels below 20 mg/dL, and therefore compatible with a normal life, although during intercurrent illnesses bilirubin levels can raise in both. The serum bilirubin concentration can be reduced by the administration of phenobarbital in most patients with CN2 but not CN1 disease, providing also a helpful tool to differentiate the two conditions [59]. Although several drugs have proved effective to slightly reduce jaundice through the reduction of the reuptake of bilirubin in the gut (calcium carbonate and orlistat), the medical management of CN1 relies mainly on phototherapy that acts by converting bilirubin into its isomers, which are excreted in the bile without the need for conjugation [60]. Patients with CN1 requires the exposure to fluorescent lamps for up to 12 h/day, but around the pubertal age thickening of the skin, increased skin pigmentation and decreased surface area in relation to body mass render this technique less effective, increasing the risk of kernicterus [61].

Liver transplantation therefore remains the definitive therapy of CN1 and is usually considered before adolescence [62]. Deciding the best timing for transplantation is challenging in these patients. If on a side, it is a general rule to postpone as much as possible surgery and exposure to immunosuppressive drugs, especially in children; on the other side, an effective control of jaundice in CN1 can become less and less consistent over the years, raising the risk of kernicterus [63]. In a report of the CN world registry published in 1996 including 57 patients, the average age at transplantation was 9.1 years. Overall brain damage developed in 26% of patients. Remarkably the age of 8 patients with and 13 without brain damage at or before transplantation was 14.3 and 5.9 years, respectively. The conclusion was that liver transplantation was performed too late in that cohort [64]. Nowadays more effective tools to control jaundice may have developed. However, despite a different response to non-surgical treatments that can allow tailoring the decisions in these patients, older age, inconsistent family compliance to phototherapy and intercurrent illnesses remain major threats to neurological integrity in CN1 patients managed conservatively, especially when the levels of bilirubin remain steadily above 25 mg/dL.

Allogeneic hepatocyte transplantation has been attempted in children with CN1, based on the concept that replacement of as little as 5% of the liver mass can reduce bilirubin down to near-normal values. Indeed this technique was able to reduce serum bilirubin levels to approximately 50% of pre-transplant levels in a child with CN1 [65]. However, in several reports, it has been shown that the beneficial effect lasts no longer than 12 months, making OLT mandatory to control the rise of bilirubin [66].

Several attempts have been carried out to accomplish gene therapy in an animal model of CN1, the Gunn rat. A normal bilirubin-UGT gene can be introduced in the diseased liver by adeno-associated vectors that are capable of correcting the phenotype through normalisation of bilirubin. This strategy is currently being tested in phase one clinical trials with promising results [67] (see also Chap. 44).

35.2.5 Primary Hyperoxaluria Type 1

Primary hyperoxaluria type 1 (PH1) is a rare, autosomal recessive disorder caused by deficiency of the liver-specific enzyme alanine/glyoxylate aminotransferase (AGT). This defect results in increased levels of serum oxalate, which is excreted by the kidney where it crystallises within renal tubules causing nephrocalcinosis and renal failure. AGT is expressed only in the liver, but PH1 does not cause any liver disease, originating a unique disease in which a structurally and functionally normal liver causes severe kidney disease and renal failure. As the glomerular filtration rate (GFR) decreases, oxalate saturates the plasma and accumulates in bone and other body tissues causing systemic oxalosis [68].

The most threatening situation occurs when PH1 presents in infancy, showing a severe phenotype and rapidly progressive renal and extrarenal oxalosis leading to renal failure and need for haemodialysis in the first year of age [69]. In these children a combined liver-kidney transplant (LKT), either simultaneous or sequential, is life-saving. Nevertheless LKT is very challenging at this age, because of the small abdominal cavity typical of a non-cirrhotic disease, the troublesome size match of two organs and the well-known haemodynamic instability of these patients [70]. If a simultaneous LKT from the same donor has the advantage of conferring a better tolerance to the kidney, the sequential procedure (first liver and then kidney transplant at a later stage) may be safer, overcoming the problems of organ size match and abdominal compartment syndrome early after transplant (Table 35.10) [71, 72].

Table 35.10 Transplantation strategies in patients with PH1 and end-stage renal disease

	Simultaneous LKT	Sequential LKT
Advantages	Better kidney tolerance if same donor for both organs	Safer in infants, reduced mortality risk
	Re-established urine output (HD often still required early after Tx)	Shorter waiting time on the list
	Re-established oxalate clearance from the body (hyperhydration required)	
Disadvantages	Longer waiting time on the list	Loss of immunological benefit because of two different donors
	Reduced patient and kidney graft survival rate	Need to continue HD till kidney transplantation is carried out
	Difficult abdominal closure, compartment syndrome	

LKT liver-kidney transplant, *Tx* transplant

However the disease has a wide spectrum of clinical expression, being sometimes diagnosed even in young adults.

When PH1 presents after infancy, patients are managed medically (pyridoxine, citrates, hydration), but once the GFR falls below a critical level of 30–60 mL/min/1.73 m^2, preemptive liver transplantation (LT) may be considered, to avoid the progression of kidney disease and the later need to combine a kidney transplant. Once GFR drops below 30 mL/min/1.73 m^2, oxalate accumulation increases exponentially, and the renal function is not salvageable after LT, obligating to perform a combined liver-kidney transplantation [73]. Table 35.11 reports the suggested guidelines for the management of patients with PH1 based on residual GFR and systemic involvement [74]. Deciding whether and when to perform a preemptive liver transplant is challenging and controversial. Probably the rate of GFR drop over time is a good marker to guide the choice of waiting or listing the patients for LT.

Table 35.11 Suggested transplantation options in pyridoxine-resistant PH1 patients according to residual GFR and systemic involvement

Tx options	Simultaneous liver + kidney	Sequential liver-kidney	Isolated kidney	Isolated liver
HD strategy	Peroperative ± postoperative according to POx and GFR	Standard HD following liver Tx aiming at POx <20 μmol/L	Preoperative and peroperative	Sometimes peroperative
GFR > 30 < 60 mL/min/1.73 m²	No	No	No	Option in carefully selected patients
GFR > 15 < 30 mL/min/1.73 m²	Yes	Option	Option if B6 response but no evidence	No
GFR < 15 mL/min/1.73 m²	Yes	Yes	Option if B6 response but no evidence	No
Infantile form (ESRD < 2 years)	Yes	Yes	No	No

POx plasma oxalate, *Tx* transplantation, *HD* haemodialysis, *GFR* glomerular filtration rate, *ESRN* end-stage renal disease. Adapted from Cochat et al. Nephrol Dial Transplant (2012) 27: 1729–1736

35.3 Liver Transplantation to Improve the Phenotype of Inborn Errors of Metabolism

35.3.1 Organic Acidurias

Organic acidurias are inborn errors of metabolism that can present acutely in early life or have a delayed presentation later in childhood. Acute presentations include ketosis, acidosis, pancytopenia and hyperammonemia. Chronic symptoms include metabolic crises, failure to thrive, hypotonia, vomiting and intellectual disability. The 'classical' organic acidurias, propionic acidemia (PA) and methylmalonic acidemia (MMA) are the most common indications for LT [75, 76]. In PA and MMA, the metabolic defect is expressed throughout the body systems, and therefore LT cannot be regarded as a cure but rather as a treatment improving their phenotype (Fig. 35.2).

LT has been utilised for *propionic acidemia (PA)* patients who have uncontrollable hyperammonemia and/or frequent metabolic decompensations or failure to thrive [17]. Despite transplanted patients do not normalise protein tolerance, they have shown a reduction of metabolic decompensations, improvement in quality of life, a significant gain in physical growth and improvement of cardiomyopathy [77–79]. Nonetheless LT appears to be a particularly risky procedure in these patients, carrying high perioperative morbidity and mortality. Charbit-Henrion described 12 patients with PA who received 16 transplants at a mean age of 4.2 years in 2 different European transplantation centres. In this cohort, collecting patients transplanted from 1999 to 2013, LT was associated with severe unexpected complications and high mortality (58%). In survivors, when present, the cardiomyopathy was resolved, and no acute metabolic decompensation occurred allowing dietary relaxation. Renal failure was present in half of the patients before LT and worsened in all of them [80]. A different outcome has been reported by another European group that described five patients transplanted between 1987 and 2008 at a median age of 1.5 years. After a mean follow-up longer than 7 years, all the children had normal graft function and a good quality of life with a protein-unrestricted diet and no further metabolic decompensations (Table 35.12) [81]. Hepatic artery thrombosis was common in both series. It is possible that the choice of transplanting at an early stage, before the development of disease-related organs injury, might be the key to better outcomes.

Liver transplantation in *methylmalonic acidemia (MMA)* has been less successful, since, though providing some enzyme replacement and reducing the frequency and severity of acute metabolic decompensations, it has proved insufficient to rescue the long-term cerebral ocular and renal complications [82, 83]. Kasahara reviewed the published literature in this field and reported on 18 children with MMA (8 males), of a median age of 20 months, who were transplanted because of frequent metabolic decompensations (18/18) and developmental delay (13/18). Seven had renal impairment. Six received a living donor LT, five a combined liver-kidney transplant. Eight patients had perioperative haemodialysis to reduce serum methylmalonic acid. After a median follow-up of 36 months, three patients died (from severe acidosis and infections), four developed renal failure and three developed severe neurological disability. Neurological and renal disease did not improve after LT [84].

Morioka described the clinical courses of seven paediatric patients with MMA undergoing living donor liver transplantation (LDLT). Serum and urinary methylmalonic acid levels were significantly decreased after LDLT, but did not normalise in any patient. However, no episode of acute metabolic decompensation or metabolic stroke was observed postoperatively. One patient died of sepsis 44 days after LDLT. The

Table 35.12 Published cases of paediatric patients transplanted for propionic acidemia

Disease	Age at LT (years)	Graft	Follow-up (months)	Alive	Complications	Metabolic crises after LT	Ref
Prop Ac	2.2	DDLLS[a]	0.2	No	PNF, HF		Charbit
Prop Ac	7.1	DDWhole	8.4	No	PTLD, HAT	No	Charbit
Prop Ac	9.0	DDWhole	255	Yes	Kidney Tx	No	Charbit
Prop Ac	1.2	DDWhole	255	Yes	No	No	Charbit
Prop Ac	1.1	DDRL	0.1	No	PNF		Charbit
Prop Ac	2.4	DDLLS[a]	206	Yes	HAT, HDF	No	Charbit
Prop Ac	1.1	DDLLS	0.1	No	PNF, HDF		Charbit
Prop Ac	1.7	DDLLS[a]	0.5	No	HAT		Charbit
Prop Ac	3.9	DDLLS	1.0	No	HF, HDF	No	Charbit
Prop Ac	6.7	DDLLS[a]	97	Yes	ARDS, HAT, HDF	No	Charbit
Prop Ac	6.5	DDLLS	0.4	No	HF		Charbit
Prop Ac	8.3	DDWhole	12.2	Yes	ARDS	No	Charbit
All	4.2 ± 3.0	7 LLSs	70 ± 106	5/12			
Prop Ac	1.8	APOLT	180	Yes	HSV, ACR	No	Vara
Prop Ac	1.1	LDLLS	137	Yes	PTLD, ACR	No	Vara
Prop Ac	0.8	LLS	87	Yes	HSV, Stroke	No	Vara
Prop Ac	7.0	LLS	59	Yes	ACR	No	Vara
Prop Ac	1.1	LLS[a]	26	Yes	HAT	No	Vara
All	2.3 ± 2.6	4 LLSs	98 ± 61	5/5			

LT liver transplantation, *DDLLS* deceased donor left lateral segment, *DDWhole* deceased donor whole liver, *DDRL* deceased donor right lobe, *APOLT* auxiliary partial liver transplantation, *LDLLS* living donor left lateral segment, *LLS* left lateral segment, *PNF* primary non-function, *HF* heart failure, *PTLD* post-transplant lymphoproliferative disease, *HAT* hepatic artery thrombosis, *HDF* haemodiafiltration, *ARDS* adult respiratory distress syndrome
[a]This patient had more than one transplant

metabolism-correcting medications being administered remained mostly unchanged after LDLT, whereas protein restriction was liberalised. After a median of 10 months of follow-up, 5/6 patients were alive. However, physical and neurodevelopmental delay were unchanged in survivors [11]. More recently Niemi described 14 patients who underwent LT ($n = 6$) or liver-kidney transplantation ($n = 8$) at a mean age of 8.2 years (range 0.8–20.7). At a mean follow-up of 3.25 ± 4.2 years, patient and liver survivals were 100% and 93%, respectively, and kidney allograft survival was 100%. There were no episodes of decompensation after transplantation. Methylmalonic acid dropped by 83% compared to pre-transplant levels. None of the patients had a further deterioration in neurodevelopmental abilities [85].

Due to the incomplete correction of the metabolic defect and the possible progression of extrahepatic disease, it is still debated whether MMA should be treated with any combination of liver and/or kidney transplantation [86].

35.3.2 Glycogen Storage Disorders

The most frequent indication for LT among disorders of carbohydrate metabolism is glycogen storage disease type 1A (GSD1A). These patients may become candidate to LT because of the development of hepatic adenomas that are known to progress to malignant lesions in a relatively large proportion of cases. LT should be considered for patients with multifocal, growing lesions that do not regress with improved dietary regimens or present imaging changes and who do not have evidence of distant metastatic disease [87]. Other indications have included growth failure and poor metabolic control. Optimal metabolic control appears to normalise growth and minimise the risk of hepatic adenomas. In case of a solitary lesion, resection may be the best surgical option [88]. Glycogen storage disease type 1B presents with frequent and often severe bacterial infections due to severe neutropenia. Liver transplantation has been found to improve in some but not all patients [89].

After liver transplantation, all GSD1A patients achieved resolution of their metabolic derangement, including correction of hypoglycaemia, lactic acidosis, hyperuricemia and hyperlipidaemia. Other benefits of transplantation include liberalisation of the diet and reduction in the risk of malignancy [90, 91]. Davies reviewed the published literature and reported on 44 children who underwent LT for different GSDs. In patients with GSD1A, 24/25 children of a mean age at OLT of 14 years survived in the long term. Their indications to LT were multiple adenomas, growth failure and poor metabolic control. Only 1/25 had HCC in the explanted liver. After LT the patients experienced good quality of life and good glycaemic control, but nephropathy, neutropenia, infections and Crohn's like disease did not resolve. Although the survival rate has improved over the past 20 years, complications in the postoperative course remain. Chronic renal failure is a well-documented complication of liver transplantation in GSD1A, with some patients progressing to renal failure within a few years after LT despite no evidence of renal disease at the time of listing [92, 93].

The same author reported on 17 children (16 males), of a mean age of 3.2 years, who underwent LT for GSD4, a condition leading to liver cirrhosis. The survival rate was 12/17 (70%). Their indications to LT were end-stage liver disease with cirrhosis and portal hypertension. After LT the quality of life was good, with full control of the disease, no progression of myopathy nor cardiomyopathy. LT appeared to be a good option for end-stage liver disease in GSD IV [92].

Other types of GSDs have been treated by LT, but the presence of significant muscular and/or cardiac manifestations makes it a less obvious choice [94].

35.3.3 Mitochondrial Disorders

Mitochondrial disorders (MDSs) are an increasingly recognised group of diseases, whose long-term outcome is generally poor. They are mainly related to mutations in genes involved in the respiratory chain, having heterogeneous phenotypes, most commonly characterised by a defect of cellular energy production (Table 35.13).

As such MDSs are systemic diseases in which organ transplantation is generally contraindicated. Those presenting with liver involvement are related to nuclear gene products (inherited with autosomal recessive pattern in 90% and autosomal dominant and X-linked pattern in 10%), responsible for mitochondrial DNA replication *(POLG1)*, maintenance of deoxyribonucleoside triphosphate (dNTP) pools *(DGUOK)* and membrane mitochondrial integrity *(MPV17)* [95, 96]. Therefore, mutations in these genes cause mitochondrial DNA depletion, characterised by hepato-cerebral forms inherited with an autosomal recessive pattern. In *Alpers syndrome* (due to mutations in POLG1), sodium valproate administered because of intractable seizures often triggers acute liver decompensation and death.

Currently, the indication for LT in mitochondrial hepatopathies is controversial. Although LT can lead to normal hepatic function, it neither stabilises nor normalises mitochondrial function in extrahepatic-affected tissues. Thus, severe systemic manifestations of mitochondrial disease are generally considered a contraindication to LT.

In patients selected for transplant, the surgical outcome in published case series has been relatively poor, with late-onset extrahepatic manifestations of mitochondrial dysfunction appearing even after initial negative screens [6]. However, good outcomes in selected patients without neurological findings have been described as well [8, 97–102].

Recent data demonstrate a 50% survival rate in a high selected group of children with MDSs who underwent liver transplantation. Remarkably, patients with mitochondrial hepatopathy and central nervous system (CNS) involvement have significantly worse post-LT survival rates than patients without CNS disease [103] (Table 35.14).

Table 35.13 Classification of primary mitochondrial hepatopathies

RC (electron transport) defects (OXPHOS)
Neonatal liver failure
Complex I deficiency
Complex IV deficiency (*SCO1* mutations)
Complex III deficiency (*BCS1L* mutations)
Co-enzyme Q deficiency
Multiple complex deficiencies (transfer and elongation factor mutations)
mtDNA depletion syndrome (*DUGOK, MPV17, POLG, SUCLG1, C10orf2/Twinkle* mutations)
Later-onset liver dysfunction or failure
Alpers-Huttenlocher disease (*POLG* mutations)
Pearson's marrow pancreas syndrome (mtDNA deletion)
Mitochondrial neurogastrointestinal encephalopathy (*TYMP* mutations)
NNH (*MPV17* mutations)

OXPHOS oxidative phosphorylation, *NNH* Navajo neurohepatopathy, *RC* respiratory chain. Adapted from Lee SL et al. J Pediatr 2013

Table 35.14 Published series of paediatric patients transplanted for mitochondrial hepatopathies

Author	N of patients (age)	Presentation	Diagnosis	Survival	Follow-up	Comments
Sokal (1999)	11 (1–7 months)	ALF	RC enzyme assay and clinical	5/11	5 months–8 years	Diarrhoea and vomiting
Durand (2001)	5 (<1 year)	ALF	RC enzyme assay and clinical	2/5	3.5 years	No extrahepatic involvement pre-LT
Dubern (2001)	5 (<1 year)	ALF	RC enzyme assay and clinical	2/5		No extrahepatic involvement pre-LT
Dimmock (2008)	10 (<10 months)	Liver failure, neurologic symptoms	DGUOK genotyping	2/10		No benefit of LT if neurologic signs
El-Hattab (2010)	10 (infancy)	Liver failure, neurologic symptoms	MPV17 genotyping	5/10; 2	4–21 years	Pts with NNH had neurologic progression post-LT
Iwama (2010)	12 (<10 months)	Liver failure	RC enzyme assay and clinical	7/12	4 months–5 years	No benefit of LT if neurologic signs
Total	53			23 (43%)		

ALF acute liver failure, *RC* respiratory chain, *LT* liver transplantation, *NNH* Navajo neurohepatopathy. Modified from Lee SL et al. J Pediatr 2013

Table 35.15 Published cases of paediatric patients transplanted for DGUOK deficiency

Disease	Age at LT (months)	Neurological signs before LT	Follow-up (years)	Alive	Neurological follow-up
DGUOK	4	Hypotonia	5	Yes	Hypotonia, good NS
DGUOK	12	Hypotonia, MR	8	Yes	Hypotonia, good NS
DGUOK	5	Hypotonia, MR nystagmus	1	Yes	Severe MR
DGUOK	9	None	23	Yes	Rhabdomyol, mild MR
DGUOK	12	None	1.5	No	Pulm H, RTA
DGUOK	1.5	Hypotonia, MR nystagmus	0.5	No	Hypotonia, severe MR
DGUOK	2	Nystagmus	1.8	No	–
DGUOK	12	Hypotonia, MR nystagmus	0.2	No	–
DGUOK	12	Hypotonia	12	Yes	ADHD, good NS
DGUOK	1	Optic dysplasia	0.2	No	Nystagmus, Pulm H
DGUOK	6	MR	1	No	Pulm H
DGUOK	3	Hypotonia	0.2	No	MOF
DGUOK	3	Nystagmus	0.2	No	–
DGUOK	17	None	1.5	Yes	Hypotonia

DGOUK deoxyguanosine kinase deficiency, *MR* mental retardation, *NS* neurological status, *Pulm H* pulmonary hypertension, *RTA* renal tubular acidosis, *ADHD* attention-deficit hyperactivity disorder, *MOF* multi-organ failure. Adapted from Grabhorn et al, Liver Transpl 2014

Nonetheless Parikh recently described 35 patients from 17 mitochondrial disease centres across North America, the United Kingdom and Australia, who had a liver, kidney or heart transplantation because of mitochondrial disorders. Excluding patients with POLG-related disease, short-term post-transplant survival approached or met outcomes seen in non-mitochondrial disease transplant patients. Remarkably many patients did not have a mitochondrial disease considered or diagnosed prior to transplantation. The authors suggested to consider with caution the option of transplantation in these patients, with the exception of polymerase gamma (POLG)-related disease which has generally a poor outcome [104].

The choice of LT for mitochondrial disorders raises considerable practical and ethical questions that remain unsolved. In general it is important to always consider this condition in cryptogenic disorders developing liver failure associated with high lactate levels and extrahepatic manifestations, especially neuromuscular impairment which is commonly progressive despite transplantation [105]. Patients with deoxyguanosine kinase deficiency (DGUOK) may have a better outcome than those affected by POLG deficiency [106] (Table 35.15).

35.3.4 Other Rare Inborn Errors of Metabolism

Ethylmalonic encephalopathy (EE) is a rare autosomal recessive neurometabolic disorder of infancy presenting with wide clinical heterogeneity. EE is clinically characterised by neurodevelopmental delay and regression, prominent pyramidal and extrapyramidal signs, recurrent petechiae, orthostatic acrocyanosis and chronic diarrhoea. Biochemical changes observed in patients with EE are ethylmalonic acid (EMA) aciduria, sometimes with mild elevations of short-chain acylglycines in the urine organic acid profile (ethylmalonic acid, methylsuccinic acid, isobutyrylglycine and isovalerylglycine), increased levels of plasma C4- and C5-acylcarnitines and elevated plasma lactate [107].

EE is caused by mutations in the ETHE1 gene, responsible for the catabolism of hydrogen sulphide (H2S). Chronic management of this disease includes combined use of antibiotics and N-acetylcysteine (NAC), which is aimed at lowering the chronic H2S load, but the patients remain at risk of acute decompensations. In a single case report, living-related transplantation performed at 7 months of age provided a great improvement of the biochemical defect, with rapid normalisation of thiosulfate biochemical derangement. No new brain lesions were detected at MRI scan [108]. However, further experiences and long-term outcome data are needed to confirm the utility of LT in EE.

Neuroblastoma-amplified sequence deficiency (NBAS) causes the defective synthesis of a protein involved in the transport between the endoplasmic reticulum and Golgi apparatus. This condition causes a clinical picture of recurrent acute liver failure (RALF) [109]. The disease is characterised by episodes of raised transaminases, severe coagulopathy and encephalopathy during febrile illnesses. In undiagnosed children LT was performed and seemed to be successful in abolishing the risk of recurrent episodes. Thus LT may be an option when episodes of ALF are particularly frequent or severe [110].

Wolcott-Rallison syndrome is characterised by infantile diabetes, skeletal dysplasia, renal disease and recurrent liver failure. This condition is due to mutations in EIF2AK3 gene [111]. Treatment is only supportive and liver transplantation appears to provide complete protection against RALF. A combined liver-pancreas or liver-kidney-pancreas transplantation has been carried out successfully in these patients, with resolution of RALF, renal failure and diabetes [112–114].

S-adenosylhomocysteine hydrolase deficiency (SAHHD) is a muscle disease associated with high blood levels of methionine and creatine kinase (CK), characterised by microcephaly, developmental delay, growth failure and coagulopathy. SAHHD results in an a defect in the methionine pathway with an abnormal SAM/SAH ratio inhibiting transmethylation reactions throughout the organ systems [115]. In a single case report, liver transplantation resulted in resolution of the coagulopathy and an improvement of MRI and increased head growth. The significant increase in hepatic methylation products and improvement of the SAM/SAH ratio due to the liver correction in turn facilitated cerebral methyltransferase activity [116]. Remarkably, LT impacted on cerebral intracellular processes, overcoming the common problem of crossing the blood-brain barrier to improve neurological outcome of metabolic diseases expressed in the central nervous system.

Infantile Refsum disease (IRD) is a peroxisomal disorder characterised by retinitis pigmentosa, sensorineural deafness, severe neurodevelopmental delay and chronic liver disease.

Biochemically IRD presents with elevated very long-chain fatty acid, plasminogen and phytanic acid levels. Early liver transplantation seems to have a significant metabolic benefit, with normalisation of phytanic acid levels and improvement in very long-chain fatty acids. The results on neurological and ophthalmological outcome suggest a stabilisation of the disease more than an improvement [117].

35.4 Further Issues

35.4.1 Domino Liver Transplant

When the inborn error of liver metabolism does not cause structural hepatic derangement, there is the possibility of using the explanted liver as a domino transplant. In domino LT the liver of the recipient is used to transplant another patient with a different disease, with the expectation that the disease will not be clinically expressed because it is compensated by the extrahepatic enzymatic activity of the recipient (Fig. 35.4) [53]. The major paediatric experience has been with organs from patients with MSUD which have been used successfully in a range of paediatric disorder, including other metabolic defects. No recipient metabolic consequence after prolonged follow-up of up to 10 years has been observed [41]. Domino organs from patients with familial hypercholesterolemia, MMA and PA have also been used successfully [118]. On the contrary, organs from patients with acute porphyria and oxalosis rapidly produced severe disease in the recipients [119]. Domino LT has been used also with livers from patients affected by familial amyloid polyneuropathy.

A recent study showed that, after a median of 7 years after the procedure, domino LT with these livers was associated with the risk of developing de novo systemic amyloidosis and amyloid neuropathy in up to 23% of transplant recipients. Neuropathy was preceded by asymptomatic amyloid deposition in various tissues [119].

The domino concept has also been applied to hepatocyte transplantation where cells from the liver of a patient with GSD type I were infused in a patient with severe phenylketonuria. This resulted in an improvement in metabolic control that unfortunately was not sustained [120].

35.4.2 Auxiliary Partial Liver Transplant

In auxiliary partial liver transplantation (APOLT), a partial liver graft is implanted in an orthotopic position after leaving behind a part of the native liver for the potential advantage of immunosuppression withdrawal or future gene therapy [121]. This is only recommended when the defect does not cause liver disease and a partial correction is likely to be effective. The major advantage of auxiliary liver transplantation is that the native liver is retained as a 'safety net' if the graft fails or if gene therapy becomes available. The major disadvantage of the procedure is that the surgical technique is highly complex, with the need to preferentially divert portal venous blood flow to the graft by native portal vein banding [122]. In experienced hands this can be very effective, and long-term stable graft function can be accomplished [123].

So far APOLT has been used in Crigler-Najjar syndrome and highly selected cases of UCDs or PA [121, 124].

The potential of auxiliary transplant has been boosted by the concept of the 'domino auxiliary'. In this technique the auxiliary transplant comes from a domino procedure. In the first reported case, the explanted left lobe of a child with PA undergoing elective transplant was implanted as an auxiliary in a child with Crigler-Najjar syndrome type I with complete correction of the metabolic defect [125]. This raises the possibility of the elective transfer of left lobes between patients with differing metabolic diseases, without impacting on the cadaveric donor pool [126].

35.4.3 Hepatocyte Transplantation

Liver cell transplantation (LCT), also called hepatocyte transplantation, has been used to offer an alternative to organ transplantation in patients with inborn errors of metabolism [127]. In patients with liver-based IEM, this transfer of enzyme activity can be regarded as a sort of gene therapy.

Because of its minimally invasive nature, LCT is especially attractive for small children in which organ transplan-

Table 35.16 Case reports of liver cell transplantation in inborn errors of liver metabolism

Diagnosis	Age	Author	Centre	Outcome
Crigler-Najjar I	10 years	Fox 1998	Omaha	Partial recovery, LT
GSD Ia	47 years	Muraca 2002	Padova	Partial recovery
OTC	Neonate	Horslen 2003	Omaha	Marginal improvement, LT
Refsum	4 years	Sokal 2003	Brussels	Partial recovery
OTC	Neonate	Mitry 2004	London	Partial recovery, LT
Crigler-Najjar I	8 years	Darwish 2004	Brussels	Partial recovery, LT
OTC	14 months	Darwish 2004	Brussels	Recovery, planned LT
Argininosuccinuria	3 years	Darwish 2004	Brussels	Partial recovery
Factor VII deficiency	3 months	Dhawan 2004	London	Partial recovery, LT
Factor VII deficiency	2 years	Dhawan 2004	London	Partial recovery, LT
PFIC 2	18 months	Dhawan 2005	London	Portal hypertension, LT
PFIC 2	3 years	Dhawan 2005	London	No effect
Crigler-Najjar I	NA	Dhawan 2005	London	NA
Crigler-Najjar I	9 years	Ambrosino 2005	Padova	Partial recovery, LT

OTC ornithine transcarbamylase deficiency, *GSD* glycogen storage disease, *PFIC* progressive familial intrahepatic cholestasis, *NA* not available

tation is challenging or in those defects in which the metabolic derangement is easily corrected by a limited delivery of normal enzymatic activity. Over the past two decades, several case reports and series have been published, with the invariable outcome of a temporary efficacy, lasting generally no longer than 12 months [65, 66, 128–133]. Table 35.16 reports the first cases published in the medical literature. Recently, Meyburg et al. reported a series of UCD patients who showed a favourable metabolic stabilisation and were bridged to liver transplantation after allogeneic liver cells transplantation [134]. Hepatocyte transplantation is discussed in depth in Chap. 43.

35.4.4 Heterozygous Donors

Considerations for the source of the donor liver include whether to use deceased or living-related grafts. The majority of IMDs are inherited in an autosomal recessive pattern, in which case parents are obligate carriers. The reduction of enzymatic activity observed in carriers relative to individuals with two functional gene copies suggests that deceased donors' livers are more suitable organs, particularly for conditions with significant extrahepatic manifestations. Nevertheless, living-related donor LT using obligate carriers has been employed successfully in situations when cadaveric donors were unavailable [94].

Parents of patients with A1ATD, Wilson's disease, genetic hemochromatosis and familial hypercholesterolemia with LDL receptor defects have successfully been living donors for LT [135]. In the specific case of OTC, only unaffected fathers should be considered as donors, avoiding heterozygous asymptomatic mothers [136]. In general, for IEMs expressed also outside of the liver, the best option remains a graft from a donor who is not carrying any mutation previously associated with the disease.

35.4.5 Outcomes

LT for IMDs has an expected survival following elective transplantation greater than 95% and of greater than 82% at 1 and 10 years, respectively [8]. For classical MSUD patient graft survival may even reach 100%.

In general, the outcome of LT for IMDs is comparable or even superior to that of patients transplanted for a cirrhotic liver disease. Improved survival in metabolic patients undergoing transplantation may be related to the presence of normal anatomy and the possibility to perform surgery electively during periods of relative clinical stability [5, 10]. The improved outcomes have also been attributed to the healthier clinical status of patients with IMDs at the time of transplantation, many of whom do not have portal hypertension or other sequelae of long-term liver dysfunction [7, 78].

Since the biochemical derangements observed in this patient population are variable and complex and, in some instances, render patients susceptible to metabolic decompensation from intra- and perioperative stress, LT should be performed only in centres in which considerable paediatric transplantation experience is coupled with expert management of IMDs [6].

References

1. Fisch RO, McCabe ER, Doeden D, et al. Homotransplantation of the liver in a patient with hepatoma and hereditary tyrosinemia. J Pediatr. 1978;93(4):592–6.
2. Largilliere C, Houssin D, Gottrand F, et al. Liver transplantation for ornithine transcarbamylase deficiency in a girl. J Pediatr. 1989;115(3):415–7.
3. Fagiuoli S, Daina E, D'Antiga L, et al. Monogenic diseases that can be cured by liver transplantation. J Hepatol. 2013;59(3):595–612.
4. Mazariegos G, Shneider B, Burton B, et al. Liver transplantation for pediatric metabolic disease. Mol Genet Metab. 2014;111(4):418–27.

5. Stevenson T, Millan MT, Wayman K, et al. Long-term outcome following pediatric liver transplantation for metabolic disorders. Pediatr Transplant. 2010;14(2):268–75.
6. Arnon R, Kerkar N, Davis MK, et al. Liver transplantation in children with metabolic diseases: the studies of pediatric liver transplantation experience. Pediatr Transplant. 2010;14(6):796–805.
7. Kayler LK, Rasmussen CS, Dykstra DM, et al. Liver transplantation in children with metabolic disorders in the United States. Am J Transplant. 2003;3(3):334–9.
8. Mc Kiernan PJ. Recent advances in liver transplantation for metabolic disease. J Inherit Metab Dis. 2017;40(4):491–5.
9. Fujisawa D, Nakamura K, Mitsubuchi H, et al. Clinical features and management of organic acidemias in Japan. J Hum Genet. 2013;58(12):769–74.
10. Sze YK, Dhawan A, Taylor RM, et al. Pediatric liver transplantation for metabolic liver disease: experience at King's College Hospital. Transplantation. 2009;87(1):87–93.
11. Morioka D, Kasahara M, Horikawa R, et al. Efficacy of living donor liver transplantation for patients with methylmalonic acidemia. Am J Transplant. 2007;7(12):2782–7.
12. McKiernan PJ, Preece MA, Chakrapani A. Outcome of children with hereditary tyrosinaemia following newborn screening. Arch Dis Child. 2015;100(8):738–41.
13. Haberle J, Boddaert N, Burlina A, et al. Suggested guidelines for the diagnosis and management of urea cycle disorders. Orphanet J Rare Dis. 2012;7:32.
14. Unsinn C, Das A, Valayannopoulos V, et al. Clinical course of 63 patients with neonatal onset urea cycle disorders in the years 2001–2013. Orphanet J Rare Dis. 2016;11(1):116.
15. Wakiya T, Sanada Y, Mizuta K, et al. Living donor liver transplantation for ornithine transcarbamylase deficiency. Pediatr Transplant. 2011;15(4):390–5.
16. Muelly ER, Moore GJ, Bunce SC, et al. Biochemical correlates of neuropsychiatric illness in maple syrup urine disease. J Clin Invest. 2013;123(4):1809–20.
17. Meyburg J, Hoffmann GF. Liver transplantation for inborn errors of metabolism. Transplantation. 2005;80(1 Suppl):S135–7.
18. McBride KL, Miller G, Carter S, et al. Developmental outcomes with early orthotopic liver transplantation for infants with neonatal-onset urea cycle defects and a female patient with late-onset ornithine transcarbamylase deficiency. Pediatrics. 2004;114(4):e523–6.
19. Ah Mew N, Krivitzky L, McCarter R, et al. Clinical outcomes of neonatal onset proximal versus distal urea cycle disorders do not differ. J Pediatr. 2013;162(2):324–9.e1.
20. Perito ER, Rhee S, Roberts JP, et al. Pediatric liver transplantation for urea cycle disorders and organic acidemias: United Network for Organ Sharing data for 2002–2012. Liver Transpl. 2014;20(1):89–99.
21. Morioka D, Kasahara M, Takada Y, et al. Current role of liver transplantation for the treatment of urea cycle disorders: a review of the worldwide English literature and 13 cases at Kyoto University. Liver Transpl. 2005;11(11):1332–42.
22. Rahayatri TH, Uchida H, Sasaki K, et al. Hyperammonemia in ornithine transcarbamylase-deficient recipients following living donor liver transplantation from heterozygous carrier donors. Pediatr Transplant. 2017;21(1).
23. Yu L, Rayhill SC, Hsu EK, et al. Liver transplantation for urea cycle disorders: analysis of the United Network for Organ Sharing Database. Transplant Proc. 2015;47(8):2413–8.
24. Brassier A, Gobin S, Arnoux JB, et al. Long-term outcomes in ornithine transcarbamylase deficiency: a series of 90 patients. Orphanet J Rare Dis. 2015;10:58.
25. Batshaw ML, Tuchman M, Summar M, et al. A longitudinal study of urea cycle disorders. Mol Genet Metab. 2014;113(1–2):127–30.
26. Gallagher RC, Lam C, Wong D, et al. Significant hepatic involvement in patients with ornithine transcarbamylase deficiency. J Pediatr. 2014;164(4):720–25.e6.
27. Vara R, Dhawan A, Deheragoda M, et al. Liver transplantation for neonatal-onset citrullinemia. Pediatr Transplant. 2018;22(4):e13191.
28. Todo S, Starzl TE, Tzakis A, et al. Orthotopic liver transplantation for urea cycle enzyme deficiency. Hepatology. 1992;15(3):419–22.
29. Ishida T, Hiroma T, Hashikura Y, et al. Early neonatal onset carbamoyl-phosphate synthase 1 deficiency treated with continuous hemodiafiltration and early living-related liver transplantation. Pediatr Int. 2009;51(3):409–10.
30. Huang HP, Chien YH, Huang LM, et al. Viral infections and prolonged fever after liver transplantation in young children with inborn errors of metabolism. J Formos Med Assoc. 2005;104(9):623–9.
31. Tuchman M. Persistent a citrullinemia after liver transplantation for carbamylphosphate synthetase deficiency. N Engl J Med. 1989;320(22):1498–9.
32. Kasahara M, Sakamoto S, Shigeta T, et al. Living-donor liver transplantation for carbamoyl phosphate synthetase 1 deficiency. Pediatr Transplant. 2010;14(8):1036–40.
33. Robberecht E, Maesen S, Jonckheere A, et al. Successful liver transplantation for argininosuccinate lyase deficiency (ASLD). J Inherit Metab Dis. 2006;29(1):184–5.
34. Newnham T, Hardikar W, Allen K, et al. Liver transplantation for argininosuccinic aciduria: clinical, biochemical, and metabolic outcome. Liver Transpl. 2008;14(1):41–5.
35. Marble M, McGoey RR, Mannick E, et al. Living related liver transplant in a patient with argininosuccinic aciduria and cirrhosis: metabolic follow-up. J Pediatr Gastroenterol Nutr. 2008;46(4):453–6.
36. Ozcay F, Baris Z, Moray G, et al. Report of 3 patients with urea cycle defects treated with related living-donor liver transplant. Exp Clin Transplant. 2015;13(Suppl 3):126–30.
37. Szymanska E, Kalicinski P, Pawlowska J, et al. Polish experience with liver transplantation and post-transplant outcomes in children with urea cycle disorders. Ann Transplant. 2017;22:555–62.
38. Ranucci G, Martinelli D, Maiorana A, Liguori A, Liccardo D, Candusso M, Cotugno G, Taurisano R, Grimaldi C, Goffredo B, Semeraro M, Cairoli S, Pariante R, Tortor F, Spada M, Torre G, Dionisi Vici C. The impact of liver transplantation on plasma and CSF amino acids in patients with argininosuccinic aciduria. J Pediatr Gastroenterol Nutr Geneve. 2018:634.
39. Kido J, Matsumoto S, Mitsubuchi H, et al. Early liver transplantation in neonatal-onset and moderate urea cycle disorders may lead to normal neurodevelopment. Metab Brain Dis. 2018;33(5):1517–23.
40. Wendel U, Saudubray JM, Bodner A, et al. Liver transplantation in maple syrup urine disease. Eur J Pediatr. 1999;158(Suppl 2):S60–4.
41. Mazariegos GV, Morton DH, Sindhi R, et al. Liver transplantation for classical maple syrup urine disease: long-term follow-up in 37 patients and comparative United Network for Organ Sharing Experience. J Pediatr. 2012;160(1):116–21.e1.
42. Mohan N, Karkra S, Rastogi A, et al. Living donor liver transplantation in maple syrup urine disease—case series and world's youngest domino liver donor and recipient. Pediatr Transplant. 2016;20(3):395–400.
43. Matsunami M, Fukuda A, Sasaki K, et al. Living donor domino liver transplantation using a maple syrup urine disease donor: a case series of three children—the first report from Japan. Pediatr Transplant. 2016;20(5):633–9.
44. Diaz VM, Camarena C, de la Vega A, et al. Liver transplantation for classical maple syrup urine disease: long-term follow-up. J Pediatr Gastroenterol Nutr. 2014;59(5):636–9.

45. Feier F, Schwartz IV, Benkert AR, et al. Living related versus deceased donor liver transplantation for maple syrup urine disease. Mol Genet Metab. 2016;117(3):336–43.
46. Suryawan A, Hawes JW, Harris RA, et al. A molecular model of human branched-chain amino acid metabolism. Am J Clin Nutr. 1998;68(1):72–81.
47. Kamei A, Takashima S, Chan F, et al. Abnormal dendritic development in maple syrup urine disease. Pediatr Neurol. 1992;8(2):145–7.
48. Strauss KA, Mazariegos GV, Sindhi R, et al. Elective liver transplantation for the treatment of classical maple syrup urine disease. Am J Transplant. 2006;6(3):557–64.
49. Zinnanti WJ, Lazovic J, Griffin K, et al. Dual mechanism of brain injury and novel treatment strategy in maple syrup urine disease. Brain. 2009;132(Pt 4):903–18.
50. Al-Shamsi A, Baker A, Dhawan A, et al. Acute metabolic crises in maple syrup urine disease after liver transplantation from a related heterozygous living donor. JIMD Rep. 2016;30:59–62.
51. Barshop BA, Khanna A. Domino hepatic transplantation in maple syrup urine disease. N Engl J Med. 2005;353(22):2410–1.
52. Khanna A, Hart M, Nyhan WL, et al. Domino liver transplantation in maple syrup urine disease. Liver Transpl. 2006;12(5):876–82.
53. Celik N, Squires RH, Vockley J, et al. Liver transplantation for maple syrup urine disease: a global domino effect. Pediatr Transplant. 2016;20(3):350–1.
54. Mayorandan S, Meyer U, Gokcay G, et al. Cross-sectional study of 168 patients with hepatorenal tyrosinaemia and implications for clinical practice. Orphanet J Rare Dis. 2014;9(107):014–0107.
55. McKiernan P. Liver transplantation for hereditary tyrosinaemia type 1 in the United Kingdom. Adv Exp Med Biol. 2017;959:85–91.
56. Vajro P, Strisciuglio P, Houssin D, et al. Correction of phenylketonuria after liver transplantation in a child with cirrhosis. N Engl J Med. 1993;329(5):363. https://doi.org/10.1056/NEJM199307293290517.
57. Crigler JF Jr, Najjar VA. Congenital familial nonhemolytic jaundice with kernicterus. Pediatrics. 1952;10(2):169–80.
58. Sneitz N, Bakker CT, de Knegt RJ, et al. Crigler-Najjar syndrome in the Netherlands: identification of four novel UGT1A1 alleles, genotype-phenotype correlation, and functional analysis of 10 missense mutants. Hum Mutat. 2010;31(1):52–9.
59. Sleisenger MH. Nonhemolytic unconjugated hyperbilirubinemia with hepatic glucuronyl transferase deficiency: a genetic study in four generations. Trans Assoc Am Physicians. 1967;80:259–66.
60. Itoh S, Onishi S. Kinetic study of the photochemical changes of (ZZ)-bilirubin IX alpha bound to human serum albumin. Demonstration of (EZ)-bilirubin IX alpha as an intermediate in photochemical changes from (ZZ)-bilirubin IX alpha to (EZ)-cyclobilirubin IX alpha. Biochem J. 1985;226(1):251–8.
61. Lund HT, Jacobsen J. Influence of phototherapy on the biliary bilirubin excretion pattern in newborn infants with hyperbilirubinemia. J Pediatr. 1974;85(2):262–7.
62. Pett S, Mowat AP. Crigler-Najjar syndrome types I and II. Clinical experience—King's College Hospital 1972–1978. Phenobarbitone, phototherapy and liver transplantation. Mol Aspects Med. 1987;9(5):473–82.
63. Sokal EM, Silva ES, Hermans D, et al. Orthotopic liver transplantation for Crigler-Najjar type I disease in six children. Transplantation. 1995;60(10):1095–8.
64. van der Veere CN, Sinaasappel M, McDonagh AF, et al. Current therapy for Crigler-Najjar syndrome type 1: report of a world registry. Hepatology. 1996;24(2):311–5.
65. Fox IJ, Chowdhury JR, Kaufman SS, et al. Treatment of the Crigler-Najjar syndrome type I with hepatocyte transplantation. N Engl J Med. 1998;338(20):1422–6.
66. Ambrosino G, Varotto S, Strom SC, et al. Isolated hepatocyte transplantation for Crigler-Najjar syndrome type 1. Cell Transplant. 2005;14(2–3):151–7.
67. Ronzitti G, Bortolussi G, van Dijk R, et al. A translationally optimized AAV-UGT1A1 vector drives safe and long-lasting correction of Crigler-Najjar syndrome. Mol Ther Methods Clin Dev. 2016;3:16049.
68. Cochat P, Rumsby G. Primary hyperoxaluria. N Engl J Med. 2013;369(7):649–58.
69. Harambat J, van Stralen KJ, Espinosa L, et al. Characteristics and outcomes of children with primary oxalosis requiring renal replacement therapy. Clin J Am Soc Nephrol. 2012;7(3):458–65.
70. Sasaki K, Sakamoto S, Uchida H, et al. Two-step transplantation for primary hyperoxaluria: a winning strategy to prevent progression of systemic oxalosis in early onset renal insufficiency cases. Pediatr Transplant. 2015;19(1):E1–6.
71. Compagnon P, Metzler P, Samuel D, et al. Long-term results of combined liver-kidney transplantation for primary hyperoxaluria type 1: the French experience. Liver Transpl. 2014;20(12):1475–85.
72. Khorsandi SE, Samyn M, Hassan A, et al. An institutional experience of pre-emptive liver transplantation for pediatric primary hyperoxaluria type 1. Pediatr Transplant. 2016;20(4):523–9.
73. Kemper MJ, Nolkemper D, Rogiers X, et al. Preemptive liver transplantation in primary hyperoxaluria type 1: timing and preliminary results. J Nephrol. 1998;11(Suppl 1):46–8.
74. Cochat P, Hulton SA, Acquaviva C, et al. Primary hyperoxaluria type 1: indications for screening and guidance for diagnosis and treatment. Nephrol Dial Transplant. 2012;27(5):1729–36.
75. Kolker S, Valayannopoulos V, Burlina AB, et al. The phenotypic spectrum of organic acidurias and urea cycle disorders. Part 2: the evolving clinical phenotype. J Inherit Metab Dis. 2015;38(6):1059–74.
76. Shchelochkov OA, Carrillo N, Venditti C. Propionic acidemia. In: Adam MP, Ardinger HH, Pagon RA, Wallace SE, Bean LJH, Stephens K, Amemiya A, editors. . Seattle: GeneReviews®; 1993.
77. Rajakumar A, Kaliamoorthy I, Reddy MS, et al. Anaesthetic considerations for liver transplantation in propionic acidemia. Indian J Anaesth. 2016;60(1):50–4.
78. Kayler LK, Merion RM, Lee S, et al. Long-term survival after liver transplantation in children with metabolic disorders. Pediatr Transplant. 2002;6(4):295–300.
79. Arrizza C, De Gottardi A, Foglia E, et al. Reversal of cardiomyopathy in propionic acidemia after liver transplantation: a 10-year follow-up. Transpl Int. 2015;28(12):1447–50.
80. Charbit-Henrion F, Lacaille F, McKiernan P, et al. Early and late complications after liver transplantation for propionic acidemia in children: a two centers study. Am J Transplant. 2015;15(3):786–91.
81. Vara R, Turner C, Mundy H, et al. Liver transplantation for propionic acidemia in children. Liver Transpl. 2011;17(6):661–7.
82. Sakamoto R, Nakamura K, Kido J, et al. Improvement in the prognosis and development of patients with methylmalonic acidemia after living donor liver transplant. Pediatr Transplant. 2016;20(8):1081–6.
83. Spada M, Calvo PL, Brunati A, et al. Early liver transplantation for neonatal-onset methylmalonic acidemia. Pediatrics. 2015;136(1):e252–6.
84. Kasahara M, Horikawa R, Tagawa M, et al. Current role of liver transplantation for methylmalonic acidemia: a review of the literature. Pediatr Transplant. 2006;10(8):943–7.
85. Niemi AK, Kim IK, Krueger CE, et al. Treatment of methylmalonic acidemia by liver or combined liver-kidney transplantation. J Pediatr. 2015;166(6):1455–61.e1.
86. Sloan JL, Manoli I, Venditti CP. Liver or combined liver-kidney transplantation for patients with isolated methylmalonic acidemia: who and when? J Pediatr. 2015;166(6):1346–50.

87. Lerut JP, Ciccarelli O, Sempoux C, et al. Glycogenosis storage type I diseases and evolutive adenomatosis: an indication for liver transplantation. Transpl Int. 2003;16(12):879–84.
88. Reddy SK, Kishnani PS, Sullivan JA, et al. Resection of hepatocellular adenoma in patients with glycogen storage disease type Ia. J Hepatol. 2007;47(5):658–63.
89. Karaki C, Kasahara M, Sakamoto S, et al. Glycemic management in living donor liver transplantation for patients with glycogen storage disease type 1b. Pediatr Transplant. 2012;16(5):465–70.
90. Chiche L, David A, Adam R, et al. Liver transplantation for adenomatosis: European experience. Liver Transpl. 2016;22(4):516–26.
91. Reddy SK, Austin SL, Spencer-Manzon M, et al. Liver transplantation for glycogen storage disease type Ia. J Hepatol. 2009;51(3):483–90.
92. Davis MK, Weinstein DA. Liver transplantation in children with glycogen storage disease: controversies and evaluation of the risk/benefit of this procedure. Pediatr Transplant. 2008;12(2):137–45.
93. Maya Aparicio AC, Bernal Bellido C, Tinoco Gonzalez J, et al. Fifteen years of follow-up of a liver transplant recipient with glycogen storage disease type Ia (Von Gierke disease). Transplant Proc. 2013;45(10):3668–9.
94. Oishi K, Arnon R, Wasserstein MP, et al. Liver transplantation for pediatric inherited metabolic disorders: considerations for indications, complications, and perioperative management. Pediatr Transplant. 2016;20(6):756–69.
95. Cui H, Li F, Chen D, et al. Comprehensive next-generation sequence analyses of the entire mitochondrial genome reveal new insights into the molecular diagnosis of mitochondrial DNA disorders. Genet Med. 2013;15(5):388–94.
96. Dames S, Chou LS, Xiao Y, et al. The development of next-generation sequencing assays for the mitochondrial genome and 108 nuclear genes associated with mitochondrial disorders. J Mol Diagn. 2013;15(4):526–34.
97. Iwama I, Baba Y, Kagimoto S, et al. Case report of a successful liver transplantation for acute liver failure due to mitochondrial respiratory chain complex III deficiency. Transplant Proc. 2011;43(10):4025–8.
98. Sokal EM, Sokol R, Cormier V, et al. Liver transplantation in mitochondrial respiratory chain disorders. Eur J Pediatr. 1999;158(2):S81–4.
99. Dubern B, Broue P, Dubuisson C, et al. Orthotopic liver transplantation for mitochondrial respiratory chain disorders: a study of 5 children. Transplantation. 2001;71(5):633–7.
100. Durand P, Debray D, Mandel R, et al. Acute liver failure in infancy: a 14-year experience of a pediatric liver transplantation center. J Pediatr. 2001;139(6):871–6.
101. El-Hattab AW, Li F-Y, Schmitt E, et al. MPV17-associated hepatocerebral mitochondrial DNA depletion syndrome: new patients and novel mutations. Mol Genet Metab. 2010;99(3):300–8.
102. Dimmock DP, Dunn JK, Feigenbaum A, et al. Abnormal neurological features predict poor survival and should preclude liver transplantation in patients with deoxyguanosine kinase deficiency. Liver Transpl. 2008;14(10):1480–5.
103. Lee WS, Sokol RJ. Mitochondrial hepatopathies: advances in genetics, therapeutic approaches, and outcomes. J Pediatr. 2013;163(4):942–8.
104. Parikh S, Karaa A, Goldstein A, et al. Solid organ transplantation in primary mitochondrial disease: proceed with caution. Mol Genet Metab. 2016;118(3):178–84.
105. Sasaki K, Sakamoto S, Uchida H, et al. Liver transplantation for mitochondrial respiratory chain disorder: a single-Center experience and excellent marker of differential diagnosis. Transplant Proc. 2017;49(5):1097–102.
106. Grabhorn E, Tsiakas K, Herden U, et al. Long-term outcomes after liver transplantation for deoxyguanosine kinase deficiency: a single-center experience and a review of the literature. Liver Transpl. 2014;20(4):464–72.
107. Pigeon N, Campeau PM, Cyr D, et al. Clinical heterogeneity in ethylmalonic encephalopathy. J Child Neurol. 2009;24(8):991–6.
108. Dionisi-Vici C, Diodato D, Torre G, et al. Liver transplant in ethylmalonic encephalopathy: a new treatment for an otherwise fatal disease. Brain. 2016;139(Pt 4):1045–51.
109. Haack TB, Staufner C, Kopke MG, et al. Biallelic mutations in NBAS cause recurrent acute liver failure with onset in infancy. Am J Hum Genet. 2015;97(1):163–9.
110. Staufner C, Haack TB, Kopke MG, et al. Recurrent acute liver failure due to NBAS deficiency: phenotypic spectrum, disease mechanisms, and therapeutic concepts. J Inherit Metab Dis. 2016;39(1):3–16.
111. Julier C, Nicolino M. Wolcott-Rallison syndrome. Orphanet J Rare Dis. 2010;5:29.
112. Tzakis AG, Nunnelley MJ, Tekin A, et al. Liver, pancreas and kidney transplantation for the treatment of Wolcott-Rallison syndrome. Am J Transplant. 2015;15(2):565–7.
113. Rivera E, Gupta S, Chavers B, et al. En bloc multiorgan transplant (liver, pancreas, and kidney) for acute liver and renal failure in a patient with Wolcott-Rallison syndrome. Liver Transpl. 2016;22(3):371–4.
114. Elsabbagh AM, Hawksworth J, Khan KM, et al. World's smallest combined en bloc liver-pancreas transplantation. Pediatr Transplant. 2018;22(1).
115. Baric I. Inherited disorders in the conversion of methionine to homocysteine. J Inherit Metab Dis. 2009;32(4):459–71.
116. Strauss KA, Ferreira C, Bottiglieri T, et al. Liver transplantation for treatment of severe S-adenosylhomocysteine hydrolase deficiency. Mol Genet Metab. 2015;116(1–2):44–52.
117. Matsunami M, Shimozawa N, Fukuda A, et al. Living-donor liver transplantation from a heterozygous parent for infantile refsum disease. Pediatrics. 2016;137(6).
118. Khanna A, Gish R, Winter SC, et al. Successful domino liver transplantation from a patient with methylmalonic acidemia. JIMD Rep. 2016;25:87–94.
119. Popescu I, Dima SO. Domino liver transplantation: how far can we push the paradigm? Liver Transpl. 2012;18(1):22–8.
120. Stephenne X, Debray FG, Smets F, et al. Hepatocyte transplantation using the domino concept in a child with tetrabiopterin nonresponsive phenylketonuria. Cell Transplant. 2012;21(12):2765–70.
121. Rela M, Muiesan P, Vilca-Melendez H, et al. Auxiliary partial orthotopic liver transplantation for Crigler-Najjar syndrome type I. Ann Surg. 1999;229(4):565–9.
122. Rela M, Bharathan A, Palaniappan K, et al. Portal flow modulation in auxiliary partial orthotopic liver transplantation. Pediatr Transplant. 2015;19(3):255–60.
123. Reddy MS, Rajalingam R, Rela M. Revisiting APOLT for metabolic liver disease: a new look at an old idea. Transplantation. 2017;101(2):260–6.
124. Rela M, Battula N, Madanur M, et al. Auxiliary liver transplantation for propionic acidemia: a 10-year follow-up. Am J Transplant. 2007;7(9):2200–3.
125. Govil S, Shanmugam NP, Reddy MS, et al. A metabolic chimera: two defective genotypes make a normal phenotype. Liver Transpl. 2015 Nov;21(11):1453–4. https://doi.org/10.1002/lt.24202.
126. D'Antiga L, Colledan M. Surgical gene therapy by domino auxiliary liver transplantation. Liver Transpl. 2015;21(11):1338–9. https://doi.org/10.1002/lt.24326.
127. Iansante V, Mitry RR, Filippi C, et al. Human hepatocyte transplantation for liver disease: current status and future perspectives. Pediatr Res. 2018;83(1–2):232–40.
128. Muraca M, Gerunda G, Neri D, et al. Hepatocyte transplantation as a treatment for glycogen storage disease type

1a. Lancet. 2002;359(9303):317–8. https://doi.org/10.1016/S0140-6736(02)07529-3.
129. Horslen SP, McCowan TC, Goertzen TC, et al. Isolated hepatocyte transplantation in an infant with a severe urea cycle disorder. Pediatrics. 2003;111(6 Pt 1):1262–7.
130. Sokal EM, Smets F, Bourgois A, et al. Hepatocyte transplantation in a 4-year-old girl with peroxisomal biogenesis disease: technique, safety, and metabolic follow-up. Transplantation. 2003;76(4):735–8.
131. Mitry RR, Dhawan A, Hughes RD, et al. One liver, three recipients: segment IV from split-liver procedures as a source of hepatocytes for cell transplantation. Transplantation. 2004;77(10):1614–6.
132. Darwish AA, Sokal E, Stephenne X, et al. Permanent access to the portal system for cellular transplantation using an implantable port device. Liver Transpl. 2004;10(9):1213–5.
133. Dhawan A, Mitry RR, Hughes RD, et al. Hepatocyte transplantation for inherited factor VII deficiency. Transplantation. 2004;78(12):1812–4.
134. Meyburg J, Opladen T, Spiekerkotter U, et al. Human heterologous liver cells transiently improve hyperammonemia and ureagenesis in individuals with severe urea cycle disorders. J Inherit Metab Dis. 2018;41(1):81–90.
135. Morioka D, Takada Y, Kasahara M, et al. Living donor liver transplantation for noncirrhotic inheritable metabolic liver diseases: impact of the use of heterozygous donors. Transplantation. 2005;80(5):623–8.
136. Rahayatri TH, Uchida H, Sasaki K, et al. Hyperammonemia in ornithine transcarbamylase-deficient recipients following living donor liver transplantation from heterozygous carrier donors. Pediatr Transplant. 2017;21(1). doi: https://doi.org/10.1111/petr.12848.

Immune Tolerance After Liver Transplantation

Sandy Feng and Alberto Sanchez-Fueyo

Abbreviations

CNI	Calcineurin inhibitor
DC	Dendritic cell
DSA	Donor-specific antibody
HCV	Hepatitis C virus
HLA	Human leukocyte antigen
IFN-γ	Interferon gamma
iNKTs	Invariant natural killer T cells
IS	Immunosuppression
LPS	Lipopolysaccharide
LSEC	Liver sinusoidal endothelial cell
MHC	Major histocompatibility complex
MLR	Mixed lymphocyte reaction
NK	Natural killer
PBMC	Peripheral blood mononuclear cell
PD-1	Programmed cell death protein 1
pDC	Plasmacytoid dendritic cell
PD-L1	Programmed death-ligand 1
TLR	Toll-like receptor
Tregs	Regulatory T cells

> **Key Points**
> - In contrast to what happens when non-liver allografts are transplanted into experimental animal models, and when liver transplants are performed in humans, in many animal models, liver allografts are spontaneously accepted. Following transplantation, these recipients develop a very robust state of donor-specific tolerance.
> - In animal models, spontaneous liver allograft tolerance is characterized both by the depletion of recipient T cells recognizing donor alloantigens and by the development of immunoregulatory mechanisms.
> - Prospective, multicenter clinical trials of immunosuppression withdrawal have shown that selected adult and pediatric liver transplant recipients are spontaneously tolerant, most commonly defined according to both biochemical and histological criteria assessed 1 year after complete discontinuation of all immunosuppression.
> - Donor-specific antibodies (DSA) which have been associated with chronic graft injury in both adult and pediatric liver transplant recipients are not prohibitive of successful immunosuppression withdrawal. Patients with DSA prior to initiating withdrawal and those who develop DSA during withdrawal have stopped immunosuppression and maintained stable graft biochemistry and histology during follow-up.
> - Until there is a reliable biomarker of tolerance, liver biopsy is an essential assessment for both eligibility prior to initiating immunosuppression withdrawal and for tolerance after successful discontinuation of immunosuppression.
> - Current efforts to induce liver transplant tolerance are centered around administration of immunomodulatory cell products, most commonly ex vivo expanded, autologous, regulatory T cells (Tregs) of either polyclonal or donor specificity, with or without conditioning with a depleting agent.
> - Although multiple biomarkers of liver transplant tolerance have been described in the literature, none of them have been adequately validated and proven to be useful in the identification of patients who can safely stop their immunosuppression.

S. Feng (✉)
Division of Transplantation, Department of Surgery, University of California San Francisco, San Francisco, CA, USA
e-mail: Sandy.Feng@ucsf.edu

A. Sanchez-Fueyo
Institute of Liver Studies, King's College, London, London, UK
e-mail: sanchez_fueyo@kcl.ac.uk

> **Research Needed in the Field**
> - Specific mechanisms underlying spontaneous tolerance based in the host immune system and/or within the liver allograft itself should be identified in humans. Whether these mechanisms are also relevant as well to patients who maintain stable liver function on minimal doses of immunosuppression (IS) needs to be established.
> - International prospective clinical trials aiming to validate previously described biomarkers of tolerance are currently underway. Efforts to identify, test, and validate additional new markers remain worthwhile.
> - Approaches to induce tolerance, including the administration of various cellular therapy products with immunomodulatory effects, should be tested for safety and efficacy either in de novo or pre-existing liver transplant recipients.

36.1 The Tolerogenic Nature of Liver Immunobiology

In addition to its metabolic, detoxifying, and synthetic functions, the liver acts as a unique immunological organ designed to detect and eliminate pathogens derived from the gut, without eliciting undesirable, destructive immune responses against food-derived antigens and intestinal bacterial degradation products [1]. The liver's anatomy and its detailed microscopic architecture are critical to ensure the effective clearance of pathogens translocating from the gut into the portal venous system [2]. The liver receives its blood supply both from an arterial and a venous system, with the venous blood representing 80% of the overall flow into the liver. On entering the liver, the arterial and portal vein blood flows mix in the liver sinusoids, a unique capillary bed of very narrow vascular channels lined by the liver sinusoidal endothelial cells (LSEC) that channel blood from the portal tracts into the central vein. This intrahepatic blood flow has low oxygen pressure and a velocity that is much slower than other capillary systems. Furthermore, the LSECs have transcellular fenestrations, arranged in the so-called sieve plates that occupy 6–10% of the sinusoidal surface area. This feature facilitates the bi-directional transfer of small substrates between the sinusoidal blood and the space of Disse and also allows interactions between the hepatocytes and circulating T cells (Fig. 36.1). In addition to being capable, as any other endothelial cell, of presenting endogenous antigens on major histocompatibility complex (MHC) class I molecules to CD8+T cells, the LSECs can cross-present exogenous antigens on MHC-I and MHC-II molecules to both CD4+ and CD8+ T cells. The sinusoidal lumens are occupied by the Kupffer cells, a large contingent of liver-resident, immobile macrophages that represent 90% of all tissue-resident macrophages and that express MHC-I and II molecules, toll-like receptors (TLRs), costimulatory molecules, and complement and antibody receptors. Kupffer cells are extremely efficient at surveilling the sinusoidal blood in quest of pathogens that may have crossed the intestinal epithelial barrier and entered the bloodstream. The sinusoids also contain the body's largest pool of two populations of innate lymphocytes, the natural killer (NK) cells and the invariant natural killer T cells (iNKTs). Although these two immune cell populations are activated by different ligands and exert distinct effector functions, they both have the capacity to screen for pathogens and to identify pathology. As such, they contribute to the liver's immune surveillance role. Hepatocytes, which are the main parenchymal cell type, also express a variety of immune receptors (including MHC-I and under inflammatory conditions also MHC-II) and are capable of detecting pathogens and presenting their antigens to T cells. The liver also contains various subpopulations of dendritic cells (DCs), preferentially located in portal tracts and around central veins, that are very efficient at internalizing and presenting exogenous antigens to T cells. Altogether, the liver microanatomy is clearly organized so as to maximize interactions between the portal blood contents and a large repertoire of cells with variable immune properties. The preferential enrichment in phagocytes and other innate immune cells and the strategic position of the liver downstream of the gut together suggest that the preeminent immune function of the liver is to act as a filter that effectively removes gut-derived pathogens and associated molecules before they reach the systemic circulation and the secondary lymphoid organs.

A potential risk of the microcirculatory architecture and immune sentinel role of the liver described above is the development of harmful adaptive immune responses against foreign but nonpathogenic antigens such as molecules derived from food or commensal gut bacteria. The balance between effective innate immune responses toward pathogens without the development of pathogenic T cell-mediated responses against innocuous stimuli is achieved by a microenvironment that favors immunological tolerance. Thus, antigen presentation taking place in the liver by either professional (e.g., DCs and macrophages) or nonprofessional (e.g., hepatocytes and LSECs) antigen-presenting cells results in T cell activation and proliferation, but not in the development of cytopathic effector functions. This state of intrahepatic adaptive immune hyporesponsiveness is maintained by a variety of different mechanisms. The one that has been studied more extensively is the phenomenon of "endotoxin tolerance", which involves the de-sensitization of TLR4 receptors expressed on liver antigen presenting cells to bacterial lipopolysaccharide (LPS) as a result of the continuous LPS exposure provided by gut-derived portal blood

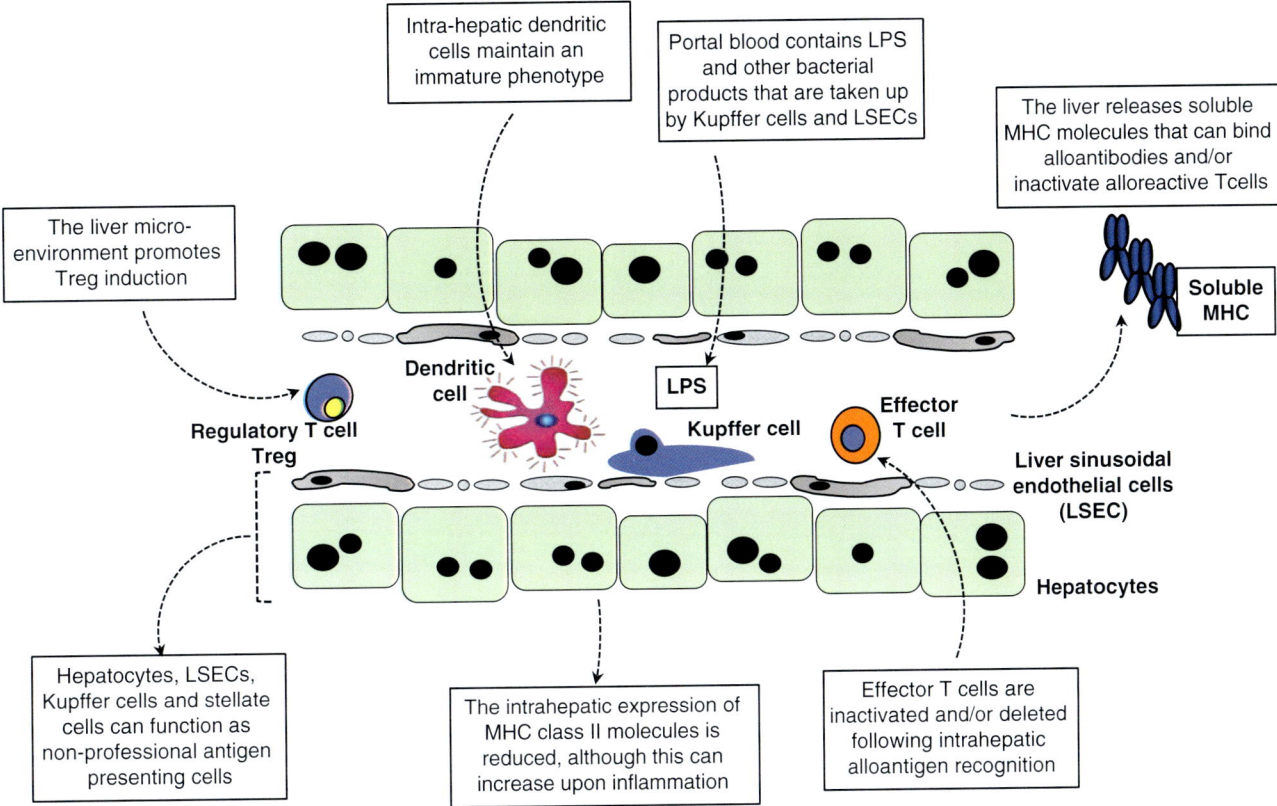

Fig. 36.1 Mechanisms of spontaneous liver allograft tolerance: The liver contains multiple subsets of DCs, which are professional antigen-presenting cells, but that tend to maintain an immature and non-immunogenic phenotype. Kupffer cells, LSEC, stellate cells, and hepatocytes can also act as nonprofessional antigen-presenting cells but tend to deliver suboptimal T cell priming and induce dysfunctional T cells. Continuous exposure to LPS by cells expressing TLR4, such as Kupffer cells and LSEC, results in downregulation of costimulatory molecules and production of immunosuppressive cytokines. Spontaneous liver allograft tolerance requires the presence of Tregs, whose generation is promoted by the liver microenvironment. The liver releases substantial amounts of MHC molecules (particularly class I) which can exert immunomodulatory properties

flow. TLRs recognize conserved bacterial and viral motifs and typically activate pro-inflammatory signaling pathways. The most studied TLR is TLR4 which, in response to LPS binding, activates a number of pro-inflammatory mediators. Continuous exposure to low levels of gut-derived LPS, however, results in upregulation of TLR4 signaling inhibitors that block the production of pro-inflammatory cytokines while maintaining the secretion of immunosuppressive mediators such as interleukin 10 and transforming growth factor-β. TLR4 hyporesponsiveness and the immunosuppressive cytokine microenvironment that results from it disrupt the signaling pathways of other TLRs and are closely linked to a number of phenomena that dampen T cell responses such as blockade of DC maturation, low expression of costimulatory molecules, and promotion of T cell exhaustion through upregulation of inhibitory receptors such as programmed cell death protein 1 (PD-1), T cell immunoglobulin and mucin domain 3, and cytotoxic T lymphocyte antigen 4. The latter is amplified by the expression of the ligand of PD-1 (PD-L1) by LSECs.

36.2 The Liver Tolerance Effect in Transplantation Models

The liver's unique environment is distinctly apparent in the setting of liver transplantation as it is responsible for the spontaneous acceptance of liver allografts observed in many animal models. This was first demonstrated in pigs [3] and subsequently in rats [4] (in which spontaneous tolerance or rejection occur depending on the donor-recipient strain combination) and then in mice [5]. Animals spontaneously accepting MHC-mismatched liver allografts develop donor-specific tolerance, which allows them to accept skin grafts from the same donor without the need for therapeutic immunosuppression (IS). Rodent models of spontaneous liver allograft tolerance have been particularly useful in providing mechanistic information. A key aspect of the development of spontaneous liver allograft tolerance is the observation that, shortly after transplantation, recipient lymphocytes infiltrate the transplanted liver and accumulate in the portal and central areas

[6]. Liver-infiltrating lymphocytes become activated and induce a mild degree of parenchymal damage with increased serum aminotransferases. However, instead of destroying the graft, they are gradually cleared from the liver by a phenomenon that likely involves lymphocyte apoptosis and/or T cell degradation within hepatocyte lysosomes (suicidal emperipolesis) [7, 8]. Both parenchymal (e.g., LSECs, hepatocytes) and non-parenchymal (e.g., DCs, NKT cells) cells are involved in these mechanisms, as well as specific cell subsets of the recipient immune system. Thus, at least in the mouse model, if recipient CD4+CD25+forkhead box protein 3 (FOXP3)+ regulatory T cells (Tregs) are depleted before transplantation using an anti-CD25 antibody, the development of tolerance is blocked, and the allograft is destroyed by the recipient immune system [9]. In this regard, spontaneous liver transplant tolerance is similar to what occurs in multiple animal models in which tolerance to other organs is therapeutically induced [10]. In animal models, demonstration of donor-specific immune unresponsiveness in vivo, typically obtained by challenging the tolerant recipient with a same-donor or third-party graft, is considered as a hallmark of allograft tolerance. Somehow paradoxically, this is often difficult to prove in vitro when employing mixed lymphocyte reactions (MLR) or cytotoxicity assays. For instance, in the setting of spontaneous liver allograft tolerance in rats and mice, MLR assays fail to identify decreased anti-donor reactivity, a phenomenon that has been called *split tolerance* [11]. The observation that spontaneously tolerant animal recipients retain anti-donor immune responses is very relevant to the immune monitoring of human liver transplant recipients and suggests that the depletion of alloreactive T cells that is observed in animal models of spontaneous does not result in the complete deletion of the alloreactive repertoire [12]. The lack of correlation between tolerance, donor-specific MLR responses, and deletion of alloreactive T cells has also been reported among kidney transplant recipients who have undergone tolerance induction through the establishment of mixed donor-recipient hematopoietic chimerism [13].

36.3 Important Definitions of Tolerance in the Clinical Setting

As we shift to consideration of tolerance in the clinical setting, it is first necessary to establish definitions for important terms. *Tolerance* is currently used to denote a state whereby a transplanted organ remains healthy in the complete absence of IS for 1 year or more. Historically, the state of the organ was simply evaluated biochemically, most commonly using liver tests. However, recognizing that normal liver tests can belie significant histopathology, liver biopsy is now expected as part of the adjudication of tolerance [14, 15]. Tolerance in the clinical setting is *operational,* as it connotes a functional state. *Spontaneous tolerance* most commonly refers to a tolerant state that was attained without special treatment(s) and unveiled by stopping IS. This contrasts with *induced tolerance* whereby patients stop IS after receiving treatment designed to achieve tolerance. Implicit in these definitions is that the recipient is unresponsive to donor antigens but remains responsive to non-donor antigens. Such donor-specific hyporesponsiveness or unresponsiveness, compared to a third party, has however not been consistently demonstrated.

36.4 History of Immunosuppression Withdrawal in Transplantation

Although the liver is widely regarded as the "most tolerogenic" organ among those transplanted, the first reports of apparently stable organ function—based on laboratory assessment—in the absence of IS emerged more than 40 years ago in kidney transplantation. Owens and colleagues reported on four recipients of living donor kidney transplants who appeared to maintain stable graft function after stopping IS for 17–52 months [16]. This sentinel report prompted national surveys identifying patients who had discontinued IS with variable success [16, 17]. Some in the community were understandably intrigued by the possibility of continued allograft function without IS, urging a "wait and see" approach, whereby IS would be restarted only in response to rejection. However, John S. Najarian, Chief of Transplantation at the University of Minnesota, sounded an alarm against such a "dangerous" and "extremely controversial" approach. Citing four graft losses resulting from irreversible rejection among five patients who stopped IS, he strongly advocated that transplant physicians restart IS for kidney transplant recipients immediately upon gaining knowledge that IS has been discontinued.

After this brief spate of reports of spontaneous tolerance in kidney transplant recipients, there was essential silence regarding purported "spontaneous tolerance" for kidney transplant recipients for several decades. However, several decades later, reports of IS discontinuation with maintenance of stable allograft function among liver transplant recipients began to emerge. These clinical experiences reflected a popular mechanism of operational tolerance that had been explored in animal models and widely discussed. Thomas E. Starzl and colleagues noted that long-term liver transplant recipients were donor-recipient chimeras not only in the allograft but often in the peripheral blood, skin, lymph nodes, and other organs. The detection of multi-lineage chimerism, indicating migration and survival of donor cells from the allograft into multiple recipient tissues, was much more striking in liver recipients, compared to other organ transplant recipients, leading them to suggest that this phenomenon may explain the tolerogenic nature of the liver [18–20]. Moreover, they also suggested that chimerism might be, in essence, a biomarker indicative of permissive conditions for IS withdrawal.

Multiple features of common clinical practice corroborated the impression that the liver was less vulnerable to permanent damage from either cellular or humoral alloimmune responses. Liver transplants have always been performed without any attention to allosensitization and without prospective crossmatching. In spite of this seemingly "cavalier" approach, acute, antibody-mediated rejection has been rare [21, 22]. Acute cellular rejection occurred frequently but was readily reversed without clear long-term sequelae [23, 24]. Moreover, with the substitution of tacrolimus for cyclosporine as the mainstay of IS regimens, acute cellular rejection rates dropped, and chronic rejection essentially disappeared [6, 25]. These clinical observations, in combination with data from large and small animal models confirming the unique tolerogenic nature of the liver, have spurred interest in IS withdrawal among several transplant centers.

36.5 Earliest Reports of Immunosuppression Withdrawal for Liver Transplant Recipients

The earliest publications regarding liver transplant recipients who were no longer taking IS emanated from the University of Pittsburgh [26–28] (Table 36.1). The first series, published in 1993, comprised of six patients (accounting for 15% of all liver transplant recipients followed for more than 10 years) who stopped IS on their own volition [26]. However, as one was described as remaining on prednisone (10 mgs/day) with a failing graft (secondary to recurrent chronic active hepatitis), he/she will not be considered to be tolerant. The remaining five tolerant patients stopped IS approximately 1, 2, 9, 10, and 11 years after transplant and had been off 13, 11, 10, 5, and 7 years, respectively. They maintained "normal liver function," although it does not seem as if any biopsies were available to attest to the histological status of the allograft.

The second series, published in 1994 also from Pittsburgh [27], comprised of seven children who developed conditions necessitating discontinuation of IS very early after transplantation: five had posttransplant lymphoproliferative disorder, while two had severe hepatitis C virus (HCV) infection; one patient suffered from both conditions (Table 36.1). Four of the seven had a prior history of one, two, or multiple episodes of acute cellular rejection. IS was stopped 0.5–1.3 years after transplant, and six of the seven (86%) remained off for 1.3–2.8 years with an unremarkable liver biopsy at the end of the reported follow-up. One of the seven (14%) was considered non-tolerant, able to stay off IS for only 0.9 months with a biopsy showing both acute cellular rejection and HCV. Notably, both patients with HCV died after retransplantation. In considering this seminal publication, several issues deserve mention as they portend important considerations for future studies (Table 36.2). First, in the words of the authors themselves, "the early timing of tolerance and the association with life-threatening viral infections differentiate these patients from those who had the IS withdrawn systematically" [26]. Second, availability of histological assessment in addition to clinical and biochemical assessment to evidence tolerance at the end of follow-up is a clear strength of the study. Third, the authors performed in vitro MLR assays and concluded that tolerant subjects were immunocompetent. However, donor-specific hyporesponsiveness, determined by differential responses to donor versus third-party antigens, was identified in only two of the six tolerant subjects.

In 1995, the third publication emerged from Pittsburgh [28] on a distinct and larger cohort of patients, both adult and pediatric, who specifically underwent physician-directed,

Table 36.1 Three earliest publications of IS withdrawal in liver transplant recipients

Year	First author (reference)	Description of cohort	Time since transplant	Liver biopsy Pre-wean	Liver biopsy Post-wean	Outcome: Successful/attempted	Duration off of IS
1993	Starzl [26]	Non-compliant subjects	1–11 years	NA	NA	NA	5–13 years
1994	Tsakis [27]	IS stopped because of every contraindication to ongoing IS: posttransplant lymphoproliferative disease ($n = 4$), hepatitis C ($n = 2$), and both posttransplant lymphoproliferative disease and hepatitis C ($n = 1$)	0.5–1.3 years	No	Yes	6/7	1.3–2.8 years
1995	Ramos [28]	Prospectively weaned Subjects must (1) be without rejection for ≥ 1 year; (2) be medically compliant; (3) have IS-related complication; (4) have cooperative primary physician	≥ 5 years required; Actual: 10.25 ± 4.3 years	Yes	No	16/59[a]	3–19 months

IS immunosuppression, *NA* not applicable
[a] Among 59 patients who initiated immunosuppression withdrawal, 16 subjects were off of medications for 3–19 months, 28 were still withdrawing, and 15 had experienced rejection

Table 36.2 Important considerations regarding trials of immunosuppression withdrawal

Prior to initiation of withdrawal	During withdrawal until the assessment of tolerance	Assessment of tolerance	Follow-up after tolerance assessment

Were specific inclusion/exclusion criteria specified?
• Living and/or deceased donor recipients
• Transplant indication
• Time after transplant
• Acceptable liver test thresholds
• Current IS regimen: number of medications, medication dose, or trough levels
• Eligibility biopsy
  – Central or local pathologist assessment
	• Was there a clearly specified algorithm for IS withdrawal?
	• What was the frequency of laboratory assessments?
	• Were there thresholds of laboratory values that mandated liver biopsy?
	• Was a second attempt at IS withdrawal allowed after an episode of rejection?
		• Was tolerance formally adjudicated?
		• If so, when relative to the last IS dose?
		• Were there formal criteria to adjudicate tolerance?
		  – Biochemical
		  – Histological
		  – Mechanistic
			• For how long were tolerant subjects followed?
			• For how long were non-tolerant subjects followed?
			• How were they followed?
			  – Biochemically
			  – Histologically
			  – Mechanistically

stepwise weaning of IS (Table 36.1). It is similarly worthwhile to present this report in some detail as again, it foreshadows important issues related to future series (Table 36.2). The investigators prospectively evaluated 72 long-term, stable liver transplant recipients for IS weaning. Eligibility criteria were clearly specified: subjects had to (a) be ≥5 years after transplant, (b) without rejection for ≥1 year, (c) be medically compliant, (d) experience complication(s) related to chronic IS, (e) have the cooperation of their primary physician, and (f) undergo a baseline liver biopsy that shows no evidence of rejection or severe hepatic disease. Thirteen of the evaluated subjects were disqualified (6 secondary to biopsy findings), leaving 59 subjects (20 were 12–20 years of age, 39 were 21–68 years of age) who initiated withdrawal 10.25 ± 4.3 years after transplant. All subjects were on prednisone, a calcineurin inhibitor (CNI), and/or azathioprine: 15 (25.4%) were on CNI monotherapy, 32 (59.4%) were on a two-drug regimen, and 12 (20.3%) were on a three-drug regimen. The order of drug withdrawal was azathioprine followed by prednisone followed by CNI; subjects failing a corticotrophin stimulation test were considered off of prednisone if dose was less than 5 mg/day. IS dose reductions were considered monthly, albeit not mandated. Liver tests (ALT, AST, GGT, and bilirubin) were checked weekly to biweekly.

At the time of publication, 16 of the 59 subjects (27.1%) had been off of medications for 3–19 months (although two were on prednisone at a dose of <5 mg/day), 28 subjects (47.4%) were still weaning, and 15 (25.4%) had experienced rejection and thus failed withdrawal. Success rates appeared to vary with transplant indication and initial IS regimen although the significant proportion of subjects still weaning make it difficult to draw definitive conclusions. Among those transplanted for biliary atresia, success rates appeared high ($n = 16$; eight off drug, three rejected, and five still weaning). In contrast, success rates appeared lower for those transplanted for primary biliary cirrhosis ($n = 9$; one off drug, three rejected, and five still weaning) or alpha-1-antitrypsin deficiency ($n = 9$; one off drug, one rejected, and seven still weaning). Success rates appeared high for those on tacrolimus monotherapy ($n = 6$; four off drug, one rejected, one still weaning), prednisone+azathioprine ($n = 10$; seven off drug, one rejected, two still weaning), and cyclosporine monotherapy ($n = 9$; four off drug, one rejected, and four still weaning). Interestingly, those on tacrolimus monotherapy were earliest after transplantation (5.4 ± 1.8 years), those on prednisone+azathioprine were the longest after transplantation (16.0 ± 4.3 years), and those on cyclosporine monotherapy were in between (9.7 ± 2.8 years). Success rates appeared low for those on CNI-based two- or three-drug regimens ($n = 34$; 1 off drug, 11 rejected, 22 still withdrawing).

Of the 15 episodes of rejection, 12 were biopsy-proven, while 3 were clinical in that biopsies were nondiagnostic for rejection but subjects were nevertheless treated. Histologically, ten subjects were classified as having minimal to mild rejection and two subjects with moderate to severe rejection. Subjects received methylprednisolone, one gram intravenously, followed by a 6-day oral prednisone cycle from 200 mgs to 10 mgs/day. One subject required two courses of pulse corticosteroids and developed herpes keratitis that was successfully treated; this was considered the only serious complication of the trial.

In considering the results of this trial, the authors suggested that "a significant percentage of appropriately selected long-surviving liver recipients can unknowingly achieve drug-free graft acceptance. Such attempts should not be contemplated until 5–10 years post-transplantation and then only with careful case selection, close monitoring, and prompt reinstitution of IS when necessary" [28]. These conclusions were also supported by the sobering results of attempting cyclosporine withdrawal to improve renal insufficiency in 12 patients early after transplantation (3 ± 1 years) on a triple-drug regimen [29]. Six subjects (50%) experienced acute rejection; all were treated with intravenous corticosteroid pulse, but two required additional treatment with OKT3. In total, three subjects developed ductopenic rejection and ultimately two died of sepsis.

Subsequent to these sentinel publications suggesting that some liver transplant recipients were indeed spontaneously tolerant of their allografts, additional reports of IS withdrawal for diverse populations and indications emerged from multiple other centers (Tables 36.3, 36.4, and 36.5). The rigor with which IS was withdrawn and tolerance was assessed varied greatly, highlighting the need for prospective, multicenter trials.

36.6 Single Center Reports of Immunosuppression Withdrawal for Adult Liver Transplant Recipients

In addition to ongoing reports from Pittsburgh as they continued to pursue spontaneous tolerance [30, 31], four European adult transplant centers—Kings' College [32, 33], Murcia [34, 35], Tor Vergata [36, 37], and Pamplona [38]—have published results (Table 36.3); three additional single center trials are listed in ClinicalTrials.gov, but no publications are as yet available (Table 36.4). The experiences encompassed small numbers of disparate subjects, weaned and followed according to different protocols. Taken together, however, important messages emerged. First, and perhaps most importantly, these reports confirmed the waning enthusiasm to include subjects transplanted for autoimmune liver disease such as autoimmune hepatitis, primary biliary cirrhosis, and primary sclerosing cholangitis, because of high rates of rejection, occurrence of recurrent disease, and potential to precipitate other autoimmune conditions. Second, subjects with HCV were recognized as a distinct group with the possible benefit of slowing recurrent disease and fibrosis progression that can result in graft failure and need for re-transplantation. Of course, the current availability of highly efficacious antiviral therapeutics has lessened the relevance of these goals. Third, although inclusion/exclusion criteria for elective weaning often did not exclude subjects within 5 years of transplant, the majority of enrolled subjects were indeed more than 5 years after transplant. With this general homogeneity, time after transplantation did not consistently correlate with the success or failure of withdrawal. Indeed, there were no clinical factors that were consistently associated with spontaneous tolerance across the reports. Fourth, physician-directed, gradual IS dose reduction appeared safe. The rapid identification of allograft dysfunction, facilitated by frequent assessment of liver tests followed by expeditious liver biopsy leading to the diagnosis and treatment of acute rejection, appeared to limit allograft injury. Fifth, liver biopsy was variably utilized for the assessment of either eligibility or tolerance. In its absence, the histological status of the allograft, both prior to and after weaning, was unknown, raising questions as to whether success rates would have been different in that inappropriate patients were allowed to wean and/or identified as tolerant.

36.7 Single Center Reports of Immunosuppression Withdrawal for Pediatric Liver Transplant Recipients

There has been a parallel thread of single center reports regarding IS withdrawal in pediatric liver transplant recipients (Table 36.5) [39–44]. As many were from Asian centers, recipients of living donor liver transplant dominated. In considering the reports focused on elective, physician-directed IS withdrawal, the largest and most notable experience from Kyoto University Hospital deserves more detailed consideration [42, 45–48]. Encouraged by the outcomes of stopping IS for toxicities and contraindications, Kyoto established a protocol to wean all stable long-term patients that they were following, defined as recipients more than 2 years posttransplant, without an episode of rejection in the preceding year, and with normal graft function (Fig. 36.2). The final retrospective analysis of the entire experience was last published in 2012 [47]. In total, between June 1990 and April 2008, 670 pediatric patients underwent living donor liver transplantation, and 537 were alive at the time of analysis. Nearly two-thirds ($n = 347$; 65%) were never weaned nor assessed for weaning predominantly because of inadequate follow-up (27%), unstable liver tests (25%), recent rejection episode (13%), too early after transplant (11%), the lack of a cooperative local physician (8%), re-transplantation (5%), or other reasons. Among the remaining 190, 132 were electively withdrawn with 50 (38%) spontaneously tolerant; 58 were nonelectively withdrawn with 34 (59%) spontaneously tolerant (Table 36.5).

The Kyoto experience, covered in multiple publications over more than 10 years, offers several important lessons for IS withdrawal to identify spontaneously tolerant subjects. First, since the transplant center established a protocol to systematically wean all eligible patients as their standard of care, these reports describe the largest cohort of electively weaned patients. The cohort was comprised exclusively of pediatric recipients of living donor grafts, most often from parental donors (one human leukocyte antigen (HLA) haplotype matched); questions regarding relevance to adult and/or deceased donor recipients are naturally raised. Second, in 2003, the Kyoto group instituted a protocol to perform surveillance biopsies 1, 2, 5, and 10 years after transplant, even if all liver tests were normal [46, 48]. Features of acute or chronic rejection, bridging fibrosis, or progression of fibrosis compared to a previous biopsy prompted escalation or reintroduction IS. They reported that spontaneously tolerant patients exhibited higher fibrosis stage than those maintained

Table 36.3 Published single center trials of IS withdrawal for adult liver transplant recipients

Center Reference (year)	Important inclusion/ exclusion criteria	Time since transplant	Outcome Successful/ attempted	Liver biopsy Pre-wean	Liver biopsy Post-wean	Duration off of IS	Comments

Pittsburgh[a] 1997 [30] 2007 [31]	• ≥2 years without rejection
	• Compliant
	• Cooperative local physician
	• Subjects transplanted for viral hepatitis and autoimmune disease were included
		• >5 years required; Actual 8.4 ± 4.4 years	18/95 19%[b]	Yes	Not all subjects	• 1997 publication: 10 months–4.8 years
						• 2007 publication
						  – 12 remain off IS with normal graft function
						  – 6 died: none with acute or chronic rejection
							• 31 subjects <21 years old; 68 subjects >21 years old
							• Two underwent combined liver-kidney transplant
							• Two subjects died of unrelated causes
							• Subjects on prednisone+azathioprine ($p = 0.0007$) and those on tacrolimus-based IS ($p = 0.003$) were more likely to be off drug at 1 year than those on cyclosporine-based IS

King's College 1998 [32] 2007 [33]	• None stated but 7 of 18 subjects had autoimmune liver disease
	• Subjects must be suffering side effect initiated or aggravated by IS
		• >5 years required; Actual median (range) 7 (5–11) years	5/18 28%	No	After 8–24 months	• 1998 publication: not clearly stated but follow-up biopsy performed 8–24 months after withdrawal
						• 2007 publication: 10 years after withdrawal, three of five tolerant subjects restarted IS for acute rejection, chronic rejection/ re-transplantation, and kidney transplantation
							• Systemic chimerism was not associated with successful IS withdrawal
							• Subjects with immunologic or viral transplant indication appear more likely to fail IS withdrawal
							• IS withdrawal precipitated systemic complications:
							  Two of three subjects with PBC complained of arthralgia which was self-limited
							  – One of three subjects with PSC had flare of ulcerative colitis
							  – Three subjects developed gout
							  – One subject developed psoriasis
							• Benefit of IS withdrawal was unclear

Murcia 2003 [34]	None stated but no subjects transplanted for viral hepatitis or autoimmune liver disease	• >2 years required • Actual 62 ± 25 months	3/9 33%	Yes	After 2 months	17–24 months off IS	Endothelial cell chimerism was not associated with successful IS withdrawal

Study	Inclusion criteria	Duration of weaning	Rejection during weaning	Protocol biopsy	Follow-up	Outcomes
Murcia 2008 [35]	• Stable for ≥2 years • ≥1 year without rejection • Excluded subjects transplanted for viral hepatitis, cancer, and autoimmune liver disease	Mean ± SD: 59 ± 26.7 months	Elective 3/10 30%	Yes	After 2 months	Median (range) 47 (43–48) months off of IS	• No baseline factors (age, sex, IS regimen or dosing, liver tests, past history of acute rejection, or time since transplant) were associated with successful withdrawal • Stopping IS improved renal function and lower blood pressure, serum glucose, and total cholesterol levels • Non-tolerant subjects had worse renal function at end of follow-up
	None stated but no subjects transplanted for viral hepatitis or autoimmune liver disease	Mean ± SD: 22.6 ± 5.6 months	Nonelective: 6: IS toxicity 4: non-compliance 5/10 50%	No		Median (range) 60 (10–132) months off of IS	
Tor Vergata 2006 [36] 2008 [37]	• HCV RNA positive • Biopsy-proven recurrent HCV • Compliant	• >12 months required • Actual 63.5 ± 20.1 months	8/34 24%	Yes	Yes annual	• Mean initial total follow-up: 45.5 ± 5.8 months • Subsequent follow-up: 78 months	• Independent predictors of successful withdrawal: – Low cyclosporine trough levels during first posttransplant week ($p = 0.004$) – Steroid-free initial IS ($p < 0.008$) • Time after transplant was not a predictor • Tolerant compared to non-tolerant subject has slower fibrosis progression during initial study that did not persist with longer follow-up
Pamplona 2013 [38]	• ≥1 year without rejection • Excluded subjects transplanted for viral hepatitis and autoimmune liver disease • Required metabolic or malignant toxicity of IS or high risk of de novo cancer	• >3 years required • Actual median 112 months	15/24 63%	No	No	• Median (IQR): 14 (8.5–22.5) months – Two subjects <6 months – Ten subjects >12 months	• Tolerant compared to non-tolerant subjects – Were farther out from transplant (156 vs. 71 months, $p < 0.003$) and – Had lower median phytohemagglutinin stimulation index (7.49 vs. 41.73, $p < 0.01$)

HCV hepatitis C virus, *IQR* interquartile range, *IS* immunosuppression, *PBC* primary biliary cirrhosis

[a]Includes subjects reported by Ramos HC et al. [28]

[b]25 (26%) rejected, 37 (39%) still weaning, and 12 (13%) withdrawn from weaning protocol secondary to non-compliance, recurrent PBC, pregnancy, and kidney transplantation

Table 36.4 Unpublished single center trials of IS withdrawal for adult liver transplant recipients

Year started NCT number	Center PI	Title	Status in clinicaltrials.gov	Excluded diagnoses	Comments
2010 NCT01198314	Seoul Choi	Withdrawal of immunosuppression in long-term stable liver transplant recipients	Unknown	Transplants for hepatitis C and autoimmune liver disease	Required time after transplant not specified
2014 NCT02062944	Northwestern Levitsky	Sirolimus withdrawal	Recruiting	Transplants for viral hepatitis or autoimmune liver disease	Enrolled subjects must be ≥3 years after living or deceased donor liver transplant and ≥3 months of stable SRL monotherapy
2015 NCT02541916	Toronto Levy	Liver immune tolerance marker utilization study (LITMUS)	Active; not recruiting	Hepatitis B or C viremia	• Enrolled subjects will be tested for a peripheral blood biomarker of tolerance derived in a preclinical setting • Subject exhibiting the tolerance biomarker will then be weaned

on IS (1.6 ± 1.2 vs. 0.9 ± 0.8; $p < 0.01$) [48]. However, patients off of IS compared to those maintained on IS differed in other respects. Tolerant patients were younger at transplant (1.0 ± 1.7 vs. 4.2 ± 4.5 years; $p < 0.01$) and longer since transplant (121.2 ± 42.8 vs. 52.2 ± 22.4 months; $p < 0.01$). Therefore, the explanatory power of differences in IS dosing relative to these other factors is impossible to determine. The final important concept to emerge from the Kyoto experience is the possible role of antibodies—both auto- and alloantibodies—in chronic graft injury that may be exacerbated by minimization and/or discontinuation of IS [49].

Over the past decade, there has been a burgeoning body of literature examining the potential role of antibodies, both autoantibodies and DSA in chronic allograft injury that, in theory, may be exacerbated by IS minimization or discontinuation. Nearly all reports suffer some or all features of suboptimal study design, including single center, cross-sectional, and/or retrospective. However, associations have consistently emerged. Traditional autoantibodies—antinuclear, anti-smooth muscle, and anti-liver-kidney microsomal antibodies—in conjunction with increased gamma globulins are well-known markers of recurrent or de novo autoimmune hepatitis that can certainly damage allografts [50]. However, even without a formal diagnosis of autoimmune hepatitis, the presence of non-organ specific autoantibodies has been associated with the finding termed "idiopathic posttransplant hepatitis" [51, 52]. More recently, DSA and, in particular, DSA against donor HLA class II antigens have been identified by many groups to be a risk factor for chronic rejection [53–55] and fibrosis [45, 49, 56, 57] in both adult and pediatric liver recipients. It is notable, though, that the presence of DSA even of high mean fluorescence intensity does not appear to be prohibitive for successful IS withdrawal [58]. Moreover, neither its presence nor its development inevitably portends progressive allograft fibrosis or damage [59, 60]. As such, the presence and/or development of DSA may be a marker of the host alloimmune system, rather than the direct agent of graft injury. Alternatively, it is also possible that liver allografts have variable vulnerability to damage that might be caused by DSA. A healthy allograft with its full complement of defense mechanisms against immune-mediated damage may maintain its histological health. In contrast, an allograft already under attack by other insults will be vulnerable to damage by DSA. This has been extended as the "two-hit hypothesis" [61] and must yet be proven.

36.8 Prospective, Multicenter Clinical Trials of IS Withdrawal for Adult and Pediatric Liver Transplant Recipients

The plethora of single center reports of successful IS withdrawal have motivated prospective, multicenter clinical trials for both adult and pediatric liver transplant recipients (Tables 36.6 and 36.7) [58, 62]. These trials address many of the gaps and weaknesses of the single center reports (Table 36.2). Inclusion and exclusion criteria for elective IS withdrawal are clearly delineated. In general, the trials enroll either adult or pediatric recipients, exclude autoimmune etiologies of liver disease, specify a minimum time after transplant, set explicit thresholds for liver tests, limit IS exposure (number of agents and/or dosing), and require clinical stability with the absence of rejection for a period of time prior to enrollment. Perhaps most importantly, the multicenter trials have uniformly required liver biopsy, often evaluated by a central pathologist, as the final eligibility

Table 36.5 Published single center trials of IS withdrawal for pediatric liver transplant recipients

Center Year (reference)	Time interval: transplant → start of IS withdrawal	Outcome Successful/attempted/%	Liver biopsy to determine Eligibility	Liver biopsy to determine Tolerance	Duration off of IS	Clinical factors associated with successful IS withdrawal	Comments
Kyoto 2001 [42] 2009 [48] 2011 [46] 2012 [47] 2012 [52] 2014 [49]	>2 years required	Elective: 50/132/38% Nonelective: 34/58/59%	No	No[a]	Unclear	• No early rejection • Higher early (1 week after transplant) tacrolimus trough levels • HLA-A matching • HLA-B **mismatching**	• Analyses of factors associated with successful withdrawal were based on 84 tolerant and 50 non-tolerant subjects (24 rejectors and 26 with fibrosis) • Importance of surveillance biopsies to follow subjects off of IS • Detection of progressive fibrosis associated with IS discontinuation and improved by reinstitution of "minimal maintenance" IS • Identified association between progressive fibrosis and antibodies, both DSA and α-angiotensin 2 type 1 receptor antibodies
Stanford 2004 [39]	Median (range) to • PTLD: 235 (21–2743) days • EBV infection: 298 (18–1658)	8/38/21%	No	No	1535.5 ± 623 days		• IS withdrawal undertaken for PTLD (n = 19) and EBV infection (n = 31) • 19/19 PTLD and 19/31 EBV infection patients stopped IS • 21 subjects had acute rejection mean ± standard deviation 107.43 ± 140 days (range 7–476 days) after stopping IS • Two rejectors required re-transplantation for chronic rejection – One had chronic rejection prior to PTLD and IS withdrawal
Seoul 2009 [40]	Median (range) 45 (14–60) months	5/5/100%	No	No[b]	Median (range) 32 (14–82) months		• Non-compliant patients with tacrolimus trough levels <1 ng/mL (n = 4) • PTLD (n = 1)

Stanford 2010 [43]	5.52 ± 4.85 years	18/Unknown/NA	No	No	7.6 ± 3.4 years	Young age at transplant	• 89 subjects with normal liver tests
							  – 18 tolerant: (6 stopped IS for PTLD)
							  – 27 minimal IS
							  – 44 acute or chronic rejection >1 year after transplant

Tokyo 2013 [44]	>2 years required	Unknown	No	No	Unknown[c]	• Female • Higher prevalence of α-HLA antibodies after transplant • Lower MFI of α-HLA antibodies	• 51 living donor liver transplant recipients with primary grafts • 40/51 (78.4%) had sera available for HLA antibody testing pre-transplant and 3 weeks posttransplant – 17 tolerant and 23 non-tolerant • Nearly all α-HLA antibodies identified were not donor specific

(continued)

Table 36.5 (continued)

Center Year (reference)	Time interval: transplant → start of IS withdrawal	Outcome Successful/ attempted/%	Liver biopsy to determine Eligibility	Tolerance	Duration off of IS	Clinical factors associated with successful IS withdrawal	Comments
Taipei 2015 [41]	• >1 year required • Actual median (range) 2.03 (1.38–3.69) years	5/16[d]/31%	Yes	Yes	Range 24.6–42.8 months	• Metabolic liver disease ($p = 0.039$) • Shorter time since transplant ($p = 0.028$)	

DSA donor-specific antibody, *EBV* Epstein-Barr virus, *IS* immunosuppression, *MFI* mean fluorescence intensity, *PTLD* posttransplant lymphoproliferative disease

[a]Institution of a surveillance biopsy protocol in January 2003 led to biopsies of 29 subjects off of IS. None had features of acute or chronic rejection, but some showed increased fibrosis

[b]Two patients underwent biopsy 32 and 64 months after IS withdrawal: no evidence of chronic rejection

[c]For tolerant subjects, overall follow-up since transplant was 4571.9 ± 544.7 days. Time from transplant to stopping IS and time off of IS are unknown

[d]Sixteen patients initiated IS withdrawal; 15 pts completed per protocol follow-up

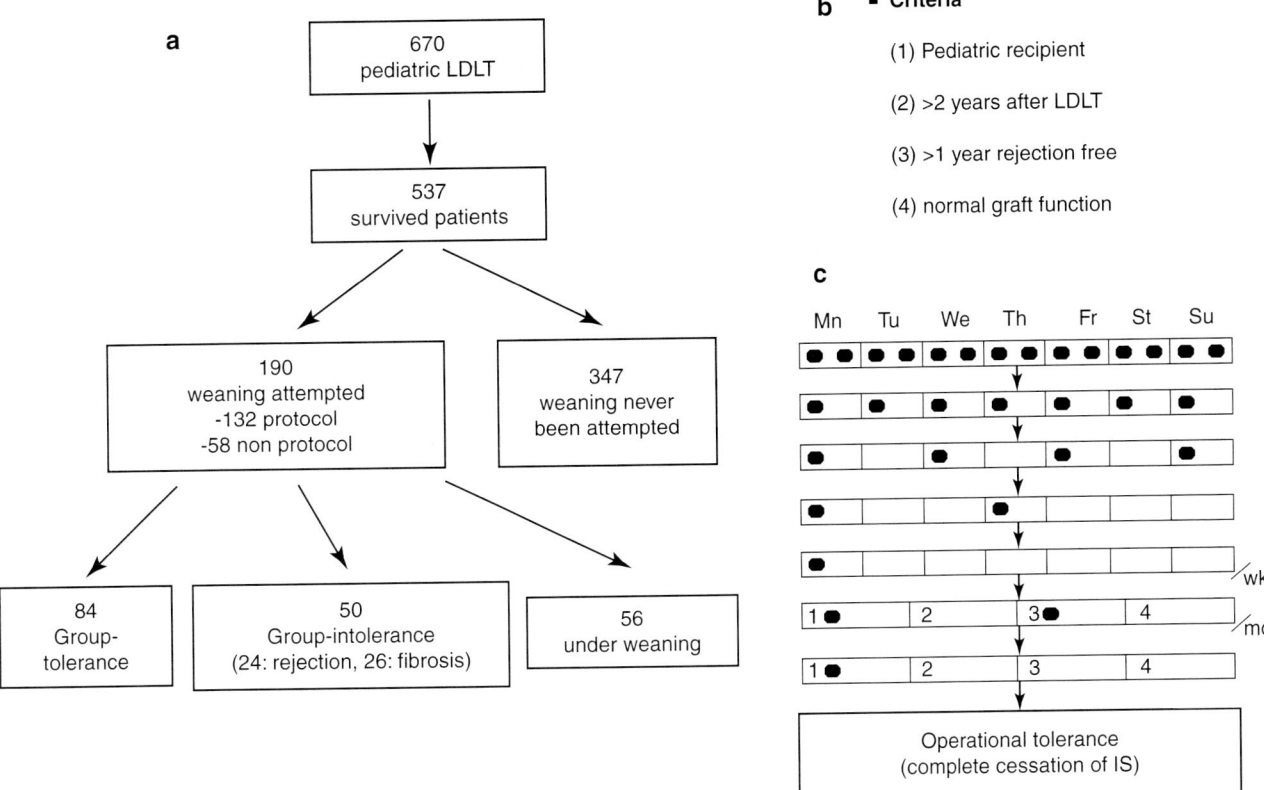

Fig. 36.2 Immunosuppression withdrawal protocol conducted at Kyoto University. The Kyoto University experience with IS withdrawal is unique in that there was a protocol to wean all stable long-term patients followed at their transplant center. (**a**) Of the 670 transplanted between June 1990 and April 2008, 537 survived. A total of 190 patients attempted IS withdrawal: 132 were weaned electively, while 58 were weaned nonelectively. At the time of publication, 56 subjects were still weaning, while 134 had completed weaning: 84 succeeded, while 50 failed as a result of either rejection ($n = 24$) or progressive fibrosis ($n = 26$). (**b**) Key criteria to select appropriate patients for elective weaning. (**c**) Algorithm for tacrolimus dose reduction: at intervals of 3–6 months, frequency of tacrolimus administration was reduced from the starting point of twice daily to once daily to once, 4 days per week to once, 2 days per week to once, weekly to once, and every other week prior to discontinuation

assessment prior to initiating IS withdrawal. Biopsies were typically scored for any evidence of acute or chronic rejection as well as for the presence and severity of inflammation and fibrosis. Notably, biopsy assessment for the three most recent trials—iWITH, OPTIMAL, and LIFT (Table 36.7)—are harmonized. All three trials utilize the same histological criteria for both eligibility and tolerance adjudication biopsies (Tables 36.8 and 36.9) that were derived from the Banff Working Group on Liver Allograft Pathology [14].

In addition to specifying characteristics of the enrolled population, the prospective multicenter trials also stipulated an algorithm for IS dose reduction and the frequency of concomitant laboratory assessments. Although protocols allowed site investigators to perform a biopsy at any time, laboratory thresholds mandating liver biopsy were defined. These "for cause" or "indication" biopsies were reviewed by the local physicians and local pathologists to guide clinical management. However, trial reporting and publication relied on central pathology assessments with respect to the diagnosis and severity of acute rejection. Notably, none of the withdrawal protocols specified how allograft dysfunction (elevated liver tests in the absence of a diagnosis of acute rejection) or acute rejection would be treated. Treatment decisions were left to physicians caring for the subjects.

For those who successfully discontinued IS, tolerance was adjudicated in a varied manner and at different times in the early clinical trials (Table 36.6). In AWISH, eligible and appropriately randomized subjects started on the 56-week weaning protocol between 1 and 2 years after deceased donor liver transplant. Tolerance was determined by biochemical criteria 6 months after the last medication dose. Liver biopsies were required at 24 and 36 months after liver transplantation, irrespective of the status of IS withdrawal, and, as such, were not timed to the time of tolerance determination. As for WISP-R, tolerance was similarly determined by laboratory criteria at 1 year after the last medication dose. Protocol liver biopsies were required 4–8 weeks, followed by 2, 4, and finally 7 years after stopping IS. Therefore, although biopsy did not figure in tolerance adjudication, the availability of multiple biopsies years after stopping IS con-

Table 36.6 Early multicenter clinical trials of IS withdrawal for adult and pediatric liver transplant recipients

Year started Reference(s) Trial name Principal investigator	Adult/ pediatric	Clinical trial identifier	Living or deceased donor transplant	Time interval: transplant → initiation of withdrawal	Liver biopsy Central or local[a] Eligibility	Liver biopsy Central or local[a] Tolerance	IS cessation to tolerance assessment	Outcome of IS withdrawal Attempted/ Successful/%	Primary endpoint
2005 None **AWISH** *Shaked*	Adult	NCT00135694	Deceased	1–2 years	Yes Central	No[b]	6 months	Unpublished	Proportion of subjects who develop any one of the following within 24 months of randomization to IS withdrawal or standard of care: • Death or graft loss • Grade 4 secondary malignancy • Grade 4 opportunistic infection • Grade 3 or higher viral hepatitis or • Grade 2 or higher decrease in GFR
2005 [62] **No name** *Sanchez-Fueyo*	Adult	NCT00647283	Deceased	>3 years	Yes Local	Yes Local	1 year	102/41/40%	Development of operational tolerance defined as successful IS drug cessation maintained for at least 12 months with stable graft function and no histopathological evidence of acute or chronic rejection
2006 [58, 59] **WISP-R** *Feng*	Pediatric	NCT00320606	Living[c]	>4 years	Yes Local	No[d]	1 year	20/12/60%	Proportion of participants who are successfully withdrawn from IS, which is defined as those who remain off IS for at least 1 year

[a]Central or local indicates whether eligibility and tolerance determination were performed by the central or a local (at the subject's site) pathologist
[b]Tolerance assessed 6 months after the last IS dose
[c]Only recipients of parental living donor liver transplants
[d]Tolerance assessed solely by liver tests 1 year after the last IS dose. Liver biopsies performed 4–8 weeks, 2, 4, and 7 years after stopping IS

Table 36.7 Recent/ongoing multicenter clinical trials of IS withdrawal for adult and pediatric liver transplant recipients

Year started Name Principal investigator	Adult/ pediatric	Clinical trial identifier	Living or deceased donor transplant	Interval: transplant →initiation of withdrawal	Liver biopsy Central or local[a] Eligibility	Liver biopsy Central or local[a] Tolerance	Time of tolerance assessment	Primary endpoint
2012 iWITH Feng	Pediatric	NCT01638559	Living or deceased	>4 years	Yes Central	Yes Central	1 year	Proportion of subjects with stable liver tests and liver histology 12 months after complete IS withdrawal, compared to study enrollment
2015 OPTIMAL Markmann	Adult	NCT02533180	Living or deceased	>6 years; If 3–6 years, recipient must be >50 years old	Yes Central	Yes Central	1 year	Proportion of subjects with stable liver tests and liver histology 12 months after complete IS withdrawal, compared to study enrollment
2015 LIFT Sanchez-Fueyo	Adult	NCT02498977	Deceased		Yes Central	Yes Central	1 year	

[a]Central or local indicates whether eligibility and tolerance determination were performed by the central or a local (at the subject's site) pathologist

Table 36.8 Histological criteria to assess eligibility to initiate IS withdrawal

Feature	Criteria
Portal inflammation and interface activity	Preferably absent but minimal to focal mild portal mononuclear inflammation may be present. Interface necroinflammatory activity is absent or equivocal/minimal and, if present, involves a minority of portal tracts
Centrizonal/perivenular inflammation	Preferably absent but minimal to focal mild perivenular mononuclear inflammation may be present. Perivenular necroinflammatory activity is absent or equivocal/minimal and, if present, involves a minority of terminal hepatic venules
Bile duct changes	No lymphocytic bile duct damage, ductopenia, and biliary epithelial senescence changes, unless there is an alternative, non-immunologic explanation (e.g., biliary strictures)
Fibrosis	Ishak Stage 3 (i.e., not more than occasional portal-to-portal bridging). Perivenular fibrosis should be less than "moderate," according to Banff criteria
Arteries	Negative for obliterative or foam cell arteriopathy

Table 36.9 Histological criteria to assess spontaneous tolerance: comparison of biopsy obtained 52 weeks after the last IS dose to the eligibility biopsy

Feature	Criteria
Portal inflammation and interface activity	Similar/identical to pre-withdrawal biopsy with preferably absent or minimal to focal mild, portal mononuclear inflammation. Interface necroinflammatory activity is absent or equivocal/minimal and, if present, involves a minority of portal tracts
Centrizonal/perivenular inflammation	Similar/identical to pre-withdrawal biopsy with minimal or no perivenular necroinflammatory activity
Bile duct changes	Similar/identical to pre-withdrawal biopsy, without new-onset biliary epithelial cell senescence changes and/or ductopenia involving >10% of portal tracts
Fibrosis	Similar/identical to pre-withdrawal biopsy, without progressive portal/periportal or perivenular fibrosis or architectural distortion unless there is an alternative explanation (≤1 point on Ishak scale)
Arteries	Negative for obliterative or foam cell arteriopathy

firmed the tolerance phenotype. The more recent portfolio of withdrawal trials is harmonious with respect to tolerance adjudication, utilizing both biochemical and histological criteria at the 1-year drug-free time-point. The criteria for biopsy review, however, formalized a logical and important concept for tolerance trials—the requirement for histological stability over time as determined by a central pathologist. Therefore, in addition to the absence of findings suggestive of acute and/or chronic rejection, the biopsy must not show evidence of graft injury that might reflect an active alloimmune response [14]. The requirement for the two sequential biopsies to be similar or essentially identical sets a high bar that aims to ensure the patient and graft health and longevity.

36.9 Tolerance Induction Trials in Pediatric Liver Transplant Recipients: Hematopoietic Chimerism

Beyond weaning IS to uncover spontaneous tolerance, there is, perhaps surprisingly, a modest experience with tolerance induction for pediatric liver transplant recipients [63–70]. In total, there have been ten reported cases of children who have undergone nonsimultaneous liver and hematopoietic stem cell transplantation with the same donor for both the liver and the bone marrow grafts. Nine donors were related, nearly all haploidentical, while one was an unrelated but HLA-identical donor. Eight patients achieved liver transplant tolerance (Table 36.10), while two did not (Table 36.11). Notably, all six patients who underwent successful stem cell transplantation and achieved complete donor chimerism were able to undergo subsequent liver transplantation and stop IS soon thereafter. The interval between stem cell and liver transplantation ranged widely, from 1 month to 10 years. In contrast, only two of the four patients who underwent liver transplantation first followed by stem cell transplantation with the same donor achieved tolerance. Both patients rejected the bone marrow graft. One patient experienced autologous myeloid recovery and has been maintained on IS with apparently normal liver function; the other patient ultimately died of sepsis and multi-system organ failure in spite of autologous rescue stem cell transplantation.

These cases together show that these protocols are feasible, given the availability of an appropriate living donor for both the stem cell and the liver grafts, and can treat liver and hematologic/oncologic disease. T cell macrochimerism was achieved at a high rate which then translated directly into robust liver allograft tolerance. However, the majority of patients (seven of ten) received a fully myeloablative conditioning regimen; one did not receive any conditioning, while the regimen was not specified in the remaining two (Tables 36.10 and 36.11). The conditioning regimen likely accounts for the donor-recipient macrochimerism as well as the significant toll of infection, both bacterial and viral, and graft-versus-host disease. This has informed a conclusion that the equipoise of this tolerance induction approach did not appear favorable for patients solely requiring liver transplantation alone, without a hematologic or oncologic indication for allogeneic stem cell transplantation [63].

36.10 Tolerance Induction Trials in Adult Liver Transplant Recipients: Hematopoietic Chimerism

Several strategies to induce tolerance for adult liver transplant recipients have been tested over the past decade with limited success (Table 36.12). The group in Miami conducted a trial enrolling two cohorts of liver transplant recipients 3 or more years after transplant: those who received, between days 0 and 100 posttransplant, one or more infusions of unmanipulated donor bone marrow prepared from vertebral bodies early after transplant ($n = 45$) and those who did not receive any donor bone marrow cells ($n = 59$) [71, 72]. None of the patients received any T cell depleting agents for induction. Moreover, those who received donor bone marrow did not receive or undergo any conditioning. Nevertheless, two of these patients developed a skin rash, were diagnosed with mild graft-versus-host disease, and responded to treatment with steroids. The administration of donor bone marrow did not increase either donor hematopoietic macrochimerism or success rates of IS withdrawal.

There has been a single report of two patients treated with a non-myeloablative conditioning regimen prior to donor stem cell infusion [73]. This aggressive tolerance induction protocol enrolled patients with cancer otherwise ineligible for deceased donor liver transplantation. Both patients received cyclophosphamide and anti-thymocyte globulin followed by donor stem cell infusion. After hematopoietic reconstitution which took 40 and 55 days, they underwent living donor liver transplantation with standard IS which was stopped 90 and 28 days after transplantation. Both patients remained off of IS: the first patient until 370 days after transplantation when he died of recurrent cancer and the second patient until 270 days after transplant, the end of follow-up. The first patient demonstrated donor chimerism through 21 days after stem cell infusion, while the second never showed any donor cells.

36.11 Impressions of Hematopoietic Chimerism as a Strategy for Tolerance Induction in De Novo Liver Transplant Recipients

Overall, considering the combined experiences of the pediatric and adult patients described in the preceding sections, the liver transplant community has not enthusiastically pursued donor hematopoietic chimerism as an approach to tolerance induction. Particularly since the degree and duration of chimerism appear to be somewhat proportional to the intensity of the conditioning regimen, there is substantial concern that an efficacious preparative regimen will incur unacceptable toxicity in patients who typically have portal hypertension and/or cholestasis. Furthermore, success—the achievement of durable donor macrochimerism—incurs the potentially devastating toxicity of graft-versus-host disease. Interestingly, the current portfolio of tolerance induction trials has a unique trial utilizing *autologous* stem cell transplantation to control the allo- and/or autoimmune response (NCT02549586). The protocol enrolls liver transplant recipients suffering recurrent episodes of rejection and/or recur-

Table 36.10 Cases of pediatric liver and hematopoietic stem cell transplants that achieved liver tolerance

Year	First author (reference)	Indication/age[a] Liver	Indication/age[a] BMT	Donor information	Conditioning	Chimerism outcome	IS withdrawal	Time after LDLT/liver status	Comments
2000	Matthes-Martin [64]	**Acute liver failure secondary to FHL/4 months**	FHL (6 months)	Related haploidentical	Myeloablative	• Donor lymphocyte infusion day 43 after HSCT → complete donor chimerism • GvHD (skin) treated with steroids	2 months after	3 months/normal	Biopsy 44 days after HSCT → no rejection
2005	Mellgren [65]	Liver veno-occlusive disease/25 months	*AML/22 months*	Father	Myeloablative	Complete donor chimerism	1 month after LDLT	2 years/normal	
2006	Shimizu [68]	Chronic liver GvHD/7 years	*ALL/4 years*	Related haploidentical	Not specified	Complete donor chimerism	1 month after LDLT	8 months/normal	Conditioning regimen not specified biopsy 2 months after LDLT → no rejection
2010	Schiller [67]	Chronic liver GvHD; hepato-pulmonary syndrome/10.5 years	*SCID/6 months*	Sister	Not specified	Complete donor chimerism	Immediately after LDLT	1 year/normal	Conditioning regimen not specified
2012	Englert [66]	Chronic liver GvHD; cirrhosis/5 years	*ALL/2 years*	Unrelated; HLA-matched	Myeloablative	Complete donor chimerism	6 months after LDLT	3 years/normal	
2012	Granot [69]	Chronic liver GvHD/9 years	*JCML/2.5 years*	Father	Myeloablative	Complete donor chimerism	Immediately after LDLT	7 years/normal	Multiple liver biopsies early after LDLT showed steatosis and cholestasis
2016	Hartleif [63]	Acute liver failure 2° to systemic adenovirus infection/11 months	*SCID/10 months*	Related haploidentical	None	• Complete donor chimerism • Severe GvHD (skin+intestine) 1 month after LDLT treated with cyclosporine+infliximab+ etanercept+steroids	22 months after LDLT	7 years/normal function and histology	Did not receive any conditioning regimen
		Hepatoblastoma/1 year	AML/10 years	Related haploidentical	Myeloablative	• Complete donor chimerism	Immediately after HSCT	14 years/normal	

[a]***Bold and italics*** indicates first transplant performed

Table 36.11 Cases of pediatric liver and hematopoietic stem cell transplants that did not achieve liver tolerance

Year	First author (reference)	Indication/age[a]		Donor information	Conditioning	Chimerism outcome	IS withdrawal	Time after LDLT/liver status	Comments
		Liver	BMT						
2011	Mali [70]	**ALF/10 years**	Aplastic anemia/10 years; 20 days after LDLT	Related haploidentical	Myeloablative	• BM rejection day 20 after HSCT • 3% donor chimerism 90 days after HSCT	Never	10 months/normal	Autologous myeloid recovery
2016	Hartleif [63]	**Hepatoblastoma/5 years**	Metastatic tumor/5.5 years	Related haploidentical	Myeloablative	BM rejection 45 days after HSCT; pt previously had intestinal GvHD treated with steroids+infliximab+tacrolimus	Never	Not applicable	Autologous rescue stem cell transplant → adenovirus sepsis → MSOF → death 55 days after HSCT

ALL acute lymphoblastic leukemia, *AML* acute myeloid leukemia, *CNI* calcineurin inhibitor, *FHL* familial hemophagocytic lymphohistiocytosis, *GvHD* graft-versus-host disease, *HSCT* hematopoietic stem cell transplantation, *JCML* juvenile chronic myelogenous leukemia, *LDLT* living donor liver transplantation, *SCID* severe combined immunodeficiency

Bold and italics indicates first transplant performed

[a]

Table 36.12 Published trials of tolerance induction (inclusive of IS complete withdrawal) in adult liver transplant recipients

Center First author Year (reference)	Intervention	Time interval: transplant → initiation of withdrawal	Liver biopsy Prior to IS withdrawal	Liver biopsy After stopping IS	Withdrawal outcome: successful/ attempted	Comments
Erasmus/Ghent Donckier 2004 [73]	• Non-myeloablative conditioning regimen of cyclophosphamide and anti-thymocyte globulin followed by donor stem cell infusion • Liver transplant after hematopoietic reconstitution: 40–55 days after stem cell infusion • Immunosuppression after liver transplant: tacrolimus in patient 1; rapamycin in patient 2	90 days patient 1 28 days patient 2	No	No	2/2	• Living donor liver transplants • Patients with cancer ineligible for deceased donor liver transplantation • No severe toxicity from conditioning regimen • No graft-versus-host disease after stem cell infusion • Transient microchimerism in one patient only • Pt 1: tumor recurrence detected 120 days after transplant; died 370 days after transplant • Pt 2: tumor recurrent suspected 215 days after transplant; still alive 270 days after transplant
Miami Tryphonopoulous 2005 [72] 2010 [71]	• **Group 1** (n = 45): 1–5 infusions of donor bone marrow cells within 100 days of transplant; • **Group 2** (n = 59): no donor bone marrow infusions	>3 years	No	After 6 months	23/104	• Deceased donor liver transplants • No difference in donor hematopoietic chimerism between groups • No difference in success rates of withdrawal between groups
Ochsner Eason 2005 [77]	• Anti-thymocyte globulin, mycophenolate, and tacrolimus at time of transplant • Tacrolimus monotherapy by 2 weeks after transplant	>6 months	No	No	1/18	• Deceased donor liver transplants • Included HCV liver disease • No enrolled subjects had autoimmune liver disease
Erasmus/Ghent Donckier 2006 [73]	• High dose anti-thymocyte globulin, sirolimus, and steroids at time of transplant • Donor-derived stem cells on posttransplant day 7	18–213 days	No	No	2/3	• Living donor recipients only • Limited exclusively to patients with advanced liver cancer and without any other curative options who were ineligible for liver transplantation under the center's standard protocol • Two patients died of recurrent HCC 356 and 561 days after transplant, after being off IS for 319 and 533 days, respectively

(continued)

Table 36.12 (continued)

Center First author Year (reference)	Intervention	Time interval: transplant → initiation of withdrawal	Liver biopsy Prior to IS withdrawal	Liver biopsy After stopping IS	Withdrawal outcome: successful/attempted	Comments
Western Ontario Assy 2007 [115]	Randomization to placebo or ursodeoxycholic acid immediately prior to IS withdrawal	>2 years	No	No	2/26	• Deceased donor liver transplants • No differences in success rates of withdrawal between groups
Erasmus/Ghent Donckier 2009 [79]	• High dose anti-thymocyte globulin and steroids • Sirolimus on posttransplant day 7	2 months	No	No	0/3	• Deceased donor liver transplants • Excluded HCV and autoimmune liver disease
Hokkaido Todo 2016 [60]	• Steroids, tacrolimus, and MMF • Cyclophosphamide on posttransplant day 5 • Donor-specific regulatory T cell infusion on posttransplant day 13	6 months	Yes	After 1 year	7/10	• Living donor recipients • Splenectomy at time of liver transplant • Biopsy every 3 months during withdrawal • Three non-tolerant subjects were all transplanted for autoimmune liver disease

rent autoimmune liver disease to receive a myeloablative conditioning regimen followed by autologous stem cell infusion. This trial piggybacks on the growing experience in the context of severe autoimmune disease such as multiple sclerosis and systemic sclerosis showing that the transplant results in a qualitatively different, reconstituted immune system. Safety and efficacy have yet to be published.

36.12 Tolerance Induction Trials in Adult Liver Transplant Recipients: Depletion of Effector Cells/Enhancement of Regulatory Cells

The majority of tolerance induction trials have explored an approach to tolerance first articulated by Sir Roy Calne in the late 1990s, based on observations derived from preclinical models of liver transplantation in rats and pigs. The theory centers on depletion of recipient T cells at time of liver transplantation to abort the immediate, aggressive anti-donor response, thereby promoting a tolerogenic engagement of the recipient's immune system by the graft's non-parenchymal cells and passenger leukocytes [74–76]. This effect can be further enhanced by minimizing exposure to CNIs, achieved by dose reduction or complete avoidance by substitution with alternative agents such as the mechanistic target of rapamycin inhibitors. Three trials, 1 conducted in the United States with 18 subjects [77] and 2 conducted in Belgium with 3 patients each [78, 79], demonstrated limited success (Tables 36.12 and 36.13). The lack of efficacy of this approach is further accentuated if one also considers the results of a similarly designed trial with the goal of IS minimization rather than withdrawal [80]. Compared to a cohort that received standard IS of corticosteroids and tacrolimus ($n = 16$), the cohort that received the experimental arm of anti-thymocyte globulin followed by low-dose tacrolimus ($n = 21$) experienced a significantly higher incidence of rejection during the study (66.7% vs. 31.2%; $p = 0.033$). Notably, the higher rate of rejection began within the first 3 months, prior to IS reduction (52.4% vs. 25%, $p = 0.09$) and continued thereafter (61.9% vs. 6.2%, $p = 0.001$).

More recently, a trial conducted in Japan harnessing the immunomodulatory capability of an ex vivo-generated Treg-enriched cell product has achieved impressive success, inducing tolerance in seven of ten subjects early after living donor liver transplantation (Table 36.12) [60]. The product is manufactured by co-culturing recipient lymphocytes and splenocytes (prepared after splenectomy performed during the transplant procedure) with irradiated donor lymphocytes in the presence of costimulatory blockade. Under these conditions, the total number of lymphocytes decreases, contributing to a substantial increase in frequency of Tregs. After 2 weeks, the culture product is washed and immediately infused into recipients on the 13th posttransplant day. At the time of transplant, enrolled subjects were initiated on standard triple IS with corticosteroids, tacrolimus, and mycophenolate mofetil consistent with standard of care. However, in preparation for the cellular product infusion, subjects also received a single dose of cyclophosphamide on posttransplant day 5 given with the specific aim of eliminating rapidly proliferating, alloantigen-activated, anti-donor recipient T cells and thereby "make space" for the cellular product infused 8 days later. On the heels of these promising results, two groups are enrolling de novo or pre-existing liver trans-

Table 36.13 Completed but unpublished trials of tolerance induction (inclusive of complete IS withdrawal) in adult liver transplant recipients

Year initiated	Principal investigator	Clinical trial identifier	Intervention	Time interval: transplant → initiation of withdrawal	Outcome: successful/attempted	Comments
2005	Multicenter/Thistlethwaite	NCT00166556	Alemtuzumab induction followed by tacrolimus monotherapy	1–2 years	Unknown	Excluded HCV and autoimmune liver disease

plant recipients to receive different Treg products, infused with or without prior depletion/conditioning. There are additional trials in the planning stages testing not only various Treg preparations (Table 36.14) but also other immunomodulatory cells such as tolerogenic DCs [81], mesenchymal stromal cells [82–84], and chimeric antigen receptor Tregs [85]. It is exciting to think that the next decade may indeed witness substantial progress in inducing and/or accelerating tolerance for liver transplant recipients.

36.13 Proposed Biomarkers of Tolerance (Table 36.15)

It is evident, from all of the efforts to either identify spontaneous tolerance or to induce tolerance, that a tolerance biomarker would be tremendously useful to select the most appropriate subjects for IS withdrawal. However, the identification of robust biomarkers of tolerance faces a number of challenges, derived from the small cohorts of tolerant transplant recipients available and from the difficulty of adjusting for the confounding factor of pharmacological IS when employing cross-sectional case-control study designs (i.e., studies in which drug-free tolerant recipients are compared to transplant recipients on IS). Attempts at developing immune-related biomarkers have been focused on addressing four major questions: (1) Do tolerant recipients exhibit signs of donor-specific immune hyporesponsiveness? (2) Is there evidence of immune regulation? (3) Is it possible to predict the outcome of IS drug withdrawal? (4) Can we safely discontinue IS by developing biomarkers of early allograft damage?

36.14 Biomarkers of Donor-Specific Hyporesponsiveness (Table 36.15)

Although donor-specific hyporesponsiveness is considered a hallmark of transplantation tolerance, the data derived from rodent models of spontaneous liver allograft tolerance suggest that spontaneous liver allograft tolerance is not necessarily associated with decreased anti-donor lymphocyte reactivity as assessed with currently available in vitro assays. This is still an open question, given that only two studies evaluating donor-specific immune responses in human-tolerant recipients have been reported. The first study described the results of MLR assays performed on 13 spontaneously tolerant liver recipients, who displayed donor-specific hyporesponsiveness which was not present prior to transplantation [86]. The second, more recent, study is the clinical trial inducing tolerance by infusion of autologous suppressor/anergic lymphocytes into ten splenectomized liver transplant recipients conditioned with cyclophosphamide (Table 36.12). Out of the seven recipients who achieved tolerance, five displayed donor-specific hyporesponsiveness in an enzyme-linked immunospot IFN-γ assay, and four did so in a conventional MLR assay [60]. Intriguingly, in another report, peripheral blood mononuclear cells (PBMCs) from tolerant recipients displayed a reduced but non-specific proliferative response following phytohemagglutinin stimulation as compared with non-tolerant patients before drug weaning was initiated [38].

36.15 Biomarkers of Immune Regulation or Exhaustion (Table 36.15)

A number of flow cytometric studies have attempted to identify evidence of active immunoregulatory networks in blood. A study that included samples from both adult and pediatric recipients with spontaneous tolerance described an increased number of plasmacytoid DCs (pDCs), a subtype of DCs expressing coregulatory markers that promote tolerance through the induction of Tregs [87]. The same group reported that, compared to patients on maintenance IS, tolerant recipients exhibited a higher PD-L1/CD86 ratio in circulating pDCs [88]. Canonically, γδ T cells are considered nonconventional T cells that participate in both innate and adaptive immunity. In healthy controls, the Vδ2+ subtype dominates, accounting for the majority of circulating γδ T cells; the ratio of circulating Vδ1+ to Vδ2+ γδ T cells is therefore typically <1.0. A Japanese cohort of pediatric spontaneously tolerant liver transplant recipients were noted to display an increased frequency of CD4+CD25+ Tregs, B cells, and a higher ratio of Vδ1+ to Vδ2+ γδ T cells [89]. This altered ratio of circulating γδ T cells in spontaneously tolerant recipients has been confirmed in three additional studies [62, 90, 91]. Furthermore, gene expression studies have revealed that the main transcriptional differences between tolerant and non-tolerant recipients are genes preferentially expressed in NK

Table 36.14 Currently enrolling trials of tolerance induction (inclusive of complete IS withdrawal) in adult and pediatric liver transplant recipients

Year initiated	Center Principal investigator	Clinical trial identifier	Title	Conditioning regimen Cellular product	Time interval: transplant → initiation of IS withdrawal	Comments
2014	King's College Sanchez-Fueyo	NCT02166177	Safety and Efficacy Study of Regulatory T Cell Therapy in Liver Transplant Patients (ThRIL)	• Rabbit thymoglobulin • Autologous polyclonal regulatory T cells	12 months after transplant	
2015	Multicenter Feng	NCT02474199	Donor-Alloantigen-Reactive Tregs (darTregs) for Calcineurin Inhibitor (CNI) Reduction (ARTEMIS)	• None • Autologous, donor alloreactive regulatory T cells	2–6 years after transplant	• Living donor recipients only • Primary endpoint: 75% CNI reduction • Secondary endpoint: complete immunosuppression withdrawal
2015	Ottawa and Toronto Levy	NCT02549586	Autologous Hematopoietic Stem Cell Transplantation for Allogeneic Organ Transplant Tolerance (ASCOTT)	• Myeloablative conditioning regimen with busulfan, cyclophosphamide, and anti-thymocyte globulin • Autologous CD34+ stem cells	Enrollment at least 3 months after liver transplant 6 months after stem cell transplant and sirolimus therapy	• Liver transplant for alcohol-induced, genetic or an autoimmune liver disease • Must have condition that might be ameliorated by stem cell transplantation and/or IS withdrawal such as evidence of recurrent autoimmune disease, repeated rejection episodes, and/or IS toxicity unresponsive to conventional management and of sufficient severity to warrant inclusion in the study by the investigator
2017	Beth Israel Deaconess Strom	NCT02739412	Efficacy of Low Dose, SubQ Interleukin-2 (IL-2) to Expand Endogenous Regulatory T-Cells in Liver Transplant Recipients	• Not applicable • No cellular product given • Induction of endogenous Tregs with subcutaneous injections of low-dose IL-2	2–4 years after transplant	
2017	King's College Sanchez-Fueyo	NCT02949492	Low-dose IL-2 for Treg Expansion and Tolerance (LITE)		2–6 years after transplant	Age < 50 years at time of enrollment

and γδ T cells [62, 91, 93]. While the Vδ1+ to Vδ2+ γδ T cell ratio is, to date, the only biomarker that has been employed in a prospective clinical trial to enrich for potentially tolerant liver recipients [90], it should be emphasized that circulating Vδ1+ T cells are increased in most immunosuppressed liver and kidney recipients. Moreover, there is a clear association between past viral infections, particularly cytomegalovirus and Vδ1 T cell expansion, raising some concerns about its specificity for liver allograft tolerance [92].

A further problem in many of these cross-sectional studies arises from the confounding effects of IS, given that tolerant patients off IS are compared to non-tolerant patients on IS. CNIs, for instance, are known to promote the apoptosis of Tregs and reduce their number in the circulation. Not entirely surprisingly, the original observations in cross-sectional studies of an increased number of Tregs in tolerant recipients have now been attributed to the consequences of their successful CNI discontinuation [62]. It should be noted, however, that in a small study from Spain, the increase in Tregs that is typically observed following the discontinuation of CNIs was only seen in those patients who eventually become tolerant, while in patients who rejected during weaning, the reduction in CNIs did not result in the expected increase in Tregs [35].

Co-expression of negative costimulatory receptors on CD8+ T cells, a hallmark of T cell exhaustion, was reported in association with operational tolerance in HCV-infected liver recipients [90]. Whether similar mechanisms are operative in non-HCV recipients is currently being investigated (OPTIMAL; NCT02533180; Table 36.7). In a retrospective cross-sectional study, tolerant recipients exhibited increased

Table 36.15 Proposed peripheral blood and liver tissue-based biomarkers of tolerance

First author (reference)	Marker	Conclusions	Study design	Patients
Mazariegos [87]	mDC/pDC ratio	pDC/mDC ratio was increased in tolerant and minimal immunosuppression recipients, compared to patients on immunosuppression and to healthy individuals	Cross-sectional case-control	6 tolerant 23 undergoing drug weaning 11 on immunosuppression 13 healthy controls
Tokita [88]	PD-L1/CD86 ratio on DC subsets	Increased PD-L1/CD86 ratio on pDC (but not mDC) subset in tolerant compared to immunosuppressed recipients	Cross-sectional case-control	13 tolerant 18 undergoing drug weaning 12 on immunosuppression
Li [89]	PBMC immunophenotyping	Tolerant compared to immunosuppressed recipients showed increased Treg and B cell frequency, increased Vδ1/Vδ2 γδ T cell ratio, and decreased NK cell frequency	Cross-sectional case-control	12 tolerant 19 on immunosuppression
Li [94]	• Liver tissue PCR gene expression • Liver tissue immunostaining	FoxP3 expression FoxP3+ cells were higher in tolerant compared to immunosuppressed or healthy control liver biopsies. Highest levels were detected in liver samples with chronic rejection	Cross-sectional case-control	28 tolerant 7 chronic rejectors 29 on immunosuppression 12 healthy controls
Martinez-Llordella [91]	• PBMC immunophenotyping • PBMC microarray/PCR gene expression	• Confirmation of increased Treg and Vδ1/Vδ2 γδ T cell ratio in tolerant recipients • Description of 628 genes differentially expressed between tolerant and non-tolerant recipients	Cross-sectional case-control	16 tolerant 16 non-tolerant (failed weaning) 10 healthy controls
Martinez-Llordella [93]	• PBMC immunophenotyping • PBMC microarray/PCR gene expression	Identification of three gene signatures enriched in natural killer and γδ T cells that discriminated between tolerant and non-tolerant recipients	Cross-sectional case-control	28 tolerant 33 non-tolerant (failed weaning) 19 on immunosuppression 16 healthy controls;
Li [97]	PBMC gene expression	Identification of a 13-gene expression signature enriched in NK cells that discriminated between tolerant and non-tolerant recipients	Cross-sectional case-control	16 tolerant 19 non-tolerant 22 conventional immunosuppression 20 low immunosuppression 6 healthy controls

Bohne [96]	• PBMC immunophenotyping
	• PBMC microarray/PCR gene expression
	• Liver tissue immunostaining
	• Liver tissue microarray/PCR gene expression
		• Identification of liver tissue gene expression signatures predictive of drug withdrawal outcome
		• Comparison between liver- and PBMC-derived predictive signatures
		• Tolerant and non-tolerant differed in iron homeostasis markers
			Longitudinal	75 undergoing drug withdrawal
				   33 successfully weaned
				   42 rejectors

Pons [35]	• PBMC immunophenotyping • PBMC PCR gene expression	Liver recipients successfully weaned but not patients eventually rejecting increased circulating Tregs and FoxP3 transcript levels during drug weaning	Longitudinal	12 undergoing drug withdrawal 5 tolerant + 7 rejectors

(continued)

Table 36.15 (continued)

First author (reference)	Marker	Conclusions	Study design	Patients
Bohne [90]	• PBMC immunophenotyping • PBMC PCR gene expression • Liver tissue immunostaining • Liver tissue microarray/PCR gene expression	Assessment of the usefulness of blood Vδ1/Vδ2 γδ T cell ratio as a marker to select liver recipients for prospective immunosuppression withdrawal Identification of increased type-1 IFN-stimulated genes and genes involved in immunoexhaustion in the liver tissue of tolerance HCV-infected recipients	Longitudinal	32 HCV-infected recipients undergoing drug withdrawal 17 tolerant + 15 rejectors
Bonaccorsi-Riani [114]	Liver tissue and whole blood microarray/PCR gene expression	Description of signatures of rejection in whole blood and liver tissue Identification of blood *CXCL10* transcript level as an early marker of rejection in recipients undergoing drug weaning	Longitudinal	55 rejectors during drug withdrawal
Garcia de la Garza [38]	Stimulation index after in vitro phytohemagglutinin stimulation of PBMCs	Successfully weaned patients exhibited decreased non-specific immunoreactivity at baseline	Longitudinal	24 undergoing drug withdrawal 15 successfully weaned 9 rejectors
Todo [116]	Donor-specific immune responses assessed by ELISpot and mixed lymphocyte reactions	Out of seven tolerant recipients, donor-specific hyporesponsiveness was observed in five by ELISpot IFN-γ assay and four by conventional mixed lymphocyte reaction assay	Tolerance induction	Ten de novo liver transplant recipients Undergoing splenectomy + cyclophosphamide + donor-reactive cellular product Seven tolerant + three rejectors

ELISpot enzyme-linked immunospot assay, *mDC* myeloid dendritic cell, *pDC* plasmacytoid dendritic cell, *PD-L1* programmed death-ligand 1, *DC* dendritic cell, *PBMC* peripheral blood mononuclear cell, *PCR* polymerase chain reaction

FOXP3+ T cells in their grafts [94]. In a longitudinal study in which liver biopsies from tolerant recipients were analyzed before and after drug withdrawal, a transient Treg-enriched inflammatory infiltrate was observed following IS discontinuation [95] which is reminiscent of what has been observed in animal models of spontaneous liver allograft tolerance.

36.16 Biomarkers to Predict Successful Immunosuppression Withdrawal or the Presence of Tolerance (Table 36.15)

High-throughput gene expression profiling has been employed to develop signatures predictive of IS withdrawal outcome, both in PBMCs [93, 96, 97] and liver tissue [96]. Side-by-side comparisons showed liver tissue-derived transcriptional signatures to be more robust, accurate, and reproducible biomarkers of tolerance than those derived from PBMCs. The intragraft expression profile, enriched predominantly in genes involved in iron homeostasis, did not overlap with genes identified from PBMCs [96]. A number of studies have attempted to identify tolerance-related signatures in blood common to liver and kidney transplant recipients. In kidney transplantation, spontaneous operational tolerance has been consistently associated with enrichment in B cell-related transcripts, probably reflecting an increase in the number of circulating transitional B cells in tolerant recipients [98–106]. No such findings have been observed in liver patients [107]. However, this literature will likely need to be revisited in light of a recent report that linked the tolerance-related B cell-specific signatures described in kidney transplantation to the confounding effects of immunosuppressive drugs [108].

36.17 Biomarkers to Predict Rejection or the Absence of Tolerance (Table 36.15)

Finally, multiple publications have described associations between acute rejection following liver, kidney, heart, or intestine transplantation and molecular changes in allograft tissue, serum, PBMCs, and fluids draining the graft (e.g., urine, bile, bronchoalveolar lavage) [109–113]. Molecular perturbations may precede clinically apparent rejection and even histological changes [109]. An alternative to the use of predictive signatures of tolerant to select patients for drug withdrawal is to derive and validate biomarkers capable of identifying early (subclinical) alloimmune-mediated graft damage, once drug withdrawal has been initiated and before clinically evidence rejection occurs. A recent report suggests that measurement of CXCL10 transcript levels in whole blood might be a viable approach to do so in the setting of liver transplantation [114] although further work is needed before this can be clinically implemented.

References

1. Kubes P, Jenne C. Immune responses in the liver. Annu Rev Immunol. 2018;36:247–77.
2. Demetris AJ, Bellamy CO, Gandhi CR, Prost S, Nakanuma Y, Stolz DB. Functional immune anatomy of the liver-as an allograft. Am J Transplant. 2016;16(6):1653–80.
3. Calne RY, Sells RA, Pena JR, Davis DR, Millard PR, Herbertson BM, et al. Induction of immunological tolerance by porcine liver allografts. Nature. 1969;223(5205):472–6.
4. Houssin D, Gigou M, Franco D, Bismuth H, Charpentier B, Lang P, et al. Specific transplantation tolerance induced by spontaneously tolerated liver allograft in inbred strains of rats. Transplantation. 1980;29(5):418–9.
5. Qian S, Demetris AJ, Murase N, Rao AS, Fung JJ, Starzl TE. Murine liver allograft transplantation: tolerance and donor cell chimerism. Hepatology. 1994;19(4):916–24.
6. Randomised trial comparing tacrolimus (FK506) and cyclosporin in prevention of liver allograft rejection. European FK506 Multicentre Liver Study Group. Lancet. 1994;344(8920):423–8.
7. Steger U, Denecke C, Sawitzki B, Karim M, Jones ND, Wood KJ. Exhaustive differentiation of alloreactive CD8+ T cells: critical for determination of graft acceptance or rejection. Transplantation. 2008;85(9):1339–47.
8. Wong YC, McCaughan GW, Bowen DG, Bertolino P. The CD8 T-cell response during tolerance induction in liver transplantation. Clin Transl Immunology. 2016;5(10):e102.
9. Li W, Kuhr CS, Zheng XX, Carper K, Thomson AW, Reyes JD, et al. New insights into mechanisms of spontaneous liver transplant tolerance: the role of Foxp3-expressing CD25+CD4+ regulatory T cells. Am J Transplant. 2008;8(8):1639–51.
10. Hall BM. CD4+CD25+ T regulatory cells in transplantation tolerance: 25 years on. Transplantation. 2016;100(12):2533–47.
11. Dahmen U, Qian S, Rao AS, Demetris AJ, Fu F, Sun H, et al. Split tolerance induced by orthotopic liver transplantation in mice. Transplantation. 1994;58(1):1–8.
12. Qian S, Lu L, Li Y, Fu F, Li W, Starzl TE, et al. Apoptosis of graft-infiltrating cytotoxic T cells: a mechanism underlying "split tolerance" in mouse liver transplantation. Transplant Proc. 1997;29(1–2):1168–9.
13. Morris H, DeWolf S, Robins H, Sprangers B, LoCascio SA, Shonts BA, et al. Tracking donor-reactive T cells: evidence for clonal deletion in tolerant kidney transplant patients. Sci Transl Med. 2015;7(272):272ra10.
14. Banff Working Group on Liver Allograft Pathology. Importance of liver biopsy findings in immunosuppression management: biopsy monitoring and working criteria for patients with operational tolerance. Liver Transpl. 2012;18(10):1154–70.
15. Demetris AJ, Isse K. Tissue biopsy monitoring of operational tolerance in liver allograft recipients. Curr Opin Organ Transplant. 2013;18(3):345–53.
16. Owens ML, Maxwell JG, Goodnight J, Wolcott MW. Discontinuance of immunosuppression in renal transplant patients. Arch Surg. 1975;110(12):1450–1.
17. Zoller KM, Cho SI, Cohen JJ, Harrington JT. Cessation of immunosuppressive therapy after successful transplantation: a national survey. Kidney Int. 1980;18(1):110–4.
18. Starzl TE, Demetris AJ, Murase N, Ildstad S, Ricordi C, Trucco M. Cell migration, chimerism, and graft acceptance. Lancet. 1992;339(8809):1579–82.
19. Starzl TE, Demetris AJ, Trucco M, Ramos H, Zeevi A, Rudert WA, et al. Systemic chimerism in human female recipients of male livers. Lancet. 1992;340(8824):876–7.
20. Thomson AW, Lu L, Wan Y, Qian S, Larsen CP, Starzl TE. Identification of donor-derived dendritic cell progenitors in bone marrow of spontaneously tolerant liver allograft recipients. Transplantation. 1995;60(12):1555–9.
21. Del Bello A, Congy-Jolivet N, Danjoux M, Muscari F, Kamar N. Donor-specific antibodies and liver transplantation. Hum Immunol. 2016;77(11):1063–70.
22. Demetris AJ, Zeevi A, O'Leary JG. ABO-compatible liver allograft antibody-mediated rejection: an update. Curr Opin Organ Transplant. 2015;20(3):314–24.
23. Rodriguez-Peralvarez M, Rico-Juri JM, Tsochatzis E, Burra P, De la Mata M, Lerut J. Biopsy-proven acute cellular rejection as an efficacy endpoint of randomized trials in liver transplantation: a systematic review and critical appraisal. Transpl Int. 2016;29(9):961–73.
24. Wiesner RH, Demetris AJ, Belle SH, Seaberg EC, Lake JR, Zetterman RK, et al. Acute hepatic allograft rejection: incidence, risk factors, and impact on outcome. Hepatology. 1998;28(3):638–45.
25. Jain A, Mazariegos G, Pokharna R, Parizhskaya M, Kashyap R, Kosmach-Park B, et al. The absence of chronic rejection in pediatric primary liver transplant patients who are maintained on tacrolimus-based immunosuppression: a long-term analysis. Transplantation. 2003;75(7):1020–5.
26. Starzl TE, Demetris AJ, Trucco M, Murase N, Ricordi C, Ildstad S, et al. Cell migration and chimerism after whole-organ transplantation: the basis of graft acceptance. Hepatology. 1993;17(6):1127–52.
27. Tzakis AG, Reyes J, Zeevi A, Ramos H, Nour B, Reinsmoen N, et al. Early tolerance in pediatric liver allograft recipients. J Pediatr Surg. 1994;29(6):754–6.
28. Ramos HC, Reyes J, Abu-Elmagd K, Zeevi A, Reinsmoen N, Tzakis A, et al. Weaning of immunosuppression in long-term liver transplant recipients. Transplantation. 1995;59(2):212–7.
29. Sandborn WJ, Hay JE, Porayko MK, Gores GJ, Steers JL, Krom RA, et al. Cyclosporine withdrawal for nephrotoxicity in liver transplant recipients does not result in sustained improvement in kidney function and causes cellular and ductopenic rejection. Hepatology. 1994;19(4):925–32.
30. Mazariegos GV, Reyes J, Marino IR, Demetris AJ, Flynn B, Irish W, et al. Weaning of immunosuppression in liver transplant recipients. Transplantation. 1997;63(2):243–9.
31. Mazariegos GV, Sindhi R, Thomson AW, Marcos A. Clinical tolerance following liver transplantation: long term results and future prospects. Transpl Immunol. 2007;17(2):114–9.
32. Devlin J, Doherty D, Thomson L, Wong T, Donaldson P, Portmann B, et al. Defining the outcome of immunosuppression withdrawal after liver transplantation. Hepatology. 1998;27(4):926–33.
33. Girlanda R, Rela M, Williams R, O'Grady JG, Heaton ND. Long-term outcome of immunosuppression withdrawal after liver transplantation. Transplant Proc. 2005;37(4):1708–9.
34. Pons JA, Yelamos J, Ramirez P, Oliver-Bonet M, Sanchez A, Rodriguez-Gago M, et al. Endothelial cell chimerism does not influence allograft tolerance in liver transplant patients

after withdrawal of immunosuppression. Transplantation. 2003;75(7):1045–7.
35. Pons JA, Revilla-Nuin B, Baroja-Mazo A, Ramirez P, Martinez-Alarcon L, Sanchez-Bueno F, et al. FoxP3 in peripheral blood is associated with operational tolerance in liver transplant patients during immunosuppression withdrawal. Transplantation. 2008;86(10):1370–8.
36. Tisone G, Orlando G, Cardillo A, Palmieri G, Manzia TM, Baiocchi L, et al. Complete weaning off immunosuppression in HCV liver transplant recipients is feasible and favourably impacts on the progression of disease recurrence. J Hepatol. 2006;44(4):702–9.
37. Orlando G, Manzia T, Baiocchi L, Sanchez-Fueyo A, Angelico M, Tisone G. The Tor Vergata weaning off immunosuppression protocol in stable HCV liver transplant patients: the updated follow up at 78 months. Transpl Immunol. 2008;20(1–2):43–7.
38. Garcia de la Garza R, Sarobe P, Merino J, Lasarte JJ, D'Avola D, Belsue V, et al. Immune monitoring of immunosuppression withdrawal of liver transplant recipients. Transpl Immunol. 2015;33(2):110–6.
39. Hurwitz M, Desai DM, Cox KL, Berquist WE, Esquivel CO, Millan MT. Complete immunosuppressive withdrawal as a uniform approach to post-transplant lymphoproliferative disease in pediatric liver transplantation. Pediatr Transplant. 2004;8(3):267–72.
40. Lee JH, Lee SK, Lee HJ, Seo JM, Joh JW, Kim SJ, et al. Withdrawal of immunosuppression in pediatric liver transplant recipients in Korea. Yonsei Med J. 2009;50(6):784–8.
41. Lin NC, Wang HK, Yeh YC, Liu CP, Loong CC, Tsai HL, et al. Minimization or withdrawal of immunosuppressants in pediatric liver transplant recipients. J Pediatr Surg. 2015;50(12):2128–33.
42. Takatsuki M, Uemoto S, Inomata Y, Egawa H, Kiuchi T, Fujita S, et al. Weaning of immunosuppression in living donor liver transplant recipients. Transplantation. 2001;72(3):449–54.
43. Talisetti A, Hurwitz M, Sarwal M, Berquist W, Castillo R, Bass D, et al. Analysis of clinical variables associated with tolerance in pediatric liver transplant recipients. Pediatr Transplant. 2010;14(8):976–9.
44. Waki K, Sugawara Y, Mizuta K, Taniguchi M, Ozawa M, Hirata M, et al. Predicting operational tolerance in pediatric living-donor liver transplantation by absence of HLA antibodies. Transplantation. 2013;95(1):177–83.
45. Miyagawa-Hayashino A, Yoshizawa A, Uchida Y, Egawa H, Yurugi K, Masuda S, et al. Progressive graft fibrosis and donor-specific human leukocyte antigen antibodies in pediatric late liver allografts. Liver Transpl. 2012;18(11):1333–42.
46. Ohe H, Li Y, Nafady-Hego H, Kayo W, Sakaguchi S, Wood K, et al. Minimal but essential doses of immunosuppression: a more realistic approach to improve long-term outcomes for pediatric living-donor liver transplantation. Transplantation. 2011;91(7):808–10.
47. Ohe H, Waki K, Yoshitomi M, Morimoto T, Nafady-Hego H, Satoda N, et al. Factors affecting operational tolerance after pediatric living-donor liver transplantation: impact of early post-transplant events and HLA match. Transpl Int. 2012;25(1):97–106.
48. Yoshitomi M, Koshiba T, Haga H, Li Y, Zhao X, Cheng D, et al. Requirement of protocol biopsy before and after complete cessation of immunosuppression after liver transplantation. Transplantation. 2009;87(4):606–14.
49. Ohe H, Uchida Y, Yoshizawa A, Hirao H, Taniguchi M, Maruya E, et al. Association of anti-human leukocyte antigen and anti-angiotensin II type 1 receptor antibodies with liver allograft fibrosis after immunosuppression withdrawal. Transplantation. 2014;98(10):1105–11.
50. Kerkar N, Yanni G. 'De novo' and 'recurrent' autoimmune hepatitis after liver transplantation: a comprehensive review. J Autoimmun. 2016;66:17–24.
51. Evans HM, Kelly DA, McKiernan PJ, Hubscher S. Progressive histological damage in liver allografts following pediatric liver transplantation. Hepatology. 2006;43(5):1109–17.
52. Miyagawa-Hayashino A, Haga H, Egawa H, Hayashino Y, Uemoto S, Manabe T. Idiopathic post-transplantation hepatitis following living donor liver transplantation, and significance of autoantibody titre for outcome. Transpl Int. 2009;22(3):303–12.
53. O'Leary JG, Kaneku H, Susskind BM, Jennings LW, Neri MA, Davis GL, et al. High mean fluorescence intensity donor-specific anti-HLA antibodies associated with chronic rejection postliver transplant. Am J Transplant. 2011;11(9):1868–76.
54. Wozniak LJ, Hickey MJ, Venick RS, Vargas JH, Farmer DG, Busuttil RW, et al. Donor-specific HLA antibodies are associated with late allograft dysfunction after pediatric liver transplantation. Transplantation. 2015;99(7):1416–22.
55. Grabhorn E, Binder TM, Obrecht D, Brinkert F, Lehnhardt A, Herden U, et al. Long-term clinical relevance of de novo donor-specific antibodies after pediatric liver transplantation. Transplantation. 2015;99(9):1876–81.
56. Egawa H, Miyagawa-Hayashino A, Haga H, Teramukai S, Yoshizawa A, Ogawa K, et al. Non-inflammatory centrilobular sinusoidal fibrosis in pediatric liver transplant recipients under tacrolimus withdrawal. Hepatol Res. 2012;42(9):895–903.
57. O'Leary JG, Demetris AJ, Philippe A, Freeman R, Cai J, Heidecke H, et al. Non-HLA antibodies impact on C4d staining, stellate cell activation and fibrosis in liver allografts. Transplantation. 2017;101(10):2399–409.
58. Feng S, Ekong UD, Lobritto SJ, Demetris AJ, Roberts JP, Rosenthal P, et al. Complete immunosuppression withdrawal and subsequent allograft function among pediatric recipients of parental living donor liver transplants. JAMA. 2012;307(3):283–93.
59. Feng S, Demetris AJ, Spain KM, Kanaparthi S, Burrell BE, Ekong UD, et al. Five-year histological and serological follow-up of operationally tolerant pediatric liver transplant recipients enrolled in WISP-R. Hepatology. 2017;65(2):647–60.
60. Todo S, Yamashita K, Goto R, Zaitsu M, Nagatsu A, Oura T, et al. A pilot study of operational tolerance with a regulatory T-cell-based cell therapy in living donor liver transplantation. Hepatology. 2016;64(2):632–43.
61. Kim PT, Demetris AJ, O'Leary JG. Prevention and treatment of liver allograft antibody-mediated rejection and the role of the 'two-hit hypothesis'. Curr Opin Organ Transplant. 2016;21(2):209–18.
62. Benitez C, Londono MC, Miquel R, Manzia TM, Abraldes JG, Lozano JJ, et al. Prospective multicenter clinical trial of immunosuppressive drug withdrawal in stable adult liver transplant recipients. Hepatology. 2013;58(5):1824–35.
63. Hartleif S, Lang P, Handgretinger R, Feuchtinger T, Fuchs J, Konigsrainer A, et al. Outcomes of pediatric identical living-donor liver and hematopoietic stem cell transplantation. Pediatr Transplant. 2016;20(7):888–97.
64. Matthes-Martin S, Peters C, Konigsrainer A, Fritsch G, Lion T, Heitger A, et al. Successful stem cell transplantation following orthotopic liver transplantation from the same haploidentical family donor in a girl with hemophagocytic lymphohistiocytosis. Blood. 2000;96(12):3997–9.
65. Mellgren K, Fasth A, Saalman R, Olausson M, Abrahamsson J. Liver transplantation after stem cell transplantation with the same living donor in a monozygotic twin with acute myeloid leukemia. Ann Hematol. 2005;84(11):755–7.
66. Englert C, Ganschow R. Liver transplantation in a child with liver failure due to chronic graft-versus-host disease after allogeneic hematopoietic stem cell transplantation from the same unrelated living donor. Pediatr Transplant. 2012;16(7):E325–7.

67. Schiller O, Avitzur Y, Kadmon G, Nahum E, Steinberg RM, Nachmias V, et al. Nitric oxide for post-liver-transplantation hypoxemia in pediatric hepatopulmonary syndrome: case report and review. Pediatr Transplant. 2011;15(7):E130–4.
68. Shimizu T, Kasahara M, Tanaka K. Living-donor liver transplantation for chronic hepatic graft-versus-host disease. N Engl J Med. 2006;354(14):1536–7.
69. Granot E, Loewenthal R, Jakobovich E, Gazit E, Sokal E, Reding R. Living related liver transplant following bone marrow transplantation from same donor: long-term survival without immunosuppression. Pediatr Transplant. 2012;16(1):E1–4.
70. Mali VP, Tan PL, Aw M, Loh LD, Quak SH, Madhavan K, et al. Mismatched bone marrow transplantation for severe aplastic anaemia after liver transplantation for associated acute liver failure. Ann Acad Med Singapore. 2011;40(9):420–1.
71. Tryphonopoulos P, Ruiz P, Weppler D, Nishida S, Levi DM, Moon J, et al. Long-term follow-up of 23 operational tolerant liver transplant recipients. Transplantation. 2010;90(12):1556–61.
72. Tryphonopoulos P, Tzakis AG, Weppler D, Garcia-Morales R, Kato T, Madariaga JR, et al. The role of donor bone marrow infusions in withdrawal of immunosuppression in adult liver allotransplantation. Am J Transplant. 2005;5(3):608–13.
73. Donckier V, Troisi R, Toungouz M, Colle I, Van Vlierberghe H, Jacquy C, et al. Donor stem cell infusion after non-myeloablative conditioning for tolerance induction to HLA mismatched adult living-donor liver graft. Transpl Immunol. 2004;13(2):139–46.
74. Calne R, Davies H. Organ graft tolerance: the liver effect. Lancet. 1994;343(8889):67–8.
75. Sriwatanawongsa V, Davies HS, Calne RY. The essential roles of parenchymal tissues and passenger leukocytes in the tolerance induced by liver grafting in rats. Nat Med. 1995;1(5):428–32.
76. Starzl TE, Murase N, Abu-Elmagd K, Gray EA, Shapiro R, Eghtesad B, et al. Tolerogenic immunosuppression for organ transplantation. Lancet. 2003;361(9368):1502–10.
77. Eason JD, Cohen AJ, Nair S, Alcantera T, Loss GE. Tolerance: is it worth the risk? Transplantation. 2005;79(9):1157–9.
78. Donckier V, Craciun L, Lucidi V, Buggenhout A, Troisi R, Rogiers X, et al. Acute liver transplant rejection upon immunosuppression withdrawal in a tolerance induction trial: potential role of IFN-gamma-secreting CD8+ T cells. Transplantation. 2009;87(9 Suppl):S91–5.
79. Donckier V, Troisi R, Le Moine A, Toungouz M, Ricciardi S, Colle I, et al. Early immunosuppression withdrawal after living donor liver transplantation and donor stem cell infusion. Liver Transpl. 2006;12(10):1523–8.
80. Benitez CE, Puig-Pey I, Lopez M, Martinez-Llordella M, Lozano JJ, Bohne F, et al. ATG-Fresenius treatment and low-dose tacrolimus: results of a randomized controlled trial in liver transplantation. Am J Transplant. 2010;10(10):2296–304.
81. Ezzelarab M, Thomson AW. Tolerogenic dendritic cells and their role in transplantation. Semin Immunol. 2011;23(4):252–63.
82. Casiraghi F, Perico N, Remuzzi G. Mesenchymal stromal cells for tolerance induction in organ transplantation. Hum Immunol. 2018;79(5):304–13.
83. Detry O, Vandermeulen M, Delbouille MH, Somja J, Bletard N, Briquet A, et al. Infusion of mesenchymal stromal cells after deceased liver transplantation: a phase I-II, open-label, clinical study. J Hepatol. 2017;67(1):47–55.
84. Hartleif S, Schumm M, Doring M, Mezger M, Lang P, Dahlke MH, et al. Safety and tolerance of donor-derived mesenchymal stem cells in pediatric living-donor liver transplantation: the MYSTEP1 study. Stem Cells Int. 2017;2017:2352954.
85. Lamarche C, Levings MK. Guiding regulatory T cells to the allograft. Curr Opin Organ Transplant. 2018;23(1):106–13.
86. Takatsuki M, Uemoto S, Inomata Y, Sakamoto S, Hayashi M, Ueda M, et al. Analysis of alloreactivity and intragraft cytokine profiles in living donor liver transplant recipients with graft acceptance. Transpl Immunol. 2001;8(4):279–86.
87. Mazariegos GV, Zahorchak AF, Reyes J, Chapman H, Zeevi A, Thomson AW. Dendritic cell subset ratio in tolerant, weaning and non-tolerant liver recipients is not affected by extent of immunosuppression. Am J Transplant. 2005;5(2):314–22.
88. Tokita D, Mazariegos GV, Zahorchak AF, Chien N, Abe M, Raimondi G, et al. High PD-L1/CD86 ratio on plasmacytoid dendritic cells correlates with elevated T-regulatory cells in liver transplant tolerance. Transplantation. 2008;85(3):369–77.
89. Li Y, Koshiba T, Yoshizawa A, Yonekawa Y, Masuda K, Ito A, et al. Analyses of peripheral blood mononuclear cells in operational tolerance after pediatric living donor liver transplantation. Am J Transplant. 2004;4(12):2118–25.
90. Bohne F, Londono MC, Benitez C, Miquel R, Martinez-Llordella M, Russo C, et al. HCV-induced immune responses influence the development of operational tolerance after liver transplantation in humans. Sci Transl Med. 2014;6(242):242ra81.
91. Martinez-Llordella M, Puig-Pey I, Orlando G, Ramoni M, Tisone G, Rimola A, et al. Multiparameter immune profiling of operational tolerance in liver transplantation. Am J Transplant. 2007;7(2):309–19.
92. Puig-Pey I, Bohne F, Benitez C, Lopez M, Martinez-Llordella M, Oppenheimer F, et al. Characterization of gamma delta T cell subsets in organ transplantation. Transpl Int. 2010;23(10):1045–55.
93. Martinez-Llordella M, Lozano JJ, Puig-Pey I, Orlando G, Tisone G, Lerut J, et al. Using transcriptional profiling to develop a diagnostic test of operational tolerance in liver transplant recipients. J Clin Invest. 2008;118(8):2845–57.
94. Li Y, Zhao X, Cheng D, Haga H, Tsuruyama T, Wood K, et al. The presence of Foxp3 expressing T cells within grafts of tolerant human liver transplant recipients. Transplantation. 2008;86(12):1837–43.
95. Taubert R, Danger R, Londono MC, Christakoudi S, Martinez-Picola M, Rimola A, et al. Hepatic infiltrates in operational tolerant patients after liver transplantation show enrichment of regulatory T cells before proinflammatory genes are downregulated. Am J Transplant. 2016;16(4):1285–93.
96. Bohne F, Martinez-Llordella M, Lozano JJ, Miquel R, Benitez C, Londono MC, et al. Intra-graft expression of genes involved in iron homeostasis predicts the development of operational tolerance in human liver transplantation. J Clin Invest. 2012;122(1):368–82.
97. Li L, Wozniak LJ, Rodder S, Heish S, Talisetti A, Wang Q, et al. A common peripheral blood gene set for diagnosis of operational tolerance in pediatric and adult liver transplantation. Am J Transplant. 2012;12(5):1218–28.
98. Braud C, Baeten D, Giral M, Pallier A, Ashton-Chess J, Braudeau C, et al. Immunosuppressive drug-free operational immune tolerance in human kidney transplant recipients: part I. Blood gene expression statistical analysis. J Cell Biochem. 2008;103(6):1681–92.
99. Newell KA, Asare A, Kirk AD, Gisler TD, Bourcier K, Suthanthiran M, et al. Identification of a B cell signature associated with renal transplant tolerance in humans. J Clin Invest. 2010;120(6):1836–47.
100. Pallier A, Hillion S, Danger R, Giral M, Racape M, Degauque N, et al. Patients with drug-free long-term graft function display increased numbers of peripheral B cells with a memory and inhibitory phenotype. Kidney Int. 2010;78(5):503–13.
101. Sagoo P, Perucha E, Sawitzki B, Tomiuk S, Stephens DA, Miqueu P, et al. Development of a cross-platform biomarker signature to detect renal transplant tolerance in humans. J Clin Invest. 2010;120(6):1848–61.
102. Brouard S, Mansfield E, Braud C, Li L, Giral M, Hsieh SC, et al. Identification of a peripheral blood transcriptional biomarker

panel associated with operational renal allograft tolerance. Proc Natl Acad Sci U S A. 2007;104(39):15448–53.
103. Chesneau M, Michel L, Dugast E, Chenouard A, Baron D, Pallier A, et al. Tolerant kidney transplant patients produce B cells with regulatory properties. J Am Soc Nephrol. 2015;26(10):2588–98.
104. Newell KA, Asare A, Sanz I, Wei C, Rosenberg A, Gao Z, et al. Longitudinal studies of a B cell-derived signature of tolerance in renal transplant recipients. Am J Transplant. 2015;15(11):2908–20.
105. Baron D, Ramstein G, Chesneau M, Echasseriau Y, Pallier A, Paul C, et al. A common gene signature across multiple studies relate biomarkers and functional regulation in tolerance to renal allograft. Kidney Int. 2015;87(5):984–95.
106. Roedder S, Li L, Alonso MN, Hsieh SC, Vu MT, Dai H, et al. A three-gene assay for monitoring immune quiescence in kidney transplantation. J Am Soc Nephrol. 2015;26(8):2042–53.
107. Lozano JJ, Pallier A, Martinez-Llordella M, Danger R, Lopez M, Giral M, et al. Comparison of transcriptional and blood cell-phenotypic markers between operationally tolerant liver and kidney recipients. Am J Transplant. 2011;11(9):1916–26.
108. Rebollo-Mesa I, Nova-Lamperti E, Mobillo P, Runglall M, Christakoudi S, Norris S, et al. Biomarkers of tolerance in kidney transplantation: are we predicting tolerance or response to immunosuppressive treatment? Am J Transplant. 2016;16(12):3443–57.
109. Anglicheau D, Suthanthiran M. Noninvasive prediction of organ graft rejection and outcome using gene expression patterns. Transplantation. 2008;86(2):192–9.
110. Reeve J, Einecke G, Mengel M, Sis B, Kayser N, Kaplan B, et al. Diagnosing rejection in renal transplants: a comparison of molecular- and histopathology-based approaches. Am J Transplant. 2009;9(8):1802–10.
111. Strehlau J, Pavlakis M, Lipman M, Shapiro M, Vasconcellos L, Harmon W, et al. Quantitative detection of immune activation transcripts as a diagnostic tool in kidney transplantation. Proc Natl Acad Sci U S A. 1997;94(2):695–700.
112. Sarwal M, Chua MS, Kambham N, Hsieh SC, Satterwhite T, Masek M, et al. Molecular heterogeneity in acute renal allograft rejection identified by DNA microarray profiling. N Engl J Med. 2003;349(2):125–38.
113. Suthanthiran M, Schwartz JE, Ding R, Abecassis M, Dadhania D, Samstein B, et al. Urinary-cell mRNA profile and acute cellular rejection in kidney allografts. N Engl J Med. 2013;369(1):20–31.
114. Bonaccorsi-Riani E, Pennycuick A, Londono MC, Lozano JJ, Benitez C, Sawitzki B, et al. Molecular characterization of acute cellular rejection occurring during intentional immunosuppression withdrawal in liver transplantation. Am J Transplant. 2016;16(2):484–96.
115. Assy N, Adams PC, Myers P, Simon V, Minuk GY, Wall W, et al. Randomized controlled trial of total immunosuppression withdrawal in liver transplant recipients: role of ursodeoxycholic acid. Transplantation. 2007;83(12):1571–6.
116. Todo S, Yamashita K. Anti-donor regulatory T cell therapy in liver transplantation. Hum Immunol. 2018;79(5):288–93.

Long-Term Outcome and Transition

Marianne Samyn

Key Points
- Long-term patient and graft survival post paediatric liver transplantation is excellent; however presence of fibrosis and inflammation in protocol liver biopsies is common.
- Complications related to long-term immunosuppression use are renal impairment and malignancy with an increased prevalence of metabolic syndrome noted in children.
- Adherence to treatment is a challenge in particular for young people, impacting on long-term outcome.
- Overall patient wellness has become an important factor of patient care, and the effects of liver disease and liver transplantation on growth, cognition and mental health cannot be underestimated.
- Providing a holistic, multidisciplinary model of care for young people beyond the transition from paediatric to adult services is essential to ensure further successful long-term outcome.

Research Needed in the Field
- Expanding knowledge regarding the concept of idiopathic post-transplant hepatitis and fibrosis and the use of non-invasive markers to assess graft function.
- Metabolic syndrome, associated with cardiovascular complications requires more research focussing on nutrition and body composition both pre- and post liver transplantation.
- Longitudinal studies addressing the impact of chronic liver disease on pubertal development and cognition.

M. Samyn (✉)
Paediatric Liver, GI and Nutrition Centre, King's College Hospital NHS Foundation Trust, London, UK
e-mail: marianne.samyn@nhs.net

37.1 Introduction

Since the first series of liver transplants by Thomas Starzl and colleagues in 1963 advances in surgical techniques, immunosuppressive management and peri- and postoperative care have contributed to the success of the programme [1]. Long-term, up to 20-year survival rates in children are now available with patient survival up to 79% and graft survival up to 64%, which is significantly better compared to adult outcomes (21–52%) [2]. Long-term complications in paediatric liver transplantation associated with re-transplantation and late mortality include chronic graft dysfunction and immunosuppression-related complications such as renal dysfunction and malignancies, either lymphoproliferative disorders or de novo malignancies [3]. Evaluation of serial post liver transplant protocol biopsies has demonstrated common features of fibrosis and non-specific inflammation even in the absence of abnormal liver function tests, and this continues to provide a challenge with regard to aetiology and management [4].

In contrast to younger children, long-term post-transplant outcomes for adolescents and young people are inferior to both younger and older age cohorts. Whereas lifestyle-related challenges including suboptimal adherence to treatment are more prevalent in this age cohort, other factors impacting on outcome are disparities on the waiting lists and application of listing criteria developed on the background of adult liver pathologies [5]. Other aspects related to patient wellness such as growth and puberty, cognition and health-related quality of life are impaired in the post liver transplant setting. Transition from paediatric to adult care is a particularly challenging period for patients but also for their parents and healthcare professionals. Unfortunately, its timing tends to be determined by chronological age rather than neurocognitive developmental stage. New information illustrating ongoing brain development well in to the mid-20s supports the importance of providing an appropriate, holistic care package for young people age 10–24 years in order to improve not only patient and graft survival but health-related quality of life [6].

This chapter will aim to address the various aspects of long-term outcome post liver transplantation in childhood including patient and graft survival, medical complications and then move on to discuss issues particular to young people including adolescence, adherence, mental health and transition from paediatric to adult health services.

37.2 Patient and Graft Survival

Over the last three and a half decades, liver transplantation has transformed the prognosis for children with end-stage liver disease and those presenting with fulminant liver failure. The introduction of cyclosporine as immunosuppressive agent, improved surgical techniques and re-transplantation contributed to improved 1-year patient survival from 71% after 1983 to 86% after 1988 in a series of 100 children transplanted between 1983 and 1990 [7]. Since, has led of tacrolimus as an alternative calcineurin inhibitor to cyclosporine has led to further improvement in survival. Current 1-year post LT in the UK is 97.1% for those electively listed and 86.1% for patients presenting with fulminant hepatic failure (NHSBT 2017).

Recently large paediatric liver transplant centres in Europe, the USA and Japan have reported on long-term survival, up to 20-year post liver transplantation, with patient and graft survival rates between 69–79.9% and 53–64%, respectively [2, 8–10]. Busuttil et al. found that patients <18 years and who were nonurgently listed exhibited superior long-term survival in cohort of 2662 recipients with overall 15-year patient survival of 64% and graft survival of 55% [11]. In adults, complications as recurrence of the original disease, cardiovascular complications and malignancy are linked with death and graft loss and definitely contribute to the overall inferior 20-year patient (34.5–52.5%) and graft (31.5–46.6%) survival compared to children [8, 12]. For cultural reasons, living-related donation is the main donor source of organ donation in Japan with excellent long-term survival data in particular for children with biliary atresia (84.8%) [13]. The challenges affecting outcome in this setting were ABO incompatibility, recipient age, aetiology of the liver disease and transplant era.

Predictors of patient survival in a cohort of 806 children were found to be renal function, mechanical ventilation at time of transplantation and aetiology of liver disease, whereas graft survival was associated with weight, transplantation era and renal replacement therapy and for those requiring re-transplantation, indicated in 21% of children, warm ischaemia time and time between primary liver transplantation and re-transplantation [9]. The main indications for re-transplantation were hepatic artery thrombosis (27%), chronic rejection (22%), primary non-function (20%) and portal vein thrombosis (17%). This is in contrast to an earlier report by Jain et al. where only 1.2% of 1000 LT recipients including 166 children required re-transplantation for rejection [8]. Re-transplantation was only required in 3.3% of 2224 paediatric living-related donor recipients in Japan and associated with inferior outcome [13].

More relevant in the context of long-term outcome is late graft loss and late mortality, defined as more than 1-year post liver transplantation. Analysis of the SPLIT database showed superior 5-year patient and graft survival for 872 children surviving the first year after transplant (94.2% and 89.2%, respectively) compared to overall database (82 and 72%) [3]. Rejection, either acute or chronic, was the most common cause of late graft loss in 48.5% of the patients followed by sequelae of hepatic artery thrombosis and biliary strictures in 20%. Independent factors associated with late graft loss were malignancy as indication for LT, occurrence of steroid resistant rejection, surgery within 30 days of LT and more than 5 hospital admissions during the first post-transplant year. Martinelli et al. noted similar indications for re-transplantation for 9 out 26 patients requiring re-transplantation more than 5 years after LT (chronic rejection $n = 4$, complications of hepatic artery thrombosis and biliary complications $n = 5$) in a cohort of 128 patients with long-term follow-up [2].

Late mortality for patients in the SPLIT database was caused by malignancy, infection, multisystem organ failure and post-transplant lymphoproliferative disorder (PTLD) in the majority of the cases, and presentation with fulminant hepatic failure, tumours as indications for LT, low weight and frequent readmission during the first year post LT were found to be independently associated with late mortality [3].

Of importance and relevant to this chapter is the inferior patient and graft survival for those transplanted between the ages of 12 and 17 years irrespective of the type of solid organ [5, 14]. Also young adults, aged 18–24 years, have poor waitlist and post-transplant outcomes compared to older and younger populations [5]. This suggests that young people are a particular vulnerable group of patients who will require specialised developmentally appropriate care. We will elaborate on this topic further in the chapter.

37.2.1 Graft Status

Routine monitoring of graft function includes serum aminotransferase and γ-glutamyl transferase activity. Martinelli et al. found that in 43% of long-term post LT survivors, at least one of these levels was outside normal limits and associated with reduced-size or split liver transplantation and past episode(s) of acute rejection [2].

Serial protocol liver biopsies have allowed us to get more insight into graft function in particular in asymptomatic patients with normal biochemistry. More than two thirds of 10-year post liver transplant biopsies (69–73%) are reported as abnormal [4]. The most common features are graft inflammation and fibrosis seen in up to 64% and 91%, respectively, of 10-year post-transplant liver biopsies in a series of 158 patients [15]. The aetiology of graft inflammation, also labelled as idiopathic post-transplant hepatitis (IPTH), remains largely unexplained; however, its relation with the presence of auto/alloantibodies, de novo class II donor-specific HLA antibodies and previous episodes of rejection suggests an immune-mediated process [4]. Hepatitis E infection has also been linked with post LT inflammation. Evans et al. found a correlation between degree of inflammation and fibrosis stage, and of concern is the increase in the prevalence and severity of fibrosis over time [15]. A recent long-term analysis of the histopathology of failed liver grafts at time of re-transplantation has shown a decline of features of chronic rejection and increase in IPTH in particular in paediatric explants [16]. Routine protocol liver biopsies are an essential part of long-term post liver transplant management, and further research into non-invasive investigations to monitor graft function such as transient elastography and MRI are being assessed in larger patient cohorts [17].

37.3 Long-Term Complications

37.3.1 Medical Complications

37.3.1.1 Renal Disease

Chronic kidney disease (CKD) is a well-recognised complication of solid organ and haematopoietic stem cell transplantation impacting on morbidity and mortality. The percentage of patients developing CKD post liver transplantation in children varies between 26 and 86% depending on the definition used, and up to 8% of children are estimated to develop end-stage renal disease [18]. Calcineurin inhibitors (CNI) and cyclosporine in particular are considered to be the key contributor to CKD post transplantation, and the nephrotoxic effect correlates with drug serum levels and treatment duration. The pattern of renal impairment observed is characterised by early deterioration during the first year post transplantation followed by a period of stabilisation and further progress during long-term follow-up. Risk factors associated with CKD post liver transplantation are the presence of renal disease prior to transplant, associated with the underlying liver disease (e.g., Alagille syndrome, ciliopathies) or in the context of hepato-renal syndrome, as well as older age at transplant [19]. Post liver transplantation, aside the use of CNI, a glomerular filtration rate of <70 mL/min/1.73m^2 at 1-year post liver transplantation was associated with development of CKD. More recently, the presence of hypertension 1 year after cardiac and liver transplantation in adults was found to be a modifiable risk factor for deteriorating renal function between 1 and 5 years post transplantation in contrast to the type or dose of CNI [20].

The practice recommendations for monitoring of renal function in paediatric non-renal transplant recipients suggest regular monitoring of renal function by means of glomerular filtration rate [21]. Whereas estimation of GFR by inulin clearance is gold standard, in practice this test is cumbersome and expensive. Serum creatinine is less reliable in children compared to adults as it is influenced by age and muscle mass. Newer small molecular mass proteins such as Cystatin C have been evaluated post liver transplantation and are now included in formulae such adapted by Schwartz and Zappitelli and can be used in this setting [22–24]. Regular monitoring of blood pressure is also recommended as well as screening for the presence of proteinuria. Collaboration with paediatric nephrologist is advisable especially in those patients who are at risk of developing CKD post LT and those who develop evidence of decreasing GFR during post LT follow-up [21, 25]. Renal sparing immunosuppressive regimens with induction of interleukin-2 blockers at time of transplantation or introduction of other agents such as mycophenolate mofetil and rapamycin during follow-up can be considered [25].

37.3.1.2 Malignancy

Solid organ transplant recipients are at risk of developing malignancy with a linear increase in incidence over time to up to 20% after 10 years of immunosuppression [26]. The most common types of malignancy are viral-mediated cancers with EBV-associated post-transplant lymphoproliferative disorder (PTLD) seen in about 50% of paediatric cases. The cumulative incidence in paediatric liver transplantation estimated between 2 and 10% [27]. Currently, a consensus towards the diagnosis and management of PTLD is lacking. Whereas monitoring of EBV viraemia is recommended, the interpretation of the results and indications for further investigations and timing of treatment is unclear. Lowering immunosuppression is considered first line of management, and other treatments aimed to reducing B cell mass such as monoclonal antibody treatment with rituximab with or without more intensive chemotherapy regimens can be required [28].

Of relevance for those transplanted during adolescence is the risk of developing other malignancies such as non-melanoma skin cancer and Kaposi sarcoma, more commonly seen in adults post liver transplantation [29]. Yearly dermatology follow-up is recommended.

37.3.1.3 Metabolic Syndrome

In adults liver transplant recipients, post-transplant metabolic syndrome (MS) including obesity, hypertension, dyslipidaemia and diabetes mellitus is well described and linked with poorer outcomes. It is estimated that out of 21–58% of adults who are overweight post liver transplantation, 43–58% will develop MS [30]. Data in children are lacking; however, in the USA, the prevalence of obesity in paediatric liver transplant recipients is between 10 and 67% and similar to the general population. Pre-transplant obesity is a risk factor for post-transplant obesity. Whereas MS is more commonly seen in the early post-transplant period, 5–10 years post transplant, the prevalence remains higher in comparison with the general population and is associated with an increased risk of cardiovascular disease in adulthood and death [30]. Recently, Perito et al. found a similar prevalence of MS in 83 children post LT compared to matched peers, even when adjusted for overweight/obesity and oral glucocorticoid use (36% vs 32%, respectively) [31]. Interestingly, but confirming what has been reported in adults was that post liver transplant children with a normal weight were at higher risk than the control group of developing MS (7% vs 1%, respectively). A novel finding in the study was the high prevalence of impaired glucose tolerance, considered to be a prediabetic state, and this was linked with duration of CNI exposure. Fasting glucose levels did not correlate with impaired glucose tolerance, and Hba1c was normal in all patients and are therefore not helpful. Routine screening for MS should be included in the routine follow-up protocols of paediatric LT patients to avoid long-term cardiovascular complications.

37.3.2 Nonadherence

Adherence is defined as "the extent to which a person's behavior, (taking medication, following a diet, and/or executing lifestyle changes) corresponds with agreed recommendations from a health care provider" [32]. Nonadherence (NA) to medications in children, adolescents and adults has been demonstrated to be the most important risk factor for late acute rejection and other adverse outcomes in the transplant setting [33]. The prevalence is estimated between 15 and 40% depending on the method used to measure adherence and threshold set for considering someone to be nonadherent [34].

Adherence to treatment is difficult to measure with no "gold standard" measurement technique. Commonly used methods are either subjective, relying on self-report or assessment of the health provider, whereas objective methods such as electronic monitoring are more precise but cumbersome and expensive. In the transplant setting, the medication level variability index (MLVI) obtained by calculating the standard deviation of consecutive immunosuppressive measurements indicates the degree in variability of immunosuppressive medication, typically tacrolimus. Levels between 1.8 and 3.5 have been shown to be associated with late acute rejection episodes in children, adolescents and adults [35].

Nonadherence tends to be multifactorial with a range of potential factors involved including treatment and illness demands, social, psychological and developmental factors as well as factors related to healthcare providers. Risk factors for NA such as female gender, lower socio-economic status, younger age and single parent households have previously been suggested; however, de Oliveira et al. demonstrated that in a group of children less than 12 years, MLVI levels >2 was more prevalent in families with higher income [36]. One of the challenges with regard to investigate NA in populations is the paucity of randomised control trials and the lack of engagement of nonadherent patients who are also likely to have poorer engagement with the treatment centres [37].

When assessing NA, trying to distinguish between unintentional and intentional NA is important. In contrast to unintentional NA, most commonly related to forgetfulness, intentional NA tends to be deliberate and is largely associated with patient and a more formal psychosocial assessment and targeted counselling are required to address it.

An important aspect of NA is its fluctuating nature, and this was illustrated in the "The Medication Adherence in Children Who Had a Liver Transplant" (MALT) prospective multisite study where 400 paediatric and adolescent liver transplant recipients with ranging post LT status were monitored for 2 years [38]. Interestingly, 23.8% of patients changed their adherence status, defined by MLVI >2 (nonadherent) and MLVI <2 (adherent), during the study period, from adherent to nonadherent in 9.9% and vice versa in 13.9%. Patients who were nonadherent during the first year were likely to remain nonadherent.

Managing NA implies continuous assessment of adherence, and therefore this needs to be incorporated in our daily practice. The importance of assessing barriers impacting on adherence both in patients and in caregivers was demonstrated by Eaton et al. with caregivers who disclosed NA expressing more emotional distress [39].

Health professionals should routinely review medication regimes and assess whether they can be simplified with regard to frequency and type of preparation. As patients grow up, liquid preparations should be changed to tablet/capsules and the slow release form of tacrolimus considered if appropriate. We reported on a fourfold decrease in biopsy-proven acute rejection in a cohort of 129 adults and young people ($n = 15$) treated with a once daily regimen compared to a group ($n = 60$) taking twice daily tacrolimus [40]. An improvement in MLVI was also noted.

Assessment of adherence should be approached in a non-judgemental fashion and where multidisciplinary input and support can help to encourage disclosure and address the various barriers to adherence in both the patient and parents/caregivers. In young people, NA is considered to be relatively developmentally appropriate, and one should keep in mind that it does not reflect distrust in healthcare professionals or equally rejection on the part of the adolescent. Both the adolescent stage of development and the process of transition from paediatric to adult health services have been associated with higher prevalence of NA, and this will be addressed further in the chapter [41, 42].

37.3.3 Patient Wellness

With excellent long-term patient survival post paediatric liver transplantation into adulthood, patient wellness and quality of life have become more relevant. Recent research implying that neurodevelopmental changes during adolescence which continue into the mid-20s has led to a better understanding of the challenges faced by adolescents and young adults in general. In this part of the chapter, we will be discussing some of these challenges in more detail in particular related to young people post liver transplantation.

37.3.3.1 Growth and Puberty

Data on growth and puberty development in children and young people with chronic liver disease and following liver transplantation remain scarce which is disappointing as the reciprocal interaction between puberty and chronic illness is relevant on a biological, psychological and social level [43, 44]. A study by Viner et al. in 1999 reported on 105 children, who demonstrated catch-up growth up to 7 years post LT with mean height on 11th centile at liver transplantation and 27th centile when they reached final height. Steroid use, graft dysfunction and re-transplantation were associated with poor linear growth [45]. Similarly, a study in 98 Australian and Japanese children found the mean height attained at 15 years post liver transplantation was on the 26th centile and height at liver transplantation determined final height. Children with growth impairment showed better growth rates however failed to catch up with those with less growth impairment at LT [46]. These studies suggest ongoing growth long-term post liver transplantation which was not confirmed by Loeb et al. who reported no further catch-up growth between 2 and 10 years post transplant [47]. The largest series comes from the studies of pediatric liver transplantation (SPLIT) registry where 20% out of a total of 892 liver transplant patients between 8 and 18 years had linear growth impairment at their last follow-up [48].

In children and adults with chronic liver disease, standard measures of height and weight are known to underestimate the degree of malnutrition compared to body composition analyses. In keeping with the results in adults, Ee et al. found that body cell mass in children reduced further following liver transplantation despite normalisation of height and weight, suggesting weight increase was related to increase in fat mass rather than body cell mass. Linear growth impairment was associated with greater reduction in body cell mass, and on multivariate analysis, older age at liver transplantation predicted reduced body cell mass [49]. Further research in this field is required in particular in the context of the risk of developing sarcopenic obesity, diabetes and metabolic syndrome with increasing age.

Pubertal delay is common in young people with chronic conditions but its prevalence in those with chronic liver disease not well documented. It is known that end-stage liver disease alters the normal physiology of the hypothalamic-pituitary-gonadal axis and disturbs oestrogen metabolism affecting sexual function. In a survey of 64 women with liver disease, 28% had irregular menses and 30% amenorrhoea prior to LT and of those <46 years 95% observed a normal menstrual cycle within the first year of LT [50]. Post LT in children, Mohammad et al. found that after median follow-up of 5.8 year after LT, only 61% of girls and 58% of boys aged 16–18 years had reached Tanner 5 pubertal stage compared to 100% of a normative population with growth impairment occurring in 11% of Tanner 5 subjects [48]. Another study found a transient delay in puberty and menarche post LT in a smaller cohort of patients [45]. The psychological impact of both pubertal and growth delay cannot be ignored, and the use of recombinant growth hormone in the post-transplant setting was associated with a positive effect on linear growth and also on psychosocial well-being [51]. We found that a cohort of young people with liver disease ($n = 80$, 30% post liver transplantation) had a poorer body image perception compared to the general population, not related to having a surgical scar or perceived side effects of immunosuppressive medication.

It is likely that the effect of growth and pubertal delay in our patients with liver disease and post liver transplantation will have a long-standing impact on their outcome well beyond the age of paediatric care.

37.3.3.2 Cognitive Function

There is evidence of poorer cognitive ability in children with chronic liver disease, particularly in those with conditions manifesting in the first years of life [52]. Although improvement is noted post liver transplant, this does not normalise, and poorer cognitive ability and associated academic achievement have been evidenced in this population and attributed to multiple factors including poor nutritional status, underlying liver disease, intensive care support and calcineurin levels as well as environmental factors such as parental education and household status [53–55]. Of relevance for young people requiring liver transplantation during adolescence are the findings of Afshar et al. who reported that longer time on the waiting list and older age at liver transplantation were predictive of poor cognitive outcome. This is of relevance in the context of known disparity on the waiting list and inferior post LT outcome of young people as mentioned earlier [5, 56].

A recent literature review on cognitive function in children with liver disease located 25 studies including 1913 children and young people; 67% of the studies reporting on cognitive function in children with chronic liver disease reported low average and abnormal cognition, and this was 82% in the post LT studies ($n = 19$). Forty-two percent of children required special educational support which is likely to affect independent management of their health condition in their adult life. The authors concluded that the knowledge on risk factors for poor neurodevelopment in children with liver disease is limited and raised concern about the lack of long-term follow-up [57].

In adults with chronic liver disease, the concept of covert or minimal hepatic encephalopathy (CHE) is well described, and diagnostic criteria including a combination of psychometric and neurophysiological tests are validated. In contrast, in children limited information is available with regard to the prevalence of CHE and its relation with the cognitive deficits seen in children with chronic liver disease and post liver transplantation [58–60]. Research in this field is complicated by the challenge of assessing neurocognition in very young children and the lack of validated tests in older children including psychometric testing and neuroimaging. The consequences of CHE on long-term socio-economic achievements is in particular relevant for adults surviving post liver transplantation, and adult data have shown a significant difference in employment in those with CHE versus those without CHE (15% versus 50%). Overall employment data in adults, post liver transplantation, are disappointing, ranging between 22 and 55% [61]. Younger age at LT, male gender, higher education and employment prior to transplantation as well as good functional status are associated with employment [61, 62]. Educational needs are now considered to make out an integral part of clinical care, and efforts should be made to optimise cognitive function and academic performance in children and young people with chronic liver disease and post liver transplantation.

37.3.3.3 Health-Related Quality of Life and Mental Health

With improvement in long-term patient outcome, enhancing health-related quality of life (HRQoL) has become more important and its assessment a vital outcome parameter in evaluating success of paediatric LT. The World Health Organization defines quality of life as a "state of complete physical, mental, and social well-being, and not merely the absence of disease or infirmity." Quality of life tools have now been adapted for children and young people post liver transplantation and with chronic liver disease. A systemic review by Parmar et al. summarised that HRQoL in paediatric LT is impaired compared to that of the general population but similar to other chronic conditions and solid organ transplant recipients. Predictors of poor HRQoL include older age at LT, poor adherence to medication and sleep disturbance which are all particularly relevant to young people [63]. Mental health is an important aspect of quality of life. When screening a cohort of 187 young people attending the multidisciplinary transition service at our centre, out of 51 young people post liver transplantation, 9.8% screened positive for a major depressive disorder and 17.7% had a probable anxiety disorder which was similar to a group with autoimmune liver disease and a group with other liver conditions [64]. Higher levels of depression and anxiety were associated with specific illness and treatment beliefs, rather than with perceived understanding of illness or treatment control. Similar to the HRQoL findings, fatigue and sleep difficulties as well as financial concerns, worry, problems at work/school and low self-esteem caused distress in young people. For several of these concerns, psychological interventions are highly effective and should be considered more routinely with their efficacy assessed. Post-traumatic stress disorder is also a well-recognised mental health concern in the post-transplant setting [65]. The higher prevalence of mental health problems in young people with liver disease and its close relationship with physical health provide further evidence for the need to provide holistic care as standard for this age group.

37.3.3.4 Transition from Paediatric to Adult-Centred Health Services

Recent scientific evidence confirms that adolescence is unique period, distinct from childhood and adulthood with particular neurodevelopmental characteristics and continuing into the mid-20s. This has led to consideration of an expanded and more inclusive definition of adolescence corresponding more closely to adolescent growth by extending the age range from 10–19 years to 10–24 years [66]. It is estimated that this cohort, defined by the WHO as "young people," currently makes up 25% of the world population.

Outcome data in the transplant setting support the relevance of considering young people as a distinct group of patients as those aged between the ages of 12 and 17 years have inferior survival compared to younger and older cohorts irrespective of the type of organ transplanted [14], and young adults aged 18–24 years are more likely to experience disparities on the waitlist for liver transplantation and with worse outcomes compared to other age groups [5].

For young people with healthcare needs, a major if not the most important challenge during adolescence is the historical organisation of healthcare provision for young people, based on chronological age rather than stage of development and young people being obliged to move from paediatric to adult healthcare providers amongst all other transitions occurring in their lives including transition in mental healthcare and social care settings. Most paediatric services are not allowed to look after young people aged over 18 years, and some turn away new patients presenting over the age of

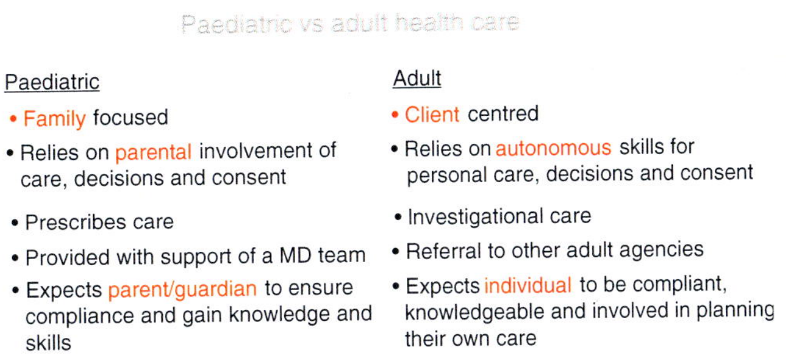

Paediatric vs adult health care

Paediatric	Adult
• Family focused	• Client centred
• Relies on parental involvement of care, decisions and consent	• Relies on autonomous skills for personal care, decisions and consent
• Prescribes care	• Investigational care
• Provided with support of a MD team	• Referral to other adult agencies
• Expects parent/guardian to ensure compliance and gain knowledge and skills	• Expects individual to be compliant, knowledgeable and involved in planning their own care

Fig. 37.1 Differences in care provision of paediatric service versus adult services

Table 37.1 Key components of transition

Key components of transition:
Early preparation, proactive approach
Treating the young person as a young person
Individualised and flexible
Communication within and between agencies
Include family, friends and partners
Routine adherence management

16 years. The difference between paediatric and adult healthcare provision are significant and illustrated in Fig. 37.1.

Following on from the original definition of transition by the adolescent health society in 1993, the academy of pediatrics formulated the following in 2002: "The goal of transition in health care for young adults with special health care needs is to maximise lifelong functioning and potential through the provision of high-quality developmentally appropriate health care services that continue uninterrupted at the individual move from adolescence to adulthood" [67, 68].

The statement of Dr. Koop in 1989 that "our concerns are not amenable to a quick fix" has been confirmed as despite concerted programme and policy efforts, in addition to investments, meaningful change in healthcare transition (HCT) has unfortunately not been made [69]. Whereas HCT has been recognised as an important health goal worldwide, a lack of agreement remains of what constitutes a successful outcome of transition process amongst young people with special healthcare needs [70, 71].

HCT is a challenging period for all involved, including patients, parents/carers and health professionals and associated with increased rates of nonadherence, poorer clinical outcomes and increased mortality [42]; however, one might argue that this is more inherent to the characteristics of the population rather than the transition process per se as better outcome has been shown for those supported by a multidisciplinary team during transition compared to young people who did not [5, 72].

HCT entails more than handing over patients from one service to another, and the focus should be on providing appropriate care for young people irrespective of whether they are looked after in paediatric or adult services. Different models of HCT service provision are possible and dependent on various factors such as location of paediatric and adult services (co-located or not), access to a multidisciplinary team of health professionals, adolescent inpatient facilities, patient load, etc. Figure 37.2 shows a model of care as provided at our centre for patients aged 12–25 years. Health professionals with no additional multidisciplinary support or adolescent facilities can still strive to provide better, holistic care for young people. The key components of a young people's service are listed in Table 37.1.

An essential tool that can facilitate engagement with young people in a clinic setting and identify psychosocial needs is the HEADSS tool, a short psychosocial screening interview instrument which was initially conceived by Berman in 1973 and then more regularly used from 1982 in a High Risk Youth programme in LA, USA [73]. The HEADSS interview addresses the major areas of adolescent psychosocial stress and has been proven to be a useful screening profile in the clinical setting. In order to address the issues relevant to our patient population including adherence to treatment, we adapted the tool which is illustrated in Fig. 37.2. The impact of psychosocial stressors on clinical care and nonadherence to treatment can be significant. A case note review of 34 patients attending our liver transition clinic who were referred to the clinical psychologist and social worker because of concerns of nonadherence demonstrated a high prevalence of intentional nonadherence (35%) or a combination of intentional and unintentional nonadherence (50%). The most common presenting problem for these young people was relationship difficulties, and a third of patients disclosed a history of childhood abuse, unknown to the clinical team [74]. As mentioned previously, young people with liver conditions including liver transplantation report a high prevalence of mental health problems; hence enquiring about mood and mental health should be part of the clinical setting [64].

In developed countries, the median age at first sexual intercourse is 16 years, and 20–30% of young people report sexual intercourse before the age of 15. Comprehensive sexual education including discussion about contraception, pregnancy and sexually transmitted disorder is therefore essential for young people with chronic liver disease and post liver transplantation.

In the context of cognitive function and quality of life post LT, enquiring about education and employment is helpful and can also help to identify those young people with learning difficulties and ensure the receive additional support to manage their condition where needed.

The provision of HCT services and research on this topic has mainly been driven by paediatric healthcare providers. In 2015, a national survey of adult transplant hepatologists on transitional care after liver transplantation in the USA provided interesting information on the perception of adult healthcare providers [75]. Thirty-two percent of respondents did not have a transition strategy at their centre, and only

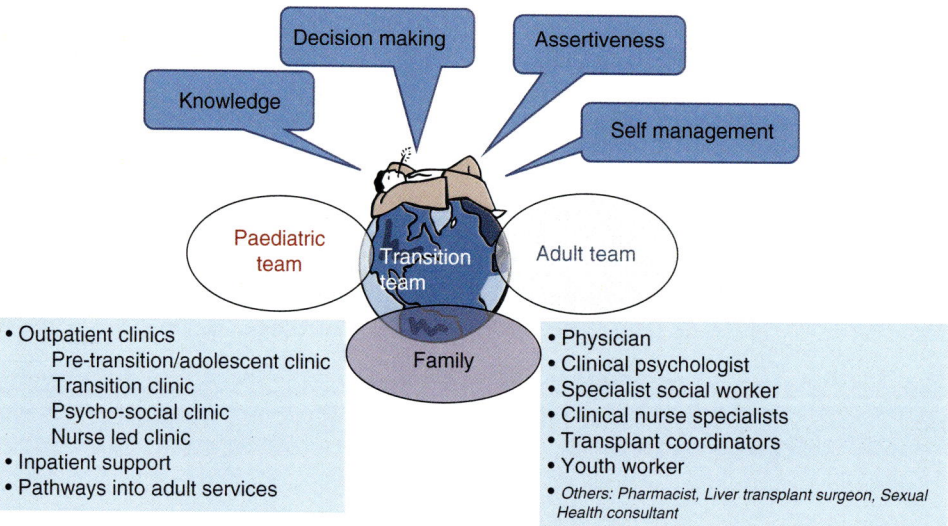

Fig. 37.2 Example of care model for multidisciplinary service provision for young people (12–25 years)

16% had a formal transition programme. A third of the patients were found not to have adequate knowledge about their condition and two thirds attending the appointment accompanied by their parent/guardian. Whereas the majority of adult transplant hepatologists were confident with their own skills to manage young people, poor adherence to treatment and lack of ability from the young people to manage their condition independently were the most common patient barriers. Issues related to the dependent relationship of patients and families with the paediatric provider, inadequate communication from and lack of confidence from the paediatric provider were perceived as barriers to transition.

The relationship between parents/carers and young people is a complex one and changes significantly during adolescence with a drive of the young person to become more independent and relationships with peers becoming more important. However, with delayed timing of role transitions in todays' society including completion of education, marriage and parenthood, young people continue to rely on parental support longer [66]. A significant proportion of the young people and parents/carers we are looking after have a long-standing relationship with the paediatric care providers. During transition parents/carers are expected to move on from a management role to a more supportive role and failure to do so is perceived as a major barrier to transition by adult health professionals [75]. Transition programmes should acknowledge the needs of parents/carers, address them and support them in their new role rather than exclude them [76]. Considering 42% of children post liver transplantation require special educational support, young people are more likely to struggle with the development of the appropriate skills to manage their condition and parental support will remain essential during this process.

Schwartz et al. described that a combination of autonomy, appropriate for the young person's developmental stage, family management styles and self-management were important ingredients for a successful transition from paediatric to adult healthcare settings [77].

The concept of self-management skills and its relation with clinical outcomes is interesting. A study of 48 young people post LT aged between 11 and 20 years demonstrated an increased perception of responsibility with older age; however, this did not transplant into a measurable impact on adherence or health outcome [78]. This was echoed in a large multisite prospective study of 400 liver transplant recipients aged 9–17 years, and the authors suggest that indiscriminate promotion of self-management by adolescents might not be advisable [79]. A challenge for health professionals is how to measure self-management skills as adolescent reports only might be reliable and determine the optimum timing for a young person's readiness to take on more responsibility.

Young people are heavily influenced by social media, and peer support and newer techniques of communication and information delivery such as mobile phone technology should be encouraged [80].

In keeping with the survey results of adult transplant hepatologists in the USA, knowledge with regard to childhood liver diseases is limited, and in the UK, this topic is currently not included in the training curriculum. In particular for rare, often genetic conditions with multisystem involvement such as Alagille syndrome and genetic cholestatic disorders, paediatricians should be encouraged to share their experience with adult colleagues [81, 82].

37.4 Conclusion

Over the last 20 years, patient and graft survival post paediatric liver transplantation has improved significantly with young people now surviving into adulthood. Aside from the long-term medical complications inherent to transplantation, the major challenges for young people such as nonadherence to treatment, mental health problems and transition from paediatric to adult health service should be addressed whilst appreciating that neurodevelopment is ongoing during this period and will impact on behaviour and management of health condition. An open-minded, holistic and non-judgemental approach from both paediatric and adult health professionals with support from a multidisciplinary team and parents/carers should be encouraged to ensure better long-term outcome for young people.

References

1. Starzl TE, Marchioro TL, Vonkaulla KN, Hermann G, Brittain RS, Waddell WR. Homotransplantation of the liver in humans. Surg Gynecol Obstet. 1963;117:659–76.
2. Martinelli J, Habes D, Majed L, Guettier C, Gonzales E, Linglart A, et al. Long-term outcome of liver transplantation in childhood: a study of 20-year survivors. Am J Transplant. 2018;18(7):1680–9.
3. Soltys KA, Mazariegos GV, Squires RH, Sindhi RK, Anand R, SPLIT Research Group. Late graft loss or death in pediatric liver transplantation: an analysis of the SPLIT database. Am J Transplant. 2007;7(9):2165–71.
4. Kelly D, Verkade HJ, Rajanayagam J, McKiernan P, Mazariegos G, Hubscher S. Late graft hepatitis and fibrosis in pediatric liver allograft recipients: current concepts and future developments. Liver Transpl. 2016;22(11):1593–602.
5. Ebel NH, Hsu EK, Berry K, Horslen SP, Ioannou GN. Disparities in waitlist and posttransplantation outcomes in liver transplant registrants and recipients aged 18 to 24 years: analysis of the UNOS database. Transplantation. 2017;101(7):1616–27.
6. Darcy A, Samyn M. Looking after young people with liver conditions: understanding chronic illness management in the context of adolescent development. Clin Liver Dis. 2017;9(5):103–6.
7. Salt A, Noble-Jamieson G, Barnes ND, Mowat AP, Rolles K, Jamieson N, et al. Liver transplantation in 100 children: Cambridge and King's College Hospital series. BMJ. 1992;304(6824):416–21.
8. Jain A, Singhal A, Fontes P, Mazariegos G, DeVera ME, Cacciarelli T, et al. One thousand consecutive primary liver transplants under tacrolimus immunosuppression: a 17- to 20-year longitudinal follow-up. Transplantation. 2011;91(9):1025–30.
9. Venick RS, Farmer DG, Soto JR, Vargas J, Yersiz H, Kaldas FM, et al. One thousand pediatric liver transplants during thirty years: lessons learned. J Am Coll Surg. 2018;226(4):355–66.
10. Kasahara M, Umeshita K, Sakamoto S, Fukuda A, Furukawa H, Sakisaka S, et al. Living donor liver transplantation for biliary atresia: an analysis of 2085 cases in the registry of the Japanese Liver Transplantation Society. Am J Transplant. 2018;18(3):659–68.
11. Busuttil RW, Farmer DG, Yersiz H, Hiatt JR, McDiarmid SV, Goldstein LI, et al. Analysis of long-term outcomes of 3200 liver transplantations over two decades: a single-center experience. Ann Surg. 2005;241(6):905–16; discussion 916–8.
12. Schoening WN, Buescher N, Rademacher S, Andreou A, Kuehn S, Neuhaus R, et al. Twenty-year longitudinal follow-up after orthotopic liver transplantation: a single-center experience of 313 consecutive cases. Am J Transplant. 2013;13(9):2384–94.
13. Kasahara M, Umeshita K, Inomata Y, Uemoto S, Japanese Liver Transplantation Society. Long-term outcomes of pediatric living donor liver transplantation in Japan: an analysis of more than 2200 cases listed in the registry of the Japanese Liver Transplantation Society. Am J Transplant. 2013;13(7):1830–9.
14. Dharnidharka VR, Lamb KE, Zheng J, Schechtman KB, Meier-Kriesche HU. Across all solid organs, adolescent age recipients have worse transplant organ survival than younger age children: a US national registry analysis. Pediatr Transplant. 2015;19(5):471–6.
15. Evans HM, Kelly DA, McKiernan PJ, Hubscher S. Progressive histological damage in liver allografts following pediatric liver transplantation. Hepatology. 2006;43(5):1109–17.
16. Neves Souza L, de Martino R, Sanchez-Fueyo A, Rela M, Dhawan A, O'Grady J, et al. Histopathology of 460 liver allografts removed at retransplantation: a shift in disease patterns over 27 years. Clin Transplant. 2018;32(4):e13227.
17. Fitzpatrick E, Dhawan A. Scanning the scars: the utility of transient elastography in young children. J Pediatr Gastroenterol Nutr. 2014;59(5):551.
18. Hingorani S. Chronic kidney disease after liver, cardiac, lung, heart-lung, and hematopoietic stem cell transplant. Pediatr Nephrol. 2008;23(6):879–88.
19. LaRosa C, Baluarte HJ, Meyers KE. Outcomes in pediatric solid-organ transplantation. Pediatr Transplant. 2011;15(2):128–41.
20. Morath C, Opelz G, Dohler B, Zeier M, Susal C. Influence of blood pressure and calcineurin inhibitors on kidney function after heart or liver transplantation. Transplantation. 2018;102(5):845–52.
21. Filler G, Melk A, Marks SD. Practice recommendations for the monitoring of renal function in pediatric non-renal organ transplant recipients. Pediatr Transplant. 2016;20(3):352–63.
22. Schwartz GJ, Munoz A, Schneider MF, Mak RH, Kaskel F, Warady BA, et al. New equations to estimate GFR in children with CKD. J Am Soc Nephrol. 2009;20(3):629–37.
23. Zappitelli M, Parvex P, Joseph L, Paradis G, Grey V, Lau S, et al. Derivation and validation of cystatin C-based prediction equations for GFR in children. Am J Kidney Dis. 2006;48(2):221–30.
24. Samyn M, Cheeseman P, Bevis L, Taylor R, Samaroo B, Buxton-Thomas M, et al. Cystatin C, an easy and reliable marker for assessment of renal dysfunction in children with liver disease and after liver transplantation. Liver Transpl. 2005;11(3):344–9.
25. Aw MM, Samaroo B, Baker AJ, Verma A, Rela M, Heaton ND, et al. Calcineurin-inhibitor related nephrotoxicity-reversibility in paediatric liver transplant recipients. Transplantation. 2001;72(4):746–9.
26. Buell JF, Gross TG, Thomas MJ, Neff G, Muthiah C, Alloway R, et al. Malignancy in pediatric transplant recipients. Semin Pediatr Surg. 2006;15(3):179–87.
27. McLin VA, Allen U, Boyer O, Bucuvalas J, Colledan M, Cuturi MC, et al. Early and late factors impacting patient and graft outcome in pediatric liver transplantation: summary of an ESPGHAN monothematic conference. J Pediatr Gastroenterol Nutr. 2017;65(3):e53–9.
28. Gross TG, Orjuela MA, Perkins SL, Park JR, Lynch JC, Cairo MS, et al. Low-dose chemotherapy and rituximab for posttransplant lymphoproliferative disease (PTLD): a Children's Oncology Group Report. Am J Transplant. 2012;12(11):3069–75.
29. Durand F. How to improve long-term outcome after liver transplantation? Liver Int. 2018;38(Suppl):134–8.
30. Rothbaum Perito E, Lau A, Rhee S, Roberts JP, Rosenthal P. Posttransplant metabolic syndrome in children and adolescents after liver transplantation: a systematic review. Liver Transpl. 2012;18(9):1009–28.
31. Perito ER, Lustig RH, Rosenthal P. Metabolic syndrome components after pediatric liver transplantation: prevalence and the impact of obesity and immunosuppression. Am J Transplant. 2016;16(6):1909–16.
32. World Health Organization. Adherence to long-term therapies: evidence for action. Geneva: World Health Organization; 2003.

33. Shemesh E, Shneider BL, Savitzky JK, Arnott L, Gondolesi GE, Krieger NR, et al. Medication adherence in pediatric and adolescent liver transplant recipients. Pediatrics. 2004;113(4):825–32.
34. Dobbels F, Van Damme-Lombaert R, Vanhaecke J, De Geest S. Growing pains: non-adherence with the immunosuppressive regimen in adolescent transplant recipients. Pediatr Transplant. 2005;9(3):381–90.
35. Christina S, Annunziato RA, Schiano TD, Anand R, Vaidya S, Chuang K, et al. Medication level variability index predicts rejection, possibly due to nonadherence, in adult liver transplant recipients. Liver Transpl. 2014;20(10):1168–77.
36. de Oliveira JTP, Kieling CO, da Silva AB, Stefani J, Witkowski MC, Smidt CR, et al. Variability index of tacrolimus serum levels in pediatric liver transplant recipients younger than 12 years: non-adherence or risk of non-adherence? Pediatr Transplant. 2017;21(8) https://doi.org/10.1111/petr.13058. Epub 2017 Oct 15.
37. Shemesh E, Mitchell J, Neighbors K, Feist S, Hawkins A, Brown A, et al. Recruiting a representative sample in adherence research- The MALT multisite prospective cohort study experience. Pediatr Transplant. 2017;21(8) https://doi.org/10.1111/petr.13067. Epub 2017 Oct 6.
38. Shemesh E, Duncan S, Anand R, Shneider BL, Alonso EM, Mazariegos GV, et al. Trajectory of adherence behavior in pediatric and adolescent liver transplant recipients: the medication adherence in children who had a liver transplant cohort. Liver Transpl. 2018;24(1):80–8.
39. Eaton CK, Gutierrez-Colina AM, Quast LF, Liverman R, Lee JL, Mee LL, et al. Multimethod assessment of medication nonadherence and barriers in adolescents and young adults with solid organ transplants. J Pediatr Psychol. 2018;43(7):789–99.
40. Considine A, Tredger JM, Heneghan M, Agarwal K, Samyn M, Heaton ND, et al. Performance of modified-release tacrolimus after conversion in liver transplant patients indicates potentially favorable outcomes in selected cohorts. Liver Transpl. 2015;21(1):29–37.
41. Kiberd JA, Acott P, Kiberd BA. Kidney transplant survival in pediatric and young adults. BMC Nephrol. 2011;12:54.
42. Harden PN, Walsh G, Bandler N, Bradley S, Lonsdale D, Taylor J, et al. Bridging the gap: an integrated paediatric to adult clinical service for young adults with kidney failure. BMJ. 2012;344:e3718.
43. Michaud PA, Suris JC, Viner R. The adolescent with a chronic condition. Part II: healthcare provision. Arch Dis Child. 2004;89(10):943–9.
44. Suris JC, Michaud PA, Viner R. The adolescent with a chronic condition. Part I: developmental issues. Arch Dis Child. 2004;89(10):938–42.
45. Viner RM, Forton JT, Cole TJ, Clark IH, Noble-Jamieson G, Barnes ND. Growth of long-term survivors of liver transplantation. Arch Dis Child. 1999;80(3):235–40.
46. Ee LC, Beale K, Fawcett J, Cleghorn GJ. Long-term growth and anthropometry after childhood liver transplantation. J Pediatr. 2013;163(2):537–42.
47. Loeb N, Owens JS, Strom M, Farassati F, Van Roestel K, Chambers K, et al. Long-term follow-up after pediatric liver transplantation: predictors of growth. J Pediatr Gastroenterol Nutr. 2018;66(4):670–5.
48. Mohammad S, Grimberg A, Rand E, Anand R, Yin W, Alonso EM, et al. Long-term linear growth and puberty in pediatric liver transplant recipients. J Pediatr. 2013;163(5):1354–60.e1–7.
49. Ee LC, Hill RJ, Beale K, Noble C, Fawcett J, Cleghorn GJ. Long-term effect of childhood liver transplantation on body cell mass. Liver Transpl. 2014;20(8):922–9.
50. Mass K, Quint EH, Punch MR, Merion RM. Gynecological and reproductive function after liver transplantation. Transplantation. 1996;62(4):476–9.
51. Janjua HS, Mahan JD. The role and future challenges for recombinant growth hormone therapy to promote growth in children after renal transplantation. Clin Transpl. 2011;25(5):E469–74.
52. Stewart SM, Uauy R, Kennard BD, Waller DA, Benser M, Andrews WS. Mental development and growth in children with chronic liver disease of early and late onset. Pediatrics. 1988;82(2):167–72.
53. Stewart SM, Hiltebeitel C, Nici J, Waller DA, Uauy R, Andrews WS. Neuropsychological outcome of pediatric liver transplantation. Pediatrics. 1991;87(3):367–76.
54. Gilmour S, Adkins R, Liddell GA, Jhangri G, Robertson CM. Assessment of psychoeducational outcomes after pediatric liver transplant. Am J Transplant. 2009;9(2):294–300.
55. Sorensen LG, Neighbors K, Martz K, Zelko F, Bucuvalas JC, Alonso EM, et al. Longitudinal study of cognitive and academic outcomes after pediatric liver transplantation. J Pediatr. 2014;165(1):65–72.e2.
56. Afshar S, Porter M, Barton B, Stormon M. Intellectual and academic outcomes after pediatric liver transplantation: relationship with transplant-related factors. Am J Transplant. 2018;18(9):2229–37.
57. Rodijk LH, den Heijer AE, Hulscher JB, Verkade HJ, de Kleine RHJ, Bruggink JLM. Neurodevelopmental outcomes in children with liver diseases: a systematic review. J Pediatr Gastroenterol Nutr. 2018;67(2):157–68.
58. Srivastava A, Chaturvedi S, Gupta RK, Malik R, Mathias A, Jagannathan NR, et al. Minimal hepatic encephalopathy in children with chronic liver disease: prevalence, pathogenesis and magnetic resonance-based diagnosis. J Hepatol. 2017;66(3):528–36.
59. Kyrana E, Dhawan A. Minimal hepatic encephalopathy in children, uncommon or unrecognised? Time to act. J Hepatol. 2017;66(3):478–9.
60. Razek AA, Abdalla A, Ezzat A, Megahed A, Barakat T. Minimal hepatic encephalopathy in children with liver cirrhosis: diffusion-weighted MR imaging and proton MR spectroscopy of the brain. Neuroradiology. 2014;56(10):885–91.
61. Huda A, Newcomer R, Harrington C, Keeffe EB, Esquivel CO. Employment after liver transplantation: a review. Transplant Proc. 2015;47(2):233–9.
62. Huda A, Newcomer R, Harrington C, Blegen MG, Keeffe EB. High rate of unemployment after liver transplantation: analysis of the United Network for Organ Sharing database. Liver Transpl. 2012;18(1):89–99.
63. Parmar A, Vandriel SM, Ng VL. Health-related quality of life after pediatric liver transplantation: a systematic review. Liver Transpl. 2017;23(3):361–74.
64. Hames A, Matcham F, Joshi D, Heneghan MA, Dhawan A, Heaton N, et al. Liver transplantation and adolescence: the role of mental health. Liver Transpl. 2016;22(11):1544–53.
65. Supelana C, Annunziato RA, Kaplan D, Helcer J, Stuber ML, Shemesh E. PTSD in solid organ transplant recipients: current understanding and future implications. Pediatr Transplant. 2016;20(1):23–33.
66. Sawyer M, Azzopardi P, Wicknemarathne D, Patton G. The age of adolescence. Lancet. 2018;2(3):223.
67. American Academy of Pediatrics, American Academy of Family Physicians, American College of Physicians-American Society of Internal Medicine. A consensus statement on health care transitions for young adults with special health care needs. Pediatrics. 2002;110(6 Pt 2):1304–6.
68. Blum RW, Garell D, Hodgman CH, Jorissen TW, Okinow NA, Orr DP, et al. Transition from child-centered to adult healthcare systems for adolescents with chronic conditions. A position paper of the Society for Adolescent Medicine. J Adolesc Health. 1993;14(7):570–6.
69. Scal P. Improving health care transition services: just grow up, will you please. JAMA Pediatr. 2016;170(3):197–9.

70. Fair C, Cuttance J, Sharma N, Maslow G, Wiener L, Betz C, et al. International and interdisciplinary identification of health care transition outcomes. JAMA Pediatr. 2016;170(3):205–11.
71. Williams R, Alexander G, Aspinall R, Bosanquet J, Camps-Walsh G, Cramp M, et al. New metrics for the Lancet Standing Commission on Liver Disease in the UK. Lancet. 2017;389(10083):2053–80.
72. Sagar N, Leithead JA, Lloyd C, Smith M, Gunson BK, Adams DH, et al. Pediatric liver transplant recipients who undergo transfer to the adult healthcare service have good long-term outcomes. Am J Transplant. 2015;15(7):1864–73.
73. Cohen E, MacKenzie R, Yates G. HEADSS, a psychosocial risk assessment instrument: implications for designing effective intervention programs for runaway youth. J Adolesc Health. 1991;12(7):539.
74. Hames A, Malan J. Whose problem is it? Improving adherence in young adults. Rotterdam: Ethical Legal and Psychosocial Aspects of Transplantation (ELPAT) Congress; 2013.
75. Heldman MR, Sohn MW, Gordon EJ, Butt Z, Mohammed S, Alonso EM, et al. National survey of adult transplant hepatologists on the pediatric-to-adult care transition after liver transplantation. Liver Transpl. 2015;21(2):213–23.
76. Samyn M. Parents and carers of young people with liver transplantation: lost in transition? Pediatr Transplant. 2017;21(1) https://doi.org/10.1111/petr.12855. Epub 2016 Dec 15.
77. Schwartz LA, Tuchman LK, Hobbie WL, Ginsberg JP. A social-ecological model of readiness for transition to adult-oriented care for adolescents and young adults with chronic health conditions. Child Care Health Dev. 2011;37(6):883–95.
78. Bilhartz JL, Lopez MJ, Magee JC, Shieck VL, Eder SJ, Fredericks EM. Assessing allocation of responsibility for health management in pediatric liver transplant recipients. Pediatr Transplant. 2015;19(5):538–46.
79. Annunziato RA, Bucuvalas JC, Yin W, Arnand R, Alonso EM, Mazariegos GV, et al. Self-management measurement and prediction of clinical outcomes in pediatric transplant. J Pediatr. 2018;193:128–133.e2.
80. Coad J, Toft A, Claridge L, Ferguson J, Hind J, Jones R, et al. Using mobile phone technology to support young liver transplant recipients moving to adult services. Prog Transplant. 2017;27(2):207–18.
81. Joshi D, Gupta N, Samyn M, Deheragoda M, Dobbels F, Heneghan MA. The management of childhood liver diseases in adulthood. J Hepatol. 2017;66(3):631–44.
82. Dhawan A, Samyn M, Joshi D. Young adults with paediatric liver disease: future challenges. Arch Dis Child. 2017;102(1):8–9.

Neurodevelopment and Health Related Quality of Life of the Transplanted Child

Vicky Lee Ng and Jessica Woolfson

"I'm happy when everything we do in the OR works. I'm pretty unhappy if it fails. But we have to guard against being happy when the operation is only a technical success. **The long haul is what counts.***"*

—Thomas Starzl, 1978

Key Points
- The prevalence of neurodevelopmental (ND) impairments and cognitive deficits, as assessed by various age-specific tools, is increased in paediatric recipients of liver transplantation.
- Risk factors for impaired ND outcomes post-liver transplant include young age of disease onset, longer duration of illness, hyperammonaemia and use of neurotoxic medications.
- ND deficits, particularly executive function, persist over time and can interfere with functioning.
- HRQOL is an important patient-reported outcome post-paediatric LT, with studies to date utilizing both disease-specific and generic HRQOL measures.
- Risk factors for impaired HRQOL post-paediatric liver transplant include time since transplant, household factors, medication adherence and sleep disturbances.

Research Needed in the Field
- Prospective, multicentre studies to determine risk factors and evaluate impact of interventions on ND deficits and lower HRQOL outcomes after paediatric liver transplant
- Longitudinal studies to determine trajectory of ND delays and lower HRQOL scores over time and impact on functional outcomes after paediatric liver transplantation, such as school performance, medical adherence and transition to adult care
- Studies that evaluate the impact of interventions and their timing on ND and HRQOL outcomes

38.1 Introduction

Liver transplantation (LT) is a well-established life-saving treatment for infants and children with end-stage liver disease caused by a number of aetiologies, as well as hepatic malignancy, and metabolic conditions. Since the first paediatric LT pioneered by Thomas Starzl in 1963, many medical and surgical innovations and developments have enhanced pre-, peri- and post-transplant management and contributed to the overarching goal of durable long-term outcomes. The current European LT [1] and American Liver Transplant Registries [2] reveal 1-year, 5-year and 10-year survival rates of over 90%, 85% and 60%, respectively.

With long-term survival now the rule rather than the exception, management has appropriately shifted to include a focus on improving the quality of life years restored by life-saving LT in infants, children and adolescents. Patient-reported outcomes (PROs) such as health-related quality of life (HRQOL) and neurodevelopment (ND) are important outcome metrics for clinical care teams taking care of post-LT patients and their families. Most paediatric LT recipients are under 5 years of age at the time of transplantation, during a period of important brain development. There has been a recent focus on identifying potential risk factors and potential interventions to improve durable outcomes after paediatric LT [3–8].

This chapter will be divided into two sections. The first section will address definitions, assessment tools, risk factors, and potential interventions on ND and school performance in patients who undergo LT as an infant, child or adolescent. This will be followed by a review of evaluation tools, risk factors and strategies to enhance HRQOL outcomes after paediatric LT. Both sections will address limitations to the current literature and propose areas of future research.

V. L. Ng (✉) · J. Woolfson
The Hospital for Sick Children, University of Toronto, Toronto, ON, Canada
e-mail: vicky.ng@sickkids.ca; jessica.woolfson@sickkids.ca

38.2 Part I: Neurodevelopmental Outcomes After Liver Transplantation

38.2.1 Definitions

Neurodevelopmental (ND) outcomes of paediatric LT include children's cognitive function, academic achievement, school performance and behavioural problems [9]. Cognitive functioning refers to the ability to process, understand and learn information, which can be compromised in disease states [10]. Cognitive function is crucial in all developmental stages and for educational achievement. Early literature has focused mainly on early development and intellectual ability (IQ) [11]. Developmental delay occurs when acquisition of skills or milestones lag behind established normal ranges for age. IQ is an intelligence score that reflects the age-graded level of performance as derived from a normative population, with an IQ score of 100 indicative of normal level performance for that age group and intellectual disability being an index score of <70 or 2SD below the mean. Cognitive functioning affects the acquisition, organization, retention, understanding or use of information. Academic achievement and school functioning are important domains that can and should be assessed outside of IQ alone. ND deficits can present as learning disabilities, including impairments with arithmetic or reading. Cognitive function is a predictor of educational achievement and future occupational outcomes and health behaviours [12].

Research exploring other ND domains include motor and visuospatial skills. Another ND domain is executive functioning (EF), an umbrella term for the skills involved in mental control and self-regulation, including attention, planning, problem-solving, reasoning, working memory, inhibition and initiation and response selection and multitasking. These are required to manage oneself and resources in order to achieve goals, particularly in an academic setting. EF assessment is relevant for school-aged children towards identification of strategies aiding behavioural regulation and school performance [3] especially in adolescents as they assume responsibility for self-managing illness and transition to adult care [13].

ND also includes domains of visuospatial functioning. Visuospatial and constructive function are needed for copying tasks and attention to detail for everyday life activities such as drawing, buttoning shirts, constructing models and putting together unassembled furniture [14]. Visual perceptual analysis and attention to detail are required for facial recognition and social perception, and visual scanning skills are needed for activities of daily living, such as controlling motor vehicles [15, 16].

38.2.2 Assessment Tools

Multiple age-specific assessment tools have been utilized to assess ND outcomes in paediatric LT recipients (Table 38.1) and chosen by clinical teams based on patient age, country of origin and the ND domain of interest. ND assessment tools used most commonly in multicentre studies are the Wechsler Intelligence Scale for Children (WISC), Wide Range Achievement Test (WRAT) and Behaviour Rating Inventory of Executive Function (BRIEF) (Table 38.1) to assess IQ, academic performance and EF, respectively.

38.2.3 Neurodevelopmental Outcomes After Liver Transplantation

38.2.3.1 Multicentre Studies

Paediatric LT recipients are at higher risk of ND deficits than healthy age-matched norms. The functional outcome group (FOG) is an international multicentre study focusing on ND outcomes in children aged 5–7 years who had undergone LT at one of the 20 sites within the Studies of Paediatric Liver Transplantation (SPLIT) network, a longitudinal registry comprised of 45 liver transplant programmes in the USA and Canada prospectively collecting comprehensive pre- and post-transplant medical data from paediatric LT candidates and recipients [17]. A total of 140 patients 2 years post-LT underwent initial ND testing with the WPPS-III, WRAT-4, Bracken Basic Concept Scale-Revised (BBCS-R) and BRIEF (FOG-1) in a 4-year period of June 2005 and December 2009 [18]. A score of 71–85 consistent with mild to moderate delay (defined as an IQ 1–2 standard deviations below the mean) was seen in 26% of paediatric LT recipients which was significantly more than 14% expected. Serious delay (IQ < 70) was seen in 4% of the study cohort, a frequency twice expected from the general population. Learning disabilities (LD) occurred in reading (19%), math (13%) or both (6%). Significantly more patients (25%) had reading and/or math LD in contrast to 7% of expected. EF deficits were reported by both parents and teachers, particularly lower working memory abilities compared to the normative population [18]. A follow-up study (FOG-2) in 2014 [4] retested 93 paediatric LT recipients (65% of the FOG-1 cohort) between the ages of 7 and 9 years old. At this second time point, 29% of patients had an IQ score 71–85 (over twice the 14% expected), and 7% had an IQ <70 (over three times the 2% expected). Although deficits in math and EF persisted over time, this study found that reading improved and was no longer different from test norms [4].

Table 38.1 Tools to assess neurodevelopment

Tool	Age range	Domains
Bayley Scales of Infant Development (BSID)	1–42 months	Development – Cognitive – Language – Motor – Social-emotional – Adaptive behaviour
Beery-Buktenica Developmental Test of Visual-Motor Integration (Beery-VMI)	>2 years	Visual and motor abilities – Visual perception – Motor coordination – Visual-motor integration
Behaviour Assessment for Children (BASC)	>2 years	Emotional and behavioural status – Activities of daily living – Functional communication – Adaptability – Hyperactivity, attention problems – Aggression, conduct disorder – Depression, withdrawal – Leadership, social skills – Learning problems
Bracken Basic Concept Scale (BBCS)	3–6 years and 11 months	Cognitive and language development – Receptive comprehension of basic concepts – Verbally label basic concepts
Behaviour Rating Inventory of Executive Function (BRIEF)	5–18 years	Executive function and self-regulation – Behaviour regulation (i.e. inhibit, shift, emotional control) – Metacognition (initiate, memory, organization, monitoring, planning) – Global executive composition
Child Behaviour Checklist (CBCL)	6–18 years	Emotional and behavioural status – Anxiety/depression – Somatic complaints – Social issues – Attention and thought problems – Rule-breaking and aggressive behaviour
Children's Depression Inventory (CDI)	7–17 years	Signs of depression – Negative mood and self-esteem – Interpersonal problems – Ineffectiveness – Anhedonia
Clinical Evaluation of Language Fundamentals (CELF)	5–8 years, 5–21 years, 8–21 years	Language and communication skills Detects language disorders – Sentence comprehension, formation, recall, assembly – Linguistic concepts – Word structure and classes – Directions – Word definitions – Structured writing – Reading comprehension, understanding spoken paragraphs – Pragmatic profile and activities
Conner's Continuous Performance Test (CPT)	>8 years	Attention and ADHD – Inattentiveness – Impulsivity – Sustained attention – Vigilance

(Continued)

Table 38.1 (continued)

Tool	Age range	Domains
Conner's Parent Rating Scale (CPR)	6–18 years	ADHD - Hyperactivity/impulsivity - Inattention-learning issues - Executive function - Defiance/aggressive behaviour - Peer/family relationships
Delis-Kaplan Executive Function System (D-KEFS)	>6 years	Verbal and non-verbal EF - Spatial
Developmental Test of Visual Perception (DTVP)	4 years to 12 years 11 months	Visual perception and visual-motor integration skills
Five to Fifteen Questionnaire (FTF)	5–15 years	ADHD - Memory - Learning - Language - Executive function - Motor skills - Perception - Social skills - Emotional/behavioural problems
Griffiths Mental Ability Scale (GMDS)	0–2 years, 2–8 years	Development - Gross motor skills - Personal-social - Language - Eye and hand coordination - Performance - Practical reasoning
Kaufman Assessment Battery for Children (K-ABC)	3–18 years	Cognitive and processing skills - Sequential processing - Simultaneous processing - Learning ability-planning ability
Minnesota Child Development Inventory	3–72 months	Development - General - Gross and fine motor - Expressive language - Comprehension-conceptual - Situation comprehension - Self-help
Movement Assessment Battery for Children (M-ABC)	3–16 years 11 months	Motor impairment
A Developmental Neuropsychology Assessment (NEPSY)	3–16 years	Cognition - Attention and EF - Language and communication - Sensorimotor functions - Visuospatial functions - Learning and memory - Social perception
The Piers-Harris Self-Concept Scale (PHCSCS)	7–18 years	Self-perception-popularity - Physical appearance and attributes - Freedom from anxiety - Intellectual and school status - Behavioural adjustment - Happiness and satisfaction
Rey Complex Figure Test (RCFT)	>6 years	Visuospatial ability and memory

Table 38.1 (continued)

Tool	Age range	Domains
Test of Attentional Performance (TAP)	>5 years	Alertness
		– Vigilance
		Attention
		– Covert attention shift
		– Divided attention
		– Sustained attention
		Eye movement
		– Visual field/neglect
		– Visual scanning
		Flexibility
		Cross-modal integration
		Go/NoGo
		Incompatibility
		Working memory
Test of Memory and Learning (TOMAL)	>5 years	Memory
		– Verbal
		– Non-verbal
		– Composite
		– Delayed, free and associative recall
		– Learning
		– Attention and concentration
		– Sequential
School Attendance and Academic Performance Survey (SAAPS)	8–18 years	School attendance
		School performance and educational outcomes
		Parental concerns regarding development and behaviour
Stanford-Binet Intelligence Scale (SBIS)	>2 years	Cognition
		– Knowledge
		– Quantitative reasoning
		– Visual-spatial processing
		– Working memory
		– Fluid reasoning
Wechsler Individual Achievement Test (WIAT)	>4 years	Achievement test and academic skills-reading
		– Math
		– Writing
		– Oral language
Wechsler Intelligence Scale for Children (WISC)	6–16 years	Cognitive development and intelligence quotient
		– Verbal comprehension
		– Visual spatial
		– Fluid reasoning
		– Working memory
		– Processing speed
		Can identify learning disabilities
Wechsler Preschool and Primary Scale of Intelligence (WPPSI)	2 years 6 months to 7 years 7 months	Cognitive development
		– Verbal IQ
		– Performance IQ
		– Full Scale IQ
		– Processing speed quotient
		– General language composite
Wide Range Achievement Test (WRAT)	>5 years	Basic academic skills-math
		– Spelling
		– Reading
		– Comprehension
Wide Range Assessment of Memory and Learning (WRAML)	>5 years	Memory and new learning
		– Verbal memory
		– Visual memory
		– Attention-concentration
		– General memory

(Continued)

Table 38.1 (continued)

Tool	Age range	Domains
Woodcock-Johnson Tests of Achievement (WJ)	>2 years	Achievement and intellectual ability - Reading - Mathematics - Writing - Oral language abilities - Academic knowledge
Vineland Adaptive Behaviour Scale (VABS)	0–18 years	Adaptive behaviour - Communication - Daily living skills - Socialization - Motor skills - Maladaptive behaviour
Vineland Social Maturity Scale (VSMS)	>0 year	Adaptive behaviour - Community skills - Self-help ability, eating, dressing - Locomotion and occupation skills - Self-direction - Socialization skills

Table 38.2 Multicentre studies and patient characteristics for ND outcomes in paediatric liver transplant recipients

Author (year)	Number of patients	Country	Age range	ND domains/ assessment test	Outcomes
Sorensen 2015 [20]	36	USA and Canada	6–16 years PALF	BVMI-6 WISC-IV CPT-2 BRIEF CDI-2	Decreased attention, EF, inhibition, metacognition, motor coordination, visual perception No difference in IQ from population norms
Sorensen 2014 [4]	144	USA and Canada	7–9 years	WISC-IV WRAT-4 BRIEF	Lower IQ, reading, math, working memory scores and EF
Sorensen 2011 [18]	144	USA and Canada	5–7 years	WPPSI-3 BBCS-R WRAT-4 BRIEF	Lower IQ, reading, math, processing speed, language, school readiness and EF, high rates of learning disabilities
Gilmour 2010 [19]	823	USA and Canada	6–18 years	SAAPS	More missed school compared to LD and special education requirements compared to healthy norms

School performance and educational outcomes are impacted by LT and can serve as a marker for ND deficits. A longitudinal analysis by the SPLIT research consortium that surveyed school functioning in 823 paediatric LT recipients between the ages of 6 and 18 years from 39 centres revealed LD in 17.4% of participants, over twice the normative population rate [19]. There was a prevalence of special education requirements in 34% of the LT population, which suggests patients experience a broad range of academic difficulties outside of LD. Furthermore, 33% of LT recipients missed more than 2 weeks of school in the proceeding school year which likely influences school performance and academic achievement.

ND outcomes were also evaluated by the National Institutes of Health-funded Paediatric Acute Liver Failure (PALF) study group with data available on children who underwent LT at paediatric LT programmes in the USA and Canada for the indication of acute liver failure [20]. IQ, visuospatial/visuomotor skills, attention and EF were evaluated in 36 participants at an interval of 3.8 years from the time of PALF (Table 38.2). This study revealed average IQ and visuospatial scores; impaired ND subdomain scores in EF, attention and motor coordination skills; and difficulty with sustained attention. There was no difference in ND variables between patients who survived spontaneously ($n = 13$) and those who received LT ($n = 23$). Teachers reported more problems with inhibition, initiation, memory and organization. A score of >65 on the BRIEF is considered to be of clinically significant concern, and 26% of patients scored >65 on the BRIEF compared to 7% of expected norms [19].

PALF has a different pathogenesis and effect on the brain than children transplanted for chronic or end-stage liver disease (ESLD). The impact of inflammatory response, oxidative stress, change in neurotransmitter function and autoregulation of cerebral blood flow and metabolism is different in ALF [21, 22]. Deficits in motor speed and control are observed in hepatic encephalopathy [23] and 25% of the PALF patients HE (14% Grade 3 or 4) [20]. Finally, the PALF study also included patients who had spontaneous resolution on their ALF and did not undergo LT.

Paediatric LT recipients have more ND deficits compared to healthy norms, particularly in the domains of EF across all aetiologies. Intellectual impairment and LDs are reported in LT survivors with ESLD but not in patients with PALF, which suggests that the pathophysiology of these two distinct conditions may play a role in long-term effects on the brain and its development.

38.2.3.2 Single-Centre Studies

Multiple single-centre cross-sectional studies reporting on subject cohorts ranging from 0 to 23 years post-paediatric LT recipients have demonstrated IQ scores between 85 and 100 (low-normal range) [5, 7, 24–28]. Noteworthy is the finding that 10–18% participants have reported IQ scores <70 (defined as mental disability range) at 1–17 years post-paediatric LT [5, 7, 24, 28].

There are only four longitudinal studies, evaluating IQ scores pre- and post-LT in the same patient cohort. In a study now almost 20 years old, mean IQ scores in a single-centre cohort of 50 children with mixed primary aetiologies (age 6–23 years) were unchanged at follow-up 3–9 years following paediatric LT [24]. The three other studies found similarly no differences in IQ pre- and post-LT 1 year after in various indications for LT [29], as well as specifically MSUD [30] and biliary atresia (BA) [8].

ND delay in domains outside of cognition is also more common in paediatric recipients of liver transplant compared to the normal population [6, 8, 24, 29]. General developmental delays are common prior to transplantation, and delay has been reported to carry over into the post-transplant period [16, 24, 29, 31]. Skills in the motor subdomain are more commonly delayed in LT recipients [32, 33]. Ascites, hepatomegaly and surgery decrease abdominal muscle strength and balance which are integral in the development of gross motor skills [8]. Delayed language (expressive and receptive) and social skills, including eye-hand coordination in LT recipients in children transplanted between 0 and 5 years, have been reported 1–12 years in follow-up [7, 31].

Paediatric LT recipients exhibit lower school performance and academic achievement, with increased associations with LD in several single-centre studies [6, 24, 29]. Math and reading scores are lower compared to population norms [24]. Kennard et al. [24] report 38% of 50 paediatric LT recipients 3–9 years post-LT required special education services, and Fouquet et al. [34] reported 31% of 80 paediatric patients who received LT for BA had delayed school performance during a 10-year follow-up study. In a small study of 18 LT recipients, 17% required full-time special education services, twice the amount of the population norms [33]. However, academic achievement is better than predicted by LT recipient IQ scores [24]. Academic achievement is also influenced by other factors such as school absenteeism as well as other ND deficits, such as those in EF and attention.

EF deficits including attention, inhibition and processing speed post-transplant have been reported in 6–21-year-old paediatric LT recipients in Australia, Germany and the USA [13, 35, 36, 37]. EF has been shown to be related to treatment adherence in patients undergoing SOT [38]. In a large single-centre study of 137 paediatric LT recipients [36], reaction times, errors and omissions on the Test of Attentional Performance (TAP) standardized test for attention were significantly below population mean 7–14 years after LT. These deficits were highly correlated with the WISC and K-ABC, which assess for intellectual capabilities [36]. Ee et al. [35] reported 13 LT recipients had greater difficulties in EF, particularly self-regulation, planning, organization and problem-solving compared to their siblings. A Finnish study [33] of 18 paediatric LT recipients was not revealing for any significant differences in EF or language skills compared to a normative population; however, this small group, which included 22% multi-organ transplants with a large age range, also demonstrated a mean higher IQ [94] than other single-centre studies.

Visuospatial and constructive functions have been reported below the population mean in several studies [6, 39, 40]. Lower scores were seen in 18 paediatric LT recipients compared to healthy normed values [33]. Visuospatial impairments may underlie arithmetic difficulties [6, 24, 39]. Visual perceptual analysis and attention to detail are lower in several studies [6, 37]. Decreased visual scanning was present in 13 LT recipients compared to 6 healthy siblings [35].

38.2.4 Impact of Time Since LT on ND

A major limitation of most studies evaluating ND outcomes following paediatric LT is the one-time ND evaluation of populations of paediatric LT recipients with variable follow-up periods. Studies that include serial ND assessment at different time points post-paediatric LT would enable evaluation of the trajectory of ND over time and thereby help to not only predict outcomes over time but also provide timing as to when intervention would be most beneficial. A total of nine studies with more than one ND assessment time point were found, with variable findings as follows: Four studies describe ND improvement or catch-up post-transplant [8, 30, 41, 42]; however three of these were in only metabolic patients [30, 41, 42]. Five studies describe persistence of functional deficits over time [4, 24, 29, 31, 32]. Table 38.3 highlights key ND assessment findings from three single-centre studies evaluating infants and children 3–48 months post-LT at less than 2 years old [8, 31, 41]. In a study of 40 BA patients who were transplanted at <2 years of age, mental and psychomotor development scores returned to pre-LT scores at 12 months post-LT, which were both greater than the 3-month post-LT values [8]. In 33 metabolic patients who underwent LT or combined liver and renal transplant at less than 42 months, psychomotor and mental scores returned to pre-LT levels at 1 year after being decreased at earlier 3 months post-transplant evaluation [41]. Psychomotor scores increased at 2 years post-LT, but there were no significant changes in mental scores, and they were lower compared to BA patients [41]. Van Mourik et al. [31] followed 25 patients who underwent LT at <12 months of age for 4 years post-LT. They reported a decrease in social skills, coordination and language in the first year post-LT and then normalization to pre-LT scores that persisted over the 4-year study period. Thevenin et al. [42] observed catch-up of ND scores in 34 infants who underwent LT or intestinal/multivisceral transplant between 12 and 15 months of age and were followed 7–10 months after LT. After initial recovery, intellectual and ND abilities have been reported as stable several years after paediatric LT [6, 29, 31]. There are reports of improvement, as seen with IQ score elevation in patients with underlying metabolic disease [30] and improved psychomotor skills several 3–5 years after LT, particularly in children transplanted at <24 months of age [29] and metabolic patients [41]. Almaas et al. [32] did not find improvement in motor skills 1 and 4 years after transplant, but the 35 study patients were older (4–12 years) which may suggest a window period for optimal motor catch-up. There were also no differences in ND scores >3 years post-LT compared to pre-transplant function [24, 31].

ND assessment in the FOG1 and FOG2 studies demonstrated that cognitive, EF and math deficits persisted over time [4, 18]. Reading scores improved from time point 1 to 2; however, study limitations articulated that the study's reading task used was too rudimentary and likely not sensitive enough to capture reading difficulties at later grades [4]. Almost half (42%) of their study participants required special education or support at school. This is comparable to Gilmour et al. [19], which also found 34% of a cohort of 823 paediatric LT recipients (aged 6–18 years) required special education services. Academic difficulties requiring support suggest that ND impairment persists over time.

38.2.5 Risk Factors/Aetiology

Table 38.4 provides pre-, peri- and post-transplant factors likely contributory to the pathophysiology of ND deficits seen in survivors of paediatric LT. Children with ESLD are vulnerable to ND delay given exposure to numerous risk factors including malnutrition from chronic liver disease, metabolic derangements and exposure to neurotoxic medications which may negatively impact the growing brain. These young patients are often most sick and vulnerable during a crucial stage of brain development.

38.2.5.1 Pre-transplant Factors

Underlying Liver Disease/Primary Aetiology

The most common indications for paediatric liver transplantation include biliary atresia, acute liver failure and metabolic liver conditions. IQ scores were higher in 31 biliary atresia patients compared to other aetiologies ($n = 12$) at mean 3 years post-LT [6]. Theorized explanations include the natural history of BA is well known resulting in patients being transplanted at a different stage of ESLD versus other liver diseases [6].

In the PALF study, IQ scores in PALF survivors were no different than those seen in age- and gender-matched normative population [20]. Potential explanations include the lack of chronicity in patients who are confirmed to have PALF and have different disease mechanisms [21, 22].

Inborn errors of metabolism such as maple syrup urine disease (MSUD), urea cycle defects (UCD) and Wilson's disease are known to directly affect the brain from neurotoxic effects of substances that accumulate from respective enzyme deficiencies or copper accumulation [43, 44], and more severe ND and intellectual impairments have been reported [5, 41, 45–47].

Age of Onset and Duration of Illness

At median 4.9 years after transplant, patients who receive LT at <12 months of age were at increased risk of ND impairment [18], following on a prior 1989 study [48]. Longer duration of illness is a risk factor for specific ND deficits post-LT, including low intelligence [15, 28, 33], more EF deficits [36] and ND delays [26]. Earlier age of onset and longer duration of illness may provide a longer exposure time to neurotoxic effects of underlying liver disease and may have a greater effect on the brain, particularly at a more vulnerable time of development compared to older children.

Age at Transplant

Younger age at LT may improve ND outcomes because it corrects underlying liver disease and ameliorates the mechanisms that contribute to ND delay. In metabolic disorders, LT prior to significant ND impairment is beneficial with better

Table 38.3 Single-centre studies and patient characteristics for ND outcomes in paediatric liver transplant recipients

Author (year)	Number of patients	Country	Age range	ND domains/ assessment test	Outcomes
Gutierrez-Colina 2017 [13]	57 (22 LT, 18 kidney transplant, 17 heart transplant)	USA	12–21 years	BRIEF	Worse EF deficits
Lee 2017 [28]	43 (28 LT, 15 kidney transplant)	Korea	3–18 years	WPPSI-III / VSMS / CPT	Lower intelligence and more intellectual delay
Almaas 2015 [32]	35	Norway	4–12 years	M-ABC	Lower motor scores including ball skills, balance
Ee 2014 [35]	13	Australia	6–17 years	WISC-IV, WIAT-II, WRAML, RCFT, BRIEF, DKEFS, CPR, CBCL	Decreased EF including visual scanning, inhibition, comprehension, memory and attention
Robertson 2013 [27]	33	Canada	<3 years	WPPSI-III, Beery-VMI	IQ and visuomotor integration lower than population norms, but within 0.5 standard deviation
Kaller 2013 [5]	64	Germany	6–18 years	WISC-IV	Worse in verbal comprehension, perceptual reasoning, processing speed and total IQ
Haavisto 2011 [33]	18	Finland	7–16 years	WISC-III, NEPSY-II, FTF	Decreased performance IQ, visuospatial/visuoconstructive function, social perception, motor skills, memory, earning, social skills. No difference in EF and language
Kaller 2010 [9]	25	Germany	5–12 years	K-ABC CBCL	IQ below population mean (low-normal range)
Kaller 2010 [36]	137	Germany	7–14 years	K-ABC, WISC-III, TAP	Attention and EF in low normal range but significantly lower than population mean
Gilmour 2009 [6]	30	Canada	0–18 years	BSID-II, WPPSI-R, WIAT, BVMI, VABS, Beery	Decreased IQ scores and school performance
Kaller 2005 [26]	44	Germany	5–13 years	K-ABC	Lower cognition
Adeback 2003 [25]	21	Sweden	4–17 years	WISC-III, WPPSI-R, PHCSCS	Decreased verbal IQ, performance IQ and total IQ
Schulz 2003 [37]	29	Germany	6–13 years	K-ABC	Lower sequential processing
Gritti 2001 [44]	16	Italy	4–11 years (metabolic)	CAT, WISC-R, WIPPSI	Decreased IQ
van Mourik 2000 [31]	25	United Kingdom	<5 years	GMDS	Temporary reduction in social skills and language in first year post-LT, catch up to pre-LT values at 5 years follow up
Kennard 1999 [24]	50	USA	6–23 years	BSID, SBIS, WPPSI-R, WISC-R, WJ-R	Lower average IQ and academic performance, more learning disabilities
Wayman 1997 [8]	40	USA	<2 years	BSID	Low-average range for mental and psychomotor development, 1/3 with developmental delay
Zitelli 1988 [29]	65	USA	N/A	BSID, SBIS, WPPSI, WISC-R, VABS ($n = 24$)	More school delay learning disabilities

Table 38.4 Risk factors that impact neurodevelopmental outcomes in paediatric liver transplant recipients

Risk factor	Outcomes
Genetic/metabolic liver disease	Lower IQ, more severe cognitive impairments [5, 9, 30, 42, 43, 45–47]
Biliary atresia	Better ND outcomes [6]
PALF	Normal IQ, EF deficits [20]
Onset of liver disease at age <1 years	Lower IQ [48]
	Remain delayed post-LT [40]
	Increase risk of ND delay if <12 months [18]
Longer duration of pre-LT disease duration	Lower IQ [9, 15, 26, 28, 33]
	More ND deficits [26]
	More EF and attention deficits [36]
Younger age at transplant	Better ND recovery (metabolics) [34, 42, 49]
	Less ND delay if LT <15 months vs. >15 months [26]
	Better ND prognosis [37]
	Better EF and attention [36]
	No difference [24]
	No difference if LT <12 months vs. >12–36 months [27]
	Decreased ND scores if <6 months at LT [8]
	More language delay if younger [7]
Growth failure	Decreased IQ [8, 11]
	Increased ND deficits/delays [4–6, 8, 26, 31, 32, 37]
	Impaired visual-motor integration [8]
	Lower sequential processing [5, 6]
	Lower language skills [4]
	No association [9]
Hyperammonaemia	Low performance IQ [6]
	No difference [8, 20]
Hyperbilirubinaemia	Speech and language delay [7]
	No difference [8]
Hypoalbuminaemia	Delayed ND [8]
Elevated creatinine	Delayed motor skills [32]
Living donor graft	Higher achievement scores [3, 26, 37]
	Better EF and attention [22, 36]
	No difference [9]
Intraoperative blood transfusion	ND delay [4]
Longer warm ischemic time	Poor ND outcome [27]
Inotropic use	Poor ND outcome [27]
Longer duration of hospitalization	Language delay [7]
	Poor ND outcome [5, 8]
Increased ICU days	Speech and language delay [7]
Cyclosporine use	Slower motor speed [40]
	Increased support at school [19]
Calcineurin inhibitor use	High levels = poor verbal IQ scores [19]
	No difference [5, 8, 9]
Single parent home	Worse ND outcomes [4]
No parental college education	Worse ND outcomes [4]

ND outcomes and recovery post-LT [34, 41, 49]. Early LT is less clearly advantageous in other populations. Several small studies have reported that transplant at a younger age was associated with better ND prognosis [37] and less ND delay [26], including less EF deficits [36]. Other single-centre studies found that age of transplant did not impact ND scores [24, 27]. However, Robertson et al. [27] found no difference in children transplanted at <12 months vs. 12–36 months, which could still be considered overall an "early" time of LT, and this study contained a large number of PALF survivors which could affect results.

Conversely, reports exist to support LT at older age groups are more advantageous. Wayman et al. [8] found that children who had undergone transplantation during the first 6 months of life demonstrated decreased ND scores, and Krull et al. [7] reported larger language delays with earlier age of LT. LT at a young age could adversely interfere with acquisition of skills that often develop during this time period. Although mixed findings can be attributed to a number of small, heterogenous studies, there may be a particular window for age for better ND outcomes post-liver transplantation.

Malnutrition and Growth Failure

Malnutrition is common in paediatric ESLD and is independently associated with ND delay [50–52]. One multicentre study found that patients with weight z-scores >2 SDs below the 50th percentile at LT were predicted to have IQ score almost 6 points lower and were three times more likely to have a lower score than patients without growth failure [4]. Six single-centre studies also similarly found that growth failure or poor nutritional status (low weight and/or height or muscle mass) was associated with poor cognitive outcomes including developmental delay and decreased cognitive scores [5, 6, 8, 26, 31, 37].

Hyperammonaemia

Ammonia is a cerebrotoxin that accumulates in the circulation in liver failure and ESLD. Chronic hyperammonaemia induces neuroinflammation and mediates cognitive impairment in animal models [53], but its role in ND outcomes in paediatric LT is not fully elucidated. Patients with minimal or clinical HE present with different levels of cognitive impairment, including psychomotor slowing, intellectual dysfunction and decreased memory and visuoconstructive abilities [54–56]. Common indications for paediatric LT in which ammonia may be contributory to ND outcomes include metabolic liver conditions and fulminant liver failure. ND delays are observed in children with urea cycle defects who experience hyperammoaemia crises [45]. Children with fulminant liver failure enrolled in the multi-centre PALF study and who survived with native liver had normal IQ suggesting multifactorial contributors [20].

Hyperbilirubinaemia

Increased pre-transplant bilirubin levels were associated with speech and language delays in a prospective study by Krull et al. [7]. However, Wayman et al. [8] did not find that bilirubin levels were statistically different between delayed and normally developing children post-liver transplant. Discrepancies may be explained by small, single-centre studies with heterogenous populations.

38.2.5.2 Intraoperative Factors

Operative and Graft Factors

Blood transfusion volume during liver transplantation was predictor of ND delay [4]. This may be a marker for surgical complications and hypoxia/poor perfusion, or a massive transfusion itself could cause neurological injury. This multicentre study did not find any association with operative time and cold ischaemia time with IQ. Longer warm ischemic time and post-operative inotropic use adversely predicted ND outcome [27]. Living donor graft had better ND outcomes [3, 36, 37] and EF [36], potentially related to shorter ischemic time. Kaller et al. [9] did not find that type of donor graft was associated with ND scores, which may be due to small study sample size.

38.2.5.3 Post-transplant Factors

Immunosuppression Medication

Calcineurin inhibitor (CNI) neurotoxicity is well-described [57]. Elevated CNI levels were associated with poor verbal IQ scores in one multicentre study [19]. Conversely, three single-centre studies did not find that type of immunosuppressive regimen was related to cognitive abilities after transplantation, although trough levels were specifically evaluated [5, 8, 9].

Duration of Hospitalization

Prolonged hospitalization during childhood is an independent risk factor for ND delay [58]. It impairs communication and language development between child and caregiver. Longer duration of hospitalization and ICU stay was associated with more language delay in paediatric patients post-LT [5, 7, 8].

Household Factors

Single-parent home at time of LT predicted an IQ that was ten points lower than patients with two adult care providers [4]. Lower parental education (high school or lower) was associated with worse ND outcome [4]. LT is a critical life event that involves the whole family; therefore a supportive and functional home environment is likely protective against ND impairments. Transplant recipients when compared with their siblings had no difference between the groups with regard to intellect, cognition, academic function or learning; however LT recipients did have more EF deficits [35]. Household factors may play a contributing role to ND outcomes post-transplant but are likely not a primary or isolated cause of deficits; genetics may also play a role.

38.2.6 Interventions

ND assessment with standardized assessment tools is important during routine clinical follow-up [5, 18, 25]. However, there are no clear specific interventions that have been described. Individualized intervention is considered to be of benefit [5, 7, 18, 25]. A small Canadian study [3] recommends the following clinical interventions: regular school attendance, recreational-based physical activity in pre- and post-transplanted children, provisional information provided to families about ND outcomes post-transplant, liaising the healthcare team with the school and family and early rehabilitation support. To date, there have been no studies to examine ND before and after a specific intervention.

38.2.7 Limitations

In the last two decades, ND outcomes are an important outcome metric in studies assessing impact of paediatric LT. Limitations include the fact that the majority of studies are cross-sectional, with a heterogenous mixture of patients including broad age ranges and often small sample sizes (commonly ranging from 20 to 60 patients). As well, utilization of different tools geared at different ages with an attempt to then collapse the results to form meaningful conclusions has resulted in mixed findings regarding risk factors for ND delay post-LT limiting generalizability [59]. Longitudinal prospective studies systematically assessing ND pre- and post-transplant are lacking and needed. Even more so, there are yet to be any published studies that examine ND outcomes after a standardized intervention has occurred.

38.2.8 Future Research

Further research is needed in several areas: firstly, a closer examination of pre-transplant status and demographic and operative factors that impact ND outcome and put patients at a greater risk of deficits; secondly, determination to what effect they are modifiable; thirdly, longitudinal, multicentre, prospective studies with longer follow-up of ND outcomes to determine if deficits change over time and to further elucidate post-transplant risk factors; fourthly, more research to focus on EF and attention, as they may be good candidates for intervention [4]; and finally, evaluation of interventions in the household, school and medical environment which may change/improve the outcome of ND deficits post-transplant and examining ND before and after such intervention.

38.3 Part II: Health-Related Quality of Life After Liver Transplantation

38.3.1 Definitions

Patient-reported outcomes (PROS) are measures that convey information reported directly by the patient that is not filtered by an observer or clinician. Self-reports should ideally be gathered; however for those who cannot self-report due to age or ND delay, proxy-reported outcomes by the primary caregiver (most often a parent) are utilized in paediatric outcome studies. Health-related quality of life (HRQOL) is a multidimensional construct that provides a more comprehensive evaluation than disease parameters alone of the impact of an illness and its treatment on functioning and well-being. It encompasses the aspects of overall quality of life that affects health (both physical and mental), which includes health perceptions and their correlates, including health risk and conditions, functional status, social support and socioeconomic status. HRQOL is an important PROS that is related to disease status and influenced by many risk factors.

38.3.2 Assessment Tools

HRQOL can be assessed using both generic and disease-specific measures (Table 38.5). Generic measures allow for the assessment of common dimensions among both healthy and chronically ill children and allow for comparison across populations. However, these may be insensitive to disease-specific issues.

HRQOL can be measured by child self-report or parental/guardian proxy. Since children's responses may fluctuate over time, HRQOL in paediatric populations should include child and parental reports [60]. The Child Health Questionnaire Forms for child self-report and parental report (CHQ CF-87 and PF-50) are used frequently in single-centre studies, although more recent and multi-studies favour the Paediatric Quality of Life Inventory (PedsQL). The PedsQL was designed as a brief, easy-to-administer patient self-reported and parent/caregiver proxy report to measure HRQOL in healthy children and adolescents and those with acute and chronic health conditions. The PedsQL Condition- and Disease-Specific Modules were designed to complement the generic score scales and provide greater measurement sensitivity in designated clinical populations. Varni et al. [61] showed the PedsQL Cognitive Functioning Scale to be feasible, reliable and valid specifically for paediatric LT recipients, with utility as a tool for assessment of EF.

The development of transplant-specific measures provides a more thorough comprehensive understanding of the child's experience and parent perception regarding the impact of organ transplantation. More recently, two validated disease-specific questionnaires were developed to address this critical need: the Paediatric Quality of Life Inventory Transplant Module (PedsQL TM) and the Paediatric Liver Transplant Quality of Life Questionnaire (PeLTQL) [62]. Their domains are described in Table 38.5.

The PedsQL TM was shown to be a feasible, reliable tool in paediatric organ transplant [60]. Transplant-specific symptoms or problems correlated with generic HRQOL, supporting construct validity. There was moderate agreement between child self-report and parental proxy report [60]. The PeLTQL is the first paediatric liver transplant-specific HRQOL tool created following rigorous tool development methodology with item generation and item reduction phases completed in North America, England and Australia. Psychometric property testing phase revealed the PeLTQL to be a non-stigmatizing opportunity to screen paediatric LT recipients for depression and anxiety [62]. The PeLTQL is currently available in over ten languages in addition to English [www.peltql.com].

38.3.3 HRQOL After Paediatric Liver Transplantation

38.3.3.1 Multicentre Studies

Table 38.6 summarizes findings from several multicentre studies evaluating HRQOL in paediatric LT recipients. PedsQL results from 873 SPLIT subjects between the ages of 2 and 18 years and more than 1-year post-LT revealed lower HRQOL by patient and parent report compared with matched healthy controls in all areas, with school functioning being the most significantly impaired domain [63]. Lower total HRQOL and general health scores have also been reported in various groups of paediatric LT recipients compared to both healthy norms (age 1–18 years), >1 year from time of transplant, including 1 study of >10-year survivors, all from North America [64–66], as well as children of other disease groups [67]. Physical functioning [65, 66] and psychosocial [66] subdomains were noted to have lower scores.

38.3.3.2 Single-Centre Studies

Tables 38.7 and 38.8 summarize results from single-centre studies evaluating HRQOL after paediatric LT, with multiple reports confirming lower total HRQOL in paediatric LT recipients compared to healthy population [68–79]. In addition, specific domains with lower scores include physical

Table 38.5 Tools to assess HRQOL in paediatric liver transplant recipients

Assessment tool	Ages	Domains
Cantril's Self-Anchoring Scale		Individual perception of present life, life during past year, life when it was the best global QOL assessment
Child Health Quality Questionnaire (CHQ)	Parent Form (PF) 50—for parents of children >5 years Child Form (CF) 87—for self-completion children >10 years	General health perception, physical functioning, role-physical, behaviour, mental health, role-emotional, parent impact-emotional and time, family cohesion and activities, bodily pain, self-esteem, family activities
Infant Toddler Quality of Life Questionnaire (ITQOL)	2 months–5 years	Global health, physical abilities, growth and development, discomfort and pain, getting along with others, general health perception, change in health, mental health, parental impact-emotional and time, family cohesion
Medical Outcomes Study Social Support Survey (MOS-SSS)		Emotional/informational support, tangible support, affectional support, positive social interaction
Modified Transplant Symptom Occurrence and Symptom Distress Scale (MTSOSD)		Medication complications and side effects
Paediatric Liver Transplant Quality of Life Tool (PeLTQL)	8–17 years, at least 1 years post-LT for child and parent	Emotional, psychological functioning, social functioning, physical health, current treatments and interventions, future health status
Peds Quality of Life Inventory (PedsQL)	Self-report 5–18 years Parental Proxy report 2–18 years	Physical functioning, emotional functioning, social functioning, school functioning. Summary scores for total scale, physical health, psychosocial health, and physical health
PedsQL Transplant Module (PedsQL TM)		About my medicines (adherence, side effects), my transplant and others (social relationships). Pain and hurt, worry, treatment anxiety. How I look, communication
PedsQL Family Impact Module	Parent report	Physical, emotional, social, and cognitive functioning; communication, worry, family daily activities and family relationships
Paediatric Sleep Questionnaire	Parent report 2–18 years	Sleep-telated breathing disorder (SRBD) index (snoring, sleepiness, behaviour); periodic limb movements during sleep including restless leg symptoms and growing pains (PLMS/RLS)
Short Form Health Survey (SF-36)		Physical functioning, role limitations due to physical health, bodily pain, general health perceptions, vitality, social functioning, role limitations due to emotional problems and mental health
The D Instrument of HRQOL	15D:>16 years 16D: 12–15 years 17D:8–11 years	Mobility, vision, hearing, breathing, sleeping, eating, speech, elimination, usual activities, mental function, discomfort and symptoms, depression, distress, vitality, sexual activity

Table 38.6 Multicentre studies and patient characteristics for HRQOL outcomes in paediatric liver transplant recipients

Author (year)	Number of patients	Country	Age	Time from LT	Domains/test	Outcome
Feldman et al. (2016) [65]	262	USA/Canada	1–18 years	1–2 years	PedsQL4	Lower physical function scores
Sorensen et al. (2015) [20]	36 PALF (23 LT)	USA/Canada	6–16 years	>1 years	PedsQL4 MF5	Lower HRQOL
Ng et al. (2012) [64]	167	USA/Canada	NR	>10 years	PedsQL4	Lower HRQOL
Limbers et al. (2011) [67]	873	USA/Canada	2–18 years	>1 years	PedsQL	Lower school functioning than other chronic disease
Alonso et al. (2010) [63]	873	USA/Canada	2–18 years	>1 years	PedsQL4	Lower HRQOL significantly school functioning
Alonso et al. (2008) [66]	102	USA/Canada	2–18 years	2 years	ITQOL CHQ-PF50 FAQ	Lower HRQOL, no physical or psychosocial difference in 2–5 years

Table 38.7 Single-centre studies and patient characteristics for HRQOL outcomes in paediatric liver transplant recipients <18 years of age at time of assessment

Author (year)	Number of patients	Country	Age	Time from LT	Domains/test	Outcome
Kikuchi et al. (2018) [70]	75	Japan	5–18 years	>3 months	PedsQL PedsQL TM	Higher HRQOL vs. USA, low school functioning
Vandekerckhove et al. (2016) [71]	24	Belgium	6–16 years	>6 months	PedsQL4	Lower HRQOL but not physical or emotional function
He et al. (2015) [72]	51	China	2–10 years	>6 months	PedsQL PedsQL TM Sleep Questionnaire	Lower HRQOL with poor sleep
Anderson et al. (2014) [39]	47	USA	2–17 years	>6 months	PedsQL PedsQL-FIM Sleep Questionnaire	Lower HRQOL with poor sleep
Haavisto et al. (2013) [73]	74 (14 LT, 44 kidney transplant, 16 heart transplant)	Finland	6–16	>1 year	15D–17D Child Behaviour Checklist Youth Self-Report and Teacher Report form for psychosocial adjustment	Lower HRQOL 8–11 years; teenagers had similar scores to healthy norms
Gritti et al. (2013) [74]	33	Italy	6–18 years	3–12 years	CHQ-CF87 CHQ-PF50	Lower general health perception scores
Alba et al. (2013) [75]	49	Chile	2–18 years	>3 years	PedsQL4	HRQOL better <4 years HRQOL in school-aged children poor
Denny et al. (2012) [76]	30	Australia	3–16 years	>1 year	PedsQL3 PedsQL TM FAQ	Lower HRQOL with decreased family function
Fredericks et al. (2012) [77]	47	USA	2–17 years	>6 months	PedsQL4 Sleep Questionnaire	Lower HRQOL with poor sleep
Dehghani et al. (2012) [78]	50	Iran	1–18 years	6 months–8 years	CHQ-CF87 CHQ-PF50	Lower HRQOL except behaviour (parental) and physical (self)
Sanchez et al. (2010) [79]	54	South America	5–18 years	>1 year	CHQ-PF50	Decreased HRQOL
Taylor et al. (2009) [80]	55	UK	12–18 years	>6 months	CHQ-CF87 MTSOS Piers-Harris Self-Concept Scale CDI	Decreased HRQOL except social behaviour and family cohesion
Fredericks et al. (2008) [81]	28	USA	12–18 years	1 months to 17 years	CHQ-CF87 CHQ-PF50 PedsQL	Decreased HRQOL
Fredericks et al. (2007) [82]	38	USA	2–16 years	1–64 months	CHQ-PF50 PedsQL CBCL BSI FAD	Decreased HRQOL especially school functioning
Sundaram et al. (2007) [83]	36	USA	11–18 years	>1 year	CHQ-CF87 CHQ-PF50	Decreased HRQOL except psychosocial. Lower physical (parental report only)
Cole et al. (2004) [84]	45	USA	<5 years	NR	ITQOL CHQ-PF50 FAQ	Increased global HRQOL scores first 6 months after transplant

Table 38.7 (continued)

Author (year)	Number of patients	Country	Age	Time from LT	Domains/test	Outcome
Alonso et al. (2003) [85]	55	USA	5–17 years	>2 years	PF50	Decreased general health, physical scores, more family disruption
Bucavalas et al. (2003) [86]	77	USA	5–18 years	6 months to 15 years	PedsQL4 CHQ-PF50	Decreased HRQOL
Midgley et al. (2000) [87]	51	USA	>2 years	3 years	LT Disability Scale Health utilities Index Mark II	Decreased HRQOL Mild functional deficits in 90% transplanted group

Table 38.8 Single-centre studies and patient characteristics for HRQOL outcomes in paediatric liver transplant recipients with <10-year follow-up

Author (year)	Number of patients	Country	Age	Time from LT	Domains/test	Outcome
Konidis et al. (2015) [81]	27	Canada	15–25 years	>15 years	PedsQL SF-36 ITQOL	Decreased in HRQOL in 18–25 years Comparable to healthy norms in <18 years
Sullivan et al. (2014) [82]	24	USA	>20 years	>20 years	SF-12	Physical HRQOL scores lower
Mohammed et al. (2012) [71]	171	USA	18–22 years	>20 years	PedsQL4 PedsQL Cognitive Functioning Scale PedsQL3-TM SF-36	Decreased HRQOL
Kosola et al. (2012) [80]	57	Finland	3.5–35 years	2–23 years	PedsQL4 SF-36	Lower school function 7–17 years, lower general health and physical function in adults
Devine et al. (2011) [89]	16	USA	>11 years	11–22 years	CHQ-CF87 CHQ-PF50	No difference in HRQOL between two time points (1–2 years apart)
Duffy et al. (2010) [74]	30	USA	>20 years	>20 years	SF-36 MOS-SSS Liver disease QOL	HRQOL decreased except mental scales
Avitzur et al. (2004) [88]	28	Canada	11–31 years	>10 years	Cantril's Self-Anchoring Scale	HRQOL lower in adults vs. children/teens

function [71, 72, 78–82], school functioning [68, 77, 79, 80, 83] and emotional/psychosocial functioning [79, 81].

38.3.4 Impact of Time Since Liver Transplantation on HRQOL

A major limitation of most studies evaluating HRQOL outcomes following paediatric LT is the one-time HRQOL evaluation of populations of paediatric LT recipients at different ages at the time of LT with variable follow-up periods. The majority HRQOL studies have focused on the early post-LT period with follow-up of several months to years (Tables 38.6, 38.7, and 38.8). Only 11 study publications on HRQOL describe follow-up beyond 10 years in paediatric LT (Table 38.9).

At 1-year follow-up, HRQOL scores from 45 patients who received LT at <5 years of age [84] improved further from those evaluated at 6-month follow-up. Time elapsed from LT is associated with increase in HRQOL scores during childhood [29, 79, 85, 86]. Younger children tend to have similar HRQOL scores to the general population. In a multi-centre study of 873 patients, Alonso et al. [66] found no difference in physical or psychosocial scores in children aged 2–5 years with normative controls.

HRQOL subdomain scores were lower in school functioning for school-aged children (8–11 years [87]; 7–17 years [70]). In >10-year survivors, physical functioning scores are lower than the general population [71, 74, 81, 82]. HRQOL is reported to be decreased in young adults (18–25 years) compared to teenagers and children [80, 81, 88]. This may improve in later adulthood: Duffy et al. (2010) [74] surveyed 68 20-year LT survivors and found they scored significantly in HRQOL when compared to the general population but better when compared to patients with chronic liver disease. This study, however, included paediatric and adult LT recipients.

There are limited longitudinal studies that explore HRQOL over multiple time points. One single-centre study

Table 38.9 Risk factors that impact health-related quality of life outcomes in paediatric liver transplant recipients

Risk factor	Outcome
Non-modifiable	
Male gender	Lower HRQOL [75, 95]
	Higher HRQOL [84]
Underlying diagnosis	No difference [66, 85]
Congenital liver disease	Lower HRQOL scores [73]
Biliary atresia	Better physical scores [65]
Younger age at LT	No difference [66, 85]
	Lower physical scores and behaviour [92, 94]
	Lower HRQOL scores [79, 86, 93, 95]
Graft type-living donor	No difference [78, 84, 85]
	Improved HRQOL [95]
Shorter duration from transplant	Lower HRQOL scores [71, 73, 74, 76, 84, 86, 91]
	Lower physical scores [74]
	More family adjustments [76]
	No difference [79, 85, 95]
Household factors	
Single parent	Lower HRQOL scores [70, 95]
Lower parental income	Lower HRQOL scores [92]
No maternal college education	Lower HRQOL scores [86, 91]
Family conflict	Worse HRQOL scores [80]
Live far from LT centre	Worse social functioning [70, 75]
Modifiable	
Severity of LD (PELD > 15)	Lower HRQOL scores [95]
Poor growth	Lower physical function scores [65]
	Increased global health score [84]
	Lower HRQOL scores [86, 95]
	No difference [72, 85]
Increased number of hospitalized days	Lower HRQOL scores [86, 90, 95]
	No difference [85]
More medications	Lower HRQOL scores [70]
Low tac levels	Lower HRQOL scores [81, 82, 96]
Anti-HTN medications	Lower physical abilities [71]
Seizure medications	Lower HRQOL scores [95]
Poor adherence to medications	Lower HRQOL scores [81, 82, 92]
Poor transplant related health (i.e. PTLD, rejection, abnormal LFTs, re-operation)	Decreased physical function scores [65]
	Decreased HRQOL [70, 93, 95]
Comorbidities	
Psychiatric/mental illness	Lower HRQOL scores [73, 83, 91]
Neurological disorder	Lower HRQOL scores [73]
Other chronic illness	Lower HRQOL scores [80]
Diabetes	Lower HRQOL scores [95]
Recipient unemployment and/or decreased education level	Lower HRQOL scores [90]
	Lower physical scores [88]
Sleep disturbances	Lower HRQOL scores [39, 72, 77]

by Devine et al. [89] followed 66 transplanted adolescents (20 LT) and assessed HRQOL at 2 time points (T1 = baseline (4 months to 16.5 years post-transplant, T2 = 18 months after T1). They showed no difference between T1 and T2 with regard to HRQOL scores in patients between the ages of 11 and 20 years old.

38.3.5 Risk Factors

Similar to ND outcomes, pre-, peri- and post-transplant factors likely contribute to HRQOL outcomes. Some of these risk factors are modifiable, which provides an opportunity for potential intervention. This can include medical, personal and family or environmental factors.

38.3.5.1 Non-modifiable Factors

Sex

Alonso et al. [86] reported that male sex was associated with lower HRQOL scores, and Alba et al. [70] found lower scores in physical and social functioning of adolescent males compared to females. Conversely, Cole et al. [84] found that general and global health perceptions were higher in males. Discrepancies may be due to patient age and duration from LT.

Primary Liver Condition

In two different multicentre studies, Feldman et al. [65] found higher physical HRQOL score subjects with biliary atresia compared to all other indications for paediatric LT, whereas Ng et al. [64] did not find a difference in HRQOL with regard to aetiology of liver disease, nor did Alonso et al. [90].

Age at Transplant

Although age at LT is a non-modifiable variable, it may be important in informing strategies to adopt during the post-transplant journey by clinical care teams towards enhancing outcomes. Younger age at LT was associated with lower HRQOL scores in several single-centre studies [73, 74, 79], in particular lower physical scores and behaviour [69, 88]. However, age at LT was not a variable impacting HRQOL in the PeLTQL tool development study [62]. Utilizing PROMs in ongoing surveillance of recipients of LT performed at the youngest age spectrum may help optimize durable outcomes. Discrepancies in these findings may be due to the duration of time from transplant in which each study was performed.

Time Since LT

Lower HRQOL scores were found in patients of various ages with shorter durations from the time of LT [68, 79, 80, 84, 87]. This included lower physical scores [69] and more family adjustments [91]. Alonso et al. [86] did not note a difference in HRQOL scores from the time of transplant, although the median interval from LT was more than 3 years and many children had survived LT for more than 10 years. This may be that the immediate post-transplant period is still fraught with frequent healthcare visits, lab work, changes to medication and higher risk of complications.

Household Factors
Variables associated with lower HRQOL include single-parent household [83, 86], lower parental income [89], lower maternal education (less than college) [79, 80], family conflict [75] and living further distance from a LT centre [70, 83]. This may be related to poor family supports and coping mechanisms, as well as decreased access to resources.

38.3.5.2 Modifiable Factors

Peri- and Post-operative Course
Severity of liver disease as measured by a PELD score >15 was associated with lower PedsQL scores at a median of 3.7 years post-LT [86]. Growth failure [65, 79, 84, 86], days hospitalized [71, 79, 86] and complications such as reoperation and rejection [65, 74, 83, 86] have also been associated with lower HRQOL scores. Co-morbidities, particularly neuropsychiatric and other chronic illness, have also been identified as risk factors for lower HRQOL in paediatric LT recipients [75, 78, 80, 85, 86].

Medication
The greater the number of prescribed medication types was related to lower transplant-specific HRQOL in a Japanese study of 75 patients with a mean age of 9 years who were transplanted for BA [83]. The need for medications to manage co-morbidities, such as hypertension or seizures, has been associated with lower HRQOL scores [68, 86]. Non-adherence to medications and medical regimens is associated with lower HRQOL [89, 76, 77, 89, 92].

Non-adherence to tacrolimus, as determined by trough tacrolimus blood levels and self-report, was present in 40% of 25 adolescents (mean age 15.1, mean time from LT 7.5 years) and predictive of poorer HRQOL compared to adherent subjects [76]. Non-adherence to tacrolimus was related to lower HRQOL, more limitations in school and social activities and decreased family cohesion in a study of 38 paediatric patients, less than 5 years from LT [77]. Frequency of medication side effects is a barrier to adherence and is also associated with poorer physical and mental health HRQOL for paediatric transplant recipients [92]. Poor adherence can lead to more post-LT complications such as hospitalizations, live biopsies and rejection and has been associated with family conflict and poorer mental health and general health perceptions, which also negatively affect HRQOL [76, 77].

Sleep Disturbances
Lower HRQOL scores are seen in paediatric LT recipients with sleep disturbances compared to healthy children, as assessed by the Paediatric Sleep Questionnaire (PSQ) in three studies. PSQ scores correlated with PedsQL total and domain scores [93–95].

38.3.6 Interventions

Targeted interventions with peer-to-peer mentoring [96] and novel adherence interventions [76] with evaluation of physical and psychosocial well-being [97] have been reported. Outpatient-based, cross-age peer-mentoring programme for LT recipients resulted in an increase in adherence as measured by tacrolimus blood levels and improvement of scores on the Developmentally Based Skills Checklist and Short Form 36 (SF-36) HRQOL survey, in a study of 26 LT recipients [96]. Clinical programmes for IS medication adherence using tacrolimus blood levels have shown success for improving adherence and decreasing rejection in paediatric LT recipients [98]. Reed-Knight et al. [99] found 94% of adolescent recipients of solid organ transplantation expressed some level of interest in receiving mental health services. Perceived need for mental health services was inversely related to self- and parental reports of HRQOL. Access to mental health services in transplant recipients may be a potential interventional tool to improve HRQOL. The pre-transplant period may serve as a pivotal time point for interventions.

38.3.7 Limitations

HRQOL is an important patient-reported outcome metric to assess in all patients who have undergone LT. To date, most studies have been single centre and cross-sectional, comprised of small sample sizes, utilized varying HRQOL tools (not always widely recognized and more often generic than disease-specific) and challenged by the often needed use of parental proxy reporting especially for the younger-aged LT recipients [100]. The literature is lacking in longitudinal prospective studies evaluating the impact of changes in HRQOL over time and understanding on why deficits persist. As well, despite the common finding of impaired HRQOL following paediatric LT, there is a paucity of studies evaluating intervention strategies on HRQOL in the post-transplant period [101].

38.3.8 Further Research

Further research is needed in several areas: firstly, examination of pre-, peri- and post-transplant factors that impact HRQOL; secondly, identification of interventions and their timing that may improve HRQOL scores within this population; thirdly, longitudinal, multicentre, prospective studies with measures of HRQOL at more than one time point to explore how HRQOL changes over time; and fourthly, more research to focus on adherence and how it affects HRQOL, as this may be a good candidate for intervention.

References

1. Adam R, Karam V, Delvart V, O'Grady J, Mirza D, Klempnauer J, et al. Evolution of indications and results of liver transplantation in Europe. A report from the European Liver Transplant Registry (ELTR). J Hepatol. 2012;57:675–88.
2. Kim WR, Lake JR, Smith JM, Schladt DP, Skeans MA, Harper AM, et al. OPTN/SRTR 2016 annual data report: liver. Am J Transplant. 2018;1:172–253.
3. Gold A, Rogers A, Cruchley E, Rankin S, Parmar A, Kamath BM, et al. Assessment of school readiness in chronic cholestatic liver disease: a pilot study examining children with and without liver transplantation. Can J Gastroenterol Hepatol. 2017;2017:9873945. https://doi.org/10.1155/2017/9873945.
4. Sorensen LG, Neighbors K, Martz K, Zelko F, Bucuvalas JC, Alonso EM. Longitudinal study of cognitive and academic outcomes after pediatric liver transplantation. J Pediatr. 2014;165:65–72.
5. Kaller T, Langguth N, Petermann F, Ganschow R, Nashan B, Schulz KH. Cognitive performance in pediatric liver transplant recipients. Am J Transplant. 2013;13:2956–65.
6. Gilmour S, Adkins R, Liddell GA, Jhangri G, Robertson CM. Assessment of psychoeducational outcomes after pediatric liver transplant. Am J Transplant. 2009;9:294–300.
7. Krull K, Fuchs C, Yurk H, Boone P, Alonso E. Neurocognitive outcome in pediatric liver transplant recipients. Pediatr Transplant. 2003;7:111–8.
8. Wayman KI, Cox KL, Esquivel CO. Neurodevelopmental outcome of young children with extrahepatic biliary atresia 1 year after liver transplantation. J Pediatr. 1997;131:894–8.
9. Kaller T, Boeck A, Sander K, Richterich A, Burdelski M, Ganschow R, et al. Cognitive abilities, behaviour and quality of life in children after liver transplantation. Pediatr Transplant. 2010;14:496–503.
10. Sorensen LG. Neuropsychological functioning and health-related quality of life in pediatric liver disease: the sum of our perspectives is greater than each alone. Curr Opin Pediatr. 2016;28:644–52.
11. Fredericks EM, Zelikovsky N, Aujoulat I, Hames A, Wray J. Post-transplant adjustment: the later years. Pediatr Transplant. 2014;18:675–88.
12. Ferguson DM, Horwood LJ, Ridder EM. Show me the child at seven II: childhood intelligence and later outcomes in adolescence and young adulthood. J Child Psychol Psychiatry. 2005;56:850–8.
13. Gutierrez-Colina AM, Reed-Knight B, Eaton C, Lee J, Loiselle Rich K, Mee L, et al. Transition readiness, adolescent responsibility, and executive functioning among pediatric transplant recipients: caregivers' perspectives. Pediatr Transplant. 2017;21(3). https://doi.org/10.1111/petr.12898.
14. Mervis CB, Robinson BR, Pani JR. Visuosaptial construction. Am J Hum Genet. 1999;65:1222–9.
15. Del Giudice E, Grossi D, Angelini R, Cristani A, Latte F, Fragassi N, et al. Spatial cognition in children. I. Development of drawing-related (visuospatial and constructional) abilities in preschool and early school years. Brain Dev. 2000;22:362–7.
16. Klonoff PS, Olson KC, Talley MC, Husk KL, Myles SM, Gehrels JA, et al. The relationship of cognitive retraining to neurological patients driving status: the role of process variables and compensation training. Brain Inj. 2010;24:63–73.
17. SPLIT Research Group. Studies of pediatric liver transplantation (SPLIT) year 2000 outcomes. Transplantation. 2001;72:463–76.
18. Sorensen LG, Neighbors K, Martz K, Zelko F, Bucuvalas JC, Alonso EM. Cognitive and academic outcomes after pediatric liver transplantation: functional outcomes group (FOG) results. Am J Transplant. 2011;11:303–11.
19. Gilmour SM, Sorensen LG, Anand R, Yin W, Alonso EM. School outcomes in children registered in the studies for pediatric liver transplant (SPLIT) consortium. Liver Transpl. 2010;16:1041–8.
20. Sorensen LG, Neighbors K, Zhang S, Limbers CA, Varni JW, Ng VL, et al. Neuropsychological functioning and health-related quality of life: pediatric acute liver failure study group results. J Pediatr Gastroenterol Nutr. 2015;60(1):75–83.
21. Srivastava A, Yadav SK, Borkar VV, Yadav A, Yachha SK, Thomas MA, et al. Serial evaluation of children with ALF with advanced MRI, serum proinflammatory cytokines, thiamine, and cognition assessment. J Pediatr Gastroenterol Nutr. 2012;55:580–6.
22. Seyan AS, Hughes RD, Shawcross DL. Changing the face of hepatic encephalopathy: role of inflammation and oxidative stress. World J Gastroenterol. 2010;16:3347–57.
23. Alonso EM, Squires RH, Whitington PF. Acute liver failure in children. In: Suchy FJ, Sokol RJ, Balisteri WF, editors. Liver disease in children. 3rd ed. Cambridge: Cambridge University Press; 2007. p. 71–96.
24. Kennard BD, Stewart SM, Phelan-McAuliffe D, Waller DA, Bannister M, Fioravani V, et al. Academic outcome in long-term survivors of pediatric liver transplantation. J Dev Behav Pediatr. 1999;20:17–23.
25. Adebäck P, Nemeth A, Fischler B. Cognitive and emotional outcome after pediatric liver transplantation. Pediatr Transplant. 2003;7:385–9.
26. Kaller T, Schulz KH, Sander K, Boeck A, Rogiers X, Burdelski M. Cognitive abilities in children after liver transplantation. Transplantation. 2005;79:1252–6.
27. Robertson CM, Dinu IA, Joffe AR, Alton GY, Yap JY, Asthana S, et al. Neurocognitive outcomes at kindergarten entry after liver transplantation at >3 yr of age. Pediatr Transplant. 2013;17:621–30.
28. Lee JM, Jung YK, Bae JH, Yoon SA, Kim JH, Choi Y, et al. Delayed transplantation may affect intellectual ability in children. Pediatr Int. 2017;59:1080–6.
29. Zitelli BJ, Miller JW, Gartner JC Jr, Malatack JJ, Urbach AH, Belle SH, et al. Changes in life-style after liver transplantation. Pediatrics. 1988;82:173–80.
30. Shellmer DA, DeVito Dabbs A, Dew MA, Noll RB, Feldman H, Strauss KA, et al. Cognitive and adaptive functioning after liver transplantation for maple syrup urine disease: a case series. Pediatr Transplant. 2011;15:58–64.
31. van Mourik ID, Beath SV, Brook GA, Cash AJ, Mayer AD, Buckels JA, et al. Long-term nutritional and neurodevelopmental outcome of liver transplantation in infants aged less than 12 months. J Pediatr Gastroenterol Nutr. 2000;30:269–75.
32. Almaas R, Jensen U, Loennecken MC, Tveter AT, Sanengen T, Scholz T, et al. Impaired motor competence in children with transplanted liver. J Pediatr Gastroenterol Nutr. 2015;60:723–8.
33. Haavisto A, Korkman M, Törmänen J, Holmberg C, Jalanko H, Qvist E. Visuospatial impairment in children and adolescents after liver transplantation. Pediatr Transplant. 2011;15:184–92.
34. Fouquet V, Alves A, Branchereau S, Grabar S, Debray D, Jacquemin E, et al. Long-term outcome of pediatric liver transplantation for biliary atresia: a 10-year follow-up in a single center. Liver Transpl. 2005;11:152–60.
35. Ee LC, Llyod O, Beale K, Fawcett J, Cleghorn GJ. Academic potential and cognitive functioning of long-term survivors after childhood liver transplantation. Pediatr Transplant. 2014;18:272–9.

36. Kaller T, Langguth N, Ganschow R, Nashan B, Schulz KH. Attention and executive functioning deficits in liver-transplanted children. Transplantation. 2010;90:1567–73.
37. Schulz KH, Wein C, Boeck A, Rogiers X, Burdelski M. Cognitive performance of children who have undergone liver transplantation. Transplantation. 2003;75:1236–40.
38. Gutiérrez-Colina AM, Eaton CK, Lee JL, Reed-Knight B, Loiselle K, Mee LL, et al. Executive functioning, barriers to adherence, and nonadherence in adolescent and young adult transplant recipients. J Pediatr Psychol. 2016;41:759–67.
39. Stewart SM, Hiltebeitel C, Nici J, Waller DA, Uauy R, Andrews WS. Neuropsychological outcome of pediatric liver transplantation. Pediatrics. 1991;87:367–76.
40. Yssaad-Fesselier R, Lion-François L, Herbillon V, Rivet C, Brunet AS, Yantren H, et al. Intellectual and visuo-spatial assessment in long-term pediatric liver transplantation for biliary atresia. Transplantation. 2009;87:1427–8.
41. Stevenson T, Millan MT, Wayman K, Berquist WE, Sarwal M, Johnston EE, et al. Long-term outcome following pediatric liver transplantation for metabolic disorders. Pediatr Transplant. 2010;14:268–75.
42. Thevenin DM, Baker A, Kato T, Tzakis A, Fernandez M, Dowling M. Neurodevelopmental outcomes for children transplanted under the age of 3 years. Transplant Proc. 2006;38:1692–3.
43. Frota NAF, Caramelli P, Barbosa ER. Cognitive impairment in Wilson's disease. Dement Neuropsychol. 2009;3:16–21.
44. Msall M, Monahan PS, Chapanis N, Batshaw ML. Cognitive development in children with inborn errors of urea synthesis. Acta Paediatr Jpn. 1988;30:435–41.
45. Kim IK, Niemi AK, Krueger C, Bonham CA, Concepcion W, Cowan TM, et al. Liver transplantation for urea cycle disorders in pediatric patients: a single-center experience. Pediatr Transplant. 2013;17:158–67.
46. Iwański S, Seniów J, Leśniak M, Litwin T, Członkowska A. Diverse attention deficits in patients with neurologically symptomatic and asymptomatic Wilson's disease. Neuropsychology. 2015;29:25.
47. Arguedas D, Stewart J, Hodgkinson S, Batchelor J. A neuropsychological comparison of siblings with neurological versus hepatic symptoms of Wilson's Disease. Neurocase. 2015;21:154–61.
48. Stewart SM, Uauy R, Waller DA, Kennard BD, Benser M, Andrews WS. Mental and motor development, social competence, and growth one year after successful pediatric liver transplantation. J Pediatr. 1989;114:574–81.
49. McBride KL, Miller G, Carter S, Karpen S, Goss J, Lee B. Developmental outcomes with early orthotopic liver transplantation for infants with neonatal-onset urea cycle defects and a female patient with late-onset ornithine transcarbamylase deficiency. Pediatrics. 2004;114:523–6.
50. Bartosh SM, Thomas SE, Sutton MM, Brady LM, Whitington PF. Linear growth after pediatric liver transplantation. J Pediatr. 1999;135:624–31.
51. Gorman KS. Malnutrition and cognitive development: evidence from experimental/quasi-experimental studies among the mild-to-moderately malnourished. J Nutr. 1995;125:2239S–44S.
52. Levitsky DA, Strupp BJ. Malnutrition and the brain: changing concepts, changing concerns. J Nutr. 1995;125:2212S–20S.
53. Rodrigo R, Cauli O, Gomez-Pinedo U, Agusti A, Hernandez-Rabaza V, Garcia-Verdugo JM, et al. Hyperammonemia induces neuroinflammation that contributes to cognitive impairment in rats with hepatic encephalopathy. Gastroenterology. 2010;139:675–84.
54. Amodio P, Del Piccolo F, Marchetti P, Angeli P, Iemmolo R, Caregaro L, et al. Clinical features and survival of cirrhotic patients with subclinical cognitive alterations detected by the number connection test and computerized psychometric tests. Hepatology. 1999;29:1662–7.
55. Weissenborn K, Heidenreich S, Ennen J, Rückert N, Hecker H. Attention deficits in minimal hepatic encephalopathy. Metab Brain Dis. 2001;16:13–9.
56. Weissenborn K, Heidenreich S, Giewekemeyer K, Rückert N, Hecker H. Memory function in early hepatic encephalopathy. J Hepatol. 2003;39:320–5.
57. Patchell RA. Neurological complications of organ transplantation. Ann Neurol. 1994;36:688–703.
58. Kerr NJ. The effect of hospitalization on the developmental tasks of childhood. Nurs Forum. 1979;18:108–30.
59. Alonso EM, Sorensen LG. Cognitive development following pediatric solid organ transplantation. Curr Opin Organ Transplant. 2009;14:522–5.
60. Weissberg-Benchell J, Zielinski TE, Rodgers S, Greenley RN, Askenazi D, Goldstein SL, et al. Pediatric health-related quality of life: feasibility, reliability and validity of the PedsQL transplant module. Am J Transplant. 2010;10:1677–85.
61. Varni JW, Limbers CA, Sorensen LG, Neighbors K, Martz K, Bucuvalas JC, et al. PedsQL™ cognitive functioning scale in pediatric liver transplant recipients: feasibility, reliability, and validity. Qual Life Res. 2011;20:913–21.
62. Ng V, Nicholas D, Dhawan A, Yazigi N, Ee L, Stormon M, et al. Development and validation of the pediatric liver transplantation quality of life: a disease-specific quality of life measure for pediatric liver transplant recipients. J Pediatr. 2014;165:547–55.
63. Alonso EM, Limbers CA, Neighbors K, Martz K, Bucuvalas JC, Webb T, et al. Cross-sectional analysis of health-related quality of life in pediatric liver transplant recipients. J Pediatr. 2010;156:270–6.
64. Ng VL, Alonso EM, Bucuvala JC, Cohen G, Limbers CA, Varni JW, et al. Health status of children alive 10 years after pediatric liver transplantation performed in the US and Canada: report of the studies of pediatric liver transplantation experience. J Pediatr. 2012;160:820–6.
65. Feldman AG, Neighbors K, Mukherjee S, Rak M, Varni JW, Alonso EM. Impaired physical function following pediatric LT. Liver Transpl. 2016;22:495–504.
66. Alonso EM, Neighbors K, Barton FB, McDiarmid SV, Dunn SP, Mazariegos GV, et al. Health-related quality of life and family function following pediatric liver transplantation. Liver Transpl. 2008;14:460–8.
67. Limbers CA, Neighbors K, Martz K, Bucuvalas JC, Webb T, Varni JW, et al. Health-related quality of life in pediatric liver transplant recipients compared with other chronic disease groups. Pediatr Transplant. 2011;15:245–53.
68. Vandekerckhove K, Coomans I, De Bruyne E, De Groote K, Panzer J, De Wolf D, et al. Evaluation of exercise performance, cardiac function, and quality of life in children after liver transplantation. Transplantation. 2016;100:1525–31.
69. Gritti A, Pisano S, Salvati T, Di Cosmo N, Iorio R, Vajro P. Health-related quality of life in pediatric liver transplanted patients compared with a chronic liver disease group. Ital J Pediatr. 2013;11:39–55.
70. Alba A, Uribe M, Hunter B, Monzón P, Ferrada C, Heine C, et al. Health-related quality of life after pediatric liver transplant: single-center experience in Chile. Transplant Proc. 2013;45:3728–30.
71. Mohammad S, Hormaza L, Neighbors K, Boone P, Tierney M, Azzam RK, et al. Health status in young adults two decades after pediatric liver transplantation. Am J Transplant. 2012;12:1486–95.
72. Dehghani SM, Imanieh MH, Honar N, Haghighat M, Astaneh B, Bahador A, et al. Evaluation of quality of life in children six months after liver transplantation. Middle East J Dig Dis. 2012;4:158–62.
73. Sanchez C, Eymann A, De Cunto C, D'Agostino D. Quality of life in pediatric liver transplantation in a single-center in South America. Pediatr Transplant. 2010;14:332–6.

74. Duffy JP, Kao K, Ko CY, Farmer DG, McDiarmid SV, Hong JC, et al. Long-term patient outcome and quality of life after liver transplantation: analysis of 20-year survivors. Ann Surg. 2010;252:652–61.
75. Taylor RM, Franck LS, Gibson F, Donaldson N, Dhawan A. Study of the factors affecting health-related quality of life in adolescents after liver transplantation. Am J Transplant. 2009;9:1179–88.
76. Fredericks EM, Magee JC, Opipari-Arrigan L, Shieck V, Well A, Lopez MJ. Adherence and health-related quality of life in adolescent liver transplant recipients. Pediatr Transplant. 2008;12:289–99.
77. Fredericks EM, Lopez MJ, Magee JC, Shieck V, Opipari-Arrigan L. Psychological functioning, nonadherence and health outcomes after pediatric liver transplantation. Am J Transplant. 2007;7:1974–83.
78. Sundaram SS, Landgraf JM, Neighbors K, Cohn RA, Alonso EM. Adolescent health-related quality of life following liver and kidney transplantation. Am J Transplant. 2007;7:982–9.
79. Bucuvalas JC, Britto M, Krug S, Ryckman FC, Atherton H, Alonso M, et al. Health-related quality of life in pediatric liver transplant recipients: a single-center study. Liver Transpl. 2003;9:62–71.
80. Kosola S, Lampela H, Lauronen J, Mäkisalo H, Jalanko H, Qvist E, et al. General health, health-related quality of life and sexual health after pediatric liver transplantation: a nationwide study. Am J Transplant. 2012;12:420–7.
81. Konidis SV, Hrycko A, Nightingale S, Renner E, Lilly L, Therapondos G, et al. Health-related quality of life in long-term survivors of paediatric liver transplantation. Paediatr Child Health. 2015;20:189–94.
82. Sullivan KM, Radosevich DM, Lake JR. Health-related quality of life: two decades after liver transplantation. Liver Transpl. 2014;20:649–54.
83. Kikuchi R, Mizuta K, Urahashi T, Sanada Y, Yamada N, Onuma E, et al. Quality of life after living donor liver transplant for biliary atresia in Japan. Pediatr Int. 2018;60:183–90.
84. Cole CR, Bucuvalas JC, Hornung RW, Krug S, Ryckman FC, Atherton H, et al. Impact of liver transplantation on HRQOL in children less than 5 years old. Pediatr Transplant. 2004;8:222–7.
85. Midgley DE, Bradlee TA, Donohoe C, Kent KP, Alonso EM. Health-related quality of life in long-term survivors of pediatric liver transplantation. Liver Transpl. 2000;6:333–9.
86. Alonso EM, Martz K, Wang D, Yi MS, Neighbors K, Varni JW, et al. Factors predicting health-related quality of life in pediatric liver transplant recipients in the functional outcomes group. Pediatr Transplant. 2013;17:605–11.
87. Haavisto A, Korkman M, Sintonen H, Holmberg C, Jalanko H, Lipsanen J, et al. Risk factors for impaired quality of life and psychosocial adjustment after pediatric heart, kidney, and liver transplantation. Pediatr Transplant. 2013;17:256–65.
88. Avitzur Y, De Luca E, Cantos M, Jimenez-Rivera C, Jones N, Fecteau A, et al. Health status ten years after pediatric liver transplantation—looking beyond the graft. Transplantation. 2004;78:566–73.
89. Devine KA, Reed-Knight B, Loiselle KA, Simons LE, Mee LL, Blount RL. Predictors of long-term health-related quality of life in adolescent solid organ transplant recipients. J Pediatr Psychol. 2011;36:891–901.
90. Alonso EM, Neighbors IC, Mattson C, Sweet E, Ruch-Ross H, Berry C, et al. Functional outcomes of pediatric liver transplant. JPGN. 2003;37:150–60.
91. Denny B, Beyerle K, Kienhuis M, Cora A, Gavidia-Payne S, Hardikar W. New insights into family functioning and quality of life after pediatric liver transplantation. Pediatr Transplant. 2012;16:711–5.
92. Simons LE, Anglin G, Warshaw BL, Mahle WT, Vincent RN, Blount RL. Understanding the pathway between the transplant experience and health-related quality of life outcomes in adolescents. Pediatr Transplant. 2008;12:187–93.
93. He K, Shen C, Chen X, Han L, Xi Z, Zhou T, et al. Health-related quality of life and sleep among Chinese children after living donor liver transplantation. Pediatr Transplant. 2015;19:547–54.
94. Andersen MN, Dore-Stites D, Gleit R, Lopez MJ, Fredericks EM. A pilot study of the association between sleep disturbance in children with liver transplants and parent and family health-related quality of life. J Pediatr Psychol. 2014;39:735–42.
95. Fredericks EM, Dore-Stites D, Calderon SY, Well A, Eder SJ, Magee JC, et al. Relationship between sleep problems and health-related quality of life among pediatric liver transplant recipients. Liver Transpl. 2012;18:707–15.
96. Jerson B, D'Urso C, Arnon R, Miloh T, Iyer K, Kerkar N, et al. Adolescent transplant recipients as peer mentors: a program to improve self-management and health-related quality of life. Pediatr Transplant. 2013;17:612–20.
97. Anthony SJ, Annunziato RA, Fairey E, Kelly VL, So S, Wray J. Waiting for transplant: physical, psychosocial, and nutritional status considerations for pediatric candidates and implications for care. Pediatr Transplant. 2014;18:423–34.
98. Shemesh E, Annunziato RA, Shneider B, Dugan CA, Warshaw J, Kerkar N, et al. Improving adherence to mediations in pediatric liver transplant recipients. Pediatr Transplant. 2008;12:316–23.
99. Reed-Knight B, Loiselle KA, Devine KA, Simons LE, Mee LL, Blount RL. Health-related quality of life and perceived need for mental health services in adolescent solid organ transplant recipients. J Clin Psychol Med Settings. 2013;20:88–96.
100. Parmar A, Vandriel SM, Ng VL. Health-related quality of life after pediatric liver transplantation: a systematic review. Liver Transpl. 2017;23:361–74.
101. Gritti A, Di Sarno AM, Comito M, De Vincenzo A, De Paola P, Vajro P. Psychological impact of liver transplantation on children's inner worlds. Pediatr Transplant. 2001;5:37–43.

Part III

Paediatric Hepatology Across the World

"The mission of us doctors is twofold:
Love for the Truth, tender care of the sick ones"

(Anonymous)

Pediatric Liver Disease in Latin America

Daniel D'Agostino, Maria Camila Sanchez, and Gustavo Boldrini

Key Points
- Hepatitis A virus (HAV) has been reported as the main cause of ALF in more than 58% of cases in Argentinean children. Disease rates decreased sharply after initiating the vaccination program in 2005.
- It has been estimated that 7–12 million Latin Americans carry HBV chronic infection. Seroprevalence for HCV is between 1 and 2%, genotype 1 being the most common.
- With the exception of Mexico, Latin America is considered a low endemic region for HEV. The most frequent HEV genotype found in South America is genotype 3.
- Geographical variations and the different subtypes of HLA are at different relative risks in liver autoimmune disease. In South America there is a predominance of HLA DR1.
- NAFLD is having a very high magnitude as described in the rest of the world. Hispanic children have a higher prevalence of NAFLD than African-American children, despite the fact that obesity rates in the two populations are similar.
- Biliary atresia is the most frequent etiology to neonatal cholestasis. The use of stool color cards has improved the awareness of the disease.
- Drug prescription patterns differ from those in European or North American countries, apart from being associated with high incidence of self-medication. A Spanish-Latin American DILI (SLATINDILI) Registry was created in late 2011 to identify hepatotoxicity cases induced by drugs, herbals, and dietary supplements.
- Due to a delay in diagnosis and unavailability of liver transplantation, a significant proportion of children develop end-stage liver disease and its complications. Biliary atresia accounts for 40–45% of etiology to liver transplantation. Delay in referral is an ongoing problem in South America, leading to the first cause of liver transplantation in the region.

Research Needed in the Field
- A Latin American registry should be started under the leadership of the SLAGHNP/LAPSGHAN to establish the PLD epidemiology and select adequate complementary tests to confirm diagnosis.
- The use of the new generation of DAAs for the treatment of hepatitis C.
- Diagnosis and management of Pediatric NAFLD.
- Identification of hepatotoxicity cases induced by drugs, herbals, and dietary supplements in LA, with detailed information and samples for genetic studies with the Spanish-Latin American DILI (SLATINDILI) Registry.

D. D'Agostino (✉) · M. C. Sanchez · G. Boldrini
School of Medicine, USAL University, Buenos Aires, Argentina

Division of Pediatric GI and Hepatology, Pediatric Liver and Intestinal Transplantation Program, Hospital Italiano, Buenos Aires, Argentina

Department of Pediatrics, Hospital Italiano, Buenos Aires, Argentina
e-mail: daniel.dagostino@hiba.org.ar;
mariacamila.sanchez@hiba.org.ar; gustavo.boldrini@hiba.org.ar

39.1 Introduction

LA is a conglomerate of adjacent countries whose official languages (Spanish and Portuguese) evolved from Latin. This region includes countries from Central and South America plus the Spanish-speaking islands of the Caribbean. The region has a population of more than 650 million, its largest countries being Brazil, Mexico, Argentina, and Colombia. The conglomerate of countries in LA shows different levels of medical complexity. There are factors that lead to different medical developments even within one same country. As there are no official records of such complexities, it is very difficult to make a general statistics that comprises the whole number of diseases affecting the population. The registries of different pathologies are scarce because few countries keep regular records.

The society representing pediatric gastroenterologists, hepatologists, and nutritionists is the Latin American Society of Pediatric Gastroenterology, Hepatology and Nutrition (SLAGHNP/LAPSGHAN).

It is important to develop research and follow-up local programs on liver disease, because its rapid progression will be a concern in public health in the near future. A Latin American registry should be started under the leadership of the SLAGHNP/LAPSGHAN to establish the liver disease epidemiology and select adequate complementary guidelines to confirm diagnosis, follow-up, and proper treatment.

39.2 Viral Hepatitis in Latin America

39.2.1 Hepatitis A

Hepatitis A virus (HAV) infection is one of the most frequently reported vaccine preventable diseases worldwide, with an estimated 1.5 million clinical cases occurring each year [1]. The most severe complication of HAV infection is acute liver failure (ALF), which is characterized by a rapid deterioration in liver function and a high fatality rate [2]. In Argentina, HAV infection has been reported to be the main cause of ALF in more than 58% of cases in children [3]. It was estimated that ALF occurred in 0.4% of cases of acute hepatitis caused by HAV infection in children aged 1–18 years from 1981 to 1996 [4]. A high incidence outbreak of HAV infection occurred during 2003–2004, when the incidence increased from 70.5 cases per 100,000 people in 2002 to 139 and 172.7 cases per 100,000 people in 2003 and 2004, respectively [5]. The incidence was higher in children aged 1–4 years and 10–14 years compared with older children and adults [6]. HAV-associated ALF was reported to account for 20% of LTs in children in Argentina [4]. A one-dose hepatitis A vaccine universal immunization (UI) program aimed at children aged 12 months was implemented in Argentina in 2005. In the private market, which represents approximately 12% of the birth cohort, children received two doses of the vaccine at 12–18 months of age. The impact of this immunization policy on the incidence of HAV infection was assessed in a study that analyzed HAV infection rates reported to the National Diseases Surveillance System in Argentina (SINAVE) since 1995 [7]. Overall vaccine coverage in 2006 was 98% for the single dose. Disease rates decreased sharply after initiating the vaccination program; the annual incidence of HAV infection for 2007 was 10.2 per 100,000, representing an 88.0% reduction compared with the average incidence for the period 1998–2002 (P 0.001). Reductions were seen in all age groups and all regions in Argentina, even though only children aged 12 months received the hepatitis A vaccine, showing a marked herd immunity effect. After the introduction of UI against HAV in 2005, only 27.7% (18/65) of FHF cases were caused by HAV infection (Fig. 39.1).

In addition to the introduction of a vaccination program, socioeconomic development, including improved sanitation and health education, also reduced HAV transmission. Six years after implementation of this country-wide single-dose program, no hepatitis A cases have been detected among vaccinated individuals, whereas among the unvaccinated, a number of cases have occurred, confirming continued circulating of hepatitis A virus in the Argentinean population. The actual incidence of hepatitis A in Argentina in 2016 is 0.11/10,000 (423 cases), mainly occurred in young adults unimmunized (Fig. 39.2). Interestingly, only 11 countries (6%) in the region have incorporated two doses of the vaccine in their programs, while in Argentina a single-dose immunization schedule for children aged ≥1 year is still being recommended. Protective anti-hepatitis A virus antibody levels after a single dose of inactivated hepatitis A vaccine can persist for almost 11 years and increase or reappear after booster vaccination [6].

39.2.2 Hepatitis B

Worldwide hepatitis B virus (HBV) infection is a major health problem. More than 2 billion people have been infected with HBV, and about 350 million individuals remain chronically infected; they constitute an enormous virus pool, a source of infection for susceptible hosts, and, most importantly, a population with high morbidity and mortality due to chronic liver disease, including hepatocellular carcinoma (HCC) [8]. Hepatitis B virus (HBV) has a remarkably complex evolutionary history. At least eight genotypes (A–H) with distinct geographical allocations and phylodynamic behaviors have been described. The information on the HBV epidemiology in Latin American countries is scanty and fragmentary, but it has been estimated that 7–12 million Latin Americans carry HBV chronic infection [9].

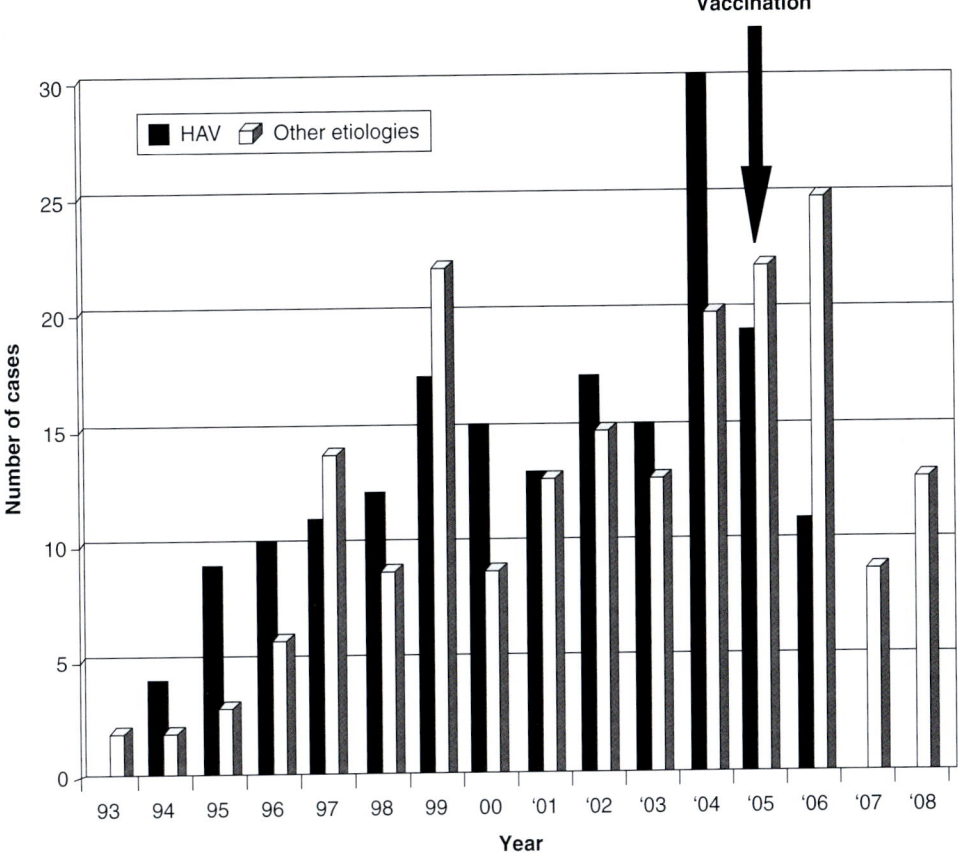

Fig. 39.1 Number of ALF cases caused by HAV and other etiologies each year in Argentina

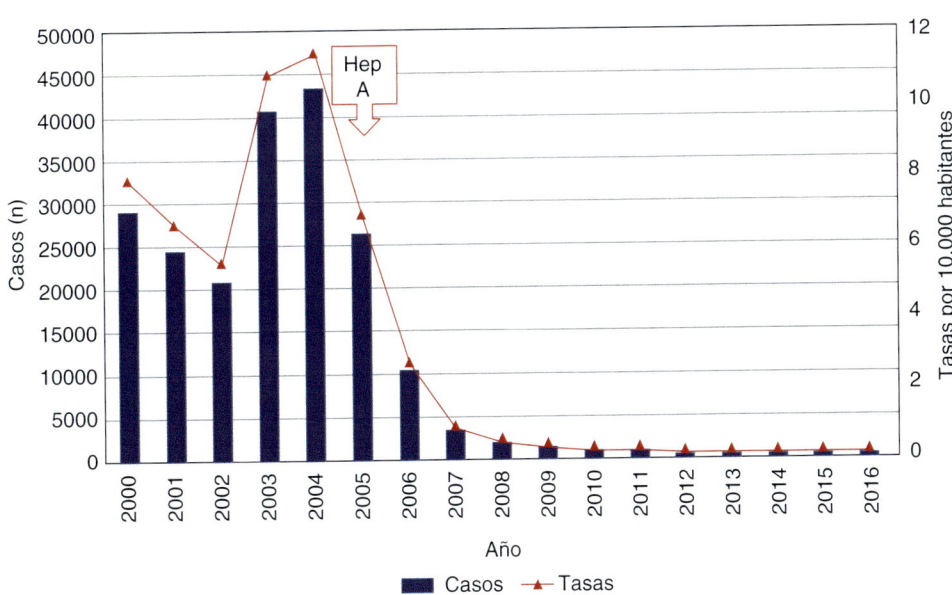

Fig. 39.2 Hepatitis A cases before and after the implementation of a single-dose program in Argentina

The rate of HBsAg-positive subjects varies between countries with the highest values being detected in the 20–40 age class as a possible consequence of a major role played by horizontal transmission [10, 11]. In addition, countries with a low HBV endemicity show a high rate of anti-HBc positivity in HBsAg-negative subjects, a clue to the more extensive exposure to HBV in the past. A slight decline in the HBsAg-positive prevalence was observed from 1990 to 2005 in Andean Latin American countries, whereas a slight increase was reported in southern Latin America. In the same period,

HBV genotypes F and H predominate in indigenous populations in Latin America, whereas genotypes A and D have been introduced from European and African Populations. Four subgenotypes of HBV genotype F (F1–F4) have been identified, predominating in Central America and frequent in Amerindians in all countries of South America and HBV genotype H in Amerindians and in Mestizos in Mexico. Genotypes F and H show a close phylogenetic relationship, suggesting an introduction of F/H ancestral strains before European colonization. Argentina has areas with different prevalence, low Buenos Aires, and others with high prevalence. Differences in pathogenesis and the probability of becoming a chronic carrier depend on the age at which hepatitis B virus (HBV) infection is acquired, ranging from 82% in infants less than 6 months of age to 15–30% in older children. HBV genotypes from 22 pediatric patients from 2 Argentinean areas that differ in prevalence were determined. Phylogenetic analysis shows a clear difference between the genotype distribution in Buenos Aires, a low prevalence area, and that found in other areas (Entre Ríos Province) with a high prevalence. The sequences of the Buenos Aires group were allocated to genotypes A (36%), D (9%), and F (55%) and demonstrated that the distribution of these genotypes virus in the acute and chronic course of infections could be an expression of the genotype. Genotype F and subgenotype 1b were the most prevalent and were over represented in acute and chronic HBeAg infections (56.1%).

Hepatitis B (HBV) infections remain endemic in many parts of the world, causing disease that can readily be prevented by vaccination. Although universal vaccination of infants against HBV and Hib has been recommended by the World Health Organization (WHO) since 1992 and 1996, respectively, an appropriate combination of vaccines and difficulties with vaccine supply have been identified as key factors contributing to this slow uptake. Unfortunately, the universal vaccination programs remain unaffordable for most South American countries. Where applied, however, they have achieved important epidemiological results (in the Colombian Amazon, the rate of HBsAg positivity dropped from 9% to 2% in children after 8 years of application) [12, 13]. The development of new DTPw-based combination vaccines is essential for the success of current and future childhood mass vaccination programs in countries where resources are limited [14]. Combining DTPw vaccines with HBV and Hib performs a key role in increasing vaccine coverage rates in line with WHO targets. Combined diphtheria-tetanus-whole cell pertussis (DTPw) vaccines remain the cornerstone of childhood vaccination programs in Latin America and many other parts of the world [15, 16]. A randomized, partially blind, multicenter study in three countries in Latin America (Argentina, Chile, and Nicaragua) between August 2004 and September 2005 was performed. A total of 585 subjects were enrolled and received primary vaccination (439 in the DTPw-HBV/Hib group and 146 in the *Tritanrix*™-HBV/Hib group). The study conclusion was the development of new DTPw-based combination vaccines is essential for the success of current and future childhood mass vaccination programs in countries where resources are limited [17]. Combining DTPw vaccines with HBV and Hib performs a key role in increasing vaccine coverage rates in line with WHO targets.

HBsAg prevalence:

Countries <2% low prevalence
Mexico, Honduras, Nicaragua, Costa Rica, Panamá, Uruguay, Chile, Argentina, Peru, northern Colombia
Intermediate prevalence (> 2%, < 8%)
Central America: Guatemala, El Salvador, Honduras, Haiti, Dominican Republic, Puerto Rico, Ecuador, French Guiana, Suriname, south Brazil
High prevalence (> 8%)
Northern Brazil, southern Colombia, Peru, northern Bolivia

39.2.3 Hepatitis C

Hepatitis C infection (HCV) is a global burden disease, and it represents a world health problem since there is no vaccine currently available. The infection is less prevalent in children than in adults. Vertical transmission is the main route of virus acquisition. Children represent a small but important portion of those infected with the HCV, and our understanding of the disease is limited in the Latin American pediatric population. HCV differs in children with regard to transmission, rates of clearance, natural history, and treatment [18]. According to the World Health Organization (WHO), 170 million people have chronic hepatitis C. In Latin America, seroprevalence for HCV is between 1 and 2%. In Brazil those with chronic hepatitis C account for 1.5 million. The most common genotypes in Argentina, Peru, Chile, and Brazil are 1 and less 2 and 3. Among children, up to 1992, parenteral transmission was the most prevalent, and after this period, the vertical transmission prevailed representing 80% of the infected. In a significant percentage of cases, it is not possible to identify the form of viral acquisition. A systematic review about the vertical transmission rate between 1992 and 2003 showed 1.7% of positive results among children whose mother was anti-HCV positive, regardless of a rate 4.3% when the mother was positive RNA-VHC, and 19.4% in the coinfection with HIV NA-VHC [19, 20]. In 2008, 98 blood samples of students aged 4–14 years old in the municipal network of Santos (Brazil) showed a 2.8% prevalence of anti-HCV. The prevalence of 0.02% of anti-HCV was low and much lower than the estimates for the Brazilian population, which ranges between 1 and 2%. According to the Ministry of Health in

2001, the positive anti-HCV in the general population of Brazil is of 1.38%, being 0.75% for the age group between 10 and 19 years old. According to the report of the study group of the Brazilian Society of Hepatology, with data from the States of Amazonas, Bahia, and Mato Grosso, anti-HCV in the population of students was of 0.20%, and none of the children in day care facilities had anti-HCV [21].

The mechanisms leading to liver cell injury, inflammation, and fibrosis are still under study in children. Staging liver fibrosis is considered to be an essential because it provides prognostic information and, in many cases, assists in therapeutic decision. HCV-positive pediatric population differs from the adult population in that it presents a higher rate of spontaneous elimination of the virus and less progression to fibrosis. Mechanisms leading to liver damage in chronic hepatitis are being discussed, but both the immune system and the virus are involved. However, liver injury in pediatric would be largely associated with a viral cytopathic effect mediated by apoptosis, while in adults it would be mainly associated with an exacerbated immune response [22]. Continued monitoring of liver fibrosis in pediatric patients will help to establish its role in predicting clinical outcomes. There was an interesting study which compared biopsies of adults with pediatric patients in Argentina that measured the markets of fibrosis. The results in children were a moderate and advanced fibrosis 64% and 20%, respectively, while 54% and 23% in adults. This pediatric population (22 children) had as well 36% moderate and severe steatosis and 90% of bile duct damage [23].

Determining candidacy for treatment of chronic HCV in a child or adolescent is often controversial. The current standard of care includes pegylated interferon once weekly in combination with ribavirin twice daily. A large multicenter pediatric study in Latin American have proven the superiority of achieving sustained virologic response (SVR), defined as being HCV RNA negative 6 months after completion of treatment, with combination therapy compared to interferon alone. Predictors of high rates of SVR include genotypes 2 and 3 (>80% SVR) and low viral load in children with genotype 1 (<60,000 IU/mL) [24]. The biochemical and virologic response is accompanied by histologic improvement in patients with SVR in these trials, and interferon was well tolerated in children. There is no evidence with the new generation of DAAs for the treatment of hepatitis in Latin American children yet.

Table 39.1 HEV genotypes reported for LA

Genotype	Region	Species		
		Human	Swine	Others[a]
Genotype 1	Uruguay	x		
	Venezuela	x		
	Cuba	x		
	Mexico	x		
Genotype 2	Mexico	x	x	
Genotype 3	Argentina	x	x	
	Brazil	x	x	
	Bolivia	x		
	Cuba	x		
	Venezuela	x		
	Mexico	x	x	x
	Uruguay	x		
	Chile	x		
	Costa Rica	x	x	

[a]Host or developed in chickens, deer, rodent, and other mammals

39.2.4 Hepatitis E

Hepatitis E virus (HEV) was not recognized as a new virus-causing hepatic disease until 1980, which is the main reason for the limited information on this viral disease [25]. Two HEV epidemiological profiles have been described: hyperendemic regions, defined as waterborne outbreaks or confirmed HEV infection in 25% of sporadic non-A, non-B hepatitis, and low endemic regions defined as confirmed HEV infection in <25% of sporadic non-A, non-B hepatitis. Latin America (LA), with the exception of Mexico, is considered to be a low endemic region. However this epidemiologic situation is partially known due to the lack of proper registry in several countries of the territory. Studies performed in LA countries between 1987 and 2006 showed a seroprevalence of HEV IgG antibodies from 0.15 to 9.6% in children <20 years [26, 27]. One study performed from 2012 to 2013 in Argentina showed an overall prevalence of anti-HEV IgG antibodies of 15.4% [28]. Reports of molecular characterization of HEV strains from LA are very scarce. The most frequent HEV genotype found in South America is the genotype 3. Yet genotypes 1 and 2 have been isolated in Uruguay, Venezuela, Cuba, and Mexico [29, 30] (Table 39.1).

Seroprevalence studies indicate that most HEV infections in healthy children are asymptomatic. In immunosuppressed patients, however, chronic HEV infection has been documented in both bone marrow and solid organ transplant pediatric recipients. In Brazil, there was a case of chronic HEV infection in a liver transplanted child was reported [31], showing that HEV should be further investigated and incorporated into the differential diagnosis of hepatitis and acute cellular rejection among liver transplant pediatric patients.

39.3 Autoimmune Hepatitis in Latin America

Autoimmune hepatitis (AIH) is an inflammatory, chronic hepatic process of unknown etiology, affecting mainly females. Due to its spontaneous evolution, if not treated, it may progress to cirrhosis in most cases.

A recent study in pediatric patients reported an incidence of 0.4 case per 100,000 children [32].

The biochemical and serological features are elevated transaminase, hypergammaglobulinemia and circulating autoantibodies, and a histologic picture of interface hepatitis. According to serum autoantibodies on diagnosis, two types of autoimmune hepatitis are found: type 1 positive for antinuclear (ANA) and/or smooth muscle antibodies (SMA), and/or soluble liver antigen (SLA), and type 2 with anti-liver kidney microsomal type 1 (anti-LKM 1) and/or anti-liver cytosol type 1 antibodies (anti-LC1). Treatments used for autoimmune hepatitis include prednisone and azathioprine, being effective in 80% of patients. Almost 20% of patients do not react to the conventional treatment, requiring another alternative therapy to preventing the progression of the disease.

There is limited bibliography published about AIH in Latin America regarding its prevalence among different pediatric ages, laboratory and clinical presentations, and its treatments.

Hypergammaglobulinemia is a diagnostic feature of AIH, but other immunoglobulins may be altered as well. The IgA deficiency and complement 4a, genetically conditioned, can be associated with the IAH. A Brazilian study reported that IgA deficiency is more frequent in patients with autoimmune hepatitis type 2 and it is genetically linked to HLA DR1 and DR7, whereas a second study demonstrated low levels of complement 4a in the pediatric population [33]. A third study showed increased IgE serum levels and sought to compare clinical and histological features according to IgE levels in AIH type [34].

There is a genetic predisposition in AIH linked with human leukocyte antigens (HLA). Geographical variations and the different subtypes of HLA contribute to different relative risks of different ethnic groups. In Europe and the USA, the haplotypes of HLA DRB1 and DRB1/0301/0401 are strongly associated with HAI type 1, while the presence of DR1501 seems to be protective [35, 36]. In studies conducted in South America (Argentina and Brazil), HLA haplotypes were analyzed in a population of pediatric and adult patients and showed a predominance of HLA DR1 1301 [37, 38] and to a lesser extent with DR3 and DR4. The DR3 association with autoimmune hepatitis type 2 is described in all ethnic groups [39, 40].

Research carried out in Argentina reported that the early onset of type 1 autoimmune hepatitis has a strong genetic influence according to the role of human leukocyte antigens and killer cell immunoglobulin-like receptor (HLA and KIR) genes. This study showed that the human KIR is known to be associated with susceptibility to autoimmune diseases. It was demonstrated that in pediatric autoimmune hepatitis (PAH), the increased frequency of the functional form of KIR2DS4-Full Length (KIR2DS4-FL), in combination with HLA-DRB1*1301, revealed a strong synergistic effect and suggested a stronger genetic influence for the early onset type 1 autoimmune [41].

The clinical features at the onset of the disease vary from asymptomatic to severe hepatitis and liver failure. It is a complex polygenic multifactorial disease produced by the interplay of environmental and etiological factors in patients with a genetic predisposition to develop autoimmune diseases.

The histologic involvement of AIH is characterized by an infiltration of lymphocytes, plasma cells, and eosinophils at the level of the portal space, with dissemination toward the right hepatic lobe (2 and 3), infiltration of the hepatocytes of the periphery, and erosion of the limiting plate, which is what has been called interface hepatitis. It has also been described as common emperipolesis, which is the presence of lymphocytes or intact plasma cells inside a hepatocyte. By the death and destruction of hepatocytes, the collapse of connective tissue is observed. Liver regeneration gives rise to the formation of rosettes (hepatocytes surrounding a biliary canaliculus in the periportal area). The severity of hepatitis interface is similar in IAH types 1 and 2; however, cirrhosis is more frequent in type 1. The presence of a few plasma cells does not rule out the disease.

Forty percent of the responders to the treatment have frequent episodes of recurrence that require an alternative treatment to prevent the progression of the disease to liver failure and the need for transplant. The therapeutic alternatives in the cases of non-responders are currently based on immunosuppressive drugs such as mycophenolate mofetil, calcineurin inhibitors, rapamycin, and anti-CD20 which are used in posttransplantation to prevent cellular rejection. Cyclosporine (CsA) is a potent immunosuppressive therapy that has been used effectively in both children and adults with HAI. In pediatrics it has been shown to induce remission in AIH types 1 and 2 when administered as an initial treatment, as was demonstrated in an Argentinian group that used it for a period of 6 months and continued with low doses of prednisone and azathioprine. The authors concluded that CsA showed a superiority to standard combination therapies and that the adverse effects of this drug—with the levels that were used—may be important but that in the majority of patients were mild and transient [42, 43].

AIH is considered a T-cell–mediated autoimmune disease. Because B cells have been shown to play a significant role in several T-cell–mediated autoimmune diseases, some of these disorders could respond to anti-CD20 monoclonal antibodies (rituximab). This was demonstrated in a recent study carried out in Argentina. Two cases of refractory AIH have been successfully treated with rituximab (375 mg/m^2 weekly for 4 doses) as rescue therapy, but its use should be restricted to specialized centers because of potentially severe side effects. Those who conducted this research stated that the treatment with rituximab contributes to diminish the number of patients eventually needing liver transplantation [44, 45].

Liver transplantation in IAH is indicated in patients with acute liver failure or those patients who develop end-stage liver disease. Some pediatric patients with AIH recover after LF with immunosuppressive therapy; liver transplantation could be avoided or delayed.

39.4 Fatty Liver in Latin America

Nonalcoholic fatty liver disease (NAFLD) is defined by hepatic fat infiltration of more than 5% of hepatocytes and nonalcoholic steatohepatitis. NASH is characterized by macrovesicular steatosis (the fat globules vary in size from very small to nearly filling the hepatocyte), ballooning degeneration with or without Mallory bodies, with lobular or portal inflammation, with or without fibrosis. Diagnosis of NASH requires a liver biopsy and careful histology examination by an expert pathologist.

Over the last decades, with increased obesity, NAFLD and NASH have been considered a common cause of liver disease and have emerged as the leading cause of chronic liver disease in children and adolescents. Obesity is a nutritional disorder in developed countries, which becomes to be a generalized problem worldwide, especially in Latin America and, above all, in the Caribbean, where 23% of adults and 7% of preschool children are overweight.

In Latin America, Mexico is the country with the highest obesity, followed by Venezuela with 30.8%, Argentina with 29.4%, and Chile with 29.1%. In 2013, more than 42 million children younger than 5 years of age worldwide were overweight; of them, more than 80% lived in developing countries. In Buenos Aires, an interesting study showed that in 11,391 normal child population, the overweight were 14.29%, obesity 9.25%, and morbid obesity 0.68%. Brazil increased this population weight from 4.1% in 1974 (6–18 years of age) to 22.1% in 2005 (7–10 years of age) with added overweight and obesity; in Costa Rica in 2003 (7–12 years old), the overweight were 34.5% and obesity 26.2%; Mexico went from 17.9% of overweight and 9% of obesity in 2006 (5–11 years of age) to 20.2% and 14.6% in 2012, respectively, and 21.3% of overweight and 11% and 9% of obesity (12–19 years of age) to 21.6% and 13.3%, respectively, in the same period [46, 47].

A larger consumption of low-cost, industrial food rich in fat, sugar and salt plus a decrease in physical activity with sedentary life turned out in overweight and obesity pattern. Between 5 and 10% of the pediatric population in LA may be experiencing NAFLD/NASH due to overweight. Reflecting the extreme increase in obesity among adolescents, this age group is also the most vulnerable for developing NAFLD.

The different prevalence in Latin America could be related to several factors as the interaction of genetic and environmental factors especially type of diet, exercise choice, socioeconomic status, and lifestyles in diverse countries.

Parents play a very important role in obesity etiology: socioeconomic level, education level, parental employment status, and obesity familial.

In an interesting study conducted in San Diego (USA), out of 742 autopsies done between 1993 and 2003 in the 2- to 19-year-old population. The prevalence of fatty liver adjusted for age, gender, race, and ethnicity was estimated to be 9.6%, although the autopsy cohort was understandably biased relative to the general population due to overrepresentation with older teen Hispanic males. Multivariate analysis showed that older age, male gender, overweight, and Hispanic ethnicity were independent predictors of fatty liver in this cohort [48]. In pediatrics, obesity is the main risk factor. In 41 adolescents, who had an average of 59 BMI, 83% had NAFLD and 20% met histological criteria for NASH. In Latin America, the data are lower possibly due to different conditions. In Cuba, in a study of 44 obese children aged 4–16 years, 48% had fatty liver, and in Venezuela studies show an average prevalence of 65% among overweight and obese children [49]. Different ethnic groups have also shown varying prevalence of fatty liver. Hispanic children have a higher prevalence of NAFLD than African-American children, despite the fact that the obesity rates in the two populations are similar [50].

39.5 Neonatal Cholestasis in Latin America

The diagnosis of cholestasis in neonates has advanced considerably during recent decades due to growing insight into pathophysiological mechanisms and remarkable methodological and technical developments in diagnostic procedures as well as therapeutic and preventive approaches. In spite of these advances in Latin America, the situation remains significantly different due to lack of resources and difficulties in diagnosis. There are no solid data about the exact percentages of frequencies of the common etiological causes of cholestasis in Latin America; in general, data come from single centers or multicenter studies from an individual country, excluding Latin America as a whole.

Biliary atresia (BA) is the most common cause of cholestasis in neonates and the most common indication for pediatric liver transplantation. There is marked variation in incidence of BA ranging from about 1 in 5–10,000 live births in Taiwan [51] to about 1 in 15–20,000 in mainland Europe and North America [52]. Unfortunately, in Latin America, there is a lack of data on incidence of BA. The etiology of biliary atresia is not defined, but the pathogenic mechanisms of the disease are closely linked to a strong immune response directed to the bile duct [52, 53].

The clinical phenotype is produced by a fibrosing and inflammatory process that obstructs the lumen of extrahepatic bile ducts and disrupts the flow of bile into the duodenum, which finalizes with the fibrosis and obliteration of the biliary tract and eventual development of biliary cirrhosis with portal hypertension and liver failure. If not treated surgically, toddlers may die after 2–3 years of the disease [54, 55].

In Brazil Carvalho et al. reviewed the clinical presentation, treatment, and outcome of 513 children with biliary atresia. The data were obtained from large clinical centers in different geographical regions of Brazil. In general, the clinical presentation with direct hyperbilirubinemia, high gamma-glutamyltranspeptidase, and a histopathology with ductal proliferation and plugs was typical in the cohort. The mean age at diagnosis and portoenterostomy was 82.6 ± 32.8 days, with surgery performed in 76.4% of the infants. In those infants treated with portoenterostomy, the 4-year survival with the native liver was 36.8%, with higher survival at 54% if the portoenterostomy was performed in infants ≤60 days of age. The combination of portoenterostomy and liver transplantation increased the overall survival to 73.4%. However, only 46.6% of all patients underwent transplantation—a low rate compared to other countries, in which access to transplantation increases to ≥60% of children [56]. The study also identifies two areas for future improvement. First, there is almost 2 weeks separating the age at onset of symptoms (12.3 ± 17 days) and the age at portoenterostomy (82.6 ± 32.8 days). While the reasons for such delay in diagnosis and surgical intervention were not obvious, they may have been related to community awareness of the disease, recognition by primary care physicians, and access to specialized care. Pediatric hepatologists have partnered with the Brazilian Society of Pediatrics and the Brazilian Health Ministry to increase community awareness by the incorporation of a stool color card in the Child health Booklet distributed by the Ministry to the parents of every neonate. The second area for improvement relates to the use of liver transplantation to improve survival when the child develops advanced liver disease. In the centers participating in the study, survival of children treated with portoenterostomy and later with liver transplantation increased in the 2000s to 77.6%. Despite this success, only 46.6% of the patients underwent liver transplantation [57].

The best outcome still remains linked to an early diagnosis and surgical treatment. In this regard, between 1999 and 2002, a single center of Argentina (The National Hospital Prof. Alejandro Posadas) conducted a prospective, observational study, which used tool screening method with colorimetric characteristics. Out of a total of 12,484 children, 4239 (33.9%) went to the first month visit with the color card. We identified 18 patients with pale or acholic stools, of whom only 4 manifested cholestatic disease (Alagille syndrome, luetic hepatitis, transient neonatal cholestasis, and biliary lithiasis). Although no cases of BA were identified, the screening test proved to be useful for the detection of other causes of neonatal cholestasis. After the screening with colorimetric cards, the center mentioned above has succeeded in the early diagnosis of biliary atresia and its early surgical intervention [58] (Table 39.2).

The scarce data published in Latin America show the urgent need of an early diagnosis and treatment as well as the evaluation of the results observed in the short- and long-term follow-up. Due to differences in socioeconomic, cultural, and extensive geographic areas that exist in Latin America, it is important to achieve a greater awareness in the pediatric hepatologists with the support of medical societies (SLAGHNP/LAPSGHAN) and funds for research.

39.6 Hepatotoxicity by Drugs and Substances

Drug- and substance-induced hepatotoxicity is known internationally as drug-induced liver injury (DILI). Liver injury induced by drugs, herbs, dietary supplements, or products to enhance athletic performance is nowadays a major problem affecting the general population and patients with underlying conditions and also falls within the scope of physicians, who are responsible for indicating different treatments, the pharmaceutical industry, and regulatory agencies. DILI accounts for 10–20% of cases of acute liver failure and liver transplant. In western countries, most DILI cases are associated with antibiotics, anticonvulsant agents, and psychotropic agents. In Asian countries, herbs and dietary supplements are the most common causes of DILI. In the USA and Europe, intrinsic hepatotoxicity accounts for 7–15% of acute liver failure cases and is the most common cause of discontinuation of a market-approved drug. In Latin America the information about hepatotoxicity is obtained from data provided by the reporting system and publications in scientific journals. Therefore, the actual quantification is quite likely only the "top of the iceberg."

Table 39.2 Colorimetric cards, comparative with different authors

Author	Year	Countries	Population	BA[a]	Others	Kasai days
Matsui	95	Japan	17,641	2/3		35 years 69
Chen	06	Taiwan	119,973	29/30	11	29 < 90
Hsiao	08	Taiwan	422,264	75		84% (<60)
Ramonet	13	Argentina	12,484	2	4[b]	38/42

[a]Biliary atresia
[b]Neonatal hepatitis [2], Alagille S, and syphilis

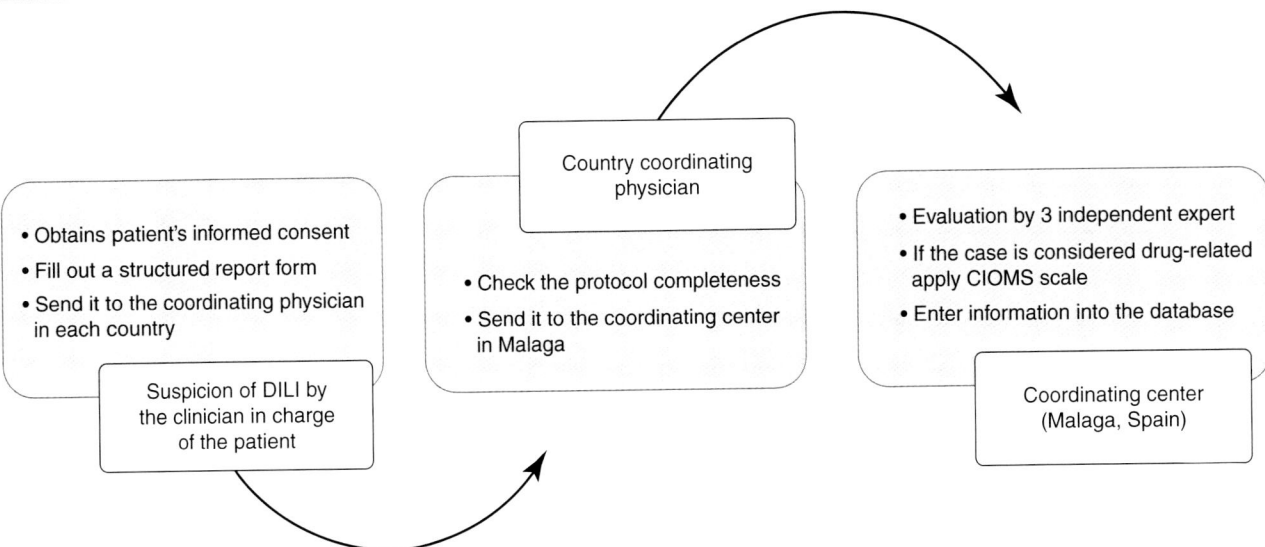

Fig. 39.3 Flow chart depicting the process for case enrollment at the Latin American drug-induced liver injury (DILI)

In the field of pediatrics, drug-induced hepatotoxicity accounts for 20% of acute liver failure cases, 14% of which have been reported in association with acetaminophen. At present, more than 1000 drugs and substances have been reported to cause hepatotoxicity among children and adults. The wide range of clinical manifestations, the multiple number of causative agents, and the lack of specific diagnostic tests make diagnosis even much more complicated [59]. As opposed to countries, such as Spain, Iceland, Japan, and the USA where registries and multicenter networks for conducting studies on DILI have existed for several years, Latin America (LA) had not set up this collaborative strategy until only 4 years ago [60]. Consequently, epidemiological data on DILI in the literature came almost exclusively from the reporting of either isolated cases or small series of subjects. Latin America is a continent comprising 23 countries, showing significant demographic growth in the last few years, and characterized by drug prescription patterns that differ from those in European or North American countries, apart from being associated with high incidence of self-medication. Like in Asia and Africa, throughout Latin America, there is a large market for herbs and supplements as an important side of folk medicine, since these products are more accessible and affordable. According to the necessity to explore in Latin America the issue of DILLI and indentify hepatotoxicity cases induced by drugs and herbals and dietary, the Spanish-Latin America DILLI Registry was created. This has been available in the web site (www.slatindili.uma.es) since 2011. With aimed to prospectively identify hepatotoxicity cases induced by drugs and herbals and dietary supplements (HDS) in LA, with detailed information and samples for genetic studies. Thus, the Spanish-Latin American DILI (SLATINDILI) Registry available online www.slatindili.uma.es was created by the end of 2011, after an initiative of and with the ongoing support from the Spanish DILI group [61–63] (Fig. 39.3).

Table 39.3 Networking therapeutic classes and individual agents with progression to ALF (acute liver failure) or OLT (orthotopic liver transplantation) published in Latin America (LA) during 1996–2012 [51]

Therapeutic class	n %	ALF/OLT n %	Individual agent
NSAIDs and antirheumatic drugs	62 (32)	16 (26)	Nimesulide, piroxicam, diclofenac, naproxen
Anti-infectious	37 (19)	11 (30)	Nitrofurantoin, isoniazid, trovafloxacin, clarithromycin
Genitourinary system and sex hormones	34 (18)	14 (22)	Progesterone, cyproterone acetate, flutamide
Antineoplastic and immunomodulators	10 (5)	2 (3)	Imatinib, tamoxifen
Anticonvulsants	7 (4)	3	Valproic acid, phenytoin
Cardiovascular system	6 (3)	1	Methyldopa
Antivirals	5 (3)	1	Nevirapine
Anesthetics	5 (3)	5	Halothane
Antithyroid	5 (3)	4	Propylthiouracil
Other groups	20	5	Ketoconazole, griseofulvin, disulfiram, mycophenolato

More than 250 patients enrolled throughout LA during the last 5 years are clear evidence that DILI registry is successfully working up to now. NetworkMain therapeutic classes and individual agents with progression to ALF (acute liver failure) or OLT (orthotopic liver transplantation) were published in Latin America (LA) during 1996–2012 [64] (Table 39.3).

Table 39.4 Pediatric liver transplant in LA

Country	Year started	Number of centers	Number of LT	LT pmp	Living donor	Survival 1 year (%)	Survival 5- years (%)
Brazil	1985	27	2824	13.9	1209	90.3–90.5	67.2–83.6
Argentina	1986	10	1070	25.1	340	80–87	74
Mexico	1994	5	247	1.9	49	85	75
Chile	1993	4	230	12.7	65	80	73
Colombia	1991	4	207	4.1	48	ND	ND
Peru	2001	1	20	0.6	11	ND	ND
Venezuela	2004	1	ND	ND	29	100	ND
Cube	2005	1	27	2.4	ND	87	ND

ND no published data

39.7 Liver Transplant in Latin America

LT has had a slow and difficult growth. The first attempts were made in Brazil in 1968, in Chile in 1969, and in Peru in 1973. It was not until the 1980s that other programs were developed in the region: Colombia (1979), Chile (1985), Brazil (1985), Mexico (1985), Cuba (1986), and Argentina (1988) [65]. In 1980, the Latin American Transplantation Society was founded, and in 1989, the Latin America Transplantation Registry was started, which was an attempt to publish data on transplantation activity in LA [66]. However, transplant registries are still scarce because few countries keep a regular record of donations and transplantation availabilities through the websites of national organizations.

Most LA countries have transplantation laws defining brain death criteria, consent forms, living donor restrictions, restrictions on economic benefits from donations, and cadaveric organ allocation. Organ trafficking is penalized. Eight countries have adopted presumed consent for retrieval, the last of them being Argentina in 2005 [67]. Economic and social disparities are also responsible for the drawbacks in transplantation activities in LA. There is a lack of governmental support, and not all of the countries provide universal health coverage for transplantation.

Pediatric LT is limited in LA, with only eight countries reporting transplantation. Brazil, Argentina, Mexico, and Colombia keep the best records of the number of pediatric LT performed (Table 39.1). These countries have also the highest number of transplants. However, websites for national organizations are not user-friendly, and the information is usually restricted to the number of transplants performed. None of the websites provide data on waiting list mortality or posttransplant survival. Social and economic disparities within the countries can explain the concentration of LT in centers located in regions with higher economic power. Comparing the governmental health expenditures in proportion to the GDP, LA countries spend between 10 and 15%, while European countries, the USA, Canada, and Australia spend more than 20% [68]. There is a shortage of governmental support by each country's national organization, especially regarding the pediatric population, makes it difficult to report on the outcomes of pediatric LT in LA, even though countries such as Brazil and Argentina are closer to achieving volumes and results comparable to North American and European countries. Currently, among LA countries, only Argentina and Brazil rank in the top 20 countries in LTs performed overall 5–9.9 pmp [69]. The other countries have a poor representation in the ranking, below five LT pmp. There is still a high offering of marginal livers that are not amenable to splitting or even to be used as reduced liver grafts. The suboptimal management of donors is another contributing factor for the low utilization of deceased donors. Pediatric patients depend on the availability of living donors and, particularly in Sao Paulo, Brazil, represent most of the pediatric LT performed. From those countries that perform pediatric LT in LA, only Cuba does not have records of live donation. In Brazil, LDLT represents 53.4% of the pediatric LT [70]. Countries with very high HDI, such as Japan, the USA, and Canada, have national registries or collaborative research groups that allow for adequate assessment of pediatric LT activity, including quality assessments, that results in the implementation of practices toward quality improvement of centers performing LT [71]. From the centers in LA that reported survival rates, these are similar to the European and North American data [72–74] (Table 39.4).

Acknowledgment To our families, colleagues, and patients; to Josefina Martinelli, who has greatly contributed to the writing of this chapter; and to the ones who trusted us to represent Latin America in this book.

References

1. Website [Internet]. [cited 2017 Nov 21]. http://www.who.int/docstore/wer/pdf/2000/wer7505.pdf. Accessed 13 Apr 2010.
2. Yeung LTF, Roberts EA. Current issues in the management of paediatric viral hepatitis. Liver Int. 2010;30(1):5–18.
3. Ciocca ME, Ramonet MD, Cuarterolo ML, López SI, Speranza AM, Gómez S, et al. O0062 Acute liver failure in children: experi-

ence with 210 patients. J Pediatr Gastroenterol Nutr. 2004;39(Suppl 1):S31.
4. Ciocca M. Clinical course and consequences of hepatitis A infection. Vaccine. 2000;18:S71–4.
5. Vacchino MN. Incidence of Hepatitis A in Argentina after vaccination. J Viral Hepat. 2008;15:47–50.
6. Ott JJ, Wiersma ST. Single-dose administration of inactivated hepatitis A vaccination in the context of hepatitis A vaccine recommendations. Int J Infect Dis. 2013;17(11):e939–44.
7. Poovorawan Y. Single-dose hepatitis A vaccination: comparison of different dose levels in adolescents. Vaccine. 1996;14(12):1092–4.
8. Lavanchy D. Hepatitis B virus epidemiology, disease burden, treatment, and current and emerging prevention and control measures. J Viral Hepat. 2004;11(2):97–107.
9. Devesa M, Pujol FH. Hepatitis B virus genetic diversity in Latin America. Virus Res. 2007;127(2):177–84.
10. Alvarado-Mora MV, Pinho JRR. Epidemiological update of hepatitis B, C and delta in Latin America. Antivir Ther. 2013;18(3 Pt B):429–33.
11. Roman S, Jose-Abrego A, Fierro NA, Escobedo-Melendez G, Ojeda-Granados C, Martinez-Lopez E, et al. Hepatitis B virus infection in Latin America: a genomic medicine approach. World J Gastroenterol. 2014;20(23):7181–96.
12. Braga WSM, Castilho M da C, Borges FG, Martinho AC de S, Rodrigues IS, Azevedo EP, et al. Prevalence of hepatitis B virus infection and carriage after nineteen years of vaccination program in the Western Brazilian Amazon. Rev Soc Bras Med Trop. 2012;45(1):13–7.
13. de la Hoz F, Perez L, de Neira M, Hall AJ. Eight years of hepatitis B vaccination in Colombia with a recombinant vaccine: factors influencing hepatitis B virus infection and effectiveness. Int J Infect Dis. 2008;12(2):183–9.
14. Wenger J. Vaccines for the developing world: current status and future directions. Vaccine. 2001;19(13–14):1588–91.
15. Prymula R, Plisek S. Clinical experience with DTPw-HBV and DTPw-HBV/Hib combination vaccines. Expert Opin Biol Ther. 2008;8(4):503–13.
16. Arístegui J, Usonis V, Coovadia H, Riedemann S, Win KM, Gatchalian S, et al. Facilitating the WHO expanded program of immunization: the clinical profile of a combined diphtheria, tetanus, pertussis, hepatitis B and Haemophilus influenzae type b vaccine. Int J Infect Dis. 2003;7(2):143–51.
17. Espinoza F, Tregnaghi M, Gentile A, Abarca K, Casellas J, Collard A, et al. Primary and booster vaccination in Latin American children with a DTPw-HBV/Hib combination: a randomized controlled trial. BMC Infect Dis. 2010;10:297.
18. Gower E, Estes C, Blach S, Razavi-Shearer K, Razavi H. Global epidemiology and genotype distribution of the hepatitis C virus infection. J Hepatol. 2014;61(1):S45–57.
19. Khaderi S, Shepherd R, Goss JA, Leung DH. Hepatitis C in the pediatric population: transmission, natural history, treatment and liver transplantation. World J Gastroenterol. 2014;20(32):11281–6.
20. Checa Cabot CA, Stoszek SK, Quarleri J, Losso MH, Ivalo S, Peixoto MF, et al. Mother-to-child transmission of hepatitis C virus (HCV) among HIV/HCV-coinfected women. J Pediatr Infect Dis Soc. 2013;2(2):126–35.
21. Ciaccia MCC, Moreira RC, Lemos MF, Oba IT, Porta G. Epidemiological, serological and molecular aspects of hepatitis B and C in children and teenagers of municipal daycare facilities schools and schools in the city of Santos. Rev Bras Epidemiol. 2014;17(3):588–99.
22. Valva P, Gismondi MI, Casciato PC, Galoppo M, Lezama C, Galdame O, et al. Distinctive intrahepatic characteristics of paediatric and adult pathogenesis of chronic hepatitis C infection. Clin Microbiol Infect. 2014;20(12):O998–1009.
23. Gismondi MI, Turazza EI, Grinstein S, Galoppo MC, Preciado MV. Hepatitis C virus infection in infants and children from Argentina. J Clin Microbiol. 2004;42(3):1199–202.
24. Wirth S, Ribes-Koninckx C, Calzado MA, Bortolotti F, Zancan L, Jara P, et al. High sustained virologic response rates in children with chronic hepatitis C receiving peginterferon alfa-2b plus ribavirin. J Hepatol. 2010;52(4):501–7.
25. Schmid R. History of viral hepatitis: a tale of dogmas and misinterpretations. J Gastroenterol Hepatol. 2001;16(7):718–22.
26. Alvarez-Muñoz MT, Torres J, Damasio L, Gómez A, Tapia-Conyer R, Muñoz O. Seroepidemiology of hepatitis E virus infection in Mexican subjects 1 to 29 years of age. Arch Med Res. 1999;30(3):251–4.
27. Villalba MCM, Montalvo Villalba MC, Guan M, Pérez A, Corredor MB, Frometa SS, et al. Seroprevalence of antibodies to hepatitis E virus in two large communities in Havana, Cuba. Trans R Soc Trop Med Hyg. 2010;104(12):772–6.
28. Munné MS, Altabert NR, Otegui MLO, Vladimirsky SN, Moreiro R, Espul MP, et al. Updating the knowledge of hepatitis E: new variants and higher prevalence of anti-HEV in Argentina. Ann Hepatol. 2014;13(5):496–502.
29. Munné MS, Vladimirsky S, Otegui L, Castro R, Brajterman L, Soto S, et al. Identification of the first strain of swine hepatitis E virus in South America and prevalence of anti-HEV antibodies in swine in Argentina. J Med Virol. 2006;78(12):1579–83.
30. dos Santos DRL, Vitral CL, de Paula VS, Marchevsky RS, Lopes JF, Gaspar AMC, et al. Serological and molecular evidence of hepatitis E virus in swine in Brazil. Vet J. 2009;182(3):474–80.
31. Passos-Castilho AM, Porta G, Miura IK, Pugliese RPS, Danesi VLB, Porta A, et al. Chronic hepatitis E virus infection in a pediatric female liver transplant recipient. J Clin Microbiol. 2014;52(12):4425–7.
32. Deneau M, Kyle Jensen M, Holmen J, Williams MS, Book LS, Guthery SL. Primary sclerosing cholangitis, autoimmune hepatitis, and overlap in utah children: epidemiology and natural history. Hepatology. 2013;58(4):1392–400.
33. Liang T. Immunology and liver Edited by K.-H. Meyer zum Büschenfelde, J.H. Hoofnagle, and M. Manns, 474 pp. Dordrecht, The Netherlands: Kluwer Academic Publishers, 1993. $115. Hepatology. 1994;20(3):766–7.
34. Porta G, Schneidwind KDR, Ribeiro CMF, Miura IK, Pugliese RPS, Baggio VL, et al. P0338 Autoimmune hepatitis type 1 in children is associated to high IGE levels. J Pediatr Gastroenterol Nutr. 2004;39(Suppl 1):S185.
35. Czaja AJ, Doherty DG, Donaldson PT. Genetic bases of autoimmune hepatitis. Dig Dis Sci. 2002;47(10):2139–50.
36. Donaldson PT, Doherty DG, Hayllar KM, McFarlane IG, Johnson PJ, Williams R. Susceptibility to autoimmune chronic active hepatitis: human leukocyte antigens DR4 and A1-B8-DR3 are independent risk factors. Hepatology. 1991;13(4):701–6.
37. Fainboim L, Marcos Y, Pando M, Capucchio M, Reyes GB, Galoppo C, et al. Chronic active autoimmune hepatitis in children. Hum Immunol. 1994;41(2):146–50.
38. Pando M, Larriba J, Fernandez GC, Fainboim H, Ciocca M, Ramonet M, et al. Pediatric and adult forms of type I autoimmune hepatitis in argentina: evidence for differential genetic predisposition. Hepatology. 1999;30(6):1374–80.
39. Yoshizawa K, Umemura T, Ota M. Genetic background of autoimmune hepatitis in Japan. J Gastroenterol. 2010;46(S1):42–7.
40. Oliveira LC, Porta G, Marin MLC, Bittencourt PL, Kalil J, Goldberg AC. Autoimmune hepatitis, HLA and extended haplotypes. Autoimmun Rev. 2011;10(4):189–93.
41. Podhorzer A, Paladino N, Cuarterolo ML, Fainboim HA, Paz S, Theiler G, et al. The early onset of type 1 autoimmune hepatitis has a strong genetic influence: role of HLA and KIR genes. Genes Immun. 2016;17(3):187–92.

42. Alvarez F, Ciocca M, Cañero-Velasco C, Ramonet M, Davila MTG, Cuarterolo M, et al. Short-term cyclosporine induces a remission of autoimmune hepatitis in children. J Hepatol. 1999;30(2):222–7.
43. Cuarterolo M, Ciocca M, Velasco CC, Ramonet M, González T, López S, et al. Follow-up of children with autoimmune hepatitis treated with cyclosporine. J Pediatr Gastroenterol Nutr. 2006;43(5):635–9.
44. D'Agostino D, Costaguta A, Alvarez F. Successful treatment of refractory autoimmune hepatitis with rituximab. Pediatrics. 2013;132(2):e526–30.
45. Terziroli Beretta-Piccoli B, Mieli-Vergani G, Vergani D. Autoimmune hepatitis: standard treatment and systematic review of alternative treatments. World J Gastroenterol. 2017;23(33):6030–48.
46. Website [Internet]. [cited 2018 Mar 7]. Organización de las Naciones Unidas para la Alimentacióny la Agricultura (FAO). Panorama de la SeguridadAlimentaria y Nutricional en América Latina y el Caribe 2013. http://www.fao.org/docrep/019/i3520s/i3520s.pdf. Accessed 5 May 2016.
47. WHO. Obesity and overweight. 2018 Feb 9 [cited 2018 Mar 7]. http://www.who.int/mediacentre/factsheets/fs311/en/.
48. Schwimmer JB, Deutsch R, Kahen T, Lavine JE, Stanley C, Behling C. Prevalence of fatty liver in children and adolescents. Pediatrics. 2006;118(4):1388–93.
49. Pontiles de Sánchez M, Morón de Salim A, Rodríguez de Perdomo H, Perdomo Oramas G. Prevalence of no alcohol fatty liver disease (NAFLD) in a population of obese children in Valencia, Venezuela. Arch Latinoam Nutr. 2014;64(2):73–82.
50. Quirós-Tejeira RE, Rivera CA, Ziba TT, Mehta N, Smith CW, Butte NF. Risk for nonalcoholic fatty liver disease in Hispanic youth with BMI > or =95th percentile. J Pediatr Gastroenterol Nutr. 2007;44(2):228–36.
51. Chiu C-Y, Chen P-H, Chan C-F, Chang M-H, Wu T-C. Biliary atresia in preterm infants in Taiwan: a nationwide survey. J Pediatr. 2013;163(1):100–3.e1.
52. Jimenez-Rivera C, Jolin-Dahel KS, Fortinsky KJ, Gozdyra P, Benchimol EI. International incidence and outcomes of biliary atresia. J Pediatr Gastroenterol Nutr. 2013;56(4):344–54.
53. Santos JL, Choquette M, Bezerra JA. Cholestatic liver disease in children. Curr Gastroenterol Rep. 2010;12(1):30–9.
54. De Bruyne R, Van Biervliet S, Vande Velde S, Van Winckel M. Clinical practice: neonatal cholestasis. Eur J Pediatr. 2011;170(3):279–84.
55. Sokol RJ, Mack C, Narkewicz MR, Karrer FM. Pathogenesis and outcome of biliary atresia: current concepts. J Pediatr Gastroenterol Nutr. 2003;37(1):4–21.
56. de Carvalho E, dos Santos JL, da Silveira TR, Kieling CO, Silva LR, et al. Biliary atresia: the Brazilian experience. J Pediatr. 2010;86(6):473–9.
57. Bezerra JA. Biliary atresia in Brazil: where we are and where we are going. J Pediatr [Internet]. 2010;86(6). https://doi.org/10.2223/jped.2057.
58. Ramonet M. Early detection of neonatal cholestasis by stool color card screening. Arch Argent Pediatr. 2013;111(2):135–9.
59. Drug-, herb- and dietary supplement-induced liver injury. Arch Argent Pediatr [Internet]. 2017;115(6). https://doi.org/10.5546/aap.2017.eng.e397.
60. Andrade RJ, Lucena MI, Fernández MC, Pelaez G, Pachkoria K, García-Ruiz E, et al. Drug-induced liver injury: an analysis of 461 incidences submitted to the Spanish registry over a 10-year period. Gastroenterology. 2005;129(2):512–21.
61. Lucena MI, Cohen H, Hernández N, Bessone F, Dacoll C, Stephens C, et al. Hepatotoxicidad, un problema global con especificidades locales: hacia la creación de una Red Hispano Latinoamericana de Hepatotoxicidad. Gastroenterol Hepatol. 2011;34(5):361–8.
62. Bessone F, Hernandez N, Dávalos M, Paraná R, Schinoni MI, Lizarzabal M, et al. Building a Spanish-Latin American network on drug induced liver injury: much to get from a joint collaborative initiative. Ann Hepatol. 2012;11(4):544–9.
63. Bessone F, Hernandez N, Lucena MI, Andrade RJ, Latin Dili Network Latindilin And Spanish Dili Registry. The Latin American DILI registry experience: a successful ongoing collaborative strategic initiative. Int J Mol Sci. 2016;17(3):313.
64. Hernández N, Bessone F, Sánchez A, di Pace M, Brahm J, Zapata R, et al. Profile of idiosyncratic drug induced liver injury in Latin America: an analysis of published reports. Ann Hepatol. 2014;13(2):231–9.
65. Hepp J, Innocenti FA. Liver transplantation in Latin America: current status. Transplant Proc. 2004;36(6):1667–8.
66. Santiago Delpin EA, García VD, Casadei D, Pereyra LT. The evolution of transplantation societies in Latin America. Transplant Proc. 1999;31(7):2933–4.
67. Mizraji R, Alvarez I, Palacios RI, Fajardo C, Berrios C, Morales F, et al. Organ donation in Latin America. Transplant Proc. 2007;39(2):333–5.
68. Website [Internet]. [cited 2017 Nov 21]. World Health Organization (WHO) World. www.who.org. Accessed 1 Oct 2014.
69. Website [Internet]. [cited 2017 Nov 21]. International registry in organ donation and Transplantation (IroDat). www.irodat.org. Accessed 1 Oct 2014.
70. Website [Internet]. [cited 2017 Nov 21]. AssociacIo Brasileira de Transplantes de Orgaos (ABTO). www.abto.org.br. Accessed 10 Dec 2014.
71. Englesbe MJ, Kelly B, Goss J, Fecteau A, Mitchell J, Andrews W, et al. Reducing pediatric liver transplant complications: a potential roadmap for transplant quality improvement initiatives within North America. Am J Transplant. 2012;12(9):2301–6.
72. Neto JS, Pugliese R, Fonseca EA, Vincenzi R, Pugliese V, Candido H, et al. Four hundred thirty consecutive pediatric living donor liver transplants: variables associated with posttransplant patient and graft survival. Liver Transpl. 2012;18(5):577–84.
73. Website [Internet]. [cited 2017 Nov 21]. Ardiles V, Ciardullo MA, D'Agostino D, et al. Langenbecks. Arch Surg. 2013;398:79. https://doi.org/10.1007/s00423-012-1020-y.
74. Acuña C, Zuleta R, Dalmazzo R, Valverde C, Uribe M, Alba A, et al. Pediatric liver transplantation experience and outcome in Chile. Transplant Proc. 2013;45(10):3724–5.

Pediatric Liver Disease in the African Continent

Mortada H. F. El-Shabrawi and Naglaa M. Kamal

Key Points
- There is a high burden of PLD in Africa as it includes the worldwide spectrum and extends to some peculiar PLD for Africa.
- Infectious causes are very prevalent including a wide spectrum of viral, bacterial, protozoal, and helminthic causes.
- NAFLD is having a very high magnitude especially in North Africa approaching the worldwide magnitude.
- Joined local governmental and international organization efforts are needed to succeed in the battle against PLD.

Research Needed in the Field
- Diagnosis and management of pediatric NAFLD
- Long-term effects of DAAs
- Vaccinations against African endemic infections

40.1 Introduction

Pediatric liver diseases (PLD) are diverse with a worldwide distribution. Discussion of liver diseases in children was detailed in this book (Chap. 1 through Chap. 22).

In the African continent, PLD follow the worldwide spectrum, but it has its special peculiarities with a lot of confiders affecting its pattern. The main objective of this chapter is to highlight these peculiarities and uncover the hidden iceberg of the problem.

Indeed, liver disease in the pediatric age group in Africa is a major problem with infectious causes being the most common as reported by Mackenjee and Coovadia in 1984 [1]. Hepatitis B infection (HBV) and *Schistosoma mansoni* (*S. mansoni*) infestation were the most important causative agents [1]. Over the past 25 years, there have been a lot of changes in the epidemiological pattern of PLD in Africa as a result of an appreciable effort in the prevention and control programs against infectious aetiological factors.

Although infectious causes are still on the top of the iceberg of African PLD, their incidence and prevalence decreased, and their pattern changed from HBV and *S. mansoni* to include other causes like hepatitis C virus (HCV) and human immunodeficiency virus (HIV) in different combinations of coinfections. Nonalcoholic fatty liver disease (NAFLD) which is now considered the most common PLD worldwide has been reported to have an almost similar high prevalence in Africa.

The submerged worldwide PLD, metabolic, inherited, and autoimmune causes, became as important cause of liver disease in children in Africa as in developed countries. It is crucial to know the true epidemiological pattern of PLD in Africa in order to plan preventive and therapeutic policies; however, it is frustrating that physicians are, to date, crippled by the lack of resources essential for definitive disease diagnosis and commencement of affordable treatment as well as the paucity of proper training programs, which make the diagnosis and management of these diseases a real problem.

To all who taught us the emerging science of Pediatric Hepatology, to all colleagues who made this science advance, and to all lovely infants and children who are the beneficiaries of this advance (*Mortada HF El-Shabrawi and Naglaa M Kamal*).

To the soul of my beloved father who died of cirrhosis secondary to chronic hepatitis C, 15 years ago before the advent of DAAs for HCV treatment. May Allah rest him in his mercy and dwell him in his spaciousness (*Naglaa M Kamal*).

M. H. F. El-Shabrawi · N. M. Kamal (✉)
Faculty of Medicine, Cairo University, Cairo, Egypt
e-mail: melshabrawi@kasralainy.edu.eg;
Nagla.kamal@kasralainy.edu.eg

Every effort should be done to improve the lives of these children. The success achieved in prevention and control campaigns of infectious causes of liver disease in African children warrants continuous honest effort to sustain achievements and decrease infectious causes even more while, at the same time, working on local national and continent-wide long-term plans for better diagnosis and management of all causes of liver diseases.

40.2 Pediatric Liver Disease in Africa

40.2.1 Africa Peculiarities

Indeed, the publications from Africa are much less than from the developed countries with most of the data for North Africa coming from Egyptian and Tunisian researches, while most of the data from sub-Saharan Africa (SSA) are coming from South Africa and Nigeria. In view of the available African literature and our personal expertise, African continent PLD peculiarities will be discussed in this chapter.

40.2.1.1 Cholestatic Disorders of Infancy

Neonatal cholestatic disorders may be as high as 1 in 2500 live births with revolutionary change in the incidence of their aetiologies and management as a result of recent advances in hepatology research. In developed countries, idiopathic neonatal giant cell hepatitis (INGCH) is no more on the top of the list as many patients who were diagnosed with INGCH proved to have identifiable diseases like alpha-one-antitrypsin (α_1–AT) deficiency, newly discovered inborn errors of metabolism, and progressive familial intrahepatic cholestasis (PFIC) [2]. Biliary atresia (BA) still retains its position with 1 in 8,000 to 1 in 21,000 live birth incidence [3]. BA and other disorders of the extrahepatic biliary tree and genetic and familial cholestasis are discussed in details in Chaps. 5 and 11, respectively.

In spite of these advances in developed countries, in Africa the situation remains significantly different due to lack of resources and difficulties in diagnosis. Consequently, still many patients have no identifiable aetiology, and INGCH remains the top diagnosis. There is no solid data about the exact percentages of frequencies of the common aetiological causes of cholestasis from Africa with most data coming from single centers without any wide continent or even individual country multicenter studies.

In a report released from South Africa 27 years ago, intrahepatic cholestatic disorders accounted for 68% of causes of cholestasis with no identifiable aetiology in the majority of them which were labeled as INGCH with relatively good prognosis. Syphilis, urinary tract infection, and septicemia made up 30% of intrahepatic causes with favorable prognosis. HIV infection was hardly known at the time of the report.

Metabolic disorders accounted for 12% only. The remaining 32% were due to extrahepatic causes and were almost entirely due to BA with late referral causing poor outcome of Kasai portoenterostomy [4]. Ten years ago, the same discouraging results of Kasai were reported by a Nigerian report attributed to late presentation, delayed referral, and diagnostic difficulties [5].

Similarly, a large percentage of cholestasis of no identifiable aetiology (12.7%) were reported from North Africa by a Tunisian work group from a single center 10 years ago. They reported an 8.5 cases/year incidence of cholestasis. Extrahepatic causes constituted 21.3% of cases with 13.8% of BA which seemed lower than the worldwide incidence. They explained that as false low incidence due to the large number of cholestatic patients who lost follow-up before extensive work-up. Intrahepatic causes attributed to 65.9% of causes; none had α_1–AT deficiency [6]. After an average follow-up of 6 years, 28% of their patients had portal hypertension (PH), 14.8% had hepatocellular insufficiency, 20% lost follow-up, and 14.8% died. They attributed this poor prognosis in their cohort to delayed diagnosis and difficulties in medical and surgical management [6].

An Egyptian report highlighted the association of cytomegalovirus (CMV) and reovirus type 3 infections in neonates and the development of cholestasis [7].

Costly and technically advanced investigations are needed to confirm diagnosis in genetic and metabolic diseases. This causes diagnostic delay in Africa where most of these diagnostic tests are sent to specialized laboratories with a consequent delay that reflects on outcome. The situation is worse when financial constrains interfere with this process altogether. African investigators usually try to depend on constellation of clinical findings along with the feasible investigations to build their diagnoses and start patients' treatment accordingly. PFIC is an example, and although liver histology is important, it is not specific for diagnosis, and genotyping is conclusive [8]. Few reports were published on PFIC genetics from Africa [8].

Choledochal cyst was reported as a relatively rare cause of cholestasis in Africa by a Nigerian group who reported three patients over an 18-year period [9]. Diseases like hereditary hemochromatosis (HHC) are rare in natives of Africans [10].

40.2.1.2 Infectious Liver Diseases

Infectious agents affecting the liver are diverse, including viral, bacterial, protozoal, helminthic, and others. Africa is endemic for many infectious pathogens which make the possibility of concomitant infections by more than one pathogen, a common finding with the resultant combined deleterious outcome on health and complexity in management. Frequently encountered associations are the coinfections of HIV, HCV, and HBV in different combinations or in combination with the highly endemic malaria or tuberculosis infections. Schistosomiasis and malaria is a common association in SSA. HCV is, and its coinfection with schistosomiasis was, a very important infectious example in Egypt.

I. **Viral Hepatitis (also refer to Chap. 7)**

Viral hepatitis is a global health problem with subsequent acute and/or chronic inflammation of the liver. It can be caused by both hepatotropic and nonhepatotropic viruses.

1. **Hepatotropic Viruses:**

Eight distinct hepatotropic viruses have been described so far: hepatitis A, B, C, D, E, G, TT, and SEN viruses [11]. Hepatitis A and E viruses are the main causes of viral hepatitis; they are enterally transmitted and do not lead to chronic liver disease (CLD) except HEV in the immunocompromised. Hepatitis B, C, and D viruses are parenterally transmitted and lead to chronic liver disease, cirrhosis, and hepatocellular carcinoma (HCC). Hepatitis D and E are rare in children ([12] Kelly developing]).

Chronic hepatitis B, C, and D affect 550 million people all over the world [13, 14]; among them 100 million are estimated to be infected with HBV or HCV in the African continent. In Africa, screening of viral hepatitis and access to medical care and treatment are not readily available with severely constrained financial resources and insufficiency of well-trained health-care workers [15]. Indeed, this silent killer is overshadowed by other naturally endemic more stigmatizing infectious diseases in Africa like HIV, TB, and malaria. Actually, chronic viral hepatitis poses a greater threat to mortality than TB or malaria worldwide with 1.4 million human mortality in 2010 [16].

A report from the European Association for the Study of the Liver (EASL) in 2014 warned about the expected jumping increase in the magnitude of CLD in Africa in the near future owing to the high burden of chronic viral hepatitis B and C [15]. It highlighted the urgent need for global awareness, vision, and strategies for mass continent eradication of this dramatic neglected burden of chronic viral hepatitis in Africa. Organized governmental and institutional effort for the screening of infected people followed by initiation of treatment especially after the advent of highly effective oral antiviral agents is warranted [15].

It is of notice to admit that the burden of disease generated by chronic viral hepatitis has been completely ignored by the international health agenda over the past few decades. Likewise, funding for chronic viral hepatitis has been by no means significant in Africa. It is estimated that 41% of the world's population live in countries where no public funding is available for viral hepatitis B/C treatment [15]. Only until recently has the World Health Organization (WHO) expressed any strong interest to fight the burden of chronic viral hepatitis with the first resolution on viral hepatitis adopted in 2010 [17] and a second one voted in 2014.

The WHO guidelines for the screening, care, and treatment of HBV and HCV have been developed very recently [18]. These international guidelines are of critical importance for governments helping them in shaping their local health policies, supporting access for viral hepatitis screening and treatment, and integrating that in their local healthcare systems. A good solution for the deficient global funding for viral hepatitis is streamlining screening, care, and treatment of viral hepatitis within the concurrent HIV, TB, or malaria programs in Africa [15]. Incidentally, public health policy makers are now becoming more willing to develop and reinforce horizontal approaches of health programs. Thus, the feasibility and evaluation of such approaches are vital in providing care to persons infected with viral hepatitis [15].

However, an essential prerequisite for all of the aforementioned effort to pay off is the efficient targeting of the African population to indulge them in the battle against chronic viral hepatitis. Mass education and awareness campaigns about chronic viral hepatitis problem, factors mitigating its progression, and required preventive measures should be carried on.

- *Hepatitis A virus (HAV):*

– *Epidemiological aspects of HAV in Africa:*

Acute viral hepatitis A is prevalent worldwide especially in the developing world. HAV is considered an environmental virus as its transmission is associated and propagated by lack of access to clean drinking water, poor sanitation, and bad hygienic conditions [11, 19, 20]. Information on HAV infection in Africa is limited. According to a WHO report in 2009 [20], most of the African continent remains a high-endemicity region, with the exception of some privileged populations in some areas, such as the white people in South Africa. In the 1990s, only 30–40% of white adults in South Africa were anti-HAV positive (seropositive) by the age of 20 years, rising to 60% by the age of 40–49 years, while almost all black children were seropositive by the age of 12 years and almost 100% of black adults were seropositive before the age of 20 years [21, 22].

SSA has some of the highest anti-HAV prevalence rates in the world, and nearly all older children and adults are naturally immunized. North Africa has an intermediate level of HAV endemicity [11].

Early studies in the 1980s showed nearly universal HAV immunity also in many African countries; 100% of children were seropositive by the age of 10 years in Algeria, and nearly 100% of adults in Morocco were seropositive [20]. In Tunisia, a large study performed in three different regions in

2007 showed 84.0%, 90.5%, and 91.7% HAV seroprevalence in three groups with a mean age of 6.94, 12.84, and 20.71 years, respectively [23].

Over the past 10 years, a significant pan-continent improvement in sanitation and access to clean water was achieved. Being a part of the United Nations post-2015 Sustainable Development Goals [24], better achievement in water, hygiene, and sanitation is expected by African countries.

It is promising that in recent studies from some African countries, a general decline in HAV infection was suggested by authors [25, 26] with urban areas transitioning to low HAV infection rates [20], while high rates are still prevalent in rural areas [19, 27, 28]. It appears that, even within the same country, low and intermediate areas may be mixed with high endemicity areas, with a series of local epidemics [12].

An Egyptian study reported a 27.3% prevalence of HAV infection in children from high socioeconomic classes compared to 81% in those of lower social class [11]. Almost the same findings were detected in a Tunisian study with 21.3% and 87.7% seroprevalence in children living in urban and rural areas, respectively [29].

With these changes in epidemiology, there will be a growing decrease in natural immunity against HAV [30] increasing the number of children and adolescents who are susceptible to HAV infection. It is of notice that the current compulsory infant/childhood vaccination strategy in most African countries doesn't include HAV vaccination under the presumption that natural immunity is gained early in life [20, 25], while infection is asymptomatic. This presents new challenges for HAV control [20, 25] with the possibility of clinical disease and potential epidemics which in turn put high burden on the individuals and the fragile health-care systems.

Indeed, the possible shift in HAV epidemiology with most HAV infections occurring late in childhood and adulthood where symptoms are severe is not well understood in Africa, but it is wise that decision-makers follow closely the epidemiological trends of HAV and review vaccination strategies. The economic and individual burden of HAV infection can be mitigated by vaccination programs that correspond to the epidemiological pattern of the disease [31].

- **Hepatitis B virus (HBV):**

– *Epidemiological aspects of HBV in Africa:*

HBV infection is a serious problem worldwide [32–34]. Approximately 2 billion infected people are alive, of whom 350 million have chronic infection and about 1 million die per year [35–37]. HBV infection is endemic worldwide, but its prevalence differs greatly among regions [38, 39]. Africa is a high prevalence region [40] especially SSA [41] which is considered a hyperendemic region with more than 8% of the population infected with HBV [42–45] which is considered the cause of 44% of cirrhotic liver disease and 47% of HCC patients in SSA [46].

Although most SSA countries are classified as hyperendemic for HBV, seroprevalence varies among different countries with Nigeria being the highest in SSA and indeed the world [13]. The pooled seroprevalence of HBV in Nigeria was 14%. It was 11.5% for children and 14.1% for pregnant women. HBV seroprevalence is 10% in South Africa [47], 5–10% in Ghana, 8–20% in Cameroon, 12% in Benin, and 12% in Chad [48–50].

HBV seroprevalence is lower in North Africa which is considered a region of intermediate endemicity. Egypt is an example with 2–8% seroprevalence, and nearly 2–3 million Egyptians are HBV chronic carriers [51–53].

The magnitude of the problem of HBV infection is much more in the pediatric population as age is the key factor determining the risk of chronic infection which increases with younger age. Chronicity is common following acute infection in neonates (90%) and young children under the age of 5 years (20–60%) but occurs rarely (<5%) when infection is acquired in adulthood [54]. Worldwide, the majority of persons with chronic hepatitis B (CHB) infection were infected at birth or in early childhood [54]. CHB in childhood has a 25% lifetime risk of premature death from complications of CLD including cirrhosis and HCC [55]. In Africa, the incidence of HCC is high in infected children and young male adults [54].

– *Methods of transmission among African population*

In hyperendemic populations, primary HBV infections occur mainly during infancy and early childhood with most CHB occurring before the age of 2 years [56]. Perinatal transmission from HBV surface antigen (HBsAg) carrier mothers to their infants is a very important route of transmission leading to chronicity in hyperendemic areas and worldwide [57]. Around 90% of the infants of seropositive mothers carrying HBV e antigen (HBeAg) became HBsAg carriers [58], irrespective of high or low HBsAg and/or the HBeAg carrier rate in the population. Horizontal transmission from highly infectious family members such as elder siblings is common, particularly in Africa [12]. In parts of Africa such as rural Senegal, horizontal infection occurs very early; 25% of children are infected by the age of 2 years, which reaches 80% by the age of 15 years [59]. Parenteral transmission from improperly sterilized syringes or other contaminated instruments and improper screening for blood/blood products remains a problem in the developing world [60, 61].

– *Management issues in Africa:*

In-depth management to halt the problem of chronic viral hepatitis in Africa requires working on two levels concomitantly. The first level is prevention of new infections by executing different modes of acquiring infections, while the second level is screening of currently infected persons and implementing national mass treatment [15].

HBV immunization has been available since 1982 and has been shown to be highly effective in reducing the prevalence of HBsAg in children worldwide [62] and accordingly the burden of CLD and HCC in those born after 1984 [63, 64]. With the support of the WHO, most African countries included HBV vaccine in their expanded programs of immunization to all children. However, the achieved coverage is only 79% for Africa as a whole [65].

Aiming to decrease HBV mother-to-child transmission (perinatal and horizontal) with subsequent high (90%) child chronic carrier rate:

1. The WHO-AFRO recommended the first dose of HBV vaccination to be given as soon as possible within the first 24 h after birth [18]; however, its implementation is still poor [66] with only 23% coverage. All remaining countries should implement it as it has 90–95% effectiveness [18].
2. Some African countries, Cameroon, Mauritania, and Rwanda, have established national guidelines on HBV mother-to-child transmission; however, all African countries should have their national guidelines [15].
3. Pregnant women in Africa should be systematically screened for HBsAg, but currently screening is not yet routine [15].

Infants born to HBsAg-positive mothers should be bathed carefully soon after birth to remove potentially infected maternal blood or secretions, and a 0.5 mL of both HBV vaccine and immunoglobulin (Ig) should be given intramuscularly simultaneously at two distant injection sites using two different syringes [2]. HBV-Ig should be given as soon as possible after birth and preferably within 12 h. Its efficacy after 12 h and before 48 h is presumed but unproved [2]. The second and third doses of vaccine are given at 1–2 and 6 months, while for preterm infants whose birth weighs less than 2 kg, the initial vaccine dose is not counted and they follow their usual vaccination schedules with the required three doses of HBV vaccine given at their scheduled times [2]. This regimen protected 95% of infants born to HBsAg-/HBeAg-positive mothers from developing the chronic carrier state; the efficacy is lower for maternal carriers with very high viral serum HBV DNA load (>108 IU/mL) [67–69].

Nosocomial transmission is another major route of viral hepatitis transmission in Africa. The WHO estimates that 24% of blood donations in low-income countries are not systematically screened for HBV/HCV. This highlights the importance of emphasizing the application of infection control policies and practices in all health-care facilities to ensure prevention of transmission of blood-borne infections [70].

Halting transmission of HBV requires effective treatment of chronically infected subjects, but this is compromised by the limited liver-oriented care in most of Africa, including medical staff, laboratory prognostic indicators, and the potent nucleos(t)ide analogs (tenofovir, entecavir) [15]. The US Food and Drug Administration (FDA) approved tenofovir in children above 12 years old, while entecavir was approved for those 2–12 years old [15]. Unfortunately, drug cost is one of the main barriers for access to treatment in Africa. The price of generic tenofovir has been negotiated to as low as €26 per year of treatment, which has been made possible mainly from funds. It is essential to establish global funding mechanisms [71].

- **Hepatitis C virus:**

    – *Epidemiological aspects of HCV in Africa:*

    It is estimated that 185 million people worldwide are infected with HCV [2]. HCV is steadily becoming the second cause for HCC [72]. In Africa, HCV infection is highly endemic [73]. The highest prevalence of HCV is in SSA (5.3%) [74]. Egypt has one of the highest HCV seroprevalences worldwide with a recent estimation of 14.7% in subjects aged 15–59 years [75] which rises up to 50% in some rural areas [76]. In 2011, 5.8% HCV seroprevalence was detected among healthy Egyptian children with a proportionate increase with age: from 0% in children aged 6–7 years to 16% in those of 15 years old. HCV viremia was detected in 75% of the studied children. This reflects the extremely high HCV seroprevalence among Egyptian children [77]. East and Central African countries, such as Burundi, Cameroon, and Gabon, are also highly endemic for HCV with a prevalence reaching 11%, 13%, and 5%, respectively [78]. Estimates can reach up to 50% in HIV-infected persons, intravenous (IV) drug abusers, those with multiple transfusions, male homosexuals, and others [79, 80].

    – *Epidemiology of HCV genotypes in Africa:*

    The distribution of HCV genotypes in Africa varies by subregions with a considerable HCV subtype diversity [15]. Genotypes 1, 2, and 3 are predominant in West Africa [81], genotype 4 in Central Africa, and genotype 5 in Southern Africa [82]. In Egypt, the principal genotype is 4 [83] with approximately 90% of Egyptian isolates belonging to a single subtype, 4a [84, 85].

    – *Methods of transmission among African population*

    Prior to the 1990s, the principal routes of HCV infection worldwide were blood transfusion, unsafe injection procedures, and IV drug abuse. In developing countries, insufficient screenings of blood, blood products, and parenteral exposure continue to be the major causes of HCV transmission [86]. Intrafamilial transmission may occur, but specific immune responses may be protective against household infection in some children [87].

Barakat and El-Bashir found that the main risk factors for HCV infection among Egyptian children were blood transfusion, IV injections, surgical intervention, dental treatment, and circumcision for boys by informal health-care providers [77].

The WHO estimates that two million new HCV infections worldwide result from unsafe injections each year [88]. Transmission of HCV through unsafe use and reuse of injection equipment in hospitals [89] or medical or dental procedures is still a threat in many African countries [90]. These routes of transmission pose serious concern, as further transmission can occur within households [87, 91].

The prime illustration of such transmission is the national campaign to eradicate schistosomiasis in Egypt, practiced in the 1960s until the early 1980s, using reusable syringes for parenteral antischistosomal therapy (PAT), whereby antimony potassium tartrate had had a major role in the HCV epidemic in Egypt [92]. This represents the world's largest iatrogenic transmission of blood-borne pathogens [92].

Furthermore, HCV is less prevalent in countries neighboring Egypt despite sharing the same sociomedical conditions and similar strains. On the other hand, other countries with high endemicity for schistosomiasis similar to Egypt don't have the same high magnitude of HCV problem which is probably because schistosomiasis control in these countries was less population and geographically intensive compared with the mass PAT campaign carried out in Egypt.

Similar scenarios were repeated from the Cameroon [93] and Gabon [94] involving campaigns against malaria.

Silent and hidden epidemics of HCV have been recently identified among IV drug user from several SSA capitals, such as Dakar or Dar es Salaam [95, 96].

– *Management issues in Africa:*

In order to fight the problem of CHC in Africa, HCV screening must be coupled with highly effective treatment [97]. The revolutional HCV treatment using the direct-acting antiviral (DAA) agents provides high sustained virological response (SVR) rates with short and well-tolerated, but highly expensive, regimens [98, 99]. African countries are resource-limited which make accessibility to these DAAs almost impossible.

To date, the only African country which succeeded in negotiating reduced prices of Sofosbuvir is Egypt, while other resource-limited countries have initiated discussions, but no agreements have been signed so far [15]. Indeed Egypt has a long-term commitment to HCV treatment, as evidence by their previous involvement with Peg-interferon/ribavirin [100].

A real success story in HCV management has been achieved by Egypt through the collaborative efforts of the government and medical community in mass screening of HCV carried free of charge followed by treatment. To date, more than 1,000,000 HCV-infected patients have been treated in Egypt, and the project is still ongoing.

In August 2017, the first study on the safety and effectiveness of DAAs in HCV management in adolescents using ledipasvir-sofosbuvir was carried out by Balistreri and his group on HCV genotype 1 infection and proved both safe and effective [101]. A breakthrough pilot study has been just released in November 2017 from Egypt by El-Shabrawi and his group on HCV genotype 4 management in adolescents with the less costly shortened 8-week course for those who achieved very rapid SVR using the far less costly combination of sofosbuvir/daclatasvir therapy [102].

A number of innovative diagnostic tools have been recently developed that could significantly improve screening and liver assessment at a low cost. Point-of-care (POC) tests for HBsAg and HCV antibodies are now available for facilitated use at the community level. Their performance has been validated in both Europe and SSA [15]. In Gambia, good sensitivity and specificity of two HBsAg POC tests have been observed [103].

Some companies are developing POC devices to quickly quantify viral load at a lower cost while adapted to the local African environment. HCV core antigen can be adapted for HCV screening in Africa [104].

– *Combined HCV and schistosomiasis infection:*

The association of HCV and schistosomiasis is very common especially in endemic areas with very high transmission of both infections. Egypt is the most important example in Africa.

This association poses unique clinical, virological, and histological patterns:

1. Clinically: HCV infection causes a more severe and irreversible form of liver disease than infection with *Schistosoma mansoni* alone [105]. Complications of cirrhosis were more common in patients with both diseases than in those with either disease alone with more patients in Child-Pugh class C, higher incidence of upper gastrointestinal hemorrhage and renal impairment, and higher mortality rate [85, 106, 107].
2. Virologically: dual infections of HCV and schistosomiasis display significant influence on host immune response due to cytotoxic shift pattern alteration as schistosomiasis induces Th2 cytokine profile with increased interleukins 4 and 10, and it downregulates the stimulatory effect of HCV on Th1 cytokines with the resultant diminished host capacity to clear the virus and HCV persistence with

HCV-RNA titers [108, 109]. Not only that but it was reported that those with combined infection have lower response rate to antiviral therapy with interferon than those with HCV infection alone [110].

3. Histologically: schistosomiasis-HCV coinfection possibly has a synergistic effect especially on hepatic fibrosis with more rapid progression which might be explained by the altered immunologic response and fibrogenesis signals [111].

– *HCV in patients with hemoglobinopathies:*

CHC is a major cause of liver morbidity and mortality among patients with hemoglobinopathies. Progression of liver fibrosis in those patients is strongly related to the severity of iron overload and the presence of CHC. Effective iron chelation therapy and HCV infection eradication may prevent liver complications. A recent Italian study highlighted the safety and efficacy of DAAs in patients with hemoglobinopathies, CHC, and advanced liver fibrosis. The 12-week SVR was 93.5% approaching that of cirrhotic patients without hemoglobinopathies. Significant reductions in serum ferritin at 12 weeks to levels similar to those with hemoglobinopathies without CHC, who adhered to chelation therapy and had no iron overload were also reported [112].

- **Hepatitis D virus (HDV):**

– *Epidemiological aspects and modes of HDV transmission in Africa:*

HDV is a satellite of HBV and requires it for proliferation. About one-fourth of chronic HBV carriers in Africa are suspected to be coinfected with HDV. It has been hypothesized by some studies that HDV might have originated in Africa [113, 114]. Nevertheless, the true origin and emergence of HDV remain unclear [115].

While HBV seroprevalence is very high across SSA and early childhood transmission is thought to be the most important route of infection [116], much less is known about HDV seroprevalence in the region [115].

In 2014, Andernach and his group detected highly variable prevalence of HDV, 0–27.3% in asymptomatic carriers and 1.3–50% in liver patients, in their participating cohorts from Burkina Faso, Nigeria, Chad, and the Central African Republic (CAR) [115]. HDV seemed to be much more common in CLD patients in the CAR than in similar cohorts in Nigeria, whereas less prevalence was detected in children from CAR compared to a similar cohort from Burkina Faso: 2.9% compared to 20.5%, respectively [115]. It was surprising that in spite of this high prevalence in children in Burkina Faso, the prevalence in their mothers was much lower [115]. Children were ten times higher in seroprevalence compared to their mothers, despite similar HBsAg prevalence, excluding vertical transmission as an important route of infection and favoring horizontal transmission [115].

Various HDV antibody rates among HBsAg-positive individuals were detected from other African countries: Cameroon (17.6%), Gabon (15.6–70.6%), Mauritania (14.7–33.1%), Mozambique (0%), Nigeria (0–12.5%), and Senegal (3.2%) [116–127].

– *Epidemiology of HDV genotypes in Africa:*

HDV genotypes showed also wide variability in Africa. Clades 1, 5, 6, and 7 were detected in Cameron [117], while clades 1, 7, and 8 were isolated in Gabon [118, 119], and clades 1 and 5 were reported from Mauritania [120–122]. Clade 1 dominated in all cohorts [113, 115, 128]. On the amino acid level, almost all clade 1 strains revealed a serine at position 202 in the HDAg, which is thought to be characteristic of African clade 1 strains [129].

– *HDV liver disease:*

Coinfection of HBV and HDV results in fulminant hepatitis more often than with HBV infection alone, and superinfection of HBV with HDV is associated with chronic HDV in up to 80% of carriers [116] and adds considerably to the high burden of CLD [116, 130].

– *Management issues:*

Concurrent infection of HBV and HDV complicates viral treatment, as regimens against HBV do not affect HDV replication. Furthermore, HDV infection suppresses HBV replication [22–24] and reduces HBV DNA in the serum to often undetectable levels, thus complicating the diagnosis and cogenotyping of HBV and HDV strains.

- **Hepatitis E virus (HEV):**

– *Epidemiological aspects in Africa:*

HEV is a major cause of epidemic waterborne hepatitis in tropical and subtropical countries in areas with poor sanitary conditions. The infection is endemic in the Middle East and Northern and Western Africa [131, 132]. It is considered the second most common cause of sporadic hepatitis in these areas [133].

In most countries, HEV seroprevalence tends to be low in early childhood with few studies released from Africa [134]. In Ghana, it was 4.4% in children aged 6–18 years [135]. In Sierra Leone, 8% seroprevalence in children aged 6–12 years was detected [136]. In Egypt, it was 36.2% in 0–4 years, 64.7% in 5–9 years, 75.6% in 10–14 years, and 75.5% in

15–19 years [137]. Egypt is a hyperendemic area for HEV with one of the highest HEV seroprevalences in young children, suggesting that most HEV in Egypt is acquired early in life [136]. HEV is a significant cause of acute sporadic hepatitis in young Egyptian children, causing 12% of acute hepatitis in children aged 1–13 years in one study [138] and 22% of acute hepatitis in children <10 years of age in another [139].

– *Modes of transmission:*

Most HEV infections in endemic areas are due to enteral transmission, usually due to fecal contamination of drinking water [134]. Parenteral transmission of HEV through blood transfusion [140] has also been documented, as has HEV transmission from mother to infant [141].

– *Epidemiology of HEV genotypes in Africa:*

Hepatitis E virus is a single-stranded RNA virus that is the sole member of the genus *Hepevirus* in the family *Hepeviridae*. It has four genotypes and one serotype. Genotype 1 is the major cause of both epidemic and sporadic hepatitis in HEV-endemic countries of Asia and Africa, whereas genotype 2 has been associated with HEV outbreaks in Mexico and Western Africa [134].

– *HEV liver disease:*

In endemic countries, HEV is a major cause of acute sporadic hepatitis as well as epidemic outbreaks of hepatitis related to fecal contamination of drinking water during heavy rainfall or floods [142, 143]. Most HEV infections in childhood are asymptomatic [134]. HEV infections peak in early adulthood [144] with more severe course with protracted coagulopathy and cholestasis and are associated with a higher mortality rate, especially in pregnant women [140, 145] and in those with underlying liver disease such as cirrhosis [146]. Chronic HEV has been detected in immunocompromised patients. Vertical transmission has also been reported. An Egyptian study reported 17% HEV viremia (HEV-RNA) in neonates of mothers infected in their third trimester [147]. It is not clear to what degree widespread asymptomatic HEV infections earlier in life leading to immunity contribute to the fact that large epidemics of enterally transmitted hepatitis have not been demonstrated in Egypt [136, 140].

2. Nonhepatotropic Viruses:

The nonhepatotropic viruses include measles virus, parvovirus B19, rubella virus, adenovirus, echovirus, coxsackie virus, varicella zoster virus, cytomegalovirus, EpsteinBarr virus, human herpesvirus 6, herpes simplex types 1 and 2, HIV, and viral hemorrhagic fevers' group of viruses [12].

• *Human immunodeficiency virus:*

– *Epidemiological aspects and modes of transmission to children in Africa:*

In 2012, 25 million people who constitute 71% of the global HIV infections were estimated to be from SSA. South Africa alone accounted for 31% of HIV deaths in SSA. South Africa remains the epicenter of the HIV pandemic, compounded by the fact that only 36% of HIV-positive patients in South Africa have access to antiretroviral (ARV) treatment [148]. Mozambique has the fifth highest prevalence of HIV in the world, with 11.5% of the population infected with HIV [149].

Not only that but also among the 3.2 million children (aged 0–14 years) with HIV infection worldwide, almost 90% are from SSA [150]. The great majority of cases of acquired immune deficiency syndrome (AIDS) in children are the result of vertical transmission from an infected mother. Mothers who are HIV positive have a one in four risk of infecting their babies. Other infections (e.g., HBV and HCV) may be transmitted to the newborn more efficiently when the mother is coinfected with HIV [151].

– *Epidemiology of HIV types in Africa:*

HIV-1 in humans resulted from at least four cross-species transmissions of simian immunodeficiency viruses (SIVs) from chimpanzees and gorillas in West Central Africa, while HIV-2 viruses resulted from at least eight independent transmissions of SIVs infecting sooty mangabeys in West Africa only, where one of these transmissions (HIV-1 group M) is responsible for the global epidemic [152].

– *HIV liver disease:*

As described above, 90% of HIV-infected children worldwide are from SSA which adds to the burden of CLD in children in Africa. HIV infection can cause acute or chronic hepatitis, nonimmune hydrops with hepatitis, cholestatic hepatitis [153], hepatosplenomegaly, and conjugated hyperbilirubinemia [151, 154].

Liver dysfunction is common in children with HIV infection due to:

1. HIV itself [155].
2. HBV/HCV coinfection [155].
3. Associated opportunistic infections such as *Mycobacterium avium-intracellulare*, CMV or lymphomas, and Kaposi sarcoma, which may develop in HIV patients [155].
4. Recurrent/chronic infection of the biliary tree with cryptosporidiosis or other organisms with a clinical picture resembling sclerosing cholangitis [156].

5. Myocarditis/congestive cardiac failure can occur in HIV-infected patients and lead to abnormal liver function tests and fibrosis of the central vein [157].
6. Drug-induced liver disease due to antiretroviral therapy [155].

– *Management issues:*

Perinatal transfer of HIV may be reduced to 8% by administering oral zidovudine antenatally or intravenously during labor to the mother and oral zidovudine to the baby until 6 weeks old [157]. The long-term medical outlook for children with HIV has improved considerably in countries that can afford the cost of triple treatment with nucleoside analogs, non-nucleoside analogs, and protease inhibitors [158]. Another advance in antiviral treatments is the nucleoside reverse transcriptase inhibitor tenofovir which is capable of producing synergistic effects against HIV when combined with other antiretroviral agents [159].

– *HBV and HIV coinfections:*

Globally, an estimated 5–10% of people infected with HIV are coinfected with HBV as they share common risk factors [160].

In SSA, an estimated three million CHB patients are dually HIV infected [161]. HIV coinfection increases the risk of CHB and accelerates HBV-related liver disease progression [162]. However, there are limited data on HIV-HBV epidemiology in SSA, particularly among children. Most SSA countries incorporated HBV vaccine into childhood immunization programs, but some reports suggest that CHB remains relatively common among HIV-infected children [163].

In urban Zambia, among those screened for HBV, approximately 10.5% of pediatric HIV-infected patients had CHB, with slightly lower prevalence among those born since HBV immunization began. HIV-HBV prevalence of 1.2–12.1% has been reported from other SSA countries [164–174]. Other studies reported HIV-HBV prevalence of 0 to >28.4% in SSA [165, 175–210].

In children coinfected with HIV and HBV, it is conceivable that impaired cytotoxic, HBV-specific, T-cell function may result in a lesser degree of hepatocyte damage despite ongoing HBV replication. Whether HIV infection-related decline in immune competence is associated with reduced liver injury is possible but uncertain. There is an increased risk of HBV-related acute liver failure observed in adults coinfected with HIV.

Tenofovir and emtricitabine have efficacy against both HBV and HIV and would be the initial treatment of choice [211].

– *HCV and HIV coinfections:*

In SSA, the pooled HCV-HIV coinfection prevalence was 5.73%. The highest estimates were in Tanzania, Burkina Faso, Cameroon, and Kenya which are countries of moderate HIV prevalence, while countries with the highest HIV prevalence, South Africa, Botswana, Zimbabwe, Zambia, Mozambique, and Malawi, were all estimated to have low to moderate levels of HCV coinfection. These differences suggest that risk behaviors responsible for HCV transmission might be quite dissociated from those associated with HIV transmission in some regions, such as Central Africa. Furthermore, regional differences might be partly explained by risk behaviors that are specific to one area (e.g., scarification or specific medical practices) [212].

HCV viral load is higher in HCV-HIV-coinfected patients compared to those with HCV infection alone [213]. Children with HIV and HCV coinfection need to be treated early, while immune competence of the host is preserved. For HCV/HIV coinfection, combination therapy with pegylated interferon/ribavirin is recommended and safe, but the response is less good than in patients infected with HCV alone. Little is known of the way in which HIV affects the course of HCV in children [211].

– *Combined HIV and HEV infections:*

In two HIV cohorts in Ghana and Cameroon, acute or chronic HEV infections did not play a role in liver pathology. A better understanding of the epidemiology- and genotype-specific characteristics of HEV infections in HIV patients in SSA is needed [214].

- **Viral hemorrhagic fevers:**

Viral hemorrhagic fevers are caused by viruses which are endemic in Africa and are characterized by fever, circulatory collapse, and hemorrhage. There may be diffuse organ involvement with jaundice, hepatomegaly, and severe hepatocellular damage and necrosis. They include yellow fever, dengue fever, dengue hemorrhagic fever and dengue shock syndrome, Lassa fever, and Marburg and Ebola viruses (Table 40.1).

The pathophysiology of diseases caused by these viruses is diffuse capillary leakage, increased vascular permeability, thrombocytopenia, and abnormalities in hemostasis [242].

II. Bacterial Infectious Diseases of the Liver:

Many bacteria can affect the liver causing hepatitis, hepatomegaly, liver abscess, or fulminant hepatic failure. Table 40.2 summarizes the most important bacterial infections of the liver in Africa which include but not limited to *Salmonella typhi*, *Mycobacterium tuberculosis*, *Listeria monocytogenes*, *Leptospira interrogans serovar icterohaemorrhagiae*, and

Table 40.1 Viral hemorrhagic fevers

Viral hemorrhagic fever	Epidemiology	Aetiology		Mode of transmission	Incubation period	Diagnosis	Treatment	Remark
		Causative agent	Animal reservoir					
Yellow fever [211]	Endemic in West and Central Africa [211]	RNA *Flaviviridae* [211]	Mosquitoes [211]	Mosquito-borne [211]	3–6 days [211]	**Clinical picture:** [211] **Mild form:** usually in endemic areas, fever, proteinuria, leukopenia, occasionally jaundice **Severe form:** 3–4 days of fever, rigors, headache, followed by transient improvement for less than 24 h before the onset of cutaneous and gastrointestinal hemorrhage and renal failure **Others:** jaundice may become apparent during recovery. Death might occur in 5% of cases, usually 7–10 days after the onset of symptoms. Africans were found to be at a reduced risk of death from yellow fever [215–217]	Supportive [211]	Live attenuated vaccine is available and effective [211]

					Clinical picture:	
Dengue fever, Dengue hemorrhagic fever (DHF), Dengue shock syndrome (DSS)	#Endemic in most of African countries [218] #Children are most frequently infected [12, 211]	RNA *Flaviviridae* [12, 211]	Mosquitoes; *Aedes aegypti* [218]	Mosquito-borne [218]	4–8 days [12, 211]	**Clinical picture:** **Mild form:** usually in endemic areas, mild febrile illness [12, 211] **Severe form:** less prevalent in Africa due to innate genetic resistance [219, 220] and less prevalence of NAFLD **Dengue fever:** biphasic fever, myalgia, arthralgia, severe headache, retro-orbital pain, rash, leucopenia, lymphadenopathy, hepatomegaly in almost all patients (79–100%) [12, 211] **Others:** hepatitis with elevation in aminotransferase enzymes is common [221] which peaks by 2nd week, with gradual normalization by the 3rd–4th week of illness [12, 211] Clinically, patients can have hepatomegaly, with complaints of hepatic tenderness. Jaundice is less common (15–62%), except in those with DHF or DSS [222] Acute liver failure is uncommon [12, 211] **DHF:** high-grade fever, thrombocytopenia, **hemorrhagic phenomena, increased vascular leakage with** weak rapid pulse, **narrow pulse pressure < 20 mmHg, hypotension, cold, clammy skin and restlessness** [12, 211] **DSS may develop:** a protein-losing shock syndrome with **b**leeding complications. Myocarditis with a congested liver and ascites, pleural effusion, fulminant hepatitis with encephalopathy, and Reye syndrome have been reported [223] DHF is graded from I to IV, with DSS showing typical signs of circulatory failure [12] Hypoxia/ischemia resulting from the prolonged shock and metabolic acidosis may be responsible for the severity of hepatic dysfunction [12] The dengue virus could become a more serious contributor in acute liver disease than initially assumed, requiring fast diagnosis and appropriate management [12] **Investigations:** 1. Dengue virus IgM, IgG enzyme-linked immunosorbent assay 2. The liver histology demonstrates centrilobular necrosis, fatty change, Kupffer cell hyperplasia, acidophilic bodies, and monocyte infiltration of the portal tract [12, 211]	#Supportive #Hepatic involvement is self-limited, although a few patients may develop hepatic failure #Recovery is usual within 48 h, except for DHF or DSS #The case fatality rate of DHF and DSS is 5% and 10%, respectively, but can decline to 1% with appropriate treatment and can reach 100% with type 2 dengue virus [12, 211]	#Incidence increased dramatically worldwide due to *Aedes aegypti* spread [218] and in part due to NAFLD pandemic [224] which could explain the association between DHF and higher socioeconomic status [225] #No available vaccine [218]

(continued)

Table 40.1 (continued)

Viral hemorrhagic fever	Epidemiology	Aetiology			Incubation period	Diagnosis	Treatment	Remark
		Causative agent	Animal reservoir	Mode of transmission				
Lassa fever	Unlike most viral hemorrhagic fevers, which are recognized only when outbreaks occur, Lassa fever is endemic in Sierra Leone, Guinea, Liberia, and other West African countries, with an estimated tens of thousands of cases annually [226]	RNA *Arenaviridae* [211]	Rats [227]	1. Exposure to rats' excreta [227, 228] 2. Human-to-human transmission through direct contact with infected blood or bodily secretions [227]	7–17 days	**Clinical picture** [211]: **Mild form:** usually in endemic areas, mild febrile illness **Severe form:** persistent fever, pharyngitis with tonsillar exudate, lethargy, gastrointestinal symptoms, and maculopapular rash In the second week, encephalopathy, circulatory collapse, and diffuse hemorrhage into the skin and organs may develop **Investigations** [211]: isolation of the virus from the throat, urine, or blood OR: detection of specific Lassa antibodies in the second week of illness by immunofluorescence	1. Strict isolation 2. Intravenous ribavirin may be effective in reducing the mortality, but even with ribavirin treatment, there was a high rate of fatalities [227]	#Endemic in rats [211]
Rift valley fever	Large parts of sub-Saharan and North Africa [229, 230] An outbreak in Southern Mauritania in 2012 resulted in 200 human deaths [231]	RNA *Bunyaviridae* [232]	Mosquitoes [232]	Mosquito-borne [232, 233]	3–6 days [234]	**Clinical picture: Mild form:** flu-like illness [232] **Severe form:** occasionally progresses to acute hepatitis, hemorrhagic fever, encephalitis, or ocular disease with a significant death rate [235]	#Supportive [232] #Efforts to discover effective antiviral drugs are underway [232]	No available vaccine [232]

					Clinical picture:	#Supportive [236]	#Nucleic acid-based products, recombinant vaccines, and antibodies appear to be less suitable for the treatment [236]
Marburg and Ebola viruses	#Outbreaks occur in certain regions of equatorial Africa at irregular intervals #In 2014, the biggest outbreak occurred in West Africa: Guinea, Sierra Leone, Liberia, and Nigeria caused by a new variant of Zaire ebolavirus and affected more than 2600 people [236]	RNA *Filoviridae* [237]	Bats [238]	Direct contact with infected body fluid and likely enter the human body via breaks in the skin or through mucosal surfaces [237, 238]	2–21 days [237]	They are among the most virulent pathogens for humans and great apes causing severe hemorrhagic fever and death within a matter of days After an initial flu-like illness, massive hepatocellular necrosis and disseminated intravascular coagulation with multi-organ failure [237] with a high mortality rate of up to 90% [239–241]	#Licensed antiviral agents are currently not available [236] #Recently, BCX4430, a promising synthetic adenosine analog with high in vitro and in vivo activity against filoviruses and other RNA viruses, has been described. It inhibits viral RNA polymerase activity when administered as late as 48 h after infection [236]	

Table 40.2 Bacterial liver disease

Infectious disease	Epidemiology	Aetiology	Pathophysiology of liver injury	Diagnosis of liver involvement	Treatment
Typhoid (enteric fever)	A major health problem in Africa [12]	*Salmonella* species (food-borne) [12]	#Endotoxin → consumptive coagulopathy, complement depletion, arteritis → hepatocytes damage [12] #Direct invasion of the hepatocyte by the organism → liver insult [12] #Typhoid bacilli are filtered by the liver and Kupffer cells and excreted in the bile [243]	**Clinical picture:** **General:** acute systemic bacterial illness with fever, toxic manifestations, malaise, and anorexia [244] **Gastrointestinal (GI):** nausea, vomiting, diarrhea/constipation, abdominal pain, GI bleeding and hepato/splenomegaly. Acute typhoid cholecystitis is rare [12] **Liver involvement:** Hepatitis resembling that of viral hepatitis. Hepatic manifestations are more severe in relapses or infections by multidrug-resistant organism [12] 1. Hepatomegaly (23–90%) [12] 2. Jaundice (1–16%) which occurs at the peak of fever unlike in viral hepatitis where jaundice is usually followed by a decrease in fever [12] 3. Hepatic encephalopathy has been rarely reported [245] **Investigations:** Hepatic transaminases: elevated with alanine aminotransferase (ALT)/lactate dehydrogenase (LDH) ratio of < 4, while it is 4 in viral hepatitis [246] Liver biopsy: mild hepatitis, parenchymatous degeneration, peripheral infiltration by mononuclear cells, and central necrosis, with characteristic granulomatous collections of mononuclear cells called typhoid/Mallory nodules [12]	#Multidrug-resistant strains necessitate treatment with [12]: third-generation cephalosporins (IV ceftriaxone or cefotaxime 100 mg/kg/day, oral cefuroxime 10 mg/kg/day) or quinolones (ciprofloxacin or ofloxacin IV 10 mg/kg/day or oral 20 mg/kg/day). #Maintenance of adequate hydration and dietary intake is essential [12] #Treatment is continued for 5 days after fever settles [12] #Hospital admission is required for complications, for toxicity, and for hydration/nutrition [12] #Hepatomegaly and jaundice usually resolve within the first 7–10 days with appropriate therapy, whereas the transaminases resolve within 2–3 weeks [12]

Table 40.2 (continued)

Infectious disease	Epidemiology	Aetiology	Pathophysiology of liver injury	Diagnosis of liver involvement	Treatment
Tuberculosis (TB)	A major health problem in Africa [12]	*Mycobacterium tuberculosis* (airborne) [12]	Liver involvement is seen in miliary and congenital TB or as a result of the hepatotoxicity of antituberculous drugs [12]	**Liver involvement:** • lPrimary hepatobiliary TB is associated with fever, abdominal pain, and hepatomegaly [12] • Hepatomegaly is found in 60% of children with abdominal or disseminated TB [247] • Recurrent obstructive jaundice (30%) [248] • Liver calcification [248] • TB cholangitis [248] • Bile duct strictures and lymph nodes at the porta hepatis [248] • Liver abscess [248] **Investigations:** • Hepatic aminotransferases: elevation is usual [12] • Liver biopsy: caseating granulomas [12]	• Streptomycin may be needed along with ethambutol and ciprofloxacin, which are safe for the liver [12] • If the patient is compliant, treatment is usually successful [12]
Leptospirosis	Important endemic but neglected bacterial zoonosis in Africa with a prevalence of 2.3–19.8% among different African countries [249–257]	• *Leptospira interrogans serovar ictero-hemorrhagiae* [258] • A spirochete [258] • Transmission via skin abrasions or mucous membranes during swimming, veterinarians or farm workers on exposure to contaminated water by infected animal urine [258] #Person-to-person spread is rare [258]	• Damage of the endothelium of small blood vessels [259] • Seeding of the organism in the meninges, liver, or kidneys [259]	**Clinical features** **Incubation period:** 1–2 weeks [211] **Subclinical form:** majority of cases [211] **Mild form:** mild flu-like illness with fever and myalgia for 1 week, with severity relating to the number of infecting organisms and the immune status of the host [211] **Severe form:** less than 10% → Weil disease → severe systemic disease → fever, headache, myalgia, extensive vasculitic rash, renal failure, myocarditis, pneumonitis, and circulatory collapse [260] **Liver involvement:** Hepatitis, jaundice, and hepatomegaly Fulminant liver failure may occur [258] **Investigations:** • Transaminases : mild elevation [211] • Serum leptospire-specific antibodies: IgM or a rising titer of IgG [211] • PCR and culture [261] • Dark-ground microscopy: detection of leptospires in blood and urine during the bacteremic and organ involvement phases, respectively [211]	#Antibiotics: most patients recover without long-term sequelae [211]: 1. Penicillin G (200,000–250,000 U/kg/day IV every 4 h for 7 days given within 4–7 days of onset 2. Tetracycline or erythromycin is also effective ##In those with liver failure, support with the molecular adsorbent recirculating system can lead to a successful outcome [262]

(continued)

Table 40.2 (continued)

Infectious disease	Epidemiology	Aetiology	Pathophysiology of liver injury	Diagnosis of liver involvement	Treatment
Bartonellosis	• Human seroprevalence is high in HIV patients [211] • In South Africa, 10% [263] – 22.5% [264] prevalence was reported in HIV patients and 9.5% in healthy volunteers [264] • A 4.5% human seroreactivity was reported from Congo [265] • Many studies reported veterinarians to be at risk [266, 267]	• *Bartonella* species, *Henselae* or *B. quintana*, fastidious bacteria, almost all reported cases in children linked to likely transmission from cats by bites or scratches [268] • The organism has been isolated from cats, dogs, and some other animals from South Africa [269], Ethiopia [270], Namibia [268], Zimbabwe [271], Gabon [272], Ghana, Algeria [273], Morocco [274], Tunisia [275], and most other African countries	Potentially, *Bartonella* spp. can infect erythrocytes, endothelial cells, pericytes, CD34(+) progenitor cells, various macrophage-type cells, including microglial cells, dendritic cells, and circulating monocytes in vitro, the clinical and pathological manifestations of bartonellosis appear to be very diverse [276]	**Clinical picture:** #**Liver involvement:** can occur in both immunosuppressed and immunocompetent children [211] #Endocarditis: 9.5% of endocarditis in a Tunisian report [275] and 3% of blood culture-negative endocarditis in a multicenter study from France, England, Canada, and South Africa [277] #Adult reports of: 1. Isolated splenic peliosis; multiple cyst-like blood-filled cavities within the parenchyma of the spleen; in an adult South African HIV patient [278] 2. Neurological disease with headache, seizures, and neurocognitive affection in a veterinarian [266] 3. Two females with *vulval bacillary angiomatosis* [279] **Laboratory:** Antibodies specific to different *Bartonella* species [211] Specific staining of biopsy material or culture [211] **Histopathology:** two types: either vascular proliferative cystic blood-filled spaces with foci of necrosis within the liver and spleen or a necrotizing granulomatous type [211] **Imaging:** Ultrasonography reveals low attenuation lesions within the liver and spleen. A giant, solitary hepatic granuloma, mimicking a hepatic tumor, has also been described [280]	Antibiotics: dramatic response to erythromycin, doxycycline [211], or telithromycin [281]

Table 40.2 (continued)

Infectious disease	Epidemiology	Aetiology	Pathophysiology of liver injury	Diagnosis of liver involvement	Treatment
Listeriosis	High prevalence in most African countries with reports from South Africa [282], Ethiopia [283, 284], Nigeria [285, 286], Egypt [287], Tunisia [288], and others	#*Listeria monocytogenes* [283] #Intracellular bacterium [289] #Food-borne: contaminated milk and dairy products [283] Contaminated fishery products and poultry were also reported [290] #Human infection from animal sources occurs as an occupational hazard especially in farmers, butchers, poultry workers, and veterinary surgeons [284]	Has amazing capacity to escape the host immune barriers and survive, replicate, and spread from one cell to the next [289]	**Clinical:** Can cause sepsis, meningitis, perinatal infection, and severe invasive illness with up to 30% mortality. It is second only to salmonellosis among the most frequent causes of death due to a food-borne illness [283] **Liver involvement:** usually in immunosuppressed children Hepatitis picture with fever, raised transaminases, and jaundice Hepatic abscess may form [211] **Laboratory:** Isolating *Listeria* organisms from blood cultures [211] An Egyptian report revealed positive ascitic fluid culture for *Listeria monocytogenes* in 24.4% of adult cirrhotic patients admitted with spontaneous bacterial peritonitis [287]	Antibiotics: Ampicillin 200–400 mg/kg/day IV for 14 days is usually effective [211]

Bartonella henselae. The first three organisms can also cause liver abscess.

Legionella pneumophila and *Salmonella typhi* can cause hepatitis resembling viral hepatitis, while granulomatous hepatitis may be caused by brucellosis and tuberculosis with fever and hepatosplenomegaly in which jaundice is uncommon and transaminases are only mildly elevated, but alkaline phosphatase is typically raised [211].

Tuberculous liver abscess usually occurs in children in endemic areas. Liver function tests may be normal. It should be suspected if abscess tap revealed sterile yellowish fluid, with negative immunodiagnostic tests for amebiasis and failure of response to combined therapy with antibiotics and antiprotozoal agents. Biopsy from the wall of the abscess may show caseating granulomas or acid-fast bacilli [12].

On the other hand, anti-TB medications, especially combination therapy isoniazid/rifampicin or isoniazid/pyrazinamide, can themselves cause hepatotoxicity in 3–10%, with fulminant hepatitis in 0.6% of cases. Malnutrition, underlying liver disease, HIV infection, and disseminated TB have been reported as risk factors. Follow-up of liver transaminases every 2–3 weeks for the first 8 weeks of therapy is crucial. The development of jaundice, hepatomegaly, transaminases >2 times the normal, or serum bilirubin >2 mg/dL in the absence of fever usually indicates toxicity and needs to switch to streptomycin/ethambutol combination [12].

III. **Protozoal Infectious Diseases of the Liver:**

Refer to Table 40.3.

IV. **Helminthic Infectious Diseases of the Liver:**

Many worms can infect the liver including [211]:

1. Cestodes (tapeworms): *Echinococcus multilocularis* and *Echinococcus granulosus*
2. Nematodes (roundworms): *Ascaris lumbricoides*, *Toxocara canis*, and *Toxocara cati*
3. Trematodes (flukes): *Schistosoma mansoni* and *Fasciola hepatica*

They can lead to a wide range of liver diseases, the type and severity of which depend not only on the type of worm but also on the intensity of the infection and the host response. Simultaneous infection with more than one type of worm may occur. Children are particularly at risk, as infection may occur following close contact with infected animals, ingestion of infected soil, or contaminated food [211]. Table 40.4 summarizes the most important worms causing liver disease in African children.

In this context, it is of importance to acknowledge the great success achieved by Egypt in its battle against schistosomiasis using mass chemotherapy by praziquantel coupled

Table 40.3 Protozoal liver infections

Disease	Epidemiology	Aetiology	Pathophysiology of liver disease	Diagnosis of liver involvement	Treatment	Remark
Malaria	Endemic in sub-Saharan Africa [12]	#**Causative agent:** *Plasmodium falciparum, P. vivax, P. malariae,* and *P. ovale* [291] #**Animal reservoir:** mosquitoes [12] #**Mode of transmission:** #Mosquito-borne [291] #Blood transfusion and shared needles [291] #Transplacental spread is uncommon [291]	#Infected mosquito → bite human → sporozoite passage into the bloodstream → selectively invade hepatocytes → initiate the exoerythrocytic stage of development → Parasite division → Hepatocyte rupture → Merozoites releases → invade erythrocytes → develop into micro- and macrogametes [291] #Some authors state that merozoites use liver vitamin A as a membrane destabilizer to invade the red blood cells. The characteristic features of hemolysis, anemia, and other symptoms of malaria are manifestations of an endogenous form of vitamin A intoxication caused by the parasites [292]	**Clinical picture:** #Continuous fever, gastrointestinal complaints (nausea, vomiting, and diarrhea), headache, lethargy, myalgia, and delirium [291] #Neurologic complications, with *P. falciparum,* include seizures and coma; renal failure may occur [291] **Liver involvement:** #Jaundice and tender hepatomegaly are common in pediatrics (68%) [12] #Jaundice usually unconjugated reflecting hemolysis [291], but may be conjugated, with *P. falciparum* more than *P. vivax* [12] #Mild elevation of hepatic aminotransferases [293] #In neonates, infection is usually severe [294] with cholestasis #Hepatic failure is uncommon [295] #Deaths caused by malarial disease are most common in children 1–5 years of age [296] #No reported chronic hepatitis or cirrhosis [12] #Tropical splenomegaly: in hyperendemic regions due to an aberrant immunological response to *Plasmodium* → hyperreactive massive splenomegaly and usually significant hepatomegaly [12] #Blackwater fever: sudden massive intravascular hemolysis in a previously infected individual with *P. falciparum* followed by fever with or without rigors, loin pain, hemoglobinuria, jaundice, bilious vomiting, circulatory collapse, and acute renal failure. Fulminant hepatic failure has also been reported [12] Cholestasis may occur, but hepatotoxicity may also be due to the toxic effects of antimalarial agents, such as amodiaquine, pyrimethamine, and sulfadoxine [12]	#Treatment varies from region to region, depending on resistance. Chloroquine, sulfadoxine/pyrimethamine, and quinine may be used [12] #Chloroquine phosphate, 10 mg/kg loading, followed by 5 mg/kg at 6, 24, and 48 h [301] #Quinidine hydrochloride is the parenteral drug of choice; however, significant side effects limit its use to emergent situations when oral medications cannot be tolerated [12] #Icterus/liver enlargement rapidly improve after treatment [12] #Although relapse of disease may occur in individuals infected with *P. vivax* and *P. ovale,* hepatic abnormalities in treated patients typically resolve completely [300, 302]	#Sub-Saharan Africans, coexistence with malaria parasites over millennia may have created evolutionary-adaptive pressures, first, to conserve and prevent vitamin A deficiency by reducing the hepatic metabolism of vitamin A and, second, to reduce the severity of malaria symptoms by lowering vitamin A stores in the liver and sequestering it in the lower extremities, thereby reducing parasite ingestion of vitamin A [218, 292] #Sulfadoxine/pyrimethamine may cause severe intravascular hemolysis in G6PD patients [12]

Investigations: #Thin and thick peripheral blood smears prepared with Giemsa stain → detection of malarial organisms [291] #Liver biopsy: fatty change, hepatocytes necrosis, nuclear vacuolation, and mononuclear cell infiltration. Kupffer cell hyperplasia with dark brown granules of malarial pigment or parasitized red blood cells and iron in cases of *P. falciparum* [297]. Sinusoids are congested with red blood cells [298]. Portal tract infiltration by lymphocytes may occur in chronic cases. If shock has occurred, centrilobular necrosis may be present [299] Immunofluorescence staining → intense deposition within the reticuloendothelial elements [300] #Tropical splenomegaly: elevated malarial polyclonal IgM antibody. Liver histology demonstrates normal hepatocytes, with numerous lymphocytes in dilated sinusoids and enlarged Kupffer cells. Malarial pigment is usually absent [12]	#In severe and complicated *P. falciparum* malaria → maintain circulatory volume and start quinine salt 10 mg/kg/8 h IV in 5% dextrose for 7 days, irrespective of the chloroquine resistance status of the area OR: artemisinin derivatives, such as [12]: • Artemisinin 10 mg/kg/24 h IV for 5 days, with a double divided dose on day 1 • Artesunate 1 mg/kg (two doses) IM</IV at an interval of 4–6 h on day 1 and then 1 mg/kg once daily for 5 days • Artemether 1.6 mg/kg (two doses) IM at an interval of 4–6 h on day 1 and then 1.6 mg/kg once daily for 5 days [12]

(continued)

Table 40.3 (continued)

Disease	Epidemiology	Aetiology	Pathophysiology of liver disease	Diagnosis of liver involvement	Treatment	Remark
Visceral leishmaniasis or Kala-azar	Endemic throughout the Mediterranean Basin, as well as parts of Africa [303, 304]	**#Causative agent:** *Leishmania donovani* [303, 304] **#Animal reservoir:** sandfly [303, 304] **#Mode of transmission:** sandfly bites [303, 304]	Sandfly bites → inoculate the organism → phagocytosis by dermal macrophages → proliferate → rupture of infected macrophages → organism spread to reticuloendothelial cells within the liver, spleen, bone marrow, lymph nodes, kidneys, and intestine [303, 304]	**Clinical picture:** After an incubation period of up to several months → fever, failure to thrive, anemia, hepatosplenomegaly, diarrhea, and bleeding diathesis [291] **Investigations:** #Laboratory: elevations of serum aminotransferase and alkaline phosphatase; hypoalbuminemia and prolongation of prothrombin times may be noted with more advanced disease [293] #Serology and PCR [305, 306] #Imaging: ultrasonography or CT: Nodular hepatosplenic lesions [307] #Liver biopsy: the hepatic lesion in older children and adults is characterized by Kupffer cell hyperplasia, many of which contain parasites. Portal tract infiltration with eosinophils, lymphocytes, and plasma cells may occur, as may granuloma formation. Fibrin ring granulomas have been reported [308] Infants may demonstrate significant hepatocellular necrosis [309] Bone marrow biopsy often demonstrates the presence of Leishman-Donovan bodies [291]	#Stibogluconate sodium, 20 mg/kg/day intravenously or intramuscularly for 20–28 [310] #Repeated treatment may be required [291] #Alternative therapy: meglumine antimoniate, pentamidine, or amphotericin B [291]	Prognosis of untreated leishmaniasis is poor [291]

Amebiasis with amebic liver abscess	Africa is highly endemic zones of amebiasis	**Causative organism:** *Entamoeba histolyticum* [311]	Trophozoites can remain as commensal, without causing evident intestinal damage, or they can be virulent destroying the muco-epithelial barrier of the human colon by first crossing the mucus and then killing host cells, triggering inflammation and subsequently causing amebiasis (intestinal/extraintestinal) [311]	**Clinical picture of amebic liver abscess:** Abdominal pain (90%), nausea (85%), right upper quadrant tenderness (67%), and less likely respiratory symptoms (24%). Jaundice and hepatomegaly may be associated [211] **Investigations:** #Although there may be no detectable abnormality, the majority of patients have leukocytosis, raised transaminases, and alkaline phosphatase with reduced serum albumin [211] #Immunological tests: antibodies to *Entamoeba histolyticum* by indirect hemagglutination assay, complement fixation, or indirect fluorescence [211] Imaging: U/S can detect liver abscesses of 1 cm or more in diameter as hypoechoic area with ring enhancement. CT can be used for confirmation and more precise localization of the lesion [312, 313] Microbiology: amebic abscess may be diagnosed by negative bacterial culture of abscess aspiration and positive serology [211]	Metronidazole [314] Paromomycin [315]

(continued)

Table 40.3 (continued)

Disease	Epidemiology	Aetiology	Pathophysiology of liver disease	Diagnosis of liver involvement	Treatment	Remark
Toxoplasmosis	The most widespread zoonotic infection. In Africa it gained special concern due to the AIDS epidemic with fatal toxoplasma encephalitis [316]	**Causative organism:** *Toxoplasma gondii* [316] **Mode of transmission:** 1. Oral ingestion of oocysts contaminated food or water [316] 2. Transplacental transmission 3. Solid organ transplantation [317, 318]	*Intracellular protozoan:* in immunocompetent, usually asymptomatic or only mild symptoms, while in immunocompromised persons, cause severe diseases [316]	**Clinical picture** in immunocompetent, usually asymptomatic or only mild symptoms, such as fever and malaise, although up to 10% will present with cervical lymphadenopathy or ocular disease [317]. In immunocompromised persons, such as HIV patients, toxoplasmosis is the most frequent severe neurologic infection (toxoplasmic encephalitis) [319, 320]. Hepatitis may be the only indicator of infection. Serious disease is primarily related to hepatic and central nervous system involvement [321]. Manifestations of congenital infection: purpura, microcephaly, chorioretinitis, intracranial calcification, and meningoencephalitis. Most infants with congenital toxoplasmosis have hepatosplenomegaly, but jaundice may be variable [151] **Investigations** [151]: Serology: specific IgM or rising IgG Plain abdominal X-ray: hepatic microcalcifications of the necrotic lesions Liver biopsy: generalized hepatitis with areas of hepatocytes necrosis. Intracellular bile stasis and periportal infiltration with histiocytes, lymphocytes, granulocytes, and eosinophils *Toxoplasma* organisms may be seen in the liver using fluorescent antibody staining	Mothers known to be infected during pregnancy may be treated with sulfadiazine and pyrimethamine or spiramycin (an investigational drug) in an attempt to prevent congenital infection. Infants with documented infection may be treated with pyrimethamine and sulfadiazine with folinic acid added to prevent hematologic toxicity of therapy. Although further cellular invasion may be prevented, preexisting damage and intracellular organisms may not be influenced by this regimen [151]	#In sub-Saharan Africa, it is overshadowed by other endemic infections especially Malaria and AIDS [316] #It is described as an environmental disease promoted by poor environmental sanitation, overcrowding, poverty, and poor hygiene [322, 323] which are all fulfilled in Africa

Table 40.4 Helminthic liver infections

Infectious disease	Epidemiology	Aetiology	Pathophysiology of liver involvement	Diagnosis	Treatment
Ascariasis	• The most prevalent human helminths [12] • Highest among children and in areas with poor sanitation [291]	• *Ascaris lumbricoides* [12] • A nematode [12] • Infection occurs via ingestion of contaminated food or water by embryonated eggs [291]	• Dead migrating larvae → stimulate granuloma formation [324] • Adult worm enters the ampullary orifice from the duodenum → either blocks the duct or advances into the common bile duct, the hepatic ducts, the cystic duct, the gallbladder, or the pancreatic duct. This is less common in children due to the smaller size of the ductal system, which makes it difficult for the worms to enter [325]	Clinical picture: • Usually asymptomatic [12] • Heavy infestation → intestinal obstruction [12] Hepatobiliary and pancreatic ascariasis: • Mild hepatic abnormalities may be associated with dead migrating larvae [193] • Adult worm impaction in the duct system → picture of obstructive jaundice, cholangitis, cholecystitis, pancreatitis [324, 326], and liver abscess formation [327] Rupture of abscesses into the peritoneal or pleural cavities may then follow [291] • Other reported complications include perforation of the common bile duct and pylephlebitis of the hepatic or portal veins (or both) [291] • The worms either move from the ducts or die there → a nidus for bile duct calculi [12] Investigations: • Stool analysis: eggs or mature worms [328] • Transaminases: usually normal [326] but may be elevated in duct ascariasis • Imaging: US [329], CT [330, 331], and MRCP may detect the worms and abscess formation • Upper endoscopy/ERCP can demonstrate the worm [332, 333]	• Oral anthelmintics [334]: Albendazole 400 mg PO once (200 mg below 2 years) or Mebendazole 100 mg bid PO × 3 days or 500 mg once or Ivermectin 150–200 mcg/kg PO once Effective in 90% of cases. A second course may be given if the patient is not cured by 3 weeks after treatment Biliary ascariasis [291]: • Conservative management for cholangitis and pancreatitis + oral anthelmintics to paralyze the worms, which are then expelled by the peristaltic activity of the intestine • If failure of response or failure to expel the worm within 3 weeks of treatment → ERCP → worm extraction [329, 335, 336] • Surgical: for hepatic abscess, common bile duct and gallbladder perforation [291]

(continued)

Table 40.4 (continued)

Infectious disease	Epidemiology	Aetiology	Pathophysiology of liver involvement	Diagnosis	Treatment
Intestinal/hepatosplenic schistosomiasis	Middle East and Africa [211]	*Schistosoma mansoni* [337] infection occurs by direct skin penetration by the cercariae, previously released from a snail host [291]	Hepatic involvement occurs as a result of the host's immunologic response to ova deposited in the portal venous system → granulomatous lesions around the ovum [338] Giant cells and fibrosis become prominent after the death of the ovum Destruction of small portal radicles → periportal fibrosis [337] → presinusoidal portal hypertension [339] Fibrosis and thrombophlebitis of larger portal branches → pipestem fibrosis [340]	Clinical picture: Hepatic disease: hepatosplenomegaly and portal hypertension with its manifestations and complications [339] Investigations: 1. Detection of the ova in stools or in rectal biopsy material [211] 2. May have picture of hypersplenism [291] 3. Eosinophilia and hyperglobulinemia [291] 4. Serum aminotransferase levels are generally not markedly elevated, but serum alkaline phosphatase levels may be increased [293] 5. Serologic studies may be useful [337] 6. Ultrasonography allows detection and grading of periportal fibrosis, accurate measurement of liver and spleen size, and measurement of portal vein size, as well as detection of intra-abdominal varices [338, 341]. CT may suggest the presence of periportal fibrosis [342]; MRI may also be of use [343] 7. Liver biopsy: periportal fibrosis, granulomas, schistosome eggs [337, 338] 8. Upper endoscopy: for varices [291]	1. One-day two-dose course of praziquantel 208 40–60 mg/kg/day [291] 2. Mild periportal fibrosis may resolve in children after effective therapy [344] 3. Management of portal hypertension and bleeding varices [339, 345]
Toxocariasis or visceral larva migrans	High in developing countries [346] Exposure to it is prevalent across the African continent [347], but little is known about its seroprevalence, e.g., Ghana 53.5% [346], Nigeria 21.5% [348] to 30.4% [349]	• *T. canis/cati* [350] • Nematode [291] • Definitive hosts (cats and dogs) [346] • Humans get infected by ingestion of embryonated eggs containing the infective larva [346]	These parasites cannot develop into adult forms in humans and are restricted to larval forms [346] which penetrate the intestinal wall and migrate via lymphatics and venous circulation, most commonly, to the liver and lung Other affected organs include the eye, heart, and central nervous system [291] causing local or systemic inflammatory reactions in the affected organ [351] Early pathologic findings in the liver consist of larvae surrounded by eosinophils; later findings include granulomas composed of epithelioid cells, giant cells, lymphocytes, and fibroblasts [298]	Clinical picture of liver involvement: fever, hepatosplenomegaly [211] Investigations: Peripheral blood eosinophilia [211] Serologic confirmation [211] Imaging: CT/MRI, multiple low-density lesions [352]	Anthelmintics, albendazole, thiabendazole (25 mg/kg/day for 5 days), and mebendazole [353] Corticosteroid may be added in pulmonary or ocular disease [291]

Hydatid disease	- Endemic in the Mediterranean Basin and parts of Africa [184] - The worm has been isolated from different animals in Africa [334] - Tunisia is a hyperendemic country for human echinococcosis [334]	- *Echinococcus granulosus* [211] - Cystode [211] - Human infection occurs by ingestion of the ova excreted by infected canines/dogs who acquire infection via consumption of sheep liver or intestine containing hydatid cysts [291]	- Ingested eggs in the duodenum → embryo → penetrates the intestinal mucosa → portal circulation → lodge in the liver or lung [291] - Hepatic involvement is marked by the development of "cysts" within the hepatic parenchyma [354] surrounded by a fibrous capsule elaborated by the host - An acellular, hyalinized layer forms the exocyst, underlaid by a germinal layer. Extrusions of the germinal layer form brood capsules which contain protoscolices [291] Hydatid sand, composed of separated brood cysts and protoscolices, floats within the main cyst cavity. Septation may occur, as may formation of daughter cysts [355]	Clinical picture: - Infection is common in childhood, although symptoms may not occur for many years. Although in adult series, involvement of the liver occurs 3 times more frequently, involvement of the lung is noted frequently in children. Simultaneous involvement of the liver and lung may occur [291] - Mainly in lung involvement, the liver may be also involved or both involved simultaneously. Other sites in 10% of children include the brain, bones, genitourinary tract, eyes, spleen, and heart [291] Hepatic hydatid cyst: - Hepatic cysts are usually slow-growing and lead to asymptomatic hepatomegaly but may become manifest due to secondary infection or because of the increase of their size [211] with subsequent compression of the surrounding tissues or rupture: Porta hepatis compression → jaundice [291] Hepatic vein compression → Budd-Chiari syndrome [291] Cyst rupture into the biliary tract → Cholangitis [291] Cyst rupture into the pericardial, peritoneal, or pleural cavities may occur [356] Anaphylaxis may occur on the release of cyst fluid [291] Investigations: - Serological diagnosis is highly sensitive [211] - Elevated s.ALP, ALT, AST and eosinophilia [291] - X-ray abdomen: calcification of the cyst wall is seldom apparent in children - U/S, CT, MRI can diagnose, classify, and identify complications and plan management [356–360] - ERCP detects daughter cysts in the biliary tree following the rupture of a primary hepatic cyst [356, 361]	- Radical surgery (pericystectomy and partial liver resection) with pre- and postoperative administration of albendazole [362], 15 mg/kg/day divided into 2 doses, oral for 1–6 months [363], is the best treatment option [362]. Mebendazole can be used, but albendazole is better as it has better absorption [362] - Percutaneous drainage [puncture, aspiration, injection of scolicidal solutions 190,200–202, re-aspiration (PAIR)] [355, 362–366] combined with albendazole therapy is a safe and effective alternative especially in asymptomatic patients [310, 367] - Anthelmintics alone can't fully eliminate the cysts [362] but can be used in cases of unresectable hepatic lesions for 1–6 months to reduce cyst size [356] - Conservative surgical treatment with the removal of the cyst content, sterilization of the residual cavity, and partial cyst resection is an option when radical surgery is difficult as in cysts located close to major biliovascular channels. Omentoplasty is effective in preventing postoperative complications following conservative surgery [362] - ERCP can be used in cases of ruptured cyst into the biliary tract to inject scolicidal agents [368] and to remove daughter cysts in the biliary tree [369]

with a vigorous media campaign with the resultant marvelous decrease in schistosomiasis morbidity and prevalence [370].

Combined Schistosoma mansoni and malaria infections:
Recently, it was reported that in the majority of schoolchildren in schistosomiasis-endemic areas, the mechanism underlying hepatosplenomegaly is not periportal fibrosis. Recent clinical and immunological evidence revealed an associated chronic malarial infection with subsequent proinflammatory Th1 response rather than a pro-fibrotic Th2 response with the resultant inflammatory HSM without periportal fibrosis. This type of HSM is not benign, with both dilation of the portal system and stunting of growth being associated [371].

Other helminthes affecting the liver which have worldwide distribution with some reports released from Africa include the following.

3. Fascioliasis: liver fluke:

Recently, reports have been released from Egypt about fascioliasis as an emerging disease. It has been endemic in certain villages in the Nile Delta of Egypt, but its overall prevalence in Egypt is unknown [372]. It is caused by a trematode named *Fasciola hepatica* with worldwide distribution [291]. Sheep and cattle are the primary hosts. Humans get infected after ingesting contaminated aquatic plants [373]. In the human, metacercariae penetrate the intestinal wall to the peritoneal cavity and then penetrate the hepatic capsule and migrate through the hepatic parenchyma until reaching the bile ducts, where they persist [374] causing biliary and parenchymal damage. Clinical presentation of human fascioliasis ranges from asymptomatic cases to tender hepatomegaly, cholangitis, hepatitis, and hepatic focal lesions [372]. Both US and CT may help to delineate these abnormalities [374, 375]. Eosinophilia is common [291]. Diagnosis rests on serology and demonstration of ova in the stool [368]. Endoscopic retrograde cholangiography (ERCP) may also be useful in the biliary phase of disease, both as a diagnostic (identification of eggs and intact flukes; visualization of flukes radiographically) and therapeutic (removal of flukes after sphincterotomy) measure [376]. Treatment is with triclabendazole 10 mg/kg given once, and some authors recommend it for two consecutive days [377]. Because the availability of this drug may be an issue, bithionol, 30–50 mg/kg on alternate days for 10–15 doses, may also be used [301, 378].

4. Capillariasis:

It is caused by *Capillaria hepatica* which is a nematode that affects rodents, cats, and dogs but may affect the human liver in a way similar to toxocariasis. Fever, hepatomegaly, and eosinophilia are the main symptoms. Diagnosis is generally made through the demonstration of organisms in liver biopsy [193]. Albendazole and mebendazole are effective treatments [310, 379, 380].

40.3 Nonalcoholic Fatty Liver Disease (NAFLD) and Steatohepatitis (NASH) in African Children
(See Also Chap. 15)

NAFLD has a wide spectrum ranging from simple steatosis, or NASH with or without fibrosis, to cirrhosis and its complications [381, 382]. It is now considered the most common form of PLD due to a steep increase in its prevalence over the past 20 years secondary to the childhood obesity pandemic [383]. Generally, 3–11% of the pediatric population [384, 385] are affected which increase up to 46% in overweight and obese children and adolescents [383].

The prevalence of hepatic steatosis varies among different ethnic groups; however there is limited data on the prevalence of NAFLD in Africa in general [386] and in children/adolescents in particular. Not only studies on African children/adolescents are scarce, but also those available were carried out on a small number of patients with no multicenter studies. In fact, all published data were from North Africa by Egyptian investigators who reported an estimated NAFLD prevalence of 15.8% [387] and 38.5% [388] in the general population of schoolchildren and in overweight/obese children, respectively. NAFLD in Egyptian children was significantly associated with waist circumference [387], insulin resistance (IR) [387, 388], and dyslipidemia [387, 388]. The low-density lipoprotein cholesterol was found to be the only sensitive predictor (independent variable) in both uni- and multivariate logistic regression analyses for NAFLD among obese Egyptian children [388]. Genetic polymorphism in obese Egyptian children with NAFLD was investigated, and the microsomal triglyceride transfer protein G/G and the manganese superoxide dismutase T/T genotypes were found to be significantly more prevalent among obese children with NASH and may be responsible for such a phenotype [389].

To the best of our knowledge, no studies have been published from any other African population on pediatric NAFLD, and one Nigerian study estimated the prevalence to be about 9% in adults [390].

On the other hand, African-Americans have been extensively studied by American investigators in comparison with Hispanics and Caucasians where NAFLD was more prevalent in Hispanics followed by Caucasians and last by African-Americans [391]. In spite of the different socioeconomic, environmental, and other risk factors, those studies may give indirect clues about SSA population as they share the same African ancestry's genetic background. African-Americans, despite showing a similar or even higher degree of IR than

Caucasians and Hispanics, have a lower prevalence of NAFLD [392] and a lower propensity for the development of NASH [393]. This dissociation suggests that this group tends to accumulate less intrahepatic fat even in the presence of IR [386]. Gene polymorphisms could explain these paradoxes as they have low prevalence (0.186) of patatin-like phospholipase containing domain 3 gene which is the most important gene involved in determining hepatic steatosis [394].

In spite of that, once NAFLD develops, NASH occurs as frequently, and as severe, as in Caucasian patients. Therefore, African-Americans with NAFLD should be screened for NASH with the same degree of clinical resolve as in Caucasian patients [395].

40.4 Other Chronic Liver Diseases in African Children

Other causes of pediatric CLD in Africa are similar to those worldwide; they include the following.

- *Fibrocystic liver disease (refer also to Chap. 9):*

They include congenital hepatic fibrosis, Caroli disease/syndrome, choledochal cyst, and others. Some reports were released from Tunisia [396] with the largest series released from Egypt [397]. It included 50 patients from both pediatric and adult population. Most cases were types I and IV-A [397].

- *Gallstone disease (refer also to Chap. 10):*

Clear differences in gallstone disease frequency exist among ethnic backgrounds. The frequency is exceedingly low among East and West African natives [398].

A prospective analysis of ultrasonographic (U/S) examinations of the gallbladder (GB) in 161 African children with sickle cell anemia (SCA) revealed cholelithiasis in 7 cases (4.2%), biliary sludge in 7.5%, and wall thickening in 8.1%. The age range of patients studied was 2.5 months to 16 years. The youngest age for development of cholelithiasis was 10 years, while biliary sludge was noted earliest at 5 years. GB wall thickening appeared as early as 4 years. Dietary and environmental factors are probably responsible for the low incidence of cholelithiasis in Africans with SCA [399].

- *Metabolic, genetic, and familial liver disease (refer also to Chaps. 12 and 14):*

Although only scarce African reports are available about these entities, we believe that these diseases are much more prevalent than reported. This is attributed to the high degree of consanguinity and sometimes the sole in tribe marriage which allow propagation and magnification of the offending genes of those inherited diseases generation after generation. It seems that those patients die early in life without diagnosis, even those who live don't have access to health-care facilities, and even if they get that access, it would be not the required highly qualified properly equipped up-to-date medical care facility needed to diagnose those diseases. Diagnosis is usually based on clinical picture and liver histopathology, as the specific enzyme assays and the confirmatory molecular genetic testing are rarely available. The needed multidisciplinary care team, the very expensive special formulas, and orphan medications in most occasions are another obstacle. After all this long journey of continuous effort by the medical team, parental refusal to believe in the documented diagnosis, reluctance to stick to management plan, and resistance to avoid consanguineous marriage are a commonly faced scenario which needs to put extra effort on health education and genetic counseling.

Scattered reports, mainly clinical and occasionally genetic, are available in the literature from African countries, mostly from Egypt, on *Wilson's disease, progressive familial intrahepatic cholestasis, glycogen storage disease, tyrosinemia, familial hemophagocytic lymphohistiocytosis, variegate porphyria, Niemann-Pick disease, galactosemia, α1-antitrypsin deficiency, Gaucher disease, and others.*

– *Wilson's disease (WD):*

From North Africa, WD was reported from Tunisia [396, 400] and Egypt [401, 402]. Egyptian studies reported a 13-year clinical experience with 54 pediatric patients with WD and the molecular genetics of 19 of them [401, 402]. Consanguinity was present in most families with more than one affected siblings. Most patients presented with hepatic symptom (61%), followed by neurologic symptoms (9.3%) and then hepato-neurological manifestations (5.5%). Family screening uncovered 13 presymptomatic patients (24% of their cohort). Increased urinary copper concentrations before/after D-penicillamine challenge were found in all patients, low serum ceruloplasmin in 97%, and Kayser-Fleischer ring in 31.5%. They treated their cohort with D-penicillamine and zinc sulfate with improvement of hepatic symptoms, but neurologic symptoms remained stationary. Three patients with fulminant and end-stage WD underwent liver transplantation [401].

Molecular genetic testing of the ATP7B gene was carried out in 19 of their patients which identified 2 novel (p.A1074A in 16% of patients, p.T1076I in another 16%) and 3 previously published mutations. The most common European mutation (p.H1069Q) was detected in only 5% of patients, and the p.P1273Q and p.A1003A mutations were detected in 10 and 26% of patients, respectively. They recommended screening of exons 14 and 18 of the ATP7B gene in suspected WD Egyptian children especially those without hepatic manifestations [402].

– *Progressive familial intrahepatic cholestasis (PFIC):*

PFIC was reported from North Africa, Tunisia [396], and Egypt [403] with a focus about an approach to diagnose them on clinical basis with the aid of gamma-glutamyl transpeptidase level where low-normal levels are detected in types 1 and 2 with diarrhea associated in type 1. They also reported that exon 6, 8, and 9 mutations of ABCB4 gene are not common among Egyptian children with PFIC3 [403].

– *Glycogen storage disease (GSD):*

Type III GSD is the most common type in North Africa. It is an autosomal recessive disorder caused by deficiency of glycogen debrancher enzyme [404]. Most of reported Egyptian children have doll facies and progressive abdominal distention with huge soft hepatomegaly and recurrent attacks of convulsions which were sometimes misdiagnosed as seizure disorders. Hypertriglyceridemia, hyperlactacidemia, hyperuricemia, and elevated creatine kinase are usually there. Uncooked corn starch is essential to prevent hypoglycemia [405]. A nice regimen was followed by the Egyptian investigators in tailoring the intervals between raw cornstarch doses for each patient according to patient's fasting tolerance which seemed very beneficial with the improvement of linear growth velocity and reduction of hypoglycemic seizures as well as the size of the liver [406].

Although hepatic manifestations were the main presenting symptoms in the previously mentioned Egyptian cohort but owing to the clinical variability characteristic of GSD III with liability to involve skeletal and cardiac muscles, 28 Egyptian children diagnosed by enzymatic assay were screened for skeletal and cardiac muscle involvement [407]. Seventeen patients (61%) had myopathic changes, three of them had associated neuropathic changes, and seven had associated left ventricular (LV) hypertrophy. Two patients had LV hypertrophy without skeletal muscle involvement. Despite the mild degrees of affection in pediatric age group, they recommended to perform prospective annual screening using electromyography (EMG) and echocardiography in order to augment dietary therapy regimen to prevent progression to life-threatening complications with advancing age [407].

– *Hereditary tyrosinemia type I (HT1):*

HT1 is an autosomal recessive disorder resulting from the deficiency of fumarylacetoacetase caused by mutations in the fumarylacetoacetate hydrolase (FAH) gene [408]. It is an increasingly recognized inborn error of metabolism among Tunisian [396] and Egyptian [409, 410] children. The largest study from Africa was an Egyptian study carried out over a period of 3 years and included 22 children who were suspected by markedly elevated serum alpha fetoprotein (αFP) levels and diagnosed by quantification of succinylacetone (SA) in dry blood spots. Infants with focal hepatic lesions and hepatomegaly were more common, 13 and 5 patients, respectively, and younger, 3.25 vs. 10 months, than those with rickets at presentation. The orphan drug nitisinone (2-[2-nitro-4-trifluoromethylbenzoyl]-1,3-cyclohexanedione) or NTBC was effective but very expensive, and liver transplantation was done in three of their patients despite adequate response to NTBC because of financial issues [409]. This very high cost of NTBC urged the Egyptian investigators to study the effect of doses lower than recommended in HT1 management. The recommended average dose of NTBC is 1 mg/kg/day. In four of their patients, they tried lower doses and followed them up for 12–27 months. They found that with NTBC doses of 0.55–0.65 mg/kg/day, SA was undetectable and αFP steeply dropped, with appreciable catch-up growth, healing of active rickets, and normalization of liver functions. They concluded that this cost-effective dose may allow the treatment of HT1 children from economically underprivileged countries, but longer follow-up periods might be still needed [410].

Regarding molecular genetic testing of those patients, a joint study was carried out between Egypt and other Middle East countries with detection of 11 novel and 6 previously described pathogenic mutations. All of them were homozygous and no founder mutation detected [408].

– *Familial hemophagocytic lymphohistiocytosis (FHLH):*

This is a life-threatening potentially treatable clinical syndrome with liver involvement varying from mild dysfunction to severe fulminant liver failure (ALF) [411]. A case series of four neonates with FHLH was published from Egypt. They presented with ALF and fulfilled the international criteria of FHLH diagnosis. Positive consanguinity and previous sibling death were reported in three of them [411].

– *Variegate Porphyria (VP):*

Aetiology: VP is an autosomal dominant hepatic porphyria due to deficient activity of PROTO-oxidase enzyme of heme pathway [412].

Epidemiology: It is particularly common in South Africa, where 3 of every 1,000 whites have the disorder [412]. Most are descendants of a couple who emigrated from Holland to South Africa in 1688 [413].

Clinical Features [412–414]
- Homozygous dominant VP is rare and presents early in childhood.
- It may present with neurologic symptoms, photosensitivity, or both.

- Acute attacks are similar to those in acute intermittent porphyria (AIP) with abdominal pain, nausea, vomiting, anxiety, restlessness, insomnia, paresis, and hyponatremia. Attacks are generally milder than in AIP and less often fatal.
- Blistering skin manifestations are identical to those in porphyria cutanea tarda (PCT) but are more difficult to treat and usually of longer duration.
- Chronic, low-grade abnormalities in liver function tests are common, and the risk of HCC is increased without an increase in serum αFP. Therefore, hepatic imaging is recommended at least yearly for early detection of these tumors.

Diagnosis
- Urine: high aminolevulinate synthase, porphobilinogen, coproporphyrin III [412].
- Stool: high fecal protoporphyrin, coproporphyrin III [412].
- Plasma: high porphyrin levels are increased [321, 322].
- Assays of PROTO-oxidase activity [412].
- PROTO-oxidase mutation [415].

Treatment
- Acute attacks are treated as in AIP: narcotic analgesics for abdominal pain, phenothiazines for nausea/vomiting/anxiety/restlessness/chloral hydrate, or low doses of short-acting benzodiazepines for insomnia/restlessness. IV carbohydrate loading for mild attacks without paresis, hyponatremia, or other severe symptoms. IV hemin should be started early for severe attacks and for mild attacks that do not respond to carbohydrate loading within 1–2 days [412, 416].
- Avoid sun exposure [412].
- Wear protective clothing [412].
- Treat skin lesions [412].
- β-Carotene, phlebotomy, and chloroquine are not helpful [412].

– *Niemann-Pick type B (NP-B)*:

NP-B is pan-ethnic, but highest incidence is Arabs and North Africans [417]. It is non-neuronopathic disease with visceral involvement, mainly hepatosplenomegaly during childhood. Pulmonary involvement is the main cause of morbidity [418].

Hereditary hemochromatosis is rare in natives of Africa [10, 419].

- *Liver tumors and nodular lesions (also refer to Chap. 19):*

Pediatric malignant liver tumors, hepatoblastoma (HB), and HCC are uncommon worldwide, representing 0.5–2% of childhood malignancies. This pattern is different in Africa as a result of infectious factors like HBV and HIV [420].

In Africa, outcomes also differ due to limitations imposed by comorbidities and lack of resources, both human and material, for major liver resection. While HB and HCC can be readily distinguished on clinical and biochemical grounds, there is a high incidence of sarcomatous tumors that mandate biopsy. HCC in African children is a lethal condition and is usually associated with HBV [421] which integrates into the genome of tumor cells [422, 423]. It is promising that aggressive HBV vaccination programs have decreased HCC in African children [420, 424, 425].

Sarcomatous tumors are often resectable but have a high rate of local recurrence. HB is a surgically curable tumor in many patients [421]. Other liver tumors include vascular tumors, lymphomas, and endodermal sinus tumor. Vascular tumors included hemangioendotheliomas, angiosarcoma, and Kaposi sarcoma-like tumors. AIDS appears to increase the prevalence of vascular tumors, presumably the result of an increase in Kaposi-like sarcoma [420].

Resection for benign liver tumors can be safely accomplished and augments institutional experience with major liver surgery [421].

- *Portal hypertension (PH) (also refer to Chap. 17):*

PH with subsequent variceal bleeding is an important, rather common cause of morbidity and mortality in pediatric CLD in Africa owing to the high endemicity of *S. Mansoni*, malaria, HBV, HCV, neglected BA, and other causes of cirrhotic and noncirrhotic increase of portal blood pressure. Extrahepatic portal vein obstruction (EHPVO) is an important cause of PH worldwide and in Africa.

Some studies proposed predictive U/S criteria for diagnosis of PH in areas where endoscopic diagnosis is not feasible due to the shortage of resources [426].

Management of PH and upper GI hemorrhage includes endoscopic injection sclerotherapy (EIS), endoscopic band ligation (EBL), and the use of propranolol.

The largest study worldwide on different management options of EHBVO was published from Africa by an Egyptian work group on 169 pediatric patients, aged 1 month–12 years. Hematemesis was a presenting symptom in 58%, splenomegaly was present in 87%, esophageal varices were present in 94%, and fundal varices were present in 23%. Possible risk factors, in the form of umbilical catheterization, umbilical sepsis, and exchange transfusion, were elicited in 18% of patients. Propranolol significantly reduced bleeding episodes ($p < 0.001$). Both EIS and EBL were effective in the management of bleeding varices and for primary and secondary prophylaxis; however, EIS was associated with the development of secondary gastric varices ($p = 0.03$) [427].

This large study of children with EHPVO demonstrates the efficacy of propranolol in the reduction of gastrointestinal bleeding in those children [427].

- *Liver and systemic illness (also refer to Chap. 13):*

The liver is commonly affected in the course of any systemic illness. Almost all infections, drugs, intoxications, body organ failure, cardiovascular, circulatory, renal, autoimmune diseases, diabetes, hyperlipidemia, and others can affect the liver.

– *Liver and diabetes mellitus (DM):*

Children with type 1 DM frequently suffer with hepatic abnormalities. An Egyptian study carried out on 692 diabetic children revealed a prevalence of 8.7% of hepatic abnormalities among the studied cohort. Clinical hepatomegaly (1.9%), elevated ALT (3.9%), anti-HCV antibodies (3.6%), and abnormal hepatic U/S (4.5%) were the mostly encountered. Forty percent of anti-HCV positive children were HCV-RNA positive. Glycogenic hepatopathy was diagnosed in three cases by liver biopsy. Abnormalities were reversible in 50% of patients after proper glycemic control. A 4- to 8-week therapeutic trial of proper glycemic control is recommended prior to more invasive diagnostic procedures [428]. NAFLD is another sequel (refer to NAFLD in Africa).

Liver and hyperlipidemia: refer to NAFLD in Africa.

– *Liver and SCA:*

SCA is highly prevalent in Africa. The hepatic affection in SCA can be manifested clinically, biochemically, ultrasonographically, and histopathologically.

Clinical Presentation
1. Conjugated jaundice secondary to intrahepatic cholestasis [429].
2. Hepatomegaly secondary to extramedullary hematopoiesis, chronic viral hepatitis due to repeated blood transfusion with inadequate screening, or vascular occlusion [430].
3. Hepatic right upper quadrant syndrome (hepatic crisis) which is a self-limited mild form of vascular occlusion that remits with IV hydration and analgesia [430].
4. Acute hepatic sequestration syndrome (AHSS) which is a potentially lethal intrahepatic vaso-occlusion, sequestration, and ischemia with liver cell failure [430]. This AHSS should be urgently treated by partial red blood cell exchange transfusion to reduce the number of sickled cells [430]. Simple blood transfusions may lead to hyperviscosity syndrome [431].

Biochemical indices: high alkaline phosphatase and conjugated bilirubin in the presence of normal transaminases and synthetic functions. This picture was seen in 12% of cases of a Nigerian study carried out on children with homozygous SCA. This picture is compatible with intrahepatic cholestasis in the presence of actively functioning liver cells and excludes liver damage [432].

Imaging: U/S adequately assess the liver and GB [399] (refer to gallstone disease in Africa).

Liver histopathology: sinusoidal distension, hemosiderosis, erythrophagocytosis, portal triaditis, cholestasis, focal necrosis, focal fibrosis, extramedullary erythropoiesis, and fatty changes. A study on 58 Nigerian SCA liver specimens at autopsy from patients 3–45 years old revealed the previous findings with sinusoidal distension, hemosiderosis, and erythrophagocytosis in nearly all specimens. The livers from the older patients (30–45 years) showed severe hemosiderosis, chronic inflammation, pigment stones, and fatty change [432].

– *Liver and thalassemia:*

Thalassemia is especially prevalent in North Africa and the Mediterranean Basin. The repeated blood transfusion in these patients carries the risk of transfusion-associated hepatitis. Children with thalassemia and HCV are more likely to develop progressive liver disease, due to the coexistence of hepatic iron overload. Significant fibrosis and cirrhosis are more common at an earlier age [*refer to HCV in patients with hemoglobinopathies*].

- *Vascular liver disease (also refer to Chap. 18):*

– *Veno-occlusive disease (VOD):*

Aetiology in Africa: VOD is a form of hepatic venous obstruction associated in Africa with ingestion of toxins (pyrrolizidine alkaloids) found in food or herbal teas with subsequent toxic injury to the sinusoidal endothelium, leading to occlusion of centrilobular veins and hepatic venules, sinusoidal congestion, and hepatocyte necrosis [433].

Epidemiology in Africa: South Africa and the Middle East [434].

Clinical features: are similar to those in Budd-Chiari syndrome, with a rapid onset of painful hepatomegaly and ascites. If the child survives the acute stage, cirrhosis and portal hypertension may develop [434].

Treatment: largely supportive and includes the administration of diuretics and *N*-acetylcysteine. Thrombolytic therapy is of limited benefit, but defibrotide, a drug with antithrombotic and thrombolytic properties, has shown promise in uncontrolled studies [435]. Low-dose heparin and ursodeoxycholic acid may have prophylactic roles [436, 437].

– *VOD and hematopoietic stem cell transplantation (HSCT):*

VOD/sinusoidal obstruction syndrome (SOS) can occur as a serious, early complication of HSCT, severe and very severe forms of which are associated with a high mortality rate. Risk factors in Africa include iron overload in thalassaemia patients, some hereditary metabolic disorders due to consanguinity, and infection with HBV or HCV [438]. The onset is usually manifest by jaundice, abdominal pain, ascites, and weight gain within 1 month of grafting, but one-third of patients are asymptomatic [434, 438].

Recommendations include prophylaxis with defibrotide and/or ursodeoxycholic acid in patients at an increased risk of VOD/SOS and treatment with defibrotide for patients with severe/very severe forms [438].

- *African herbal traditional medicine and liver disease:*

Traditional herbal medicines are widely used in Africa especially SSA and the Middle East with a strong belief of patients in traditional medicine practitioners to the extent that, in most instances, patients first seek medical advice with them before doctors with a false fixed belief of the perceived benefits of the herbs and being harmless [439].

In the 1990s an estimated 80% of Ugandans living in rural villages used traditional healers for primary health care [440]. Herbal hepatotoxicity has been recognized for many years, and new agents are constantly being identified [439, 441]. Some potentially hepatotoxic traditional herbal medicines used in Uganda and sub-Saharan Africa include *Hoodia gordonii* [442], kava [443], *Phytolacca dioica* [444], and herbs from the Asteraceae family [445].

The varied manifestations of liver injury include steatosis, acute and chronic hepatitis, hepatic fibrosis, zonal or diffuse hepatic necrosis, bile duct injury, veno-occlusive disease [refer also to vascular liver disease in Africa], and acute liver failure requiring liver transplantation and carcinogenesis [439]. Ingestion of plants containing pyrrolizidine alkaloids caused outbreaks of veno-occlusive liver disease in Egypt and South Africa [446, 447]. Pyrrolizidine alkaloids are inert until dehydrogenation by cytochrome P450 3A4 (CYP3A4) in the liver [448], where reactive toxic pyrrolic and *N*-oxide metabolites directly damage liver sinusoidal endothelial cells and hepatocytes [449]. Pyrroles cause chromosomal damage in a dose-dependent manner, resulting in an inflammatory response that culminates in fibrin deposition [445, 449, 450].

Patients usually use these herbs along with their prescribed conventional medicines; potential interactions between them may interfere with patient management. Concurrent use of such products is not often disclosed unless specifically sought after and can lead to perpetuation of the liver injury [441].

Current analytic methods such as high-performance liquid chromatography, gas chromatography-mass spectrometry, and immunoassays can provide identification of the toxins in these plants. In most cases of plant poisoning, treatment continues to be only of symptoms, with few specific antidotes available [439, 451]. Counseling about herb use should be part of routine health counseling, continued public education, and physician awareness, and more pharmaceutic quality control is required to tackle this growing problem.

References

1. Mackenjee MK, Coovadia HM. Chronic liver disease in black children in Durban, South Africa. Ann Trop Paediatr. 1984;4(3):165–9.
2. Suchy FJ. Approach to the infant with cholestasis. In: Suchy FJ, Sokol RJ, Balistreri WF, editors. Liver disease in children. 3rd ed: Cambridge University Press; 2007. p. 179–89.
3. Nio M, Ohi R, Miyano T, et al. Five- and 10-year survival rates after surgery for biliary atresia: a report from the Japanese Biliary Atresia Registry. J Pediatr Surg. 2003;38:997–1000.
4. Motala C, Ireland JD, Hill ID, Bowie MD. Cholestatic disorders of infancy—aetiology and outcome. J Trop Pediatr. 1990;36(5):218–22.
5. Mshelbwala PM, Sabiu L, Lukong CS, Ameh EA. Management of biliary atresia in Nigeria: the ongoing challenge. Ann Trop Paediatr. 2007;27(1):69–73.
6. Bouyahia O, Khelifi I, Mazigh SM, Gharsallah L, Chaouachi B, Hamzaoui M, Barsaoui S, Ben Becher S, Bousnina S, Boukthir S, El Gharbi AS. Cholestasis in infants: a study of the Children's Hospital of Tunisia. Tunis Med. 2008;86(2):128–35.
7. Amer OT, Abd El-Rahman HA, Sherief LM, Hussein HF, Zeid AF, Abd El-Aziz AM. Role of some viral infections in neonatal cholestasis. Egypt J Immunol. 2004;11(2):149–55.
8. Giovannoni I, Santorelli FM, Candusso M, Di Rocco M, Bellacchio E, Callea F, Francalanci P. Two novel mutations in African and Asian children with progressive familial intrahepatic cholestasis type 3. Dig Liver Dis. 2011;43(7):567–70.
9. Akinyinka OO, Falade AG, Akinbami FO, Alli T, Atalabi M, Irabor D, Ogunbiyi O, Faweya AG, Madarikan BA, Onojobi-Daniel A, Johnson AO. Choledochal cysts in African infants: a report of 3 cases and a review of the literature. Trop Gastroenterol. 2005;26(1):34–6.
10. Olynyk JK, Cullen DJ, Aquilia S, et al. A population-based study of the clinical expression of the hemochromatosis gene. N Engl J Med. 1999;341:718–24.
11. Franco E, Meleleo C, Serino L, Sorbara D, Zaratti L. Hepatitis A: epidemiology and prevention in developing countries. World J Hepatol. 2012;4(3):68–73.
12. Quak S-H, Sibal A, Chang M-H. Liver disease in the developing world. In: Kelly D, editor. Diseases of the liver and biliary system in children. 3rd ed: Wiley-Blackwell Publishing; 2008. p. 553–76.
13. Ott JJ, Stevens GA, Groeger J, Wiersma ST. Global epidemiology of hepatitis B virus infection: new estimates of age-specific HBsAg seroprevalence and endemicity. Vaccine. 2012;30:2212–9.
14. Mohd Hanafiah K, Groeger J, Flaxman AD, Wiersma ST. Global epidemiology of hepatitis C virus infection: new estimates of age-specific antibody to HCV seroprevalence. Hepatology. 2013;57:1333–42.
15. Lemoine M, Eholié S, Lacombe K. Reducing the neglected burden of viral hepatitis in Africa: strategies for a global approach. J Hepatol. 2015;62(2):469–76.
16. Lozano R, Naghavi M, Foreman K, Lim S, Shibuya K, Aboyans V, et al. Global and regional mortality from 235 causes of death for 20

16. age groups in 1990 and 2010: a systematic analysis for the Global Burden of Disease Study 2010. Lancet. 2012;380:2095–128.
17. WHO. Viral hepatitis Report by the Secretariat. http://apps.who.int/gb/ebwha/pdf_files/WHA63/A63_15-en.pdf. Last accessed 20 Nov 2017.
18. WHO. Guidelines for the prevention, care and treatment of persons with chronic hepatitis B infection March 2015. http://apps.who.int/iris/bitstream/10665/154590/1/9789241549059_eng.pdf. Last accessed 29 Nov 2017.
19. Jacobsen K, Koopman JS. The effects of socioeconomic development on worldwide hepatitis A virus seroprevalence patterns. Int J Epidemiol. 2005;34(3):600–9.
20. WHO. The global prevalence of hepatitis A virus infection and susceptibility: a systematic review. whqlibdoc.who.int/hq/2010/WHO_IVB_10.01_eng.pdf. Last accessed 28 Nov 2017.
21. Tufenkeji H. Hepatitis A shifting epidemiology in the Middle East and Africa. Vaccine. 2000;18(Suppl 1):S65–7.
22. Johnston L. Hepatitis A and B—a brief overview. SA Pharm J. 2010;77:40–5.
23. Rezig D, Ouneissa R, Mhiri L, Mejri S, Haddad-Boubaker S, Ben Alaya N, Triki H. [Seroprevalences of hepatitis A and E infections in Tunisia]. Pathol Biol (Paris). 2008;56:148–53.
24. Post-2015 sustainable development agenda. https://sustainabledevelopment.un.org/post2015. Last accessed 2 Dec 2017.
25. Jacobsen KH. Hepatitis A virus in West Africa: is an epidemiological transition beginning? Niger Med J. 2014;55(4):279–84.
26. Wasley A, Fiore A, Bell BP. Hepatitis A in the era of vaccination. Epidemiol Rev. 2006;28(1):101–11.
27. Mohd Hanafiah K, Jacobsen KH, Wiersma ST. Challenges to mapping the health risk of hepatitis A virus infection. Int J Health Geogr. 2011;10:57.
28. Jacobsen KH, Wiersma ST. Hepatitis A virus seroprevalence by age and world region, 1990 and 2005. Vaccine. 2010;28(41):6653–7.
29. Letaief A, Kaabia N, Gaha R, Bousaadia A, Lazrag F, Trabelsi H, Ghannem H, Jemni L. Age-specific seroprevalence of hepatitis a among school children in central Tunisia. Am J Trop Med Hyg. 2005;73:40–3.
30. Hadler SC. Global impact of hepatitis A infection: changing patterns. In: Hollinger FB, Lemon SM, Margolis H, editors. Viral hepatitis and liver disease. Baltimore: Williams & Wilkins; 1991. p. 14–20.
31. Kanyenda TJ, Abdullahi LH, Hussey GD, Kagina BM. Epidemiology of hepatitis A virus in Africa among persons aged 1-10 years: a systematic review protocol. Syst Rev. 2015;4:129.
32. Liu J, Fan D. Hepatitis B in China. Lancet. 2007;369:1582–3.
33. Torpy JM, Burke AE, Golub RM. JAMA patient page. Hepatitis B. JAMA. 2011;305:1500.
34. Yang SG, Wang B, Chen P, Yu CB, Deng M, Yao J, Zhu CX, Ren JJ, Wu W, Ju B, Shen JF, Chen Y, Li MD, Ruan B, Li L. Effectiveness of HBV vaccination in infants and prediction of HBV prevalence trend under new vaccination plan: findings of a large-scale investigation. PLoS One. 2012;7(10):e47808.
35. Liaw YF, Chu CM. Hepatitis B virus infection. Lancet. 2009;373:582–92.
36. Dienstag JL. Hepatitis B virus infection. N Engl J Med. 2008;359:1486–500.
37. Kane M. Global programme for control of hepatitis B infection. Vaccine. 1995;13(Suppl 1):S47–9.
38. Lee WM. Hepatitis B virus infection. N Engl J Med. 1997;337:1733–45.
39. Edmunds WJ, Medley GF, Nokes DJ, O'Callaghan CJ, Whittle HC, et al. Epidemiological patterns of hepatitis B virus (HBV) in highly endemic areas. Epidemiol Infect. 1996;117:313–25.
40. Lok AS, McMahon BJ. Chronic hepatitis B (AASLD practice guidelines). Hepatology. 2001;34:1225–41.
41. Peebles K, Nchimba L, Chilengi R, Bolton Moore C, Mubiana-Mbewe M, Vinikoor MJ. Pediatric HIV-HBV coinfection in Lusaka, Zambia: prevalence and short-term treatment outcomes. J Trop Pediatr. 2015;61(6):464–7.
42. Ola SO, Odaibo GN. Alfa-feto protein, HCV and HBV infections in Nigerian patients with primary hepatocellular carcinoma. Niger Med Pract. 2007;51:33–5.
43. Lesi OA, Kehinde MO, Omilabu SA. Prevalence of the HBeAg in Nigerian patients with chronic liver disease. Nig Q Hosp Med. 2004;14:1–4.
44. Ndububa DA, Ojo OS, Adetiloye VA, Durosinmi MA, Olasode BJ, Famurewa OC, et al. Chronic hepatitis in Nigerian patients: a study of 70 biopsy-proven cases. West Afr J Med. 2005;24:107–11.
45. Musa BM, Bussell S, Borodo MM, Samaila AA, Femi OL. Prevalence of hepatitis B virus infection in Nigeria, 2000-2013: a systematic review and meta-analysis. Niger J Clin Pract. 2015;18(2):163–72.
46. Perz JF, Armstrong GL, Farrington LA, Hutin YJ, Bell BP. The contributions of hepatitis B virus and hepatitis C virus infections to cirrhosis and primary liver cancer worldwide. J Hepatol. 2006;45:529–38.
47. Firnhaber C, Reyneke A, Schulze D, Malope B, Maskew M, MacPhail P, et al. The prevalence of hepatitis B co-infection in a South African urban government HIV clinic. S Afr Med J. 2008;98:541–4.
48. Dongdem JT, Kampo S, Soyiri IN, Asebga PN, Ziem JB, Sagoe K. Prevalence of hepatitis B virus infection among blood donors at the Tamale Teaching Hospital, Ghana (2009). BMC Res Notes. 2012;5:115.
49. Fomulu NJ, Morfaw FL, Torimiro JN, Nana P, Koh MV, William T. Prevalence, correlates and pattern of Hepatitis B among antenatal clinic attenders in Yaounde-Cameroon: is perinatal transmission of HBV neglected in Cameroon? BMC Pregnancy Childbirth. 2013;13:158.
50. WHO. Hepatitis B Global Infection rate. 2006. http://www.pkids.org/files/pdf/phr/02-09.globalhbv.pdf. Last accessed 11 Dec 2017.
51. Attia MA. Prevalence of hepatitis B and C in Egypt and Africa. Antivir Ther. 1998;3:1–9. PMID: 10726051.
52. El-Zayadi A, Hepatitis B. Virus infection the Egyptian situation. Arab J Gastroenterol. 2007;8:94–8.
53. WHO/UNICEF immunization summary. Geneva, Switzerland: World Health Organization; 2007. http://whqlibdoc.who.int/hq/2007/who_ivb_2007_eng.pdf. Last accessed 26 Nov 2017.
54. WHO. Guidelines for the prevention, care and treatment of persons with chronic hepatitis b infection (March 2015). http://apps.who.int/iris/bitstream/10665/154590/1/9789241549059_eng.pdf. Last accessed 28 Nov 2017.
55. McMahon BJ. The natural history of chronic hepatitis B virus infection. Semin Liver Dis. 2004;24(Suppl 1):17–21.
56. Bhave S, Bavdekar A, Madan Z, et al. Evaluation of immunogenicity and tolerability of a live attenuated hepatitis a vaccine in Indian children. Indian Pediatr. 2006;43:983–7.
57. Mast EE, Weinbaum CM, Fiore AE, Alter MJ, Bell BP, Finelli L, Rodewald LE, Douglas JM, Janssen RS, Ward JW. A comprehensive immunization strategy to eliminate transmission of hepatitis B virus infection in the United States: recommendations of the Advisory Committee on Immunization Practices (ACIP) Part II: immunization of adults. MMWR Recomm Rep. 2006;55:1–33; quiz CE1-4.
58. Stevens CE, Beasley RP, Tsui J, Lee WC. Vertical transmission of hepatitis B antigen in Taiwan. N Engl J Med. 1975;292:771–4.
59. Feret E, Larouze B, Diop B, et al. Epidemiology of hepatitis B virus infection in the rural community of Tip, Senegal. Am J Epidemiol. 1987;125:140–9.

60. Beasley RP, Hwang LY, Lin CC, et al. Incidence of hepatitis B virus infection in preschool children in Taiwan. J Infect Dis. 1982;146:198–204.
61. Hsu SC, Chang MH, Ni YH, et al. Horizontal transmission of hepatitis B virus in children. J Pediatr Gastroenterol Nutr. 1993;292:771–4.
62. WHO. Viral hepatitis policy and practice: report of a survey of WHO Member States, 2010. http://www.who.int/immunization/topics/hepatitis_b_survey_2010/en/. Last accessed 1 Dec 2017.
63. Chiang CJ, Yang YW, You SL, Lai MS, Chen CJ. Thirty-year outcomes of the national hepatitis B immunization program in Taiwan. JAMA. 2013;310:974–6.
64. Peto TJ, Mendy ME, Lowe Y, Webb EL, Whittle HC, Hall AJ. Efficacy and effectiveness of infant vaccination against chronic hepatitis B in the Gambia Hepatitis Intervention Study (1986–90) and in the nationwide immunization program. BMC Infect Dis. 2014;14:7.
65. GAVI. 2010. http://www.gavialliance.org/support/nvs/hepb/.
66. WHO. Global immunization data. http://www.who.int/immunization/monitoring_surveillance/global_immunization_data.pdf. Last accessed 2 Dec 2017.
67. Wong VC, Ip HM, Reesink HW, Lelie PN, Reerink-Brongers EE, Yeung CY, Ma HK. Prevention of the HBsAg carrier state in newborn infants of mothers who are chronic carriers of HBsAg and HBeAg by administration of hepatitis-B vaccine and hepatitis-B immunoglobulin. Double-blind randomized placebo-controlled study. Lancet. 1984;1:921–6.
68. Mast EE, Margolis HS, Fiore AE, Brink EW, Goldstein ST, Wang SA, Moyer LA, Bell BP, Alter MJ. A comprehensive immunization strategy to eliminate transmission of hepatitis B virus infection in the United States: recommendations of the Advisory Committee on Immunization Practices (ACIP) part 1: immunization of infants, children, and adolescents. MMWR Recomm Rep. 2005;54:1–31.
69. Wiseman E, Fraser MA, Holden S, Glass A, Kidson BL, Heron LG, Maley MW, Ayres A, Locarnini SA, Levy MT. Perinatal transmission of hepatitis B virus: an Australian experience. Med J Aust. 2009;190:489–92.
70. Rutala WA, Weber DJ. Healthcare Infection Control Practices Advisory Committee (HICPAC). Guideline for disinfection and sterilization in healthcare facilities, 2008. http://stacks.cdc.gov/view/cdc/11560/.
71. http://www.stridesarco.com/pdf/pressrelease/2013/Strides_Arcolab_Product_Approval_PR_August_1_2013.pdf. Last accessed 24 June 2014.
72. Hainaut P, Boyle P. Curbing the liver cancer epidemic in Africa. Lancet. 2008;371:367–8.
73. El-Shabrawi MH, Kamal NM. Burden of pediatric hepatitis C. World J Gastroenterol. 2013;19(44):7880–8.
74. Uhanova J, Tate RB, Tataryn DJ, Minuk GY. A population based study of the epidemiology of hepatitis C in a North American population. J Hepatol. 2012;57:736–42.
75. Guerra J, Garenne M, Mohamed MK, Fontanet A. HCV burden of infection in Egypt: results from a nationwide survey. J Viral Hepat. 2012;19:560–7.
76. Kamal SM, Nasser IA. Hepatitis C genotype 4: what we know and what we don't yet know. Hepatology. 2008;47:1371–83.
77. Barakat SH, El-Bashir N. Hepatitis C virus infection among healthy Egyptian children: prevalence and risk factors. J Viral Hepat. 2011;18:779–84.
78. Madhava V, Burgess C, Drucker E. Epidemiology of chronic hepatitis C virus infection in sub-Saharan Africa. Lancet Infect Dis. 2002;2:293–302.
79. Nelson PK, Mathers BM, Cowie B, Hagan H, Des Jarlais D, Horyniak D, et al. Global epidemiology of hepatitis B and hepatitis C in people who inject drugs: results of systematic reviews. Lancet. 2011;378:571–83.
80. Barth RE, Huijgen Q, Taljaard J, Hoepelman AI. Hepatitis B/C and HIV in sub-Saharan Africa: an association between highly prevalent infectious diseases. A systematic review and meta-analysis. Int J Infect Dis. 2010;14:e1024–31.
81. Pybus OG, Barnes E, Taggart R, Lemey P, Markov PV, Rasachak B, Syhavong B, Phetsouvanah R, Sheridan I, Humphreys IS, Lu L, Newton PN, Klenerman P. Genetic history of hepatitis C virus in East Asia. J Virol. 2009;83:1071–82.
82. Lemoine M, Thursz M. Hepatitis C a global issue: access to care and new therapeutic and preventive approaches in resource-constrained areas. Semin Liver Dis. 2014;34:89–97.
83. Global surveillance and control of hepatitis C. Report of a WHO Consultation organized in collaboration with the Viral Hepatitis Prevention Board, Antwerp, Belgium. J Viral Hepat. 1999;6:35–47.
84. Ray SC, Arthur RR, Carella A, Bukh J, Thomas DL. Genetic epidemiology of hepatitis C virus throughout Egypt. J Infect Dis. 2000;182(3):698–707.
85. Kamal S, Madwar M, Bianchi L, Tawil AE, Fawzy R, Peters T, Rasenack JW. Clinical, virological and histopathological features: long-term follow-up in patients with chronic hepatitis C co-infected with S. mansoni. Liver. 2000;20(4):281–9.
86. Esmat G, Hashem M, El-Raziky M, El-Akel W, El-Naghy S, El-Koofy N, El-Sayed R, Ahmed R, Atta-Allah M, Hamid MA, El-Kamary SS, El-Karaksy H. Risk factors for hepatitis C virus acquisition and predictors of persistence among Egyptian children. Liver Int. 2012;32:449–56.
87. Hashem M, El-Karaksy H, Shata MT, Sobhy M, Helmy H, El-Naghi S, Galal G, Ali ZZ, Esmat G, Abdelwahab SF, Strickland GT, El-Kamary SS. Strong hepatitis C virus (HCV)-specific cell-mediated immune responses in the absence of viremia or antibodies among uninfected siblings of HCV chronically infected children. J Infect Dis. 2011;203:854–61.
88. Hauri A, Hutin Y, Armstrong G. Contaminated injections in health care settings. In: Ezzati M, Mopez A, Rodgers A, Murray C, editors. Comparative quantification of health risks, 2. Geneva: WHO; 2004. p. 1803–50.
89. Okwen MP, Ngem BY, Alomba FA, Capo MV, Reid SR, Ewang EC. Uncovering high rates of unsafe injection equipment reuse in rural Cameroon: validation of a survey instrument that probes for specific misconceptions. Harm Reduct J. 2011;8:4.
90. Kandeel AM, Talaat M, Afifi SA, El-Sayed NM, Abdel Fadeel MA, Hajjeh RA, et al. Case control study to identify risk factors for acute hepatitis C virus infection in Egypt. BMC Infect Dis. 2012;12:294.
91. Paez Jimenez A, Sharaf Eldin N, Rimlinger F, El-Daly M, El-Hariri H, El-Hoseiny M, et al. HCV iatrogenic and intrafamilial transmission in Greater Cairo, Egypt. Gut. 2010;59:1554–60.
92. Frank C, Mohamed MK, Strickland GT, Lavanchy D, Arthur RR, Magder LS, El Khoby T, Abdel-Wahab Y, Aly Ohn ES, Anwar W, Sallam I. The role of parenteral antischistosomal therapy in the spread of hepatitis C virus in Egypt. Lancet. 2000;355:887–91.
93. Pepin J, Labbe AC, Mamadou-Yaya F, Mbelesso P, Mbadingai S, Deslandes S, et al. Iatrogenic transmission of human T cell lymphotropic virus type 1 and hepatitis C virus through parenteral treatment and chemoprophylaxis of sleeping sickness in colonial Equatorial Africa. Clin Infect Dis. 2010;51:777–84.
94. Njouom R, Caron M, Besson G, Ndong-Atome GR, Makuwa M, Pouillot R, et al. Phylogeography, risk factors and genetic history of hepatitis C virus in Gabon, central Africa. PLoS One. 2012;7:e42002.
95. Raguin G, Lepretre A, Ba I, Ndoye I, Toufik A, Brucker G, et al. Drug use and HIV in West Africa: a neglected epidemic. Tropical Med Int Health. 2011;16:1131–3.

96. Bowring AL, Luhmann N, Pont S, Debaulieu C, Derozier S, Asouab F, et al. An urgent need to scale-up injecting drug harm reduction services in Tanzania: prevalence of blood-borne viruses among drug users in Temeke District, Dar-es-Salaam, 2011. Int J Drug Policy. 2013;24:78–81.

97. Wedemeyer H, Duberg AS, Buti M, Rosenberg WM, Frankova S, Esmat G, et al. Strategies to manage hepatitis C virus (HCV) disease burden. J Viral Hepat. 2014;21:60–89.

98. Chhatwal J, Wang X, Ayer T, Kabiri M, Chung RT, Hur C, Donohue JM, Roberts MS, Kanwal F. Hepatitis C Disease Burden in the United States in the era of oral direct-acting antivirals. Hepatology. 2016;64(5):1442–50.

99. Gane EJ, Hyland RH, An D, Svarovskaia E, Pang PS, Brainard D, Stedman CA. Efficacy of ledipasvir and sofosbuvir, with or without ribavirin, for 12 weeks in patients with HCV genotype 3 or 6 infection. Gastroenterology. 2015;149(6):1454–61.

100. Callaway E. Hepatitis C drugs not reaching poor. Nature. 2014;508:295–6.

101. Balistreri WF, Murray KF, Rosenthal P, Bansal S, Lin CH, Kersey K, Massetto B, Zhu Y, Kanwar B, German P, Svarovskaia E, Brainard DM, Wen J, Gonzalez-Peralta RP, Jonas MM, Schwarz K. The safety and effectiveness of ledipasvir-sofosbuvir in adolescents 12-17 years old with hepatitis C virus genotype 1 infection. Hepatology. 2017;66(2):371–8.

102. El-Shabrawi M, Abdo AM, El-Khayat H, Yakoot M. Shortened 8 weeks course of dual sofosbuvir/daclatasvir therapy in adolescent patients, with chronic hepatitis C infection. J Pediatr Gastroenterol Nutr. 2018;66(3):425–7.

103. Njai HF, Shimakawa Y, Ferguson L, Sanneh B, Dalessandro U, Njie N, et al. Performance of two rapid tests of hepatitis B surface antigen for screening hepatitis B virus (HBV) infection in the rural communities of The Gambia. J Hepatol. 2014;60:S522.

104. Tagny CT, Mbanya D, Murphy EL, Lefrere JJ, Laperche S. Screening for hepatitis C virus infection in a high prevalence country by an antigen/antibody combination assay versus a rapid test. J Virol Methods. 2014;199:119–23.

105. Angelico M, Renganathan E, Gandin C, Fathy M, Profili MC, Refai W, De Santis A, Nagi A, Amin G, Capocaccia L, Callea F, Rapicetta M, Badr G, Rocchi G. Chronic liver disease in the Alexandria governorate, Egypt: contribution of schistosomiasis and hepatitis virus infections. J Hepatol. 1997;26(2):236–43.

106. Koshy A, al-Nakib B, al-Mufti S, Madda JP, Hira PR. Anti-HCV-positive cirrhosis associated with schistosomiasis. Am J Gastroenterol. 1993;88(9):1428–31.

107. Gad A, Tanaka E, Orii K, Rokuhara A, Nooman Z, Serwah AH, Shoair M, Yoshizawa K, Kiyosawa K. Relationship between hepatitis C virus infection and schistosomal liver disease: not simply an additive effect. J Gastroenterol. 2001;36(11):753–8.

108. El-Kady IM, El-Masry SA, Badra G, Halafawy KA. Different cytokine patterns in patients coinfected with hepatitis C virus and Schistosoma mansoni. Egypt J Immunol. 2004;11(1):23–9.

109. El-Kady IM, Lotfy M, Badra G, El-Masry S, Waked I. Interleukin (IL)-4, IL-10, IL-18 and IFN-gamma cytokines pattern in patients with combined hepatitis C virus and Schistosoma mansoni infections. Scand J Immunol. 2005;61(1):87–91.

110. El-Shazly Y, Abdel-Salam AF, Abdel-Ghaffar A, Mohran Z, Saleh SM. Schistosomiasis as an important determining factor for the response of Egyptian patients with chronic hepatitis C to therapy with recombinant human alpha-2 interferon. Trans R Soc Trop Med Hyg. 1994;88(2):229–31.

111. Attallah AM, Abdallah SO, Albannan MS, Omran MM, Attallah AA, Farid K. Impact of hepatitis C virus/Schistosoma mansoni coinfection on the circulating levels of HCV-NS4 protein and extracellular-matrix deposition in patients with different hepatic fibrosis stages. Am J Trop Med Hyg. 2016;95(5):1044–50.

112. Origa R, Ponti ML, Filosa A, Galeota Lanza A, Piga A, Saracco GM, Pinto V, Picciotto A, Rigano P, Madonia S, Rosso R, D'Ascola D, Cappellini MD, D'Ambrosio R, Tartaglione I, De Franceschi L, Gianesin B, Di Marco V, Forni GL, Italy for THAlassemia and hepatitis C Advance—Società Italiana Talassemie ed Emoglobinopatie (ITHACA-SITE). Treatment of hepatitis C virus infection with direct-acting antiviral drugs is safe and effective in patients with hemoglobinopathies. Am J Hematol. 2017;92(12):1349–55.

113. Radjef N, Gordien E, Ivaniushina V, Gault E, Anais P, Drugan T, Trinchet JC, Roulot D, Tamby M, Milinkovitch MC, Dény P. Molecular phylogenetic analyses indicate a wide and ancient radiation of African hepatitis delta virus, suggesting a delta virus genus of at least seven major clades. J Virol. 2004;78:2537–44.

114. Taylor J, Pelchat M. Origin of hepatitis delta virus. Future Microbiol. 2010;5:393–402.

115. Andernach IE, Leiss LV, Tarnagda ZS, Tahita MC, Otegbayo JA, Forbi JC, Omilabu S, Gouandjika-Vasilache I, Komas NP, Mbah OP, Muller CP. Characterization of hepatitis delta virus in sub-Saharan Africa. J Clin Microbiol. 2014;52(5):1629–36.

116. WHO. Hepatitis B fact sheet (WHO/CDS/CSR/LYO/2002.2). http://www.who.int/csr/disease/hepatitis/HepatitisB_whocdscsrlyo2002_2.pdf. Last accessed 3 Dec 2017.

117. Foupouapouognigni Y, Noah DN, Sartre MT, Njouom R. High prevalence and predominance of hepatitis delta virus genotype 1 infection in Cameroon. J Clin Microbiol. 2011;49:1162–4.

118. Makuwa M, Mintsa-Ndong A, Souquiere S, Nkoghé D, Leroy EM, Kazanji M. Prevalence and molecular diversity of hepatitis B virus and hepatitis delta virus in urban and rural populations in northern Gabon in central Africa. J Clin Microbiol. 2009;47:2265–8.

119. Makuwa M, Caron M, Souquiere S, Malonga-Mouelet G, Mahe A, Kazanji M. Prevalence and genetic diversity of hepatitis B and delta viruses in pregnant women in Gabon: molecular evidence that hepatitis delta virus clade 8 originates from and is endemic in central Africa. J Clin Microbiol. 2008;46:754–6.

120. Mansour W, Malick FZ, Sidiya A, Ishagh E, Chekaraou MA, Veillon P, Ducancelle A, Brichler S, Le Gal F, Lo B, Gordien E, Lunel-Fabiani F. Prevalence, risk factors, and molecular epidemiology of hepatitis B and hepatitis delta virus in pregnant women and in patients in Mauritania. J Med Virol. 2012;84:1186–98.

121. Mansour W, Bollahi MA, Hamed CT, Brichler S, Le Gal F, Ducancelle A, Lô B, Gordien E, Rosenheim M, Lunel F. Virological and epidemiological features of hepatitis delta infection among blood donors in Nouakchott, Mauritania. J Clin Virol. 2012;55:12–6.

122. Lunel-Fabiani F, Mansour W, Amar AO, Aye M, Le Gal F, Malick FZ, Baïdy L, Brichler S, Veillon P, Ducancelle A, Gordien E, Rosenheim M. Impact of hepatitis B and delta virus co-infection on liver disease in Mauritania: a cross sectional study. J Infect. 2013;67:448–57.

123. Cunha L, Plouzeau C, Ingrand P, Gudo JP, Ingrand I, Mondlane J, Beauchant M, Agius G. Use of replacement blood donors to study the epidemiology of major blood-borne viruses in the general population of Maputo, Mozambique. J Med Virol. 2007;79:1832–40.

124. Nwokediuko SC, Ijeoma U. Seroprevalence of antibody to HDV in Nigerians with hepatitis B virus-related liver diseases. Niger J Clin Pract. 2009;12:439–42.

125. Olal SO, Akere A, Otegbayo JA, Odaibo GN, Olaleye DO, Afolabi NB, Bamgboye EA. Are patients with primary hepatocellular carcinoma infectious of hepatitis B, C and D viruses? Afr J Med Med Sci. 2012;41(Suppl):187–91.

126. Onyekwere CA, Audu RA, Duro-Emmanuel F, Ige FA. Hepatitis D infection in Nigeria. Indian J Gastroenterol. 2012;31:34–5.

127. Diop-Ndiaye H, Touré-Kane C, Etard JF, Lô G, Diaw P, Ngom-Gueye NF, Gueye PM, Ba-Fall K, Ndiaye I, Sow PS, Delaporte E, Mboup S. Hepatitis B, C seroprevalence and delta viruses in

HIV-1 Senegalese patients at HAART initiation (retrospective study). J Med Virol. 2008;80:1332–6.
128. Le Gal F, Gault E, Ripault MP, Serpaggi J, Trinchet JC, Gordien E, Dény P. Eighth major clade for hepatitis delta virus. Emerg Infect Dis. 2006;12:1447–50.
129. Le Gal F, Badur S, Hawajri NA, Akyüz F, Kaymakoglu S, Brichler S, Zoulim F, Gordien E, Gault E, Dény P. Current hepatitis delta virus type 1 (HDV1) infections in central and eastern Turkey indicate a wide genetic diversity that is probably linked to different HDV1 origins. Arch Virol. 2012;157:647–59.
130. Smedile A, Rosina F, Saracco G, Chiaberge E, Lattore V, Fabiano A, Brunetto MR, Verme G, Rizzetto M, Bonino F. Hepatitis B virus replication modulates pathogenesis of hepatitis D virus in chronic hepatitis D. Hepatology. 1991;13:413–6.
131. Mushahwar IK. Hepatitis E virus: molecular virology, clinical manifestations, diagnosis, transmission, epidemiology, prevention. J Med Virol. 2008;80:646–58.
132. Aggarwal R, Jameel S. Hepatitis E. Hepatology. 2011;54:2218–26.
133. Emerson SU, Purcell RH. Running like water—the omnipresence of hepatitis E. N Engl J Med. 2004;351:2367–8.
134. Verghese VP, Robinson JL. A systematic review of hepatitis E virus infection in children. Clin Infect Dis. 2014;59(5):689–97.
135. Martinson FE, Marfo VY, DeGraaf J. Hepatitis E virus seroprevalence in children living in rural Ghana. West Afr J Med. 1999;18:76–9.
136. Hodges M, Sanders E, Aitken C. Seroprevalence of hepatitis markers; HAV, HBV, HCV and HEV amongst primary school children in Freetown, Sierra Leone. West Afr J Med. 1998;17:36–7.
137. Fix AD, Abdel-Hamid M, Purcell R, et al. Prevalence of antibodies to hepatitis E in two rural Egyptian communities. Am J Trop Med Hyg. 2000;62:519–23.
138. Hyams KC, McCarthy MC, Kaur M, et al. Acute sporadic hepatitis E in children living in Cairo, Egypt. J Med Virol. 1992;37:274–7.
139. El-Zimaity DMT, Hyams KC, Imam IZE, et al. Acute sporadic hepatitis E in an Egyptian pediatric population. Am J Trop Med Hyg. 1993;48:372–6.
140. Khurroo MS. Discovery of hepatitis E: the epidemic non-A, non-B hepatitis 30 years down the memory lane. Virus Res. 2011;161:3–14.
141. Colson P, Coze C, Galian P, Mireille H, De Micco P, Tamalet C. Transfusion-associated hepatitis E, France. Emerg Infect Dis. 2007;13:648–9.
142. Arora NK, Panda SK, Nanda SK, et al. Hepatitis E infection: study of an outbreak. J Gastroenterol Hepatol. 1999;14:572–7.
143. Guthmann JP, Klovstad H, Boccia D, et al. A large outbreak of hepatitis E among a displaced population in Darfur, Sudan, 2004: the role of water treatment methods. Clin Infect Dis. 2006;42:1685–91.
144. Arankalle VA, Tsarev SA, Chadha MS, et al. Age-specific prevalence of antibodies to hepatitis A and E in Pune, India, 1982 and 1992. J Infect Dis. 1995;171:447–50.
145. Labrique AB, Shikdar SS, Krain LJ, et al. Hepatitis E: a vaccine-preventable cause of maternal deaths. Emerg Infect Dis. 2012;18:1401–4.
146. Hooks SB, Billings CJ, Herrera JL. Hepatitis E virus infection. Pract Gastroenterol. 2009;33:11–7.
147. El Sayed Zaki M, El Aal AA, Badawy A, El-Deeb DR, El-Kheir NY. Clinicolaboratory study of mother-to-neonate transmission of hepatitis E virus in Egypt. Am J Clin Pathol. 2013;140(5):721–6.
148. Naicker P, Sayed Y. Non-B HIV-1 subtypes in sub-Saharan Africa: impact of subtype on protease inhibitor efficacy. Biol Chem. 2014;395(10):1151–61.
149. Vermund SH, Blevins M, Moon TD, José E, Moiane L, Tique JA, Sidat M, Ciampa PJ, Shepherd BE, Vaz LME. Poor clinical outcomes for HIV infected children on antiretroviral therapy in rural Mozambique: need for program quality improvement and community engagement. PLoS One. 2014;9(10):e110116.
150. Theodoratou E, McAllister DA, Reed C, Adeloye DO, Rudan I, Muhe LM, Madhi SA, Campbell H, Nair H. Global, regional, and national estimates of pneumonia burden in HIV-infected children in 2010: a meta-analysis and modelling study. Lancet Infect Dis. 2014;14(12):1250–8.
151. Rosenthal P. Neonatal hepatitis and congenital infections. In: Suchy FJ, Sokol RJ, Balistreri WF, editors. Liver disease in children. 3rd ed: Cambridge University Press; 2007. p. 232–46.
152. Peeters M, Jung M, Ayouba A. The origin and molecular epidemiology of HIV. Expert Rev Anti-Infect Ther. 2013;11(9):885–96.
153. Persaud D, Bangaru B, Greco MA, et al. Cholestatic hepatitis in children infected with the human immunodeficiency virus. Pediatr Infect Dis J. 1993;12:492–8.
154. Hadžić N. Liver disease in immunodeficiencies. In: Suchy FJ, Sokol RJ, Balistreri WF, editors. Liver disease in children. 3rd ed: Cambridge University Press; 2007. p. 513–30.
155. Beath SV. The liver in systemic illness. In: Kelly D, editor. Diseases of the liver and biliary system in children. 3rd ed: Wiley-Blackwell Publishing; 2008. p. 381–403.
156. Lefkowitch JH. Pathology of AIDS-related liver disease. Dig Dis. 1994;12:321–30.
157. Hardman TC, Purdon SD. The cardiological complications associated with HIV infection and acquired immune deficiency syndrome (AIDS). Br J Cardiol. 2002;9:593–9.
158. Connor EM, Sperling RS, Gelber R, et al. Reduction of maternal–infant transmission of human immunodeficiency virus type 1 with zidovudine treatment. N Engl J Med. 1994;331:1173–80.
159. Palella FJ, Delaney KM, Moorman AC, et al. Declining morbidity and mortality among patients with advanced HIV infection. N Engl J Med. 1998;338:853–60.
160. Stabinski L, O'Connor S, Barnhart M, Kahn RJ, Hamm TE. Prevalence of HIV and hepatitis B virus co-infection in SSA and the potential impact and program feasibility of hepatitis B surface antigen screening in resource-limited settings. J Acquir Immune Defic Syndr. 2015;68(Suppl 3):S274–85.
161. Puoti M, Manno D, Nasta P, et al. Hepatitis B virus and HIV coinfection in low-income countries: unmet needs. Clin Infect Dis. 2008;46:367–9.
162. Hoffmann CJ, Thio CL. Clinical implications of HIV and hepatitis B co-infection in Asia and Africa. Lancet Infect Dis. 2007;7:402–9.
163. Peebles K, Nchimba L, Chilengi R, Moore CB, Mubiana-Mbewe M, Vinikoor MJ. Pediatric HIV–HBV coinfection in Lusaka, Zambia: prevalence and short-term treatment outcomes. J Trop Pediatr. 2015;61:464–7.
164. Rouet F, Chaix ML, Inwoley A, et al. Frequent occurrence of chronic hepatitis B virus infection among west African HIV type-1—infected children. Clin Infect Dis. 2008;46:361–6.
165. Anigilaje EA, Olutola A. Prevalence and clinical and immunoviralogical profile of human immunodeficiency virus-hepatitis B coinfection among children in an antiretroviral therapy programme in Benue State, Nigeria. ISRN Pediatr. 2013;2013:932697.
166. Ikpeme EE, Etukudo OM, Ekrikpo UE. Seroprevalence of HBV and HIV co-infection in children and outcomes following highly active antiretroviral therapy (HAART) in Uyo, South-South Nigeria. Afr Health Sci. 2013;13:955–61.
167. Telatela SP, Matee MI, Munubhi EK. Seroprevalence of hepatitis B and C viral co-infections among children infected with human immunodeficiency virus attending the paediatric HIV care and treatment center at Muhimbili National Hospital in Dar-es-Salaam, Tanzania. BMC Public Health. 2007;7:6.
168. Mutwa PR, Boer KR, Rusine JB, et al. Hepatitis B virus prevalence and vaccine response in HIV-infected children and adolescents

on combination antiretroviral therapy in Kigali, Rwanda. Pediatr Infect Dis J. 2013;32:246–51.
169. Dziuban EJ, Marton SA, Hughey AB, et al. Seroprevalence of hepatitis B in a cohort of HIV-infected children and adults in Swaziland. Int J STD AIDS. 2013;24:561–5.
170. Chakraborty R, Rees G, Bourboulia D, et al. Viral coinfections among African children infected with human immunodeficiency virus type 1. Clin Infect Dis. 2003;36:922–4.
171. Durowaye MO, Ernest SK, Ojuawo IA. Prevalence of HIV co-infection with Hepatitis B and C viruses among children at a tertiary hospital in Ilorin, Nigeria. Int J Clin Med Res. 2014;1:42–7.
172. Katusiime C, Kambugu A. Hepatitis B virus infection in adolescents and young adults with human immunodeficiency virus infection in an urban clinic in a resource-limited setting. J Int AIDS Soc. 2012;15 (Suppl 4):18060–301.
173. Nwolisa E, Mbanefo F, Ezeogu J, et al. Prevalence of hepatitis B co-infection amongst HIV infected children attending a care and treatment centre in Owerri, Southeastern Nigeria. Pan Afr Med J. 2013;14:89.
174. Sadoh AE, Sadoh WE, Iduoriyekemwen NJ. HIV coinfection with hepatitis B and C viruses among Nigerian children in an antiretroviral treatment programme. S Afr J Child Health. 2011;5:7–10.
175. Day SL, Odem-Davis K, Mandaliya KN, et al. Prevalence, clinical and virologic outcomes of hepatitis B virus co-infection in HIV-1 positive Kenyan women on antiretroviral therapy. PLoS One. 2013;8:e59346.
176. Ayuk J, Mphahlele J, Bessong P. Hepatitis B virus in HIV-infected patients in northeastern South Africa: prevalence, exposure, protection and response to HAART. S Afr Med J. 2013;103:330–3.
177. Ladep NG, Agaba PA, Agbaji O, et al. Rates and impact of hepatitis on human immunodeficiency virus infection in a large African cohort. World J Gastroenterol. 2013;19:1602–10.
178. Mayaphi SH, Roussow TM, Masemola DP, et al. HBV/HIV co-infection: the dynamics of HBV in South African patients with AIDS. S Afr Med J. 2012;102(3 pt 1):157–62.
179. Franzeck FC, Ngwale R, Msongole B, et al. Viral hepatitis and rapid diagnostic test based screening for HBsAg in HIV-infected patients in rural Tanzania. PLoS One. 2013;8:e58468.
180. Ramos JM, Toro C, Reyes F, et al. Seroprevalence of HIV-1, HBV HTLV-1 and Treponema pallidum among pregnant women in a rural hospital in Southern Ethiopia. J Clin Microbiol. 2011;51:83–5.
181. Manyazewal T, Sisay Z, Biadgilign S, et al. Hepatitis B and hepatitis C virus infections among antiretroviral-naive and -experienced HIV coinfected adults in Addis Abba, Ethiopia. Int J Infect Dis. 2012;16:96.
182. Harania RS, Karuru J, Nelson M, Stebbing J. HIV, hepatitis B and hepatitis C coinfection in Kenya. AIDS. 2008;22:1221–2.
183. Pirillo MF, Bassani L, Germinario EA, et al. Seroprevalence of hepatitis B and C viruses among HIV-infected pregnant women in Uganda and Rwanda. J Med Virol. 2007;79:1797–801.
184. Rusine J, Ondoa P, Asiimwe-Kateera B, et al. High seroprevalence of HBV and HCV infection in HIV-infected adults in Kigali, Rwanda. PLoS One. 2013;8:e63303.
185. Mutwa PR, Boer KR, Rusine JB, et al. Hepatitis B virus prevalence and vaccine response in HIV-infected children and adolescents on combination antiretroviral therapy in Kigali, Rwanda. Pediatr Infect Dis J. 2013;32:246–51.
186. Patel P, Davis S, Tolle M, et al. Prevalence of hepatitis B and hepatitis C coinfections in an adult HIV centre population in Gaborone, Botswana. Am J Trop Med Hyg. 2011;85:390–4.
187. Rabenau HF, Lennemann T, Kircher C, et al. Prevalence- and genderspecific immune response to opportunistic infections in HIV-infected patients in Lesotho. Sex Transm Dis. 2010;37:454–9.
188. De Paschale M, Manco MT, Belvisi L, et al. Prevalence of markers of hepatitis B virus infection or vaccination in HBsAg-negative subjects. Blood Transfus. 2012;10:344–50.
189. Ilboudo D, Simpore J, Ouermi D, et al. Towards the complete eradication of mother-to-child HIV/HBV coinfection at Saint Camille Medical Centre in Burkina Faso, Africa. Braz J Infect Dis. 2010;14:219–24.
190. Bado G, Penot P, N'Diaye MD, et al. Hepatitis B seroprevalence in HIVinfected patients consulting in a public day care unit in Bobo Dioulasso, Burkina Faso. Med Mal Infect. 2013;43:202–7.
191. Ouermi D, Simpore J, Belem AM, et al. Co-infection of Toxoplasma gondii with HBV in HIV-infected and uninfected pregnant women in Burkina Faso. Pak J Biol Sci. 2009;12:1188–93.
192. Kouanfack C, Aghokeng AF, Mondain AM, et al. Lamivudine-resistant HBV infection in HIV-positive patients receiving antiretroviral therapy in a public routine clinic in Cameroon. Antivir Ther. 2012;17:321–6.
193. Zoufaly A, Onyoh EF, Tih PM, et al. High prevalence of hepatitis B and syphilis co-infections among HIV patients initiating antiretroviral therapy in the north-west region of Cameroon. Int J STD AIDS. 2012;23:435–8.
194. Onyoh EF. High prevalence of hepatitis B and syphilis co-infection among newly diagnosed HIV patients in the northwest region of Cameroon. Tropical Med Int Health. 2012;17:12.
195. Jobarteh M, Malfroy M, Peterson I, et al. Seroprevalence of hepatitis B and C virus in HIV-1 and HIV-2 infected Gambians. Virol J. 2010;7:230.
196. Sagoe KW, Agyei AA, Ziga F, et al. Prevalence and impact of hepatitis B and C virus co-infections in antiretroviral treatment naive patients with HIV infection at a major treatment center in Ghana. J Med Virol. 2012;84:6–10.
197. Geretti AM, Patel M, Sarfo FS, et al. Detection of highly prevalent hepatitis B virus coinfection among HIV-seropositive persons in Ghana. J Clin Microbiol. 2010;48:3223–30.
198. Obi RK, Nwanebu FC, Ohalete CN, et al. A prospective study of three blood-borne viral pathogens among pregnant women attending ante-natal care in Owerri, Nigeria. J Public Health Epidemiol. 2012;4:226–9.
199. Salami T, Babatope I, Adewuyi G, et al. Hepatitis B and HIV co-infection-experience in a rural/suburban health center in Nigeria. J Microbiol Biotechnol Res. 2012;2:841–4.
200. Okocha EC, Oguejiofor OC, Odenigbo CU, et al. Prevalence of hepatitis B surface antigen seropositivity among HIV-infected and non-infected individuals in Nnewi, Nigeria. Niger Med J. 2012;53:249–53.
201. Adekunle AE, Oladimeji AA, Temi AP, et al. Baseline CD4+ T lymphocyte cell counts, hepatitis B and C viruses seropositivity in adults with Human Immunodeficiency Virus infection at a tertiary hospital in Nigeria. Pan Afr Med J. 2011;9:6.
202. Sadoh AE, Sadoh WE. Some laboratory features of HIV infected Nigerian children co-infected with hepatitis B and C. Ann Biomed Sci. 2012;11:29–39.
203. Tremeau-Bravard A, Ogbukagu IC, Ticao CJ, et al. Seroprevalence of hepatitis B and C infection among the HIV-positive population in Abuja, Nigeria. Afr Health Sci. 2012;12:312–7.
204. Adesina O, Oladokun A, Akinyemi O, et al. Human immunodeficiency virus and hepatitis B virus coinfection in pregnancy at the University College Hospital, Ibadan. Afr J Med Med Sci. 2010;39:305–10.
205. Lesi OA, Kehinde MO, Oguh DN, et al. Hepatitis B and C virus infection in Nigerian patients with HIV/AIDS. Niger Postgrad Med J. 2007;14:129–33.
206. Adewole OO, Anteyi E, Ajuwon Z, et al. Hepatitis B and C virus coinfection in Nigerian patients with HIV infection. J Infect Dev Ctries. 2009;3:369–75.

207. Otegbayo JA, Taiwo BO, Akingbola TS, et al. Prevalence of hepatitis B and C seropositivity in a Nigerian cohort of HIV-infected patients. Ann Hepatol. 2008;7:152–6.
208. Olokoba A, Olokoba L, Salawu F, et al. Hepatitis B virus and human immunodeficiency virus co-infection in North-Eastern Nigeria. Int J Trop Med. 2008;34:73–5.
209. Balogun TM, Emmanuel S, Ojerinde EF. HIV, Hepatitis B and C viruses' coinfection among patients in a Nigerian tertiary hospital. Pan Afr Med J. 2012;12:100.
210. Diop-Ndiaye H, Toure-Kane C, Etard JF, et al. Hepatitis B, C seroprevalence and delta viruses in HIV-1 Senegalese patients at HAART initiation (retrospective study). J Med Virol. 2008;80:1332–6.
211. Davison S, Boxall EH. Infective disorders of the liver. In: Kelly D, editor. Diseases of the liver and biliary system in children. 3rd ed: Wiley-Blackwell Publishing; 2008. p. 129–68.
212. Rao VB, Johari N, du Cros P, Messina J, Ford N, Cooke GS. Hepatitis C seroprevalence and HIV co-infection in sub-Saharan Africa: a systematic review and meta-analysis. Lancet Infect Dis. 2015;15:819–24.
213. Matthews-Greer JM, Caldito GC, Adley SD, Willis R, Mire AC, Jamison RM, McRae KL, King JW, Chang WL. Comparison of hepatitis C viral loads in patients with or without human immunodeficiency virus. Clin Diagn Lab Immunol. 2001;8(4):690–4.
214. Feldt T, Sarfo FS, Zoufaly A, Phillips RO, Burchard G, van Lunzen J, Jochum J, Chadwick D, Awasom C, Claussen L, Drosten C, Drexler JF, Eis-Hübinger AM. Hepatitis E virus infections in HIV-infected patients in Ghana and Cameroon. J Clin Virol. 2013;58(1):18–23.
215. Kiple K, King V. Another dimension to the black diaspora: diet, disease and racism. Cambridge: Cambridge University Press; 1981.
216. Quaresma JA, Barros VL, Pagliari C, Fernandes ER, Guedes F, Takakura CF, et al. Revisiting the liver in human yellow fever: virus-induced apoptosis in hepatocytes associated with TGF-beta, TNF-alpha and NK cells activity. Virology. 2006;345(1):22–30.
217. Rowland M, Plackett TP, Smith R. Yellow fever vaccine-associated viscerotropic disease. Milit Med. 2012;177:467–9.
218. Mawson AR. Retinoids, race and the pathogenesis of dengue hemorrhagic fever. Med Hypotheses. 2013;81:1069–74.
219. Halstead SB, Streit TG, Lafontant J, Putvatana R, Russel K, Sun W, et al. Haiti: absence of dengue hemorrhagic fever despite hyperendemic dengue virus transmission. Am J Trop Med. 2001;65(3):180–3.
220. Sierra B, Kouri G, Guzman MG. Race: a risk factor for dengue hemorrhagic fever. Arch Virol. 2007;52:533–43.
221. Nguyen TL, Nguyen TH, Tieu NT. The impact of dengue haemorrhagic fever on liver function. Res Virol. 1997;148:273–7.
222. Mohan B, Patwari AK, Anand VK. Hepatic dysfunction in childhood dengue infection. J Trop Pediatr. 2000;46:40–3.
223. Nimmannitya S, Thisyakorn U, Hemsrichart V. Dengue haemorrhagic fever with unusual manifestations. Southeast Asian J Trop Med Public Health. 1987;18:398–406.
224. Lazo M, Clark JM. The epidemiology of nonalcoholic fatty liver disease: a global perspective. Semin Liver Dis. 2008;28(4):339–50.
225. Figueiredo MA, Rodrigues LC, Barreto ML, Lima JW, Costa MC, Morato V, et al. Allergies and diabetes as risk factors for dengue hemorrhagic fever: results of a case control study. PLoS Negl Trop Dis. 2010;4(6):e699.
226. Richmond JK, Baglole DJ. Lassa fever: epidemiology, clinical features, and social consequences. BMJ. 2003;327:1271–5.
227. Shaffer JG, Grant DS, Schieffelin JS, Boisen ML, Goba A, Hartnett JN, Levy DC, Yenni RE, Moses LM, Fullah M, Momoh M, Fonnie M, Fonnie R, Kanneh L, Koroma VJ, Kargbo K, Ottomassathien D, Muncy IJ, Jones AB, Illick MM, Kulakosky PC, Haislip AM, Bishop CM, Elliot DH, Brown BL, Zhu H, Hastie KM, Andersen KG, Gire SK, Tabrizi S, Tariyal R, Stremlau M, Matschiner A, Sampey DB, Spence JS, Cross RW, Geisbert JB, Folarin OA, Happi CT, Pitts KR, Geske FJ, Geisbert TW, Saphire EO, Robinson JE, Wilson RB, Sabeti PC, Henderson LA, Khan SH, Bausch DG, Branco LM, Garry RF, Viral Hemorrhagic Fever Consortium. Lassa fever in post-conflict sierra leone. PLoS Negl Trop Dis. 2014;8(3):e2748.
228. Monath TP, Newhouse VF, Kemp GE, Setzer HW, Cacciapuoti A. Lassa virus isolation from Mastomys natalensis rodents during an epidemic in Sierra Leone. Science. 1974;185:263–5.
229. Balkhy HH, Memish ZA. Rift Valley fever: an uninvited zoonosis in the Arabian peninsula. Int J Antimicrob Agents. 2003;21:153–7.
230. Daubney R, Hudson JR, Garnham PC. Enzootic hepatitis or rift valley fever. An undescribed virus disease of sheep cattle and man from east Africa. J Pathol Bacteriol. 1931;34:545–79.
231. Digoutte JP, Peters CJ. General aspects of the 1987 Rift Valley fever epidemic in Mauritania. Res Virol. 1989;140:27–30.
232. Mudhasani R, Kota KP, Retterer C, Tran JP, Whitehouse CA, Bavari S. High content image-based screening of a protease inhibitor library reveals compounds broadlyactive against Rift Valley fever virus and other highly pathogenic RNA viruses. PLoS Negl Trop Dis. 2014;8(8):e3095.
233. Patrican LA, Bailey CL. Ingestion of immune blood meals and infection of Aedes fowleri, Aedes mcintoshi, and Culex pipiens with Rift Valley fever virus. Am J Trop Med Hyg. 1989;40:534–40.
234. Rudolph KE, Lessler J, Moloney RM, Kmush B, Cummings DA. Incubation periods of mosquito-borne viral infections: a systematic review. Am J Trop Med Hyg. 2014;90(5):882–91.
235. Laughlin LW, Meegan JM, Strausbaugh LJ, Morens DM, Watten RH. Epidemic Rift Valley fever in Egypt: observations of the spectrum of human illness. Trans R Soc Trop Med Hyg. 1979;73:630–3.
236. Stock I. Marburg and Ebola hemorrhagic fevers—pathogens, epidemiology and therapy. Med Monatsschr Pharm. 2014;37(9):324–30.
237. Rougeron V, Feldmann H, Grard G, Becker S, Leroy EM. Ebola and Marburg haemorrhagic fever. J Clin Virol. 2015;64:111–9.
238. Messaoudi I, Amarasinghe GK, Basler CF. Filovirus pathogenesis and immune evasion: insights from Ebola virus and Marburg virus. Nat Rev Microbiol. 2015;13(11):663–76.
239. Towner JS, Sealy TK, Khristova ML, Albarino CG, Conlan S, Reeder SA. Newly discovered ebola virus associated with hemorrhagic fever outbreak in Uganda. PLoS Pathog. 2008;4:e1000212.
240. Towner JS, Khristova ML, Sealy TK, Vincent MJ, Erickson BR, Bawiec DA. Marburgvirus genomics and association with a large hemorrhagic fever outbreak in Angola. J Virol. 2006;80:6497–516.
241. Towner JS, Rollin PE, Bausch DG, Sanchez A, Crary SM, Vincent M. Rapid diagnosis of Ebola hemorrhagic fever by reverse transcription-PCR in an outbreak setting and assessment of patient viral load as a predictor of outcome. J Virol. 2004;78:4330–41.
242. Raheel U, Faheem M, Riaz MN, Kanwal N, Javed F, Zaidi N, et al. Dengue fever in the Indian Subcontinent: an overview. J Infect Dev Ctries. 2011;5(4):239–47.
243. Jagdish K, Patwari AK, Sarin SK, et al. Hepatic manifestations in typhoid fever. Indian Pediatr. 1994;31:807–11.
244. Kumar R, Gupta N, Shalini. Multidrug-resistant typhoid fever. Indian J Pediatr. 2007;74:39–42.
245. Olubodun JO, Kuti JA, Adefuye BO, Talabi AO. Typhoid fever associated with severe hepatitis. Cent Afr J Med. 1994;40:262–4.
246. El Newihi HM, Alamy ME, Reynolds TB. Salmonella hepatitis: analysis of 27 cases and comparison with acute viral hepatitis. Hepatology. 1996;24:516–9.

247. Thapa BR, Yachha SK, Mehta S. Abdominal tuberculosis. Indian Pediatr. 1991;28:1093–100.
248. Alvarez SZ, Carpio R. Hepatobiliary tuberculosis. Dig Dis Sci. 1983;28:193–200.
249. Biggs HM, Bui DM, Galloway RL, Stoddard RA, Shadomy SV, Morrissey AB, et al. Leptospirosis among hospitalized febrile patients in northern Tanzania. Am J Trop Med Hyg. 2011;85(2):275–81.
250. Collares-Pereira M, Gomes AC, Prassad M, Vaz RG, Ferrinho P, Stanek G, et al. Preliminary survey of Leptospirosis and Lyme disease amongst febrile patients attending community hospital ambulatory care in Maputo, Mozambique. Cent Afr J Med. 1997;43(8):234–8.
251. de Geus A, Wolff JW, Timmer VE. Clinical leptospirosis in Kenya (1): a clinical study in Kwale District, Coast Province. East Afr Med J. 1977;54(3):115–24.
252. Forrester AT, Kranendonk O, Turner LH, Wolff JW, Bohlander HJ. Serological evidence of human leptospirosis in Kenya. East Afr Med J. 1969;46(9):497–506.
253. Hogerzeil HV, De Geus A, Terpstra WJ, Korver H, Ligthart GS. Leptospirosis in rural Ghana: part 2. Current leptospirosis. Trop Geogr Med. 1986;38(4):408–14.
254. Ismail TF, Wasfy MO, Abdul-Rahman B, Murray CK, Hospenthal DR, Abdel-Fadeel M, et al. Retrospective serosurvey of leptospirosis among patients with acute febrile illness and hepatitis in Egypt. Am J Trop Med Hyg. 2006;75(6):1085–9.
255. Murray CK, Gray MR, Mende K, Parker TM, Samir A, Rahman BA, et al. Use of patient-specific Leptospira isolates in the diagnosis of leptospirosis employing microscopic agglutination testing (MAT). Trans R Soc Trop Med Hyg. 2011;105(4):209–13.
256. Parker TM, Ismail T, Fadeel MA, Maksoud MA, Morcos M, Newire E, et al. Laboratory-based surveillance for acute febrile illness in Egypt: a focus on leptospirosis. Am J Trop Med Hyg. 2006;75(5 Suppl):18.
257. Tagoe JA, Puplampu N, Odoom SC, Abdul-Rahman B, Habashy EE, Pimentel B, et al. Serosurvey of leptospirosis among patients with acute febrile illness in Accra. Am J Trop Med Hyg. 2010;83(5 Suppl):306.
258. Allan KJ, Biggs HM, Halliday JE, Kazwala RR, Maro VP, Cleaveland S, Crump JA. Epidemiology of leptospirosis in Africa: a systematic review of a neglected zoonosis and a paradigm for 'one health' in Africa. PLoS Negl Trop Dis. 2015;9(9):e0003899.
259. Evangelista KV, Coburn J. Leptospira as an emerging pathogen: a review of its biology, pathogenesis and host immune responses. Future Microbiol. 2010;5(9):1413–25.
260. Newman RC, Cohen HL. Weil's disease in Cape Town. A case report. S Afr Med J. 1962;36(41):851–3.
261. Bourhy P, Collet L, Lernout T, Zinini F, Hartskeerl RA, Linden H, et al. Human leptospira isolates circulating in Mayotte (Indian Ocean) have unique serological and molecular features. J Clin Microbiol. 2012;50(2):307–11.
262. Covic A, Maftei ID, Gusbeth TP. Acute liver failure due to leptospirosis successfully treated with MARS dialysis. Int Urol Nephrol. 2007;39:313–6.
263. Frean J, Arndt S, Spencer D. High rate of Bartonella henselae infection in HIV-positive outpatients in Johannesburg, South Africa. Trans R Soc Trop Med Hyg. 2002;96(5):549–50.
264. Trataris AN, Rossouw J, Arntzen L, Karstaedt A, Frean J. Bartonella spp. in human and animal populations in Gauteng, South Africa, from 2007 to 2009. Onderstepoort J Vet Res. 2012;79(2):452.
265. Laudisoit A, Iverson J, Neerinckx S, Shako JC, Nsabimana JM, Kersh G, Kosoy M, Zeidner N. Human seroreactivity against Bartonella species in the Democratic Republic of Congo. Asian Pac J Trop Med. 2011;4(4):320–2.
266. Maggi RG, Mascarelli PE, Havenga LN, Naidoo V, Breitschwerdt EB. Co-infection with Anaplasma platys, Bartonella henselae and Candidatus Mycoplasma haematoparvum in a veterinarian. Parasit Vectors. 2013;6:103.
267. Kelly PJ, Matthewman LA, Hayter D, Downey S, Wray K, Bryson NR, Raoult D. Bartonella (Rochalimaea) henselae in southern Africa—evidence for infections in domestic cats and implications for veterinarians. J S Afr Vet Assoc. 1996;67(4):182–7.
268. Noden BH, Tshavuka FI, van der Colf BE, Chipare I, Wilkinson R. Exposure and risk factors to coxiella burnetii, spotted fever group and typhus group Rickettsiae, and Bartonella henselae among volunteer blood donors in Namibia. PLoS One. 2014;9(9):e108674.
269. Molia S, Kasten RW, Stuckey MJ, Boulouis HJ, Allen J, Borgo GM, Koehler JE, Chang CC, Chomel BB. Isolation of Bartonella henselae, Bartonella koehlerae subsp. koehlerae, Bartonella koehlerae subsp. bothieri and a new subspecies of B. koehlerae from free-ranging lions (Panthera leo) from South Africa, cheetahs (Acinonyx jubatus) from Namibia and captive cheetahs from California. Epidemiol Infect. 2016;144(15):3237–43. Epub 2016 July 25.
270. Kumsa B, Parola P, Raoult D, Socolovschi C. Molecular detection of Rickettsia felis and Bartonella henselae in dog and cat fleas in Central Oromia, Ethiopia. Am J Trop Med Hyg. 2014;90(3):457–62.
271. Kelly PJ, Eoghain GN, Raoult D. Antibodies reactive with Bartonella henselae and Ehrlichia canis in dogs from the communal lands of Zimbabwe. J S Afr Vet Assoc. 2004;75(3):116–20.
272. Gundi VA, Bourry O, Davous B, Raoult D, La Scola B. Bartonella clarridgeiae and B. henselae in dogs, Gabon. Emerg Infect Dis. 2004;10(12):2261–2. No abstract available.
273. Azzag N, Haddad N, Durand B, Petit E, Ammouche A, Chomel B, Boulouis HJ. Population structure of Bartonella henselae in Algerian urban stray cats. PLoS One. 2012;7(8):e43621. https://doi.org/10.1371/journal.pone.0043621. Epub 2012 Aug 30.
274. Boudebouch N, Sarih M, Beaucournu JC, Amarouch H, Hassar M, Raoult D, Parola P. Bartonella clarridgeiae, B. henselae and Rickettsia felis in fleas from Morocco. Ann Trop Med Parasitol. 2011;105(7):493–8.
275. Znazen A, Rolain JM, Hammami N, Kammoun S, Hammami A, Raoult D. High prevalence of Bartonella quintana endocarditis in Sfax, Tunisia. Am J Trop Med Hyg. 2005;72(5):503–7.
276. Breitschwerdt EB. Bartonellosis: one health perspectives for an emerging infectious disease. ILAR J. 2014;55(1):46–58.
277. Raoult D, Fournier PE, Drancourt M, Marrie TJ, Etienne J, Cosserat J, Cacoub P, Poinsignon Y, Leclercq P, Sefton AM. Diagnosis of 22 new cases of Bartonella endocarditis. Ann Intern Med. 1996;125(8):646–52.
278. Magwai MG, Andronikou S. Isolated splenic peliosis in an immunocompromised patient. S Afr J Surg. 2012;50(3):92.
279. Ramdial PK, Sing Y, Ramburan A, Dlova NC, Bagratee JS, Calonje E. Bartonella quintana-induced vulval bacillary angiomatosis. Int J Gynecol Pathol. 2012;31(4):390–4.
280. Murano I, Yoshii H, Kurashige K, Sugio Y, Tsukahara M. Giant hepatic granuloma caused by Bartonella henselae. Pediatr Infect Dis J. 2001;20:319–20.
281. Rolain JM, Maurin M, Bryskier A, Raoult D. In vitro activities of telithromycin (HMR 3647) against Rickettsia rickettsii, Rickettsia conorii, Rickettsia africae, Rickettsia typhi, Rickettsia prowazekii, Coxiella burnetii, Bartonella henselae, Bartonella quintana, Bartonellabacilliformis, and Ehrlichia chaffeensis. Antimicrob Agents Chemother. 2000;44(5):1391–3.
282. Jacobs MR, Stein H, Buqwane A, Dubb A, Segal F, Rabinowitz L, Ellis U, Freiman I, Witcomb M, Vallabh V. Epidemic listeriosis. Report of 14 cases detected in 9 months. S Afr Med J. 1978;54(10):389–92.

283. Seyoum ET, Woldetsadik DA, Mekonen TK, Gezahegn HA, Gebreyes WA. Prevalence of Listeria monocytogenes in raw bovine milk and milk products from central highlands of Ethiopia. J Infect Dev Ctries. 2015;9(11):1204–9. https://doi.org/10.3855/jidc.6211.
284. Seyoum ET, Woldetsadik DA, Mekonen TK, Gezahegn HA, Gebreyes WA. Prevalence of Listeria monocytogenes in raw bovine milk and milk products from central highlands of Ethiopia. J Infect Dev Ctries. 2015;9(11):1204–9.
285. Onyemelukwe GC, Lawande RV, Egler LJ, Mohammed I. Listeria monocytogenes in Northern Nigeria. J Infect. 1983;6(2):141–5.
286. Akpavie SO, Ikheloa JO. An outbreak of listeriosis in cattle in Nigeria. Rev Elev Med Vet Pays Trop. 1992;45(3–4):263–4.
287. El Sayed Zaki M, El Shabrawy WO, El-Eshmawy MM, Aly Eletreby S. The high prevalence of Listeria monocytogenes peritonitis in cirrhotic patients of an Egyptian Medical Center. J Infect Public Health. 2011;4(4):211–6.
288. Elbeldi A, Smaoui H, Hamouda S, Helel S, Hmaied F, Ben Mustapha I, Barsaoui S, Bousnina S, Marrakchi Z, Barbouche MR, Kechrid A. [Listeriosis in Tunis: seven cases reports]. Bull Soc Pathol Exot. 2011;104(1):58–61.
289. Stavru F, Archambaud C, Cossart P. Cell biology and immunology of Listeria monocytogenes infections: novel insights. Immunol Rev. 2011;240(1):160–84.
290. Ababouch L. Potential of Listeria hazard in African fishery products and possible control measures. Int J Food Microbiol. 2000;62(3):211–5.
291. Novak DA, Lauwers GY, Kradin RL. Bacterial, parasitic, and fungal infections of the liver. In: Suchy FJ, Sokol RJ, Balistreri WF, editors. Liver disease in children. 3rd ed: Cambridge University Press; 2007. p. 871–96.
292. Mawson AR. The pathogenesis of malaria: a new perspective. Pathog Global Health. 2013;107(3):122–9.
293. Diaz Granados CA, Duffus WA, Albrecht H. Parasitic diseases of the liver. In: Zakim D, Boyer TD, editors. Hepatology. Philadelphia: Saunders; 2003. p. 1073–108.
294. Ibhanesebhor SE. Clinical characteristics of neonatal malaria. J Trop Pediatr. 1995;41:330–3.
295. Devarbhavi H, Alvares JF, Kumar KS. Severe falciparum malaria simulating fulminant hepatic failure. Mayo Clin Proc. 2005;80:355–8.
296. Barnett ED. Malaria. In: Feigin RD, Cherry JD, Demmler GJ, Kaplan S, editors. Textbook of pediatric infectious diseases. Philadelphia: Saunders; 2004. p. 2714–40.
297. Kochar DK, Singh P, Agarwal P, et al. Malarial hepatitis. J Assoc Physicians India. 2003;51:1069–72.
298. Edington GM. Other viral and infectious diseases. In: Macsween RNM, Anthony PP, Scheuer PJ, editors. Pathology of the liver. Edinburgh: Churchill Livingstone; 1979. p. 192–220.
299. Warrell DA. Pathophysiology of severe falciparum malaria in man. Parasitology. 1987;94(Suppl):S53–76.
300. Cook GC. Liver in Malaria. Postgrad Med J. 1994;70:780–4.
301. Takafuji ET, Kirkpatrick JW, Miller RN, et al. An efficacy trial of doxycycline chemoprophylaxis against leptospirosis. N Engl J Med. 1984;310:497–500.
302. Sowunmi A. Hepatomegaly in acute falciparum malaria in children. Trans R Soc Trop Med Hyg. 1996;90:540–2.
303. Haghighi P, Rezai HR. Leishmaniasis: a review of selected topics. Pathol Annu. 1977;12(Pt 2):63–89.
304. Wittner M, Tanowitz HB. Leishmaniasis. In: Feigin RD, Cherry JD, Demmler GJ, Kaplan S, editors. Textbook of pediatric infectious diseases. Philadelphia: W. B. Saunders; 2004. p. 2730–9.
305. Katakura K, Kawazu S, Naya T, et al. Diagnosis of kala-azar by nested PCR based on amplification of the Leishmania miniexon gene. J Clin Microbiol. 1998;36:2173–7.
306. Noyes HA, Reyburn H, Bailey JW, Smith D. A nested-PCR based schizodeme method for identifying Leishmania kinetoplast minicircle classes directly from clinical samples and its application to the study of the epidemiology of Leishmania tropica in Pakistan. J Clin Microbiol. 1998;36:2877–81.
307. Bukte Y, Nazaroglu H, Mete A, Yilmaz F. Visceral leishmaniasis with multiple nodular lesions of the liver and spleen: CT and sonographic findings. Abdom Imaging. 2004;29:82–4.
308. Moreno A, Marazuela M, Yebra M, et al. Hepatic fibrin-ring granulomas in visceral leishmaniasis. Gastroenterology. 1988;95:1123–6.
309. Moragas A, Serrano A, Toran N. Acute form of visceral leishmaniasis in a 3-month-old infant. Pediatr Pathol. 1986;6:111–7.
310. American Academy of Pediatrics. Drugs for parasitic infections. In: Pickering L, editor. Red book: 2003 report of the committee on infectious diseases. Elk Grove Village: American Academy of Pediatrics; 2003. p. 744–70.
311. Thibeaux R, Weber C, Hon CC, Dillies MA, Avé P, Coppée JY, Labruyère E, Guillén N. Identification of the virulence landscape essential for Entamoeba histolytica invasion of the human colon. PLoS Pathog. 2013;9(12):e1003824.
312. Barnes PF, De Cock KM, Reynolds TN, Ralls PW. A comparison of amebic and pyogenic abscess of the liver. Medicine. 1987;66:472–83.
313. Wolfsen HC, Bolen JW, Bowen JL, Fenster LF. Fulminant herpes hepatitis mimicking hepatic abscesses. J Clin Gastroenterol. 1993;16:61–4.
314. Voldřich M, Novotný P, Tyll T, Rudiš J, Belšan T, Hedlová D, Stefanová M. [The current view of the diagnosis and management of amebiasis in the light of the authors own case reports]. Epidemiol Mikrobiol Imunol. 2014;63(3):226–31.
315. Kikuchi T, Koga M, Shimizu S, Miura T, Maruyama H, Kimura M. Efficacy and safety of paromomycin for treating amebiasis in Japan. Parasitol Int. 2013;62(6):497–501.
316. Gyang VP, Akinwale OP, Lee YL, Chuang TW, Orok A, Ajibaye O, Liao CW, Cheng PC, Chou CM, Huang YC, Fan KH, Fan CK. Toxoplasma gondii infection: seroprevalence and associated risk factors among primaryschoolchildren in Lagos City, Southern Nigeria. Rev Soc Bras Med Trop. 2015;48(1):56–63.
317. Montoya JG, Liesenfeld O. Toxoplasmosis. Lancet. 2004;363:1965–76.
318. Alvarados-Esquivel C, Estrada-Martinez S, Liesenfeld O. Toxoplasma gondii infection in workers occupationally exposed to unwashed raw fruits and vegetables: a case control seroprevalence study. Parasit Vectors. 2011;4:235.
319. Porter SB, Sande MA. Toxoplasmosis of the central nervous system in the acquired immunodeficiency syndrome. New Engl J Med. 1992;327:1643–8.
320. Assis AM, Barreto ML, Gomes GS, Prado MS, Santos NS, Santos LM, et al. Childhood anemia prevalence and associated factors in Salvador, Bahia, Brazil. Cad Saude Publica. 2004;20:1633–41.
321. Schmidt DR, Hogh B, Andersen O, et al. Treatment of infants with congenital toxoplasmosis: tolerability and plasma concentrations of sulfadiazine and pyrimethamine. Eur J Pediatr. 2005;165:19–25.
322. Jones JL, Kruszon MD, Meadey JB. Toxoplasmosis gondii infection in the USA; seroprevalence and risk factors. Am J Epidemiol. 2001;154:357–65.
323. Nissapatorn V, Azmi Noor MA, Cho SM, Fong MY, Init I, Rohela M, et al. Toxoplasmosis; Prevalence and risk factors. J Obstet Gynaecol. 2003;23:618–24.
324. Khuroo MS. Hepatobiliary and pancreatic ascariasis. Indian J Gastroenterol. 2001;20(Suppl 1):C28–32.
325. Khurroo MS, Zargar SA, Mahajan R. Hepatobiliary and pancreatic ascariasis in India. Lancet. 1990;335:1503–6.
326. Louw JH. Abdominal complications of ascariasis. Surg Rounds. 1981;4:54–65.

327. Bari S, Sheikh KA, Ashraf M, Hussain Z, Hamid A, Mufti GN. Ascaris liver abscess in children. J Gastroenterol. 2007;42:236–40.
328. Khurroo MS, Zargar SA, Mahajan R, Bhat RL, Javid G. Sonographic appearances in biliary ascariasis. Gastroenterology. 1987;93:267–72.
329. El Sheikh Mohamed AR, Al Karawi MA, Yasawy MI. Modern techniques in the diagnosis and treatment of gastrointestinal and biliary tree parasites. Hepato-Gastroenterology. 1991;38:180–8.
330. Radin DR, Vachon LA. CT findings in biliary and pancreatic ascariasis. J Comput Assist Tomogr. 1986;10:508–9.
331. Rocha MS, Costa NS, Angelo MT, et al. CT identification of ascaris in the biliary tract. Abdom Imaging. 1995;20:317–9.
332. Bhushan B, Watal G, Mahajan R, Khuroo MS. Endoscopic retrograde cholangiopancreaticographic features of pancreaticobiliary ascariasis. Gastrointest Radiol. 1988;13:327–30.
333. Reddy DN, Sriram PV, Rao GV. Endoscopic diagnosis and management of tropical parasitic infestations. Gastrointest Endosc Clin N Am. 2003;13:765–73.
334. Bharti B, Bharti S, Khurana S. Worm infestation: diagnosis, treatment and prevention. Indian J Pediatr. 2018;85(11):1017–24. https://doi.org/10.1007/s12098-017-2505-z.
335. Beckingham IJ, Cullis SN, Krige JE, et al. Management of hepatobiliary and pancreatic Ascaris infestation in adults after failed medical treatment. Br J Surg. 1998;85:907–10.
336. Pereira-Lima JC, Jakobs R, da Silva CP, et al. Endoscopic removal of Ascaris lumbricoides from the biliary tract as emergency treatment for acute suppurative cholangitis. Z Gastroenterol. 2001;39:793–6.
337. Doehring E. Schistosomiasis in childhood. Eur J Pediatr. 1988;147:2–9.
338. Bica I, Hamer DH, Stadecker MJ. Hepatic schistosomiasis. Infect Dis Clin N Am. 2000;14:583–604, viii.
339. De CK. Hepatosplenic schistosomiasis: a clinical review. Gut. 1986;27:734–45.
340. Symmers W. Note on a new form of liver cirrhosis due to the presence of ova of Bilharzia haematobium. J Pathol Bacteriol. 1903;9:237–9.
341. Lambertucci JR, Cota GF, Pinto-Silva RA, et al. Hepatosplenic schistosomiasis in field-based studies: a combined clinical and sonographic definition. Mem Inst Oswaldo Cruz. 2001;96(Suppl):147–50.
342. Palmer PE. Schistosomiasis. Semin Roentgenol. 1998;33:6–25.
343. Willemsen UF, Pfluger T, Zoller WG, et al. MRI of hepatic schistosomiasis mansoni. J Comput Assist Tomogr. 1995;19:811–3.
344. Doehring SE, Abdel RI, Kardorff R, et al. Ultrasonographical investigation of periportal fibrosis in children with Schistosomamansoni infection: reversibility of morbidity twenty-three months after treatment with praziquantel. Am J Trop Med Hyg. 1992;46:409–15.
345. Petroianu A, De Oliveira AE, Alberti LR. Hypersplenism in schistosomatic portal hypertension. Arch Med Res. 2005;36:496–501.
346. Kyei G, Ayi I, Boampong JN, Turkson PK. Sero-epidemiology of Toxocara canis infection in children attending four selected health facilities in the central region of Ghana. Ghana Med J. 2015;49(2):77–83.
347. Lötsch F, Vingerling R, Spijker R, Grobusch MP. Toxocariasis in humans in Africa—a systematic review. Travel Med Infect Dis. 2017;20:15–25.
348. Fisher AA, Laing JE, Stoeckel JE, Townsend JW. Handbook for family planning operations research design. New York: Population Council; 1998.
349. Ajayi OO, Duhlinska DD, Agwale SM, Njoku M. Frequency of human toxocariasis in Jos, Plateau State, Nigeria. Mem Inst Oswaldo Cruz. 2000;95:147–9.
350. Schantz PM. Toxocara larva migrans now. Am J Trop Med Hyg. 1989;41:21–34.
351. Gillespie SH. Human toxocariasis, a review. J Appl Bacteriol. 1987;63:473–9.
352. Azuma K, Yashiro N, Kinoshita T, et al. Hepatic involvement of visceral larva migrans due to Toxocara canis: a case report—CT and MR findings. Radiat Med. 2002;20:89–92.
353. Macpherson CN. The epidemiology and public health importance of toxocariasis: a zoonosis of global importance. Int J Parasitol. 2013;43(12–13):999–1008.
354. Sherlock S. Diseases of the liver and biliary system. 7th ed. Oxford: Blackwell Scientific; 1985.
355. Farmer PM, Chatterley S, Spier N. Echinococcal cyst of the liver: diagnosis and surgical management. Ann Clin Lab Sci. 1990;20:385–91.
356. Al Karawi MA, El Sheikh Mohamed AR, Yasawy MI. Advances in diagnosis and management of hydatid disease. Hepato-Gastroenterology. 1990;37:327–31.
357. Sayek I, Onat D. Diagnosis and treatment of uncomplicated hydatid cyst of the liver. World J Surg. 2001;25:21–7.
358. Agildere AM, Aytekin C, Coskun M, et al. MRI of hydatid disease of the liver: a variety of sequences. J Comput Assist Tomogr. 1998;22:718–24.
359. Balci NC, Sirvanci M. MR imaging of infective liver lesions. Magn Reson Imaging Clin N Am. 2002;10:121–35, vii.
360. Etlik O, Bay A, Arslan H, et al. Contrast-enhanced CT and MRI findings of atypical hepatic Echinococcus alveolaris infestation. Pediatr Radiol. 2005;35:546–9.
361. Spiliadis C, Georgopoulos S, Dailianas A, et al. The use of ERCP in the study of patients with hepatic echinococcosis before and after surgical intervention. Gastrointest Endosc. 1996;43:575–9.
362. Gomez I, Gavara C, López-Andújar R, Belda Ibáñez T, Ramia Ángel JM, Moya Herraiz Á, Orbis Castellanos F, Pareja Ibars E, San Juan Rodríguez F. Review of the treatment of liver hydatid cysts. World J Gastroenterol. 2015;21(1):124–31.
363. Geramizadeh B. Isolated peritoneal, mesenteric, and omental hydatid cyst: a clinicopathologic narrative review. Iran J Med Sci. 2017;42(6):517–23.
364. Golematis BC, Peveretos PJ. Hepatic hydatid disease: current surgical treatment. Mt Sinai J Med. 1995;62:71–6.
365. Schipper HG, Kager PA. Diagnosis and treatment of hepatic echinococcosis: an overview. Scand J Gastroenterol Suppl. 2004;50–5.
366. Agaoglu N, Turkyilmaz S, Arslan MK. Surgical treatment of hydatid cysts of the liver. Br J Surg. 2003;90:1536–41.
367. Khuroo MS, Dar MY, Yattoo GN, Zargar SA, Javaid G, Khan BA, Boda MI. Percutaneous drainage versus albendazole therapy in hepatic hydatidosis: a prospective, randomized study. Gastroenterology. 1993;104:1452–9.
368. Hillyer GV, Soler-de GM, Rodriguez PJ, et al. Use of the Falcon assay screening test—enzyme-linked immunosorbent assay (FAST-ELISA) and the enzyme-linked immunoelectrotransfer blot (EITB) to determine the prevalence of human fascioliasis in the Bolivian Altiplano. Am J Trop Med Hyg. 1992;46:603–9.
369. Sciume C, Geraci G, Pisello F, et al. Treatment of complications of hepatic hydatid disease by ERCP: our experience. Ann Ital Chir. 2004;75:531–5.
370. WHO. International strategies for tropical disease treatments Experiences with praziquantel. 1998. http://apps.who.int/medicinedocs/pdf/whozip48e/whozip48e.pdf. Last accessed on 4 Dec 2017.
371. Ndeffo Mbah ML, Skrip L, Greenhalgh S, Hotez P, Galvani AP. Impact of Schistosoma mansoni on malaria transmission in Sub-Saharan Africa. PLoS Negl Trop Dis. 2014;8(10):e3234.
372. Mekky MA, Tolba M, Abdel-Malek MO, Abbas WA, Zidan M. Human fascioliasis: a re-emerging disease in Upper Egypt. Am J Trop Med Hyg. 2015;93(1):76–9.

373. Jones EA, Kay JM, Milligan HP, Owens D. Massive infection with Fasciola hepatica in man. Am J Med. 1977;63:836–42.
374. MacLean JD, Graeme-Cook FM. Case records of the Massachusetts General Hospital. Weekly clinicopathological exercises. Case 12-2002. A 50-year-old man with eosinophilia and fluctuating hepatic lesions. N Engl J Med. 2002;346:1232–9.
375. Cosme A, Ojeda E, Poch M, et al. Sonographic findings of hepatic lesions in human fascioliasis. J Clin Ultrasound. 2003;31:358–63.
376. Sezgin O, Altintas E, Disibeyaz S, et al. Hepatobiliary fascioliasis: clinical and radiologic features and endoscopic management. J Clin Gastroenterol. 2004;38:285–91.
377. el-Morshedy H, Farghaly A, Sharaf S, Abou-Basha L, Barakat R. Triclabendazole in the treatment of human fascioliasis: a community-based study. East Mediterr Health J. 1999;5(5):888–94.
378. Abdul HS, Contreras R, Tombazzi C, et al. Hepatic fascioliasis: case report and review. Rev Inst Med Trop Sao Paulo. 1996;38:69–73.
379. Choe G, Lee HS, Seo JK, et al. Hepatic capillariasis: first case report in the Republic of Korea. Am J Trop Med Hyg. 1993;48:610–25.
380. Terrier P, Hack I, Hatz C, et al. Hepatic capillariasis in a 2-year old boy. J Pediatr Gastroenterol Nutr. 1999;28:338–40.
381. Younossi ZM, Stepanova M, Rafiq N, Makhlouf H, Younoszai Z, Agrawal R, Goodman Z. Pathologic criteria for nonalcoholic steatohepatitis: interprotocol agreement and ability to predict liver-related mortality. Hepatology. 2011;53:1874–82.
382. Matteoni CA, Younossi ZM, Gramlich T, Boparai N, Liu YC, McCullough AJ. Nonalcoholic fatty liver disease: a spectrum of clinical and pathological severity. Gastroenterology. 1999;116:1413–9.
383. Schwimmer JB, Deutsch R, Kahen T, Lavine JE, Stanley C, Behling C. Prevalence of fatty liver in children and adolescents. Pediatrics. 2006;118:1388–93.
384. Welsh JA, Karpen S, Vos MB. Increasing prevalence of nonalcoholic fatty liver disease among United States adolescents, 1988-1994 to 2007-2010. J Pediatr. 2013;162:496–500.e1.
385. Giorgio V, Prono F, Graziano F, Nobili V. Pediatric non alcoholic fatty liver disease: old and new concepts on development, progression, metabolic insight and potential treatment targets. BMC Pediatr. 2013;13:40.
386. Marzuillo P, Miraglia del Giudice E, Santoro N. Pediatric fatty liver disease: role of ethnicity and genetics. World J Gastroenterol. 2014;20(23):7347–55.
387. Alkassabany YM, Farghaly AG, El-Ghitany EM. Prevalence, risk factors, and predictors of nonalcoholic fatty liver diseaseamong schoolchildren: a hospital-based study in Alexandria, Egypt. Arab J Gastroenterol. 2014;15(2):76–81.
388. el-Karaksy HM, el-Koofy NM, Anwar GM, el-Mougy FM, el-Hennawy A, Fahmy ME. Predictors of non-alcoholic fatty liver disease in obese and overweight Egyptian children: single center study. Saudi J Gastroenterol. 2011;17(1):40–6.
389. El-Koofy NM, El-Karaksy HM, Mandour IM, Anwar GM, El-Raziky MS, El-Hennawy AM. Genetic polymorphisms in non-alcoholic fatty liver disease in obese Egyptian children. Saudi J Gastroenterol. 2011;17(4):265–70.
390. Onyekwere CA, Ogbera AO, Balogun BO. Non-alcoholic fatty liver disease and the metabolic syndrome in an urban hospital serving an African community. Ann Hepatol. 2011;10(2):119–24.
391. Browning JD, Szczepaniak LS, Dobbins R, Nuremberg P, Horton JD, Cohen JC, Grundy SM, Hobbs HH. Prevalence of hepatic steatosis in an urban population in the United States: impact of ethnicity. Hepatology. 2004;40:1387–95.
392. Park YW, Zhu S, Palaniappan L, Heshka S, Carnethon MR, Heymsfield SB. The metabolic syndrome: prevalence and associated risk factor findings in the US population from the Third National Health and Nutrition Examination Survey, 1988-1994. Arch Intern Med. 2003;163:427–36.
393. Santoro N, Feldstein AE, Enoksson E, Pierpont B, Kursawe R, Kim G, Caprio S. The association between hepatic fat content and liver injury in obese children and adolescents: effects of ethnicity, insulin resistance, and common gene variants. Diabetes Care. 2013;36:1353–60.
394. Romeo S, Kozlitina J, Xing C, Pertsemlidis A, Cox D, Pennacchio LA, Boerwinkle E, Cohen JC, Hobbs HH. Genetic variation in PNPLA3 confers susceptibility to nonalcoholic fatty liver disease. Nat Genet. 2008;40:1461–5.
395. Bril F, Portillo-Sanchez P, Liu IC, Kalavalapalli S, Dayton K, Cusi K. Clinical and histologic characterization of nonalcoholic steatohepatitis in African American patients. Diabetes Care. 2018;41(1):187–92. pii: dc171349.
396. Chaabouni M, Bahloul S, Ben Romdhane W, Ben Saleh M, Ben Halima N, Chouchene C, Ben Hmad A, Zroud N, Kammoun T, Karray A. Epidemiological, etiological and evolutionary aspects of children cirrhosis in a developing country: experience of the pediatric department of SFAX University hospital, Tunisia. Tunis Med. 2007;85(9):738–43.
397. Gadelhak N, Shehta A, Hamed H. Diagnosis and management of choledochal cyst: 20 years of single center experience. World J Gastroenterol. 2014;20(22):7061–6.
398. Heubi JE. Diseases of the gallbladder in infancy, childhood, and adolescence. In: Suchy FJ, Sokol RJ, Balistreri WF, editors. Liver disease in children. 3rd ed: Cambridge University Press; 2007. p. 346–65.
399. Nzeh DA, Adedoyin MA. Sonographic pattern of gallbladder disease in children with sickle cell anaemia. Pediatr Radiol. 1989;19(5):290–2.
400. Amri F, Pousse H, Gueddiche MN, Radhouane M, Sfar MT, Kharrat H, Essoussi AS, Harbi A. Cirrhosis and cirrhogenic diseases in Tunisian children. Multicenter study of 65 cases. Pediatrie. 1992;47(6):473–5.
401. El-Karaksy H, Fahmy M, El-Raziky MS, El-Hawary M, El-Sayed R, El-Koofy N, El-Mougy F, El-Hennawy A, El-Shabrawi M. A clinical study of Wilson's disease: the experience of a single Egyptian Paediatric Hepatology Unit. Arab J Gastroenterol. 2011;12(3):125–30.
402. El-Mougy FA, Sharaf SA, Elsharkawy MM, Mandour IA, El-Essawy RA, Eldin AM, Helmy HM, Soliman DH, Selim LH, Sharafeldin HM, Mogahed EA, El-Karaksy HM. Gene mutations in Wilson disease in Egyptian children: report on two novel mutations. Arab J Gastroenterol. 2014;15(3–4):114–8.
403. Fathy M, Kamal M, Al-Sharkawy M, Al-Karaksy H, Hassan N. Molecular characterization of exons 6, 8 and 9 of ABCB4 gene in children with Progressive Familial Intrahepatic Cholestasis type 3. Biomarkers. 2016;21(7):573–7.
404. Ghishan FK, Zawaideh M. Inborn errors of carbohydrate metabolism. In: Suchy FJ, Sokol RJ, Balistreri WF, editors. Liver disease in children. 3rd ed: Cambridge University Press; 2007. p. 595–625.
405. El-Karaksy H, Anwar G, El-Raziky M, Mogahed E, Fateen E, Gouda A, El-Mougy F, El-Hennawy A. Glycogen storage disease type III in Egyptian children: a single centre clinico-laboratory study. Arab J Gastroenterol. 2014;15(2):63–7.
406. El-Karaksy H, El-Raziky MS, Anwar G, Mogahed E. The effect of tailoring of cornstarch intake on stature in children with glycogen storage disease type III. J Pediatr Endocrinol Metab. 2015;28(1–2):195–200.
407. Mogahed E, Girgis M, Sobhy R, Elhabashy H, Abdelaziz O, El-Karaksy H. Skeletal and cardiac muscle involvement in children with glycogen storage disease type III. Eur J Pediatr. 2015;174:1545–8.

408. Imtiaz F, Rashed MS, Al-Mubarak B, Allam R, El-Karaksy H, Al-Hassnan Z, Al-Owain M, Al-Zaidan H, Rahbeeni Z, Qari A, Meyer BF, Al-Sayed M. Identification of mutations causing hereditary tyrosinemia type I in patients of Middle Eastern origin. Mol Genet Metab. 2011;104(4):688–90.
409. El-Karaksy H, Fahmy M, El-Raziky M, El-Koofy N, El-Sayed R, Rashed MS, El-Kiki H, El-Hennawy A, Mohsen N. Hereditary tyrosinemia type 1 from a single center in Egypt: clinical study of 22 cases. World J Pediatr. 2011;7(3):224–31.
410. El-Karaksy H, Rashed M, El-Sayed R, El-Raziky M, El-Koofy N, El-Hawary M, Al-Dirbashi O. Clinical practice. NTBC therapy for tyrosinemia type 1: how much is enough? Eur J Pediatr. 2010;169(6):689–93.
411. Abdullatif H, Mohsen N, El-Sayed R, El-Mougy F, El-Karaksy H. Haemophagocytic lymphohistiocytosis presenting as neonatal liver failure: a case series. Arab J Gastroenterol. 2016;17(2):105–9.
412. Desnick RJ, Astrin H, Anderson KE. Heme biosynthesis and the porphyrias. In: Suchy FJ, Sokol RJ, Balistreri WF, editors. Liver disease in children. 3rd ed: Cambridge University Press; 2007. p. 677–93.
413. Meissner P, Hift RJ, Corrigall A. Variegate porphyria. In: Kadish KM, Smith K, Guilard R, editors. Porphyrin handbook, part II. San Diego: Academic; 2003. p. 93–120.
414. Schmitt C, Gouya L, Malonova E, et al. Mutations in human CPO gene predict clinical expression of eitherhepatic hereditary coproporphyria or erythropoietic harderoporphyria. Hum Mol Genet. 2005;14:3089–98.
415. Stenson PD, Ball EV, Mort M, et al. Human Gene Mutation Database (HGMD): 2003 update. Hum Mutat. 2003;21:577–81.
416. Anderson KE, Bloomer JE, Bonkovsky HL, et al. Recommendations for the diagnosis and treatment of the acute porphyrias. Ann Intern Med. 2005;142:439–51.
417. Simonaro CM, Desnick RJ, McGovern MM, et al. The demographics and distribution of type B Niemann-Pick disease: novel mutations lead to new genotype/phenotype correlations. Am J Hum Genet. 2002;71:1413–9.
418. Schuchman EH, Desnick RJ. Niemann-Pick disease types A and B: acid sphingomyelinase deficiencies. In: Scriver CR, Beaudet AL, Sly WS, et al., editors. The metabolic and molecular bases of inherited disease. New York: McGraw-Hill; 2001. p. 3589–610.
419. Knisely AS, Narkewicz MR. Iron storage disorders. In: Suchy FJ, Sokol RJ, Balistreri WF, editors. Liver disease in children. 3rd ed: Cambridge University Press; 2007. p. 661–76.
420. Moore SW, Davidson A, Hadley GP, Kruger M, Poole J, Stones D, Wainwright L, Wessels G. Malignant liver tumors in South African children: a national audit. World J Surg. 2008;32(7):1389–95.
421. Hadley GP, Govender D, Landers G. Primary tumours of the liver in children: an African perspective. Pediatr Surg Int. 2004;20(5):314–8.
422. Pontisso P, Morsica G, Ruvoletto MG, et al. Latent hepatitis B virus infection in childhood hepatocellular carcinoma. Analysis by polymerase chain reaction. Cancer. 1992;69:2731–5.
423. Cheah PL, Looi LM, Lin HP, Yap SF. A case of childhood hepatitis B virus infection related primary hepatocellular carcinoma with short malignant transformation time. Pathology. 1991;23:66–8.
424. Chang MH. Decreasing incidence of hepatocellular carcinoma among children following universal hepatitis B immunization. Liver Int. 2003;23:309–14.
425. Montesano R. Hepatitis B immunization and hepatocellular carcinoma: the Gambia Hepatitis Intervention Study. J Med Virol. 2002;67:444–6.
426. Jaka H, Koy M, Liwa A, Kabangila R, Mirambo M, Scheppach W, Mkongo E, McHembe MD, Chalya PL. A fibreoptic endoscopic study of upper gastrointestinal bleeding at Bugando Medical Centre in northwestern Tanzania: a retrospective review of 240 cases. BMC Res Notes. 2012;5:200.
427. El-Karaksy HM, El-Koofy N, Mohsen N, Helmy H, Nabil N, El-Shabrawi M. Extrahepatic portal vein obstruction in Egyptian children. J Pediatr Gastroenterol Nutr. 2015;60(1):105–9.
428. El-Karaksy HM, Anwar G, Esmat G, Mansour S, Sabry M, Helmy H, El-Hennawy A, Fouad H. Prevalence of hepatic abnormalities in a cohort of Egyptian children with type 1 diabetes mellitus. Pediatr Diabetes. 2010;11(7):462–70.
429. Isichei UP. Liver function and the diagnostic significance of biochemical changes in the blood of African children with sickle cell disease. J Clin Pathol. 1980;33:626–30.
430. Norris WE. Acute hepatic sequestration in sickle cell disease. J Natl Med Assoc. 2004;96(9):1235–9.
431. Sheehy TW. Sickle cell hepatopathy. South Med J. 1977;70:533–8.
432. Aken'ova YA, Olasode BJ, Ogunbiyi JO, Thomas JO. Hepatobiliary changes in Nigerians with sickle cell anaemia. Ann Trop Med Parasitol. 1993;87(6):603–6.
433. Zuckerman M, Steenkamp V, Stewart MJ. Hepatic veno-occlusive disease as a result of a traditional remedy: confirmation of toxic pyrrolizidine alkaloids as the cause, using an in vitro technique. J Clin Pathol. 2002;55(9):676–9.
434. Millar AJW. Surgical disorders of the liver and bile ducts and portal hypertension. In: Kelly D, editor. Diseases of the liver and biliary system in children. 3rd ed: Wiley-Blackwell Publishing; 2008. p. 433–74.
435. Chopra R, Eaton JD, Grassi A, et al. Defibrotide for the treatment of hepatic veno-occlusive disease: results of the European compassionate-use study. Br J Haematol. 2000;111:1122–9.
436. DeLeve LD, Shulman HM, McDonald GB. Toxic injury to hepatic sinusoids: sinusoidal obstruction syndrome (veno-occlusive disease). Semin Liver Dis. 2002;22:27–42.
437. Attal M, Huguet F, Rubie H, et al. Prevention of hepatic venoocclusive disease after bone marrow transplantation by continuous infusion of low-dose heparin: a prospective, randomized trial. Blood. 1992;79:2834–40.
438. Al Jefri AH, Abujazar H, Al-Ahmari A, Al Rawas A, Al Zahrani Z, Alhejazi A, Bekadja MA, Ibrahim A, Lahoucine M, Ousia S, Bazarbachi A. Veno-occlusive disease/sinusoidal obstruction syndrome after haematopoietic stem cell transplantation (Middle East/North Africa regional consensus on prevention, diagnosis and management). Bone Marrow Transplant. 2017;52(4):588–91.
439. Calitz C, du Plessis L, Gouws C, Steyn D, Steenekamp J, Muller C, Hamman S. Herbal hepatotoxicity: current status, examples, and challenges. Expert Opin Drug Metab Toxicol. 2015;11(10):1551–65.
440. Hamill FA, Apio S, Mubiru NK, Mosango M, Bukenya-Ziraba R, et al. Traditional herbal drugs of southern Uganda, I. J Ethnopharmacol. 2000;70:281–300.
441. Chitturi S, Farrell GC. Herbal hepatotoxicity: an expanding but poorly defined problem. J Gastroenterol Hepatol. 2000;15(10):1093–9.
442. Dara L, Hewett J, Lim JK. Hydroxycut hepatotoxicity: a case series and review of liver toxicity from herbal weight loss supplements. World J Gastroenterol. 2008;14:6999–7004.
443. Teschke R, Fuchs J, Bahre R, Genthner A, Wolff A. Kava hepatotoxicity: comparative study of two structured quantitative methods for causality assessment. J Clin Pharm Ther. 2010;35:545–63.
444. Ashafa AO, Sunmonu TO, Afolayan AJ. Toxicological evaluation of aqueous leaf and berry extracts of Phytolacca dioica L. in male Wistar rats. Food Chem Toxicol. 2010;48:1886–9.
445. Asres K, Sporer F, Wink M. Identification and quantification of hepatotoxic pyrrolizidine alkaloids in the Ethiopian medicinal plant Solanecio gigas (Asteraceae). Pharmazie. 2007;62:709–13.
446. Chen Z, Huo JR. Hepatic veno-occlusive disease associated with toxicity of pyrrolizidine alkaloids in herbal preparations. Neth J Med. 2010;68:252–60.

447. Ridker PM, McDermott WV. Comfrey herb tea and hepatic veno-occlusive disease. Lancet. 1989;1:657–8.
448. Prakash AS, Pereira TN, Reilly PE, Seawright AA. Pyrrolizidine alkaloids in human diet. Mutat Res. 1999;443:53–67.
449. Chen T, Mei N, Fu PP. Genotoxicity of pyrrolizidine alkaloids. J Appl Toxicol. 2010;30:183–96.
450. Yeong ML, Wakefield SJ, Ford HC. Hepatocyte membrane injury and bleb formation following low dose comfrey toxicity in rats. Int J Exp Pathol. 1993;74:211–7.
451. Stewart MJ, Steenkamp V, Zuckerman M. The toxicology of African herbal remedies. Ther Drug Monit. 1998;20(5):510–6.

Pediatric Liver Disease in the Asian Continent

Anshu Srivastava and Rishi Bolia

Abbreviations

AATD	α₁-antitrypsin deficiency
ACLD	Acute on chronic liver disease
ACLF	Acute-on-chronic liver failure
AIH	Autoimmune hepatitis
ALA	Amoebic liver abscess
ALF	Acute liver failure
ALT	Alanine aminotransferase
APASL	Asian Pacific Association for the Study of the Liver
ATT	Antitubercular therapy
AVH	Acute viral hepatitis
BA	Biliary atresia
BCS	Budd–Chiari syndrome
BMI	Body mass index
CAM	Complementary and alternative medicine
CBD	Common bile duct
CHC	Chronic hepatitis C
CLD	Chronic liver disease
CNNA	Culture-negative neutrocytic ascites
CTLN-2	Citrullinemia type II
DAA	Directly acting antivirals
DDLT	Deceased donor liver transplantation
DHF	Dengue haemorrhagic fever
DILI	Drug-induced liver injury
EHPVO	Extrahepatic portal venous obstruction
ERCP	Endoscopic retrograde cholangiopancreatography
ESLD	End-stage liver disease
FTTDCD	Failure to thrive and dyslipidemia caused by citrin deficiency
HAV	Hepatitis A virus
HBeAg	Hepatitis B e antigen
HBsAg	Hepatitis B surface antigen
HBV	Hepatitis B virus
HCC	Hepatocellular carcinoma
HCV	Hepatitis C virus
HEV	Hepatitis E virus
HV	Hepatic veins
ICC	Indian childhood cirrhosis
IPH	Idiopathic portal hypertension
IVC	Inferior vena cava
LDLT	Living donor liver transplantation
LFT	Liver function tests
MARS	Molecular adsorbent recirculating system
MCT	Medium-chain triglyceride
MLPVB	Mesenterico-left portal vein bypass
NAFLD	Non-alcoholic fatty liver disease
NC	Neonatal cholestasis
NCPF	Non-cirrhotic portal fibrosis
NICCD	Neonatal intrahepatic cholestasis caused by citrin deficiency
PAIR	Percutaneous aspiration injection and re-aspiration
PFIC	Progressive familial intrahepatic cholestasis
PHT	Portal hypertension
PLA	Pyogenic liver abscess
SBP	Spontaneous bacterial peritonitis
SEAR	South-East Asia Region
TIPSS	Transjugular intrahepatic portosystemic shunt
UTI	Urinary tract infection
WD	Wilson's disease

A. Srivastava · R. Bolia
Department of Pediatric Gastroenterology, Sanjay Gandhi Postgraduate Institute of Medical Sciences, Lucknow, India

Key Points
- Hepatitis A virus (HAV) is the most common cause of acute viral hepatitis (AVH). Other infections like dengue, leptospirosis, scrub typhus, etc. mimic AVH in clinical presentation.

- Liver abscess has a high incidence among children in this region.
- Hydatid disease (echinococcosis) is endemic mainly in northern China and India.
- Biliary atresia accounts for 22–45% of all cases of neonatal cholestasis. Delay in referral is an ongoing problem in South and East Asia which has improved by use of stool colour cards.
- Alpha-1 antitrypsin deficiency is extremely uncommon in Asia, while neonatal intrahepatic cholestasis caused by citrin deficiency (NICCD) is being increasingly recognized as a cause of cholestasis of infancy in East Asia.
- Extrahepatic portal vein obstruction (EHPVO) with its associated complications of variceal bleeding, portal biliopathy, colopathy, growth failure, etc. is the most common cause of portal hypertension.
- Hepatitis B is endemic in Southeast Asia, with ~75% of people with chronic HBV in the world being from Southeast Asia and Western Pacific regions.
- Due to a delay in diagnosis and non-availability of liver transplantation, a significant proportion of children develop end-stage liver disease and its complications.
- Liver transplantation, which is mainly living donor, is not accessible to a large proportion of the population because of financial constraints.

Research Needed in the Field
- Collaborative research between developing and developed nations to study the complete disease spectrum including complications of end-stage liver disease and thereafter formulate best practice guidelines applicable across the world
- Genetic testing for metabolic liver disease to determine mutations prevalent in different geographical areas

South and East Asia host half of the world's population with India and China alone constituting over 36% of it [1]. About one third of all child deaths in the world occur in WHO South-East Asia region (SEAR) which is home to nearly 2/3 of the world's malnourished children [2, 3]. The population density, ethnicity and economic status differ between the various countries in this region as well as in different areas of the specific country.

Liver diseases are an important cause of morbidity and mortality. The prevalence and spectrum of liver diseases in this region are different from what is seen in the west. Malnutrition, unsafe water and inadequate sanitation, high prevalence of infections including viral hepatitis, socio-economic disparity, a different genetic make-up and poor access to healthcare, are the most important reasons for these differences [4]. A shortage of trained healthcare workers has further compounded this problem. Southeast Asia has 4.3 health workers per 1000 population, compared with the USA, where there are 24.8 healthcare workers per 1000 population [5]. Lack of awareness and limitations of access and availability of advanced healthcare often leads to delay in diagnosis and presentation with advanced liver disease with its attendant complications.

Literature to be considered for inclusion in this chapter was based on a systematic search of two common electronic databases (PubMed and Google Scholar). Publications from the year 2000 and beyond have been included. The search was restricted to reports written in English. Data from the following countries was included—India, Pakistan, Bangladesh, Sri Lanka, Nepal, Bhutan, the Maldives, Myanmar, Malaysia, Thailand, Singapore, Taiwan, Vietnam, North Korea, South Korea, Hong Kong, Indonesia, the Philippines, Cambodia and China (Fig. 41.1). Data from secondary sources, such as WHO and government reports and statistics, were also searched and included.

In the following sections, we have dealt with different group of liver diseases like acute hepatitis and liver failure, chronic liver disease and its complications, neonatal cholestasis and hepatobiliary infections separately, giving the epidemiology in this region and highlighting the differences between the aetiology, clinical presentation and outcome of these conditions as compared to the "west".

41.1 Acute Hepatitis and Acute Liver Failure

Acute hepatitis is a nonspecific term that refers to an acute inflammation of the liver resulting from a wide range of aetiologies. Depending on the aetiology, acute hepatitis may show a self-limiting course or recovery in response to treatment or withdrawal of the offending agent. It may also result in a fulminant course leading to acute liver failure (ALF). There are considerable differences in the aetiology of ALF between Asia and the west. Paracetamol overdose and metabolic diseases, which are the commonest identifiable cause of ALF in the UK, Canada and the USA, are less commonly seen in Southeast Asia [6]. The most common ALF aetiology here is viral hepatitis (hepatitis A virus), which is often associated with a poor outcome (Table 41.1).

41.1.1 Acute Viral Hepatitis (AVH)

Hepatitis A virus (HAV) is the most common cause of AVH. Studies from India and Nepal have shown that HAV, HEV and HBV account for 64–85%, 8–16% and 5–14% of

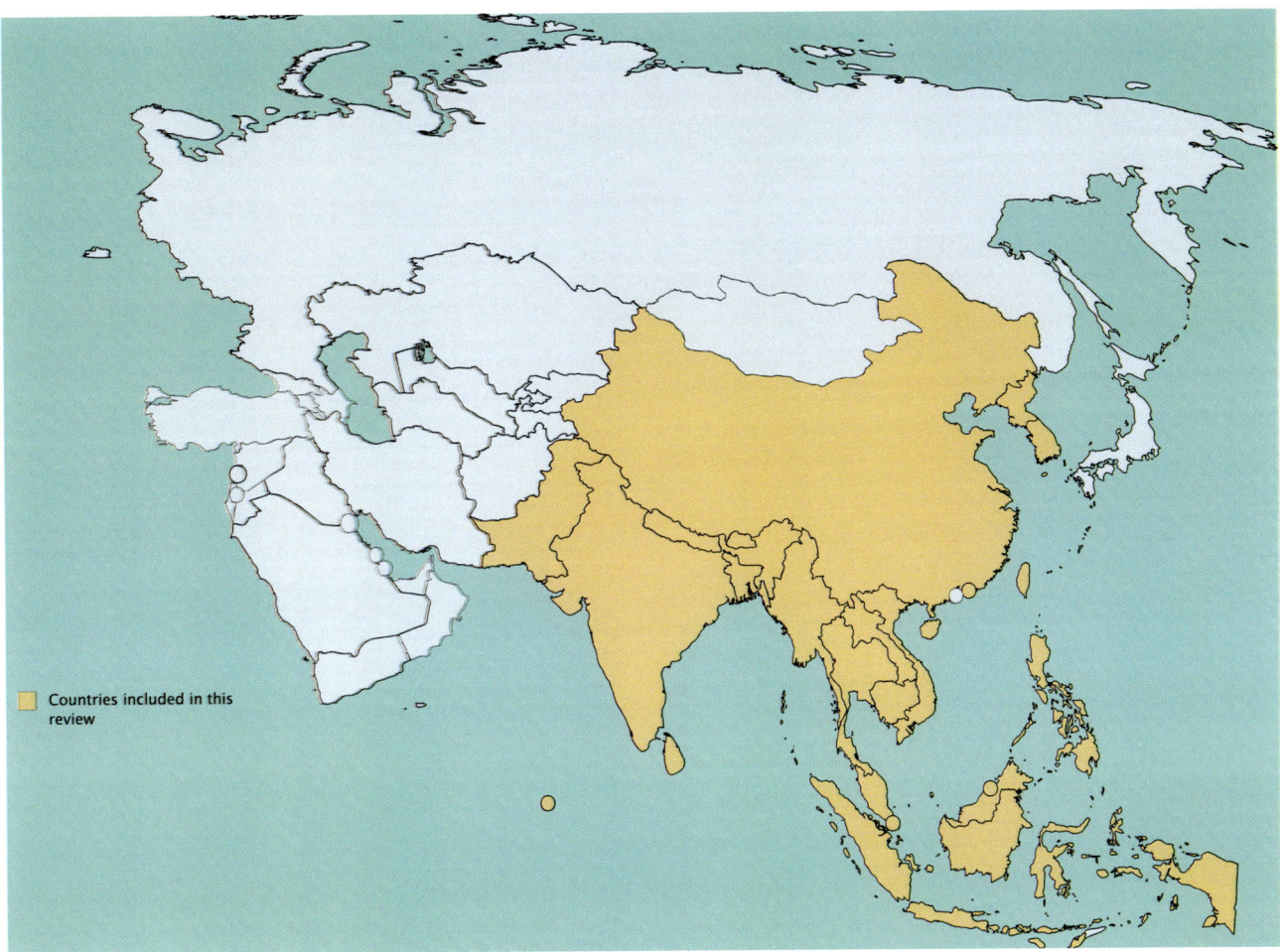

Fig. 41.1 Map of Asia showing the countries included in this review

Table 41.1 Aetiology and outcome of acute liver failure

Country (year)	Most common aetiology (%) (reference)	Number (n) of cases Age group	Outcome[a] (mortality)	Other common causes
Bangladesh (2009)	Viral hepatitis (34.5%) [7]	n = 35 0–18 years	34%[b]	Wilson's disease 31%
Vietnam (2008)	Hepatitis A (28.6%)[c] [8]	n = 33 3 months–15 years	–	–
Pakistan (2010)	Hepatitis A (56%) [9]	n = 50 1–15 years	60%	HBV 18%, Wilson's disease 8%
Philippines (2012)	Hepatitis A (19.2%) [10]	n = 27 0–18 years	84.6%	HBV 3.8%
India (2013)	Hepatitis A (49.4–58%) [11–13]	n = 43–97 <18 years	25–45.3%	HBV 4.6–14.4% HEV 4.6–27%
Thailand (2013)	Dengue (18–34.3%) [14, 15]	n = 11, 40 1–15 years	45–68.6%	HBV 9% Wilson's disease 9%
China (2014)	DILI (25%) [16]	n = 32 ≤12 years	58%	CMV 18.7% Indeterminate 47%

[a]Mortality without transplantation, *DILI* drug-induced liver injury, *HBV* hepatitis B virus, *HEV* hepatitis E virus, *CMV* cytomegalovirus
[b]Additional 23% left hospital with risk bond
[c]Hepatitis A (HAV IgM positive)

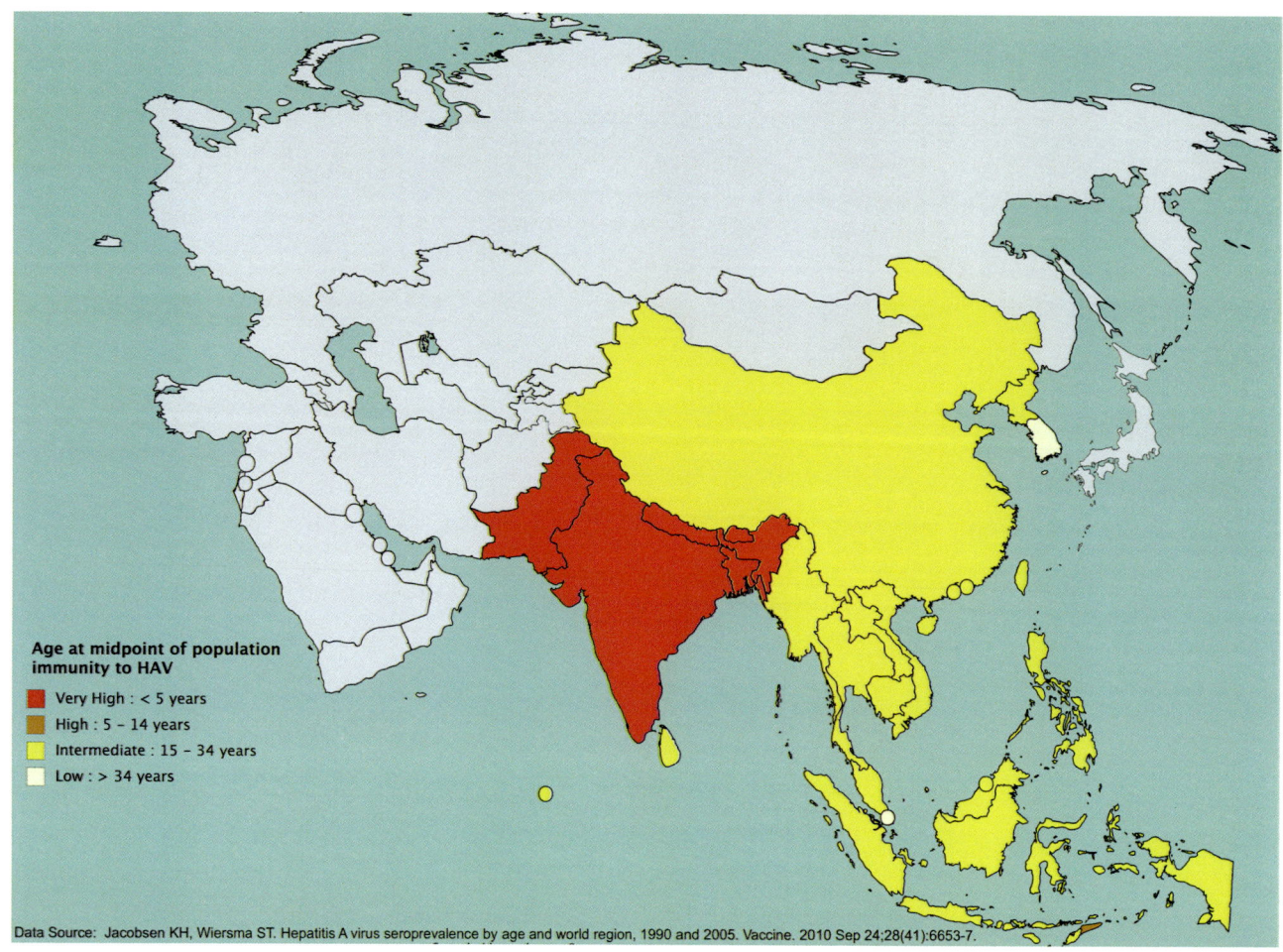

Fig. 41.2 Risk map of HAV immunity in South, East and Southeast Asia

all AVH in children, respectively [17–20]. The typical presentation is of a prodrome followed by the appearance of jaundice and then recovery over 4–6 weeks. Prolonged cholestasis, relapsing hepatitis (with clear improvement between two icteric periods), acute pancreatitis, thrombocytopenia, transient ascites and intravascular haemolysis due to G6PD deficiency are the atypical manifestations seen in children with AVH [17, 18, 20, 21]. Ascites has been reported in 10–22% cases of sporadic AVH in children. These children with AVH and ascites, are mostly younger, have compromised biosynthetic liver functions irrespective of viral aetiology and show complete recovery in follow-up [22]. Presence of ascites in an AVH case suggests either AVH alone or an underlying asymptomatic chronic liver disease (CLD) with superimposed AVH (also known as acute on chronic liver disease [ACLD]). Proper evaluation (both for aetiology and underlying CLD) and follow-up till complete recovery is required to differentiate between the two entities.

The endemicity of hepatitis A in the SEAR ranges from low (<50% exposed by the age of 30 years) in the eastern areas to high (90% exposed by the age of 10 years) in the southern areas [23] (Fig. 41.2). The overall annual number of acute hepatitis A cases is estimated to be ~400,000 with 800 deaths [24]. In recent years an epidemiological transition is being seen in this region with a number of countries shifting from high to moderate and from moderate to low endemicity. The changes have resulted from improvement in sanitation and quality of drinking water, reflecting socio-economic progress. This shifting from high to intermediate endemicity, paradoxically, leads to higher disease incidence of hepatitis A as infections occur in the older age groups in whom reported rates of clinically evident hepatitis A are higher [25]. This also highlights the importance of use of vaccine against HAV in preventing the infection and associated morbidity.

Hepatitis E virus (HEV) infection is the second common cause of AVH. The seroprevalence of HEV as determined by presence of IgG HEV ranges from 0.3 to 17% in children <10 years of age and 1.3–25% in 11–20 years old in this region [26]. The clinical features and transmission are similar to HAV. However HEV infection can lead to a chronic carrier state with chronic hepatitis in immune-suppressed children with solid organ transplants [27].

Co-infection with multiple viruses, especially hepatitis A and E, is observed in some patients with acute viral hepatitis; however it has not been shown to produce more severe disease [17].

41.1.2 Drug-Induced Hepatitis

Acute hepatitis is the most common manifestation of drug-induced liver injury (DILI). In the west paracetamol is the leading cause of DILI. In contrast, the leading cause in children in India is antitubercular therapy (ATT, combination of three hepatotoxic drugs [isoniazid, rifampicin and pyrazinamide], 56%) and antiepileptics (phenytoin and carbamazepine, 41%) [28]. ATT-induced hepatotoxicity is seen in 5–28% patients and can vary from transient asymptomatic elevation in the liver enzymes to icteric hepatitis to fulminant liver failure. Isoniazid is the most commonly incriminated drug [29]. Most of the ATT-induced liver injury is seen in the first 2 months of therapy although it can occur any time. Twenty-five percent of all ATT-related DILI have ALF, and these patients have a worse outcome (mortality of ~70%) in comparison to ALF related to AVH [30]. Regular monitoring for symptoms and liver function tests (LFT) can lead to early detection of liver injury and timely stoppage of ATT. Strict caution and guidelines need to be followed for reintroducing ATT in patients with DILI and also while prescribing ATT to children with CLD [31].

41.1.3 Toxin-Induced Hepatitis

"Mushroom (genus – *Amanita phalloides*) poisoning" is another cause of ALF reported from this part of the world [32]. Most of the cases present with nausea, vomiting and diarrhoea following ingestion, which are labelled and treated as food poisoning. Hepatic injury is seen after 48–96 h of ingestion and progresses to ALF with high mortality (~66%, 13/18 children) [32]. Silymarin, penicillin G and plasmapheresis/molecular adsorbent recirculating system (MARS) for removal of toxin have been reported to improve the outcome [33]. Suicidal or accidental poisoning with rodenticides containing yellow phosphorous ("Ratol"—3% yellow phosphorous) is an important cause of ALF in India. Toxic cardiomyopathy and rhabdomyolysis with renal failure are often associated in this condition [34].

41.1.4 Other Infections Associated with Jaundice and Deranged Liver Function Tests (LFT)

A clinical presentation like ALF can be seen in various tropical infections, and these conditions may mimic ALF. Malarial hepatopathy due to *Plasmodium falciparum* infection may have jaundice, anaemia, splenomegaly and altered sensorium [35]. A similar presentation can also be seen in dengue [36, 37], typhoid, leptospirosis and scrub typhus [38, 39]. The major differentiating feature between AVH and these infections is that fever subsides after appearance of jaundice in AVH, while it continues in other infections. However, one should remember that simultaneous infections are not uncommon, for example, hepatitis A infection and enteric fever occurring together as both have feco-oral transmission [40].

Dengue fever is a major challenge to public health in Southeast Asia and has been reported from every country in this region except DPR Korea [41]. Dengue infection is the most important cause of ALF in children in Thailand [14]. In a study on 312 patients from Laos, it was the second most common cause for acute hepatitis (after HAV) [42]. Liver injury is more common in children with severe dengue, i.e. dengue haemorrhagic fever (DHF) [43]. Reported case fatality rates for the region are approximately 1%, but in India, Indonesia and Myanmar, focal outbreaks away from the urban areas have reported case fatality rates of 3–5%. The peak of the disease is seen from June to September, generally around the rainy season [44]. In a study from Thailand comparing patients with DHF and other causes of liver failure, it was found that DHF patients had significantly higher AST than ALT [37]. Other pointers towards a diagnosis of dengue would be presence of rash, leucopoenia, arthralgia, myalgia, a positive tourniquet test and thrombocytopenia.

41.2 Hepatobiliary Infections

Liver abscess (Fig. 41.3a–c) in the paediatric population has become relatively uncommon in developed countries, but it continues to have a high incidence among children in developing countries. Incidence varies from ~724 per 100,000 admissions in Brazil, 78.9 per 100,000 paediatric admissions in South India and down to 25 and 20 cases per 100,000 admissions in the USA and Taiwan [45].

Pyogenic liver abscess (PLA) is much more common in children than amoebic liver abscess (ALA). The incidence of ALA is decreasing [45]. *Staphylococcus aureus* is the most common isolated pathogen of paediatric PLA both in developed and developing countries. However, *Klebsiella pneumoniae* (*K. pneumoniae*) has recently been reported as the leading cause of PLA in Taiwan [46]. Chaudhary et al. have reported 154 children (mean age of 6.7 years) with PLA over a 5-year period from a single centre in North India [47]. Nearly 25% cases settled with medical therapy alone, 55% required percutaneous drainage (aspiration or catheter drainage) and 20% needed open surgical drainage. The mortality rate in LA has now been reduced to <5% [47, 48].

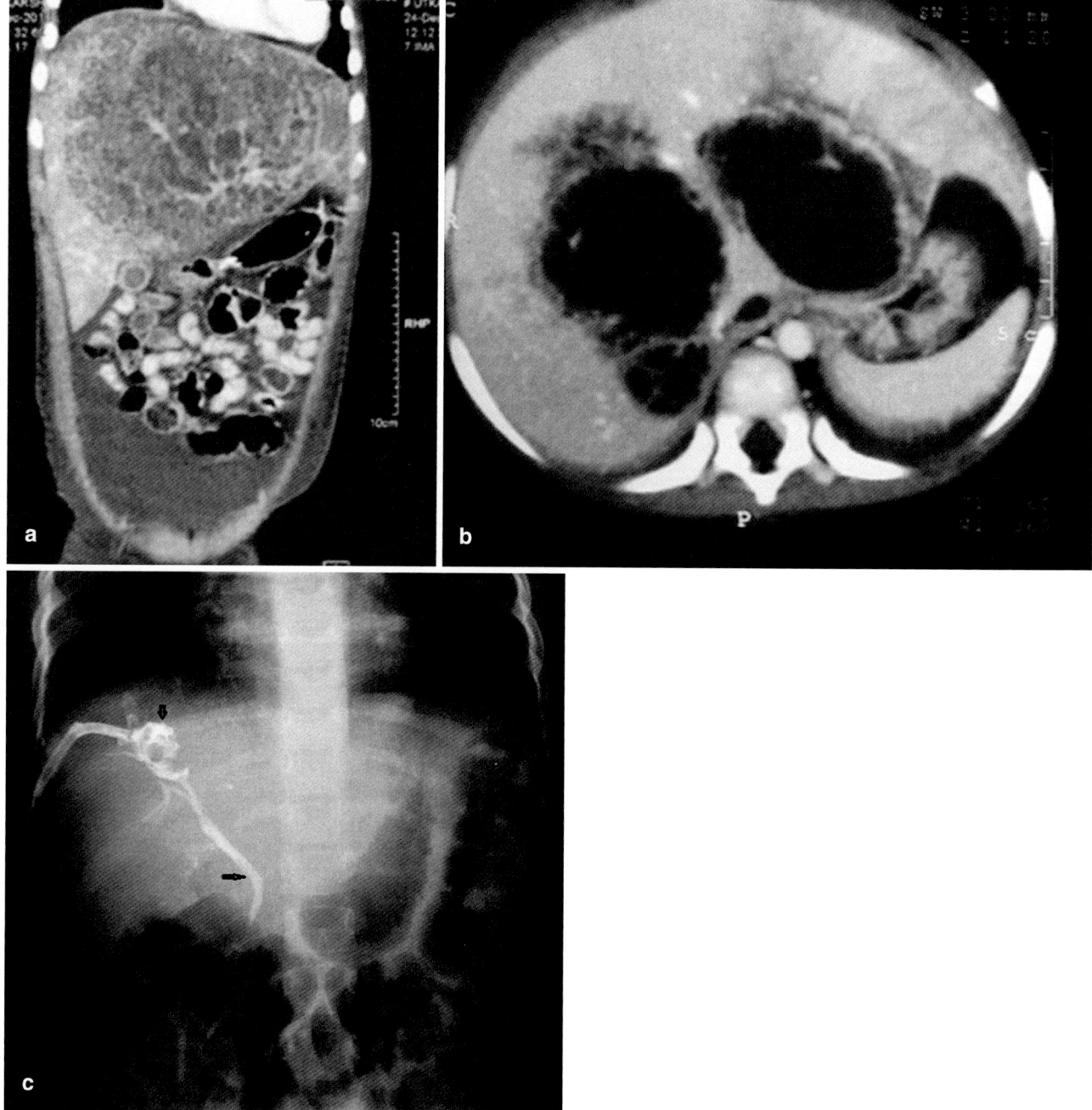

Fig. 41.3 (a) Contrast-enhanced computed tomography (CECT) showing a large multiloculated pyogenic liver abscess with impending rupture with ascites. (b) Contrast-enhanced computed tomography (CECT) of two large liver abscesses with liquefied contents with two other adjacent smaller multiloculated abscesses. (c) Cavitogram in patient with liver abscess with percutaneous catheter drainage showing communication of the liver abscess with the biliary tree. Solid arrow showing the common bile duct, and other arrow showing the abscess cavity

Underlying immunodeficiency especially chronic granulomatous disease is seen commonly in children with PLA from the west [49]. On the other hand, in developing countries increased frequency of helminthic infections and malnutrition is thought to predispose children towards PLA, and they do not commonly have any overt immunodeficiency [45]. The clinical presentation of PLA and ALA is similar except that multiloculated abscess on USG is a feature of PLA, and drainage is less often required in ALA [48].

Rare cases of liver abscess due to tuberculosis and ascariasis have been reported from the Indian subcontinent [50, 51]. Ascariasis is endemic in the Indian subcontinent and Pakistan [52]. In Kashmir, in northern India, ascariasis is the most common parasitic infestation and accounts for 50–60% of paediatric admissions in the surgical emergency department. Hepatobiliary and pancreatic ascariasis accounts for about 10% of such admissions [53]. Ultrasound abdomen shows presence of worms in gall bladder/common bile duct (CBD) and confirms the diagnosis. Complications include obstructive jaundice, cholangitis, cholecystitis, acute pancreatitis and hepatic abscesses. Medical therapy (albendazole, antibiotics) and extraction of worms from CBD on endoscopic retrograde cholangiopancreatography (ERCP) were successful in 97% cases in a large series of 214 cases from India [53].

In Asia, hydatid disease (Echinococcosis) (Fig. 41.4) is endemic mainly in the Middle East, India and northern China [54]. But it is seen in other parts of Asia as well. A high prevalence has also been documented in Nepal [55]. The highest prevalence is found in rural areas where older animals are slaughtered. Most often children have cystic echinococcosis (caused by *E. granulosus*) which involves the liver and lung, and they present with hepatomegaly, pain and fever. Around 20% are asymptomatic and detected incidentally [56]. Treatment may be summarized into four basic modalities: antiparasitic drugs (albendazole), percutaneous aspiration injection and re-aspiration (PAIR), surgery and non-intervention (watch and wait) [57]. Alveolar echinococcosis caused by *E. multilocularis* is an aggressive disease described mostly from north and northwest China [58]. Invasion of contagious structures and brain metastasis can occur, and surgical resection along with albendazole is essential for therapy.

41.3 Neonatal Cholestasis

Cholestasis is defined as impaired bile formation or flow resulting in accumulation of various substances (bilirubin, bile acids and cholesterol, etc.) which are normally excreted in bile. Neonatal cholestasis (NC) was seen in 0.3–2.8% neonates in the South East Asia Regional Neonatal-Perinatal Database [59]. Presence of conjugated hyperbilirubinemia is the hallmark of NC and differentiates it from the more common condition of unconjugated hyperbilirubinemia in neonates/infants. The prevalence of neonatal cholestasis and the common causes in South, East and Southeast Asia have been summarized in Table 41.2.

41.3.1 Biliary Atresia

Of the various aetiologies of NC, the thrust is on early diagnosis and management of potentially treatable conditions, commonest of which is biliary atresia (BA). Studies on aetiology of NC from Bangladesh, India, Nepal, Indonesia, Malaysia, Taiwan and China have shown that biliary atresia (BA) accounts for 22–45% of all NC cases [62–66]. BA is a condition where prompt diagnosis and early intervention are essential for a good outcome. Delay in referral is a major problem encountered in this region. In a study from Malaysia, 45% of patients with NC were referred after 60 days of life [65]. The average age at diagnosis of BA was 88.6 days in

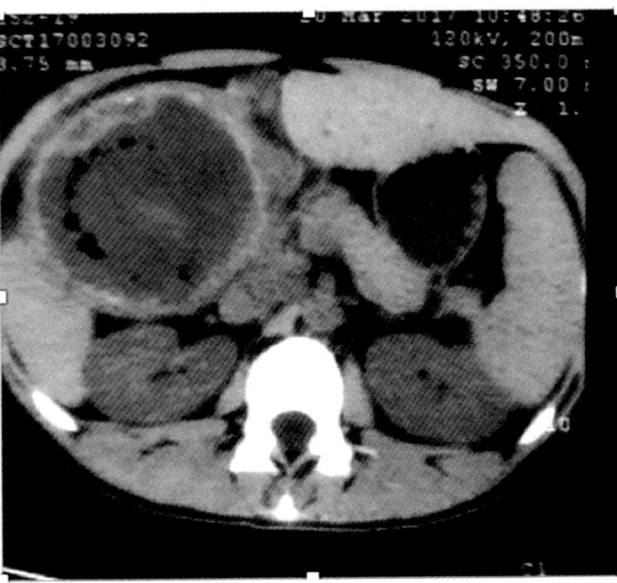

Fig. 41.4 Contrast-enhanced computed tomography (CECT) showing hydatid cyst of the liver with membranes and air in the cyst. This child had spontaneous rupture of hydatid cyst into the biliary tree and underwent ERCP with extraction of membranes from common bile duct and stenting of CBD

Table 41.2 Aetiology of neonatal cholestasis

Country, year, number of cases	Prevalence [59]	Common causes and frequency (percentage)
Bangladesh [60] (2005) n = 62	–	Neonatal hepatitis (TORCH)—35.5%, biliary atresia—25.8%
India [61] (2010) n = 410	0.3%	Biliary atresia—30%, choledochal cyst 4.6% TORCH and other infections—16.3%, unknown 30.7%
Indonesia	0.07–2.8%	–
Nepal	0.03%	–
Thailand [62] (2005) n = 252	1.8%	Idiopathic neonatal hepatitis (INH) 23% Extrahepatic biliary atresia 22.2% TPN-related cholestasis 18.3%
Malaysia [63] (2010) n = 146		Idiopathic neonatal hepatitis (38%) Biliary atresia (29%)
Taiwan [64] (2014) n = 256		Biliary atresia (35.9%), neonatal hepatitis (26%) PFIC (11.3%), NICCD (5.5%)

TORCH Toxoplasma gondii, rubella, cytomegalovirus and herpes simplex virus, *TPN* total parenteral nutrition, *PFIC* progressive familial intrahepatic cholestasis, *NICCD* neonatal intrahepatic cholestasis caused by citrin deficiency

Thailand [66]. Lack of awareness among medical and public health workers is an important reason for the delay. Educating healthcare workers, creation of simple guidelines and the yellow alert programme have led to some improvement in referral age in India [67]. To promote the early diagnosis of BA, a universal screening system using an infant stool colour card was established in 2002 in Taiwan [68]. This simple innovation led to significant improvement in the outcome of infants with BA. The proportion of children subjected to Kasai portoenterostomy at an age of <60 days increased from 49.4 to 65.7% ($p < 0.02$), 5-year jaundice-free survival rate with native liver increased from 27.3 to 64.3% ($p < 0.001$), and the 5-year overall survival rate increased from 55.7 to 89.3% ($p < 0.001$) in cohorts who were diagnosed before and after the use of universal screening stool card [68].

41.3.2 α_1-Antitrypsin Deficiency (AATD)

The prevalence of AATD varies in different geographical regions, being the highest in Northern and Western Europe with a mean gene frequency of Z allele of 0.014 among Caucasians. The gene frequency in data available from seven countries (Indonesia, Malaysia, Singapore, the Philippines, Thailand, Vietnam, New Guinea) in Southeast Asia is low (0.0036). It is 0 in China and 0.0061 in South Korea [69]. Nearly 10–15% of individuals with PiZZ AAT phenotype develop liver injury, which may take the form of neonatal cholestasis syndrome, asymptomatic derangement of liver function tests or compensated or decompensated chronic liver disease during childhood. In studies from the West, AAT deficiency has been reported in 0.5–2% of children with CLD and 5–15% of those with NC [70]. In comparison, AATD is extremely uncommon in Asia. In a study from Bangladesh, 1 of 62 (1.6%) infants with NC had AAT deficiency [60]. In a prospective study from Malaysia, no cases of AAT deficiency were identified on evaluation of 114 consecutive patients with liver diseases [71]. Similar results were obtained in studies from the Philippines and India [61, 72].

41.3.3 Neonatal Intrahepatic Cholestasis Caused by Citrin Deficiency (NICCD)

This entity is being increasingly recognized as a cause of cholestasis of infancy in East Asia. It was first described by Ohura et al. in 2001 [73]. NICCD occurs due to mutation in SLC25A13 gene located at chromosome 7q21.3. Nearly 81 mutations have been described; the frequency of individual mutations varies from country to country [74]. Majority of reported cases are in Japanese and East Asian populations, including Taiwanese, Korean and Chinese [75]. The carrier frequency is 1/63, 1/65, 1/108 and 1/110 in the Chinese, Japanese, Korean and Thai population, respectively [76].

Citrin deficiency has a different presentation at different ages which includes neonatal intrahepatic cholestasis caused by citrin deficiency (NICCD) in infants, failure to thrive and dyslipidemia caused by citrin deficiency (FTTDCD) in young children and adult onset citrullinemia type II (CTLN-2) [77]. NICCD patients present with NC in the first few months of life, with a chubby face, hepatomegaly (fatty liver) and failure to thrive. Liver dysfunction with hypoalbuminemia, coagulopathy, with or without hypoglycaemia, high plasma citrulline, methionine, tyrosine, threonine and/or arginine is seen. Patients with NICCD are sometimes confused with those with galactosemia and tyrosinemia. In two studies from Taiwan and China, citrin deficiency was the cause of neonatal cholestasis in 10.4 and 11% of intrahepatic NC [64, 78]. The symptoms in most children with NICCD resolve by 12 months of age. However, a small group may develop progressive liver failure and need transplantation. Therapy is with lactose (galactose)-restricted and medium-chain triglyceride (MCT)-supplemented formula and fat-soluble vitamin supplementation.

Younger children with citrin deficiency often develop a fondness for protein-/lipid-rich food and dislike for carbohydrates by 2 years of age. This gives a clue to the likely diagnosis when one is evaluating a nonobese child with fatty liver. These cases can also present with recurrent pancreatitis. Some patients may develop CTLN 2 as adults, usually after the first decade, and present with fatty liver and neurological manifestations due to hyperammonemia which is often fatal [79].

Confirmation of diagnosis requires DNA sequencing analysis to detect mutation in the SLC25A13 gene. As the majority of infants with NICCD recover, they are often wrongly diagnosed as idiopathic neonatal hepatitis. Citrin deficiency should be kept in mind in children with NC or fatty liver across all populations [80].

41.3.4 Progressive Familial Intrahepatic Cholestasis (PFIC)

In recent years, PFIC is increasingly being recognized as a cause of NC and also of cholestatic jaundice in older infants from this region [81, 82]. PFIC accounted for 8 and 11% of all NC in studies from India and Taiwan [64, 81]. The mutations reported in Taiwanese patients were different from that reported in the western population [83]. High index of suspicion and inclusion of GGT in liver function testing is useful. However, non-availability of immunohistochemistry and genetic analysis at most places is a major limitation in confirming the diagnosis of PFIC from this region.

41.4 Non-cirrhotic Portal Hypertension (NCPHT)

This includes a group of liver disorders characterized by clinically significant portal hypertension (PHT) with preserved liver function [84]. Extrahepatic portal venous obstruction (EHPVO) and non-cirrhotic portal fibrosis (NCPF) are the two main aetiologies of NCPHT which are more often seen in the developing world [84]. The aetiology of PHT in children varies from country to country. In the west, cirrhosis is the most common cause, while in the developing world, EHPVO is most common [85]. In a large study of 517 children with PHT from India, EHPVO was seen in 54%, cirrhosis in 39%, congenital hepatic fibrosis (CHF) in 3%, NCPF in 2% and Budd–Chiari syndrome (BCS) in 2% cases [85]. Similarly, EHPVO accounted for 73% and NCPF for 11% of all cases of non-cirrhotic PHT, in a study of predominantly young adults from China [86].

41.4.1 Extrahepatic Portal Venous Obstruction (EHPVO)

As per the Asian Pacific Association for the Study of the Liver (APASL) consensus, EHPVO is defined as "a vascular disorder of liver, characterized by obstruction of the extrahepatic portal vein (PV) with or without involvement of intra-hepatic PV radicles or splenic or superior mesenteric veins" [87]. Extensive work has been done and published on EHPVO from India. The various factors linked causatively to EHPVO include umbilical sepsis/catheterization, portal pyemia after intra-abdominal sepsis and various prothrombotic states. However, the aetiology remains idiopathic in more than 70% cases. As majority of these patients belong to the lower socio-economic strata and disease seems to be declining in the last decade even in the developing world, it suggests that infection plays an important role.

EHPVO generally presents with variceal bleeding and/or splenomegaly [85, 88]. The bleeding episodes are recurrent and often related to febrile illnesses. Historically, variceal bleed was the main concern in EHPVO, but with the availability of effective medications and endotherapy (Fig. 41.5a, b), variceal bleed is effectively controlled, and mortality has become a rarity. The presence of PHT, development of portosystemic collaterals and reduced hepatic blood flow are responsible for the various complications seen in EHPVO patients. These include growth failure, poor quality of life, portal biliopathy (Fig. 41.6a, b), colopathy/enteropathy (Fig. 41.7a, b), minimal hepatic encephalopathy, hepato-pulmonary syndrome, recurrence of bleed due to secondary gastric varices, autonomic dysfunction and liver dysfunction [84, 89–91]. Shunt surgery (portosystemic shunts, meso-Rex bypass) offers a single one-time definitive procedure for alleviating the portal hypertension. The only curative therapy for EHPVO is the creation of a physiological shunt, i.e. mesenterico-left PV bypass (MLPVB) or Rex shunt which maintains the hepatic portal blood flow and reduces the portal hypertension as well. Various non-physiological shunts which bypass the portal blood either totally (nonselective, e.g. mesocaval or proximal splenorenal) or partially (selective, e.g. distal splenorenal) into systemic circulation have been used for treatment of EHPVO for a long time. The timing and choice of surgical shunt depends on various factors like favourable anatomy, technical expertise and availability of interventional radiology support [91, 92].

41.4.2 Non-cirrhotic Portal Fibrosis (NCPF)

This disorder of presinusoidal portal hypertension occurs due to involvement of small and medium branches of the portal vein and is also referred to as idiopathic portal hypertension (IPH), hepatoportal sclerosis or obliterative venopathy in literature [84]. NCPF is diagnosed in a child presenting with portal hypertension (splenomegaly/varices) with preserved liver functions, patent portal and hepatic veins and liver histology showing typical changes of preserved lobular architecture, phlebosclerosis, periportal fibrosis, aberrant vessels in portal tract and absence of cirrhosis [84, 93].

Typically NCPF has been described in older children generally in their early second decade, with an average age of 11 and 13.8 years at diagnosis in two series from India [94, 95]. However, it can occur in children as young as 5 years [95]. Most cases present with splenomegaly and or variceal bleed, and the diagnosis is made after exclusion of EHPVO and cirrhosis. Most cases have moderate to massive splenomegaly, and the liver may be normal, enlarged or slightly shrunken. Management centres around control of variceal bleed followed by secondary prophylaxis until eradication and supportive therapy for complications like anaemia, hypersplenism, splenic infarct and post bleed ascites, etc. Screening for transfusion-acquired hepatitis B/C and vaccination against hepatitis B should always be done in children with NCPHT.

Congenital hepatic fibrosis which primarily affects the renal and hepatobiliary system is another important cause of NCPHT which has been reported from around the world including Southeast Asia in children [85, 96].

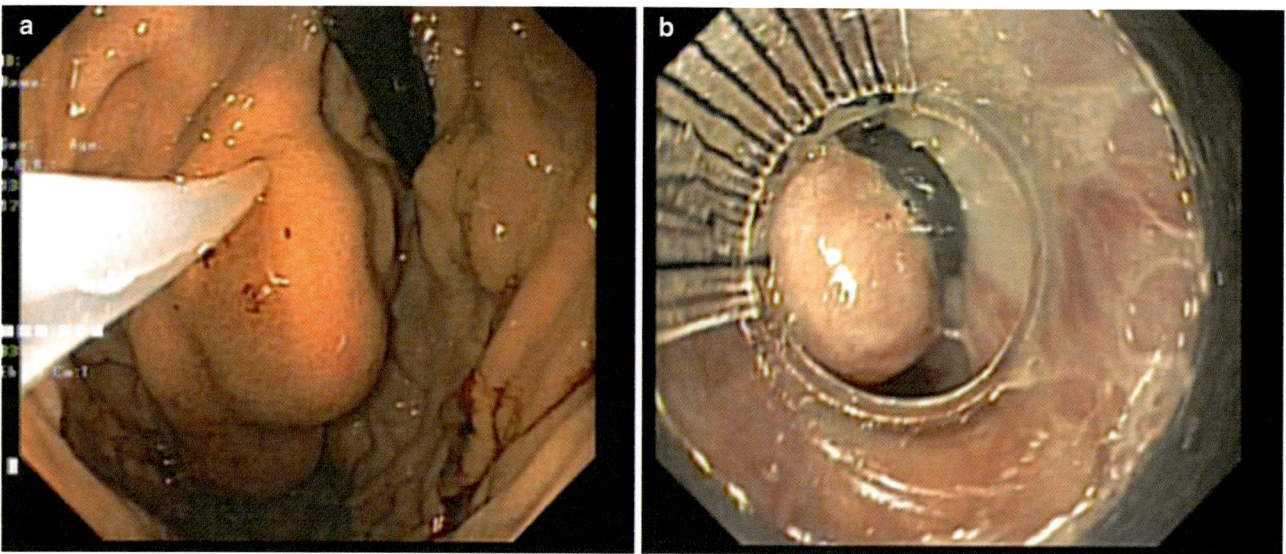

Fig. 41.5 (a) Upper gastrointestinal endoscopy showing large fundal varices (scope in retroversion position) with sclerotherapy needle in situ for glue injection in a child with extrahepatic portal venous obstruction with gastric variceal bleed. (b) Upper gastrointestinal endoscopy showing endoscopic variceal ligation (EVL) of large oesophageal varices (band seen in black) and cylinder of multi-band ligator being seen

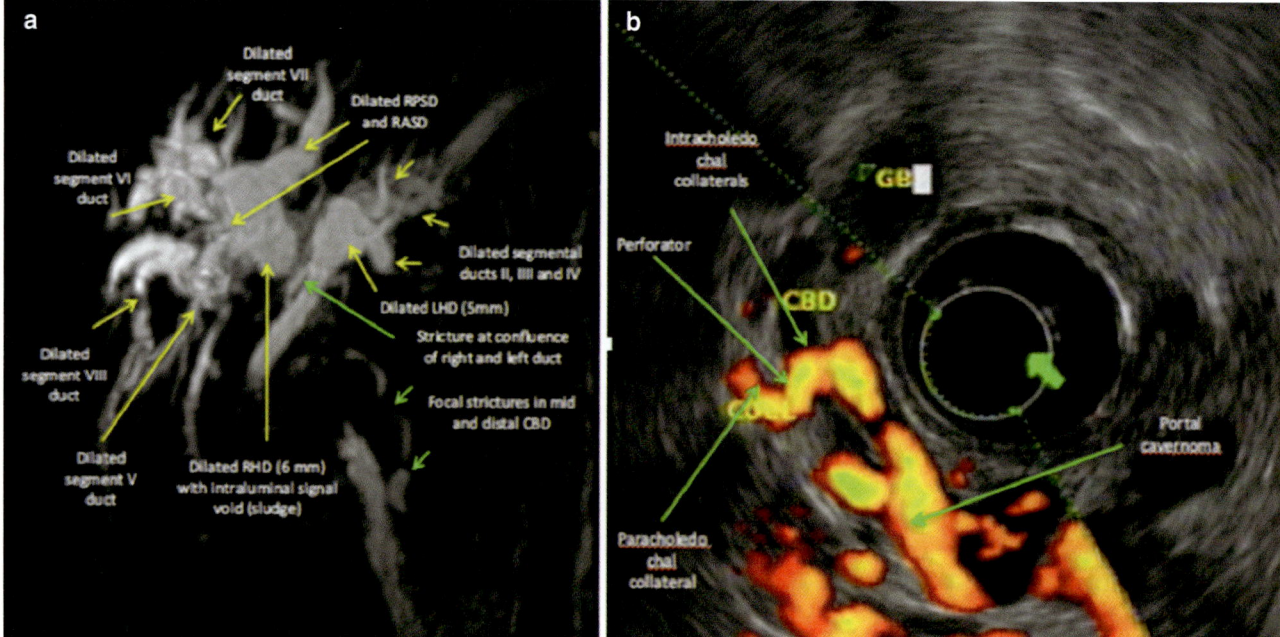

Fig. 41.6 (a) Magnetic resonance cholangiopancreatography (MRCP) showing portal biliopathy in a child with extrahepatic portal venous obstruction. (b) Endoscopic ultrasound showing intra- and paracholedochal collaterals in a patient with EHPVO and portal biliopathy

41.5 Chronic Liver Disease and Its Complications

Chronic liver disease (CLD) refers to a spectrum of disease ranging from chronic hepatitis to cirrhosis with or without decompensation. The aetiology of CLD includes a wide range of genetic and acquired disorders, and it varies among infants, younger children and adolescents. The aetiology also varies between the west and Asian countries, with BA, AATD and autoimmune hepatitis (AIH) being more common in the west and hepatitis B/C and Wilson's disease (WD) in Asia. The proportion of cryptogenic cases may be

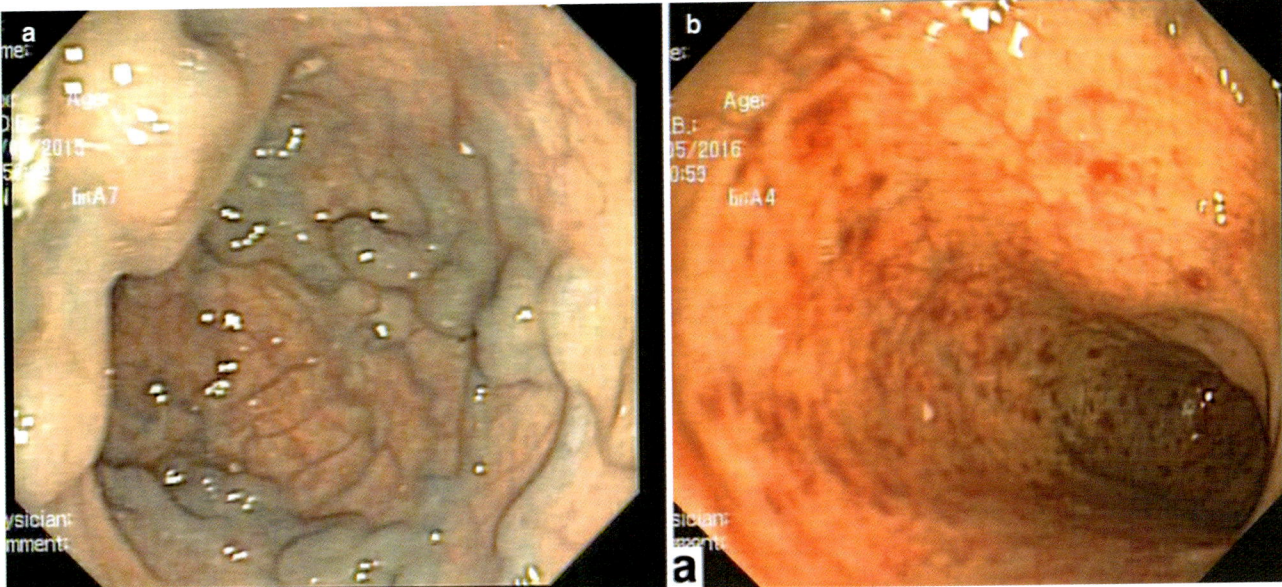

Fig. 41.7 (a) Colonoscopy showing rectal varices in a child with extrahepatic portal venous obstruction. (b) Colonoscopy showing changes of portal hypertensive colopathy in a child with extrahepatic portal venous obstruction

higher in the developing world due to lack of extensive testing mostly for metabolic liver diseases. The few available studies on the aetiology of CLD as an all-inclusive group are shown in Table 41.3.

41.5.1 Hepatitis B

Low- and middle-income countries have the maximum burden of hepatitis B virus (HBV)-related disease and its complications. Nearly 25% subjects who get HBV in childhood develop cirrhosis or hepatocellular carcinoma (HCC) in adulthood [101]. Hepatitis B is endemic in Southeast Asia, with ~75% of people with chronic HBV in the world being from Southeast Asia and Western Pacific regions [102]. The hepatitis B prevalence as per WHO 2013 estimates was 10.8% for Vietnam, 8.7% for Laos, 6.4% for Thailand, 4.1% for Cambodia and 3.4% for Myanmar [103]. China has a prevalence ranging from 7.9 to 8.7% [104, 105]. India, Pakistan and Bangladesh have a prevalence ranging from 2 to 8% in different population groups, while in Sri Lanka it is <1% [106–108] (Fig. 41.8). The overall seroprevalence of hepatitis B in SEAR region in the young age group of 0–14 years is 1.2–1.4% [109]. The HBV genotypes reported from the different countries are as follows—*India* (A, C, D), *Pakistan* (D), *China* (B, C), *Indonesia* (B, C), *Vietnam* (B, C), *Hong Kong* (B, C), *the Philippines* (B, C), *Thailand* (B, C), *Taiwan* (B) *and South Korea* (C) [101].

The introduction of the hepatitis B vaccine has led to a substantial reduction of chronic hepatitis B infection in these countries where infection is transmitted in early childhood.

Table 41.3 Aetiology of chronic liver disease in children

	India [97] (2016) 3 months–18 years (n = 499)	China [98] (2004) (biopsy based, n = 1020, 0–16 years)	Pakistan [99, 100] (2004, n = 55, 1–14 years and 2011, n = 60, <12 years)
Cholestatic including biliary atresia	17.6%	0.1% (BA)	6.7%
Chronic hepatitis B and hepatitis C	22.8% (includes Hep B and C)	75.4% 12.9%	5–24% 31.6%
NAFLD	9.8%	NA	NA
Autoimmune	11.2%	0.7%	1.7–16%
Wilson's disease	11.4%	1.9%	6.7–16%
Other MLD	11.4%		8.3%
HVOTO and cryptogenic	15.6%	0.1%	35–44%

NAFLD non-alcoholic fatty liver disease, *MLD* metabolic liver disease, *HVOTO* hepatic vein outflow tract obstruction

Within 10 years of launching the vaccination programme against HBV, the hepatitis B surface antigen (HBsAg) carrier rate of Taiwanese children decreased tenfold, from approximately 10 to 1%. This was accompanied by a four fold reduction in HCC incidence rate in 6–9-year-olds. This demonstrated for the first time that a mass vaccination programme can reduce cancer incidence in humans [110]. In China, chronic HBV carrier rate in children fell from 10% in the year 1992 to 1–2% in 2006, after initiation of universal infant vaccination programme, thus preventing ~30 million

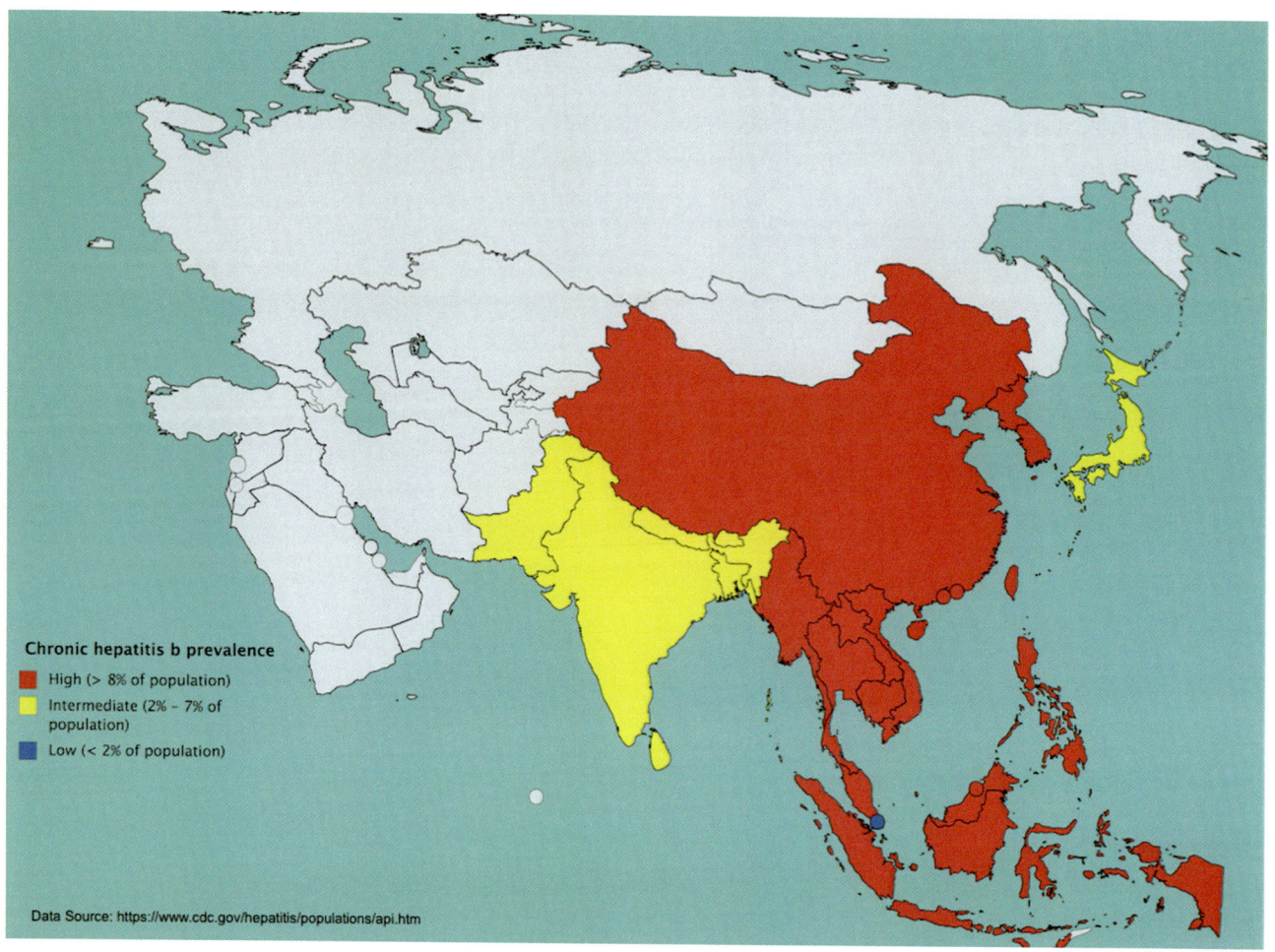

Fig. 41.8 Chronic hepatitis B prevalence in South, East and Southeast Asia

new HBV infections [111]. However, gaps still exist in coverage of hepatitis B vaccination, particularly in rural areas, with fewer than 21% of newborns in Laos receiving their first dose of vaccine on time [112].

Transmission of HBV from carrier mothers to their babies and unsafe injection practices are the two main routes of infection in these areas [113]. Nearly 75% of children with chronic HBV in this region are clinically asymptomatic and HBeAg (hepatitis B e antigen) positive. However a small proportion may present with chronic liver disease and even HCC at the first presentation [113]. Most children with vertical transmission of HBV are in the "immune-tolerant phase" with normal liver function in infancy and childhood. However, a very small subset of infants born to HBV-positive mothers are at risk of developing fulminant hepatitis (FH) with a high mortality of nearly 50%. Younger age of onset (age <7 months) of hepatitis and negative maternal HBeAg were associated with FH on multivariate analysis in a study of 41 infants [114]. Most of these babies with FH received only the HBV vaccine and not the HBV immunoglobulin at birth. The necessity of following all children born to HBsAg-carrier mothers and screening them for HBV infection at 9–18 months of age cannot be overemphasized.

Keeping in mind the disease burden of HBV, a "Global Health Sector Strategy on Viral Hepatitis, 2016–2021" was adopted by the World Health Assembly in 2016 [115]. It aims to reduce new hepatitis infections by 90% and deaths by 65% by the year 2030. Mass implementation of HBV vaccination, reducing maternal–child transmission by screening and appropriate antiviral therapy in mother, providing for sterile injections and ensuring access to newer oral antivirals for patients with chronic HBV will be required for achieving the target.

41.5.2 Hepatitis C

Nearly 11 million of the ~150 million total subjects with chronic hepatitis C (CHC) are children less than 15 years of age [116]. The prevalence of CHC varies among the different countries of this region. In general population the highest prevalence is seen in East Asia (China, Hong Kong, Macau,

North Korea, Taiwan) of 3.7% (3.1–4.5%), followed by South Asia (Bangladesh, Bhutan, India, Nepal, Pakistan) of 3.4% (2.6–4.4%) and Southeast Asia (Indonesia, Cambodia, Laos, Sri Lanka, the Maldives, Myanmar, Mauritius, Malaysia, the Philippines, Thailand, Vietnam) of 2.0% (1.7–2.3%) as per analysis in 2005 [117]. World over, genotype 1 is most prevalent, especially in the Western world. Genotype 3 is the second most common worldwide and more often seen in South Asia, while genotypes 2 and 6 are mainly seen in East Asia [116].

Inadequate screening of transfusion products and use of unsterile needles and syringes are the major routes of hepatitis C virus (HCV) transmission in the developing world which is reflected in the high anti-HCV seropositivity to the tune of 40% in multi-transfused children from this region [118]. Vertical transmission from mother to baby and intravenous drug abuse in adolescents are the other modes of transmission.

Because of the asymptomatic nature of chronic hepatitis B and hepatitis C, most infected people are not aware of their status until years later when they have symptoms of cirrhosis or liver cancer [117]. HCC is a dreaded complication of CHB and CHC; it typically affects children in the second decade of life and is often locally advanced or metastatic at diagnosis [119]. These children have a poor prognosis in absence of a transplant which is again not available to a majority from the developing world.

The WHO global health sector strategy on viral hepatitis has planned for an increase in diagnosis of chronic viral hepatitis C infection, with 30% of infected people knowing their status by 2020 and 90% by 2030 [115]. The availability of potent directly acting antivirals (DAA) for therapy of CHC and the reduction in the prices of these medications in low and lower-middle income countries would lead to provision of cost-effective therapy and reduction of overall HCV-related mortality and morbidity both in paediatric and adult populations.

41.5.3 Budd–Chiari Syndrome

Budd–Chiari syndrome (BCS) is caused by occlusion of the hepatic veins (HVs) and/or supra-hepatic inferior vena cava (IVC). It excludes veno-occlusive disease and cardiac conditions such as constrictive pericarditis and right-sided heart failure. BCS is labelled as "primary BCS" when obstruction occurs due to thrombus, webs or endophlebitis and as "secondary BCS" when obstruction is due to an extra-luminal lesion such as tumour, abscess or cyst that either invades the lumen or causes extrinsic compression.

BCS is an uncommon disease in children, more common in Asia than the West. In India, BCS accounts for 7.4% of all paediatric chronic liver disease in comparison to only 0.1% of all liver disease cases seen at King's College, London [120, 121].

Table 41.4 Site of block, prevalence of prothrombotic conditions and success of radiological intervention in children with Budd–Chiari syndrome

Country	Year, number of cases	Type of block	Prothrombotic condition (%)	Success of radiological interventions (%)
Nepal [123]	2014, n = 168 (only membranous occlusion of IVC taken)	IVC: 100%	-NA-	-NA-
India [120, 124, 125]	2014, n = 46; 2014, n = 13; 2016, n = 25	HV: 69, 72, 96% Both HV and IVC: 4, 24, 31% IVC: 0–4%	69, 75, 77%	Technical success 100%
Pakistan [126]	2015, n = 25 (both children and adults)	HV: 56%	84%	–
China [127]	2016, n = 35 (<25 years old)	HV: 60% Both HV and IVC: 37% IVC: 3%	91%	

Type of block: *HV* only hepatic veins, *Both HV and IVC* both hepatic vein and inferior vena cava, *IVC* only inferior vena cava

Previously, it was believed that BCS in the West is characterized by a thrombotic obstruction of the hepatic veins sparing the inferior vena cava (IVC), related to underlying prothrombotic conditions, while the Asian variant was characterized by a non-thrombotic, fibrous, obstruction of the IVC [122]. However, recent publications have shown that isolated HV obstruction is the most common type even in India as shown in Table 41.4.

Ascites with hepatomegaly and tortuous abdominal and/or back veins is the classical presentation of BCS in children. Nearly 85% cases had ascites and hepatomegaly, 70% had splenomegaly and prominent veins and 35% had variceal bleed in the largest series from India, comprising of 46 cases [124]. Doppler ultrasound provides clues to the diagnosis of BCS by showing blocked HV/IVC, caudate lobe hypertrophy and intrahepatic collaterals.

Complete prothrombotic workup should be done in all BCS cases. Sequential use of increasingly invasive therapy, starting with medical therapy (anticoagulation, supportive therapy for PHT complications), followed by radiological intervention and then liver transplantation, has been recommended in adults [128]. However, there are no evidence-based guidelines in children. Hepatic venogram is essential for planning the type of radiological intervention, i.e. angioplasty, stenting or transjugular intrahepatic portosystemic shunt (TIPSS). Paediatric literature has shown that anticoagulation alone has high failure rate of 66% [125], and angioplasty has lower patency rates than stenting or TIPSS in children in follow-up [124, 125]. Strict monitoring for adequacy of anticoagulation and patency of stent is essential to avoid fatal bleeds (intracranial) and stent blockage, and this adds to the complexity of management in children. Serial alpha-fetoprotein and USG monitoring is required for detection of HCC. Radiological intervention (HV stenting or TIPSS) (Fig. 41.9) improves liver function, portal hypertension and growth in children. Liver transplantation should be reserved for fulminant liver failure or ESLD which is not amenable to or fails radiological intervention.

Various Asian studies that have described the type of block, prevalence of prothrombotic conditions (%) and success of radiological interventions (%) have been summarized in Table 41.4.

41.5.4 Wilson's Disease

Wilson's disease is an autosomal recessive disorder of copper metabolism which has been reported from this entire region. One of the largest series in the world of 282 cases (mean age of 15.9 ± 8.1 years) has been described from India [129]. A positive family history was noted in 47%, consanguinity in 54% cases and the mean duration of symptoms at diagnosis was 28.0 ± 36.6 months in this series [129]. The study highlighted that the need of multiple tests, including liver copper estimation and genetic analysis to confirm the diagnosis, causes delay in diagnosis and initiation of treatment of WD in the developing world. In addition, need of lifelong therapy and follow-up is a problem in the economically underprivileged children.

There are indications that the incidence of Wilson's disease in South and East Asia is higher than the western world. Mass screening for Wilson's disease, based on the measurement of ceruloplasmin level, suggested a frequency of ~1:3600 in Korea [130]. Genetic testing showed that the prevalence of WD was ~1:3000 in Korean population and ~1 in 5400 in Hong Kong Han Chinese [131, 132]. In Malaysia, the prevalence of WD is thought to be lower in the Malay population in comparison to the Indian and Chinese [133].

The confirmation of diagnosis requires genetic testing for mutations in the ATP7B gene, which spans 21 exons. Until now >500 different mutations have been described, with each study describing novel mutations in different populations. Thus, testing for a limited number of ATP7B mutations in a control population is likely to be of limited value, and direct sequence analysis of the entire ATP7B coding region is the best way. This was highlighted by a recent study from the UK, in which the calculated frequency of individuals predicted to carry two pathogenic mutations was 1:7026, which was significantly higher than the classical reported WD prevalence of 1:30,000 [134]. Further evidence from large population studies of various ethnic groups with direct sequencing of the ATP7B gene is required to confirm whether there is a true difference in the prevalence of WD between the east and west.

Various mutations have been shown to be more common in different ethnic populations. The p.R778L (c.2333G > T) is one of the common mutations in Chinese (mainland), Taiwanese, Hong Kong, Japanese and Korean patients, while

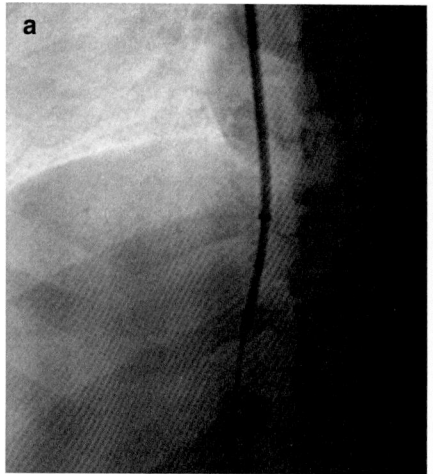
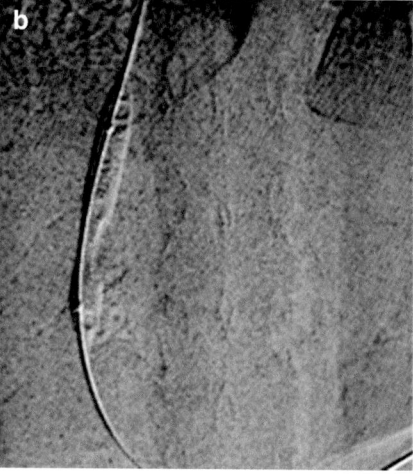
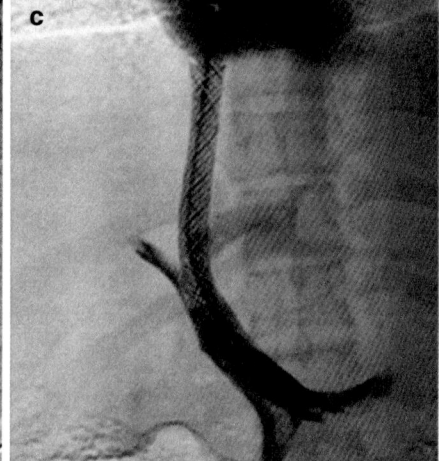

Fig. 41.9 Modified transjugular intrahepatic portosystemic shunt in a patient with Budd–Chiari syndrome. (**a**) Colapinto needle across the inferior vena cava (IVC) wall towards the right portal bifurcation. (**b**) 8 mm balloon dilatation of liver parenchymal tract. (**c**) Post-stenting venogram shows good flow across the stent

in India (western, southern and eastern) the p.C271* was most common [135, 136]. Based on the frequency and location of common mutations, various authors have advised stepwise screening, first for exons 2, 8, 12, 13 and 16 which cover 70% of mutations in Chinese and exons 2, 8, 13, 14 and 18 which cover ~80% of mutations in Indian patients [132, 136]. Patients who do not have any mutations in these exons can thereafter be subjected to sequencing of all exons.

D-Penicillamine is the most common copper chelator used for treatment of WD globally and in Asia. Trientine which is recommended in patients who are intolerant of penicillamine is not available in most countries across Asia [135].

41.5.5 Indian Childhood Cirrhosis

Indian childhood cirrhosis (ICC) is a unique liver disease which was endemic in India. In the classical description, children between 6 months and 5 years of age were affected with most being around 2 years. The initial clinical presentation was with intermittent fever, irritability and a decreased appetite which gradually progressed to hepatosplenomegaly, ascites, jaundice, gastrointestinal bleeding, encephalopathy and death mostly within a period of few months. A hard palpable liver with sharp leafy margin was the hallmark [137]. After initially being described in India, this condition was later documented sporadically in children of non-Indian origin in other countries [138]. The unique histologic findings of ICC, which included ballooned hepatocytes with Mallory hyaline inclusions, aggressive intralobular pericellular fibrosis, increase in intrahepatic copper and poor regeneration, made this condition stand out from the rest of paediatric liver diseases. A positive family history was seen in nearly a third of cases. Initially it was believed to be caused due to hepatotoxic effect of excess dietary copper, but epidemiologic, clinical and morphological data from recent large, well-controlled studies failed to incriminate exogenous copper in causing a toxic injury or the copper overloading of liver in ICC [138]. The exact aetiopathogenesis of this disease is still elusive. A genetic susceptibility which induces an abnormality of copper homeostasis following toxic injury by a yet unidentified factor is thought to lead to both ICC and ICC like disease. The disease has also been reported in older children between 6 and 15 years of age from India and labelled as "atypical copper cirrhosis" as it was not fitting the classical age description [139, 140]. The disease in older children also appears to have a slightly better outcome. The disease is now thought to have virtually disappeared from the country, with only sporadic cases being reported [139]. The ascribed current decline in ICC could either be due to missing a diagnosis because of the atypical presentation in older children and non-availability of a liver histology or due to a true reduction in incidence secondary to time-related economic and sociocultural changes.

41.5.6 Non-alcoholic Fatty Liver Disease

Non-alcoholic fatty liver disease (NAFLD) is an important cause of liver disease worldwide. The disease spectrum can vary from elevated transaminases to cirrhosis. Pathogenesis is related to obesity, insulin resistance, oxidative stress, lipotoxicity and resultant inflammation in the liver progressing to fibrosis. The prevalence of NAFLD varies, based on the method used for diagnosis (imaging, raised transaminases, histology). The studies on prevalence of NAFLD from this region are shown in Table 41.5.

Rural populations from Asian countries have a lower prevalence of NAFLD, though in metropolitan areas the prevalence of NAFLD is rising rapidly [145]. NAFLD accounts for a relatively lower proportion of patients with raised transaminases in the East as viral hepatitis is responsible for a high proportion of cases in this region [147, 148]. However, metabolic syndrome is strongly associated with elevated alanine aminotransferase (ALT) concentration, when only non-viral elevation in ALT is considered [144].

A recent meta-analysis of NAFLD in children and adolescents between 1 and 19 years showed that NAFLD prevalence does not vary by geographical region in the general population, but in obese population, the prevalence was

Table 41.5 Country-wise prevalence of non-alcoholic fatty liver disease in children

Country (year, reference)	Diagnostic method	Age group evaluated	Total subjects (n)	Prevalence of NAFLD (%)
India (2012, [141])	USG	5–12 y	100	3% (general population)
India (2016, [142])	USG	11–15 y	100	62% (overweight and obese)
Taiwan (2011, [143])	USG	12–13 y	220	16% (normal weight), 50.5% (overweight), 63.5% (obese)
Korea (2005, [144])	LFT (ALT>40U/L)	10–19 y	1594	3.6% (boys) 2.8% (girls)
China (2015, [145])	USG	7–18 y	7229	General population 7.5% (boys), 2.5% (girls), obese (44.8%)
Pakistan (2009, [146])	USG	6–11 y	93	7.5% (obese boys); none in obese girls and normal weight children

LFT liver function test, *USG* ultrasonography, *NAFLD* non-alcoholic fatty liver disease, *y* years

higher in Asia than in Europe, Middle East/North Africa and North America [149]. Overall in children, NAFLD prevalence is higher in males compared to females and increases incrementally with increase in body mass index (BMI).

Whether residing in the East or the West, Asians seem to be at a higher risk than their Caucasian and African American counterparts. There is a strong genetic predisposition for the development of NAFLD in Asians. The PNPLA3 rs738409 G-allele was associated with NAFLD and a higher ALT level in Chinese children, and it had a strong association with moderate-to-severe steatosis [150]. Similarly, the risk of NAFLD increased 5.84 times (2.59–13.1) in Taiwanese children with GG genotype in comparison to PNPLA3 rs738409 CC genotype [143]. According to the National Center for Biotechnology Information human SNP database, the G allele frequency is 0.344 in Han Chinese, 0.233 in Europeans and 0.125 in Africans [151]. This suggests that Asians have a much higher genetic susceptibility to NAFLD than Europeans and Africans.

Among adults, the South Asian phenotype of NAFLD appears to differ from that which is seen in developed nations. South Asian patients with NAFLD appear to have lower BMI and obesity rates (lean NAFLD) which is also called as the Asian Paradox and attributed to ethnic variations in visceral fat distribution [152].

41.5.7 Complications of Chronic Liver Disease

The natural history of end-stage liver disease (ESLD) in terms of prevalence of complications (ascites, spontaneous bacterial peritonitis, variceal bleeding, renal failure and hepatic encephalopathy) and response to therapy is different in children as compared to adults. The literature is limited and mostly from the developing world as majority of children are transplanted early in the West. In contrast, delay in diagnosis and non-availability of liver transplantation for a significant proportion of children with ESLD in the developing world gives a unique though unfortunate opportunity to study the natural history, progression and outcome of chronic liver disease.

Malnutrition is a big problem in CLD children especially those who are younger or with cholestatic liver disease. It can affect the outcome even after liver transplant, and all measures should be taken to actively target and prevent this complication [153]. Nearly 62% children with CLD had moderate to severe undernutrition, and 40% had failure to thrive in a recent study from Indonesia [154].

Advances in endoscopic techniques have drastically improved the outcome of variceal bleeding in children. The feasibility, effectiveness and safety of endoscopic band ligation for oesophageal varices and glue (cyanoacrylate) injection for gastric varices (Fig. 41.5a, b) have been shown in children with both chronic liver disease and EHPVO [155, 156].

Information regarding prevalence, precipitants and outcome of hepatic encephalopathy in children with CLD is limited. In a small study of CLD children with HE, ~75% children showed complete and 13% had partial response to lactulose [157].

Spontaneous bacterial peritonitis (SBP) has been reported in 29–43% children with chronic liver disease with only half of them being symptomatic [158, 159]. Most of this data has come from the developing world, i.e. Asia, Africa and South America [160]. In the largest study from India, about 25% children with ascitic fluid infection (AFI) had a poor in-hospital outcome with advanced liver disease (higher Child Pugh score) and GI bleeding being its predictors. The mortality and recurrence rate of AFI over 1 year in CLD children with SBP/culture-negative neutrocytic ascites (CNNA) was 24% and 27%, respectively [158].

Children with decompensated chronic liver disease (DCLD) have immune dysfunction which places them at an increased risk of infections like SBP, urinary tract infection (UTI), bacteraemia, pneumonia, etc. Nearly half of the children with DCLD were found to have infection in a study from India, and biomarkers like procalcitonin and CRP were useful for early diagnosis of infection [161]. The growing antibiotic resistance with emergence of multiresistant bacteria (MRB) is a serious problem [162].

A subset of children with CLD decompensate following an acute insult which is labelled as acute-on-chronic liver failure (ACLF). EASL and APASL have defined ACLF in adults. However there are differences in the two definitions, infections are included as acute insult in the EASL but not in the APASL definition [163]. Limited studies from India on ACLF as per the APASL definition have shown that infection with hepatotropic viruses (hepatitis E virus, hepatitis A virus, etc.), drug-induced liver injury (including complementary and alternative medicine) and flare of underlying disease are the most common acute insults in children [97, 164]. CLD was diagnosed for the first time in a large proportion during their presentation with a superimposed acute insult. Children with ACLF have a higher mortality which is often contributed by multiorgan failure [164]. Prognostic scores like the paediatric chronic liver failure sequential organ failure (pCLIF SOFA) score help in assessment, enabling timely interventions [165]. High index of suspicion, prompt diagnosis of infections coupled with judicious use of sensitive antibiotics, ICU care and organ support are required to improve the outcome in these children.

41.6 Liver Transplantation

Living donor liver transplantation (LDLT) developed in East Asia in the 1990s to overcome the shortage of grafts for children due to the scarcity of deceased donors. It was intro-

Table 41.6 Indications and type of liver transplantation in children

Country (year, reference)	Number of cases	LDLT	Indications			
			BA	ALF	MLD	Tumour
India (2011, [166]) (2013, [167])	28 ~350 (estimate)	92.8% ~95%	53.5% ~75% (cholestatic liver disease, mainly BA)	3.5%	14.2%	3.5%
Thailand (2015, [168])	24		Most common			
China (2010, [169])	337	63.8%	25.4%		39.2% (35.4% WD 2.2% GSD)	5.9%
Korea (2013, [170])	534	84.6%	57.7%	10.3%	5.1% WD 1.9% GSD	2.8%
Singapore (2012, [171])	81	65.4%	65.4%	7.4%	DNA	DNA

LDLT living donor liver transplant, *BA* biliary atresia, *ALF* acute liver failure, *MLD* metabolic liver diseases, *WD* Wilson's disease, *GSD* glycogen storage disease, *DNA* details not available

duced in Japan and later spread to Korea, Taiwan, Hong Kong and other Asian countries. While deceased donor liver transplantation (DDLT) constitutes more than 90% of transplants in the western world, in Asian countries, most transplants are LDLT. DDLT is uncommon because of cultural, religious and political reasons in this region.

In the SPLIT registry from the USA comprising of 1187 paediatric liver transplantations, the most common indication for liver transplant was biliary atresia (41.6%) followed by acute liver failure (12.2%). The common indications for liver transplantation and the proportion of LDLT in the total transplants from Southeast Asia are shown in Table 41.6.

The outcome following LDLT in eastern countries has been quite satisfactory when compared to their western counterparts. The survival rates after LDLT are similar to those of DDLT; however, biliary complications are higher after LDLT and contribute significantly to the morbidity. These complications, which occur in around 25–30% patients, are the Achilles heel of LDLT and have remained constant [172].

Cadaveric organ donation is showing encouraging trends from some countries such as South Korea and China, but other countries such as Japan and India have not made any significant progress in this direction [173]. In addition liver transplantation is still not accessible to large proportions of economically underprivileged patients in India and other developing countries as the facility is primarily available in the private sector hospitals. The need of the hour is to design strategies to fill the gap between demand and availability of organ for liver transplant and make it accessible for all.

41.7 Conclusions and Future Directions

Liver diseases are an important cause of morbidity and mortality in South, East and Southeast Asia. The aetiology and profile are quite different from the west. Viral hepatitis is one of the most important causes for acute and chronic liver disease, the absolute burden of which has increased between 1990 and 2013 unlike the other communicable diseases [174]. The diversity in genetics is responsible for the variation in prevalence of certain metabolic conditions. Scarcity of state-of-the-art investigative facilities, delayed presentation to the experts with advanced disease and non-availability of liver transplantation at many centres are the major limitations to a good patient outcome.

There is a need for collaborative work between the developing and developed nations including exchange training programmes for better understanding of the complete disease spectrum and providing optimal patient care. It is also pertinent to make all-inclusive management guidelines, which outline a plan of management even in resource-constrained situations. Advancements in the field of science and increased global travel have made this world a small place, and physicians need to be aware of the various liver conditions even if they are not managing them regularly.

References

1. World Population Prospects: The 2017 Revision, Key Findings and Advance Tables. United Nations Department of Economic and Social Affairs/Population Division [Internet]. [cited 2017 Jul 8]. https://esa.un.org/unpd/wpp/Publications/Files/WPP2017_KeyFindings.pdf.
2. Child and adolescent health and development [Internet]. [cited 2017 Jul 17]. http://www.searo.who.int/entity/child_adolescent/topics/child_health/en/.
3. United Nations Children's Fund, World Health Organization TWB. Levels and trends in child malnutrition. UNICEF-WHO-The World Bank joint child malnutrition estimates. [Internet]. UNICEF, New York; WHO, Geneva; The World Bank, Washington, DC. 2012 [cited 2017 Sep 3]. www.who.int/nutgrowthdb/jme_unicef_who_wb.pdf. Accessed 3 Sept 2017.
4. The World Health Report 2006—working together for health [Internet]. [cited 2017 Jun 17]. www.who.int/whr/2006/en/.

5. Dhillon PK, Jeemon P, Arora NK, Mathur P, Maskey M, Sukirna RD, et al. Status of epidemiology in the WHO South-East Asia region: burden of disease, determinants of health and epidemiological research, workforce and training capacity. Int J Epidemiol. 2012;41(3):847–60.
6. Squires RH, Shneider BL, Bucuvalas J, Alonso E, Sokol RJ, Narkewicz MR, et al. Acute liver failure in children: the first 348 patients in the pediatric acute liver failure study group. J Pediatr. 2006;148(5):652–8.
7. Mazumder MW, Karim AB, Rukunuzzaman M, Rahman MA. Aetiology and outcome of acute liver failure in children: experience at a Tertiary Care Hospital of Bangladesh. Mymensingh Med J. 2016;25(3):492–4.
8. PL H, Trong KH, Tran TT, Huy TTT, Abe K. Detection of hepatitis A virus RNA from children patients with acute and fulminant hepatitis of unknown etiology in Vietnam: genomic characterization of Vietnamese HAV strain. Pediatr Int. 2008;50(5):624–7.
9. Latif N, Mehmood K. Risk factors for fulminant hepatic failure and their relation with outcome in children. J Pak Med Assoc. 2010;60(3):175–8.
10. Bravo LC, Gregorio GV, Shafi F, Bock HL, Boudville I, Liu Y, et al. Etiology, incidence and outcomes of acute hepatic failure in 0-18 year old Filipino children. Southeast Asian J Trop Med Public Health. 2012;43(3):764–72.
11. Kaur S, Kumar P, Kumar V, Sarin SK, Kumar A. Etiology and prognostic factors of acute liver failure in children. Indian Pediatr. 2013;50(7):677–9.
12. Srivastava A, Yachha SK, Poddar U. Predictors of outcome in children with acute viral hepatitis and coagulopathy. J Viral Hepat. 2012;19(2):e194–201.
13. Poddar U, Thapa BR, Prasad A, Sharma AK, Singh K. Natural history and risk factors in fulminant hepatic failure. Arch Dis Child. 2002;87(1):54–6.
14. Poovorawan Y, Chongsrisawat V, Shafi F, Boudville I, Liu Y, Hutagalung Y, et al. Acute hepatic failure among hospitalized Thai children. Southeast Asian J Trop Med Public Health. 2013;44(1):50–3.
15. Poovorawan Y, Hutagalung Y, Chongsrisawat V, Boudville I, Bock HL. Dengue virus infection: a major cause of acute hepatic failure in Thai children. Ann Trop Paediatr. 2006;26(1):17–23.
16. Zhao P, Wang C-Y, Liu W-W, Wang X, Yu L-M, Sun Y-R. Acute liver failure in Chinese children: a multicenter investigation. Hepatobiliary Pancreat Dis Int. 2014;13(3):276–80.
17. Kumar A, Yachha SK, Poddar U, Singh U, Aggarwal R. Does co-infection with multiple viruses adversely influence the course and outcome of sporadic acute viral hepatitis in children? J Gastroenterol Hepatol. 2006;21(10):1533–7.
18. Poddar U, Thapa BR, Prasad A, Singh K. Changing spectrum of sporadic acute viral hepatitis in Indian children. J Trop Pediatr. 2002;48(4):210–3.
19. Chadha MS, Walimbe AM, Chobe LP, Arankalle VA. Comparison of etiology of sporadic acute and fulminant viral hepatitis in hospitalized patients in Pune, India during 1978-81 and 1994-97. Indian J Gastroenterol. 2003;22(1):11–5.
20. Kc S, Sharma D, Poudyal N, Basnet BK. Acute Viral Hepatitis in Pediatric Age Groups. JNMA J Nepal Med Assoc. 2014;52(193):687–91.
21. Kumar KJ, Kumar HCK, Manjunath VG, Anitha C, Mamatha S. Hepatitis A in children- clinical course, complications and laboratory profile. Indian J Pediatr. 2014;81(1):15–9.
22. Yachha SK, Goel A, Khanna V, Poddar U, Srivastava A, Singh U. Ascitic form of sporadic acute viral hepatitis in children: a distinct entity for recognition. J Pediatr Gastroenterol Nutr. 2010;50(2):184–7.
23. Jacobsen KH. The global prevalence of hepatitis A virus infection and susceptibility: a systematic review. Geneva: World Health Organization; 2010. 428 p.
24. http://hepcasia.com/wp-content/uploads/2015/03/who_searo_viral-hepatitis-report.pdf [Internet]. [cited 2017 Jun 14]. http://hepcasia.com/wp-content/uploads/2015/03/who_searo_viral-hepatitis-report.pdf.
25. Van Effelterre T, Marano C, Jacobsen KH. Modeling the hepatitis A epidemiological transition in Thailand. Vaccine. 2016;34(4):555–62.
26. Verghese VP, Robinson JL. A systematic review of hepatitis E virus infection in children. Clin Infect Dis. 2014;59(5):689–97.
27. Fischler B, Baumann U, Dezsofi A, Hadzic N, Hierro L, Jahnel J, et al. Hepatitis E in children: a position paper by the ESPGHAN Hepatology Committee. J Pediatr Gastroenterol Nutr. 2016;63(2):288–94.
28. Devarbhavi H, Karanth D, Prasanna KS, Adarsh CK, Patil M. Drug-induced liver injury with hypersensitivity features has a better outcome: a single-center experience of 39 children and adolescents. Hepatology. 2011;54(4):1344–50.
29. Donald PR. Antituberculosis drug-induced hepatotoxicity in children. Pediatr Rep. 2011;3(2):e16.
30. Devarbhavi H, Singh R, Patil M, Sheth K, Adarsh CK, Balaraju G. Outcome and determinants of mortality in 269 patients with combination anti-tuberculosis drug-induced liver injury. J Gastroenterol Hepatol. 2013;28(1):161–7.
31. Dhiman RK, Saraswat VA, Rajekar H, Reddy C, Chawla YK. A guide to the management of tuberculosis in patients with chronic liver disease. J Clin Exp Hepatol. 2012;2(3):260–70.
32. Jan MA, Siddiqui TS, Ahmed N, Ul Haq I, Khan Z. Mushroom poisoning in children: clinical presentation and outcome. J Ayub Med Coll Abbottabad. 2008;20(2):99–101.
33. Ozçay F, Baskin E, Ozdemir N, Karakayali H, Emiroglu R, Haberal M. Fulminant liver failure secondary to mushroom poisoning in children: importance of early referral to a liver transplantation unit. Pediatr Transplant. 2006;10(2):259–65.
34. Saraf V, Pande S, Gopalakrishnan U, Balakrishnan D, Menon RN, Sudheer OV, et al. Acute liver failure due to zinc phosphide containing rodenticide poisoning: clinical features and prognostic indicators of need for liver transplantation. Indian J Gastroenterol. 2015;34(4):325–9.
35. Khan W, Zakai HA, Umm-E-Asma. Clinico-pathological studies of Plasmodium falciparum and Plasmodium vivax - malaria in India and Saudi Arabia. Acta Parasitol. 2014;59(2):206–12.
36. Kumar R, Tripathi P, Tripathi S, Kanodia A, Venkatesh V. Prevalence of dengue infection in north Indian children with acute hepatic failure. Ann Hepatol. 2008;7(1):59–62.
37. Chongsrisawat V, Hutagalung Y, Poovorawan Y. Liver function test results and outcomes in children with acute liver failure due to dengue infection. Southeast Asian J Trop Med Public Health. 2009;40(1):47–53.
38. Chanta C, Triratanapa K, Ratanasirichup P, Mahaprom W. Hepatic dysfunction in pediatric scrub typhus: role of liver function test in diagnosis and marker of disease severity. J Med Assoc Thai. 2007;90(11):2366–9.
39. Dass R, Deka NM, Duwarah SG, Barman H, Hoque R, Mili D, et al. Characteristics of pediatric scrub typhus during an outbreak in the North Eastern region of India: peculiarities in clinical presentation, laboratory findings and complications. Indian J Pediatr. 2011;78(11):1365–70.
40. Karanth SS, Bhat R, Gupta A. Refractory hypocalcemia precipitated by dual infection with typhoid fever and hepatitis A in a patient with congenital hypoparathyroidism. Asian Pac J Trop Med. 2012;5(8):667–8.

41. http://apps.who.int/iris/bitstream/10665/44188/1/9789241547871_eng.pdf [Internet]. [cited 2017 Jul 21]. http://apps.who.int/iris/bitstream/10665/44188/1/9789241547871_eng.pdf.
42. Syhavong B, Rasachack B, Smythe L, Rolain J-M, Roque-Afonso A-M, Jenjaroen K, et al. The infective causes of hepatitis and jaundice amongst hospitalised patients in Vientiane, Laos. Trans R Soc Trop Med Hyg. 2010;104(7):475–83.
43. Martínez Vega R, Phumratanaprapin W, Phonrat B, Dhitavat J, Sutherat M, Choovichian V. Differences in liver impairment between adults and children with dengue infection. Am J Trop Med Hyg. 2016;94(5):1073–9.
44. Schwartz E, Weld LH, Wilder-Smith A, von Sonnenburg F, Keystone JS, Kain KC, et al. Seasonality, annual trends, and characteristics of dengue among ill returned travelers, 1997-2006. Emerg Infect Dis. 2008;14(7):1081–8.
45. Mishra K, Basu S, Roychoudhury S, Kumar P. Liver abscess in children: an overview. World J Pediatr. 2010;6(3):210–6.
46. Hsu Y-L, Lin H-C, Yen T-Y, Hsieh T-H, Wei H-M, Hwang K-P. Pyogenic liver abscess among children in a medical center in Central Taiwan. J Microbiol Immunol Infect. 2015;48(3):302–5.
47. Roy Choudhury S, Khan NA, Saxena R, Yadav PS, Patel JN, Chadha R. Protocol-based management of 154 cases of pediatric liver abscess. Pediatr Surg Int. 2017;33(2):165–72.
48. Srivastava A, Yachha SK, Arora V, Poddar U, Lal R, Baijal SS. Identification of high-risk group and therapeutic options in children with liver abscess. Eur J Pediatr. 2012;171(1):33–41.
49. Muorah M, Hinds R, Verma A, Yu D, Samyn M, Mieli-Vergani G, et al. Liver abscesses in children: a single center experience in the developed world. J Pediatr Gastroenterol Nutr. 2006;42(2):201–6.
50. Bhatt GC, Nandan D, Singh S. Isolated tuberculous liver abscess in immunocompetent children—report of two cases. Pathog Glob Health. 2013;107(1):35–7.
51. Bari S, Sheikh KA, Ashraf M, Hussain Z, Hamid A, Mufti GN. Ascaris liver abscess in children. J Gastroenterol. 2007;42(3):236–40.
52. Alam J, Wazir MD, Muhammad Z. Biliary Ascariasis in children. J Ayub Med Coll Abbottabad. 2001;13(2):32–3.
53. Malik AH, Saima BD, Wani MY. Management of hepatobiliary and pancreatic ascariasis in children of an endemic area. Pediatr Surg Int. 2006;22(2):164–8.
54. Huizinga WKJ, Grant CSDAS. In: Morris PJWWC, editor. Oxford textbook of surgery. 2nd ed. Oxford: Oxford University Press; 2000. p. 3298–305.
55. Ghartimagar D, Ghosh A, Shrestha MK, Talwar OP, Sathian B. 14 years hospital based study on clinical and morphological spectrum of hydatid disease. JNMA J Nepal Med Assoc. 2013;52(190):349–53.
56. Oral A, Yigiter M, Yildiz A, Yalcin O, Dikmen T, Eren S, et al. Diagnosis and management of hydatid liver disease in children: a report of 156 patients with hydatid disease. J Pediatr Surg. 2012;47(3):528–34.
57. Chai J, Menghebat, Jiao W, Sun D, Liang B, Shi J, et al. Clinical efficacy of albendazole emulsion in treatment of 212 cases of liver cystic hydatidosis. Chin Med J (Engl). 2002;115(12):1809–13.
58. Yang YR, Sun T, Li Z, Zhang J, Teng J, Liu X, et al. Community surveys and risk factor analysis of human alveolar and cystic echinococcosis in Ningxia Hui Autonomous Region, China. Bull World Health Organ. 2006;84(9):714–21.
59. South East Asia Regional Neonatal-Perinatal Database [Internet]. [cited 2017 Jul 14]. http://www.newbornwhocc.org/pdf/SEAR_NPD-Final_report.PDF.
60. Bazlul Karim ASM, Kamal M. Cholestatic jaundice during infancy: experience at a tertiary-care center in Bangladesh. Indian J Gastroenterol. 2005;24(2):52–4.
61. Arora NK, Arora S, Ahuja A, Mathur P, Maheshwari M, Das MK, et al. Alpha 1 antitrypsin deficiency in children with chronic liver disease in North India. Indian Pediatr. 2010;47(12):1015–23.
62. Aanpreung P, Laohapansang M, Ruangtrakool R, Kimhan J. Neonatal cholestasis in Thai infants. J Med Assoc Thai. 2005;88(Suppl 8):S9–15.
63. Lee WS, Chai PF, Boey CM, Looi LM. Aetiology and outcome of neonatal cholestasis in Malaysia. Singapore Med J. 2010;51(5):434–9.
64. Lu F-T, Wu J-F, Hsu H-Y, Ni Y-H, Chang M-H, Chao C-I, et al. γ-Glutamyl transpeptidase level as a screening marker among diverse etiologies of infantile intrahepatic cholestasis. J Pediatr Gastroenterol Nutr. 2014;59(6):695–701.
65. Lee WS. Pre-admission consultation and late referral in infants with neonatal cholestasis. J Paediatr Child Health. 2008;44(1–2):57–61.
66. Wongsawasdi L, Ukarapol N, Visrutaratna P, Singhavejsakul J, Kattipattanapong V. Diagnostic evaluation of infantile cholestasis. J Med Assoc Thai. 2008;91(3):345–9.
67. Mathiyazhagan G, Jagadisan B. Referral patterns and factors influencing age at admission of infants with cholestasis in India. Indian J Pediatr. 2017;84(8):591–6.
68. Lien T-H, Chang M-H, Wu J-F, Chen H-L, Lee H-C, Chen A-C, et al. Effects of the infant stool color card screening program on 5-year outcome of biliary atresia in Taiwan. Hepatology. 2011;53(1):202–8.
69. de Serres FJ. Worldwide racial and ethnic distribution of alpha1-antitrypsin deficiency: summary of an analysis of published genetic epidemiologic surveys. Chest. 2002;122(5):1818–29.
70. Moyer V, Freese DK, Whitington PF, Olson AD, Brewer F, Colletti RB, et al. Guideline for the evaluation of cholestatic jaundice in infants: recommendations of the North American Society for Pediatric Gastroenterology, Hepatology and Nutrition. J Pediatr Gastroenterol Nutr. 2004;39(2):115–28.
71. Lee WS, Yap SF, Looi LM. alpha1-Antitrypsin deficiency is not an important cause of childhood liver diseases in a multi-ethnic Southeast Asian population. J Paediatr Child Health. 2007;43(9):636–9.
72. Tan JJ, Cutiongco-dela Paz EM, Avila JMC, Gregorio GV. Low incidence of alpha 1-antitrypsin deficiency among Filipinos with neonatal cholestatis. J Paediatr Child Health. 2006;42(11):694–7.
73. Ohura T, Kobayashi K, Tazawa Y, Nishi I, Abukawa D, Sakamoto O, et al. Neonatal presentation of adult-onset type II citrullinemia. Hum Genet. 2001;108(2):87–90.
74. Song Y-Z, Zhang Z-H, Lin W-X, Zhao X-J, Deng M, Ma Y-L, et al. SLC25A13 gene analysis in citrin deficiency: sixteen novel mutations in East Asian patients, and the mutation distribution in a large pediatric cohort in China. PLoS One. 2013;8(9):e74544.
75. Lu YB, Kobayashi K, Ushikai M, Tabata A, Iijima M, Li MX, et al. Frequency and distribution in East Asia of 12 mutations identified in the SLC25A13 gene of Japanese patients with citrin deficiency. J Hum Genet. 2005;50(7):338–46.
76. Treepongkaruna S, Jitraruch S, Kodcharin P, Charoenpipop D, Suwannarat P, Pienvichit P, et al. Neonatal intrahepatic cholestasis caused by citrin deficiency: prevalence and SLC25A13 mutations among Thai infants. BMC Gastroenterol. 2012;12:141.
77. Saheki T, Song Y-Z. Citrin deficiency. GeneReviews(®). Available from http://www.ncbi.nlm.nih.gov/books/NBK1181/. Accessed 5 Jan 2018.
78. Chen R, Wang X-H, Fu H-Y, Zhang S-R, Abudouxikuer K, Saheki T, et al. Different regional distribution of SLC25A13 mutations in Chinese patients with neonatal intrahepatic cholestasis. World J Gastroenterol. 2013;19(28):4545–51.
79. Ngu HL, Zabedah MY, Kobayashi K. Neonatal intrahepatic cholestasis caused by citrin deficiency (NICCD) in three Malay children. Malays J Pathol. 2010;32(1):53–7.

80. Vitoria I, Dalmau J, Ribes C, Rausell D, García AM, López-Montiel J, et al. Citrin deficiency in a Romanian child living in Spain highlights the worldwide distribution of this defect and illustrates the value of nutritional therapy. Mol Genet Metab. 2013;110(1–2):181–3.
81. Agarwal S, Lal BB, Rawat D, Rastogi A, Bharathy KGS, Alam S. Progressive Familial Intrahepatic Cholestasis (PFIC) in Indian children: clinical spectrum and outcome. J Clin Exp Hepatol. 2016;6(3):203–8.
82. Lee WS, Chai PF, Looi LM. Progressive familial intrahepatic cholestasis in Malaysian patients—a report of five cases. Med J Malaysia. 2009;64(3):216–9.
83. Chen H-L, Liu Y-J, Su Y-N, Wang N-Y, Wu S-H, Ni Y-H, et al. Diagnosis of BSEP/ABCB11 mutations in Asian patients with cholestasis using denaturing high performance liquid chromatography. J Pediatr. 2008;153(6):825–32.
84. Khanna R, Sarin SK. Non-cirrhotic portal hypertension—diagnosis and management. J Hepatol. 2014;60(2):421–41.
85. Poddar U, Thapa BR, Rao KLN, Singh K. Etiological spectrum of esophageal varices due to portal hypertension in Indian children: is it different from the West? J Gastroenterol Hepatol. 2008;23(9):1354–7.
86. Wu J, Li Z, Wang Z, Han X, Ji F, Zhang WW. Surgical and endovascular treatment of severe complications secondary to noncirrhotic portal hypertension: experience of 56 cases. Ann Vasc Surg. 2013;27(4):441–6.
87. Sarin SK, Sollano JD, Chawla YK, Amarapurkar D, Hamid S, Hashizume M, et al. Consensus on extra-hepatic portal vein obstruction. Liver Int. 2006;26(5):512–9.
88. Hanif FM, Soomro GB, Akhund SN, Luck NH, Laeeq SM, Abbas Z, et al. Clinical presentation of extrahepatic portal vein obstruction: 10-year experience at a tertiary care hospital in Pakistan. J Transl Intern Med. 2015;3(2):74–8.
89. Yadav SK, Srivastava A, Srivastava A, Thomas MA, Agarwal J, Pandey CM, et al. Encephalopathy assessment in children with extra-hepatic portal vein obstruction with MR, psychometry and critical flicker frequency. J Hepatol. 2010;52(3):348–54.
90. Krishna YR, Yachha SK, Srivastava A, Negi D, Lal R, Poddar U. Quality of life in children managed for extrahepatic portal venous obstruction. J Pediatr Gastroenterol Nutr. 2010;50(5):531–6.
91. Shneider BL, de Ville de Goyet J, Leung DH, Srivastava A, Ling SC, Duché M, et al. Primary prophylaxis of variceal bleeding in children and the role of MesoRex Bypass: summary of the Baveno VI Pediatric Satellite Symposium. Hepatology. 2016;63(4):1368–80.
92. Lal R, Sarma SM, Gupta MK. Extrahepatic portal venous obstruction: what should be the mainstay of treatment? Indian J Pediatr. 2017;84(9):691–9.
93. Sarin SK, Kumar A, Chawla YK, Baijal SS, Dhiman RK, Jafri W, et al. Noncirrhotic portal fibrosis/idiopathic portal hypertension: APASL recommendations for diagnosis and treatment. Hepatol Int. 2007;1(3):398–413.
94. Sood V, Lal BB, Khanna R, Rawat D, Sharma CB, Alam S. Non-cirrhotic Portal Fibrosis in Pediatric Population. J Pediatr Gastroenterol Nutr. 2017;64(5):748–53. https://doi.org/10.1097/MPG.0000000000001485.
95. Poddar U, Thapa BR, Puri P, Girish CS, Vaiphei K, Vasishta RK, et al. Non-cirrhotic portal fibrosis in children. Indian J Gastroenterol. 2000;19(1):12–3.
96. Parkash A, Cheema HA, Malik HS, Fayyaz Z. Congenital hepatic fibrosis: clinical presentation, laboratory features and management at a tertiary care hospital of Lahore. J Pak Med Assoc. 2016;66(8):984–8.
97. Alam S, Lal BB, Sood V, Rawat D. Pediatric acute-on-chronic liver failure in a specialized liver unit: prevalence, profile, outcome, and predictive factors. J Pediatr Gastroenterol Nutr. 2016;63(4):400–5.
98. Zhang H-F, Yang X-J, Zhu S-S, Zhao J-M, Zhang T-H, Xu Z-Q, et al. Pathological changes and clinical manifestations of 1020 children with liver diseases confirmed by biopsy. Hepatobiliary Pancreat Dis Int. 2004;3(3):395–8.
99. Hanif M, Raza J, Qureshi H, Issani Z. Etiology of chronic liver disease in children. J Pak Med Assoc. 2004;54(3):119–22.
100. Tahir A, Malik FR, Ahmad I, Akhtar P. Aetiological factors of chronic liver disease in children. J Ayub Med Coll Abbottabad. 2011;23(2):12–4.
101. Nannini P, Sokal EM. Hepatitis B: changing epidemiology and interventions. Arch Dis Child. 2017;102(7):676–80.
102. Lesmana LA, Leung NW, Mahachai V, Phiet PH, Suh DJYG. Hepatitis B: overview of the burden of disease in the Asia-Pacific region. Liver Int. 2006;26:3–10.
103. Schweitzer A, Horn J, Mikolajczyk RT, Krause G, Ott JJ. Estimations of worldwide prevalence of chronic hepatitis B virus infection: a systematic review of data published between 1965 and 2013. Lancet (London, England). 2015;386(10003):1546–55.
104. Luo Z, Xie Y, Deng M, Zhou X, Ruan B. Prevalence of hepatitis B in the southeast of China: a population-based study with a large sample size. Eur J Gastroenterol Hepatol. 2011;23(8):695–700.
105. Zeng F, Guo P, Huang Y, Xin W, Du Z, Zhu S, et al. Epidemiology of hepatitis B virus infection: results from a community-based study of 0.15 million residents in South China. Sci Rep. 2016;6:36186.
106. Jafri W, Jafri N, Yakoob J, Islam M, Tirmizi SFA, Jafar T, et al. Hepatitis B and C: prevalence and risk factors associated with seropositivity among children in Karachi, Pakistan. BMC Infect Dis. 2006;6:101.
107. Rukunuzzaman M, Afroza A. Clinical, biochemical and virological profile of chronic hepatitis B virus infection in children. Mymensingh Med J. 2012;21(1):120–4.
108. Khan MAN. Epidemiology of hepatitis B in SAARC countries. In: Sarin SKOK, editor. Hepatitis B and C: carrier to cancer. New Delhi: Harcourt; 2002. p. 19–23.
109. Ott JJ, Stevens GA, Groeger J, Wiersma ST. Global epidemiology of hepatitis B virus infection: new estimates of age-specific HBsAg seroprevalence and endemicity. Vaccine. 2012;30(12):2212–9.
110. Chang MH, Chen CJ, Lai MS, Hsu HM, Wu TC, Kong MS, et al. Universal hepatitis B vaccination in Taiwan and the incidence of hepatocellular carcinoma in children. Taiwan Childhood Hepatoma Study Group. N Engl J Med. 1997;336(26):1855–9.
111. Zhou Y, Wu C, Zhuang H. Vaccination against hepatitis B: the Chinese experience. Chin Med J (Engl). 2009;122(1):98–102.
112. Parry J. At last a global response to viral hepatitis. Bull World Health Organ. 2010;88(11):801–2.
113. Satapathy SK, Garg S, Chauhan R, Malhotra V, Sakhuja P, Sharma BC, et al. Profile of chronic hepatitis B virus in children in India: experience with 116 children. J Gastroenterol Hepatol. 2006;21(7):1170–6.
114. Tseng Y-R, Wu J-F, Kong M-S, Hu F-C, Yang Y-J, Yeung C-Y, et al. Infantile hepatitis B in immunized children: risk for fulminant hepatitis and long-term outcomes. PLoS One. 2014;9(11):e111825.
115. WHO. Global Health Sector Strategy on Viral Hepatitis 2016–2021 [Internet] [cited 2017 July 17]. http://apps.who.int/iris/bitstream/10665/246177/1/WHO-HIV-2016.06-eng.pdf.
116. Sokal E, Nannini P. Hepatitis C virus in children: the global picture. Arch Dis Child. 2017;102(7):672–5.
117. Mohd Hanafiah K, Groeger J, Flaxman AD, Wiersma ST. Global epidemiology of hepatitis C virus infection: new estimates of age-specific antibody to HCV seroprevalence. Hepatology. 2013;57(4):1333–42.

118. Chanpong GF, Laras K, Sulaiman HA, Soeprapto W, Purnamawati S, Sukri N, et al. Hepatitis C among child transfusion and adult renal dialysis patients in Indonesia. Am J Trop Med Hyg. 2002;66(3):317–20.
119. Kelly D, Sharif K, Brown RM, Morland B. Hepatocellular carcinoma in children. Clin Liver Dis. 2015;19(2):433–47.
120. Alam S, Khanna R, Mukund A. Clinical and prothrombotic profile of hepatic vein outflow tract obstruction. Indian J Pediatr. 2014;81(5):434–40.
121. Nobre S, Khanna R, Bab N, Kyrana E, Height S, Karani J, et al. Primary Budd-Chiari Syndrome in Children. King's College Hospital Experience. J Pediatr Gastroenterol Nutr. 2017;65(1):93–6.
122. Martens P, Nevens F. Budd-Chiari syndrome. United Eur Gastroenterol J. 2015;3(6):489–500.
123. Shrestha SM, Shrestha S. Hepatic vena cava syndrome: a common cause of liver cirrhosis in children in Nepal. Trop Gastroenterol. 2014;35(2):85–95.
124. Kathuria R, Srivastava A, Yachha SK, Poddar U, Baijal SS. Budd-Chiari syndrome in children: clinical features, percutaneous radiological intervention, and outcome. Eur J Gastroenterol Hepatol. 2014;26(9):1030–8.
125. Sharma VK, Ranade PR, Marar S, Nabi F, Nagral A. Long-term clinical outcome of Budd-Chiari syndrome in children after radiological intervention. Eur J Gastroenterol Hepatol. 2016;28(5):567–75.
126. Tasneem AA, Soomro GB, Abbas Z, Luck NH, Hassan SM. Clinical presentation and predictors of survival in patients with Budd Chiari syndrome: experience from a tertiary care hospital in Pakistan. J Pak Med Assoc. 2015;65(2):120–4.
127. Zhou W-J, Cui Y-F, Zu M-H, Zhang Q-Q, Xu H. Budd-Chiari syndrome in young Chinese: clinical characteristics, etiology and outcome of recanalization from a single center. Cardiovasc Intervent Radiol. 2016;39(4):557–65.
128. Valla D-C. Primary Budd-Chiari syndrome. J Hepatol. 2009;50(1):195–203.
129. Taly AB, Meenakshi-Sundaram S, Sinha S, Swamy HS, Arunodaya GR. Wilson disease: description of 282 patients evaluated over 3 decades. Medicine (Baltimore). 2007;86(2):112–21.
130. Hahn SH, Lee SY, Jang Y-J, Kim SN, Shin HC, Park SY, et al. Pilot study of mass screening for Wilson's disease in Korea. Mol Genet Metab. 2002;76(2):133–6.
131. Park H-D, Ki C-S, Lee S-Y, Kim J-W. Carrier frequency of the R778L, A874V, and N1270S mutations in the ATP7B gene in a Korean population. Clin Genet. 2009;75(4):405–7.
132. Mak CM, Lam C-W, Tam S, Lai C-L, Chan L-Y, Fan S-T, et al. Mutational analysis of 65 Wilson disease patients in Hong Kong Chinese: identification of 17 novel mutations and its genetic heterogeneity. J Hum Genet. 2008;53(1):55–63.
133. Mohamed R, Tan CT, Wong NW. Wilson's disease—a review of cases at University Hospital, Kuala Lumpur. Med J Malaysia. 1994;49(1):49–52.
134. Coffey AJ, Durkie M, Hague S, McLay K, Emmerson J, Lo C, et al. A genetic study of Wilson's disease in the United Kingdom. Brain. 2013;136.(Pt 5):1476–87.
135. Zhang YWZ. Wilson's disease in Asia. Neurol Asia. 2011;16(2):103–9.
136. Aggarwal A, Chandhok G, Todorov T, Parekh S, Tilve S, Zibert A, et al. Wilson disease mutation pattern with genotype-phenotype correlations from Western India: confirmation of p.C271* as a common Indian mutation and identification of 14 novel mutations. Ann Hum Genet. 2013;77(4):299–307.
137. Tanner MS, Portmann B. Indian childhood cirrhosis. Arch Dis Child. 1981;56(1):4–6.
138. Nayak NC, Chitale AR. Indian childhood cirrhosis (ICC) & ICC-like diseases: the changing scenario of facts versus notions. Indian J Med Res. 2013;137(6):1029–42.
139. Patra S, Vij M, Kancherala R, Samal SC. Is Indian childhood cirrhosis an extinct disease now?—An observational study. Indian J Pediatr. 2013;80(8):651–4.
140. Ramakrishna B, Date A, Kirubakaran C, Raghupathy P. Atypical copper cirrhosis in Indian children. Ann Trop Paediatr. 1995;15(3):237–42.
141. Chaturvedi K, Vohra P. Non-alcoholic fatty liver disease in children. Indian Pediatr. 2012;49(9):757–8.
142. Pawar SV, Zanwar VG, Choksey AS, Mohite AR, Jain SS, Surude RG, et al. Most overweight and obese Indian children have nonalcoholic fatty liver disease. Ann Hepatol. 2016;15(6):853–61.
143. Lin Y-C, Chang P-F, Hu F-C, Yang W-S, Chang M-H, Ni Y-H. A common variant in the PNPLA3 gene is a risk factor for non-alcoholic fatty liver disease in obese Taiwanese children. J Pediatr. 2011;158(5):740–4.
144. Park HS, Han JH, Choi KM, Kim SM. Relation between elevated serum alanine aminotransferase and metabolic syndrome in Korean adolescents. Am J Clin Nutr. 2005;82(5):1046–51.
145. Zhang X, Wan Y, Zhang S, Lu L, Chen Z, Liu H, et al. Nonalcoholic fatty liver disease prevalence in urban school-aged children and adolescents from the Yangtze River delta region: a cross-sectional study. Asia Pac J Clin Nutr. 2015;24(2):281–8.
146. Ramzan M, Ali IMA. Sonographic assessment of hepatic steatosis (fatty liver) in School Children of Dera Ismail Khan City (NWFP) Pakistan. Pak J Nutr. 2009;8(6):797–9.
147. Clark JM, Brancati FL, Diehl AM. The prevalence and etiology of elevated aminotransferase levels in the United States. Am J Gastroenterol. 2003;98(5):960–7.
148. Madan K, Batra Y, Panda SK, Dattagupta S, Hazari S, Jha JK, et al. Role of polymerase chain reaction and liver biopsy in the evaluation of patients with asymptomatic transaminitis: implications in diagnostic approach. J Gastroenterol Hepatol. 2004;19(11):1291–9.
149. Anderson EL, Howe LD, Jones HE, Higgins JPT, Lawlor DA, Fraser A. The prevalence of non-alcoholic fatty liver disease in children and adolescents: a systematic review and meta-analysis. PLoS One. 2015;10(10):e0140908.
150. Shang X-R, Song J-Y, Liu F-H, Ma J, Wang H-J. GWAS-identified common variants with nonalcoholic fatty liver disease in chinese children. J Pediatr Gastroenterol Nutr. 2015;60(5):669–74.
151. Database of Single Nucleotide Polymorphisms. dbSNP accession:ss48413901 [Internet]. [cited 2017 Aug 27]. http://www.ncbi.nlm.nih.gov/projects/SNP/snp_ss.cgi?ss=ss48413901.
152. Singh S, Kuftinec GN, Sarkar S. Non-alcoholic fatty liver disease in South Asians: a review of the literature. J Clin Transl Hepatol. 2017;5(1):76–81.
153. Leonis MA, Balistreri WF. Evaluation and management of end-stage liver disease in children. Gastroenterology. 2008;134(6):1741–51.
154. Widodo AD, Soelaeman EJ, Dwinanda N, Narendraswari PP, Purnomo B. Chronic liver disease is a risk factor for malnutrition and growth retardation in children. Asia Pac J Clin Nutr. 2017;26(Suppl 1):S57–60.
155. Oh SH, Kim SJ, Rhee KW, Kim KM. Endoscopic cyanoacrylate injection for the treatment of gastric varices in children. World J Gastroenterol. 2015;21(9):2719–24.
156. Kang KS, Yang HR, Ko JS, Seo JK. Long-term outcomes of endoscopic variceal ligation to prevent rebleeding in children with esophageal varices. J Korean Med Sci. 2013;28(11):1657–60.
157. Sharma P, Sharma BC. Profile of hepatic encephalopathy in children with cirrhosis and response to lactulose. Saudi J Gastroenterol. 2011;17(2):138–41.
158. Srivastava A, Malik R, Bolia R, Yachha SK, Poddar U. Prevalence, clinical profile, and outcome of ascitic fluid infection in children with liver disease. J Pediatr Gastroenterol Nutr. 2017;64(2):194–9.

159. Vieira SMG, Matte U, Kieling CO, Barth AL, Ferreira CT, Souza AF, et al. Infected and noninfected ascites in pediatric patients. J Pediatr Gastroenterol Nutr. 2005;40(3):289–94.
160. El-Shabrawi MHF, El-Sisi O, Okasha S, Isa M, Elmakarem SA, Eyada I, et al. Diagnosis of spontaneous bacterial peritonitis in infants and children with chronic liver disease: a cohort study. Ital J Pediatr. 2011;37:26.
161. Bolia R, Srivastava A, Marak R, Yachha SK, Poddar U. Role of procalcitonin and C-reactive protein as biomarkers of infection in children with liver disease. J Pediatr Gastroenterol Nutr. 2016;63(4):406–11.
162. Bolia R, Srivastava A, Marak R, Yachha SK, Poddar U. Prevalence and impact of bacterial infections in children with liver disease—a prospective study. J Clin Exp Hepatol. 2018;8(1):35–41. https://doi.org/10.1016/j.jceh.2017.08.007.
163. Bajaj JS. Defining acute-on-chronic liver failure: will East and West ever meet? Gastroenterology. 2013;144(7):1337–9.
164. Lal J, Thapa BR, Rawal P, Ratho RK, Singh K. Predictors of outcome in acute-on-chronic liver failure in children. Hepatol Int. 2011;5(2):693–7.
165. Bolia R, Srivastava A, Yachha SK, Poddar U. Pediatric CLIF-SOFA score is the best predictor of 28-day mortality in children with decompensated chronic liver disease. J Hepatol. 2018;68(3):449–55. https://doi.org/10.1016/j.jhep.2017.10.001.
166. Rao S, D'Cruz AJ, Aggarwal R, Chandrashekar S, Chetan G, Gopalakrishnan G, et al. Pediatric liver transplantation: a report from a pediatric surgical unit. J Indian Assoc Pediatr Surg. 2011;16(1):2–7.
167. Sibal A, Bhatia V, Gupta S. Fifteen years of liver transplantation in India. Indian Pediatr. 2013;50(11):999–1000.
168. Nonthasoot B, Sirichindakul B, Suphapol J, Taesombat W, Sutherasan M, Nivatvongs S. Orthotopic liver transplantation at King Chulalongkorn Memorial Hospital: a report. J Med Assoc Thai. 2015;98(Suppl 1):S127–30.
169. Zhou J, Shen Z, He Y, Zheng S, Fan J. The current status of pediatric liver transplantation in Mainland China. Pediatr Transplant. 2010;14(5):575–82.
170. Kim JM, Kim KM, Yi N-J, Choe YH, Kim MS, Suh KS, et al. Pediatric liver transplantation outcomes in Korea. J Korean Med Sci. 2013;28(1):42–7.
171. Mali VP, Aw M, Quak SH, Loh DL, Prabhakaran K. Vascular complications in pediatric liver transplantation; single-center experience from Singapore. Transplant Proc. 2012;44(5):1373–8.
172. Soejima Y, Taketomi A, Yoshizumi T, Uchiyama H, Harada N, Ijichi H, et al. Biliary strictures in living donor liver transplantation: incidence, management, and technical evolution. Liver Transpl. 2006;12(6):979–86.
173. Shukla A, Vadeyar H, Rela M, Shah S. Liver transplantation: east versus west. J Clin Exp Hepatol. 2013;3(3):243–53.
174. Stanaway JD, Flaxman AD, Naghavi M, Fitzmaurice C, Vos T, Abubakar I, et al. The global burden of viral hepatitis from 1990 to 2013: findings from the Global Burden of Disease Study 2013. Lancet (London, England). 2016 10;388(10049):1081–8.

Part IV
Future Perspectives

"I know that I know nothing"

(Socrates, 470–399 BC)

Next-Generation Sequencing in Paediatric Hepatology

Lorenzo D'Antiga

Key Points
- With the introduction of next-generation sequencing, the diagnosis of genetic diseases has become extremely efficient and widely available.
- Whole exome sequencing is currently replacing targeted sequencing for children with a clear-cut phenotype, as well as those with a complex phenotype, due to its cost-effectiveness.
- Virtual panels oriented by the phenotype are used to confirm a diagnosis, whereas the clinical exome sequencing with variant filtering is adopted for more complex clinical conditions.
- NGS may not detect copy number variants; therefore other tools should also be considered in puzzling cases.
- In paediatric hepatology, NGS is making a paradigm shift in the approach to several clinical patterns of disease, such as infantile cholestasis, storage disorders, acute liver failure and non-alcoholic fatty liver disease.

Research Needed in the Field
- Further clarify the indications to test a proband and the relatives, based on level of clinical suspicion.
- Understand better how to combine the use of biochemistry and enzymatic tests in conjunction with NGS.
- Improve the ability of NGS to detect copy number variations.
- Evaluate the role of NGS as a screening tool in acute illness.
- Find a more reliable tool to determine the pathogenicity of point variants.
- Define how to report negative tests and incidental findings.

42.1 Introduction

Genetic testing has been rapidly evolving in the last few years [1]. In the 1970s, several techniques were developed to determine the individual order of bases of the genetic code. Among these the most efficient, which has become the gold standard in clinical laboratories, was described by Frederick Sanger [2].

Sanger technique has proven enormously successful due to its great precision, cost-effectiveness and low error rate, as shown by its use to sequence the 3.2 billion bases of the Human Genome Project. However, since it has been developed to sequence only one individually amplified DNA molecule at a time, it is unsuitable for large-scale projects [3]. Thus, until recently, a genetic test aimed at answering a question arisen from a specific clinical suspicion, pointing towards a selected genetic target. This gene-centred approach, although very reliable to detect single mutations, was inefficient and expensive, since it often required several attempts to make a diagnosis.

Over the past decade, next-generation sequencing (NGS) has grown remarkably as far as platform, technology and bioinformatics, allowing its widespread use in clinical settings. In the recent years, the introduction of NGS has accomplished the simultaneous analysis of a large number of genes, up to whole exome sequencing (WES) or even whole genome sequencing (WGS) (Fig. 42.1).

Nowadays it is possible to sequence the complete human genome within a few hours at relatively low cost, using widely available technologies that are becoming increasingly powerful, and whose limitations are more interpretative than technical [4].

Progresses of DNA sequencing and genotyping array technology allow the detection of variants, deletions and

L. D'Antiga (✉)
Paediatric Hepatology, Gastroenterology and Transplantation, Hospital Papa Giovanni XXIII, Bergamo, Italy
e-mail: ldantiga@asst-pg23.it

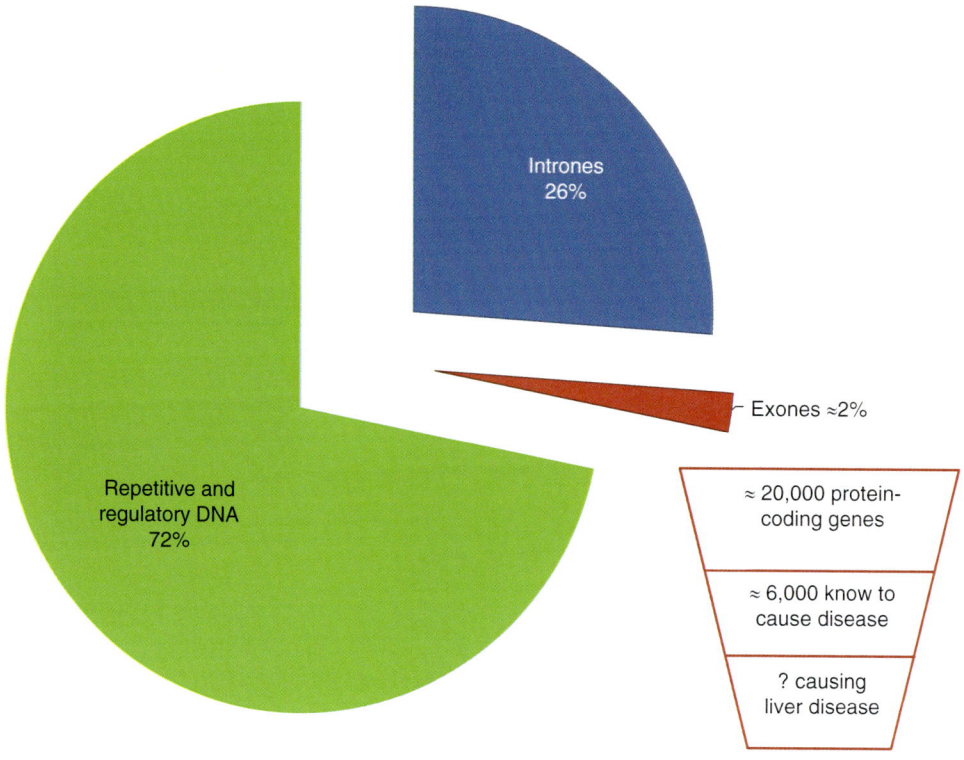

Fig. 42.1 The entire protein-coding sequence of an individual (the "exome") represents only 2% of the entire genome and encodes for some 20,000 proteins, of whom approximately 6000 have been associated to human diseases

duplications at genome level. Among these techniques, targeted gene sequencing (TGS) and WES are particularly useful to retrieve point mutations that are causative of monogenic disorders (MDs) [5].

There is no doubt that genetic testing may relevantly contribute to a prompt identification of patients with a MD. Nevertheless, it is illusory to think that the recognition of a genetic defect can fully characterize the clinical features of a Mendelian condition [6]. Indeed, environmental factors, usually referred to as epigenetic modifiers, deeply affect the phenotypic expression of MDs [7–9]. In this complex setting, a deeper knowledge of genomic variants represents the main stride towards the understanding of the determinants of genotype-phenotype match in MDs [10]. Besides, the availability of rapid mutation detection in disease-related locuses can offer the opportunity to bump into unexpected clinical pictures for a certain gene variant. More broadly, WES and WGS have an inherent potential for the discovery of novel disease-causing mutations, when applied to selected cases having homogeneous phenotypes.

NGS is rapidly expanding, and its applicability is well ahead the current clinical use. Since approximately 20% of the paediatric liver transplants (LT) are performed in children with MDs affecting the liver [11], the opportunity to simultaneously look for a group of related genes is of great help in this setting [12].

42.2 Next-Generation Sequencing

Massively parallel or "next-generation" sequencing has made it possible to generate large amounts of sequence data analysed simultaneously, thus providing variant information down to single-base resolution in a rapid, cost-effective and high-throughput fashion on the scale of the whole human genome. Enrichment techniques by either solid or liquid capture hybridization or amplicon methods allow to rapidly isolate candidate regions of interest (ROI) ranging from hundreds of kilobases in size to the entire protein-coding sequence of an individual (the "exome") [13].

NGS involves three fundamental steps: sample preparation, sequencing and data analysis [14]. The process starts with deoxyribonucleic acid (DNA) extraction usually from peripheral blood samples. In capture hybridization techniques, the sample is digested by mechanical disruption or by transposomes fragmenting the DNA; the fragments are then ligated to adapters which consist of short oligonucleotides of known sequences that are used as priming sites for amplification, indexed by polymerase chain reaction (PCR) and enriched by hybridization with specific probes for the ROI. Alternatively, in amplicon-based methods, the ROIs are either selected by targeting with primers or amplicons are created with targeted probes. The number of samples analysed simultaneously depends on the throughput of the instrument and on the size of the ROI. Successful

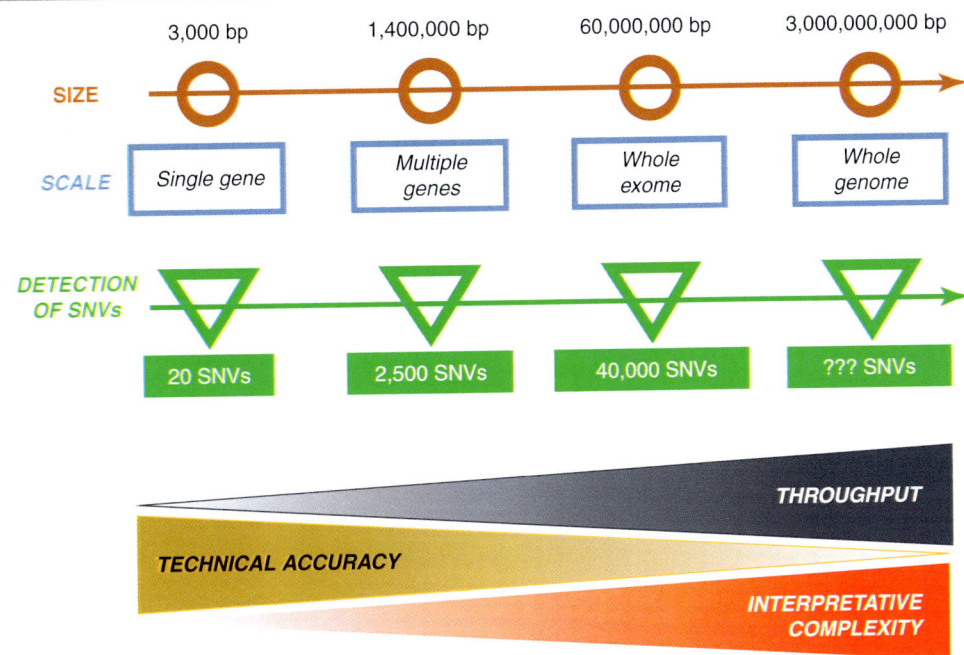

Fig. 42.2 Total number of variants (SNVs and indels) upon stepwise expansion of analysed genomic portions, expressed as base pairs and sequencing strategy (from targeted genes to whole genome). In the bottom part of the figure, it is shown the correlation among the platform throughput, the technical accuracy and the interpretative complexity. While the technical accuracy decreases, the amount of data and its complexity raise exponentially. *SNV* single-nucleotide variant

sequencing is highly dependent on the efficiency of the enrichment procedure and depends also on the type of bases of the ROI. The amount of reads is not uniformly distributed on the analysed region. In general, the higher the number of genes, the less accurate the coverage; the bigger the number of variants, the more difficult the interpretation (Fig. 42.2) [15].

Following sequencing, data analysis involves further steps, including base calling, read alignment, variant calling and variant annotation (Fig. 42.3). The genomic position of these variations is annotated to evaluate their significance: chromosomal position, base change, zygosity, gene or region involved, position in the gene (e.g. intron, exon, untranslated region), protein or transcript effect (missense, synonymous, introduction of a stop codon, splicing), population frequency reported on available databases and pathogenicity prediction [16–18]. This information may include also the presence of the variant in public databases, the degree of evolutionary conservation of the encoded nucleotide and a prediction of whether the variant is pathogenic due its potential impact on protein function using computer-based algorithms [19, 20].

42.3 NGS Strategies

42.3.1 Targeted Gene Sequencing (TGS)

The use of targeted panels has the advantage to be focused on a limited number of suspected diseases, has a better coverage of the genes of interest and is time- and cost-saving when it comes to reporting. Similarly to Sanger sequencing, this technique is suitable as a confirmation of a clinical suspicion based on signs, symptoms and biochemical tests. In paediatric hepatology, TGS is particularly indicated to characterize genetic cholestatic disorders, most commonly presenting early in life with conjugated hyperbilirubinemia, or to identify different disease subtypes causing a similar metabolic derangement, such as glycogen storage disorders, mitochondrial disorders and non-alcoholic fatty liver disease [21–24]. In defined conditions or syndromes, clinical features and biochemical markers can guide the investigation towards a specific pathway or group of genes responsible for a given phenotype. In these cases, a TGS analysis has proven efficient and cost-effective [25]. Table 42.1 reports a list of common monogenic disorders of the liver that can be detected by targeted NGS techniques.

In our institution, we have developed a customized TGS panel that—at the time of writing—comprises the locuses of interest of 31 genes related to the 28 most common genetic disorders affecting the liver. Due to the high cost-effectiveness and technical handiness, the panel has been designed to include the most common monogenic liver diseases irrespective of the clinical phenotype, such as genetic cholestatic disorders, inborn errors of metabolism or defects causing chronic liver disease. In our centre, TGS yielded a detection rate of 57% in the setting of cholestasis of infancy.

Except from Alagille syndrome, all diseases included in our panel are inherited in an autosomal recessive manner and are characterized by homozygous or double heterozygous mutations. For this reason, the availability of the DNA of the parents is essential to confirm that the two variants are located on different alleles [26].

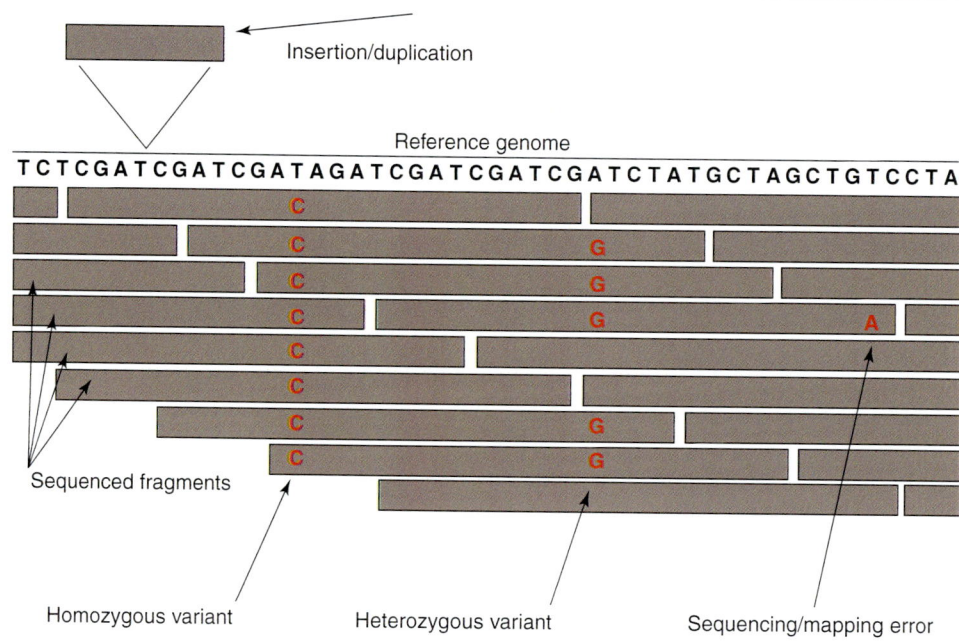

Fig. 42.3 Individual reads (brown rectangles) aligned to the reference genome of an healthy individual. The coverage for each genomic position is the number of reads that overlap at that position. Ideally the number of reads should be more than 50. Bases that match the reference sequence have been omitted. The arrows show examples of homozygous and heterozygous single-nucleotide variants, as well as the inability of NGS to recognize copy number variations such as insertions or duplications, which cannot be aligned to the reference genome

Table 42.1 Most common liver based monogenic disorders

Disease name	Defective protein	OMIM	Gene	Locus	Pointers to the diagnosis
Neonatal/infantile cholestasis					
Progressive familial intrahepatic cholestasis type 1 (PFIC 1)	FIC1	211600	ATP8B1[a]	18q21.31	– Low GGT – Short stature – Diarrhoea
Progressive familial intrahepatic cholestasis type 2 (PFIC 2)	Bile salt export pump (BSEP)	601847	ABCB11[a]	2q31.1	– Low GGT
Progressive familial intrahepatic cholestasis type 3 (PFIC 3)	Multidrug resistance protein 3	602347	ABCB4[a]	7q21.12	– High GGT – Early portal hypertension
Progressive, familial intrahepatic cholestasis type 4 (PFIC 4)	Tight junction protein 2	615878	TJP2[a]	9q21.11	– Low GGT
Progressive, familial intrahepatic cholestasis type 5 (PFIC 5)	Farnesoid X-activated receptor	617049	NR1H4	12q23.1	– Low GGT
Myosin VB-associated cholestasis	Myosin VB	606540	MYO5B	18q21.1	– Low GGT
Alagille syndrome	Jagged-1, Notch2	118450 610205	JAG1[a] NOTCH2[a]	20p12.2 1p12	– High GGT – Peculiar face – Bile duct paucity
Alpha-1 antitrypsin deficiency	Alpha-1-antitrypsin	613490	SERPINA1[a]	14q32.13	– Low serum A1AT – Steatosis
Bile acid synthesis defects: Δ4-3-oxosteroid-5β-reductase deficiency	Δ4-3-oxosteroid-5β-reductase	235555	AKR1D1[a]	7q33	– Low GGT – Normal serum primary bile acids – No itching
Bile acid synthesis defects: 3β-hydroxy-Δ5-C27-steroid dehydrogenase deficiency (3βHSD)	3β-hydroxy-Δ5-C27-steroid dehydrogenase	607765	HSD3B7[a]	16p11.2	– Low GGT – Normal serum primary bile acids – No itching
Bile acid synthesis defects: Oxysterol 7α-hydroxylase deficiency	Oxysterol 7α-hydroxylase	613812	CYP7B1[a]	8q12.3	– Low GGT – Normal serum primary bile acids – No itching
Familial hypercholanemia due to amidation defects (BAAT)	– Bile acid-CoA:amino acid N-acyltransferase	602938	BAAT[a]	9q31.1	– Low GGT – High serum primary bile acids (unconjugated) – Itching
Arthrogryposis-renal dysfunction-cholestasis (ARC) syndrome	VPS33B protein VIPAR protein	208085 613404	VPS33B[a], VIPAR[a]	15q26.1 14q24.3	– Low GGT – Arthrogryposis
Transaldolase deficiency	TALDO	606003	TALDO1[a]	11p15.5	– Low GGT – Hepatosplenomegaly

Table 42.1 (continued)

Disease name	Defective protein	OMIM	Gene	Locus	Pointers to the diagnosis
Neonatal sclerosing cholangitis (NISCH)	Claudin-1	607626	CLDN1	3q28	– Neonatal sclerosing cholangitis – Ichthyosis
Neonatal sclerosing cholangitis	Doublecortin domain-containing protein 2	605755	DCDC2	6p22.3	– Neonatal sclerosing cholangitis
Citrin deficiency (NICCD)	CMC2	605814	SLC25A13[a]	7q21.3	– Mild cholestasis, fatty changes – Elevated citrullin – Resolves by 6-12 months with MCT-based formula
Niemann Pick A,B	SMPD1	257200 607616	SMPD1[a]		– Early hepatosplenomegaly – Progressive developmental delay – Pulmonary involvement
Niemann Pick C	NPC1 NPC2	257220 607625	NPC1[a] NPC2[a]	18q11.2 14q24.3	– Early hepatosplenomegaly – Progressive developmental delay
Gaucher disease	Glucosylceramidase	230800	GBA[a]	1q22	– Early hepatosplenomegaly – Pancytopenia
Chronic liver disease and/or portal hypertension					
Congenital hepatic fibrosis	Fibrocystin	263200	ARPKD[a]	6p12.3-p12.2	– Hepatosplenomegaly – Polycystic kidney – Normal liver function
LAL-deficiency (mild form)	Lysosomal acid lipase	278000	LIPA[a]	10q23.31	– Microvescicular steatosis – Raised cholesterol level
Congenital defects of glycosylation 1b	Phosphomannose isomerase	602579	MPI[a]	15q24.1	– Chronic diarrhea – Low antithrombin III – Non cirrhotic portal hypertension – Normal mental status
Wilson disease	Copper-transporting ATPase 2	277900	ATP7B[a]	13q14.3	– Low ceruloplasmin – Fatty liver – Neurologic symptoms later in life
Acute liver failure					
Galactosemia	GAL-1-PUT	230400	GALT[a]	9p13.3	– Triggered by galactose in diet – Hypoglycaemia – E.Coli sepsis – Renal tubular dysfunction
Tyrosinemia	Fumarylacetoacetase	276700	FAH[a]	15q25.1	– Triggered by tyrosine in diet – Renal tubular dysfunction – Rickets – Early cirrhosis and HCC
Hereditary fructose intolerance	Fructose-bisphosphate aldolase B	229600	ALDOB[a]	9q31.1	– Triggered by fructose/sucrose in diet – Hypoglycaemia – Vomiting, shock
MCAD deficiency	Medium-chain specific acyl-CoA dehydrogenase	201450	ACADM[a]	1p31.1	– Reye-like presentation – Fatty liver
Mitochondrial DNA Depletion sdr (POLG)	DNA polymerase subunit gamma-1	203700	POLG[a]	15q26.1	– Intractable epilepsy – Triggered by valproate – Severe encephalopathy, lactic acidosis
Mitochondrial DNA Depletion sdr (DGUOK)	Deoxyguanosine kinase	251880	DGUOK[a]	2p13.1	– Hypoglycaemia – Neurological involvement – Lactic acidosis
Mitochondrial DNA Depletion sdr (MPV17)	Mpv17	256810	MPV17[a]	2p23.3	– Hypoglycaemia – Neurological involvement
Ornithine transcarbamylase (OTC) deficiency	Ornithine carbamoyltransferase	311250	OTC[a]	Xp11.4	– Male subjects – Hyperammonemia – Encephalopathy
Recurrent acute liver failure (RALF)	Neuroblastoma-amplified sequence	616483	NBAS	2p24.3	– Triggered by fever – Recurrent ALF episodes

[a]genes included in the targeted NGS panel at our Institution

42.3.2 Whole Exome Sequencing (WES)

Despite targeted NGS has proven cost-effective, rapid progresses in capture designs have allowed all protein-coding regions to be sequenced without significant raise of costs. For this reason, the interest is rapidly shifting towards WES.

The use of WES is recommended to improve the diagnostic yield in cases of an uncertain or compound phenotype, with a likely inheritable background but no clear pointers to the diagnosis.

A tight liaison between the laboratory geneticist and the clinician is necessary to ascertain the correct diagnosis from WES, that involves filtering of gene candidates, on the basis of phenotypic features disclosed by previous clinical investigations, and type of Mendelian inheritance ascertained from parents sequencing [27].

A relevant aspect of WES is that previous experiences have shown incomplete capture of target regions, with 40% of targeted bases and 20% of known disease-causing sites resulting poorly covered [28, 29]. It is therefore clear that a critical phase in the WES is the enrichment phase, requiring further technical improvements [30]. However technical advances are remarkably increasing the coverage and the precision of WES; thus many laboratories are shifting towards this technique allowing to evaluate targeted regions but also offering the possibility to assess the bioinformatically stored data of the entire exome at a later stage. In our centre, we are shifting towards sequencing the whole exome even when we aim at evaluating only targeted genes.

42.3.3 Clinical Exome Sequencing (CES)

In several cases, WES does not allow to point to the genetic diagnosis, since most of generated data falls on genes not yet associated with human diseases and thus not includible in a clinical genetic report. In these cases, and especially when the clinical manifestations are not clear, CES represents a good alternative and a good compromise between cost, time and detection rate. This analysis includes all genes associated with known diseases (the "mendeliome"). The clinical exome used in our centre, at the time of writing, includes 4813 disease genes reported in the Human Gene Mutation Database (HGMD) and OMIM (Online Mendelian Inheritance in Man).

42.3.4 Whole Genome Sequencing (WGS)

WGS sequences all bases in the genome and offers a resolution that is not reachable by other sequencing methods, allowing to study coding and noncoding regions [31]. WGS has also the advantage of detecting structural rearrangements of part of the genome, otherwise visible only with karyotype or array-CGH, such as chromosomal translocations or inversions or dosage. Nevertheless, WGS is more expensive and less feasible than WES in daily practice, since it produces more than 100 Gb of data per single test; thus a huge effort is required to perform bioinformatic analysis and store safely all gathered information [32].

42.4 Interpretation of the Results and Reporting

Case Scenario The second child of healthy and unrelated parents presented at birth with facial dysmorphisms, preauricular pits, anomalous pulmonary venous return, jaundice, acholic stools, hypospadia and hydronephrosis, intestinal malrotation and anocutaneous fistula. The child was hypotonic and showed poor sucking, developmental delay and thinning of the corpus callosum at brain MRI. Investigations of conjugated jaundice demonstrated that the child was affected by biliary atresia and underwent a successful Kasai portoenterostomy. Whole exome sequencing did not reveal any known genetic condition. Due to the complex clinical picture, a microdeletion/microduplication syndrome was suspected, and array-CGH and multiplex ligation-dependent probe amplification (MLPA) were run in parallel, demonstrating a duplication of chromosome 22, consistent with the diagnosis of Cat eye syndrome, known to be associated with biliary atresia.

Genetic testing is usually performed to confirm a clinical phenotype linked to a known genetic disease, suggested by specific clinical and biochemical investigation. However, especially in unusual and rare cases, a discrepancy between genetic test and clinical significance often occurs [33]. For this reason, it is very important to have a hypothesis of the type of inheritance on the basis of the family history (autosomal dominant or recessive, sporadic condition or X-linked transmission), so that the NGS strategy and reporting can be tailored to the specific case.

Each test performed by NGS generates thousands to millions of base pairs of DNA and detects lots of variants, the number depending on the size of the ROIs (Fig. 42.2). All these data must be filtered and interpreted, with the help of storage facilities, bioinformatic technologies and disease databases. Remarkably, most of the detected variants have not been definitely linked to a disease (VUS, variants of unknown significance), and therefore inevitable incidental findings may lead to divert from the diagnosis.

Mendelian rules represent a simplification of the real contribution of missense mutations to the patient's phenotype. In general, there are variants that have been associated with particular diseases, other identified as intermediate contributors to the phenotype and other considered modifiers of a given condition. Indeed, there are probably no fully penetrant alleles, and many variants are likely to contribute to every disease at a variable extent, making the genotype-phenotype match unpredictable in most cases.

Among variants, those causing a stop codon or a truncating protein can be considered likely to be causative of a disease, whereas variants related to missense mutations (having variable effects on different proteins) are unpredictable as far as post-transcriptional effect on function. Aspects supporting the pathogenicity of a variant causing a missense mutation are (1) the previous report in human genome databases, (2) minor allele frequency (MAF) in the general population (the higher the frequency, the lower the probability to be causal in rare diseases) [34], (3) evidence of being causative in published literature, (4) co-segregation with the disease within the same family, (5) de novo variant in a sporadic condition and (6) biostatistical prediction models.

In specialized centre, after filtering, the remaining variants are classified in accordance to the most recent guidelines [35]. Only variants associated with the patient phenotype that are present in HGMD Professional 2013.4 (https://portal.biobase international.com/hgmd/pro/start.php) and/or ClinVar (http://www.ncbi.nlm.nih.gov/clinvar/) are included in the final report as "pathogenic mutations". Variants found in genes implicated in the patient phenotype and classified as potentially pathogenic by the American College of Medical Genetics (ACMG) that have not been previously described, or those present in HGMD without any functional validation, should be reported as VUS needing further investigations [36].

It is important to consider that, although exceedingly effective in identifying single-nucleotide variants, substitution and insertion/deletion of few nucleotides, NGS is not accurate for other genomic variations, such as copy number, structural rearrangements (translocation and inversion) or partial rearrangements of a gene. Furthermore, the most commonly adopted NGS strategies are not able to detect triplet expansion or methylation status of a given genomic region.

42.5 Monogenic Liver Diseases in Children

Nearly half of chronic liver disorders presenting in childhood have a genetic cause, and approximately 20% of LT in children are performed as a consequence of liver-based MDs [11]. If we exclude biliary atresia (the main indication to paediatric LT) and autoimmune liver disease, most of the remaining conditions causing progressive hepatopathy in childhood are inheritable. It is therefore clear that, in this setting, a powerful instrument to discover pathogenic variants bears a tremendous revolutionary power in the clinical management of a child presenting with liver disease [37].

Although most skilled clinicians would regard NGS as a very inelegant diagnostic tool, the opportunity to get straight to the diagnosis with a simple peripheral blood sample, avoiding invasive procedures and complex biochemical tests, is undoubtedly appealing. NGS entails a paradigm shift in clinical approach to suspect genetic liver disease: from the classical scenario, in which hypotheses rise from clinical and biochemical data and lead to genetic confirmation, to a new one, in which candidate disease-associated variants are filtered on a probabilistic basis and are finally matched with the clinical picture. Besides, biochemical and enzymatic tests often do not provide faster reports, require special investigative equipment and expert interpretation, and their reliability is affected by the stage of the disease. A major advantage of the NGS in paediatric hepatology is that it overcomes possible laboratory pitfalls. In fact, in the subclinical/early phase, clinical and biochemical hallmarks may be absent or insufficient to make the diagnosis until a trigger (diet, oxidative stress, infections) produces a consistent (and sometimes irreversible) metabolic derangement [38]. Similarly, at the other end of the spectrum, in a child with end-stage liver disease or with acute decompensation, looking for a specific metabolite pattern can be tricky; in fulminant liver failure, genetic testing may represent the only way to achieve a diagnosis of a metabolic condition [39]. NGS will never replace biochemical and enzymatic tests in the management of MDs, but it may act as a bundle tool able to provide a fast and reliable diagnosis, especially in unclear phenotypic presentations. Reciprocal confirmation between genetic and biochemical diagnosis is recommended, when feasible. Table 42.2 reports some clinical hints to the suspicion of MDs in patients presenting with or having an ongoing liver disease.

42.6 NGS in Cholestasis of Infancy

Case Scenario A female infant with negative family history, presented at 4 months of age with cholestasis and bile duct paucity on liver histology. Further clinical workup revealed a posterior embryotoxon, a peripheral pulmonary stenosis and butterfly vertebrae at spine x-ray. A cholestasis NGS panel including Jag1 and Notch2 genes was carried out but revealed no mutations in the genes responsible for Alagille syndrome. Given the strong clinical suspicion, multiplex ligation-dependent probe amplification (MLPA) was also performed and demonstrated an heterozygous de novo total deletion of JAG1. The array-CGH analysis performed to define the extension of the deletion showed that the patient had a heterozygous 20p12.2 deletion of 140 kb including only JAG1 gene.

Cholestatic liver disease affects approximately 1/2500 term infants and is most commonly due to biliary atresia (up

Table 42.2 Pointers to the diagnosis of genetic liver disease

Medical history (consanguinity, previous affected siblings, dietary triggers, provocative symptoms, hypoglycaemia, acidosis, neurological symptoms, rhabdomyolysis)	Tyrosinaemia, Galactosaemia, Fructosaemia, Urea cycle defects, Fatty acid oxidation defects, Mitochondrial cytopathies
Hydrops fetalis	Lysosomal storage disorders, Wolman disease, Congenital defects of glycosilation
Neonatal cholestasis	A1ATD, PFIC, Galactosaemia, Tyrosinaemia, Niemann Pick C, Inborn errors of bile acid, Cystic fibrosis, Ciliopathies
Cholestasis with low GGT	PFIC 1, 2 and 4, Bile acid defects, ARC, TALDO
Fatty liver early in life	Hereditary fructose intolerance, fatty acid oxidation defects, LAL deficiency, mitochondrial cytopathies
Isolated hepatomegaly	Glycogen storage disease, LAL deficiency, Fatty acid oxidation defects, Mucopolysaccharidosis
Hepatosplenomegaly	All lysosomal storage disorders, congenital hepatic fibrosis
Neonatal cholestasis with splenomegaly	Niemann Pick C, Gaucher disease
Chronic liver disease	A1ATD, Wilson disease, Glycogen Storage Disease 3 and 4
Liver failure	Tyrosinaemia, Galactosaemia, Fructosaemia, Urea cycle defects, Fatty acid ox defects, Wilson disease, mitochondrial cytopathies

A1ATD alpha-1 antitrypsin deficiency, *CF* cystic fibrosis, *GGT* gamma-glutamyl transpeptidase, *NICCD* neonatal idiopathic cholestasis due to citrin deficiency, *PFIC* progressive familial intrahepatic cholestasis, *NP-C* Niemann-Pick type C disease, *ARC* arthrogryposis renal dysfunction and cholestasis syndrome, *TALDO* transaldolase deficiency, *LAL* lysosomal acid lipase

to 40% of cases) [40]. In the past, up to 60% of infants with neonatal cholestasis and a histological pattern of giant cell hepatitis were classified as "idiopathic neonatal hepatitis". This term is now used much less frequently because modern tools allowed to recognize specific genetic syndromes; as a consequence, the rate of infants diagnosed with "neonatal idiopathic cholestasis" has dropped to less than 20% of all infants presenting with conjugated jaundice [41]. Conversely—in the early NGS era—a genetic cause is being identified in about 40% of the children with intrahepatic (non-biliary atresia) cholestasis; thus this technique represents a very powerful tool to recognize these disorders, expected to further reduce the percentage of "idiopathic" cases [22, 42].

Progressive familial intrahepatic cholestasis (PFIC)—a group of disorders caused by a disturbance of the bile transport through the canalicular membrane—accounts for more than 10% of the children with neonatal cholestasis. PFICs are almost uniquely associated with low gamma-glutamyl transpeptidase (GGT) serum level (only the rare inborn errors of bile acid synthesis/conjugation—having the hallmark of low/normal serum primary bile acids—share this feature) and are indistinguishable on clinical ground one from the other [43–48] (Table 42.1).

Dröge and co-workers studied 427 patients with suspected inherited cholestasis; 149 patients carried at least 1 disease-causing mutation in FIC1, BSEP or MDR3, respectively. Overall, 154 different mutations were identified, of which 25 were novel. All 13 novel missense mutations were disease-causing according to bioinformatics analyses and homology modelling. One or more common polymorphisms were found in the three genes of patients without disease-causing mutations. Minor allele frequencies of common polymorphisms in BSEP (p.V444A) and MDR3 (p.I237I) were significantly overrepresented in patients without disease-causing mutation, indicating that these common variants may contribute to cholestasis development [49].

The most important value of applying NGS in the field of early-onset cholestasis is the opportunity to rapidly identify the defect causing *low-GGT PFICs (PFIC1, PFIC2, PFIC4* and the recently discovered *PFIC5* and *Myosin VB-associated cholestasis)* [50, 51]. Indeed each defect bears the risk of different complications before and after transplantation (such as severe post-LT diarrhoea, steatosis and graft loss in *PFIC1* and the risk of HCC in the native liver or recurrent immune-mediated disease after LT in *PFIC2*) [52–56]. Thus, genetic characterization is the crossroad for an aware decision-making about possible medical, surgical bile acid lowering treatment (e.g. biliary diversion) or towards transplantation.

The diagnosis of other MDs presenting with infantile cholestasis may be very difficult without genetic testing. Some examples are given by patients with bile acid conjugation defects (such as *familial hypercholanemia* due to BAAT deficiency) having a defect of amidation of primary bile acid that requires mass spectrometry or specific liver immunostaining to be revealed [57]. *Citrin deficiency* (neonatal-onset type II citrullinemia) may present clinically with prolonged jaundice and failure to thrive but with otherwise non-specific histology and liver tests and a normal serum amino acid profile. In all these patients, NGS has proven a very effective tool to disclose rare types of genetic cholestasis [58, 59].

Alagille syndrome (AS) is commonly diagnosed on clinical ground, based on historical clinical criteria described by Alagille in 1975 [60]. Almost all the genetically confirmed cases in our experience had a previous suspicion. Nevertheless, due to the variable penetrance of this autosomal dominant condition, AS has a wide spectrum of clinical disease expression and severity; for this reason, many such patients not fulfilling the classical clinical criteria remain undiagnosed, unless JAG1 and NOTCH2 disease-causing variations are regularly looked for [61]. Being aware of such condition before a LT is offered is important, since it allows to identify and possibly treat coexisting pulmonary artery stenosis or intracranial vascular malformations at risk of potentially devastating complications [62]. Remarkably, 5–7% of AS patients have a partial or complete deletion of JAG1, which may not be detected by NGS. Thus, when the clinical suspicion is high and NGS is not diagnostic, a more specific test for deletions, such as multiplex ligation-dependent probe amplification (MLPA), is recommended.

In some inborn errors of metabolism causing severe liver disease early after birth, NGS overcomes the problem of securing the diagnosis in patients already started on a substrate-free diet. This is especially the case of *galactosaemia* and *hereditary fructose intolerance*, in which the marker metabolite rapidly disappears and a challenge with the putative causative substrate is harmful [63].

Lysosomal storage disorders (such as *Niemann-Pick Type B and C, Gaucher disease, Lysosomal acid lipase deficiency*) are hallmarked by splenomegaly and can present with neonatal cholestasis [64]. Although the standard diagnosis is usually made by enzymatic testing, this type of assay is not widely available and needs centralization to specialized laboratory, with some time lapse before the diagnosis can be made. NGS may not offer faster results but has the advantage to make the diagnosis and define the genotypic signature of the condition (often corresponding to different predicted outcomes) and can be particularly useful to the paediatric hepatologist as part of a NGS panel for patients presenting early in life with cholestasis [65].

Alpha-1 antitrypsin (A1AT) deficiency (A1ATD) can present early in life with completely acholic stools and histological features mimicking biliary atresia; for this reason, A1ATD should be ruled out before performing a liver biopsy and a direct cholangiography. In most patients, a borderline or frankly low serum A1AT level is a good pointer to the diagnosis, although, since A1AT is an acute phase reactant, during inflammation its serum level can be found in the normal range, and the condition may be overlooked [66]. A1ATD genetic signature should be therefore obtained either by isoelectrofocusing (giving the detailed A1AT phenotype) or genotyping in unclear cases [67].

At our institution, infants with conjugated hyperbilirubinemia undergo a stepwise evaluation in which a NGS expanded panel for genetic liver diseases (*Bergamo Liver Panel*) acquires a pivotal role to the diagnosis. Figure 42.4 illustrates this novel approach, which is currently under evaluation in a prospective study. In this algorithm stool colour, liver biopsy pattern and GGT level are the main crossroads,

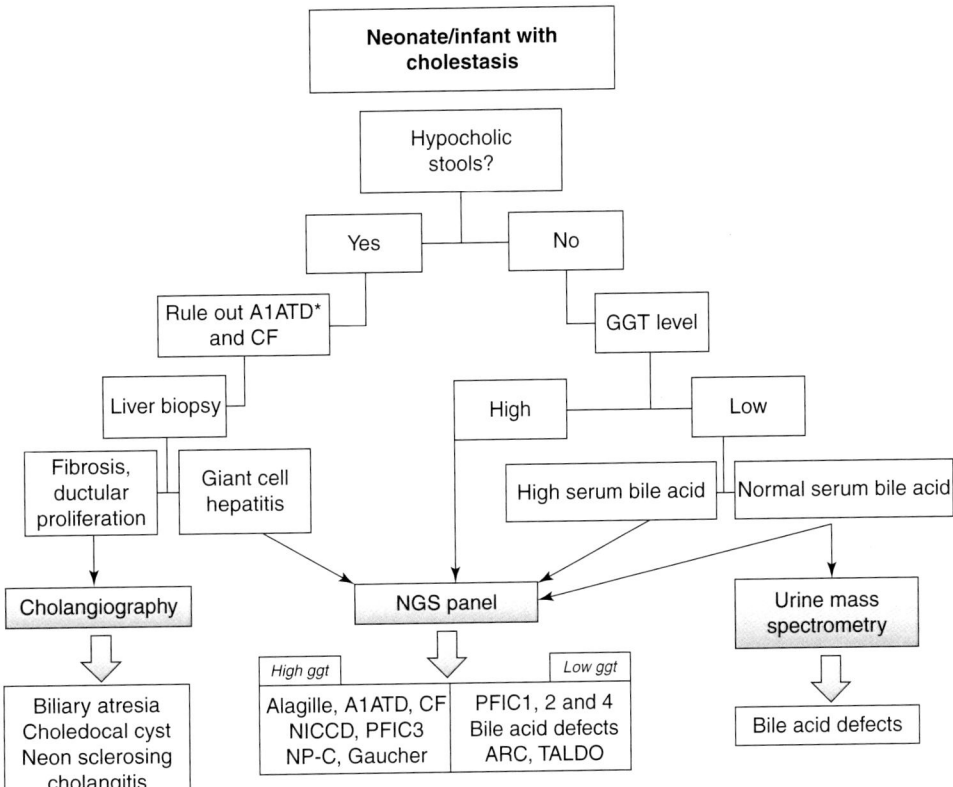

Fig. 42.4 Algorithm adopted in Bergamo for the diagnostic workup of cholestatic infants. *A1ATD* alpha-1 antitrypsin deficiency, *CF* cystic fibrosis, *GGT* gamma-glutamyl transpeptidase, *NICCD* neonatal idiopathic cholestasis due to citrin deficiency, *PFIC* progressive familial intrahepatic cholestasis, *NP-C* Niemann-Pick type C disease, *ARC* arthrogryposis, renal dysfunction and cholestasis syndrome, *TALDO-D* transaldolase deficiency. *In infants with acholic stools, A1AT is tested in serum before Kasai portoenterostomy, whereas its genetic testing is included in the NGS panel we use if histology shows giant cell hepatitis

whereas intraoperative cholangiogram and NGS lead to the conclusive diagnosis. Preliminary results show that—in this paediatric LT setting—the detection rate of genetic causes of infantile cholestasis is around 50%, and that NGS is cost-effective when compared with a traditional stepwise diagnostic approach based on clinical and biochemical pointers.

The genes included in the *Bergamo Liver Panel* are indicated in Table 42.1 with an asterisk.

42.7 NGS in Acute Liver Failure

Case Scenario A full-term girl of adequate weight was born to non-consanguineous parents. Soon after birth, she developed cholestasis with normal GGT, elevated serum bile acids and AST > ALT. She had a rapid deterioration towards liver failure with coagulopathy, ascites, hyperammonaemia, hypoglycaemia and renal failure. She appeared severely hypotonic, and concomitant findings were Coombs-negative haemolytic anaemia and central hypothyroidism requiring L-thyroxine. The child was therefore listed and underwent a successful liver transplant.

The extensive biochemical workup could not confirm any known cause of neonatal cholestasis/liver failure. The clinical exome sequencing on the girl-parent trio revealed that she was compound heterozygote for two mutations in the ATP7B gene causing Wilson's disease (WD) (p.His1069Gln + p.Gln7fs); the mother was homozygote for p.His1069Gln, and the father was heterozygote for p.Gln7fs. Biochemical and histology testing confirmed WD both in the child and in the mother, who was already cirrhotic. The team assumed that the girl's picture was the result of an in utero *copper overload of a WD foetus in a WD untreated mother and that only NGS could diagnose a disease that would have never been looked for at this age.*

The cause of acute liver failure (ALF) in children can be determined in approximately half of patients, whereas in the other half, the condition remains indeterminate. An underlying MD causing severe metabolic derangements is identified in 10–28% of children with ALF [68, 69], largely depending on the diagnostic capabilities of the centre. Genetic causes of ALF and possible clinical and biochemical features are depicted in Fig. 42.5.

The earlier the presentation of ALF, the higher the suspicion for an inherited metabolic disease (IMD) should be maintained. The management of a child with ALF is challenging. Children with ALF are often listed for LT before a diagnosis is achieved. Reaching a timely diagnosis, however, is of great importance in this scenario, because IMD may respond to medical treatment, and—conversely—some of them represent relative contraindications to LT [70, 71]. The importance of a rapid genetic diagnosis is even greater considering that—during acute decompensation—appropriate biochemical and histological evaluations can be unfeasible or ineffective because of the patient instability and the numerous confounders produced by severe organ injury. In this setting, in the next future NGS will probably represent a pillar in the management of ALF, effectively identifying underlying IMDs, provided the turnaround time is fast enough to impact on decision to transplant or not.

The genetic causes of ALF are *galactosaemia, fructosemia, mitochondrial depletion syndromes (MDSs), tyrosinaemia type 1*, rarely forms of congenital glycosylation defect

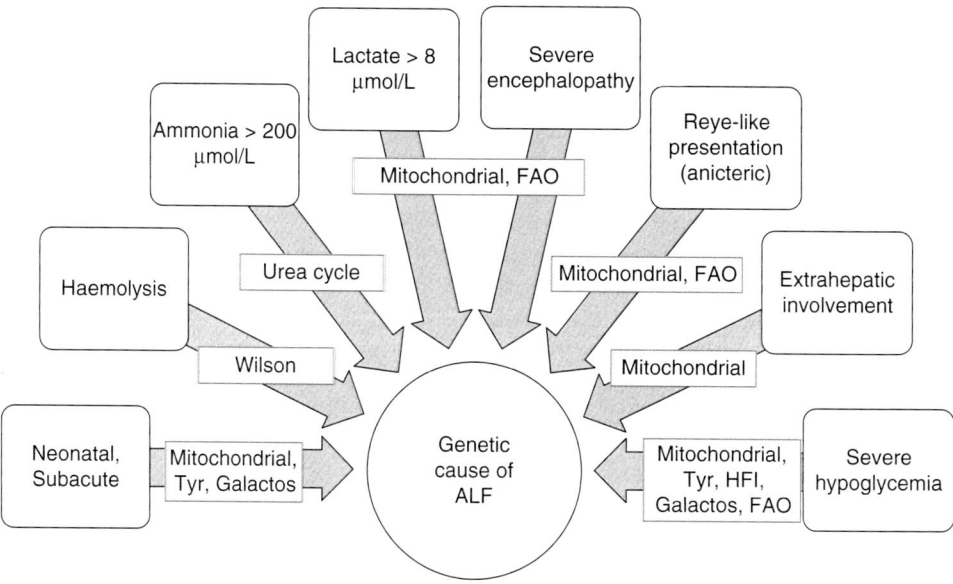

Fig. 42.5 Genetic causes of acute liver failure and possible clues for their identification. *ALF* acute liver failure, *TYR* tyrosinaemia; Galactos, galactosaemia, *FAO* fatty acid oxidation defects, *HFI* hereditary fructose intolerance

(*CDG*, *especially CDG-1a*) and of *fatty acids oxidation defects*, *often presenting with a Reye-like picture*; in males in the postneonatal period, *ornithine transcarbamylase deficiency* should be considered. In older children, a relatively common cause is *Wilson disease*.

Galactosaemia and *fructosemia* have been already mentioned among the causes of infantile cholestasis and ALF. These diseases respond dramatically to the substrate-free diet (galactose and fructose, respectively), but challenging a fragile infant with these sugars to make the definite diagnosis is unadvisable.

Tyrosinaemia type 1 is easily diagnosed observing the plasma amino acid profile and urine succinylacetone. Low-protein diet and nitisinone help in disease control, and postpone LT.

Mitochondrial disorders (*MDSs*) are mainly related to mutations in genes involved in the respiratory chain, having heterogeneous phenotypes, most commonly characterized by a defect of cellular energy production. As such, they are systemic diseases in which organ transplantation is generally contraindicated. Those presenting with liver involvement are related to nuclear gene products (inherited with autosomal recessive pattern in 90% and autosomal dominant and X-linked pattern in 10%), responsible for mitochondrial DNA replication (*POLG1*), maintenance of deoxyribonucleoside triphosphate (dNTP) pools (*DGUOK*) and membrane mitochondrial integrity (*MPV17*) [72, 73]. Therefore, mutations in these genes cause mitochondrial DNA depletion, characterized by hepato-cerebral forms inherited with an autosomal recessive pattern. In *Alpers syndrome* (due to mutations in POLG1), sodium valproate administered because of intractable seizures often triggers acute liver decompensation and death. The histological changes on liver biopsy include fatty degeneration, bile duct proliferation, fibrosis and lobular collapse [74], but NGS may warrant a rapid confirmation of the diagnosis, which is therefore relevant for the management of these patients.

Undoubtedly, the wide clinical and biochemical heterogeneity of MDSs represents a diagnostic challenge. The complex contribution of nuclear and mitochondrial genes on mitochondrial function and integrity, associated with the occurrence of heteroplasmy (random mixture of mitochondria with normal and mutant DNA in different tissues), makes the clinical phenotype very unpredictable. Enzymatic assays on muscle biopsy are time-consuming, while a low enzymatic activity on liver biopsy could be secondary. In this scenario TGS can be very effective in the suspicion of such defects, since these are caused by mutations in very few genes [75]. Remarkably, NGS helps to discriminate cases of acutely ill children in which mitochondrial DNA depletion was secondary to acute liver injury [23]. Genetic information, neurologic status and ethical considerations should be part of the evaluation of these children.

A complete list of the genes associated with ALF is in Table 42.1.

42.8 Conclusion

Diagnosing a genetic disease used to be a fine art for few, and pursuing it with single genetic testing is a complex process. NGS allows the detection of a large number of variants in clusters of genes and is becoming a widely available and standardized technique that, combined with biochemical data and phenotype examination, may rapidly lead to the correct diagnosis of all known monogenic liver diseases. NGS will never replace biochemical testing that is central to establish the clinical phenotype and guide the patient management and follow-up but represents a great tool to make the diagnosis in difficult situations, providing information on genotype-phenotype match, offering diagnostic confirmation to the clinical picture.

This strategy has been successfully implemented in our centre, and now it's fully integrated into the care of patients with neonatal/infantile cholestasis or unexplained liver disease. However, it is of even greater importance in the paediatric LT setting when used to unmask genetic causes of ALF. Its use may reduce the time to diagnosis and the number of invasive tests or procedures, facilitate decision-making and fill the gap of the laboratory diagnostics in certain situations. With the growing adoption of CES, WES and WGS, in the next years, it will be important to optimize and standardize a diagnostic procedure that combines clinical phenotype, genetic testing and biochemical tests. In this perspective NGS can operate a Copernican revolution, turning upside-down the bedside-to-bench approach to the diagnosis of an inherited condition.

Remarkably, the use of NGS should go along full awareness of its limitations and cost. Whereas a panel-based method is useful to confirm a diagnosis suggested by clinical and biochemical findings, and represents a quite reliable tool, WES may be challenging like finding a needle in a haystack, because of the huge number of variants detected. In both cases, but vital in WES, a strong interaction between the clinician and the geneticist is required to identify the diagnosis and confirm it on clinical ground. A further relevant issue is that currently the turnaround time might not be sufficiently rapid to have an impact on clinical decision, especially in acute presentations.

Several challenges remain to be faced with this fascinating new instrument, such as the choice of NGS techniques in different clinical scenarios, the selection criteria to test a patient, the filtering strategy in WES and WGS and how to report negative results or VUS. Nevertheless, it is likely that, due to cost-effectiveness, in the future whole genome sequencing will replace targeted sequencing, but only selected "virtual" panels of genes, chosen depending on the patient phenotype, will be analysed; this will offer the possibility to assess the bioinformatically stored data of the entire exome/genome at a later stage.

The inclusion of NGS in diagnostic processes will soon lead to a paradigm shift in medicine, changing completely our approach to the patient as well as our understanding of factors affecting genotype-phenotype match.

References

1. Antonarakis SE, Beckmann JS. Mendelian disorders deserve more attention. Nat Rev Genet. 2006;7(4):277–82.
2. Sanger F, Nicklen S, Coulson AR. DNA sequencing with chain-terminating inhibitors. Proc Natl Acad Sci U S A. 1977;74(12):5463–7.
3. Metzker ML. Sequencing technologies—the next generation. Nat Rev Genet. 2010;11(1):31–46.
4. Stranneheim H, Wedell A. Exome and genome sequencing: a revolution for the discovery and diagnosis of monogenic disorders. J Intern Med. 2016;279(1):3–15. Epub 2015/08/08.
5. Kuhlenbaumer G, Hullmann J, Appenzeller S. Novel genomic techniques open new avenues in the analysis of monogenic disorders. Hum Mutat. 2011;32(2):144–51. Epub 2011/02/01.
6. Bush WS, Oetjens MT, Crawford DC. Unravelling the human genome-phenome relationship using phenome-wide association studies. Nat Rev Genet. 2016;17(3):129–45.
7. Mann DA. Epigenetics in liver disease. Hepatology. 2014;60(4):1418–25.
8. Portela A, Esteller M. Epigenetic modifications and human disease. Nat Biotechnol. 2010;28(10):1057–68.
9. Szelinger S, Malenica I, Corneveaux JJ, Siniard AL, Kurdoglu AA, Ramsey KM, et al. Characterization of X chromosome inactivation using integrated analysis of whole-exome and mRNA sequencing. PLoS One. 2014;9(12):e113036. Epub 2014/12/17.
10. Nicastro E, Loudianos G, Zancan L, D'Antiga L, Maggiore G, Marcellini M, et al. Genotype-phenotype correlation in Italian children with Wilson's disease. J Hepatol. 2009;50(3):555–61. Epub 2009/01/03.
11. Sze YK, Dhawan A, Taylor RM, Bansal S, Mieli-Vergani G, Rela M, et al. Pediatric liver transplantation for metabolic liver disease: experience at King's College Hospital. Transplantation. 2009;87(1):87–93.
12. Nicastro E, D'Antiga L. Next generation sequencing in pediatric hepatology and liver transplantation. Liver Transpl. 2018;24(2):282–93. Epub 2017/10/29.
13. Couderc R, Jonard L, Louha M. Next generation sequencing: the technology we need in pediatric laboratories? Clin Biochem. 2011;44(7):514–5. Epub 2011/11/01.
14. Rehm HL, Bale SJ, Bayrak-Toydemir P, Berg JS, Brown KK, Deignan JL, et al. ACMG clinical laboratory standards for next-generation sequencing. Genet Med. 2013;15(9):733–47.
15. Rizzo JM, Buck MJ. Key principles and clinical applications of "next-generation" DNA sequencing. Cancer Prev Res. 2012;5(7):887–900.
16. Kingsmore SF, Saunders CJ. Deep sequencing of patient genomes for disease diagnosis: when will it become routine? Sci Transl Med. 2011;3(87):87ps23.
17. Brookes AJ, Robinson PN. Human genotype-phenotype databases: aims, challenges and opportunities. Nat Rev Genet. 2015;16(12):702–15.
18. Christenhusz GM, Devriendt K, Van Esch H, Dierickx K. Focus group discussions on secondary variants and next-generation sequencing technologies. Eur J Med Genet. 2015;58(4):249–57. Epub 2015/02/11.
19. Casanova J-L, Conley ME, Seligman SJ, Abel L, Notarangelo LD. Guidelines for genetic studies in single patients: lessons from primary immunodeficiencies. J Exp Med. 2014;211(11):2137–49.
20. Ng SB, Nickerson DA, Bamshad MJ, Shendure J. Massively parallel sequencing and rare disease. Hum Mol Genet. 2010;19(R2):R119–R24.
21. Wang J, Cui H, Lee NC, Hwu WL, Chien YH, Craigen WJ, et al. Clinical application of massively parallel sequencing in the molecular diagnosis of glycogen storage diseases of genetically heterogeneous origin. Genet Med. 2013;15(2):106–14. Epub 2012/08/18.
22. Togawa T, Sugiura T, Ito K, Endo T, Aoyama K, Ohashi K, et al. Molecular genetic dissection and neonatal/infantile intrahepatic cholestasis using targeted next-generation sequencing. J Pediatr. 2016;171:171–7.e1–4. Epub 2016/02/10.
23. McKiernan P, Ball S, Santra S, Foster K, Fratter C, Poulton J, et al. Incidence of primary mitochondrial disease in children younger than 2 years presenting with acute liver failure. J Pediatr Gastroenterol Nutr. 2016;63(6):592–7. Epub 2016/08/03.
24. Ravi Kanth VV, Sasikala M, Sharma M, Rao PN, Reddy DN. Genetics of non-alcoholic fatty liver disease: from susceptibility and nutrient interactions to management. World J Hepatol. 2016;8(20):827–37.
25. Jones MA, Rhodenizer D, da Silva C, Huff IJ, Keong L, Bean LJ, et al. Molecular diagnostic testing for congenital disorders of glycosylation (CDG): detection rate for single gene testing and next generation sequencing panel testing. Mol Genet Metab. 2013;110(1–2):78–85. Epub 2013/06/29.
26. Sakai R, Sifrim A, Vande Moere A, Aerts J. TrioVis: a visualization approach for filtering genomic variants of parent-child trios. Bioinformatics. 2013;29(14):1801–2. Epub 2013/05/10.
27. Rabbani B, Mahdieh N, Hosomichi K, Nakaoka H, Inoue I. Next-generation sequencing: impact of exome sequencing in characterizing Mendelian disorders. J Hum Genet. 2012;57(10):621–32.
28. Bamshad MJ, Ng SB, Bigham AW, Tabor HK, Emond MJ, Nickerson DA, et al. Exome sequencing as a tool for Mendelian disease gene discovery. Nat Rev Genet. 2011;12(11):745–55.
29. Sulonen A-M, Ellonen P, Almusa H, Lepistö M, Eldfors S, Hannula S, et al. Comparison of solution-based exome capture methods for next generation sequencing. Genome Biol. 2011;12(9):1–18.
30. Niroula A, Vihinen M. Variation interpretation predictors: principles, types, performance and choice. Hum Mutat. 2016;37(6):579–97. Epub 2016/03/19.
31. Jarinova O, Ekker M. Regulatory variations in the era of next-generation sequencing: implications for clinical molecular diagnostics. Hum Mutat. 2012;33(7):1021–30. Epub 2012/03/21.
32. Belkadi A, Bolze A, Itan Y, Cobat A, Vincent QB, Antipenko A, et al. Whole-genome sequencing is more powerful than whole-exome sequencing for detecting exome variants. Proc Natl Acad Sci U S A. 2015;112(17):5473–8.
33. Lemke AA, Bick D, Dimmock D, Simpson P, Veith R. Perspectives of clinical genetics professionals toward genome sequencing and incidental findings: a survey study. Clin Genet. 2013;84(3):230–6. Epub 2012/11/21.
34. Derkach A, Chiang T, Gong J, Addis L, Dobbins S, Tomlinson I, et al. Association analysis using next-generation sequence data from publicly available control groups: the robust variance score statistic. Bioinformatics. 2014;30(15):2179–88. Epub 2014/04/16.

35. Matthijs G, Souche E, Alders M, Corveleyn A, Eck S, Feenstra I, et al. Guidelines for diagnostic next-generation sequencing. Eur J Hum Genet. 2016;24(1):2–5.
36. May T, Zusevics KL, Strong KA. On the ethics of clinical whole genome sequencing of children. Pediatrics. 2013;132(2):207–9. Epub 2013/07/10.
37. Fagiuoli S, Daina E, D'Antiga L, Colledan M, Remuzzi G. Monogenic diseases that can be cured by liver transplantation. J Hepatol. 2013;59(3):595–612. Epub 2013/04/13.
38. Blok MJ, van den Bosch BJ, Jongen E, Hendrickx A, de Die-Smulders CE, Hoogendijk JE, et al. The unfolding clinical spectrum of POLG mutations. J Med Genet. 2009;46(11):776–85.
39. Sallie R, Katsiyiannakis L, Baldwin D, Davies S, O'Grady J, Mowat A, et al. Failure of simple biochemical indexes to reliably differentiate fulminant Wilson's disease from other causes of fulminant liver failure. Hepatology. 1992;16(5):1206–11. Epub 1992/11/01
40. Fawaz R, Baumann U, Ekong U, Fischler B, Hadzic N, Mack CL, et al. Guideline for the evaluation of cholestatic jaundice in infants: joint recommendations of the North American Society for Pediatric Gastroenterology, Hepatology, and Nutrition and the European Society for Pediatric Gastroenterology, Hepatology, and Nutrition. J Pediatr Gastroenterol Nutr. 2017;64(1):154–68. Epub 2016/07/19.
41. Balistreri WF, Bezerra JA. Whatever happened to "neonatal hepatitis"? Clin Liver Dis. 2006;10(1):27–53.
42. Grammatikopoulos T, Sambrotta M, Strautnieks S, Foskett P, Knisely AS, Wagner B, et al. Mutations in DCDC2 (doublecortin domain containing protein 2) in neonatal sclerosing cholangitis. J Hepatol. 2016;65(6):1179–87. Epub 2016/07/30.
43. Balistreri WF, Bezerra JA, Jansen P, Karpen SJ, Shneider BL, Suchy FJ. Intrahepatic cholestasis: summary of an American Association for the Study of Liver Diseases single-topic conference. Hepatology. 2005;42(1):222–35. Epub 2005/05/18.
44. Lu F-T, Wu J-F, Hsu H-Y, Ni Y-H, Chang M-H, Chao C-I, et al. γ-Glutamyl transpeptidase level as a screening marker among diverse etiologies of infantile intrahepatic cholestasis. J Pediatr Gastroenterol Nutr. 2014;59(6):695–701.
45. Davit-Spraul A, Gonzales E, Baussan C, Jacquemin E. Progressive familial intrahepatic cholestasis. Orphanet J Rare Dis. 2009;4(1):1–12.
46. Sambrotta M, Strautnieks S, Papouli E, Rushton P, Clark BE, Parry DA, et al. Mutations in TJP2 cause progressive cholestatic liver disease. Nat Genet. 2014;46(4):326–8.
47. Setchell KDR, Heubi JE, Shah S, Lavine JE, Suskind D, Al–Edreesi M, et al. Genetic defects in bile acid conjugation cause fat-soluble vitamin deficiency. Gastroenterology. 2013;144(5):945–55.e6.
48. Riello L, D'Antiga L, Guido M, Alaggio R, Giordano G, Zancan L. Titration of bile acid supplements in 3beta-hydroxy-Delta 5-C27-steroid dehydrogenase/isomerase deficiency. J Pediatr Gastroenterol Nutr. 2010;50(6):655–60. Epub 2010/04/20.
49. Droge C, Bonus M, Baumann U, Klindt C, Lainka E, Kathemann S, et al. Sequencing of FIC1, BSEP and MDR3 in a large cohort of patients with cholestasis revealed a high number of different genetic variants. J Hepatol. 2017;67(6):1253–64. Epub 2017/07/25
50. Gomez-Ospina N, Potter CJ, Xiao R, Manickam K, Kim MS, Kim KH, et al. Mutations in the nuclear bile acid receptor FXR cause progressive familial intrahepatic cholestasis. Nat Commun. 2016;7:10713. Epub 2016/02/19.
51. Qiu YL, Gong JY, Feng JY, Wang RX, Han J, Liu T, et al. Defects in myosin VB are associated with a spectrum of previously undiagnosed low gamma-glutamyltransferase cholestasis. Hepatology. 2017;65(5):1655–69. Epub 2016/12/28.
52. Knisely AS, Strautnieks SS, Meier Y, Stieger B, Byrne JA, Portmann BC, et al. Hepatocellular carcinoma in ten children under five years of age with bile salt export pump deficiency. Hepatology. 2006;44:478–86.
53. Iannelli F, Collino A, Sinha S, Radaelli E, Nicoli P, D'Antiga L, et al. Massive gene amplification drives paediatric hepatocellular carcinoma caused by bile salt export pump deficiency. Nat Commun. 2014;5:3850. Epub 2014/05/14.
54. Nicastro E, Stephenne X, Smets F, Fusaro F, de Magnee C, Reding R, et al. Recovery of graft steatosis and protein-losing enteropathy after biliary diversion in a PFIC 1 liver transplanted child. Pediatr Transplant. 2012;16(5):E177–82. Epub 2011/06/16.
55. Jara P, Hierro L, Martínez-Fernández P, Alvarez-Doforno R, Yánez F, Diaz MC, et al. Recurrence of bile salt export pump deficiency after liver transplantation. N Engl J Med. 2009;361(14):1359–67.
56. Shneider BL. Liver transplantation for progressive familial intrahepatic cholestasis: the evolving role of genotyping. Liver Transpl. 2009;15(6):565–6.
57. Hadzic N, Bull LN, Clayton PT, Knisely AS. Diagnosis in bile acid-CoA: amino acid N-acyltransferase deficiency. World J Gastroenterol. 2012;18(25):3322–6. Epub 2012/07/12.
58. Chen S-T, Su Y-N, Ni Y-H, Hwu W-L, Lee N-C, Chien Y-H, et al. Diagnosis of neonatal intrahepatic cholestasis caused by citrin deficiency using high-resolution melting analysis and a clinical scoring system. J Pediatr. 2012;161(4):626–31.e2.
59. Herbst SM, Schirmer S, Posovszky C, Jochum F, Rödl T, Schroeder JA, et al. Taking the next step forward—diagnosing inherited infantile cholestatic disorders with next generation sequencing. Mol Cell Probes. 2015;29(5):291–8.
60. Alagille D, Odievre M, Gautier M, Dommergues JP. Hepatic ductular hypoplasia associated with characteristic facies, vertebral malformations, retarded physical, mental, and sexual development, and cardiac murmur. J Pediatr. 1975;86(1):63–71. Epub 1975/01/01.
61. Li L, Dong J, Wang X, Guo H, Wang H, Zhao J, et al. JAG1 mutation spectrum and origin in Chinese children with clinical features of Alagille syndrome. PLoS One. 2015;10(6):e0130355. Epub 2015/06/16.
62. Emerick KM, Krantz ID, Kamath BM, Darling C, Burrowes DM, Spinner NB, et al. Intracranial vascular abnormalities in patients with Alagille syndrome. J Pediatr Gastroenterol Nutr. 2005;41(1):99–107. Epub 2005/07/02.
63. McKiernan PJ. Neonatal cholestasis. Semin Neonatol. 2002;7(2):153–65.
64. Yerushalmi B, Sokol RJ, Narkewicz MR, Smith D, Ashmead JW, Wenger DA. Niemann-pick disease type C in neonatal cholestasis at a North American Center. J Pediatr Gastroenterol Nutr. 2002;35(1):44–50.
65. Gotti G, Marseglia A, De Giacomo C, Iascone M, Sonzogni A, D'Antiga L. Neonatal jaundice with splenomegaly: not a common pick. Fetal Pediatr Pathol. 2016;35(2):108–11. Epub 2016/02/06.
66. Lang T, Muhlbauer M, Strobelt M, Weidinger S, Hadorn HB. Alpha-1-antitrypsin deficiency in children: liver disease is not reflected by low serum levels of alpha-1-antitrypsin—a study on 48 pediatric patients. Eur J Med Res. 2005;10(12):509–14. Epub 2005/12/17.
67. Snyder MR, Katzmann JA, Butz ML, Wiley C, Yang P, Dawson DB, et al. Diagnosis of alpha-1-antitrypsin deficiency: an algorithm of quantification, genotyping, and phenotyping. Clin Chem. 2006;52(12):2236–42. Epub 2006/10/21
68. Squires RH Jr, Shneider BL, Bucuvalas J, Alonso E, Sokol RJ, Narkewicz MR, et al. Acute liver failure in children: the first 348 patients in the pediatric acute liver failure study group. J Pediatr. 2006;148(5):652–8.e2.
69. Hegarty R, Hadzic N, Gissen P, Dhawan A. Inherited metabolic disorders presenting as acute liver failure in newborns and young children: King's College Hospital experience. Eur J Pediatr. 2015;174(10):1387–92.
70. Gallagher RC, Lam C, Wong D, Cederbaum S, Sokol RJ. Significant hepatic involvement in patients with ornithine transcarbamylase deficiency. J Pediatr. 2014;164(4):720–5 e6. Epub 2014/02/04.

71. Staufner C, Haack TB, Kopke MG, Straub BK, Kolker S, Thiel C, et al. Recurrent acute liver failure due to NBAS deficiency: phenotypic spectrum, disease mechanisms, and therapeutic concepts. J Inherit Metab Dis. 2016;39(1):3–16. Epub 2015/11/07.
72. Cui H, Li F, Chen D, Wang G, Truong CK, Enns GM, et al. Comprehensive next-generation sequence analyses of the entire mitochondrial genome reveal new insights into the molecular diagnosis of mitochondrial DNA disorders. Genet Med. 2013;15(5):388–94. Epub 2013/01/05.
73. Dames S, Chou LS, Xiao Y, Wayman T, Stocks J, Singleton M, et al. The development of next-generation sequencing assays for the mitochondrial genome and 108 nuclear genes associated with mitochondrial disorders. J Mol Diagn. 2013;15(4):526–34. Epub 2013/05/15.
74. Spinazzola A, Invernizzi F, Carrara F, Lamantea E, Donati A, DiRocco M, et al. Clinical and molecular features of mitochondrial DNA depletion syndromes. J Inherit Metab Dis. 2008;32(2):143–58.
75. Menezes MJ, Riley LG, Christodoulou J. Mitochondrial respiratory chain disorders in childhood: Insights into diagnosis and management in the new era of genomic medicine. Biochim Biophys Acta Gen Subj. 2014;1840(4):1368–79.

Cell Therapy in Acute and Chronic Liver Disease

Massimiliano Paganelli

Abbreviations

ALF	Acute liver failure
cGMP	Current good manufacturing practice
EpCAM	Epithelial cell adhesion molecule
ESC	Embryonic stem cells
iPSC	Induced pluripotent stem cell
LCT	Liver cell transplantation
MSC	Multipotent mesenchymal stromal cell
PHH	Primary human hepatocyte
PSC	Pluripotent stem cell
VEGF	Vascular endothelial growth factor

> **Key Points**
> - Cell therapy aims at treating children and adults with liver failure or inborn errors of liver metabolism through the transplantation of cells performing liver-specific functions.
> - Although still experimental, liver cell transplantation has been performed for more than 20 years in several centers around the world and is now considered a safe procedure.
> - At present, hepatocytes isolated from donors' livers (primary human hepatocytes) are the cells of choice, but they suffer from some major limitations.
> - Clinical results obtained so far are encouraging, but several problems need to be addressed to improve the feasibility and efficacy of the procedure.
> - Several stem cells are being explored as alternative sources of hepatocyte-like cells for liver cell transplantation, with the promise to overcome current limitations.

Research Needed in the Field
- Improving the engraftment of transplanted cells and finding clinically relevant approaches to address the lack of selective advantage and regeneration stimuli are crucial steps required to increase the efficacy of liver cell transplantation.
- A better understanding of the process leading to the rejection of transplanted cells is needed to prolong their life span and decrease the number of infusions required to see and maintain an effect.
- Standardization of the procedure among centers is needed to compare clinical trials and improve available clinical protocols.
- The efficacy of stem cell-derived hepatocyte-like cells depends on the improvement of in vitro differentiation protocols in terms of maturity of the obtained cells, reproducibility, and cell yield.
- Particular attention should be dedicated to proving the safety of iPSC-derived hepatocyte-like cells (which could soon allow autologous cell therapy) and the development of biomaterials and new tissue engineering approaches, which hold the promise to allow allogeneic transplantation without immunosuppression.

M. Paganelli (✉)
Pediatric Gastroenterology, Hepatology and Nutrition, Sainte-Justine University Hospital Center, Montreal, QC, Canada

Hepatology & Cell Therapy Laboratory, Sainte-Justine Research Center, Montreal, QC, Canada

Department of Pediatrics, Université de Montréal, Montreal, QC, Canada
e-mail: m.paganelli@umontreal.ca

43.1 Introduction

Cirrhosis and chronic liver failure are the common outcomes of most progressive liver diseases. The loss of the liver's synthetic and detoxifying functions entails major systemic complications such as ascites, hepatic encephalopathy, and gastrointestinal bleeding, among others. Additionally, almost 10% of all non-cancer, liver-related deaths are due to acute liver failure (ALF), which is an extremely severe, progressive syndrome resulting from a sudden insult on the liver exceeding the organ's innate regenerative capacity. ALF in children and adolescents has a poor outcome, with only 50% of patients surviving with their native liver [1–3]. Moreover, there is a significant number of liver conditions, such as inborn errors of liver metabolism, that do not lead to liver failure but entail severe hepatic and extrahepatic consequences. Although individually rare, when considered together, liver-based metabolic diseases represent more than 10% of pediatric liver transplants [4]. A treatment is available for only a few of such conditions. In all cases the treatment reduces the symptoms and improves the prognosis, but does not cure the disease. The standard of care for acute and chronic liver failure, as for most inborn errors of liver metabolism, is liver transplantation, but only 65% of pediatric patients are transplanted within 2 years from the registration on the waiting list [5]. Children with ALF need to be transplanted within days from the diagnosis, before their disease becomes irreversibly too severe (20% die waiting for a donor) [1, 3]. Infants are at even greater risk of death, with almost half dying before transplantation and 50% of those receiving a transplant dying postoperatively [6]. The outcome of children with inborn errors of liver metabolism is far better, but such patients have very low priority on the waiting list and often develop systemic complications while waiting for an organ [7]. Furthermore, liver transplantation has major limitations: besides entailing a still significant short-term mortality and morbidity risk, it requires lifelong immunosuppression and is often complicated by severe long-term hepatic and extrahepatic problems. Such high risks seem disproportioned for the many metabolic liver diseases that are characterized by a single enzyme deficiency but a normal liver parenchyma, as well as for many patients with ALF who would need just a temporary replacement of liver functions while their own liver regenerates. Several alternative approaches based on partial liver transplantation or extracorporeal detoxifying devices have been developed over the years to temporarily replace liver functions, with only partially satisfactory results [8–12]. Nevertheless, experience with auxiliary partial liver transplantation proved that liver functions can be successfully restored provided a sufficient mass of healthy donor hepatocytes is supplied. This concept led to the hypothesis that hepatocytes could be administered not only within a graft but as single cells. The field of liver cell transplantation (LCT) has hence been developing for the past two decades and, although still considered experimental, has shown increasing potential not only as a bridge to but as an alternative to liver transplantation. Nevertheless, several questions need to be answered, and obstacles overcome before such an approach might find its place in daily clinical practice.

43.2 Cell Sources

The success of LCT for liver disease is determined, above all, by the functionality of the employed cells. Not only do they need to be effective in performing the functions to be replaced, but they have to be readily available in sufficient amounts upon patients' presentation, rapidly functional upon administration, of predictable quality and, most importantly, safe. Primary human hepatocytes (PHHs) isolated from donors' livers were the first to show an efficacy in treating liver disease and are still considered the gold standard to compare any other cell source to. Several alternative sources, notably fetal and neonatal PHHs and hepatocytes derived from the differentiation of stem cells of varied origin, have been explored over the years, with promising results (Fig. 43.1 and Table 43.1).

43.2.1 Primary Human Hepatocytes

Transplantation of hepatocytes digested from donors' livers to treat metabolic liver diseases and liver failure was first described in experimental animals in the 1970s [13, 14]. After 15 years spent on improving isolation and perfusion protocols [15], with proof-of-concept safety and efficacy assessed with autologous hepatocyte transplantation [16], the first clinical trials were conducted in 1994 and 1997 in patients with fulminant liver failure using fetal and adult PHHs [17, 18]. The first children treated with PHHs received autologous transplantation of cells transduced with a retroviral vector carrying the LDL receptor gene to treat familial hypercholesterolemia [19]. The first administration of allogeneic PHHs to a child was described in 1998 to treat Crigler-Najjar syndrome type I [20]. Since then, several cases using freshly isolated and cryopreserved PHHs have been reported for diverse inborn errors of liver metabolism, for ALF, and in patients with cirrhosis [21–23].

The suspension of liver cells is obtained through two-step collagenase digestion of donors' livers [24–26]. After cannulation of the portal or hepatic veins and clamping of

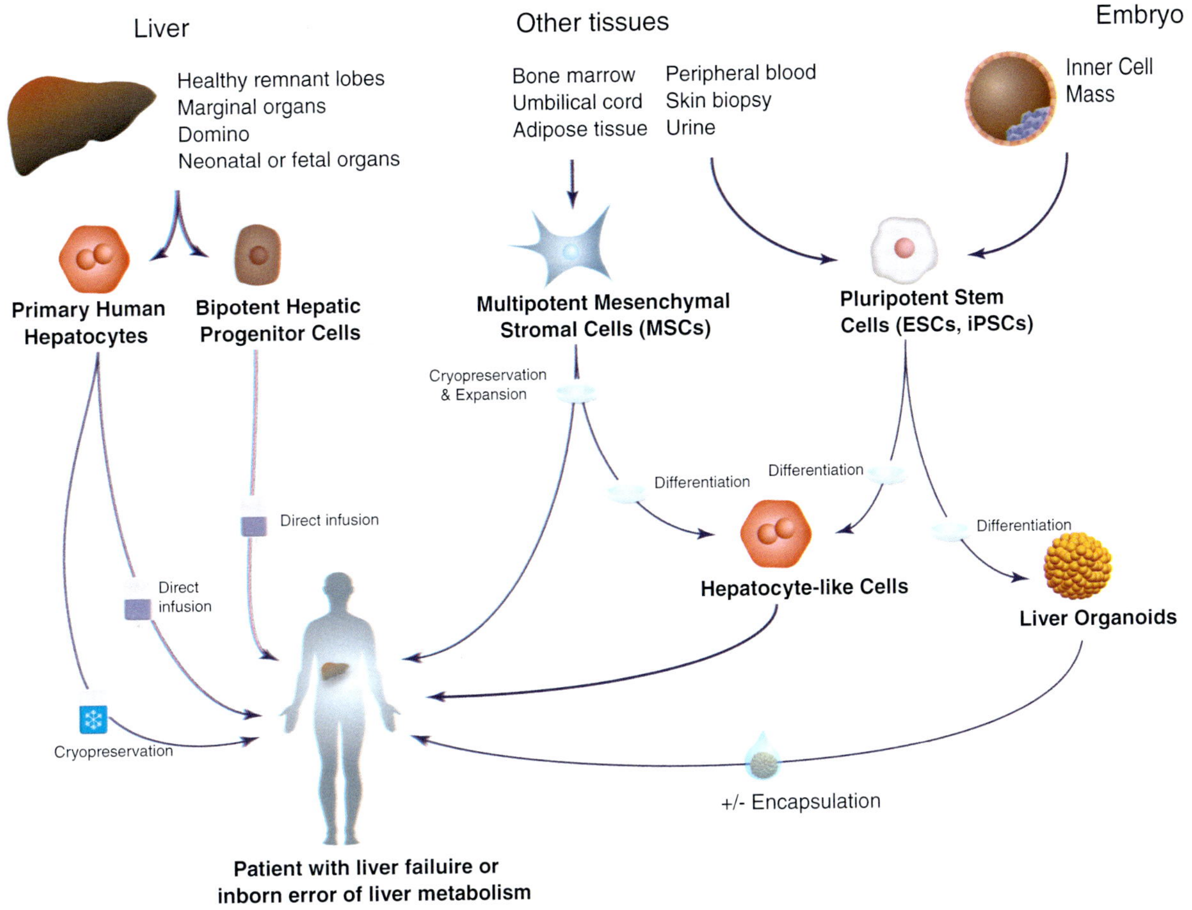

Fig. 43.1 Available cell sources for liver cell transplantation. Besides primary human hepatocytes (PHHs), several cell sources have been explored over the years as possible candidates for liver cell transplantation: bile duct-derived bipotent progenitor cells, multipotent mesenchymal stromal cells (MSCs), and hepatocyte-like cells or organoids derived from MSCs, embryonic stem cells (ESCs) or induced pluripotent stem cells (iPSCs)

the other vessels, the organ is washed for 20 min with calcium-free buffered solution supplemented with the chelating agent EGTA at 37 °C, in order to remove blood. Subsequently, the tissue is perfused with calcium-containing buffered solution supplemented with collagenase and proteases for about 10 min to digest the extracellular matrix. The liver capsule is then opened, and the cell suspension is released and passed through strainers to remove remaining cell aggregates. After multiple centrifugations at low speed to remove non-parenchymal cells, the obtained suspension is mostly ($\approx$95%) composed of hepatocytes. The entire procedure has to be conducted in a clean room following strict protocols in compliance with current good manufacturing practice (cGMP) standards. The obtained PHHs are then tested to assess their viability and exclude the presence of any infectious agents. At this point the cells can either be used for LCT or cryopreserved for future use.

Livers made available for digestion are mostly adult organs rejected for transplantation because of reduced quality (patients on ECMO, non-heartbeating donors, long cold ischemia time). Remnant tissues from unused split livers or liver reductions can also be used to obtain liver cells for transplantation. Although organs from marginal donors (severe steatosis, older donors, ischemia time >14 h) can be an attractive source of cells, the quality of obtained hepatocytes is often suboptimal [25, 27, 28]. Organ shortage is therefore the major limitation to the use of PHHs for LCT. Liver transplantation is still the treatment of choice for end-stage liver disease as well as for inborn errors of liver metabolism and many tumors. The widening of indications for liver transplantation, the acceptance of marginal donors, and the increased use of split liver transplants further reduced the pool of organ available for digestion. Since not enough donors are avail-

Table 43.1 Available cell sources for liver cell transplantation: advantages and disadvantages

Cell source	Advantages	Disadvantages	Clinical studies
PHHs			
Adult, freshly-isolated	• Gold standard for metabolic functions	• Scarce availability, organ shortage • Variability between donors • Unsuited for urgent LCT or repeated infusions • Poor engraftment, rejection	Yes
Adult, cryopreserved	• Easy storage and shipment	• Reduced metabolic functions • Variability between donors • Short life span • Poor engraftment, rejection	Yes
Neonatal	• Better stability upon cryopreservation • Isolated from otherwise discarded organs	• Scarce availability • Short life span • Poor engraftment, rejection	Yes
Fetal	• Isolated from otherwise discarded organs • Possible expansion in the recipient's liver posttransplant • Low immunogenicity, no immunosuppression	• Scarce availability • Low cell yield • Risk of tumor formation to be determined	Yes
Bipotent hepatic progenitor cells	• Possible expansion in the recipient's liver posttransplant • Low immunogenicity, no immunosuppression • Can be isolated from the gallbladder	• Need for in vivo differentiation: unsuited for ALF or acute decompensations • Efficacy and safety still to be demonstrated	Limited (preliminary report, short-term data)
MSCs			
Undifferentiated	• Availability and expansion • Easy storage and shipment • Reassuring safety profile	• Need for in vivo differentiation: unsuited for ALF or acute decompensations • Not effective in clinical trials or reported cases • Concerns about the risk of thrombosis	Yes
MSC-derived hepatocyte-like cells or progenitors	• Availability and expansion • Easy storage and shipment • Reassuring safety profile	• Poor liver functions upon transdifferentiation in vitro • Need for in vivo maturation: unsuited for ALF or acute decompensations	No
PSCs (ESCs and iPSCs)			
Undifferentiated		• Not to be used: risk of ectopic tissue formation	No
PSC-derived hepatocyte-like cells	• iPSCs are easily available through non-invasive procedures (more difficult for ESCs) • Unlimited self-renewal • Consistent quality across populations • Autologous transplantation possible: iPSCs from patients with liver failure or metabolic liver disease (post-genome editing), no need for immunosuppression	• Need for in vivo maturation: unsuited for ALF or acute decompensations • Potential risk of ectopic tissue formation	No
Liver organoids	• Availability, expansion, consistency • Better differentiation in vitro	• Need for in vivo maturation: unsuited for ALF or acute decompensations • Potential risk of ectopic tissue formation	No
Encapsulated organoids and tissues	• Availability, expansion, consistency • Full maturation in vitro • Stability over time and cryopreservation • Immunoisolation: no need for immunosuppression upon allogeneic transplantation • Reduced risk of tumor formation	• Long-term efficacy and safety in vivo still to be demonstrated	No

Abbreviations: *PHH* primary human hepatocytes, *MSC* multipotent mesenchymal stromal cell, *PSC* pluripotent stem cell, *ESC* embryonic stem cells, *iPSC* induced pluripotent stem cell, *ALF* acute liver failure, *LCT* liver cell transplantation

able to satisfy the demand for liver transplantation, organs left for PHH isolation are rare and often of insufficient quality.

Accurate donor selection and current isolation protocols allow to obtain a good viability and metabolic activity of freshly isolated PHHs, although an important and poorly predictable variability in the quality of obtained cells is observed between comparable donors. PHHs are available for LCT within 6–8 h from the procurement of the organ. Results of post-manipulation sterility tests are usually not available at the time of transplantation, which raises potential safety concerns. Strict compliance to cGMP helps reducing the risks of cell contamination.

Although the best efficacy of LCT has been reported with freshly isolated PHHs, transplantation of fresh PHHs is logistically complex. Having a suitable donor readily available to isolate PHHs when a patient presents with fulminant liver failure is unlikely. Furthermore, up to 80–90% of transplanted cells reaching the liver sinusoids are rapidly cleared because of sinusoidal events [29, 30]. Since the amount of cells that can be administered over a single infusion is limited, multiple infusions over several days are often required to reach a sufficient efficacy (see below), which makes the use of freshly isolated PHHs hardly feasible.

Cryopreservation of PHHs allows considering LCT for patients with fulminant or acute-on-chronic liver failure or acute decompensations of metabolic disorders, increasing the safety of the procedure while allowing multiple infusions over days or weeks. Nevertheless, cryopreservation affects the viability and metabolic function of hepatocytes, with the result that the thawed cells have a significantly reduced efficacy upon transplantation and are often not suitable for clinical use. The detrimental effect of freezing on PHH metabolic functions has been widely studied, and several protocols have been developed to limit cryodamage [31–34]. Despite the significant improvements made over the last 20 years, cryopreserved hepatocytes are still of significantly poorer quality compared to freshly isolated cells. Nevertheless, at least transient successful replacement of liver functions has been reported in patients with ALF and metabolic liver diseases using cryopreserved PHHs [18, 22, 35–37]. The most important determinant of cell quality after thawing is still the quality of the initial cell suspension used, which brings us back to the importance of selecting suitable organs and to the problem of organ shortage. Overall, many adults and children have been transplanted with either freshly isolated or cryopreserved PHHs over the last 25 years for diverse indications [21–23]. The efficacy and safety of such an approach are described below.

43.2.2 Alternative Sources of Primary Hepatocytes

Organ shortage is the major limitation to the use of adult PHHs for LCT. Alternative sources have been explored over the years. Fetal and neonatal hepatocytes are promising alternatives because they are isolated from organs that are not suitable for liver transplantation. The use of donated livers from the first gestational trimester is limited by the low yield of the isolation (many livers would be required to perform LCT even in a single newborn), the immaturity of the obtained parenchymal cells, and the high percentage of hematopoietic cells. Effective isolation and transplantation of a significant amount of viable PHHs with high proliferative capacity from fetuses of 18–22 weeks has been reported [38]. Nevertheless, the obtained cell suspension contains an important ratio of mesenchymal and hematopoietic cells that are transplanted with the hepatocytes. This further increases the already theoretical risk of tumor formation that is intrinsic to fetal cell transplantation [39]. Moreover, liver-specific functions start to be performed at levels comparable to adult hepatocytes later during fetal development, with many functions (drug metabolism, biotransformation, transport) being significantly reduced or different compared to the liver at birth [40]. Nevertheless, ammonia detoxification into urea is performed by fetal hepatocytes already at the end of the second trimester of gestation, and the cells have been shown to mature within the recipient's liver upon transplantation [41]. LCT using fetal PHHs has been described for patients with fulminant hepatic failure and end-stage liver disease, with encouraging results especially for the treatment of hepatic encephalopathy [17, 38, 42].

Neonatal livers, which are not routinely used for transplantation, provide a high yield of good-quality hepatocytes [43, 44]. Although some of cytochrome P450 and UDP-glucuronosyltransferase enzymes are less expressed, neonatal hepatocytes show an activity of CYP3A4 enzyme (which implicated in the metabolism of antirejection drugs such as tacrolimus) that is comparable to adult PHHs. Neonatal PHHs have metabolic and ureogenic activities comparable to adult cells while showing a significantly greater capacity to withstand cryopreservation [43, 44]. Moreover, the cell suspension obtained from neonatal livers is almost exclusively composed of diploid hepatocytes still capable of proliferation and contains a greater proportion of epithelial cell adhesion molecule (EpCAM)-positive hepatic progenitor cells [43, 45]. This implies a greater potential of neonatal PHHs to proliferate within the recipient's liver upon LCT and allows to overcome some of the known limitations of hepatocyte transplantation such as the cells' limited life span and the need for a regenerative stimulus (see below) [46, 47].

Cryopreserved neonatal PHHs were shown safe and at least partially effective in reducing hyperammonemia in patients with urea cycle defects and supporting survival in children with ALF [44, 48].

The concept of domino liver transplant describes the use of a liver explanted from donors with a metabolic liver disease to transplant patients with a different condition [49]. Many inborn errors of liver metabolism are characterized by the deficiency of a single enzyme, with all other liver-specific functions being normally performed by a normal parenchyma [7]. Over the years more than 1200 domino transplants have been performed worldwide [50]. Such an approach allows to expand the pool of organs available for transplantation. The risk of recurrence of the donor's disease in the recipient is significant. Nevertheless, careful selection and coupling of donors and recipients allow to either avoid or delay the appearance of symptoms of the donor's disease in recipients. The same concept is being assessed for LCT. Isolation of PHHs from diseased livers provides more than satisfactory cell yield and quality [51]. Moreover, the amount of donor cells transplanted (5–10% of the theoretical liver mass) is not sufficient to cause symptoms of the donor's disease in the recipient (whose hepatocytes are able to provide the single enzymatic function missing in such cells), while it is enough to replace other lacking liver-specific functions. The first case of domino LCT was reported in 2012 [52]. Such an approach is promising and might allow to overcome, at least partially, the shortage of organs available for LCT.

43.2.3 Stem and Progenitor Cells as an Alternative Cell Source for Transplantation

Stem cells, characterized by easier availability, high expansion potential, and resistance to cryopreservation, are promising candidates to overcome part of the limitations of PHHs. Several stem cells have been explored as a potential source of hepatocytes over the years. Such cells are very different in terms of availability, self-renewal capacity, differentiation potential, and safety profile. Two different approaches can be pursued: transplanting hepatic progenitor cells capable to initially proliferate and then differentiate to mature hepatocytes within the recipient's liver or expanding the stem cells in vitro, to differentiate them into functional hepatocytes and then transplant the latter into the patient.

The first approach implies the availability of a sufficient amount of cells capable of differentiating only into hepatocytes upon transplantation within the liver, in order not to constitute a risk of tumor or ectopic tissue formation. Such cells require time to proliferate and differentiate in vivo and cannot be used in patients needing an immediate effect (like fulminant or acute-on-chronic liver failure or decompensated metabolic liver diseases). Moreover, since a precise characterization of such hepatic progenitors is well defined in rodents but lacking in humans, the availability of such cells is very limited, and they have a reduced expansion potential in vitro. As discussed above, EpCAM+ cells isolated from fetal livers possess a good differentiation potential and seem to have a very low immunogenicity (minimal HLA class I and II antigen expression, immunomodulatory properties through Fas-mediated apoptosis) [53–55]. EpCAM+ bipotent bile duct cells, which can be obtained from a liver biopsy of an adult liver or from the gallbladder, are stable upon expansion in vitro and can efficiently differentiate into hepatocytes upon transplantation and are interesting candidates for LCT [53, 56–58]. Transplantation of such bipotent progenitors obtained from the fetal livers was described in 27 patients with liver cirrhosis, who showed some clinical improvement and no reported side effects [59, 60]. Remarkably, the patients showed prolonged effects despite being transplanted without any immunosuppression. These results are promising, although long-term safety and definitive proof of lasting efficacy and lack of rejection of such an approach are still to be demonstrated.

Multipotent mesenchymal stromal cells (MSC, formerly referred to as mesenchymal stem or stem/progenitor cells) can be isolated from the bone marrow, umbilical cord, liver, adipose tissue, etc. [61]. Although they are not progenitor cells and they do not possess all the characteristics of stem cells (they are heterogeneous populations of plastic-adherent cells with limited self-renewal potential), MSCs can be easily expanded in vitro and have been extensively used to generate hepatocyte-like cells upon transplantation within the liver [62–64]. These cells have a stable phenotype, immunomodulatory properties, and a good safety profile, but they are not easily available (especially when derived from adult livers) [65, 66]. Nevertheless, adipose tissue or bone marrow-derived MSCs can allow autologous LCT, virtually eliminating the need for immunosuppression. MSCs were shown capable to partially restore liver functions upon LCT in preclinical models, although whether such an effect is more attributable to the cells' immunomodulatory activity than to their potential to transdifferentiate into hepatocytes is still controversial [67, 68]. Several patients with cirrhosis and metabolic liver disease have already been treated with autologous or allogeneic MSC transplantation (see below) [69–73].

Whereas the concept of transplanting hepatic progenitor cells with the hope to have an in vivo expansion and differentiation is fascinating, it precludes the use of LCT in patients needing urgent replacement of liver functions. It also raises safety concerns in terms of control of the differentiation (bipotent progenitors spontaneously differentiate into cholangiocytes as well) and tumor formation (because of the low immunogenicity of cells with high replicative potential). Therefore, most groups have been focusing on the use of stem cells as a "cell factory" to produce hepatocytes for LCT. Stem cells of various origins can be easily expanded in vitro and subsequently differentiated to liver cells following established protocols. The obtained terminally differentiated hepatocyte-like cells can then be transplanted into the recipient and provide rapid replacement of liver functions. Transdifferentiation of MSCs upon culture in specific conditions with the sequential addition of liver-specifying growth factors over 3–4 weeks leads to the acquisition of the morphology and many of the markers and functions specific to the hepatocyte [62, 63, 74–78]. Nevertheless, such hepatocyte-like cells are significantly less effective than hepatocytes (either freshly isolated or cryopreserved) in performing most of the functions needed by patients with liver failure or metabolic liver diseases.

Over the last 10 years, research focus moved to pluripotent stem cells (PSC), such as embryonic stem cells (ESC) and induced pluripotent stem cells (iPSC), as a potential source of hepatocytes. PSCs have a distinct phenotype, can self-renew indefinitely and can be terminally differentiated into derivatives of all three germ layers. ESCs, which are isolated from the inner mass of a blastocyst, are not easily available, and their use has raised ethical concerns. Twelve years ago Kazutoshi Takahashi and Shinya Yamanaka described a method to reprogram somatic cells into PSCs through the transduction of four transcription factors [79, 80]. Since then, iPSCs have been obtained from somatic cells of many different tissues and are routinely and reproducibly generated in research labs around the world from skin fibroblasts and peripheral blood mononuclear cells. iPSCs are comparable to ESCs in terms of self-renewal and differentiation potential, while being much more easily available. Various differentiation protocols mimicking liver organogenesis have been described for both ESCs and iPSCs [81–86]. Growth factors and small molecules are sequentially supplemented to the culture media over a 4-week period to guide the cells through the stages of primitive streak, definitive endoderm, posterior foregut, and eventually hepatoblasts (bipotent hepatic progenitors) and hepatocytes [83, 87, 88]. At the end of the process, PSC-derived hepatocyte-like cells perform many hepatocyte-specific functions but are more similar to fetal than to adult hepatocytes [89]. Nevertheless, such cells can efficiently engraft within the recipient liver upon transplantation and mature in vivo over a few weeks to achieve the functionality of adult hepatocytes [82]. As discussed above, this implies a very promising potential of these cells to treat chronic conditions and metabolic liver diseases but a less-than-optimal expected efficacy in treating patients with acute or acute-on-chronic liver failure [88]. Since iPSCs can be easily reprogrammed from small peripheral blood samples, we are now capable of generating iPSCs-derived hepatocytes from any patient in a few months. This opens the way to autologous LCT for chronic liver diseases. Even more interesting, currently available methods for genome editing (CRISPR/Cas9, etc.) allow correcting the disease-causing mutation in iPSCs from patients with metabolic liver diseases. Such edited cells can be differentiated into healthy hepatocyte-like cells and theoretically be used for autologous LCT, thus treating the patient's disease without the need for immunosuppression. Unfortunately, safety concerns need to be addressed before PSC-derived hepatocyte-like cells can be tested in clinical trials. Indeed, PSCs tend to form teratomas when transplanted into immunosuppressed mice. Although the absence of ectopic tissue formation has been proven upon proper differentiation of PSCs into hepatocytes, and no tumors were reported in the first clinical trials of PSC-derived cells for non-hepatic indications, several strategies are currently being pursued to assure the safety of the approach (see below) [88, 90, 91].

Direct reprogramming (or transdifferentiation) of human fibroblasts into hepatocyte-like cells has been accomplished by the transduction of several transcription factors [92, 93]. Generation of multipotent progenitor cells capable of in vitro expansion and subsequent differentiation into hepatocyte-like cells was also accomplished with a similar technique [94]. The obtained cells showed liver-specific functions in vitro, but satisfying maturation was only achieved upon transplantation into the liver of immunocompromised mice. This approach might be interesting because it might address the safety concerns related to the use of PSCs. Nevertheless, better maturation of the cells in vitro is needed if a future use in patients with ALF or decompensation of a metabolic disease is envisaged.

Several approaches have been studied to improve the quality of ESC- and iPSC-derived hepatocyte-like cells. The interaction between hepatocytes and non-parenchymal cells in the liver was shown to be crucial for liver development [95]. The recreation of such cell-to-cell interactions between iPSC-derived hepatocytes and endothelial or mesenchymal cells induces a significant maturation of liver cells [96–100]. Over the last few years, liver organoids and engineered liver tissues have become a powerful tool to produce mature hepatocytes in vitro for both disease modeling and future LCT [98, 101–104]. We and others have been working on further improving the quality of iPSC-derived hepatocytes through the use of polymers and hydrogels of different origins in order to recreate a 3D microenvironment to support maturation and cell-to-cell interactions [100, 105–110]. Hydrogels were also shown to provide immunoisolation to the embedded cells or tissues (see below), thus protecting the cells from rejection after transplantation, virtually eliminating the need for immunosuppression, and protecting the recipient form the risk of tumor formation [44, 96, 111–113].

43.3 Indications and Patient Selection

As mentioned above, patients with ALF need prompt replacement of liver functions for the time needed for a suitable donor to become available for liver transplantation. LCT has the potential to restore, at least partially, liver functions and prevent the progression of hepatic encephalopathy, cerebral edema, and coagulopathy while preventing multi-organ failure. LCT can theoretically support the patient for the time needed by his liver to regenerate, thus virtually eliminating the need for organ transplantation for at least some of the adults and children affected by ALF [18, 21, 22, 114]. In case of full recovery, transplanted PHHs can be eliminated by simple withdrawal of the immunosuppression.

Although rare in children, acute-on-chronic liver failure, which consists in the acute decompensation of patients with underlying cirrhosis, is responsible for tens of thousands of hospitalizations every year only in the USA and a severe prognosis (up to 50% mortality rate). Such patients might benefit from LCT as a bridge to transplantation or to the restoration of pre-crisis conditions [21, 22].

So far, the best results were obtained when LCT was used to treat inborn errors of liver metabolism (see below). Transplanted cells can restore the single liver function lacking because of a genetic disease. At present, liver transplantation for metabolic liver diseases allows achieving excellent long-term survival with minimal morbidity. But in the future, once the still existing limitations of the techniques are overcome, LCT might even be preferable to liver transplantation for all those conditions characterized by the deficiency of a single enzyme and normal liver parenchyma [7]. LCT has already been reported for glycogen storage disease type Ia and Ib, Crigler-Najjar type I syndrome, infantile Refsum's disease, urea cycle defects, phenylketonuria, factor VII deficiency, familial hypercholesterolemia, and primary hyperoxaluria (see below) [19, 20, 35, 36, 48, 52, 115–126]. In children with inborn errors of liver metabolism, LCT can treat acute decompensation, prevent extrahepatic sequelae, improve the quality of life, and bridge to liver transplantation (for which these patients have low priority on the waiting list) or to upcoming alternative treatments (gene therapy). LCT has also been tried in children with metabolic conditions causing parenchymal injury and progressive liver disease (α1-antitrypsin deficiency, BSEP deficiency, tyrosinemia type I) [118, 120, 122]. Although some benefit was observed, it is important to note that for such conditions, LCT cannot prevent the progression of the disease or the development of tumors.

Cell transplantation can also be indicated in newborns and infants with liver failure who are too young or undernourished for organ transplantation. In this case, LCT might allow supporting liver functions for the time needed for the patients to become eligible for liver transplantation.

43.4 Clinical Procedure

Over the last 20 years, LCT has evolved into a safe procedure that is routinely performed in several centers around the world. LCT has not spread to all liver centers yet because still hindered by the limitations of PHHs and the safety concerns of stem cell-derived products. Nonetheless, a few groups have worked hard to establish a clinical procedure that in the future might be easily exported to any liver transplant center.

43.4.1 Dose and Route of Administration

The total amount of liver cells to be transplanted to treat metabolic liver diseases is considered to be 5–10% of the theoretical liver mass ($2-4 \times 10^8$ cells/kg of body weight). Such a quantity is needed because only a small fraction of such cells engraft and survive within the recipient body (see below) [127, 128]. Less cells are needed to transiently replace liver functions in patients with fulminant liver failure (2–3% of the liver mass).

The liver is the most studied site for cell engraftment upon LCT. We discussed of the importance of the environment for the maturation and survival of liver cells. Administration of the cells through the portal venous system allows them to engraft within the liver parenchyma and takes advantage of the paracrine signals and cell-to-cell contacts of the liver niche. Several techniques have been described to access the portal venous system: percutaneous transhepatic injection into the portal vein is a safe and minimally invasive procedure, but it is not suitable for repeated administrations (which are almost always needed for LCT); catheterization of the portal vein through permanent catheters (Broviac or port-a-cath) is more cumbersome and invasive, but it allows safer repeated infusions; catheterization of the umbilical vein provides direct and safe access to the portal system in newborns [129]. Malformations or venous thrombosis must be excluded by Doppler ultrasound before the procedure, and the portal venous pressure has to be monitored during each administration. In order to prevent portal hypertension and thrombosis, the number of cells to be infused has to be limited to $30-100 \times 10^6$/kg of body weight, with an infusion rate <8 mL/kg/h and no less than 2–6 h interval between the doses [39].

Intrasplenic administration through the splenic artery is an interesting alternative for LCT, especially for patients with fulminant liver failure or cirrhosis (because of the systemic inflammatory state, capillarization of the sinusoids, and preexisting portal hypertension) [18, 37, 130–133].

Transplantation into the peritoneal cavity has also been assessed in experimental animals and in a few patients [13,

14, 17, 44, 96, 112]. The lack of the liver niche will reduce in vivo maturation of the cells and shorten their life span. Encapsulation of the cells with hydrogels seems effective in addressing both limitations, supporting the survival of the cells, and preventing rejection [44, 96, 112]. The simplicity of access of the intraperitoneal site could allow a more widespread use of LCT once the ideal cell source will be identified.

43.4.2 Anticoagulation

Although portal thrombosis has been only rarely reported after LCT, administration of a large amount of cells within the hepatic sinusoids poses a potential risk of thrombus formation. Transient increase of portal venous pressure is often registered during LCT. Patients with fulminant liver failure are considered at increased risk of portal thrombosis. Moreover, the tissue factor-dependent procoagulant activity of PHHs might have a significant impact on the engraftment and survival of transplanted cells [134]. Heparin is therefore added to the cell suspension before infusion, while D-dimer concentration and portal flow by Doppler ultrasound are measured before and after each infusion. Additional anticoagulation has been used in patients with metabolic liver disorders to prevent thrombus formation upon transplantation of MSCs [135].

43.4.3 Immunosuppression

Rejection is the main cause of the short life span of transplanted cells [136, 137]. Although the liver is an immune-privileged organ, single cells seem to be more immunogenic. Once injected through the portal venous system, the cells migrate within the sinusoids, where they form cell emboli [138]. Adhesion proteins on the surface of transplanted cells, which are normally hidden within the parenchyma, trigger the cytolytic clearance of the cells by the innate immune system within the sinusoids [138, 139]. Moreover, tissue factor expressed on the hepatocyte surface activates the coagulation and complements cascades, triggering what has been defined as "instant blood-mediated inflammatory reaction," which results in cell destruction [134, 140, 141].

Patients undergoing allogeneic LCT receive an immunosuppressive regimen comparable to the one administered after liver transplantation. A single dose of methylprednisolone is injected before the infusion, followed by oral tacrolimus treatment. No studies have been conducted to establish the dose of tacrolimus needed. Through levels of 10 ng/mL for the first month, 8 ng/mL until month 3 and 6 ng/mL onward are usually considered acceptable [26]. Close monitoring of rejection risk might improve engraftment and extend the effect of LCT [136]. Emergence of donor-specific antibodies (DSA) was associated to the loss of transplanted cells [137]. Nevertheless, new biomarkers are needed to improve the prevention and treatment post-LCT rejection.

The use of hepatocyte-like cells differentiated from patient-derived stem cells, in which the disease-causing mutation has been preventively corrected by genome editing, might soon allow autologous LCT for metabolic liver diseases, thus eliminating the need for immunosuppression.

MSCs seem to have immunomodulatory properties. Co-transplantation of liver cells with MSCs or endothelial cells is being assessed as a potential approach to reduce immunogenicity and improve the success of LCT. New approaches using biomaterials to encapsulate the transplanted cells or organoids and isolate them from the recipient's immune system are currently being assessed. Preliminary preclinical and very early clinical results show that encapsulated liver cells and organoids can be safely transplanted without eliciting measurable allogeneic rejection, at least on the short term [44, 96, 111–113].

43.5 Efficacy and Safety of LCT in Children

So far, more than 40 patients have received either adult or fetal allogeneic PHH transplantation for drug-induced, idiopathic, or viral ALF, worldwide [21, 22]. Of the 14 children reported in the English literature (7.6 ± 5.6 years of age), 2 survived without needing further intervention, while 5 were successfully bridged to liver transplantation [17, 18, 44, 118, 142, 143]. Reduction of plasma ammonia levels was noted in most treated patients, with approximately half of them showing a measurable improvement of hepatic encephalopathy. Among described adult cases, most patients showed a reduction of ammonia levels, about 20% of them recovered without needing further intervention, and 15% were successfully bridged to liver transplantation, with the remaining cases dying of multi-organ failure or sepsis. Overall, no clear benefit on survival could be demonstrated so far with PHHs in patients with ALF.

Very few children have received LCT for chronic or acute-on-chronic liver failure. All the three patients reported showed an improvement of hepatic encephalopathy for several weeks upon intrasplenic injection of PHHs, and two of them were successfully bridged to liver transplantation [18, 143].

As discussed above, best results with PHHs were obtained when LCT was performed in patients with metabolic liver diseases [23]. So far, more than 40 newborns, infants, children, and adolescents have received PHHs for several inborn errors of liver metabolism (5.9 ± 4.6 infusions per patient on average, from 1.5 ± 0.7 donors/patient) [19, 20, 35, 36, 48, 52, 115–120, 122–126]. Eleven of the 12 patients with

Crigler-Najjar type I syndrome showed a significant reduction of serum bilirubin levels (up to 50%). Seven of the ten with known outcome received a liver transplant 4–48 months after LCT, one is on the waiting list for transplantation, and one is treated with phototherapy 1 year after LCT. Only one patient showed no improvement after LCT. Sixteen patients (2.3 ± 3.1 years of age) received several PHH infusions for urea cycle defects (ornithine transcarbamylase deficiency, argininosuccinate lyase deficiency, carbamoyl phosphate synthetase I deficiency, citrullinemia). All but one showed reduced ammonia levels post-LCT, with increased urea levels and protein tolerance. Two children of 14 and 42 months of age showed psychomotor improvement, and two were reported neurologically normal (one after subsequent liver transplantation). The effect of LCT was limited to a few months: of the 13 children with a known outcome, 8 were listed for or underwent liver transplantation 7.9 ± 4.7 months after LCT, 1 was alive with his own liver 3 months post-LCT, and 4 died. Two of these four patients died because of complications of hyperammonemia (1.5 and 4 months post-LCT), while two children of 5 and 12 years died because of sepsis (unrelated to the procedure). Efficacy was measurable in most of the described patients suffering from other metabolic conditions but always limited to a few months despite repeated infusions over several weeks. Therefore, although PHH transplantation results in reduced exacerbations and extrahepatic sequelae and allows more permissive diets, liver transplantation is still required to treat the disease.

The studies conducted to date were very heterogeneous and almost never included a control group. Large multicenter trials with clear and measurable outcomes and greater standardization of cell isolation protocols, quality controls, administered dose, and transplantation procedure would be needed to fully assess the efficacy of PHHs. But several unsolved problems (cell quality, engraftment, long-term cell survival, etc.) need to be addressed before such studies can successfully be carried out. Whereas the efficacy of PHH transplantation needs to be improved, the safety of the procedure is very reassuring, with no patient having experienced major complications.

Several patients with cirrhosis and end-stage liver disease have already received allogeneic infusions of MSCs (mostly isolated from the bone marrow). Although some clinical improvement was noted for a few patients, no measurable beneficial effect was registered [69, 70]. Transplantation of liver-derived MSCs was reported in a few pediatric patients with inborn errors of liver metabolism (hemophilia A, ornithine transcarbamylase deficiency, and glycogen storage disease 1a), with a reassuring short-term safety profile but very limited efficacy [71–73].

No clinical trials have been conducted or approved yet to assess the effect of PSC-derived hepatocyte-like cells.

43.6 Unsolved Problems

Several aspects of LCT still need to be addressed and improved for this approach to become a real alternative to liver transplantation. Most of the identified problems are a consequence of the limitations of PHHs and will probably be solved once a better alternative cell source will be identified.

43.6.1 Engraftment of Transplanted Cells

One of the most crucial determinants of LCT efficacy is the successful engraftment of transplanted cells within the target organ. Unfortunately, more than 70% of such cells are rapidly cleared by the reticuloendothelial system within a few hours, while the remaining cells are progressively destroyed by both the innate and adaptive immune responses over weeks or months, despite immunosuppression (see above). Upon reaching the sinusoids, transplanted liver cells cause an ischemic injury which activates the reticuloendothelial system, endothelial cells, and hepatic stellate cells [30, 144]. The innate immune response together with sinusoidal events (oxidative stress, inadequate or absent adhesion to the endothelium, cytokine-mediated cytotoxicity) is responsible for the rapid loss of the majority of transplanted cells. Among the mostly deleterious locally acting vasoactive molecules released, vascular endothelial growth factor (VEGF) helps permeabilize the endothelial cells, thus allowing some of the injected liver cells to migrate into the parenchyma (16–20 h from LCT) [138, 145]. Subsequent integration of transplanted cells within the liver parenchyma requires 1–5 days and is facilitated by hepatic stellate cells [146]. Once integrated, transplanted cells acquire the gene expression profile of adjacent recipient's cells, which is determined by their position within the liver lobule.

Several approaches are being pursued to improve the engraftment of transplanted cells. Multiple drugs are being studied to pre-treat patients prior to LCT in order to inhibit the inflammatory cascade (anti-TNFα agents), disrupt the endothelial barrier (cyclophosphamide or doxorubicin), modify sinusoidal responses (ET-1 receptor blocker darusentan, prostacyclin, or nitroglycerine), or activate hepatic stellate cells (celecoxib or naproxen) [30, 128, 138, 147, 148]. Interventions on donor cells are also being considered. Nevertheless, repurposing an already approved drug would allow a faster transition to the clinical practice.

Knowing whether transplanted cells localize only within the target organ (the liver, spleen, or the abdominal cavity) or spread throughout the body has important implications for the safety of the procedure [131]. Accurate monitoring of delivered cells in vivo would also be useful to assess engraftment and rejection. Unfortunately, assessment of the biodistribution of transplanted cells has been particularly challenging in humans. Radiolabeling with Indium-111 or 99 m-technetium proved effective for short-term tracking of the transplanted cells [72, 73, 126, 149]. Several approaches to allow long-term tracking of the cells are being developed and assessed in animal models.

43.6.2 Selective Advantage and Regenerative Stimulus

Once integrated within the liver, adult PHHs do not proliferate unless liver regeneration is stimulated. This happens only in patients with active parenchymal disease and continuous hepatocyte injury, whereas most of inborn errors of liver metabolism are characterized by healthy hepatocytes. Moreover, even when such a stimulus is present, transplanted cells do not have any selective advantage compared to host hepatocytes. The result is that expansion of the pool of transplanted, healthy liver cells does not occur, with significant repopulation of the liver without external intervention being virtually impossible. This, together with the limited engraftment of the cells and their progressive rejection, impedes the treatment of diseases requiring large amounts of healthy cells or the replacement of host hepatocytes. In certain conditions, like tyrosinemia type I, BSEP deficiency or Wilson's disease, transplanted liver cells have an advantage over resident hepatocytes, but the persistence of host cells constitutes a risk for progressive fibrosis/cirrhosis or tumor formation. Several approaches have been assessed to stimulate the selective proliferation of transplanted hepatocytes, but most of them are not suitable for clinical application [39]. Some of such approaches have already been used in humans: partial hepatectomy is considered safe, but its efficacy is still unclear; portal vein embolization is routinely used in case of large liver resections and showed a good efficacy in animals undergoing LCT; partial irradiation of the native liver before LCT, which unlike partial hepatectomy or portal vein embolization provides both a regenerative stimulus and a selective advantage to donor cells, was shown effective in preclinical models and safe but only partially effective, in two infants with urea cycle defects and one adult with phenylketonuria [39, 136, 137, 150].

Fetal and neonatal PHHs suspensions, which contain more EpCAM+ progenitor cells, might allow to increase the repopulation of the recipient's liver (see above), although such cells will not have a selective advantage over host hepatocytes. Stem or progenitor cells or stem cell-derived liver cells are promising candidates to overcome the limitation of the lack of regenerative stimulus. Nevertheless, new methods to provide a selective advantage to transplanted cells need to be developed before fascinating approaches such as autologous LCT with edited, patient-derived iPSCs (see above) can be successfully implemented.

43.6.3 Safety of Stem and Progenitor Cells and of Stem Cell-Derived Hepatocytes

As discussed above, every cell population that has self-renewal capabilities has the potential to generate tumors upon transplantation, especially if the recipient is immunosuppressed. No major concerns exist about bipotent progenitors in terms of tumor formation, but their long-term safety still needs to be proved [60]. Indeed, these cells have a limited proliferation potential and can differentiate only to cholangiocytes or hepatocytes but are present only in very small amounts and within a very defined niche in the adult human liver. Multipotent MSCs are physiologically present in the body and can differentiate into somatic cells of several tissues, and their self-renewal is limited (they rapidly achieve senescence). As discussed above, MSCs are already used in several medical applications, and their efficacy, but not their safety, is the concern [65, 66, 70, 151, 152]. On the contrary, concerns exist about the use of PSCs, because of their tendency to form teratomas upon injection into immunocompromised mice [153]. PSCs (either ESCs or iPSCs) can give rise to every tissue of the body and can self-renew indefinitely. Although they cannot be used in their undifferentiated state, PSCs are currently considered the most promising source of liver cells for LCT. The question is whether the risk of ectopic tissue or tumor formation persists once PSCs are differentiated in vitro into hepatocyte-like cells. Significant resources are being dedicated by researchers working on different organs to address this question. Whereas a solid amount of data is available to show that terminally differentiated cells derived from PSCs do not constitute a risk for tumor formation, doubts still exist about the persistence of residual undifferentiated cells throughout the differentiation process and their tumorigenicity [88, 91]. Several approaches have been developed and are being assessed to eliminate residual undifferentiated cells, but whether this is needed is still unclear [154–157]. Moreover, PSCs (as other stem cells) can acquire and expand epigenetic aberrations and cancer-associated mutations upon long-term culture [158, 159]. Careful genetic and epigenetic characterization of the cells before their use to produce hepatocyte-like cells for LCT is therefore crucial, and standards need to be set by scientific societies and regulatory agencies in view of upcoming clinical trials [160].

Encapsulation of stem cell-derived hepatocytes or liver organoids using finely tuned biomaterials is a promising approach to avoid the spread of potentially tumorigenic cells throughout the recipient's body. Moreover, such a technology provides immunoisolation to the embedded cells (see above), thus eliminating the need and added risk of immunosuppression [96, 113].

43.7 Perspectives

LCT is a fascinating experimental therapeutic option that, despite the big progresses made over the last almost 25 years, is still hampered by significant unsolved problems that hamper its widespread application. The main focus of current research is finding an alternative, easily available, consistent, and safe liver cell population capable of in vivo expansion and mature, liver-specific metabolic functions upon cryopreservation and thawing. Improvement of cell engraftment and tracking and adequate prevention of rejection would also be needed. Such cells would finally turn LCT into a real alternative to liver transplantation for many patients with ALF or inborn errors of liver metabolism, while improving survival and the quality of life of patients with acute-on-chronic liver failure or end-stage liver disease.

Extracorporeal liver support devices have been available for some years. The two commercially available systems use molecular adsorption and dialysis to purify the blood from toxic compounds that cannot be detoxified from the patient's failing liver. Clinical trials in patients with liver failure have shown no significant benefit of either of the two systems on standard therapy [11, 12, 161, 162]. In order to improve the efficacy of the approach, several bioartificial liver devices have been developed over the last 20 years to incorporate porcine or human liver cells [163–165]. The efficacy of such extracorporeal devices still needs to be improved for them to be considered as an alternative or even a bridge to liver transplantation. Nevertheless, once a suitable source of mature liver cells will be identified, bioartificial livers might become a very interesting therapeutic option for patients with acute or acute-on-chronic liver failure, as well as for those with end-stage liver disease who are not eligible for transplantation.

Autologous transplantation of liver cells differentiated from edited patient-derived stem cells, in which the disease-causing mutation has been corrected by genome editing, is another very promising approach that is developing fast (see above). Although safety issues and the problem of selective advantage upon transplantation still need to be properly addressed, this technology might be disruptive for children with metabolic liver disease. Nevertheless, it is likely that current progresses in gene therapy might soon deliver a safe, clinically suitable method to correct disease-causing mutations directly in vivo, thus eliminating the need for cell transplantation for patients with metabolic liver diseases.

Thanks to recent advances in tissue engineering and biomaterial sciences, it is becoming feasible to generate complex liver organoids and tissues with functions comparable to the human liver [103, 104, 110, 113, 166]. Such stem cell-derived liver tissues reach full maturity in vitro and show liver functions comparable to the liver, which are stable long-term and upon cryopreservation [110, 113]. Although still far from any clinical application, such approaches have the potential to change the way we treat liver disease.

References

1. Squires RH, Shneider BL, Bucuvalas J, et al. Acute liver failure in children: the first 348 patients in the pediatric acute liver failure study group. J Pediatr. 2006;148:652–8.
2. Lu BR, Zhang S, Narkewicz MR, Belle SH, Squires RH, Sokol RJ, Pediatric Acute Liver Failure Study Group. Evaluation of the liver injury unit scoring system to predict survival in a multinational study of pediatric acute liver failure. J Pediatr. 2013;162:1010–6. e1–4.
3. Lee WM, Todd Stravitz R, Larson AM. AASLD position paper: the management of acute liver failure: update 2011. 2011. https://doi.org/10.1002/hep.25551.
4. Sze YK, Dhawan A, Taylor RM, Bansal S, Mieli-Vergani G, Rela M, Heaton N. Pediatric liver transplantation for metabolic liver disease: experience at King's college hospital. Transplantation. 2009;87:87–93.
5. Organ Procurement and Transplantation Network. Competing risk percentage with deceased donor transplant at specific time points for registrations listed: 2003–2014; 2018.
6. Durand P, Debray D, Mandel R, Baujard C, Branchereau S, Gauthier F, Jacquemin E, Devictor D. Acute liver failure in infancy: a 14-year experience of a pediatric liver transplantation center. J Pediatr. 2001;139:871–6.
7. Sokal EM. Liver transplantation for inborn errors of liver metabolism. J Inherit Metab Dis. 2006;29:426–30.
8. van Hoek B, de Boer J, Boudjema K, Williams R, Corsmit O, Terpstra OT. Auxiliary versus orthotopic liver transplantation for acute liver failure. EURALT Study Group European Auxiliary Liver Transplant Registry. J Hepatol. 1999;30:699–705.
9. Faraj W, Dar F, Bartlett A, Melendez HV, Marangoni G, Mukherji D, Vergani GM, Dhawan A, Heaton N, Rela M. Auxiliary liver transplantation for acute liver failure in children. Ann Surg. 2010;251:351–6.
10. Weiner J, Griesemer A, Island E, et al. Longterm outcomes of auxiliary partial orthotopic liver transplantation in preadolescent children with fulminant hepatic failure. Liver Transpl. 2016;22:485–94.
11. Lexmond WS, Van Dael CML, Scheenstra R, Goorhuis JF, Sieders E, Verkade HJ, Van Rheenen PF, Kömhoff M. Experience with molecular adsorbent recirculating system treatment in 20 children listed for high-urgency liver transplantation. Liver Transpl. 2015;21:369–80.
12. Bourgoin P, Merouani A, Phan V, Litalien C, Lallier M, Alvarez F, Jouvet P. Molecular absorbent recirculating system therapy (MARS®) in pediatric acute liver failure: a single center experience. Pediatr Nephrol. 2014;29:901–8.
13. Matas AJ, Sutherland DE, Steffes MW, Mauer SM, Sowe A, Simmons RL, Najarian JS. Hepatocellular transplantation for metabolic deficiencies: decrease of plasms bilirubin in Gunn rats. Science. 1976;192:892–4.
14. Sutherland DE, Numata M, Matas AJ, Simmons RL, Najarian JS. Hepatocellular transplantation in acute liver failure. Surgery. 1977;82:124–32.
15. Gupta S, Chowdhary JR. Hepatocyte transplantation: back to the future. Hepatology. 1992;15:156–62.
16. Mito M, Kusano M. Hepatocyte transplantation in man. Cell Transplant. 1993;2:65–74.

17. Habibullah CM, Syed IH, Qamar A, Taher-Uz Z. Human fetal hepatocyte transplantation in patients with fulminant hepatic failure. Transplantation. 1994;58:951–2.
18. Strom SC, Fisher RA, Thompson MT, Sanyal AJ, Cole PE, Ham JM, Posner MP. Hepatocyte transplantation as a bridge to orthotopic liver transplantation in terminal liver failure. Transplantation. 1997;63:559–69.
19. Grossman M, Rader DJ, Muller DW, Kolansky DM, Kozarsky K, Clark BJ, Stein EA, Lupien PJ, Brewer HB, Raper SE. A pilot study of ex vivo gene therapy for homozygous familial hypercholesterolaemia. Nat Med. 1995;1:1148–54.
20. Fox IJ, Chowdhury JR, Kaufman SS, Goertzen TC, Chowdhury NR, Warkentin PI, Dorko K, Sauter BV, Strom SC. Treatment of the crigler–najjar syndrome type I with hepatocyte transplantation. N Engl J Med. 1998;338:1422–7.
21. Fisher RA, Strom SC. Human hepatocyte transplantation: worldwide results. Transplantation. 2006;82:441–9.
22. Smets F, Najimi M, Sokal EM. Cell transplantation in the treatment of liver diseases. Pediatr Transplant. 2008;12:6–13.
23. Khan Z, Strom SC. Hepatocyte transplantation in special populations: clinical use in children. Methods Mol Biol. 2017;1506:3–16.
24. Seglen P. Preparation of isolated rat liver cells. Methods Cell Biol. 1976;13:29–83.
25. Mitry RR, Hughes RD, Aw MM, Terry C, Mieli-Vergani G, Girlanda R, Muiesan P, Rela M, Heaton ND, Dhawan A. Human hepatocyte isolation and relationship of cell viability to early graft function. Cell Transplant. 2003;12:69–74.
26. Coppin L, Sokal E, Stephenne X. Hepatocyte transplantation in children methods. Mol Biol. 2017;1506:295–315.
27. Bhogal RH, Hodson J, Bartlett DC, et al. Isolation of primary human hepatocytes from normal and diseased liver tissue: a one hundred liver experience. PLoS One. 2011;6:e18222–8.
28. Sagias FG, Mitry RR, Hughes RD, Lehec SC, Patel AG, Rela M, Mieli-Vergani G, Heaton ND, Dhawan A. N-Acetylcysteine improves the viability of human hepatocytes isolated from severely Steatotic donor liver tissue. Cell Transplant. 2010;19:1487–92.
29. Rajvanshi P, Kerr A, Bhargava KK, Burk RD, Gupta S. Studies of liver repopulation using the dipeptidyl peptidase IV-deficient rat and other rodent recipients: cell size and structure relationships regulate capacity for increased transplanted hepatocyte mass in the liver lobule. Hepatology. 1996;23:482–96.
30. Krohn N, Kapoor S, Enami Y, Follenzi A, Bandi S, Joseph B, Gupta S. Hepatocyte transplantation-induced liver inflammation is driven by cytokines-chemokines associated with neutrophils and kupffer cells. Gastroenterology. 2009;136:1806–17.
31. Stephenne X, Najimi M, Ngoc DK, Smets F, Hue L, Guigas B, Sokal EM. Cryopreservation of human hepatocytes alters the mitochondrial respiratory chain complex 1. Cell Transplant. 2007;16:409–19.
32. Stephenne X, Najimi M, Sokal EM. Hepatocyte cryopreservation: is it time to change the strategy? World J Gastroenterol. 2010;16:1–14.
33. Terry C, Dhawan A, Mitry RR, Lehec SC, Hughes RD. Optimization of the cryopreservation and thawing protocol for human hepatocytes for use in cell transplantation. Liver Transpl. 2010;16:229–37.
34. Terry C, Hughes RD, Mitry RR, Lehec SC, Dhawan A. Cryopreservation-induced nonattachment of human hepatocytes: role of adhesion molecules. Cell Transplant. 2007;16:639–47.
35. Stephenne X, Najimi M, Smets F, Reding R, de Goyet J de V, Sokal EM. Cryopreserved liver cell transplantation controls ornithine transcarbamylase deficient patient while awaiting liver transplantation. Am J Transplant. 2005;5:2058–61.
36. Lee K-W, Lee J-H, Shin SW, et al. Hepatocyte transplantation for glycogen storage disease type Ib. Cell Transplant. 2007;16:629–37.
37. Bilir BM, Guinette D, Karrer F, Kumpe DA, Krysl J, Stephens J, McGavran L, Ostrowska A, Durham J. Hepatocyte transplantation in acute liver failure. Liver Transpl. 2000;6:32–40.
38. Gridelli B, Vizzini G, Pietrosi G, et al. Efficient human fetal liver cell isolation protocol based on vascular perfusion for liver cell-based therapy and case report on cell transplantation. Liver Transpl. 2012;18:226–37.
39. Puppi J, Strom SC, Hughes RD, et al. Improving the techniques for human hepatocyte transplantation: report from a consensus meeting in London. Cell Transplant. 2012;21:1–10.
40. Suchy FJ. Functional development of the liver. In: Suchy FJ, Sokol RJ, Balistreri WF, editors. Liver disease in children. 4th ed. Cambridge: Cambridge University Press; 2014. p. 10–23.
41. Cantz T, Zuckerman DM, Burda MR, Dandri M, Göricke B, Thalhammer S, Heckl WM, Manns MP, Petersen J, Ott M. Quantitative gene expression analysis reveals transition of fetal liver progenitor cells to mature hepatocytes after transplantation in uPA/RAG-2 mice. Am J Pathol. 2010;162:37–45.
42. Pietrosi G, Vizzini G, Gerlach J, et al. Phases I-II matched case-control study of human fetal liver cell transplantation for treatment of chronic liver disease. Cell Transplant. 2015;24:1627–38.
43. Tolosa L, Pareja-Ibars E, Donato MT, Cortés M, López S, Jiménez N, Mir J, Castell JV, Gómez-Lechón MJ. Neonatal livers: a source for the isolation of good-performing hepatocytes for cell transplantation. Cell Transplant. 2014;23:1229–42.
44. Lee CA, Dhawan A, Iansante V, et al. Cryopreserved neonatal hepatocytes may be a source for transplantation: evaluation of functionality toward clinical use. Liver Transpl. 2018;24:394–406.
45. Guidotti J-E, Brégerie O, Robert A, Debey P, Bréchot C, Desdouets C. Liver cell polyploidization: a pivotal role for binuclear hepatocytes. J Biol Chem. 2003;278:19095–101.
46. Suzuki A, Taniguchi H, Zheng YW, et al. Proliferative and functional ability of transplanted murine neonatal hepatocytes in adult livers. Transplant Proc. 2000;32:2370–1.
47. Brilliant KE, Mills DR, Callanan HM, Hixson DC. Engraftment of syngeneic and allogeneic endothelial cells, hepatocytes and cholangiocytes into partially hepatectomized rats previously treated with mitomycin C. Transplantation. 2009;88:486–95.
48. Meyburg J, Das AM, Hoerster F, et al. One liver for four children: first clinical series of liver cell transplantation for severe neonatal urea cycle defects. Transplantation. 2009;87:636–41.
49. Popescu I, Dima SO. Domino liver transplantation: how far can we push the paradigm? Liver Transpl. 2011;18:22–8.
50. Dept of Transplantation Surgery, Karolinska University Hospital Huddinge, Stockholm, Sweden. Domino liver transplant registry; 2017. http://www.fapwtr.org/about/dltr.htm. Accessed 5 Jun 2018.
51. Gramignoli R, Tahan V, Dorko K, et al. New potential cell source for hepatocyte transplantation: discarded livers from metabolic disease liver transplants. Stem Cell Res. 2013;11:563–73.
52. Stéphenne X, Debray FG, Smets F, et al. Hepatocyte transplantation using the domino concept in a child with tetrabiopterin nonresponsive phenylketonuria. Cell Transplant. 2012;21:2765–70.
53. Cardinale V, Wang Y, Carpino G, et al. Multipotent stem/progenitor cells in human biliary tree give rise to hepatocytes, cholangiocytes, and pancreatic islets. Hepatology. 2011;54:2159–72.
54. Schmelzer E, Zhang L, Bruce A, et al. Human hepatic stem cells from fetal and postnatal donors. J Exp Med. 2007;204:1973–87.
55. Riccio M, Carnevale G, Cardinale V, et al. The Fas/Fas ligand apoptosis pathway underlies immunomodulatory properties of human biliary tree stem/progenitor cells. J Hepatol. 2014;61:1097–105.

56. Huch M, Gehart H, van Boxtel R, et al. Long-term culture of genome-stable bipotent stem cells from adult human liver. Cell. 2015;160:299–312.
57. Carpino G, Cardinale V, Gentile R, et al. Evidence for multipotent endodermal stem/progenitor cell populations in human gallbladder. J Hepatol. 2014;60:1194–202.
58. Semeraro R, Carpino G, Cardinale V, et al. Multipotent stem/progenitor cells in the human foetal biliary tree. J Hepatol. 2012;57:987–94.
59. Khan AA, Shaik MV, Parveen N, et al. Human fetal liver-derived stem cell transplantation as supportive modality in the management of end-stage decompensated liver cirrhosis. Cell Transplant. 2010;19:409–18.
60. Cardinale V, Carpino G, Gentile R, et al. Transplantation of human fetal biliary tree stem/progenitor cells into two patients with advanced liver cirrhosis. BMC Gastroenterol. 2014;14:231–5.
61. Horwitz E, Le Blanc K, Dominici M, Mueller I, Slaper-Cortenbach I, Marini F, Deans R, Krause D, Keating A. Clarification of the nomenclature for MSC: the International Society for Cellular Therapy position statement. Cytotherapy. 2005;7:393–5.
62. Campard D, Lysy PA, Najimi M, Sokal EM. Native umbilical cord matrix stem cells express hepatic markers and differentiate into hepatocyte-like cells. Gastroenterology. 2008;134:833–48.
63. Najimi M, Khuu DN, Lysy PA, Jazouli N, Abarca J, Sempoux C, Sokal EM. Adult-derived human liver mesenchymal-like cells as a potential progenitor reservoir of hepatocytes? Cell Transplant. 2007;16:717–28.
64. Aurich I, Mueller LP, Aurich H, et al. Functional integration of hepatocytes derived from human mesenchymal stem cells into mouse livers. Gut. 2007;56:405–15.
65. Scheers I, Maerckx C, Ngoc Khuu D, Marcelle S, Decottignies A, Najimi M, Sokal E. Adult derived human liver progenitor cells in long term culture maintain appropriate gatekeeper mechanisms against transformation. Cell Transplant. 2012;21(10):2241–55.
66. Scheers I, Lombard C, Paganelli M, Campard D, Najimi M, Gala J-L, Decottignies A, Sokal E. Human umbilical cord matrix stem cells maintain multilineage differentiation abilities and do not transform during long-term culture. PLoS One. 2013;8:e71374.
67. Kuo TK, Hung S-P, Chuang C-H, Chen C-T, Shih Y-RV, Fang S-CY, Yang VW, Lee OK. Stem cell therapy for liver disease: parameters governing the success of using bone marrow mesenchymal stem cells. Gastroenterology. 2008;134:2111–21, 2121. e1–3.
68. Banas A, Teratani T, Yamamoto Y, Tokuhara M, Takeshita F, Osaki M, Kawamata M, Kato T, Okochi H, Ochiya T. IFATS collection: in vivo therapeutic potential of human adipose tissue mesenchymal stem cells after transplantation into mice with liver injury. Stem Cells. 2008;26:2705–12.
69. Mohamadnejad M, Alimoghaddam K, Bagheri M, Ashrafi M, Abdollahzadeh L, Akhlaghpoor S, Bashtar M, Ghavamzadeh A, Malekzadeh R. Randomized placebo-controlled trial of mesenchymal stem cell transplantation in decompensated cirrhosis. Liver Int. 2013;33:1490–6.
70. Moore JK, Stutchfield BM, Forbes SJ. Systematic review with meta-analysis: to assess the effects of autologous stem cell therapy for patients with liver disease. Aliment Pharmacol Ther. 2014;39:673–85.
71. Sokal EM, Stephenne X, Ottolenghi C, Jazouli N, Clapuyt P, Lacaille F, Najimi M, de Lonlay P, Smets F. Liver engraftment and repopulation by in vitro expanded adult derived human liver stem cells in a child with ornithine carbamoyltransferase deficiency. JIMD Rep. 2014;13:65–72.
72. Defresne F, Tondreau T, Stephenne X, Smets F, Bourgois A, Najimi M, Jamar F, Sokal EM. Biodistribution of adult derived human liver stem cells following intraportal infusion in a 17-year-old patient with glycogenosis type 1A. Nucl Med Biol. 2014;41:371–5.
73. Sokal EM, Lombard CA, Roelants V, et al. Biodistribution of liver-derived mesenchymal stem cells after peripheral injection in a hemophilia a patient. Transplantation. 2017;101:1845–51.
74. Lee K-D, Kuo TK-C, Whang-Peng J, Chung Y-F, Lin C-T, Chou S-H, Chen J-R, Chen Y-P, Lee OK-S. In vitro hepatic differentiation of human mesenchymal stem cells. Hepatology. 2004;40:1275–84.
75. Banas A, Teratani T, Yamamoto Y, Tokuhara M, Takeshita F, Quinn G, Okochi H, Ochiya T. Adipose tissue-derived mesenchymal stem cells as a source of human hepatocytes. Hepatology. 2007;46:219–28.
76. Ishii K, Yoshida Y, Akechi Y, et al. Hepatic differentiation of human bone marrow-derived mesenchymal stem cells by tetracycline-regulated hepatocyte nuclear factor 3beta. Hepatology. 2008;48:597–606.
77. Paganelli M, Dallmeier K, Nyabi O, Scheers I, Kabamba B, Neyts J, Goubau P, Najimi M, Sokal EM. Differentiated umbilical cord matrix stem cells as a new in vitro model to study early events during hepatitis B virus infection. Hepatology. 2013;57:59–69.
78. Paganelli M, Nyabi O, Sid B, et al. Downregulation of Sox9 expression associates with hepatogenic differentiation of human liver mesenchymal stem/progenitor cells. Stem Cells Dev. 2014;23:1377–91.
79. Takahashi K, Yamanaka S. Induction of pluripotent stem cells from mouse embryonic and adult fibroblast cultures by defined factors. Cell. 2006;126:663–76.
80. Takahashi K, Tanabe K, Ohnuki M, Narita M, Ichisaka T, Tomoda K, Yamanaka S. Induction of pluripotent stem cells from adult human fibroblasts by defined factors. Cell. 2007;131:861–72.
81. Hay DC, Zhao D, Fletcher J, et al. Efficient differentiation of hepatocytes from human embryonic stem cells exhibiting markers recapitulating liver development in vivo. Stem Cells. 2008;26:894–902.
82. Basma H, Soto Gutiérrez A, Yannam GR, et al. Differentiation and transplantation of human embryonic stem cell–derived hepatocytes. Gastroenterology. 2009;136:990–999.e4.
83. Si-Tayeb K, Noto FK, Nagaoka M, Li J, Battle MA, Duris C, North PE, Dalton S, Duncan SA. Highly efficient generation of human hepatocyte-like cells from induced pluripotent stem cells. Hepatology. 2009;51:297–305.
84. Rashid ST, Corbineau S, Hannan N, et al. Modeling inherited metabolic disorders of the liver using human induced pluripotent stem cells. J Clin Invest. 2010;120:3127–36.
85. Hannan NRF, Segeritz C-P, Touboul T, Vallier L. Production of hepatocyte-like cells from human pluripotent stem cells. Nat Protoc. 2013;8:430–7.
86. Shan J, Schwartz RE, Ross NT, Logan DJ, Thomas D, Duncan SA, North TE, Goessling W, Carpenter AE, Bhatia SN. Identification of small molecules for human hepatocyte expansion and iPS differentiation. Nat Chem Biol. 2013;9:514–20.
87. Loh KM, Ang LT, Zhang J, et al. Efficient endoderm induction from human pluripotent stem cells by logically directing signals controlling lineage bifurcations. Cell Stem Cell. 2014;14:237–52.
88. Takayama K, Akita N, Mimura N, et al. Generation of safe and therapeutically effective human induced pluripotent stem cell-derived hepatocyte-like cells for regenerative medicine. Hepatol Commun. 2017;1:1058–69.
89. Baxter M, Withey S, Harrison S, et al. Phenotypic and functional analyses show stem cell-derived hepatocyte-like cells better mimic fetal rather than adult hepatocytes. J Hepatol. 2015;62:581–9.
90. Song WK, Park K-M, Kim H-J, Lee JH, Choi J, Chong SY, Shim SH, Del Priore LV, Lanza R. Treatment of macular degeneration using embryonic stem cell-derived retinal pigment epithelium: preliminary results in Asian patients. Stem Cell Rep. 2015;4:860–72.

91. Mandai M, Watanabe A, Kurimoto Y, et al. Autologous induced stem-cell–derived retinal cells for macular degeneration. N Engl J Med. 2017;376:1038–46.
92. Huang P, Zhang L, Gao Y, et al. Direct reprogramming of human fibroblasts to functional and expandable hepatocytes. Cell Stem Cell. 2014;14:370–84.
93. Du Y, Wang J, Jia J, et al. Human hepatocytes with drug metabolic function induced from fibroblasts by lineage reprogramming. Cell Stem Cell. 2014;14:394–403.
94. Zhu S, Rezvani M, Harbell J, Mattis AN, Wolfe AR, Benet LZ, Willenbring H, Ding S. Mouse liver repopulation with hepatocytes generated from human fibroblasts. Nature. 2014;508:93–7.
95. Si-Tayeb K, Lemaigre FP, Duncan SA. Organogenesis and development of the liver. Dev Cell. 2010;18:175–89.
96. Song W, Lu Y-C, Frankel AS, An D, Schwartz RE, Ma M. Engraftment of human induced pluripotent stem cell-derived hepatocytes in immunocompetent mice via 3D co-aggregation and encapsulation. Sci Rep. 2015;5:1–13.
97. Berger DR, Ware BR, Davidson MD, Allsup SR, Khetani SR. Enhancing the functional maturity of induced pluripotent stem cell-derived human hepatocytes by controlled presentation of cell-cell interactions in vitro. Hepatology. 2015;61:1370–81.
98. Takebe T, Sekine K, Enomura M, et al. Vascularized and functional human liver from an iPSC-derived organ bud transplant. Nature. 2013;499:481–4.
99. Zinchenko YS, Culberson CR, Coger RN. Contribution of non-parenchymal cells to the performance of micropatterned hepatocytes. Tissue Eng. 2006;12:2241–1251.
100. Li CY, Stevens KR, Schwartz RE, Alejandro BS, Huang JH, Bhatia SN. Micropatterned cell–cell interactions enable functional encapsulation of primary hepatocytes in hydrogel microtissues. Tissue Eng A. 2014;20:2200–12.
101. Ohashi K, Yokoyama T, Yamato M, et al. Engineering functional two- and three-dimensional liver systems in vivo using hepatic tissue sheets. Nat Med. 2007;13:880–5.
102. Takebe T, Zhang R-R, Koike H, Kimura M, Yoshizawa E, Enomura M, Koike N, Sekine K, Taniguchi H. Generation of a vascularized and functional human liver from an iPSC-derived organ bud transplant. Nat Protoc. 2014;9:396–409.
103. Nagamoto Y, Takayama K, Ohashi K, Okamoto R, Sakurai F, Tachibana M, Kawabata K, Mizuguchi H. Transplantation of a human iPSC-derived hepatocyte sheet increases survival in mice with acute liver failure. J Hepatol. 2016;64:1068–75.
104. Takebe T, Sekine K, Kimura M, et al. Massive and reproducible production of liver buds entirely from human pluripotent stem cells. Cell Rep. 2017;21:2661–70.
105. Du C, Narayanan K, Leong MF, Wan ACA. Induced pluripotent stem cell-derived hepatocytes and endothelial cells in multi-component hydrogel fibers for liver tissue engineering. Biomaterials. 2014;35:6006–14.
106. Stevens KR, Miller JS, Blakely BL, Chen CS, Bhatia SN. Degradable hydrogels derived from PEG-diacrylamide for hepatic tissue engineering. J Biomed Mater Res. 2015;103:3331–8.
107. Saheli M, Sepantafar M, Pournasr B, Farzaneh Z, Vosough M, Piryaei A, Baharvand H. Three-dimensional liver-derived extracellular matrix hydrogel promotes liver organoids function. J Cell Biochem. 2018;119:4320–33.
108. Shi X-L, Zhang Y, Gu J-Y, Ding Y-T. Coencapsulation of hepatocytes with bone marrow mesenchymal stem cells improves hepatocyte-specific functions. Transplantation. 2009;88:1178–85.
109. Underhill GH, Chen AA, Albrecht DR, Bhatia SN. Assessment of hepatocellular function within PEG hydrogels. Biomaterials. 2007;28:256–70.
110. Raggi C, M'Callum M, Mangahas C, Cohen Z, Shikanov A, Paganelli M. Human stem cell-derived encapsulated liver tissue as an effective, consistent and long-lasting in vitro tool for drug testing and development. Hepatology. 2017;66:148A.
111. No Da Y, Jeong GS, Lee S-H. Immune-protected xenogeneic bio-artificial livers with liver-specific microarchitecture and hydrogel-encapsulated cells. Biomaterials. 2014;35:8983–91.
112. Jitraruch S, Dhawan A, Hughes RD, Filippi C, Soong D, Philippeos C, Lehec SC, Heaton ND, Longhi MS, Mitry RR. Alginate microencapsulated hepatocytes optimised for transplantation in acute liver failure. PLoS One. 2014;9:e113609–23.
113. Raggi C, M'Callum MA, Mangahas C, Selleri S, Beauséjour C, Shikanov A, Haddad E, Paganelli M. Safety of stem cell-derived encapsulated liver tissue to treat liver failure: immune-isolation and absence of foreign body reaction or tumor formation upon transplantation without immunosuppression. Cytotherapy. 2018;20:S19.
114. Schneider A, Attaran M, Meier PN, Strassburg C, Manns MP, Ott M, Barthold M, Arseniev L, Becker T, Panning B. Hepatocyte transplantation in an acute liver failure due to mushroom poisoning. Transplantation. 2006;82:1115–6.
115. Lysy P-A, Najimi M, Stephenne X, Bourgois A, Smets F, Sokal E-M. Liver cell transplantation for crigler-najjar syndrome type I: update and perspectives. World J Gastroenterol. 2008;14:3464–70.
116. Sokal EM, Smets F, Bourgois A, et al. Hepatocyte transplantation in a 4-year-old girl with peroxisomal biogenesis disease: technique, safety, and metabolic follow-up. Transplantation. 2003;76:735–8.
117. Stéphenne X, Najimi M, Sibille C, Nassogne M-C, Smets F, Sokal EM. Sustained engraftment and tissue enzyme activity after liver cell transplantation for argininosuccinate lyase deficiency. Gastroenterology. 2006;130:1317–23.
118. Strom SC, Chowdhury JR, Fox IJ. Hepatocyte transplantation for the treatment of human disease. Semin Liver Dis. 1999;19:39–48.
119. Dhawan A, Mitry RR, Hughes RD, et al. Hepatocyte transplantation for inherited factor VII deficiency. Transplantation. 2004;78:1812–4.
120. Dhawan A, Mitry RR, Hughes RD. Hepatocyte transplantation for liver-based metabolic disorders. J Inherit Metab Dis. 2006;29:431–5.
121. Muraca M, Gerunda G, Neri D, Vilei M-T, Granato A, Feltracco P, Meroni M, Giron G, Burlina AB. Hepatocyte transplantation as a treatment for glycogen storage disease type 1a. Lancet. 2002;359:317–8.
122. Ribes-Koninckx C, Ibars EP, Agrasot MÁC, Bonora-Centelles A, Miquel BP, Carbó JJV, Aliaga ED, Pallardó JM, Gomez-Lechon M-J, Castell JV. Clinical outcome of hepatocyte transplantation in four pediatric patients with inherited metabolic diseases. Cell Transplant. 2012;21:2267–82.
123. Hughes RD, Mitry RR, Dhawan A, Lehec SC, Girlanda R, Rela M, Heaton ND, Muiesan P. Isolation of hepatocytes from livers from non-heart-beating donors for cell transplantation. Liver Transpl. 2006;12:713–7.
124. Beck BB, Habbig S, Dittrich K, et al. Liver cell transplantation in severe infantile oxalosis—a potential bridging procedure to orthotopic liver transplantation? Nephrol Dial Transplant. 2012;27:2984–9.
125. Mitry RR, Dhawan A, Hughes RD, et al. One liver, three recipients: segment IV from split-liver procedures as a source of hepatocytes for cell transplantation. Transplantation. 2004;77:1614–6.
126. Bohnen NI, Charron M, Reyes J, Rubinstein W, Strom SC, Swanson D, Towbin R. Use of indium-111-labeled hepatocytes to determine the biodistribution of transplanted hepatocytes through portal vein infusion. Clin Nucl Med. 2000;25:447–50.
127. Wang L-J, Chen YM, George D, Smets F, Sokal EM, Bremer EG, Soriano HE. Engraftment assessment in human and mouse liver tissue after sex-mismatched liver cell transplantation by real-time

127. quantitative PCR for Y chromosome sequences. Liver Transpl. 2002;8:822–8.
128. Forbes SJ, Gupta S, Dhawan A. Cell therapy for liver disease: from liver transplantation to cell factory. J Hepatol. 2015;62:S157–69.
129. Darwish AA, Sokal E, Stephenne X, Najimi M, de Goyet J de V, Reding R. Permanent access to the portal system for cellular transplantation using an implantable port device. Liver Transpl. 2004;10:1213–5.
130. Ponder KP, Gupta S, Leland F, Darlington G, Finegold M, DeMayo J, Ledley FD, Chowdhury JR, Woo SL. Mouse hepatocytes migrate to liver parenchyma and function indefinitely after intrasplenic transplantation. Proc Natl Acad Sci U S A. 1991;88:1217–21.
131. Rajvanshi P, Fabrega A, Bhargava KK, Kerr A, Pollak R, Blanchard J, Palestro CJ, Gupta S. Rapid clearance of transplanted hepatocytes from pulmonary capillaries in rats indicates a wide safety margin of liver repopulation and the potential of using surrogate albumin particles for safety analysis. J Hepatol. 1999;30:299–310.
132. Wang F, Zhou L, Ma X, Ma W, Wang C, Lu Y, Chen Y, An L, An W, Yang Y. Monitoring of intrasplenic hepatocyte transplantation for acute-on-chronic liver failure: a prospective five-year follow-up study. Transplant Proc. 2014;46:192–8.
133. Strom SC, Fisher RA, Rubinstein WS, et al. Transplantation of human hepatocytes. Transplant Proc. 1997;29:2103–6.
134. Stéphenne X, Vosters O, Najimi M, Beuneu C, Dung KN, Wijns W, Goldman M, Sokal EM. Tissue factor-dependent procoagulant activity of isolated human hepatocytes: relevance to liver cell transplantation. Liver Transpl. 2007;13:599–606.
135. Stephenne X, Nicastro E, Eeckhoudt S, Hermans C, Nyabi O, Lombard C, Najimi M, Sokal E. Bivalirudin in combination with heparin to control mesenchymal cell procoagulant activity. PLoS One. 2012;7:e42819–3.
136. Soltys KA, Setoyama K, Tafaleng EN, et al. Host conditioning and rejection monitoring in hepatocyte transplantation in humans. J Hepatol. 2017;66:987–1000.
137. Jorns C, Nowak G, Nemeth A, et al. De novo donor-specific HLA antibody formation in two patients with Crigler-Najjar syndrome type I following human hepatocyte transplantation with partial hepatectomy preconditioning. Am J Transplant. 2015;16:1021–30.
138. Gupta S, Rajvanshi P, Sokhi R, Slehria S, Yam A, Kerr A, Novikoff PM. Entry and integration of transplanted hepatocytes in rat liver plates occur by disruption of hepatic sinusoidal endothelium. Hepatology. 1999;29:509–19.
139. Olszewski WL, Interewicz B, Durlik M, Rudowska A, Mecner B. Early loss of transplanted autologous hepatocytes-lysis by leukocytes in vivo and in vitro. Transplant Proc. 2001;33:651–3.
140. Gustafson EK, Elgue G, Hughes RD, Mitry RR, Sanchez J, Haglund U, Meurling S, Dhawan A, Korsgren O, Nilsson B. The instant blood-mediated inflammatory reaction characterized in hepatocyte transplantation. Transplantation. 2011;91:632–8.
141. Lee CA, Dhawan A, Smith RA, Mitry RR, Fitzpatrick E. Instant blood-mediated inflammatory reaction in hepatocyte transplantation: current status and future perspectives. Cell Transplant. 2016;25:1227–36.
142. Soriano HE, Wood RP, Kang DC, Pediatric CO, Finegold MJ, Darlington GJ, Ferry G. Hepatocellular transplantation (HCT) via portal vein catheter in a patient with fulminant liver failure. Pediatr Res. 1996;39:127.
143. Soriano HE, Wood RP, Kang DC, Ozaki CF, Finegold MJ, BF C, Reid BS, Ferry GD. Hepatocellular transplantation (HCT) in children with fulminant liver failure (FLF). Hepatology. 1997;26(S):443A.
144. Enami Y, Bandi S, Kapoor S, Krohn N, Joseph B, Gupta S. Hepatic stellate cells promote hepatocyte engraftment in rat liver after prostaglandin-endoperoxide synthase inhibition. Gastroenterology. 2009;136:2356–64.
145. Slehria S, Rajvanshi P, Ito Y, Sokhi RP, Bhargava KK, Palestro CJ, McCuskey RS, Gupta S. Hepatic sinusoidal vasodilators improve transplanted cell engraftment and ameliorate microcirculatory perturbations in the liver. Hepatology. 2002;35:1320–8.
146. Benten D, Kumaran V, Joseph B, Schattenberg J, Popov Y, Schuppan D, Gupta S. Hepatocyte transplantation activates hepatic stellate cells with beneficial modulation of cell engraftment in the rat. Hepatology. 2005;42:1072–81.
147. Bahde R, Kapoor S, Bandi S, Bhargava KK, Palestro CJ, Gupta S. Directly acting drugs prostacyclin or nitroglycerine and endothelin receptor blocker bosentan improve cell engraftment in rodent liver. Hepatology. 2013;57:320–30.
148. Bahde R, Kapoor S, Viswanathan P, Spiegel H-U, Gupta S. Endothelin-1 receptor a blocker darusentan decreases hepatic changes and improves liver repopulation after cell transplantation in rats. Hepatology. 2014;59:1107–17.
149. Cheng K, Benten D, Bhargava K, Inada M, Joseph B, Palestro C, Gupta S. Hepatic targeting and biodistribution of human fetal liver stem/progenitor cells and adult hepatocytes in mice. Hepatology. 2009;50:1194–203.
150. Dagher I, Boudechiche L, Branger J, et al. Efficient hepatocyte engraftment in a nonhuman primate model after partial portal vein embolization. Transplantation. 2006;82:1067–73.
151. Houlihan DD, Newsome PN. Critical review of clinical trials of bone marrow stem cells in liver disease. Gastroenterology. 2008;135:438–50.
152. Pan X-N. Bone marrow-derived mesenchymal stem cell therapy for decompensated liver cirrhosis: a meta-analysis. World J Gastroenterol. 2014;20:14051–8.
153. Gropp M, Shilo V, Vainer G, et al. Standardization of the teratoma assay for analysis of pluripotency of human ES cells and biosafety of their differentiated progeny. PLoS One. 2012;7:e45532–10.
154. Tomizawa M, Shinozaki F, Sugiyama T, Yamamoto S, Sueishi M, Yoshida T. Survival of primary human hepatocytes and death of induced pluripotent stem cells in media lacking glucose and arginine. PLoS One. 2013;8:e71897–10.
155. Khatib El MM, Ohmine S, Jacobus EJ, et al. Tumor-free transplantation of patient-derived induced pluripotent stem cell progeny for customized islet regeneration. Stem Cells Transl Med. 2016;5:694–702.
156. Katsukawa M, Nakajima Y, Fukumoto A, Doi D, Takahashi J. Fail-safe therapy by gamma-ray irradiation against tumor formation by human-induced pluripotent stem cell-derived neural progenitors. Stem Cells Dev. 2016;25:815–25.
157. Parr CJC, Katayama S, Miki K, Kuang Y, Yoshida Y, Morizane A, Takahashi J, Yamanaka S, Saito H. MicroRNA-302 switch to identify and eliminate undifferentiated human pluripotent stem cells. Sci Rep. 2016;6:32532.
158. Weissbein U, Plotnik O, Vershkov D, Benvenisty N. Culture-induced recurrent epigenetic aberrations in human pluripotent stem cells. PLoS Genet. 2017;13:e1006979–16.
159. Merkle FT, Ghosh S, Kamitaki N, et al. Human pluripotent stem cells recurrently acquire and expand dominant negative P53 mutations. Nature. 2017;545:229–33.
160. Andrews PW, Ben-David U, Benvenisty N, et al. Assessing the safety of human pluripotent stem cells and their derivatives for clinical applications. Stem Cell Reports. 2017;9:1–4.
161. Khuroo MS, Khuroo MS, Farahat KLC. Molecular adsorbent recirculating system for acute and acute-on-chronic liver failure: a meta-analysis. Liver Transpl. 2004;10:1099–106.
162. Kribben A, Gerken G, Haag S, et al. Effects of fractionated plasma separation and adsorption on survival in patients with acute-on-chronic liver failure. Gastroenterology. 2012;142:782–789.e3.
163. Ellis AJ, Hughes RD, Wendon JA, Dunne J, Langley PG, Kelly JH, Gislason GT, Sussman NL, Williams R. Pilot-controlled trial

of the extracorporeal liver assist device in acute liver failure. Hepatology. 1996;24:1446–51.
164. Demetriou AA, Brown RS Jr, Busuttil RW, et al. Prospective, randomized, multicenter, controlled trial of a bioartificial liver in treating acute liver failure. Ann Surg. 2004;239:660–70.
165. Glorioso JM, Mao SA, Rodysill B, et al. Pivotal preclinical trial of the spheroid reservoir bioartificial liver. J Hepatol. 2015;63:388–98.
166. Tatsumi K, Okano T. Hepatocyte transplantation: cell sheet Technology for Liver Cell Transplantation. Curr Transplant Rep. 2017;4:184–92.

Gene Therapy in Pediatric Liver Disease

Andrès F. Muro, Lorenzo D'Antiga, and Federico Mingozzi

Key Points

- Liver gene therapy mediated by rAAV vectors has shown safety and efficacy as an alternative to liver transplantation.
- First evidence of long-term safety and efficacy of rAAV-mediated liver gene transfer in humans comes from the hemophilia A and B trials.
- Novel therapeutic protocols are being tested to overcome immunological hurdles such as pre-existing antibodies and cellular responses directed against the AAV capsid.
- The use of relevant animal models was key for the generation and improvement of therapeutic vectors and protocols and for the deeper understanding of disease mechanisms.
- The use of engineered endonucleases allows for the permanent and site-specific modification of the hepatocyte genome, altering metabolic pathways, inserting therapeutic genes into "safe-harbor loci" or editing diseased genes.

Research Needed in the Field

- Improve strategies to allow administration of AAV gene therapy to seropositive patients.
- Develop efficient strategies to block immune responses against AAV capsid antigens, in order to allow readministration of the therapeutic vector in case of loss of efficacy over time.
- Development of less immunogenic delivery vectors, which could be efficiently (re)administered to larger proportions of the population. In this respect, the development of efficient non-viral delivery methods could be a potentially viable approach.
- An important challenge is the improvement in the gene editing/targeting rate by the development of highly efficient and more specific endonucleases with transient activity and low off-target effects.

44.1 Introduction

44.1.1 Expectations on Gene Therapy for Monogenic Disorders

Gene therapy reached high popularity in the mid-1990s, when preclinical and proof-of-concept studies (especially in congenital immunodeficiencies) were accomplished and published [1, 2]. While the scientific community was trying to translate these preliminary reports into clinical trials, the death of a young adult treated for ornithine transcarbamylase deficiency with an adenoviral vector brought the field into a period of obscurity and uncertainty [3]. The following optimism derived from the clinical success in the treatment of X-linked severe combined immunodeficiency [4] was soon turned down by the occurrence of leukemia in 5 of 20 patients

A. F. Muro (✉)
Mouse Molecular Genetics Laboratory, International Center for Genetic Engineering and Biotechnology (ICGEB), Padriciano, Trieste, Italy
e-mail: muro@icgeb.org

L. D'Antiga
Paediatric Hepatology, Gastroenterology and Transplantation, Hospital Papa Giovanni XXIII, Bergamo, Italy
e-mail: ldantiga@asst-pg23.it

F. Mingozzi (✉)
INSERM, Évry, France

Genethon, Évry, France
e-mail: fmingozzi@genethon.fr

secondary to insertional mutagenesis [5, 6]. Meanwhile, further concerns were raised by the growing evidence of vector-induced immune responses jeopardizing this treatment strategy [7].

In recent years, preclinical experiments have been definitely translated into successful clinical trials in different inherited disorders, such as Leber's congenital amaurosis [8–10], X-linked adrenoleukodystrophy [11], metachromatic leukodystrophy [12], and hemophilia B [13–15]. In 2012 the European Medicines Agency (EMA) granted the authorization to marketing alipogene tiparvovec (Glybera®), a gene therapy treatment for lipoprotein lipase deficiency. Two more gene therapies for inherited diseases were recently approved; in 2016 the EMA approved Strimvelis, an ex vivo gene therapy approach for the treatment of ADA-SCID, and in 2017 the Food and Drug Administration (FDA) approved Luxturna, an AAV gene therapy to treat a rare form of congenital blindness.

Numerous interventional clinical trials on gene therapy mainly applied on cancer but also on monogenic disease are currently ongoing worldwide. Most of them are in the first phase of drug development (phase 1 and 1/2) to investigate safety and efficacy of these novel drugs (Fig. 44.1), although as the field of gene therapy is reaching maturity the number of phase III trials is increasing (source: ClinicalTrials.gov).

44.1.2 The Challenge of Treating Monogenic Disorders of the Liver

Several human diseases have a genetic basis, some caused by chromosomal abnormalities or mutations at multiple loci, while most caused by mutations of a single gene (Online Mendelian Inheritance in Man; 2017). Monogenic diseases (MDs) affect a substantial population, estimated by the World Health Organization, to amount approximately to 10 out of 1000 births (http://www.who.int/genomics/public/geneticdiseases/en/). Since nearly half of pediatric chronic liver disorders have a genetic cause and approximately 20% of pediatric liver transplantations are performed in children with MDs, the pediatric hepatologist is frequently challenged by inherited conditions, often orphan of a definitive cure (Fig. 44.2) [16].

Ideally, the goal of treatment for MDs is to revert the disease manifestations to a normal or non-harmful phenotype. In the last decades, several different approaches have been adopted for monogenic diseases, including substrate elimination diets, pharmacologic interventions to allow alternative pathway excretion of toxic metabolites, oral replacement of enzymatic cofactors, and the use of chelation to enhance excretion. A major step forward has been represented by enzyme replacement treatment (ERT) in those MDs caused by enzyme deficiency or dysfunction. However, ERT is usually extremely expensive and has to be maintained lifelong and, therefore, its cost-effectiveness may be questioned [17]. Furthermore, development of humoral immune responses in ERT in some case may lead to loss of efficacy over time.

So far organ transplantation (including auxiliary partial liver transplantation) has been used very effectively as "surgical gene therapy" and currently is the standard treatment for a variety of life-threatening MDs, offering often a cure, sometimes the improvement of the clinical phenotype [18]. Two key concepts that should guide this choice of treatment is whether there is extrahepatic expression of the enzymatic defect and parenchymal damage (Table 44.1).

Patients with MDs confined to the liver, such as Crigler-Najjar syndrome type 1 (CN1), Wilson's disease (WD), hereditary hemochromatosis, alpha-1 antitrypsin deficiency (A1ATD), and some urea cycle defects, can be cured by LT, either using an organ from a deceased donor or also by living donation from heterozygous relatives [19].

Patients with liver MDs expressed largely extrahepatically, such as defects of branched chain amino acids propionic acidemia (PA), methylmalonic acidemia, and maple syrup urine disease (MSUD), have been treated by LT with variable success. In these conditions, LT is intended to provide a source of continuous enzyme replacement to improve the phenotype, rather than correcting it completely [20].

In case of gene therapy, an appropriate timing is crucial, for several reasons. For instance, ornithine transcarbamylase deficiency may present acutely soon after birth, during childhood, or in adulthood (more frequently in hemizygous females). However during acute metabolic crises (for instance, in the neonatal-onset disease), the liver suffers from an acute toxic injury that causes liver necrosis and regeneration, a condition unsuitable for effective episomal gene transfer with non-integrative vectors (Fig. 44.3).

Another relevant aspect of gene therapy with vectors that do not integrate in the host genome relates to the fact that the liver grows progressively throughout childhood; therefore gene therapy delivered soon after birth (often an ideal timing to correct the disease early) ends up with loss of efficacy caused by the loss of episomal vector DNA in the transduced cells in a rapidly growing liver mass (Fig. 44.4) [21–23].

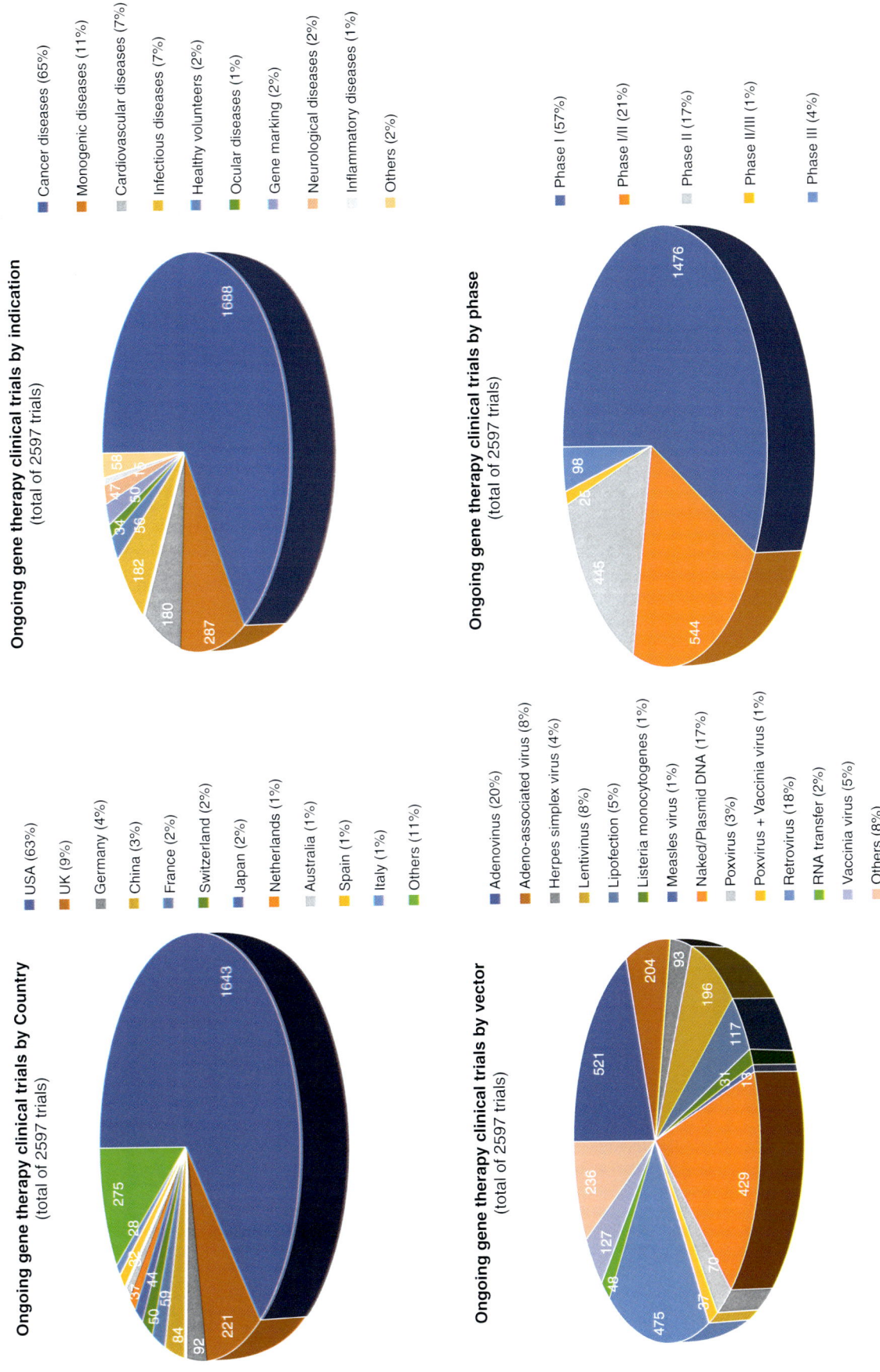

Fig. 44.1 Ongoing clinical trials according to country, indication, and type of vector (data retrieved from http://www.wiley.com//legacy/wileychi/genmed/clinical/, 2018)

Fig. 44.2 Indications to 626 pediatric liver transplants performed in Bergamo. *LT* liver transplantation, *WD* Wilson's disease, *HUS* hemolytic uremic syndrome, *UCD* urea cycle defects, *OA* organic acidemias, *GSD* glycogen storage disease, *PH* primary hyperoxaluria, *CN1* Crigler-Najjar type 1, *PFIC* progressive familial intrahepatic cholestasis

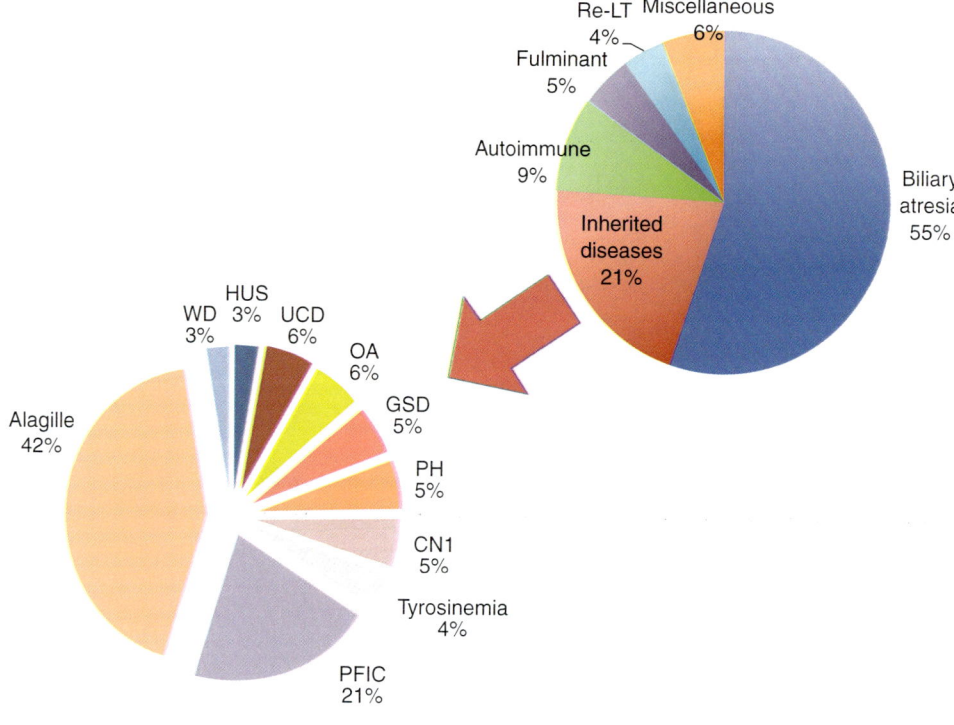

Table 44.1 Examples of monogenic disorders classified according to the extent of either liver or systemic dysfunction

Monogenic diseases with primary hepatic expression and parenchymal damage
Wilson's disease
Hereditary hemochromatosis
Tyrosinemia type 1
Alpha-1 antitrypsin deficiency
Argininosuccinic aciduria (ASL)
Glycogen storage disease type I (adenoma/hepatocellular carcinoma)
Progressive familial intrahepatic cholestasis (intestinal expression of the disease in PFIC1)
Monogenic diseases with primary hepatic expression without significant parenchymal damage
Urea cycle disorders (except ASL)
Crigler-Najjar syndrome (some fibrosis in adulthood)
Familial amyloid polyneuropathy
Atypical hemolytic uremic syndrome-1
Primary hyperoxaluria type 1
Acute intermittent porphyria
Coagulation defects
GSD type Ia (in metabolic control)
Homozygous familial hypercholesterolemia
Monogenic diseases with both hepatic and extrahepatic expression
Organic acidurias (propionic acidemia, methylmalonic acidemia)
Maple syrup urine disease
Alagille syndrome
Cystic fibrosis
Erythropoietic protoporphyria
Lysosomal storage disorders (Gaucher, Niemann-Pick, lysosomal acid lipase deficiency)

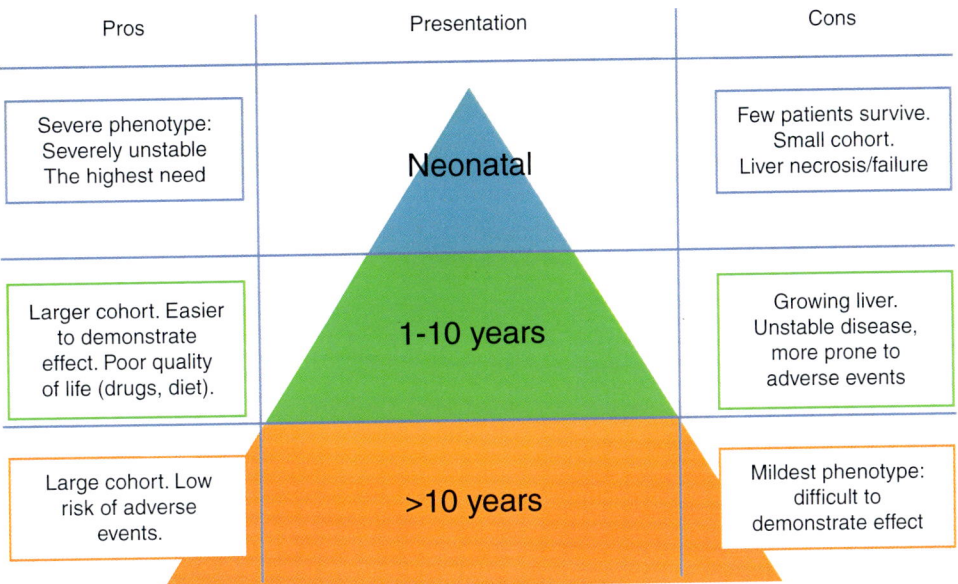

Fig. 44.3 Pros and cons of gene therapy applied at different ages in ornithine transcarbamylase deficiency

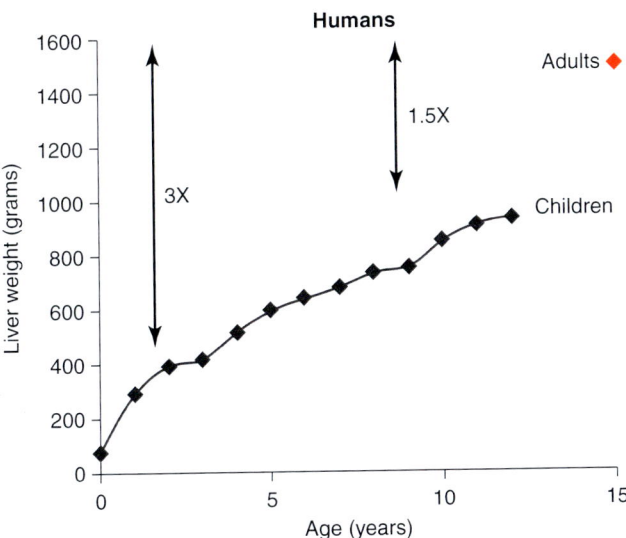

Fig. 44.4 Increase of liver weight by age in humans (modified from [24, 25])

44.2 Gene Therapy and Liver Gene Therapy

The liver carries out a wide variety of vital functions, including metabolism of proteins, lipids, and carbohydrates; synthesis of plasma proteins, such as albumin and clotting factors; formation and secretion of bile; and detoxification of body metabolites such as ammonia and bilirubin. Mutations of genes responsible for these functions result in many different disorders, most of them with very severe consequences [16, 26].

While the understanding of the molecular causes of most liver disorders has observed considerable progress over the past years, the development of therapies has been limited and mostly represented by enzyme replacement therapies (ERT). Consequently, liver transplantation remains the unique therapeutic option for most liver diseases, with important long-term risks, costs, and limitations. These concerns and shortcomings emphasize the clinical need to find alternative therapies to cure liver-related disorders.

Any strategy of liver regenerative medicine should take advantage of the experience gained with liver transplantation, which allowed challenging the capacity of a fully corrected organ to control each different MD. It is quite obvious that a disease having a phenotype expressed in extrahepatic tissues and that is not fully corrected by organ transplantation is unlikely to be successfully treated by a strategy able to target only part of the liver mass and replace only part of its enzymatic activity.

One attractive approach for the treatment of liver disorders is gene therapy. This procedure can be defined as the delivery of a nucleic acid into specific diseased cells in order to achieve long-term therapeutic benefit.

One relevant issue is represented by the presence/absence of liver parenchymal damage in the liver of the targeted disease and the phase of its course. In liver-based MDs characterized by a structurally normal liver, genes encoding enzymes that allow the regulation of complex metabolic pathways or circulating proteins may be more easily targeted, since the liver structure and the hepatocyte function are otherwise normal. In these conditions, the replacement of a defective protein with one producing the wild-type (normal) protein may successfully treat or prevent the systemic manifestations. In fact, the human syndromes amenable to liver gene therapy by gene replacement are, principally, monogenic recessive diseases with primary hepatic expression without liver damage, which can be cured by liver transplantation (Table 44.2). In such situations, the diseased phenotype can be corrected by the delivery of the therapeutic vector to hepatocytes. This strategy is likely to be much more challenging in MDs characterized by liver parenchymal damage and hepatic injury, since this represents a clear architectural limitation to cell correction by gene therapy using an non-integrative therapeutic cassette, bearing an increased risk of toxicity and loss of efficacy due to ongoing regeneration. Some of these diseases may require the permanent modification of the genome to avoid loss of the therapeutic DNA.

Several publications have reported proof-of-concept studies for adeno-associated virus (AAV)-based gene therapy in animal models of various inherited liver disorders, such as urea cycle defects, glycogen storage disease type Ia, organic acidurias, homozygous familial hypercholesterolemia, phenylketonuria, long-chain fatty acid oxidation disorders, progressive familial intrahepatic cholestasis, and primary hyperoxaluria type I [27]. A new era for gene therapy is therefore open, and this strategy seems to be back to the bedside to offer a concrete option to treat monogenic diseases of the liver on a large scale. Table 44.2 reports the best-suited diseases to be treated by gene therapy for liver-based MDs.

44.2.1 Vectors for Gene Replacement Therapy

Gene therapy by gene replacement consists in the addition of new genes to a patient's cells to replace missing or malfunctioning ones.

The first obstacle that gene therapy has to overcome is the efficient delivery of the transgene expression cassette to the target organ, by means of a vector containing the genetic material. An ideal vector should result in the efficient transduction of the target tissue/cell, leading to a sufficient, long-lasting, and safe expression of the therapeutic transgene [28]. The transgene expression cassette is commonly composed of (1) the therapeutic transgene, which may be a codon-optimized cDNA to achieve higher transgene expression; (2) a liver-specific enhancer/promoter, to determine high levels and liver-specific transgene expression; and (3) the presence an intron downstream of the promoter and a polyadenylation sequence downstream of the transgene to guarantee correct pre-mRNA processing and stability (Fig. 44.5).

The transgene expression cassette can be delivered by means of different methods/platforms, such as (a) naked

Table 44.2 Best-suited diseases for gene therapy initial approaches

Favorable features
Single-gene defects
Single organ involvement
Animal model available for preclinical proofs of concept
Therapeutic goal modest; an increase in plasma levels of 2–10% of physiologic levels would be sufficient to ameliorate the phenotype (i.e., hemophilia, Crigler-Najjar syndrome)
Efficacy can be assessed by validated routine laboratory assay
No advanced disease
Wide range of levels is likely to be efficacious and nontoxic

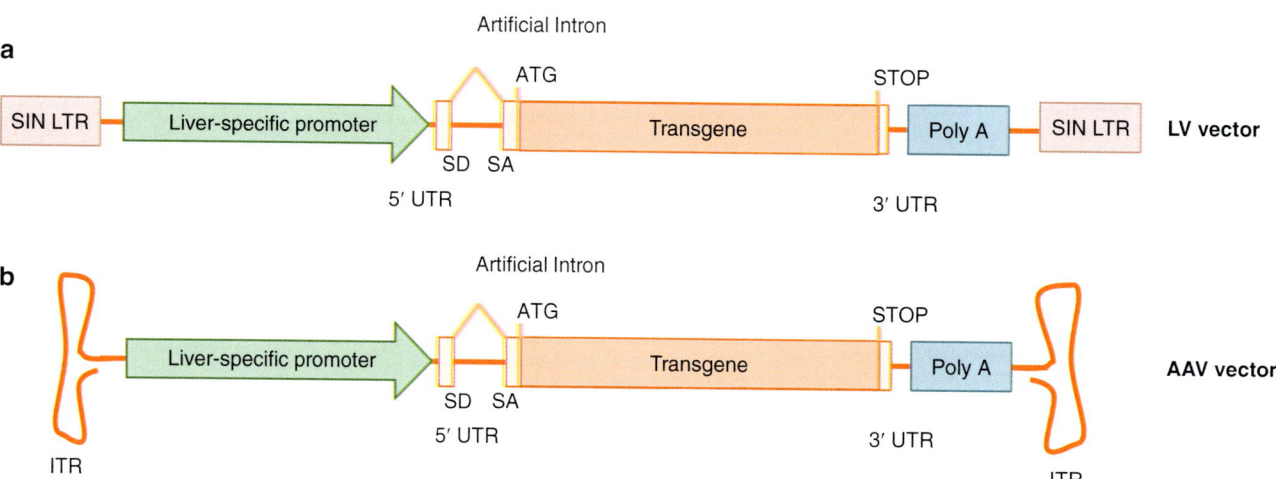

Fig. 44.5 Scheme of a therapeutic cassette based on self-inactivating lentiviral and AAV vector genomes. The therapeutic gene is transcribed under the control of a tissue-specific promoter, in our case a liver-specific one (green). The 5′ UTR contains an artificial intron to improve mRNA processing and transport to the cytoplasm. The transgene is often encoded by a codon-optimized version of the cDNA, to improve mRNA translatability. The transcribed mRNA is polyadenylated to improve mRNA stability and translation. Panels **a** and **b** shows the architecture of the construct in the case of AAV and LV vectors, respectively. The AAV vector contains an inverted terminal repeat (ITR) at each end, while the last generation of LV vectors contains self-inactivating (SIN) LTRs (SIN-LTR), in which the strong viral promoters are removed. The transgene, thus, is transcribed from its own promoter

Table 44.3 Ideal features for a gene therapy vector

Optimal vector features
Efficient transfection with a single infusion
Simple way of administration (i.e., peripheral vein)
Known molecular mechanism, delivery, expression, safety, tested in animal models
Low immunogenicity, both humoral and cellular
Low risk of DNA integration with activation of a pro-oncogene (insertional mutagenesis)
Vector persistence, function maintained over time (transfect stem cell or progenitors)

DNA, as either plasmids or mini-circles; (b) non-viral synthetically produced engineered nanoparticles, such as liposomes and polymers; or (c) viral vectors in which the viral genome is replaced by the transgene expression cassette. Table 44.3 lists the ideal features of vectors to be used in gene therapy for liver-based MDs.

44.2.2 Viral Vectors

While naked DNA gene transfer and liposome nanoparticles present numerous advantages in terms of ease of production, costs of the vector, and low immunogenicity compared to some viral approaches, these methods still require further optimization to be efficiently translated to the clinics [29]. The use of recombinant viral vectors represents today the most efficient approach for introducing genetic material into diseased tissues or cells, and, consequently, they have been the most frequently used delivery vectors in gene therapy studies, both at the preclinical and clinical level.

However, the use of viral vectors as delivery tools presents some limitations:

1. The presence of pre-existing anti-capsid neutralizing antibodies in those patients exposed to the virus from which the vector is derived. These antibodies can prevent the efficient transduction of the target organ.
2. Transduced cells are presented as "non-self" by the HLA complex, potentially raising an immune response that may result in their elimination. In addition, the generation of antivirus antibodies may also prevent the readministration of the viral vector in case of loss of therapeutic efficacy over time.
3. The vector DNA, containing strong gene promoters driving expression of the therapeutic cassette, can integrate into the host genome. This may result in misregulation of proto-oncogenes by insertional mutagenesis or transactivation, leading to tumorigenesis.

Below, a brief description of the most commonly used recombinant viral vectors is provided. These include vectors derived from adenovirus, retro- and lentivirus, and adeno-associated virus.

44.2.2.1 Retroviral and Lentiviral Vectors

Retroviruses are enveloped and ssRNA-based viral particles, which randomly integrate into the infected cell chromatin after conversion of their RNA into double-stranded DNA, providing long-term expression. The recombinant viral DNA genome has two long terminal repeats (LTR) at both ends, while the coding sequences for the *gap*, *pol*, and *env* viral proteins are replaced with the transgene of interest.

The ability of the vector to integrate into the host genome can be adopted to maintain the transgene information in a self-renewing context but could lead to insertional mutagenesis. However, under certain circumstances and with some specific integrating vectors, the integrated genome can lead to proto-oncogene transactivation and tumor development.

Gamma-retroviruses are unable to transduce nondividing cells as the nuclear membrane prevents retroviral vectors from entering the nucleus [30] and are more often considered for ex vivo gene therapy. Due to the high risk of genotoxicity as a result of integrational mutagenesis [31, 32], these vectors are generally not used in clinical trials. Self-inactivating versions of gamma-retrovirus were recently successfully tested in the clinic [33].

Lentiviruses (LV) are able to infect both dividing and nondividing cells because of the active transport of the pre-integration complex into the nucleus through the nucleopore [34]. The risk of pro-oncogene transactivation has been significantly reduced by the development of safer third-generation LV vectors, bearing self-inactivating (SIN) LTRs, in which the strong viral promoters present in the LTRs are deleted during the reverse-transcription process and the therapeutic transgene is expressed from an internal promoter [35] (Fig. 44.5a). The LV safer profile is associated with their preference to integrate in downstream regions within transcribed genes and the low preference to integrate in the 5′ regions of genes, at or upstream of the transcription start site, and in DNAse I-sensitive sites [36]. This, however, does not completely eliminate the associated risks, as strong enhancer-promoter elements are included in the vector constructs.

LV-based gene transfer has been extensively studied in humans in the context of ex vivo gene transfer trials [11, 12, 37, 38] and in some in vivo applications [39–41]. While no clinical data on liver gene transfer with LV vectors is available, recent published work has demonstrated the feasibility of the approach in a large-animal model of gene transfer for hemophilia [42–44].

44.2.2.2 Adenoviral Vectors

Adenoviruses are non-enveloped double-stranded DNA viruses, capable of transducing dividing and nondividing cells. Adenoviral vectors have a 36 kb genome, and recombinant adenovirus have a large cargo capacity to accommodate long transgenes. Viral DNA remains episomal, enabling long-lasting transgene expression in the transduced cells. Viral vectors based on adenovirus initially offered the potential of highly efficient, therapeutic in vivo gene delivery. However, important concerns on their further use were raised in 1999 after a young patient died following systemic inflammation and multi-organ failure, in a clinical trial to treat ornithine transcarbamylase deficiency [3]. Consequently, much of the focus of research and development of viral vectors has shifted toward the development of novel vectors that could combine low genotoxicity and immunogenicity with highly efficient delivery, such as lentivirus and adeno-associated virus for ex vivo and in vivo gene therapy, respectively.

44.2.2.3 Adeno-Associated Viral Vectors

Adeno-associated viruses (AAV) are nonpathogenic human parvoviruses with a 4.7 kb single-stranded genome, containing two inverted terminal repeats (ITR) at the extremities, and the *rep* and *cap* genes, which contain different ORFs and translation start sites [45]. In recombinant AAV vectors, a therapeutic expression cassette of about 5 kb is inserted between the ITRs in place of *rep* and *cap viral* genes (Fig. 44.5b). The resulting gene transfer vector can transduce both dividing and nondividing cells, with stable transgene expression for years in the absence of helper virus in postmitotic tissues [13, 46, 47].

Although wild-type AAV serotype-2 (AAV2) is capable of *rep*-dependent integration in the AAVS1-specific genomic locus, gene therapy AAV vectors are not capable of site-selective genomic integration [48]. Instead, after entry into the cell and second-strand synthesis, recombinant AAV forms high-molecular-weight concatemers or circular DNA that persist extrachromosomally in nondividing cells. The genomic integration of recombinant AAV vectors occurs at a low frequency into random sites [49, 50]. Reports of genotoxicity following AAV gene transfer in mice are contrasting [51–54]. While the risk appears to be minimal, also based on multi-year data in large-animal models [46, 55] and humans [13, 55] (Nathwani, personal communication to FM) treated with AAV vectors, long-term follow-up of patients will be required to address potential concerns of a link between wild-type AAV and hepatocellular carcinoma [56].

Several naturally occurring AAV serotypes have been identified, and countless AAV variants have been engineered in the lab [57, 58]. These AAV variants present unique immunological and gene delivery properties, with the viral capsid determining species and target cell tropism through interaction with a diversity of cell surface receptors/co-receptors [27, 59, 60].

Recombinant AAV vectors have emerged as the most promising gene delivery systems for gene therapy of monogenic liver disorders, having an excellent benefit-risk ratio [27, 61, 62]. However, they still have important limitations (reviewed in [63]), such as (a) pre-existing humoral immunity toward some serotypes, which limits the enrolment of patients in the gene therapy trials [64]; (b) the limited carrying capacity of AAV (5 kb), which limits their use in cases of large genes [65]; (c) the progressive loss of AAV viral genomes and expression over time in concert with hepatocyte proliferation [21–23], observed during liver growth in pediatric subjects or in the context of specific liver disease states causing hepatocyte proliferation; and (d) the immunogenicity of capsid proteins, which triggers generation of neutralizing antibodies that prevent the readministration of the therapeutic vector.

44.2.3 RNA Interference

RNA interference (RNAi) is an endogenous cellular mechanism for controlling gene expression. This is mediated by small interfering RNAs (siRNAs) of 21–22 nucleotides in length (dsRNA), promoting the cleavage of target messenger RNA (mRNA) with exactly complementary sequences by means of the RNA-induced silencing complex (RISC). Synthetic siRNAs versions can be introduced into cells and used to silence specific genes. In fact, siRNAs are routinely used in laboratory to silence genes in tissue culture cells. In addition, they can be also used in vivo as potent therapeutic drugs to silence disease-causing genes (Table 44.4).

Two paradigmatic conditions in which RNAi proved its efficacy are hypercholesterolemia and α-1 antitrypsin deficiency. Since null mutations of the PCSK9 receptor results in the reduction of plasma cholesterol (see Sect. 44.5.3.1 and Fig. 44.9 for a detailed description), a possible therapy is the reduction in PCSK9 mRNA levels by RNAi. In fact, delivery

Table 44.4 Comparison between gene therapy, RNAi, and gene editing approaches

Gene therapy by gene addition/replacement	RNAi	Gene editing
Restoration of the missing activity by viral/non-viral transduction of the therapeutic cDNA	Targeted repression of defective genes by knockdown of the diseased mRNA	Precise targeted modifications of the genome sequences, which are transmitted to daughter cells
Random addition of exogenous DNA into the genome (lentiviral vectors). Risk of insertional mutagenesis and tumorigenesis	Can be only used when gene knockdown is beneficial	Can be used to knockout endogenous genes, to correct the mutated gene or to insert a gene into a safe-harbor locus
Loss of viral DNA associated to cell duplication (AAV vectors). In this case requires readministration of therapeutic vector (not possible yet due to immune response generated by the first administration)	Transient effect. Requires multiple treatments Difficult to fully repress gene expression	Requires nucleases. Risks of off-target mutagenesis (lower with mRNA or protein delivery, or self-inactivating systems)

of lipidoid nanoparticles containing siRNA reduced PCSK9 mRNA levels by 50–70% in mice, rats, and nonhuman primates (NHP), with a rapid reduction of serum cholesterol levels of up to 50–60% of WT levels [66]. These results were essential for the development of a clinical trial in patients having high levels of LDL cholesterol in plasma [67, 68].

α-1 antitrypsin deficiency (AATD) is caused by the pathological accumulation of the PiZ isoform, encoded by a mutant allele of α-1 antitrypsin. Then, an approach based on the delivery of siRNA to hepatocytes of PiZ mice (see description of mice in Sect. 44.5.3.2 below) was effective to reduce the production of the PiZ toxic variant. This treatment ceased liver disease progression in short-term treatments, reverted the liver disease in long-term treatments, and prevented the development of the disease in young animals [69]. Administration of siRNA to NHP was also effective to decrease AAT production [69], paving the way to its application to patients in ongoing clinical trials (http://arrowheadpharma.com).

44.3 Animal Models of Liver Diseases and Gene Replacement-Mediated Therapeutic Approaches

Animal models are a powerful tool to study the pathophysiology of disease and to design effective therapies. In the last years, a number of small-animal models of liver syndromes have been generated, recapitulating the main features of human diseases. These strains proved to be fundamental for the development and optimization of novel gene therapy approaches, many of which conducted to successful clinical trials. AAV gene therapy vectors have been successfully used in numerous preclinical studies of liver-based monogenic diseases [62], for example, hemophilia A and B, acute and intermittent porphyria, Crigler-Najjar syndrome, ornithine transcarbamylase deficiency (examples are discussed below; see Table 44.5 for a more comprehensive list). For some of these diseases, proof-of-concept studies of AAV gene transfer were successfully translated to human trials [13–15, 70–73].

44.3.1 Hemophilia

Hemophilia A and B are monogenic X-linked disorders caused by deficiency of coagulation factor VIII (hemophilia A) or factor IX (hemophilia B) [74]. The incidence of hemophilia A is 1 in 5000 male live births, and that of hemophilia B is 1 in 30,000. Hemophilia is characterized by uncontrolled bleeding episodes mostly into soft tissues, joints, and muscles, which can be life-threatening in the case of intracranial bleeds [75]. Most hemophilia patients are severely affected, with less than 1% of residual factor activity. Increasing the levels of the missing coagulation factor to >5% by infusion of the recombinant clotting factors is sufficient to prevent spontaneous and life-threatening episodes [76].

The potential of liver gene therapy for hemophilia has been recently demonstrated in clinical trials in patients [13–15, 55, 72, 77]. These results were the consequence of the fruitful collaboration among numerous research groups for more than a decade, with the optimization of protocols and vectors in mouse and dog models of hemophilia A and B [78–83], including studies in hemophilia B mice and dogs with the hyperactive FIX Padua variants [84–87]. Importantly, a number of mouse models of hemophilia B have been generated bearing either null mutations (i.e., CRIM negative) or missense mutations resulting in the production of the defective FIX protein (i.e., CRIM positive). These models allowed detailed studies on the role of the genetic background in the overall risk of anti-FIX inhibitory antibody formation in protein replacement and gene therapy [62, 82].

Several studies were also published by Nathwani and colleagues in nonhuman primates (NHP), mice, and rats, using a self-complementary AAV8 vector encoding for FIX (scAAV8-FIX). In these studies, doses of 2×10^9 vg/mouse (~1×10^{11} vg/kg) resulted in circulating FIX transgene levels of 100% or normal, or 5000 ng/mL, while in rats and NHP a dose 10- to 100-fold higher of the same vector was necessary to obtain similar therapeutic effects [88–90] suggesting that AAV vectors exhibit a markedly different tropism for NHPs and human hepatocytes vs. mouse liver. More recently, this finding was confirmed using a human-mouse chimeric liver mouse model [58, 91].

44.3.2 Crigler-Najjar Syndrome

The Crigler-Najjar syndrome type I (CNSI) is a recessively inherited disorder caused by mutations in the UGT1A1 gene. It is characterized by severe unconjugated hyperbilirubinemia since birth, with accumulation of bilirubin in serum and lipophilic tissues, especially the brain [92]. Affected patients have a lifelong risk of developing bilirubin encephalopathy, which may lead to severe and permanent brain damage, and death by kernicterus if untreated. The disease is temporarily treated with phototherapy, but orthotopic liver transplantation is required in the long term [16, 93], a very risky procedure with several limitations.

A key animal model of this paradigmatic liver inherited disorder is the Gunn rat [94]. Gunn rats bear a spontaneous mutation in the exon 4 of the Ugt1 locus creating an in-frame premature stop codon, resulting in a nonlethal model of the Crigler-Najjar syndrome [95]. Despite the fact that these animals do not fully recapitulate all features of the Crigler-Najjar

Table 44.5 Examples of monogenic liver diseases with preclinical studies in animal models

Disease name	Gene symbol	Condition	Gene name	Estimated incidence	Mechanism of disease	Clinical features	Is OLT effective?	Current therapies	Animal models (ref)	Gene therapy approach (ref)
Acute intermittent porphyria	HMBS	Autosomal dominant	Hydroxymethylbilane synthase	1:50,000	Accumulation of aminolevulinic acid (ALA) and porphobilinogen (PBG)	Life-threatening acute neurological attacks (caused by recurrent nerve damage) with severe abdominal pain, hypertension, tachycardia, nausea, motor weakness, and transient psychosis	[112] Yes?	OLT, IV administration of hemin	[203]	[107–110, 204]
Alpha-1 antitrypsin deficiency	SERPINA1	Autosomal recessive	Alpha-1 antitrypsin	1:1500–1:3500	Absence of antitrypsin in the lung; presence of toxic aggregates in hepatocytes	Lung disease or emphysema, chronic obstructive lung disease (loss of function). Liver scarring or cirrhosis, pathological accumulation of unsecreted PiZ AAT (gain of function)	Yes	IV infusion of recombinant factor	[205]	[69, 206–210]
Citrullinemia type I (neonatal)	ASS	Autosomal recessive	Argininosuccinate synthase	1:57,000 (represent 13% of urea cycle patients)	Defects to dispose ammonia, resulting from proteins breakdown	Hyperammonemia with lethargy, poor feeding, vomiting or irritability, and tachypnea. Respiratory alkalosis, cerebral edema, seizures, loss of reflexes, hypothermia, apnea, coma, and death	Partially	OLT, diet, ammonia scavengers	[211, 212]	[213–215]
Crigler-Najjar syndrome	UGT1A1	Autosomal recessive	Uridine diphosphate glucuronosyl transferase 1A1	1:1,000,000	Accumulation of unconjugated bilirubin	Severe brain damage and death by kernicterus	Yes	OLT, phototherapy	[103, 104, 216]	[22, 97, 98, 100, 104, 105, 200, 217–228]
Familial hypercholesterolemia	LDLR	Autosomal dominant	LDL receptor	1:500 (het); 1:1250,000–1:1,000,000 for homo	Increase in LDL levels	Premature atherosclerosis, coronary artery disease	Yes	Statins, ezetimibe, lomitapide, diet, exercise, etc.	[229, 230]	[229, 231–237]

Hemophilia A	F.VIII	X-linked/recessive	Coagulation factor VIII	1:10,000	Defect in coagulation—lack of coagulation factor VIII	Bleeding following an injury, frequent spontaneous bleeding episodes, often into their joints and muscles. Life-threatening in the case of intracranial bleeds	Yes	ERT	[82, 238]	[129, 239–241]
Hemophilia B	F.IX	X-linked/recessive	Coagulation factor IX	1:25,000	Defect in coagulation—lack of coagulation factor IX	Bleeding following an injury, frequent spontaneous bleeding episodes, often into their joints and muscles. Life-threatening in the case of intracranial bleeds	Yes	ERT	[82, 242–245]	[42, 43, 79, 84, 189, 196, 197, 246–248]
Maple syrup urine disease (MSU)	BCKDHA (E1a), BCKDHB (E1b) or DBT (E2)	Autosomal recessive	Branched-chain hydroxy acids and keto acids (BCKA) Decarboxylase alpha subunit; BCKA decarboxylase beta subunit; dihydrolipoyl transacylase	1:185,000–290,000 (1:176 in Mennonites)	Inability to metabolize branched amino acids elevated branched amino acids in plasma	Frequent neonatal lethality, retarded mental development, severe neurological manifestations (encephalopathy, vacuolization and edema of the basal ganglia, brain stem and cerebrum, lack of dendritic development in cortex, and dysmyelination)	[249] Yes	OLT, dietary restriction of Leu, Ile and Val	[250, 251]	–
Methylmalonic acidemia	MUT, MMAA or MMAB	Autosomal recessive	Methylmalonyl-CoA mutase	1:120,000	Methylmalonic acidemia	Developmental retardation and chronic metabolic acidosis, hepatomegaly, and coma	Poor correction. Combined liver + kidney	Medical treatment, diet	[252]	[253–258]

(continued)

Table 44.5 (continued)

Disease name	Gene symbol	Condition	Gene name	Estimated incidence	Mechanism of disease	Clinical features	Is OLT effective?	Current therapies	Animal models (ref)	Gene therapy approach (ref)
Ornithine transcarbamylase deficiency (OTC)	OTC	X-linked/recessive	Ornithine transcarbamylase	1:15,000–70,000	Ammonia accumulation	Toxic effects of ammonia accumulation in the CNS: brain edema. Liver is the only site of complete urea cycle	Yes	OLT, ammonia scavengers, diet restriction	[259–261]	[115, 118–120, 122–127, 191, 261–264]
Progressive familial intrahepatic cholestasis (pfic1 to 3)	ATP8B1, ABCB11, and ABCB4	Autosomal recessive		1:50,000–1:100,000	Defects in transport of aminophospholipid, bile acid or phosphatidylcholine	Jaundice, growth failure, hepatomegaly, splenomegaly Hepatocellular injury and cholestasis, acute liver failure, fibrosis	Yes	Choleretic drugs, biliary diversion	[265, 266]	–
Propionic acidemia (PA)	PCCA/PCCB	Autosomal recessive	Propionyl CoA carboxylase	1:100,000 (in the USA); up to 1:1000 in high-risk populations	Defects to metabolize odd-chain fatty acids and some amino acids; acidemia	Metabolic acidosis, hyperglycinemia, ketosis, hyperammonemia with elevated levels of propionyl carnitine in the blood; serious brain injury; death	Partially	Medical treatment, diet	[267, 268]	[267, 269, 270]
Tyrosinemia type 1 (TT1)	FAH	Autosomal recessive	Fumarylacetoacetate dehydrogenase	1:100,000–120,000 (1:1846 in selected populations)	Accumulation of fumarylacetoacetate, resulting in mutagenic, cytostatic, and acutely apoptotic events	Deficiency in the metabolism of Tyr and Phe. Increased HCC risk and liver failure	Yes	NTBC, dietary tyrosine restriction	[271–274]	[187, 188, 201, 275–279]

Wilson's disease	ATP7B	Autosomal recessive	Copper-transporting P-type ATPase	1:7000	Increased intracellular copper concentrations, oxidative stress, free radical formation, and mitochondrial dysfunction	Liver pathologies as well as neurological and psychiatric abnormalities Cell death in the liver, brain, and other organs	Yes	Copper chelants, zinc	[280–283]	[284, 285]
Wolman disease	LIPA (LAL)	Autosomal recessive	Lysosomal acid lipase	1:100,000–500,000	Accumulation of triglycerides and cholesterol esters in lysosomes	Hepatic and adrenal failure, hepatosplenomegaly, diarrhea, and vomit leading to feeding difficulties, growth retardation, and cachexia	Partially	BM transplantation; ERT	[286]	[287]

syndrome, such as neonatal lethality, they were used to test numerous gene therapy approaches, ranging from naked plasmid administration to chimeric oligonucleotides, adenoviral-, lentiviral-, and AAV-vectors [96–100]. Crigler-Najjar syndrome, in spite of being very rare (incidence 0.6–1 per 10^6 live newborns), is a very attractive target for the development of gene therapy approaches as the genetic defect affects only the liver, without causing damage to the parenchyma, and correction is obtained both in humans and rodents by restoring 5–10% of enzyme activity, lowering plasma bilirubin to safe levels [101–103]. In addition, monitoring the efficacy of the treatment is rather simple, by determining bilirubin in blood and bilirubin conjugates in bile. Recently, a mouse model bearing the same point mutation of the Gunn rat was generated, and, remarkably, these mice presented neonatal lethality, more closely mimicking all features of the human syndrome [103, 104]. Long-term phenotypic correction was obtained by neonatal delivery of an AAV8 vector expressing the UGT1A1 transgene under the control of a liver-specific promoter [22]. Another recent study of adult administration of the same UGT1A1 transgene packaged into an AAV9 vector resulted in bilirubin levels similar to WT mice, suggesting the feasibility of the approach, at least in mice [105]. The optimization of the UGT1A1 expression cassette allowed successful treatment adult Gunn rats and neonate Ugt1$^{-/-}$ mice at relatively low vector doses, resulting in the long-term correction of the phenotype [100], supporting the use of this vector in a clinical trial for Crigler-Najjar syndrome.

44.3.3 Acute Intermittent Porphyria

Acute intermittent porphyria is an autosomal dominant inborn error of heme biosynthesis. Patients have life-threatening acute intermittent neurological attacks when hepatic heme synthesis is activated. Current treatments have important limitations, and the severe and recurrent porphyria attacks can be cured only by liver transplantation [106].

Gene therapy experiments in animal models [107–110] and clinical approaches by liver transplantation [111, 112] predicted the potential correction of acute intermittent porphyria (AIP) in patients. However, in spite of a dose tenfold higher than the one administered to hemophilia B patients [13, 55], severe AIP patients treated with a single intravenous dose of an AAV5 vector expressing a codon-optimized version of the human PBGD cDNA did not show a clear clinical benefit or a change in biochemical endpoints after viral transduction [71]. The reasons of the lack of benefits could be related to the lower transduction efficiency of the human liver by AAV5, compared to AAV8, as observed in NHP [90, 113], or to the requirement of higher levels of enzyme activity to rescue the phenotype, compared to what predicted by the studies in the animal models of the disease. Nevertheless, this first-in-human trial of AAV5 gene transfer showed clear evidences of safety and represented a stepping stone for other trials of gene transfer for hemophilia A and B, in which clear evidence of liver transduction was demonstrated [13, 14, 70, 71, 73].

44.3.4 Ornithine Transcarbamylase Deficiency

Ornithine transcarbamylase (OTC) deficiency is the most prevalent urea cycle disorder, affecting the catabolism of amino acids. It is caused by mutations in the X-linked OTC gene, which encodes for a mitochondrial enzyme OTC. Similarly to other urea cycle disorders, OTC deficiency results in hyperammonemia in the neonatal period. Unless immediately treated with ammonia scavengers, hemodialysis to remove ammonia, and specific diet, severe hemizygotes die of hyperammonemic coma, and survivors may develop neurological impairment. Orthotopic liver transplantation remains the treatment of choice for OTC deficiency.

Similarly to Crigler-Najjar syndrome, OTCD is an ideal model to develop liver-targeted gene therapy strategies: the liver has normal parenchyma, liver transplantation fully rescues the disease, the efficacy of the therapy can be easily assessed by measuring specific metabolites' levels in plasma or urine with routine biochemical analysis, and only a fraction of the WT enzyme activity is required to rescue the phenotype.

The Spf^{Ash} strain of mice bears a spontaneous point mutation at the donor splice site of exon 4 of the X-linked OTC gene that results in about a 20-fold reduction in *OTC* mRNA, protein, and enzyme activity [114], modeling the late-onset form of OTC deficiency in humans. More than two decades ago, adult Spf^{Ash} and Spf/Y mice were corrected by administration of recombinant adenovirus expressing the human OTC cDNA [115–120], providing preclinical support for the treatment of late-onset OTC deficiency patients. The use of a recombinant adenoviral vector, however, resulted in the tragic death of a patient due to a systemic inflammatory response [3, 121]. Safer gene transfer protocols based on AAV vectors have been recently developed, resulting in long-term correction of adult Spf^{Ash} mice [122]. Of note, loss of therapeutic efficacy was observed when mice were treated with AAV vectors as newborns, due to dilution of the therapeutic effect consequent to liver growth [123].

However, since the presence of residual OTC activity in these mice was a concern to assess the capacity of the gene therapy approaches to cure severe forms of the disease, residual OTC activity was knocked-down by AAV-mediated shRNA delivery [124]. In this model, AAV-mediated gene transfer was effective in adult Spf^{Ash} mice, but it was insufficient to prevent hyperammonemia in neonatal Spf^{Ash} mice, therefore, supporting the clinical translation of the approach only into adult patients [124, 125].

Additional preclinical data, in support of a clinical trial using AAV-mediated gene transfer into OTC deficiency patients, was provided by the group of Dr. J. Wilson who showed the increase in OTC activity and sustained expression using a codon-optimized human OTC cDNA in adult Spf^{Ash} mice [126, 127].

44.3.5 Animal models of liver diseases and therapeutic approaches: Concluding Remarks

The possibility to generate animal models of human syndromes, accompanied by the improvement in efficacy and safety of gene therapy approaches, resulted in several successfully liver gene transfer clinical trials [13–15, 70–73]. The most common approaches tested to date consisted in the replacement of the mutated gene responsible for the disease [79, 100, 104] (see Table 44.5 for other examples). However, as the field has gained more confidence in the liver gene transfer platform, a number of new approaches has been explored, including the use of truncated proteins [128], hyperactive enzymes [84], cofactors with longer plasma half-life [129], or secretable enzymes [130]. Some of these approached have been successfully translated to the clinic [15]. Several additional strategies, in which gene transfer is used to transform the liver in a factory for circulating enzymes that are then taken up by diseased organs [130, 131], are being tested and have the potential to transform the way protein therapeutics are delivered. Overall, the use of animal models is a "sine qua non" condition in the gene therapy field to generate preclinical data demonstrating safety and efficacy of these novel therapeutic approaches and to address current limitations of gene therapy [63].

44.4 Liver Gene Transfer in the Clinic

The liver is a particularly attractive organ for the development of gene-based therapeutic approaches for a number of reasons, including the fact that it is one of the body's major biosynthetic organs. Furthermore, studies in small- and large-animal models and in humans have demonstrated that it is possible to target hepatocytes with high efficiency using AAV vectors administered intravenously, obtaining multi-year transgene expression. From an immunological perspective, it is established that expression of a transgene in hepatocytes induces antigen-specific tolerance mediated by regulatory T cells [132–135], thus minimizing the risk of development of detrimental immune responses against the therapeutic transgene.

To date, liver gene transfer with AAV vectors has been tested in the clinic only for few indications, although the emerging results in the context of gene therapy for hemophilia A and B are extremely promising [13–15, 70–73].

In hemophilia, initial results in the dog model of the disease provided a strong rationale for targeting the liver to express the therapeutic factor IX (FIX) transgene [79]. Accordingly, in the first AAV-FIX liver trial, a single-stranded AAV2 vector carrying the human FIX transgene expressed under the control of a liver-specific promoter was administered through the hepatic artery in severe hemophilia B patients [72]. This trial has been particularly important for the field of in vivo gene transfer, as it demonstrated for the first time that it was possible to transduce the human liver with AAV vectors, leading to therapeutic levels of transgene expression. What was not anticipated by studies in preclinical animal models was the fact that liver expression in humans was not sustained. Specifically, following vector administration, an immune response directed against capsid proteins resulted in clearance of the transduced hepatocytes by CD8+ T cells and loss of expression [72, 136] (vide infra). An additional potential issue highlighted by this trial was that pre-existing immunity to AAV in humans in the form of neutralizing antibodies completely prevented liver transduction [72]. Following the results obtained in the AAV2-FIX trial, a second trial was initiated in which a self-complementary AAV8 vector encoding for a codon-optimized version of the FIX transgene was administered intravenously to target the liver of seronegative hemophilia B subjects [13, 14]. In this study, a short course of immunosuppression was used to block potentially detrimental immune responses triggered by the viral vector. This approach successfully demonstrated that it was possible to target the liver via the administration of an AAV8 vector delivered through a peripheral vein. Additionally, it showed that transient immunosuppression could be safely applied with gene transfer to avoid detrimental immune responses and leading to long-term expression of the transgene product. Despite their small size, these initial studies represented the fundaments of the recent clinical success in gene transfer for hemophilia A and B [13–15, 44, 70, 71, 73]. The experience AAV in humans has resulted in important knowledge on the safety and efficacy of liver gene transfer and allowed testing of strategies to achieve the goal of safe and long-term correction for a number of genetic and metabolic diseases. Moving forward, aside from extending the success of AAV vector-mediated liver gene transfer, the main goal for the field will be to ensure consistency and predictability of results across large patient populations.

44.4.1 Immunogenicity of AAV Vectors in Humans

One key concept when discussing immune responses to AAV vectors is that the viral *capsid* in AAV vectors is identical or nearly identical to the capsid of the wild-type virus to which humans are naturally exposed [137–139]. Thus, it is expected that the host immune responses triggered by vector administration will be similar to those associated with a natural

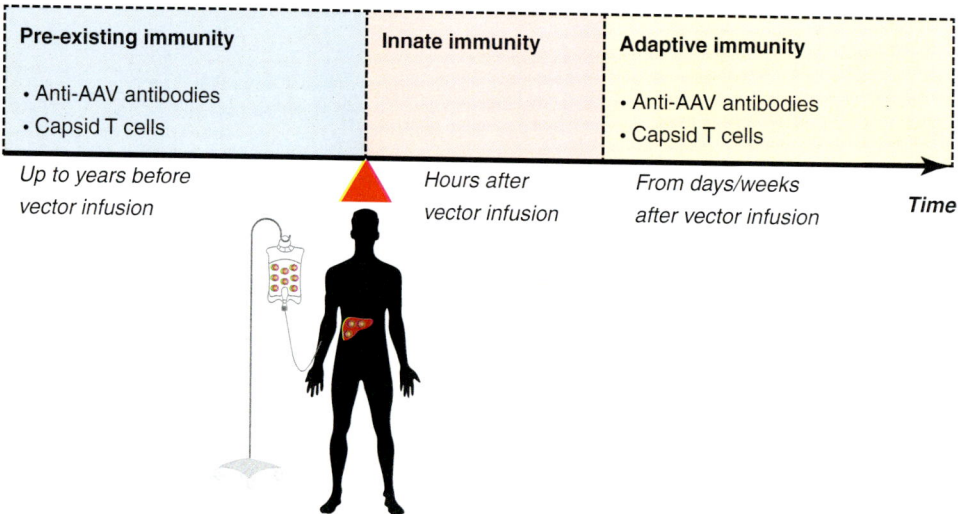

Fig. 44.6 Interaction of AAV vectors with the host immune system. Humans are exposed to wild-type AAV early in life, resulting in both humoral- and cell-mediated immunity to the AAV capsid. Thus, in gene therapy, except when naïve young children are treated, AAV vectors are administered in a context of pre-existing immunity. Starting from the moment the AAV vector is infused, recognition of the capsid and the vector genome by the innate immune system results in a chain of events that brings to the formation anti-AAV antibodies and, in some cases, activation of capsid T cells

infection with AAV, although the quantity of viral particles administered and their route of administration may contribute to the unique features on immune responses observed in gene transfer with AAV vectors (Fig. 44.6).

44.4.1.1 T-Cell Responses to AAV Vectors

Early liver gene transfer trials showed that cell-mediated immunity directed against the AAV capsid can play an important role in term of both safety and efficacy. In particular, in the first clinical trial in which an AAV2 vector was introduced into the liver of severe hemophilia B subjects [72], upon AAV gene transfer to liver, two subjects developed a transient and asymptomatic elevation of liver enzymes associated with loss of FIX transgene expression around week 4 after vector delivery. These observations were associated with the expansion of capsid-specific CD8+ T cells, which likely were responsible for the immune rejection of transduced hepatocytes [136]. A similar set of observations was also made in the context of several additional trials (reviewed in [140]); in some of these studies, timely intervention with oral corticosteroids was key to ablate the detrimental effect of the ongoing immune response on transgene expression [13–15], while in other trials, this approach was not efficacious [140]. Notably, results from both the trials conducted to date highlight important differences in the biology of AAV vectors of different serotypes, both in terms of doses required to obtain therapeutic efficacy and relative potential toxicities triggered by vector administration.

One important aspect of T-cell-mediated immune responses to AAV is that they seem to be detected in a dose-dependent fashion, a result consistent with published in vitro antigen presentation data [141, 142]. Above a certain threshold of capsid antigen load, activation of capsid-specific T cells may result in hepatotoxicity and loss of transgene expression, in some cases. It is not entirely clear at this point what other triggers influence AAV vector immunogenicity, as, for example, in some cases large doses of vector were administered to patients and increase in liver enzymes observed was not associated with immune responses directed to the AAV capsid [13, 14, 70, 71, 73]. The influence of vector doses and manufacturing on the immunogenicity of AAV vectors are currently a matter of debate, as the presence of contaminants deriving from the process used for AAV manufacturing (e.g., host cell DNA contaminants, plasmid DNA, etc.) is also a possible dose-dependent factor potentially influencing the safety profile of AAV vectors.

44.4.1.2 Humoral Immunity to AAV Vectors

The impact of neutralizing antibodies (NAb) directed against AAV on vector transduction has been first evidenced in the first AAV2-FIX liver gene transfer trial [72], in which one subject enrolled in the high vector dose cohort (2×10^{12} vg/kg) had a NAb titer to AAV2 of 1:2 and expressed peak levels of F.IX transgene of ~11% of normal, while another subject in the same dose cohort with a pre-treatment NAb titer of 1:17 did not have any detectable circulating FIX following vector administration. These results were also confirmed in preclinical studies, which showed that even low NAb titers can completely block transduction of the liver following AAV8 vector administration [143]. After exposure to wild-type AAV, a significant proportion of individuals develop humoral immunity against the capsid, usually starting around 2 years of age [138, 144, 145]. Thus, the window of time in which the majority of humans appears to be naïve to anti-AAV antibodies is narrow. Additionally, due to the high prevalence of anti-AAV antibodies in humans, and the cross-reactivity of these antibodies across AAV serotypes [137, 138, 144, 146, 147], anti-AAV neutralizing antibodies can have a profound impact on the efficacy of gene transfer and should be carefully measured prior to enrollment of perspective subjects in clinical trials. The issue of anti-AAV neutralizing antibodies is reviewed in Mingozzi and High, 2017 [148].

44.5 Advances in Correcting the Hepatocyte Genome In Vivo

The application of gene replacement therapy mediated by the delivery of AAV into the liver [13, 14] faces potential limitations such as the loss of genome copies—consequent to the episomal nature of the AAV DNA and its dilution/loss during hepatocyte duplication—especially when considering gene transfer in infants [21, 23, 103].

Genome editing, a possible alternative to gene addition to correct disease-causing mutations, is defined as the specific and permanent modification of the genome in a living organism. This is achieved by the insertion, deletion, or replacement of DNA at a precise site in the genome of a living organism or cell. Then, the corrected/edited genome is then transmitted to the daughter cells after proliferation, without loss of genetic information or therapeutic efficacy.

Genome editing has been a long-standing goal of gene therapy, but its application was initially limited by the low frequency of spontaneous homologous recombination [149, 150]. Accordingly, early attempts to rely on spontaneous rate of homologous recombination for the correction of mutations were only partially successful. For example, gene targeting in vivo by AAV8-mediated delivery resulted in frequencies of gene correction of about ~2.0×10^{-4} recombination events per hepatocyte in a mouse model of mucopolysaccharidosis (Sly syndrome) [151], far from any therapeutic application.

44.5.1 DNA Repair Mechanisms and Gene Editing

The ability to increase homologous recombination (HR) to therapeutic levels was discovered by M. Jasin's lab, who demonstrated that generation of double-strand breaks (DSBs) in the target genomic region results in the increase of more than two orders of magnitude in HR rate [152–154].

DSBs normally occur during the cell cycle, and cells have developed two main DNA repair pathways: (a) nonhomologous end joining (NHEJ), which is an error-prone mechanism active during all phases of the cell cycle, that may result in gene mutations by insertions and/or deletions (INDELs) (Fig. 44.7c) and (b) homology-directed repair (HDR), a high-fidelity DNA repair mechanism active after DNA replication in late S/G2 phases [155], that requires the presence of a homologous sequence acting as a template (Fig. 44.7d, e) [156].

44.5.2 Gene Editing with Engineered Endonucleases

With the progressive emergence of site-specific engineered endonucleases [157, 158], it became possible to take advantage of these cellular DNA repair pathways to introduce the desired modifications in the genome. These platforms enabled targeted and efficient modification of genes, making gene therapy by genome engineering one of the fastest growing fields [158]. The main platforms currently used are zinc finger endonucleases (ZFNs), transcriptional activator-like effector nucleases (TALENs), and, more recently, the clustered regularly interspaced palindromic repeats (CRISPR)/Cas9 system [159]. The introduction of a site-specific double-stranded break (DSB) in the genomic DNA can be followed by HDR-mediated efficient replacement of the desired sequence when a DNA donor template is present, or can result in gene disruption by NHEJ repair, with the introduction of small insertions or deletions [156] (Fig. 44.7).

44.5.2.1 Zinc Finger Nucleases

ZFNs are artificial, engineered endonucleases comprised of DNA-binding domain modules derived from a class of eukaryotic transcription factors (zinc finger proteins) fused to a non-specific DNA-cleavage domain of the FokI restriction endonuclease [160, 161]. Each zinc finger module recognizes a nucleotide triplet, and multiple zinc fingers (typically up to six) are joined together to target, virtually, any desired DNA sequence in the genome, making them ideal candidates for gene repair. Since the FokI DNA-cleavage domain must dimerize to be active, two ZFNs are required to generate a DSB (Fig. 44.8a).

Importantly, the first clinical trial of liver gene editing using ZFN is ongoing, in patients suffering from Hunter diseases (mucopolysaccharidosis type II, MPS II). A few patients have already been treated, but no data is available to date. Other clinical trials using ZFN will soon start, for hemophilia B and MPSI, both based on the insertion of a correct copy of the affected gene in the albumin gene, in a minority of hepatocytes.

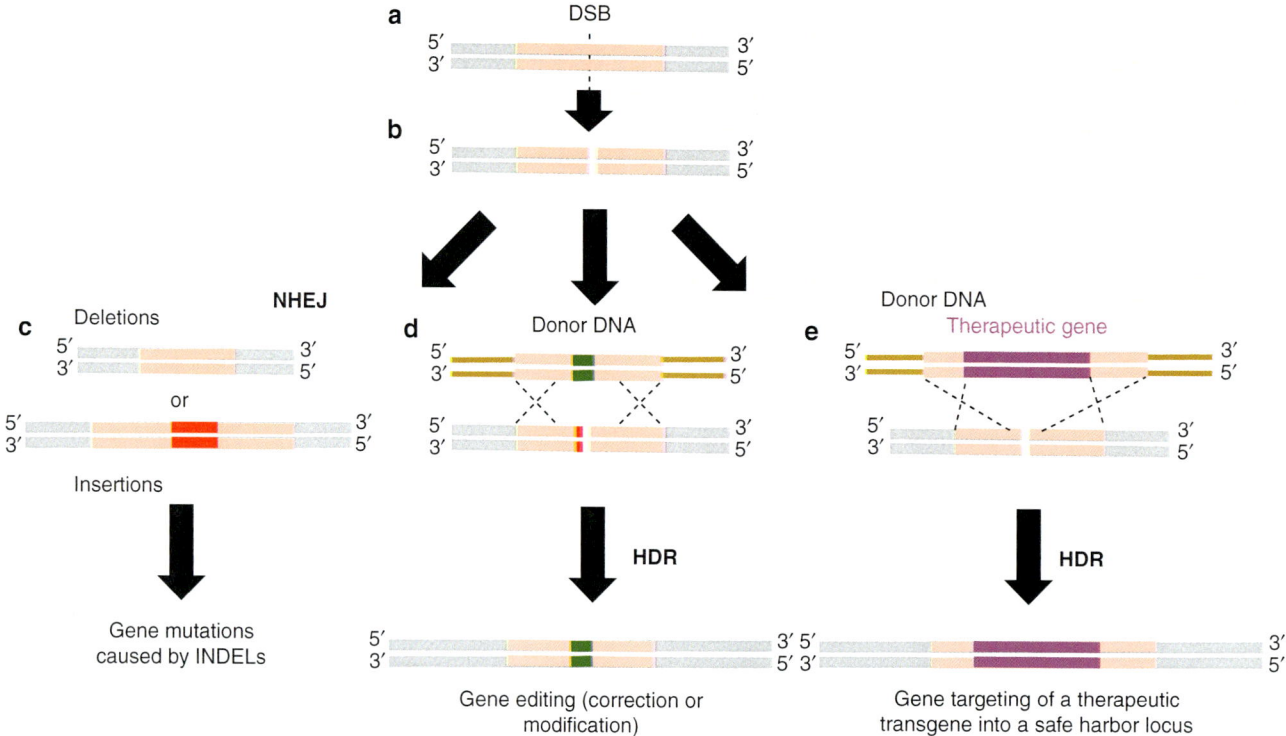

Fig. 44.7 Overview of possible genome-editing outcomes after the induction of a double-strand break (DSB). The generation of DSB (**a**, **b**) can be repaired by error-prone nonhomologous end joining (NHEJ) (**c**) or by the precise homology-directed repair (HDR) mechanism (**d**, **e**). In the presence of donor DNA having homology regions (orange), it is possible to edit the existing gene (**d**) or to introduce a transgene (purple) in the desired genomic region (**e**). Plasmid DNA of the donor construct is indicated by ochre thinner lines

44.5.2.2 Transcription Activator-Like Effector Nucleases (TALEN)

TALENs have generated much interest because of their simple design, high rates of cleavage activity, and almost limitless target range, making them viable options for a wide range of applications. Similarly to ZFNs, TALENs are chimeric enzymes composed by two independent domains: a DNA recognition derived from TALE proteins and a FokI nuclease domain [162]. TALEs are proteins produced by bacteria that bind to DNA sequences in the plant genome-activating transcription. The DNA recognition domain is composed of several modules made up of 33–35 aa [163]. Each module binds one single nucleotide with specificity dictated by two hypervariable residues (repeat variable di-residue, RVD) (Fig. 44.8b). The choice of each single domain and their combination let to target a desired sequence [164, 165]. Like ZFNs, TALENs must be also be used as dimers to generate DSBs. In spite of the simplicity in their design and apparently being more specific than ZFNs [166], the use of TALENs in gene editing was limited by the almost simultaneous development of the simpler and more versatile CRISPR/Cas9 platforms.

44.5.2.3 CRISPR/Cas9 System

RNA-guided nucleases (RGN) have revolutionized the ability of editing the genome of several organisms and, in particular, the clustered regularly interspaced short palindromic repeats (CRISPR)/Cas system has played a major role in this mean. The CRISPR/Cas systems were developed by bacteria and archaea as a kind of an adaptive immune system to protect themselves from invading foreign nucleic acids [167, 168].

The CRISPR/Cas type II system has been studied and characterized to develop genome-editing tools and strategies in eukaryotes due to its higher simplicity. It requires only two elements to specify Cas9 activity: the Cas9 nuclease for DNA cleavage and the single-guide RNA (sgRNA). The sgRNA has about 80–85 nt in length and is responsible for DNA recognition (20 nt that base-pair to the target DNA) and binding to the nuclease [169] (Fig. 44.8c).

The target site should contain, in addition to the 20 bases of homology with the sgRNA, a protospacer adjacent motif (PAM) at the 3′ of the target sequence, which is not present in the sgRNA. Consequently, any sequence in the genome can be potentially targeted, provided that the target sequence

are very easily produced; and (c) various sgRNAs can be delivered simultaneously, thus having multiple targets.

44.5.2.4 Limitations in the Use of Engineered Endonucleases

Genome editing has the advantage of permanently modifying the hepatocyte genome, assuring long-term correction even during hepatocyte proliferation, extensively occurring in neonatal/pediatric age and certain disease states, in which episomal vectors would otherwise be lost (Table 44.4). However, major concerns need to be addressed before their safe and efficient translation into the clinic. In fact, the clinical application of nucleases has several theoretical limitations: (a) the off-target activity of the nucleases, which can result in mutations and rearrangements leading to tumors; (b) immunogenicity of the nucleases used for gene editing and, in some cases, the presence of pre-existing immunity to the nucleases of bacterial origin; (c) low efficiency of homologous recombination in vivo in quiescent cells; and (d) when the delivery of nucleases to the target organ is mediated by AAV, the potential insertion of the DNA encoding for the nucleases (which has potent tissue-specific gene promoters) into the host genome, with the risk of insertional mutagenesis and transactivation of nearby genes, and tumor development.

To limit the risks of off-targets, different groups are working on the generation of high-fidelity Cas9 variants with more efficient on-target specificity, which reduced off-target rate to almost undetectable levels, still maintaining robust on-target cleavage [170–172]. Safety could be also increased by the temporal expression of the endonucleases in the target tissues, by means of mRNA/protein delivery, self-targeting versions and/or drug-controlled activity, in order to minimize long-term undesired effects [173–177]. Thus, application of high-fidelity endonucleases in a temporary manner will result in a significant reduction of the risks associated to gene editing, paving the way to their application in the clinic.

Additionally, genome-editing approaches require further improvements in their overall efficiency, especially in post-mitotic cells such as the adult liver, in which the mitotic index is less than 1% and the HDR repair system is less active, representing a major challenge in the field.

The further development of these technologies may result in potential therapies for many rare human disorders such as inborn errors of metabolism with no current available alternatives, for which just a low level of gene correction could be sufficient to reduce the accumulation of toxic metabolic products to safe levels. Some examples are described below.

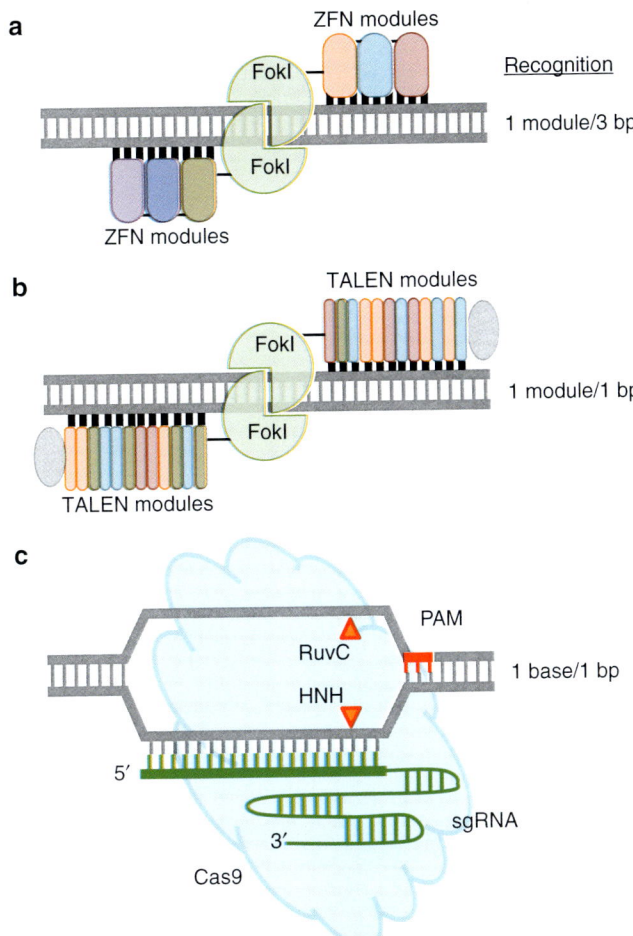

Fig. 44.8 Scheme of the main programmable engineered nucleases. Each monomer of the zinc finger nucleases (ZFN) is composed of zinc finger modules (each one recognizing three bases of the DNA), linked to a FokI endonuclease domain (**a**). The active ZFN is a dimer, due to the requirement of the FokI endonuclease. Each monomer of transcription activator-like effector nucleases (TALEN) is composed of several modules, each one recognizing a single base in the DNA (**b**). Similarly to the ZFN, they act as dimers. The clustered regularly interspaced short palindromic repeats (CRISPR)/Cas system is composed of a single-guide RNA (sgRNA) having 20 bases of homology with the target sequence and the Cas9 endonuclease, which has 2 active sites (HNH and RuvC). The protospacer adjacent motif (PAM) is adjacent to the homology region, but is not present in the sgRNA

is flanked by the specific PAM motif (Fig. 44.8c). CRISPR/Cas9 systems derived from different bacteria differ in the recognized PAM sequence.

The advantages of the CRISPR/Cas9 system versus ZFN and TALENs reside on the fact that (a) a single endonuclease is required, which is always the same (the Cas9 nuclease); thus no protein engineering is needed; (b) targeting depends on the canonical base-pairing rules, and the short sgRNAs

44.5.3 Gene Editing Approaches to Cure Mouse Models of Liver Diseases

44.5.3.1 Reprogramming Metabolic Pathways by Gene Inactivation

Hypercholesterolemia brings up an excellent example of the potentiality of reprogramming metabolic pathways by gene inactivation. Binding of proprotein convertase subtilisin/kexin type 9 (PCSK9) to the LDL receptor targets the receptor for lysosomal degradation, instead of receptor recycling to the plasma membrane, thus reducing LDL clearance from plasma (Fig. 44.9). Individuals with loss-of-function mutations in the PCSK9 gene presented a significant reduction of LDL-C levels (up to 80%) as well as CHD risk (88%) with no adverse clinical consequences [178–181]. Reduction of atherosclerosis was also observed in a Pcsk9 knockout mouse model [182]. These results provided, thus, strong support to therapeutic approaches based on the disruption of the PCSK9 gene by genome editing in cases of hypercholesterolemia. Loss-of-function mutations of the endogenous mouse Pcsk9 gene were introduced in vivo by CRISPR/Cas9 with high efficiency, reducing blood cholesterol levels [183]. The approach was also effective in chimeric liver-humanized mice bearing human hepatocytes in which the human PCSK9 gene was permanently inactivated by an in vivo CRISPR/Cas9 approach [184].

Gene knock-out mediated by CRISPR/Cas9 can be also used to inactivate a gene in a disease-associated pathway rendering the phenotype benign. This approach was applied in a hereditary tyrosinemia type I (HT-I, or FAH deficiency) mouse model, having a null mutation of the fumarylacetoacetate hydrolase (Fah) gene. When the Hpd (hydroxyphenylpyruvate dioxygenase) gene was deleted by in vivo treatment with CRISPR/Cas9, edited (Fah$^{-/-}$/Hpd$^{-/-}$) hepatocytes displayed a growth advantage over non-edited (Fah$^{-/-}$) hepatocytes and replaced the entire liver in only a few weeks. Inactivation of the Hpd gene rerouted the tyrosine catabolism, converting hepatocytes from HT-I to the benign HT-III [185]. Thus, reprogramming of metabolic pathways has the potential to overcome difficulties associated with editing a critical disease-causing gene and can be explored as an option for treating other diseases.

44.5.3.2 Editing of Genes That Confer Growth Advantage (Fah and Pizz)

Some liver diseases are caused by the intracellular accumulation of a toxic metabolite or gene product, leading to organ failure, as it happens in hereditary tyrosinemia or alpha-1 antitrypsin deficiency (AATD). In these specific cases, wild-type hepatocytes have a growth advantage over the mutated ones, allowing the repopulation of the diseased liver by heterologous hepatocyte transplantation.

For example, fumarylacetoacetate hydrolase (FAH) deficiency causes accumulation of toxic metabolites in hepatocytes, such as fumarylacetoacetate, resulting in severe liver damage and increased risk of developing hepatocellular carcinoma [186]. In spite of low gene repair frequencies by spontaneous recombination (which ranged from 1/6300 to 1/11,600 Fah$^+$ clones per hepatocyte in Fah^{5981SB} mice treated with AAV vectors carrying a wild-type genomic sequence for repairing the mutated Fah gene), the edited hepatocytes outcompeted their mutated counterparts, expanding the healthy "corrected" hepatocyte population and recovering a normal phenotype [187]. Much higher frequencies of gene repair were obtained after the systemic delivery of a donor oligonucleotide plus the CRISPR-Cas9 system into a mouse model of HT, bearing a one-base splicing mutation (Fah$^{-/-}$ mice). In this case, the proportion of corrected hepatocytes

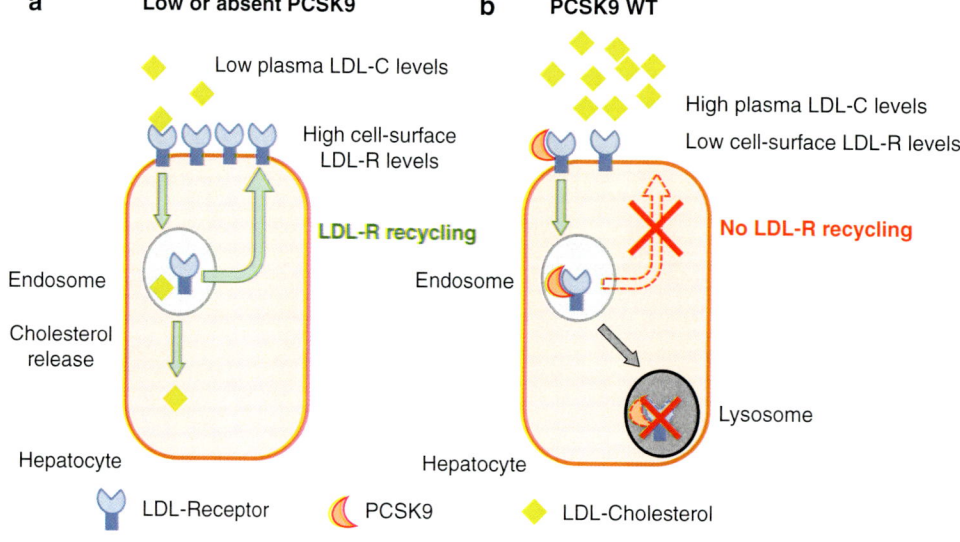

Fig. 44.9 Modifying a metabolic pathway by gene inactivation. In the absence of PCSK9 (**a**), cell surface levels of the LDL receptor (LDL-R) are high and circulating levels of LDL-cholesterol (LDL-C) low. The LDL-R is recycled back to the cell surface after delivery of the LDL-C to acidic endosomes. In the presence of PCSK9 (**b**), the LDL-R levels in the cell surface are low, and circulating levels of LDL-C high. The LDL-R complexed with PCSK9 is targeted to degradation in the lysosome

with initial expression of the wild-type Fah protein was in the range of ~1/250 liver cells which expanded, 1 month after injection, up to 33.5% of total hepatocytes [188]. These proof-of-principle experiments suggest that CRISPR-Cas9-mediated genome editing has potential for correction of human genetic diseases. However, further experimentation is still required to exclude the risks of HCC development by the presence of toxic metabolites in non-corrected hepatocytes or by off-target nuclease activities.

Similarly, in α-1 antitrypsin deficiency (AATD), one frequent pathologic allele, known as PiZ (p. E342K), results in protein misfolding and aggregation within the hepatocyte endoplasmic reticulum, with a loss of function in the lungs (deficiency of antiprotease activity) and a gain of function in the liver (accumulation of toxic PiZ aggregates). These patients, in addition of developing panacinar emphysema in the lungs, hepatocyte aggregate accumulation results in hepatocellular damage, fibrosis and cirrhosis, with an increased risk for hepatocellular carcinoma over time. Correction of PIZ hepatocytes by targeting a promoterless cDNA, without nucleases, into the albumin locus to mouse model of AATD, expressing the PiZ variant, results in the selective expansion of genome-edited hepatocytes, consequent to their survival advantage, with the improvement of the liver phenotype [189, 190]. In this case, the low frequency of spontaneous recombination is compensated by the growth advantage of the corrected hepatocytes. However, improvements in gene targeting efficiency or delivery strategies are required for other diseases that do not present selective advantage of corrected cells.

44.5.3.3 Correction of Hepatocytes That Do Not Present Growth Advantage

Recently, the feasibility to correct a point mutation in a gene-causing disease, in which the corrected cells show no growth advantage, was demonstrated by the successful application of the CRISPR/Cas9 platform to correct the OTC gene in spf^{ash} mice [191] (see Sect. 44.3.4 for a description of the animal model). Neonatal administration of two AAVs, one carrying the Cas9 endonuclease, and the second one carrying both the sgRNA and the donor DNA, resulted in the reversion of the mutation in about 10% of hepatocytes increasing survival when challenged with a high-protein diet. Importantly, in those animals the levels of Cas9 decreased over time, consequent to liver growth and viral DNA dilution.

However, when adult Spf^{Ash} mice were treated, the efficiency of gene correction in adult OTC-deficient mice was lower and, unexpectedly, resulted in a more severe phenotype than the initially present with the subtle mutation, with diminished protein tolerance and lethal hyperammonemia on a chow diet. This was caused by the generation of large deletions that ablated residual expression from the endogenous *Otc* gene by means of Cas9 endonuclease activity not followed by HR-mediated correction, a correction mechanism less active in non-replicating cells [191].

These results, on one hand, provide evidence for efficacy of an in vivo gene editing therapeutic approach in a neonate animal model of a lethal human disease, in which the corrected hepatocytes do not have any selective advantage. On the other hand, they confirm that homologous recombination in adults is a major challenge in the field. In fact, gene editing in adults still needs further improvements to increase homologous recombination rate to therapeutic levels, limiting the concerns of INDEL generation or chromosomal rearrangements in the target locus by error-prone NHEJ-mediated DSB repair.

Importantly, the correction of disease-causing mutations requires a specific setup for each case, suggesting that the application of this approach may be limited to specific diseases in which just a few mutations are responsible for the diseased phenotype.

44.5.3.4 Correction of the Genetic Defect by Targeting a "Safe-Harbor Locus"

An alternative methodology overcoming these concerns is based in the insertion of a therapeutic cDNA into a "safe-harbor locus" to correct the genetic defect. In this way, a single therapeutic approach can be applied to correct most existing mutations in that diseased gene. A safe-harbor locus can be defined as a gene/chromosomal location in which the insertion of a transgene has no aberrant physiologic consequences and the transgene can be expressed at the levels necessary to achieve therapeutic efficacy. Different loci have been tested so far in mice, such as the Rosa26 [30, 192] and the *PPP1R12C* loci, also referred as *AAVS1*, which is the integration site of wild-type adeno-associated virus (AAV) into the human genome [193–195]. Recently, the albumin gene was identified as a suitable candidate locus for inserting therapeutic genes in hepatocytes. In fact, albumin is expressed at high levels in hepatocytes, which guarantees both liver specificity and high expression of the therapeutic cDNA for the duration of life.

Using these platforms, different approaches were designed to treat preclinical models of hemophilia B, ornithine transcarbamylase deficiency, tyrosinase deficiency, Crigler-Najjar syndrome type I, and other syndromes.

The group of K. High pioneered genome editing of coagulation factor IX deficiency (hemophilia B) using ZFNs. In their first approach, they used ZFNs to correct mutated hFIX cDNA inserted in the Rosa26 locus of neonate and adult mice [196, 197]. In these mice, the endogenous murine FIX gene is inactive [196]. This strategy resulted in phenotypic correction of hemophilia B with the production of up to 4–6% of normal hFIX levels in plasma in neonates [196] and up to 25% of normal hFIX levels in adults [197].

In a second approach, a promoterless WT hFIX cDNA (lacking the first exon) was inserted in the first intron of the endogenous albumin locus with the use of ZFNs. Targeted recombination resulted in the production of a hybrid mRNA, under the transcriptional control of the robust albumin promoter, in which the first albumin exon is fused in frame with the hFIX ORF. In spite that the hybrid mAlb-hF9 mRNA represented a small fraction (0.5%) of total wild-type mAlb transcript, circulating hFIX reached supraphysiological levels of FIX with the higher AAV doses, with no significant effect on albumin production [198]. The same strategy was applied for the functional correction of hemophilia A phenotype in hemophilia A mice with a donor DNA encoding a truncated variant of hFVIII, and for the production of functional GBA lysosomal enzyme in WT animals, setting the basis for a systemic treatment of the non-neuronal forms of lysosomal storage diseases, such as Gaucher and Fabry diseases. Sangamo Therapeutics is presently applying this strategy in a phase I/II clinical trial for MPSII and hemophilia B.

The major challenges to clinical translation of genome-editing technologies regard specificity and safety of these approaches. Specificity is one of the main safety concerns, due to the permanent nature of the genetic modifications. Deleterious nuclease-generated off-target mutations could result in cells with oncogenic potential, leading to the expansion of edited cells and tumor formation. In addition, off-target insertional mutagenesis of both transgene and endonuclease vectors may lead to transactivation of nearby genes, including oncogenes, by the strong gene promoters driving expression of nucleases and transgenes in the vectors, potentially resulting in tumor formation [31, 32, 51, 53]. Therefore, even low levels of off-target mutagenesis may have devastating consequences. Other concerns are related to potential immunogenicity of the endonuclease [199].

To prevent most of the abovementioned concerns, the group of M. Kay developed a targeting strategy without the use of nucleases [189]. This approach, based on the spontaneous insertion of the therapeutic cDNA just upstream of the albumin stop codon, results in a fused mRNA that is translated into two separated proteins: albumin and the therapeutic protein, in this case coagulation factor IX [189] (Fig. 44.10). Treatment of neonatal and adult mice with AAV vectors delivering the targeting construct resulted in about 0.5% of recombined hepatocytes. This low recombination frequency

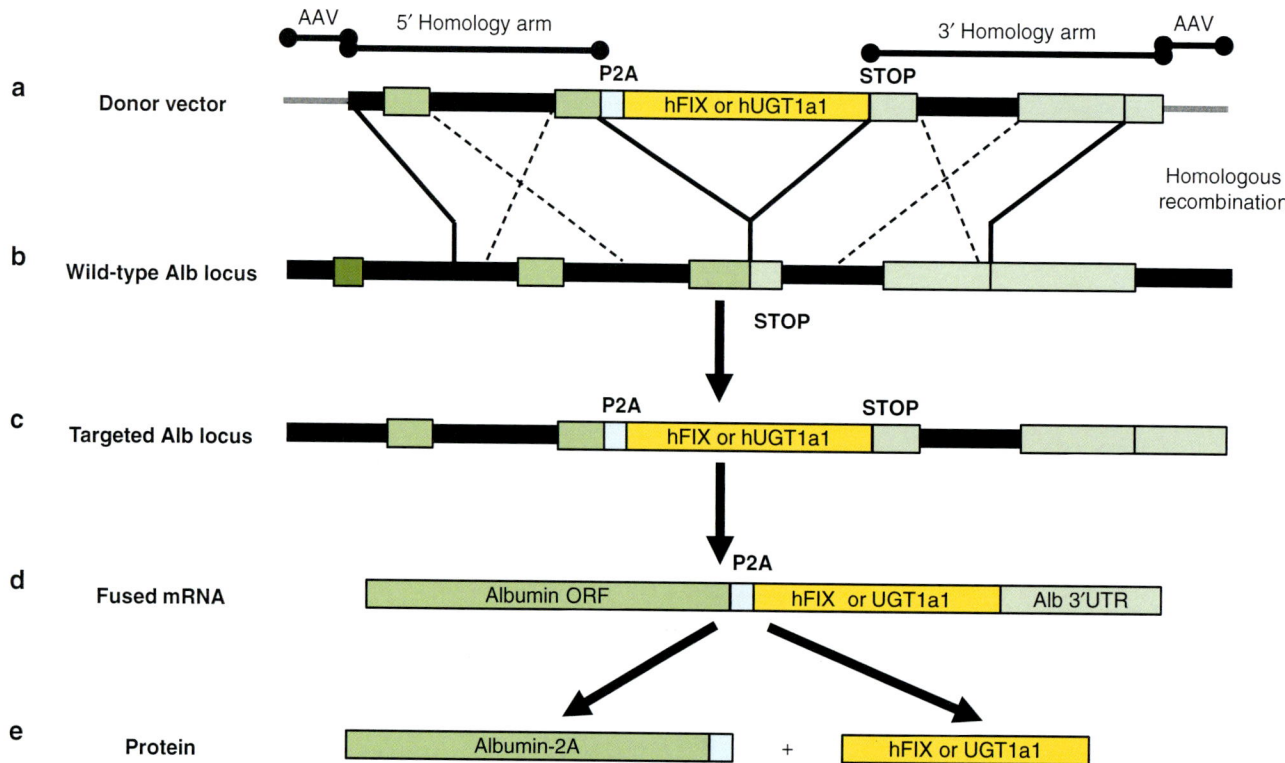

Fig. 44.10 Strategy for gene targeting in the albumin locus. Vector design and experimental scheme. The donor vector (**a**) (AAV8) has regions of homology (5′ and 3′ homology arms) that allow site-specific recombination into the wild-type albumin locus (**b**). The donor vector contains the hFIX or the WT human UGT1A1 cDNAs, preceded by the 2A-peptide, and flanked by albumin gene homology arms. Site-specific recombination (**c**) results in a targeted locus that is transcribed under the control of the endogenous albumin promoter. Then, a fused "chimeric bi-cistronic" mRNA (**d**) is transcribed and is translated into two separate proteins (**e**). Rectangles represent exons; thick black lines, introns, and intergenic regions; thin gray lines, extragenic DNA sequences. Modified from Barzel et al. [189]

was compensated by the robust production of coagulation factor IX (under the control of the albumin promoter), reaching up to 20% of WT circulating plasma levels in humans, potentially enough to rescue the severe hemophilia B phenotype. Recombinant hepatocytes, which do not have any growth advantage, were able to transmit the edited albumin locus to daughter hepatocytes, supporting long-term protection.

The same approach was applied to a lethal mouse model of Crigler-Najjar syndrome type I, resulting in the complete rescue of neonatal lethality and cerebellar and behavioral abnormalities, with stable low plasma bilirubin levels even 12 months after AAV delivery [200] (Fig. 44.10). Although this strategy may not be widely applicable owing to the low absolute targeting rate, this and future improved strategies should be also considered for therapeutic applications.

An approach conferring a selective advantage to the recombinant hepatocytes that, therefore, can be selectively expanded, was recently developed by the group of M. Grompe, reaching supraphysiological levels of human FIX in mice [201]. However, this method requires temporary treatment of patients with a hepatotoxic drug, raising ethical and safety concerns that may require further studies before its potential translation into the clinics.

44.5.4 Gene Editing: Concluding Remarks

Many of the inherited metabolic disorders of the liver are caused by a single-gene mutation (Online Mendelian Inheritance in Man; *2017*) and present neonatal or pediatric onset. To date, the only effective curative treatment for many of these diseases is liver transplantation [16], which holds several risks and shortcomings [202]. Gene therapy approaches mediated by viral transduction of the therapeutic gene to neonates and juvenile patients still have important limitations, such as vector loss during cell proliferation, in the case of AAV vectors, or insertional mutagenesis caused by the integration of the vector, in the case of lentiviral vectors (concern also present in adult delivery). Therefore, the possibility to stably correct or edit the genome is a very promising therapeutic alternative that has emerged in the recent years. However, these procedures still present important challenges that need to be addressed before their extensive application to patients suffering from genetic diseases of the liver.

References

1. Blaese RM, Culver KW, Miller AD, Carter CS, Fleisher T, Clerici M, et al. T lymphocyte-directed gene therapy for ADA- SCID: initial trial results after 4 years. Science. 1995;270(5235):475–80.
2. Bordignon C, Notarangelo LD, Nobili N, Ferrari G, Casorati G, Panina P, et al. Gene therapy in peripheral blood lymphocytes and bone marrow for ADA- immunodeficient patients. Science. 1995;270(5235):470–5.
3. Raper SE, Chirmule N, Lee FS, Wivel NA, Bagg A, Gao GP, et al. Fatal systemic inflammatory response syndrome in a ornithine transcarbamylase deficient patient following adenoviral gene transfer. Mol Genet Metab. 2003;80(1–2):148–58.
4. Cavazzana-Calvo M, Hacein-Bey S, de Saint Basile G, Gross F, Yvon E, Nusbaum P, et al. Gene therapy of human severe combined immunodeficiency (SCID)-X1 disease. Science. 2000;288(5466):669–72.
5. Hacein-Bey-Abina S, von Kalle C, Schmidt M, Le Deist F, Wulffraat N, McIntyre E, et al. A serious adverse event after successful gene therapy for X-linked severe combined immunodeficiency. N Engl J Med. 2003;348(3):255–6.
6. Mukherjee S, Thrasher AJ. Gene therapy for PIDs: progress, pitfalls and prospects. Gene. 2013;525(2):174–81.
7. Mingozzi F, High KA. Immune responses to AAV in clinical trials. Curr Gene Ther. 2007;7(5):316–24.
8. Russell S, Bennett J, Wellman JA, Chung DC, Yu ZF, Tillman A, et al. Efficacy and safety of voretigene neparvovec (AAV2-hRPE65v2) in patients with RPE65-mediated inherited retinal dystrophy: a randomised, controlled, open-label, phase 3 trial. Lancet. 2017;390(10097):849–60.
9. Bainbridge JW, Smith AJ, Barker SS, Robbie S, Henderson R, Balaggan K, et al. Effect of gene therapy on visual function in Leber's congenital amaurosis. N Engl J Med. 2008;358(21):2231–9.
10. Maguire AM, Simonelli F, Pierce EA, Pugh EN Jr, Mingozzi F, Bennicelli J, et al. Safety and efficacy of gene transfer for Leber's congenital amaurosis. N Engl J Med. 2008;358(21):2240–8.
11. Cartier N, Hacein-Bey-Abina S, Bartholomae CC, Veres G, Schmidt M, Kutschera I, et al. Hematopoietic stem cell gene therapy with a lentiviral vector in X-linked adrenoleukodystrophy. Science. 2009;326(5954):818–23.
12. Biffi A, Montini E, Lorioli L, Cesani M, Fumagalli F, Plati T, et al. Lentiviral hematopoietic stem cell gene therapy benefits metachromatic leukodystrophy. Science. 2013;341(6148):1233158.
13. Nathwani AC, Reiss UM, Tuddenham EG, Rosales C, Chowdary P, McIntosh J, et al. Long-term safety and efficacy of factor IX gene therapy in hemophilia B. N Engl J Med. 2014;371(21):1994–2004.
14. Nathwani AC, Tuddenham EG, Rangarajan S, Rosales C, McIntosh J, Linch DC, et al. Adenovirus-associated virus vector-mediated gene transfer in hemophilia B. N Engl J Med. 2011;365(25):2357–65.
15. George LA, Sullivan SK, Giermasz A, Rasko JEJ, Samelson-Jones BJ, Ducore J, et al. Hemophilia B gene therapy with a high-specific-activity factor IX variant. N Engl J Med. 2017;377(23):2215–27.
16. Fagiuoli S, Daina E, D'Antiga L, Colledan M, Remuzzi G. Monogenic diseases that can be cured by liver transplantation. J Hepatol. 2013;59(3):595–612.
17. Lachmann RH. Enzyme replacement therapy for lysosomal storage diseases. Curr Opin Pediatr. 2011;23(6):588–93.
18. D'Antiga L, Colledan M. Surgical gene therapy by domino auxiliary liver transplantation. Liver Transplant. 2015;21(11):1338–9.
19. Kasahara M, Sakamoto S, Horikawa R, Koji U, Mizuta K, Shinkai M, et al. Living donor liver transplantation for pediatric patients with metabolic disorders: the Japanese multicenter registry. Pediatr Transplant. 2014;18(1):6–15.
20. Vara R, Turner C, Mundy H, Heaton ND, Rela M, Mieli-Vergani G, et al. Liver transplantation for propionic acidemia in children. Liver Transplant. 2011;17(6):661–7.
21. Wang L, Wang H, Bell P, McMenamin D, Wilson JM. Hepatic gene transfer in neonatal mice by adeno-associated virus serotype 8 vector. Hum Gene Ther. 2012;23(5):533–9.
22. Bortolussi G, Zentilin L, Vanikova J, Bockor L, Bellarosa C, Mancarella A, et al. Life-long correction of hyperbilirubinemia

22. with a neonatal liver-specific AAV-mediated gene transfer in a lethal mouse model of Crigler Najjar syndrome. Hum Gene Ther. 2014;25(9):844–55.
23. Cunningham SC, Dane AP, Spinoulas A, Logan GJ, Alexander IE. Gene delivery to the juvenile mouse liver using AAV2/8 vectors. Mol Ther. 2008;16(6):1081–8.
24. Coppoletta JM, Wolbach SB. Body length and organ weights of infants and children: a study of the body length and normal weights of the more important vital organs of the body between birth and twelve years of age. Am J Pathol. 1933;9(1):55–70.
25. Garby L, Lammert O, Kock KF, Thobo-Carlsen B. Weights of brain, heart, liver, kidneys, and spleen in healthy and apparently healthy adult Danish subjects. Am J Hum Biol. 1993;5(3):291–6.
26. Hansen K, Horslen S. Metabolic liver disease in children. Liver Transplant. 2008;14(4):391–411.
27. Junge N, Mingozzi F, Ott M, Baumann U. Adeno-associated virus vector-based gene therapy for monogenetic metabolic diseases of the liver. J Pediatr Gastroenterol Nutr. 2015;60(4):433–40.
28. Kay MA, Glorioso JC, Naldini L. Viral vectors for gene therapy: the art of turning infectious agents into vehicles of therapeutics. Nat Med. 2001;7(1):33–40.
29. Hardee CL, Arevalo-Soliz LM, Hornstein BD, Zechiedrich L. Advances in non-viral DNA vectors for gene therapy. Genes. 2017;8(2):65.
30. Miller DG, Adam MA, Miller AD. Gene transfer by retrovirus vectors occurs only in cells that are actively replicating at the time of infection. Mol Cell Biol. 1990;10(8):4239–42.
31. Hacein-Bey-Abina S, Garrigue A, Wang GP, Soulier J, Lim A, Morillon E, et al. Insertional oncogenesis in 4 patients after retrovirus-mediated gene therapy of SCID-X1. J Clin Invest. 2008;118(9):3132–42.
32. Hacein-Bey-Abina S, Von Kalle C, Schmidt M, McCormack MP, Wulffraat N, Leboulch P, et al. LMO2-associated clonal T cell proliferation in two patients after gene therapy for SCID-X1. Science. 2003;302(5644):415–9.
33. Ribeil JA, Hacein-Bey-Abina S, Payen E, Magnani A, Semeraro M, Magrin E, et al. Gene therapy in a patient with sickle cell disease. N Engl J Med. 2017;376(9):848–55.
34. Suzuki Y, Craigie R. The road to chromatin—nuclear entry of retroviruses. Nat Rev Microbiol. 2007;5(3):187–96.
35. Naldini L. Ex vivo gene transfer and correction for cell-based therapies. Nat Rev Genet. 2011;12(5):301–15.
36. Kotterman MA, Chalberg TW, Schaffer DV. Viral vectors for gene therapy: translational and clinical outlook. Annu Rev Biomed Eng. 2015;17:63–89.
37. Aiuti A, Biasco L, Scaramuzza S, Ferrua F, Cicalese MP, Baricordi C, et al. Lentiviral hematopoietic stem cell gene therapy in patients with Wiskott-Aldrich syndrome. Science. 2013;341(6148):1233151.
38. Cavazzana-Calvo M, Payen E, Negre O, Wang G, Hehir K, Fusil F, et al. Transfusion independence and HMGA2 activation after gene therapy of human beta-thalassaemia. Nature. 2010;467(7313):318–22.
39. Campochiaro PA, Lauer AK, Sohn EH, Mir TA, Naylor S, Anderton MC, et al. Lentiviral vector gene transfer of endostatin/angiostatin for macular degeneration (GEM) study. Hum Gene Ther. 2017;28(1):99–111.
40. Dalkara D, Goureau O, Marazova K, Sahel JA. Let there be light: gene and Cell therapy for blindness. Hum Gene Ther. 2016;27(2):134–47.
41. Palfi S, Gurruchaga JM, Ralph GS, Lepetit H, Lavisse S, Buttery PC, et al. Long-term safety and tolerability of ProSavin, a lentiviral vector-based gene therapy for Parkinson's disease: a dose escalation, open-label, phase 1/2 trial. Lancet. 2014;383(9923):1138–46.
42. Cantore A, Annoni A, Lui T, Bartolaccini S, Biffi M, Russo F, et al. Liver-directed gene therapy for hemophilia B with immune stealth lentiviral vectors. Blood. 2017;130(Suppl 1):605.
43. Cantore A, Ranzani M, Bartholomae CC, Volpin M, Valle PD, Sanvito F, et al. Liver-directed lentiviral gene therapy in a dog model of hemophilia B. Sci Transl Med. 2015;7(277):277ra28.
44. Milani M, Annoni A, Bartolaccini S, Biffi M, Russo F, Di Tomaso T, et al. Genome editing for scalable production of alloantigen-free lentiviral vectors for in vivo gene therapy. EMBO Mol Med. 2017;9(11):1558–73.
45. Cotmore SF, Tattersall P. Parvoviruses: small does not mean simple. Annu Rev Virol. 2014;1(1):517–37.
46. Niemeyer GP, Herzog RW, Mount J, Arruda VR, Tillson DM, Hathcock J, et al. Long-term correction of inhibitor-prone hemophilia B dogs treated with liver-directed AAV2-mediated factor IX gene therapy. Blood. 2009;113(4):797–806.
47. Buchlis G, Podsakoff GM, Radu A, Hawk SM, Flake AW, Mingozzi F, et al. Factor IX expression in skeletal muscle of a severe hemophilia B patient 10 years after AAV-mediated gene transfer. Blood. 2012;119(13):3038–41.
48. Smith RH. Adeno-associated virus integration: virus versus vector. Gene Ther. 2008;15(11):817–22.
49. Kaeppel C, Beattie SG, Fronza R, van Logtenstein R, Salmon F, Schmidt S, et al. A largely random AAV integration profile after LPLD gene therapy. Nat Med. 2013;19(7):889–91.
50. Nakai H, Wu X, Fuess S, Storm TA, Munroe D, Montini E, et al. Large-scale molecular characterization of adeno-associated virus vector integration in mouse liver. J Virol. 2005;79(6):3606–14.
51. Donsante A, Miller DG, Li Y, Vogler C, Brunt EM, Russell DW, et al. AAV vector integration sites in mouse hepatocellular carcinoma. Science. 2007;317(5837):477.
52. Li H, Malani N, Hamilton SR, Schlachterman A, Bussadori G, Edmonson SE, et al. Assessing the potential for AAV vector genotoxicity in a murine model. Blood. 2011;117(12):3311–9.
53. Chandler RJ, LaFave MC, Varshney GK, Trivedi NS, Carrillo-Carrasco N, Senac JS, et al. Vector design influences hepatic genotoxicity after adeno-associated virus gene therapy. J Clin Invest. 2015;125(2):870–80.
54. Chandler RJ, LaFave MC, Varshney GK, Burgess SM, Venditti CP. Genotoxicity in mice following AAV gene delivery: a safety concern for human gene therapy? Mol Ther. 2016;24(2):198–201.
55. Nathwani AC, Rosales C, McIntosh J, Rastegarlari G, Nathwani D, Raj D, et al. Long-term safety and efficacy following systemic administration of a self-complementary AAV vector encoding human FIX pseudotyped with serotype 5 and 8 capsid proteins. Mol Ther. 2011;19(5):876–85.
56. Nault JC, Datta S, Imbeaud S, Franconi A, Mallet M, Couchy G, et al. Recurrent AAV2-related insertional mutagenesis in human hepatocellular carcinomas. Nat Genet. 2015;47(10):1187–93.
57. Asokan A, Schaffer DV, Samulski RJ. The AAV vector toolkit: poised at the clinical crossroads. Mol Ther. 2012;20(4):699–708.
58. Lisowski L, Dane AP, Chu K, Zhang Y, Cunningham SC, Wilson EM, et al. Selection and evaluation of clinically relevant AAV variants in a xenograft liver model. Nature. 2014;506(7488):382–6.
59. Wu Z, Asokan A, Samulski RJ. Adeno-associated virus serotypes: vector toolkit for human gene therapy. Mol Ther. 2006;14(3):316–27.
60. Pillay S, Meyer NL, Puschnik AS, Davulcu O, Diep J, Ishikawa Y, et al. An essential receptor for adeno-associated virus infection. Nature. 2016;530(7588):108–12.
61. Hastie E, Samulski RJ. Recombinant adeno-associated virus vectors in the treatment of rare diseases. Expert Opin Orphan Drugs. 2015;3(6):675–89.

62. Mingozzi F, High KA. Therapeutic in vivo gene transfer for genetic disease using AAV: progress and challenges. Nat Rev Genet. 2011;12(5):341–55.
63. Colella P, Ronzitti G, Mingozzi F. Emerging issues in AAV-mediated in vivo gene therapy. Mol Ther Methods Clin Dev. 2018;8:87–104.
64. Mingozzi F, High KA. Immune responses to AAV vectors: overcoming barriers to successful gene therapy. Blood. 2013;122(1):23–36.
65. Dong JY, Fan PD, Frizzell RA. Quantitative analysis of the packaging capacity of recombinant adeno-associated virus. Hum Gene Ther. 1996;7(17):2101–12.
66. Frank-Kamenetsky M, Grefhorst A, Anderson NN, Racie TS, Bramlage B, Akinc A, et al. Therapeutic RNAi targeting PCSK9 acutely lowers plasma cholesterol in rodents and LDL cholesterol in nonhuman primates. Proc Natl Acad Sci U S A. 2008;105(33):11915–20.
67. Fitzgerald K, Frank-Kamenetsky M, Shulga-Morskaya S, Liebow A, Bettencourt BR, Sutherland JE, et al. Effect of an RNA interference drug on the synthesis of proprotein convertase subtilisin/kexin type 9 (PCSK9) and the concentration of serum LDL cholesterol in healthy volunteers: a randomised, single-blind, placebo-controlled, phase 1 trial. Lancet. 2014;383(9911):60–8.
68. Fitzgerald K, White S, Borodovsky A, Bettencourt BR, Strahs A, Clausen V, et al. A highly durable RNAi therapeutic inhibitor of PCSK9. N Engl J Med. 2017;376(1):41–51.
69. Guo S, Booten SL, Aghajan M, Hung G, Zhao C, Blomenkamp K, et al. Antisense oligonucleotide treatment ameliorates alpha-1 antitrypsin-related liver disease in mice. J Clin Invest. 2014;124(1):251–61.
70. Rangarajan S, Walsh L, Lester W, Perry D, Madan B, Laffan M, et al. AAV5-factor VIII gene transfer in severe hemophilia A. N Engl J Med. 2017;377:2519–30.
71. D'Avola D, Lopez-Franco E, Sangro B, Paneda A, Grossios N, Gil-Farina I, et al. Phase I open label liver-directed gene therapy clinical trial for acute intermittent porphyria. J Hepatol. 2016;65(4):776–83.
72. Manno CS, Pierce GF, Arruda VR, Glader B, Ragni M, Rasko JJ, et al. Successful transduction of liver in hemophilia by AAV-factor IX and limitations imposed by the host immune response. Nat Med. 2006;12(3):342–7.
73. Miesbach W, Meijer K, Coppens M, Kampmann P, Klamroth R, Schutgens R, et al. Gene therapy with adeno-associated virus vector 5-human factor IX in adults with hemophilia B. Blood. 2018;131(9):1022–31.
74. Mannucci PM, Tuddenham EG. The hemophilias—from royal genes to gene therapy. N Engl J Med. 2001;344(23):1773–9.
75. Soucie JM, Nuss R, Evatt B, Abdelhak A, Cowan L, Hill H, et al. Mortality among males with hemophilia: relations with source of medical care. The Hemophilia Surveillance System Project Investigators. Blood. 2000;96(2):437–42.
76. White GC 2nd, Rosendaal F, Aledort LM, Lusher JM, Rothschild C, Ingerslev J, et al. Definitions in hemophilia. Recommendation of the scientific subcommittee on factor VIII and factor IX of the scientific and standardization committee of the International Society on Thrombosis and Haemostasis. Thromb Haemost. 2001;85(3):560.
77. Rangarajan S, Walsh L, Lester W, Perry D, Madan B, Laffan M, et al. AAV5-factor VIII gene transfer in severe hemophilia A. N Engl J Med. 2017;377(26):2519–30.
78. Jiang H, Pierce GF, Ozelo MC, de Paula EV, Vargas JA, Smith P, et al. Evidence of multiyear factor IX expression by AAV-mediated gene transfer to skeletal muscle in an individual with severe hemophilia B. Mol Ther. 2006;14(3):452–5.
79. Mount JD, Herzog RW, Tillson DM, Goodman SA, Robinson N, McCleland ML, et al. Sustained phenotypic correction of hemophilia B dogs with a factor IX null mutation by liver-directed gene therapy. Blood. 2002;99(8):2670–6.
80. Sabatino DE, Armstrong E, Edmonson S, Liu YL, Pleimes M, Schuettrumpf J, et al. Novel hemophilia B mouse models exhibiting a range of mutations in the factor IX gene. Blood. 2004;104(9):2767–74.
81. Arruda VR. Toward gene therapy for hemophilia A with novel adenoviral vectors: successes and limitations in canine models. J Thromb Haemost. 2006;4(6):1215–7.
82. Sabatino DE, Nichols TC, Merricks E, Bellinger DA, Herzog RW, Monahan PE. Animal models of hemophilia. Prog Mol Biol Transl Sci. 2012;105:151–209.
83. Arruda VR, Doshi BS, Samelson-Jones BJ. Novel approaches to hemophilia therapy: successes and challenges. Blood. 2017;130(21):2251–6.
84. Crudele JM, Finn JD, Siner JI, Martin NB, Niemeyer GP, Zhou S, et al. AAV liver expression of FIX-Padua prevents and eradicates FIX inhibitor without increasing thrombogenicity in hemophilia B dogs and mice. Blood. 2015;125(10):1553–61.
85. Finn JD, Nichols TC, Svoronos N, Merricks EP, Bellenger DA, Zhou S, et al. The efficacy and the risk of immunogenicity of FIX Padua (R338L) in hemophilia B dogs treated by AAV muscle gene therapy. Blood. 2012;120(23):4521–3.
86. Cantore A, Nair N, Della Valle P, Di Matteo M, Matrai J, Sanvito F, et al. Hyperfunctional coagulation factor IX improves the efficacy of gene therapy in hemophilic mice. Blood. 2012;120(23):4517–20.
87. Monahan PE, Sun J, Gui T, Hu G, Hannah WB, Wichlan DG, et al. Employing a gain-of-function factor IX variant R338L to advance the efficacy and safety of hemophilia B human gene therapy: preclinical evaluation supporting an ongoing adeno-associated virus clinical trial. Hum Gene Ther. 2015;26(2):69–81.
88. Graham T, McIntosh J, Work LM, Nathwani A, Baker AH. Performance of AAV8 vectors expressing human factor IX from a hepatic-selective promoter following intravenous injection into rats. Genet Vaccines Ther. 2008;6:9.
89. Nathwani AC, Gray JT, McIntosh J, Ng CY, Zhou J, Spence Y, et al. Safe and efficient transduction of the liver after peripheral vein infusion of self-complementary AAV vector results in stable therapeutic expression of human FIX in nonhuman primates. Blood. 2007;109(4):1414–21.
90. Nathwani AC, Gray JT, Ng CY, Zhou J, Spence Y, Waddington SN, et al. Self-complementary adeno-associated virus vectors containing a novel liver-specific human factor IX expression cassette enable highly efficient transduction of murine and nonhuman primate liver. Blood. 2006;107(7):2653–61.
91. Vercauteren K, Hoffman BE, Zolotukhin I, Keeler GD, Xiao JW, Basner-Tschakarjan E, et al. Superior in vivo transduction of human hepatocytes using engineered AAV3 capsid. Mol Ther. 2016;24(6):1042–9.
92. Crigler JF Jr, Najjar VA. Congenital familial nonhemolytic jaundice with kernicterus. Pediatrics. 1952;10(2):169–80.
93. Strauss KA, Robinson DL, Vreman HJ, Puffenberger EG, Hart G, Morton DH. Management of hyperbilirubinemia and prevention of kernicterus in 20 patients with Crigler-Najjar disease. Eur J Pediatr. 2006;165(5):306–19.
94. Cornelius CE, Arias IM. Animal model of human disease. Crigler-Najjar syndrome. Animal model: hereditary nonhemolytic unconjugated hyperbilirubinemia in Gunn rats. Am J Pathol. 1972;69(2):369–72.
95. Iyanagi T, Emi Y, Ikushiro S. Biochemical and molecular aspects of genetic disorders of bilirubin metabolism. Biochim Biophys Acta. 1998;1407(3):173–84.
96. Miranda PS, Bosma PJ. Towards liver-directed gene therapy for Crigler-Najjar syndrome. Curr Gene Ther. 2009;9(2):72–82.

97. Seppen J, Bakker C, de Jong B, Kunne C, van den Oever K, Vandenberghe K, et al. Adeno-associated virus vector serotypes mediate sustained correction of bilirubin UDP glucuronosyltransferase deficiency in rats. Mol Ther. 2006;13(6):1085–92.
98. Montenegro-Miranda PS, Pichard V, Aubert D, Ten Bloemendaal L, Duijst S, de Waart DR, et al. In the rat liver, adenoviral gene transfer efficiency is comparable to AAV. Gene Ther. 2014;21(2):168–74.
99. Kren BT, Parashar B, Bandyopadhyay P, Chowdhury NR, Chowdhury JR, Steer CJ. Correction of the UDP-glucuronosyltransferase gene defect in the gunn rat model of Crigler-Najjar syndrome type I with a chimeric oligonucleotide. Proc Natl Acad Sci U S A. 1999;96(18):10349–54.
100. Ronzitti G, Bortolussi G, van Dijk R, Collaud F, Charles S, Leborgne C, et al. A translationally optimized AAV-UGT1A1 vector drives safe and long-lasting correction of Crigler-Najjar syndrome. Mol Ther Methods Clin Dev. 2016;3:16049.
101. Fox IJ, Chowdhury JR, Kaufman SS, Goertzen TC, Chowdhury NR, Warkentin PI, et al. Treatment of the Crigler-Najjar syndrome type I with hepatocyte transplantation. N Engl J Med. 1998;338(20):1422–6.
102. Sneitz N, Bakker CT, de Knegt RJ, Halley DJ, Finel M, Bosma PJ. Crigler-Najjar syndrome in the Netherlands: identification of four novel UGT1A1 alleles, genotype-phenotype correlation, and functional analysis of 10 missense mutants. Hum Mutat. 2010;31(1):52–9.
103. Bortolussi G, Baj G, Vodret S, Viviani G, Bittolo T, Muro AF. Age-dependent pattern of cerebellar susceptibility to bilirubin neurotoxicity in vivo. Dis Model Mech. 2014;7(9):1057–68.
104. Bortolussi G, Zentilin L, Baj G, Giraudi P, Bellarosa C, Giacca M, et al. Rescue of bilirubin-induced neonatal lethality in a mouse model of Crigler-Najjar syndrome type I by AAV9-mediated gene transfer. FASEB J. 2012;26(3):1052–63.
105. Bockor L, Bortolussi G, Iaconcig A, Chiaruttini G, Tiribelli C, Giacca M, et al. Repeated AAV-mediated gene transfer by serotype switching enables long-lasting therapeutic levels of hUgt1a1 enzyme in a mouse model of Crigler-Najjar syndrome type I. Gene Ther. 2017;24(10):649–60.
106. Fontanellas A, Avila MA, Berraondo P. Emerging therapies for acute intermittent porphyria. Expert Rev Mol Med. 2016;18:e17.
107. Unzu C, Sampedro A, Mauleon I, Gonzalez-Aparicio M, Enriquez de Salamanca R, Prieto J, et al. Helper-dependent adenoviral liver gene therapy protects against induced attacks and corrects protein folding stress in acute intermittent porphyria mice. Hum Mol Genet. 2013;22(14):2929–40.
108. Paneda A, Lopez-Franco E, Kaeppel C, Unzu C, Gil-Royo AG, D'Avola D, et al. Safety and liver transduction efficacy of rAAV5-cohPBGD in nonhuman primates: a potential therapy for acute intermittent porphyria. Hum Gene Ther. 2013;24(12):1007–17.
109. Yasuda M, Bishop DF, Fowkes M, Cheng SH, Gan L, Desnick RJ. AAV8-mediated gene therapy prevents induced biochemical attacks of acute intermittent porphyria and improves neuromotor function. Mol Ther. 2010;18(1):17–22.
110. Unzu C, Sampedro A, Mauleon I, Alegre M, Beattie SG, de Salamanca RE, et al. Sustained enzymatic correction by rAAV-mediated liver gene therapy protects against induced motor neuropathy in acute porphyria mice. Mol Ther. 2011;19(2):243–50.
111. Soonawalla ZF, Orug T, Badminton MN, Elder GH, Rhodes JM, Bramhall SR, et al. Liver transplantation as a cure for acute intermittent porphyria. Lancet. 2004;363(9410):705–6.
112. Singal AK, Parker C, Bowden C, Thapar M, Liu L, McGuire BM. Liver transplantation in the management of porphyria. Hepatology. 2014;60(3):1082–9.
113. Davidoff AM, Gray JT, Ng CY, Zhang Y, Zhou J, Spence Y, et al. Comparison of the ability of adeno-associated viral vectors pseudotyped with serotype 2, 5, and 8 capsid proteins to mediate efficient transduction of the liver in murine and nonhuman primate models. Mol Ther. 2005;11(6):875–88.
114. Hodges PE, Rosenberg LE. The spfash mouse: a missense mutation in the ornithine transcarbamylase gene also causes aberrant mRNA splicing. Proc Natl Acad Sci U S A. 1989;86(11):4142–6.
115. Kiwaki K, Kanegae Y, Saito I, Komaki S, Nakamura K, Miyazaki JI, et al. Correction of ornithine transcarbamylase deficiency in adult spf(ash) mice and in OTC-deficient human hepatocytes with recombinant adenoviruses bearing the CAG promoter. Hum Gene Ther. 1996;7(7):821–30.
116. Ye X, Robinson MB, Batshaw ML, Furth EE, Smith I, Wilson JM. Prolonged metabolic correction in adult ornithine transcarbamylase-deficient mice with adenoviral vectors. J Biol Chem. 1996;271(7):3639–46.
117. Ye X, Robinson MB, Pabin C, Quinn T, Jawad A, Wilson JM, et al. Adenovirus-mediated in vivo gene transfer rapidly protects ornithine transcarbamylase-deficient mice from an ammonium challenge. Pediatr Res. 1997;41(4 Pt 1):527–34.
118. Batshaw ML, Robinson MB, Ye X, Pabin C, Daikhin Y, Burton BK, et al. Correction of ureagenesis after gene transfer in an animal model and after liver transplantation in humans with ornithine transcarbamylase deficiency. Pediatr Res. 1999;46(5):588–93.
119. Raper SE, Wilson JM, Yudkoff M, Robinson MB, Ye X, Batshaw ML. Developing adenoviral-mediated in vivo gene therapy for ornithine transcarbamylase deficiency. J Inherit Metab Dis. 1998;21(Suppl 1):119–37.
120. Zimmer KP, Bendiks M, Mori M, Kominami E, Robinson MB, Ye X, et al. Efficient mitochondrial import of newly synthesized ornithine transcarbamylase (OTC) and correction of secondary metabolic alterations in spf(ash) mice following gene therapy of OTC deficiency. Mol Med. 1999;5(4):244–53.
121. Raper SE, Yudkoff M, Chirmule N, Gao GP, Nunes F, Haskal ZJ, et al. A pilot study of in vivo liver-directed gene transfer with an adenoviral vector in partial ornithine transcarbamylase deficiency. Hum Gene Ther. 2002;13(1):163–75.
122. Moscioni D, Morizono H, McCarter RJ, Stern A, Cabrera-Luque J, Hoang A, et al. Long-term correction of ammonia metabolism and prolonged survival in ornithine transcarbamylase-deficient mice following liver-directed treatment with adeno-associated viral vectors. Mol Ther. 2006;14(1):25–33.
123. Cunningham SC, Spinoulas A, Carpenter KH, Wilcken B, Kuchel PW, Alexander IE. AAV2/8-mediated correction of OTC deficiency is robust in adult but not neonatal Spf(ash) mice. Mol Ther. 2009;17(8):1340–6.
124. Cunningham SC, Kok CY, Dane AP, Carpenter K, Kizana E, Kuchel PW, et al. Induction and prevention of severe hyperammonemia in the spfash mouse model of ornithine transcarbamylase deficiency using shRNA and rAAV-mediated gene delivery. Mol Ther. 2011;19(5):854–9.
125. Cunningham SC, Kok CY, Spinoulas A, Carpenter KH, Alexander IE. AAV-encoded OTC activity persisting to adulthood following delivery to newborn spf(ash) mice is insufficient to prevent shRNA-induced hyperammonaemia. Gene Ther. 2013;20(12):1184–7.
126. Wang L, Wang H, Morizono H, Bell P, Jones D, Lin J, et al. Sustained correction of OTC deficiency in spf (ash) mice using optimized self-complementary AAV2/8 vectors. Gene Ther. 2012;19(4):404–10.
127. Wang L, Morizono H, Lin J, Bell P, Jones D, McMenamin D, et al. Preclinical evaluation of a clinical candidate AAV8 vector for ornithine transcarbamylase (OTC) deficiency reveals functional enzyme from each persisting vector genome. Mol Genet Metab. 2012;105(2):203–11.

128. Murillo-Sauca O, Moreno D, Gazquez C, Barberia M, Cenzano I, Solchaga SM, et al. Gene therapy optimization for Wilson's disease. J Hepatol. 2018;68:S83.
129. McIntosh J, Lenting PJ, Rosales C, Lee D, Rabbanian S, Raj D, et al. Therapeutic levels of FVIII following a single peripheral vein administration of rAAV vector encoding a novel human factor VIII variant. Blood. 2013;121(17):3335–44.
130. Puzzo F, Colella P, Biferi MG, Bali D, Paulk NK, Vidal P, et al. Rescue of Pompe disease in mice by AAV-mediated liver delivery of secretable acid alpha-glucosidase. Sci Transl Med. 2017;9(418).
131. Ferla R, Claudiani P, Cotugno G, Saccone P, De Leonibus E, Auricchio A. Similar therapeutic efficacy between a single administration of gene therapy and multiple administrations of recombinant enzyme in a mouse model of lysosomal storage disease. Hum Gene Ther. 2014;25(7):609–18.
132. Mingozzi F, Liu YL, Dobrzynski E, Kaufhold A, Liu JH, Wang Y, et al. Induction of immune tolerance to coagulation factor IX antigen by in vivo hepatic gene transfer. J Clin Invest. 2003;111(9):1347–56.
133. Mingozzi F, Hasbrouck NC, Basner-Tschakarjan E, Edmonson SA, Hui DJ, Sabatino DE, et al. Modulation of tolerance to the transgene product in a nonhuman primate model of AAV-mediated gene transfer to liver. Blood. 2007;110(7):2334–41.
134. Dobrzynski E, Mingozzi F, Liu YL, Bendo E, Cao O, Wang L, et al. Induction of antigen-specific CD4+ T-cell anergy and deletion by in vivo viral gene transfer. Blood. 2004;104(4):969–77.
135. Cao O, Dobrzynski E, Wang L, Nayak S, Mingle B, Terhorst C, et al. Induction and role of regulatory CD4+CD25+ T cells in tolerance to the transgene product following hepatic in vivo gene transfer. Blood. 2007;110(4):1132–40.
136. Mingozzi F, Maus MV, Hui DJ, Sabatino DE, Murphy SL, Rasko JE, et al. CD8(+) T-cell responses to adeno-associated virus capsid in humans. Nat Med. 2007;13(4):419–22.
137. Boutin S, Monteilhet V, Veron P, Leborgne C, Benveniste O, Montus MF, et al. Prevalence of serum IgG and neutralizing factors against adeno-associated virus (AAV) types 1, 2, 5, 6, 8, and 9 in the healthy population: implications for gene therapy using AAV vectors. Hum Gene Ther. 2010;21(6):704–12.
138. Erles K, Sebokova P, Schlehofer JR. Update on the prevalence of serum antibodies (IgG and IgM) to adeno-associated virus (AAV). J Med Virol. 1999;59(3):406–11.
139. Veron P, Leborgne C, Monteilhet V, Boutin S, Martin S, Moullier P, et al. Humoral and cellular capsid-specific immune responses to adeno-associated virus type 1 in randomized healthy donors. J Immunol. 2012;188(12):6418–24.
140. Vandamme C, Adjali O, Mingozzi F. Unraveling the complex story of immune responses to AAV vectors trial after trial. Hum Gene Ther. 2017;28(11):1061–74.
141. Finn JD, Hui D, Downey HD, Dunn D, Pien GC, Mingozzi F, et al. Proteasome inhibitors decrease AAV2 capsid derived peptide epitope presentation on MHC class I following transduction. Mol Ther. 2010;18(1):135–42.
142. Pien GC, Basner-Tschakarjan E, Hui DJ, Mentlik AN, Finn JD, Hasbrouck NC, et al. Capsid antigen presentation flags human hepatocytes for destruction after transduction by adeno-associated viral vectors. J Clin Invest. 2009;119(6):1688–95.
143. Jiang H, Couto LB, Patarroyo-White S, Liu T, Nagy D, Vargas JA, et al. Effects of transient immunosuppression on adenoassociated, virus-mediated, liver-directed gene transfer in rhesus macaques and implications for human gene therapy. Blood. 2006;108(10):3321–8.
144. Calcedo R, Morizono H, Wang L, McCarter R, He J, Jones D, et al. Adeno-associated virus antibody profiles in newborns, children, and adolescents. Clin Vaccine Immunol. 2011;18(9):1586–8.
145. Li C, Narkbunnam N, Samulski RJ, Asokan A, Hu G, Jacobson LJ, et al. Neutralizing antibodies against adeno-associated virus examined prospectively in pediatric patients with hemophilia. Gene Ther. 2012;19(3):288–94.
146. Calcedo R, Vandenberghe LH, Gao G, Lin J, Wilson JM. Worldwide epidemiology of neutralizing antibodies to adenoassociated viruses. J Infect Dis. 2009;199(3):381–90.
147. Mingozzi F, Chen Y, Edmonson SC, Zhou S, Thurlings RM, Tak PP, et al. Prevalence and pharmacological modulation of humoral immunity to AAV vectors in gene transfer to synovial tissue. Gene Ther. 2013;20(4):417–24.
148. Mingozzi F, High KA. Overcoming the host immune response to adeno-associated virus gene delivery vectors: the race between clearance, tolerance, neutralization, and escape. Annu Rev Virol. 2017;4(1):511–34.
149. Russell DW, Hirata RK. Human gene targeting by viral vectors. Nat Genet. 1998;18(4):325–30.
150. Sedivy JM, Sharp PA. Positive genetic selection for gene disruption in mammalian cells by homologous recombination. Proc Natl Acad Sci U S A. 1989;86(1):227–31.
151. Miller DG, Wang PR, Petek LM, Hirata RK, Sands MS, Russell DW. Gene targeting in vivo by adeno-associated virus vectors. Nat Biotechnol. 2006;24(8):1022–6.
152. Rouet P, Smih F, Jasin M. Introduction of double-strand breaks into the genome of mouse cells by expression of a rare-cutting endonuclease. Mol Cell Biol. 1994;14(12):8096–106.
153. Rouet P, Smih F, Jasin M. Expression of a site-specific endonuclease stimulates homologous recombination in mammalian cells. Proc Natl Acad Sci U S A. 1994;91(13):6064–8.
154. Smih F, Rouet P, Romanienko PJ, Jasin M. Double-strand breaks at the target locus stimulate gene targeting in embryonic stem cells. Nucleic Acids Res. 1995;23(24):5012–9.
155. Ceccaldi R, Rondinelli B, D'Andrea AD. Repair pathway choices and consequences at the double-strand break. Trends Cell Biol. 2016;26(1):52–64.
156. Shibata A, Jeggo PA. DNA double-strand break repair in a cellular context. Clin Oncol. 2014;26(5):243–9.
157. Cox DB, Platt RJ, Zhang F. Therapeutic genome editing: prospects and challenges. Nat Med. 2015;21(2):121–31.
158. Carroll D. Genome engineering with targetable nucleases. Annu Rev Biochem. 2014;83:409–39.
159. Gaj T, Gersbach CA, Barbas CF 3rd. ZFN, TALEN, and CRISPR/Cas-based methods for genome engineering. Trends Biotechnol. 2013;31(7):397–405.
160. Urnov FD, Rebar EJ, Holmes MC, Zhang HS, Gregory PD. Genome editing with engineered zinc finger nucleases. Nat Rev Genet. 2010;11(9):636–46.
161. Li L, Wu LP, Chandrasegaran S. Functional domains in Fok I restriction endonuclease. Proc Natl Acad Sci U S A. 1992;89(10):4275–9.
162. Li T, Huang S, Jiang WZ, Wright D, Spalding MH, Weeks DP, et al. TAL nucleases (TALNs): hybrid proteins composed of TAL effectors and FokI DNA-cleavage domain. Nucleic Acids Res. 2011;39(1):359–72.
163. Cermak T, Doyle EL, Christian M, Wang L, Zhang Y, Schmidt C, et al. Efficient design and assembly of custom TALEN and other TAL effector-based constructs for DNA targeting. Nucleic Acids Res. 2011;39(12):e82.
164. Deng D, Yan C, Pan X, Mahfouz M, Wang J, Zhu JK, et al. Structural basis for sequence-specific recognition of DNA by TAL effectors. Science. 2012;335(6069):720–3.
165. Morbitzer R, Romer P, Boch J, Lahaye T. Regulation of selected genome loci using de novo-engineered transcription activator-like effector (TALE)-type transcription factors. Proc Natl Acad Sci U S A. 2010;107(50):21617–22.

166. Mussolino C, Morbitzer R, Lutge F, Dannemann N, Lahaye T, Cathomen T. A novel TALE nuclease scaffold enables high genome editing activity in combination with low toxicity. Nucleic Acids Res. 2011;39(21):9283–93.
167. Wiedenheft B, Sternberg SH, Doudna JA. RNA-guided genetic silencing systems in bacteria and archaea. Nature. 2012;482(7385):331–8.
168. Fineran PC, Charpentier E. Memory of viral infections by CRISPR-Cas adaptive immune systems: acquisition of new information. Virology. 2012;434(2):202–9.
169. Jinek M, Chylinski K, Fonfara I, Hauer M, Doudna JA, Charpentier E. A programmable dual-RNA-guided DNA endonuclease in adaptive bacterial immunity. Science. 2012;337(6096):816–21.
170. Kleinstiver BP, Pattanayak V, Prew MS, Tsai SQ, Nguyen NT, Zheng Z, et al. High-fidelity CRISPR-Cas9 nucleases with no detectable genome-wide off-target effects. Nature. 2016;529(7587):490–5.
171. Slaymaker IM, Gao L, Zetsche B, Scott DA, Yan WX, Zhang F. Rationally engineered Cas9 nucleases with improved specificity. Science. 2016;351(6268):84–8.
172. Casini A, Olivieri M, Petris G, Montagna C, Reginato G, Maule G, et al. A highly specific SpCas9 variant is identified by in vivo screening in yeast. Nat Biotechnol. 2018;36:265–71.
173. Kim S, Kim D, Cho SW, Kim J, Kim JS. Highly efficient RNA-guided genome editing in human cells via delivery of purified Cas9 ribonucleoproteins. Genome Res. 2014;24(6):1012–9.
174. Liang X, Potter J, Kumar S, Zou Y, Quintanilla R, Sridharan M, et al. Rapid and highly efficient mammalian cell engineering via Cas9 protein transfection. J Biotechnol. 2015;208:44–53.
175. Ramakrishna S, Kwaku Dad AB, Beloor J, Gopalappa R, Lee SK, Kim H. Gene disruption by cell-penetrating peptide-mediated delivery of Cas9 protein and guide RNA. Genome Res. 2014;24(6):1020–7.
176. Yin H, Song CQ, Dorkin JR, Zhu LJ, Li Y, Wu Q, et al. Therapeutic genome editing by combined viral and non-viral delivery of CRISPR system components in vivo. Nat Biotechnol. 2016;34(3):328–33.
177. Petris G, Casini A, Montagna C, Lorenzin F, Prandi D, Romanel A, et al. Hit and go CAS9 delivered through a lentiviral based self-limiting circuit. Nat Commun. 2017;8:15334.
178. Cohen J, Pertsemlidis A, Kotowski IK, Graham R, Garcia CK, Hobbs HH. Low LDL cholesterol in individuals of African descent resulting from frequent nonsense mutations in PCSK9. Nat Genet. 2005;37(2):161–5.
179. Cohen JC, Boerwinkle E, Mosley TH Jr, Hobbs HH. Sequence variations in PCSK9, low LDL, and protection against coronary heart disease. N Engl J Med. 2006;354(12):1264–72.
180. Hooper AJ, Marais AD, Tanyanyiwa DM, Burnett JR. The C679X mutation in PCSK9 is present and lowers blood cholesterol in a southern African population. Atherosclerosis. 2007;193(2):445–8.
181. Zhao Z, Tuakli-Wosornu Y, Lagace TA, Kinch L, Grishin NV, Horton JD, et al. Molecular characterization of loss-of-function mutations in PCSK9 and identification of a compound heterozygote. Am J Hum Genet. 2006;79(3):514–23.
182. Denis M, Marcinkiewicz J, Zaid A, Gauthier D, Poirier S, Lazure C, et al. Gene inactivation of proprotein convertase subtilisin/kexin type 9 reduces atherosclerosis in mice. Circulation. 2012;125(7):894–901.
183. Ding Q, Strong A, Patel KM, Ng SL, Gosis BS, Regan SN, et al. Permanent alteration of PCSK9 with in vivo CRISPR-Cas9 genome editing. Circ Res. 2014;115(5):488–92.
184. Wang X, Raghavan A, Chen T, Qiao L, Zhang Y, Ding Q, et al. CRISPR-Cas9 targeting of PCSK9 in human hepatocytes in vivo-brief report. Arterioscler Thromb Vasc Biol. 2016;36(5):783–6.
185. Pankowicz FP, Barzi M, Legras X, Hubert L, Mi T, Tomolonis JA, et al. Reprogramming metabolic pathways in vivo with CRISPR/Cas9 genome editing to treat hereditary tyrosinaemia. Nat Commun. 2016;7:12642.
186. Russo P, O'Regan S. Visceral pathology of hereditary tyrosinemia type I. Am J Hum Genet. 1990;47(2):317–24.
187. Paulk NK, Wursthorn K, Wang Z, Finegold MJ, Kay MA, Grompe M. Adeno-associated virus gene repair corrects a mouse model of hereditary tyrosinemia in vivo. Hepatology. 2010;51(4):1200–8.
188. Yin H, Xue W, Chen S, Bogorad RL, Benedetti E, Grompe M, et al. Genome editing with Cas9 in adult mice corrects a disease mutation and phenotype. Nat Biotechnol. 2014;32(6):551–3.
189. Barzel A, Paulk NK, Shi Y, Huang Y, Chu K, Zhang F, et al. Promoterless gene targeting without nucleases ameliorates haemophilia B in mice. Nature. 2015;517(7534):360–4.
190. Borel F, Tang Q, Gernoux G, Greer C, Wang Z, Barzel A, et al. Survival advantage of both human hepatocyte xenografts and genome-edited hepatocytes for treatment of alpha-1 antitrypsin deficiency. Mol Ther. 2017;25(11):2477–89.
191. Yang Y, Wang L, Bell P, McMenamin D, He Z, White J, et al. A dual AAV system enables the Cas9-mediated correction of a metabolic liver disease in newborn mice. Nat Biotechnol. 2016;34(3):334–8.
192. Connelly JP, Barker JC, Pruett-Miller S, Porteus MH. Gene correction by homologous recombination with zinc finger nucleases in primary cells from a mouse model of a generic recessive genetic disease. Mol Ther. 2010;18(6):1103–10.
193. DeKelver RC, Choi VM, Moehle EA, Paschon DE, Hockemeyer D, Meijsing SH, et al. Functional genomics, proteomics, and regulatory DNA analysis in isogenic settings using zinc finger nuclease-driven transgenesis into a safe harbor locus in the human genome. Genome Res. 2010;20(8):1133–42.
194. Hockemeyer D, Soldner F, Beard C, Gao Q, Mitalipova M, DeKelver RC, et al. Efficient targeting of expressed and silent genes in human ESCs and iPSCs using zinc-finger nucleases. Nat Biotechnol. 2009;27(9):851–7.
195. Kotin RM, Linden RM, Berns KI. Characterization of a preferred site on human chromosome 19q for integration of adeno-associated virus DNA by non-homologous recombination. EMBO J. 1992;11(13):5071–8.
196. Li H, Haurigot V, Doyon Y, Li T, Wong SY, Bhagwat AS, et al. In vivo genome editing restores haemostasis in a mouse model of haemophilia. Nature. 2011;475(7355):217–21.
197. Anguela XM, Sharma R, Doyon Y, Miller JC, Li H, Haurigot V, et al. Robust ZFN-mediated genome editing in adult hemophilic mice. Blood. 2013;122(19):3283–7.
198. Sharma R, Anguela XM, Doyon Y, Wechsler T, DeKelver RC, Sproul S, et al. In vivo genome editing of the albumin locus as a platform for protein replacement therapy. Blood. 2015;126(15):1777–84.
199. Chew WL, Tabebordbar M, Cheng JK, Mali P, Wu EY, Ng AH, et al. A multifunctional AAV-CRISPR-Cas9 and its host response. Nat Methods. 2016;13(10):868–74.
200. Porro F, Bortolussi G, Barzel A, De Caneva A, Iaconcig A, Vodret S, et al. Promoterless gene targeting without nucleases rescues lethality of a Crigler-Najjar syndrome mouse model. EMBO Mol Med. 2017;9(10):1346–55.
201. Nygaard S, Barzel A, Haft A, Major A, Finegold M, Kay MA, et al. A universal system to select gene-modified hepatocytes in vivo. Sci Transl Med. 2016;8(342):342ra79.
202. Adam R, Karam V, Delvart V, O'Grady J, Mirza D, Klempnauer J, et al. Evolution of indications and results of liver transplantation in Europe. A report from the European Liver Transplant Registry (ELTR). J Hepatol. 2012;57(3):675–88.
203. Lindberg RL, Porcher C, Grandchamp B, Ledermann B, Burki K, Brandner S, et al. Porphobilinogen deaminase deficiency in mice

causes a neuropathy resembling that of human hepatic porphyria. Nat Genet. 1996;12(2):195–9.
204. Unzu C, Sampedro A, Mauleon I, Vanrell L, Dubrot J, de Salamanca RE, et al. Porphobilinogen deaminase over-expression in hepatocytes, but not in erythrocytes, prevents accumulation of toxic porphyrin precursors in a mouse model of acute intermittent porphyria. J Hepatol. 2010;52(3):417–24.
205. Carlson JA, Rogers BB, Sifers RN, Finegold MJ, Clift SM, DeMayo FJ, et al. Accumulation of PiZ alpha 1-antitrypsin causes liver damage in transgenic mice. J Clin Invest. 1989;83(4):1183–90.
206. Cruz PE, Mueller C, Cossette TL, Golant A, Tang Q, Beattie SG, et al. In vivo post-transcriptional gene silencing of alpha-1 antitrypsin by adeno-associated virus vectors expressing siRNA. Lab Invest. 2007;87(9):893–902.
207. Chiuchiolo MJ, Crystal RG. Gene therapy for Alpha-1 antitrypsin deficiency lung disease. Ann Am Thorac Soc. 2016;13(Suppl 4):S352–69.
208. Conlon TJ, Cossette T, Erger K, Choi YK, Clarke T, Scott-Jorgensen M, et al. Efficient hepatic delivery and expression from a recombinant adeno-associated virus 8 pseudotyped alpha1-antitrypsin vector. Mol Ther. 2005;12(5):867–75.
209. Morral N, Parks RJ, Zhou H, Langston C, Schiedner G, Quinones J, et al. High doses of a helper-dependent adenoviral vector yield supraphysiological levels of alpha1-antitrypsin with negligible toxicity. Hum Gene Ther. 1998;9(18):2709–16.
210. Schiedner G, Morral N, Parks RJ, Wu Y, Koopmans SC, Langston C, et al. Genomic DNA transfer with a high-capacity adenovirus vector results in improved in vivo gene expression and decreased toxicity. Nat Genet. 1998;18(2):180–3.
211. Patejunas G, Bradley A, Beaudet AL, O'Brien WE. Generation of a mouse model for citrullinemia by targeted disruption of the argininosuccinate synthetase gene. Somat Cell Mol Genet. 1994;20(1):55–60.
212. Perez CJ, Jaubert J, Guenet JL, Barnhart KF, Ross-Inta CM, Quintanilla VC, et al. Two hypomorphic alleles of mouse Ass1 as a new animal model of citrullinemia type I and other hyperammonemic syndromes. Am J Pathol. 2010;177(4):1958–68.
213. Chandler RJ, Tarasenko TN, Cusmano-Ozog K, Sun Q, Sutton VR, Venditti CP, et al. Liver-directed adeno-associated virus serotype 8 gene transfer rescues a lethal murine model of citrullinemia type 1. Gene Ther. 2013;20(12):1188–91.
214. Kok CY, Cunningham SC, Carpenter KH, Dane AP, Siew SM, Logan GJ, et al. Adeno-associated virus-mediated rescue of neonatal lethality in argininosuccinate synthetase-deficient mice. Mol Ther. 2013;21(10):1823–31.
215. Ye X, Whiteman B, Jerebtsova M, Batshaw ML. Correction of argininosuccinate synthetase (AS) deficiency in a murine model of citrullinemia with recombinant adenovirus carrying human AS cDNA. Gene Ther. 2000;7(20):1777–82.
216. Gunn CH. Hereditary acholuric jaundice in a new mutant strain of rats. J Hered. 1934;29:137–9.
217. Toietta G, Mane VP, Norona WS, Finegold MJ, Ng P, McDonagh AF, et al. Lifelong elimination of hyperbilirubinemia in the Gunn rat with a single injection of helper-dependent adenoviral vector. Proc Natl Acad Sci U S A. 2005;102(11):3930–5.
218. Seppen J, van der Rijt R, Looije N, van Til NP, Lamers WH, Oude Elferink RP. Long-term correction of bilirubin UDPglucuronyltransferase deficiency in rats by in utero lentiviral gene transfer. Mol Ther. 2003;8(4):593–9.
219. Seppen J, van Til NP, van der Rijt R, Hiralall JK, Kunne C, Elferink RP. Immune response to lentiviral bilirubin UDP-glucuronosyltransferase gene transfer in fetal and neonatal rats. Gene Ther. 2006;13(8):672–7.
220. Pastore N, Nusco E, Piccolo P, Castaldo S, Vanikova J, Vetrini F, et al. Improved efficacy and reduced toxicity by ultrasound-guided intrahepatic injections of helper-dependent adenoviral vector in Gunn rats. Hum Gene Ther Methods. 2013;24(5):321–7.
221. Flageul M, Aubert D, Pichard V, Nguyen TH, Nowrouzi A, Schmidt M, et al. Transient expression of genes delivered to newborn rat liver using recombinant adeno-associated virus 2/8 vectors. J Gene Med. 2009;11(8):689–96.
222. Montenegro-Miranda PS, Paneda A, ten Bloemendaal L, Duijst S, de Waart DR, Aseguinolaza GG, et al. Adeno-associated viral vector serotype 5 poorly transduces liver in rat models. PLoS One. 2013;8(12):e82597.
223. Nguyen TH, Bellodi-Privato M, Aubert D, Pichard V, Myara A, Trono D, et al. Therapeutic lentivirus-mediated neonatal in vivo gene therapy in hyperbilirubinemic Gunn rats. Mol Ther. 2005;12(5):852–9.
224. Schmitt F, Remy S, Dariel A, Flageul M, Pichard V, Boni S, et al. Lentiviral vectors that express UGT1A1 in liver and contain miR-142 target sequences normalize hyperbilirubinemia in Gunn rats. Gastroenterology. 2010;139(3):999–1007, 07 e1–2.
225. Nguyen TH, Aubert D, Bellodi-Privato M, Flageul M, Pichard V, Jaidane-Abdelghani Z, et al. Critical assessment of lifelong phenotype correction in hyperbilirubinemic Gunn rats after retroviral mediated gene transfer. Gene Ther. 2007;14(17):1270–7.
226. Wang X, Sarkar DP, Mani P, Steer CJ, Chen Y, Guha C, et al. Long-term reduction of jaundice in Gunn rats by nonviral liver-targeted delivery of sleeping beauty transposon. Hepatology. 2009;50(3):815–24.
227. Nguyen N, Bonzo JA, Chen S, Chouinard S, Kelner MJ, Hardiman G, et al. Disruption of the ugt1 locus in mice resembles human Crigler-Najjar type I disease. J Biol Chem. 2008;283(12):7901–11.
228. Greig JA, Nordin JML, Draper C, Bell P, Wilson JM. AAV8 gene therapy rescues the newborn phenotype of a mouse model of Crigler-Najjar. Hum Gene Ther. 2018;29(7):763–70.
229. Ishibashi S, Brown MS, Goldstein JL, Gerard RD, Hammer RE, Herz J. Hypercholesterolemia in low density lipoprotein receptor knockout mice and its reversal by adenovirus-mediated gene delivery. J Clin Invest. 1993;92(2):883–93.
230. Powell-Braxton L, Veniant M, Latvala RD, Hirano KI, Won WB, Ross J, et al. A mouse model of human familial hypercholesterolemia: markedly elevated low density lipoprotein cholesterol levels and severe atherosclerosis on a low-fat chow diet. Nat Med. 1998;4(8):934–8.
231. Lebherz C, Gao G, Louboutin JP, Millar J, Rader D, Wilson JM. Gene therapy with novel adeno-associated virus vectors substantially diminishes atherosclerosis in a murine model of familial hypercholesterolemia. J Gene Med. 2004;6(6):663–72.
232. Lebherz C, Sanmiguel J, Wilson JM, Rader DJ. Gene transfer of wild-type apoA-I and apoA-I Milano reduce atherosclerosis to a similar extent. Cardiovasc Diabetol. 2007;6:15.
233. Chen SJ, Sanmiguel J, Lock M, McMenamin D, Draper C, Limberis MP, et al. Biodistribution of AAV8 vectors expressing human low-density lipoprotein receptor in a mouse model of homozygous familial hypercholesterolemia. Human gene therapy. Clin Dev. 2013;24(4):154–60.
234. Chen SJ, Rader DJ, Tazelaar J, Kawashiri M, Gao G, Wilson JM. Prolonged correction of hyperlipidemia in mice with familial hypercholesterolemia using an adeno-associated viral vector expressing very-low-density lipoprotein receptor. Mol Ther. 2000;2(3):256–61.
235. Kassim SH, Li H, Bell P, Somanathan S, Lagor W, Jacobs F, et al. Adeno-associated virus serotype 8 gene therapy leads to significant lowering of plasma cholesterol levels in humanized mouse models of homozygous and heterozygous familial hypercholesterolemia. Hum Gene Ther. 2013;24(1):19–26.
236. Kassim SH, Li H, Vandenberghe LH, Hinderer C, Bell P, Marchadier D, et al. Gene therapy in a humanized mouse model

237. Somanathan S, Jacobs F, Wang Q, Hanlon AL, Wilson JM, Rader DJ. AAV vectors expressing LDLR gain-of-function variants demonstrate increased efficacy in mouse models of familial hypercholesterolemia. Circ Res. 2014;115(6):591–9.
238. Bi L, Lawler AM, Antonarakis SE, High KA, Gearhart JD, Kazazian HH Jr. Targeted disruption of the mouse factor VIII gene produces a model of haemophilia A. Nat Genet. 1995;10(1):119–21.
239. Chavez CL, Keravala A, Chu JN, Farruggio AP, Cuellar VE, Voorberg J, et al. Long-term expression of human coagulation factor VIII in a tolerant mouse model using the phiC31 integrase system. Hum Gene Ther. 2012;23(4):390–8.
240. Merlin S, Cannizzo ES, Borroni E, Bruscaggin V, Schinco P, Tulalamba W, et al. A novel platform for immune tolerance induction in hemophilia A mice. Mol Ther. 2017;25(8):1815–30.
241. Monahan PE, Lothrop CD, Sun J, Hirsch ML, Kafri T, Kantor B, et al. Proteasome inhibitors enhance gene delivery by AAV virus vectors expressing large genomes in hemophilia mouse and dog models: a strategy for broad clinical application. Mol Ther. 2010;18(11):1907–16.
242. Lozier JN, Dutra A, Pak E, Zhou N, Zheng Z, Nichols TC, et al. The Chapel Hill hemophilia A dog colony exhibits a factor VIII gene inversion. Proc Natl Acad Sci U S A. 2002;99(20):12991–6.
243. Evans JP, Brinkhous KM, Brayer GD, Reisner HM, High KA. Canine hemophilia B resulting from a point mutation with unusual consequences. Proc Natl Acad Sci U S A. 1989;86(24):10095–9.
244. Mauser AE, Whitlark J, Whitney KM, Lothrop CD Jr. A deletion mutation causes hemophilia B in Lhasa Apso dogs. Blood. 1996;88(9):3451–5.
245. Wang L, Zoppe M, Hackeng TM, Griffin JH, Lee KF, Verma IM. A factor IX-deficient mouse model for hemophilia B gene therapy. Proc Natl Acad Sci U S A. 1997;94(21):11563–6.
246. Mingozzi F, Schuttrumpf J, Arruda VR, Liu Y, Liu YL, High KA, et al. Improved hepatic gene transfer by using an adeno-associated virus serotype 5 vector. J Virol. 2002;76(20):10497–502.
247. Arruda VR, Schuettrumpf J, Herzog RW, Nichols TC, Robinson N, Lotfi Y, et al. Safety and efficacy of factor IX gene transfer to skeletal muscle in murine and canine hemophilia B models by adeno-associated viral vector serotype 1. Blood. 2004;103(1):85–92.
248. Nichols TC, Whitford MH, Arruda VR, Stedman HH, Kay MA, High KA. Translational data from adeno-associated virus-mediated gene therapy of hemophilia B in dogs. Hum Gene Ther Clin Dev. 2015;26(1):5–14.
249. Wendel U, Saudubray JM, Bodner A, Schadewaldt P. Liver transplantation in maple syrup urine disease. Eur J Pediatr. 1999;158(Suppl 2):S60–4.
250. Homanics GE, Skvorak K, Ferguson C, Watkins S, Paul HS. Production and characterization of murine models of classic and intermediate maple syrup urine disease. BMC Med Genet. 2006;7:33.
251. Johnson MT, Yang HS, Magnuson T, Patel MS. Targeted disruption of the murine dihydrolipoamide dehydrogenase gene (Dld) results in perigastrulation lethality. Proc Natl Acad Sci U S A. 1997;94(26):14512–7.
252. Chandler RJ, Sloan J, Fu H, Tsai M, Stabler S, Allen R, et al. Metabolic phenotype of methylmalonic acidemia in mice and humans: the role of skeletal muscle. BMC Med Genet. 2007;8:64.
253. Chandler RJ, Venditti CP. Pre-clinical efficacy and dosing of an AAV8 vector expressing human methylmalonyl-CoA mutase in a murine model of methylmalonic acidemia (MMA). Mol Genet Metab. 2012;107(3):617–9.
254. Carrillo-Carrasco N, Chandler RJ, Chandrasekaran S, Venditti CP. Liver-directed recombinant adeno-associated viral gene delivery rescues a lethal mouse model of methylmalonic acidemia and provides long-term phenotypic correction. Hum Gene Ther. 2010;21(9):1147–54.
255. Chandler RJ, Venditti CP. Long-term rescue of a lethal murine model of methylmalonic acidemia using adeno-associated viral gene therapy. Mol Ther. 2010;18(1):11–6.
256. Chandler RJ, Venditti CP. Adenovirus-mediated gene delivery rescues a neonatal lethal murine model of mut(0) methylmalonic acidemia. Hum Gene Ther. 2008;19(1):53–60.
257. Senac JS, Chandler RJ, Sysol JR, Li L, Venditti CP. Gene therapy in a murine model of methylmalonic acidemia using rAAV9-mediated gene delivery. Gene Ther. 2012;19(4):385–91.
258. Wong ES, McIntyre C, Peters HL, Ranieri E, Anson DS, Fletcher JM. Correction of methylmalonic aciduria in vivo using a codon-optimized lentiviral vector. Hum Gene Ther. 2014;25(6):529–38.
259. Hulbert LL, Doolittle DP. Abnormal skin and hair: a sex-linked mutation in the house mouse. Genetics. 1971;68:s29.
260. Cupp MB. Sparse-fur, sf. *Mouse News Lett.* 1958;19:37
261. Wang L, Bell P, Morizono H, He Z, Pumbo E, Yu H, et al. AAV gene therapy corrects OTC deficiency and prevents liver fibrosis in aged OTC-knock out heterozygous mice. Mol Genet Metab. 2017;120(4):299–305.
262. Bell P, Wang L, Chen SJ, Yu H, Zhu Y, Nayal M, et al. Effects of self-complementarity, codon optimization, transgene, and dose on liver transduction with AAV8. Hum Gene Ther Methods. 2016;27(6):228–37.
263. Brunetti-Pierri N, Clarke C, Mane V, Palmer DJ, Lanpher B, Sun Q, et al. Phenotypic correction of ornithine transcarbamylase deficiency using low dose helper-dependent adenoviral vectors. J Gene Med. 2008;10(8):890–6.
264. Mian A, McCormack WM Jr, Mane V, Kleppe S, Ng P, Finegold M, et al. Long-term correction of ornithine transcarbamylase deficiency by WPRE-mediated overexpression using a helper-dependent adenovirus. Mol Ther. 2004;10(3):492–9.
265. Paulusma CC, Groen A, Kunne C, Ho-Mok KS, Spijkerboer AL, Rudi de Waart D, et al. Atp8b1 deficiency in mice reduces resistance of the canalicular membrane to hydrophobic bile salts and impairs bile salt transport. Hepatology. 2006;44(1):195–204.
266. Wang R, Salem M, Yousef IM, Tuchweber B, Lam P, Childs SJ, et al. Targeted inactivation of sister of P-glycoprotein gene (spgp) in mice results in nonprogressive but persistent intrahepatic cholestasis. Proc Natl Acad Sci U S A. 2001;98(4):2011–6.
267. Guenzel AJ, Hofherr SE, Hillestad M, Barry M, Weaver E, Venezia S, et al. Generation of a hypomorphic model of propionic acidemia amenable to gene therapy testing. Mol Ther. 2013;21(7):1316–23.
268. Miyazaki T, Ohura T, Kobayashi M, Shigematsu Y, Yamaguchi S, Suzuki Y, et al. Fatal propionic acidemia in mice lacking propionyl-CoA carboxylase and its rescue by postnatal, liver-specific supplementation via a transgene. J Biol Chem. 2001;276(38):35995–9.
269. Hofherr SE, Senac JS, Chen CY, Palmer DJ, Ng P, Barry MA. Short-term rescue of neonatal lethality in a mouse model of propionic acidemia by gene therapy. Hum Gene Ther. 2009;20(2):169–80.
270. Chandler RJ, Chandrasekaran S, Carrillo-Carrasco N, Senac JS, Hofherr SE, Barry MA, et al. Adeno-associated virus serotype 8 gene transfer rescues a neonatal lethal murine model of propionic acidemia. Hum Gene Ther. 2011;22(4):477–81.
271. Culiat CT, Klebig ML, Liu Z, Monroe H, Stanford B, Desai J, et al. Identification of mutations from phenotype-driven ENU mutagenesis in mouse chromosome 7. Mamm Genome. 2005;16(8):555–66.
272. Aponte JL, Sega GA, Hauser LJ, Dhar MS, Withrow CM, Carpenter DA, et al. Point mutations in the murine fumarylacetoacetate hydrolase gene: animal models for the human genetic disorder hereditary tyrosinemia type 1. Proc Natl Acad Sci U S A. 2001;98(2):641–5.
273. Grompe M. Fah knockout animals as models for therapeutic liver repopulation. Adv Exp Med Biol. 2017;959:215–30.

274. Hickey RD, Lillegard JB, Fisher JE, McKenzie TJ, Hofherr SE, Finegold MJ, et al. Efficient production of Fah-null heterozygote pigs by chimeric adeno-associated virus-mediated gene knockout and somatic cell nuclear transfer. Hepatology. 2011;54(4):1351–9.
275. Held PK, Olivares EC, Aguilar CP, Finegold M, Calos MP, Grompe M. In vivo correction of murine hereditary tyrosinemia type I by phiC31 integrase-mediated gene delivery. Mol Ther. 2005;11(3):399–408.
276. Overturf K, Al-Dhalimy M, Ou CN, Finegold M, Tanguay R, Lieber A, et al. Adenovirus-mediated gene therapy in a mouse model of hereditary tyrosinemia type I. Hum Gene Ther. 1997;8(5):513–21.
277. Montini E, Held PK, Noll M, Morcinek N, Al-Dhalimy M, Finegold M, et al. In vivo correction of murine tyrosinemia type I by DNA-mediated transposition. Mol Ther. 2002;6(6):759–69.
278. Paulk NK, Pekrun K, Zhu E, Nygaard S, Li B, Xu J, et al. Bioengineered AAV capsids with combined high human liver transduction in vivo and unique humoral Seroreactivity. Mol Ther. 2018;26(1):289–303.
279. Hickey RD, Mao SA, Glorioso J, Elgilani F, Amiot B, Chen H, et al. Curative ex vivo liver-directed gene therapy in a pig model of hereditary tyrosinemia type 1. Sci Transl Med. 2016;8(349):349ra99.
280. Schilsky ML, Stockert RJ, Sternlieb I. Pleiotropic effect of LEC mutation: a rodent model of Wilson's disease. Am J Phys. 1994;266(5 Pt 1):G907–13.
281. Wu J, Forbes JR, Chen HS, Cox DW. The LEC rat has a deletion in the copper transporting ATPase gene homologous to the Wilson disease gene. Nat Genet. 1994;7(4):541–5.
282. Buiakova OI, Xu J, Lutsenko S, Zeitlin S, Das K, Das S, et al. Null mutation of the murine ATP7B (Wilson disease) gene results in intracellular copper accumulation and late-onset hepatic nodular transformation. Hum Mol Genet. 1999;8(9):1665–71.
283. Theophilos MB, Cox DW, Mercer JF. The toxic milk mouse is a murine model of Wilson disease. Hum Mol Genet. 1996;5(10):1619–24.
284. Merle U, Encke J, Tuma S, Volkmann M, Naldini L, Stremmel W. Lentiviral gene transfer ameliorates disease progression in Long-Evans cinnamon rats: an animal model for Wilson disease. Scand J Gastroenterol. 2006;41(8):974–82.
285. Murillo O, Luqui DM, Gazquez C, Martinez-Espartosa D, Navarro-Blasco I, Monreal JI, et al. Long-term metabolic correction of Wilson's disease in a murine model by gene therapy. J Hepatol. 2016;64(2):419–26.
286. Du H, Duanmu M, Witte D, Grabowski GA. Targeted disruption of the mouse lysosomal acid lipase gene: long-term survival with massive cholesteryl ester and triglyceride storage. Hum Mol Genet. 1998;7(9):1347–54.
287. Du H, Heur M, Witte DP, Ameis D, Grabowski GA. Lysosomal acid lipase deficiency: correction of lipid storage by adenovirus-mediated gene transfer in mice. Hum Gene Ther. 2002;13(11):1361–72.